Community and Public Health Nursing

Promoting the Public's Health

Community and Public Health Nursing

Promoting the Public's Health

TENTH EDITION

Cherie Rector, PhD, RN, PHN
Professor Emeritus
Department of Nursing
California State University, Bakersfield
Bakersfield, California

Mary Jo Stanley, PhD, RN, CNS, CNE
Professor
Director, School of Nursing
California State University, Stanislaus
Turlock, California

Vice President, Nursing Segment: Julie K. Stegman
Manager, Nursing Education and Practice Content: Jamie Blum
Acquisitions Editor: Michael Kerns
Senior Development Editor: Meredith L. Brittain
Editorial Coordinator: Ashley Pfeiffer
Marketing Manager: Brittany Clements
Editorial Assistant: Molly Kennedy
Senior Production Project Manager: Alicia Jackson
Manager, Graphic Arts & Design: Steve Druding
Art Director: Jennifer Clements
Manufacturing Coordinator: Karin Duffield
Prepress Vendor: SPi Global

Tenth edition

9 8 7 6 5 4 3 2 1

Printed in China

Cataloging in Publication data available on request from publisher
ISBN: 978-1-9751-2304-8

shop.lww.com

CCS1220

With love, to my husband, my children, and my grandchildren.

—Cherie Rector

To my husband and three sons—you make my heart smile. You are the steady seas in which I sail; thank you for your unwavering support.

—Mary Jo Stanley

ABOUT THE AUTHORS

Dr. Cherie Rector, PhD, RN, PHN, is a native Californian and an Emeritus Professor in the Department of Nursing at California State University, Bakersfield. While there, she served as lead faculty in community health nursing, Director of the School Nurse Credential Program and the RN to BSN Program, helping to develop and revise curriculum in those areas. She also developed an online curriculum for the RN to BSN program, and taught in-person, distance learning, and online courses in graduate and undergraduate programs. Prior to that, she served in an administrative position as Director of Allied Health and the Disabled Students Program at College of the Sequoias. She has also been the Coordinator of the School Nurse Credential Program and the RN to BSN Program at California State University, Fresno, overseeing curriculum development in those areas, for both online and in-person classes. Undergraduate teaching areas have included community health nursing, foundations/health assessment, health teaching, leadership, and capstone classes; in addition, she has taught graduate courses in community health nursing, research, vulnerable populations, family theories, interprofessional development, and school nursing. She has served as a consultant to school districts and hospitals in the areas of child health, research, and evidence-based practice; has served on various state, local, and national boards and task forces; and has had leadership roles in professional nursing organizations. Over the course of her career, Dr. Rector has practiced in community health and school nursing settings and in acute care neonatal nursing. Her grants, research, publications, and presentations have focused largely on child and adolescent health, school nursing, public health nursing, nursing education, and program development for underrepresented students. She earned an associate degree in nursing from College of the Sequoias and a BSN from the Consortium of the California State Universities, Long Beach. She completed a master's degree in nursing (Clinical Nurse Specialist, Community Health) and a school nurse credential from California State University, Fresno. Her PhD in educational psychology is from the University of Southern California. She is an active member of the American Public Health Association (PHN Section), the Western Institute of Nursing, Sigma Theta Tau, and the Association of Community Health Nursing Educators.

Dr. Mary Jo Stanley, PhD, RN, CNS, CNE, is a Professor and Director of the School of Nursing at California State University, Stanislaus. Prior to this role, she served as the RN-BSN Program Director, helping create online curriculum and instruction for the program. Previous positions in academia include coordinator for the second degree prelicensure program at the University of Colorado, Colorado Springs; in addition to this role, she also coordinated community health placements for RN-BSN students overseeing curriculum in those areas. At the University of Northern Colorado, Dr. Stanley coordinated summer community health clinical placements revising and updating curriculum. Undergraduate teaching areas have included community health, leadership and management, health assessment, foundations, health promotion, health education, capstone practicum, and professional roles; in addition, she has taught graduate classes in nursing education, contemporary practices, and nursing research and has served as graduate project Chair for Masters of Science in Nursing students. Dr. Stanley has consulted for online instruction and is a certified online course reviewer. Over the course of Dr. Stanley's career, she has practiced in community and school health settings, and in acute care in the ICU and PACU. Her research, publications, presentations, and grants have focused on educational development, strategies for teaching, and community health. She earned a Bachelor of Science in Nursing, Master of Science in Nursing, Clinical Nurse Specialist, and School Nurse Credential from San Jose State University. She completed her PhD in nursing with an emphasis on education from the University of Northern Colorado and is a Certified Nurse Educator (CNE). She is an active member of the Association of Community Health Nursing Educators and Sigma Theta Tau International.

CONTRIBUTORS

CONTRIBUTORS TO THE 10TH EDITION

Sheila Adams-Leander, RN, PhD, CCC
Associate Professor
School of Nursing
Milwaukee School of Engineering
Milwaukee, Wisconsin
Online Faculty for Doctorate of Nursing Practice Program
College of Nursing and Health Professions
Grand Canyon University
Phoenix, Arizona
Chapter 5, Transcultural Nursing

Peggy H. Anderson, DNP, MS, RN
Associate Teaching Professor
Undergraduate Program Coordinator
Brigham Young University
College of Nursing
Provo, Utah
Chapter 20, School-Age Children and Adolescents

Anne Watson Bongiorno, RN, PHD, APRN-BC, CNE
Professor
Department of Nursing
SUNY Plattsburgh
Plattsburgh, New York
Chapter 4, Evidence-Based Practice and Ethics

Yezenia Cadena-Malek, RN, BSN, MSHS
Health Promotion Educator
Army Public Health Nursing/Health Promotion
Department of Preventive Medicine
JBSA Fort Sam Houston
San Antonio, Texas
Chapter 8, Communicable Disease

Denise Cummins, DNP, RN, WHNP-BC
Assistant Teaching Professor
College of Nursing
Brigham Young University
Provo, Utah
Chapter 12, Planning, Implementing, and Evaluating Community/Public Health Programs

Heide R. Cygan, DNP, RN, PHNA-BC
Assistant Professor
Department of Community, Systems and Mental Health Nursing
College of Nursing
Rush University
Chicago, Illinois
Chapter 13, Policy Making and Advocacy

Beverly A. Dandridge, MSN, FNP, MSAJS, CAPT, USPHS
Department of Homeland Security
USPHS Commissioned Corps Liaison
Washington, District of Columbia
Chapter 17, Disasters and Their Impact
Chapter 28, Public Settings

Mary Ann Drake, PhD, RN, CNE
Professor
Department of Nursing
Webster University
Saint Louis, Missouri
Chapter 14, Family as Client

Rachell A. Ekroos, PhD, APRN, FNP-BC, AFN-BC, FAAN
Chief Executive Officer
Center for Forensic Nursing Excellence International
Las Vegas, Nevada
Chapter 18, Violence and Abuse

Naomi E. Ervin, PhD, RN, PHCNS-BC, FNAP, FAAN
Retired Professor
Shelby, Michigan
Chapter 15, Community as Client

Deborah S. Finnell, RN, DNS, CARN-AP, FAAN
Professor Emerita
Johns Hopkins School of Nursing
Baltimore, Maryland
Chapter 25, Behavioral Health in the Community

Lakisha Nicole Flagg, DrPH, MS, MPH, RN, APHN-BC, CPH
Strategy, Policy, and Communications Program Manager
Louisiana Department of Health's Bureau of Family Health
Adjunct Faculty
Graduate Program
Texas Tech University Science Center
Lubbock, Texas
Chapter 15, Community as Client

Carmen George, DNP, MSN, BSN, WHNP-BC
Assistant Professor of Nursing School of Nursing University of Nevada
Las Vegas
Chapter 19, Maternal–Child Health

Patricia (Trish) Hanes, PhD, MSN, MAED, MS-DPEM, RN, CNE, NEMAA, CSSGB
Professor Emeritus
School of Nursing
Azusa Pacific University
Azusa, California
Chapter 3, History and Evolution of Public Health Nursing

Lenore Hernandez, PhD, MSN, RN, CNS, APRN-BCADM, CDE
Clinical Nurse Specialist in Diabetes
Department of Medicine
Northern California Veterans Healthcare Administration
Martinez, California
Chapter 23, Working With Vulnerable People

Judith L. Hold, EdD, RN
Assistant Professor of Nursing
Wellstar School of Nursing
Kennesaw State University
Kennesaw, Georgia
Chapter 21, Adult Health

Ezra C. Holston, PhD, MSN, RN
Assistant Director
Utah State University
Department of Nursing and Health Professions
Logan, Utah
Chapter 14, Family as Client

Vanessa Amore Jones, DNP, APRN, FNP-C
Director of Graduate Nursing Studies
Assistant Professor, DNP Program Coordinator
University of North Georgia
Dahlonega, Georgia
Chapter 21, Adult Health

Betty C. Jung, MPH, RN, MCHES
Director for Public Health Expertise Network of Mentors
Adjunct Lecturer
Department of Public Health
Southern Connecticut State University
New Haven, Connecticut
Chapter 7, Epidemiology in the Community

Mary Lashley, PhD, RN, PHNCS, BC, CNE
Professor
Department of Nursing
Towson University
Towson, Maryland
Allentown, Pennsylvania
Chapter 26, Working With the Homeless

Angelique Lawyer, MSN, MPH, PHNA-BC
Public Health Consultant
Gaia Public Health Solutions
Chapel Hill, North Carolina
Chapter 29, Private Settings

Jeanne M. Leffers, PhD, RN, FAAN
Professor Emeritus
University of Massachusetts, Dartmouth
North Dartmouth, Massachusetts
Chapter 9, Environmental Health and Safety

Colleen Marzilli, PhD, DNP, MBA, RN-BC, CCM, PHNA-BC, CNE, NEA-BC, FNAP
Coordinator Concurrent ADN/BSN Program
Coordinator CONHS International Programs
Associate Professor
School of Nursing
The University of Texas at Tyler
Tyler, Texas
Chapter 10, Communication, Collaboration, and Technology

Ruth McDermott-Levy, PhD, MPH, RN, FAAN
Associate Professor and Director
Center for Global & Public Health
M. Louise Fitzpatrick College of Nursing
Villanova University
Villanova, Pennsylvania
Chapter 9, Environmental Health and Safety

Charlene Niemi, PhD, RN, PHN, CNE
Assistant Professor
Nursing Program
California State University, Channel Islands
Camarillo, California
Chapter 24, Clients With Disabilities

Carol Pochron, MSN, RN
Adjunct Instructor
Department of Nursing
DeSales University
Center Valley, Pennsylvania
Adjunct Instructor
Department of Nursing
Moravian College
Bethlehem, Pennsylvania
Board Member of Parish Nurse Coalition of the Greater Lehigh Valley
Per Diem Nurse
Department of Hospice
Lehigh Valley Health Network
Allentown, Pennsylvania
Chapter 29, Private Settings

Cherie Rector, PhD, RN, PHN
Professor Emeritus
Department of Nursing
California State University, Bakersfield
Bakersfield, California
Chapter 1, Introduction: The Journey Begins
Chapter 4, Evidence-Based Practice and Ethics
Chapter 6, Structure and Economics of Community/Public Health Services
Chapter 10, Communication, Collaboration, and Technology

Judith M. Scott, PhD, RN
Assistant Professor
Helen and Arthur E. Johnson Beth-El College of Nursing and Health Sciences
University of Colorado Colorado Springs
Colorado Springs, Colorado
Chapter 22, Older Adults

Mary Jo Stanley, PhD, RN, CNS, CNE
Professor
Director, School of Nursing
California State University, Stanislaus
Turlock, California
Chapter 28, Public Settings
Chapter 29, Private Settings
Chapter 30, Home Health and Hospice Care

Rebecca E. Sutter, DNP, APRN, BC-FNP
Mason and Partners Clinic Co-Director
Associate Professor of Nursing
School of Nursing
College of Health and Human Services
George Mason University
Fairfax, Virginia
Chapter 23, Working With Vulnerable People

Susan M. Swider, PhD, PHNA-BC, FAAN
Director, DNP Tracks in Advanced Public Health Nursing
Transformative Leadership: Population Health
Department of Community Systems and Mental Health Nursing
College of Nursing
Rush University
Chicago, Illinois
Chapter 13, Policy Making and Advocacy

Dana Todd, PhD, APRN
Professor
School of Nursing and Health Professions
Murray State University
Murray, Kentucky
Chapter 2, Public Health Nursing in the Community
Chapter 11, Health Promotion Through Education
Chapter 19, Maternal–Child Health

Lauren Traveller, DNP, APRN, FNP-C
Assistant Professor of Nursing
Southern Utah University
Cedar City, Utah
Chapter 18, Violence and Abuse

Katharine West, DNP, MPH
Associate Faculty
College of Nursing, Southern California Campus
University of Phoenix
Ontario, California
Chapter 16, Global Health Nursing

Robin M. White, PhD, MSN, RN
Director of BSN Nursing Program
Associate Professor
University of Tampa Nursing Program
Tampa, Florida
Chapter 27, Rural, Migrant, and Urban Health

Elizabeth Wright, MSN, APRN, CNE
Assistant Professor Nursing
Post Licensure Division
Indiana Wesleyan University
Marion, Indiana
Chapter 30, Home Health and Hospice Care

CONTRIBUTORS TO THE 9TH EDITION

Sheila Adams-Leander, RN, PhD
Associate Professor
Milwaukee School of Engineering University
Milwaukee, Wisconsin
Chapter 5

Peggy H. Anderson, DNP, MS, RN
Associate Teaching Professor
Brigham Young University
College of Nursing
Provo, Utah
Chapter 22

Barbara Blake, RN, PhD, ACRN, FAAN
Professor
Kennesaw State University
Kennesaw, Georgia
Chapter 23

Anne Bongiorno, PhD, APHN-BC
Associate Professor
State University of New York, Plattsburgh
Plattsburgh, New York
Chapter 4

Bonnie Callen, PhD, RN, PHCNS-BC
Associate Professor (Retired)
University of Tennessee, Knoxville
Knoxville, Tennessee
Chapter 24

Beverly A. Dandridge, MSN, FNP, MSAJS, CCHP
CAPT, USPHS Commissioned Corps
Department of Homeland Security
USPHS Commissioned Corps Liaison
Washington, District of Columbia
Chapters 17 and 30

Janna L. Dieckmann, PhD, RN
Associate Professor
University of North Carolina at Chapel Hill
Chapel Hill, North Carolina
Chapter 26

Rebecca Doughty, MN, RN, PhD(c)
Director of Health Services
Spoken Public Schools
Spokane, Washington
Chapter 30

Mary Ann Drake, PhD, RN, CNE
Professor
Webster University
St. Louis, Missouri
Chapter 18

Naomi Ervin, PhD, RN, PHCNS-BC, FNAP, FAAN
Adjunct Professor
Madonna University
Livonia, Michigan
Chapter 25

Deborah S. Finnell, DNS, PHMHP-BC, CARN-AP, FAAN
Associate Professor
Johns Hopkins School of Nursing
Baltimore, Maryland
Chapter 27

MAJ Lakisha N. Flagg, DrPH, MS, CPH, APHN-BC
Chief, Army Public Health Nursing
Brooke Army Medical Center
Joint Base San Antonio Fort Sam Houston, Texas
San Antonio, Texas
Chapter 15

Ezra C. Holston, PhD, RN
Assistant Professor
University of Tennessee, Knoxville
Knoxville, Tennessee
Chapter 19

Barbara Joyce, PhD, RN, CNS, ANEF
Associate Professor
Helen and Arthur E. Johnson Beth-El College of Nursing & Health Sciences
University of Colorado Colorado Springs
Colorado Springs, Colorado
Chapter 20

Betty C. Jung, MPH, RN, MCHES
Program Director
Public Health Expertise Network of Mentors
Adjunct Lecturer
Southern Connecticut State University
New Haven, Connecticut
Chapter 7

Katherine Laux Kaiser, PhD, RN, PHCNS-BC
Professor
University of Nebraska Medical Center
College of Nursing
Omaha, Nebraska
Chapter 21

Mary Lashley, PhD, RN, PHNCS-BC
Professor
Towson University
Towson, Maryland
Chapter 28

Angelique Lawyer, MSN, MPH, APHN-BC, RN
Nurse Consultant, Chief Surgeon's Office
National Guard Bureau
Arlington, Virginia
Chapter 31

Jeanne M. Leffers, PhD, RN, FAAN
Professor Emeritus
University of Massachusetts, Dartmouth
North Dartmouth, Massachusetts
Chapter 9

Karin L. Lightfoot, PhD, MSN, RN-BC, PHN
Assistant Professor
California State University, Chico
Chico, California
Chapters 8 and 14

Colleen Marzilli, PhD, DNP, MBA, RN-BC, CCM, APHN-BC, CNE
Assistant Professor
The University of Texas at Tyler
Tyler, Texas
Chapter 10

Debra J. Millar, MSN, RN, APHN-BC
Assistant Professor
California State University, Stanislaus
Turlock, California
Chapters 12 and 16

Mary Ellen Miller, PhD, RN, APHN-BC
Associate Professor
Director, Bridging the Gaps Lehigh Valley Affiliate
DeSales University
Center Valley, Pennsylvania
Chapter 31(Lead)

Margaret Oot-Hayes, PhD, RN
Professor
Regis College
Weston, Massachusetts
Chapter 30

Judith M. Paré, PhD, RN
Dean, School of Nursing and Behavioral Sciences
Becker College
Worcester, Massachusetts
Chapter 29

Carol Pochron, MSN, RN
Adjunct Professor
DeSales University
Center Valley, Pennsylvania
Chapter 31

Cherie Rector, PhD, RN, PHN
Professor Emeritus
Department of Nursing
California State University, Bakersfield
Bakersfield, California
Chapters 1, 2, and 29

Annmarie Donahue Samar, PhD, PHCNS-BC, NEA-BC, RN
Professor
Framingham State University
Framingham, Massachusetts
Chapter 10

Lisabeth M. Searing, PhD, RN
Assistant Professor
Illinois Wesleyan University
Bloomington, Illinois
Chapter 6

Bryan W. Sisk, RN, BSN, MPH
Associate Director Patient Care Services
Nurse Executive
Central Texas Veterans Health Care System
Temple, Texas
Veteran's Content Expert Contributor

Susan M. Swider, PhD, APHN-BC, FAAN
Professor, Department of Community, Systems and Mental Health Nursing
Program Director, DNP in Advanced Public Health Nursing and Leadership to Enhance Population Health Outcomes
Rush University
College of Nursing
Chicago, Illinois
Chapter 13

Gloria Ann Jones Taylor, PhD, RN
Professor
Kennesaw State University
Kennesaw, Georgia
Chapter 23

Dana Todd, PhD, APRN
Associate Professor
Murray State University
Murray, Kentucky
Chapters 3, 11, and 21

Kristine D. Warner, PhD, MPH, RN
Assistant Dean and Managing Director
MEPN Program
University of California, San Francisco
San Francisco, California
Chapter 2

Robin M. White, PhD, MSN, RN
Assistant Professor
University of Tampa
Tampa, Florida
Chapter 29

Marjory D. Williams, PhD, RN
Associate Chief Nursing Service, Education and Research
Central Texas Veterans Health Care System
Temple, Texas
Veteran's Content Expert Contributor

Elizabeth Wright, MSN, RN
Assistant Professor of Nursing
Indiana Wesleyan University
Marion, Indiana
Chapter 32

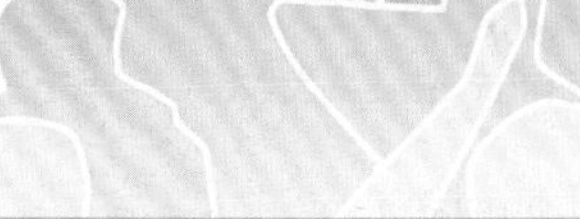

REVIEWERS

Barbara Blackford, MSN, RN-CNE
Assistant Professor
Marian University
Indianapolis, Indiana

Anne Bongiorno, PhD, APHN-BC, CNE
Professor
SUNY Plattsburgh
Plattsburgh, New York

Kelly Brittain, PhD, RN
Associate Professor
Michigan State University
College of Nursing
East Lansing, Michigan

Esther Brown, EdD, RN, FCN-BC, ThB
Associate Professor
Widener University
Chester, Pennsylvania

Angeline Bushy, PhD, RN, FAAN
Professor, Bert Fish Eminent Chair
University of Central Florida
College of Nursing
Daytona Beach, Florida

Adelita G. Cantu, PhD, RN
Associate Professor
University of Texas at San Antonio
School of Nursing
San Antonio, Texas

Holly Cassells, PhD, RNC
Chair, Graduate Nursing Program
University of the Incarnate Word
San Antonio, Texas

Stephanie Chung, PhD, RN
Assistant Professor
Georgian Court University
Lakewood, New Jersey

Jennifer Cooper, DNP, MSN
Assistant Professor
Hood College
Frederick, Maryland

Joan Creed, DNP, RN, CCM
Clinical Assistant Professor
University of South Carolina
Columbia, South Carolina

Margaret C. Delaney, EdD, APRN, PNP-BC
Instructor
Benedictine University
Lisle, Illinois

Kathie DeMuth, MSN, RN
Assistant Professor
Bellin College
Green Bay, Wisconsin

Christina DesOrmeaux, PhD, RN
Assistant Clinical Professor
The Cizik School of Nursing
The University of Texas Health Science Center at Houston
Houston, Texas

Kathleen Dever, EdD, MS, RN
Associate Professor
Wegmans School of Nursing
St. John Fisher College
Rochester, New York

Lisa J. Fardy, DNP, MSN, MPH, RN, PHCNS-BC
Associate Professor of Nursing and Public Health
Regis College
Weston, Massachusetts

Cindy Farris, PhD, MSN, MPH, CNE
Assistant Professor
Florida Gulf Coast University
Fort Myers, Florida

Jackie Gillespie, MN, RN, Retired CNE
Nursing Educator (Retired)
Clemson University School of Nursing
Clemson, South Carolina

Patty Nolan Goldsmith, MS, RN, PHNA-BC
Senior Lecturer
University of Arizona
College of Nursing
Tucson, Arizona

Dawn M. Goodolf, PhD, RN
Associate Professor
Moravian College
Bethlehem, Pennsylvania

Donna S. Guerra, EdD, MSN, RN
Clinical Assistant Professor
University of Alabama in Huntsville
Huntsville, Alabama

Susan Harrington, PhD, RN
Associate Professor
Grand Valley State University
Grand Rapids, Michigan

Tammy Kiser, DNP, RN
Assistant Professor of Nursing
James Madison University
Harrisonburg, Virginia

Alexis Koenig, EdD, MSN, RN, CNE, CCHP
Associate Professor
East Stroudsburg University
East Stroudsburg, Pennsylvania

Julie A. Kruse, PhD, RN
Associate Professor
Oakland University
School of Nursing
Rochester, Michigan

Kimberly Lacey, DNSc, MSN, RN, CNE
Professor
Southern Connecticut State University
New Haven, Connecticut

Barbara Whitman Lancaster, DNP, APN, WHNP-BC
Assistant Professor
Middle Tennessee State University
Murfreesboro, Tennessee

Erica Lemberger, DNP, FNP-BC, AFN-BC, RN, SANE A/P
Associate Professor
Spalding University
Louisville, Kentucky

Amanda Jean Madrid, RN, MSN, PHN-BC
Assistant Professor
California Baptist University
Riverside, California

Aimee McDonald, PhD, RN
Assistant Professor
William Jewell College
Liberty, Missouri

Cindy McZeal, MSN, PHN, RN
Program Coordinator
California State University Los Angeles
Los Angeles, California

Sandra E. Monk, PhD, RN, CHPN
Assistant Professor
Shorter University
Rome, Georgia

Geraldine Moore, EdD, RN, BC, AE-C
Professor
Molloy College
Barbara H. Hagan School of Nursing and Health Sciences
Rockville Centre, New York

Linda Morgan, PhD, MSN, RN, PHN
Associate Professor
Reinhardt University
Waleska, Georgia

Susan A. Natale, PhD, RN, NEA-BC
Associate Professor
Curry College
Milton, Massachusetts

Sabita Persaud, PhD, RN, PHNA-BC
Associate Professor
Notre Dame of Maryland
Baltimore, Maryland

Tami J. Pobocik, PhD, RN
Associate Professor
Saginaw Valley State University
University Center, Michigan

Pamela Rafferty-Semon, MSN-Ed, RN
Associate Lecturer
Kent State University
Kent, Ohio

Mary Jean Ricci, MSN, RN-BC
Director of Clinical Education, Assistant Professor of Nursing, Chair of Population Health
Drexel University
Philadelphia, Pennsylvania

Diane Riff, DNP, APRN, NP-C
Associate Professor
University of Louisville
Louisville, Kentucky

Kathleen Rindahl, DNP, RN, FNP-C
Associate Professor
Fresno State University
School of Nursing
Fresno, California

Ronna Schrum, DNP, RN, CRNP
Assistant Professor
Frostburg State University
Frostburg, Maryland

Kathleen F. Tate, EdD, MSN, MBA, RN, CNE
Associate Professor of Nursing
Northwestern State University
Shreveport, Louisiana

Antionella Upshaw, PhD, RN, BS
Assistant Professor
Southern University and A&M College
Baton Rouge, Louisiana

Maria Warnick, MSN, CRNP
Assistant Director
Gwynedd Mercy University
Gwynedd Valley, Pennsylvania

Rita West, DNSc, RN, NEA-BC
Assistant Professor
Baptist College of Health Sciences
Memphis, Tennessee

Lori A. Wheeler, PhD, RN
Assistant Professor
Thomas Jefferson University
Philadelphia, Pennsylvania

Kathlene H. Williams, MS, RN, CNE
Assistant Professor of Nursing
McNeese State University
Lake Charles, Louisiana

Debra Windle, PHN, MSN, CNS
Nursing Faculty
California State University Long Beach
Long Beach, California

Pamela J. Worrell-Carlisle, PhD, RN
Assistant Professor
School of Nursing
Georgia Southern University
Statesboro, Georgia

Amy Yakos, MSN, RN-BC, CEN
Clinical Lecturer
Ball State University
Muncie, Indiana

PREFACE

The 10th edition of *Community and Public Health Nursing: Promoting the Public's Health* provides undergraduate nursing students an introduction to community/public health and population-focused nursing in the community. Community settings may include public health departments, community-based organizations, schools, correctional facilities, industries, and businesses. The textbook introduces students to key populations with whom they may work in community settings and to commonly occurring situations in which they may find themselves as new nurses in the community and in other settings.

Community/public health nursing skills provide new nurses with a broader focus of patient care (e.g., families, aggregates, communities, populations), not just individual patients. Even if new graduates plan on employment in acute care settings (which is often the most familiar setting for them), a public health and population focus is useful there. A recent example of how this is helpful is the COVID-19 pandemic, which has burdened many hospitals as they sought to provide care for patients and to find adequate PPE, staff, and bed space. This pandemic brought to the forefront the importance of public health in ensuring our nation's health and prosperity. It is important for acute care nurses to have an understanding of their patients' unique circumstances and how to best join with patients and their families in working to prevent disease and further complications, and to promote better health. To help students gain a holistic view of the patient, throughout this book students are provided with examples and information that will broaden their knowledge of patients and enable them to provide more effective nursing care—wherever they may be employed.

The purpose of this book is to give undergraduate students a solid, basic grounding in public health principles and community/public health nursing practice. It is our hope to generate an interest in this important nursing specialty and that some graduates will join us in working to prevent disease, promote health, and protect at-risk populations.

Chapters reflect contributors' and reviewers' broad spectrum of views and expertise, coalescing into a carefully edited and cohesive textbook with a shared community/public health vision.

NEW TO THIS EDITION

This edition reflects a continuing effort to communicate in a user-friendly style with nursing students who are entering the world of community/public health nursing for the first time. We focus on showing the connection between community/public health population-focused nursing and the practice of acute care nursing, providing students with examples and information that will broaden their knowledge of their patients and enable them to provide more effective nursing care wherever they may choose to practice. We also point out to students that population-focused care is not only unique to public health but also important in acute care settings (e.g., infection control, programs to reduce length of stays or readmission rates), and many hospital systems recognize the need for more community-based options. Health care reform has changed the landscape for patients and providers, and health care is becoming even more community-based. Population-focused tools and interventions are not only important in community/public health nursing—they are needed in acute care, as infection rates continue to rise, and nurse-sensitive outcome indicators are closely monitored.

Expanded and new content in this 10th edition includes the following:

- **Healthy People 2030:** Content from the updated framework informs readers about this decade's health goals and objectives for various population groups.
- **Ten essential public health services:** Content is added throughout the text and an exercise in each of the end-of-chapter Active Learning Exercises sections asks students to consider and apply these essentials.
- **LGBTQ, veteran, and refugee populations:** Coverage has been expanded as follows:
  - We have included specific sections on these vulnerable groups in Chapter 23, Working With Vulnerable People.
  - LGBTQ content is incorporated throughout the textbook and in some features in an effort to help nursing students to better comprehend and address the needs of this population.
  - Veteran's health content is the focus of some features (e.g., some of the Stories From the Field and Perspectives boxes) and critical thinking activities to better explore this population and the role of the community/public health nurse (C/PHN) in serving them.
- **Streamlining of content:** To better represent population and aggregate health:
  - Reading-intensive text has been converted into more concise, bulleted lists.
  - More graphics and infographics have been included to help students understand basic concepts.
  - The Summary at the end of each chapter is a bulleted list that clearly reinforces key points and concepts.
  - Some supplemental material has been moved to thepoint.lww.com/Rector10e.

Special Boxes in This Book: This section of this book's front matter, found immediately following the

Table of Contents, makes it easier to find the features and stories that bring the theoretical content in the text to life.

Organization of This Book

For the 10th edition, the content has been streamlined into 7 units and 30 chapters.

Unit 1, "Foundations of Community/Public Health Nursing," covers fundamental principles and background about community/public health nursing.

- Chapter 1, "The Journey Begins: Introduction," discusses basic public health concepts of health, illness, wellness, community, aggregate, population, and levels of prevention. The chapter introduces leading health indicators, along with *Healthy People 2030* goals and objectives.
- Chapter 2, "Public Health Nursing in the Community," explains roles and settings for community/public health nursing, the three primary functions of public health, and the 10 essential public health services. Standards of practice are also discussed.
- Chapter 3, "History and Evolution of Public Health Nursing," examines the stages of public health nursing's rich and meaningful history, its nursing leaders, the evolution of nursing education, and the social influences that have shaped our current practice. Features highlighting historical landmarks and C/PHN experiences during different time periods, along with historical photos and resources, bring this history to life.
- Chapter 4, "Evidence-Based Practice and Ethics," considers values, ethical principles, and ethical decision-making in community/public health nursing and acute care settings. The chapter also introduces quality and safety, evidence-based practice, research principles, and the use of systematic reviews to improve practice.
- Chapter 5, "Transcultural Nursing," defines cultural principles, highlighting the importance of cultural diversity and the need for cultural sensitivity. Information presented includes cultural assessment and folk remedies, as well as complementary and alternative medicine.

Unit 2, "Community/Public Health Essentials," covers the structure of community/public health within the overall health system infrastructure and introduces the basic public health tools of epidemiology, communicable disease control, and environmental health.

- Chapter 6, "Structure and Economics of Community/Public Health Services," examines the economics of health care and compares U.S. outcomes with those of other countries, while also discussing the private and government health insurance options. It also examines the functions of official health agencies and their organizational structures, as well as landmark legislation and policies related to public health.
- Chapter 7, "Epidemiology in the Community," highlights basic concepts of epidemiology and different methods of epidemiologic investigation and research, along with the C/PHN's role in epidemiology.
- Chapter 8, "Communicable Disease," presents a population focus on communicable disease control and immunization programs, highlighting vaccine hesitancy and effective approaches with clients. The chapter also discusses communicable disease investigations and common communicable diseases often seen in C/PHN practice.
- Chapter 9, "Environmental Health and Safety," reviews environmental health concepts and assessments, the precautionary principle, having an ecologic perspective, and the use of an upstream approach to reduce environmental risks.

Unit 3, "Community/Public Health Nursing Toolbox," includes common tools used by the community/public health nurse to ensure effective practice.

- Chapter 10, "Communication, Collaboration, and Technology," discusses communication, collaboration, working with groups, contracting with clients, and the C/PHN's use of motivational interviewing and OARS, as well as informatics and health technology. Technologies examined include Big Data, EHRs, mHealth, and GIS, among others, and examples of technology applications are provided.
- Chapter 11, "Health Promotion Through Education," presents health education, the three types of learning, health promotion and change, along with learning theories and models, as well as a description of teaching in the community.
- Chapter 12, "Planning, Implementing, and Evaluating Community/Public Health Programs," focuses on identifying problems and planning and developing community health programs. The chapter examines designing interventions and evaluating outcomes, along with social marketing approaches and grant funding.
- Chapter 13, "Policy Making and Advocacy," concludes this unit with an explanation of the C/PHN's role in political advocacy, policy analysis, and policy making, highlighting examples of C/PHN and community involvement in addressing policy issues.

Unit 4, "The Health of Our Population," further expands the focus of the community/public health nurse.

- Chapter 14, "Family as Client," examines the family as the C/PHN's client and discusses methods of family assessment. Conceptual frameworks and application of the nursing process to family health help promote healthy families. Home visiting protocols are discussed, along with contracting and referrals.
- Chapter 15, "Community as Client," applies the nursing process to communities as clients (contrasted to individual patient focus in acute care). The chapter presents models and frameworks for community assessment and discusses different types of assessments, along with sources of data, community diagnoses, and community development.
- Chapter 16, "Global Health Nursing," presents global health principles and data methods of international organizations. Topics covered include international agencies, nongovernmental organizations, and various foundations, along with global health problems/

practices as well as global service-based learning and the ethical considerations involved.

- Chapter 17, "Disasters and Their Impact," examines preparedness with a closer look at disasters, terrorism, mass casualty events, and war. Phases of a disaster and disaster management are covered, along with disaster plans and treatment for survivors. Also discussed is the C/PHN's role in emergency preparedness, disaster management, preventive measures against terrorism, and *Healthy People 2030* objectives.
- Chapter 18, "Violence and Abuse," encompasses violence across the life span, including child abuse, elder abuse, community violence, and intimate partner violence. Crisis intervention is also included.

Unit 5, "Aggregate Populations," introduces the family as an aggregate, along with other aggregates with whom the C/PHN routinely works.

- Chapter 19, "Maternal–Child Health," covers common issues, concerns, and interventions for maternal–child health clients and their infants (e.g., complications of pregnancy and childbirth, teen pregnancy, STIs, substance abuse), including health services for mothers and infants through preschool.
- Chapter 20, "School-Age Children and Adolescents," examines physical and emotional health problems affecting children and adolescents (e.g., diabetes, asthma, injuries, communicable disease, substance abuse, preventive programs), along with learning problems and disabilities.
- Chapter 21, "Adult Health," discusses the leading causes of death, genomic risks, environmental factors, and health care needs of the adult population. The chapter also presents the effects of chronic illness and the C/PHN's role in working with adults to provide early detection, education, and rehabilitation.
- Chapter 22, "Older Adults," covers the unique issues facing the older client (e.g., common myths, preventive measures, health services, end-of-life care) and the C/PHN's role in working with this population.

Unit 6, "Vulnerable Populations," provides information about client groups that are often aggregated by public health departments.

- Chapter 23, "Working With Vulnerable People," describes vulnerable populations, contributing factors, and helpful models or frameworks related to vulnerability. The chapter also discusses social determinants of health and the socioeconomic gradient leading to health disparities, along with the C/PHN's role.
- Chapter 24, "Clients With Disabilities," covers issues related to disabilities, the role of Healthy People and legislation (e.g., ADA, IDEA) in meeting the needs of the disabled population. It reinforces the importance of the C/PHN's role with this population.
- Chapter 25, "Behavioral Health in the Community," addresses behavioral health issues (e.g., mental health, substance use) and the C/PHN's role in focusing on these problems using frameworks and screening tools.
- Chapter 26, "Working With the Homeless," covers the homeless population and problems associated with homelessness (e.g., poverty, lack of affordable health care and housing, mental illness, addictions, financial troubles, health problems). The chapter also examines the C/PHN role as an advocate and case manager.
- Chapter 27, "Rural, Migrant, and Urban Communities," encompasses the challenges and common problems facing these populations. It also explores issues of social justice, medically underserved populations, and frontier nursing.

Unit 7, "Settings for Community/Public Health Nursing," examines public and private settings in more depth, as well as home health and hospice nursing.

- Chapter 28, "Public Settings," describes practice options in government-sponsored agencies, such as state and local public health departments, public schools, correctional facilities, and the U.S. Public Health Service.
- Chapter 29, "Private Settings," includes a focus on C/PHN opportunities in private agencies (e.g., nurse-led health centers, faith-based nursing, occupational health, entrepreneurship).
- Chapter 30, "Home Health and Hospice Care," discusses the important roles of home health and hospice/palliative care nursing, especially given our aging population.

The appendix presents the Quad Council Tier 1 Community/Public Health Nursing Competencies.

Features of the Text

The 10th edition of *Community and Public Health Nursing: Promoting the Public's Health* includes key features from previous editions as well as new features, including the following:

- **Evidence-Based Practice** boxes supplement current research cited throughout the text, incorporating specific research examples pertinent to chapter content and explaining how they can be applied to achieve optimal client, aggregate, and population outcomes. Thought-provoking questions challenge students' understanding of evidence-based concepts and the application of EBP/research in community/public health nursing practice.
- **Stories From the Field** (titled From the Case Files in the ninth edition) boxes present a scenario/case study, followed by student-centered, application-based questions that focus on the nursing process. Students are challenged to reflect on assessment and intervention in typical, yet challenging, examples of public health nursing as it is used in practice. Questions ask students to apply chapter content to examples that highlight client situations.
- **Levels of Prevention Pyramid** boxes, unique to this text in their complexity and comprehensiveness, enhance understanding of the levels of prevention concepts that are basic to public/community health nursing. Each box addresses a chapter topic, describing

nursing actions at each of the three levels of prevention. We place primary prevention (rather than tertiary prevention) at the pyramid's base to reflect its importance as a foundation for health.

- *Healthy People 2030* boxes highlight pertinent goals and objectives to promote health related to specific populations or problems.
- **Perspectives** (titled Voices From the Community/Student Voices in the ninth edition) boxes provide stories (viewpoints) from a variety of sources. Perspectives may be from nursing students, novices or experienced public health nurses, faculty members, policy makers, or clients. These short features are designed to promote critical thinking, help students reflect on commonly held misconceptions about public/community health nursing, and recognize the link between skills learned in this specialty practice and other practice settings, especially acute care hospitals.
- **What Do *You* Think?** boxes provoke thought or stir discussion on subject matter that is often unique to public health, similar to how instructors might stop and ask a thought-provoking question during lecture. These features encourage the reader to pause and more deeply consider an issue.
- **QSEN: Focus on Quality** boxes highlight quality and safety concepts. These include QSEN (Quality and Safety Education for Nurses) concepts related to environmental health and disasters, patient-centered care (family/community; empowerment), teamwork/collaboration (communication; system barriers), EBP/QI/ethics, and data (e.g., tracking the homeless).
- **Population Focus** boxes help refocus student attention to chapter concepts from a population-focused viewpoint. Although chapter content generally contains population-based information, in selected chapters an additional focus on population is needed. Current case studies or examples of effective population-based interventions help make the concept of population-based health more evident and understandable to students.
- **C/PHN Use of the Nursing Process** boxes allow students to see how assessment, diagnosis, planning, intervention, and evaluation are used within the context of community/public health situations as presented in selected chapters.
- **Learning Objectives** and **Key Terms** sharpen the reader's focus and provide a quick guide for mastering the chapter content.
- The **Introduction** section presents the chapter topic, and the bulleted **Summary** section provides an overview of material covered, serving as a concise and focused review.
- A **References** list at the end of each chapter provides current research as well as classic sources that offer a broad base of authoritative information for furthering knowledge on each chapter's subject matter.
- **Active Learning Exercises** (titled Activities to Promote Critical Thinking in the ninth edition) challenge students, foster critical thinking, and promote application of chapter content. They often include active involvement in solving community health problems in the form of Internet activities, small group work, and interviews with clients, key community informants, or experts. One of the exercises in each chapter is a thought question related to the 10 essential public health services to promote evaluation and application in community/public health nursing.
- **Additional assessment tools** are provided throughout the chapters (and on thePoint) to enhance student assessment skills with individuals, families, or aggregates/populations.

A COMPREHENSIVE PACKAGE FOR TEACHING AND LEARNING

To further facilitate teaching and learning, a carefully designed ancillary package has been developed to assist faculty and students.

RESOURCES FOR INSTRUCTORS

Tools to assist with teaching this text are available upon its adoption on thePoint® at http://thePoint.lww.com/Rector10e.

- An **e-Book** gives you access to the book's full text and images online.
- The **Test Generator** lets you put together exclusive new tests to help assess students' understanding of the material. Test questions are mapped to chapter learning objectives and page numbers.
- An extensive collection of materials is provided for each book chapter:
  - **Pre-Lecture Quizzes** (and answers) are quick, knowledge-based assessments that allow you to check students' reading comprehension.
  - **PowerPoint Presentations** provide an easy way for you to integrate the textbook with your students' classroom experience, either via slide shows or handouts. Multiple-choice and true/false questions are integrated into the presentations to promote class participation and allow you to use i-clicker technology.
  - **Assignments** (and suggested answers) include group, written, clinical, and Web assignments.
  - **Case Studies** with related questions (and suggested answers) give students an opportunity to apply their knowledge to a client case similar to one they might encounter in practice.
- An **Image Bank** lets you use the photographs and illustrations from this textbook in your PowerPoint slides or as you see fit in your course.
- Sample **Syllabi** provide guidance for structuring your community and public health nursing course.
- A **QSEN Competency Map** identifies content and special features in the book related to competencies identified by the QSEN Institute.
- A **BSN Essentials Competency Map** identifies book content related to the BSN Essentials.

Contact your sales representative or check out LWW.com/Nursing for more details and ordering information.

RESOURCES FOR STUDENTS

An exciting set of resources is available to help students review material and become even more familiar with vital concepts. Students can access all these resources on thePoint® at http://thePoint.lww.com/Rector10e, using the codes printed on the inside front cover of their textbooks.

- **NCLEX-Style Review Questions** for each chapter help students review important concepts and practice for NCLEX.
- **Podcasts** educate students about community health topics.
- **Journal Articles** offer access to current articles relevant to each chapter and available in Wolters Kluwer journals to familiarize students with nursing literature.
- **Supplemental Materials** offer additional information to accompany the textbook content.
- **Links to Videos** enable examination of thought-provoking issues related to vulnerable populations.
- **Learning Objectives** help readers identify important chapter content and focus their reading.

A COMPREHENSIVE, DIGITAL, INTEGRATED COURSE SOLUTION: LIPPINCOTT® COURSEPOINT+

The same trusted solution, innovation, and unmatched support that you have come to expect from *Lippincott CoursePoint+* is now enhanced with more engaging learning tools and deeper analytics to help prepare students for practice. This powerfully integrated digital learning solution combines learning tools, case studies, virtual simulation, real-time data, and the most trusted nursing education content on the market to make curriculum-wide learning more efficient and to meet students where they're at in their learning. And now, it's easier than ever for instructors and students to use, giving them everything they need for course and curriculum success!

Lippincott CoursePoint+ for Rector & Stanley: Community and Public Health Nursing, 10th edition, includes the following:

- Engaging course content provides a variety of learning tools to engage students of all learning styles.
- A more personalized learning approach gives students the content and tools they need at the moment they need it, giving them data for more focused remediation and helping to boost their confidence.
- Powerful tools students need to learn the critical thinking and clinical judgment skills that will help them become practice-ready nurses, including:
    - **Video Cases** help students anticipate what to expect as a nurse, with detailed scenarios that capture their attention and integrate clinical knowledge with community and public health concepts that are critical to real-world nursing practice. By watching the videos and completing related activities, students will flex their problem-solving, prioritizing, analyzing, and application skills to aid both in NCLEX preparation and preparation for practice.
    - **Interactive Modules** help students quickly identify what they do and do not understand, so they can study smartly. With exceptional instructional design that prompts students to discover, reflect, synthesize, and apply, students actively learn. SmartSense remediation links to the eBook are integrated throughout.
    - **Lippincott Clinical Experiences: Community, Public, and Population Health Nursing** (also available for separate purchase), codeveloped with nursing educators Jone Tiffany, DNP, RN, CNE, CHSE, ANEF, and Barbara Hoglund, EdD, MSN, FNP-BC, CNE, offers clinical experiences that consistently expose students to diverse settings, situations, and populations. As students immerse themselves in a safe and engaging virtual environment, they are exposed to the real-life application of key community, public, and population health concepts. Students make observations, hold virtual conversations, triage at a disaster scene, do research online, conduct interviews, and more. The students' virtual experience is enhanced by surrounding curricula, including suggested readings, active learning assignments, and assessments, which are designed to assist with their knowledge acquisition and enhance their critical thinking skills. Additional real-world clinical assignments can also supplement or replace current clinical activities or Practicum. These clinicals get students thinking about their communities through a community health lens and looking at larger public health and population health issues. Reporting tools track students' learning and progress.
- Unparalleled reporting provides in-depth dashboards with several data points to track student progress and help identify strengths and weaknesses.

Unmatched support includes training coaches, product trainers, and nursing education consultants to help educators and students implement CoursePoint+ with ease.

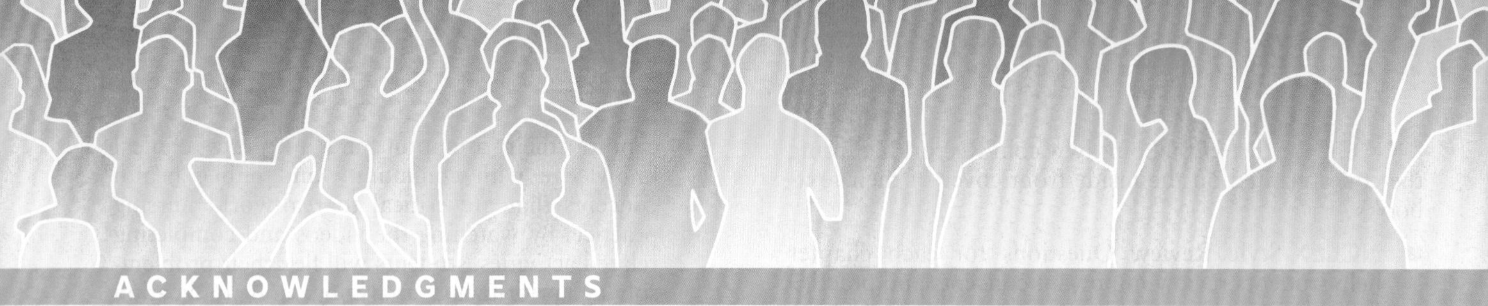

ACKNOWLEDGMENTS

This book continues as an evolving work in progress. Our goal is to continually update and improve it, incorporating input from nursing students, faculty, and public health nurses. We welcome and encourage feedback. We thank the reviewers for their thoughtful critiques and suggestions, and the contributors (past and present) who have shared their time and expertise.

We especially want to thank Meredith Brittain, senior development editor, who gave careful attention to detail, as well as the big picture, in producing our final product. Her efforts are greatly appreciated, and the textbook is a testament to her focus on precision and detail. We would also like to recognize freelance development editor David Payne for his careful editing and helpful observations. We recognize the diligent work of our acquisitions editors, Christina Burns and Michael Kerns, who guided us through this process from start to finish. We also thank others at Wolters Kluwer for their support, including Ashley Pfeiffer and Alicia Jackson.

Appreciation is also given to Charlene Niemi, PhD, RN, PHN, CNE, for her work assisting us in finalizing and editing several chapters and pitching in on short notice to revise and update chapter sections when needed. Family, friends, and colleagues were also instrumental in providing moral support and encouragement. It is our hope that nursing students and faculty will find our efforts meaningful.

CONTENTS

SPECIAL BOXES IN THIS BOOK

C/PHN USE OF THE NURSING PROCESS

EVIDENCE-BASED PRACTICE

HEALTHY PEOPLE 2030

LEVELS OF PREVENTION PYRAMID

PERSPECTIVES

POPULATION FOCUS

QSEN: FOCUS ON QUALITY

STORIES FROM THE FIELD

WHAT DO *YOU* THINK?

UNIT 1

Foundations of Community/ Public Health Nursing

CHAPTER 1

The Journey Begins: Introduction

"For a community to be whole and healthy, it must be based on people's love and concern for each other."

—Millard Fuller (1935–2009), Founder, Habitat for Humanity

KEY TERMS

Aggregate
Community
Community health
Community health nursing
Geographic community
Health
Health continuum
Health promotion
Illness
Population
Population focused
Primary prevention
Public health
Public health nursing
Secondary prevention
Tertiary prevention
Wellness

LEARNING OBJECTIVES

Upon mastery of this chapter, you should be able to:

1. Explain the concepts of community, population, aggregate, and public health.
2. Give specific examples of nursing interventions that differentiate the three levels of prevention.
3. Describe three benefits that community/public health nursing experience can provide to those working in acute care nursing.
4. Identify examples of how the eight characteristics of community/public health nursing can be applied.

INTRODUCTION

Opportunities and challenges in nursing are boundless and rapidly changing. You have spent a lot of time and effort learning how to care for individual patients in medical–surgical and other acute care–oriented nursing specialties. You have provided nursing care in familiar acute care settings for the very ill, both young and old, but always with other professionals at your side. Now you are entering a unique and exciting area of nursing—community/public health.

As one of the oldest specialty nursing practices, public health nursing offers unique challenges and opportunities. Public health nursing is community based and population focused. A nurse entering this field will encounter the complex challenge of working with populations rather than just individual clients and the opportunity to carry on the heritage of early public health nursing efforts with the benefit of modern advances. In doing so, there are the challenges of:

- Expanding nursing's focus from the individual and family to communities and populations
- Determining the needs of populations at risk and designing interventions to specifically address them
- Learning the complexities of a constantly changing health care system

Operating within an environment of rapid change and increasingly complex challenges, this nursing specialty holds the potential to shape the quality of community health services and improve the nation's health.

Now you are being asked to leave that familiar acute care setting and go out into the community—into homes, schools, recreational facilities, work settings, parishes, and even street corners that are commonplace to your clients and unfamiliar to you. Here, in the community, you will:

- Find few or no monitoring devices or charts full of laboratory data
- Have no professional and allied health workers next to you to assist you
- Use the nontangible skills of listening, assessing, planning, teaching, coordinating, evaluating, and referring
- Draw on the skills you have learned throughout your acute care setting experiences (e.g., behavioral health and women's, children's, and adult health nursing) and begin to "think on your feet" in new and exciting situations

Often, your practice will be solo, and you will need to combine creativity, ingenuity, intuition, and resourcefulness along with these skills. Talk about boundless opportunities and challenges! (see Box 1-1).

You may feel that this new setting is too demanding and be anxious about how you will perform in it. But perhaps, just perhaps, you will find that it is rewarding, that it constantly challenges you, interests you, and allows you to work holistically with clients of all ages, at

BOX **1-1** PERSPECTIVES

A Nursing Student Viewpoint on Community/Public Health Nursing

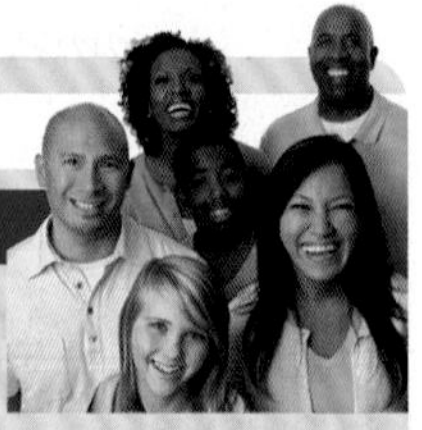

I was really terrified when I got to my community/public health rotation and found that I had to go knock on people's doors! I was close to graduating and felt comfortable in the hospital (the routines and machines). Now, I had to actually find apartments in an area of the city where I never go! And, was unclear about my tasks. I had minimal equipment—a baby scale, a blood pressure cuff, a stethoscope, a thermometer, and a paper tape measure. I was assigned a 16-year-old mother with a 4-month-old baby. I don't even have children! What can I tell her? She is a teenager who "knows it all." My clinical instructor told me to "build a relationship with her" and to "gain trust and rapport," difficult to do when you are scared to death. But I needed this class to finish nursing school, so I drove over there and knocked on her door.

The apartment building was disheveled. When she answered the door, she seemed uninterested—or maybe a little defensive. I told her who I was and why I was there, and she motioned me inside pointing toward the baby, propped up on the tattered couch. I spent the next 15 weeks visiting Anna and her baby every Thursday—weighing and measuring the baby, doing *Ages & Stages Questionnaires* and sharing the results with Anna about developmental milestones, getting her appointments for immunizations, listening to her story of abuse and abandonment, and I began to realize that what I was doing was actually exciting and rewarding. By the end of my rotation, I was going to miss Anna and little José! I had provided education on baby-proofing her apartment, finding resources for food and clothing, and getting birth control. We even talked about how she could finish high school.

After graduation, I took a job in the ED and thought of Anna and José when young mothers would bring in their sick babies. I used C/PHN skills in "connecting" with a teen mom to ensure follow through with antibiotics and antipyretics we were prescribing for her baby's high fever and serious infection. One day, I glanced up from my paperwork to see Anna and José. She looked so relieved to see me! She was frantic with worry about the serious burn José had on his right hand. The other nurses were mumbling about "child abuse" and how "irresponsible teen mothers always were." Anna had left José with a neighbor while she went to an appointment about GED. The older woman was not used to dealing with a busy toddler, and Jose was able to reach the handle of a pan of refried beans. The team treated José's burn, and I gave Anna instructions for follow-up care. The bond we had developed was still there. She trusted me, and I knew that she would follow through with the instructions. The other nurses who were making comments about Anna did not know her circumstances. I feel that I am a more effective ED nurse because of the things I learned during my C/PHN rotation. Someday, when I get tired of the hospital, I may work as a public health nurse. You never know!

Madison, age 24

all stages of illness and wellness, and that it absolutely demands the use of your critical thinking skills. And some of you may decide, when you finish your community/public health nursing course, that you have found your career choice. Even if you are not drawn away from acute care nursing, your community/public health nursing experience will give you:

- Deeper understanding of the people for whom you provide care—where and how they live, the family and cultural dynamics at play, and the problems they will face when discharged from your care
- A realization that clients are not only individuals or families, but also aggregates, communities, and populations, giving you an expanded view of nursing
- Knowledge of myriad community agencies and resources to better assist you in providing a continuum of care for your clients

Finding out begins with understanding the concepts of community and health. This chapter provides an overview of these basic concepts, the components of public health practice, and the salient characteristics of contemporary community/public health nursing practice, so that you can enter this specialty area of nursing in concert with its intentions. The opportunities and challenges of community/public health nursing will become even more apparent as the chapter progresses. We begin by discussing community health and how it provides the context for community/public health nursing practice.

COMMUNITY HEALTH

Human beings are social creatures. We generally live out our lives in the company of other people. An Eskimo is part of a small, tightly knit community of close relatives; a rural Mexican may live in a small village with hardly more than 200 members. In contrast, someone from New York City might be a member of many overlapping communities, such as professional societies, a political party, a religious group, a cultural society, a neighborhood, and the city itself. Even those who try to escape community membership always begin their lives in some type of group, and they usually continue to depend on groups for material and emotional support.

We can draw two important conclusions from this fact:

- Communities are an essential and permanent feature of the human experience.
- As systems theory reminds us, just as a whole is greater than the sum of its parts, so the health of a community is more than the sum of the health of its individual citizens.

Systems theory proposes that systems are open and that there is interaction between systems and their environment (Bertalanffy, 1968). A community that achieves a high level of wellness is composed of healthy citizens, functioning in an environment that protects and promotes health. The communities in which people reside and work have a profound influence on our collective health and well-being (Scott et al., 2018). For instance, do you suppose that green space in a city can influence health? In a population-based study of 1,680 urban adults living in a deprived area of the United Kingdom, the overall prevalence of psychological distress was 22.7%. However, for those living near adequate green spaces, there was a 54% reduction in risk of psychological distress (Pope et al., 2018). Healthier communities can be created.

Before going further, it would be helpful to distinguish between the concepts of community health and public health. Although both are organized community efforts aimed at the promotion, protection, and preservation of the public's health, community health has been defined as "the health status of a defined group of people"....and the "private and public (governmental)" actions taken to "promote, protect, and preserve their health" (McKenzie, Pinger, & Seabert, 2018, p. 6). **Community health** is the identification of needs, along with the protection and improvement of collective health, within a geographically defined area.

- A more comprehensive definition is a "multi-sector and multi-disciplinary collaborative enterprise that uses public health science, evidence-based strategies, and other approaches to engage and work with communities in a culturally appropriate manner, to optimize the health and quality of life of all persons who live, work, or are otherwise active in a defined community or communities" (Goodman, Bunnell, & Posner, 2014, p. 5).

To understand the nature and significance of community health, it is necessary to more closely examine the concepts of community and of health, which are covered in the following sections. The remainder of this section focuses on public health.

Public health is a broader concept and often goes beyond community boundaries, dealing with populations around the world. Public health, as a specialty of nursing practice, seeks to provide organizational structure, a broad set of resources, and the collaborative activities needed to accomplish the goal of an optimally healthy community. When you work in hospitals or other acute care settings, your primary focus is the individual patient. Patients' families are often viewed as ancillary, and little thought is given to the world outside the hospital. Public health, however:

- Broadens the focus of care to families, aggregates, communities, and populations
- Views the community as the recipient of service and health as the product
- Is concerned with the interchange between population groups and their total environment and with the impact of that interchange on collective health

The terms community health nurse and public health nurse are combined throughout this text (C/PHN).

Although many believe that health and illness are issues concerning only individuals, evidence indicates that they are also community issues and that the world is a community. Many types of professionals are involved in public health, forming a complex team, such as:

- A city planner designing an urban renewal project
- A social worker providing counseling about child abuse or working with adolescent substance abusers

- A physician treating clients affected by a sudden outbreak of hepatitis and assisting public health epidemiologists and public health nurses (PHNs) to find the source
- Those working in prenatal clinics, programs providing meals for older adults, genetic counseling centers, and educational programs for early detection of cancer

The professional nurse is an integral member of this team, a linchpin and a liaison between physicians, social workers, government officials, and law enforcement officers. Community/public health nurses (C/PHNs) work in every conceivable kind of community agency, from a state public health department to a community-based advocacy group. Their duties range from examining infants in a well-baby clinic to teaching older adult stroke victims in their homes to planning community and population-focused interventions (e.g., marketing campaigns to reduce tobacco use). They also carry out epidemiologic research and engage in health policy analysis and decision-making. Despite its breadth, however, public health nursing is a specialized practice, generally requiring a bachelor's degree, and certification is needed in some states. There is currently no national nursing certification for public health nursing (only renewals), but one is available specifically for public health professionals (including PHNs) through the National Board of Public Health Examiners (American Association of Colleges of Nursing, 2019). Together, we will examine the unique contribution made by this nursing specialty to our health care system.

Historically, as a practice specialty, public health has been associated primarily with the efforts of official or government entities—for example, federal, state, or local tax-supported health agencies that target a wide range of health issues. In contrast, private health efforts or nongovernmental organizations (NGOs), such as those of the American Lung Association or the American Cancer Society, work toward solving selected health problems. The latter augments the former. Currently, community health practice encompasses both approaches and works collaboratively with all health agencies and efforts, public or private, which are concerned with the public's health. In this text, community health practice refers to a focus on specific, designated communities. It is a part of the larger public health effort and recognizes the fundamental concepts and principles of public health as its birthright and foundation for practice. In the IOM's landmark publication, *The Future of the Public's Health* (1998), the mission of public health is defined simply as "fulfilling society's interest in assuring conditions in which people can be healthy" (p. 7). See Box 1-2.

Winslow's classic 1920 definition of public health still holds true and forms the basis for our understanding of community health in this text:

> **Public health** is "the science and art of preventing disease, prolonging life, and promoting health through the organized efforts and informed choices of society, organizations, public and private communities, and individuals" (CDC, 2017c, para 1).

A more recent and concise definition of public health is:

- "Public health promotes and protects the health of people and the communities where they live, learn work and play" (American Public Health Association, 2018, para. 1).

A Web site sponsored by the Association of Schools of Public Health with support from Pfizer Public Health, *What Is Public Health?* (ASPH, 2018), provides some interesting videos and information about this topic and also proffers this definition:

BOX **1-2** PERSPECTIVES

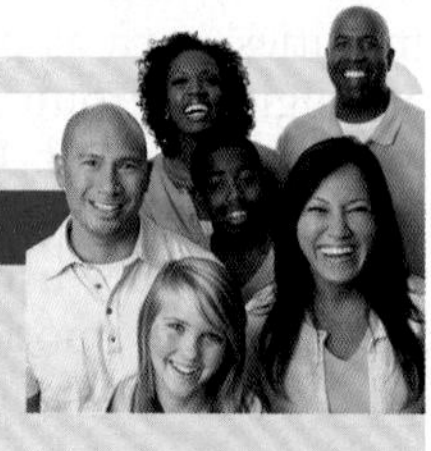

A Public Health Nursing Instructor Viewpoint

When I first introduce the topic of public health, many students don't understand why they have to take this "different" class; they are accustomed to acute care settings, and public health nursing seems so foreign to them. So, I ask students "Why do people end up being hospitalized?" Typical answers include "They needed surgery," "They had an accident," and the like.

Then, I tell them the story of 4-year-old Jackson:

"Why is Jackson in the hospital? (Because he has asthma and pneumonia.)

What caused the asthma and pneumonia? (He got a cold and it got worse, resulting in pneumonia, exacerbated by his asthma.)

Why did it get worse? (Because he lives in a poor neighborhood.)

How does that cause more problems? (Because he is exposed to more asthma triggers, [such as air pollution, mold, dust mites/cockroach allergens, and cigarette smoke] which exacerbate his asthma when he gets an upper respiratory infection—often leading to pneumonia.)

Why is he living there? (Because his family is poor and can only afford an apartment in a crowded building located in an area of town near factories and highways. The building is poorly maintained.)

Why can't his parents work harder so they can move to a better place? (Because he lives with his mother and 3 siblings, and she works two jobs. That income only covers rent, food, and a few bills.)

Why can't his mom get a better job? (Because she doesn't have the skills and education needed to get a higher paying job.) But why...?"

And then they become more aware of why this class is important and begin to comprehend how complicated social and economic issues affect health.

Adapted from Federal, Provincial and Territorial Advisory Committee on Population Health (ACPH) (1999).

- "Public health protects and improves the health of individuals, families, communities, and populations, locally and globally" (para. 1). Examples of global public health issues include "improving access to health care, controlling infectious disease, and reducing environmental hazards, violence, substance abuse, and injury" (para. 3).
- "Public health professionals focus on preventing disease and injury by promoting healthy lifestyles" (para. 2).

One of the challenges public health practice faces is to remain responsive to the community's health needs. As a result, its structure is complex; numerous health services and programs are currently available or will be developed. Examples include health education, family planning, accident prevention, environmental protection, immunization, nutrition, early periodic screening and developmental testing, school programs, mental health services, occupational health programs, and the care of vulnerable populations. The Department of Homeland Security, for example, is a community health and safety agency established in the aftermath of the terrorist attacks on New York City and Washington, DC, on September 11, 2001. See Chapter 6.

The core public health functions have been delineated as assessment, policy development, and assurance. These are discussed in more detail in Chapter 2.

THE CONCEPT OF COMMUNITY

The concepts of community and health together provide the foundation for understanding community health. Broadly defined, a **community** is a collection of people who share some important feature of their lives (Fig. 1-1). In this text, the term community refers to a collection of people who interact with one another and whose common interests or characteristics form the basis for a sense of unity or belonging.

- A community can be a society of people holding common rights and privileges (e.g., citizens of a town), sharing common interests (e.g., a community of farmers), or living under the same laws and regulations (e.g., a prison community).
- The function of any community includes its members' collective sense of belonging and their shared identity, values, norms, communication, and common interests and concerns (Anderson & McFarlane, 2019).

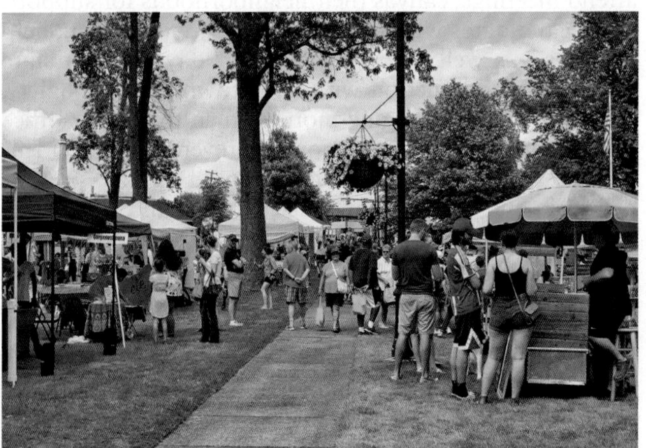

FIGURE 1-1 There are many different types of communities.

Some communities—for example, a tiny village in Appalachia—are composed of people who share almost everything. They live in the same location, work at a limited type and number of jobs, attend the same churches, and make use of the sole health clinic with its visiting physician and nurse. Other communities, such as members of Mothers Against Drunk Driving (MADD), are large, scattered, and composed of individuals who share only a common interest and involvement in a certain goal. Although most communities of people share many aspects of their experience, it is useful to identify three types of communities that have relevance to community health practice: geographic, common interest, and health problem or solution. Unit 4 contains more in-depth information about the community as client.

Geographic Community

A community that is defined by its geographic boundaries is called a **geographic community**. A city, town, or neighborhood is a geographic community.

Consider the community of Hayward, Wisconsin. Located in northwestern Wisconsin, it is set in a wooded environment, far removed from any urban center and in a climatic zone characterized by extremely harsh winters. With a population of approximately 2,300, it is considered a rural community. The population fluctuates with the seasons: summers bring hundreds of tourists and seasonal residents. Hayward is a social system as well as a geographic location. The families, schools, hospital, churches, stores, and government institutions are linked in a complex network. This community, like others, has an informal power structure. It has a communication system that includes gossip, the newspaper, the "co-op" store bulletin board, radio, television, and social media. In one sense, then, a community consists of a collection of people located in a specific place and is made up of institutions organized into a social system.

A few miles south are other communities, including Northwoods Beach and Round Lake; these, along with Hayward and other towns and isolated farms, form a larger community called Sawyer County. If a nurse worked for a health agency serving only Hayward, that community would be of primary concern; however, if the nurse worked for the Sawyer County Health Department, this larger community would be the focus. A PHN employed by the State Health Department in Madison, Wisconsin, would have an interest in Sawyer County and Hayward, but only as part of the larger community of Wisconsin.

Frequently, a single part of a city can be treated as a community. Cities are often broken down into census tracts, or neighborhoods. In New York City, the neighborhood called Harlem is a community, as is the Haight-Ashbury district of San Francisco.

In community health, identifying a geographic area as a community is useful because it:

- Provides a clear target for the analysis of health needs
- Makes available data, such as morbidity and mortality figures, that can augment assessment studies to form the basis for planning health programs

- Facilitates mobilizing community members for action and forming groups to carry out intervention and prevention efforts that address needs specific to that community, such as shelters for battered women, work site safety programs in local hazardous industries, or improved sexual health education in the schools
- Helps in gaining the support of politically powerful individuals and resources present in a geographic community

On a larger scale, the world can be considered as a global community. Indeed, it is very important to view the world this way. Borders of countries change with political upheaval.

Communicable diseases are not aware of arbitrary political boundaries. A person can travel around the world in <24 hours, and so can diseases, such as Zika virus, Ebola, or COVID-19. Global pandemics require cooperation and information sharing among affected nations. Political uprisings in the Middle East have an impact on people in Western countries. Floods or tsunamis in Southeast Asia or volcanic eruptions in Iceland have meaning for other national economies. The world is one large community that needs to work together to ensure a healthy today and a healthier and safer tomorrow. Globalization raises an expectation of health for all, for if good health is possible in one part of the world, the forces of globalization should allow it elsewhere and everyone then enjoys the benefits (World Health Organization, 2020b). We learn more about global health in Chapter 16.

Common-Interest Community

A community also can be defined by a common interest or goal. A collection of people, even if they are widely scattered geographically, can have an interest or goal that binds the members together. This is known as a *common-interest community.*

The members of a church in a large metropolitan area and families who have lost members to suicide are both common-interest communities. Sometimes, within a certain geographic area, a group of people may develop a sense of community by promoting their common interest. Individuals with disabilities who are scattered throughout a large city may emerge as a community through a common interest in promoting adherence to federal guidelines for wheelchair access, parking spaces, elevators, or other services for those with disabilities. The residents of an industrial community may develop a common interest in air or water pollution issues, whereas others who work but do not live in the area may not share that interest. Communities form to protect the rights of children, stop violence against women, promote sensible gun laws, clean up the environment, develop a smoke-free environment, or provide support for social and structural change (e.g., Black Lives Matter). The kinds of shared interests that lead to the formation of communities vary widely.

Common-interest communities whose focus is a health-related issue can join with community health agencies to promote their agendas. The single-minded commitment that characterizes such communities can be a mobilizing force for action. Many successful prevention and health promotion efforts, including improved services and increased community awareness of specific problems, have resulted from the work of common-interest communities.

Moms Demand Action is a current example. It began in response to the Sandy Hook school shooting in 2012, when Shannon Watts, a mother of five children, looked for an organization like Mothers Against Drunk Drivers that addressed the gun violence problem in America and the lack of regulations around gun sales in many places (see more on violence and abuse in Chapter 18). She couldn't find one, so she started a Facebook page that got instant and overwhelming responses from other mothers across the country. She had previously worked for 15 years as a communications executive, and even though she was now a stay-at-home mom, she felt passionately about the need for mothers to bring a new narrative to the public debate on guns. She has now organized a grassroots network of mothers to promote gun violence prevention and work together with Mayors Against Illegal Guns to enact common sense gun legislation at the local, state, and national levels (Everytown for Gun Safety Action Fund, 2020; Karlis, 2018).

While supporting the second amendment, Moms Demand Action seeks to counter the powerful influence of the gun lobby and fight the public health crisis of gun violence. Stating that "seven American children or teens are shot and killed every day," this organization seeks "sensible gun laws and policies" to protect families and children (Karlis, 2018, para. 5). After the Parkland, Florida high school shooting, a related organization, Students Demand Action, was organized and now has over 50,000 volunteers who are working to register new voters and raise awareness. Moms Demand Action has over 6 million members and volunteers who attend city and county government meetings and state legislative hearings and question lawmakers on their views about gun legislation.

Watts feels that they are successful because "a gun extremist's love will never match a mother's love for her child" (Karlis, 2018, para. 30). It is important for women to be involved, as Watts notes that "if you compare women in America to our peers in high-income countries, we're 16 times more likely to be shot" (Karlis, 2018, para. 30). But it's not just mothers who are active in Moms Demand Action. Men also take time to march, attend meetings, canvas their neighborhoods for support, assist candidates who favor sensible gun legislation, help fundraise, as well as attend advocacy days at their state capitols. In conjunction with Everytown for Gun Safety, they are also encouraging more women to run for office and hope to ensure legislation to prevent child accidental gun deaths, strengthen background checks, prevent domestic abusers from owning firearms, and strengthen gun trafficking laws (Moms Demand Action, 2018). You can learn more about their successful lobbying and legislation at https://momsdemandaction.org/about/victories/

Community of Solution

A type of community encountered frequently in community/public health practice is a group of people who come together to solve a problem that affects all of them. This type of community is known as a *community of solution.*

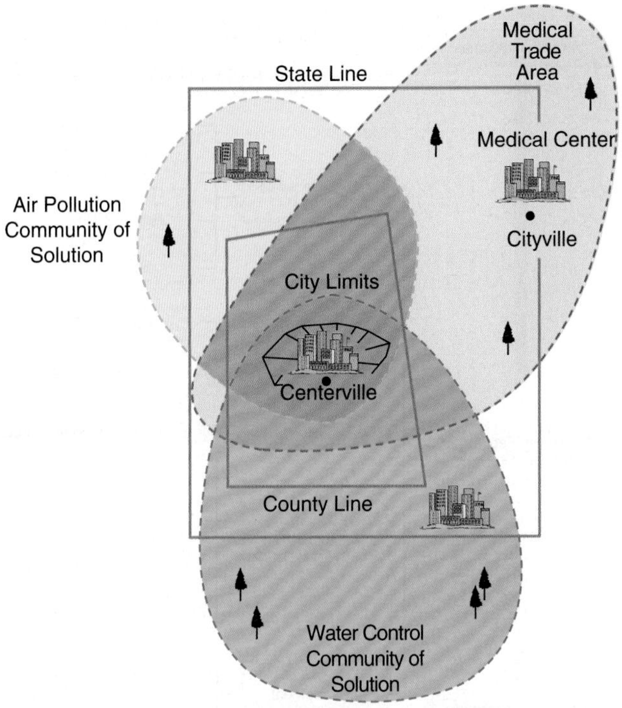

FIGURE 1-2 A city's communities of solution. State, county, and city boundaries (*solid lines*) may have little or no bearing on health solution boundaries (*dashed lines*).

The shape of this type of community varies with the nature of the problem, the size of the geographic area affected, and the number of resources needed to address the problem.

For example, a water pollution problem may involve several counties whose agencies and personnel must work together to control upstream water supply, industrial waste disposal, and city water treatment. This group of counties forms a community of solution focusing on a health problem. Figure 1-2 depicts some communities of solution related to a single city.

In recent years, communities of solution have formed in many cities to address the spread of diseases and have worked with community members to assess public safety and security and create plans to make the community a safer place in which to live. Recently, Flint, Michigan was faced with a growing water crisis involving high levels of lead and an outbreak of Legionnaire's disease, eventually leading to criminal charges being brought against state and city officials for "misconduct in office, conspiracy, and willful neglect of duty" (Kennedy, 2016, para. 71). Public health agencies, social service groups, schools, citizens, and media personnel banded together to create public awareness of the dangers and to promote preventive behaviors. See Chapter 9.

Governments can create communication barriers, so better coordination between community partners and governmental authorities and sharing of technology and knowledge are critical components in communities of solution. Stout, Howard, Lewis, McPherson, and Schall (2017), working with the Institute for Healthcare Improvement, reported on several successful projects initiated and completed by communities of solution in the United States, Africa, and South America. These included multi-year initiatives with the following goals:

- To reduce mortality by 66% in those younger than age 5
- To assist 186 communities in supplying permanent housing to over 106,000 homeless people
- To help establish local health assemblies that promote public health initiatives in a poor, remote country in which a 5th grade education is the highest level of education available to residents of 36 small, isolated villages (initiatives included providing community health workers, immunizations, malaria detection and treatment, midwives providing family planning, establishing nursery schools, building secondary schools with science curricula to increase the numbers of health care providers, establishing eco-tourism to help with road building and improve economic growth)

As you can see, a community of solution is an important conduit for change in community/public health.

Populations and Aggregates

Population health is a foundation of community/public health practice (National Quality Forum, 2018). The three types of communities just discussed underscore the meaning of the concept of community: in each instance, a collection of people chose to interact with one another because of common interests, characteristics, or goals. The concept of population has a different meaning.

In this text, the term **population** refers to all of the people occupying an area or to all of those who share one or more characteristics (Anderson & McFarlane, 2019).

- In contrast to a community, a population is made up of people who do not necessarily interact with one another and do not necessarily share a sense of belonging to that group.
- A population may be defined geographically, such as the population of the United States or a city's population.
- This designation of a population is useful in community/public health for epidemiologic study and for collecting demographic data for purposes such as health planning.
- A population also may be defined by common qualities or characteristics, such as the older adult population, the homeless population, or a particular racial or ethnic group.
- In community/public health, this meaning becomes useful when a specific group of people (e.g., homeless individuals) is targeted for intervention; the population's common characteristics (e.g., the health-related problems of homelessness) become a major focus of the intervention.

In this text, the term **aggregate** refers to a mass or grouping of distinct individuals who are considered as a whole and who are loosely associated with one another. It is a broader term that encompasses many different-sized groups. Both communities and populations are types of aggregates. Unit 5 discusses community/public health nursing with aggregates, and Unit 6 discusses vulnerable populations. In Unit 7, we will examine the different settings for community/public health nursing.

The aggregate focus, or a concern for groupings of people in contrast to individual health care, is a distinguishing feature of community/public health practice. C/PHNs may work with aggregates such as pregnant and parenting teens, older adults with diabetes, or gay men with HIV/AIDS.

Because of community/public health nursing's focus on communities, aggregates, and families, new nursing and health care delivery systems may develop that are more profitable and effective in preventing health problems that require expensive hospitalizations. Community/public health workers, including C/PHNs, must clearly define the community targeted for study and intervention and understand its complexity before assessing its needs and designing interventions to address them. To help define the community, the C/PHN should answer the following questions:

- Who makes up the community?
- Where are they located, and what are their characteristics?
- What are the characteristics of the people in terms of age, gender, race, socioeconomic level, and health status?
- How does the community interact with other communities?
- What is its history? What are its resources?
- Is the community undergoing rapid change, and, if so, what are the changes?

These questions, as well as the tools needed to assess a community for health purposes, are discussed in detail in Chapter 15.

THE CONCEPT OF HEALTH

Health, in the abstract, refers to a person's physical, mental, and spiritual state; it can be positive (as being in good health) or negative (as being in poor health).

- The World Health Organization (WHO) offers a positive explanation of health as "a state of complete physical, mental, and social wellbeing and not merely the absence of disease or infirmity" (WHO, 2020a, para. 1).
- Building on this classic definition, our definition of **health** in this text is as follows: a holistic state of well-being, which includes soundness of mind, body, and spirit.

Health is determined by more than just medical care. It is influenced by various factors—location of home, education, income, diet, exercise, accessibility of health care, and health behaviors (County Health Rankings, 2018). See Figure 1-3 for the County Health Rankings Model. Likewise, the WHO (2020a) has outlined the prerequisites for health as "peace, shelter, education, food, income, a stable eco-system, sustainable resources, social justice, and equity" (para. 5).

Community health practitioners place a strong emphasis on **wellness**, which includes this definition of health but also incorporates the capacity to develop a person's potential to lead a fulfilling and productive life—one that can be measured in terms of quality of life. Today, our health is greatly affected by our lifestyles, preventive measures we take, and risk behaviors in which we engage (Saint Onge & Krueger, 2017). We are increasingly aware of the strong relationship of health to environment (Box 1-3), although this concept is not new (Thompson & Schwartz Barcott, 2017).

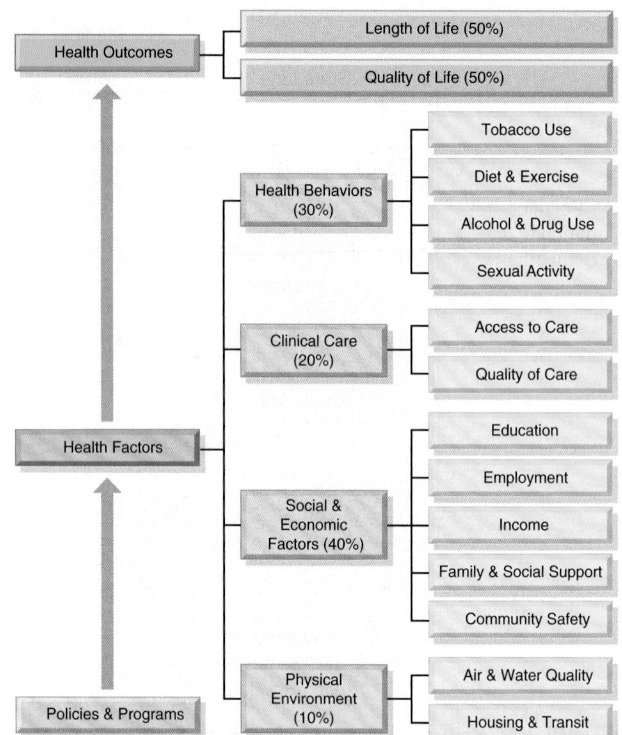

FIGURE 1-3 County Health Rankings Model demonstrates how many factors lead to health outcomes. (Courtesy of University of Wisconsin Population Health Institute. County Health Rankings & Roadmaps 2019. https://www.countyhealthrankings.org/county-health-rankings-model. County Health Rankings Model © 2014 UWPHI. Used with permission.)

BOX 1-3 WHAT DO *YOU* THINK?

The Link Between Personal Health and the Environment

Life expectancy increased from 47.3 years in 1900 to 76.8 years in 2000, and it is estimated that about 25 years of this growth can be attributed to public health advances (e.g., infectious disease control/prevention). The remainder of the gain is the result of improvements in prevention and therapeutic interventions (e.g., lifestyle behaviors, medical advances).

1. *Do you think there is a direct link between your health and your environment?*
2. *If your answer is Yes, then how? If it is No, then what else might explain the findings?*

Source: CDC (2011).

Over 150 years ago, Florence Nightingale explored the relationship between health/illness and the environment. She believed that a person's health was greatly influenced by ventilation, noise, light, cleanliness, diet, and a restful bed (Nightingale, 1859/1992). As is well documented, the built environment, or man-made structures and surroundings in a community (e.g., highways and bike paths, parks and open spaces, public buildings, and housing developments), significantly affects the health of individuals, aggregates, and populations (CDC, 2017a; Hankey & Marshall, 2017; Mueller et al., 2017). Nightingale's model, along with others, is explained in Chapter 15, and the environment's relationship to health is discussed in more detail in Chapter 9.

Culture also shapes our view of health. Some cultures see health as the freedom from and absence of evil and illness as punishment for being bad or doing evil or a result of witchcraft (Iheanacho et al., 2016). Many individuals come from families in which beliefs regarding health and illness are heavily influenced by religion, superstition, folk beliefs, or "old wives' tales." C/PHNs commonly encounter such beliefs when working with various groups in the community. Chapter 5 explores these beliefs more thoroughly for a better understanding of how health beliefs influence every aspect of a person's life, as well as principles of transcultural nursing in the community.

The Health Continuum: Wellness—Illness

Western societies often exhibit a polarized or "either/or" way of thinking about health: either people are healthy and well or they are ill. Yet, wellness is a relative concept, not an absolute, and **illness** is a state of being *relatively* unhealthy. The study of factors affecting health and illness is known as epidemiology and is discussed in Chapter 7. There are many levels and degrees of wellness and illness, from a robust 75-year-old woman who is fully active and functioning at an optimal level of wellness to a 75-year-old man with end-stage renal disease whose health is characterized as frail. Someone recovering from pneumonia may be mildly ill, whereas a teenage boy with functional limitations because of episodic depression may be described as mildly well. The continuum, however, can change.

Because healthiness involves a range of degrees from optimal health at one end to total disability or death at the other (Fig. 1-4), it often is described as a **health continuum**. This health continuum applies not only to individuals but also to families and communities. A nurse might speak of a "family in crisis," meaning one that is experiencing a relative degree of illness or altered functioning, or of a healthy family, meaning one that exhibits many wellness characteristics, such as effective communication and conflict resolution, as well as the ability to effectively work together and use resources appropriately. More information on working with families and communities is included in Chapters 14 and 15.

Likewise, a community, as a collection of people, may be described in terms of degrees of wellness or illness. The health of an individual, family, group, or community moves back and forth along this continuum throughout the lifespan. Healthy people make healthy communities and a healthy society.

The Declaration of Alma Ata, which took place in 1978, noted that health is a "fundamental human right" and that the level of health must be raised for all countries in order for any society to improve their health (WHO, 2020d, para. 2).

By thinking of health relatively, as a matter of degree, the scope of nursing practice can be broadened to focus on preventing illness or disability as well as promoting wellness. Traditionally, most health care has focused on treatment of acute and chronic conditions at the illness end of the continuum. Gradually, the emphasis is shifting to focus on the wellness end of the continuum, as outlined in the government document, *Healthy People 2030* (U.S. Department of Health and Human Services [USDHHS], Office of Disease Prevention and Health Promotion [ODPHP], 2020). The vision for *Healthy People 2030* is for everyone to reach their "full potential" and enjoy "well-being" throughout their lives (para.10). This effort aims to improve the health of American citizens by establishing objectives and benchmarks that can be monitored over time. There have been Healthy People objectives for 2000, 2010, 2020, and now for 2030. A main foundational principle is that a population's health and well-being are a prerequisite to securing a flourishing and equitable society. The mission, foundational principles, and five overarching goals of *Healthy People 2030* were used to guide further planning (USDHHS, 2020).

The goals overarch topics and objectives (Box 1-4). The objectives are stated in measurable terms that specify

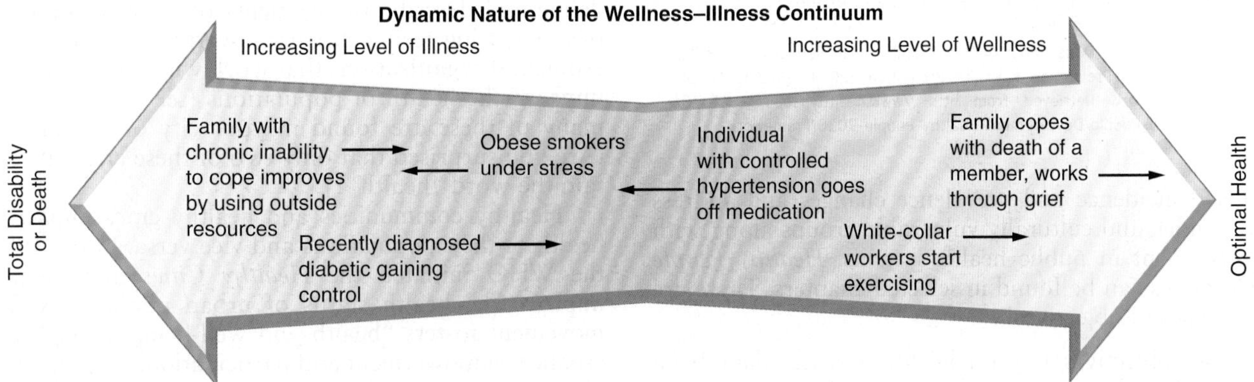

FIGURE 1-4 The health continuum. A person's relative health is usually in a state of flux, either improving or deteriorating. This diagram of the wellness–illness continuum shows several examples of people in changing states of health.

BOX 1-4 *HEALTHY PEOPLE 2030*

Issues in Community/Public Health Nursing

Mission

To promote, strengthen, and evaluate the Nation's efforts to improve the health and well-being of all people.

Foundational Principles

Foundational principles explain the thinking that guides decisions about Healthy People 2030.

- Health and well-being of all people and communities are essential to a thriving, equitable society.
- Promoting health and well-being and preventing disease are linked efforts that encompass physical, mental, and social health dimensions.
- Investing to achieve the full potential for health and well-being for all provides valuable benefits to society.
- Achieving health and well-being requires eliminating health disparities, achieving health equity, and attaining health literacy.
- Healthy physical, social, and economic environments strengthen the potential to achieve health and well-being.
- Promoting and achieving the Nation's health and well-being is a shared responsibility that is distributed across the national, state, tribal, and community levels, including the public, private, and not-for-profit sectors.
- Working to attain the full potential for health and well-being of the population is a component of decision-making and policy formulation across all sectors.

Healthy People 2030 Overarching Goals

- Attain healthy, thriving lives and well-being, free of preventable disease, disability, injury, and premature death.
- Eliminate health disparities, achieve health equity, and attain health literacy to improve the health and well-being of all.
- Create social, physical, and economic environments that promote attaining full potential for health and well-being for all.
- Promote healthy development, healthy behaviors, and well-being across all life stages.
- Engage leadership, key constituents, and the public across multiple sectors to take action and design policies that improve the health and well-being of all.

Reprinted from U.S. Department of Health and Human Services (USDHHS). Office of Disease Prevention & Health Promotion. (2019). *Healthy People 2030: Framework.* Retrieved from https://www.healthypeople.gov/2020/About-Healthy-People/Development-Healthy-People-2030/Framework

targeted incidence and prevalence changes and address age, gender, and culturally vulnerable groups along with improvement in public health systems. *Healthy People 2030* boxes can be found in selected chapters. There are three types of objectives:

- Core objectives rely on health statistics data from established sources (e.g., U.S. Census, surveys, datasets) for accurate assessment of progress meeting targets.
- Developmental objectives are selected from "high priority areas without reliable baseline data, but with established evidence-based interventions" (Association for State and Territorial Health Officers, 2019, para. 4).
- Research objectives are areas for potential studies without consistent evidence-based interventions.

Progress toward the *Healthy People 2020* objectives was mixed at the midcourse review, with only 21.1% of the 1,054 measurable objectives meeting or exceeding targeted goals. Some improvement was noted in 19.1%, but 11.1% actually reported worse outcomes on proposed goals (USDHHS, 2017). *Healthy People 2020* and *Healthy People 2030* emphasize that the health of an individual is linked to the health of the larger community and that this larger community's health is related to the health of the corresponding state and ultimately our nation (Artiga & Hinton, 2018; CDC, 2018a; USDHHS, 2019). See Figure 1-5. The recommended leading health indicators for *Healthy People 2030* are an outcomes metric for measuring progress toward national public health goals. The main topic areas under which the leading health indicators are organized are compared in Box 1-5.

- Probably the most commonly recognized metric for the health of a nation is the life expectancy of its citizens. Life expectancy in the United States dropped from 78.7 years for a child born in 2015 to 78.6 for 2016 (Kochanek, Murphy, Jiaquan, & Arias, 2017).
- We now have a lower life expectancy than other developed nations. For instance, we are below the average life expectancy of 80.3 years for the nations of Canada, France, Germany, Japan, Mexico, and the United Kingdom (Donnelly, 2018).

Community characteristics of health have been described by the Centers for Disease Control and Prevention (CDC) as health-related quality of life indicators. Two sources of community-level health indicators include the County Health Rankings and Roadmaps and the Prevention Status Reports (CDC, 2017b). Compare your county's ratings with those of others in your state. Many indicators of community health have been used over the years, such as income distribution, unemployment rates, number of health professionals, and lifestyle choices. Health Resources in Action (2013) sought to define and describe the elements of healthy communities by getting feedback from government and nongovernmental organizations that work with communities to improve the health of populations (see Box 1-6). How many of these are found in your city or community? (Are you surprised that only two of these elements contain the word "health"?)

Healthy communities and healthy cities impact the health of their populations and vice versa. In the 1980s, the WHO initiated the *Healthy Cities* movement to improve the health status of urban populations. This movement fosters "health and well-being through governance, empowerment and participation, creating urban places for equity and community prosperity, and investing in people for a peaceful planet" (WHO, Regional Office for Europe, 2018, p. 3).

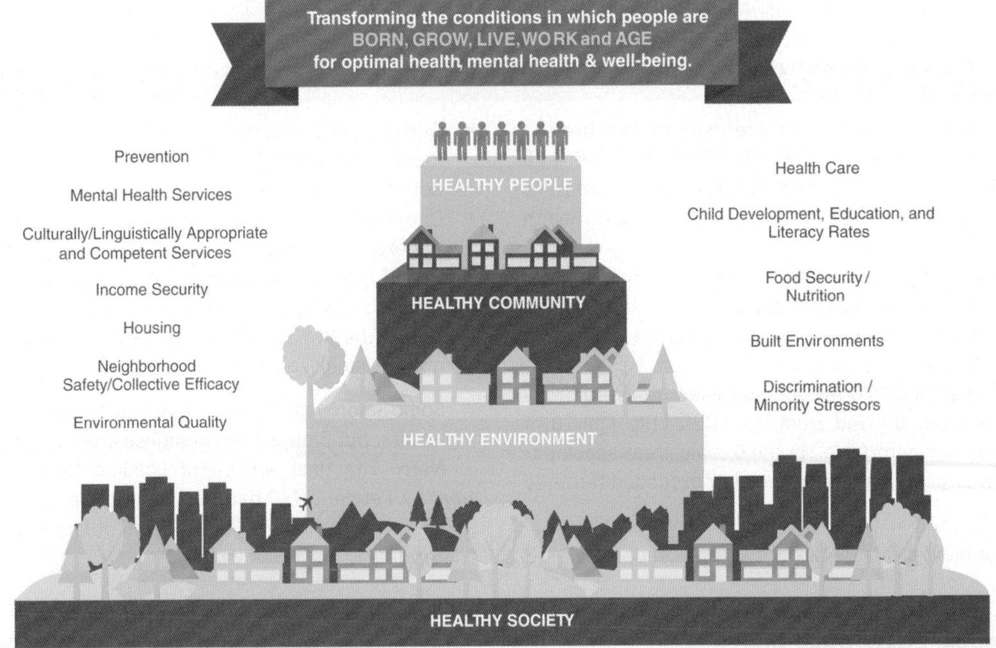

FIGURE 1-5 The health of the individual is related to community, state, and national health. (From California Department of Public Health (CDPH). (August 2015). *Portrait of promise: The California statewide plan to promote health and mental health equity.* Report to the legislature and the people of California by the Office of Health Equity, CDPH. (p. 18). Retrieved from https://www.cdph.ca.gov/Programs/OHE/CDPH%20Document%20Library/ADA%20Approved%20POP%20Report.pdf#search=social%20determinants%20of%20health%20graphic)

Health as a State of Being

Health refers to a state of being, including many different qualities and characteristics.

- An individual might be described as energetic, outgoing, enthusiastic, beautiful, caring, loving, and intense. Together, these qualities become the essence of a person's existence; they describe a state of being.
- A geographic community, such as a neighborhood, might be characterized as congested, deteriorating, unattractive, dirty, and disorganized, all of which suggest diminishing degrees of vitality.
- A population, such as workers involved in a massive layoff, might be characterized as banding together to provide support and share resources to effectively seek new employment. Such a community shows signs of healthy adaptation and positive coping.

Health involves the total person or community. All of the dimensions of life affecting everyday functioning determine an individual's or a community's health, including physical, psychological, spiritual, economic, and sociocultural experiences. All of these factors must be considered when dealing with the health of an individual or community. The approach should be holistic, including not only physical and emotional status but also the status of home, family, and work.

When considering an aggregate or group of people in terms of health, it becomes useful for intervention purposes to speak of the "health of a community" (Fig. 1-6). With aggregates as well as individuals, health as a state of being does not merely involve that group's physical state but also includes psychological, spiritual, and socioeconomic factors.

As an example, the health of the population on the island of Puerto Rico, an American territory, was dramatically changed on September 20, 2017 when Hurricane Maria directly hit the island with winds of 155 miles per hour (nearly category 5) and stayed over the island for more than 30 hours (Fig. 1-7; Abbasi, 2018; Meyer, 2017). Two weeks earlier, Hurricane Irma had hit the island, and while much milder than Maria, it had already caused serious problems with the power system (Zorrilla, 2017). Flooding occurred in coastal areas, and an estimated 472,000 homes were seriously damaged (over 87,000 completely destroyed). It is estimated that 440,000 of the 3.4 million inhabitants were without power to their homes for 6 months. Most of Puerto Rico's 69 hospitals were without fuel for generators. Three to four days after landfall, only three of the major hospitals were managing to function.

Many patients with surgical emergencies had to be sent to the U.S. mainland for treatment. One in seven people on the island have diabetes, and people threw out insulin after the storm due to lack of refrigeration. Pharmacies couldn't function for several weeks, dialysis centers had no access to electricity or water for several days, and physicians were unable to reopen their offices in rural areas for a few months due to lack of access to electronic medical records (Abbasi, 2018; Alcorn, 2017). There are still serious concerns about the effects on the mental health of survivors of having lived through such a destructive event (Lybarger, 2018). Many found the response of the federal government to be slow and deficient (Alcorn, 2017; Zorrilla, 2017).

The official death toll was estimated at 64, but one Harvard study put the number of deaths between

BOX 1-5 *HEALTHY PEOPLE 2030*

Proposed Leading Health Indicators

The leading health indicators (LHIs) are used to measure the health of the nation. For Healthy People 2020, there were 26 objectives/indicators arranged under 12 general topic areas. As a group, the leading health indicators reflect the major health concerns in the United States.

Healthy People 2030 has proposed 18 topic areas and 34 measures of health/objectives. A comparison of the Healthy People 2020 and the recommended Healthy People 2030 topic areas is shown below.

The Healthy People 2020 midcourse review assessed progress toward the goals derived from the 2020 LHIs. Only 8 of the 26 objectives/indicators (i.e., in the 6 topic areas accompanied by an asterisk in the below table) met or exceeded targeted goals, as follows:

- Both Environmental Quality targets were exceeded.
- One of the two Injury and Violence targets was exceeded (decreased homicide rate).
- Both Maternal, Infant, and Child Health targets were met.
- One of the four Nutrition, Physical Activity, and Obesity targets was exceeded (aerobic and strengthening age 18 and over).
- One of the two Substance Abuse targets was exceeded (adolescents' use of alcohol or illicit drugs in past 30 days).
- One of the two Tobacco targets was exceeded (9th to 12th graders smoking in past 20 days).

Some improvement was shown in 8 additional objectives/indicators, but 3 objectives demonstrated worse outcomes.

Note: The final version of Leading Health Indicators for *Healthy People 2030* had not been completed by the August 2020 rollout of *Healthy People 2030* objectives and are due at a later date.

Healthy People 2020 Topic Areas	Recommended Healthy People 2030 Topic Areas
Access to Health Services	Access to Health Services
Clinical Preventive Services	Clinical Preventive Services
Injury and Violence*	Injury
Environmental Quality*	Environmental Quality
Maternal, Infant, and Child Health*	Maternal, Infant, and Child Health
Mental Health	Mental Health
Nutrition, Physical Activity, and Obesity*	Obesity
Oral Health	Oral Health
Reproductive and Sexual Health	Reproductive and Sexual Health
Social Determinants	Social Determinants
Substance Abuse*	Substance Abuse
Tobacco*	Tobacco
	Health Care System Quality
	Health Care Access
	Social Capital/Civic Engagement
	Serious Illness
	Determinants of Health Equity
	General Health, Health-Related Quality, or Well-being

*One or two objectives met or exceeded target.
Source: NASEM (2020); ODPHP (2016).

800 and 8,500. The Puerto Rican government updated the death toll estimate in 2018 to 1,427 (Kishore et al., 2018; Robles, 2018). A study done later that year by George Washington University and the University of Puerto Rico (Milken Institute, 2018) estimated deaths of between 2,658 and 3,290. Survivors must deal with serious environmental threats and the loss of their homes and businesses. Environmental hazards include sewage-contaminated drinking water or well water from Superfund sites (recognized by the federal government as extremely contaminated), along with mud contaminated by diesel and fuel oil used in power plants. Mold exposure is also problematic, and people lived in temporary tents or shelters for many months after the event. There were literally tons of downed trees and manmade debris, leading to trash and pollution problems for months and years to come. All of these things continue to affect the health of Puerto Ricans (Newkirk II, 2017). Many dimensions of health were significantly affected by this crisis. We examine disaster and bioterrorism in Chapter 17.

BOX 1-6 Qualities of a Healthy Community

- Equity and justice (few disparities)
- Low poverty levels indicating that jobs are available (a generally good economy)
- Education
- Health care and services to prevent illness
- Environment that is sustainable and wide-ranging community participation that is fair and inclusive
- Employ environmental strategies
- Participation across multiple sectors
- Capability to examine and address their own health problems
- Collaborative strategies
- Housing/shelter
- Civic engagement
- Public policy that focus on health
- Availability of healthy food
- Safety
- Ability to have active lives
- Transportation
- Empowered residents
- Healthy child development
- Data are employed to guide and evaluate programs

Adapted from Health Resources in Action (2013).

Subjective and Objective Dimensions of Health

Health involves both *subjective* and *objective* dimensions; that is, it involves both how people feel (subjective) and how well they can function in their environment (objective).

Subjectively, a healthy person is one who feels well and who experiences the sensation of a vital, positive state. Healthy people are full of life and vigor, capable of physical and mental productivity. They feel minimal discomfort and displeasure with the world around them. People experience varying degrees of vitality and well-being, and the state of feeling well fluctuates. Some mornings we wake up feeling more energetic and enthusiastic than we do on other mornings. How people feel varies day by day, even hour by hour; nonetheless, how they feel overall is a strong indicator of their overall state of health.

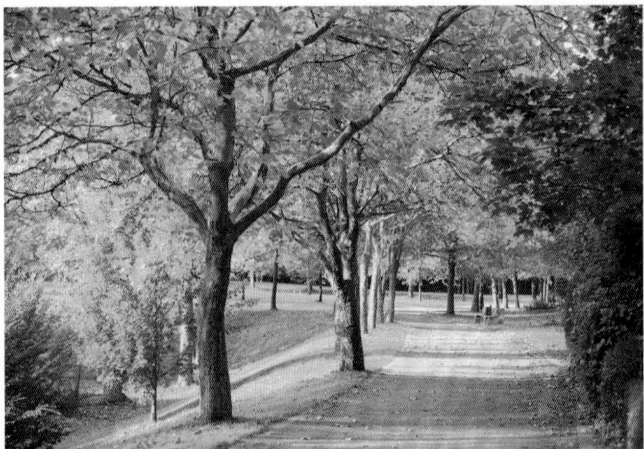

FIGURE 1-6 Healthy communities promote the health of their inhabitants.

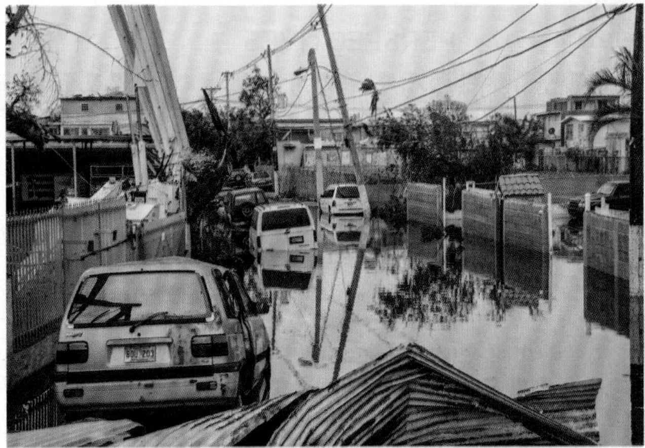

FIGURE 1-7 San Juan, Puerto Rico after Hurricane Maria.

Health also involves the objective dimension of ability to function. A healthy individual or community carries out necessary activities and achieves enriching goals. Unhealthy people not only feel unwell, but they are limited, to some degree, in their ability to carry out daily activities.

Indeed, levels of illness or wellness are measured largely in terms of ability to function (van Puffelen et al., 2015). A person confined to bed is often labeled sicker than an ill person managing self-care. A family that meets its members' needs is healthier than one that has poor communication patterns and is unable to provide adequate physical and emotional resources. A community actively engaged in crime prevention or in policing of industrial wastes shows signs of healthy functioning. The degree of functioning is directly related to the state of health (Box 1-7).

The ability to function can be observed. A man dresses and feeds himself and goes to work. Despite financial limitations, a family supports its members through an emotional crisis. A community provides adequate resources and services for its members. These performances, to some degree, can be regarded as indicators of health status.

The actions of an individual, family, or community are motivated by their values. Some activities, such as walking and taking care of personal needs, are functions valued by most people. In assessing the health of individuals and communities, the C/PHN can observe people's ability to function but also must know their values, which may contrast sharply with those of the nurse. The influence of values on health is examined more closely in Chapter 4.

- The subjective dimension (feeling well or ill) and the objective dimension (functioning) together provide a clearer picture of people's health. When they feel well and demonstrate functional ability, they are close to the wellness end of the health continuum.

BOX 1-7 PERSPECTIVES

Voices from the Community

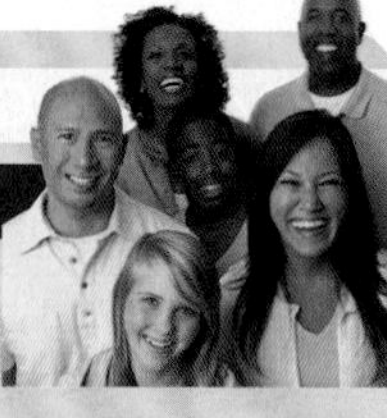

I never thought much about being healthy or not, now that you ask. I keep busy, I cook like I'm expecting company, I have a good appetite. I really think all these so-called healthy things people suggest are fads, just so someone can get rich—like tofu and low fat this and that. Don't give me margarine, only butter, ... and skim milk, it's like drinking water! I work in my garden, I read, and I eat fresh foods. And don't talk to me about my smoking, it's the one pleasure I have left.

Bettie, age 81

- Even those with a disease, such as arthritis or diabetes, may feel well and perform well within their capacity. These people can be considered healthy or closer to the wellness end of the continuum. Figure 1-8 depicts the relationships between the subjective and objective views of health.

Continuous and Episodic Health Care Needs

Community/public health practice encompasses care for populations in all age groups with birth-to-death developmental health care needs. These *continuous needs* may include, for example, assistance with providing a toddler-proof home, help in effectively dealing with the progressive emancipation of preteens and teenagers, anticipatory guidance for reducing and managing the stress associated with retirement, or help coping with the death of an aged parent. These are developmental events experienced by most people, and they represent typical life occurrences. The C/PHN has the skills to work at the individual, family, and group level to meet these needs.

In addition, populations may have a one-time, specific, negative health event, such as an illness or injury that is not an expected part of life. These *episodic needs* might derive from a head injury incurred from an automobile crash or a diagnosis of tuberculosis or another communicable disease. In reaction to such an event in 2016, the CDC raised its Emergency Operations Center's response level for Zika virus outbreaks in the Americas to its highest alert status (Level 1). Although most cases were then found in South American and the Caribbean, there was concern about spread due to travel to the U.S. mainland. In 2018, the level was reduced to 2, with 452 symptomatic Zika cases having been reported in the United States in 2017 (only seven of which were deemed to be acquired by local mosquito-borne transmission in Texas and Florida). In 2018, preliminary data revealed just 74 Zika cases acquired by local mosquito-borne transmission (CDC, 2018b, 2018c). By early October 2019, ten cases were reported; none were acquired locally (CDC, 2019). In a response to a novel coronavirus (COVID-19) pandemic, on March 13, 2020, a nationwide emergency was declared by President Trump (Federal Emergency Management Agency, n.d.). Chapter 7 discusses epidemiology in regard to COVID-19. Find more information on communicable diseases in Chapter 8 and on the public health system in Chapter 6.

In a given day, the C/PHN may interact with clients having either continuous or episodic health care needs or both. For example, how do middle-aged adults, planning their retirement and preparing for the death of an aged parent, deal with their adult child's AIDS diagnosis? Or, how do parents of a teenager confront their child's drug dependence? Complex situations such as these may be positively influenced by the interaction with and services of the C/PHN.

COMPONENTS OF COMMUNITY/PUBLIC HEALTH PRACTICE

Community/public health practice can best be understood by examining two basic components—promotion of health and prevention of health problems. The levels of prevention are a key to community/public health practice.

Promotion of Health

Promotion of health is recognized as one of the most important components of public health and community health practice. **Health promotion** includes all efforts that seek to move people closer to optimal well-being or higher levels of wellness.

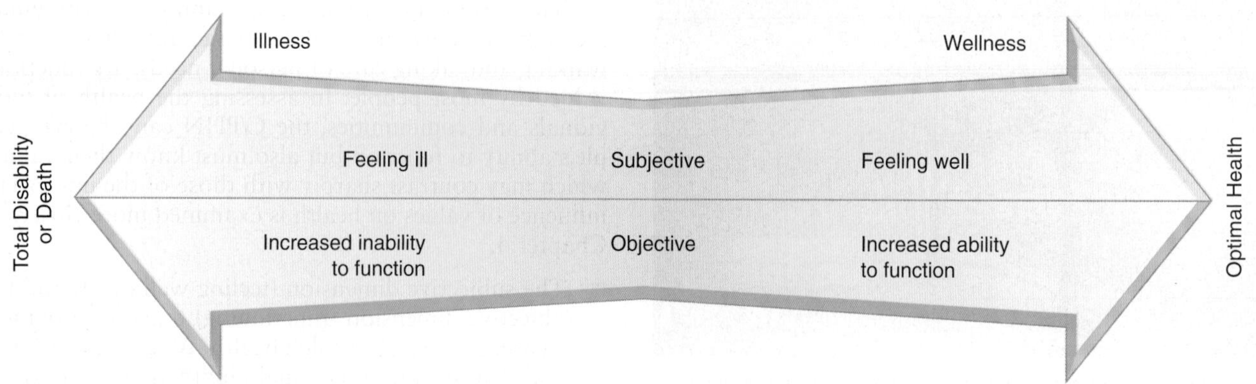

FIGURE 1-8 Subjective and objective views of the wellness–illness continuum.

Nursing, in particular, has a social mandate for engaging in wellness and health promotion (Salmond & Echevarria, 2017). Health promotion programs and activities include many forms of health education—for example, teaching the dangers of drug use, demonstrating healthful practices such as regular exercise, and providing more health-promoting options such as heart-healthy menu selections.

Community health promotion, then, encompasses the development and management of wellness promotion and preventive health care services that are responsive to community health needs. Wellness programs in schools and industry are examples. Demonstration of such healthful practices as eating nutritious foods and exercising more regularly often is performed and promoted by individual health workers. In addition, groups and health agencies that support a smoke-free environment, encourage physical fitness programs for all ages, or demand that food products be properly labeled underscore the importance of these practices and create public awareness.

The goal of health promotion is to raise levels of wellness for individuals, families, populations, and communities (WHO, 2020c, 2020e). Public health efforts promote health, ensuring healthy lives and promoting well-being for all age groups. In this country, during the 1980s, the U.S. Public Health Service published the Surgeon General's Report, *Healthy People*, and continued with goals and objectives each decade since then to address the health of the nation.

This report:

- Provided vision and an agenda for significantly reducing preventable death and disability nationwide, enhancing quality of life, and greatly reducing disparities in the health status of populations
- Emphasized the need for individuals to assume personal responsibility for controlling and improving their own health destiny
- Challenged society to find ways to make good health available to vulnerable populations whose disadvantaged state placed them at greater risk for health problems
- Called for an intensified shift in focus from treating preventable illness and functional impairment to concentrating resources and targeting efforts that promote health and prevent disease and disability

The Institute of Medicine's 2002 hallmark report, *The Future of the Public's Health in the 21st Century*, notes that the majority of health care spending, "as much as 95%," focuses on "medical care and biomedical research," whereas evidence suggests that "behavior and environment are responsible for over 70% of avoidable mortality" and that health care is only one of many "determinants of health" (p. 2).

The implications of this national agenda for health have far-reaching consequences for persons engaged in health care. For centuries, health care has focused on the illness end of the health continuum, but health professionals can no longer justify concentrating most of their efforts exclusively on treating the sick and injured. We now live in an age when it is not only possible to promote health and prevent disease and disability, but it is our mandate and responsibility to do so. For more on health promotion, see Chapter 11.

Prevention of Health Problems

Prevention of health problems constitutes a major part of community/public health practice. Prevention means anticipating and averting problems or discovering them as early as possible to minimize potential disability and impairment. It is practiced on three levels in community/public health: primary, secondary, and tertiary prevention (Lenartowicz, 2018). These concepts recur throughout the chapters of this text, in narrative format and in the Levels of Prevention Pyramids, because they are basic to community/public health nursing (Box 1-8).

Primary prevention precludes the occurrence of a health problem; it includes measures taken to keep illness or injuries from occurring. It is applied to a generally healthy population and precedes disease or dysfunction. Primary prevention involves anticipatory planning and action on the part of community/public health professionals, who must project themselves into the future, envision potential needs and problems, and then design programs to counteract them so that they never occur. The concepts of primary prevention and planning for the future are foreign to many social groups, who may resist on the basis of conflicting values.

Examples of primary prevention activities by a C/PHN include:

- Providing childhood vaccinations and yearly flu shots
- Encouraging older people to install and use safety devices (e.g., grab bars by bathtubs, handrails on steps) to prevent injuries from falls
- Teaching young adults healthy lifestyle behaviors, so that they can make them habitual behaviors for themselves and their children
- Working through a local health department in consultation with a school district to help control and prevent communicable diseases such as measles, pertussis, or varicella by providing regular immunization programs and vaccine oversight
- Instructing a group of overweight individuals on how to follow a well-balanced diet while losing weight to prevent nutritional deficiency (Box 1-8)
- Teaching safe sex practices or the dangers of smoking/vaping and substance abuse
- Serving on a fact-finding committee exploring the effects of a proposed toxic waste dump on the outskirts of town

Because it is our view that this is where most of the emphasis should be placed in the health care system, we use it as the base of our pyramid, instead of the usual placement of tertiary prevention as the base (Leavell & Clark, 1953).

Secondary prevention involves efforts to detect and treat existing health problems at the earliest possible stage, when intervention is most likely to be effective in controlling or eradicating it. This is the goal behind testing of water and soil samples for contaminants and hazardous chemicals in the field of community environmental health.

BOX **1-8** LEVELS OF PREVENTION PYRAMID

Link Between Poor Diet, Inactivity, and Obesity

SITUATION: Poor nutritional habits and inactivity are leading to obesity and a greater incidence of type 2 diabetes among children and adults.

GOAL: Using the three levels of prevention, avoid or promptly diagnose and treat, negative health conditions, and improve population health.

Tertiary Prevention

Rehabilitation	***Prevention***	
	Health Promotion and Education	***Health Protection***
▪ If diabetic, encourage weight, blood pressure, and cholesterol maintenance, along with good glucose control to prevent complications of diabetes. ▪ Reassess data to determine effectiveness of interventions.	▪ Teach children and families the importance of maintaining a healthy weight through proper diet and exercise. Promote awareness of dangers of obesity and diabetes through use of PSAs and billboards.	▪ Provide weight loss support. ▪ Provide access to periodic health care to check A_1C levels and foot and eye exams.

Secondary Prevention

Early Diagnosis	***Prompt Treatment***
▪ Encourage weight loss in obese populations to prevent development of type 2 diabetes. Provide screening programs for high-risk groups. ▪ Refer clients with high glucose or other problems (e.g., hypertension, high cholesterol) to primary care provider or diabetes clinics.	▪ Initiate educational and incentive programs to improve dietary practices. ▪ Teach clients (individuals or families) on a one-to-one basis to modify dietary practices and activity levels.

Primary Prevention

Health Promotion and Education	***Health Protection***
▪ Provide nutrition educational programs to promote awareness at schools, work sites, etc. ▪ Encourage restaurants and schools to offer healthy menu items. ▪ Recommend nutrition classes offered at neighborhood centers or health care facilities	▪ Promote physical fitness, nutritional, and wellness activities. ▪ Work with local entities to provide easier access to fresh fruits and vegetables, as well as provide bike paths and walking clubs, and to reduce easy access to sodas, tax high-calorie foods.

Examples of secondary prevention activities by a C/PHN include:

- Conducting community hypertension and cholesterol screening programs to help identify high-risk individuals and encourage early treatment to prevent heart attacks or stroke
- Encouraging breast and testicular self-examination, regular mammograms, and Pap smears for early detection of possible cancers and providing skin testing for tuberculosis
- Assessing for early signs of child abuse in a family, emotional disturbances among widows, or alcohol and drug abuse among adolescents

Tertiary prevention attempts to reduce the extent and severity of a health problem to its lowest possible level, so as to minimize disability and restore or preserve function. The individuals involved have an existing illness or disability whose impact on their lives is lessened through tertiary prevention. See more on clients living with disabilities in Chapter 24.

Examples include:

- Treatment and rehabilitation of persons after a stroke to reduce impairment
- Postmastectomy exercise programs to restore functioning
- Early treatment and management of diabetes to reduce problems or slow their progression

In community/public health, the need to reduce disability and restore function applies equally to families, groups, communities, and individuals. Many groups form for rehabilitation and offer support and guidance for those recuperating from some physical or mental disability. Examples include:

- Alcoholics Anonymous
- Halfway houses for psychiatric patients discharged from acute care settings
- Ostomy clubs
- Drug rehabilitation programs

In broader community health practice, tertiary prevention is used to minimize the effects of an existing unhealthy community condition. Examples of such prevention are:

- Insisting that businesses provide wheelchair access
- Warning urban residents about the dangers of a chemical spill
- Recalling a contaminated food or drug product
- Preventing injuries among survivors and volunteers during rescue in an earthquake, fire, hurricane, mass casualty incident due to gun violence, or even a terrorist attack

Health assessment of individuals, families, and communities is an important part of all three levels of preventive practice. Health status must be determined to anticipate problems and select appropriate preventive measures. C/PHNs working with young parents who themselves have been victims of child abuse can institute early treatment for the parents to prevent abuse and foster adequate parenting of their children. If the assessment of a community reveals inadequate facilities and activities to meet the future needs of its growing senior population, agencies and groups can collaborate to develop the needed resources.

Health problems are most effectively prevented by maintenance of healthy lifestyles and healthy environments. To these ends, community/public health practice directs many of its efforts to providing safe and satisfying living and working conditions, nutritious food, and clean air and water (Ali & Katz, 2018).

CHARACTERISTICS OF COMMUNITY/PUBLIC HEALTH NURSING

As a specialty field of nursing, community/public health nursing adds public health knowledge and skills that address the needs and problems of communities and aggregates and focuses care on communities and vulnerable populations. Community/public health nursing is grounded in both public health science and nursing science, which makes its philosophical orientation and the nature of its practice unique. It has been recognized as a subspecialty of both fields. Recognition of this specialty field continues with a greater awareness of the important contributions made by community/public health nursing to improve the health of the public.

Knowledge of the following elements of public health is essential to community/public health nursing (ANA, 2013; Quad Council Coalition Competency Review Task Force, 2018):

- Priority of preventive, protective, and health-promoting strategies over curative strategies (see Chapters 11 and 12)
- Means for measurement and analysis of community health problems, including epidemiologic concepts and biostatistics (see Chapter 7)
- Influence of environmental factors on aggregate health (see Chapter 9)
- Principles underlying management and organization for community health, because the goal of public health is accomplished through organized community efforts (see Chapters 6, 12, and 15)
- Public policy analysis and development, along with health advocacy and an understanding of the political process (see Chapters 6 and 13)

Confusion over the meaning of "community health nursing" arises when it is defined only in terms of where it is practiced. Because health care services have shifted from the hospital to the community, many nurses in other specialties now practice in the community. Examples of these practices include home health care, community mental health, geriatric nursing, long-term care, and occupational health. Although C/PHNs today practice in the same or similar settings, the difference often lies in applying the public health principles to large groups and communities of people—or having a population focus within the community one serves (Fig. 1-9).

For nurses moving into this field of nursing, it requires a shift in focus—from individuals to a broader focus on aggregates and populations. Nursing and other theories undergird its practice, and the nursing process is one of its basic tools. See Chapters 14 and 15 for more details.

Community/public health nursing, then, as a specialty of nursing, combines nursing science with public health science to formulate a community-based and population-focused practice (Anderson & McFarlane, 2019). "Public health nursing practice focuses on population health through continuous surveillance and assessment of the multiple determinants of health with the intent to promote health and wellness; prevent disease, disability, and premature death; and improve neighborhood quality of life" (Box 1-9; ANA, 2013, p. 2). Examples of community/public health nursing include:

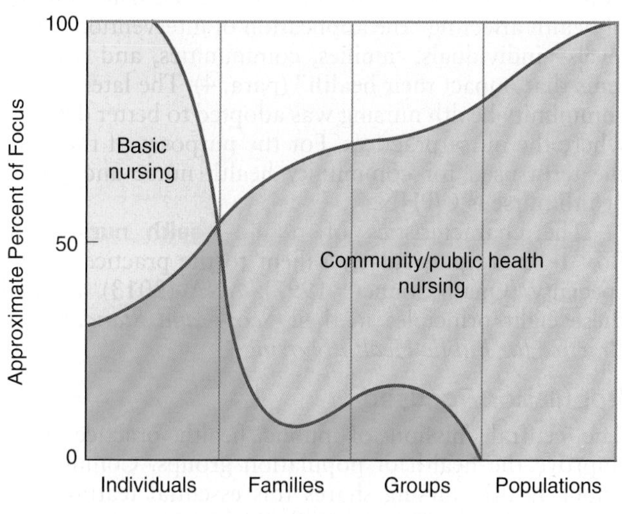

FIGURE 1-9 Difference in client focus between basic nursing and community/public health nursing.

BOX 1-9 The Definition and Practice of Public Health Nurses

Public health nursing is the practice of promoting and protecting the health of populations using knowledge from nursing, social, and public health sciences (para. 2).

Key characteristics of practice include (1) a focus on the health needs of an entire population, including inequities and the unique needs of subpopulations; (2) assessment of population health using a comprehensive, systematic approach; (3) attention to multiple determinants of health; (4) an emphasis on primary prevention; and (5) application of interventions at all levels—individuals, families, communities, and the systems that impact their health (para. 4).

The baccalaureate degree in nursing (BSN) is recommended for entry-level public health nurses (para. 12).

Reprinted from American Public Health Association (APHA) Public Health Nursing Section. (2013). *The definition and practice of public health nursing.* Washington, DC: APHA. Used with permission.

- Developing a program for providing food and shelter for homeless individuals sleeping in a park based on one's concern for this population
- Collaborating to institute an educational program on vaping in the local school system
- Assessing the needs of older people in retirement homes to ensure necessary services and provide health instruction and support

C/PHNs use primary, secondary, and tertiary interventions (levels of prevention) that are evidence-based and develop programs and services that help achieve health for all.

During the first 70 years of the 20th century, community health nursing was known as public health nursing. The PHN section of the American Public Health Association's (2013) definition of a PHN is someone who promotes and protects the health of populations and who is prepared at the baccalaureate level. The PHN also makes systematic and comprehensive assessments of population health and examines the many social determinants of health affecting "the application of interventions at all levels—individuals, families, communities, and the systems that impact their health" (para. 4). The later title of community health nursing was adopted to better describe where the nurse practices. For the purposes of this text, the term used for community health nurse and public health nurse is C/PHN.

The characteristics of **public health nursing** in Box 1-10 are particularly salient to the practice of this specialty (Quad Council, 1997). ANA (2013) adapted these eight principles in their *Scope and Standards of Practice for Public Health Nursing*.

BOX 1-10 Key Characteristics of Public Health Nursing

1. The main focus is "systematic and comprehensive" population health care (para. 2).
2. Population health must remain a focus when providing care to individuals, families, and aggregates.
3. Primary prevention takes precedence, prioritizing health promotion and disease prevention.
4. Clients are collaborative partners in planning, policy-making, and developing strategies and programs.
5. Interventions are instituted to "create healthy environments" and affect the social and economic conditions of populations, permitting them to flourish (para. 2).
6. There is an ongoing obligation to "actively identify and reach out to all who might benefit from a...service" (para. 2).
7. Allocated resources must support growth in "maximum population health benefit," utilizing evidence-based practice and quality improvement (para. 2)
8. Population health is most efficiently achieved "through collaboration with members of other professions," stakeholders, and organizations (para. 2).

Source: Quad Council (1997).

Population Focused

The central mission of public health practice is to improve the health of population groups. Community/public health nursing shares this essential feature with public health practice: it is **population focused**, meaning that it is concerned for the health status of population groups and their environment and prevention of disease (Association of Public Health Nurses, 2018).

A population may consist of older adults living throughout the community or of Syrian refugees clustered in one section of a city. It may be a scattered group with common characteristics, such as people at high risk of developing diabetes or battered women living throughout a county. It may include all people living in a neighborhood, district, census tract, city, state, or province.

Working with individuals and families as aggregates has been common for community health nursing; however, such work must expand to incorporate a population-oriented focus, a feature that distinguishes community/public health nursing specialties. Basic nursing focuses on individuals, and community/public health nursing focuses on aggregates, but the many variations in community needs and nursing roles inevitably cause some overlap.

A population-oriented focus requires the assessment of relationships. When working with groups and communities, the nurse does not consider individuals separately but rather in context—that is, in relationship to the rest of the community.

When an outbreak of hepatitis occurs, for example, the C/PHN does more than just work with others to treat it. The nurse tries to stop the spread of the infection, locate possible sources, and prevent its recurrence in the community. As a result of their population-oriented focus, C/PHNs seek to discover possible groups with a common health need, such as expectant mothers, or groups at high risk for development of a common health problem (e.g., obese children at risk for type 2 diabetes, victims of child abuse). C/PHNs continually look for problems in the environment that influence community health and seek ways to increase environmental quality. They work to prevent health problems and promote healthier lifestyles, such as promoting school-based education about nutrition and physical activity or exercise programs for groups of seniors (Fig. 1-10).

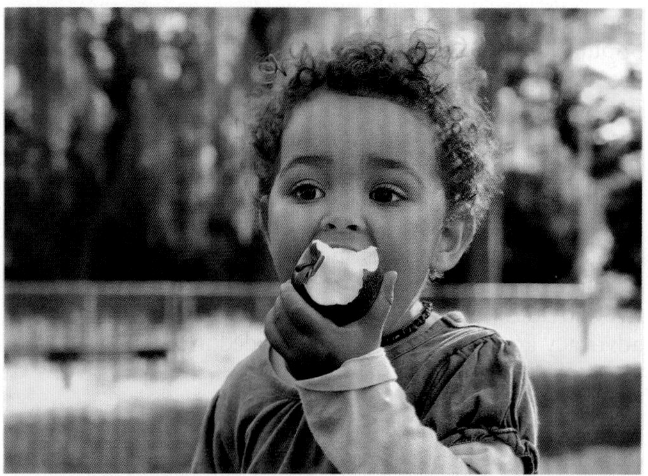

FIGURE 1-10 Healthy eating habits can begin in childhood.

The Greatest Good for the Greatest Number of People

A population-oriented focus involves a new outlook and set of attitudes. Individualized care is important, but prevention of aggregate problems in community/public health nursing practice reflects more accurately its philosophy and benefits more people. The community or population at risk is the client. Furthermore, because C/PHNs are concerned about several aggregates at the same time, service will, of necessity, be provided to multiple and overlapping groups. The ethical theory of utilitarianism promotes the greatest good for the greatest number. Further discussion of ethical principles in community/public health nursing can be found in Chapter 4.

Clients as Equal Partners

The goal of public health, increasing both the years and quality of healthy life and eliminating health disparities for populations, requires a partnership effort. Just as learning cannot take place in schools without student participation, the goals of public health cannot be realized without consumer participation. Community/public health nursing's efforts toward health improvement only go so far.

Clients' health status and health behavior will not change unless people accept and apply the proposals (developed in collaboration with clients) presented by the C/PHN. C/PHNs can encourage individuals' participation by promoting their autonomy rather than permitting dependency. For example, older persons attending a series of nutrition or fitness classes can be encouraged to take the initiative and develop health or social programs on their own. Independence and feelings of self-worth are closely related. By treating people as independent adults, with trust and respect, C/PHNs promote self-reliance and the ability to function independently. Autonomy is an important objective of public health, as is equality (Knight, 2016), and these are discussed in more detail in Chapter 4.

Frequently, consumers are intimidated by health professionals and are uninformed about health and health care. They do not know what information to seek and are hesitant to act assertively. For example, a migrant worker brought her 2-year-old son, who had symptoms resembling those of scurvy, to a clinic. Recognizing a vitamin C deficiency, the physician told her to feed the boy large quantities of orange juice but gave no further explanation. Several weeks later, she returned to the clinic, but the child was much worse. After questioning her, the nurse discovered that the mother had been feeding the child large amounts of an orange soft drink, not understanding the difference between that beverage and orange juice. Obviously, the quality of care is affected when the consumer does not understand and cannot participate in the health care process.

Health literacy, or "the degree to which an individual has the capacity to obtain, process, and understand basic health information and services needed to make appropriate health decisions," is an important concept that is discussed more fully in Chapter 10 (CDC, 2019, para. 1).

When people believe that their health, and that of the community, is their own responsibility, not just that of health professionals, they will take a more active interest in promoting it. The process of taking responsibility for developing one's own health potential is called self-care. As people maintain their own lives, health, and well-being, they are engaging in self-care. Some examples of self-care activities at the aggregate level include building safe playgrounds, developing teen employment opportunities, and providing senior exercise programs.

When people's ability to continue self-care activities falls below their need, they experience a self-care deficit. At this point, nursing may appropriately intervene. However, nursing's goal is to assist clients to return to or reach a level of functioning at which they can attain optimal health and assume responsibility for maintaining it (Alligood, 2018; Schulman-Green, Jaser, Park, & Whittemore, 2016; Zandiyeh, Hedayati, & Zare, 2015). To this end, C/PHNs foster their clients' sense of responsibility by treating them as adults capable of managing their own affairs. Nurses can encourage people to negotiate health care goals and practices, develop their own programs, contact their own resources (e.g., support groups, transportation services), identify and implement lifestyle changes that promote wellness, and learn how to monitor their own health.

When planning for the health of communities, for example, partnerships must be established, and the values and priorities of the community incorporated into program planning, data collection and interpretation, and policymaking. More information on program planning is given in Chapter 12.

Prioritizing Primary Prevention

In community/public health nursing, the promotion of health and prevention of illness are a first-order priority. Less emphasis is placed on curative care.

Some corrective actions always are needed, such as cleanup of a toxic waste dump site, or stricter enforcement of day care standards, but community health best serves its constituents through preventive and health-promoting actions (Ali & Katz, 2018; Anderson & McFarlane, 2019). These include services to mothers and infants, prevention of environmental pollution, school health programs, senior citizens' fitness classes, and "workers' right-to-know" legislation that warns against hazards in the workplace.

Another distinguishing characteristic of community/public health nursing is its emphasis on positive health, or wellness (Anderson & McFarlane, 2019). Medicine and acute care nursing have dealt primarily with the illness end of the health continuum. In contrast, community health nursing always has had a primary charge to prevent health problems from occurring and to promote a higher level of health.

C/PHNs concentrate on the wellness end of the health continuum in a variety of ways. They teach proper nutrition or family planning, promote immunizations among preschool children, encourage regular physical and dental checkups, assist with starting exercise classes or physical fitness programs, and promote healthy interpersonal relationships. Their goal is to help the community reach its optimal level of wellness.

This emphasis on wellness changes the role of community/public health nursing from a reactive to a proactive stance. It places a greater responsibility on C/PHNs to find opportunities for intervention. In clinical nursing and medicine, individual patients seek out professional assistance because they have health problems. They present their problems to the health care practitioner for diagnosis and treatment. C/PHNs, in contrast, seek out potential health problems in the community. They identify high-risk groups and institute preventive programs. C/PHNs visit clients in their homes and other settings (Fig. 1-11).

For example, they watch for early signs of child neglect or abuse and intervene when any occur, often long before a request for help is made. They look for possible environmental hazards in the community, such as smoking in public places or lead-based paint in older housing units, and work with appropriate authorities to correct them. A wellness emphasis requires taking initiative and making sound judgments, which are characteristics of effective community/public health nursing.

Selecting Interventions That Create Healthy Conditions in Which Populations May Thrive

With our population focus, it is prudent for C/PHNs to design interventions for the whole community, not limiting it only to those individuals seeking service or the poor and vulnerable, but promoting the health of entire populations and working to prevent "disease, injury and premature death" (ANA, 2013, p. 3).

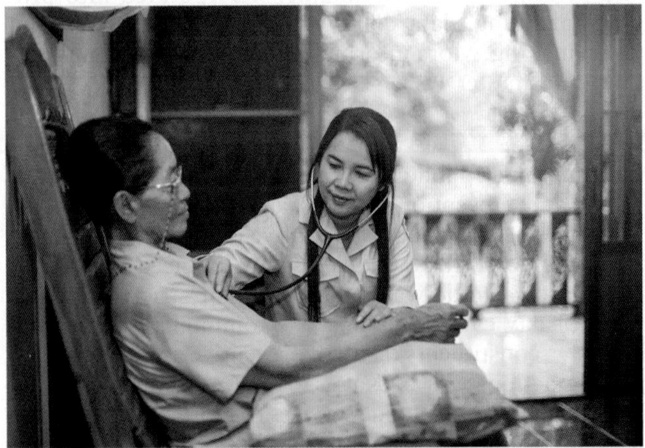

FIGURE 1-11 A C/PHN visits a client's home.

Advocacy for our clients (individuals, families, aggregates, communities, or populations) is an essential function of community/public health nursing. We want to create healthy environments for our clients so that they can thrive and not simply survive, and we do this by having a proactive stance toward trends in health care and society, ever changing public concerns, and work with policy and legislative activities (ANA, 2013). More information about health advocacy and policymaking is provided in Chapter 13.

Actively Reaching Out

We know that some clients are more prone to develop disability or disease because of their vulnerable status (e.g., poverty, no access to health care, homelessness). Outreach efforts are needed to promote the health of these clients and to prevent disease.

In acute care and primary health care settings, like emergency rooms or physician offices, clients come to you for service. However, in community/public health, nurses must focus on the whole population—not just those who come to us for services—and seek out clients wherever they may be (ANA, 2013). Like Lillian Wald and her Henry Street Settlement, C/PHNs must learn about the populations they serve and be willing to search out those most at risk. You can learn more about the rich history of community/public health nursing in Chapter 3. Unit 6 covers vulnerable populations.

Optimal Use of Available Resources

It is our duty to wisely use the resources we are given. For most state and local public health agencies, budgets are critically stressed. The use of documented evidence as a basis for community/public health nursing practice promotes more efficient and cost-effective strategies in health promotion (ANA, 2013; Quad Council, 2018). Tertiary health care has gotten the largest percentage of our health care dollar, leaving decreased funds for primary and secondary services. The lack of regular sources of health care sends many people to expensive emergency departments for treatment (IOM, 2002; Siekman & Hilger, 2018).

It is vital that C/PHNs ground their practice in research and evidence (see Chapter 4) and use that information to educate policy makers about best practices (see Chapter 13). Using personnel and resources effectively and prudently will pay off in the long run.

Interprofessional Collaboration

C/PHNs must work in cooperation with other team members, coordinating services and addressing the needs of population groups. This interprofessional collaboration among health care workers, other professionals and organizations, and clients is essential for establishing effective services and programs.

Individualized efforts and specialized programs, when planned in isolation, can lead to fragmentation and gaps in health services. Interprofessional collaboration is an even greater necessity when working with population groups, especially those from vulnerable or at-risk segments. Collaboration improves client outcomes, staff communication, and the quality of care (Lage, Rusinak, Carr, Grabowski, & Ackerly, 2015).

Collaboration involves working with members of other professions on community advisory boards and health planning committees to develop needs assessment surveys and to contribute toward policy development efforts. In addition to partnering with the population, other groups the C/PHN collaborates with include:

- Academic institutions, and others conducting research
- Businesses and pertinent industries
- Community organizations, coalitions, and advocacy groups
- Community service agencies such as schools, law enforcement, urban planning, and emergency response
- Faith-based organizations
- Health care providers and facilities
- Legislative, regulatory, and policymaking bodies
- Local, state, and federal public health organizations
- Members of the public health team, such as epidemiologists, social workers, health promotion specialists, nutritionists, environmental health workers, and health educators (ANA, 2013, p. 15)

Interprofessional collaboration requires clarification of each team member's role, a primary reason for C/PHNs to fully understand the nature of their practice. When planning a city-wide immunization program with a community group, for example, nurses need to explain the ways in which they might contribute to the program's objectives. They can share their knowledge of the public's preference about times and locations for the program, meet with various local agencies and organizations (e.g., health insurance companies, local hospitals) to gain financial support, help to organize and give immunizations, and influence planning for follow-up programs. Collaboration is discussed further in Chapter 10.

Another component includes development of policies to promote and protect the health of clients. Meeting with local legislators and providing testimony to local, state, and national bodies are common methods of ensuring enactment of effective health policies.

Client participation is promoted when people serve as partners on the health care team. An aim of community/public health nursing is to collaborate *with* people rather than do things *for* them.

As consumers of health services are treated with respect and trust, confidence and skill in self-care are gained. Thus, promoting their own health and that of their community as their contribution to health programs becomes increasingly valuable. C/PHNs encourage the involvement of health care consumers by soliciting their ideas and opinions, by inviting them to participate on health boards and committees, and by finding ways to promote their participation in decisions affecting their collective health. By assessing the needs of community, based partly upon the population's perceptions, the C/PHN can discover the most pressing health needs and work toward more effective interventions. Community assessment and intervention are explored in depth in Chapters 12 and 15.

SUMMARY

- Community health is defined as the identification of needs and the protection and improvement of collective health within a geographically defined area.
- A community is a collection of people who share some common interest or goal. Three types of communities were discussed: geographic, common-interest, and health problem-solving communities.
- *Health* is an abstract concept that includes all of the many characteristics of a person, family, or community, whether physical, psychological, social, or spiritual.
- People have levels of illness or wellness known as the *health continuum*.
- Health has both subjective and objective dimensions: the subjective involves how well people feel; the objective refers to how well they are able to function.
- Health care needs may be continuing, as with developmental concerns that occur over a person's lifetime, or episodic, occurring unexpectedly throughout a lifetime.
- Eight important characteristics of public health nursing practice are the client is the population; the primary obligation is to achieve the greatest good for the greatest number of people; working with clients as equal partners; primary prevention is the priority; focus on strategies that create healthy environmental, social, and economic conditions; actively identify and reach out to all who might benefit; make optimal use of available resources and create new evidence-based strategies; and collaborate with a variety of professions, populations, organizations, and other stakeholders to promote and protect the health of populations (ANA, 2013).

ACTIVE LEARNING EXERCISES

1. Debate similarities and differences between community/public health nursing and acute care nursing. Give examples of how public health principles are relevant for nurses working in hospitals (e.g., population health, epidemiology).
2. Identify specific examples of each of the three types of communities in your area (geographic, interest, solution). Discuss any local needs that are not being met (e.g., substance abuse, transportation) and how they might be addressed. Who should be involved as community members in addressing interventions?
3. Discuss the levels of prevention (primary, secondary, tertiary). Review your County Health Ranking and list three health issues found in your community. Decide on one primary, one secondary, and one tertiary intervention to address one of these health issues.
4. Using the eight characteristics of public health nursing outlined in this chapter, give specific examples of how a community/public health nurse might demonstrate four characteristics in addressing common health issues in your area.

REFERENCES

Abbasi, J. (August 1, 2018). Hurricane Maria and Puerto Rico: A physician looks back at the storm. *JAMA, Medical News & Perspectives*. Retrieved from https://jamanetwork.com/journals/jama/fullarticle/2696323

Alcorn, T. (October 7, 2017). Puerto Rico's health system after Hurricane Maria. *The Lancet World Report*, 10103(PE24). Retrieved from https://www.thelancet.com/journals/lancet/article/PIIS0140-6736(17)32591-6/fulltext

Ali, A., & Katz, D. L. (2018). Disease prevention and health promotion: How integrative medicine fits. *American Journal of Preventive Medicine, 49*(5 Suppl 3), S230–S240.

Alligood, M. R. (2018). *Nursing theorists and their work* (9th ed.). St. Louis, MO: Elsevier.

American Association of Colleges of Nursing. (2019). *Certification for public health nursing*. Retrieved from https://www.aacnnursing.org/Population-Health-Nursing/Certification-for-Public-Health-Nursing

American Nurses Association (ANA). (2013). *Public health nursing: Scope and standards of practice* (2nd ed.). Silver Springs, MD: Author.

American Public Health Association (APHA). (2018). *What is public health?* Retrieved from https://www.apha.org/what-is-public-health

American Public Health Association (APHA) Public Health Nursing Section. (2013). *The definition and practice of public health nursing*. Washington, DC: APHA.

Anderson, E. T., & McFarlane, J. (2019). *Community as partner: Theory and practice in nursing* (8th ed.). Philadelphia, PA: Lippincott Williams & Wilkins.

Artiga, S., & Hinton, E. (May 2018). *Beyond healthcare: The role of social determinants in promoting health and health equity*. Henry J. Kaiser Family Foundation. Retrieved from http://files.kff.org/attachment/issue-brief-beyond-health-care

Association of Public Health Nurses (APHN). (2018). *What is a PHN?* Retrieved from http://www.phnurse.org/What-is-Public-Health

Association of Schools of Public Health (ASPH). (2018). *Discover: What is public health?* Retrieved from http://www.aspph.org/discover/

Association for State and Territorial Health Officers. (April 2019). From Healthy People 2020 to Healthy People 2030. *ASTHO Brief*. Retrieved from https://www.astho.org/ASTHOBriefs/From-Healthy-People-2020-to-Healthy-People-2030/

Bertalanffy, L. V. (1968). *General systems theory: Foundations, development, applications*. New York: George Braziller, Inc.

Centers for Disease Control (CDC). (2011). Ten great public health achievements—United States, 2001—2010. *Morbidity and Mortality Weekly, 60*(19), 619–623. Retrieved from https://www.cdc.gov/mmwr/preview/mmwrhtml/mm6019a5.htm

Centers for Disease Control and Prevention (CDC). (2017a). *CDC research on SDOH: Neighborhood and the built environment*. Retrieved from https://www.cdc.gov/socialdeterminants/neighborhood/

Centers for Disease Control and Prevention (CDC). (2017b). *Community health assessment: Data & benchmarks*. Retrieved from https://www.cdc.gov/stltpublichealth/cha/data.html

Centers for Disease Control and Prevention (CDC). (2017c). *Introduction to public health*. Retrieved from https://www.cdc.gov/publichealth101/public-health.html

Centers for Disease Control and Prevention (CDC). (2018a). *Healthy People 2020: About healthy people*. Retrieved from https://www.healthypeople.gov/2020/About-Healthy-People

Centers for Disease Control & Prevention (CDC). (2018b). Zika virus. *CDC Newsroom*. Retrieved from https://www.cdc.gov/media/dpk/diseases-and-conditions/zika-virus/dpk-zika-virus.html

Centers for Disease Control & Prevention (CDC). (2018c). *Zika virus: 2018 case counts in the US*. Retrieved from https://www.cdc.gov/zika/reporting/2018-case-counts.html

Centers for Disease Control & Prevention (CDC). (October 3, 2019). *Zika virus: 2019 case counts in the US*. Retrieved from https://www.cdc.gov/zika/reporting/2019-case-counts.html

Centers for Disease Control and Prevention (CDC). (2019). *What is health literacy?* Retrieved from https://www.cdc.gov/healthliteracy/learn/index.html

County Health Rankings. (2018). *What is health?* Retrieved from http://www.countyhealthrankings.org/what-is-health

Donnelly, G. (February 9, 2018). Here's why life expectancy in the U.S. dropped again this year. *Fortune*. Retrieved from http://fortune.com/2018/02/09/us-life-expectancy-dropped-again/

Everytown for Gun Safety Action Fund. (2020). *About Moms Demand Action for gun sense in America*. Retrieved from https://everytown.org/moms/

Federal Emergency Management Agency (FEMA). (n.d.). *COVID-19 disaster declarations*. Department of Homeland Security. Retrieved from https://www.fema.gov/coronavirus/disaster-declarations

Federal, Provincial, and Territorial Advisory Committee on Population Health. (1999). *Toward a healthy future: Second report on the health of Canadians*. Ottawa, Canada: Minister of Public Works and Government Services Canada.

Goodman, R. A., Bunnell, R., & Posner, S. F. (2014). What is "community health"? Examining the meaning of an evolving field in public health. *Preventive Medicine, 67*(Suppl 1), 58–61.

Hankey, S., & Marshall, J. D. (2017). Urban form, air pollution, and health. *Current Environmental Health Reports, 4*(4), 491–503.

Health Resources in Action. (July 25, 2013). *Defining healthy communities*. Boston, MA: Author. Retrieved from https://hria.org/wp-content/uploads/2016/10/defininghealthycommunities.original.pdf

Iheanacho, T., Kapadia, D., Ezeanolue, C. O., Osuji, A. A., Ogidi, A. G., Ike, A., ... Ezeanolue, E. E. (2016). Attitudes and beliefs about mental illness among church-based lay health workers: Experience from a prevention of mother-to-child HIV transmission trial in Nigeria. *International Journal of Cultural Mental Health, 9*(1), 1–13.

Institute of Medicine. (1998). *The future of public health*. Washington, DC: National Academy Press.

Institute of Medicine. (2002). *The future of the public's health in the 21st century*. Washington, DC: National Academy Press.

Karlis, N. (April 22, 2018). *How Shannon Watts became the NRA's number one enemy*. Retrieved from https://www.salon.com/2018/04/22/how-shannon-watts-became-the-nras-number-one-enemy/

Kennedy, M. (April 20, 2016). *Lead-laced water in Flint: A step-by-step look at the makings of a crisis*. Retrieved from https://www.npr.org/sections/thetwo-way/2016/04/20/465545378/lead-laced-water-in-flint-a-step-by-step-look-at-the-makings-of-a-crisis

Kishore, N., Margues, D., Mahmud, A., Kiang, M. V., Rodriguez, I., Fuller, A., ... Buckee, C. O. (2018). Mortality in Puerto Rico after Hurricane Maria. *New England Journal of Medicine, 379*(2), 162–170.

Knight, R. (2016). Empirical population and public health ethics: A review and critical analysis to advance robust empirical-normative inquiry. *Health (London), 20*(3), 274–290.

Kochanek, K. D., Murphy, S. L., Xu, J., & Arias, E. (2017). *Mortality in the United States, 2016* (NCHS Data Brief, No. 293). Retrieved from https://www.cdc.gov/nchs/data/databriefs/db293.pdf

Lage, D. E., Rusinak, D., Carr, D., Grabowski, D. C., & Ackerly, D. C. (2015). Creating a network of high-quality skilled nursing facilities: Preliminary data on the postacute care quality improvement experiences of an accountable care organization. *Journal of the American Geriatric Society, 63*(4), 804–808.

Leavell, H., & Clark, E. (1953). *Textbook of preventive medicine*. New York: McGraw-Hill.

Lenartowicz, M. (2018). *Prevention of disease in the elderly*. Merck Manual: Professional Version. Retrieved from https://www.merckmanuals.com/professional/geriatrics/prevention-of-disease-and-disability-in-the-elderly/prevention-of-disease-in-the-elderly

Lybarger, J. (2018). Mental health in Puerto Rico. *Monitor on Psychology, 49*(5), 20.

McKenzie, J. F., Pinger, R. R., & Seabert, D. M. (2018). *An introduction to community and public health* (9th ed.). Burlington, MA: Jones & Bartlett Learning.

Meyer, R. (October 4, 2017). What's happening with the relief effort in Puerto Rico? A timeline of the unprecedented catastrophe of hurricane Maria. *The Atlantic*. Retrieved from https://www.theatlantic.com/science/archive/2017/10/what-happened-in-puerto-rico-a-timeline-of-hurricane-maria/541956/

Milken Institute. (August 27, 2018). *Ascertainment of the estimated excess mortality from hurricane Maria in Puerto Rico*. George Washington University and the University of Puerto Rico. Retrieved from https://prstudy.publichealth.gwu.edu/sites/prstudy.publichealth.gwu.edu/files/reports/Acertainment%20of%20the%20Estimated%20Excess%20Mortality%20from%20Hurricane%20Maria%20in%20Puerto%20Rico.pdf

Moms Demand Action. (November 7, 2018). *Everytown unveils five-point action plan and campaign to break the pattern of gun violence after gun sense majorities elected in the US House of Representatives, key governorships and statehouses*. Retrieved from https://momsdemandaction.org/everytown-unveils-five-point-action-plan-and-campaign-to-breakthepattern-of-gun-violence-after-gun-sense-majorities-elected-in-u-s-house-of-representatives-key-governorships-and-statehouses/

Mueller, N., Rojas-Rueda, D., Basagana, X., Cirach, M., Cole-Hunter, T., Dadvand, P., ... Nieuwenhuljsen, M. (2017). Urban and transport planning related exposures and mortality: A health impact assessment for cities. *Environmental Health Perspectives, 125*(1), 89–96.

National Academy of Sciences, Engineering, and Medicine (NASEM). (2020). *Leading health indicators 2030: Advancing health, equity, and well-being*. Washington, DC: National Academies Press. doi: 10.17226/25682.

National Quality Forum. (2018). Pre*vention and population health*. Retrieved from http://www.qualityforum.org/ProjectDescription.aspx?projectID=86178

Newkirk, V. R., II. (October 18, 2017). Puerto Rico's environmental catastrophe. *The Atlantic*. Retrieved from https://www.theatlantic.com/politics/archive/2017/10/an-unsustainable-island/543207/

Nightingale, F. (1859/1992). *Notes on nursing: What it is, and what it is not* [Commemorative edition]. Philadelphia, PA: Lippincott Williams & Wilkins.

Office of Disease Prevention and Health Promotion (ODPHP). (2016). *Healthy People 2020: Midcourse review*. Retrieved from https://www.cdc.gov/nchs/data/hpdata2020/CHIV_LHI.pdf

Pope, D., Tisdall, R., Middleton, J., Verma, A., van Ameijden, E., Birt, C., & Macherianakis, N. G. (2018). Quality of and access to green space in relation to psychological distress: Results from a population-based cross-sectional study as part of the EURO-URHIS 2 project. *European Journal of Public Health, 28*(1), 35–38.

Quad Council. (1997). *Tenets of public health nursing*. Retrieved from http://www.quadcouncilphn.org/documents-3/1997-tenets-of-public-health-nursing/

Quad Council Coalition Competency Review Task Force. (2018). *Community/public health nursing competencies*. Retrieved from http://www.quadcouncilphn.org/documents-3/2018-qcc-competencies/

Robles, F. (August 9, 2018). Puerto Rican government acknowledges hurricane death toll of 1,427. *The New York Times*. Retrieved from https://www.nytimes.com/2018/08/09/us/puerto-rico-death-toll-maria.html

Saint Onge, J. M., & Krueger, P. M. (2017). Health lifestyle behaviors among U.S. adults. *SSM-Population Health, 3*, 89–98.

Salmond, S. W., & Echevarria, M. (2017). Healthcare transformation and changing roles for nursing. *Orthopedic Nursing, 36*(1), 12–25.

Schulman-Green, D., Jaser, S. S., Park, C., & Whittemore, R. (2016). A metasynthesis of factors affecting self-management of chronic illness. *Journal of Advanced Nursing, 72*(7), 1469–1489.

Scott, S. B., Munoz, E., Mogle, J. A., Gamaldo, A. A., Smyth, J. M., Almeida, D. M., & Sliwinski, M. J. (2018). Perceived neighborhood characteristics predict severity and emotional response to daily stressors. *Social Science & Medicine, 200*, 262–279.

Siekman, N., & Hilger, R. (2018). High users of healthcare: Strategies to improve care, reduce costs. *Cleveland Clinic Journal of Medicine, 85*(1), 25–31. Retrieved from https://www.mdedge.com/ccjm/article/155213/practice-management/high-users-healthcare-strategies-improve-care-reduce-costs

Stout, S., Howard, P., Lewis, N., McPherson, M., & Schall, M. (2017). *Foundations of a community of solutions*. SCALE 1.0 synthesis reports. Cambridge, MA: Institute for Healthcare Improvement. Retrieved from https://www.100mlives.org/wp-content/uploads/2017/07/Foundations-of-Community-of-Solutions-Approach-7.10.17.pdf

Thompson, M. R., & Schwartz Barcott, D. (2017). The concept of exposure in environmental health for nursing. *Journal of Advance Nursing, 73*(16), 1315–1330.

U.S. Department of Health and Human Services (USDHHS). (2019). *Healthy People 2020. Leading health indicators*. Retrieved from https://www.cdc.gov/nchs/healthy_people/hp2020/hp2020_indicators.htm

U.S. Department of Health and Human Services (USDHHS), National Center for Health Statistics. (April 20, 2017). *Healthy People 2020 midcourse review*. Retrieved from https://www.cdc.gov/nchs/healthy_people/hp2020/hp2020_midcourse_review.htm

U.S. Department of Health and Human Services (USDHHS), Office of Disease Prevention and Health Promotion (ODPHP). (2020). *Healthy People 2030 framework*. Retrieved from https://www.healthypeople.gov/2020/About-Healthy-People/Development-Healthy-People-2030/Proposed-Framework

van Puffelen, A. L., Heijmans, M. J., Rijken, M., Rutten, G. E., Nijpels, G.; Discourse Study Group. (2015). Illness perceptions and self-care behaviours in the first years of living with type 2 diabetes: Does the presence of complications matter? *Psychology & Health, 30*(11), 1274–1287.

World Health Organization (WHO). (2020a). *Constitution of WHO: Principles*. Retrieved from http://www.who.int/about/mission/en/

World Health Organization (WH0). (2020b). *Globalization and health*. Retrieved from http://www.who.int/trade/globalization_resource/en/

World Health Organization (WHO). (2020c). *Health promotion: Promoting healthier populations*. Retrieved from http://www.who.int/healthpromotion/en/

World Health Organization (WHO). (2020d). *Social determinants of health: WHO called to return to the Declaration of Alma Ata*. Retrieved from http://www.who.int/social_determinants/tools/multimedia/alma_ata/en/

World Health Organization (WHO). (2020e). *The Ottawa Charter for health promotion*. Retrieved from http://www.who.int/healthpromotion/conferences/previous/ottawa/en/

World Health Organization (WHO), Regional Office for Europe. (February 13, 2018). *Copenhagen Consensus of Mayors: Healthier and happier cities for all*. Retrieved from http://www.euro.who.int/__data/assets/pdf_file/0003/361434/consensus-eng.pdf?ua=1

Zandiyeh, Z., Hedayati, B., & Zare, E. (2015). Effect of public health nurses' educational intervention on self-care of the patients with type 2 diabetes. *Journal of Education and Health Promotion, 4*, 88.

Zorrilla, C. D. (2017). The view from Puerto Rico—Hurricane Maria and its aftermath. *New England Journal of Medicine, 377*, 1901–1803.

CHAPTER 2

Public Health Nursing in the Community

"One good community nurse will save a dozen policemen."

—Herbert Hoover

KEY TERMS

Advocate
Assessment
Assurance
Case management
Clinician
Collaborator
Educator
Leader
Manager
Policy development

LEARNING OBJECTIVES

Upon mastery of this chapter, you should be able to:

1. Identify the three core public health functions basic to community/public health nursing.
2. Differentiate among seven different roles of the community/public health nurse.
3. Discuss the seven roles within the framework of public health nursing functions.
4. Explain the importance of each role for influencing people's health.
5. Describe seven settings in which a community/public health nurse might practice.
6. Identify principles of effective nursing practice in the community.

INTRODUCTION

Historically, community and public health nurses (C/PHNs) have engaged in many professional roles. Nurses in this professional specialty have provided care to the sick, taught positive health habits and self-care, advocated on behalf of needy populations, developed and managed health programs, provided leadership, and collaborated with other professionals and consumers to implement changes in health services. Although the practice settings may have differed, the essential goal of the C/PHN has always been a healthier community. The home certainly has been one site for practice, but so too have public health clinics, schools, factories, and other community-based locations. Today, the roles and settings of community/public health nursing practice have expanded even further, offering a wide range of professional opportunities.

This chapter examines how the conceptual foundations and core functions of community/public health practice are integrated into the various roles and settings of community/public health nursing. It provides an opportunity to gain greater understanding about how and where this nursing specialty is practiced. Moreover, it will expand awareness of the many existing and future possibilities for C/PHNs to improve the public's health. As you read through this chapter, think about client populations that you may have encountered in the acute care setting and consider your role with these same populations in a community setting. You may just discover a community/public health nursing specialty area that you have never considered.

CORE PUBLIC HEALTH FUNCTIONS

The various roles and settings for practice hinge on three primary core functions of public health—assessment, policy development, and assurance—and are applied at three levels of service—individual, family, and community (Institute of Medicine, 1988, 2002; CDC, 2018). Essential services that are linked to these core functions are also covered below.

Assessment

An essential first function in public health, assessment, means that the C/PHN must first gather and analyze information that will affect the health of the people to be served. **Assessment** is *the systematic collection, assembly, analysis, and dissemination of information about the health of a community*. Health needs, risks, environmental conditions, political agendas, and financial and other resources need to be assessed (Schneider, 2017). Data may be gathered in many ways (e.g., interviewing people in the community, conducting surveys, gathering information from public records, applying research).

The C/PHN is typically both trusted and valued by clients, agencies, and private providers. Trust placed in the nurse can often be attributed to demonstrating consistency, honesty, and dependability, and to an ongoing presence in the community. Although securing and maintaining the trust of others are pivotal to all nursing practice, they are even more critical when working in the community. Trust can afford a nurse access to client populations that may be difficult to engage. In the capacity of a trusted professional, C/PHNs gather relevant client data that enable them to identify strengths, weaknesses, and needs. It is important to recognize that as difficult as it may be for the nurse to gain the trust and respect of the community, if ever lost, these may not be easily reinstated.

At the community level, nurses perform assessment both formally and informally as they identify and interact with key community leaders. With families, the nurse can evaluate family strengths and areas of concern in the immediate living environment and in the neighborhood. At the individual level, the nurse identifies people within the family in need of services and evaluates their functional capacity using specific assessment measures and a variety of tools. Assessment of communities and families as the initial step in the nursing process is discussed more fully in Chapters 14 and 15.

Policy Development

Policy development is enhanced by the synthesis and analysis of information obtained during assessment to create comprehensive public health policy (Schneider, 2017). At the community level, the nurse provides leadership in convening and facilitating community groups to evaluate health concerns and develop a plan to address those concerns. Often, the nurse recommends specific training and programs to meet identified health needs of target populations (see Chapter 12) and raises the awareness of key policy makers about factors such as health regulations and budget decisions that negatively affect the health of the community (see Chapter 13).

With families, the nurse recommends new programs or increased services based on identified needs. Additional data may be needed to detect trends in groups or clusters of families, so that effective intervention strategies can be employed with these families.

At the individual level, the nurse assists in the development of standards for individual client care, recommends or adopts risk classification systems to assist with prioritizing individual client care, and participates in establishing criteria for opening, closing, or referring individual cases.

Assurance

Assurance is the pledge to our constituents that services necessary to achieve agreed-upon goals are provided by encouraging the actions of others (public or private) or requiring action through regulation or provision of direct services (Schneider, 2017). These activities often consume most of the C/PHN's time. Nurses perform the assurance function at the community level when they provide services to target populations, improve quality assurance activities (e.g., Quality and Safety Education for Nurses/QSEN), maintain safe levels of communicable disease surveillance and outbreak control, and collaborate with community leaders in the preparation of a community emergency preparedness plan. In addition, they participate in outcomes research, provide expert consultation, promote evidence-based practice, ensure competence and currency, and provide services within the community based on standards of care. QSEN features are found in later chapters.

Essential Services

To more clearly articulate the services that are linked to the core functions of assessment, policy development, and assurance, the Public Health Functions Steering Committee developed a list of 10 essential public health services in 1994 (Centers for Disease Control & Prevention [CDC], 2018). This initial effort to define the service components of the core functions provided an organized service delivery plan for public health providers across the country. A model depicting the relationships between the core functions and the essential services was eventually developed (Box 2-1). In March 2020, proposed revisions to the 10 essential public health services were distributed for comment; the final version was launched in September 2020 (CDC, 2020). Some of the changes included more emphasis on communication, equity, diversity, quality improvement, updating terminology, and use of more active language (Public Health National Center for Innovations, 2020).

BOX 2-1 Public Health Nursing Within the Core Public Health Functions Model

- This model includes assessment, policy development, and assurance surrounding the 10 essential services. Monitor Health; Diagnose and Investigate; Inform, Educate, and Empower; Mobilize Community Partnerships; Develop Policies; Enforce Laws; Link to Services; Assure Competent Workforce; Evaluate; Research and System Management are at the center of the model, as they are related to each essential service.
  - *Assessment* is the systematic collection, assembly, analysis, and dissemination of information about the health of a community.
  - *Policy development* uses the scientific information gathered during assessment to create comprehensive public health policies.
  - *Assurance* is the pledge to constituents that services necessary to achieve agreed-upon goals are provided by encouraging actions of others (private or public), requiring action through regulation, or providing service directly
- The community/public health nurse or C/PHN health nurse carries out these core functions and essential services at the individual, family, and community levels.

Source: Centers for Disease Control and Prevention (2018); Institute of Medicine (1988, 2002).

As illustrated in Box 2-1, this model shows the types of services necessary to achieve the core functions of assessment, policy development, and assurance. It also emphasizes the circular or ongoing nature of the process. The placement of equity in the center of the model represents the need to address health inequities, barriers, and discrimination in all public health services (Public Health National Center for Innovations, 2020).

As you review this model, think about what types of services might be provided in each category, depending on whether you are focusing on an individual, a family, or a community. It is not necessary for the C/PHN to personally provide all of the listed services. Working in collaboration with an interdisciplinary team, the nurse can support the efforts of others to achieve improved health in the community. What is important is that the team members all recognize their respective roles and work toward the same goal. A description of the original 10 essential services is found in Box 2-2. An example applying the 10 essential services to environmental health can be found at https://www.cdc.gov/nceh/ehs/10-essential-services/index.html.

STANDARDS OF PRACTICE

In 2008, the American Association of Colleges of Nursing (AACN) published the revised *The Essentials of Baccalaureate Education for Professional Nursing Practice*, a major step in providing clear guidelines as to what constitutes professional nursing education. This document provides nine essentials that are expected outcomes for baccalaureate nursing education (2019). This document is currently under revision. AACN developed a supplemental resource, *Public Health: Recommended Baccalaureate Competencies and Curricular Guidelines for Public Health Nursing*, to enhance population-focused activities associated with each of the nine essentials (2013), and it is also undergoing revision (2019). These documents clearly articulate the growing need to prepare nurses to assume roles in the community setting.

Community/public health nursing practice is further defined by specific standards developed under the auspices of the American Nurses Association (ANA) in collaboration with the Quad Council of Public Health Nursing Organizations (ANA, 2013), which is now the Council of Public Health Nursing Organizations (CPHNO). The CPHNO is composed of representatives from the Alliance of Nurses for Healthy Environments; the American Public Health Association, Public Health Nursing Section (APHA-PHN); the Association of Community Health Nursing Educators (ACHNE); and the Association of Public Health Nurses. These four organizations represent academics and professional practitioners, providing a broad spectrum of views regarding professional practice in the field of community/public health nursing. *Public Health Nursing: Scope and Standards of Practice* (ANA, 2013) , which is now the Council of Public Health Nursing Organizations (CPHNO). The CPHNO provides guidance as to what constitutes public health nursing and how it can be differentiated from other nursing specialties. The standards of care it outlines are consistent with the nursing process and include assessment, population diagnosis and priorities, outcomes identification, planning, implementation, and evaluation. This document is an important reference for all those practicing in the community. It provides the basis for evaluating an individual's performance in this field and is used by many employers to assess job performance. The C/PHN also provides nursing services based on other standards developed by the ANA, such as:

- Code of Ethics for Nurses with Interpretive Statements (2015a)
- Nursing's Social Policy Statement (2010)
- Nursing: Scope and Standards of Practice (2015b)

BOX 2-2 Ten Essential Public Health Services

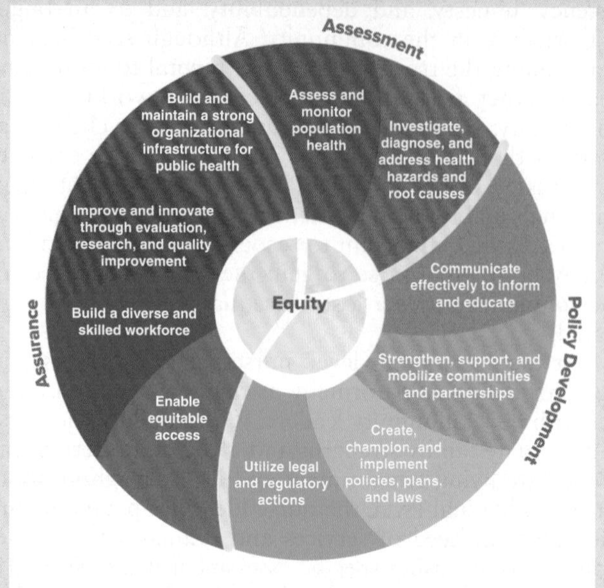

1. Assess and monitor population health status, factors that influence health, and community needs and assets.
2. Investigate, diagnose, and address health problems and hazards affecting the population.
3. Communicate effectively to inform and educate people about health, factors that influence it, and how to improve it.
4. Strengthen, support, and mobilize communities and partnerships to improve health.
5. Create, champion, and implement policies, plans, and laws that impact health.
6. Utilize legal and regulatory actions designed to improve and protect the public's health.
7. Assure an effective system that enables equitable access to the individual services and care needed to be healthy.
8. Build and support a diverse and skilled public health workforce.
9. Improve and innovate public health functions through ongoing evaluation, research, and continuous quality improvement.
10. Build and maintain a strong organizational infrastructure for public health.

Reprinted from CDC. (2020). 10 essential public health services (revised, 2020). Retrieved from https://www.cdc.gov/publichealthgateway/publichealthservices/essentialhealthservices.html

Each of these documents provides essential information regarding sound general nursing practice. When combined with *Public Health Nursing: Scope and Standards of Practice* (ANA, 2013), they provide the C/PHN with a clear understanding of accepted practice in this nursing specialty.

ACHNE, in addition to their collaboration with ANA, published the updated *Essentials of Baccalaureate Nursing Education for Entry-Level Community/Public Health Nursing* in 2010 (Education Committee of ACHNE). This document builds on previous versions and is consistent with both the *Essentials* document (AACN, 2008) and the scope and standards of public health nursing practice (ANA, 2013). It describes core professional values as well as knowledge and basic competencies. Core values of professional behavior emphasize community/population as client, prevention, partnership, healthy environment, and diversity (ACHNE, Education Committee, 2010). An emphasis of *Healthy People 2030* (USDHHS, 2020) is to create and support a competent public and personal health care workforce, and it includes professional competencies required for sound practice (see Box 2-3).

The Quad Council of Public Health Nursing Organizations (which is now the CPHNO) updated its own document, *Community/Public Health Nursing (C/PHN) Competencies*, in 2018. The competencies include eight domains (pp. 36–40):

1. Assessment and analytic skills
2. Policy development/program planning skills
3. Communication skills
4. Cultural competency skills
5. Community dimensions of practice skills
6. Public health sciences skills
7. Financial planning, evaluation, and management skills
8. Leadership and systems thinking skills

The competencies consist of three tiers of practice, beginning with the C/PHN generalist in tier one, followed by the C/PHN manager overseeing programs in tier two, and ending with C/PHN administrator practice skills requiring higher-level education and authority in tier three (Quad Council Coalition, 2018). The tier one public health nursing competencies are listed in this book in the appendix and also on the inside back cover.

With specific standards of practice and clear competencies to achieve, the C/PHN can integrate the core functions of assessment, policy development, and assurance, as well as the 10 essential services, throughout all of the various roles and community settings of practice.

ROLES OF C/PHNS

Just as the health care system is continually evolving, community/public health nursing practice evolves to remain effective with the clients it serves. Over time, the role of the C/PHN has broadened. This breadth is reflected in the description of public health nursing from the APHA-PHN (2013):

> Public health nursing ... focuses on improving the population health by emphasizing prevention and attending to multiple determinants of health. Often used interchangeably with community health nursing, [it] includes advocacy, policy development, and planning.... Public health nursing action occurs through community applications of theory, evidence, and a commitment to health equity (para. 3).

BOX 2-3 *HEALTHY PEOPLE 2030*

Selected Public Health Infrastructure Objectives

Core and Developmental Objectives	
PHI-01, 02, 03, D07	Increase the proportion of state, tribal, and territorial public health agencies that are accredited.
PHI-04, 05, 06, D01, D02	Increase the proportion of state, local, tribal, and territorial public health agencies that use Core Competencies for Public Health Professionals in continuing education for personnel.
PHI-04, 05, D06	Increase the proportion of state, local, tribal and territorial jurisdictions that have a health improvement plan.
Research Objectives	
PHI-R04	Monitor and understand the public health workforce—composition, enumeration, gaps, and needs.
PHI-R05	Monitor the education of the public health workforce—degrees conferred, schools and programs of public health, and related disciplines and curricula.
PHI-R06	Enhance the use and capabilities of informatics in public health.
PHI-R08	Explore financing of the public health infrastructure.
PHI-R09	Explore the impact of community health assessment and improvement planning efforts.
PHI-R10	Explore the impact of accreditation and national standards.

PHI, public health infrastructure.
Reprinted from U. S. Department of Health & Human Services. (2020). *Public health infrastructure.* Retrieved from https://health.gov/healthypeople/objectives-and-data/browse-objectives/public-health-infrastructure

C/PHNs wear many hats while conducting day-to-day practice. This chapter examines seven major roles of the C/PHN: clinician, educator, advocate, manager, collaborator, leader, and researcher. It also describes the factors that influence the selection and performance of those roles.

Clinician Role

- The most familiar role of the C/PHN is that of clinician or care provider. Different from such a role in the acute care setting, the **clinician** role in community/public health means that the nurse ensures health services are provided not just to individuals and families but also to groups and populations. Nursing service is still designed for the special needs of clients; however, when those clients compose a group or population, clinical practice takes different forms.
- It requires different skills to assess collective needs and tailor service accordingly. For instance, one C/PHN might visit older residents in a seniors' high-rise apartment building. Another might serve as the clinic nurse in a rural prenatal clinic that serves migrant farm workers. These are opportunities to assess the needs of aggregates and design appropriate services.

For C/PHNs, the clinician role involves certain emphases that are different from those of basic nursing. Three clinician emphases, in particular, are useful to consider here: holism, health promotion, and skill expansion.

Holistic Practice

- Most clinical nursing seeks to be broad and holistic. In community health, however, a holistic approach means considering the broad range of interacting needs—physical, emotional, social, spiritual, and economic—that affect the collective health of the "client" as a large system rather than as an individual (Dossey & Keegan, 2016).
- In community/public health, the client is a composite of people whose relationships and interactions with each other must be considered in totality. Holistic practice must emerge from this systems perspective (Fig. 2-1).

For example, when working with a group of pregnant teenagers living in a juvenile detention center, the nurse would consider the girls' relationships with one another, their parents, the fathers of their unborn children, and the detention center staff. The nurse would evaluate their ages, developmental needs, and peer influences, as well as their knowledge of pregnancy, delivery, and issues related to the choice of keeping or giving up their babies. The girls' reentry into the community and their future plans for school or employment would also be considered. Holistic service would go far beyond the physical condition of pregnancy and childbirth. It would incorporate consideration of pregnant adolescents in this community as a population at risk. What factors contributed to these girls' situations, and what preventive efforts could be instituted to protect these or other teens from future pregnancies? The clinician role of the C/PHN involves holistic practice from an aggregate perspective.

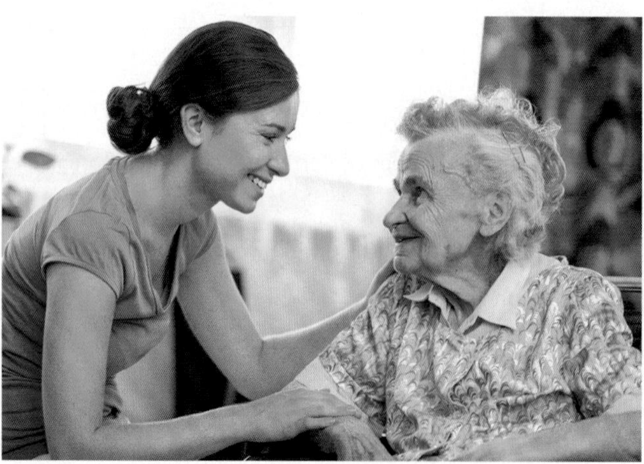

FIGURE 2-1 C/PHN student visiting an elderly client in her home.

Focus on Wellness

- The clinician role in community/public health also is characterized by its focus on promoting wellness. As discussed in Chapter 1, the C/PHN provides service along the entire range of the health continuum, but especially emphasizes promotion of health and prevention of illness.
- The C/PHN may provide education to healthy aggregate populations (e.g., schoolchildren, pregnant mothers). Effective services also include seeking out clients who are at risk for poor health and offering preventive and health-promoting services, rather than waiting for them to come for help after problems arise.

Nurses identify groups and populations who are vulnerable to certain health threats, and they design preventive and health-promoting programs to address these threats in collaboration with the community (Murdaugh, Parsons, & Pender, 2019). Examples include immunization of preschoolers, family planning programs, blood pressure screening, and prevention of behavioral problems in adolescents. Protecting and promoting the health of vulnerable populations is an important component of the clinician role and is addressed extensively in the chapters in Unit 6, which cover vulnerable aggregates.

Expanded Skills

Nursing requires multiple skills, including observation, listening, communication and counseling, and integrates psychological and sociocultural factors into practice.

- Additionally, environmental and community-wide considerations—such as problems caused by pollution, violence and crime, drug abuse, unemployment, poverty, homelessness, and limited funding for health programs—have created a need for stronger skills in assessing the needs of groups and populations and intervening at the community level (CDC, 2019).
- The clinician role in population-based nursing also requires skills in collaboration with consumers and other professionals, community organization and development, research, program evaluation, administration, leadership, and skill in epidemiology and biostatistics, as well as an ability to effect change (ANA, 2013). These skills are addressed in greater detail in later chapters.

Educator Role

A second important role of the C/PHN is that of **educator** or health teacher. Health teaching, a widely recognized part of nursing practice, is legislated through nurse practice acts and is one of the major functions of the C/PHN (ANA, 2013).

The educator role is especially useful in promoting the public's health for at least two reasons:

1. Community clients are usually not acutely ill and can absorb and act on health information. For example, a class of expectant parents, unhampered by significant health problems, can grasp the relationship of diet to fetal development. They understand the value of specific exercises to the childbirth process, are motivated to learn, and are more likely to perform those exercises. Thus, the educator role has the potential for finding greater receptivity and providing higher-yield results.
2. A wider audience can be reached. With an emphasis on populations and aggregates, the educational efforts of community/public health nursing are appropriately targeted to reach many people. Instead of limiting teaching to one-on-one or small groups, the nurse has the opportunity and mandate to develop educational programs based on community needs that seek a community-wide impact.

Whereas nurses in acute care often teach patients one-on-one, focusing on issues related to their illness and hospitalization, C/PHNs go beyond these topics to educate people in a variety of areas. Community-living clients need and want to know about issues such as family planning, weight control, smoking cessation, and stress reduction. Aggregate-level concerns also include such topics as environmental safety, sexual discrimination and harassment at school or work, violence, and drugs. C/PHN teaching addresses questions such as: What foods and additives are safe to eat? How can people organize the community to work for reduction of gun violence? What are health consumers' rights? Topics C/PHNs teach extend from personal and family health to environmental health and community organization. The emphasis throughout the health teaching process continues to be on illness prevention and health promotion (Rhodes, Visker, Cox, Forsyth, & Woolman, 2017). Telehealth (which is discussed in Chapter 10) is useful when needing to reach distant clients or groups. Health teaching as a tool for community/public health nursing practice is discussed in detail in Chapter 11.

Advocate Role

The issue of clients' rights is important in health care. Every patient or client has the right to receive just, equal, and humane treatment.

The role of the nurse includes client advocacy, which is highlighted in the ANA *Code of Ethics for Nurses with Interpretive Statements* (2015a), *Nursing's Social Policy Statement* (2010), and *Nursing's Social Policy Statement: Understanding the Profession from Social Contract to Social Covenant* (Fowler, 2016). Our current health care system is often characterized by fragmented and depersonalized services, and many clients—especially the poor, the disadvantaged, those without health insurance, and people with language barriers—frequently are denied their rights. They become frustrated, confused, discouraged, and unable to cope with the system on their own. The C/PHN often acts as an **advocate** for clients, pleading their cause or acting on their behalf. Clients may need someone to explain which services to expect and which services they ought to receive, to make referrals as needed, or to guide them through the complexities of the system and ensure the satisfaction of their needs. This is particularly true for minorities and disadvantaged groups (Fig. 2-2; Kalaitzidis & Jewell, 2015; Lassi & Bhutta, 2015; Nsiah, Siakwa, & Ninnoni, 2019).

Advocacy Goals

Client advocacy has two underlying goals:

1. Help clients gain greater independence or self-determination. Until clients can research the needed information and access health and social services for themselves, the C/PHN acts as an advocate for them by showing them what services are available, those to which they are entitled, and how to obtain them.
2. Make the system more responsive and relevant to the needs of clients (Byers, 2015; Nsiah et al., 2019). By calling attention to inadequate, inaccessible, or unjust care, C/PHNs can facilitate change (see Chapter 13).

Consider the experience of the Merrill family. Sarah Merrill has three small children. Early one Tuesday morning, the baby, Samuel, suddenly started to cry. Nothing would comfort him. Sarah went to a neighbor's apartment, called the local clinic, and was told to come in the next day. When she arrived, she was told that the clinic did not take appointments and was too busy to see any more patients that day. Sarah's neighbor reassured her that "sometimes babies just cry." For the rest of the day and night, Samuel cried incessantly. On Wednesday, Sarah and her children made the 45-minute bus ride to the clinic and waited 3 hours in the crowded reception room; the wait was punctuated by interrogations from

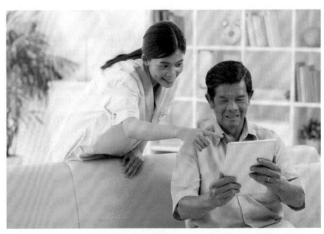

FIGURE 2-2 Like nurses working in every type of setting, C/PHNs are advocates for their clients.

clinic workers. Sarah's other children were restless, and the baby was crying. Finally, they saw the physician. Samuel had an inguinal hernia that could have strangulated and become gangrenous. The doctor admonished Sarah for waiting so long to bring the baby in. Immediate surgery was necessary. Someone at the clinic told Sarah that Medicaid would pay for it. Someone else told her that she was ineligible. At this point, all of her children were crying. Sarah had been up most of the night. She was frantic and confused and felt that no one cared. This family needed an advocate.

Advocacy Actions

The advocate role incorporates four characteristic actions: being assertive, taking risks, communicating and negotiating well, and identifying resources and obtaining results. Let's consider how a C/PHN might have taken each of these actions in the case of the Merrill family.

1. *Advocates must be assertive.* Fortunately, in the Merrill's dilemma, the clinic had a working relationship with the City Health Department and contacted Tracy Lee, a C/PHN liaison with the clinic, when Sarah broke down and cried. Tracy took the initiative to identify the Merrill's needs and find appropriate solutions. She contacted the Department of Social Services and helped the Merrill family to establish eligibility for coverage of surgery and hospitalization costs. She helped Sarah arrange for the baby's hospitalization and care for the other children.
2. *Advocates must take risks—go "out on a limb" if need be—for the client.* Tracy was outraged by the kind of treatment received by the Merrill family: the delays in service, the impersonal care, and the surgery that could have been planned as elective rather than as an emergency. She wrote a letter describing the details of the Merrill's experience to the clinic director, the chairman of the clinic board, and the nursing director. This action resulted in better care for the Merrill family and a series of meetings aimed at changing clinic procedures and providing better telephone screening.
3. *Advocates must communicate and negotiate well by bargaining thoroughly and convincingly.* Tracy stated the problem clearly and politely, yet firmly argued for its solution.
4. *Advocates must identify and obtain resources for the client's benefit.* By contacting the most influential people in the clinic and appealing to their desire for quality service, Tracy was able to facilitate change and hopefully improve service for other patients.

Advocacy at the population level incorporates the same goals and actions. Whether the population is homeless people, battered women, or migrant children, the C/PHN in the advocate role speaks and acts on their behalf. The goals remain the same: to promote clients' self-determination and to shape a more responsive system (Dickson & Lobo, 2018; Dworkin & Sood, 2016). Advocacy for large aggregates, such as those with inadequate health care coverage or access to care, means changing national policies and laws (see Chapter 13).

Manager Role

C/PHNs, like all nurses, engage in the role of managing health services (Kagan, Schachaf, Rapaport, Livine, & Madjar, 2017). The management process, like the nursing process, incorporates a series of problem-solving activities or functions: planning, organizing, leading, and controlling and evaluating.

- As a **manager**, the nurse helps achieve clients' goals by assessing their needs, planning and organizing to meet those needs, directing and leading to achieve results, and controlling and evaluating the progress to ensure that goals are met.
- The nurse serves as a manager when overseeing client care as a case manager, supervising ancillary staff, managing caseloads, running clinics, or conducting community health needs assessment projects.

Nurse as Planner

The first function in the management process is planning. A planner sets the goals and direction for the organization or project and determines the means to achieve them.

- Planning includes defining goals and objectives, determining the strategy for reaching them, and designing a coordinated set of activities for implementing and evaluating them, which tends to include broader, more long-range goals (Gordon, 2018).
- Planning may be strategic. An example of *strategic planning* is setting 2-year agency goals to reduce opioid abuse in the county by 10%.
- Planning may be operational, focusing more on short-term planning needs. An example of *operational planning* is setting 6-month objectives to implement a new computer system for client record keeping.

The concepts of planning with individuals, families, and communities are discussed further in Chapters 12, 14, and 15.

Nurse as Organizer

The second function of the manager role is that of organizer. This involves designing a structure within which people and tasks function to reach the desired objectives. A manager must arrange matters so that the job can be done. People, activities, and relationships have to be assembled to put the plan into effect. In the process of organizing, the nurse manager provides a framework for the various aspects of service, so that each runs smoothly and accomplishes its purpose (Feetham & Doering, 2015; Weatherford, Bower, & Vitello-Cicciu, 2018).

Nurse as Leader

In the manager role, the C/PHN also must act as a leader. As a **leader**, the nurse directs, influences, or persuades others to effect change that will positively impact people's health and move them toward a goal (Rosa, 2016; Weatherford et al., 2018).

- The leading function includes persuading and motivating people, directing activities, ensuring effective two-way communication, resolving conflicts, and coordinating the plan.

- Coordination means bringing people and activities together, so that they function in harmony while pursuing desired objectives.

Transformational and authentic leadership is characterized by the ability of leaders to inspire change and demonstrate empathy and leads to increased job satisfaction and performance (Lee, Chiang, & Kuo, 2019). Change management strategies are necessary to achieve the Triple Aim of improving population health, reducing health care costs, and providing improved patient outcomes (Shirey & White-Williams, 2015).

Nurse as Controller and Evaluator

The fourth management function is to control and evaluate projects or programs. A controller monitors the plan and ensures that it stays on course. In this function, the C/PHN must realize that plans may not proceed as intended and may need adjustments or corrections to reach the desired results or goals and must judge outcomes against original goals and objectives (Swider, Levin, & Reising, 2017).

An example of the controlling and evaluating function is evident in a program started in several preschool day care centers. The goal of the project is to reduce the incidence of illness among the children through intensive health education on prevention that addresses both the physical health and emotional health of the children with staff, parents, and children. At first, staff closely monitored the application of the prevention principles in day-to-day care, and the two C/PHNs managing the project were pleased with the progress of the classes. After several weeks, however, staff became busy and did not follow some plans carefully. Preventive activities, such as coughing into the shirtsleeve and washing the hands after using the bathroom and before eating, were not being closely monitored. Several children who were clearly sick had not been kept at home. Staff often overlooked quiet or reserved children and did not include them in activities. To address these problems and get the project back on course, the nurses worked with staff and parents to motivate them. They held monthly meetings with the staff, observed the classes periodically, and offered one-on-one instruction to staff, parents, and children. One activity was to establish competition between the centers for the best health record, with the promise of a photograph of the winning center's children and an article in the local newspaper. Their efforts were successful.

Management Behaviors

As managers, C/PHNs engage in many different types of behaviors. First described in a classic book by Mintzberg (1973), the management roles were grouped into three sets of behaviors: decision-making, transferring of information, and engaging in interpersonal relationships (Management at Work, 2019).

Decision-Making Behaviors. Mintzberg identified four types of decisional roles or behaviors: entrepreneur, disturbance handler, resource allocator, and negotiator.

- A manager serves in the *entrepreneur* role when initiating new projects. Starting a nurse-managed center to serve a homeless population is an example.
- C/PHNs play the *disturbance handler* role when they manage disturbances and crises—particularly interpersonal conflicts among staff, between staff and clients, or among clients (especially when being served in an agency).
- The *resource allocator* role is demonstrated by determining the distribution and use of human, physical, and financial resources.
- Nurses play the *negotiator* role when bargaining, perhaps with higher levels of administration or a funding agency, for new health policy or budget increases to support expanded services for clients (Management at Work, 2019).

Transfer of Information Behaviors. Three informational roles or behaviors include monitor, information disseminator, and spokesperson.

- The *monitor* role requires collecting and processing information, such as gathering ongoing evaluation data to determine whether a program is meeting its goals.
- In the *disseminator* role, nurses transmit the collected information to people involved in the project or organization.
- In the *spokesperson* role, nurses share information on behalf of the project or agency with outsiders (Management at Work, 2019). See Chapter 10 for more on communication.

Interpersonal Behaviors. While engaging in various interpersonal roles, the C/PHN may function as a figurehead, a leader, and a liaison.

- In the *figurehead* role, the nurse acts in a ceremonial or symbolic capacity, such as participating in a ribbon-cutting ceremony to mark the opening of a new clinic or representing the project or agency for news media coverage.
- In the *leader role*, the nurse motivates and directs people involved in the project.
- In the *liaison* role, a network is maintained with people outside the organization or project for information exchange and project enhancement (MindTools, n.d.).

Management Skills

Three basic management skills are needed for successful achievement of goals: human, conceptual, and technical.

- *Human skills* refer to the ability to understand, communicate, motivate, delegate, and work well with people (Cherry & Jacob, 2020). An example is a nursing supervisor's or team leader's ability to gain the trust and respect of staff and promote a productive and satisfying work environment. A manager can accomplish goals only with the cooperation of others. Therefore, human skills are essential to successful performance of the manager role.
- *Conceptual skills* refer to the mental ability to analyze and interpret abstract ideas for the purpose of

understanding and diagnosing situations and formulating solutions (Lalleman, Smid, Lagerwey, Oldenhof, & Schuurmans, 2015). Examples are analyzing demographic data for program planning and developing a conceptual model to describe and improve organizational function.
- *Technical skills* refer to the ability to apply special management-related knowledge and expertise to a particular situation or problem. Such skills performed by a C/PHN might include implementing a staff development program or developing a computerized management information system (Lalleman et al., 2015). See Chapter 10 on technology in community/public health nursing.

Case Management

Case management has become the standard method of managing health care in the delivery systems in the United States, and managed care organizations have become an integral part of community-oriented care.

- **Case management** is a systematic process by which a nurse assesses clients' needs, plans for and coordinates services, refers to other appropriate providers, and monitors and evaluates progress to ensure that clients' multiple service needs are met in a cost-effective manner.
- With health care reform, the importance of case management, or care coordination among an interdisciplinary team, is emphasized as a means to control costs and improve client outcomes (National Committee for Quality Assurance, 2018; Phillips & Fitzsimons, 2015).

As clients leave hospitals earlier, as families struggle with multiple and complex health problems with meager resources, as more older persons need alternatives to nursing home care, as competition and scarce resources contribute to fragmentation of services, and as the cost of health care continues to increase, there is a growing need for someone to oversee and coordinate all facets of needed service (Chait & Glied, 2018; Cook, Hall, Garvan, & Kneipp, 2015). Through case management, the nurse addresses this need in the community (Fig. 2-3).

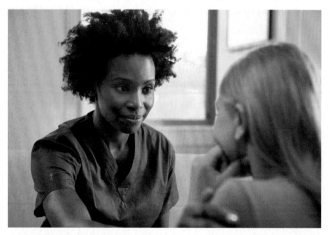

FIGURE 2-3 C/PHNs may serve as case managers for battered women and other aggregates.

The activity of case management often follows discharge planning as a part of continuity of care. When applied to individual clients, it means overseeing their transition from the hospital back into the community and monitoring them to ensure that all of their service needs are met. Case management also applies to aggregates (Young et al., 2018). In this context, it involves overseeing and ensuring that group or population health-related needs are met, particularly for those who are at high risk of illness or injury.

For example, the C/PHN may work with battered women who come to a shelter. First, the nurse must ensure that their immediate needs for safety, security, food, finances, and childcare are met. Then, the nurse must work with other professionals to provide more permanent housing, employment, ongoing counseling, and financial and legal resources for this group of women. Whether applied to families or aggregates, case management, like other applications of the manager role, uses the three sets of management behaviors and engages the C PHN as planner, organizer, leader, controller, and evaluator. See Unit 6.

Collaborator Role

C/PHNs seldom practice in isolation. They work with many people, including clients, other nurses, physicians, teachers, health educators, social workers, physical therapists, nutritionists, occupational therapists, psychologists, epidemiologists, biostatisticians, attorneys, secretaries, environmentalists, city planners, and legislators.

As members of the health team, C/PHNs assume the role of **collaborator**, which means working jointly with others in a common endeavor, cooperating as partners. Successful community/public health practice depends on this multidisciplinary collegiality and leadership (Brown, 2017).

The following examples show a C/PHN employed by the local Area Agency on Aging functioning as collaborator. Three families needed to find good nursing homes for their grandparents. The nurse met with the families, including the older adult members; made a list of desired features, such as a shower and access to walking trails; and then worked with a social worker to locate and visit several homes. The grandparents' respective physicians were contacted for medical consultation, and, in each case, the older adult member made the final selection. In another situation, the C/PHN collaborated with the city council, police department, neighborhood residents, and manager of a senior citizens' high-rise apartment building to help a group of older people organize and lobby for safer streets.

Leadership Role

C/PHNs are becoming increasingly active in the leadership role, separate from leading within the manager role mentioned earlier. The leadership role focuses on effecting change; thus, the nurse becomes an agent of change.

As leaders, C/PHNs seek to initiate changes that positively affect people's health. They also seek to influence people to think and behave differently about their health and the factors contributing to it. The role of social determinants of health, such as the availability of health services and how the physical environment affects population health, is discussed in Chapter 11 in relation to health promotion of individuals and communities.

- At the community level, the leadership role includes health planning and may involve working with a team of professionals to direct and coordinate projects, such as a campaign to restrict marketing of e-cigarettes to adolescents or to lobby legislators for improved child day care facilities.
- When nurses guide community/public health decision-making, stimulate an industry's interest in health promotion, initiate group therapy, direct a preventive program, or influence health policy, they assume the leadership role.

A broader attribute of the leadership role is that of visionary. A leader with *vision* sees what can be and leads people on a path toward that goal (Katz, 2018; Nolan et al., 2015). A leader's vision may include long- and short-term goals.

In one instance, it began as articulating the need for stronger community/public health nursing services to an underserved population in an inner-city neighborhood served by a C/PHN. In this densely populated, tenant-occupied neighborhood, drugs, crime, and violence were commonplace. One summer, an 8-year-old boy was shot and killed. The enraged immigrant families in the neighborhood felt helpless and hopeless. The nurse visited several families, and they shared their concerns with him. The nurse felt strongly about this community and offered to work with them to effect change. He gathered volunteers from neighborhood churches, and, together, they began to discuss the community's concerns. They prioritized their needs and began planning to make their community healthier. The nurse organized his workweek such that he could provide health screening and education to families in the basement of a church on one morning each week. Initially, only a few families accessed this new service. In a matter of months, however, it became recognized as a valuable community service and was expanded to a full day; the increasing volunteer group soon outgrew the space. The C/PHN worked closely with influential community members and the families being served. They determined that many more services were needed in this neighborhood, and they began to broaden their outreach and think of ways to provide the needed services.

Within a year, the group had written several grants to the city and to a private corporation in an effort to expand the voluntary services. The funding that they obtained allowed them to rent vacant storefront space, hire a part-time nurse practitioner, contract with the health department for additional community/public health nursing services, and negotiate with the local university to have medical, nursing, and social work students placed there on a regular basis. The group, under the visionary leadership of the C/PHN, planned to add a one-on-one reading program for children, a class in English as a second language for immigrant families, a mentoring program for teenagers, and dental services. Even the police department had opened a substation in the neighborhood, making their presence more visible. This C/PHN's vision filled an immediate, critical need in the short term that developed into a comprehensive community center in the long term. Violence and crime diminished, and the neighborhood became a safer place where children could play.

Researcher Role

- In the researcher role, C/PHNs engage in the systematic investigation, collection, and analysis of data for solving problems and enhancing community/public health practice. Research is an investigative process in which all C/PHNs can become involved by asking questions and looking for evidence-based solutions (Wilson, Rosemberg, Visovatti, Munro-Kramer, & Feetham, 2017).
- The ongoing need for evidence-based practice is supported by *Healthy People 2030*, as public health researchers incorporate "stakeholder engagement throughout all phases," which helps them to more accurately determine successful programs and interventions (Livingood, Bilello, Choe, & Lukens-Bull, 2018, p. 155).

C/PHNs practice the researcher role at several levels. In addition to everyday inquiries, nurses often participate in agency and organizational studies to determine such matters as practice activities, priorities, and education of C/PHNs (Livingood et al., 2018). The researcher role (at all levels) helps to determine needs, evaluate effectiveness of care, and develop a theoretic basis for community/public health nursing practice. Chapter 4 will explain this research in greater detail.

SETTINGS FOR COMMUNITY AND PUBLIC HEALTH NURSING PRACTICE

The previous section examined major C/PHN roles, which can now be placed in context by viewing the settings in which they are practiced. The sites are increasingly varied and include a growing number of nontraditional settings and partnerships with nonhealth groups. Employers of C/PHNs range from state and local health departments and home health agencies to managed care organizations, businesses and industries, and nonprofit organizations. For this discussion, these settings are grouped into seven categories: homes, ambulatory service settings, schools, occupational health settings, residential institutions, faith communities, and the community at large (domestic and international). This section provides a brief overview of the various settings. Chapters 28 and 29 will provide much more detail on specific roles and settings, including both public and private practice settings.

Homes

Since Lillian Wald and the nurses at the Henry Street Settlement first started their practice in 1893 (see Chapter 3), the most frequently used setting for community/public health nursing practice has been the home. In the home, all of the public health nursing roles are performed to varying degrees. Clients who are discharged from acute care institutions, such as hospitals or behavioral health facilities, may be referred to C/PHNs for continued care and follow-up. Here, the nurse can see clients in a family and environmental context and tailor service to the clients' unique needs (Fig. 2-4; Keeling, 2015).

For example, Mr. White, 67 years of age, was discharged from the hospital with a colostomy. Jessica Levitz, the C/PHN from the county visiting nursing agency, immediately started home visits. She met with Mr. White

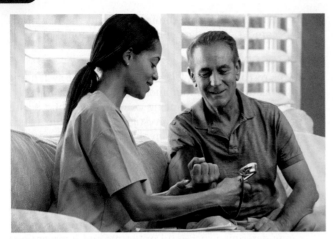

FIGURE 2-4 C/PHNs make home visits to assess and follow up with clients.

and his wife to discuss their needs as a family and to plan for Mr. White's care and adjustment to living with a colostomy. Practicing the clinician and educator roles, she reinforced and expanded on the teaching started in the hospital for colostomy care, including bowel training, diet, exercise, and proper use of equipment. As part of a total family care plan, Jessica provided some forms of physical care for Mr. White as well as counseling, teaching, and emotional support for both Mr. White and his wife. In addition to consulting with the physician and social service worker, she arranged and supervised visits from the home health aide, who gave personal care and homemaker services. She thus performed the manager, leader, and collaborator roles.

The home is also a setting for health promotion. Many C/PHN visits focus on assisting families to understand and practice healthier living behaviors. Nurses may, for example, instruct clients on parenting, infant care, child growth and development, diet, exercise, coping with stress, or managing grief and loss.

The character of the home setting is as varied as the clients served by the C/PHN. In one day, the nurse may visit a well-to-do widow in her spacious home, a middle-income family in their modest bungalow, an older transient man in his one-room fifth-story walk-up apartment, and a teen mother and her infant living in a group foster home. In each situation, the nurse can view the clients in perspective and, therefore, better understand their constraints, capitalize on their resources, and tailor health services to meet their needs.

In the home, unlike in most other health care settings, clients are on their own "turf." They feel comfortable and secure in familiar surroundings and often are better able to understand and apply health information. Client self-respect can be promoted, because the client is host and the nurse is a guest.

Sometimes, the thought of visiting in clients' homes can cause anxiety. This may be your first experience outside the acute care, long-term care, or clinic setting. Visiting clients in their own environment may make you feel uncomfortable. You may be asked to visit families in unfamiliar neighborhoods and have to walk through those neighborhoods to locate the clients' homes. Frequently, fear of the unknown is the real fear—a fear that often has been enhanced by stories from previous nursing students. This may be the same feeling as that experienced when caring for your first client, first entering the operating room, or first having a client in the intensive care unit. However, in the community, more variables exist, and the nurse should follow the specific instructions given during the clinical experience and everyday commonsense safety precautions. General guidelines for safety and making home visits are covered in detail in Chapter 14.

Changes in the health care delivery system, along with shifting health economics and service delivery (discussed in Chapter 6), are moving the primary setting for C/PHN practice away from the home. Many local public health departments are finding it increasingly difficult to provide widespread home visiting by their public health nurses.

Instead, many agencies are targeting populations that are most in need of direct intervention. Examples include families with low-birth-weight babies, clients requiring directly observed administration of tuberculosis medications, and families requiring ongoing monitoring because of identified child abuse or neglect. With limited staff and financial resources, the highest-priority clients or groups are targeted.

With skills in population-based practice, C/PHNs serve the public's health best by focusing on sites where they can have the greatest impact. At the same time, they can collaborate with various types of home care providers, including hospitals, other nurses, physicians, rehabilitation therapists, community aides, and durable medical equipment companies, to ensure continuous and holistic service. The nurse continues to supervise home care services and engage in case management. The increased demand for highly technical acute care in the home requires specialized skills that are best delivered by nurses with this expertise. Chapter 30 further examines the nurse's role in the home health and hospice settings.

Ambulatory Service Settings

Ambulatory service settings include a variety of venues for C/PHN practice in which clients require day or evening services that do not include overnight stays. Examples include the following:

- A local public health department
- A clinic offering comprehensive services in an outpatient department of a hospital or medical center
- A comprehensive community or neighborhood health center
- A specialized clinic, such as a family planning clinic or a well-child clinic, in a community location convenient for clients, such as in a church basement or a pharmacy
- A day care center, such as for those with physical disabilities or behavioral health issues
- A nurse-managed health center, often provided as a community service component of a school of nursing, with the mission of enhancing student clinical experiences while meeting identified community needs in the areas of primary health care and health promotion (see Chapter 29)
- A medical practice office, such as associated with a health maintenance organization and involving screening, referrals, case management services, counseling, health education, and group work

BOX 2-4 PERSPECTIVES

A Graduating Student's Viewpoint on Postgraduation Employment

Before entering nursing school, I spent 5 years on active duty as a corpsman in the Navy. I remembered seeing some nurses who visited our hospital wearing what looked like Navy uniforms but was told that they worked for the federal government and weren't in the Navy. I didn't think much of it until I was looking up information on the U.S. Public Health Service and the Surgeon General. Only then did it dawn on me that those nurses were part of the Commissioned Corps of the Public Health Service. I didn't even know they existed, much less what they did, so I looked around the section of the Web site dealing with nursing. It turns out that they do quite a bit—respond to disasters, provide health services to Native Americans, and even work with the federal prisons. It surprised me to find out that they hire new graduates for many of their positions. I still haven't decided what I want to do after I graduate, but I may seriously consider this option. They even have an extern program available while I'm still in school—who knows, I may be in uniform again.

Matt, age 29

See Chapter 28 for more about the U.S. Public Health Service.

- An independent nursing practice in a community nursing center that also may include home visits
- A setting associated with a selected client group, such as a migrant camp, tribal land, correctional facility, children's day care center, faith community, coal-mining community, or remote frontier area

In each ambulatory setting, all of the community/public health nursing roles are used to varying degrees (Box 2-4).

Schools

- Schools of all levels make up a major group of settings for community/public health nursing practice. Nurses from community/public health nursing agencies frequently serve private schools at elementary and intermediate levels. Public schools are served by the same agencies or by C/PHNs who are hired directly by the school system.
- The C/PHN may work with groups of students in preschool settings, such as Montessori schools or Head Start centers, as well as in vocational or technical schools, junior colleges, and college and university settings. Specialized schools, such as those for students with developmental disabilities, are another setting for community/public health nursing practice (Fig. 2-5).

C/PHNs' roles in school settings are changing. School nurses, whose primary role initially was that of clinician (for individual, family, and population health), are widening their practice to include more health education, interprofessional collaboration, and client advocacy. For example, one school had been accustomed to using the nurse as a first-aid provider and record keeper. Her duties were handling minor problems, such as headaches and cuts, and keeping track of such events as immunizations and medication administration at a local high school. This nurse sought to expand her practice and, after consultation and preparation, collaborated with a health educator and some of the teachers to offer a series of classes on personal hygiene, diet, and sexuality. She started a drop-in center for health counseling at the school and established a network of professional contacts for consultation and referral.

Nurses in school settings also assume managerial and leadership roles and recognize that the researcher role should be an integral part of their practice. The nurse's role with school-age and adolescent populations is discussed in detail in Chapters 20 and 28.

Occupational Health Settings

Business and industry provide another group of settings for community/public health nursing practice. Employee health has long been recognized as making a vital contribution to individual lives, the productivity of business, and the well-being of the entire nation. Organizations are expected to provide a safe and healthy work environment, in addition to offering insurance for health care.

More companies, recognizing the value of healthy employees, are going beyond offering traditional health benefits to supporting health promotional efforts. Some businesses, for example, offer healthy snacks, such as fruit at breaks, and promote walking or jogging during the noon hour. A few larger corporations have built exercise facilities for their employees, provide health education and wellness programs, and offer financial incentives for losing weight or staying well.

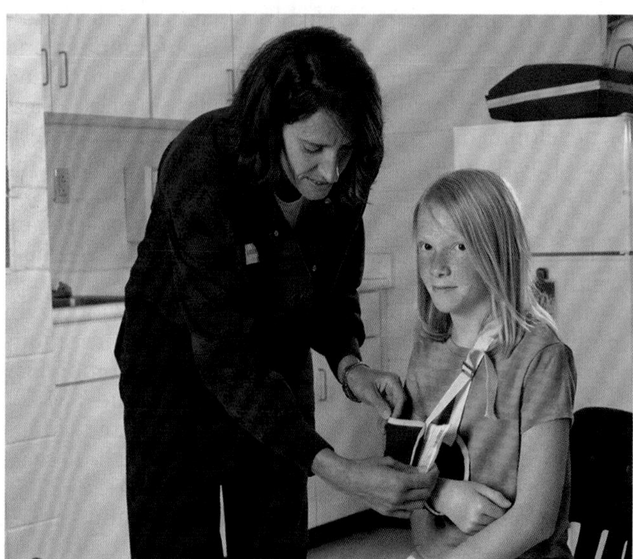

FIGURE 2-5 School nursing is another community/public health nursing role.

Occupational health settings range from industries and factories, such as an automobile assembly plant, to business corporations and even large retail sales systems. The field of occupational health offers a challenging opportunity, particularly in smaller businesses, where nursing coverage usually is not provided. Chapter 29 more fully describes the role of the nurse serving the working adult population.

Residential Institutions

Any facility where clients reside can be a setting in which community/public health nursing is practiced. Residential institutions include halfway houses, in which clients live temporarily while recovering from drug addiction, and inpatient hospice programs, in which terminally ill clients live.

Some residential settings, such as hospitals, exist solely to provide health care; others provide a variety of services and support. C/PHNs based in a community agency maintain continuity of care for their clients by collaborating with hospital personnel, visiting clients in the hospital, and planning care during and after hospitalization. Some C/PHNs serve one or more hospitals on a regular basis as a liaison with the community and by providing consultation for discharge planning and periodic in-service programs to keep hospital staff updated on community services for their clients. Other C/PHNs with similar functions are based in the hospital and serve the hospital community.

A continuing care center is another example of a residential site providing health care that may use community/public health nursing services. In this setting, residents are usually older adults; some live quite independently, whereas others become increasingly dependent and have many chronic health problems.

The nurse functions as advocate and collaborator to improve services. The nurse may, for example, coordinate available resources to meet the needs of residents and their families and help safeguard the maintenance of quality operating standards. Chapter 22 discusses the C/PHN's role with older adults. Chapter 30 discusses nursing services needed by clients after hospitalization through home care services or by families and clients in hospice programs. Sheltered workshops and group homes for children or adults with mental illness or developmental disability are other examples of residential institutions that serve clients who share specific needs.

C/PHNs also practice in settings where residents are gathered for purposes other than receiving care, where health care is offered as an adjunct to the primary goals of the institution. For example, many nurses work with camping programs for healthy children and adults offered by religious organizations and other community agencies, such as the Boy Scouts, Girl Scouts, and YMCA.

Other camp nurses work with children and adults who have chronic or terminal illnesses, through disease-related community agencies such as the American Lung Association, American Diabetes Association, and American Cancer Society. Camp nurses practice all available roles, often under interesting and challenging conditions and around the clock.

Another often-overlooked practice setting is the correctional institution. Inmates, whether incarcerated for the short or long term, have the same health care needs as the general public. The challenge to the nurse in this setting is to provide health care in an unbiased and nonjudgmental manner within the realities of the setting.

Because of the unique nature of this population, there are typically additional health and social service needs, often stemming from the reason for the incarceration in the first place (e.g., drug abuse) and that place them at increased risk for select health problems (e.g., AIDS, tuberculosis, poor nutrition). Chapter 28 discusses the role of the nurse in the correctional setting.

Residential institutions provide unique settings for the C/PHN to practice health promotion. Clients are more accessible, their needs can be readily assessed, and their interests can be stimulated. These settings offer the opportunity to generate an environment of caring and optimal quality health care provided by community/public health nursing services.

Faith Communities

Faith community nursing finds its beginnings in an ancient tradition. The beginnings of community/public health nursing can be traced to religious orders (see Chapter 3), and for centuries, religious and spiritual communities were important sources of health care.

In faith community nursing today, the practice focal point remains the faith community and the religious belief system provided by the philosophical framework. This nursing specialty may take different names, such as church-based health promotion, parish nursing, or faith community nursing practice. Whatever the service is called, it involves a large-scale effort by the church community to improve the health of its members through education, screening, referral, treatment, and group support.

The ANA, in collaboration with the Health Ministries Association, has published standards of care for faith community nursing practice in collaboration with the Health Ministries Association, Inc. (ANA, 2017). The standards act as guidelines for faith communities that plan to offer or are offering faith community nursing services. This specialty area of practice is guided by a variety of standards set up by several groups. Together, these standards provide guidance and direction for caregiving within the faith community.

When C/PHNs work as faith community nurses, they enhance accessibility to available health services in the community while meeting the unique needs of the members of that religious community, practicing within the framework of the tenets of that religion. In most situations, the nurse is a practitioner of the same religious belief system. Chapter 29 provides more detailed information about this specialty area of practice.

Community at Large

Unlike the six settings already discussed, the seventh setting for community/public health nursing practice is not confined to a specific philosophy, location, or building. When working with groups, populations, or the total community, the nurse may practice in many different

BOX 2-5 Innovative Community/Public Health Nursing Practice

In some community/public health nursing courses, students do not have access to an established agency such as a health department or community center from which to establish a client base. Student nurses and practicing C/PHNs can provide outreach services and do case finding in innovative settings such as these:

Settings	Clients	Roles of the Community Health Nurse
1. Senior centers when giving flu shots or when commodities are distributed	Older adults	Educator, clinician, advocate
2. Outside of grocery stores, department stores, movie theaters, large pharmacies (blood pressure checks and teaching/referrals; conducting surveys)	People of all ages and families	Educator, clinician, advocate, researcher
3. At parent–teacher association (PTA) meetings, sporting events, dances, and school registration (in collaboration with school nurses; answer questions, provide health information and first aid, set up immunization clinics on site; check immunization records)	Young adults, children, and teenagers	Educator, clinician, advocate, collaborator, manager
4. Outside of concerts, plays, farmer's markets, etc. (answer questions, provide information, screenings, and referrals)	People of all ages	Educator, clinician, advocate
5. Conferences or seminars (present research, provide information)	Adults	Leader, educator, clinician, researcher
6. "On the street" (engaging with clients, making referrals)	Homeless persons, passersby, transients, low-income urban dwellers	Educator, clinician, advocate
7. Truck stops (screenings, education, referrals)	Predominantly employed men	Educator, clinician, advocate
8. Mobile clinics (seeing clients, making referrals)	People of all ages	Educator, clinician, advocate

Leader's role—initiate, plan, strategize, collaborate, and cooperate with community groups to present programs that are focused on specific populations' needs.

Educator's role—teach nutrition, stress management, safety, exercise, prevention of sexually transmitted diseases, and other men and women's health issues, child home/school/play and stranger safety, and child growth and development, and provide anticipatory guidance. Have pamphlets available to support verbal information on health and safety topics, specific diseases, social security, Medicare, and Medicaid.

Clinician's role—perform blood pressure screening, height, weight, blood testing for diabetes and cholesterol, occult blood test, hearing and vision tests, scoliosis measurements, and administration of immunizations.

Advocate's role—provide information regarding community resources as needed, cut "red tape" for those who need it, answer questions, and guide people to additional resources, such as Web sites and "800" phone numbers.

Collaborator's role—join with other social service and health professionals as team members to address the needs of clients (families, aggregates, communities).

Researcher's role—investigate an issue or problem, talk with community members, collect data, analyze results, and share outcomes (disseminate).

places (Box 2-5). For example, a C/PHN, as clinician and health educator, may work with a parenting group in a church or town hall. Another nurse, as client advocate, leader, and researcher, may study the health needs of a neighborhood's older adult population by collecting data throughout the area and meeting with university researchers or resource professionals in many places. Also, a nurse may work with community-based organizations such as an LGBTQ advocacy organization or a support group for parents experiencing the violent death of a child. Again, the community at large becomes the setting for practice for a nurse who serves on health care planning committees, lobbies for health legislation at the state capital, runs for a school board position, or assists with flood relief in another state or another country (Fig. 2-6). See Box 2-5.

Although the term "setting" implies a place, remember that community/public health nursing practice is not limited to a specific site, but is a specialty of nursing that is defined by the nature of its

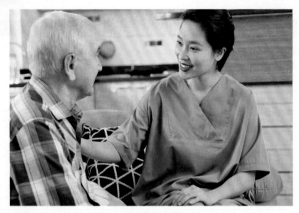

FIGURE 2-6 The C/PHN works with many different groups, including older adults.

practice, not its location, and it can be practiced anywhere. As you read through this chapter, perhaps an area of practice or a particular population captured your attention. If you are interested in tribal health, you might consider working as a U.S. Public Health Service nurse, or if you find that you are more interested in providing comprehensive health promotion programs to rural individuals, a nurse-managed health center may be of interest. Opportunities for community/public health nursing run the gamut from the American Red Cross, state and local health departments, the Peace Corps, to various international aid groups. Both private and public health agencies are actively seeking nurses with an interest in improving the health of their communities.

SUMMARY

- The various roles and settings for practice hinge on three primary functions of public health—assessment, policy development, and assurance—and are applied at three levels of service—individual, family, and community.
- Assessment is the systematic collection, assembly, analysis, and dissemination of information about the health of a community.
- Policy development involves convening and facilitating community groups to evaluate health concerns and develop a plan to address those concerns, recommending new programs or increased services based on identified needs to address the needs of families, and developing standards for individual client care.
- Assurance is the pledge to provide services to clients that are necessary to achieve agreed-upon goals by encouraging the actions of others (public or private) or requiring action through regulation or provision of direct services.
- The 10 essential public health services fall within the three core functions and represent the scope of work done by C/PHN and other public health professionals.
- Community/public health nursing practice is defined by specific standards of practice developed by organizations such as AACN, ANA, and the CPHNO (formerly the Quad Council of Public Health Nursing Organizations) in publications related to ethics, scope of practice, and core competencies.
- C/PHNs play many roles, including that of clinician, educator, advocate, manager, collaborator, leader, and researcher.
- There are many types of settings in which the C/PHN may practice. These settings can be grouped into seven major categories: homes, ambulatory service settings, occupational health settings, residential institutions, faith communities, and the community at large.
- Community/public health nursing practice is not limited to a specific site but is a specialty of nursing that is defined by the nature of its practice (i.e., population health), not solely its location.

ACTIVE LEARNING EXERCISES

1. Discuss ways in which a C/PHN can make service holistic and focused on wellness with:
   a. Preschool-age children in a day care setting
   b. A group of chemically dependent adolescents
   c. A group of older adults living in a senior high-rise building
2. Explain how at least 3 of the 10 essential public health services could be employed by a C/PHN in addressing a health risk in your community (e.g., opioid epidemic, low immunization rates, adolescent vaping, environmental hazards).
3. Think of a recent problem in your community and describe 3 of the 7 roles outlined in this chapter that you, as a C/PHN, would use to help intervene in dealing with the problem.
4. Choose one of the C/PHN roles or practice areas described in this chapter that may be of interest to you. Discuss the similarities and differences between the C/PHN roles or practice areas you chose with those chosen by other classmates.
5. Compare one of the examples used in this chapter to describe C/PHN roles (e.g., advocate for the Merrill family) to one of your client's issues. How can you apply exemplars of that role to your clinical experience?

REFERENCES

American Association of Colleges of Nursing (AACN). (2008). *The essentials of baccalaureate education for professional nursing practice*. Washington, DC: Author.

American Association of Colleges of Nursing (AACN). (2013). *Public health: Recommended baccalaureate competencies and curricular guidelines for public health nursing*. Washington, DC: Author.

American Association of Colleges of Nursing (AACN). (2019). *Revisiting AACN's essentials series: Re-envisioning nursing education (FAQs)*. Retrieved from https://www.aacnnursing.org/Portals/42/Downloads/Essentials/Essentials-Revision-Frequently-Asked-Questions.pdf

American Nurses Association (ANA). (2010). *Nursing's social policy statement: The essence of the profession*. Silver Spring, MD: Nursesbooks.org.

American Nurses Association (ANA). (2013). *Public health nursing: Scope and standards of practice* (2nd ed.). Silver Spring, MD: Nursesbooks.org.

American Nurses Association (ANA). (2015a). *Code of ethics for nurses with interpretive statements*. Silver Spring, MD: Nursesbooks.org.

American Nurses Association (ANA). (2015b). *Nursing: Scope and standards of practice* (3rd ed.). Silver Spring, MD: Nursesbooks.org.

American Nurses Association (ANA). (2017). *School nursing: Scope and standards of practice* (3rd ed.). Silver Spring, MD: Nursesbooks.org.

American Nurses Association and the Health Ministries Association. (2017). *Faith community nursing* (3rd ed.). Silver Spring, MD: Author.

American Public Health Association. (2013). *The definition and practice of public health nursing: A statement of APHA public health nursing section*. Washington, DC: American Public Health Association.

Association of Community Health Nursing Educators (ACHNE), Education Committee. (2010). Essentials of baccalaureate nursing education for entry-level community/public health nursing. *Public Health Nursing, 27*, 371–382. doi: 10.1111/j.1525-1446.2010.00867.x.

Brown, C. L. (2017). Linking public health nursing competencies and service-learning in a global setting. *Public Health Nursing, 34*(5), 485–492.

Byers, V. (2015). The challenges of leading change in health-care delivery from the frontline. *Journal of Nursing Management*, *24*(6), 449–456. doi: 10.1111/jonm.12342.

Centers for Disease Control and Prevention (CDC). (2019). *CDC research on SDOH: Neighborhood and the built environment*. Retrieved from https://www.cdc.gov/socialdeterminants/neighborhood/

Centers for Disease Control & Prevention (CDC). (2020). *10 essential public health services (revised)*. Retrieved from https://www.cdc.gov/publichealthgateway/publichealthservices/essentialhealthservices.html

Chait, N., & Glied, S. (2018). Promoting prevention under the Affordable Care Act. *Annual Review of Public Health, 39*, 507–524.

Cherry, B., & Jacob, S. R. (2020). *Contemporary nursing: Issues, trends, and management* (8th ed.). St. Louis, MO: Mosby.

Cook, C. L., Hall, A. G., Garvan, C. S., & Kneipp, S. M. (2015). A public health nursing model assists women receiving Temporary Assistance for Needy Families benefits to identify a usual source of primary care. *Care Management Journals, 16*(4), 203–207.

Dickson, E., & Lobo, M. L. (2018). Critical caring theory and public health nursing advocacy for comprehensive sexual health education. *Public Health Nursing, 35*(1), 78–84.

Dossey, B. M., & Keegan, L. (2016). *Holistic nursing: A handbook for practice* (7th ed.). Burlington, MA: Jones & Bartlett Publishers.

Dworkin, P. H., & Sood, A. B. (2016). A population health approach to system transformation for children's healthy development. *Child & Adolescent Psychiatric Clinics of North America, 25*(2), 307–317.

Feetham, S., & Doering, J. J. (2015). Career cartography: A conceptualization of career development to advance health and policy. *Journal of Nursing Scholarship, 47*(1), 70–77.

Fowler, M. (2016). *Nursing's social policy statement: Understanding the profession from social contract to social covenant*. Silver Spring, MD: American Nurses Association.

Gordon, L. (2018). The community as patient: Assessing needs for public health program planning and intervention. *Journal of the Academy of Nutrition and Dietetics, 118*(10), A157.

Institute of Medicine. (1988). *The future of public health*. Washington, DC: National Academy Press.

Institute of Medicine. (2002). *The future of the public's health in the 21st century*. Washington, DC: National Academy Press.

Kagan, I., Schachaf, S., Rapaport, Z., Livine, T., & Madjar, B. (2017). Public health nurses in Israel: A case study on a quality improvement project of nurse's work life. *Public Health Nursing, 34*(1), 78–86.

Kalaitzidis, E., & Jewell, P. (2015). The concept of advocacy in nursing: A critical analysis. *Health Care Management, 34*(4), 308–315.

Katz, J. (February 2018). How a police chief, a governor and a sociologist would spend $100 billion to solve the opioid crisis. *The New York Times*. Retrieved from https://www.nytimes.com/interactive/2018/02/14/upshot/opioid-crisis-solutions.html

Keeling, A. W. (2015). Historical perspectives on an expanded role for nursing. *Online Journal of Issues in Nursing, 20*(2), 2. Retrieved from http://ojin.nursingworld.org/MainMenuCategories/ANAMarketplace/ANAPeriodicals/OJIN/TableofContents/Vol-20-2015/No2-May-2015/Historical-Perspectives-Expanded-Role-Nursing.html

Lalleman, P. C., Smid, G. A., Lagerwey, M. D., Oldenhof, L., & Schuurmans, M. J. (2015). Nurse middle managers' dispositions of habitus: A Bourdieusian analysis of supporting role behaviors in Dutch and American hospitals. *Advances in Nursing Science, 38*(3), E1–E16.

Lassi, S. Z., & Bhutta, Z. A. (2015). Community-based intervention packages for reducing maternal morbidity and mortality and improving neonatal outcomes. *Cochrane Database Systematic Reviews, 23*(3), CD007754. doi: 10.1002/14651858.CD007754.pub3.

Lee, H., Chiang, H., & Kuo, H. (2019). Relationship between authentic leadership and nurses' intent to leave: The mediating role of work environment and burnout. *Journal of Nursing Management, 27*(1), 52–65.

Livingood, W. C., Bilello, L. A., Choe, U., & Lukens-Bull, K. (2018). Enhancing the science of discovery in public health systems and services research through participatory research methods. *Population Health Management, 21*(2), 155–162.

Management at Work. (2019). *Mintzberg's 10 managerial roles*. Retrieved from https://management.atwork-network.com/2008/04/15/mintzberg's-10-managerial-roles/

MindTools. (n.d.). *Mintzberg's management roles: Identifying the roles managers play*. Retrieved from https://www.mindtools.com/pages/videos/management-roles-transcript.htm

Mintzberg, H. (1973). *The nature of managerial work*. New York, NY: Harper & Row.

Murdaugh, C. L., Parsons, M. A., & Pender, N. J. (2019). *Health promotion in nursing practice* (8th ed.). Upper Saddle River, NJ: Prentice Hall.

National Committee for Quality Assurance. (2018). *Population health management resource guide*. Retrieved from https://www.ncqa.org/wp-content/uploads/2018/08/20180827_PHM_PHM_Resource_Guide.pdf

Nolan, A., Kennedy, S., O'Malley, A., Kirwan, M., Hughes, A., Barry, A., ... Nugent, L. (2015). Mothers' voices: Results of a survey of public health nurse-led breastfeeding support groups. *Primary Health Care, 25*(7), 26–21.

Nsiah, C., Siakwa, M., & Ninnoni, J. (2019). Registered nurses' description of patient advocacy in the clinical setting. *Nursing Open, 6*(3), 1124–1132. Retrieved from https://www.ncbi.nlm.nih.gov/pmc/articles/PMC6650676/

Phillips, M., & Fitzsimons, V. (2015). The Affordable Care Act: Impact on case managers. *Professional Case Management, 20*(6), 323–327.

Public Health National Center for Innovations. (2020). *Defining public health practice: 25 years of the 10 essential public health services*. Retrieved from https://phnci.org/uploads/resource-files/EPHS-English.pdf

Public Health National Center for Innovations. (2020). *Vetting the 10 essential public health services: Here's what you need to know*. Retrieved from https://phnci.org/journal/vetting-the-10-essential-public-health-services-heres-what-you-need-to-know

Quad Council Coalition Competency Review Task Force. (2018). *Community/public health nursing competencies*. Retrieved from http://www.quadcouncilphn.org/documents-3/2018-qcc-competencies/

Rhodes, D., Visker, J., Cox, C., Forsyth, E., & Woolman, J. (2017). Public health and school nurses' perception of barriers to HPV vaccination in Missouri. *Journal of Community Health Nursing, 34*(4), 180–189.

Rosa, W. (Ed.). (2016). *Nurses as leaders: Revolutionary visions of leadership*. New York, NY: Springer Publishing Company.

Schneider, M. J. (2017). *Introduction to public health* (5th ed.). Burlington, MA: Jones & Bartlett Learning.

Shirey, M. R., & White-Williams, C. (2015). Boundary spanning leadership practices for population health. *Journal of Advanced Nursing, 45*(9), 411–415.

Swider, S. M., Levin, P. F., & Reising, V. (2017). Evidence of public health nursing effectiveness: A realist review. *Public Health Nursing, 34*(4), 324–334.

U.S. Department of Health and Human Services (USDHHS). (2020). *Healthy people 2030: Development of the national health promotion and disease prevention objectives for 2030*. Retrieved from https://www.healthypeople.gov/2020/About-Healthy-People/Development-Healthy-People-2030

Weatherford, B., Bower, K. A., & Vitello-Cicciu, J. (2018). The CNO and leading innovation: Competencies for the future. *Nursing Administration Quarterly, 42*(1), 76–82.

Wilson, D. S., Rosemberg, M. S., Visovatti, M., Munro-Kramer, M. L., & Feetham, S. (2017). Career cartography: From stories to science and scholarship. *Journal of Nursing Scholarship, 49*(3), 336–346.

Young, A. M., Mudge, A. M., Banks, M. D., Rogers, L., Demedio, K., & Isering, E. (2018). Improving nutritional discharge planning and follow up in older medical inpatients: Hospital to home outreach for malnourished elders. *Nutrition & Dietetics, 75*(3), 283–290.

CHAPTER 3

History and Evolution of Public Health Nursing

"Our basic idea was that the nurse's peculiar introduction to the patient and her organic relationship with the neighborhood should constitute the starting point for a universal service to the region. We considered ourselves best described by the term 'public health nurses.'"

—**Lillian Wald** (1867–1940), Pioneer of Public Health Nursing

KEY TERMS

American Nurses Association (ANA)
District nursing
Frontier Nursing Service
Henry Street Settlement
Industrial nursing
National League for Nursing (NLN)
National Organization for Public Health Nursing (NOPHN)
Population health
Rural nursing
Visiting nurse associations (VNAs)

LEARNING OBJECTIVES

Upon mastery of this chapter, you should be able to:

1. Describe the four stages of community/public health nursing's development.
2. Identify the contributions of selected nursing leaders throughout history to the advancement of community/public health nursing.
3. Discuss the academic and advanced professional preparation of community/public health nurses.
4. Compare and contrast community health nursing with public health nursing.
5. Analyze the relationship between our historical roots and current nursing practice.
6. Discuss governmental landmarks in the evolution of community/public health nursing.

INTRODUCTION

You just left the home of a client who is concerned about a new family that just moved into the building where she lives. This family of six lives in an apartment with barely enough room for two. After years in this neighborhood, you are well aware of the high rents charged for apartments with peeling paint, rodents, and garbage all around the buildings. Your client is concerned that the young mother looks "worn out" and coughs all the time. She said she tried to help, but the family doesn't speak much English. She describes four young children all under the age of about 5. She's never seen the husband, but you know that most of the men in this neighborhood leave early in the morning to try to get some day work, so you are not surprised. You thank her for the information and assure your client that you will do what you can to help her new neighbors. You start thinking about how you will prepare for the visit to the family who doesn't even expect you. At the top of your planning list is trying to find someone who speaks their language; you only know a few words. You suspect without even seeing the mother what the cough means, although you hope you are wrong. Then you think about the four young children living so close together and creating so much work for a woman who isn't well. The husband may want to help his wife more, but if he doesn't work, they don't have money to pay rent and buy food. You wonder if he has the cough too.

As you read this scenario, what picture comes to mind? What language does this family speak? What disease does this young mother most likely have? Now, think about when this event might have occurred. If you thought this was a current scenario, it certainly could be, but this scenario was actually set in the early 1900s. This family emigrated from Greece and had not yet mastered the English language. The mother exhibits signs of consumption (the common name for tuberculosis at that time). Because birth control information was not available to most women, the mother was unable to effectively space out her pregnancies. The filthy and overcrowded housing, termed tenements, was typical of the time. The husband found work as a laborer where he could. Few social services were available—if there was no work, then there was no food for the family, and no money to pay the rent. The family came to America with the hope of a new start, but what they found was in many ways worse without their support system of family and friends.

Community/public health nurses (C/PHNs) in the early 20th century had to deal with many of the same issues we face today.

- We thought that tuberculosis (TB) was a disease of the past; now clients with TB, including multidrug-resistant strains, are becoming alarmingly more common (Centers for Disease Control and Prevention (CDC), 2019).
- Poverty, communicable diseases, poor housing, lack of social services, and limited access to family planning information remain as challenges to improving the health of our population (see Fig. 3-1).

As a C/PHN, you will be facing similar challenges to those faced by nurses of the past. History is exciting because we get to hear the "voices" of nurses who have gone before us and to see what they endured and the extent of their dedication and service while establishing the profession. It is also essential, for without it, we often fail to see patterns and learn from past mistakes.

- This chapter traces community/public health nursing's rich historical development, highlighting the contributions of several nursing leaders and examining the global societal influences that shaped early and evolving community/public health nursing practice.
- The final section of the chapter describes the academic and advanced professional preparation required of C/PHNs today. Nursing's past influences its present, and both guide its future in the 21st century.

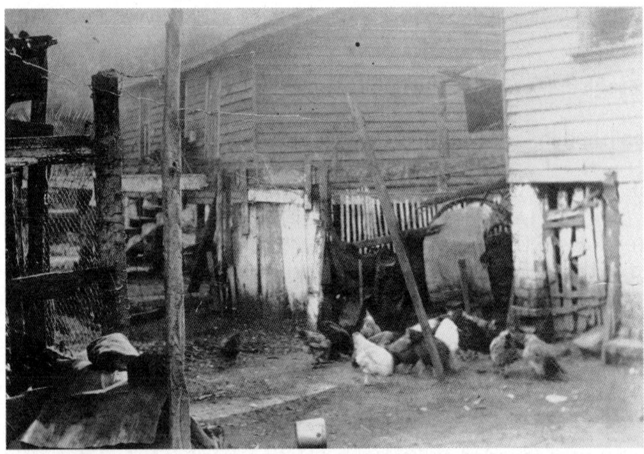

FIGURE 3-1 Public health nursing: Where inspection begins. (From the American Red Cross and U.S. Medical Department of Sanitary Service (1917–1918). Retrieved from https://commons.wikimedia.org/wiki/File:Medical_Department_-_Sanitary_Service_-_Sanitation_-_Public_health_nursing._Where_inspection_begins_-_NARA_-_45499047.jpg)

HISTORICAL DEVELOPMENT OF COMMUNITY/PUBLIC HEALTH NURSING

The history of community/public health nursing, since its recognized inception in Europe and more recently in America, encompasses continuing change and adaptation (Donahue, 2011; Keeling, Hehman, & Kirchgessner, 2018). The historical record reveals a professional nursing specialty that has been on the cutting edge of innovations in public health practice and has provided leadership to public health efforts. (See Table 3-1 for information about the four general stages that mark the development of public/community health nursing.)

See Chapter 1 for a more complete discussion of the terms *public health nurse* and *community health nurse* and Chapter 2 for descriptions and discussion of the development of public health and community health.

In the historical evolution of this specialty, a shift in thinking about the focus of practice resulted in the broader use of the term *community health nurse* to refer to the generalist practice in this specialty. The title *public health nurse* now refers not just to those working in public health agencies but also those working in many diverse community settings where population-focused nursing occurs (Edmonds, Campbell, & Gilder, 2016; Kulbok, Thatcher, Park, & Meszaros, 2012). It is important to recognize that the work of the nurse is, as it always has been, to improve the health of the whole community, however that community is defined. The term community/public health nurse (C/PHN) will generally be used throughout this text.

Early Home Care Nursing (Before Mid-1800s)

The Origins of Early Nursing

The early roots of home care nursing began with religious and charitable groups (Table 3-2; Pugh, 2001; Theofanidis & Sapountzi-Krepia, 2015):

- Deaconesses: Women in ancient Rome who cared for needy patients
- Knights Hospitaller: Warrior monks in Western Europe who protected and cared for pilgrims on their way to Jerusalem, founded in the early 11th century
- The Misericordia: A group of monks in Florence, Italy, who provided first aid care for accident victims on a 24-hour basis around the year 1244

Medieval times saw the development of various institutions devoted to the sick, including hospitals and nursing orders.

During the 17th century, nursing care for the poor expanded in Europe:

- In England, the Elizabethan Poor Law, written in 1601, provided medical and nursing care to the poor and disabled.
- In France, St. Frances de Sales organized the Friendly Visitor Volunteers in the early 1600s (Dolan, 1978).
- In 1617, St. Vincent de Paul started the Sisters of Charity in Paris, France, an organization composed of nuns and laywomen dedicated to serving the poor and needy. They emphasized preparing nurses and supervising nursing care, as well as determining causes and solutions for clients' problems, thereby laying a foundation for modern community/public health nursing (Bullough & Bullough, 1978).

TABLE 3-1 Development of Community Health Nursing

Stage	Focus	Nursing Orientation	Service Emphasis	Institutional Base (Agencies)
Early home care (before mid-1800s)	Sick poor	Individuals	Curative	Lay and religious orders
District nursing (1860–1900)	Sick poor	Individuals; preventive	Curative; beginning of organized home visiting	Voluntary; some government
Public health nursing (1900–1970)	Needy public	Families	Curative; preventive	Government; some voluntary
Emergence of community health nursing (1970–present)	Total community	Populations; illness prevention	Health promotion; practice	Many kinds; some independent

The Industrial Revolution (about 1760–1840) led to increased migration to cities. Hospitals were built in larger cities, and dispensaries were developed to provide greater access to physicians; however, medical education had no standardized curriculum until 1904 (Schwartz, Ajjarapu, Stamy, & Schwinn, 2018). Hospitals were mostly used by the indigent; for most others, nursing care was still given in the home. Public health challenges included the following:

- In both Europe and America, overcrowding and poverty led to epidemics, high infant mortality, occupational diseases and injuries, and increasing mental illness.
- Disease was rampant; mortality rates were high; and institutional conditions, especially in prisons, hospitals, and "asylums" for the insane, were deplorable.
- The sick and afflicted were kept in filthy rooms without adequate food, water, cover, or care for their physical and emotional needs (Bullough & Bullough, 1978).

Dorothea Dix (1802–1887) brought attention to the plight of the mentally ill, abused, and neglected in US jails and almshouses. Her accomplishments included the following:

- In one of the first social research efforts in the United States, she presented her firsthand accounts of the terrible situations she found to the legislatures of Massachusetts, New York, New Jersey, and Pennsylvania (Reddi, 2005).
- Through her efforts, there was an almost 10-fold increase in the number of mental institutions, and the overall care of the mentally ill improved.

TABLE 3-2 Landmarks in Nursing History: Pre-1800s

Time Frame	Landmark
Pre–middle ages	• Religious and charitable groups provided early care in the home. • Indigenous peoples used "shamans" or medicine men and women to provide care. • Little was known about disease origins.
500–1000	• The "Lady of the Manor" gave care. • Hildegard of Bingen, among other religious caregivers, provided nursing care.
650	• Hotel Dieu ("House of God") Hospital was established in Paris.
1000–1500	• Military orders, such as Knights Hospitaller of Jerusalem, cared for those returning from the Crusades. Men provided care. • St. Francis of Assisi (1182–1226) and St. Clare of Assisi (1194–1253) ministered to the sick. • The Maltese cross (shown below) was adopted as the insignia of the sick (later used on military nursing uniforms).
1500–1800	• Religious nursing orders (e.g., Sisters of Charity) were founded and extended to America, Ireland, and Britain.

Source: Donahue (2011); Nutting and Dock (1907).

- Although not trained as a nurse, Dix would, in later years, oversee the Union Army female nurses prior to resuming her efforts with the mentally ill (Desrochers, 2012).

Although few in number, both Catholic and Anglican religious nursing orders continued the work of caring for the sick poor in their homes. It was in the midst of these deplorable conditions and in response to them that Florence Nightingale began her work.

The Early Nightingale Years

"Health is not only to be well but to use well the powers we have."

—Florence Nightingale (1820–1910).

Born in 1820 into a wealthy English family, Florence Nightingale helped bring about major reforms in health care and improved the status of nursing through her extensive travel, excellent education—including training at the first school for nurses in Kaiserswerth, Germany, and determination to serve the needy (Fig. 3-2 and Table 3-3).

During the Crimean War (1854–1856) in Scutari, Nightingale observed the deplorable conditions in the military hospitals, including thousands of sick and wounded men lying in filth, without beds, clean coverings, food, water, or laundry facilities (Florence Nightingale Museum Trust, 1997; Lee, Clark, & Thompson, 2013; Woodham-Smith, 1951). In response, she organized competent nursing care and established kitchens and laundries, resulting in hundreds of lives saved. Her work further demonstrated that capable, holistic nursing intervention could prevent illness and improve the health of a population at risk—precursors to modern community/public health nursing practice (Hogan, 2015).

Nightingale's subsequent work reforming health in the military was supported by implementation of another public health strategy: the use of biostatistics. Through meticulously gathered data and statistical comparisons, Nightingale demonstrated that military mortality rates, even in peacetime, were double those of the civilian population because of the terrible living conditions in the barracks—what we describe today as evidence-based practice (Rooney, 2016).

She promoted five essential components to optimal health and healing—pure air, pure water, efficient drainage, cleanliness, and adequate lighting. Specifically, her concern was with the environment of patients, the need for keen observation, the focus on the whole patient rather than the disease, and the importance of assisting nature to bring about a cure (Nightingale, 1876, 1969; Palmer, 2001). This work led to important military reforms and

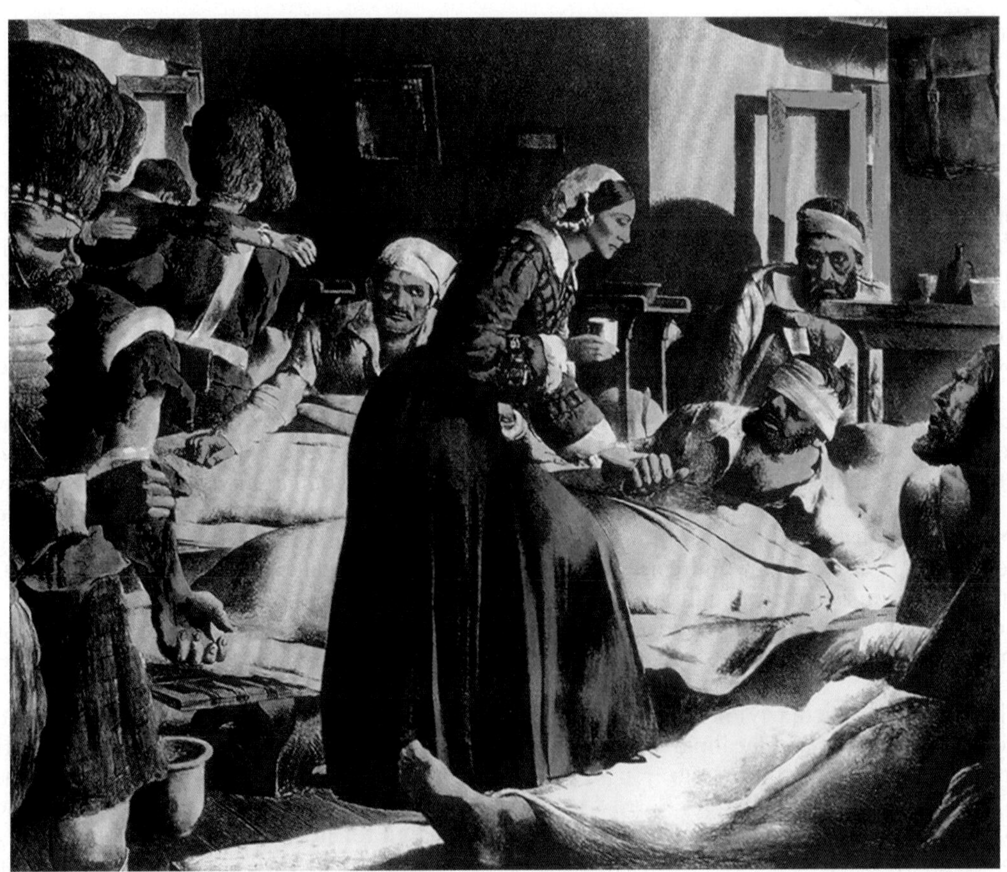

FIGURE 3-2 Florence Nightingale's concern for populations at risk, as well as her vision and successful efforts at health reform, provided a model for community health nursing today.

TABLE 3-3 Contributions of Florence Nightingale

Role	Result
Lobbyist	• Increased health standards and practice • Reformed military health care
Feminist	• Changed perceptions of women as nurses
Educator	• Developed standards of education for nursing practice • School at St. Thomas' Hospital, London, opened using Nightingale model
Military nurse	• Served in the Crimean War as nurse and administrator
Public health nurse	• Advocated holistic, population-focused care • Incorporated health promotion and disease prevention into practice model • Promoted five essential components to optimal health and healing: 1. Pure air 2. Pure water 3. Efficient drainage 4. Cleanliness 5. Adequate lighting
Author	• Wrote influential *Notes on Nursing* and *Notes on Hospitals*, among many other publications
Statistician	• Pioneered the use of statistics to change practice. • Harriet Martineau's *England and Her Soldiers* and Nightingale's *Sanitary Statistics of Native Colonial Schools and Hospitals* both incorporated her statistics and evidence-based practice to change medical and nursing care (Donahue, 2011; Rooney, 2016).
Architect	• After publication of *Notes on Hospitals*, her work became associated with long pavilion-style hospital wings, emphasizing light and ventilation (one is still visible today at St. Thomas' Hospital, London) (Richardson, 2010)
Social advocate/ reformer	• Advocated for poor and disenfranchised, especially in military • Authored *On Trained Nursing for the Sick Poor*

Source: Donahue (2011); Florence Nightingale Museum Trust (1997); Lee et al. (2013); Nightingale (1859/1969); Richardson (2010); Rooney (2016); Woodham-Smith (1951).

prioritization of hygiene (Lee et al., 2013). See Chapter 15 for more on the Nightingale model.

Miss Nightingale's concern for populations at risk included the sick at home. Her book, *Notes on Nursing: What It Is, and What It Is Not*, published in England in 1859, was written to improve nursing care in the home. It was also during this period that Nightingale clarified nursing as a woman's occupation (Evans, 2004). This gender distinction in nursing was due more to the culture of the times than as a direct exclusion of men from the practice; it was consistent with social norms of that period.

Florence Nightingale also became a skillful lobbyist for health care reform. Her exemplary influence on English politics and policy improved the quality of existing health care and set standards for future practice. Furthermore, she demonstrated how population-focused nursing works (Lee et al., 2013).

Nightingale's work, particularly her five essential components to optimal health and healing, are relevant to today's community/public health nursing:

- *Pure air* is important in reducing the transmission of airborne pathogens, such as tuberculosis (TB), which continues to be a worldwide public health threat. Drug-resistant TB strains continue to proliferate, particularly among poorer nations. In 2017, 10.4 million people were infected with TB; while 1.7 million people died. The World Health Organization (WHO, 2018) estimates that *one-quarter* of the world's population has latent TB!
- Three agencies—WHO, UNICEF, and the United States Agency for International Development (USAID)—jointly developed a document that directly reflects Nightingale's components of *pure water, efficient drainage, and cleanliness* as evidence-based practice. *Improving Nutrition Outcomes with Better Water, Sanitation, and Hygiene* gives guidelines for achieving Global Nutrition Goals for 2025 and other health goals (WHO, 2015).
- *Efficient drainage* is an issue even in first world countries as disease-bearing mosquitoes breed in stagnant water.
- *Cleanliness*, specifically hand hygiene, continues to be a topic of teaching for disease prevention; the Centers for Disease Control and Prevention (CDC, 2016) launched a "Clean Hands Count" educational campaign for health care providers and the public.
- *Adequate lighting* is relevant to nurses in the community as they assess home safety, particularly in older

adults, who may have limited vision and balance, and community safety, such as poor exterior lighting, which can cause accidents and have other safety implications (Lee et al., 2013).

District Nursing (Mid-1800s–1900)

Nightingale's Continued Influence

The next stage in the development of community/public health nursing was the formal organization of visiting nursing or **district nursing**—for example, nurses working outside hospitals in community settings, such as homes, focusing on care and health promotion (Runciman, 2014).

In 1859, William Rathbone, an English philanthropist, became convinced of the value of home nursing as a result of private care given to his wife. In 1861, with Florence Nightingale's help and advice, Rathbone opened a training school for nurses connected with the Royal Liverpool Infirmary and established a visiting nurse service for the sick poor in Liverpool.

As the service grew, visiting nurses were assigned to districts in the city—hence the name, district nursing. The names of these nurses were entered into a central register, and they were known as "Queen's Nurses," as Queen Victoria recognized the benefits of this program for her people and was a supporter (Hughes, 1902, 344) (see Fig. 3-3).

Florence Nightingale documented the need for community/public health nursing in her writings and recorded conversations:

- "Hospitals are but an intermediate stage of civilization. At present, hospitals are the only place where the sick poor can be nursed, or, indeed often the sick rich. But the ultimate object is to nurse all sick at home" (Nightingale, 1876, para. 8).
- "The aim of the district nurse is to give first-rate nursing to the sick poor at home" (Nightingale, 1876 [also cited in Mowbray (1997, p. 24)]).
- "The health visitor must create a new profession for women" (conversation with Frederick Verney, 1891 [cited in Mowbray (1997, p. 25)]).

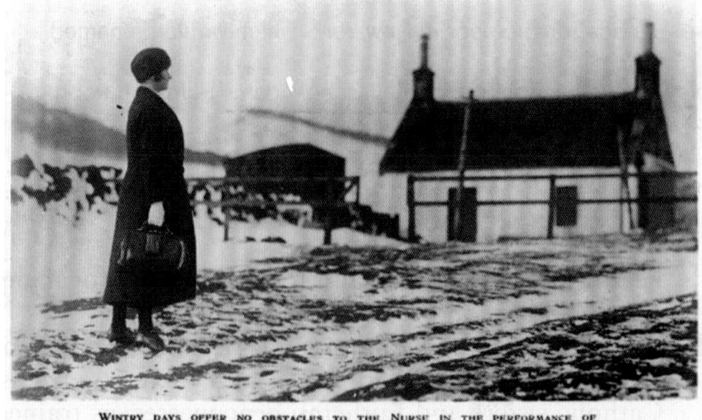
WINTRY DAYS OFFER NO OBSTACLES TO THE NURSE IN THE PERFORMANCE OF HER DUTIES.

FIGURE 3-3 A Queen's District Nurse making a call in Scotland, 1927. (Retrieved from https://www.nlm.nih.gov/exhibition/picturesofnursing/exhibition2.html)

Founding of the American Red Cross and Evolution of Disaster Nursing

In May 1881, Clara Barton and others founded the American Red Cross, modeling it after the International Red Cross, which was founded in 1863 and is responsible for more global outreach and response in its humanitarian efforts (Table 3-4). Below are some milestones in the history of the American Red Cross:

- August 1881: A chapter was founded in Dansville, New York.
- September 1881: A devastating forest fire in Michigan claimed 800 victims; this was the newly formed organization's first disaster response, setting the stage for future fire response (Hanes, 2016).
- 1898: Clara Barton went to Havana, Cuba, during the Spanish–American War with supplies for victims, the first record of Red Cross military collaboration.
- 1905: The American Red Cross was chartered by the Congress to provide relief during disasters and emergencies, support the military, help communities become more resilient, and conduct other well-known activities, such as blood collection.

Today the Red Cross continues working toward the health and betterment of our local communities and our nation by giving assistance to those in need during both small and catastrophic crises (American Red Cross, 2020).

Home Visiting Takes Root

Although district nurses primarily cared for sick individuals, they also taught cleanliness and wholesome living to their patients, even during that early period (Kalisch & Kalisch, 2004). The problems of early home care patients in the United States were numerous and complex. Thousands of European and eastern European immigrants as well as poor African Americans filled tenement housing in the poorest and most crowded slums of the large coastal cities during the late 1800s. Inadequate sanitation, unsafe and unhealthy working conditions, prejudices, and language and cultural barriers added to poverty and disease (Table 3-5; Box 3-1).

Public Health Nursing (1900–1970)

By the beginning of the 20th century, district nursing had broadened its focus to include the health and welfare of the general public, not just the poor. This new emphasis was part of a broader consciousness about public health. As demand rose, the number of private health agencies increased. These agencies supplemented the often-limited work of government health departments.

- As Bullough and Bullough point out, specialized programs (e.g., infant welfare, tuberculosis clinics, venereal disease control) were developed and "although the hospital nursing school movement emphasized the care of the sick, a small but growing number of nurses were finding employment in preventive health care" (1978, p. 143).
- In 1900, there were an estimated 200 public health nurses (PHNs); by 1912, that number had grown to 3,000 (Gardner, 1936). This was an important development:

TABLE **3-4** Landmarks in Nursing History: 1800–1900

Year	Landmark
1760–1840	The Industrial Revolution led to increased migration to cities, resulting in poverty, overcrowding, disease, mental illness, and increased mortality.
1844	Charles Dickens published *Martin Chuzzlewit*, portraying nurses as untrained, drunken, incompetent, and slovenly, which reflects the public opinion of the time.
1845	Dorothea Dix addressed the New Jersey and Pennsylvania legislatures regarding abuse and neglect of the mentally ill.
1848	The first women's rights convention in the United States was held in Seneca Falls, New York.
1849	Harriet Tubman escaped from slavery; she went on to lead many slaves to freedom through the Underground Railroad.
1850	Florence Nightingale began nursing training at the Institute of St. Vincent de Paul in Alexandria, Egypt.
1853	John Snow linked a contaminated water pump to cholera in a London epidemic.
1854	Florence Nightingale cared for the injured in the Crimean War.
1855	Mary Seacole established a boarding house to care for sick and injured soldiers in the Crimean War.
1857	Ellen Ranyard pioneered the first "district nursing" program in England.
1860	Florence Nightingale's *Notes on Nursing: What It Is, and What It Is Not* was published.
1861	The Civil War embroiled the United States until 1865. Harriet Tubman served as an unpaid nurse to wounded civilians and soldiers. Dorothea Dix was placed in charge of all female nurses in Union military hospitals.
1862	Louis Pasteur proposed the germ theory, which eventually led to the rejection of the "miasma" (bad air) theory of the origin of disease.
1865	Sojourner Truth served as a nurse for the Freedman's Relief Association during Reconstruction in Washington, DC.
1873	The first Nightingale model nursing school was established in the United States at Bellevue Hospital.
1877	Francis Root was the first public health nurse hired by the Women's Branch of the New York Mission.
1878	The Woman Suffrage Amendment was introduced in the US Congress.
1879	Mary Eliza Mahoney became the first African American to graduate from an American nursing school.
1881	Clara Barton and associates established the American Red Cross, and she became its first president.
1885	A visiting nurse association was established in Buffalo, New York.
1886	Visiting nurse associations were established in Philadelphia and Boston.
1893	Lillian Wald and Mary Brewster organized a visiting nurses service for the poor in New York, which would be named the Henry Street Settlement in 1906. *American Society of Superintendents of Training Schools for Nursing* was founded by Isabel Adams Hampton Robb (later renamed the National League for Nursing).

Source: Bowery Boys (2017); D'Antonio (2017); Donahue (2011); Keeling et al. (2018); Lewinson et al. (2017).

"it brought health care and health teaching to the public, gave nurses an opportunity for more independent work, and helped to improve nursing education" (Bullough & Bullough, 1978, p. 143).

- Around 1900, Jessie Sleet was hired by the Charity Organization Society's (COS) tuberculosis committee as a temporary district nurse in New York City (Mosley, 2007). Credited as the first Black public health nurse, Jessie Sleet was a pioneer in early public health nursing practice and forged the way for many others (Table 3-6).
- By 1910, new federal laws made states and communities accountable for the health of their citizens. Catholic sisters and Lutheran deaconesses, as trained nurses operating out of motherhouses in various cities in the United States, provided care for local communities, sometimes working with other agencies such as the Red Cross (Keeling et al., 2018).

TABLE **3-5** Some Public Health Issues of the 18th to the 20th Centuries

Communicable Diseases	Health Issues
Tuberculosis/Consumption	Lack of sanitation/hygiene
Influenza	Contaminated/lack of clean water
Measles	Infections
Mumps	Nutrition/nutritional disorders/diseases
Rubella	Food preparation, harmful additives, and storage (spoiled food)
Typhoid	Temperature: heat and cold
Diphtheria	Vermin
Cholera	Cultural, religious, and superstitious beliefs
Smallpox	Respiratory diseases
Pneumonia	Chronic illness management
Pertussis, "whooping cough"	Maternity and postpartum care
Rheumatic fever	Well baby care
Scarlet fever	Alcoholism
Meningitis	Domestic abuse
Tetanus	Medication administration
Yellow fever	Drug addiction (i.e., opiates in early medicines)
Polio	Surgical dressings/bandages (e.g., how to apply/change) Postoperative care (including illegal, as with abortions)
Conjunctivitis "pinkeye"	Household economy
Scabies, ringworm	Mental illness
Lice/typhus	Disasters
Fleas/plague	Poisoning (use of heavy metals in utensils and medicines common)
Epidemics/pandemics	Family planning/birth control
Isolation and quarantine	Trust

Source: Rosenberg (2008).

BOX **3-1** WHAT DO *YOU* THINK?

Communicable Diseases: Now vs. Then

What diseases can we treat today? Which have been eradicated worldwide? Discuss some recent outbreaks of historic diseases, including where, when, and why they occurred. Describe some new diseases that were not identified or did not occur in this time period. What are the roles of the C/PHN in health promotion and disease prevention?

Nurses Making a Difference

The role of the district nurse expanded during this stage. Lillian D. Wald (1867–1940), a leading figure in this expansion, first used the term *public health nursing* to describe this specialty (Ruel, 2014; Table 3-7). District nurses, while caring for the sick, had pioneered in health teaching, disease prevention, and promotion of good health practices. Nurses working outside of the hospital increased their knowledge and skills in specialized areas such as tuberculosis, maternal and child health, school health, and mental disorders.

TABLE 3-6 Landmarks in Nursing History: 1900–1970

Year	Landmark
1900	Jessie Sleet Scales became the first African American public health nurse in the United States.
1900	Clara Barton led her final disaster relief effort with the American Red Cross, responding to a devastating Galveston, TX, hurricane.
1901	Clara Maass died after volunteering to test for yellow fever.
1902	The New York City Board of Education hired Lina Rogers Struthers as a school nurse and began the first public school nurse program in the country.
1905	The American Red Cross received a congressional charter.
1906	The Pure Food and Drug Act was passed, prohibiting misbranding and adulteration of drugs and food.
1909	The Metropolitan Life Insurance Company provided the first insurance reimbursement for visiting nursing care, beginning industrial nursing.
1910	A public health nursing program was instituted at Teachers College, Columbia University. Florence Nightingale died and was buried in a family churchyard.
1912	The National Organization for Public Health Nursing (NOPHN) was formed, with Lillian Wald as the first president.
1914	Margaret Sanger published the monthly newsletter *The Woman Rebel* to promote contraception and was charged with distributing illegal "birth control" information.
1917	The United States entered into World War I. The 18th Amendment was passed by Congress (ushering in Prohibition).
1918	The U.S. Public Health Service established the Division of Public Health Nursing to aid the war effort. World War I armistice occurred. Worldwide influenza pandemic began. Frances Reed Elliott became the first African American nurse accepted into the American Red Cross Nursing Service.
1919	The 19th Amendment was passed by Congress, giving women the right to vote.
1920	Women voted for the first time in a presidential election.
1921	Margaret Sanger founded the American Birth Control League to distribute contraception information.
1925	The Frontier Nursing Service was established by Mary Breckinridge.
1929	The US stock market crashed (beginning of the Great Depression).
1930	The Tuskegee syphilis study began in Alabama (see Chapter 4).
1933	The 18th Amendment was repealed (Prohibition ends).
1935	The Social Security Act was signed into law.
1937	Birth control information was now legal in all but two states (Massachusetts and Connecticut).
1941	The United States entered into World War II.
1943	The Cadet Nurse Corps Program was established, providing federal funding for academic nursing education in exchange for work in "essential nursing services."
1944	The first basic program in nursing became accredited as including sufficient public health content. The Public Health Service Act authorized qualified nurses to be commissioned in the U.S. Public Health Service.
1945	World War II ended. The United Nations voted to establish the World Health Organization.

TABLE 3-6 Landmarks in Nursing History: 1900–1970 *(Continued)*

Year	Landmark
1946	The Hill-Burton Act was approved, contributing to a shift to hospital-based care with federal funding of hospitals and medical centers. The Communicable Disease Center was established (a forerunner of the Centers for Disease Control and Prevention).
1949	Lucile Petry Leone became the Chief Nurse Officer of the Public Health Service, the first nurse and first woman to achieve a flag rank in the Public Health Service or military.
1950	The United States became involved in the Korean Conflict (which ended in 1953).
1954	In the case of Brown vs. Board of Education, a landmark Supreme Court decision prohibited racial segregation in public schools.
1955	The Salk polio vaccine was introduced (the first polio epidemic in the US began in 1894, with a surge of cases noted in 1952).
1956	The Health Amendments Act provided funds to support public health nurse advanced training.
1960s	The Tuskegee syphilis study in Alabama ended.
1961	The Peace Corps was founded. The United States entered into the Vietnam War.
1965	Medicare and Medicaid were established.
1969	The National Environmental Policy Act provided first coordinated oversight effort. Based on the 1964 Surgeon General's report, passed national legislation requiring health warnings on cigarette packaging and ceasing broadcast media advertising.

Source: Donahue (2011); Keeling et al. (2008); The College of Physicians of Philadelphia (2020).

Lillian Wald's contributions to public health nursing were enormous:

- Appalled by the conditions of an immigrant neighborhood in New York's Lower East Side, she and a nurse friend, Mary Brewster, started the **Henry Street Settlement** in 1893 to provide nursing and welfare services.
- The Lower East Side was home to many poor Irish, Italian, Jewish, and Chinese immigrants, and the Henry Street Visiting Nurse Service visited many sick children and families in their homes (Bowery Boys, 2017) (Fig. 3-4).

TABLE 3-7 Lillian Wald, Public Health Nurse and Social Activist

Year	Contribution
1893	Started Henry Street Settlement to serve the poor in NYC Lower East Side; first to use the term Public Health Nurse; expanded roles of nurses; used trained nurses instead of lay people to provide care (Ruel, 2014).
1900s	Developed project to address childhood illness, reducing school absenteeism; began first school nursing program (Bullough & Bullough, 1978; Hawkins & Watson, 2003; Kalisch & Kalisch, 2004; Vessey & McGowen, 2006.
1906	Hired Miss Elizabeth Tler as first Black public health nurse to serve African American community leading to a satellite office at Stillman House (Fee & Bu, 2010).
1908	Worked to establish NYC Board of Child Hygiene (Ruel, 2014).
1909	Worked with Metropolitan Life Insurance Co. to reduce death rates by using visiting nurses to provide services to policyholders (Ruel, 2014).
1910–1912	Developed plan for national rural nursing service, which was developed with the American Red Cross to form American Red Cross Rural Nursing Service, later Town and Country Nursing Service (1913–1918), then the Bureau of Public Health Nursing. Program ended in 1947 (Ruel, 2014).
1912	Worked to establish Federal Children's Bureau; founder and first president of National Organization for Public Health Nursing (NOPHN); merged with the National League for Nursing (NLN) in 1952 (Christy, 1970; Feld, 2008; Lindenmeyer, n.d.).
1915	Wrote *The House on Henry Street* to highlight the achievements of the Henry Street Settlement (Wald, 1915).

TABLE 3-7 Lillian Wald, Public Health Nurse and Social Activist (*Continued*)

Year	Contribution
1934	Published *Windows on Henry Street* describing work and views on public health nursing (Wald, 1934). Influenced social reforms: to establish health and social policies, improvements were made in child labor and pure food laws, tenement housing, parks, city recreation centers, treatment of immigrants, and teaching of mentally handicapped children (Kalisch & Kalisch, 2004; Ruel, 2014). Emphasized illness prevention and health promotion through health teaching and nursing intervention, as well as epidemiologic methodology as early EBP (Vessey & Mc Gowen, 2006). Encouraged improved coursework at the Teachers College of Columbia University (New York) to prepare public health nurses for practice; modeled how nursing leadership, involvement in policy formation, and use of epidemiology led to improved health for the public (Ruel, 2018). Henry Street Settlement still in operation today: https://www.henrystreet.org/

Source: Bullough and Bullough (1978); Christy (1970); Donahue (2010); Fee and Bu (2010); Feld (2008); Hawkins and Watson (2003); Kalisch and Kalisch (2004); Ruel (2014); Wald (1915, 1934); Vessey and McGowen (2006).

- During one of the worst periods of depression, nurses from this organization supplied individuals and families with ice for keeping food fresh, meals, medicine, and sterilized milk; made referrals to hospitals and clinics, as needed; and "emphasized the human dignity of even the poorest" tenement families (Fee & Bu, 2010, p. 1206).

Wald's books, *The House on Henry Street* (1915) and *Windows on Henry Street* (1934), depict her work and convey her love of public health nursing (Fig. 3-5). The following Web site provides moving videos and photos of the neighborhood, Wald's *Baptism of Fire*, and *TheHouse on Henry Street*: https://www.henrystreet.org/about/our-history/exhibit-the-house-on-henry-street/

Wald's Growing Influence

Wald used her success at the Henry Street Settlement in reducing illness-caused employee absenteeism as evidence to address the issue of childhood illness and school absenteeism (Bullough & Bullough, 1978; Hawkins & Watson, 2003). In the early 1900s, medical inspectors sent home about 15 to 20 children per day from each school in New York City for health-related reasons, but no one followed up with them to make sure that they were properly treated and returned to school. Wald suggested that placing nurses in the schools would allow for follow-up on recurring cases and home visits during the periods of exclusion. She argued that the nurses could supplement the work done by local physicians,

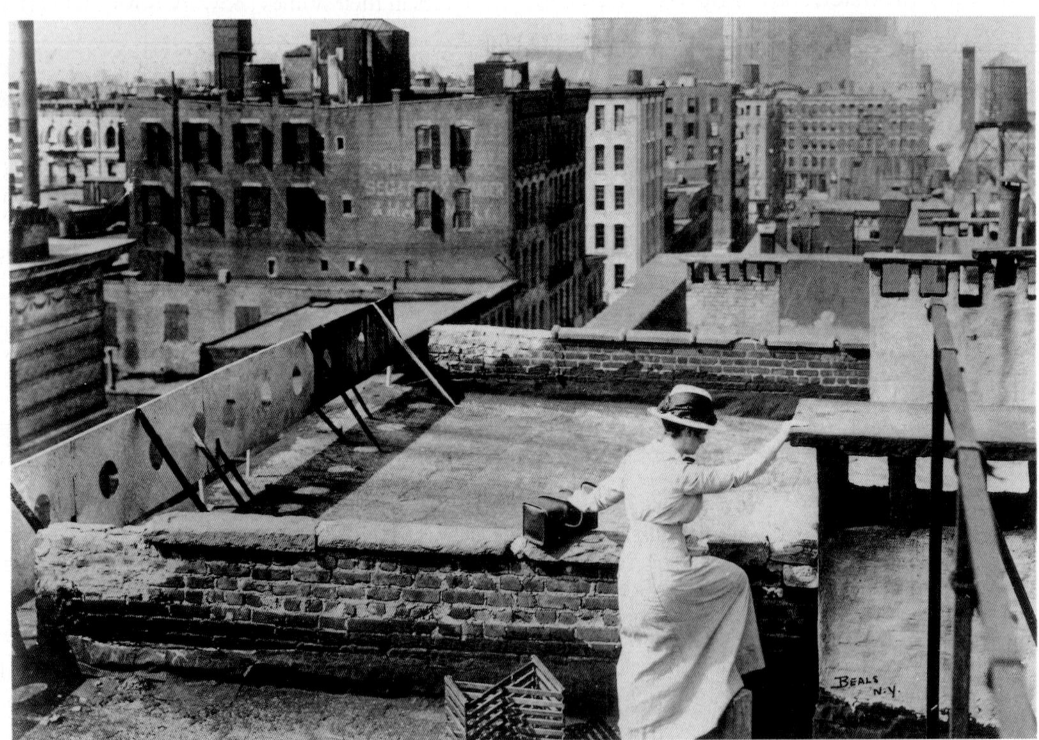

FIGURE 3-4 Iconic image of nurse crossing rooftops in New York City, 1908. (Used with permission of Visiting Nurse Service of New York.)

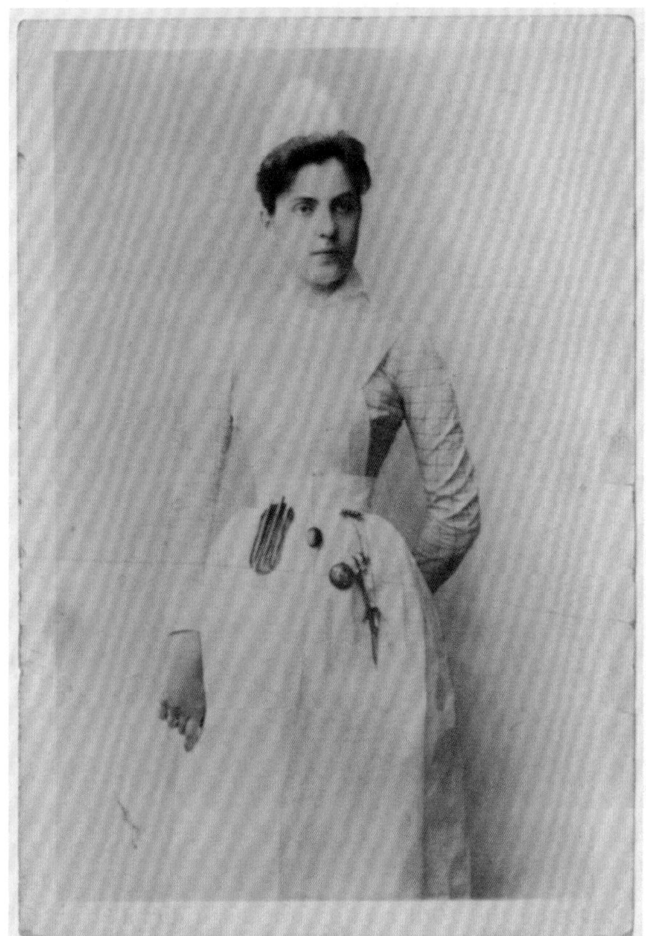

FIGURE 3-5 Lillian Wald as a student at New York Hospital Training School for Nurses, 1891. (Used with permission of the Visiting Nurse Service of New York.)

who occasionally examined the children. Offering the services of one nurse for 1 month, Wald hoped to demonstrate how effective a school nurse could be. Lina Rogers Struthers was the first school nurse appointed in this endeavor (Kalisch & Kalisch, 2004). One year after this initial experiment, the number of children sent home from the New York City schools had dropped dramatically, another example of evidence-based practice. By September 1903, only 1,000 children needed to be excluded (compared with 10,000 one year earlier); this was about a 10-fold reduction. By 1905, 44 nurses covered 181 public schools (Hawkins & Watson, 2003; Vessey & McGowen, 2006).

In 1909, Wald embarked on another visionary path. She convinced the Metropolitan Life Insurance Company that nurse intervention could reduce death rates (Hamilton, 2007; Hawkins & Watson, 2003). In collaboration with the Henry Street Settlement, the company organized the Visiting Nurse Department and provided services to policyholders in a section of Manhattan, beginning a program of **industrial nursing**. The success of this program resulted in expansion to other parts of the city and to 12 other eastern cities within a year. By 1912, the company had 589 Metropolitan nursing centers (Kalisch & Kalisch, 2004; Ruel, 2014). Industrial nurses proliferated after Wald's work with the Metropolitan Life Insurance Company in 1909 (Toering, 1919).

Another Nurse—Another Problem

As Lillian Wald worked to alleviate suffering caused by disease and poverty, Margaret Sanger began another battle. Born in 1879, she saw her own mother die at age 49, after 18 pregnancies and a long battle with tuberculosis. She attended nursing school and began working as a visiting nurse (Ruffing-Rahal, 1986).

The Comstock Act of 1873 prevented her from providing her female clients any information on contraception, despite the fact that affluent and educated Americans had reliable contraception. Even discussing contraception was prohibited (Baker, 2011). In 1912, she watched helplessly as a 28-year-old mother of three died from abortion-induced septicemia; a woman who had earlier begged her for information on preventing future pregnancies (Ruffing-Rahal, 1986). Margaret Sanger opened her first birth control clinic in Brooklyn, but 10 days later it was closed, and she was arrested (Fig. 3-6). She persisted and other clinics succeeded, resulting in the eventual formation of the International Planned Parenthood Federation (Baker, 2011).

Public Health Nursing Advances

PHNs gradually gained more autonomy in such areas as home care and instruction of good health practices to families and community groups (Figs. 3-7 and 3-8). They worked with children and families affected by polio and administered the polio vaccine, once developed, at mass immunization clinics. One account relates

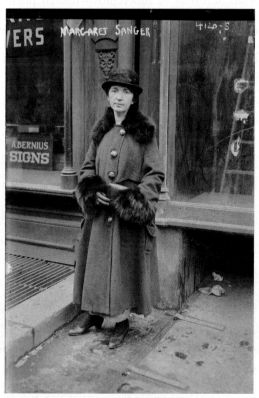

FIGURE 3-6 Margaret Sanger, thought to be standing in front of her birth control clinic.

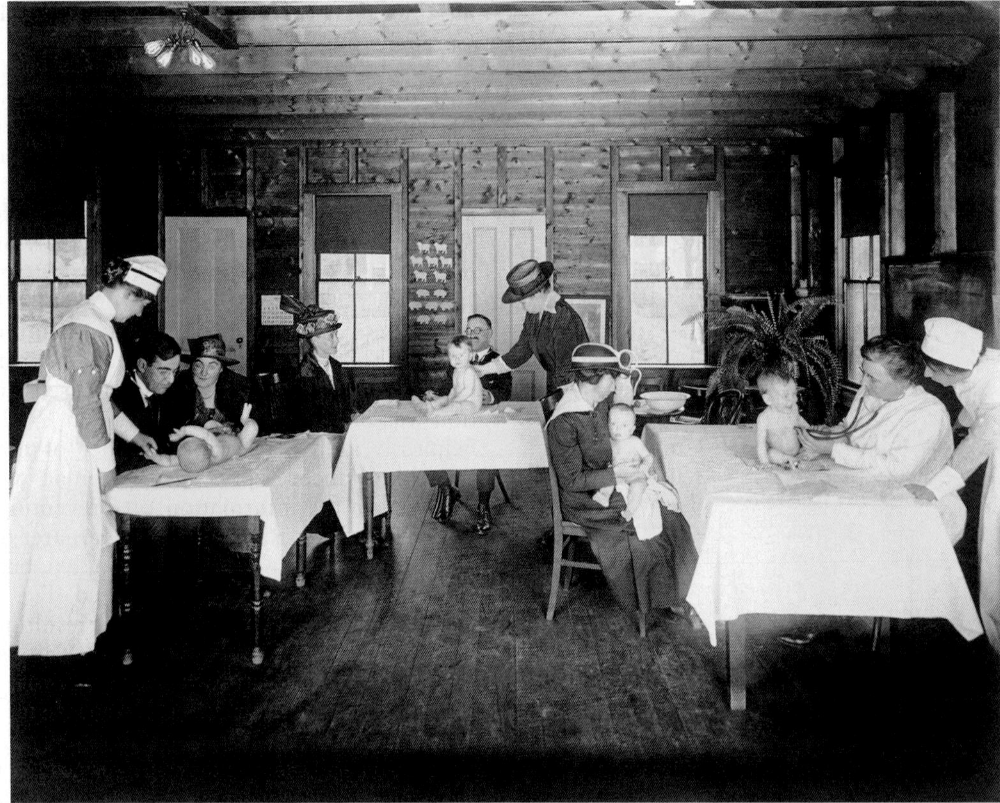

FIGURE 3-7 Well baby clinic in Framingham, Massachusetts (1920).

a single PHN's experience providing care to those living in an isolated outpost on Kodiak Island, Alaska, during an outbreak of tuberculosis-related pneumonia (Carter, 2001; Curtis, 2008; Keeling et al., 2018). Industrial nursing also expanded, with 66 US firms employing nurses by 1910 (Bullough & Bullough, 1978). Out of necessity, PHNs began keeping better records of their services and continued home visiting for those in need. They also responded to **population health** needs, as more individual care was now available at hospitals and health centers (see Box 3-2).

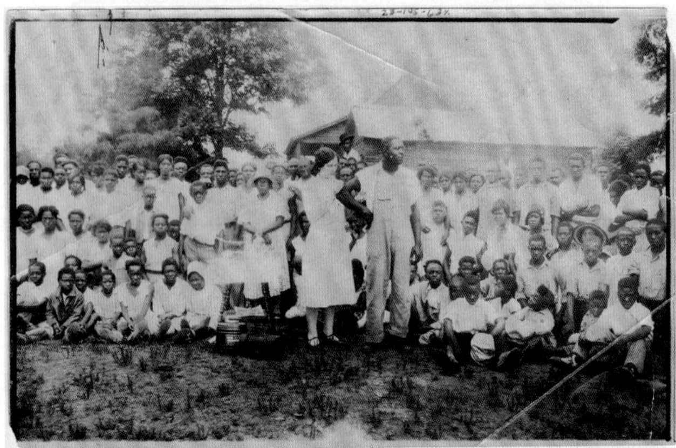

FIGURE 3-8 "Nurse Immunizing Man in Overalls in Front of a Large Group," Mississippi, ca. 1920s. (Retrieved from https://commons.wikimedia.org/wiki/File:Nurse_immunizing_man_in_overalls,_in_center_of_large_group_(16429738357).jpg)

During the 20th century, the institutional base for much of public health nursing shifted to the government.

- By 1955, 72% of the counties in the continental United States had local health departments, staffed primarily by PHNs, who emphasized health promotion and provided care for the ill at home (Erwin & Brownson, 2017).
- Some of the district nursing services, known as **visiting nurse associations (VNAs)**, remained privately funded and administered, offering their own home nursing care. In some places, city or county health departments joined administratively and financially with VNAs to provide a combination of services, such as home care of the sick and health promotion to families (Fig. 3-9).
- The Red Cross offered public health nursing services from 1912 to 1951: first via the Rural Nursing Services headed by Fannie Clement; second via the Town and Country Nursing Service, which served both rural areas and cities; and third via the Red Cross Public Health Nursing Service. The Red Cross also provided public health nursing services to families of soldiers during both World Wars (Ramsay, 2012; Sarnecky, 2018).

An innovative example of **rural nursing** was the **Frontier Nursing Service**, which was started by Mary Breckinridge (1881–1965) in 1925, to serve mountain families in Kentucky. From six outposts, nurses on horseback (see Fig. 3-10) visited remote families to deliver babies and provide food and nursing services. The work

BOX **3-2** STORIES FROM THE FIELD

New York City Public Health Nurses and the 1918 Influenza Pandemic

The 1918 influenza pandemic caused over 40 million deaths worldwide and 675,000 US deaths. The country was at war (World War I), and the American Red Cross, the U.S. Public Health Service, and health care workers were stretched thin. The epidemic began in New York City with three cases during mid-September of 1918. It spread quickly and crossed social class and income boundaries; within a few days, there were 31 new cases reported (Keeling, 2009; Keeling & Wall, 2015).

Cities across the Eastern seaboard requested assistance, and a coordinated plan for a decentralized response was set in place. Lillian Wald, who directed the Henry Street visiting nurses, had weathered epidemics on the Lower East Side of New York City before and quickly responded to this new, even more virulent threat. When making home visits, nurses found "whole families were ill ... without anyone to give them the simplest nursing care" (Keeling, 2009, p. 2735). One person described "People, desperate in their need watched from windows and doorways for the nurse. They surrounded her on the street, imploring her to go in six directions at once" (Geister, 1957, pp. 583–584).

Wald noted about 500 calls for nursing services to patients with influenza and pneumonia in the "first four days of October" and that nurses were instructed to wear masks but "31 out of ... 170 had succumbed to influenza" (Keeling, 2009, p. 2736). The Nurses' Emergency Council was organized for a citywide response, led by Lillian Wald, who requested that all who employed nurses allow them to work in caring for those afflicted by the epidemic. With this central structure, duplication of services was avoided, and services could be provided more quickly.

Wald requested automobiles for the visiting nurses to help them travel more quickly and carry "linens, pneumonia jackets, and quarts of soup"; the nurses started work early every morning and went out again at 4 PM to check on cases reported later each day (Keeling, 2009, p. 2737). They finished rounds around midnight, only to start again early the next morning. In Harlem, a nurse reported on a family of seven—"the mother has influenza, the father has lobar pneumonia, two children have measles and bronchopneumonia, and one child is only four weeks old," noting that they had no care until their case was reported to the visiting nurse association. This was a common situation across the city.

As the epidemic began to subside, the Nurses' Emergency Council discontinued central services on the 6th of November, and the Henry Street nurses opened postinfluenza clinics to address the follow-up needs of families. There were about 11,000 deaths from influenza and about 10,000 deaths from pneumonia reported in New York City over the 2-month period of the epidemic. All that the nurses could provide was comfort care—clean linens, bed baths, fluids, and monitoring. There was little help from the federal level of government; private, philanthropic, and religious organizations worked together with local government and nursing agencies to combat the deadly epidemic.

1. *How has your city or country responded to the novel coronavirus (COVID-19) pandemic? In what ways is this similar to the 1918 flu pandemic?*
2. *What disease threats are most likely to affect your community?*
3. *What resources are available?*
4. *How would public health nurses be involved?*

Source: Geister (1957); Keeling (2009); Keeling and Wall (2015).

was hard, but rewarding; it combined general public health nursing and midwifery (January, 2009). From the beginning, Breckinridge insisted on accurate record keeping; this was used to assess patient risks and treatments.

Over the years, the service has expanded to provide medical, dental, and nursing care. The Frontier Nursing Service continues today, with its remarkable accomplishments of reducing mortality rates and promoting health among this disadvantaged population, as the parent holding company for the Frontier Nursing University. It is the largest nurse–midwifery program in the United States. In addition, Mary Breckinridge Healthcare, Inc. consists of multiple rural health care agencies (Carter, 2018; Dawley, 2003) (see Box 3-3).

This public health nursing stage was characterized by service to the public, with the family targeted as a primary unit of care (Fig. 3-11). Official health agencies, which placed greater emphasis on disease prevention and health promotion, provided the chief institutional base.

- For instance, from 1928 to 1941, the East Harlem Nursing and Health Service offered "integrated family service(s)" by interdisciplinary independent PHNs to those living within an 87-city block area populated by mostly Italian immigrant and Italian American factory workers and laborers and their families (D'Antonio, 2013, p. 992).
- In New York City, 87% of babies were delivered at home, often by PHNs, and their services were in demand during the Great Depression as they worked to sustain families and address the social determinants of health that devastated them (D'Antonio, 2013).

Nurses in Military Service

Since Florence Nightingale's service to the British soldiers during the Crimean War, nurses have continued to provide service during wartime.

- Women served in many capacities (nurses, cooks, seamstresses) during the Revolutionary War.
- Clara Barton, a founder of the American Red Cross, volunteered her services during the Civil War, as did about 20,000 women of different races and classes (D'Antonio, 2010, 2013).
- In 1901, the Army Nurse Corps was established, and in 1908, the Navy Nurse Corps was added (Lineberry, 2013).
- During World War I, many new graduates responded to the pleas of the Red Cross for nurses to care for the sick and wounded and entered the Army Nurse Corps.

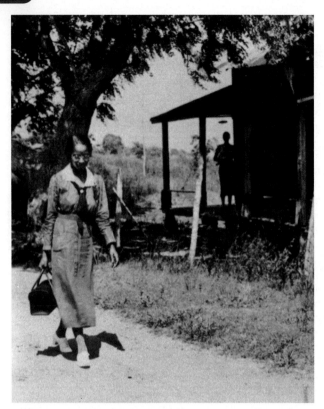

FIGURE 3-9 A public health nurse walks past a rural wooden house.

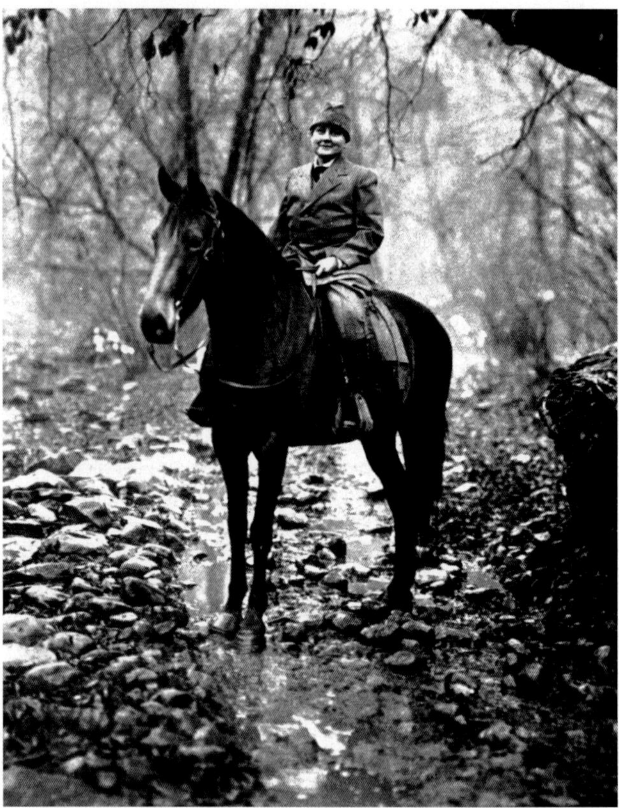

FIGURE 3-10 Mary Breckinridge on horseback. Photo Courtesy of Frontier Nursing University Archives. Used with permission.

BOX 3-3 PERSPECTIVES

Roaming Through the Hills With the Public Health Nurse (1920)

As a state nursing supervisor, I visit PHNs during a typical week providing services in rural Virginia. The first PHN's territory consisted of a mountainous area, with winding, often muddy roads. Our first visit was made on horseback: "The road straight up the mountain was winding and lovely and way below in a gorge ran a stream" on our way to Star-Chapel School. After traveling by horseback all day, we crossed a final stream to reach a house that backed up to the mountain; "the stream dashing over the rocks at the front door" where we were invited to spend the night (Webb, 2011, pp. 291–292). The family was eager to help the nurse who had cared for others during the 1918 flu epidemic.

At the school, we checked the children, and the PHN talked to them about how to prevent disease and the importance of personal hygiene. We visited two more schools on the way back home. In the southwest corner of the state, I visited another PHN, and we traveled 30 miles by logging train, which seemed to be "balanced on the peak of a mountain top" to visit a small, isolated town that desperately wants a nurse to visit schoolchildren and families (Webb, 2011, p. 292).

In another county, the PHN visits with a girl who is recovering from meningitis, and her mother brags that she wants a clean glass and washes her hands now before she eats every meal. We then travel to a log cabin where mothers and children meet every week, and the PHN weighs babies and provides health pamphlets and talks about "babies, screening houses, homemade ice boxes," and other topics of interest (Webb, 2011, p. 293). At an old stone fireplace, the women cook gingerbread and make hot cocoa. We later visited a rundown camp and found women there each having between three and eight children, along with a 14-year-old who had stopped dipping snuff, as the nurse advised. The nurse had promised her a prize, and she proudly claimed it. The PHN talked with a 12-year-old girl who refused to go to school and found that the reason was that she couldn't see, and her eyes were hurting. The mother agreed that she needed to see a specialist, but the girl would not agree to this unless her father made her go.

The PHN was disappointed to see a 4-year-old, who had agreed to stop chewing tobacco, come by to visit her with a cigarette in his mouth! Our state needs many more PHNs, and we are budgeting the money for services, but we don't have enough nurses who are willing to do this type of rural pioneer nursing. It can be very rewarding (Webb, 2011).

A silent film showing these nurses making visits on horseback during difficult conditions (begin at about the 10-minute mark) can be found at: https://collections.nlm.nih.gov/catalog/nlm:nlmuid-8600028A-vid

1. *Where are rural nurses practicing today?*
2. *How has it changed from the 1920s?*
3. *What problems continue in this population? How can current resources (e.g., technologic, pharmacologic, social, political) be effectively used by PHNs?*

Adapted from a 1920 article found in Webb (2011).

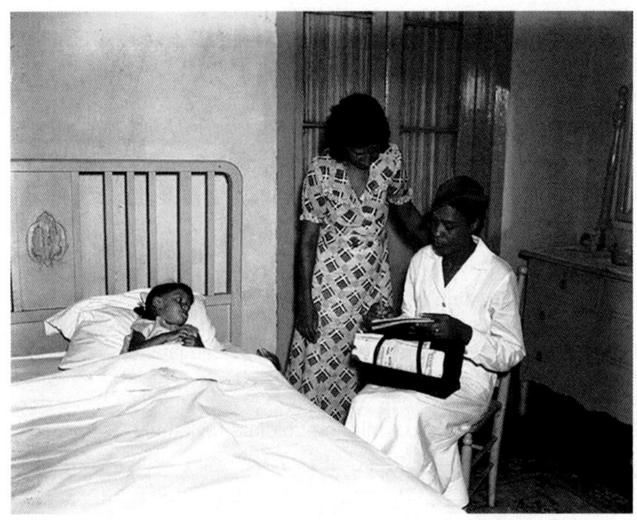

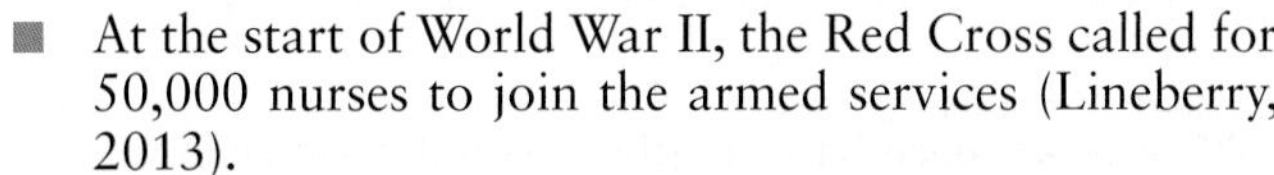

FIGURE 3-11 This Works Progress Administration (WPA) photograph shows a New Orleans public health nurse making a house call during the Great Depression, 1936. (Retrieved from https://commons.wikimedia.org/wiki/File:NurseHousecall1936.jpg)

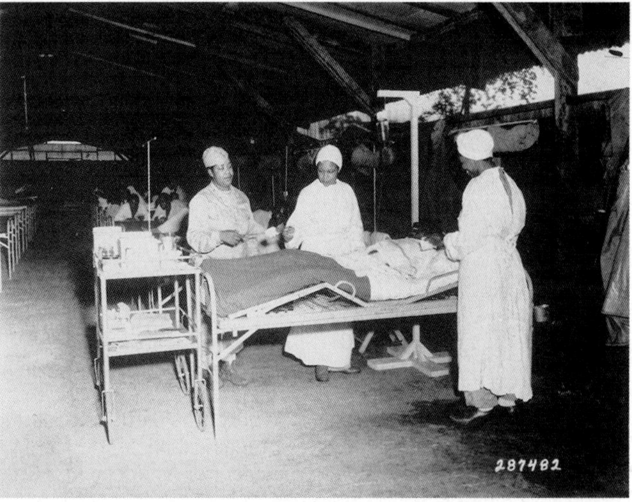

FIGURE 3-12 WW II, 1944. Surgical ward treatment at the 268th Station Hospital, Base A, Milne Bay, New Guinea. (Retrieved from https://commons.wikimedia.org/wiki/File:Surgical_ward_treatment_at_the_268th_Station_Hospital..._(5546316741).jpg)

- At the start of World War II, the Red Cross called for 50,000 nurses to join the armed services (Lineberry, 2013).
- The Cadet Nurse Corps was created in 1942 to feed the demand for nurses during World War II, but military nurses didn't receive permanent commissioned officer status until 1947 (Robinson, 2009).
- In 1945, President Franklin D. Roosevelt "desegregated nursing in the U.S. Armed Forces" (D'Antonio, 2010, p. 132).
- About 74,000 nurses served during the Second World War; some ended up behind enemy lines, in combat, and as Japanese prisoners of war (Lineberry, 2013) (see Fig. 3-12).
- Over 28,500 nurses are actively employed in the service branches under the Defense Health Agency and the U.S. Public Health Service (Military Health System Communications Office, 2018).

The Profession Evolves

By the 1920s, public health nursing was acquiring a more professional stature, in contrast to its earlier association with charity. Nursing as a whole was gaining professional status as a science, as well as an art. The formation of national nursing organizations began during this stage and contributed to nursing's professional growth.

- The American Society of Superintendents of Training Schools for Nurses in the United States and Canada:
  - Founded in 1893 by Isabel Hampton Robb
  - Purpose: to establish educational standards for nursing
  - Became the National League of Nursing Education in 1912, the forerunner of the current **National League for Nursing (NLN)**, established in 1952 (Ellis & Hartley, 2012; Stegen & Sowerby, 2019)
- The **American Nurses Association (ANA)**:
  - Developed from a meeting of nursing leaders who initiated an alumnae organization of 10 schools of nursing to form the National Associated Alumnae of the United States and Canada in 1896
  - Purpose: to promote nursing education and practice standards
  - In 1899, renamed the Nurses' Associated Alumnae of the United States and Canada
  - Canada excluded from the title in 1901, because New York, where the organization was incorporated, did not allow representation from two countries
  - Became the ANA in 1911; Canadian nurses formed a separate nursing organization (Ellis & Hartley, 2012).
- The **National Organization for Public Health Nursing (NOPHN)**:
  - Founded by Lillian Wald and Mary Gardner in 1912
  - Purpose: setting standards for PHNs (Christy, 1970; Feld, 2008; NOPHN, 1939)
  - In 1931, developed "general and specialized objectives" regarding work with individuals, families, and communities
  - In 1940, added 12 functions of PHNs (Abrams, 2004, p. 507); began using community health nurse as a more inclusive gesture
  - In 1952, merged with NLN (Abrams, 2004)

These three organizations, in particular, strengthened ties between nursing groups and improved nursing education and practice. The accomplishments of Wald and other nurse leaders reflect their concern for populations at risk and demonstrate how leadership, involvement in policy formation, and use of epidemiology led to improved health for the public (see Table 3-8 for information on famous PHNs).

The multiple problems faced by many families impelled a trend toward nursing care generalized enough

TABLE 3-8 A Partial List of Famous Nurses in the Development of US Public Health Nursing 1800–1950

Name	Years	Why This Person Is Famous
Sairey Gamp	1842–1844	Charles Dickens' (1907) fictitious stereotypical caricature of a drunken, slovenly, untrained nurse; first seen in the book *Martin Chuzzlewit*, published as serial in 1842–1844; it reflected common views of nurses.
Florence Nightingale	1820–1910	Often recognized as the "mother of modern nursing"; she was a social and health reformer who changed perceptions and practice of nursing (Keeling et al., 2018).
Mary Seacole	1805–1881	An adventurous daughter of a Scottish soldier and a Creole doctress, this Jamaican lay nurse cared for soldiers and families in her hotel in the Crimea (National Geographic, 2013).
Clara Barton	1821–1912	"Angel of the Battlefield" during US Civil War; ran the Office of Missing Soldiers for family reunification. Founder of American Red Cross, 1871 (Red Cross, 2018).
Mary Ann "Mother" Bickerdyke	1817–1901	US Civil War nurse called "Cyclone in Calico"; changed conditions in military camps. Named by Gen. W.T. Sherman as matron of military hospital in Cairo, IL; set up 300 field hospitals on 19 battlefields. Campaigned for pensions on behalf of soldiers and nurses (Keeling et al., 2018; Nursingtheory.org, 2016).
Walt Whitman	1819–1892	Famous poet; lay nurse during the US Civil War; visited more than 80,000 patients (Keeling et al., 2018).
Lillian Wald	1867–1940	Started Henry Street Settlement in NYC; used evidence-based practice to revolutionize public health nursing; health and social activist (Keeling et al., 2018).
Isabel Hampton Robb	1859–1910	Set standards for nursing practice, education, and ethics. First president of the Nurses' Associated Alumnae of the United States and Canada, (now ANA), 1897. One of the founders of the American Journal of Nursing Company. President of Association of Superintendents of Training Schools (now NLN), 1908 (AAHN, 2018).
Adelaide Nutting	1858–1948	WWI: Chairman of the Committee of Nursing of the General Medical Board of the Council of National Defense, coordinating nursing services and recruiting nurses Many other accomplishments in nursing (Spring, 2017).
Jane Delano	1862–1919	President of the Associated Alumnae and president of the Board of Directors of the American Journal of Nursing, 1908. Chairman, American Red Cross Nursing Service and second superintendent of the Army Nurse Corps, 1909. Credited for recruiting the majority of the 21,480 Army nurses who served during World War I (Sarnecky, 2018).
Clara Maass	1876–1901	Died after volunteering to be infected with yellow fever while working with the Yellow Fever Commission, headed by Maj. Walter Reed (Keeling et al., 2018).
Mary Breckinridge	1881–1965	Founder of Frontier Nursing Service, nurse midwife Used EBP and data to change rural nursing Organizations still operating today including Frontier Nursing University (Carter, 2018).

Source: AAHN (2018); Carter (2018); Dickens (1907); Keeling et al. (2018); National Geographic (2013); Nursingtheory.org (2016); Red Cross (2018); Sarnecky (2018); Spring (2017).

to meet diverse needs and provide holistic services, but there was also a call for specialization in some densely populated areas, where tuberculosis, infant care, and school children were a primary concern (Brainard, 2012; King, 2011; Ruel, 2014) (see Figs. 3-13 and 3-14).

As nursing education became increasingly rigorous, collegiate programs included public health as essential content in basic nursing curricula.

- Adelaide Nutting developed the first such course in 1912, at Teachers College in New York, in affiliation with the Henry Street Settlement.
- A group of agencies met in 1946 to establish guidelines for public health nursing, and by 1963, public health content was required for NLN accreditation in all baccalaureate degree–level nursing programs (Kulbok & Glick, 2014; Spring, 2017).

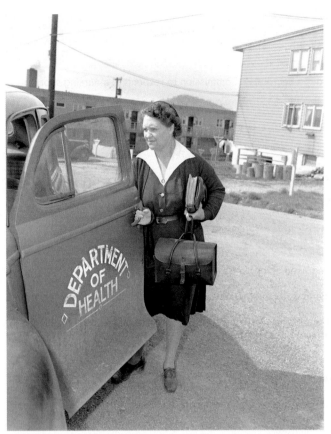

FIGURE 3-13 A public health nurse carrying the classic PHN bag in Oakridge, Tennessee, 1947. Note dark uniform, hat, and sensible shoes. (Retrieved from https://commons.wikimedia.org/wiki/File:Public_Health_Nursing_Oak_Ridge_1947_(12000263256).jpg)

- The nurse practitioner (NP) movement, starting in 1965 at the University of Colorado, was initially a part of public health nursing and emphasized primary health care to rural and underserved populations. The number of educational programs to prepare NPs increased, with some NPs continuing in public health and others moving into different clinical areas (Hawkins & Watson, 2010).

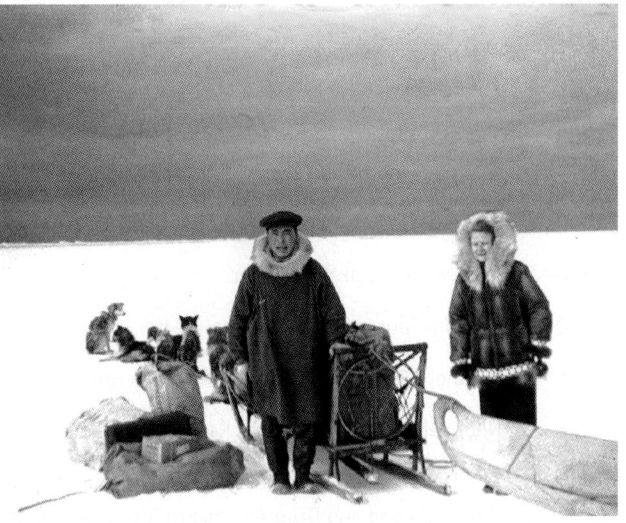

FIGURE 3-14 In Alaska in 1954, a public health nurse makes a home visit to clients, aided by an Eskimo man and his dog team. (Retrieved from https://commons.wikimedia.org/wiki/File:1956_Alaska_-_Eskimo_and_dog_team.jpg)

Community Health Nursing (1970 to the present)

The emergence of the term community health nursing heralded a new era (Table 3-9). By the late 1960s and early 1970s, while PHNs continued their work, many other nurses who were not necessarily practicing public health were based in the community. Their practice settings included community-based clinics, doctors' offices,

TABLE 3-9 Landmarks in Nursing History: 1970 and Beyond

Year	Landmark
1972	The Social Security Administration allowed Medicare coverage for those <65 years with long-term chronic disease and end-stage renal disease.
1973	US military troops left South Vietnam. In the case of Roe vs. Wade, a landmark Supreme Court decision legalized abortion.
1977	Global smallpox eradication was achieved.
1978	Drug-resistant tuberculosis was reported in Mississippi.
1979	Healthy People: The Surgeon General's Report on Health Promotion and Disease Prevention was released.
1980s	A focus on in-patient care led to decreased funding for public health services.
1980	The American Nurses Association (ANA) published *Nursing: A Social Policy Statement.*
1985	Red Cross Blood Services began testing for the HIV antibody.
1986	*Standards of Community Health Nursing Practice* was published by the ANA. The National Center for Nursing Research was created at the National Institutes of Health.

(*Continued*)

TABLE 3-9 Landmarks in Nursing History: 1970 and Beyond *(Continued)*

Year	Landmark
1988	The U.S. Department of Health and Human Services formed the Secretary's Commission to respond to a nursing shortage. IOM published *The Future of Public Health.*
1990s	Aging "Baby Boomers" created the need for improved geriatric care.
1990	The Persian Gulf War began.
1990	*Healthy People 2000: National Health Promotion and Disease Prevention Objectives.*
1991	Elizabeth Dole became the first woman president of the American Red Cross since Clara Barton.
1993	National Center for Nursing Research became the National Institute of Nursing Research.
1996	The Health Insurance Portability and Accountability Act (HIPPA) was signed into law. The U.S. Food and Drug Administration issued restrictive regulations for cigarettes and smokeless tobacco.
1997	Oregon legalized Death with Dignity, allowing terminally ill patients to end their lives with self-administered lethal injection.
1997	President Bill Clinton apologized for US government sanctions of the "Tuskegee Study of Untreated Syphilis in the Negro Male" resulting in new federal guidelines on ethical treatment of human subjects.
1999	*The Scope and Standards of Public Health Nursing Practice* published by the ANA. Targeted drug therapies for some cancers introduced (Herceptin, TyKerb).
2000s	Nurse-run clinics unable to meet Medicaid/Medicare requirements to hire physicians; many closed.
2000	*Healthy People 2000 results published; no nurses on the committee.* *Healthy People 2010: Understanding and Improving Health.* Draft sequencing of human genome completed and released to public.
2001	September 11 attacks resulted in over 3,000 deaths in New York City, Washington, and Pennsylvania. The Iraq War began.
2002	President George W. Bush signed Nurse Reinvestment Act. Hormone replacement therapy linked to increased risk of heart attack, blood clots, stroke, and breast cancer.
2003	Worldwide epidemic of severe acute respiratory syndrome (SARS).
2005	Hurricane Katrina became the most expensive disaster in US history.
2006	Medicare Part D Prescription Drug benefit implemented. *Public Health Nursing: Scope and Standards of Practice published by the ANA.* HIV cocktail drug, Atripla, and HPV vaccine, Gardasil, approved by the FDA.
2008	Barack Obama elected President, being the first African American to hold this position.
2009	*Essentials of Baccalaureate Nursing Education for Entry-Level Community/Public Health Nursing published by the Association of Community Health Nursing Educators, Education Committee.* H1N1 influenza "swine flu" outbreak declared a national emergency with over 22 million American's contracting the disease and 4,000 deaths.
2010	The Patient Protection and Affordable Care Act signed and included federal funding for nurse—family home visitation programs such as the Nurse Family Partnership to improve maternal/child health. Grant funding approved for existing school-based clinics as well as new construction. *Institute of Medicine published the Future of Nursing: Leading Change, Advancing Health.* Haiti earthquake triggered large nursing response.
2011	*The Future of Nursing: Leading Change, Advancing Health,* an Institute of Medicine report was released. Healthy People 2020 released. Medicare reimbursement to Certified Nurse—Midwives increased from 65% to 100% of the Physician Fee Schedule. National Health Service Corps (NHSC) hired over 10,000 additional nurses and other health care professionals.

TABLE **3-9** Landmarks in Nursing History: 1970 and Beyond *(Continued)*

Year	Landmark
2012	*Patient-Centered Outcomes Research Institute (PCORI)* established, with two recognized nurse leaders/researchers serving on the Board of Governors and Methodology Committee. Institute of Medicine published For the *Public's Health: Investing in a Healthier Future.*
2013	Under the Affordable Care Act, grants and scholarships expanded for nursing and other health professionals. The ANA published second edition of *Public Health Nursing: Scope and Standards of Practice.*
2014	The *Advanced Nursing Education Grant* program funded to expand the number of nurses in advanced nursing education and practice. The *Nursing Education and Loan Repayment Program* expanded to include up to 85% of loan forgiveness for registered nurses, advanced practice nurses, and faculty members working a minimum of 2 years in either critical shortage areas or accredited schools of nursing. Flint water crisis; school nurses and volunteers responded. Ebola outbreak in West Africa.
2015	Right-to-Die legislation for terminally ill patients enacted in California.
2017	*Healthy People 2020* midcourse review corrected and published; no nurse on committee.
2016	*Healthy People 2030*: Nurse Therese Richmond appointed to committee.
2020	*Healthy People 2030* released.

Source: Donahue (2011), Keeling et al. (2018), USDHHS (n.d.); American Nurses Association (2014).

worksites, and schools (Fig. 3-15). To provide a label that encompassed all nurses in the community, the ANA and others called them community health nurses. This term was not universally accepted, however, and many people—including nurses and the general public—had difficulty distinguishing community health nursing from public health nursing and determining whether community health nursing was a generalized or a specialized practice.

To help resolve this confusion, the following actions were taken:

- The ANA's Division of Community Health Nursing:
  - Developed A Conceptual Model of Community Health Nursing in 1980 to distinguish generalized preparation at the baccalaureate level from specialized preparation at the masters or postgraduate level
  - Defined the generalist as one who provides nursing service to individuals and groups of clients while keeping "the community perspective in mind" (American Nurses Association, Community Health Nursing Division, 1980, p. 9)
- In 1984, the U.S. Department of Health and Human Services, Bureau of Health Professions, Division of Nursing:
  - Convened a Consensus Conference on the Essentials of Public Health Nursing Practice and Education in Washington, DC (U.S. Department of Health and Human Services [USDHHS], Division of Nursing, 1984)
  - Identified community health nursing as the broader term, referring to all nurses practicing in the community, regardless of their educational preparation
  - Identified public health nursing as a part of community health nursing involving a generalist practice for nurses prepared with basic public health content at the baccalaureate level and a specialized practice for nurses prepared in public health at the master's level or beyond (Table 3-10)
- In 2009, the Association of Community Health Nursing Educators (ACHNE) released an updated revision of their original document, *Essentials of Baccalaureate Education for Entry-Level Community/Public Health* Nursing, noting that both terms encompass population-based practice.

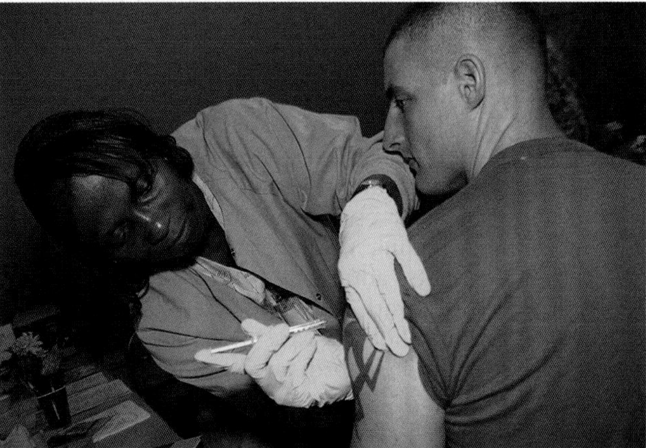

FIGURE 3-15 Germany, 2008. A nurse vaccinates a US marine at Stuttgart Army Health Clinic. (Retrieved from https://commons.wikimedia.org/wiki/File:USMC-080918-M-0884D-002.jpg)

In this text, the terms public health nursing and community health nursing are combined (C/PHN), but whichever

TABLE **3-10** Community/Public Health Nursing

Area of Practice	Sample Activities
Public health	Primary care activities, epidemiology
Disaster nursing	Nurses' roles in prevention/preparedness, response, recovery, and mitigation for/of disasters
Environmental health	Analysis of environmental hazards
Health education	Community education activities/academic education
Home health	Primary health care in residences
Hospice	End-of-life care
Midwifery	Ante- through postpartum care; women's health
Military nursing	International health relief projects
Missionary nursing	Operating clinics in underserved areas
Occupational/industrial health	Health education, safety evaluation
Ombudsman/community advocate	Work with individuals and communities to education and advocate for proper, reasonable, and timely health care
Policy formation/social justice/political activism	Serve on local boards and committees; join professional organizations
Population health	Health promotion activities for populations such as diabetes education or weight loss programs
Research	Study and disseminate information on issues relevant to PHN/CHN
Rural nursing	Home visits, immunization clinics
School nursing	Health promotion/disease tracking and prevention in schools
Visiting nurses	Provide short- or long-term care in the home
Volunteerism	Flu clinics, Disaster Management Assistance Teams (DMAT)

term is used to describe this nursing specialty, the fundamental issues and defining criteria remain the same:

- Are populations or communities the target of practice?
- Are the nurses prepared in public health and engaging in public health practice?

Finally, confusion also arose regarding the changing roles and functions of C/PHNs. Accelerated changes in health care organization and financing, technology, and social issues made increasing demands on C/PHNs to adapt to new patterns of practice. Many new kinds of community/public health services appeared. Hospital-based programs reached into the community. Private agencies proliferated, offering home care and other community-based services.

The debate over these areas of confusion continued through the 1990s, and some issues remain unresolved. Still, the direction in which public health and community health nursing must move remains clear: to care *for*, not simply *in*, the community. Public health nursing continues to mean the synthesis of nursing and the public health sciences applied to promoting and protecting the health of populations. Community health nursing, for some, refers more broadly to nursing in the community. Community health nurses are carving out new roles for themselves in primary health care. Collaboration and interdisciplinary teamwork are recognized as crucial to effective community nursing. This field of nursing is assuming responsibility as a full professional partner in community health.

Community/public health nurses:

- Work through many kinds of agencies and institutions, such as senior citizen centers, ambulatory services, mental health clinics, and family planning programs
- Conduct community needs assessment, document nursing outcomes, engage in program evaluation and quality improvement, assist in formulating public policy, and conduct community nursing research
- Seek to promote health, not just prevent illness, by applying current research evidence; promoting healthier lifestyle practices such as eating healthy diets, exercising, and maintaining social support systems; promoting healthy conditions in schools and work sites; and designing meaningful activities for children, adolescents, adults, and older adults (Kulbok et al., 2012; Milbrath & DeGuzman, 2015)
- Seek to provide holistic care by collaborating with others to offer more coordinated, comprehensive, and personalized services—a case-management approach

The 2020 Gallup Poll is an example of the current attention given to the opinions of consumers. In this poll, nursing is the most highly rated profession with

BOX **3-4** LEVELS OF PREVENTION PYRAMID

Promoting Community/Public Health Nursing

SITUATION: The general population is aware of nurses working in acute care settings or clinics, but fewer people interact regularly with population-focused, community-based nurses. As budgets are tightened, C/PHNs need to market their unique skill set and influence on health promotion and disease prevention in order to nurture this important nursing specialty.
GOAL: To clarify and enhance the community/public health nurse's role to promote greater impact of services.

Tertiary Prevention

- Promote increasing influence of the nurse through an expanded role in service delivery
- Minimize the impact of community misunderstandings of the nurse's role through education

Secondary Prevention

- Promote aggregate-level interventions
- Foster nurse involvement on community boards and other political groups

Primary Prevention

- Participate in policy formation
- Be politically active
- Assist in acquiring funding for community health programs
- Conduct research on health and nursing outcomes to enhance evidence-based practice
- Collaborate with the news media to publicize current public health issues

respect to honesty and ethics; it has held that position for 18 consecutive years. The honesty and ethical standards of nurses were rated either "high" or "very high" by 85% of respondents, ahead of physicians (65%), pharmacists (64%), police officers (54%), and members of clergy at 40% (Reinhart, 2020). And, as history has demonstrated, nursing's most effective contributions to the overall health of our nation are based in the community.

Nurses comprise the largest group of professionals in the public health workforce—about 16% or 47,000 employees in local, state, and federal agencies (Beck, Boulton, & Coronado, 2014). A study conducted 2 years later estimated a total number of full-time equivalent nurses working at state and local health departments at 40,791 (Beck & Boulton, 2016). As funding is limited in community and public health, it is important for C/PHNs to continue to demonstrate their worth. According to the U.S. Bureau of Labor Statistics (2020), job growth for registered nurses continues to be robust (with employment of registered nurses projected to grow 12% from 2018 to 2028); a significant driver of growth is the continuing recognition of the importance of preventive health care (Box 3-4).

TABLE **3-11** History of Public Health Nursing and the 10 Essential Public Health Services

Area(s)	Essential(s)	Historical Action(s)
Assessment	Assess and monitor population health	Nightingale began this work in the Crimea, and Wald continued this tradition at the Henry Street Settlement House.
Policy development	Communicate effectively to inform and educate. Create, champion, and implement policies, plans, and laws	Nightingale worked to change military policies providing better environments for soldiers' recovery. Wald ended exclusion of schoolchildren without any follow-up (school nurses hired); she promoted policies leading to the establishment of the Federal Children's Bureau.
Policy development; Assurance	Utilize legal and regulatory actions. Build a diverse and skilled workforce. Improve and innovate through evaluation, research, and quality improvement.	Wald fought to enforce pure food laws as well as child labor laws. She encouraged public health nurse preparation at the college level and founded a professional organization of public health nurses (NOPHN), which developed into the NLN, an accrediting body for schools of nursing.

Source: CDC. (2020).

SUMMARY

- Community/public health nursing developed historically through four stages.
  1. The *early home care stage* (before the mid-1800s) emphasized care to the sick poor in their homes by various lay and religious orders.
  2. The *district nursing stage* (mid-1800s) included voluntary home nursing care for the poor by specialists or "health nurses" who treated the sick and taught wholesome living to patients.
  3. The *public health nursing stage* (1900–1970) was characterized by an increased concern for the health of the general public.
  4. The *community health nursing stage* (1970 to the present) includes increased recognition of community health nursing as a specialty field, with focus on communities and populations.
- Nursing leaders contributed to development of community/public health nursing, most notably:
  - Florence Nightingale, who outlined public health nursing
  - Clara Barton, a Civil War nurse who founded the American Red Cross and shaped disaster nursing
  - Lillian Wald, who developed public health nursing, influenced legislation and policy, and instituted school and industrial nursing as new areas of public health
- Community/public health nursing encompasses many areas dealing with individuals, families, communities, and populations. Some examples include public health, disaster nursing, environmental health, health education, home health, hospice, midwifery, military nursing, missionary nursing, occupational/industrial health, ombudsman/community advocate, policy formation/social justice/political activism, population health, research, rural nursing, school nursing, visiting nurses, and volunteerism.
- Academic preparation for community/public health nursing *begins* at the baccalaureate level. The need for advanced preparation was recognized in the early 20th century, as college-level coursework was provided for this specialty.
- C/PHNs work in interdisciplinary teams in a variety of agencies with various populations to promote health.

ACTIVE LEARNING EXERCISES

1. Select one societal influence on the development of community/public health nursing and explore its continuing impact. What other events are occurring today that shape community/public health nursing practice? Using current, credible resources, support your arguments with documentation.
2. Research the life and works of a historical public health nursing leader. Using this information, determine how this practitioner might deal with a current population-based issue, such as the opioid epidemic, sexually transmitted diseases, obesity, vaping, gun violence, or child neglect and abuse.
3. Read an historical article about early public health nursing experiences. Compare these experiences with your public health clinical experiences today. What are the most striking similarities and differences?
4. Choose two areas of community/public health nursing where you might like to practice (Table 3-10). Compare and contrast those two areas describing geographic locations (e.g., international, rural), type of employment (e.g., public, private, grant funded), and job description, duties, activities areas of focus, and nursing orientation (e.g., individual, families, communities, populations). Compare your information with a classmate's selections.
5. After reviewing Box 3-11, review the 10 essential public health services (see Box 2-2) and give 4 additional examples of how they were implemented in historical community/public health settings (historical actions). Include who implemented them, what they did, where it occurred, and when. Give an example related to today's community/public health nursing practice.

thePoint: Everything You Need to Make the Grade!

thePoint® Visit http://thePoint.lww.com/Rector10e for NCLEX-style review questions, journal articles, supplemental materials, study aids for all learning styles, and more!

REFERENCES

A minimum of instruction for mothers (Editorial). (1919). *The Public Health Nurse, IX*(10), 769–770. Retrieved from https://archive.org/stream/publichealthnurs1110nati/publichealthnurs1110nati#page/n34/mode/1up

Abrams, S. E. (2004). From function to competency in public health nursing, 1931 to 2003. *Public Health Nursing, 21*(5), 507–510.

American Association for the History of Nursing (AAHN). (2018). *Isabel Adams Hampton Robb, 1860–1910*. Retrieved from https://www.aahn.org/robb

American Nurses Association, Community Health Nursing Division. (1980). *A conceptual model of community health nursing* (Publication No. CH-10 2M 5/80). Kansas City, MO: Author.

American Nurses Association. (2014, June 18). *Healthcare transformation: The affordable care act and more*. Retrieved from http://nursingworld.org/MainMenuCategories/Policy-Advocacy/HealthSystemReform/AffordableCareAct.pdf

American Red Cross. (2020). *Red Cross timeline*. Retrieved from https://www.redcross.org/about-us/who-we-are/history/significant-dates.html

Association of Community Health Nursing Educators (ACHNE). (2009). *Essentials of baccalaureate nursing education for entry level community/public health nursing*. Retrieved from https://www.achne.org/i4a/utilities/getmemberfile.cfm?file=Documents/EssentialsOfBaccalaureate_Dec_8_2009.pdf&showLink=true

Baker, J. H. (2011). *Margaret Sanger: A life of passion*. New York, NY: Hill and Wang.

Beck, A. J., & Boulton, M. L. (2016). The public health nurse workforce in U.S. state and local health departments, 2012. *Public Health Reports, 131*, 145–152.

Beck, A. J., Boulton, M. L., & Coronado, F. (2014). Public health workforce enumeration. *American Journal of Preventive Medicine, 47*(5, Suppl. 3), s306–s313.

Bowery Boys. (2018). *Henry Street Settlement and the legacy of Lillian Wald.* Retrieved from http://www.boweryboyshistory.com/2017/03/henry-street-settlement-legacy-lillian-wald.html

Brainard, A. M. (2012). The many-sided opportunity of field nursing. *Public Health Nursing*, 29(3), 283–285.

Bullough, V., & Bullough, B. (1978). *The care of the sick: The emergence of modern nursing.* New York, NY: Neale, Watson.

Carter, E. (September 20, 2018). The forgotten frontier: Nursing done in wild places. *Circulating now: From the historical collection of the National Library of Medicine.* Retrieved from https://circulatingnow.nlm.nih.gov/2018/09/20/the-forgotten-frontier-nursing-done-in-wild-places/

Carter, K. F. (2001). Trumpets of attack: Collaborative efforts between nursing and philanthropies to care for the child crippled with polio 1930 to 1959. *Public Health Nursing, 18*(4), 253–261.

Centers for Disease Control and Prevention (CDC). (2016). *Clean hands count.* Retrieved from https://www.cdc.gov/handhygiene/campaign/index.html

Centers for Disease Control and Prevention (CDC). (2019). *Data and statistics: Tuberculosis.* Retrieved from https://www.cdc.gov/tb/statistics/default.htm

Centers for Disease Control and Prevention (CDC). (2020). *10 Essential Public Health Services.* Retrieved from https://www.cdc.gov/publichealthgateway/publichealthservices/essentialhealthservices.html

Christy, T. W. (1970). Portrait of a leader: Lillian D. Wald. *Nursing Outlook, 18*(3), 50–54.

Curtis, M. (2008). Stricken village. *Public Health Nursing, 25*(4), 383–386.

D'Antonio, P. (2010). *American nursing: A history of knowledge, authority, and the meaning of work.* Baltimore, MD: Johns Hopkins University Press.

D'Antonio, P. (2013). Cultivating constituencies: The story of the East Harlem Nursing and Health Service, 1928–1941. *American Journal of Public Health, 103*(6), 988–996.

D'Antonio, P. (2017). *Nursing with a message: Public health demonstrations projects in New York City.* New Brunswick, NJ: Rutgers University Press.

Dawley, K. (2003). Origins of nurse-midwifery in the United States and its expansion in the 1940s. *Journal of Midwifery & Women's Health, 48*(2), 86–95.

Desrochers, A. (March 29, 2012). Dorothea Dix: Mental health reformer and civil war nurse. *Smithsonian Institution Archives.* Retrieved from https://siarchives.si.edu/blog/dorothea-dix-mental-health-reformer-and-civil-war-nurse

Dickens, C. (1907). *Martin Chuzzlewit.* New York, NY: Alfred A. Knopf Publishing.

Dolan, J. A. (1978). *Nursing in society: A historical perspective.* Philadelphia, PA: W. B. Saunders.

Donahue, M. P. (2011). *Nursing, the finest art: An illustrated history* (3rd ed.). Maryland Heights, MO: Mosby Elsevier.

Edmonds, J. K., Campbell, L. A., & Gilder, R. E. (2017). Public health nursing practice in the Affordable Care Act era: A national survey. *Public Health Nursing*, 34(1), 50–58. doi: 10.1111/phn.12286.

Ellis, J. R., & Hartley, C. L. (2012). *Nursing in today's world: Trends, issues, and management* (10th ed.). Philadelphia, PA: Wolters Kluwer Health/Lippincott Williams & Wilkins.

Erwin, P. C., & Brownson, R. C. (2017). *Scutchfield & Keck's principles of public health practice* (4th ed.). Boston, MA: Cengage.

Evans, J. (2004). Men nurses: A historical and feminist perspective. *Journal of Advanced Nursing*, 47, 321–328.

Fee, E., & Bu, L. (2010). The origins of public health nursing: The Henry Street Visiting Nurse Service. *American Journal of Public Health, 100*(7), 1206–1207.

Feld, M. N. (2008). *Lillian Wald: A biography.* Chapel Hill, NC: University of North Carolina Press.

Florence Nightingale Museum Trust. (1997). *The Florence Nightingale Museum's school visit pack.* London, UK: Author.

Gardner, M. S. (1936). *Public health nursing* (3rd ed.). New York, NY: Macmillan.

Geister, J. (October 1957). The flu epidemic of 1918. *Nursing Outlook, 5*, 582–584.

Hamilton, D. (2007). The cost of caring: The Metropolitan Life Insurance Company's visiting nurse service, 1909–1953. In P. D'Antonio, E. D. Baer, S. D. Rinker, & J. E. Lynaugh (Eds.), *Nurses' work: Issues across time and place* (pp. 141–164). New York, NY: Springer.

Hanes, P. (2016). Wildfire disasters and nursing. *Nursing Outlook, 51*(4), 625–645.

Hawkins, J. W., & Watson, J. C. (2010). School nursing on the Iron Range in a public health nursing model. *Public Health Nursing, 27*(6), 571–578.

Hogan, D. (September 2015). Public health nursing: A rich history. *The Florida Nurse, 10.*

Hughes, A. (1902). The origin, growth, and present status of district nursing in England. *American Journal of Nursing, 2*(5), 337–345.

January, A. M. (2009). Friday at the Frontier Nursing Service. *Public Health Nursing, 26*(2), 202–203.

Kalisch, P. A., & Kalisch, B. J. (2004). *American nursing: A history* (4th ed.). Philadelphia, PA: Lippincott Williams & Wilkins.

Keeling, A. W. (2009). "When the city is a great field hospital": The influenza pandemic of 1918 and the New York City nursing response. *Journal of Clinical Nursing, 18*, 2732–2738.

Keeling, A. W., Hehman, J. C., & Kirchgessner, J. C. (2018). *History of professional nursing in the United States: Toward a culture of health.* New York, NY: Springer.

Keeling, A. W., & Wall, B. M. (2015). *Nurses and disasters.* New York, NY: Springer Publishing Company.

King, M. G. (2011). Four responsibilities of the tuberculosis nurse, circa 1919. *Public Health Nursing*, 28(5), 469–472.

Kulbok, P. A., & Glick, D. F. (2014). "Something must be done!" Public health nursing education in the United States from 1900 to 1950. *Family & Community Health, 37*(3), 170–178.

Kulbok, P. A., Thatcher, E., Park, E., & Meszaros, P. S. (2012). Evolving public health nursing roles: Focus on community participatory health promotion and prevention. *Online Journal of Issues in Nursing, 17*(2), Manuscript 1. doi: 10.3912/OJIN.Vol17No02Man01.

Lee, G., Clark, A. M., & Thompson, D. R. (2013). Florence Nightingale—Never more relevant than today. *Journal of Advanced Nursing, 69*(2), 234–246.

Lewinson, S.B., McAllister, A., & Smith, K. M. (Eds.). (2017). *Nursing history for contemporary role development.* New York, NY: Springer.

Lindenmeyer, K. (n.d.). *Children's bureau.* Retrieved from https://socialwelfare.library.vcu.edu/programs/child-welfarechild-labor/children's-bureau/

Lineberry, C. (May 7, 2013). *A brief history of female nurses in the military, from the American Revolution to World War II.* Retrieved from http://www.huffingtonpost.com/cate-

Milbrath, G. R., & DeGuzman, P. B. (2015). Neighborhood: A conceptual analysis. *Public Health Nursing*, 32(4), 349–358.

Military Health System Communications Office. (May 8, 2018). *National nurses' week: Remembering nurses and their contributions to military medicine.* Retrieved from https://www.airforcemedicine.af.mil/News/Display/Article/1514662/national-nurses-week-remembering-nurses-and-their-contributions-to-military-med/

Mosley, M. O. (2007). Satisfied to carry the bag: Three Black community health nurses' contributions to health care reform, 1900–1937. In P. D'Antonio, E. D. Baer, S. D. Rinker, & J. E. Lynaugh (Eds.), *Nurses' work: Issues across time and place* (pp. 65–78). New York, NY: Springer.

Mowbray, P. (1997). *Florence Nightingale museum guidebook.* London, UK: The Florence Nightingale Museum Trust.

National Geographic Resource Library. (November 27, 2013). *Mary Seacole.* Retrieved from https://www.nationalgeographic.org/article/mary-seacole/

National Organization for Public Health Nursing (NOPHN). (1939). *Manual of public health nursing* (3rd ed.). New York, NY: Macmillan.

Nightingale, F. (1969). *Notes on nursing: What it is, and what it is not.* London, UK: Harrison. (Original work published 1859.)

Nightingale, F. (1876). [Letter to the editor]. *The Times* (London). Retrieved from https://www.ucl.ac.uk/bloomsbury-project/articles/archives/nightingale.pdf

Nursingtheory.org. (2016). *Mary Ann Bickerdyke, Mother Bickerdyke.* Retrieved from http://www.nursing-theory.org/famous-nurses/Mary-Ann-Bickerdyke.php

Nutting, M. A., & Dock, L. L. (1907). *A history of nursing: The evolution of nursing systems from the earliest times to the foundation of the first English and American training schools for nurses* (2 volumes). New York, NY: G. P. Putnam's Sons.

Palmer, I. S. (2001). Florence Nightingale: Reformer, reactionary, researcher. In E. C. Hein (Ed.), *Nursing issues in the 21st century: Perspectives from the literature (pp. 26–38).* Philadelphia, PA: Lippincott Williams & Wilkins.

Pugh, A. (2001). Men, monasteries, wars, and wards. *Nursing Times*, 97(44), 24–25.

Ramsay, A. G. (2012). The end of an era. *Public Health Nursing, 29*(4), 380–383.

Reddi, V. (2005). *Dorothea Lynde Dix (1802–1887).* Retrieved from http://www.truthaboutnursing.org/press/pioneers/dix.html

Reinhart, R. J. (January 6, 2020). Nurses continue to rate highest in honesty, ethics. *Gallup.* Retrieved from https://news.gallup.com/poll/274673/nurses-continue-rate-highest-honesty-ethics.aspx

Richardson, R. (2010). *Florence Nightingale and hospital design.* Retrieved from http://www.kingscollections.org/exhibitions/specialcollections/nightingale-and-hospital-design/florence-nightingale-and-hospital-design

Robinson, T. M. (2009). *Your country needs you.* Bloomington, IN: Xilbris.

Rooney, D. (2016). *Florence Nightingale: Pioneer statistician.* Retrieved from https://beta.sciencemuseum.org.uk/stories/2016/11/4/florence-nightingale-the-pioneer-statistician

Rosenberg, C. E. (2008). Siting epidemic disease: 3 centuries of American history. *Journal of Infectious Diseases, 197*(Supplement 1), S4–S6. https://doi.org/10.1086/524985. Retrieved from https://academic.oup.com/jid/article/197/Supplement_1/S4/842514

Ruel, S. R. (2014). Lillian Wald. *Home Healthcare Nurse, 32*(10), 597–600.

Ruffing-Rahal, M. (1986). Margaret Sanger: Nurse and feminist. *Nursing Outlook*, 34, 246–249.

Runciman, P. (2014). The health promotion work of the district nurse: Interpreting its embeddedness. *Primary Health Care Research & Development, 15*(1), 15–25.

Sarnecky, M. T. (2018). *Miss Jane A. Delano, 2nd Superintendent, Army Nurse Corps*. Retrieved from https://e-anca.org/History/Superintendents-Chiefs-of-the-ANC/Miss-Jane-A-Delano

Schwartz, C. C., Ajjarapu, A. S., Stamy, C. D., & Schwinn, D. A. (2018). Comprehensive history of 3-year and accelerated US medical school programs: A century in review. *Medical Education Online, 23*, 1530557. Retrieved from https://www.ncbi.nlm.nih.gov/pmc/articles/PMC6211283/pdf/zmeo-23-1530557.pdf

Spring, K. (2017). *Mary nutting*. National Women's History Museum. Retrieved from www.womenshistory.org/education-resources/biographies/mary-nutting

Stegen, A. J., &Sowerby, H. (2019). *Nursing in today's world: Trends, issues, and management* (11th ed.). Philadelphia, PA: Wolters Kluwer.

The College of Physicians of Philadelphia. (2020). *The history of vaccines: Polio*. Retrieved from https://www.historyofvaccines.org/timeline/polio

Theofanidis, D., & Sapountzi-Krepia, D. (2015). Nursing and caring: An historical overview from ancient Greek tradition to modern times. *International Journal of Caring Science, 8*(3), 791–800.

Toering, J. (1919). Nursing work in the telephone company. *The Public Health Nurse, IX*(10), 793–796. Retrieved from https://archive.org/stream/publichealthnurs1110nati/publichealthnurs1110nati#page/n34/mode/1up

U.S. Bureau of Labor Statistics. (2020). *Occupational outlook handbook: Registered nurses*. Retrieved from https://www.bls.gov/ooh/healthcare/registered-nurses.htm

U.S. Department of Health and Human Services (USDHHS), Division of Nursing. (1984). *Consensus conference on the essentials of public health nursing practice and education: Report of the conference*. Rockville, MD: Author.

U.S. Department of Health and Human Services, Office of Health Promotion and Disease Prevention. (n.d.). *Healthy people 2020*. Retrieved from https://www.healthypeople.gov/sites/default/files/HP2020Framework.pdf

Vessey, J. A., & McGowen, K. A. (2006). A successful public health experiment: School nursing. *Pediatric Nursing, 32*(213), 255–258.

Wald, L. D. (1915). *The house on Henry Street*. New York, NY: Holt.

Wald, L. D. (1934). *Windows of Henry Street*. Boston, MA: Little Brown.

Webb, B. (2011). Roaming through Virginia with the public health nurse. *Public Health Nursing, 28*(3), 291–293.

Woodham-Smith, C. (1951). *Florence Nightingale*. New York, NY: McGraw-Hill.

World Health Organization. (2015). *Improving nutrition outcomes with better water, sanitation, and hygiene*. Retrieved from http://www.who.int/water_sanitation_health/publications/washandnutrition/en/

World Health Organization. (2018). *Tuberculosis*. Retrieved from http://www.who.int/news-room/fact-sheets/detail/tuberculosis

CHAPTER 4

Evidence-Based Practice and Ethics

"Research is formalized curiosity. It is poking and prying with a purpose."

—Zora Neale Hurston (1891–1960), Novelist

We must not see any person as an abstraction. Instead, we must see in every person a universe with its own secrets, with its own treasures, with its own sources of anguish, and with some measure of triumph."

—Elie Wiesel from *The Nazi Doctors and the Nuremberg Code*

KEY TERMS

RESEARCH/EVIDENCE-BASED PRACTICE

- Community-based participatory research (CBPR)
- Evidence-based practice
- Integrative review
- Meta-analysis
- Randomized control trial (RCT)
- Research
- Scoping review
- Systematic review
- Validity

ETHICS

- Autonomy
- Beneficence
- Bioethics
- Distributive justice
- Egalitarian justice
- Ethical decision-making
- Ethical dilemma
- Ethics
- Fidelity
- Instrumental values
- Justice
- Moral
- Moral evaluations
- Nonmaleficence
- Respect
- Restorative justice
- Social justice
- Terminal values
- Value
- Value systems
- Values clarification
- Veracity

LEARNING OBJECTIVES

Upon mastery of this chapter, you should be able to:

1. Discuss the concept of evidence-based practice (EBP) in community/public health.
2. List the necessary steps in the process of EBP.
3. Analyze the potential impact of research on community/public health nursing practice.
4. Identify the community/public health nurse's role in conducting research and using research findings to improve his or her practice.
5. Describe the nature of values and value systems and their influence on community/public health nursing.
6. Articulate the impact of key values on professional decision-making.
7. Discuss the application of ethical principles to community/public health nursing decision-making.
8. Use a decision-making process with and for community/public health clients that incorporates values and ethical principles.

INTRODUCTION

As a new student in community/public health nursing, you may ask, "Can I really do something to make a difference in the lives of my clients?" You may feel shocked and discouraged by the crushing poverty and overwhelming sense of helplessness experienced by many of your clients and by the continual recurrence of problems such as substance abuse, domestic violence, unemployment, and criminal activity. For the first time in your life, you may truly confront the inequalities and injustices of our health care system. You will face many ethical dilemmas in community/public health nursing. You may ask, "Why

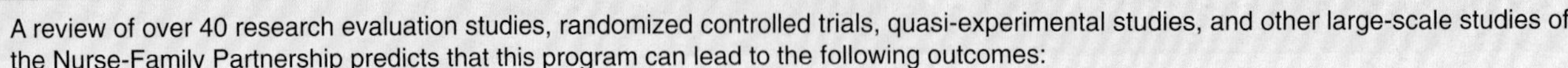
A review of over 40 research evaluation studies, randomized controlled trials, quasi-experimental studies, and other large-scale studies of the Nurse-Family Partnership predicts that this program can lead to the following outcomes:

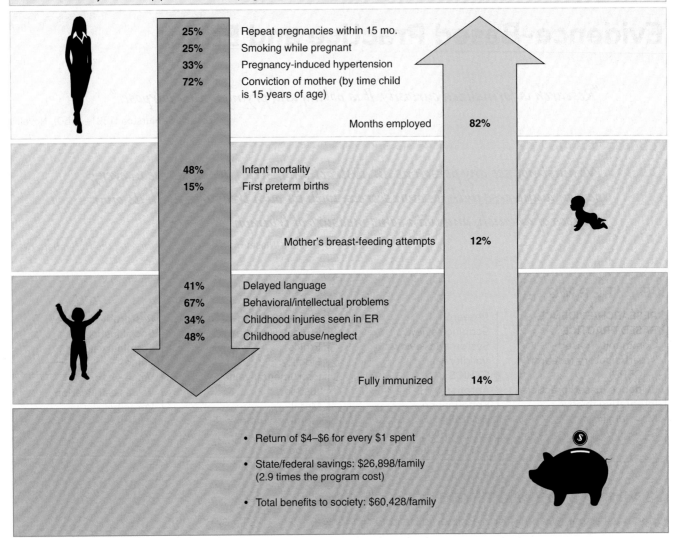

FIGURE 4-1 Research that makes a difference: the Nurse-Family Partnership. (Source: Nurse-Family Partnership. Retrieved from https://www.nursefamilypartnership.org/wp-content/uploads/2019/11/Miller-State-Specific-Fact-Sheet_US_2019.pdf; Karoly, L. A. (2017). Investing in the early years: The costs and benefits of investing in early childhood in New Hampshire. *RAND.* Retrieved from https://www.rand.org/pubs/research_reports/RR1890.html; Nurse-Family Partnership. (2019). *About us.* Retrieved from https://www.nursefamilypartnership.org/about/)

should I bother to make home visits to pregnant teens? Why should I offer smoking cessation classes at the local homeless shelter? Will it really matter?"

Recent public health nursing research validates that nursing care *does* matter and that you really *can* make a difference in the lives of your clients. For example, Nurse-Family Partnership (NFP) programs, based on research conducted by David Olds and his colleagues, are reaping results in many communities across the United States and around the world (Coalition for Evidence-Based Policy, 2015; Karoly, 2017; Mejdoubi et al., 2015; Nurse-Family Partnership, 2017, 2018). See Figure 4-1.

RESEARCH THAT MAKES A DIFFERENCE: THE NURSE-FAMILY PARTNERSHIP (NFP)

In an early longitudinal study by Olds and his research team (1997) conducted with a primarily white sample in a semirural setting over a 15-year period, regular visits by public health nurses (PHNs) to poor, unmarried women and their first-born children resulted in dramatic differences when compared with similar mothers and children in a control group. Many of the women were younger than age 19. PHNs made an average of nine prenatal visits and 23 child-related visits (until the child turned 2 years old). The effects of the intervention continued for up to 15 years after the birth of the first child.

Statistically significant differences were noted in the following outcomes:

- Fewer subsequent pregnancies and an increased percentage of live births
- Longer intervals of time between first and second births
- Fewer incidences of reported child abuse and neglect
- Fewer months on public assistance and food stamps
- Fewer reported arrests and convictions of mothers
- Less impairment from alcohol or other drug use reported by mothers

A 2014 study examining data from 1,138 women compiled over two decades (1990–2011) looked at outcome measures of maternal mortality and preventable-cause child mortality rates (Olds et al., 2014b). Four treatment interventions were examined:

- Transportation for prenatal care (control group)
- Developmental screening for infants and toddlers, as well as transportation (control group)
- Prenatal and postpartum home visiting with transportation (intervention group)
- Transportation, screening, prepregnancy/postpregnancy home visiting and infant/toddler home visiting (intervention group—NFP components)

Findings revealed the following:

- Maternal mortality rates for both control groups were higher than for those in both of the intervention groups.
- Results comparing the two control groups versus the two intervention groups were statistically significant ($p = 0.008$), indicating that the interventions were worthwhile.
- Child data, only available in groups 2 (2nd control group) and 4 (2nd intervention group), revealed statistical significance for preventable-cause child mortality rate ($p = 0.04$) for those in the group with all components of the NFP.

These and other studies are powerful evidence noting the effectiveness of a program of regular C/PHN visits to this vulnerable group. A classic study by the Olds research team examining pregnancy outcomes, childhood injuries, and repeated childbearing (Kitzman et al., 1997) was recognized by the National Institute of Nursing Research (National Institutes of Health, n.d.b) as one of 10 landmark nursing research studies.

The NFP model is based on theory and research. Olds and his colleagues have conducted repeated **randomized controlled trials (RCTs)** with different populations living in a variety of settings and contexts, over varying lengths of time (Eckenrode et al., 2010; Karoly, 2017; Kitzman et al., 2010a, 2010b; Olds et al., 2014a, 2014b; Sierau et al., 2016), and have consistently found that the NFP program results in the benefits mentioned in Figure 4-1 (NFP, 2018).

In a time of tight budgets, number crunchers may ask: do PHNs really make a difference, or can less expensive health care workers also get results? An early study by Olds et al. (2004) examined differences between PHN and paraprofessional (e.g., home aides) visitation in a large, randomized study of mostly Mexican American low-income first-time mothers.

- At the beginning of the study, no statistical differences were noted between participants in both groups.
- Two years after the end of the program, participants visited by paraprofessionals had fewer low birth weight babies and better results than did control subjects on measures of mastery and mental health, and their home environments were conducive to early learning.
- However, mothers visited by nurses showed immediate as well as long-term benefits.
  - They had longer intervals between first and second births, there were fewer incidences of domestic violence, and their home environments were found to be conducive to early learning.
  - Children of those mothers had better behavioral adaptation during testing, more advanced language scores, and better executive functioning. Others have reported similar findings (Olds et al., 2014a).

Later research found "no significant paraprofessional effects on emotional/behavioral problems" among children of mothers with fewer psychological means in a study comparing paraprofessionals to control group counterparts (p. 114). Those children visited by nurses were found to have

- Fewer emotional and behavioral problems overall at age 6 years ($p = 0.08$)
- Fewer internalizing problems at age 9 years ($p =0.08$)
- Less dysfunctional attention at age 9 years ($p = 0.07$)
- When compared with control-group counterparts, nurse-visited children exhibited better receptive language at the ages of 2, 4, and 6 years ($p = 0.01$) and better sustained attention at ages 4, 6, and 9 years ($p = 0.006$).

Olds and his fellow researchers are convinced that PHNs are the key to success.

In tough budget times, state and local agencies may be hesitant to expand programs. But the costs of PHN visits are more than offset by the large savings in both dollars and human suffering (NFP, 2017). Over the years, several think tank and policy groups have done cost–benefit analyses of the NFP, all concluding that this program reaps large returns on investment.

- The cost effectiveness of NFP was verified by Wu, Dean, Rosen, and Muennig (2017). Compiling data from RCTs and other available data, they concluded that the program was most effective with high-risk mothers—improving population health and "saving both money and lives" (p. 1586).
- Quality-adjusted life years were 0.19 higher and with additional earnings along with other reported benefits, the net gain would be $9,617 per child visited by a PHN. They estimated 100% certainty that the program would gain even higher economic benefits over costs.

When H.R. 3590 (The Patient Protection and Affordable Care Act—"Obamacare") was passed in 2010, early childhood home visitation programs were singled out as effective practices, and new grant funding to states was made available to promote these programs. The number of newly enrolled clients increased 25-fold between 2010 and 2013 (NFP National Service Office, 2015). In February 2018, additional funds were allocated to support these programs through 2020 (Maternal Child Health Bureau, n.d.).

Dr. Olds and his colleagues have encouraged replication, using the established framework undergirding their proven results. The value of this program that provides

BOX 4-1 PERSPECTIVES

An NFP Nurse Viewpoint on Public Health Nursing

I walked into the high school not sure what to expect, after all, I was used to visiting my clients in their homes. A very young looking girl walked in, noticeably pregnant and extremely shy. I tried to meet her eyes, but she kept looking down as we walked to a room. We met there every week for 6 weeks.

Several months later when my client called to tell me that her mom had physically abused her and that her brother had threatened her with a gun, I felt helpless. I listened to her and hooked her up with resources for a safe place to go. If she couldn't count on her own mom, how would she ever succeed, I wondered?

She called me a lot after that day, many times just to talk. She wanted desperately to go to school, but since leaving her mom's home, she lived too far away to walk. I gave her as many bus passes as I could to get her to school and back. I thought that would be enough, until I could speak to school officials and find her some permanent transportation. Little did I know, but I was the ONLY one who cared if this child got to school or not. I tried tirelessly to get through to case workers, school officials, and social workers. I never thought that I would have this problem; a pregnant girl who wanted to go to school and adults who didn't care. How could this girl win?

My client gave birth to her baby and continued to faithfully keep our scheduled visits. We would laugh and have fun, while covering the program curriculum. She was doing a great job of parenting her baby and growth and development was on target. The baby was thriving. She was living somewhere new and again insisted that she wanted to go to school. We found out what district she was in and they needed her to get a physical exam and records from her old school. I encouraged her but was not too sure if she could get it all done. Those types of errands are easy for most people, but for someone who has no means of transportation and little support, it is a huge ordeal.

A week later I got a phone call, it was my client. I had to ask who it was because this young lady sounded so sure of herself and assertive. I couldn't believe that it was her! When had she started to speak up and articulate like this? She was calling to tell me that she had gotten her physical and her school records, and she was just waiting to hear from the school. I told her how proud I was of her for being so responsible.

The next time I saw my client, she rushed to the door and pulled me inside. She wanted to show me something and led me to her room. There, laid out on the bed was her ROTC uniform, complete with shiny black shoes. Her grandmother was willing to help with the baby so that she could participate. She looked me right in the eyes and said in a powerful voice... "What do you think?" I told her that I had no doubt in my mind that she would do great things in life, and that I was so proud of her. She said "Ms. Jody, I don't know why you are so proud; you are the one who taught me to be this way." Amazing! I have had so many success stories and seen so many healthy moms and babies. I love working with this program. What I do can make a big difference.

Jody, RN, PHN, NFP Nurse

PHN visits to at-risk mothers and children in their homes has been validated. So, PHNs really *do* make a difference! See Box 4-1.

RESEARCH AND EVIDENCE-BASED PRACTICE

This evidence about the effectiveness of public health nursing visits could be gleaned only by conducting formal nursing research. Research in nursing is not a new phenomenon; Florence Nightingale is considered the earliest nurse researcher. She collected and analyzed data on the soldiers she cared for during the Crimean War (1859). She also employed principles of **evidence-based practice (EBP)** because she sought to enhance their care by using evidence to improve her nursing practice and patient outcomes.

This section defines the terms research and EBP, explains the need for EBP, lists and describes the steps of the EBP process, differentiates EBP implementation from research and quality improvement, discusses the need for ethical oversight of research, and presents the basic components of research that are needed to promote EBP.

Defining Research and EBP

Research is the systematic collection and analysis of data related to a particular problem or phenomenon. Research that is properly conducted and analyzed has the potential to yield valuable information that can affect the health of large groups of people. Indeed, it should guide our practice of community/public health nursing, and it often serves as the basis for changes in health care policies and programs.

According to Melnyk and Fineout-Overholt (2019), EBP in nursing means just that—systematically searching for and critically appraising and synthesizing evidence (or research findings), along with consideration of expert clinical nursing judgment and patients' wishes, in making decisions about how to care for patients or clients.

Rebar and Gersch (2015, p. 11) describe EBP as

- Reviewing the best available evidence, most often the results of research
- Using the nurse's clinical expertise
- Determining the values and cultural needs of the individual
- Determining the preferences of the individual, family, and community

Alvidrez et al. (2019) discuss evidence-based interventions in public health and recognize that some of the best available evidence includes not only that from clinical research but also from health data (e.g., immunization rates, mortality rates, health status surveys) and practice (e.g., program evaluations, reports from expert panels).

Clinical reasoning is an important component in EBP. Practice knowledge of expert clinical nurses is vital to the process and efficacy of results (Belita et al., 2018; Glynn, McVey, Wendt, & Russell, 2017). Training programs are necessary for nurses to successfully apply EBP to their practices, in the community as well as in acute care (Black, Balneaves, Garossino, Puyat, & Qian, 2015).

The Quad Council Coalition, the preeminent public health nursing alliance that has now been renamed the Council of Public Health Nursing Organizations, delineated specific proficiencies required of public health nurses. The Quad Council Coalition PHN Competencies include analytic assessment skills, basic public health science skills, and policy development/program planning skills that include research and EBP (2018). In the current national atmosphere of managed care, value-based care, and obstinately rising health care costs, the importance of conducting valid research on how health care dollars can be spent to benefit the greatest number of people is vitally important. (The Quad Council Tier 1 Community/Public Health Nursing Competencies are listed in the appendix; the Tier 2 and Tier 3 competencies are found at http://www.quadcouncilphn.org/documents-3/2018-qcc-competencies/.)

The Need for EBP

Across many different settings, from acute to community-based care, implementation of EBP guidelines or practices has been shown to improve nursing practice and client outcomes, as well as reduce costs and standardize care (Kutney-Lee et al., 2015; Lasater, Germack, Small, & McHugh, 2016; Melnyk, Fineout-Overholt, Giggleman, & Choy, 2017; Zhu, Dy, Wenzel, & Wu, 2018).

How did this more recent paradigm shift toward EBP occur? Dr. Archie Cochrane, a British epidemiologist, is widely regarded as the force behind evidence-based clinical practice in medicine (Brucker, 2016). Even though we often cling to "the way we've always done it," we certainly have ample evidence of the need for a shift to EBP in health care: the Institute of Medicine (IOM; now the National Academy of Medicine) has been studying the issues of health care quality and effectiveness since 2000 and has called for widespread and systematic changes through its seminal reports:

- *To Err Is Human: Building a Safer Health System* (IOM, 2000)
- *Crossing the Quality Chasm: A New Health System for the 21st Century* (IOM, 2001)
- *Priority Areas for National Action: Transforming Health Care Quality* (IOM, 2003)
- *The Future of the Public's Health in the 21st Century* (IOM, 2003)
- *For the Public's Health: The Role of Measurement in Action and Accountability* (IOM, 2011)
- *For the Public's Health: Investing in a Healthier Future* (IOM, 2012).

These landmark reports draw attention to the fact that we spend billions of dollars each year researching new treatments and more than a trillion dollars annually on health care, but "we repeatedly fail to translate that knowledge and capacity into clinical practice" (IOM, 2003, p. 2). As discussed in Chapter 6, the United States has a large, complex, and expensive health care system, with lower-than-expected quality and safety outcomes affecting population health.

The Future of Nursing highlights the need for nurses to work with other health professionals in "redesigning health care" by "conducting research" and improving practices through evidence-based means (IOM, 2011, pp. 7, 11).

Steps of the EBP Process

The effective practitioner uses his or her clinical judgment and expertise to reflect on the practice of community/public health nursing and determine whether safe, effective, quality, and cost-efficient care is being delivered. Problems or situations that need clarification can then be identified, and current research can be reviewed to guide needed changes in practice. Although acknowledged barriers exist, they can be overcome using available resources (Cline, Burger, Amankwah, Goldenberg, & Ghazarian, 2017). Melnyk and Fineout-Overholt (2019, p. 17) outline the steps of the EBP process:

- Step "0": Cultivate a spirit of inquiry within an EBP culture/environment.
- Step 1: Ask the burning clinical question in PICOT format (see below).
- Step 2: Search for and collect the most relevant best evidence.
- Step 3: Critically appraise the evidence for its validity, reliability, and applicability, and then synthesize that evidence.
- Step 4: Integrate the best evidence with one's clinical expertise, patient preferences, and values in making a practice decision or change.
- Step 5: Evaluate outcomes of the practice decision or change based on evidence.
- Step 6: Disseminate the outcomes of the EBP decision or change.

These steps will be explored in more detail, as well as available resources and implications for community/public health nursing practice.

Cultivating a Spirit of Inquiry

For effective change to occur, nurses must continually examine, question, and challenge current practices (Melnyk & Fineout-Overholt, 2019).

- We need to be continually curious about how we can best conduct our practice and the evidence needed to guide our clinical decision-making; we also need to be immersed in a supportive culture that sustains this curiosity.
- Asking questions such as, "Why are we doing this?" and "Is there evidence to support this practice?" demonstrates this spirit of inquiry.

Asking the Question

What if you or your colleagues doubt the effectiveness of some method in your current nursing practice and want to find out whether there is new research or evidence that may convince you to make a change? How do you begin your journey to EBP?

Melnyk and others suggest that the first step to solving the problem is "asking the burning clinical question" (2019, p. 17). This question may be about client care or effective interventions, such as

- What methods are most effective in ensuring client medication compliance with tuberculosis protocols?
- What is the best information I can give new mothers about preventing sudden infant death syndrome?

It could also be about systems approaches to population health:

- What is the most effective method of improving human papillomavirus (HPV) vaccination rates for adolescents?
- How can C/PHNs better collaborate with families, physicians, and hospitals in preventing quick readmission of heart failure patients due to poor understanding and control of symptoms?

The PICOT question is one way to develop an answerable, searchable EBP question. First, the population or problem must be specified (P) and an intervention (I) determined, then a comparison intervention or issue (C) is identified and an outcome (O) is measured over a specific period of time (T). Example:

- Ashley, a school nurse working at a Midwestern high school, noticed an increase in levels of obesity and depression among her students (***Population/Problem***) and searched for examples of EBP-based interventions that might be helpful.
- She found studies linking obesity with depression among adolescents (Goldschmidt, Wall, Loth, & Neumark-Sztainer, 2015; Hoare et al., 2014), along with a systematic review of longitudinal studies indicating a bidirectional association (Mannan, Mamun, Doi, & Clavarino, 2016). Two pretest/posttest studies with relatively small sample sizes found positive results for depression and healthy lifestyle scores using an intervention called COPE—Creating Opportunities for Personal Empowerment (***Intervention***; Hoying & Melnyk, 2016; Hoying, Melnyk, & Arcoleo, 2016).
- Further searching led to a large-scale RCT ($n = 779$) that included once-a-week sessions in a 15-week health class, integrating COPE (cognitive–behavioral skills-building intervention) and 20 minutes of physical activity (Melnyk et al., 2013). A control group participated in a Healthy Teens program consisting of general health skills that did not employ cognitive–behavioral therapy (***Comparison***).
- Testing for obesity (pedometer steps, body mass index [BMI]) and mental health outcomes (social skills, anxiety and depression scores; ***Outcome***) were completed pre- and immediately postintervention, and again at 6 months postintervention (***Time***).
- Results indicated that COPE was more effective than the comparison, with significant differences related to obesity and social skills tests, but decreases occurred in both groups for anxiety and depression at first posttest and again at 6 months (no statistical differences).

A second study of the RCT evaluated results again at 12 months postintervention (Melnyk et al., 2015) and found those in the COPE group had significantly lower BMIs, lower rates of overweight/obesity, and more average pedometer steps compared with the Healthy Teen group. For those with high depression scores, significant improvements were noted in the COPE group versus the control group. Grades were also better.

Armed with a plan and prior approval from her school nursing supervisor, Alison presented the information at a monthly school nurses meeting. A couple of other nurses wanted to join Alison in a pilot study at each of their high schools. Along with Megan, their supervisor, they developed an implementation plan and methods of evaluating outcomes. They began their COPE program in health classes the next fall and found similar outcomes to the RCTs.

They worked together to write an abstract for a state school nursing conference, and it was accepted for a poster presentation. They were busy discussing their study with many other school nurses at the poster session of their school nurses' conference and decided to try writing a manuscript for a school nursing journal. Alison and her colleagues had seen a problem, researched it, and operationalized an intervention that bore significant outcomes. They had also disseminated their research, and it all began with a question (Melnyk, 2017).

Finding the Evidence

Melnyk and Fineout-Overholt (2019) stress the importance of systematically searching for all relevant research on a clinical question of interest and critically analyzing the evidence, while keeping in mind the unique needs of the clients served, as well as current practice standards, guidelines, and ethical considerations. It is also important to gather input from expert clinicians, review big data sources such as existing federal, state, and county databases, and examine social or other media sources on your topic (Wong, Chiang, Choi, & Loke, 2016). See Chapter 10 and Levels of Evidence on thePoint.

- Excellent places to begin are **integrative** or **systematic reviews** that compile all recent studies and summarize what is known about the problem or situation. The Cochrane Collaboration (www.cochrane.org) lists systematic reviews on various topics of interest to both physicians and nurses.
- **Scoping reviews** are conducted to discover new evidence on a subject, types of evidence available in a specific area of inquiry, or to determine missing areas in a body of literature (Munn et al., 2018).
- **Meta-analysis** is a statistical method used to combine results of multiple smaller research studies (similar in content, purpose, subjects) to increase the statistical power of the overall findings (Hoffman, 2019). It may be used alone or together with systematic reviews.
  - By combining the results of many similar studies, meta-analysis affords greater statistical power and can give the researcher a more complete general perspective, especially when research on a certain issue may seem inconclusive (Melnyk & Fineout-Overholt, 2019).

  For instance, a community/public health nurse (C/PHN) working with a group of adults who have diabetes might be interested in the systematic review and meta-analysis on the importance of resistance exercise (using weights) for clients with type 2 diabetes. Findings included increased insulin sensitivity, increased muscle density, abdominal fat loss, and reduction in hemoglobin A1c levels. The best results were noted in participants using high-intensity resistance exercise (Liu et al., 2019).

- Although a C/PHN may certainly have a "hunch" that exercise is good for clients, this newer systematic review and meta-analysis of current studies provides solid evidence on which to base specific recommendations.

Other systematic reviews and meta-analysis on promoting adherence to antiretroviral therapy (ART) for human immunodeficiency virus (HIV)/acquired immunodeficiency syndrome (AIDS) clients might be helpful to a C/PHN supervisor in designing an AIDS case management program employing C/PHNs.

- A systematic review of 124 studies including a large majority of RCTs done in North America, Africa, and Europe found a "large and overall strong evidence base" for five interventions: (1) cognitive–behavioral therapy; (2) education; (3) directly observed therapy; (4) treatment supporters; and (5) active reminder devices for ART, such as text messaging (Chaiyachati, Ogbuoji, Price, Suthar, & Barnighausen, 2014, p. s199).
- A later meta-analysis of studies focusing on ART adherence among pregnant women in Africa found that there were differences in the results for those getting education, social support, and structural support. Results were higher than those with only text reminders and others with only social and structural support (Omonaiye, Nicholson, Kusljic, & Manias, 2018).
- From this evidence, a C/PHN case manager may conclude, provided the client population is similar to those studied, that medication compliance may be most effectively ensured through development of a nurse–client relationship, group support, and focused patient education on medication management skills.

Critical Appraisal of the Evidence

Collection and critical analysis of the best evidence in the literature, like that done by the school nurses above, constitute the second and third steps in the EBP process. Systematic reviews should be carefully examined to determine **validity** (Park, 2018). You can do this by asking these types of questions:

- What was the review question (specific population, intervention, etc.) and search strategy?
- Were the studies in the review properly designed and executed (were findings valid)?
- Were there similar results found in all studies?
- How reliable are the results (only minimal bias)?
    - Were sample sizes large enough and results statistically significant?
    - Were there confounding factors (e.g., outside influences that make you doubt the results; differences between groups in intervention or outcome assessment, high rates of attrition)?

It is also helpful to compare the results with those of previous research and clinical practice, and keep in mind that at least one large-scale study has found that over one third of systematic reviews neglected to fully discuss adverse events or outcomes (Melnyk & Fineout-Overholt, 2019; Parsons, Golder, & Watt, 2019). Grids outlining levels and quality of evidence in public health nursing are available in research or EBP textbooks and online.

What if no systematic reviews are available in your area of interest? Where can you find the necessary evidence needed to make good practice decisions? You can look for RCTs, meta-analysis research, program evaluation studies, systematic literature reviews, or practice guidelines, keeping in mind that several studies (or one or two large-scale, tightly controlled studies) are preferred.

Integrating the Evidence

It is important to make a decision based on your clinical expertise and knowledge of your clients' values and preferences when incorporating this information into your practice (Melnyk & Fineout-Overholt, 2019). You can do this by asking:

- How can I apply these results to my community/public health nursing practice?
- Are my clients similar to the population studied? Will it benefit my clients?
- Does this go against my client's values or preferences?
- Do I have the necessary resources?

Evidence has shown that C/PHNs have been effective with different client populations in ameliorating postpartum depression, promoting awareness, and facilitating improved family functioning in families with neglected and abused children, and the benefits of the NFP for children, mothers, and families have been consistently demonstrated (Coalition for Evidence-Based Policy, 2015; Karoly, 2017; Mejdoubi et al., 2015; Nurse-Family Partnership, 2017, 2018; Sierau et al., 2016).

The Cochrane Public Health and Health Systems Web site may yield useful systematic reviews (https://publichealth.cochrane.org). Newer research outside of public health nursing may also be applied in the community, depending on one's clinical expertise and knowledge of clients. The Cochrane Nursing Care Web site may be helpful (https://nursingcare.cochrane.org/resources). The Joanna Briggs Institute (n.d.) provides evidence-based tools for health professionals through their broad global collaboration with hospitals and universities.

For instance, a recent systematic review about the effectiveness of nicotine replacement therapy (NRT) in gaining long-term smoking cessation found 133 studies with almost 65,000 participants. When compared with no intervention or a placebo, NRTs such as transdermal patches (Fig. 4-2), gum, nasal sprays, and lozenges were found to be more helpful in increasing rates of successfully quitting smoking by 50% to 60%.

- The research was termed "high quality" and researchers felt that further research was not likely to alter these conclusions (Hartmann-Boyce, Chepkin, Ye, Bullen, & Lancaster, 2018, para. 7).
- This research might spark an interest in C/PHNs to consider promoting these products to aid in smoking cessation when providing counseling for adult clients who wish to stop smoking.

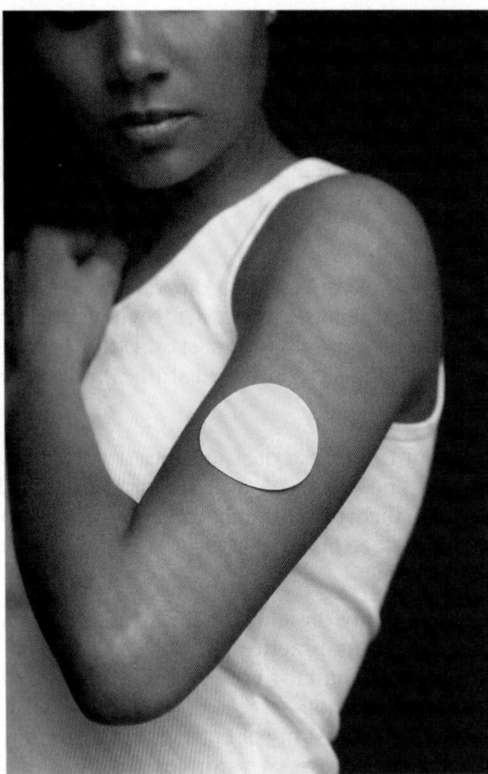

FIGURE 4-2 Recent research concludes that nicotine replacement therapy is effective in smoking cessation.

When examining population-based strategies, The Community Guide (n.d.) provides task force recommendations based on systematic reviews, along with additional resources on various topics of interest (https://www.thecommunityguide.org).

Evaluating Outcomes

A critical step of the EBP process is to evaluate any practice change. For instance, if you decide to implement findings from the systematic review on NRT smoking cessation cited above, a standardized protocol of home visits and further patient education/follow-up by C/PHNs would need to be established. Baseline and postintervention data would need to be collected to deduce any potential positive change noted. Results can vary based on specific environment, population, implementation, and other factors. Evidence can lead you to choose a course, but evaluation of your outcomes is necessary to ensure that you have achieved the best results (Melnyk & Fineout-Overholt, 2019).

The design of an evidence-based research project represents the overall plan for carrying out the study or intervention. A major consideration in selecting a particular design is to try to control as much as possible those factors that are not included but can influence the results. An example of control is easily demonstrated in a classic study by Douglas, Mallonee, and Istre (1999):

- Researchers wanted to discover the percentage of homes with functioning smoke alarms. They initially conducted a telephone survey, a commonly used method of survey research in community health and found that 71% of households reported functioning smoke alarms.
- Concerned that this might be an inflated number, they conducted an on-site survey to confirm the results. After face-to-face interviews, they found that only 66% of householders reported having functioning alarms.
- However, when researchers were actually able to go into homes and tested the smoke alarms in person, only 49% were fully functioning. By having researchers test the smoke alarms, this design controlled for inflated results of the more commonly conducted, convenient, and economical telephone survey.

Is self-report always unreliable? Results may vary, but a study of 589 12-year-olds reporting toothbrushing frequency compared with oral hygiene indices found that self-report could be used in place of levels of plaque, for instance, when studying dental caries in adolescents (Gil et al., 2015). The C/PHN must determine the most efficient, cost-effective, and reliable method of obtaining necessary data.

Once an intervention is developed, further studies can evaluate its appropriateness and, ultimately, its effectiveness. Beyond EBP implementation, other lines of clinically based research can also be designed.

Disseminating Outcomes

We need to share our results to improve the body of knowledge in community/public health nursing and provide studies that can be used in future systematic reviews. Often, C/PHNs are required to report results to stakeholders (e.g., grant-funding agencies, local or county governing bodies).

- Formal reports are often required, or scorecards may be used that compare local results with state and national data.
- We can also share outcomes information with our colleagues locally, through staff meetings, informal networking, blogs, or pertinent listserv, etc.
- When EBP outcomes are shared at state and national professional meetings or through publication in peer-reviewed journals, a wider audience can be reached, and our knowledge base is exponentially increased.

Differences Between EBP Implementation, Quality Improvement, and Research

If you have worked as a student in an acute care hospital, you have been introduced to quality or performance improvement (QI/PI) initiatives. QI/PI became even more important to health care after the IOM reports cited earlier. These approaches involve a systematic analysis of data and processes with the aim of improving the delivery of health care.

Over the last decade, the National Quality Forum (2019) has endorsed over 300 quality measures, and hospitals are now required to publicly report certain quality data indicators. The Centers for Medicare and Medicaid Services began to financially penalize hospitals by not paying for services when certain quality indicators (e.g., pressure ulcers, hospital acquired infections, readmission rates) were not met (Lasater et al., 2016). See Chapter 6.

Accrediting bodies for acute care hospitals first mandated quality care initiatives, but these are now spreading to ambulatory areas and other settings (Dunlap et al., 2016). With the push for accreditation in public health agencies, this issue is becoming even more pertinent to C/PHNs and to public health systems with a focus on population health (Gerding, DeLellis, Neri, & Dignam, 2018; Kronstadt, Beitsch, & Kaye, 2015; Thomas, Corso, & Monroe, 2015).

- Along with EBP, quality improvement (QI) is another core competency needed by all health professionals, as noted in many of the seminal national reports mentioned earlier. For those working in hospitals where QI is at the forefront, it can be difficult to discern differences between EBP, research, and QI.
- Thinking critically about practice problems is an important component of all three approaches. Reflecting on why we do things a particular way and critically thinking through a problem in a purposeful, systematic way are vital steps in the process.
- QI involves gathering and using data and methods of improving processes and procedures to determine effective nursing interventions that can improve patient outcomes and systems approaches, such as rapid-cycle testing and compliance monitoring (Balakas & Smith, 2016).
- Quality and Safety Education for Nurses (QSEN) provides guidance on using skills needed to provide improved care and outcomes (Altmiller, 2019). QSEN features are found in selected chapters of this book.

The differences between QI/PI, EBP implementation, and clinical research are sometimes unclear (Ginex, 2017). Melnyk and Fineout-Overholt (2019) note that EBP project implementation does not often involve being able to generalize findings because representative samples are not used. Rather, convenience samples of inpatients or clients are used to test initiatives for practice improvement. However, that distinction alone does not release nurses from gaining ethical approval (e.g., Institutional Review Board [IRB], Human Subjects Committee [HSC]). This is certainly required when disseminating results through publication or national presentations.

Obtain Institutional Review Board or Human Subjects Committee Approval

Whenever research is to be conducted that involves human subjects, prior approval must be gained from either an IRB or a HSC. This can be true for research studies or when measuring client outcomes elicited from EBP-implemented changes in nursing interventions (unless, perhaps, this is a QI effort that affects all clients equally and involves only one setting).

The reason for this approval is to safeguard the rights of prospective study participants (Melnyk & Fineout-Overholt, 2019). Each health department should have a committee or a gatekeeper, such as the health officer, who understands the federal guidelines for protecting subjects involved in research studies.

Sadly, one of the most egregious examples of exploitation of human subjects was a study carried out by the U.S. Public Health Service. The Tuskegee study, begun in 1932 and ended in 1972, sought to learn more about syphilis and to justify treatment services for blacks in Alabama (Centers for Disease Control and Prevention [CDC], 2015).

The 399 men with syphilis who participated in the study had agreed to be examined and treated. However, they were misled about the exact purpose of the study and were not given all of the facts; therefore, they were unable to truly give informed consent. Even after penicillin became the drug of choice for treatment of syphilis in 1947, the researchers failed to offer this treatment to the infected participants (CDC, 2015).

Later, a nurse historian found evidence that research on syphilis, also funded by the Public Health Service, was conducted in Guatemala beginning in 1946. However, these participants were purposely infected with syphilis, causing even greater outrage and a formal apology from President Barack Obama to Guatemalan President Alvaro Colom (Reverby, 2011; Rodriguez, 2013).

Questions remain regarding biospecimens from both the Guatemala and Tuskegee studies still being used in ongoing research, raising ethical concerns and issues regarding compensation to victims and their families (Rodriguez, 2013; Spector-Bagdady & Lombardo, 2018).

Because of earlier Nazi atrocities, the Nuremberg Code and the Declaration of Helsinki were adopted by the world scientific community and then revised in 1975 as a means of ensuring ethical research practices; the President's Council on Bioethics was established in 2001 after President Clinton apologized on behalf of the nation to the Tuskegee participants and their families in 1997 (Blais & Hayes, 2016; CDC, 2020).

The following ethical principles are widely viewed as basic protections for research participants (U.S. Department of Health and Human Services [USDHHS], 2016b). Freedom from harm or exploitation encompasses several aspects:

- First, no research can be done that may inflict permanent or serious harm.
- Second, the research study must be stopped if it becomes evident that harm may come to participants. Debriefing, or allowing participants to ask questions of the researcher at the conclusion of the study, as a means of protecting them from any unseen psychological harm, is also a component.
- There should be some identified benefits from participation in the research study, and any costs or risks should be clearly outlined, so that participants can more easily determine the cost–benefit ratio (referred to as *full disclosure*).
- Subjects should also be told that they are able to withdraw from the study at any time without prejudice or penalty (known as *self-determination*). Consent forms should include full disclosure of the nature of the study, the time and commitment required of subjects, the researcher's contact information, and a pledge of confidentiality (or *assurance of privacy*).

Vulnerable subjects, as determined by federal guidelines, include children; people with mental, emotional, or physical disabilities; institutionalized people (e.g., prisoners); pregnant women; and the terminally ill. Special care must be taken to ensure protection of vulnerable subjects. Data collection can only begin after approval has been obtained from the proper entities (USDHHS, 2016a).

Informed consent is an area where clear distinctions between research, EBP, and QI are problematic. If you change your practice to benefit your clients, based on the best evidence and your clinical judgment/knowledge of your clients, it would be cumbersome to ask for written consent from every patient before implementing changes. This might be part of a QI initiative or a trial EBP implementation. It is not feasible, and it is expected that professional practice changes will be made over time without consulting clients. However, clinical management oversight is expected to ensure that client rights are not violated. See Box 4-2.

Understanding Research Basics to Promote EBP

To fully integrate the principles of EBP, it is important to have a basic understanding of the research process. More in-depth information on this subject is available in nursing research texts (e.g., Polit & Beck, 2018), but a brief synopsis (Steps in the Research Process) is provided on thePoint®. EBP methods are encouraged over basic research, especially for practicing C/PHNs. Doctorally prepared nurses and public health professionals, sometimes in conjunction with practicing C/PHNs or health department staff, more often conduct traditional research studies (Balakas & Smith, 2016). Problems recently identified and studied within community/public health nursing include the following:

- Systematic review of nurse-led interventions with homeless populations (Weber, 2019)
- Systematic review of the impact of weight stigma on psychological and physiological health outcomes for overweight and obese adults (Wu & Berry, 2018)
- Qualitative meta-synthesis of PHNs' role in identifying and managing perinatal mental health problems (Noonan, Galvin, Doody, & Jomeen, 2017)
- Key informant recommendations for how to engage African American women in community-based health promotion (Holt, Johnson, & Zabler, 2018)

BOX 4-2 QSEN: FOCUS ON QUALITY

Patient-Centered Care for EBP and Ethics

Patient-Centered Care: Recognize the patient or designee as the source of control and full partner in providing compassionate and coordinated care based on respect for patient preferences, values, and needs (Cronenwett et al., 2007, p. 123).

(See https://qsen.org/competencies/pre-licensure-ksas/#quality_improvement for the knowledge, skills, and attitudes associated with this QSEN competency.)

You have all dealt with individual patients in acute care settings. Some of you have also worked closely with patient families. Now, you will be widening your lens to focus on larger groups of patients (e.g., aggregates) and communities (e.g., populations). How do these QSEN competencies apply to aggregates such as mothers addicted to drugs or to population groups such as the elderly in your community?

As health care continues to evolve, nurses are being asked to shift to systems thinking, rather than just focus on an individual patient. Leslie et al. (2018) noted that systems thinking was needed to improve the quality of health care, and that a quality health system was critical to the success of universal health care coverage around the world. We must solve the problems with quality and safety in health care. A systematic review of transitional care interventions that aimed to reduce hospital readmissions found that, to be successful, interventions needed to be flexible in response to patient needs, extend beyond the hospital stay, and include intensive discharge planning (Kansagara et al., 2016). High quality systems are patient centered and promote positive experiences for our clients. It is important that clients are treated with respect and courtesy, have their questions about care and medications answered and their needs met about requests for information or education, as well as health topics explained in a way that are easily understood (Cook et al., 2015).

For example, we will not effectively address the high rates of early readmission for heart failure patients by simply checking prescriptions before discharge for an individual patient or even giving them reminder magnets to put on their refrigerators in the hope that this will help them remember to take their medications. Studies of the effectiveness of home-based interventions reveal that they can reduce readmissions and ED visits for clinically complex patients (Coppa, Winchester, & Roberts, 2018), as well as reduce risk factors for those with recurring strokes or transient ischemic attacks (Towfight et al., 2017). Nurse home visits and disease management clinics can lower rates of all-cause mortality and hospital readmissions after heart failure hospitalizations (Van Spall et al., 2017).

We need to work with interdisciplinary teams to identify high-risk patients, prepare patients and their families for discharge, and then work with specialized programs that follow patients while they are at home to make sure they are continuing to adhere to medication and other intervention regimens (Rashid et al., 2017). Transitional care management has been shown to be effective for patients with multiple chronic conditions. Home visits by nurses reduced 30-day readmission rates, and after 6-month follow-up, the total cost of care for "highest risk patients" was significantly less (Jackson, Kasper, Williams, & DuBard, 2016, p. 163). Keeping care patient centered and demonstrating respect for our clients (individuals, families, aggregates, or populations) is a key to success.

What other problems do you see that could benefit from a broader focus on quality and safety?

Source: Cook et al. (2015); Coppa et al. (2018); Cronenwett et al. (2007); Jackson et al. (2016); Kansagara et al. (2016); Leslie et al. (2018); Rashid et al. (2017); Towfight et al. (2017); Van Spall et al. (2017).

- Early through late adolescents' evaluation of a Facebook page that provides sexual health education (Jones, Williams, Sipsma, & Patil, 2018)
- Noise concerns of residents living near fracking sites in Southwest Pennsylvania (Richburg & Slagley, 2017)
- Identifying community priorities for neighborhood livability: Engaging neighborhood residents to facilitate community assessment (Reyes & Meyer, 2020).
- Use of health care after piloting a homeless medical respite program (Biederman, Gamble, Wilson, Douglas, & Feigal, 2019)
- Association of elevated blood pressure in rural, low-income preschoolers with mother's hypertension during pregnancy (Johnson, Montgomery, & Ewell, 2018)
- Perceptions of PHNs and school nurses regarding HPV vaccination in Missouri (Rhodes, Visker, Cox, Forsyth, & Woolman, 2017)
- Using a mixed-methods approach to improve health through public housing resident and staff collaboration (Noonan, Hartman, Briggs, & Biederman, 2017)
- Individual health outcomes secondary to a nurse-led coalition-based health promotion program for underserved diverse populations (Simpson & Hass, 2019)
- Patient rationale for seeking HIV postexposure prophylaxis: qualitative study of a nurse-led program (O'Byrne, Orser, MacPherson, & Valela, 2018)
- Impact of expanded health insurance coverage for unauthorized pregnant women on prenatal care use (Atkins, Held, & Lindley, 2018)

A research question is a starting point for both traditional research and EBP methods. Although somewhat similar in purpose (to answer a question), there are fewer steps in the EBP process. Formulation of a PICOT question in EBP is a similar process to the research question outlined in the steps of the research process, especially in its specificity.

- Each of the research study titles above provides clues to the population of interest and the problem or intervention. Outcomes and time period can be discerned by reading the abstract and journal article (e.g., PICOT).
- Clear research questions, thorough review of the literature, human subjects protection, and a sound research design are factors to consider when evaluating the results of studies for incorporation into your practice.

IMPACT OF RESEARCH ON COMMUNITY/PUBLIC HEALTH AND NURSING PRACTICE

Research has the potential to have a significant impact on community/public health nursing in several ways, by affecting public policy and the community's health, the effectiveness of community/public health nursing practice in providing positive outcomes for our clients, and the status and influence of nursing as a profession.

Community/Public Health Practice and Patient Outcomes

Research, with policy or practice implications for addressing the health needs of aggregates, has been conducted on numerous topics (Ellen, Lavis, Horowitz, & Berglas, 2018). Many studies done by nurses and others have examined issues related to prevention, lifestyle change, quality of life, and health needs of specific at-risk populations (Box 4-3).

Public Policy and Community/Public Health

Research results can influence public policy, the quality of services, and, in turn, the public's health (Ellen et al., 2018). Examining the U.S. history of the paradigm change from positive feelings toward cigarette smoking to approval of tobacco control policies provides a powerful example of the use of research in changing health policies and promoting population health. This change began in a few states and has spread, to varying degrees, across all 50 states.

The Tobacco Control Scorecard was first developed in 2004. It statistically estimates the effectiveness of various policies on rates of smoking. A 2018 study updated these estimations of "policy effect size" and found that taxing cigarettes, smoke-free air laws, wide-ranging media bans, mass media campaigns, smoking cessation treatment programs, and "graphic health warnings" each play important roles in reducing rates of cigarette smoking, with large tax increases being the most powerful (Levy, Tam, Kuo, Fong, & Chaloupka, 2018, p. 454). They also noted that further research on regulation of the contents of tobacco products was necessary.

Projections about the outcomes and benefits of those policies is another research area helpful to policymakers: computer simulation models have been employed to determine which policy changes yield the most benefit in net total savings and lives saved. Michigan had enacted some tobacco control policies, yet had higher adult smoking prevalence than states with similar policies. Michigan had among the lowest in expenditures related to tobacco control.

- A study, using *SimSmoke* tobacco policy simulation model, examined the effect of tobacco control policies and found a relative reduction rate of 22% from 1993 to 2013 and a projected reduction rate of 30% by 2054.
- Of the 22% reduction, policies that raised taxes represented 44% of that reduction, smoke-free air policies 28%, and cessation treatment policies 26%. An additional 2% was associated with youth access policies.
- By 2054, about 234,000 smoking-related deaths are projected to have been prevented. If additional policies were to be enacted, it is estimated that 80,000 more lives could be saved (Levy, Huang, Havukai, & Meza, 2016).

In the United States, it is estimated that the total economic costs of smoking reach as high as $300 billion per year, split between direct medical care for adults ($170 billion) and lost productivity from premature death and second-hand smoke exposure ($156 billion). About $25.8 billion per year in taxes and legal settlements are received by states (Hall & Doran, 2016).

BOX **4-3** EVIDENCE-BASED PRACTICE

A Change of Position

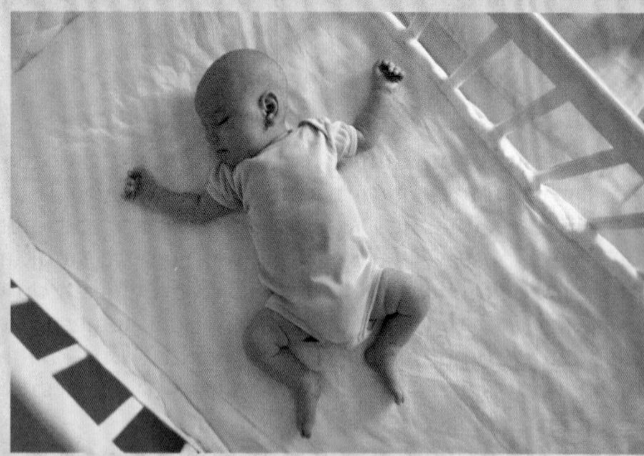

For generations, mothers were told that babies would be at risk of aspiration if they were put to sleep on their backs. Why did this change? In the late 1980s, research indicated that prone positioning of infants was related to greater incidences of sudden infant death syndrome (SIDS), according to a group at the National Institute of Child Health and Human Development (NIH) who conducted an epidemiologic study examining SIDS risk factors (Hoffman, Damus, Hillman, & Krongrad, 1988). In the early 1990s, an expert panel from the same institute and the American Academy of Pediatrics concluded that infant sleeping positioning was an important factor in prevention of SIDS, and a recommendation was made for parents to place their infants on their backs when sleeping. The *Back to Sleep* campaign began in 1994 (National Institutes of Health, n.d.a). C/PHNs have been instrumental in education about SIDS and are often sources of support for families who have lost infants to SIDS (Stastny, Keens, & Alkon, 2016).

Since then, the incidence of SIDS has continued to drop in the United States—from 130.3 deaths in 1990 to 38.0 deaths per 100,000 live births in 2016. The most dramatic drop occurred shortly after the Back to Sleep campaign was instituted (Lambert, Parks, & Shapiroi-Mendoza, 2018). Despite this decrease, SIDS is the fourth leading cause of infant death (Newberry, 2019). And there remains an ethnic difference in incidence with American Indians having a rate of 205.8 deaths and non-Hispanic Black infants 181.0, compared to lower rates for non-Hispanic Whites and for Hispanics (see charts, CDC, 2019).

The term sudden unexpected infant death (SUID) encompasses SIDS, accidental suffocation and strangulation in bed, or infant death due to unknown causes (CDC, 2019). Research continues with studies showing:

- Association of bed sharing and/or smoking with increased SUID (MacFarlane et al., 2018).
- Increased risk factors for SIDS with maternal smoking and being a twin (Friedmann, Dahdouh, Kugler, Mimran & Balayla, 2017).
- Pathology-based study of medullary astrogliosis demonstrated differences in the intensity of "glial fibrillary acidic protein staining" in specific medullar regions between infants sleeping alone or bed-sharing indicating differing mechanisms for death, such as asphyxiation with infant bed sharing (Spinelli, Byard, Van Den Heuvel, & Collins-Praino, 2018, para. 27).
- CDC monitoring from 2009 to 2015 found that between 12.2% and 33.8% of respondents reported nonsupine sleep positions, 61.4% bed sharing with infants, and 38.5% using soft bedding such as bumper pads and thick blankets. Results showed cultural and racial differences as factors (Bombard et al., 2018).
- The importance of collaborative translation of knowledge with our clients (Middlemiss, Cowan, Kildare, & Seddio, 2017). Evidence from U.S. Indian Health Services and New Zealand SIDS prevention programs show that better responses occur when we align our messages of risk, safety, and practices with cultural groups' long-held value and norms.
  - Especially with groups where bed sharing is a norm, the message focuses on keeping infant sleep spaces safe and avoiding asphyxiation, while acknowledging that some families don't adhere to the avoidance of bed sharing.
  - Families and friends are included in the conversation about safe practices to promote their ownership of the message and how it impacts infant health.
- Current recommendations from the American Academy of Pediatrics (AAP, 2016) to reduce the risk of SIDS and other sleep-related infant deaths advise parents to always
  - Place sleeping infants in a supine position (not on side or stomach) until age 1.
  - Use a firm sleeping surface (no pillows or quilts under the baby) and no sitting devices for prolonged sleep especially in infants under 4 months.
  - Keep soft objects (stuffed toys, pillows, bumper pads, blankets) away from infant's sleep area.
  - Place infant in own bed, in parent's room near parent's bed for first 6 to 12 months (no bed sharing).
  - Breast-feeding is recommended.
  - Avoid maternal smoking during and after pregnancy and infant's exposure to secondhand smoke.
  - Avoid alcohol and illicit drug use.
  - Offer a pacifier at sleep time throughout the first year of life (it has been shown to reduce the risk of SIDS).
- Avoid overheating (do not overbundle babies, watch for sweating) or cover their heads.
- Encourage "tummy time" to aid in development and reduce incidence of positional plagiocephaly (uneven, flat head).
- Get regular prenatal care.
- Immunize infants according to CDC and AAP guidelines.
- Avoid the use of commercial devices that are inconsistent with safe sleep guidelines (e.g., wedge pillows, carbon dioxide dispersion mattresses). These may be marketed as effective in reducing SIDS cases, but there is not sufficient proof of efficacy.

1. *Do your community/public health clients put their babies to sleep on their backs? If not, ask them about their concerns, including any cultural norms for sleeping arrangements.*
2. *How can you best approach them about the beneficial effects of following AAP's safe infant sleeping recommendations?*

Source: AAP (2016); Bombard et al. (2018); CDC (2019); Friedmann et al. (2017); Hoffman et al. (1988); Lambert et al. (2018); Middlemiss et al. (2017); National Institutes of Health (n.d.a); Newberry (2019); Spinelli et al. (2018); Stastny et al. (2016).

Nursing's Professional Status and Influence

Another way in which research has a significant impact on community/public health nursing is in its potential to enhance nursing's status and influence. As community/public health nursing research sheds light on the critical health needs of at-risk populations, exposes deficiencies in the health care system, demonstrates more efficient and cost-effective methods for delivering services, and documents the effectiveness of nursing interventions, the profession will gain a stronger voice and have a greater impact on health policy and programs. After all, C/PHNs have always been advocates for their clients and promoted policies that improved health.

Some examples of research that influences public health nursing's professional status include

- A scoping review of environmental health nursing research (Polivka & Chaudry, 2018)
- Evidence of public health nursing effectiveness: A realist review (Swider, Levin, & Reising, 2017)
- An academic practice partnership: Building capacity to meet sexual health education policy requirements of a public-school system (Cygan, McNaughton, Reising, & Reid, 2018)
- Fluoride varnish application, a QI project implemented in a rural pediatric practice (Gnaedinger, 2018)
- Sexually transmitted disease services and third-party payer reimbursement: Attitudes, knowledge, and current practices among 60 health departments/districts. Why does this matter to PHNs? (Kovar & Bynum, 2019)
- Development of a comprehensive infection control program for a short-term shelter serving trafficked women (Jones et al., 2019)
- A community-based participatory research (CBPR) approach to finding community strengths and challenges to prevent youth suicide and substance abuse (Holliday, Wynne Katz, Ford, & Barbosa-Leiker, 2018)
- Chicago public school nurses examine barriers to school asthma care coordination (Pappalardo et al., 2019)

These examples reflect the diversity of research studies and EBP implementation across community/public health nursing areas. From the QI project of applying fluoride varnish for a 4-month period using a protocol developed by the California Dental Association for infants and toddlers (Gnaedinger, 2018) to the large-scale survey of staff members in 60 rural and urban health departments regarding knowledge, attitudes, and billing practices for sexually transmitted disease services that has both policy and funding implications, C/PHNs are actively involved in promoting research and EBP and highlighting the importance of nursing knowledge.

The CBPR study that involves searching for the needs of a tribal community in determining programs and services that address problems on the reservation reflects the partnership and engagement of nurse researchers, community members, and other stakeholders in decision-making and developing research knowledge and interventions (Holliday et al., 2018). This exemplifies the definition of **community-based participatory research (CBPR)** as described by Jull, Giles, and Graham (2017).

Strong documentation supports the effectiveness of community/public health nursing interventions. Nurses in the community setting must provide empirical proof of their worth as professionals while serving the needs of their clients. This kind of information must be made visible if it is to influence legislators, planners, administrators, and other decision-makers in health care. As visibility increases, nursing's status and influence will grow.

The Community/Public Health Nurse's Role in Research

Community/public health nursing has a focus on health promotion and disease prevention and providing services across the lifespan where people live, work, and learn. C/PHNs also focus on the development of community capacity building for health and work with partnerships, coalitions, and policy makers to promote a healthier environment.

- C/PHNs have two important responsibilities with respect to research in community/public health: to apply research findings to practice (EBP) and to conduct or participate in nursing research.
- Because research results provide essential information for improving health policy and the delivery of health services, C/PHNs must be knowledgeable consumers of research. That is, they need to be able to critically examine research reports and apply study findings to improve the public's health.

C/PHNs have many opportunities to apply the results of other investigators' research and systematic reviews, but a necessary prerequisite is to be informed about research findings. As an essential part of their role, C/PHNs must read the journals focusing on community/public health nursing. Nursing agencies and employment sites in community/public health can encourage nurses to become more knowledgeable about research findings by subscribing to journals and circulating them among staff, by holding seminars to discuss recent research results, and by promoting nurses' application of research findings in their practice.

Although the amount of community/public health nursing research is expanding and its quality is improving, many more C/PHNs need to conduct research and participate in EBP. An increasing number of nurses have developed skill in research through advanced preparation, and they are conducting investigations related to aggregate health needs. Other C/PHNs work collaboratively with trained investigators on a variety of research projects affecting community/public health.

Whether initiated by the nurse or involving the nurse as a team member, these projects are an opportunity to influence the types of research questions that are addressed and the ways in which the research is carried out, factors that ultimately affect the community's health (Melnyk & Fineout-Overholt, 2019).

VALUES AND ETHICS IN COMMUNITY/PUBLIC HEALTH NURSING

EBP includes not only the research process but also the knowledge and long-standing values nurses bring to their practice. According to the classic treatise by Carper

(1978), this is the art of nursing. Our personal history and experiences contribute to our understanding of what it means to be a good nurse.

Values and beliefs support

- Your decisions about the right course of action to take
- How to be just and fair in dealing with others
- What outcomes you deem to be right

Nursing, like many other professions, has ethical codes that guide decision-making and provide a framework for thinking about the moral dimensions of practice issues. Nursing has had an ethical code for practice since 1910, when Gettner published "The Nightingale Pledge." This evolved into the current "Code of Ethics for Nurses," as the American Nurses Association (ANA) has updated the code to reflect current issues and ideologies. The latest document was approved in 2015 (Box 4-4). In this chapter, we consider the role of nurses in ethics and discuss recent issues that you may encounter in your community/public health practice.

The Code of Ethics for Nurses:

- Is based on the values of respect and dignity for all individual as well as society at large
- Includes a mandate to respect the values and beliefs of each individual nurse
- Provides an essential first step in ethical decision-making by helping us to explore the ethical values that shape our practice, a process called values clarification (see thePoint for resources on values and values clarification).

Just as EBP is the result of the rigorous application of scientific method, our philosophy of nursing is based on clarity about our ethical code of practice, informing a logical system for moral reasoning, which grounds practice with integrity within the context of social justice (ANA, 2015).

Nurses in public health focus their practice on providing care for populations within our community of concern. When the needs of the individual must be evaluated in light of the needs of the larger group, this can lead to ethical concerns. Using an objective ethical reasoning process assists with separating the myriad of social, political, and economic issues from the actual ethical concerns (ANA, 2010, 2015; Fowler, 2015). Consider the following situations:

- You are providing health care to a population of migrant farm workers whose housing lacks adequate sanitation and refrigeration. You recognize that this is a valid health and safety issue. However, when you report the situation to your supervisor, you are told that since these farm workers are here illegally, challenging these conditions may bring about negative consequences for the workers. What would you do?
- What if you were working in a homeless shelter and were told to evict someone who would not agree to take a tuberculin skin test? You agree that residents should comply with this demand, but would you hesitate to implement the eviction if the resident were a frail older adult or the teenage mother of a newborn?

BOX 4-4 Code of Ethics for Nurses—Provisions, Approved as of January 6, 2015

The nurse, in all professional relationships, practices with compassion and respect for the inherent dignity, worth, and uniqueness of every individual, unrestricted by considerations of social or economic status, personal attributes, or the nature of their health problems.

1. The nurse respects the unique attributes of every person, practices with compassion and respect for each person's self-worth and dignity.
2. "The nurse's primary commitment is to the patient, whether an individual, family, group, community, or population" (p. v).
3. The nurse promotes, advocates for, and strives to protect the health, safety, and rights of the patient.
4. The nurse is responsible and accountable for individual nursing practice and determines actions consistent with the nurse's obligation to provide optimum patient care, with a focus on health promotion.
5. The nurse owes the same duties to self as to others, including the responsibility to preserve integrity and safety, to "maintain competence, and to continue personal and professional growth" (p. v).
6. The nurse is a key member of the team in maintaining and improving ethical environments for both patient care and the work of nursing in the provision of safe and quality care.
7. The nurse plays a leadership role in advancement of the profession through contributions to practice, education, administration, and knowledge development and most importantly the development of health policy and nursing policy.
8. The nurse works together with "other health professionals and the public" to protect and promote human rights and diminish health disparity and improve health diplomacy in the community and globally (p. v).
9. The profession of nursing, as represented by associations and their members, is responsible for articulating nursing values, for maintaining the reliability and integrity of the nursing profession and its practice, and for shaping social policy.

Adapted from American Nurses Association (ANA) (2015).

Within the United States, many marginalized people are failed by the health care system or may go without any health care at all. At the same time, affluent individuals enjoy a plethora of health care options, including preventive screenings and health promotion classes. C/PHNs often are confronted by this disparity when making ethical decisions about client care. Social justice, human rights, and equality are hallmarks of public health nursing ethics (see more in Chapters 13, 23, and 27).

Progress in the United States often is linked to the exploitation of people in less-developed countries, and this contributes to widening disparities in health, wealth, and human rights. Distributive justice, or the fair allocation of goods and services, comes into play (discussed later in this chapter and in Chapter 23). Failure to respond to such global challenges only leads to greater poverty and deprivation, continuing conflict, escalating migration, and the spread of infectious disease, all further adding to our ethical dilemmas.

Advances in technology also contribute to ethical dilemmas. For example, electronic health records make client information readily accessible, thus raising issues of confidentiality, clients' rights, issues of empowerment, and informed consent (Vezyridis & Timmons, 2015). Sensitive information is now frequently stored electronically and may be accessed through unethical means (Davis, 2018). Technology also forces nurses to confront the issues of genetic testing and stem cell research (Box 4-5), as well as assisted suicide and euthanasia (Katz, 2015). Further ethical questions arise regarding limb transplants, such as hand transplants and the decisions about who is to receive them, as well as what happens to tissues removed during biopsy or surgery (Cooney et al., 2018). Ethical issues in nursing practice are changing at a rapid pace, especially in oncology nursing, where the benefits of genetically sound evidence-based care need to be contemplated with ethical considerations (Beamer, 2017).

Underlying every issue and influencing every ethical and professional decision are **values**. Ethics and values are inextricably intertwined in professional decision-making, because values are the criteria by which decisions are made. Ethical decision-making is central to nursing practice (Milliken, 2018). The topics of values and ethics are each covered below.

BOX 4-5 Immortal Cells, Ethical Dilemma

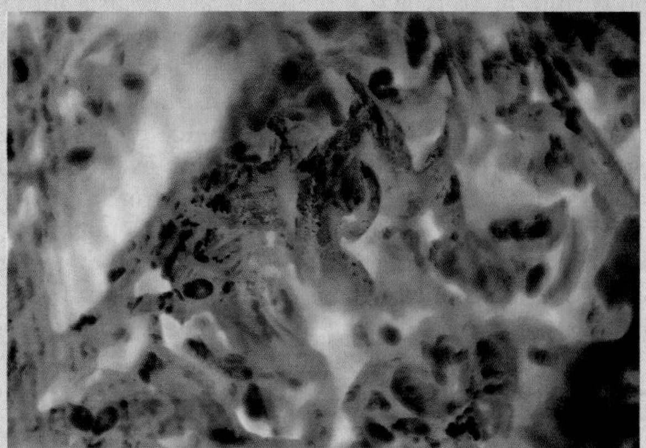

Stained HeLa cervical cancer cells under the microscope.

How would you feel if tissues or cells taken from you during surgery or a routine biopsy were subsequently used in health research without your knowledge or permission (or remuneration)? That happened to Henrietta Lacks, a black woman from Baltimore, whose cells (known as HeLa cells) were the first immortal human cells and used in the development of the field of virology. HeLa cells were tested in the first space missions to determine zero gravity's effects and were vital to the development of polio and hepatitis B vaccines, as well as chemotherapy, in vitro fertilization, cloning, and gene mapping (Skloot, 2011). These cells, taken from a biopsy of her cervix a few months before she died of cervical cancer in 1951, were useful in the development of medications for leukemia, herpes, hemophilia, and influenza. They have been used in innumerable studies around the world to test the effects of massive radiation (e.g., nuclear blasts), hormones, vitamins, steroids, tuberculosis, salmonella, and hemorrhagic fever. HeLa cells were also instrumental in many historic scientific discoveries (e.g., cigarettes caused lung cancer, how cancer cells grew differently from normal cells, how HIV infected cells) and continue to be used today in scientific research. Although this happened in the 1950s, today, it is still often considered legal for a researcher to use tissues removed from your body for scientific research without your consent. It has been considered by law to be "abandoned waste" and may be used for gain without the knowledge, consent, or reimbursement to the donor. A recent revision to the "Common Rule," a federal regulation that governs researchers and human subjects, failed to substantially change the rules on human specimen collection and use (Jaschik, 2017).

Source: Jaschik (2017); Skloot (2011); "The Immortal Life of Henrietta Lacks," produced by Oprah Winfrey et al. and released in 2017 (IMDb, 2019, retrieved from https://www.imdb.com/title/tt5686132/).

VALUES

What are values in nursing? According to Baillie (2017), these are

- Respect and dignity
- Commitment to quality of care
- Compassion
- Improving lives
- Working together for patients

Standards for Behavior

In general, moral values (Kinneging, 2016)

- Function as standards that guide actions and behavior in daily situations
- Act as a code of conduct for living one's life
- Become internalized to inform a personal code of conduct
- Undergird behavioral norms
- Act as a voice of conscience

Values often remain relatively stable over time, persisting to provide continuity to personal and social existence. Some values endure over time, but others may change as societal norms evolve (Bongiorno, 2018). Social life in the community requires standards within the individual as well as an agreement about standards among groups of individuals (Pereira, 2015). A group's culture provides a set of enduring values. We organize values into a hierarchical system in which certain values have more weight or importance than others. As an individual confronts social situations throughout life, isolated values learned in early childhood come into competition with other values, requiring a weighing of one value against another. Concern for others' welfare, for instance, competes with self-interest. Through experience and maturation, the individual integrates values learned within different contexts into systems in which each value is ordered relative to other values (Adams et al., 2018). More recent research has examined moral regulation within the framework of avoidance versus approach motivation (Lee, Padilla-Walker, & Nelson, 2015). For example, if you used duty as a basis for action, these would be proscriptive moral emotions. Duty is a consequential emotion, where you would think about concrete negative consequences to an action. For example, what would happen if you did not study well for an exam in nursing school? Prescriptive moral emotions might focus more abstractly and in a positive manner on what ought to be done; these might inspire you to study so that you can be a better nurse at the bedside. Think about which beliefs or values inspire you to do well in nursing school (Cornwall & Higgins, 2015).

Reference

- Values have a reference quality. That is, they may refer to end states of existence called **terminal values**, such as spiritual salvation, peace of mind, or world peace, or they may refer to modes of conduct called **instrumental values**, such as confidentiality, keeping promises, and honesty. Sometimes values may conflict (Husted, Husted, Scotto, & Wolf, 2015). (Go to thePoint for a figure depicting factors that influence terminal values.)
- A nurse may experience a conflict between two moral values, such as whether to act honestly (tell a client about a fatal diagnosis) or to act respectfully (honor the family's request not to tell the client).

Preference

A value may show preference for one mode of behavior over another, such as exercise over inactivity, or it may show a preference for one end state over another, such as physical fitness and leanness over sedentary lifestyle and obesity. The preferred end state, or mode of behavior, is located higher in the personal value hierarchy.

Value Systems

Value systems generally are considered organizations of beliefs that are of relative importance in guiding individual behavior (Hultman, 2017). Instead of being guided by single or isolated values, behavior at any point in time (or over a period of time) is influenced by multiple or changing clusters of values. It is important to understand how values are integrated into a person's total belief system, how values assume a place in a hierarchy of values, and how this hierarchical system changes over time.

Hierarchical System of Values

Learned values are integrated into an organized system of values, and each value has an ordered priority with respect to other values (Hultman, 2017). For example, a person may place a higher value on physical comfort than on exercising. This system of ordered priority is stable enough to reflect the continuity of someone's personality and behavior within culture and society, yet it is sufficiently flexible to allow a reordering of value priorities in response to changes in the environment or social setting (e.g., society's emphasis on physical fitness and youth) or changes based on personal experiences (e.g., diagnosis of type 2 diabetes). Behavioral change would be regarded as the visible response to a reordering of values within an individual's hierarchical value system.

Conflict Between Values in a System

Nurses often enter patient and community situations that activate several values in their system of beliefs. Because not all of the activated values are compatible with one another, conflict between values occurs.

- This conflict between values is a part of the decision-making process and resolving these value conflicts is crucial to making good decisions. C/PHNs face such conflicts of values when caring for patients whose determinants of health create a situation in which they must decide how to use scarce resources for care (Blacksher, 2015).
- This can be a struggle when patients want the freedom to choose how to live their life but don't want to suffer, either. One example is how the smoker with chronic obstructive pulmonary disease wants home health visits but refuses to quit smoking. Even within a single community agency, nurses may find that they prioritize client service or programming values differently.

Some values seem to consistently triumph over others, persisting as stronger directives for individual behavior. Providing quality health care for all without sacrificing the basic rights of a few is an ongoing ethical struggle for most people (Martin 2017; Strair, 2017). It is the hierarchical system and changes to that system of values that determine, in part, how conflicts are resolved and how decisions are made. One way to understand the influence of values on your own behavior, as well as on that of community/public health clients, and to properly prioritize them is to use various values clarification techniques in decision-making.

- **Values clarification** is a process that helps to identify the personal and professional values that guide your actions, by prompting you to examine what you believe about the worth, truth, or beauty of any object, thought, or behavior and where this belief ranks compared with your other values (see thePoint for activities to help you identify your values).
- Values clarification may be helpful for patients making decisions for treatment and screening processes, such as whether to choose a certain drug or treatment that is in keeping with the patients' lifestyle (Palacio, Kirolos, & Tamariz, 2015).

ETHICS

How is ethics defined and what is meant by the term *ethical*? The *Merriam Webster Online Dictionary* (2019) defines **ethics** as "the principles of conduct governing a group" (para. 4). Long-standing values are central to any consideration of ethics or ethical decision-making. Most nurses easily recognize the moral crisis in extreme decisions such as futile care and abortion dilemmas. Less obvious moral dilemmas often found in the routine practice of community/public health nursing are not always easy to identify or analyze from an ethical perspective. What constitutes an ethical problem is not always obvious.

- Ethics may be viewed as behaviors governed by a set of principles based on long-standing values.

- Ethics are often idealized as "what ought to be."
- **Ethical decision-making** means making a choice that is consistent with a moral code and can be justified from an ethical perspective.
- Of necessity, the decision-maker must exercise moral judgment.
- The term "**moral**" refers to conforming to a standard that is right and good.
- C/PHNs become "moral agents" by making decisions that have direct and indirect consequences for the welfare of their patient population.
- **Bioethics** refers to using ethical principles and methods of decision-making in questions involving health care issues, while keeping the centrality of the patient as the focus of practice (Vaughn, 2017).
- In public health, the population is the patient.

Public Health Ethics

Protection and promotion of health are at the core of community/public health nursing. Public health ethics is "a systematic process to clarify, prioritize, and justify possible courses of public health action based on ethical principles, values and beliefs of stakeholders, and scientific and other information" (CDC, 2017, para. 1).

- Specific ethical principles apply to public health in that we advocate for populations such as healthy communities and the equitable distribution of limited resource. Ethical decisions seek to balance individual rights and the collective good in the use of resources.
- Community/public health nursing often bases its practice on values related to preventing disease or harm and developing community input into solving problems while respecting individual rights. A major moral value is the empowerment of the disenfranchised and equal access to resources.
- Promoting health, protecting confidentiality (except in cases in which disclosure is justified), and collaborating or partnering with other community agencies are viewed as universal practices.
- Other principles include respecting diverse values or beliefs and working effectively with different cultural groups to enhance the social and physical environment while employing competent public health professionals.
- Public health is most often concerned with distribution of resources and shaping behavior and thoughts, which may include resources, such as clean water, and constraints, such as quarantine.
- We need to keep in mind the responsibility to global justice when implementing public health programs and policy (Jennings, 2015). Without care for global justice, there may be an uneasy balance between individual and public interests and rights. See Chapter 16.

A framework is applied in public health ethics inquiry. Three core functions of this inquiry include

1. Identifying and clarifying the ethical dilemma
2. Analyzing it in terms of alternative courses of action and their consequences
3. Resolving the dilemma by deciding which course of action best incorporates and balances the guiding principles and values (CDC, 2017, para. 5)

Identifying Ethical Situations

Ethics involves making evaluative judgments. To be ethically responsible in the practice of community/public health nursing, it is important to develop the ability to recognize evaluative judgments as they are made and implemented in nursing practice. Nurses must be able to distinguish between evaluative and nonevaluative judgments.

Evaluative statements involve judgments of value, rights, duties, and responsibilities. Examples are "Parents should never strike their children" and "It is the duty of every citizen to vote." Among the words to watch for are verbs such as *want, desire, refer, should,* or *ought* and nouns such as *benefit, harm, duty, responsibility, right,* or *obligation.*

Sometimes, the evaluations are expressed in terms that are not direct expressions of evaluations but clearly are functioning as value judgments. Winland-Brown et al. (2015) provide useful clinical applications of the ANA code of ethics and refer to the obligations or duties of nurses to both patient and self (see Box 4-4). Another important step is to distinguish between moral and nonmoral evaluations.

Moral evaluations refer to judgments that conform to standards of what is right and good. Moral evaluations assess human actions, institutions, or character traits rather than inanimate objects, such as parks or architectural structures. They are prescriptive–proscriptive beliefs having certain characteristics separating them from other evaluations such as aesthetic judgments, personal preferences, or matters of taste. Moral evaluations also have distinctive characteristics (Elemers, 2017):

- Morality and sociability impact social judgment. We want to be able to anticipate others' actions that could lead to benefit or harm or their skill and ability.
- Values possess universality or reflect a standpoint that applies to everyone. They are evaluations that everyone in principle ought to be able to make and understand, even if some individuals, in fact, do not.
- Moral evaluations avoid giving a special place to a person's own welfare. They have a focus that keeps others in view or at least considers one's own welfare on a par with that of others.

Moral evaluations, such as "parents should take care of their children," meet these criteria. A nonmoral evaluation, such as "Mrs. X has five children," does not evoke a moral judgment of Mrs. X but instead is an assessment of her family composition.

Resolving Moral Conflicts and Ethical Dilemmas

When judgments involve moral values, conflicts are inevitable. In clinical practice, the nurse may be faced with moral conflicts, such as the choice between preserving the welfare of one set of clients over that of others. Examples include the following:

- The nurse may have to choose whether to keep a promise of confidentiality to persons who are infected by HIV when they continue to have unprotected sex with unknowing partners.
- The nurse may have to choose between protecting the interests of colleagues or the interests of the employing institution by reporting a nurse who has made a medication error but has failed to report that error.

Each of these decisions involves an **ethical dilemma**, which occurs when moral values conflict with one another, causing the nurse to face a choice with equally attractive or undesirable alternatives (Robichaux, 2017). Ethical dilemmas create difficult decision-making, even in ordinary nursing situations.

Decision-Making Frameworks

To resolve ethical dilemmas or the conflict between moral values in community/public health nursing practice and to provide morally accountable nursing service, several frameworks for ethical decision-making have been proposed. Among these frameworks, three key steps are considered as fundamental to choosing between alternative courses of action that reflect moral reasoning (Martin, 2017). These steps separate questions of fact from questions of value, identify both clients' and nurse's value systems, and consider ethical principles and concepts (Box 4-6).

The identification of clients' values and those of other persons involved in conflict situations is an important part of ethical decision-making (Box 4-7).

An ethical decision-making framework that was first described by Guo in 2008 and that is referred to as the DECIDE model is initially useful in determining the problem and reviewing options. What is missing from this model is the patients' preference, a vital component (Nelson, 2015). For public health, patients' preference may be replaced with the harm-versus-benefit argument. The DECIDE model includes the following steps:

1. D—*Define the problem (or problems)*. What are the key facts of the situation? Who is involved? What are their rights and duties and your rights and duties?
2. E—*Ethical review*. What ethical principles have a bearing on the situation, and which principle or principles should be given priority in making a decision?
3. C—*Consider the options*. What options do you have in the situation? What alternative courses of action exist? What help, means, and methods do you need to use?
4. I—*Investigate outcomes*. Given each available option, what consequences are likely to follow from each course of action open to you? Which is the most ethical thing to do?
5. D—*Decide on action*. Having chosen the best available option, determine a specific action plan, set clear objectives, and then act decisively and effectively.
6. E—*Evaluate results*. Having initiated a course of action, assess how things progress, and when concluded, evaluate carefully whether you achieved your goals.

BOX 4-6 A Framework for Ethical Decision-Making

Step 1. Clarify the ethical dilemma.

- Whose problem is it?
- Who should make the decision?
- Who is affected by the decision?
- What ethical principles are related to the problem?

Step 2. Gather additional data.

- Have as much information about the situation as possible.
- Be up to date on any legal cases related to the ethical question.

Step 3. Identify options.

- Brainstorm with others to identify as many alternatives as possible.
- The more options identified, the more likely it is that an acceptable solution will be found.

Step 4. Make a decision (choose from the options identified).

- Determine the most acceptable option—that is, the one more feasible than others.

Step 5. Act (carry out the decision).

- It may be necessary to collaborate with others to implement the decision and identify options.

Step 6. Evaluate (after acting on a decision, evaluate its impact).

- Was the best course of action chosen?
- Would an alternative have been better? Why?
- What went right and what went wrong? Why?

Note: Although legal requirements or social expectations may sway a decision one way or another, they are extrinsic to the ethical analysis and should not be confused with right and wrong. What is legal and what is expected are not necessarily right and wrong.

Other frameworks can be used. The framework for ethical decision-making shown in Box 4-6 helps to organize thoughts and acts as a guide through the decision-making process. The steps help to determine a course of action, with heavy responsibility at the evaluation level: here the outcomes need to be judged and decisions repeated or rejected in future situations. Box 4-6 also summarizes several views in the field on ethical decision-making. This framework advocates keeping multiple values in tension before resolution of conflict and action on the part of the nurse. It suggests that it is not capable of resolution until all possible alternative actions have been explored. Three tests may be helpful to your decision-making process (Husted et al., 2015):

BOX **4-7** STORIES FROM THE FIELD

Independence Versus Safety

C/PHNs encounter value differences every day, and value differences, in turn, create ethical problems. Consider, for example, the dilemma faced by one nurse in Seattle on her first home visit to an older adult male, Mr. Bell, referred by concerned neighbors. This 82-year-old gentleman was homebound and living alone with severe arthritis under steadily deteriorating conditions. Overgrown shrubs and vines covered the yard and house, making access impossible except through the back door. A wood burning stove in the kitchen was the sole source of heat. The kitchen, along with a corner of the dining room, constituted Mr. Bell's living quarters. The remainder of the once-lovely three-bedroom home, including the bathroom, was layered with dust, unused. His bed was a cot in the dining room; his toilet, a 2-lb coffee can under the cot. Unbathed, unshaven, and existing on food and firewood brought by neighbors, Mr. Bell seemed to be living in deplorable conditions. Yet he prized his independence so highly that he adamantly refused to leave. Mr. Bell had one son living in a neighboring state but had little contact with him.

The conflict of values between Mr. Bell's choice to live independently and the nurse's value of having him in a safer living situation raises several ethical questions. When do health practitioners or family members have the right or duty to override an individual's preferences? When do neighbors' rights (Mr. Bell's home was an eyesore and his care was a source of anxiety for his neighbors) supersede one homeowner's rights? Should the nurse be responsible when family members can help but won't take action?

In this case, the nurse entering Mr. Bell's home applied her values of respect for the individual and his right to autonomy even at the risk of public safety. Not until he fell and broke a hip would he reluctantly agree to be moved into a nursing home.

1. *What are Mr. Bell's values? What are the values of neighbors who are concerned about him but feel that they can no longer care for him?*
2. *What are the nurse's values? What are the values of the nurse's employer?*
3. *What are society's values? What ethical principle does this story most exemplify?*

- Impartiality test—Did you use an objective method that examined whether the ethical principles were upheld?
- Universalizability test—Is this decision one that you can generalize to most people from a rational point of view?
- Context test—Did you examine the multiple perspectives of this issue, engage the team in your decision-making process, and consider patient preference where possible?

Final resolution of the ethical conflict occurs through a conscious choice of action, even though some values would be overridden by other stronger, presumably more moral values. Conflict resolution techniques can be helpful to the process, including developing empathy, reframing, reflective listening, and assertive messaging (Martin, 2017). Communication and conflict are discussed in Chapter 10.

Basic Values that Guide Decision-Making

When applying a decision-making framework, certain values influence community/public health nursing decisions. Three basic human values are considered key to guiding decision-making in the provider–client relationship: self-determination, well-being, and equity. The resolution may not be absolute, as there are many lenses with which to view an ethical dilemma, but using a consistent, objective method of analysis is vital (Box 4-8).

Self-Determination

The value of self-determination or individual autonomy is a person's exercise of the capacity to shape and pursue personal plans for life.

BOX **4-8** Confronting Challenges for Ethical Decision-Making in Nursing

Nurses in every specialty area regularly face ethical situations and dilemmas such as end-of-life decisions, patient privacy, or organizational policies (Rainer, Schneider, & Lorenz, 2018). It is the nature of our profession. Ethical sensitivity and awareness are important characteristics for effective nursing, and empathy is needed in order to build trust and rapport with our clients (Adams, 2018; Milliken & Grace, 2017b). As we strive to work through ethical dilemmas, we should consider some common challenges:

- Routine Actions—Nursing often values routines or "the way we have always done it." This mindset can prevent us from seeking important information and correctly considering ethical principles.
- Social Structures—Organizational constraints (e.g., procedures, policies) may limit actions and individual beliefs.
- Rule of Thumb Decision-Making—Nurses often have set ways of handling common challenges, and this may obscure the full picture in novel or complex ethical situations (e.g., cultural differences, new technologies/advances).
- Moral Disengagement—Because we are individuals, moral reasoning and self-awareness are varied. But when we or a colleague use minimizing behaviors (e.g., ignoring consequences, displacing responsibility, demeaning or labeling clients or coworkers), we need to pause and reflect on our levels of empathy and engagement and refocus our efforts.
- Situational Factors—Health care workers can have a great deal of power over clients, and the use of scientific jargon, professional detachment, and undue persuasion (piling on) can lead to unethical outcomes. Whistleblowers should be protected as they often provide a needed check to our system of health care (Niemi, 2016).

Source: Adams (2018); Milliken & Grace (2017b); Niemi (2016); Rainer et al. (2018).

Respect for self-determination:

- Is instrumentally valued because self-judgment about a person's goals and choices is conducive to an individual's sense of well-being
- Is the basis for informed consent
- Is based on the belief that better outcomes will result when autonomy is held in high regard
- Can maximize the outcomes of enhanced self-concept, enhanced health-promoting behaviors, and enhanced quality of care
- Is emphasized in the United States but does not receive the same emphasis in all societies or ethnic groups
- In health care contexts, is of such high ethical importance in U.S. society that it overrides practitioner determinations in many situations (Ryan & Deci, 2017)

Client empowerment is an approach that differs from the paternalistic approach to health care, in which decisions are made for, rather than with, the client; instead, it enables patients and professionals to work in partnership (Akpotor & Johnson, 2018). Many physicians and other health providers, including C/PHNs, fail to recognize the high value attributed to self-determination by many consumers or the differences in views of self-determination among ethnic groups. The freedom of our patients must be respected and integrated into the matrix of health care decisions in any encounter or program (Carter, Entwistle, & Little, 2015; Resnik, 2018).

The conflict between provider and consumer may be broader. When self-determination deteriorates into self-interest, it poses a major roadblock to equitable health care. Self-interest is the fulfillment of one's own desires, without regard for the greater good. Consumers mostly have to fend for themselves when they encounter the world of for-profit health care, just as they do in other commercial markets. This "buyers beware" pattern contributes to that deterioration.

When providing health care, the nurse should nurture self-determination and encourage client's personal responsibility for health care decisions. This includes informing clients of options and the reasoning behind all recommendations. Yet self-determination and personal autonomy at times are impermissible or even impossible. For example, society must impose restrictions on unacceptable client choices, such as child abuse and other abusive behaviors, or situations in which clients are not competent to exercise self-determination, as is true for certain levels of mental illness or dementia.

There are two situations in which self-determination should be restricted (Schreiber et al., 2018):

- When some objectives of individuals are contrary to the public interest or the interests of others in society (e.g., endangering others with a communicable disease)
- When a person's decision-making is so defective or mistaken that the individual is deemed legally incompetent (i.e., the person cannot fully comprehend the options, the consequences of actions related to the options, and the true costs and benefits)

Well-Being

Determining what constitutes health for people and how their well-being can be promoted often requires knowledge of clients' subjective preferences. It is generally recognized that clients may be inclined to pursue different directions in treatment procedures based on individual goals, values, and interests.

- C/PHNs should develop an understanding of each client group's needs and develop reasonable alternatives for service from which clients may choose (Box 4-9).
- When individuals are not capable of making a choice, the nurse or other surrogate decision-maker is obliged

BOX 4-9 STORIES FROM THE FIELD

A Family Living in Poverty

Contrasting value systems may be seen in many community/public health practice settings. Andrea Vargas, a C/PHN, experienced such a contrast on her first home visit to a family living in poverty. Referred by a school nurse for the children's recurring problems with head lice and staphylococcal infections, the family was living in a converted outbuilding on the outskirts of town.

Although basically clean and orderly, the living conditions were cramped, inadequate, and unsafe. Three hammocks were strung, stacked one upon the other, across the far corner of the room to accommodate the three younger children (out of a total of six). The older two children slept on the couch and the floor, while the baby slept with the single mother in the small bed. There was an old gas stove for cooking, and it was currently being used to heat the room, as the wall heater did not work. The mother did not know why it was no longer working. She seemed "stuck"—unable to muster the effort to talk with the landlord about the lack of a working heater. Even though using a gas stove to heat the room was dangerous (because of carbon monoxide), it seemed to her to be the easiest way to deal with the problem.

Andrea knew that landlords were sometimes slow to respond to the needs of low-income renters and she saw this as unjust. The mother's main pleasure in life was watching soap operas on television, and Andrea felt that the mother seemed disinterested in trying to improve her circumstances. The nurse interpreted the situation through the framework of her own value system, in which health and safety were priorities, and justice was an instrumental value. Yet the mother, who might have shared those values in the past, appeared to be incapable of advocating for her family, no longer able to cope with her situation. It is possible that environmental influences reordered the family's value system priorities. Rather than imposing her own values, Andrea chose to determine the priorities of the family, assess their needs, and begin where they were.

1. *Will she have a greater chance at success by doing this?*
2. *What needs can you identify with this family?*
3. *Where could you find assistance for this family in your community?*

to make health care decisions that promote the value of well-being. With shared decision-making, the nurse seeks not only to understand clients' needs but also to present the alternatives in a way that enables clients to choose those they prefer.

- Well-being and self-determination are two values that are intricately related when providing community/public health nursing services (Klausen, 2018; Sexton, O'Donovan, Mulryan, McCallion, & McCarron, 2017).

Equity

The third value that is important to decision-making in health care contexts is the value of equity or justice, which means being treated equally or fairly. The principle of equity implies that it is unjust (or inequitable) to treat people the same if they are, in significant respects, unalike. Equity generally means that all individuals should have the same access to health care according to benefit or needs (Box 4-10). However, effectively applying this value is often a complex enterprise and fraught with difficulties (Saniford, Vivas Consuelo, Rouse, & Bramley, 2018).

The major problem with this definition of equity is that it assumes that an adequate level of health care can be economically available to all citizens. In times of limited technical, human, and financial resources, it may be impossible to fully respect the value of equity (Cohen & Marshall, 2017; Krisberg, 2018). Choices must be made and resources allotted despite professional practice values that create ethical dilemmas that seem impossible to resolve. Many of these conflicts are reflected in current health care reform efforts that focus on access to services, quality of services, and ways to control rising costs. We also have many new genomics issues with access to care paramount in equity decisions (Rogowski & Schleidgen, 2015). The following list represents some of the most pressing aggregate health problems related to inequities in the distribution of and access to health and illness care facing patients worldwide.

- *Too many women go without preventive care.* The overall rate of infant mortality (all infant deaths before 1 year of age) is 5.1 per 1,000 in the United States. Although this rate is lower than previous rates, the disparities between the rates for populations of color and those for White non-Hispanic and White Hispanic populations remain high (Kaiser Family Foundation [KFF], 2017b).

BOX 4-10 LEVELS OF PREVENTION PYRAMID

Distributive Justice for Battered Women and Children

SITUATION: Provide distributive justice for battered women and children by changing a proposed state law that would eliminate funding for shelters for battered women and children to a law that preserves resources for this population.

GOAL: Using the three levels of prevention, avoid or promptly diagnose and treat negative health conditions and restore the fullest possible potential.

Tertiary Prevention

Rehabilitation	***Prevention***	
	Health Promotion and Education	***Health Protection***
If unable to stop the proposed law ▪ Seek volunteer services to fill the gaps in funding paid employees. ▪ Seek donations to support existing shelter buildings.	▪ Educate the public regarding the need for lost/limited services using various forms of media and/or venues.	▪ Seek private resources or grants to fund shelters. ▪ Propose a new bill to match private funding for shelters at the next legislative session.

Secondary Prevention

Early Diagnosis	***Prompt Treatment***
▪ Recognition that the proposed bill is going to pass	▪ Advocate for amendments to the proposed bill to preserve limited funding for shelters.

Primary Prevention

Health Promotion and Education	***Health Protection***
▪ Advocacy ▪ Active lobbying against the bill ▪ Garnering community support in favor of the revised bill	▪ Community understand the impact of the potential loss ▪ Put a "human face" on the problem

  - Unintended pregnancies are much higher among populations of color than among White populations. Poverty is strongly related to difficulty in accessing family planning services (Snow, Laski, & Mutumba, 2015).
  - Health care system factors such as access to care, patient preferences, and provider-related factors also impact the lack of preventive care.
- *Immunization rates for children entering kindergarten are an example of how public health works.* The median vaccination coverage among kindergarteners from 2017 to 2018 was 94.3% for measles, mumps, and rubella; 95.1% for diphtheria, tetanus, and acellular pertussis; and 93.8% for two doses of varicella (Mellerson, 2018).
  - Compliance with scheduled vaccines, which is generally high, and consistently high rates of immunization against common childhood communicable diseases are required for achieving community or herd immunity (Oxford Vaccine Group, 2018). Without high vaccination rates, we will lose the benefit of herd immunity and diseases will return, as happened in Japan in 1979 when only 10% of children were vaccinated and 13,000 cases of whooping cough and 41 deaths were reported (CDC, 2018).
  - Childhood immunization rate disparities have been dramatically reduced through multiple interventions and a strong infrastructure of vaccine services (Walsh, Doherty, & O'Neill, 2016). However, exemptions (medical, religious, personal) have been rising, with Oregon having the highest level at 7.6% and Mississippi the lowest at 2.2%. Personal belief exemptions, often related to antivaccination influence, were highest in Oregon (7.5%) and lowest in California (2.0%), where these exemptions are no longer permitted (CDC, 2018). See Chapters 8 and 20.
- *Disparities in immunization rates exist for adults along racial and ethnic lines, as well as by poverty level.* In a study comparing adults, the rate of influenza vaccination during the 2018-2019 flu season for non-Hispanic Whites was 48.7%, but for non-Hispanic Blacks and Hispanics the rates were 39.4% and 37.1%, respectively (CDC, 2019a). This may be due to the following among the Black population: lower knowledge levels about the flu vaccine, distrust of the vaccine, and barriers or missed opportunities to receive the vaccine (Quinn, 2018).
- *The uninsured are likely to go without physician care.* Differences in access to expensive, discretionary procedures emerge according to health insurance status, race, and ethnicity, as well as other sociodemographic factors.
  - The Affordable Care Act has helped to improve the numbers of previously uninsured in America, but those remaining uninsured are the working poor.
  - Over half of those without health insurance live at 200% below the poverty level, with White non-Hispanic Americans remaining more likely to be insured than people of color (Kaiser Family Foundation, 2017a).
- *Environmental hazards threaten global health.* Global trade, travel, and changing social and cultural patterns make the population vulnerable to diseases that are endemic to other parts of the world, as well as to previously unknown diseases.
  - Past influenza pandemics have highlighted the need for better preparation for future pandemics, and the novel coronavirus pandemic (COVID-19) has further emphasized that need (Desmond-Hellmann, 2020). (Patel et al., 2017).
  - Pollution of air, water, and soil to support industry contributes to pathogen mutations and threatens public health (Yu, Gunn, Wall, & Fanning, 2017).
- *Equity is tied to social justice (see below) and can be a difficult concept to truly grasp.*
  - People are socialized to see the world through the eyes of their own experience.
  - Once we can "unpack" how race, gender, income, education, age, and sexual identity influence equity and social justice, we then become allies to those who lack privilege (Adams et al., 2018).

Application of Values to Ethical Decision-Making in Community/Public Health Nursing

These key values of self-determination, well-being, and equity influence nursing practice in many ways (Ryan & Deci, 2017). The value of self-determination has implications for how C/PHNs regard the following:

- The choices of clients
- Privacy
- Informed consent
- Diminished capacity for self-determination

The value of well-being has implications for how C/PHNs seek to:

- Prevent harm and provide benefits to client populations
- Determine effectiveness of nursing services
- Weigh costs of services against real client benefits (Ryan & Deci, 2017)

The value of equity has implications for community/public health nursing in terms of its priorities for:

- Distributing health goods (macro-allocation issues)
- Deciding which populations will obtain available health goods and services (micro-allocation issues)
- Which individuals or groups have access to genetic tests (Ryan & Deci, 2017)

When a decision is based on only one value, it is more likely that conflict will emerge due to competing values. For example, deciding primarily on the basis of client well-being may conflict with decisions made on the basis of self-determination or equity. How C/PHNs balance these values may even conflict with their own personal values or the professional values of nursing as a whole. In these situations, values clarification techniques used with an ethical decision-making process may assist in producing decisions that promote the greatest well-being for clients without substantially reducing their self-determination or ignoring equity.

Ethical Principles

Based in patient-centered practice, fundamental ethical principles along with context and the nurse's knowledge provide guidance in making decisions regarding clients' care: respect, autonomy, beneficence, nonmaleficence, justice, veracity, and fidelity (Butts & Rich, 2019; Husted et al., 2015).

Respect

Respect refers to treating people as unique, equal, and responsible moral agents (Butts & Rich, 2019):

- Emphasizes one's importance as a member of the community and of the health services team
- Acknowledges community clients as valued participants in shaping their own and the community's health outcomes
- Includes treating clients as equals on the health team and holding them, as well as their views, in high regard (Akrami, & Abbasi, 2018)

Autonomy

Autonomy means freedom of choice and the exercise of people's rights (Butts & Rich, 2019). Autonomy:

- Is related to individualism and self-determination dominant values underlying this principle (Husted et al., 2015)
- Promotes individuals' and groups' rights to and involvement in decision-making as those decisions enhance their well-being and do not harm the well-being of others
- Requires nurses to make certain that clients are fully informed and that the decisions are made deliberately, with careful consideration of the consequences (Box 4-11)

Beneficence

- **Beneficence** means doing good or benefiting others.
- Is the promotion of good or taking action to ensure positive outcomes on behalf of clients (Robichaux, 2017).

BOX **4-11** STORIES FROM THE FIELD

An Older Client Gives Up

Tom Hardwick, PHN, has been assigned to monitor Mr. Jackson, an older man who was diagnosed with tuberculosis (TB; positive skin test, positive sputum and x-ray). Mr. Jackson's wife unexpectedly died recently, and he is depressed and wants to "join her." He is not eating or sleeping much. He refuses to take TB medications or his eight other medications for heart disease, thyroid insufficiency, type 2 diabetes, glaucoma, high cholesterol and triglycerides, and hypertension.

He has consistently refused any of Tom's suggestions or assistance. He does not want to see a mental health counselor, and Tom wonders if he should continue to make home visits. He has a busy caseload and needs to focus on the most pressing cases. Mr. Jackson's children feel that his depression and refusal of medications are a "temporary condition" in response to his wife's death and have asked for Tom's assistance in keeping their father healthy.

1. *Why is this an ethical dilemma?*
2. *What are the ethical principles involved?*
3. *What does Mr. Jackson value? What are his children's values? What are Tom's values?*
4. *Prioritize your values. What are the possible actions you could take?*

- Involves, in C/PHN, making decisions that actively promote clients' stated interests and their view of well-being (Husted et al., 2015).

Nonmaleficence

- **Nonmaleficence** means avoiding or preventing harm to others as a consequence of a person's own choices and actions (Butts & Rich, 2019; Robichaux, 2017):
- Involves taking steps to avoid negative consequences
- Examples include:
  - Encouraging providers to prescribe opioids within the newest guidelines
  - Promoting legislation to protect young people from e-cigarette (vaping) use

Justice

The principle of **justice** refers to treating people fairly (Butts & Rich, 2019; Husted et al., 2015).

- This includes the fair distribution of both benefits and costs among society's members
- Examples:
  - Equal access to health care
  - Equitable distribution of services to rural as well as urban populations
  - Fair distribution of resources after a disaster

Within this principle are three different views on allocation, or what constitutes the meaning of "fair" distribution.

- **Distributive justice** is the view that benefits should be given first to the disadvantaged or those who need them most (Box 4-10). Decisions based on this view particularly help the needy, although it may mean withholding goods (e.g., food stamps, Medicaid) from others who may also be deserving, but less in need (Robichaux, 2017).
- **Egalitarian justice** promotes decisions based on equal distribution of benefits to everyone, regardless of need (e.g., Medicare). See Box 4-12.
- **Restorative justice** determines that benefits should go primarily to those who have been wronged by prior injustice, such as victims of crime or racial discrimination (Robichaux, 2017).

Social justice refers to the fair and equitable distribution of wealth, economic opportunity, and access to privileges in society and is tied to human rights (Adams et al., 2018). The ANA (2016) clearly articulates the duty of nurses to ensure that client care is socially just. See Chapter 23 for more on social justice.

Veracity

The principle of **veracity** refers to telling the truth (Butts & Rich, 2019; Robichaux, 2017). This:

- Includes giving community/public health clients accurate information in a timely manner
- Involves treating clients as equals
- Expands the opportunity for greater client involvement
- Provides needed information for decision-making (Husted et al., 2015)

BOX 4-12 WHAT DO *YOU* THINK?

Predatory Drug Pricing

Other developed countries pay markedly less than the United States for prescription drugs (i.e., Japan 70%, France 59%, Denmark 29%). The prices of prescription drugs in the United States are expected to rise 6.3% per year between 2016 and 2025. The U.S. government paid about 43% of the cost of all prescriptions in 2015, yet when Medicare D (prescription drug coverage) was enacted, the legislation barred Medicare from negotiating with pharmaceutical companies to get lower costs (Olson & Sheiner, 2017).

Drug companies influenced this and other legislation that prohibits negotiating prices on drugs and medical devices, having spent over $2.5 billion over the past 10 years funding lobbyists and politicians in Congress. In fact, lobbyists outnumber the members of Congress 2 to 1 (McGreahl, 2017).

Drug manufacturers are protected by U.S. patent and intellectual property laws to protect their investment in developing a new drug—estimated as high as $2.5 billion. And they have learned to game the generic drug laws that were enacted to promote competition (i.e., antitrust laws). When their patents are about to expire, they simply make a very minor adjustment and re-patent the medication, thus avoiding generic competitors and allowing increased prices. Legislative attempts to legalize the importation of lower-price drugs from outside the United States, to reverse the ban on the government negotiating drug prices, and on increasing Medicare rebates on generic drugs have failed (Walsdorf, 2018). Our "multiple, overlapping health care systems," with government, private insurance, and private payors, have also made it difficult to maintain a consistent method of drug pricing and purchasing, making it easier for drug companies to limit access to specific medications leading to price spikes (Marciarille, 2017, p. 46).

The result of these policies and practices became very apparent when prices began to soar beginning in 2015:

- The price of an established drug, Darprim to treat toxoplasmosis (often associated with HIV/AIDS patients), rose 5,000%—from $13.50 to $750 per pill (Pianin, 2016).
- Two pharmaceutical companies—Retrophine Inc., and Rodelis Therapeutics—raised prices on some drugs 2,000% (Pianin, 2016).
- Valeant raised prices on two long-standing drugs to treat Wilson's disease, from a 30-day cost of $500 to over $24,000 (Peterson, 2016).
- The cost of a lifesaving medication for those with serious allergic reactions, EpiPens, rose to over $600 in the United States, while the United Kingdom was able to negotiate a $70 price tag (McGreahl, 2017). Mylan, a drug company making EpiPens, gave their CEO an increase in salary from $2.5 million to $18.9 million between 2007 and 2016 (Babcock, 2017).
- In the midst of a serious U.S. opioid crisis, naloxone (Narcan—used to reverse opioid overdose), in all forms except nasal spray, increased between 469% and 2,281% between 2006 and 2017. Because of drug shortages due to only one drug company selling the 0.4-mg single-dose product, sustained and dramatic price increases have resulted (Rosenberg, Schick, Chai, & Mehta, 2018).
- From 2002 to 2013, insulin prices more than tripled—from $40 to $130 a vial (Pearl, 2018). A survey of type 1 or type 2 diabetics found that 26% had used less than their prescribed insulin dose due to rising costs, and that almost half had intermittently gone without diabetes treatment ("High Cost Has 1 in 4 Diabetics," 2018; Upwell Community, 2019).

It may now be important to not only consider side effects and effectiveness of a medication but the negative impact of excessive cost. This may enable Medicare and other insurers to consider cost as well as quality in deciding which drugs to include in their formularies. For instance, physicians at Memorial Sloan-Kettering Cancer Center refused to put a new, very high-priced drug for colon cancer (Zaltrap) on their formulary because it was too expensive, and they encouraged other physicians to examine the financial strain to their patients in their decision-making process. After some publicity, the pharmaceutical company dropped the price by 50% (Buck, 2017).

1. *Do you think drug prices are problematic? State the ethical principles involved.*
2. *Do both sides of the argument have merit (drug company's costs, a consumer's inability to pay)?*
3. *Does this situation constitute an ethical dilemma?*
4. *How could you go about resolving this? Consider the rights of a few versus the rights of many.*
5. *Apply Iserson's (1999) three tests (under heading Decision-Making Frameworks).*

Source: Babcock (2017); Buck (2017); "High Cost Has 1 in 4 Diabetics" (2018); Marciarille (2017); McGreahl (2017); Olson & Sheiner (2017); Peterson (2016); Pianin (2016); Rosenberg et al. (2018); Upwell Community (2019); Walsdorf (2018).

Fidelity

Fidelity means remaining true to your word or keeping promises (Butts & Rich, 2019; Oana, 2017). It:

- Allows people to count on commitments being met, to which they have a right
- Results in the nurse earning the client's respect and trust
- When bidirectional, influences the quality of the nurse's relationship with clients, who then are more likely to share information
- Involves building trust and leads to improved decisions and better health
- When lacking, can cause community members to lose faith and interest in participation

Ethical Standards and Guidelines

As the number and complexity of ethical decisions in community health increase, so too does the need for ethical standards and guidelines to help nurses make the best choices possible.

- The ANA's *Code for Nurses with Interpretive Statements* (2015) provides a helpful guide.
- The Association of State and Territorial Directors of Nursing (n.d.), a public health nursing organization, published a text on how to incorporate ethical principles into local health department processes and provide guidelines for the C/PHN role in eliminating health inequalities.
- More health care organizations are using ethics committees or ethics rounds to deal with ethical aspects of client services (Hajibabaee, Joolaee, Cheraghi, Salari, & Rodney, 2016).
- Ethics committees also function in a variety of community/public health care settings. In public health agencies, cases of clients with complicated communicable disease diagnoses and health care provider concerns are discussed as they relate to policy, protocols, and the health and safety of the broader population (Santos et al., 2017).

Ethics and research (or EBP) are intertwined. All nurses need competency in both areas to provide quality care to those they serve.

SUMMARY

- Implementation of EBP enables C/PHNs to promote health and prevent illness among at-risk populations and to design and evaluate community-based interventions.
- EBP is essential to ensuring economical and effective interventions for our clients.
- Systematic reviews can provide direction for those who have developed a "burning clinical question."
- Research and application of EBP have a significant impact on community/public health and nursing practice by providing new knowledge that helps to shape health policy, improve service delivery, and promote the public's health.
- It offers the potential to enhance nursing's status and influence through documentation of the effectiveness of nursing interventions and broader recognition of nursing's contributions to health services.
- Nurses must learn to evaluate evidence critically, assessing the validity and applicability to their own practice. Nurses should search for current evidence and discuss EBP initiatives with colleagues and supervisors.
- A commitment to use and conduct research will move the nursing profession forward and enhance its influence on the health of at-risk populations.
- Values and ethical principles strongly influence C/PHN practice and ethical decision-making.
- *Values* are lasting beliefs that are important to individuals, groups, and cultures. A value system organizes these beliefs into a hierarchy of relative importance that motivates and guides human behavior.
- Values function as standards for behavior, as criteria for attitudes, and as standards for moral judgments, and they give expression to human needs.
- The nature of values can be understood by examining their qualities of endurance, their hierarchical arrangement, and their function as prescriptive–proscriptive beliefs and by examining them in terms of reference and preference.
- The nurse often is faced with decisions that affect client's values and involve conflicting moral values and ethical dilemmas.
- Understanding what personal values are and how they affect behavior assists the nurse in making ethical evaluations and addressing ethical conflicts in practice.
- Several frameworks for ethical decision-making that include the identification and clarification of values impinging on the making of ethical decisions were discussed in this chapter.
- Three key human values influence client health and nurse decision-making: the right to make decisions regarding a person's health (self-determination), the right to health and well-being, and the right to equal access and quality of health care.
- At times, these three key human values are affected by the value of self-interest on the part of another person or a system.
- Seven fundamental principles guide C/PHNs in making ethical decisions: respect, autonomy, beneficence, nonmaleficence, justice, veracity, and fidelity.

ACTIVE LEARNING EXERCISES

1. As a C/PHN working in a big city, you encounter a large number of children with lead poisoning due to environmental contamination. You are interested in lead abatement programs. Where can you find evidence on successful programs/outcomes, cost–benefit analysis, and policies that have been implemented in other areas? Who would need to be involved in getting this type of program instituted?
2. Select a community/public health nursing systematic review or research article and analyze its potential impact on health policy and C/PHN practice. Critique the article, using the criteria presented in this chapter. What are the main findings? How can you apply this to your community setting? What policies could be affected and how?
3. You have just completed an EBP implementation study on the effectiveness of a series of birth control classes in three high schools, and the results show a reduction in the number of pregnancies over the last year. Is this enough information to declare it a success? What else could you do to strengthen your case? Describe three ways in which you could disseminate this information to your nursing colleagues and school officials.
4. Find a community/public health study that represents efforts to "Strengthen, Support, and Mobilize

Communities and Partnerships" (1 of the 10 essential public health services; see Box 2-2) (e.g., community-based participatory research study). How would you apply the methods, interventions, and findings of that study to an issue in your community?

5. Describe where you stand on the following issues. For each statement, decide whether you strongly agree, agree, disagree, strongly disagree, or are undecided. Discuss your rationales and compare your results with a small group of classmates:
   a. Clients have the right to participate in all decisions related to their health care.
   b. Continuing education should not be mandatory to maintain licensure.
   c. Clients always should be told the truth.
   d. Nurses should be required to take relicensure examinations every 5 years.
   e. Clients should be allowed to read their health record on request.
   f. Abortion on demand should be an option available to every woman.
   g. Critically ill newborns should be allowed to die.
   h. Laws should guarantee health care for each person in this country.
6. Search local or national news for stories involving ethical dilemmas. Pick one and describe which ethical principles were involved. How was the dilemma resolved? Or, how would you go about deciding on an equitable resolution?

REFERENCES

Adams, M., et al. (2018). *Readings for diversity and social justice* (4th ed.). New York, NY: Routledge.

Adams, S. B. (2018). Empathy as an ethical imperative. *Creative Nursing, 24*(3), 166–172.

Akrami, F., & Abbasi, M. (2018). Exploring the prominence of ethical principles and moral norms in the areas of clinical practice and public health. *Annals of Medical Health Science Research, 8*, 11–15.

Akpotor, M. E., & Johnson, E. A. (2018). Client empowerment: A concept analysis. *International Journal of Caring Sciences, 11*(2), 743–750.

Altmiller, G. (2019). Care bundles, QSEN, and student learning. *Nurse Educator, 44*(1), 7–8.

Alvidrez, J., Napoles, A. M., Bernal, G., Lloyd, J., Cargill, V., Godette, D., ... Farhat, T. (2019). Building the evidence base to inform planned intervention adaptations by practitioners serving health disparity populations. *American Journal of Public Health, 109*(Suppl 1), s94–s101.

American Academy of Pediatrics (AAP). (2016). SIDS and other sleep-related infant deaths: Updated 2016 recommendations for safe sleeping environment. *Pediatrics, 138*(5), 1–12. Retrieved from https://pediatrics.aappublications.org/content/138/5/e20162938

American Nurses Association (ANA). (2010). *Nursing's social policy statement the essence of the profession*. Washington, DC: Author.

American Nurses Association (ANA). (2015). *Code for nurses with interpretive statements*. Washington, DC: Author.

American Nurses Association (ANA). (2016). *Position statement. The Nurse's Role in Ethics and Human Rights: Protecting and Promoting Individual Worth, Dignity, and Human Rights in Practice Setting*. Retrieved from https://www.nursingworld.org/~4af078/globalassets/docs/ana/ethics/ethics-and-human-rights-protecting-and-promoting-final-formatted-20161130.pdf

Association of State and Territorial Directors of Nursing (ASTDN). (n.d.). *The public health nurse's role in achieving health equity: Eliminating inequalities in health. Position Paper*. Author. Retrieved from http://phnurse.org/resources/APHN%20Health%20Equity%20Position%20Paper%2012-3-15.pdf

Atkins, D. M., Held, M. L., & Lindley, L. C. (2018). The impact of expanded health insurance coverage for unauthorized pregnant women on prenatal care utilization. *Public Health Nursing, 35*(6), 459–465.

Babcock, P. (2017). Solidarism and the EpiPen. *Ethics & Medics, 42*(2), 3–4.

Baillie, L. (2017). An exploration of the 6Cs as a set of values for nursing practice. *British Journal of Nursing, 26*(10), 558–563.

Balakas, K., & Smith, J. R. (2016). Evidence-based practice and quality improvement in nursing education. *Journal of Perinatal and Neonatal Nursing, 30*(3), 191–194.

Beamer, L. C. (2017). Ethics and genetics: Examining a crossroads in nursing through a case study. *Clinical Journal of Oncology Nursing, 21*(6), 730–737.

Belita, E., Yost, J., Squires, J. E., Ganann, R., Burnett, T., & Dobbins, M. (2018). Measures assessing attributes of evidence-informed decision-making (EIDM) competence among nurses: A systematic review protocol. *Systematic Reviews, 7*(1), 181.

Biederman, D. J., Gamble, J., Wilson, S., Douglas, C., & Feigal, J. (2019). Health care utilization following a homeless medical respite pilot program. *Public Health Nursing, 36*, 296–302. doi: 10.1111/phn.12589.

Black, A. T., Balneaves, L. G., Garossino, C., Puyat, J. H., & Qian, H. (2015). Promoting evidence-based practice through a research training program for point-of-care clinicians. *Journal of Nursing Administration, 45*(1), 14–20.

Blacksher, E. (2015). *Public health ethics. Ethics in medicine*. Retrieved from https://depts.washington.edu/bioethx/topics/public.html

Blais, K. K., & Hayes, J. S. (2016). *Professional nursing practice: Concepts and perspectives* (7th ed.). Upper Saddle River, NJ: Pearson Prentice Hall.

Bombard, J. M., Kortsmit, K., Warner, L., Shapiro-Mendoza, C., Cox, S., Kroelinger, C., ... Barfield, W. D. (2018). Vital signs: Trends and disparities in infant safe sleep practices—United States, 2009-20-15. *Morbidity and Mortality Weekly Report, 67*(1), 39–46.

Bongiorno, A. (October 2018). Voices of inclusion: Developing cultural competency through art and story. Paper presented at the 44th meeting of the Transcultural Nursing Society. San Antonio, TX.

Brucker, M. C. (2016). Applying evidence to health care with Archie Cochrane's legacy. *Nursing for Women's Health, 20*(5), 441–442.

Buck, I. D. (2017). The cost of high prices: Embedding an ethic of expense into the standard of care. *Boston College Law Review, 58*(101), 102–150.

Butts, J. B., & Rich, K. L. (2019). *Nursing ethics across the curriculum* (5th ed.). Burlington, MA: Jones & Bartlett Learning.

Carper, B. A. (1978). Fundamental patterns of knowing in nursing. *Advances in Nursing Science, 1*(1), 13–23.

Carter, S. M., Entwistle, V. A., & Little, M. (2015). Relational conceptions of paternalism: A way to rebut nanny-state accusations and evaluate public health interventions. *Public Health, 129*(8), 1021–1029.

Centers for Disease Control and Prevention (CDC). (2017). *Public health ethics*. Retrieved from https://www.cdc.gov/od/science/integrity/phethics/index.htm

Centers for Disease Control and Prevention (CDC). (2018). *What would happen if we stopped vaccinations?* Retrieved from https://www.cdc.gov/vaccines/vac-gen/whatifstop.htm

Centers for Disease Prevention & Control (CDC). (September 26, 2019a). *Flu vaccination coverage, Unites States, 2018-2019 influenza season*. Retrieved from https://www.cdc.gov/flu/fluvaxview/coverage-1819estimates.htm

Centers for Disease Control and Prevention (CDC). (2019). *Sudden unexpected infant death and sudden infant death syndrome*. Retrieved from https://www.cdc.gov/sids/data.htm

Centers for Disease Control and Prevention (CDC). (2020). *The Tuskegee timeline*. Retrieved from http://www.cdc.gov/tuskegee/timeline.htm

Chaiyachati, K. H., Ogbuoji, O., Price, M., Suthar, A., & Barnighausen, T. (2014). Interventions to improve adherence to antiretroviral therapy: A rapid systematic review. *AIDS, 28*(Suppl 2), s187–s204.

Cline, G. J., Burger, K. J., Amankwah, E. K., Goldenberg, N. A., & Ghazarian, S. R. (2017). Promoting the Utilization of Science in Healthcare (PUSH) project. *Journal for Nurses in Professional Development, 33*(3), 113–119.

Coalition for Evidence-Based Policy. (2015). *Social programs that work: Nurse-Family Partnership—top tier*. Retrieved from http://evidencebased-programs.org/1366-2/nurse-family-partnership

Cohen, B., & Marshall, S. (2017). Does public health advocacy seek to redress health inequities? A scoping review. *Health & Social Care in the Community, 25*(2), 309–328.

Cook, N., Hollar, L., Isaac, E., Paul, L., Amofah, A., & Shi, L. (2015). Patient experience in health center medical homes. *Journal of Community Health, 40*, 1155–1164.

Cooney, C. M., et al. (2018). The ethics of hand transplantation: A systematic review. *Journal of Hand Surgery, 43*(1), 84.e1–84.e15.

Coppa, D., Winchester, S. B., & Roberts, M. B. (2018). Home-based nurse practitioners demonstrate reductions in rehospitalizations and emergency department visits in a clinically complex patient population through an academic-clinical partnership. *Journal of the American Association of Nurse Practitioners, 30*(6), 335–343.

Cornwall, J., & Higgins, T. (2015). Approach and avoidance in moral psychology: Evidence for three distinct motivational levels. *Personality & Individual Differences, 86*, 139–149.

Cronenwett, L., Sherwood, G., Barnsteiner, J., Disch, J., Johnson, J., Mitchell, P., ... Warren, J. (2007). Quality and safety education for nurses. *Nursing Outlook, 55*(3), 122–131.

Cygan, H. R., McNaughton, D., Reising, V., & Reid, B. (2018). An academic practice partnership Building capacity to meet sexual health education policy requirements of a public-school system. *Public Health Nursing, 35*(5), 414–419.

Davis, J. (March 14, 2018). *Medical data of 33,000 BJC healthcare patients exposed online for 8 months*. Retrieved from https://www.healthcareit-news.com/news/medical-data-33000-bjc-healthcare-patients-exposed-online-8-months

Desmond-Hellmann, S. (April 3, 2020). Preparing for the next pandemic: The COVID-19 crisis has clear lessons for what we can do now to stop a future global health emergency. *The Wall Street Journal*. Retrieved from https://www.wsj.com/articles/preparing-for-the-next-pandemic-11585936915

Douglas, M. R., Mallonee, S., & Istre, G. R. (1999). Estimating the proportion of homes with functioning smoke alarms: A comparison of telephone survey and household survey results. *American Journal of Public Health, 89*(7), 1112–1114.

Dunlap, N. E., Ballard, D. J., Cherry, R. A., Dunagan, W. C., Ferniany, W., Hamilton, A. C., ... Walsh, K. E. (July 22, 2016). *Observations from the field: Reporting quality metrics in health care*. National Academy Press. Retrieved from https://nam.edu/wp-content/uploads/2016/07/Observations-from-the-Field-Reporting-Quality-Metrics-in-Health-Care.pdf

Eckenrode, J., Campa, M., Luckey, D., Henderson, C., Cole, R., Kitzman, H., ... Olds, D. L. (2010). Long-term effects of prenatal and infancy nurse home visitation on the life course of youths. *Archives of Pediatrics and Adolescent Medicine, 164*(1), 9–15.

Elemers, N. (2017). *Morality and the regulation of social behavior: Groups as moral anchors*. New York, NY: Routledge (Taylor & Francis Group).

Ellen, M. E., Lavis, J. N., Horowitz, E., & Berglas, R. (2018). How is the use of research evidence in health policy perceived? A comparison between the reporting of researchers and policy-makers. *Health Research, Policy, and Systems, 16*, 64. doi: 10.1186/s12961-018-0345-6.

Fowler, M. D. (2015). *Guide to nursing's social policy statement: Understanding the profession from social contract to social covenant*. Washington, DC: American Nurses Association.

Friedmann, I., Dahdouh, E. M., Kugler, P., Mimran, G., & Balayla, J. (2017). Maternal and obstetrical predictors of sudden infant death syndrome (SIDS). *Journal of Maternal-Fetal & Neonatal Medicine, 30*(19), 2315–2323.

Gerding, J. A., DeLellis, N. O., Neri, A. J., & Dignam, T. A. (2018). Environmental health program performance and its relationship with environment-related disease in Florida. *Florida Public Health Review, 15*, 1–12.

Gil, G. S., Morikava, F. S., Santin, G. C., Pintarelli, T. P., Fraiz, F. C., & Ferreira, F. M. (2015). Reliability of self-reported toothbrushing frequency as an indicator for the assessment of oral hygiene in epidemiological research on caries in adolescents: A cross-sectional study. *BMC Medical Research Methodology, 15*, 14. Retrieved from https://bmcmedresmethodol.biomed-central.com/articles/10.1186/s12874-015-0002-5

Ginex, P. K. (August 29, 2017). The difference between quality improvement, evidence-based practice, and research. *ONS Voice*. Retrieved from https://voice.ons.org/news-and-views/oncology-research-quality-improvement-evidence-based-practice

Glynn, D. M., McVey, C., Wendt, J., & Russell, B. (2017). Dedicated educational nursing unit: Clinical instructors role perceptions and learning needs. *Journal of Professional Nursing, 33*(2), 108–112.

Gnaedinger, E. A. (2018). Fluoride varnish application, a quality improvement project implemented in a rural pediatric practice. *Public Health Nursing, 35*(6), 534–540.

Goldschmidt, A. B., Wall, M. M., Loth, K. A., & Neumark-Sztainer, D. (2015). Risk factors for disordered eating in overweight adolescents and young adults. *Journal of Pediatric Psychology, 40*(10), 1048–1055.

Grace, P., Milliken, A. (2016). Educating nurses for ethical practice in contemporary health care environments. *Hastings Center Report, 46*, S13–S17. doi: 10.1002/hast.625.

Guo, K. L. (2008). DECIDE: A decision-making model for more effective decision making by health care managers. *Health Care Management, 27*(2), 118–127.

Hajibabaee, F., Joolaee, S., Cheraghi, M., Salari, P., & Rodney, P. (2016). Hospital/clinical ethics committees'notion: an overview. *Journal of Medical Ethics & History of Medicine, 9*(17), 1–9.

Hall, W., & Doran, C. (2016). How much can the USA reduce health care costs by reducing smoking? *PLOS Medicine, 3*(5), e1002021.

Hartmann-Boyce, J., Chepkin, S. C., Ye, W., Bullen, C., & Lancaster, L. (2018). Nicotine replacement therapy versus control for smoking cessation (review). *Cochrane Database of Systematic Reviews*, (5), CD000146. Retrieved from https://www.cochranelibrary.com/cdsr/doi/10.1002/14651858.CD000146.pub5/epdf/abstract

HealthDay. (December 3, 2018). *High cost has over 1 in 4 diabetics cutting back on insulin*. Retrieved from https://www.drugs.com/news/cost-has-over-1-4-diabetics-cutting-back-insulin-78801.html

Hoare, E., Millar, L., Fuller-Tyszkiewicz, M., Skouteris, H., Nichols, M., Jacka, F., ... Allender, S. (2014). Associations between obesogenic risk and depressive symptomatology in Australian adolescents: A cross-sectional study. *Journal of Epidemiology and Community Health, 68*(8), 767–772.

Hoffman, J. (2019). *Biostatistics for medical and biomedical practitioners* (2nd ed.). New York, NY: Academic Press, Elsevier.

Hoffman, H., Damus, K., Hillman, L., & Krongrad, E. (1988). Risk factors for SIDS. Results of the National Institute of Child Health and Human Development SIDS Cooperative Epidemiological Study. *Annals of the New York Academy of Sciences, 533*, 13–30.

Holliday, C. E., Wynne, M., Katz, J., Ford, C., & Barbosa-Leiker, C. (2018). A CBPR approach to finding community strengths and challenges to prevent youth suicide and substance abuse. *Journal of Transcultural Nursing, 29*(1), 64–73.

Holt, J. M., Johnson, T. S., & Zabler, B. (2018). Engaging African American women in community-based health promotion programs: Key informant recommendations. *Journal of Community Health Nursing, 35*(3), 137–147.

Hoying, J., & Melnyk, B. (2016). COPE: A pilot study with urban-dwelling minority sixth-grade youth to improve physical activity and mental health outcomes. *Journal of School Nursing, 32*(5), 347–356.

Hoying, J., Melnyk, B., & Arcoleo, K. (2016). Effects of the COPE cognitive behavioral skills building TEEN program on the healthy lifestyle behaviors and mental health of Appalachian early adolescents. *Journal of Pediatric Health Care, 30*(1), 65–72.

Hultman, K. (2017). Unleashing the power of values. *Organization Development Journal, 35*(2), 17–32.

Husted, G., Husted, J., Scotto, C., & Wolf, K. (2015). *Bioethical decision making in nursing* (5th ed.). New York, NY: Springer.

Institute of Medicine (IOM). (2000). *To err is human: Building a safer health care system*. Washington, DC: National Academies Press.

Institute of Medicine (IOM). (2001). *Crossing the quality chasm: A new health system for the 21st century*. Washington, DC: National Academies Press.

Institute of Medicine. (2003a). *Priority areas for national action: Transforming health care quality*. Washington, DC: National Academies Press.

Institute of Medicine. (2003b). *The future of the public's health in the 21st century*. Washington, DC: The National Academies Press. Retrieved from https://doi.org/10.17226/10548

Institute of Medicine. (2011a). *For the public's health: The role of measurement in action and accountability*. Washington, DC: The National Academies Press. Retrieved from https://doi.org/10.17226/13005

Institute of Medicine. (2011b). *The future of nursing: Leading change, advancing health*. Washington, DC: National Academies Press.

Institute of Medicine (IOM). (2012). *For the public's health: Investing in a healthier future*. Washington, DC: The National Academies Press.

Institute of Medicine. (2014). *Strategies for scaling effective family-focused preventive interventions to promote children's cognitive, affective, and behavioral health*. Workshop Summary. Washington, DC: The National Academies Press.

Iserson, K. V. (1999). Ethical issues in emergency medicine. *Emergency Medicine Clinics of North America, 17*(2), 283–306.

Jackson, C., Kasper, E., Williams, C., & DuBard, C. A. (2016). Incremental benefit of a home visit following discharge for patients with multiple chronic conditions receiving transitional care. *Population Health Management, 19*(3), 163–217.

Jaschik, S. (January 19, 2017). *New "Common Rule" for research. Inside Higher Education.* Retrieved from https://www.insidehighered.com/news/2017/01/19/us-issues-final-version-common-rule-research-involving-humans

Jennings, B. (2015). Relational liberty revisited: Membership, solidarity and public health ethics of place. *Public Health Ethics, 8*(1), 7–17.

Joanna Briggs Institute. (n.d.) *About us.* Retrieved from https://joannabriggs.org/about.html

Johnson, P., Montgomery, M., & Ewell, P. (2018). Elevated blood pressure in low-income, rural preschool children is associated with maternal hypertension during pregnancy. *Journal of Community Health Nursing, 35*(1), 12–18.

Jones, E., Lomis, M., Mealey, S., Newman, M., Schroder, H., Smith, A., & Wickline, M. (2019). Development of a comprehensive infection control program for a short-term shelter serving trafficked women. *Public Health Nursing, 36*(1), 53–61.

Jones, K., Williams, J., Sipsma, H., & Patil, C. (2018). Adolescent and emerging adults' evaluation of a Facebook site providing sexual health education. *Public Health Nursing, 36*, 11–17.

Jull, J., Giles, J., & Graham, I. D. (2017). Community-based participatory research and integrated knowledge translation: Advancing the co-creation of knowledge. *Implementation Science, 12*, 150. Retrieved from https://implementationscience.biomedcentral.com/track/pdf/10.1186/s13012-017-0696-3

Kaiser Family Foundation (KFF). (2017a). *Key facts about the uninsured.* Retrieved from https://www.kff.org/uninsured/fact-sheet/key-facts-about-the-uninsured-population/

Kaiser Family Foundation (KFF). (2017b). *Key health and health care indicators by race/ethnicity and state.* Retrieved from https://www.kff.org/disparities-policy/fact-sheet/key-health-and-health-care-indicators-by/

Kansagara, D., Chiovaro, J., Kagen, D., Jencks, S., Rhyne, K., O'Neil, M., … Englander, H. (2016). So many options, where do we start? An overview of the care transitions literature. *Journal of Hospital Medicine, 11*(3), 221–230.

Karoly, L. A. (2017). *Investing in the early years: The costs and benefits of investing in early childhood in New Hampshire.* RAND Corporation. Retrieved from https://www.rand.org/pubs/research-reports/RR1890.html

Katz, A. (April 2, 2015). Cancer genetics: Genetic counseling, ethical issues, and the nurse's role. *Oncology Nurses Society.* Retrieved from http://congress.ons.org/cancer-genetics-genetic-counseling-ethical-issues-and-the-nurses-role/

Kinneging, A. (2016). *Defining moral values.* Intercollegiate Review. Digital. Wilmington, DE: Intercollegiate Studies Institute. Retrieved from https://home.isi.org/defining-moral-values

Kitzman, H., Olds, D., Henderson, C., Hanks, C., Cole, R., Tatelbaum, R., et al. (1997). Effect or prenatal and infancy home visitation by nurses on pregnancy outcomes, childhood injuries, and repeated childbearing: A randomized controlled trial. *Journal of the American Medical Association, 278*(8), 644–652.

Kitzman, H., Olds, D., Henderson, C., Hanks, C., Cole, R., Arcoleo, K. J., et al. (2010a). Enduring effects of prenatal and infancy home visiting by nurses on children. *Archives of Pediatrics and Adolescent Medicine, 164*(5), 412–418.

Kitzman, H. J., Olds, D. L., Cole, R. E., Hanks, C. A., Anson, E. A., Arcoleo, K. J., … Holmberg, J. R. (2010b). Enduring effects of prenatal and infancy home visiting by nurses on children: Follow up of a randomized trial among children at age 12 years. *Archives of Pediatrics & Adolescent Medicine, 164*(5), 412–418.

Klausen, S. H. (2018). Ethics, knowledge, and a procedural approach to well-being. *Inquiry.* Retrieved from https://doi.org/10.1080/0020174X.2018.1529619

Kovar, C. L., & Bynum, S. (2019). Sexually transmitted disease services and third-party payer reimbursement: Attitudes, knowledge, and current practices among 60 health departments/districts. Why does this matter to public health nurses? *Public Health Nursing, 36*(3), 357–362. Retrieved from https://onlinelibrary.wiley.com/toc/15251446/0/0

Krisberg, K. (2018). Addressing health equity through state, regional partnerships. *Nation's Health, 48*(7), S1–S2.

Kronstadt, J., Beitsch, L. M., & Bender, K. (2015). Marshaling the evidence: The prioritized public health accreditation research agenda. *American Journal of Public Health, 105*(S2), s153–s158.

Kutney-Lee, A., Stimpfel, A. W., Sloane, D. M., Cimiotti, J. P., Quinn, L. W., & Aiken, L. H. (2015). Changes in patient and nurse outcomes associated with magnet hospital recognition. *Medical Care, 53*(6), 550–557.

Lambert, A. B., Parks, S. E., & Shapiroi-Mendoza, C. K. (2018). National and state trends in sudden unexpected infant death: 1990–2015. *Pediatrics, 141*(3), 1–7.

Lasater, K. B., Germack, H. D., Small, D. S., & McHugh, M. D. (2016). Hospitals known for nursing excellence perform better on value-based purchasing measures. *Policy & Politics in Nursing Practice, 17*(4), 177–186.

Lee, C. T., Padilla-Walker, L. M., & Nelson, L. (2015). Person-centered approach to moral motivations during emerging adulthood: Are all forms of other-orientation adaptive? *Journal of Moral Education, 44*(1), 51–63. doi: 10.1080/03057240.2014.1002460.

Leslie, H., Hirschhorn, L., Marchant, T., Doubova, S., Gueje, O, & Kruk, M. (2018). Health systems thinking: A new generation of research to improve healthcare quality. *PLoS Medicine, 15*(10), 1–4.

Levy, D., Huang, A., Havumaki, J., & Meza, R. (2016). The role of public policies in reducing smoking prevalence: Results from the Michigan *SimSmoke* tobacco policy simulation. *Cancer Causes & Control, 27*(5), 615–625.

Levy, D., Tam, J., Kuo, C., Fong, G., & Chaloupka, F. (2018). The impact of implementing tobacco control policies: The 2017 tobacco control policy scorecard. *Journal of Public Health Management & Practice, 24*(5), 448–457.

Liu, Y., Ye, W., Chen, Q., Zhang, Y., Kuo, C. H., & Korivi, M. (2019). Resistance exercise intensity is correlated with attenuation of HbA1c and insulin in patients with Type 2 Diabetes: A systematic review and meta-analysis. *International Journal of Research in Public Health, 16*(1). pii: E140.

MacFarlane, M., Thompson, J., Zuccollo, J., McDonald, G., Elder, D., Stewart, A., … Mitchell, E. (2018). Smoking in pregnancy is a key factor for sudden infant death among Maori. *Acta Paediatrica, 107*(11), 1924–1931.

Mannan, M., Mamun, A., Doi, S., & Clavarino, A. (2016). Prospective associations between depression and obesity for adolescent males and females: A systematic review and meta-analysis of longitudinal studies. *PLoS One, 11*(6), e0157240.

Marciarille, A. M. (2017). The prescription drug pricing moment: Using public health analysis to clarify the fair competition debate on prescription drug pricing and consumer welfare. *The Journal of Law, Medicine, & Ethics, 45*(S1), 45–49.

Martin, G. (2017). Views on the ethical struggle for universal, high quality, affordable health care and its relevance for gerontology. *Experimental Gerontology, 87*(Pt B), 182–189.

Maternal Child Health Bureau. (n.d.). *The maternal, infant, and early childhood home visiting program: Partnering with parents to help children succeed.* Retrieved from https://mchb.hrsa.gov/sites/default/files/mchb/MaternalChildHealthInitiatives/HomeVisiting/pdf/programbrief.pdf

McGreahl, C. (October 19, 2017). *How big pharma's money—and its politicians—feed the US opioid crisis.* Retrieved from https://www.theguardian.com/us-news/2017/oct/19/big-pharma-money-lobbying-us-opioid-crisis

Mejdoubi, J., van den Haijkant, C. M., van Leerdam, F., Heymans, M. W., Crijnen, A. M., & Hirasing, R. A. (2015). The effect of VoorZorg, the Dutch nurse-family partnership, on child maltreatment and development: A randomized controlled trial. *PLOS One, 10*(4), e0120182. doi: 10.371/journal.pone.0120182.

Mellerson, J. L. (2018). Vaccination coverage for selected vaccines and exemption rates among children in kindergarten—United States, 2017–2018 school year. *Morbidity and Mortality Weekly Report (MMWR), 67*(40), 1115–1122.

Melnyk, B. (2017). The evidence-based practice competencies related to disseminating evidence. In B. M. Melnyk, L. Gallagher-Ford, & E. Fineout-Overholt (Eds.). *Implementing the evidence-based practice competencies in healthcare: A practical guide for improving quality, safety, & outcomes.* Indianapolis, IN: Sigma Theta Tau International.

Melnyk, B., & Fineout-Overholt, E. (2019). *Evidence-based practice in nursing and healthcare: A guide to best practice* (4th ed.). Philadelphia, PA: Wolters Kluwer.

Melnyk, B. M., Fineout-Overholt, E., Giggleman, M., & Choy, K. (2017). A test of the ARCC© Model improves implementation of evidence-based practice, healthcare culture, and patient outcomes. *Worldviews on Evidence-Based Nursing, 14*(1), 5–9.

Melnyk, B., Jacobson, D., Kelly, S., Belyea, M., Shaibi, G., Small, L., Marsiglia, F. (2013). Promoting healthy lifestyles in high school adolescents: A randomized controlled trial. *American Journal of Preventive Medicine, 45*(4), 407–415.

Melnyk, B., Jacobson, D., Kelly, S., Belyea, M., Shaibi, G., Small, L., Marsiglia, F. (2015). Twelve- month effects of the COPE healthy lifestyles TEEN program on overweight and depressive symptoms in high school students. *Journal of School Health, 85*(12), 861–870.

Merriam Webster Online Dictionary. (2019). *Ethics.* Retrieved from https://www.merriam-webster.com/dictionary/ethics

Middlemiss, W., Cowan, S., Kildare, C., & Siddio, K. (2017). Collaborative translation of knowledge to protect infants during sleep: A synergy of discovery and practice. *Family Relations, 66*, 659–669.

Miller, T. R. (September 2012). *Nurse-Family Partnership home visitation: Costs, outcomes, and return on investment. Executive Summary.* Beltsville, MD: H.B.S.A., Inc.

Milliken, A. (2018). Nurse ethical sensitivity: An integrative review. *Nursing Ethics, 25*(3), 278–303.

Milliken, A., & Grace, P. (2017a). Nurse ethical awareness: The value of sharing diverse perspectives. *Nursing Ethics, 24*(5), 515–516. https://journals.sagepub.com/doi/pdf/10.1177/0969733017721534

Milliken, A., & Grace, P. (2017b). Nurse ethical awareness: Understanding the nature of everyday practice. *Nursing Ethics, 24*(5), 517–524.

Munn, Z., Peters, M., Stern, C., Tufanaru, C., McArthur, A., & Aromataris, E. (2018). Systematic review or scoping review? Guidance for authors when choosing between a systematic or scoping review approach. *BMC Medical Research Methodology, 18*, article 143. Retrieved from https://bmcmedresmethodol.biomedcentral.com/articles/10.1186/s12874-018-0611-x

National Institutes of Health. (n.d.a). *Back to Sleep public education campaign*. Retrieved from https://www.nichd.nih.gov/sids/

National Institutes of Health. (n.d.b). *Ten landmark nursing research studies*. Retrieved from https://www.ninr.nih.gov/sites/www.ninr.nih.gov/files/10-landmark-nursing-research-studies.pdf

National Quality Forum. (2019). *NQF's work in quality measurement*. Retrieved from http://www.qualityforum.org/about_nqf/work_in_quality_measurement/

Nelson, W. A. (2015). Making ethical decisions. A six-step process should guide ethical decision making in healthcare. *Health Care Executive, 30*(4), 46–48.

Newberry, J. A. (2019). Creating a safe sleep environment for the infant: What the pediatric nurse needs to know. *Journal of Pediatric Nursing, 44*(2019), 119–122.

Niemi, P. (2016). Six challenges for ethical conduct in science. *Science and Engineering Ethics, 22*, 1007–1025.

Nightingale, F. (1859/1992). *Notes on nursing: What it is, and what it is not* [Commemorative ed.]. Philadelphia, PA: Lippincott Williams & Wilkins.

Noonan, N., Galvin, R., Doody, O., & Jomeen, J. (2017). A qualitative meta-synthesis: Public health nurses' role in the identification and management of perinatal mental health problems. *Journal of Advanced Nursing, 73*(3), 545–557.

Noonan, D., Hartman, A. M., Briggs, J., & Biederman, D. J. (2017). Collaborating with public housing residents and staff to improve health: A mixed-methods analysis. *Journal of Community Health Nursing, 34*(4), 203–213.

Nurse-Family Partnership (NFP). (2017). *Nurse-Family Partnership: Outcomes, costs and return on investment in the U.S.* Retrieved from https://www.nursefamilypartnership.org/wp-content/uploads/2017/02/Miller-State-Specific-Fact-Sheet_US_20170405-1.pdf

Nurse-Family Partnership (NFP). (2018). *Overview*. Retrieved from https://www.nursefamilypartnership.org/wp-content/uploads/2018/11/Overview-2018.pdf

Nurse-Family Partnership (NFP) National Service Office. (October 2015). *National results of the maternal, infant, and early childhood home visiting program*. Retrieved from https://www.nursefamilypartnership.org/wp-content/uploads/2018/04/2015NFP_MIECHVReport_forprint-1.pdf

Oana, O. (2017). Moral education and virtue ethics- an operational framework. *Euromentor, 8*(4), 98–116.

O'Byrne, P., Orser, L., MacPherson, P., & Valela, N. (2018). The patient rationale for seeking HIV PEP: Qualitative results from a nurse-led program. *Public Health Nursing, 35*(5), 386–395.

Olds, D., Eckenrode, J., Henderson, C., Kitzman, H., Powers, J., Cole, R., … Pettitt, L. M. (1997). Long-term effects of home visitation on maternal life course and child abuse and neglect: Fifteen-year follow-up of a randomized trial. *Journal of the American Medical Association, 278*(8), 637–643.

Olds, D. L., Holmberg, J. R., Donelan-McCall, N., Luckey, D. W., Knudtson, M. D., & Robinson, J. (2014a). Effects of home visits by paraprofessionals and by nurses on children: Follow-up of a randomized trial at ages 6 and 9 years. *JAMA Pediatrics, 168*(2), 114–121.

Olds, D. L., Kitzman, H., Knudtson, M. D., Anson, E., Smith, J. A., & Cole, R. (2014b). Effect of home visiting by nurses on maternal and child mortality: Results of a 2-decade follow-up of a randomized clinical trial. *JAMA Pediatrics, 168*(9), 800–806.

Olds, D., Robinson, J., Pettitt, L., Luckey, D., Holmberg, J., Ng, R. K., et al. (2004). Effects of home visits by paraprofessionals and by nurses: Age 4 follow-up results of a randomized trial. *Pediatrics, 114*(6), 1560–1568.

Olson, P., & Sheiner, L. (April 26, 2017). *The Hutchins Center explains: Prescription drug spending*. The Brookings Institution. Retrieved from https://www.brookings.edu/blog/up-front/2017/04/26/the-hutchins-center-explains-prescription-drug-spending/

Omonaiye, O., Nicholson, P., Kusljic, S., & Manias, E. (2018). A meta-analysis of effectiveness of interventions to improve adherence in pregnant women receiving antiretroviral therapy in sub-Saharan Africa. *International Journal of Infectious Diseases, 74*, 71–82.

Oxford Vaccine Group. (2018). *Herd immunity (herd protection)*. Retrieved from http://vk.ovg.ox.ac.uk/herd-immunity

Palacio, A., Kirolos, I., & Tamariz, L. (2015). Patient values and preferences when choosing anticoagulants. *Patient Preference and Adherence, 9*, 133–138.

Pappalardo, A. A., Paulson, A., Bruscato, R., Thomas, L., Minier, M., & Martin, M. A. (2019). Chicago Public School nurses examine barriers to school asthma care coordination. *Public Health Nursing, 36*(1), 36–44.

Park, S. H. (2018). Tools for assessing fall risk in the elderly: A systematic review and meta-analysis. *Aging Clinical and Experimental Research, 30*(1), 1–16.

Parsons, R., Golder, S., & Watt, I. (2019). More than one-third of systematic reviews did not fully report the adverse events outcome. *Journal of Clinical Epidemiology, 108*, 95–101.

Patel, T. S., Cinti, S., Sun, D., Li, S., Luo, R., Wen, B., … Stevenson, J. G. (2017). Oseltamivir for pandemic influenza preparation: Maximizing the use of an existing stockpile. *American Journal of Infection Control, 45*(3), 303–305.

Pearl, R. (September 24, 2018). *The immorality of prescription drug pricing in the United States. Retrieved* from https://www.forbes.com/sites/robertpearl/2018/09/24/nostrum/#753357314fb1

Pereira, G. (2015). What do we need to be part of dialogue? From discursive ethics to critical social justice. *Critical Horizons, 16*(3), 280–298.

Peterson, M. (December 21, 2016). *How 4 drug companies rapidly raised prices on life saving drugs*. Retrieved from https://www.latimes.com/business/la-fi-senate-drug-price-study-20161221-story.html

Pianin, E. (December 21, 2016). *Outraged by spiking drug prices, Congress tiptoes around price controls*. The Fiscal Times. Retrieved from http://www.thefiscaltimes.com/2016/12/21/Outraged-Spiking-Drug-Prices-Congress-Tiptoes-Around-Price-Controls

Polit, D., & Beck, C. T. (2018). *Essentials of nursing research: Appraising evidence for nursing practice* (9th ed.). Philadelphia, PA: Wolters Kluwer.

Polivka, B., & Chaudry, R. V. (2018). A scoping review of environmental health nursing research. *Public Health Nursing, 35*(1), 10–17.

Quad Council Coalition. (2018). *Community/public health nursing (C/PHN) competencies*. Retrieved from http://www.quadcouncilphn.org/documents-3/2018-qcc-competencies/

Quinn, S. C. (2018). African American adults and seasonal influenza vaccination: Changing our approach can move the needle. *Human Vaccines & Immunotherapeutics, 14*(3), 719–723.

Rainer, J., Schneider, J. K., & Lorenz, R. A. (2018). Ethical dilemmas in nursing: An integrative review. *Journal of Clinical Nursing, 27*(19–20), 3446–3461.

Rashid, J., Leath, B., Truman, B., Atkinson, D. D., Gary, L. C., & Manian, N. (2017). Translating comparative effectiveness research into practice: Effects of interventions on lifestyle, medication adherence, and self-care for Type 2 Diabetes, hypertension, and obesity among Black, Hispanic, and Asian residents of Chicago and Houston, 2010–2013. *Journal of Public Health Management & Practice, 23*(5), 468–476.

Rebar, C., & Gersch, C. (2015). *Understanding nursing research: Using research in evidence-based practice* (4th ed.). Philadelphia, PA: Wolters Kluwer.

Resnik, D. B. (2018). Proportionality in public health regulation: The case of dietary supplements. *Food Ethics, 2*(1), 1–16.

Reverby, S. M. (2011). "Normal exposure" and inoculation syphilis: A PHS "Tuskegee" doctor in Guatemala. *The Journal of Policy History, 23*(1), 6–28.

Reyes, D., & Meyer, K. (2020). Identifying community priorities for neighborhood livability: Engaging neighborhood residents to facilitate community assessment. *Public Health Nursing, 37*(1), 87–95.

Rhodes, D., Visker, J., Cox, C., Forsyth, E., & Woolman, K. (2017). Public health and school nurses' perceptions of barriers to HPV vaccination in Missouri. *Journal of Community Health Nursing, 34*(4), 180–189.

Richburg, C. M., & Slagley, J. (2017). Noise concerns of residents living in close proximity to hydraulic fracturing sites in Southwest Pennsylvania. *Public Health Nursing, 36*, 3–10.

Robichaux, C. (Ed.). (2017). *Ethical competence in nursing practice: Competencies, skills, decision making*. New York, NY: Springer Publishing Company, LLC.

Rodriguez, M. A. (2013). First, do no harm: The US sexually transmitted disease experiments in Guatemala. *American Journal of Public Health, 103*, 2122–2126.

Rogowski, W., & Schleidgen, S. (2015). Using needs-based frameworks for evaluating new technologies: An application to genetic tests. *Health Policy, 119*(2), 147–155.

Rosenberg, M., Schick, A., Chai, G., & Mehta, S. (2018). Trends and economic drivers for United States naloxone pricing, January 2006 to February 2017. *Addictive Behaviors, 86*, 86–89.

Ryan, R. M., & Deci, E. L. (2017). *Self-determination theory: Basic psychological needs in motivation, development, and wellness*. New York, NY: The Guilford Press.

Saniford, P., Vivas Consuelo, D., Rouse, P., & Bramley, D. (2018). The trade-off between equity and efficiency in population health gain: Making it real. *Social Science & Medicine, 212*, 136–144.

Santos, J., Palumbo, F., Molsen-David, E., Willke, R., Drummond, M., Ho, A., … Thompson, D. (2017). ISPOR Code of Ethics 2017 (4th edition). *Value in Health*, 20(10), 1227–1242.

Schreiber, N., Bourgeois, J, Landry, J., Schmajuk, M., Erickson, J., … Cohen, M. A. (2018). What psychiatrists need to know about the determination of dispositional capacity. *Psychiatric Times, 35*(4). Retrieved from https://www.psychiatrictimes.com/forensic-psychiatry/what-psychiatrists-need-know-about-determination-dispositional-capacity

Sexton, E., O'Donovan, M. A., Mulryan, N., McCallion, P., & McCarron, M. (2017). Whose quality of life? A comparison of measures of self-determination and emotional wellbeing in research with older adults with and without intellectual disability. *Journal of Intellectual & Developmental Disability, 41*(4), 324–337.

Sierau, S., Dahne, V., Brand, T., Kurtz, V., von Klitzing, K., & Jungmann, T. (2016). Effects of home visitation on maternal competencies, family environment, and child development: A randomized controlled trial. *Prevention Science, 17*(1), 40–51.

Simpson, V., & Hass, Z. (2019). Individual health outcomes secondary to a nurse-led coalition-based health promotion program for underserved diverse populations. *Public Health Nursing, 36*(5), 667–675.

Skloot, R. (2011). *The immortal life of Henrietta Lacks.* New York, NY: Random House/Broadway Books.

Snow, R., Laski, L., & Mutumba, M. (2015). Sexual and reproductive health: Progress and outstanding needs. *Global Public Health, 10*(2), 149–173.

Spector-Bagdady, K., & Lombardo, P. A. (2018). From in vivo to in vitro: How the Guatemala STD experiments transformed bodies into biospecimens. *Millbank Quarterly, 96*(2), 244–271.

Spinelli, J., Byard, R., Van Den Heuvel, C., & Collins-Praino, L. E. (2018). Medullary astrogliosis in sudden infant death syndrome varies with sleeping environment: Evidence for different mechanisms of death in alone versus co-sleepers? *Journal of Child Neurology, 33*(4), 269–274.

Stastny, P. F., Keens, T. G., & Alkon, A. (2016). Supporting SIDS in families: The public health nurse SIDS home visit. *Public Health Nursing, 33*(3), 242–248.

Strair, R. (2017). Universal health care: The cost of being human. *Journal of Clinical Ethics, 28*(3), 247–249.

Swider, S. M., Levin, P. F., & Reising, V. (2017). Evidence of public health nursing effectiveness: A realist review. *Public Health Nursing, 34*(4), 324–334.

The Community Guide. (n.d.). *Your online guide to what works to promote healthy communities.* Retrieved from https://www.thecommunityguide.org

Thomas, C. W., Corso, L., Monroe, J. A. (2015). The value of the "system" in public health services and systems research. *American Journal of Public Health, 105*(s2), s147–s149.

Towfight, A., Cheng, E., Ayala-Rivera, M., McCreath, H., Sanossian, N., Dutta, T., ... Vickrey, B. (2017). Randomized controlled trial of a coordinated care intervention to improve risk factor control after stroke or transient ischemic attack in the safety net: Secondary stroke prevention by uniting community and chronic care model teams early to end disparities (SUCCEED). *BMC Neurology, 17*, 24. doi: 10.1186/s12983-017-0792-7.

Upwell Community. (2019). *True cost of diabetes.* Retrieved from https://www.upwell.com/true-cost-of-diabetes

U.S. Department of Health and Human Services (USDHHS). (2016a). *Human subjects regulations decision charts.* Retrieved from https://www.hhs.gov/ohrp/regulations-and-policy/decision-charts/index.html

U.S. Department of Health and Human Services (USDHHS). (2016b). *The Belmont report: Ethical principles and guidelines for the protection of human subjects of research.* Retrieved from http://www.hhs.gov/ohrp/policy/belmont.html

Van Spall, H., Rahman, T., Mytton, O., Ramasundarahettige, C., Ibrahim, Q., Kabali, C., ... Connolly, S. (2017). Comparative effectiveness of transitional care services in patients discharged from the hospital with heart failure: A systematic review and network meta-analysis. *European Journal of Heart Failure, 19*, 1427–1443.

Vaughn, L. (2017). *Bioethics: Principles, issues, & cases* (3rd ed.). London: Oxford University Press.

Vezyridis, P., & Timmons, S. (2015). On the adoption of personal health records: Some problematic issues for patient empowerment. *Ethics and Information Technology, 17*(2), 113–124.

Walsh, B., Doherty, E., & O'Neill, C. (2016). Since the start of the Vaccines for Children Program, uptake has increased, and most disparities have decreased. *Health Affairs, 35*(2), 356–364.

Walsdorf, A. (2018). I get by with a little help from my 750-dollar-per-tablet friends: A model act for states to prevent dramatic pharmaceutical price increases. *Minnesota Law Review*, 102, 2497–2545. Retrieved from https://www.minnesotalawreview.org/wp-content/uploads/2018/07/Walsdorf_MLR.pdf

Weber, J. J. (2019). A systematic review of nurse-led interventions with populations experiencing homelessness. *Public Health Nursing, 36*(1), 96–106.

Winland-Brown, J., Lachman, V. D., & Swanson, E. O. (2015). The new 'Code of Ethics for Nurses with Interpretive Statements' 2015: Practical clinical application, part I. *Medsurg Nursing, 24*(4), 269–271.

Wong, H. T., Chiang, V. C., Choi, K. S, & Loke, A. Y. (2016). The need for a definition of big data for nursing science: A case study of disaster preparedness. *International Journal of Environmental Research and Public Health, 13*(10), 1015.

Wu, Y. K., & Berry, D. C. (2018). Impact of weight stigma on psychological and psychological health outcomes for overweight and obese adults: A systematic review. *Journal of Advanced Nursing*, 74(5), 1030–1042. doi: 10.1111/jan.13511.

Wu, J., Dean, K. S., Rosen, Z., & Meunnig, P. A. (2017). The cost-effectiveness analysis of Nurse-Family Partnership in the United States. *Journal of Health Care for the Poor and Underserved, 28*(4), 1578–1597.

Yu, Z., Gunn, L., Wall, P., & Fanning, S. (2017). Antimicrobial resistance and its association with tolerance to heavy metals in agriculture production. *Food Microbiology, 64*, 23–32.

Zhu, J., Dy, S., Wenzel, J., & Wu, A. (2018). Association of magnet status and nurse staffing with improvements in patient experience with hospital care, 2008–2015. *Medical Care, 56*(2), 111–120.

CHAPTER 5

Transcultural Nursing

"People everywhere share common biological and psychological needs, and the function of all cultures is to fulfill such needs; the nature of the culture is determined by its function."

—Bronislaw Malinowski (1884–1942), Cultural Anthropologist

"Looking from... our high places of safety in the developed civilization, it is easy to see all the crudity and irrelevance of magic. But without its power and guidance early man could not have mastered his practical difficulties ..., nor could man have advanced to the higher stages of civilization."

—Horace Miner (1912–1993), Anthropologist

KEY TERMS

Complementary and alternative medicine (CAM)
Cultural assessment
Cultural brokering
Cultural diversity
Cultural relativism
Cultural self-awareness
Cultural sensitivity
Culture
Culture shock
Dominant values
Enculturation
Ethnic group
Ethnicity
Ethnocentrism
Ethnorelativism
Folk medicine
Home remedies
Indigenous
Intraethnic variations
Integrated health care
Majority–minority
Microculture
Minority group
Race
Subcultures
Transcultural (cross-cultural) nursing

LEARNING OBJECTIVES

Upon mastery of this chapter, you should be able to:

1. Define and explain the concept of culture.
2. Discuss the meaning of cultural diversity and its significance for community/public health nursing.
3. Describe the meaning and effects of ethnocentrism on community/public health nursing practice.
4. Identify five characteristics shared by all cultures.
5. Conduct a cultural assessment.
6. Apply principles of transcultural nursing in community health nursing practice.

INTRODUCTION

The United States is a country of immigrants. People of many different cultural groups and races built this nation. For hundreds of years, people have seen this land as a refuge from political, religious, or economic strife. **Indigenous** (or native) people were present when the early settlers arrived on these shores and when people were brought here in slavery. Refugees, fleeing poverty and hunger, as well as war and oppression, flocked to this country over the next two centuries. The citizenship of most countries around the world is an amalgamation of people who have different values, ideals, and behaviors. Many people have chosen to discover their ancestry through DNA testing as a means of drawing families closer together. Do you know the story of how your ancestors came to your country?

Although Americans have many differences, they also have much in common. In the Western culture, an individual's work and creative achievements are applauded. There is respect for one another's personal preferences about food, dress, or personal beliefs. The right to be oneself—and thereby to be different from others—is even protected by state and federal laws. Although individuality is a cherished American value, there are limits to the range of differences most Americans find acceptable. People with behavior outside the acceptable range may be labeled as socially nonconforming. For example, the US culture approves of moderate alcohol intake but not alcoholism.

The beliefs and sanctions of the dominant or majority culture are called **dominant values**. In the United States, the majority culture is non-Hispanic Whites, whose dominant values have largely included the work ethic, thrift, success, independence, initiative, privacy, cleanliness, attractive appearance, and a focus on the future. Dominant values reflect the cultural power differentials and the unearned, frequently unrecognized privileges held by Americans with White social identities (Holm, Rowe, Brady, & White-Perkins, 2017).

Awareness of dominant values is important in community/public health nursing because the values shape people's thoughts and behaviors; this awareness helps nurses answer questions such as the following:

- Why are some client behaviors acceptable to health professionals and others not?
- Why do nurses have difficulty persuading certain clients to accept new ways of thinking and acting?

Explanations for such questions can be found by examining the concept of culture, especially its influence on health, health behaviors, and community/public health nursing practice. For example:

- An emphasis on the need for milk in the diet may reflect cultural blindness, considering that people from diverse ethnic groups are often lactose intolerant and that food allergies affecting the quality of life for minority children appear to be understudied and undiagnosed (Widge, Flory, Sharma, & Herbert, 2018).
- Regardless of their own cultural backgrounds, nurses are generally educated to believe that the biomedical model is the best framework, and dominant social values are often reinforced.

However, these dominant values can and do change as a result of changing demographics and population shifts (Fig. 5-1). Current research on this issue reveals areas of concern (Box 5-1).

Awareness of dominant culture and values helps us better understand political, socioeconomic, and health care outcomes.

- Because the powerful exert control over political, economic, and social structures that influence all members of society, laws are in place prohibiting discrimination based on "race, color, religion, national origin, and sex," as well as disability (U.S. Equal Employment Opportunity Commission, n.d., para. 1).
- Governments' political decisions affecting the health of populations, beginning with deregulation and reductions in government spending in this country, have led to increased rates of poverty, inequality, incarceration, obesity, and other conditions tied to the social determinants of health (Nadasen, 2017).
- Culture so strongly influences community/public health nursing practice that the Quad Council of Public Health Nursing Organizations (which is now the Council of Public Health Nursing Organizations) incorporated it into the competency domains for community/public health nursing practice. Domain 4, cultural competency skills, focuses on individual and community needs, actions to support a diverse workforce, an organization's cultural competence, and the effect of public health policies/programs on diverse populations (Quad Council Coalition Competency Review Task Force, 2018). See Chapter 2 for Quad Council Competencies.

THE CONCEPT OF CULTURE

Culture refers to the beliefs, values, and behaviors that are shared by members of a society and provide a template or "road map" for living.

- Culture tells people what is acceptable or unacceptable in a given situation.
- Culture dictates what to do, say, or believe.
- Culture is learned. As children grow up, they learn from their parents and others around them how to interpret the world. In turn, these assimilated beliefs and values prescribe desired behavior. We think of this as learned behavior, but can culture actually impact your neurobiology (Box 5-2)?

Culture is a multifaceted concept, a way of organizing and thinking about life. Culture includes customs, law, morals, beliefs, knowledge, and habits practiced by members of a group or society. It is all of the socially inherited characteristics of a group, comprising everything that one generation can tell, convey, or hand down to the next generation. Scholars from many disciplines have defined culture in these ways:

- Learned, shared, and transmitted values, beliefs, and norms held by a group of people that guide their actions (McFarland & Wehbe-Alamah, 2018)
- A patterned response of behavior that develops from the impact of social and religious structures in a community over time, from infancy through old age, and can be apparent in a community's intellectual and artistic achievements (Giger, 2017)
- A mediating or moderating variable in business, human relations, psychology, and most human endeavors (Coyle, 2018)
- A historically transmitted pattern of meanings, closely tied with religion and ethics; an identification of those people or behaviors outside the cultural bounds (Forbes & Mahan, 2017)

Anthropologists describe culture as systems of beliefs, values, and norms of behavior found in all societies. More than simply custom or ritual, it is a way of organizing and thinking about life. It gives people a sense of security about their behavior; without having to consciously

In 109 counties, white population share fell below 50% between 2000 and 2018

US counties in which the non-Hispanic white share of the population fell below 50% from 2000 to 2018

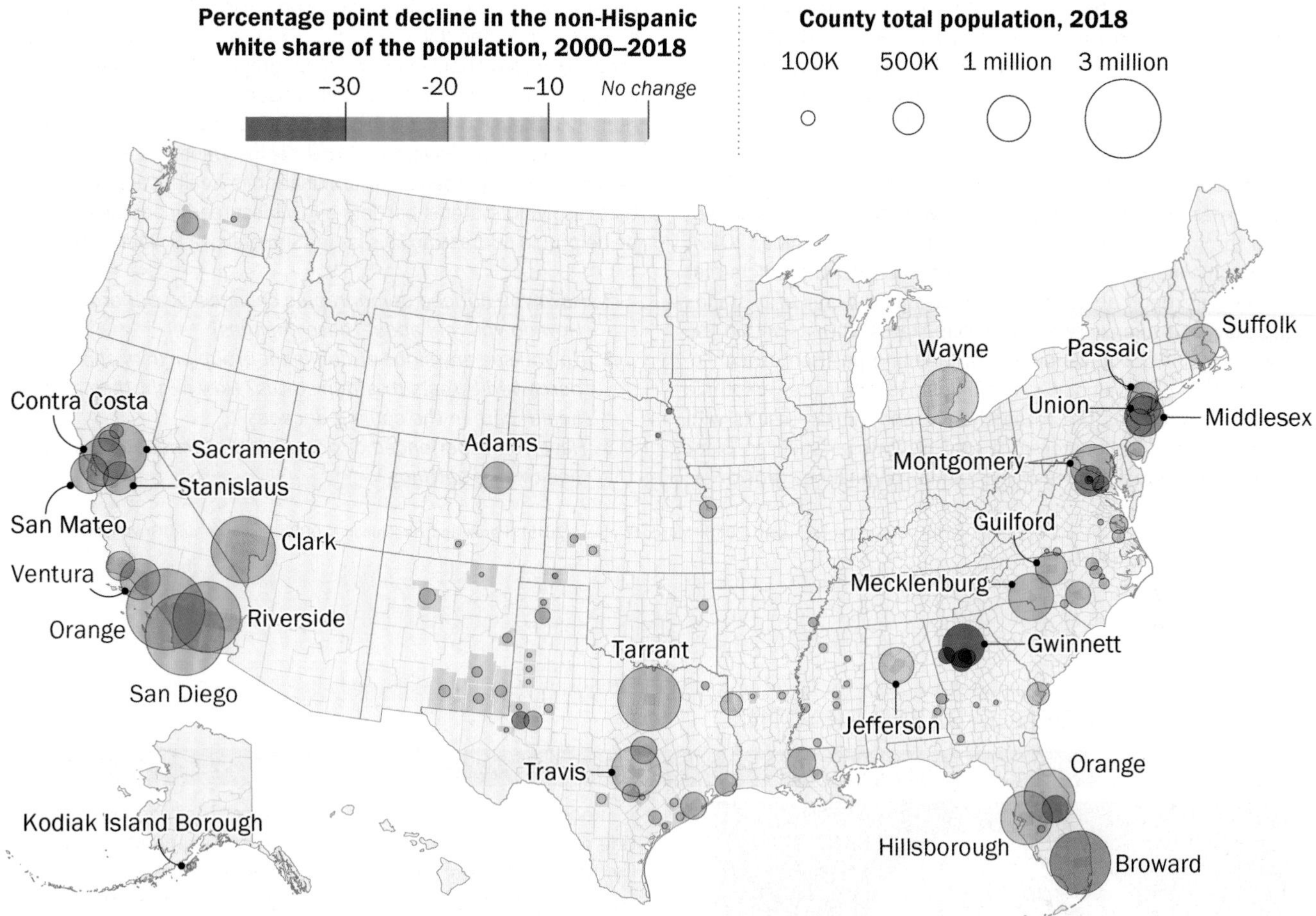

FIGURE 5-1 In 109 counties, White population share fell below 50% between 2000 and 2018: US Counties in which the non-Hispanic White share of the population fell below 50% from 2000 to 2018. (Reprinted with permission from Krogstad, J. M. (August 21, 2019). *Reflecting a Demographic Shift, 109 US Counties have become majority nonwhite since 2000.* Washington, D.C.: Pew Research Center. Retrieved from https://www.pewresearch.org/fact-tank/2019/08/21/u-s-counties-majority-nonwhite/ft_19-08-21_majorityminoritycounties_in-109-counties-white-population-share-fell-below-50-percent-2000-2018_2/)

think about it, they know how to act. For example, Spector (2017) notes that culture:

- Determines the value placed on achievement, independence, work, and leisure
- Forms the basis for the definitions of gender roles
- Influences a person's response to authority figures
- Dictates religious beliefs and practices
- Shapes child-rearing

Every community and social or ethnic group has its own culture; individual members act based on what they have learned within their culture. As anthropologist Edward Hall (1959) noted over a half-century ago, culture controls our lives and influences even the smallest elements of everyday living. It is the knowledge people use to design their own actions and, in turn, to interpret others' behavior (Spradley, McCurdy, & Shandy, 2016). For example, culture:

- Determines the appropriate distance for two people to stand when speaking to each other: non-Hispanic White Americans tolerate at least 2.5 ft, whereas Latin Americans prefer a shorter distance, as little as 18 in.
- Influences one's perception of time: non-Hispanic White Americans may expect people to be on time for appointments and think it inconsiderate to keep someone waiting, whereas those from Vietnamese, Native American, and Hispanic cultures have a more elastic perception of time and do not interpret lateness for appointments as thoughtlessness

The concept of culture must be distinguished from two other related but different concepts:

- **Race** refers to a biologically designated group of people whose distinguishing features, such as skin color or facial characteristics, are inherited.

BOX 5-1 WHAT DO *YOU* THINK?

Transition to a Majority–Minority Nation

According to projections from the U.S. Census Bureau, in a seminal article by Perez and Hirschman (2009), we will become a **majority–minority** nation by mid-century, as current minority groups gain in population while the existing majority non-Hispanic White population decreases. This is manifesting in an uneven fashion across the 50 states with the growth of the Hispanic population, especially children ages 0 to 4 (Murdock, Cline, Zey, Perez, & Wilner Jeanty, 2015). Even though some disagree with the methods used to calculate these results (Alba, 2016), research conducted by Craig and Richeson (2014) predicts that this census report about the change to majority–minority standing may lead to anxiety about "group status" threats within the former majority population and "a widening partisan divide" (p. 1189). This phenomenon is not unique to one racial or ethnic group, however, as the researchers found similar results with other groups who perceived a loss of status—such as Black Americans perceiving Hispanic/Latino population growth as threatening to their status (Richeson & Grossman, 2016). Four studies conducted by Craig and Richeson (2017) found that access to information about this demographic shift led the majority group to believe that they will encounter greater discrimination while the minority groups may encounter less discrimination. Other researchers have noted that socioeconomic status is also associated with perceived discrimination in health care and note that resolving systems barriers and widespread inequities would be helpful in addressing this issue (Stepanikova & Oates, 2017).

1. *Have you noticed demographic changes in your area? How do you feel about these changes?*
2. *Do you see any signs of dominant group anxiety and perceived threats to group status? How might they affect health care in the coming decades?*
3. *Have you experienced or observed discrimination in health care settings?*

Source: Alba (2016); Craig and Richeson (2014); Craig and Richeson (2017); Murdock et al. (2015); Perez and Hirschman (2009); Richeson and Grossman (2016); Stepanikova and Oates (2017).

BOX 5-2 EVIDENCE-BASED PRACTICE

Can Culture Affect Your Neurobiology?

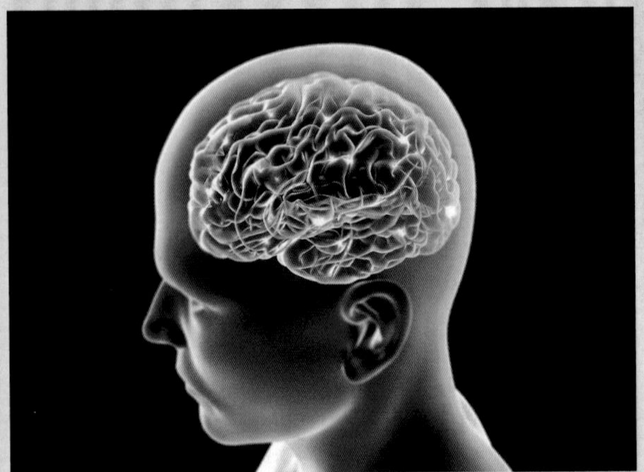

Research into the neuroscience of culture examines the interplay between culture, biological factors, physiological processes, and genetic influences.

Researchers in a 19-site longitudinal cohort study, the Adolescent Brain and Cognitive Development (ABCD) Initiative, are measuring a range of biological and behavioral processes at a time of marked change in the human brain's structure and networks (Luciana et al., 2018; Zucker et al., 2018). Over 11,000 children, ages 9 to 10 years, are enrolled in this study, which explores how neurologic developmental processes interact with culture and environment in areas such as risk taking and substance abuse. Preliminary results indicate that culture and environment have major roles influencing behavioral and neural development (Luciana et al., 2018; Zucker, et al., 2018).

Recent evidence converges to suggest that the neuropeptide oxytocin facilitates empathy, a key social cognitive capacity that affects interpersonal functioning. Culture is thought to influence the behavioral effects of oxytocin in both Chinese and Caucasian populations. In a study of 132 healthy Chinese adults, intranasal oxytocin was found to facilitate emotional empathy, similar to prior research with Caucasians (Geng et al., 2018). In another study, oxytocin was found to influence social connections and empathy with others but had a different effect in collectivistic versus individualistic cultures (group orientation vs. individual orientation). In this research, differences were noted across genders, as males were more influenced by oxytocin than females (Xu et al., 2017). This evidence is important as impaired empathy has been identified as a component of schizophrenia, autism, and personality disorders, and the oxytocin connection is of interest internationally (Montag et al. 2018).

Lastly, differences between Western and Asian cultures have been explored from a neuroscience standpoint. In a quantitative meta-analysis of 35 functional magnetic resonance imaging (fMRI) studies, researchers concluded that distinct neural networks do mediate cultural differences in both social and nonsocial processes (Han & Ma, 2014).

1. *What are your impressions of these findings?*
2. *How can this information be useful to you as a nurse working with different cultural groups?*
3. *Can this research impart a risk of stereotyping people from different groups?*

Source: Geng et al. (2018); Han and Ma (2014); Luciana et al. (2018); Montag et al. (2018); Widge et al. (2018); Wood et al. (2018); Xu et al. (2017); Zucker et al. (2018).

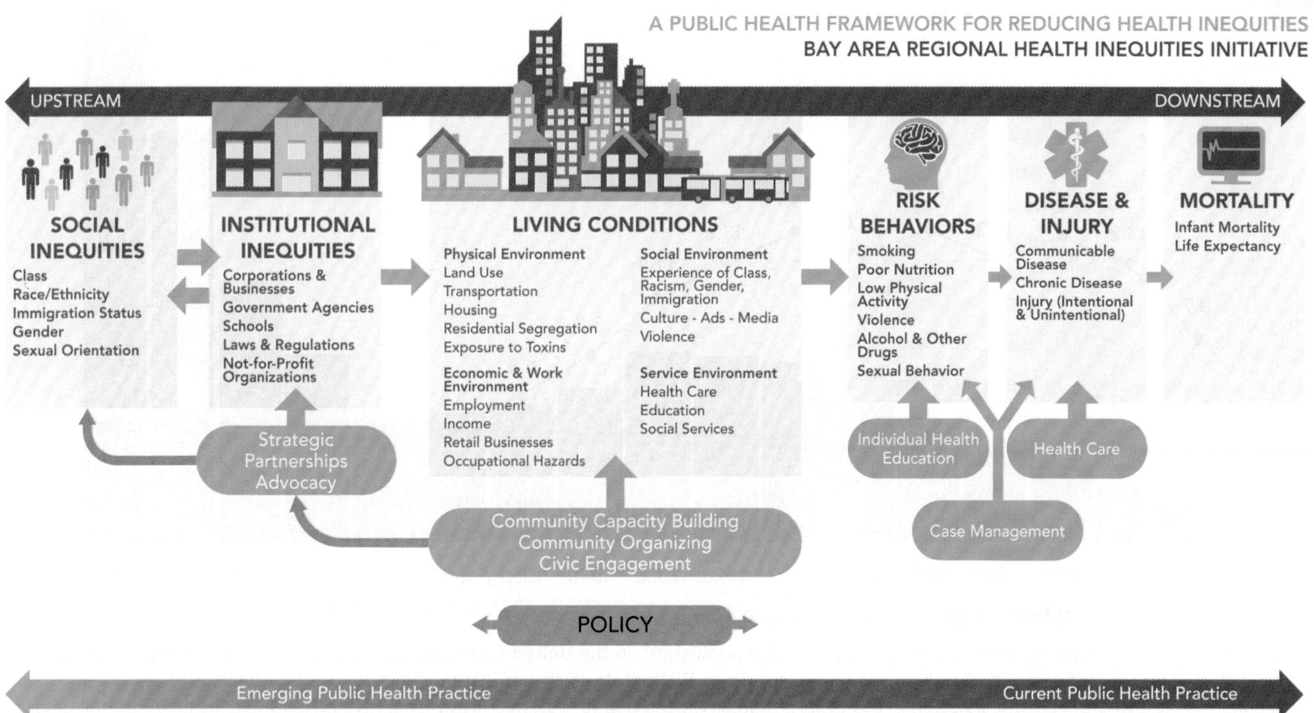

FIGURE 5-2 A public health framework for reducing health inequities. (Used with permission from Bay Area Regional Health Inequities Initiative, with updated graphics by California Department of Public Health. Retrieved from http://barhii.org/framework/)

- **Ethnic group** is an assemblage of people with common origins and a shared culture and identity; they may share a common geographic origin, race, language, religion, traditions, values, and food preferences (Spradley et al., 2016).

Race and ethnicity are factors influencing social inequality, and ultimately morbidity and mortality. See Figure 5-2.

Cultural Diversity

Cultural diversity, or *cultural plurality*, refers to the coexistence of a variety of cultural patterns within a geographic area. This diversity can occur both between and within countries and communities. Cultural diversity within communities has unique advantages and challenges. Language barriers and misunderstanding of cultural values can occur, whereas cultural practices, celebrations, and food traditions can enrich the community.

A major driver of cultural diversity in the United States has been immigration. Cultural diversity in the United States began when Native Americans were challenged by early foreign settlements. Before the mid-20th century, settlers came primarily from European countries, peaking in numbers just after the turn of the 20th century, with about 9 million immigrants admitted in the first decade. During much of that time, especially during the late 1600s through the early 1800s, Africans were enslaved and brought to the United States against their will, mostly to Southern states, where they were sold to plantation owners as property in order to labor on large plantations and farms. Slavery and cultural oppression engendered profound effects for many generations (Bellagamba, Greene, & Klein, 2017).

Immigration stayed high during the early 1900s and then dropped sharply from the 1950s to 1980s. It has risen more significantly since 2000. Immigration from non-European regions, such as Asia and South America, then steadily increased. Batalova, Blizzard, and Bolter (2020) note that the total number of immigrants from all countries in the 1990s actually exceeded the number who arrived during the first decade of the 20th century, when immigration was formerly at its peak (Fig. 5-3).

Current trends in US immigration include the following:

- A large, undocumented foreign-born population, which is difficult to count in a population census due to such factors as English language ability, literacy skills, understanding of the census, residential attachment, and legal status, which can contribute to coverage error (Jensen, Bhaskar, & Scopilliti, 2015)
- Immigrants from all regions of the world, in greater numbers from some areas than others (Fig. 5-4), becoming lawful permanent residents and, in due course, US citizens (Witsman, 2018) (Fig. 5-5)
- The fastest growing group of immigrants being people reporting two or more races, growing from 8 million in 2014 to a projected 26 million in 2060 (Fig. 5-4)
- The second-fastest growing group of immigrants being Asians, growing from 5.4% of the total population in 2014 to a projected 9.3% of the total population in 2060 (Colby & Ortman, 2015)

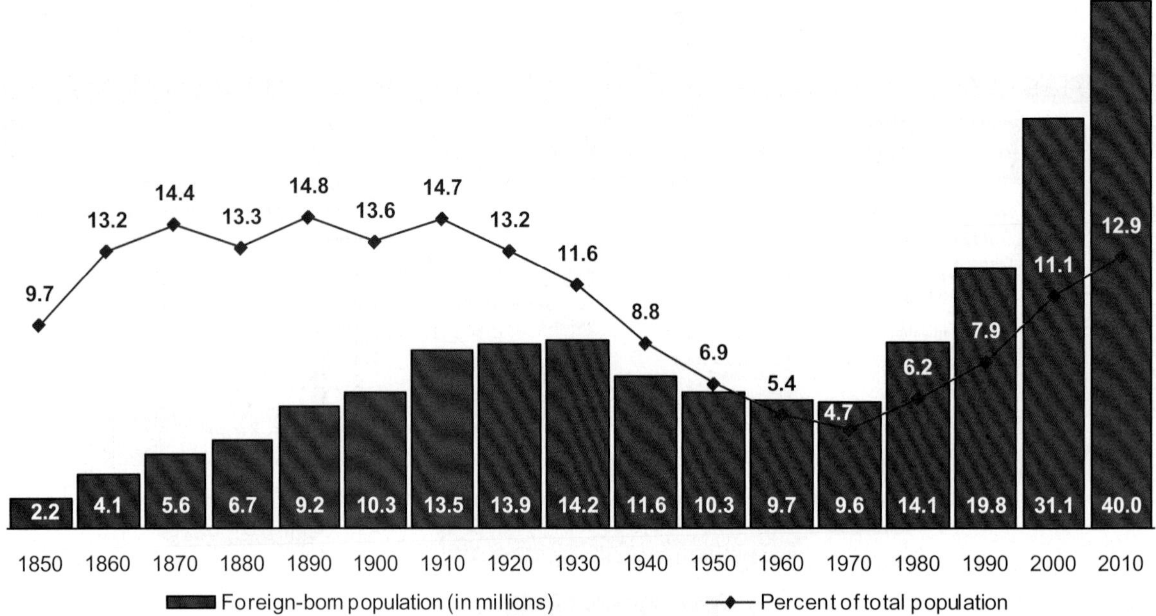

FIGURE 5-3 Foreign-born population and percent of total population, in the United States: 1850 to 2010. (Reprinted from Grieco, E. M., Trevelyan, E., Larson, L., Acosta, Y., Gambino, C., de la Cruz, P., ... Walters, N. (October 2012). *The size, place of birth, and geographic distribution of the foreign-born population in the United States: 1960-2010* (p. 19). Retrieved from https://www.census.gov/content/dam/Census/library/working-papers/2012/demo/POP-twps0096.pdf)

- Rapid growth in the Hispanic/Latino population (Box 5-3 and Table 5-1)

Undocumented or illegal immigration continues to be a controversial topic in this country. Plans to end the flow of illegal immigrants across our southwestern border include building a 700-mile border wall and legislation that penalizes employers of undocumented workers. Concerns include the following:

- In the past 20 years, many thousands of migrants are estimated to have died while crossing illegally into this country; there were 230 confirmed deaths during the first 9 months of 2014, with likely many more that were unknown (Brian & Laczko, 2018).
- Social justice is an important issue in community/public health nursing, and the national debate does not often consider the economic desperation and security concerns that drive people to put themselves in such jeopardy (see Chapters 23 and 27).

Immigration patterns are strongly influenced by immigration laws established since the 1800s:

- In 1891, medical and economic inspections were ordered at all major entry points as an influx of poor immigrants mostly from Europe led to fears of disease and contagion.
- The Immigration Act of 1924 limited immigration and allowed consideration of national origin in an effort to slow the influx of immigrants from Eastern and Southern Europe. Immigration has steadily trended upward since 1945, partly explained by changes in immigration laws.
- In 1965, quotas were ended that limited immigration of certain groups, and family-sponsored immigration, known as family migration, was officially endorsed.
- The Immigration Reform and Control Act of 1986 (Public Law 99-603) "legalized 2.7 million undocumented immigrants," and the Immigration Act of 1990 (Public Law 101-649) set numerical ceilings on certain immigrant groups, in part due to the AIDS crisis, and authorized increases for highly skilled workers or specific family members of aliens (Fairchild, 2018).

The terrorist attacks in 2001 led US President George W. Bush to suspend all immigration for 2 months. Suspicion about people from Middle Eastern countries permeated the nation—and worsened the social climate for immigrants. More recent trends include the following:

- Political upheaval, crime, and war precipitating the migration of refugees and migrants from the Middle East, South Asia, and Africa into Europe and of Central Americans into the United States, with no comprehensive effort to quickly find placements for the continual stream of people as all countries wrestle with the social and political issues
- A social climate in the United States and other countries is often characterized by ambivalence about accepting refugees and immigrants and ambiguity about their status, such that newcomers find an environment that is both welcoming and hostile
- Law enforcement practices related to immigration that result in involuntary separation of parents and children at the US border, with negative and persistent effects on the health and well-being of both children and adults (Gubernskaya & Dreby, 2017)
- Increased staffing for both border and immigration officials, broader use of drones, an average of almost one death per day at the border with Mexico, and, from 1993 to 2020, a 10-fold increase in the budget for border protection (American Immigration Council, 2020)

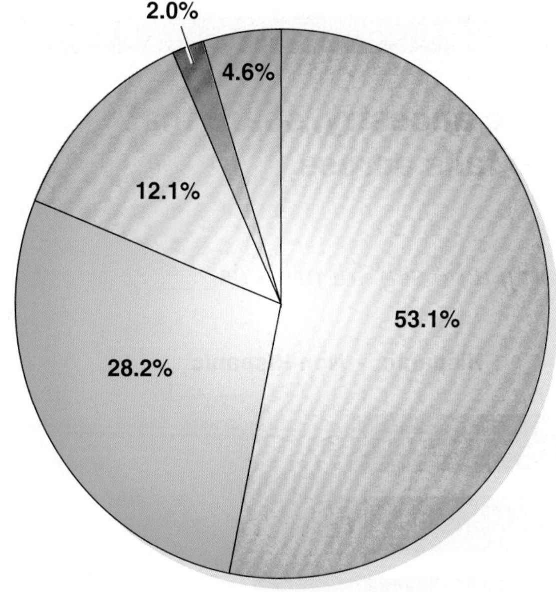

Latin America
Highest %: Mexico, El Salvador, Cuba, Dominican Republic, Guatemala

Asia
Highest %: India, Philippines, China, Vietnam, South Korea

Europe
Highest %: United Kingdom, Germany, Poland

North America
Highest %: Canada

Other (includes Africa and Oceania)
Highest %: Nigeria, Egypt, Ghana, Ethiopia

FIGURE 5-4 Percent distribution of foreign-born population by region of birth in the United States, 2010 Census. Total foreign-born population living in the United States in 2010 was 12.9% of population. These individuals are young, mostly from Latin America or Asia, and often settle in Southern or Western states. (Source: Grieco, E. M., Trevelyan, E., Larson, L., Acosta, Y., Gambino, C., de la Cruz, P., ... Walters, N. (October 2012). *The size, place of birth, and geographic distribution of the foreign-born population in the United States: 1960-2010.* Retrieved from https://www.census.gov/content/dam/Census/library/working-papers/2012/demo/POP-twps0096.pdf)

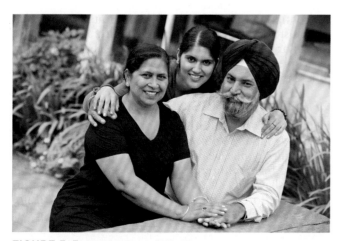

FIGURE 5-5 Sikh family now US citizens.

Although broad cultural values are shared by most large national societies, those societies contain smaller cultural groups called **subcultures**.

Subcultures:

- Are developed and preserved over time to meet the unique needs, values, and beliefs of people (McFarland & Wehbe-Alamah, 2018)
- Are aggregates of people within a society who share separate distinguishing characteristics, such as:
  - **Ethnicity** (being a member of a social group with a common racial, national, or cultural background, such as African American, Hispanic American [Merriam Webster Dictionary, 2020])
  - Occupation (e.g., farmers, physicians)
  - Socioeconomic status (e.g., working class, middle class)
  - Religion (e.g., Catholics, Muslims)
  - Geographic area (e.g., New Englanders, Southerners)
  - Age (e.g., older adults, school-age children)
  - Gender (e.g., women, men)
  - Sexual preference (e.g., gay, lesbian)
- Contain even smaller groups known as **microcultures**, consisting of people who share specific experiences or practices and who hold a special cultural knowledge unique to the subgroup, which they share with others in the community (Spradley et al., 2016), such as:
  - Recent African refugees sharing resources and housing
  - Syrian refugees (see Fig. 5-6) seeking business and entrepreneurial opportunities
  - Hmong immigrants from Southeast Asia adopting selected aspects of US culture
  - Third-generation Norwegians sharing unique food, dress, and values
- Retain some characteristics of the society of origin, as noted by the eminent anthropologist Margaret Mead (1960), such as beliefs and practices, foods, language spoken at home, holiday celebrations, and treatment of illness
- Include Native Americans, Mexican Americans, Irish Americans, Swedish Americans, Italian Americans, African Americans, Puerto Rican Americans, Chinese Americans, Japanese Americans, Vietnamese Americans, and many other ethnic groups

Furthermore, many microcultures exist in groups on the margins of mainstream culture, and acquire their own sets of beliefs and patterns for dealing with their environments. They have distinctive ways of defining the world and coping with life, such as:

- Narcotics users and transient alcoholics
- Gangs, criminals, and terrorist groups
- Appalachian people living in the mountains of Kentucky, West Virginia, Tennessee, and Virginia
- Migrant farm workers
- Urban homeless families

Ethnocentrism

There is a difference between a healthy cultural or ethnic identification and ethnocentrism. Anthropologists

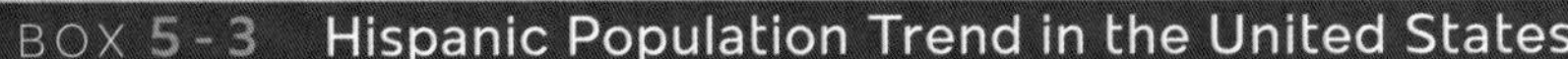

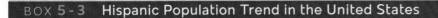

BOX 5-3 Hispanic Population Trend in the United States

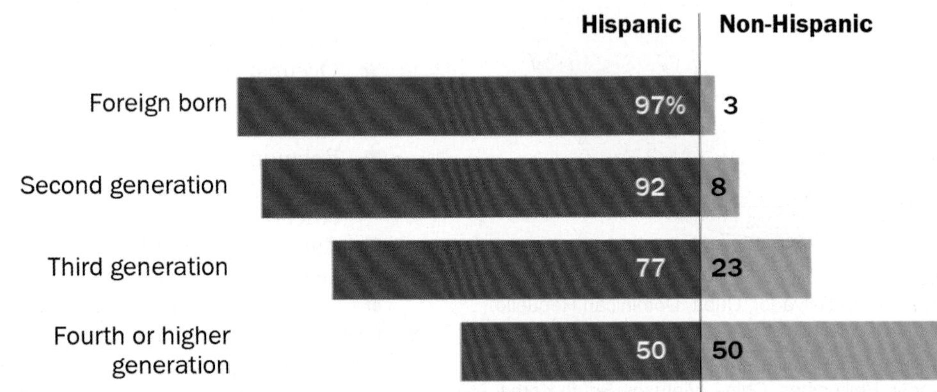

According to the U.S. Census Bureau, people of Hispanic origin identify with "Cuban," "Mexican," "South American," "Central American," or "all other Hispanic or Latino origin," regardless of race (U.S. Census Bureau, 2020, para. 1). Our Hispanic population is growing, from 12.5% of the population in the 2000 census to our most recent 2010 census figures of 16.3% of the population (Table 5-1). The 2019 population estimate for Hispanics/Latinos is 18.3% (U.S. Quick Facts, n.d.). The change in population numbers is only part of the story. The Hispanic population born in the United States is increasing, as portrayed in the figure in this box. Being first or second generation born in the United States and other factors such as intermarriage contribute to the increase in percentage of adults with Hispanic ancestry who self-identify as American. This indicates they feel a common identity with other Americans. The number of Hispanic cultural activities is diminishing, as adults reporting childhood experiences with Latino/Hispanic cultural are in decline across the generations as displayed below (Lopez, Gonzalez-Barrera, & López, 2017). Lopez et al. report that 11% of American adults with Hispanic heritage no longer identify themselves as Hispanic.

Source: Lopez et al. (2017); U.S. Census Bureau 2020, para. 1; U.S. Quick Facts (n.d.).
Figure reprinted with permission from Lopez, M. H., Gonzalez-Barrera, A., & Lopez, G. (December 20, 2017). *Hispanic identity fades across generations as immigrant connections fall away.* Washington, D.C.: Pew Research Center. Retrieved from https://www.pewresearch.org/hispanic/2017/12/20/hispanic-identity-fades-across-generations-as-immigrant-connections-fall-away/

note that **ethnocentrism** is a preference for one's own culture and belief that one's culture of origin is the best approach to life (Spradley et al., 2016). Ethnocentrism can inhibit a person's capacity for effective communication in a culturally diverse environment (Young, Haffjee, & Corsun, 2017). In turn, this can cause serious damage to interpersonal relationships and interfere with the quality and effectiveness of nursing interventions (McFarland & Wehbe-Alamah, 2018).

As shown in Figure 5-7, people can experience a developmental progression along a continuum from ethnocentrism, feeling one's own culture is best, to **ethnorelativism**—seeing all behavior in a cultural context (Blair, 2019). Some people may stop progressing and remain stagnated at one step, and others may move backward on the continuum. The left side of the continuum represents the most extreme reaction to intercultural differences: refusal or denial. On the right side is the characterization of people who show the most sensitivity to intercultural differences: incorporation.

CHARACTERISTICS OF CULTURE

In their study of culture, anthropologists and sociologists have made significant contributions to the field of community/public health. Their findings shed light on why and how culture influences behavior. Five characteristics shared by all cultures are especially pertinent to nursing's efforts to improve community health: culture is learned, it is integrated, it is shared, it is tacit, and it is dynamic.

TABLE 5-1 US Population by Race and Hispanic/Latino Origin, Census 2000 and 2010

Race and Hispanic/ Latino Origin	Census 2000, Population	Percent of Population	Census 2010, Population	Percent of Population	Percent Change, 2000–2010
Total Population	**281,421,906**	**100.0%**	**308,745,538**	**100.0%**	**+9.7%**
White	211,460,626	75.1	223,553,265	72.4	5.7
Black or African American	34,658,190	12.3	38,929,319	12.6	12.3
American Indian and Alaska Native	2,475,956	0.9	2,932,248	0.9	18.4
Asian	10,242,998	3.6	14,674,252	4.8	43.3
Native Hawaiian and other Pacific Islander	398,835	0.1	540,013	0.2	35.4
Hispanic or Latino	35,305,818	12.5	50,477,594	16.3	43.0
Some other race	15,359,073	5.5	19,107,368	6.2	24.4
Two or more races	6,826,228	2.4	9,009, 073	2.9	32.0

Adapted from Humes et al. (2011).

Culture Is Learned

Patterns of cultural behavior are acquired, not inherited. People are not born with a cultural belief system but gain it through **enculturation**, the process of learning one's culture (Fig. 5-8). Aspects one learns through enculturation include (Kottack, 2017; Spradley et al., 2016):

- Beliefs
- Dress
- Diet
- Language
- Expressions of emotions such as sadness, grief, joy, and happiness
- Smiling, laughter, and humor

Although culture is learned, each individual may experience life in a singular way, which affects the process and results of that learning. For example, rigid gender roles may be culturally taught, but an individual may approach life as transgender (Andrews, Boyle, & Collins, 2020). Because culture is learned, parts of it can be relearned. People might change certain cultural elements or adopt new behaviors or values. Some individuals and groups are more willing and able than others to try new ways and thereby influence change.

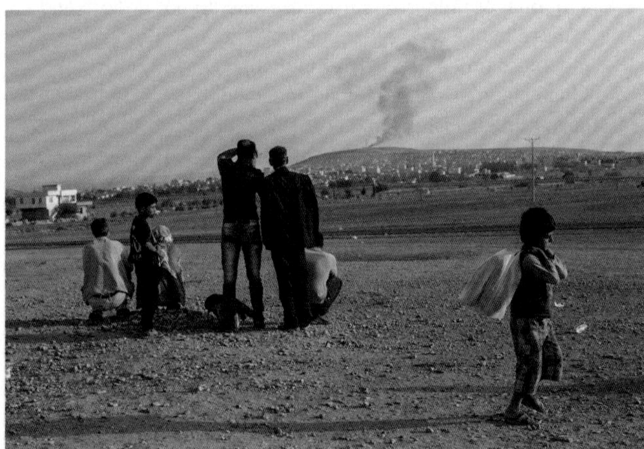

FIGURE 5-6 Syrian refugees in Turkey looking back at their burning homes.

Culture is Integrated

Culture is a functional, integrated whole, not merely an assortment of customs and traits. As in any system, all parts of a culture are interrelated and interdependent. The components of a culture, such as its social norms or religious beliefs, perform separate functions but come into harmony with each other to form an operating and cohesive whole. Therefore, each component should be viewed in light of its connection to other components and to the whole, not independently.

To provide effective nursing care, nurses may find their own cultural beliefs, and practice systems need to be adjusted or reintegrated to accommodate the cultural beliefs and practices of others. For example, a nurse may promote the need for eating three balanced meals each day based on social and cultural beliefs and values that are related to good nutrition. This is necessary for health, and health is essential for productivity in work and career, quality of life, and achieving life goals. A client's beliefs and values in these areas may not be completely congruent with the nurse's (Box 5-4).

Culture is Shared

Culture is the product of aggregate behavior, not individual habit. Certainly, individuals practice a culture, but customs are phenomena shared by all members of the

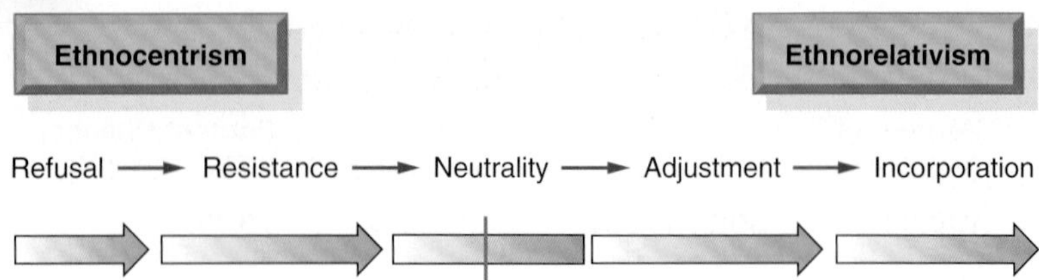

FIGURE 5-7 Cross-cultural sensitivity continuum.

group. About 50 years ago, anthropologist George Murdock explained this idea as follows (1972, p. 258):

> Culture does not depend on individuals. An ordinary habit dies with its possessor, but a group habit lives on in the survivors... transmitted from generation to generation.... From earliest childhood behavior is conditioned by the habits of those around him. He has no choice but to conform to.... his group."

Involving the ideas of what is good, right, just, and fair, a culture's values are among its most important elements. A **value** is a notion or idea designating relative worth or desirability. The normative criteria by which people justify their decisions are based on values that are more deeply rooted than behaviors and, consequently, more difficult to change. Each culture classifies phenomena into good and bad, desirable and undesirable, and right and wrong. When people respond in favor of or against some practice, they are reflecting their culture's values about that practice.

Examples of values include:

- Desirable traits: honesty, loyalty, and faithfulness
- Undesirable traits: lying, stealing, and cheating
- Eating meat: desirable and healthy versus sacrilegious or unhealthful
- Response to pain or grief: loud, vocal expressions versus silence and stoicism
- Speed and efficiency versus patience and thoughtfulness

No matter the culture, shared values give people in a specific culture stability and security and provide a standard for behavior, helping them know what to believe and how to act (Andrews et al., 2020). See Chapter 4 for more on values and ethics.

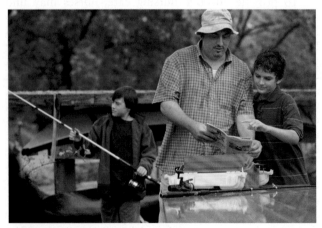

FIGURE 5-8 Family enculturation helps children acquire shared values and attitudes.

When community/public health nurses (C/PHNs) know that culture is shared, their understanding of human behavior expands, and their ability to provide effective care to members of specific cultures increases. For example, it was found that women from the Hmong culture were reluctant to get a Pap test for cervical cancer because they had to be in the lithotomy position, which they (along with women from other cultures) perceived as immodest. Realizing that this impacts women's access to cancer screening, researchers have developed a urine test that can detect cervical cancer at early stages, similar to the Pap test, making screening more accessible to underserved populations (Guerrero-Preston et al., 2016; Wood, Loftres, & Vahabi, 2018). This demonstrates that focusing on one individual's behavior may be less effective than working within the culture to promote well-being (Box 5-5).

Culture is Generally Tacit

As a guide for human interaction, culture can be **tacit**, mostly unspoken and unexpressed at the unconscious

BOX 5-4 Recognizing and Respecting the Integrated Nature of Culture in Nursing

Below are some examples of clients whose beliefs and practices may prove challenging for the nurse to respect and accommodate if not viewed in the context of their culture:

- Parents who are Jehovah's Witnesses may refuse a blood transfusion for their child. This refusal may appear irrational or uninformed to those who do not understand their religious view of accepting blood and the need for bloodless procedures. The single behavior of refusing blood transfusions, when viewed in context, is part of a larger belief system and a basic component of the family's culture (Campbell, Machan, & Fisher, 2016).
- A Muslim woman may ask to be examined by a person of the same sex. Separation of genders is integral to her cultural beliefs, and it may be uncomfortable or even traumatic to receive care from a person of the opposite sex (Mujallad & Taylor, 2016).
- A member of a Native American community may be unable to adhere to appointments for renal dialysis. Although such a client may appear to be noncompliant with care, rigid appointment scheduling may require the client to reframe the client's concept of time, violating concepts of patience and pride (Spector, 2017).

Source: Campbell et al. (2016); Mujallad and Taylor (2016); Spector (2017).

BOX 5-5 STORIES FROM THE FIELD

Being Sensitive to Cultural Beliefs and Practices

In some rural American communities, the use of catnip tea is highly valued for reducing colic in babies. Kayla, a C/PHN, was concerned about a baby not consuming enough infant formula because the mother, Josie, was giving so much catnip tea to the baby based on her friends and family having successfully used it to reduce symptoms of colic. Realizing that culture is shared, Kayla worked through informal cultural leaders—the elder women. She contacted the oldest woman in the community and discussed the cultural practice. The elder shared the group's beliefs that catnip tea is vital to the well-being of infants for the first 6 months. Together with other women in the community, they discussed concerns and babies' need for nutrients and relief from colic pain. The elders acknowledged that only 1 or 2 oz of catnip tea are needed for pain relief. This was shared with young mothers in the community, and the mothers gradually reduced the amount of tea given to their infants. This helped infants consume more formula and gain weight. Josie learned that she could give less tea and more formula, resulting in less pain and more weight gain for her baby. The C/PHN worked within the bounds of cultural tradition, and the health of the infants improved (Spector, 2017).

1. *Can you think of a similar cultural practice in your community that you may be able to approach in the same way as this C/PHN?*
2. *How would you go about researching the tradition and finding ways to incorporate the practice into your plan of care?*

Source: Spector (2017).

level. Members of a cultural group, without the need for discussion, know how to act and what to expect from one another. Culture provides an implicit set of cues for behavior, not a written set of rules. Spradley et al. (2016) explained that culture often lies below a conscious level because it is such a regular and pervasive part of the daily environment. It is like a memory bank in which knowledge is stored for recall when the situation requires it, but this recall process is mostly unconscious.

Culture:

- Teaches the proper tone of voice to use for each occasion
- Prescribes how close to stand when talking with someone familiar or unfamiliar
- Guides how one should appropriately respond to elders and based on one's gender, role, and status

All of these attitudes and behaviors become so ingrained—so tacit—that they are seldom, if ever, discussed.

Because culture is mostly tacit, realizing which of one's own behaviors may be offensive to people from other groups is difficult. It also is difficult to know the meaning and significance of other cultural practices.

- Silence is valued and expected by many Native Americans and Islamic women but may make others uncomfortable.
- Offering food to a guest in many cultures is not merely a social gesture but an important symbol of hospitality and acceptance; to refuse it, for any reason, may be an insult and a rejection.
- Touching or calling someone by their first name may be viewed as a demonstration of caring by some groups but could be seen as disrespectful and offensive to others.

C/PHNs have a twofold task in developing cultural sensitivity: we must try to learn clients' cultures and also must try to make our own culture less tacit and more explicit. Nurses bring both their professional and personal cultural history to the workplace, often developing unique values not shared with others who are not in the profession (Blais & Hayes, 2016). Cross-cultural tension can be resolved through conscious efforts to develop awareness, patience, and acceptance of cultural differences.

Culture is Dynamic

Every culture undergoes change; none is entirely static. Each culture is an amalgamation of ideas, values, and practices from many sources. This dynamic process is related to exposure to other cultural groups, and every culture is in a dynamic state of adding or deleting components. Functional aspects are retained; less functional ones are eliminated. Individuals may generate innovations within a culture and some members see advantages to changing behaviors, being willing to adopt new practices. This is important when working with communities to use new resources, such as access to the yearly flu vaccine.

When people enter a new culture, such as Sudanese refugees resettling in the United States (see Fig. 5-9), anxiety and frustration can occur. Nothing may be familiar; foods, language, expectations for dress, gestures, and even facial expressions may be misunderstood. This lack of familiarity can result in conflicted feelings that have been termed **culture shock**, leading to difficulty with interactions in the new culture (Spradley et al., 2016). Culture shock can develop with nurses providing care in unfamiliar countries and is known to affect international students studying in the United States or American students studying abroad. Serious difficulties can arise when members of a culture do not adapt to change or when culture shock is pervasive in a community (Box 5-6).

Cultural adaptation is the successful adjustment to cultural changes and often follows the process of culture shock. Examples of cultural adaptation can range from something as simple as learning to use a knife and fork to the complexities of becoming fluent in a new language. C/PHNs can facilitate cultural adaptation by explaining practices and expectations of the American health care system in the context of the original culture of their clients. For example, nurses working with recent African immigrants can explain to them the need for general health exams for all children entering school and that this does not mean their children are "in trouble."

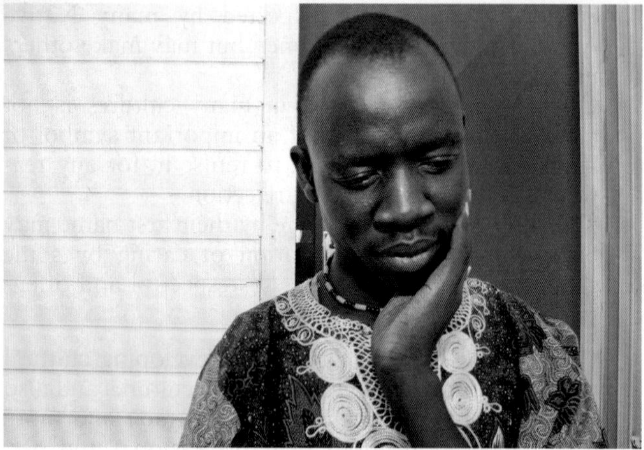

FIGURE 5-9 Sudanese man now living in the United States.

Community/public health nurses must remember the dynamic nature of culture for several reasons.

- Cultures and subcultures change over time; patience and persistence are key attributes when working toward improving health behaviors.
- Cultures change as their members see greater advantages in adopting "new ways." Describing the changes in language and context acceptable to the culture is essential. Successful nurses understand their clients' culture when delivering culturally competent care (Andrews et al., 2020).

BOX **5-6** EVIDENCE-BASED PRACTICE

Cultural Identity and Outcomes

Southeast Asian Hmong teenagers are among the first generation to be raised in the United States. Their parents had high hopes for them to restore honor and pride to a displaced people, but the teens struggle to balance their American lifestyle with Hmong traditions. They can feel overwhelming stress resulting from the generational and cultural gaps between themselves and their parents. Hmong community leaders, community health workers, school districts, law enforcement, and Hmong families have joined together to develop interventions to address these issues. A longitudinal study of Asian Americans found that 48% chose that label most of the time and that this "American identity" was often tied to positive academic and psychological adjustment (Kiang & Witkow, 2018, p. 64). Cheon, Bayless, Wang, and Yip (2018) examined ethnic/racial self-labeling among a diverse group of adolescents and noted differing patterns tied to contextual and individual influences.

1. *Can you identify a group in your community with similar issues to the Hmong parents and children?*
2. *Has your community provided any services to assist families in acculturating or adapting to their cultural change?*
3. *If you are a C/PHN working with this group, what types of assessment and interventions would be helpful?*

Source: Cheon et al. (2018); Kiang and Witkow (2018).

- Within a culture, change may occur because of certain key individuals who are receptive to new ideas and are able to influence their peers. Key individuals can adapt suggested changes to fit the cultural and group values.
- The health care culture is dynamic; Westerners are beginning to appreciate the validity of non-Western practices such as acupuncture, meditation, and the use of therapeutic herbs and spices such as turmeric and fenugreek (Canizares, Hogg-Johnson, Gignac, Glazier, & Badley, 2017).
- Our national health-related goals, the Healthy People initiative, change every 10 years. *Healthy People 2030* includes a focus on eliminating health disparities and improving health literacy (Office of Disease Prevention and Health Promotion, 2019). See Box 5-7.

ETHNOCULTURAL HEALTH CARE PRACTICES

Throughout history, people have relied on natural elements to treat misfortunes, illness, or injuries experienced by family, clan, tribe, or community members. Specialized knowledge about practices and substances (e.g., rituals, incantations, berries, plants, barks) is often held by one person in the group. This revered community leader, known as a medicine man/woman, healer, or shaman, may acquire the skills through apprenticeship or is believed to be born with them (McFarland & Wehbe-Alamah, 2018; Spector, 2017).

In this section, we present:

- An overview of the three views of health care: biomedical, magicoreligious, and holistic
- Selected folk medicines and home remedies, such as herbs, teas, and poultices
- Over-the-counter (OTC) drugs and patent medications
- Complementary or alternative therapies
- Recently developed, expensive medications
- Various self-care practices

This section concludes with the C/PHN's role and responsibilities to provide culturally competent care in relation to caring for, respecting, teaching, and treating clients from different cultures.

The World Community

Beliefs about the causes and effects of illness, health practices, and health-seeking behaviors are all influenced by a person's, a group's, or a community's perception of what causes illness and injury and what actions can best treat or cure the health problem. The three major views in the world community are biomedical, magicoreligious, and holistic health beliefs (Andrews et al., 2020).

Biomedical View

Common in Western societies, the biomedical view theorizes that all aspects of health can be understood through the sciences of biology, chemistry, physics, and mathematics. Furthermore, there is the belief that life can be manipulated by humans through physical and biochemical

BOX **5-7** *HEALTHY PEOPLE 2030*

2030 Objectives with Statistically Significant Racial/Ethnic Disparities in Leading Health Indicators at Healthy People 2020 Midcourse Review

Core Objectives	
AHS-01	Increase the proportion of people with health insurance
AHS-07	Increase the proportion of people with a usual primary care provider
C-07	Increase the proportion of adults who get screened for a colorectal cancer
HDS-04	Reduce the proportion of adults with high blood pressure
D-03	Reduce the proportion of adults with diagnosed diabetes who have an A1c value >9%
IID-06	Increase the vaccination coverage level of 4 doses of the DTaP vaccine in children by age 2
TU-01,04	Reduce current tobacco use in adults and adolescents
TU-18	Increase the proportion of smoke-free homes
IVP-03	Reduce unintentional injury deaths
IVP-09	Reduce homicides
MICH-02	Reduce the rate of all infant deaths (within 1 y).
MICH-07	Reduce preterm births
MHMD-01	Reduce the suicide rate
MHMD-06	Increase the proportion of adolescents with depression who get treatment
PA-02	Increase the proportion of adults who do enough aerobic physical activity guideline needed for substantial health benefits
NWS-03,04	Reduce the proportion of adults, children, and adolescents with obesity
OH-08	Increase the proportion of children, adolescents, and adults who use the oral health care system
FP-03,01	Reduce the proportion of unintended pregnancies; reduce pregnancies in adolescents
SU-04,05,06	Reduce the proportion of adolescents who drank alcohol alcohol, used marijuana drugs, or marijuana in the month
SU-09	Reduce the proportion of people under 21 years who engaged in binge drinking in the past month

Reprinted from U.S. Department of Health and Human Services (USDHHS). (2020). *Browse 2030 objectives.* Retrieved from https://health.gov/healthypeople/objectives-and-data/browse-objectives

processes (Andrews et al., 2020). Examples of this viewpoint include:

- Disease is the breakdown of the human machine through stress, injury, pathogens, or genetic/structural changes.
- Disease causes illness, which has a specific cause and a set of treatment requirements.
- Treatments can be aggressive including medication, surgery, and even genetic engineering.

Many health care professionals, including C/PHNs, believe this biomedical model is the only and best approach. As a result, they may have trouble understanding diverse cultures that incorporate the holistic or magicoreligious views, and clients may not receive culturally competent care. To be effective with diverse clients, C/PHNs must be knowledgeable about and accepting of a range of cultural health practices (Murcia & Lopez, 2016; Patwardhan, Mutalik, & Tillu, 2015).

Magicoreligious View

Many cultural beliefs are grounded in the magicoreligious approach, which focuses on control of health and illness by supernatural forces.

- Diseases are thought to originate from intrusion of a malevolent spirit, punishment for the deeds of ancestors, and other indications that God, the gods, or other supernatural forces are in control.
- Health is seen as a spiritual gift or reward and illness as an opportunity to be resigned to God's will (Andrews et al., 2020).
- Prayers for healing or well-being of self and others, participation in prayer groups, and requests for prayer are effective (Baldwin, Velasquez, Koenig, Salas, & Boelens, 2016; Levin, 2016).
- Death rituals connected with religious faith are designed to ease human departure from this life and help others cope with grief and loss (Roberson, Smith, & Davidson, 2018).
- Health and illness belong first to the community and then to the individual; communal activities are viewed as helpful (Andrews et al., 2020).
- Ceremonies, wearing special garments, and work with spiritual healers are important.

Religious beliefs, an individual's spirituality, and how these factors interface with wellness and healing practices are important to clients and cannot be separated from their culture. Community/public health nurses who are familiar with and respect the magicoreligious viewpoint offer culturally competent care.

Holistic View

Approaching health from a holistic standpoint, the world is viewed as seeking harmonious balance; imbalance of natural forces can create chaos and disease. Many cultural groups use a holistic approach in tandem with biomedical and magicoreligious beliefs. In this belief system, for an individual to be healthy, all facets of the individual's nature—physical, mental, emotional, and spiritual—must be in balance (Eliopoulos, 2018). The holistic viewpoint can be expressed by:

- Use of specific foods, beverages, and herbs to balance *hot or cold* disease states
- The Chinese concept of *yin and yang*, in which forces of nature are balanced
- Considering that infectious disease such as tuberculosis is not only caused by an organism but also by the environment, malnutrition, and poverty (Andrews et al., 2020; Eliopoulos, 2018)

Folk Medicine and Home Remedies

All cultures have home remedies and aspects of folk medicine. Many of us remember our mothers giving us hot herbal tea with lemon or using ointments and piling on blankets to relieve symptoms of a mild illness. Treatments as part of **Folk medicine** are verbally passed down from generation to generation and began when access to medical care was limited. Some clients may never plan to seek Western medical treatment but may share with you, the C/PHN, a practice they are using to treat a family member. Your response and actions may mean the difference between health and illness or injury. Folk practices are common in maternal and child health; some that may be encountered include (Andrews et al., 2020; Spector, 2017) the following:

- Pregnant women not reaching above their head, as doing so will cause the umbilical cord to strangle the baby
- Taping coins over a newborn's umbilical area to prevent hernias
- Giving catnip tea to infants because it soothes them
- Holding a baby upside down by the heels to "wake up the liver"
- Not letting a cat be near a sleeping baby, because it will "suck the life" out of the baby
- Using vinegar to relieve hypertension and skin irritations (Quandt, Sandberg, Grzywacz, Altizer, & Arcury, 2015)

Home remedies are individualized caregiving practices, often used before people seek advice from health care professionals. Each of us has a set of home remedies our parents used on us that we are likely to use on ourselves or our own children before or instead of calling the pediatrician. Examples include using baking soda paste on a bee sting, ice on a "cold sore," or cranberry juice to prevent a urinary tract infection.

Herbalism

Use of herbs to treat illness is a centuries-old practice that is gaining popularity in our American culture (Fig. 5-10). Clients may not consider the use of herbs to be a "medical treatment" and may not tell health care professionals about their use (Donoghue, 2018). Textbooks and other books for the general public have been published on medicinal herbs (Chevallier, 2016; Kennedy, 2017; Pizzorno, Murray, & Joiner-Bey, 2016). In an increasingly multicultural society, the source, form, and identity of many herbs, roots, barks, and liquid preparations are difficult for most C/PHNs to distinguish. A book with pictures and descriptions, botanical form, purported indications and uses, and implications for nursing management of herbs is an important tool to keep handy when interacting with clients (Barrett, 2015). Basic safety questions that C/PHNs should answer about an herb when teaching or interacting with families include:

- Is the herb contraindicated with prescription medications the client is taking?
- Is the herb harmful? Does it have negative side effects? How often is it used?
- Is the client relying on the herb, without positive health changes, and neglecting to get effective treatment from a health care practitioner?

Just because herbs are not regulated as drugs, they are not risk-free. Variations in quality, strength, processing, storage, and purity may occur, leading to unpredictable effects. For these reasons, herbs must be used only in

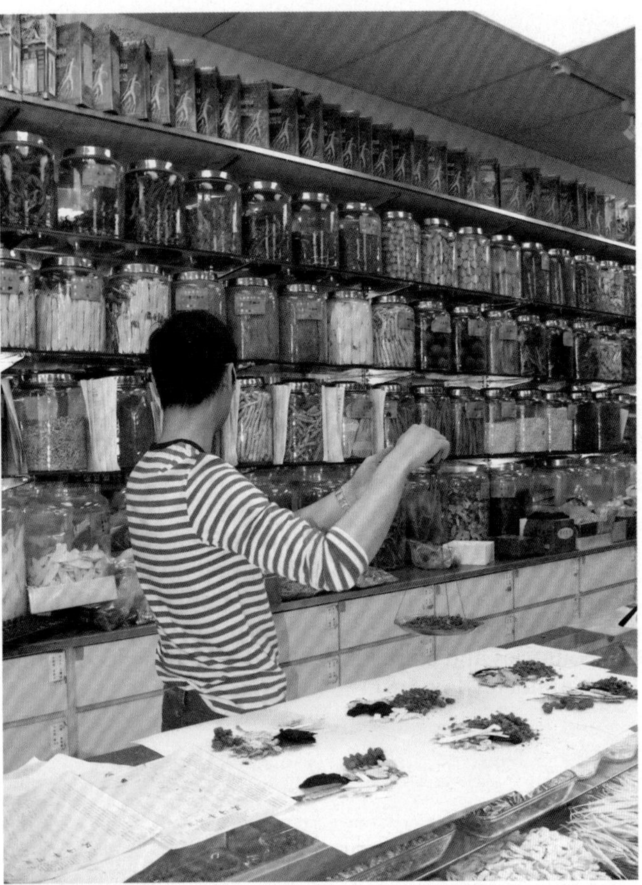

FIGURE 5-10 A Chinese herb store.

moderation and with caution, preferably with guidance by a health care practitioner (Donoghue, 2018). Examples of potentially harmful herbal supplements include Ephedra, Ginko, and Goldenseal for those persons with cardiac conditions, as these herbs can increase blood pressure and heart rate, as well as heighten the risk of bleeding (Cleveland Clinic, 2018).

Prescription and OTC Drugs

The cautions mentioned about herbs can also apply to most dietary supplements and OTC preparations. Additional concerns with these drugs include:

- Dietary supplements and OTC drugs undergo a less rigorous process of review and testing by the U.S. Food and Drug Administration than do prescription medications (USFDA, 2015).
- Many OTC drugs were once available only by prescription and remain powerful medicines.
- Herbal or dietary supplements do not have to be FDA -approved before manufacturers can sell them (USFDA, 2017).
- All drugs can have major side effects, may be contraindicated in people with certain conditions, and may not be safe to use in combination with certain other drugs.
- Many new prescription medications are so expensive that clients cannot afford to take them as prescribed. Often, older, less expensive, and more frequently used drugs work as well as the newer, more expensive ones, which are heavily marketed by drug companies to health care practitioners and consumers.

Community/public health nurses who see clients over time can assist them through medication review and instruction, advocating for them to receive a less expensive form of the same medication and reporting on the effectiveness of newly prescribed medications. Many pharmaceutical companies now have low-cost prescription assistance programs for those in need (Partnership for Prescription Assistance, 2018).

Integrated Health Care and Self-Care Practices

Complementary and alternative medicine (CAM), a multibillion-dollar industry in the United States, includes a broad array of healing resources (Donoghue, 2018). Self-care activities may include CAM, other medications, and spiritual and cultural practices.

These widely varied approaches are designed to promote comfort, health, and well-being and may include

- Therapies and treatments (juice diets, fasting, coffee enemas, and biofeedback)
- Exercise activities (T'ai chi, yoga, and dance)
- Exposure (aromatherapy, music therapy, and light therapy)
- Manipulation (acupuncture, acupressure, chiropractic, cupping ([Fig. 5-11], and reflexology).

Complementary therapies are often used in conjunction with Western medicine, an approach known as **integrated health care**, such as for pain relief during labor (Vitale & Jenner, 2018) and to improve sleep in the intensive care unit (Cho, Lee, & Hur, 2017). Complementary therapies have become so commonplace that some have suggested developing policies and guidelines for their use.

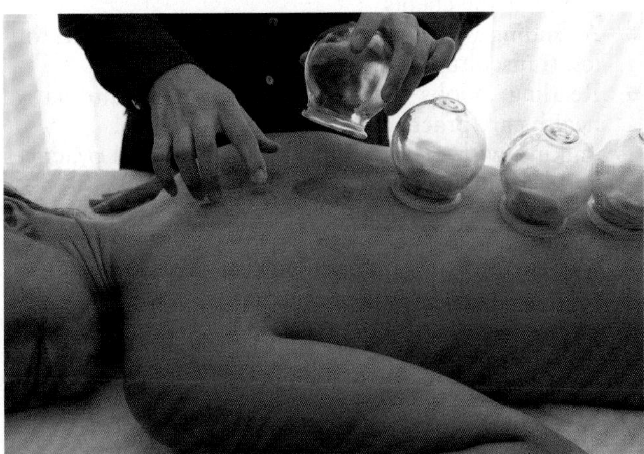

FIGURE 5-11 Cupping has been used by many cultures.

The C/PHN should be aware of the variety of therapies available and how to get information for clients while remaining objective and supportive of the client's choices. When a therapy contradicts the recommendations of the client's health care practitioner, the nurse may be able to provide the pros and cons of continuing the complementary therapy. Also, the nurse may be able to suggest therapy forms that would complement Western medicine for the client, such as music to promote relaxation and reduce stress or biofeedback for chronic pain management. Complementary and self-care practices should be uniquely chosen for each individual within the context of the client's cultural group (Lindquist & Tracy, 2018). The culturally competent nurse respects these decisions, while promoting client health.

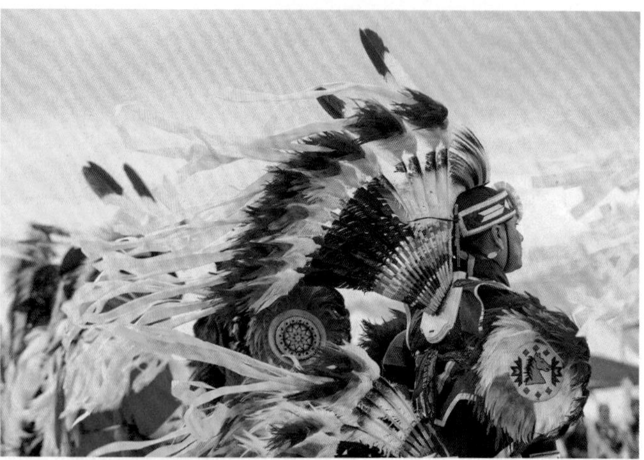

FIGURE 5-12 Nevada Paiute tribe powwow.

ROLE AND PREPARATION OF THE COMMUNITY/PUBLIC HEALTH NURSE

As a C/PHN, for you to be an effective health care advocate for clients from different cultural groups, you must be prepared to:

- Speak knowledgeably about health care practices and choices
- Assess the client or family adequately, to know what belief system motivates their choices
- Teach clients about the limits and benefits of cultural health care practices
- Individualize assessment and caregiving for the client within the client's culture, not generalize about the client based on cultural group norms

Preparation to work effectively with clients in the area of cultural health care involves developing cultural awareness and promoting sensitivity to the differences among people from diverse ethnocultural groups. You, the nurse, can prepare by:

- Performing a cultural self-assessment to identify your own beliefs and biases
- Learning from peers who are from the same cultural group as the clients
- Attending workshops or conferences on cultural topics, transcultural nursing, and cultural ethics
- Reading books on ethnocultural and alternative health care practices
- Talking with clients about their views and practices and learning from them
- Keeping an open mind and being curious about various practices
- Attending community cultural events, such as Native American powwows (Fig. 5-12), ethnic food and cultural festivals, or Cinco de Mayo celebrations

There are textbooks, novels, and articles about cultures in the community in which one practices. For example, the classic book *The Spirit Catches You and You Fall Down* (Fadiman, 1998) describes a Hmong child, her American doctors, and the collision of two cultures in California. The experience of public health nurse Karin Urso, who worked with people from many different countries and cultures, illustrates the benefits of being open-minded (Box 5-8).

BOX **5-8** PERSPECTIVES

Learning About Other Cultures

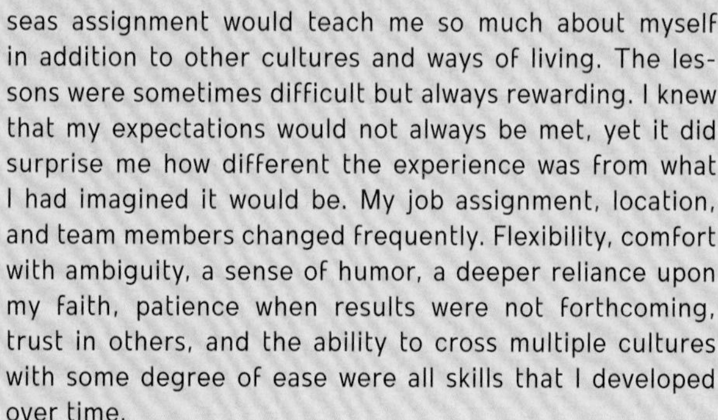

I was always interested in learning about other countries and cultures. However, I didn't realize that an overseas assignment would teach me so much about myself in addition to other cultures and ways of living. The lessons were sometimes difficult but always rewarding. I knew that my expectations would not always be met, yet it did surprise me how different the experience was from what I had imagined it would be. My job assignment, location, and team members changed frequently. Flexibility, comfort with ambiguity, a sense of humor, a deeper reliance upon my faith, patience when results were not forthcoming, trust in others, and the ability to cross multiple cultures with some degree of ease were all skills that I developed over time.

Most important to being successful at my job was to maintain the attitude of a "learner," not a "solver of problems" or "the person with all the answers." I made friends with people from all over the world who graciously accepted me into their lives, thus enriching mine. I learned that we all are different, but that every behavior has a reasonable explanation when you take the time to listen with your heart as well as with your ears. I found that I actually preferred other ways of doing and being while still maintaining those parts of my identity that were valuable to me. When I returned home, I found that my newly developed skills were still necessary—because I had changed and had to adjust to reentry into my home culture!

Karin Urso, PHN

TRANSCULTURAL COMMUNITY/PUBLIC HEALTH NURSING PRINCIPLES

Culture profoundly influences thinking and behavior and has an enormous impact on the effectiveness of health care. Just as physical and psychological factors determine clients' needs and attitudes toward health and illness, so too can culture.

- About 50 years ago Kark emphasized that "culture is perhaps the most relevant social determinant of community health" (1974, p. 149).
- Culture determines how people rear their children, react to pain, cope with stress, deal with death, and value the past, present, and future.
- Culture influences diet and eating practices, which can be difficult to change due to culture's impact (McFarland & Wehbe-Alamah, 2018; Spector, 2017).

Despite its importance, the client's culture is often misunderstood or ignored in the delivery of health care (McFarland & Wehbe-Alamah, 2018). Cultural diversity is increasing in our world, and it is essential that health care professionals are prepared to effectively work with diverse health care team members and clients (Andrews et al., 2020). Effective and culturally competent care involves:

- Avoiding ethnocentric attitudes
- Bridging cultural differences
- Developing knowledge and skill in serving multicultural clients
- Placing clients' responses to care within the context of their lives

Avoiding ethnocentrism requires the nurse to be willing to examine one's own culture carefully and to become aware that alternative viewpoints are possible. The nurse attempts to understand the meaning other people derive from their culture and appreciate their culture as important and useful to them (McFarland & Wehbe-Alamah, 2018). Ignoring consideration of clients' different cultural origins often has negative results.

- Culture is a universal experience; each person is part of some group, and that group helps to shape the values, beliefs, and behaviors that make up their culture. Even within fairly homogeneous cultural groups, subcultures and microcultures have distinctive characteristics.
- Further differences, often due to social class, socioeconomic status, age, or degree of acculturation, can be found within microcultures. These latter differences, called **intraethnic variations**, only underscore the range of culturally diverse clients served by C/PHNs.

Community/public health nursing practice with cross-cultural groups, known as **transcultural nursing**, means providing culturally sensitive nursing service to people of an ethnic or racial background different from the nurse's (Andrews et al., 2020; McFarland & Wehbe-Alamah, 2018). Principles of transcultural nursing practice can guide C/PHNs (Box 5-9):

- Develop cultural self-awareness.
- Cultivate cultural sensitivity.

BOX 5-9 Cross-Cultural Guidelines

1. C/PHNs should strive to ensure all population members receive care and services that are respectful and sensitive to their client's cultural beliefs and practices.
2. Be aware of your own belief system and values; understand and acknowledge that cultural differences may exist.
3. Develop a basic understanding and knowledge of other cultures, but do not use generalizations about other cultures to stereotype or oversimplify your ideas about another person or group. Remember there are differences within each cultural group that are influenced by individual characteristics and geographical location; therefore, never assume you understand what a person from another culture thinks or feels.
4. Demonstrate a genuine interest in the client's personal circumstances and seek to establish trust. Suspend judgments and respect the opinion of others.
5. Be aware of power imbalances and the effect on communication. Identify members who are accorded higher status and authority in family or group and respect the status hierarchy. Respect gender and age differences.
6. Do not assume that there is only one way (yours) to communicate. Keep working on ways to improve your cross-cultural communication skills. For example, avoid using jargon or slang that may not be understood cross-culturally. Use very clear and simple English.
7. Unspoken communication can be powerful; be aware and use appropriate body language.
8. Practice active listening. Try to put yourself in the other person's shoes, especially when another person's ideas or perceptions are different from your own. Be willing to step outside your comfort zone.
9. Do not assume that just because clients say they understand the information that they really do. Clarify questions and statements. Seek feedback by reframing the question in a different form to ensure understanding.
10. Apologize for cultural mistakes. Admit your own limitations and state willingness to learn from others. Show appreciation for the opportunity to learn from others.
11. Easily understood information and services should be delivered in the preferred language of the population served. Whenever possible, use interpreters who are trained in culturally competent care, and if possible, avoid using family members or friends to interpret. Look directly at the client, not the interpreter, when speaking.
12. Assess immigration history and refugee stress or trauma; with children and adolescents, assess gaps in acculturation and potential family conflicts and cause of health problems and health beliefs; assess if they have experienced discrimination, racism, or bias.
13. Practice—we get better at cross-cultural collaboration when we practice it.

Source: Douglas et al. (2014); Douglas, Pacquiao and Purnell (2018); Underwood and Kelber (2015).

- Assess the client group's culture.
- Show respect and patience while learning about other cultures.
- Examine culturally derived health practices.

Develop Cultural Self-Awareness

To avoid stereotyping, prejudice and racism, ethnocentrism, cultural imposition, and cultural conflict (a perceived threat arising from a misunderstanding of expectations between clients and nurses when either group is not aware of cultural differences), self-awareness is crucial for the nurse working with people from other cultures (Andrews et al., 2020; McFarland & Wehbe-Alamah, 2018). **Cultural self-awareness** means recognizing the values, beliefs, and practices that make up one's own culture and becoming sensitive to the impact of one's culturally based responses.

Although C/PHNs may think they are being helpful when operating from their own sets of cultural values and practices, doing so may actually have negative consequences and even cause damage to relationships with clients when cultural values differ. The nurse who has expectations for prenatal weight gain and values actions to limit weight could cause damage to a therapeutic relationship if the nurse does not take into account cultural expectations about diet during pregnancy to assure a healthy infant. To develop awareness, nurses can complete a cultural self-assessment by analyzing their own:

- Influences related to racial and ethnic background
- Verbal and nonverbal communication patterns
- Values and norms (expected cultural practices or behaviors)
- Health-related beliefs and practices

Because culture is mostly tacit, it takes conscious effort and hard work to develop true awareness of one's own cultural biases or influence. A nurse can ask selected clients to critique nursing actions in light of the clients' own culture. Developing this awareness will reward you with a more effective understanding of self and an enhanced ability to provide culturally relevant service to clients (Andrews et al., 2020; Spector, 2017). See Box 5-10 and Table 5-2.

Cultivate Cultural Sensitivity

Nurses should be aware of the significant impact of culture on behavior. **Cultural sensitivity** requires recognizing that culturally based values, beliefs, and practices influence people's health and lifestyles and need to be considered in plans for service (Browne, Hackett, & Burger, 2017; Darnell & Hickson, 2015; McFarland & Wehbe-Alamah, 2018). It also first demands self-reflection about personally held stereotypes and biases, along with self-assessment of one's own cultural influences (Marion et al., 2017). Some hints to ensure culturally sensitive care include:

- View culture as an enabler rather than a resistant force.
- Recognize feelings and reinforce dignity and worth as an individual or group.
- Take time for a pleasant conversation and build rapport.

BOX 5-10 Cultural Self-Assessment

Think about the culture of your family (parents and grandparents). Answer the following questions about your own cultural background:

- Relationship to the dominant culture—Does the dominant culture have any stereotypes, misconceptions, suspicions, or historical issues related to your family's culture? If a minority culture, what is your family's view of the dominant culture? What cultural stereotypes does your family express?
- Verbal—What is the dominant language of your family's culture? How does your family share information and feelings, explain the meaning of terms, use proverbs, and incorporate direct questioning versus silence and passivity?
- Nonverbal—Describe your family's use of eye contact, facial expressions, body movements, and touch.
- Perception of time—Is your family's culture future, present, or past oriented?
- Personal space—Describe your family's concepts of boundaries and interpersonal distance.
- Perception of family roles and organization—Who is responsible for care of the children in your family? Who makes financial and health care decisions? Describe gender roles.
- Biological variations—Describe your family's skin and hair color, susceptibility to disease, enzymatic differences, and typical growth and development.
- Diet—What are typical meals in your family? How food is used (celebrations, fasting, healing, etc.)?
- Education—Describe your family's typical learning style (visual, auditory, psychomotor; formal/informal education).
- Spirituality—What are your family's spiritual beliefs and values, spiritual practices and support, rituals and taboos?
- Health beliefs—Describe your family's understanding of the meaning of health and illness (e.g., cause, perception of symptoms/intensity, seriousness, expression of illness, need for medical attention); beliefs about death and dying; beliefs about pregnancy, labor and delivery, postpartum period, and childcare.
- Health behaviors—What activities does your family do to promote health and prevent disease? Describe their help-seeking behaviors and use of home remedies, traditional or folk healers, and magicoreligious practitioners. What status is given to health care providers?

- Involve significant family members in care.
- Reassure the client regarding confidentiality.
- Be aware of cultural diversity within the same ethnic group.
- Communicate openness, acceptance, and willingness to learn.
- When a cultural practice is unknown, ask the client to detail preferences, and then provide respectful care.
- Incorporate cultural beliefs into the plan of care.

A client's cultural values and health practices may sharply contrast with those of the nurse. Failure to recognize this contrast can lead to a communication breakdown

TABLE **5-2** Cultural Assessment Guide

Category	Sample Data
Ethnic/racial background	Countries of origin Mostly native born or US born? Reasons for emigrating if applicable Racial/ethnic identity Experience with racism or racial discrimination?
Language and communication patterns	Languages of origin Languages spoken in the home Preferred language for communication How verbal communication patterns are affected by age, sex, other? Preferences for use of interpreters Nonverbal communication patterns (e.g., eye contact, touching)
Cultural values and norms	Group beliefs and standards for male and female roles and functions Standards for modesty and sexuality Family/extended family structures and functions Values regarding work, leisure, success, time Values regarding education and occupation Norms for child-rearing and socialization Norms for social networks and supports Values regarding aging and treatment of elders Values regarding authority Norms for dress and appearance
Biocultural factors	Group genetic predisposition to health conditions (e.g., hypertension, anemia) Socioculturally associated illnesses (e.g., AIDS, alcoholism) Group attitudes toward body parts and functions Group vulnerability or resistance to health threats? Folk illnesses common to group? Group physical/genetic differences (e.g., bone mass, height, weight, longevity)
Religious beliefs and practices	Religious beliefs affecting roles, childbearing and child-rearing, health and illness? Recognized religious healers? Religious beliefs and practices for promoting health, preventing illness, or treatment of illness Beliefs and rituals regarding conception and birth Beliefs and rituals regarding death, dying, grief
Health beliefs and practices	Beliefs regarding causes of illness Beliefs regarding treatment of illness Beliefs regarding use of healers (traditional and Western) Health promotion and illness prevention practices Folk medicine practices Beliefs regarding mental health and illness Dietary, herbal, and other folk cures Food beliefs, preparation, consumption Experience with Western medicine

and ineffective care. Once differences in culture are recognized, it is important to accept and appreciate them. For example, a nurse visiting a new immigrant family can avoid the dangerous ethnocentric trap of assuming that the nurse's way is best and consequently develop a more trusting and effective relationship with the clients. As a part of developing cultural sensitivity, nurses need to understand clients' points of view. By listening, observing, and learning about other cultures, the nurse can use culturally sensitive strategies for care and avoid ethnocentrism. Nurses who attempt to understand the feelings and ideas of their clients, establish a trusting relationship and open the door to the possibility of their clients' adopting new healthy behaviors. The American Nurses Association's (2015) *Nursing: Scope and Standards of Practice* outlines a set of competencies for culturally congruent practice. See Table 5-3 for culturally related competencies for registered nurses.

Assess the Client Group's Culture

Learning the culture of the client first is critical to effective nursing practice. During a **cultural assessment** (Giger, 2017), the nurse obtains health-related information about the values, beliefs, and practices of a cultural group. There usually is a culturally based reason for clients to engage in (or avoid) certain actions. Instead of making assumptions or judging clients' behavior, the nurse first must learn about the culture that guides that behavior. For example,

TABLE 5-3 Cultural Competence

Competencies	C/PHN Actions
Knowledge of cultural groups	Identify and develop understanding of cultural groups in your practice area.
Self-reflection	Demonstrate awareness of your own cultural background, beliefs, and values; recognize how these can influence your interactions with others.
Effective communication	Apply "culturally competent verbal and nonverbal communication skills" in recognizing cultural beliefs, health care practices and values of your clients (Douglas et al., 2014, p. 112).
Cultural sensitivity	Demonstrate openness to understanding diverse clients in assessing and implementing culturally competent care.
Advocacy and empowerment	Advocate for integration of client's health care beliefs and practices; recognize ethnocentric or biased policies and empower clients to overcome barriers. Advocate for culturally competent care in your place of employment.
Multicultural health care workforce	Promote recruitment and retention of students (and employees) in nursing and other fields to achieve a more culturally balanced workforce.
Evidence-based practice	Apply EBP and research that is "most effective for the culturally diverse populations" served (p. 115). Encourage and engage in research to reduce health outcome disparities.

Source: Douglas et al. (2014).

a client might severely limit the foods she allows her child to eat, believing that many from her culture have food allergies (Widge et al., 2018).

Interviewing members of a subcultural group can provide valuable data to enhance understanding (Andrews et al., 2020). The concept of cultural diversity can be understood in a general way, but each individual group should be appreciated within its own cultural and historical context. It is not practical to deeply study all cultural groups the nurse encounters. Instead, a general cultural assessment can be accomplished by questioning key informants, observing the cultural group, and reading current professional literature. These six categories comprise a general cultural assessment:

1. *Ethnic or racial background*: Where did the group originate, and how does that influence their status and identity?
2. *Language and communication patterns*: What language is preferred, and what are the group's culturally based communication patterns?
3. *Cultural values and norms*: What are the values, beliefs, and standards regarding family roles education, child-rearing, work and leisure, aging, dying, and rites of passage?
4. *Biocultural factors:* What unique physical or genetic traits predispose this group to certain conditions or illnesses?
5. *Religious beliefs and practices*: What are the common religious beliefs, and how do they influence roles, health, and illness?
6. *Health beliefs and practices*: What are the beliefs and practices regarding illness prevention, causes, and treatment?

In practice, a thorough cultural assessment may be too time-consuming and costly. Instead, the two-phase assessment process may be used, as outlined in Table 5-4. Categories to explore in the assessment include values, beliefs, customs, and social structure components.

Show Respect and Patience While Learning About Other Cultures

When learning about other cultures, key behaviors are to demonstrate respect and to practice patience. Some behaviors that help the nurse overcome language barriers include:

- Allow enough time for communication.
- Maintain a relaxed and unhurried attitude.
- Arrange for an interpreter when needed (Fig. 5-13).

TABLE 5-4 Two-Phase Cultural Assessment Process

Phase I—Data Collection	
Step 1	Assess values, beliefs, and customs (e.g., ethnic affiliations, religion, decision-making patterns).
Step 2	Collect problem-specific cultural data (e.g., cultural beliefs and practices related to diet and nutrition).
Step 3	Make nursing diagnoses. Determine cultural factors influencing nursing intervention (e.g., child-rearing beliefs and practices that might affect nurse teaching toilet training or child discipline).
Phase II—Data Organization	
Step 1	Compare cultural data with: Standards of client's own culture (e.g., client's diet compared with cultural norms) Standards of the nurse's culture Standards of the health facility providing service
Step 2	Determine incongruities in above standards.
Step 3	Seek to modify one or more systems (client's, nurse's, or the facility's) to achieve maximum congruity.

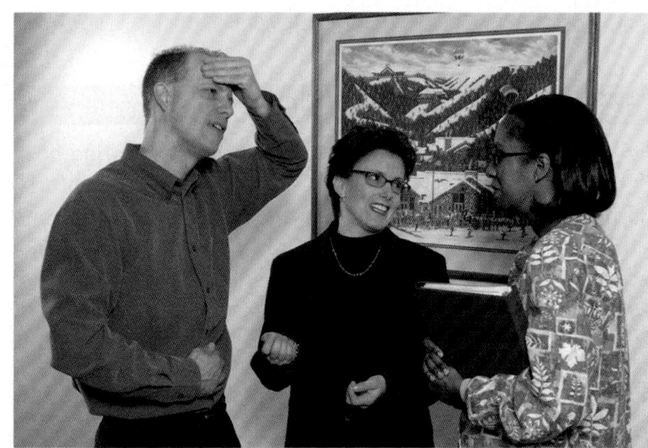

FIGURE 5-13 Hearing-impaired client helped by interpreter using sign language.

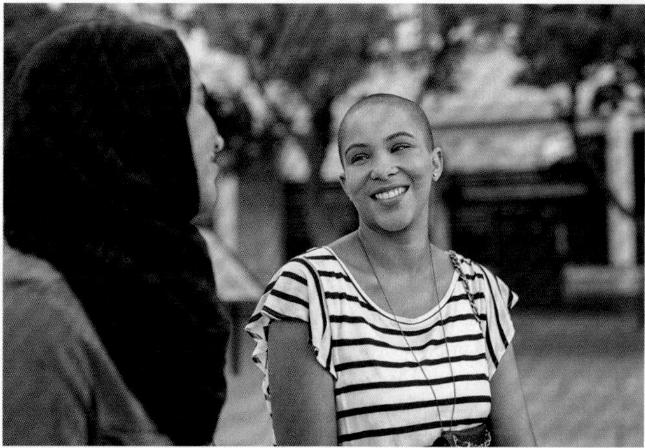

FIGURE 5-14 Building trust and rapport with your client is essential.

- Speak to the client, not the interpreter.
- Use simple language and avoid slang and jargon.
- Watch for verbal and nonverbal cues.
- Ask open-ended questions.
- Validate feelings and understanding.
- Use any words you know in the client's language.

A nurse shows respect when involving a women's group in decisions and offering them choices about health topics to cover. Respect is evident when a nurse gives positive recognition to the importance of a client's culture. Attentive listening is a way to show respect and to learn about a client's culture. The nurse arranging for an interpreter to assist with a language barrier shows respect, including for those with hearing impairment. See thePoint for best practices for working with interpreters.

A **minority group** is part of a population that differs from the majority and often receives different and unequal treatment. A message may be conveyed that their ways are inferior to those of the dominant culture, and it can be difficult for them to retain pride in their lifestyles or in themselves (McFarland & Wehbe-Alamah, 2018; Spector, 2017). This message may be implied or unintentional. In interacting with clients from a minority group, the nurse should:

- Provide personal attention: some clients may perceive efficiency and less personal attention as disrespect, which could impair their trust in health care professionals.
- Show respect: this can help break down barriers in cross-cultural communication.
- Practice cultural relativism: **cultural relativism** is recognizing and respecting alternative viewpoints and understanding values, beliefs, and practices within their cultural context (Spector, 2017).
- Be patient: it takes time to establish the nurse–client relationship, especially when working with two different cultures. Trust must be earned, and that may take weeks, months, or years. Time must be allowed for both nurse and clients to learn how to communicate with one another, to test one another's trustworthiness and to learn about one another.

Cultural brokering involves mediating or building connections between those from different cultural backgrounds to promote change (Douglas et al., 2014; Jang, 2017). Aspects of both the nurse's and the clients' cultures can, and probably will, change. When working with a family from an unfamiliar cultural background, for example, you can explain your usual method of working with clients and may modify some usual practices to adapt them to the family's culture. The family, in turn, may begin to assume the nurse's recommended health care practices. This process of building trust and rapport with your client may take several months, but time, respect, and patience all help to break down cultural barriers (Fig. 5-14).

Consider Culturally Derived Health Practices

Some traditional practices, such as customary diet, birth rituals, and certain folk remedies, may promote both physical and psychological health. Other practices, neither harmful nor health promoting, are useful in preserving the culture, security, and sense of identity of a cultural group. Some traditional practices may be directly harmful to health.

Examples of harmful practices include:

- Sole use of herbal poultices to treat an infected wound when antibiotics are needed
- "Burning" the abdomen to compensate for heat loss associated with diarrhea
- The use of Greta or Azarcon (common Hispanic home remedies for stomach discomfort), which contain lead (CDC, 2019; McFarland & Wehbe-Alamah, 2018)

Cultural health practice and aggregate health assessment can be combined to preserve accepted practices while incorporating Western medicine for full treatment efficacy. If a group has a high incidence of low-birth-weight babies, pregnancy complications, skin infections, mental illness, or other health problems, it may be helpful to learn more about the group's cultural health practices. Practices clearly damaging to health can be discussed with group leaders and healers. Knowing the group's norms for authority and decision-making can be helpful to achieve improvements while respecting traditional health practices. An example of the consequences of not clearly understanding cultural norms is found in Boxes 5-11 and 5-12.

BOX **5-11** STORIES FROM THE FIELD

The Importance of Cultural Sensitivity

In a foreign country, well-intentioned government officials, including representatives of the health ministry, identified problems related to substandard housing among a particular aggregate of native people. To assist this community, the officials spent a great deal of time, energy, and finances planning and building homes for the native group. The homes were small but modern and offered many of the conveniences that officials believed would improve the quality of life for the community.

The members of the native group were appreciative of the group's efforts and moved into their new homes. Before long, however, officials realized that one by one the community members were moving back to their "substandard" housing. When asked about their lack of appreciation for the improved lifestyle, the group informed the officials that their watering hole was their lifeline and that the houses were not only uncomfortable to them but were too far from their watering hole. Soon, all the native families had returned to living on the land, and the homes were part of a veritable ghost town in the middle of nowhere.

1. *Was the native community truly "poor," as the officials seemed to think?*
2. *Discuss your perception of the following issues: cultural imposition, cultural poverty, dignity, and spirit.*
3. *Debate with a fellow student the pros and cons of trying again to improve the native people's quality of life.*

BOX **5-12** STORIES FROM THE FIELD

Emily's New Clients

As she drove down the dirt road and parked her car next to the reservation community hall, Emily Josten felt apprehensive. The previous C/PHN had alerted her about the "difficulty of working with this population" and that she had "never gotten anywhere with them." Only through the urging of Mrs. Brown, a community aid, had a group of the women reluctantly agreed to meet with the new nurse. They would see what she had to say.

Emily walked to the far corner where a group of women sat silently in a circle. Only their eyes turned; their faces remained impassive. Mrs. Brown introduced her to the group. Emily smiled. She told them of her background and explained that she had not worked with people on the reservation before. There was a long silence. No one spoke. Emily continued, "I'd like to help you if I can, maybe with problems about care of your children when they are sick or questions about how to keep them healthy, but I don't know what you need or want." Silence fell again. She would like to learn from them, she repeated. Would they help her? Again, Emily felt an uncomfortable silence.

Then one woman began to speak. Quietly, but with deep feeling, she described several bad experiences with the previous nurse and the county social worker. Then others spoke up: "They tell us what we should do. They don't listen. They say our way is not good." Seeing Emily's interest and concern, the women continued. One of their main issues was their children's health. Another was the high incidence of accidents and injuries on the reservation. They wanted to learn how to give first aid. Other concerns were expressed. The group agreed that Emily could help them by teaching a first-aid class.

In the weeks that followed, Emily taught several classes on first aid and emergency care. She then began a series of sessions on child health. Each time, she asked the women to choose a topic or problem for discussion and then elicited from them their accustomed ways of dealing with each problem; for example, how they handled toilet training or taught their children to eat solid foods. Her goal was to learn as much as she could about their culture and to incorporate that information into her teaching, which preserved as many of their practices as possible. Emily also visited informally with the women in their homes and at community gatherings.

She learned about their way of life, their history, and their values. For example, patience was highly valued. It was important to be able to wait patiently, even if a scheduled meeting was delayed as much as 2 hours. It also was important for others to speak, which explained the women's comfort with silences during a conversation. Honesty, reliability, and generosity were viewed as important standards of behavior. These were some of the values by which they judged Emily and other professionals. Emily's honesty in keeping her promises enabled the women to trust her. Her generosity in giving her time, helping them occasionally with some household task and arranging for childcare during classes, won their respect.

The women came to accept her, and Emily was invited to eat with them and share in tribal gatherings. The women corrected and advised her on acceptable ways to speak and act. Her openness and patience to learn and her respect for them individually, and as a people, had paved the way to improving their health. At first, she felt that her progress was slow, but this slowness was an advantage. She had built a solid foundation of cross-cultural trust, and in the months that followed she saw many changes in her clients' health practices.

1. *What actions did Emily take that were culturally sensitive? Discuss ways in which you can incorporate these actions into your client care.*
2. *Discuss with another student the reasons you think the first C/PHN failed to make progress with this group of women.*
3. *Did Emily complete a cultural assessment? If your answer is "no," why not? If "yes," describe how this was done.*

SUMMARY

- Culture refers to the beliefs, values, and behaviors that are shared by members of a society and provide a template or "road map" for living.
- Culture has five characteristics:
  1. It is learned from others.
  2. It is an integrated system of customs and traits.
  3. It is shared.
  4. It is tacit, mostly unspoken.
  5. It is dynamic.
- Cultural diversity, or *cultural plurality*, refers to the coexistence of a variety of cultural patterns within a geographic area, either between cultures or within a given culture; smaller culturally distinctive groups may exist within a culture and are known as subcultures and microcultures.
- The increasing number of clients from different cultures requires that community health nurses should understand and appreciate cultural diversity.
- Ethnocentrism, or a bias toward one's own ethnic group, can create serious barriers to effective nursing care.
- Understanding cultural diversity and being sensitive to the values and behaviors of cultural groups often is the key to effective community health intervention.
- To gain acceptance, nurses strive to introduce improved health practices presented in a manner consistent with clients' cultural values.
- Nurses should be aware of and respect the three major views of health care in the world—biomedical, magicoreligious, and holistic.
- Nurses should be able to identify CAM treatments, such as folk medicine, home remedies, herbs, and other therapies; assess their clients' use of them; and, when appropriate, recommend their use.
- Five transcultural nursing principles, drawn from an understanding of the concept of culture, can guide community/public health nursing practice:
  1. Develop cultural self-awareness.
  2. Cultivate cultural sensitivity.
  3. Assess the client group's culture.
  4. Show respect and patience while learning about other cultures.
  5. Examine culturally derived health practices.

ACTIVE LEARNING EXERCISES

1. Pair up with another student from a different culture. Have a conversation about your own cultural practices (e.g., food, health, values, holidays). Complete a cultural interview and assessment of each other using a guide from this chapter. What similar patterns or themes do you notice? What are the differences? What was something new about this culture that you discovered?
2. Complete a cultural assessment of one of your clients and share the findings with your class. How do cultural values influence health behaviors, parenting, diet, social interaction, and other areas of life? How can you incorporate this information into your plan of care?
3. Consider health concerns or issues with a cultural group in your community. How could you apply 3 of the 10 essential public health services (see Box 2-2) in resolving this issue? Explain the rationale for your choices. What interventions would be most helpful? How would you ensure cultural competence and sensitivity?
4. Consider a recent high-profile event (e.g., Puerto Rico or Bahamas hurricanes, mass shooting in El Paso, TX) or a similar local event. Debate with other students whether ethnocentrism, stereotyping, and/or racism were influential factors, and give your rationale.
5. Find out if you have refugee populations in your area or state. Talk with program staff or the refugees themselves. Or, if this does not apply in your area, talk with two people from an unfamiliar cultural group. What caused them to move here? What assistance or resources are provided to them? How are they learning English? How are they finding housing and jobs? What are their hopes for the future? Have they felt welcomed or experienced discrimination? Describe four ways that C/PHNs can provide care and assistance for refugee populations.

thePoint: Everything You Need to Make the Grade!

thePoint® Visits http://thePoint.lww.com/Rector10e for NCLEX-style review questions, journal articles, supplemental materials, study aids for all learning styles, and more!

REFERENCES

Alba, R. (2016). The likely persistence of a White majority: How Census Bureau statistics gave misled thinking about the American future. *American Prospect: Longform*, *1*(11), 2016. Retrieved from http://prospect.org/article/likely-persistence-white-majority-0

American Immigration Council. (2020). *The cost of immigration enforcement and border security*. Retrieved from https://www.americanimmigrationcouncil.org/research/the-cost-of-immigration-enforcement-and-border-security

American Nurses Association (ANA). (2015). *Nursing: Scope and standards of practice* (3rd ed.). Silver Springs, MD: Nursesbooks.org.

Andrews, M., Boyle, J., & Collins, J. (2020). *Transcultural concepts in nursing care* (8th ed.). Philadelphia, PA: Wolters Kluwer, Lippincott Williams & Wilkins.

Baldwin, P. Velasquez, K., Koenig, H., Salas, R., & Boelens, P. (2016). Neural correlates of healing prayers, depression, and traumatic memories: A preliminary study. *Complementary Therapies in Medicine*, *27*, 123–129. doi: 10.1016-j.ctim.2016.07.002.

Barrett, M. (Ed.). (2015). *Handbook of clinically tested herbal remedies* (Vol. 1 & 2). New York, NY: Routledge, Taylor & Francis Group.

Batalova, J., Blizzard, J., & Bolter, B. (February 14, 2020). *Frequently requested statistics on immigrants and immigration in the United States*. Migration Policy Institute. Retrieved from https://www.migrationpolicy.org/article/frequently-requested-statistics-immigrants-and-immigration-united-states?gclid=EAIaIQobChMIoeecsKDr6AIVHz2tBh37ogAIEAAYASAAEgI6Q_D_BwE

Bellagamba, A., Greene, S. E., & Klein, M. A. (2017). *African voices on slavery and the slave trade*. New York, NY: Cambridge University Press.

Blair, K. (Ed.). (2019). *Advanced practice nursing: Core concepts for professional role development* (6th ed.). New York, NY: Springer Publishing Company.

Blais, K. K., & Hayes, J. S. (2016). *Professional nursing practice: Concepts and perspectives* (7th ed.). Upper Saddle River, NJ: Prentice Hall.

Brian, T., & Laczko, F. (2018). *Migrant deaths on world borders, January-September 2014*. Geneva, Switzerland: International Organization for Migration. Retrieved from https://www.iom.int/statements/iom-releases-new-data-migrant-fatalities-worldwide-almost-40000-2000

Browne, D. R., Hackett, S., & Burger, A. (2017). Employing community voices: Informing practice and programming through Camden Healthy Start focus groups. *Maternal & Child Health Journal*, *21*(Suppl 1), 101–106.

Campbell, Y. N., Machan, M. D., & Fisher, M. D. (2016). The Jehovah's Witness population: Considerations for preoperative optimization of hemoglobin. *AANA Journal*, *84*(3), 173–178.

Canizares, M., Hogg-Johnson, S., Gignac, M., Glazier, R., & Badley, E. (2017). Changes in the use practitioner-based complementary and alternative medicine over time in Canada: cohort and period effects. *PLoS One*, *12*(5), e0177307. doi: 10.1371/journal.pone.0177307.

Centers for Disease Control & Prevention (CDC). (2019). *Lead in foods, cosmetics, and medicines*. Retrieved from https://www.cdc.gov/nceh/lead/tips/folkmedicine.htm

Cheon, Y. M., Bayless, S. D., Wang, Y., & Yip, T. (2018). The development of ethnic/racial self-labeling: Individual differences in context. *Journal of Youth and Adolescence*, *47*(10), 2261–2278.

Chevallier, A. (2016). *Encyclopedia of herbal medicine: 550 herbs and remedies for common ailments*. New York, NY: DK Publishing.

Cho, E., Lee, M. Y., & Hur, M. H. (2017). The effects of aromatherapy on intensive care unit patients' stress and sleep quality: a nonrandomized controlled trial. *Evidence-Based Complementary and Alternative Medicine*, *2010*, 10 pages. Article ID 2856592. doi: 10.1155.2017.2856592.

Cleveland Clinic. (2018). *Herbal supplements: Helpful or harmful*. Retrieved from https://my.clevelandclinic.org/health/articles/17095-herbal-supplements-helpful-or-harmful

Colby, S., & Ortman, J. (2015). Projections of the size and composition of the United States population, 2014 to 2060. *United States Census Bureau, Current Population Reports*. Retrieved from http://www.census.gov/content/dam/Census/library/publications/2015/demo/p25-1143.pdf

Coyle, D. (2018). *Culture code: The secrets of highly successful groups*. New York, NY: Bantam Books.

Craig, M. A., & Richeson, J. A. (2014). On the precipice of a "majority-minority" America: Perceived status threat from the racial demographic shift affects White Americans' political ideology. *Psychological Science*, *25*(6), 1189–1197.

Craig, M. A., & Richeson, J. A. (2017). Information about the US racial demographic shift triggers concerns about anti-White discrimination among the prospective White "minority". *PLoS One*, *12*(9), e0185389.

Darnell, L. K., & Hickson, S. V. (2015). Culturally competent patient patient-centered nursing care. *Nursing Clinics of North America*, *50*(1), 99–108.

Donoghue, T. (2018). Herbal medications and anesthesia case management. *AANA Journal*, *86*(3), 242–248.

Douglas, M., Pacquiao, D., & Purnell, L. (Eds.). (2018). *Global applications of culturally competent health care: Guidelines for practice*. Switzerland: Springer International Publishing.

Douglas, M. K., Rosenkoetter, M., Pacquiao, D. F., Callister, L. C., Hattar-Pollara, M., Lauderdale, J., ... Purnell, L. (2014). Guidelines for implementing culturally competent nursing care. *Journal of Transcultural Nursing*, *25*(2), 109–121.

Eliopoulos, C. (2018). *Invitation to holistic health: A guide to living a balanced life*. Burlington, MA: Jones & Bartlett Learning.

Fadiman, A. (1998). *The spirit catches you and you fall down*. New York, NY: Farrar, Straus, & Giroux.

Fairchild, A. L. (2018). US immigration: A shrinking vision of belonging and deserving. *American Journal of Public Health*, *108*(5), 604–605.

Forbes, B. D., & Mahan, J. H. (Eds.). (2017). *Religion and popular culture in America* (3rd ed.). Oakland, CA: University of California Press.

Geng, Y., Zhao, W., Zhou, F., Ma, X., Yao, S., Hurlemann, R., ... Kendrick, K. (2018). Oxytocin enhancement of emotional empathy: generalization across cultures and effects on amygdala activity. *Frontiers in Neuroscience*, *12*, 512. doi: 10.3389/fnins.2018.00512.

Giger, J. N. (2017). *Transcultural nursing* (7th ed.). St. Louis, MO: Elsevier.

Gubernskaya, Z., & Dreby, J. (2017). US immigration policy and the case for family unity. *Journal on Migration and Human Security*, *5*(2), 417–430.

Guerrero-Preston, R., Valle, B., Jedlicka, A., Turaga, N., Folawiyo, O., ... Sidransky, D. (2016). Molecular triage of premalignant lesions in liquid-based cervical cytology and circulating cell free DNA from urine, using a panel of methylated human papilloma virus and host genes. *Cancer Prevention Research*, *9*(12), 915–924. doi: 10.1158/1940-6207.CAPR-16-0138.

Hall, E. T. (1959). *The silent language*. Garden City, NY: Doubleday.

Han, S., & Ma, Y. (2014). Cultural differences in human brain activity: A quantitative meta-analysis. *NeuroImage*, *99*, 293–300.

Holm, A. L., Rowe, G. M., Brady, M., & White-Perkins, D. (2017). Recognizing privilege and bias: An interactive exercise to expand health care providers' personal awareness. *Academic Medicine*, *92*(3), 360–364.

Humes, K. R., Jones, N. A., & Ramirez, R. R. (March 2011). *Overview of race and Hispanic origin: 2010*. Retrieved from http://www.census.gov/prod/cen2010/briefs/c2010br-02.pdf

Jang, S. (2017). Cultural brokerage and creative performance in multicultural teams. *Organization Science*, *28*(6), 993–1009. Retrieved from https://pubsonline.informs.org/doi/10.1287/orsc.2017.1162

Jensen, E., Bhaskar, R., & Scopilliti, M. (2015). *Demographic analysis 2010: Estimates of coverage of the foreign-born population in the American Community Survey*. Population Division, U.S. Census Bureau, Working Paper No. 103. Retrieved from http://www.census.gov/content/dam/Census/library/working-papers/2015/demo/POP-twps0103.pdf

Kark, S. L. (1974). *Epidemiology and community medicine*. New York, NY: Appleton-Century-Crofts.

Kennedy, A. (2017). *Herbal medicine: Natural remedies*. Berkeley, CA: Althea Press.

Kiang, L., & Witkow, M. R. (2018). Identifying as American among adolescents from Asian backgrounds. *Journal of Youth and Adolescence*, *47*(1), 64–76.

Kottack, C. (2017). *Cultural anthropology: Appreciating cultural diversity* (17th ed.). New York, NY: McGraw-Hill Education.

Levin, J. (2016). Prevalence and religious predictors of healing prayer use in the USA: findings from the Baylor religion Survey. *Journal of Religion and Health*, *55*, 1136–1158. doi: 10.1007/s10943-016-0240-9.

Lindquist, R., & Tracy, M. (Eds.). (2018). *Complementary and alternative therapies in nursing* (8th ed.). New York, NY: Springer Publishing Company.

Lopez, M., Gonzalez-Barrera, A., & López, G. (2017). *Hispanic identity fades across generations as immigrant connections fall away*. Retrieved from http://www.pewhispanic.org/2017/12/20/hispanic-identity-fades-across-generations-as-immigrant-connections-fall-away/

Luciana, M., Bjork, J., Nagel, B., Barch, D., Gonzalez, R., Nixon, S., & Banich, M. (2018). Adolescent neurocognitive development and impacts of substance use: Overview of the adolescent cognitive development (ABCD) baseline neurocognition battery. *Developmental Cognitive Neuroscience*, *32*, 67–79. doi: 10.1016/n.den.2018.02.006.

Marion, L., Douglas, M., Lavin, M. A., Barr, N., Thomas, E., & Bickford, C. (2017). Implementing the new ANA standard 8: Culturally congruent practice. *OJIN: Online Journal of Issues in Nursing, 22*, 1. Retrieved from http://ojin.nursingworld.org/MainMenuCategories/ANAMarketplace/ANAPeriodicals/OJIN/TableofContents/Vol-22-2017/No1-Jan-2017/Articles-Previous-Topics/Implementing-the-New-ANA-Standard-8.html

McFarland, M., & Wehbe-Alamah, H. (2018). *Culture, care, diversity, and universality: A theory of* nursing (4th ed.). New York, NY: Mc-Graw-Hill Education.

Mead, M. (1960). Cultural contexts of nursing problems. In F. C. MacGregor (Ed.), *Social science in nursing* (pp. 74–88). New York, NY: Wiley.

Merriam Webster Dictionary. (2020). *Ethnicity*. Retrieved from https://www.merriam-webster.com/dictionary/ethnicity

Montag, C., Markowetz, A., Blaszkiewicz, K., Andone, I., Lachmann, B., Sariyska, R., ... Markett, S. (2018). Facebook usage on smartphones and gray matter volume of the nucleus accumbens. *Behavioural Brain Research, 329*, 221–228. doi: 10.1016/j.bbr.2017.04.035.

Mujallad, A., & Taylor, E. J. (2016). Modesty among Muslim women: Implications for nursing care. *Medsurg Nursing*, *25*(3), 169–172.

Murcia, S., & Lopez, L. (2016). The experience of nurses in care for culturally diverse families: A qualitative meta-synthesis. *Revista latino-americana de enfermagem*, *24*, e2718.

Murdock, G. (1972). The science of culture. In M. Freilich (Ed.), *The meaning of culture: A reader in cultural anthropology* (pp. 252–266). Lexington, MA: Xerox College Publishing.

Murdock, S. H., Cline, M., Zey, M., Perez, D., & Wilner Jeanty, P. (2015). *Population change in the United States: Socioeconomic challenges and opportunities in the twenty-first century*. New York, NY: Springer.

Nadasen, P. (December 21, 2017). *Extreme poverty returns to America: The U.N. finds growing numbers of Americans are living in the most impoverished circumstances. How did we get here?* The Washington Post. Retrieved from https://www.washingtonpost.com/news/made-by-history/wp/2017/12/21/extreme-poverty-returns-to-america/?utm_term=.08d5f3176553

Office of Disease Prevention and Health Promotion. (2019). *Healthy People 2030 framework*. Retrieved from https://www.healthypeople.gov/2020/About-Healthy-People/Development-Healthy-People-2030/Framework

Partnership for Prescription Assistance. (2018). *Prescription assistance programs*. Retrieved from www.pparx.org/

Patwardhan, B., Mutalik, G., & Tillu, G. (2015). *Integrative approaches for health: Biomedical research, Ayurveda and yoga*. New York, NY: Elsevier.

Perez, A. D., & Hirschman, C. (2009). The changing racial and ethnic composition of the US population: Emerging American identities. *Population and Development Review*, *35*(1), 1–51.

Pizzorno, J., Murray, M., & Joiner-Bey, H. (2016). *The clinician's handbook of natural medicine* (3rd ed.). St. Louis, MO: Elsevier.

Quad Council Coalition Competency Review Task Force. (2018). *Community/public health nursing competencies*. Retrieved from www.quadcouncilphn.org

Quandt, S., Sandberg, J., Grzywacz, J., Altizer, K., & Arcury, T. (2015). Home remedy use among African American and White older adults. *JAMA*, *107*(2), 121–129.

Richeson, J. A., & Grossman, L. (2016). Anxiety in the guise of racism. *New Scientist*, *230*(3078), 40–41.

Roberson, K., Smith, T., & Davidson, W. (2018). Understanding death rituals. *International Journal of Childbirth Education*, *3*(33), 22–26.

Spector, R. E. (2017). *Cultural diversity in health and illness* (9th ed.). Upper Saddle River, NJ: Pearson Education.

Spradley, J., McCurdy, D., & Shandy, D. (2016). *Conformity and conflict: Readings in cultural anthropology* (15th ed.). New York, NY: Pearson.

Stepanikova, I., & Oates, G. R. (2017). Perceived discrimination and privilege in health care: The role of socioeconomic status and race. *American Journal of Preventive Medicine*, *52*(1S1), S86–S94.

Underwood, S. M., & Kelber, S. (2015). Enhancing the collection, discussion and use of family health history by consumers, nurses and other health care providers. *Nursing Clinics of North America, 50*(3), 509–529. doi: 10.1016/j.cnur.2015.05.006.

U.S. Census Bureau. (n.d.). *Quick facts, 2019: United States*. Retrieved from https://www.census.gov/quickfacts/fact/table/US/PST045219

U.S. Census Bureau. (2020). *About Hispanic origin*. Retrieved from https://www.census.gov/topics/population/hispanic-origin/about.html

Reprinted from U.S. Department of Health and Human Services (USDHHS). (2020). *Browse 2030 objectives*. Retrieved from https://health.gov/healthypeople/objectives-and-data/browse-objectives

U.S. Equal Employment Opportunity Commission. (n.d.). *Laws enforced by EEOC*. Retrieved from http://www.eeoc.gov/laws/statutes/

U.S. Food and Drug Administration (USFDA). (2015). *Drug applications for over-the-counter (OTC) drugs*. Retrieved from https://www.fda.gov/drugs/types-applications/drug-applications-over-counter-otc-drugs

U.S. Food and Drug Administration (USFDA). (2017). *Is it really 'FDA approved'?* Retrieved from https://www.fda.gov/consumers/consumer-updates/it-really-fda-approved

Vitale, A., & Jenner, M. (2018). Use of aromatherapy for discomfort in labor. *International Journal of Childbirth Education*, *33*(2), 31–35.

Widge, A. T., Flory, E., Sharma, H., & Herbert, L. J. (2018). Food allergy perceptions and health-related quality of life in a racially diverse sample. *Children, 5*(6), 70. Retrieved from https://www.ncbi.nlm.nih.gov/pmc/articles/PMC6025107/

Witsman, K. (2018). *U.S. lawful permanent residents: 2017, Department of Homeland Security Office of Immigration Statistics, annual flow report*. Retrieved from https://www.dhs.gov/sites/default/files/publications/Lawful_Permanent_Residents_2017.pdf

Wood, B., Loftres, A., & Vahabi, M. (2018). Strategies to reach marginalized women for cervical cancer screening: A qualitative study of stakeholder perspectives. *Current Oncology*, 25(1), e8–e16. Retrieved from https://www.ncbi.nlm.nih.gov/pmc/articles/PMC5832295/

Xu, X., Yao, S., Xu, L., Geng, Y., Zaho, W., ... Kendrick, K. (January 12, 2017). Oxytocin biases men but not women to restore social connections with individuals who socially exclude them. *Scientific Reports*, *7*, 40589. Retrieved from https://www.nature.com/articles/srep40589

Young, C., Haffejee, B., & Dorsun, D. (2017). The relationship between ethnocentrism and cultural intelligence. *International Journal of Intercultural Relations*, *58*, 31–41. doi: 10.1016/j.intrel.2017.04.001.

Zucker, R., Gonzalez, R., Ewing, S., Paulus, M., Arroyo, J., ... Wills, T. (2018). Assessment of culture and environment in the Adolescent Brain and Cognitive Development Study: Rationale, description of measures, and early data. *Developmental Cognitive Neuroscience*, *32*, 107–120. doi: 10.1016.j.dcn.2018.03.004.

UNIT 2

Community/Public Health Essentials

CHAPTER 6

Structure and Economics of Community/Public Health Services

"The success or failure of any government in the final analysis must be measured by the well-being of its citizens. Nothing can be more important to a state than its public health; the state's paramount concern should be the health of its people."

—Franklin Delano Roosevelt (1882–1945)

KEY TERMS

Adverse selection
Capitation
Cost sharing
Cost shifting
Cross subsidization
Diagnosis-related groups (DRGs)
Economics
Exclusive provider organization (EPO)
Fee-for-service (FFS)
Health—income gradient
Health maintenance organization (HMO)
Health reimbursement accounts (HRAs)
Health savings accounts (HSAs)
High-deductible health plans (HDHPs)
High-deductible health plans with a savings option (HDHP/SOs)
Macroeconomic theory
Managed care
Managed competition
Medicaid
Medical home
Medicare
Microeconomic theory
Moral hazard
Point-of-service (POS) plan
Preferred provider organization (PPO)
Prospective payment
Retrospective payment
Risk averse
Single-payer system
Supply and demand
Third-party payments
Underinsured
Uninsured
Universal coverage

LEARNING OBJECTIVES

Upon mastery of this chapter, you should be able to:

1. Describe the current organizational structure of the United States' health care system, including public health.
2. Explain the influence of selected legislative acts in the United States on shaping current health care policy and practice.

3. Compare and contrast different payment systems for health care services, including managed care, fee-for-service, and single-payer systems.
4. Analyze the trends and issues influencing health care economics and delivery of public health services.
5. Discuss potential health care reform measures and the potential impact on community/public health nursing.
6. Describe how health care system funding and financing influences community/public health nursing practice.

INTRODUCTION

In the United States, two systems address the health of the people who live here: the health care system and the public health system (American Public Health Association [APHA], 2019a). The United States' health system is often described as a "crazy quilt." This type of quilt is not planned; rather, it develops from scraps of fabric that are collected over many years. Similarly, health care and public health services in the United States are provided through a mix of private and public programs and institutions; each of these was created to meet specific needs at different times in history. The substantial gaps in the U.S. systems, or tears in the quilt, are intermittently patched with new programs, institutions, or funding streams. Each patch makes a complicated system even more difficult to navigate.

Nurses preparing for population-based practice need to be familiar with both systems (health care and public health): their organization, operation, and financing. To understand financing, community/public health nurses must be familiar with the economics of health care and the influence of politics on public health services. The structure and economics of community/public health care are intertwined.

- Health care economics is a specialized field of economics that describes and analyzes "value and behavior in the delivery and consumption of.... healthcare" (American Academy of Pediatrics, 2019, para. 1).
- Economic analysis evaluates the effects of health policy (Bernell, 2016). The goal of health care economics, much like that of public health, is to overcome scarcity by making good choices while providing essential services.

This chapter begins with a review of significant events that influenced the current U.S. health system. It then provides an overview of health care economics, including different payment systems used in the United States and sources of public and private funding for health care and community health services.

HISTORICAL INFLUENCES ON HEALTH CARE

For centuries, humans have battled disease. As in current times, travel historically provided an exchange of goods and knowledge; however, it also has spread disease. For instance, trade between Europe and Asia, military conquests, and Christian crusades to the Middle East brought diseases to European cities.

- The bubonic plague, known as the Black Death during the mid-1300s, was a devastating epidemic, reportedly killing between 50 and 60 million people (about 60% of the population in Europe) (Benedictow, 2005; Rosen, 2015).
- The plague "returned periodically" for almost 500 years (Cohn, 2008, p. 74). Venice and other port cities created quarantine areas outside of the city. Travelers were required to stay in these areas for a length of time, until city officials determined they were free of disease (Rosen, 2015).
- During the periods of Colonialism, Imperialism, and the Triangle Trade, extended influence furthered global health impacts (Bivins, 2007).
- Later, regulations developed to protect health, such as safety rules for miners and concern with sailors' health. Reforms during the Enlightenment period were influenced by a growing emphasis on human dignity, human rights, and the search for scientific truth (Erwin & Brownson, 2017b).
- Social and sanitary reforms increased, such as vaccination stations in London and establishment of a General Board of Health in the mid-1800s (Lewis, 1952; Richardson, 1887). See Chapters 3 and 7.

Development of the U.S. Health Care System

Early health care in the American colonies consisted of private practices, with occasional (but infrequent) governmental action for the public good (Erwin & Brownson, 2017b). Physicians had few tools at their disposal and could do little to change the course of illness (Hoffer, 2019a & Rosen, 2015).

- Until the mid-1800s, hospitals were places for the very poor to receive care, and the patients often died; those who could afford it had physicians visit them at home. During the late 1800s, scientific advances, including germ theory and sterilization, made hospitals safer, whereas industrialization led to more people living in cities and away from family members who could provide care (Kisacky, 2019).
- An emphasis on improved sanitation and working conditions stemmed from landmark reports, like Shattuck and Griscom.
- The professionalization of nursing care also occurred at this time, further contributing to the move from home-based to hospital-based care (see Chapter 3).

Early public health actions were isolated, local responses to specific problems (Rosen, 2015). The first *federal* public health action occurred in 1878, when the U.S. Congress created a federal quarantine system, enforced by the Marine Hospital Service (National Institutes of Health [NIH], 2017). With increasing travel between cities and states, local quarantines became ineffective. The coordinated strategy was successful; epidemics were quickly checked, and communities recognized the benefits of federal government action, resulting in continued growth. (See http://thepoint.lww.com/Rector10e for a table of historical milestones and legislation.)

- The Marine Hospital Service eventually became the U.S. Public Health Service, one of the seven uniformed services of the United States (USDHHS, n.d.a).

- Their first lab in a New York hospital grew into the National Institutes of Health, headquartered in Bethesda, Maryland—which now includes more than 75 institutes supporting scientists conducting research activities in every state and globally (NIH, 2019).
- Since 1854, when President Pierce vetoed legislation to address "indigent insane," many presidents, from Theodore Roosevelt to Franklin D. Roosevelt and from Richard Nixon to William Clinton, have sought some type of universal health coverage (Manchikanti, Helm, Benyamin, & Hirsch, 2017, p. 107).
- In 1900, the average amount spent on health care by individual Americans was $5 a year, which would equal just over $128 in 2020 economy. Compare that to the $11,172 spent in 2018 (Blumberg & Davidson, 2009; Centers for Medicare & Medicaid Services [CMS], 2019e; Saving.org, 2020).

Over time, events and insights contributed to improved programs and services, along with a broader recognition that individual health was affected by the health of the wider community. Our current public health system is not really a single entity, but more of a loosely affiliated network of federal, state, and local health agencies that have been chronically underfunded (Erwin & Brownson, 2017b).

Early Health Insurance

- Starting in 1929 with Baylor University Hospital in Texas, hospitals offered prepayment plans for hospital services to teachers as a way to increase hospital use. They had already been marketing the benefits of hospital childbirth to fill beds.
- Soon after, physician groups developed similar plans. These became known as Blue Cross (hospital) and Blue Shield (physician) plans, the beginning of modern insurance companies.
- The first government involvement in health insurance was in 1965, when Medicare and Medicaid were created—providing insurance for older adults and families living in poverty (Blumberg & Davidson, 2009).

Over the next five decades, in addition to the prior public health actions, legislation passed addressing health care services for targeted groups. (See http://thepoint.lww.com/Rector10e for a table of important public health actions, reports, and legislation from 1647 to 2020.) In recent years, health care reform has focused on regulating the health insurance industry, including the price for insurance and the services that are covered (Shi & Singh, 2019).

- The Patient Protection and Affordable Care Act or ACA, improved access to care by making insurance available to people who were considered "uninsurable" due to preexisting health conditions (Healthcare.gov, 2010).
- The ACA expanded Medicaid in a number of states, extending coverage to low-income individuals and families. In addition, the ACA required insurance companies to cover preventative health care visits without a copay and to cover those with preexisting conditions, improving access to care for those with insurance.
- The number percentage of **uninsured** (those lacking health insurance) had been 18% before passage of the ACA but dropped to a low of 10.9% by 2016 (Witters, 2019).
- In recent years, political disagreements about the ACA have led to weakening of some protections. Despite this, federal surveys revealed a fairly stable national rate of uninsured between 2016 and 2017 at 8.8%. However, states that did not participate in Medicaid expansion had higher rates, averaging 12.2% (Keith, 2018).
- At the end of 2018, a Gallup poll reported that the uninsured rate had increased to 13.7% (Witters, 2019). From 2016 to 2018, the number of uninsured Americans grew by 1.2 million (KFF, 2019d).

Recent Calls to Action

Formerly known as the Institute of Medicine (IOM), the Health and Medicine Division of the National Academies of Sciences, Engineering, and Medicine is an independent, nongovernmental, nonprofit organization that researches health care and public health problems (NASEM, 2017). Established in 1970, it has produced many groundbreaking reports that have advanced health care and public health services. Table 6-1 describes several of these reports.

The Healthy People initiative established science-based, 10-year goals and objectives for improving the health of everyone in the United States (Office of Disease Prevention and Health Promotion, 2019; USDHHS, 2020a). Each decade since 1979, the Healthy People goals and objectives have directed research and grant dollars to support activities that improve health. In comparison to *Healthy People 2020*, fewer, more targeted topics and objectives are found in *Healthy People 2030* (USDHHS, 2020a). See Chapters 1 and 2 for more on the development of Healthy People initiatives.

HEALTH CARE ORGANIZATIONS IN THE UNITED STATES

A blend of private and public agencies provides oversight for both the health care and public health system in the United States. The actions of these agencies often complement each other, and in recent years, the roles of private groups and government agencies have become increasingly interdependent (Turnock, 2016b).

Private Health Sector Organizations

Private groups include professional associations and nongovernmental organizations (NGOs) focusing on health-related issues. Health-related professional associations influence the quality and type of community/public health services available in the United States through the promotion of standards, research, information, and programs. Many also lobby legislators. These organizations are funded primarily through membership dues, bequests, and contributions (U.S. Department of State, n.d.).

- Health issues focused NGOs (e.g., American Cancer Society, American Diabetes Association) supply funds for research, to lobby legislators, and to educate the public. Funding is through private contributions.

TABLE 6-1 Selected Reports of the Institute of Medicine (Now the National Academy of Medicine)

Year	Title of Report	Description
1988	The Future of Public Health	■ Highlighted disarray in the current public health system ■ Called for improvements in public health infrastructure; focused on governmental responsibilities
1996	America's Health in Transition: Protecting and Improving Quality	■ Described inconsistency in access to care: some Americans lacking access to adequate care—even those with insurance—compared with others receiving care that is not necessary ■ Called for measurement, monitoring, and improvement of quality care
1999	To Err is Human: Building a Safer Health System	■ Revealed extent of deaths due to medical errors in hospitals and identified problems in systems and processes, not individual misbehavior, as the cause of errors ■ Called for increased focus on knowledge about systems that promote safety, mandatory reporting of medical errors, and development of safety standards
2001	Crossing the Quality Chasm: A New Health System for the 21st Century	■ Listed performance expectations for the health care system, aligning payment incentives with accountability and quality improvement ■ Promoted evidence-based practice and informatics
2002	The Future of the Public's Health in the 21st Century	■ Called for expanding the responsibilities of the public health system beyond governmental agencies to include private and nongovernmental entities ■ Outlined how partnerships could be formed with communities, businesses, the media, universities, and others to expand the reach of public health and achieve the *Healthy People 2010* goals
2010	The Future of Nursing: Leading Change, Advancing Health	■ Expressed the importance of nursing's role in achieving vision for health care in the Patient Protection and Affordable Care Act ■ Recommended strategies to improve nursing education, provide opportunities for leadership, and allow the scope of nursing practice to match nurses' education and training
2012	For the Public's Health: Investing in a Healthier Future	■ Noted the need for additional focus on population-based prevention rather than on clinical care ■ Called for federal spending on public health to be doubled and that minimum public health services and costs should be determined

Source: National Academies Press (2020).

- Others, such as the National Society for Autistic Children, Planned Parenthood Federation of America, and the National Council on Aging, focus on the needs of special populations.
- Some NGOs provide services and health care. These include Habitat for Humanity, the American Red Cross, and the Public Health Institute (Anbazhagan, 2016; Yale School of Public Health, 2019).
- A few agencies focus on disease prevention, such as the Trust for America's Health and the Prevention Institute. Many foundations provide grant support for health programs, research, and professional education as part of their mission (e.g., Robert Wood Johnson Foundation, Bill and Melinda Gates Foundation, National Philanthropic Trust, 2018).

Health-Related Professional Associations

Many health-related professional associations, like the National Organization for Public Health Nursing (1912–1952), have influenced the quality and type of community/public health services delivered (Bekemeier, Walker Linderman, Kneipp, & Zahner, 2015; Quad Council, 2018). See Chapter 3. Others include the following:

- American Public Health Association (APHA, 2019a), founded in 1872, maintains a prominent role in the dissemination of public health information, influence on health policy, and advocacy for the nation's health.
- Other nursing and community health organizations that have promoted quality efforts in community/public health include (APHN, n.d.; Nurse.org, 2019) the following:

- Association of Public Health Nurses (APHN) (formerly the Association of State and Territorial Directors of Nursing)
- Association of State and Territorial Health Officers (ASTHO)
- National Association of County and City Health Officials (NACCHO)
- Association for Community Health Nursing Educators (ACHNE)
- Public Health Nursing Section, American Public Health Association (APHA)
- Alliance of Nurses for Health Environments (ANHE)

Public Health Agencies

Public health agencies perform a wide variety of activities, some requiring legal authority to ensure enforcement (e.g., environmental pollution, communicable disease control, food handling). These agencies provide important data, including the collection and monitoring of vital statistics and communicable diseases. They also conduct research, provide consultation, and sometimes financially support other community/public health efforts. These activities can be grouped under one of the three core public health functions: assessment, policy development, and assurance (CDC, 2019).

Core Public Health Functions

Public health agencies perform a wide variety of activities, organized around the three core public health functions of assessment, policy development, and assurance (CDC, 2019; Table 6-2). As discussed in Chapters 1 and 2, C/PHNs practice as partners with other public health professionals within these core functions.

Table 6-3 describes the actions of some federal agencies in relation to the three core functions. States retain the primary responsibility for their citizens' health and are responsible for implementing federal policies. At the local level, a city government health agency, a county agency, or a combination of both assess, plan, and serve the health needs of their community (Goldsteen, Goldsteen, & Goldsteen, 2017). Table 6-4 compares the public health responsibilities of federal, state, and local governments related to the 10 Essentials of Public Health Services.

Federal Public Health Agencies

The federal public health responsibilities include the following:

- Policymaking and implementing legislation
- Financing public health through health care services, grants, contracts, and reimbursements to states and local public health agencies
- Protection of public health and prevention activities through surveillance, research, and regulation
- Collecting and disseminating data (national data, health statistics, surveys, research)
- Acting to assist states in mounting effective responses during public health emergencies (e.g., natural disaster, bioterrorism, emerging diseases)
- Developing public health goals in collaboration with state and local governments and other relevant stakeholders (e.g., *Healthy People 2030*)
- Building capacity for population health at federal, state, and local levels by providing resources and infrastructure
- Directly managing health care delivery through categorical grant programs (maternal–child health

TABLE 6-2 Core Public Health Functions Applied to Populations and People at Risk

Type of Services	Core Public Health Function	Description of Services
Population-wide services	Assessment	Health status monitoring and disease surveillance (community health assessments)
	Public policy	Leadership, policy, planning, and administration (Health in All Policies, collaborative partnerships)
	Assurance	▪ Investigation and control of diseases and injuries ▪ Protection of environment, workplaces, housing, food, and water ▪ Laboratory services to support disease control and environmental protection ▪ Health education and information ▪ Community mobilization for health-related issues ▪ Targeted outreach and linkage to personal services ▪ Health services quality assurance and accountability ▪ Training and education of public health professionals
Personal services and home visits for people at risk	N/A	▪ Primary care for underserved and those people not served through health care system ▪ Treatment services for targeted conditions ▪ Clinical preventive services ▪ Payments for personal services delivered by others

Source: Centers for Disease Control and Prevention (CDC) (2019).

TABLE 6-3 Examples of Federal Government Agencies' Actions Related to the Three Core Public Health Functions

Core Public Health Function	Agency	Example of Action
Assessment	Centers for Disease Control and Prevention National Center for Health Statistics	Conducts surveillance for disease outbreaks Conducts national surveys that monitor health behaviors
Policy development	Substance Abuse and Mental Health Services Administration Health Resources and Services Administration	Uses data to educate policymakers about mental health and substance use disorders Analyzes potential effects of proposed policy
Assurance	Environmental Protection Agency Indian Health Service	Evaluates safety of water for drinking Funds or provides care for underserved populations living on tribal lands

TABLE 6-4 Federal, State, and Local Activities Related to the Ten Essential Public Health Services

Essential Service	Federal	State	Local
Assess and monitor population health	Collect and disseminate information using national surveys	Collect and analyze data specific to the state	Complete community health assessments
Investigate, diagnose, and address health hazards and root causes	Maintain national surveillance systems and provide specialty laboratory services that state or local public health laboratories cannot perform	Monitor statewide health threats and report to the federal level when appropriate; perform laboratory testing to identify cause of health hazard	Identify individuals and groups who have conditions that threaten public health
Communicate effectively to inform and educate	Distribute national reports about health issues (Surgeon General examples)	Conduct media campaigns and programs on prevention; coordinate statewide health alerts	Provide educational materials supporting local programs
Strengthen, support, and mobilize communities and partnerships	Collaborate with national nongovernmental organizations	Coordinate efforts of state agencies	Establish relationships with community leaders and agencies
Create, champion, and implement policies, plans, and laws	Establish national public health goals, in collaboration with state and local health officials and public health experts	Set statewide health objective and priorities	Implement programs to meet public health goals
Utilize legal and regulatory actions	Enforce public health regulations affecting interstate commerce	Develop statewide regulations for services and the environment	Assess compliance with regulations and take appropriate action
Enable equitable access	Establish and manage national health insurance programs and insurance marketplaces (U.S. Public Health Service)	Implement federal initiatives and equitably distribute funds to communities	Address unmet needs in the community through case management and clinics
Build a diverse and skilled workforce	Provide expertise or resources when public health needs exceed state capacity; promote diversity in health professions training	Set requirements and maintain records of licensure for public health professionals	Screen, hire, and train staff
Improve and innovate through evaluation, research, and quality improvement	Disseminate evidence-based practices for public health services	Gather data and compile results of program evaluations	Determine if existing services meet the community's needs and search for innovative solutions.
Build and maintain a strong organizational infrastructure for public health	Promote adequate funding for public health programs and research	Determine solutions appropriate for specific state and provide adequate staffing for programs	Fund and implement new programs and report on effectiveness

Source: Centers for Disease Control and Prevention (CDC) (2020); Public Health Law Center (n.d.).

programs, Medicaid, Medicare, community health centers) and services (public health laboratories, Indian health clinics) (CDC, 2013; IOM, 2002)

At the national level, public health organizations can be clustered into four groups of government agencies:

- U.S. Public Health Service (USPHS) is staffed by the Commissioned Corps, which consists of over 6,700 uniformed health professionals (see Chapter 28 for more on the Commissioned Corps). Employees of the USPHS work in many different federal agencies (USDHHS, n.d.a). See Chapter 28.
- The U.S. Department of Health and Human Services (USDHHS), including the Centers for Disease Control and Prevention (CDC).
- Federal departments that oversee areas impacting health, such as the Departments of Labor, Education, Environmental Health, Agriculture, and Transportation, among others.
- Federal agencies that focus on international health concerns, such as the U.S. Agency for International Development (USAID) and the Office of International Health Affairs, are under the auspices of the U. S. Department of State (Turnock, 2016a). See Chapter 16.

Table 6-5 provides a selected list of federal agencies related to public health. Figure 6-1 represents the organizational chart for the USDHHS.

State Public Health Agencies

The state health department (SHD) is responsible for providing leadership in and monitoring of comprehensive public health needs and services in the state. SHDs promote population health, focusing on prevention and protection. They also administer federally funded programs.

General functions of SHDs include (CDC, 2013; Erwin & Brownson, 2017b) the following:

- Statewide health planning
- Intergovernmental and other agency relations
- Intrastate agency relations
- Certain statewide policy determinations
- Standards setting
- Health regulatory functions
- State laboratory services
- Surveillance and epidemiology
- Training and technical support

The Association of State and Territory Health Officials (ASTHO) surveys SHDs; the latest published data were collected in 2019 and 2016. The structure of SHDs is described in Figure 6-2. The person in charge of the SHD is generally appointed by the governor and is, most often, a physician. In fact, 64% of state health officials have a medical degree. In 2016, the leaders of four SHDs (Maryland, North Carolina, North Dakota, and Oregon) were nurses (ASTHO, 2017). By March 2020, 36 SHDs had achieved initial accreditation by the Public Health Accreditation Board (PHAB, 2020).

Marked changes occurred between 2007 and 2016. Responsibility for substance abuse programs increased from 32% to 76%, while number of SHDs that provided long-term care services decreased from 79% to 57% (ASTHO, 2017). SHDs most often provide training to local health departments (LHDs) in chronic disease and tobacco prevention and control (88%), as well as preparedness and maternal–child health (84%). Priorities also included health disparities/minority health initiatives (86%), and 59% of agencies promoted rural health programs (ASTHO, 2017).

- Between 2010 and 2019, state health agency workforce dropped by 15.3%. The largest losses were among administrative and business/finance employees. As of 2020, 25% of employees are projected to be eligible for retirement; in some states, it is as high as over 40%.
- Public health nurses comprise 7.8% of the state health agency workforce, compared to 0.1% of physician assistants/nurse practitioners and 0.6% of public health physicians. Other employees include epidemiologists/statisticians, environmental health and laboratory specialists, nutritionists and dental health professionals, as well as informatics and public information specialists.
- The largest group of employees (26.8%) work within the financial/business and administrative categories (ASTHO, 2020).

Local Public Health Departments

The primary responsibilities of LHDs are to assess the local population's health status and needs, determine how well those needs are being met, and take action toward satisfying unmet needs. Specifically, they should fulfill these core functions as follows (Erwin & Brownson, 2017b):

- Monitor local health needs and the resources for addressing them.
- Develop policy and provide leadership in advocating equitable distribution of resources and services, both public and private.
- Evaluate availability, accessibility, and quality of health services for all members of the community.
- Keep the community informed about how to access public health services.

The National Association of City and County Health Officials (NACCHO, 2017) identified 2,800 LHDs in the United States in 2016; about 90% of these had significant local governance. Most LHDs (62%) serve populations of <50,000 people. A few (6%) serve over half of the U.S. population (each catchment area serves between 50,000 and 500,000 people). A review of an earlier NACCHO report separated out data from the 20 largest LHDs in the United States (Leider, Castrucci, Hearne, & Russo, 2015). These 20 LHDs represented 1% of all LHDs but served 15% of the population.

LHDs primarily report to local government (77%), while about 16% are a unit of the SHD and 8% have a shared governance structure. Figure 6-3 shows a typical organizational chart for a LHD.

TABLE 6-5 Selected Federal Public Health Agencies of the U.S. Department of Health and Human Services

Agency	Mission, Function, or Area of Focus
USDHHS Agencies	
Administration for Children and Families (ACF)	Supports initiatives that empower families and individuals and improve access to services in order to create strong, healthy communities
Administration for Community Living (ACL)	Funds services provided by community-based organizations that enable older adults and people with disabilities of all ages to live where they choose, with the people they choose, and with the ability to participate fully in their communities
Agency for Healthcare Research and Quality (AHRQ)	Supports research on health care outcomes and costs, patient safety and medical errors, and access to effective services
Agency for Toxic Substances and Disease Registry (ATSDR)	Prevents exposure and adverse human health effects and diminished quality of life associated with exposure to hazardous substances from waste sites, unplanned releases, and other sources of pollution present in the environment
Centers for Disease Control and Prevention (CDC)	Promotes health and quality of life by preventing and controlling disease, injury, and disability
Centers for Medicare & Medicaid Services (CMS)	Administers Medicare, Medicaid, and other major programs such as the State Children's Health Insurance Program; the Medicare Prescription Drug, Improvement, and Modernization Act; and the Health Insurance Portability and Accountability Act (HIPAA)
Food and Drug Administration (FDA)	Ensures the safety of foods and cosmetics and the safety and efficacy of pharmaceuticals, biological products, and medical devices
Health Resources and Services Administration (HRSA)	Assures equitable access to comprehensive, quality health care for all
Indian Health Service (IHS)	Is the principal federal health care advocate and provider for American Indians and Alaska Natives who belong to more than 550 federally recognized tribes in 35 states
National Institutes of Health (NIH)	Provides leadership and financial support for research about ways to prevent disease, as well as the causes, treatments, and even cures for common and rare diseases
Substance Abuse and Mental Health Services Administration (SAMHSA)	Works to improve the quality and availability of prevention, treatment, and rehabilitative services in order to reduce illness, death, disability, and cost to society resulting from substance abuse and mental illnesses
Non-USDHHS Agencies	
U.S. Department of Labor, Occupational Safety and Health Administration (OSHA)	Workplace and worker safety
U.S. Department of Agriculture (USDA)	▪ Dietary guidelines ▪ Food support programs (food stamps—Supplemental Nutrition Assistance Program (SNAP) ▪ Farm-based food control (in contrast to control by the FDA, which is product-based)
Environmental Protection Agency (EPA)	Pollution control
U.S. Department of Housing and Urban Development (HUD)	Healthy Homes initiative (lead, etc.)
Federal Emergency Management Agency (FEMA)	Public health preparedness and disaster response
U.S. Department of Education (DOE)	Safe and Healthy Students program

Source: USDHHS (n.d.c, n.d.d, 2015).

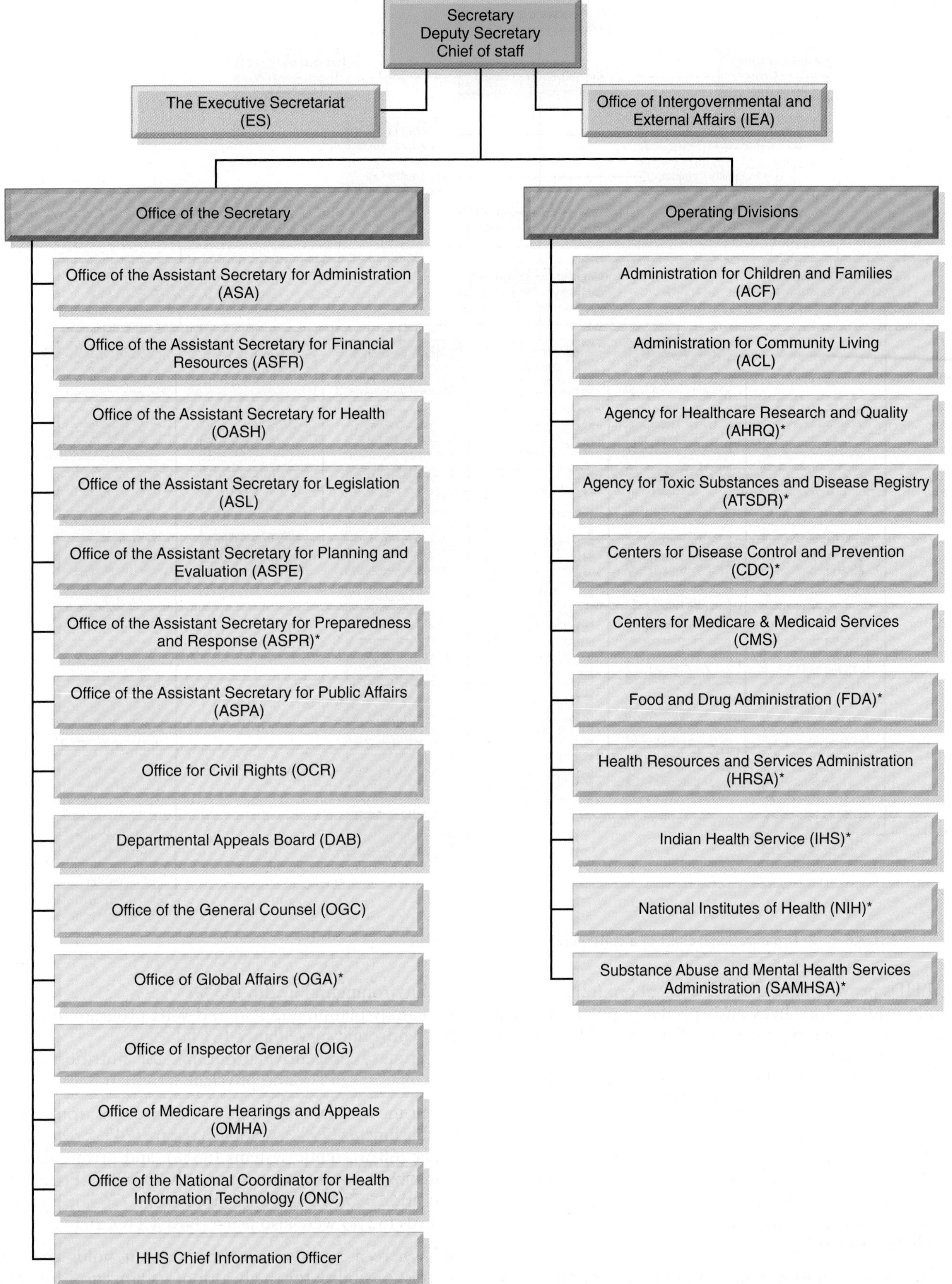

FIGURE 6-1 Department of Health and Human Services organizational chart: January 2020b. *Components of the Public Health Service. (Reprinted from U.S. Department of Health & Human Services. (2020). *HHS organizational chart*. Content created by Assistant Secretary for Public Affairs (ASPA). Last reviewed January 13, 2020. Retrieved from https://www.hhs.gov/about/agencies/orgchart/index.html)

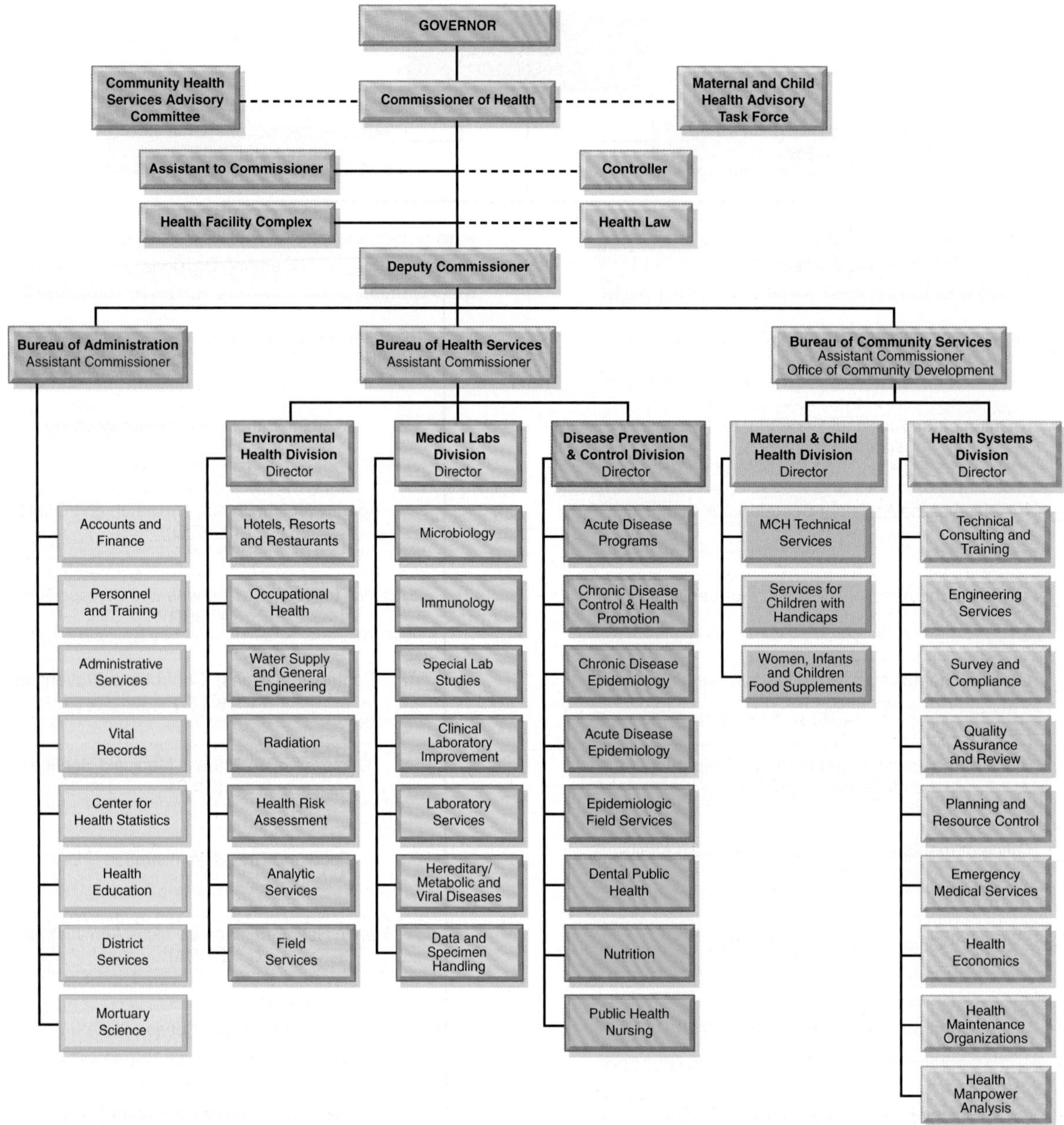

FIGURE 6-2 Organizational chart of a state public health department.

LHDs provide public health clinical programs to help people lead healthy lives and specific population-based health services within their jurisdictions. Table 6-6 lists clinical programs and services reported by more than 50% of LHDs (NACCHO, 2017). The most commonly provided clinical services were as follows:

- Adult and childhood immunizations (90%, 88%)
- TB screening and services (84%, 79%)
- Women, Infants, and Children (WIC) services (66%)
- Screening for HIV and other STDs (62%, 65%)
- Blood lead screening (61%)
- Home visits (60%)

The most common population-based programs provided include the following:

- Adult and childhood immunizations (90%, 88%)
- Communicable/infectious disease (93%)
- Environmental health (85%)
- Family planning (53%) and WIC program (66%)
- Syndromic surveillance (61%)
- Primary preventive programs for nutrition (74%), tobacco (74%), and physical activity (60%)

In the area of regulations or inspections, food service establishments (79%), schools/day care (74%), recreational water (68%), septic systems (65%), and private drinking water (60%) were most commonly reported. Food safety education (77%), nuisance abatement (76%), and vital records (62%) were also listed (NACCHO, 2017).

- Where a board of health exists, it holds the legal responsibility for the health of its citizens. More than three quarters of LHDs report to a local board of health; this is more common for small health departments compared to medium and large departments (NACCHO, 2017).

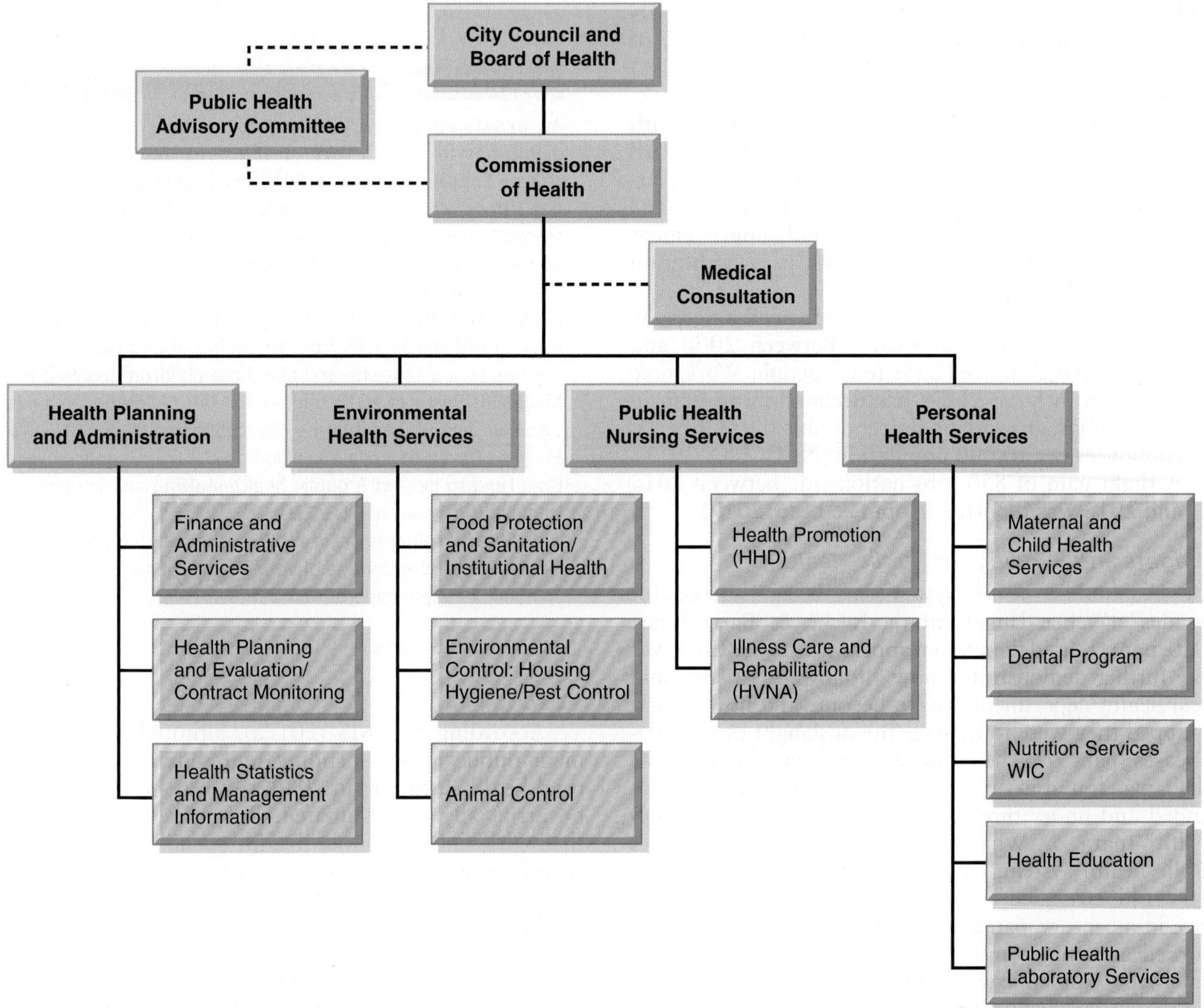

FIGURE 6-3 Organizational chart of a city public health department.

TABLE 6-6 Services Offered by Local Health Departments

% of LHDs Offering Services	Clinical Programs	Population Services
>75%	■ Adult immunizations ■ Childhood immunizations ■ Tuberculosis screening and treatment	■ Communicable/infectious disease and environmental health surveillance ■ Inspection of food service establishments ■ Food safety education ■ Nuisance abatement
50%–74%	■ Screening and treatment of sexually transmitted infections and HIV/AIDS ■ Blood lead screening ■ Blood pressure and body mass index screening ■ Women, Infants, and Children services ■ Home visits ■ Family planning	■ Maternal and child health epidemiology ■ Syndromic surveillance ■ Primary prevention for nutrition, physical activity, unintended pregnancy, and tobacco ■ Chronic disease programs ■ Septic systems regulation ■ Smoke-free ordinances enforcement ■ Private drinking water and lead inspections ■ Inspection of children's camps, hotels/motels, schools/day cares, recreational water, and body art establishments ■ Vector control ■ Vital records

Source: NACCHO (2017).

- Unlike SHDs, nearly one third of directors of LHDs are nurses, including 40% of small LHDs and 47% of rural LHDs. Nurses are less likely to lead large (9%) and urban (16%) LHDs.
- As of March 2020, 255 LHDs and 3 tribal health agencies had received initial accreditation by PHAB (2020). However, a majority of LHDs were completing prerequisite activities required by the PHAB (i.e., community health assessments and improvement plans) indicating continuing interest in accreditation (Robin & Leep, 2017).
- As in SHDs, LHDs have also experienced a decrease in staffing in the past decade. Between 2008 and 2016, LHDs employed 23% fewer people. Workforce reduction in large LHDs has declined more than in small LHDs, at a rate of almost double the number of employees per 10,000 population (NACCHO, 2017). A slight gain of 850 jobs nationwide between 2015 and 2016 was reported (Robin & Leep, 2017).

Budgets and Funding for Public Health

The U.S. public health system has been "starved for decades" (Weber, Ungar, Smith, Recht, & Barry-Jester, 2020, para. 1), and the sudden appearance of SARS-CoV-2 only further demonstrated how "hollowed-out state and local health departments" have become and how poorly equipped they were to manage the onslaught of COVID-19 cases (para. 7). The entire system, beginning with the CDC, was found in an investigative report to be "underfunded and under threat, unable to protect the nation's health" (para. 5). What had been considered a premier public health system, envied by other countries around the world, struggled to meet the crushing demands of a once-in-a-century pandemic on top of an already overworked and underfunded reality. Further, the degree to which the pandemic was politicized resulted in public health workers being "disrespected, ignored, and even vilified," leading to resignations, retirements, and occasional firings (Weber et al., 2020, para.8). In some states, as the pandemic worsened and the economy and tax revenues dwindled, workers were furloughed, had their hours cut, or their pay frozen. See What Do You Think? (Box 6-1).

- Funding for public health peaked at 3.2% of total health expenditures in 2002 after the 9/11 attacks and again in 2008 but decreased to 2.65% in 2014. While overall health spending is projected to increase by an average of 6% per year over the next 10 years, funding for public health has continued to decrease from its peak to a projected low of 2.4% by 2023 (Himmelstein & Woolhandler, 2016a).
- In 2016, the CDC's budget was $22.26 per person, and state public health agencies budgeted an average of $31.26 per person (Trust for America's Health [TFAH], 2019).
- In 2018, total U.S. health care spending was $11,172 per person and 2019 projections showed an increase to $11,559 (CMS, n.d.b, 2019e; Himmelstein & Woolhandler, 2016b). When you compare this to the per person budget of the CDC and state public health agencies, you get a real sense of the very small percentage given to public health in comparison to overall health costs.

BOX 6-1 WHAT DO *YOU* THINK?

Service Over Salaries

An investigative report found that 20% of public health employees (excluding large health departments) had salaries of $35,000 or less in 2017. Well-educated employees (i.e., those with bachelor's, master's, or PhDs) can earn substantially more working in the private sector. At times, some workers actually qualify for the very programs that they oversee, like WIC. For instance, a disease intervention specialist at the Kentucky state health department, tirelessly working to keep HIV and syphilis from spreading, found that her salary was so low that she and her three children qualified for Medicaid. Boston's 2018 budget for the police department was five time higher than its city public health department; Boston offered to move $3 million dollars from a police overtime fund to help with public health staffing and immunization clinics (Weber et al., 2020).

How can residents ensure that public health is adequately funded? What percentage of your city or county budget goes to public health compared to other services?

Source: Weber et al. (2020).

According to CMS (2017a), although U.S. government public health spending represented only 2.5% of total health spending in 2016, this number may actually be artificially overestimated. Recent research indicates that CMS inflates public health spending by including spending on behavioral health care, community health clinics, and disability-related services among other non-public health activities (Leider, 2016; Leider, Resnick, Bishai, & Scutchfield, 2018). Determining the amount of government spending on public health is difficult as the sources of funding are varied and not coordinated across levels of government (TFAH, 2019).

- Federal public health agencies are largely funded by the federal government, but about 75% of that funding ends up at the state and local levels, along with other private and public organizations.
- At the state level, federal grants and monetary support, along with state tax dollars, fund programs.
- The majority of federal grant money is provided by the Prevention and Public Health Fund created by the ACA. From its 2018 budget, $586 million of the total $800 million budget went to state and LHDs (Johnson, 2019).
- The money that makes its way to LHDs often comes through competitive grants and block grants; it is supplemented by local taxes (Congressional Research Service, 2018; Leider et al., 2018; TFAH, 2019).

The lack of consistency and transparency limits public health officials' ability to defend public health programs when budget cuts are threatened. Given that public health agencies are vital safety net services, the decreases in budgets and staffing are very challenging (Bekemeier, Singh, & Schoemann, 2018).

- The proposed 2020 federal budget originally included a 12% cut to the U.S. Department of Health and Human Services, as well as $750 million in cuts to the CDC,

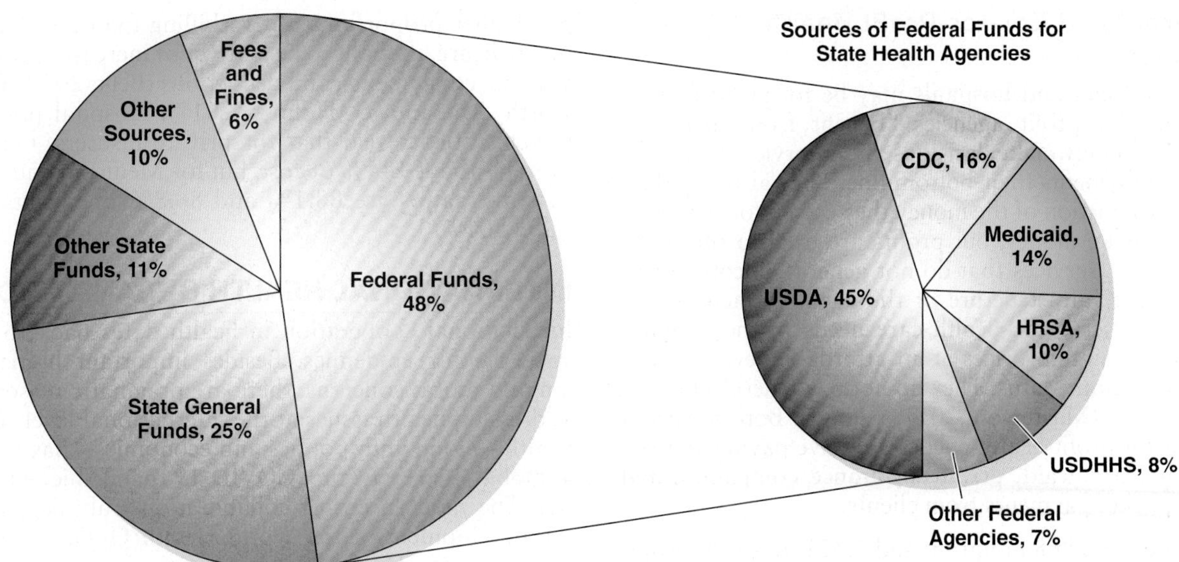

FIGURE 6-4 Funding sources for state health agencies. (Data from Association of State and Territorial Health Officials (ASTHO). (2017). *ASTHO profile of state public health: Volume four*. Retrieved from https://www.astho.org/Profile/Volume-Four/2016-ASTHO-Profile-of-State-and-Territorial-Public-Health/)

and cuts of almost $1 billion to the Health Resources and Services Administration were also included.

- There was also a 31% cut to the Environmental Protection Agency.
- These budget cuts, adding to reductions from prior years, were strongly opposed by public health organizations (APHA, 2019b).

Both ASTHO and NACCHO collect information on public health spending by state and LHDs. In 2015, federal dollars in state health agency budgets totaled $14.3 billion; the range of dollars per state was as small as $26 million and as high as $1.8 billion (ASTHO, 2017).

- About 80% of state health agencies derive 40% of their funding from federal sources. As of 2016, 56% of state health agencies were accredited.
- LHDs also receive federal funding, a portion of which are "pass through dollars," meaning the state receives the funding from the federal government but sends the money on to LHDs who provide the services.

Figure 6-4 shows the percent of state health agencies' budgets derived from state and federal sources.

- In 2015, over one third of state health agency grants, awards, and contracts were shared almost evenly between independent LHDs and community-based nonprofit agencies (ASTHO, 2017).
- In 2016, an average of 30% of LHD funding came from local taxes (NACCHO, 2017). Figure 6-5 highlights the sources of funding for LHDs.

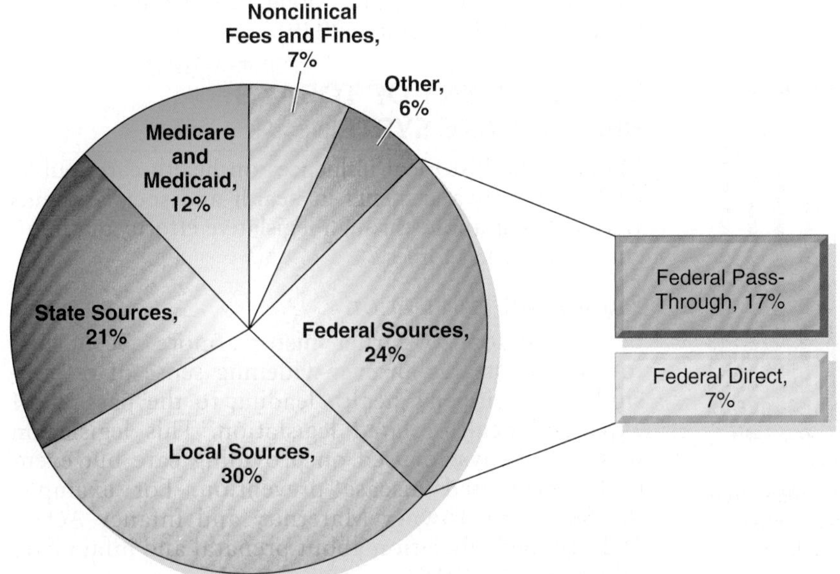

FIGURE 6-5 Funding sources for local health departments. (Data from National Association of County and City Health Officials (NACCHO). (2017). *2016 national profile of local health departments*. Retrieved from http://nacchoprofilestudy.org/wp-content/uploads/2017/10/ProfileReport_Aug2017_final.pdf)

For-Profit and Not-for-Profit Health Agencies

Health agencies and hospitals may be for-profit or not-for-profit. For-profit agencies "benefit from investors' money" and may make decisions about services offered in a way that benefits their bottom line. They also pay their investors a portion of the money they earn. Not-for-profit agencies make money, but profits are used to offset the cost of other services that do not generate income or to improve the infrastructure of the agency's facilities, as they must "serve the health care needs of the community" and maintain prices at an affordable level to keep tax their exempt status. They do not pay federal, state, or county taxes (Masterson, 2017, para. 7). Both for-profit and not-for-profit health agencies receive payments from Medicare, Medicaid, private insurance companies, and out-of-pocket payments from clients.

- There are 2,968 nonprofit and 1,322 for-profit hospitals in the United States (American Hospital Association, 2019). And, a recent study of hospital profitability found that 7 out of 10 of the most profitable U.S. hospitals were nonprofits, including Gundersen Lutheran Medical Center, Stanford Hospital and Clinics, and Louisville's Norton Hospital (Bai & Anderson, 2016).
- In a study of hospital profitability, Bai and Anderson (2016) found that 45% of hospitals were profitable, although the median hospital lost $82 per discharge.
- The top 10 hospitals earned over $163 million in total profits from patient care, and only 3 were for-profit. Nonprofits used their money to expand services, fund research, or build capital projects. Hospitals with the highest prices generally earned greater profits, making the case for a need to curb excessive fees (Belk, 2019).

Forty years ago, hospital payments were more closely aligned with billing. In 2015, U.S. hospitals billed "an average of 3 1/2 times what they received in payments" (Fig. 6-6), receiving <30% of billings on average (Belk, 2019, para. 1). Yet, profit margins over the past few years have averaged 8%. Private health insurance companies pay higher proportions of overbilling than do Medicaid or Medicare, thought to be a driver of increasing costs for policies, copayments, and deductions (Belk, 2019; Woodworth, Romano, & Holmes, 2017). Hospital payment-to-cost ratios reveal that for private insurers, hospitals average about 145% of cost, but for Medicaid and Medicare, the ratios are 88.1% and 86.8% of hospital cost (Gee, 2019).

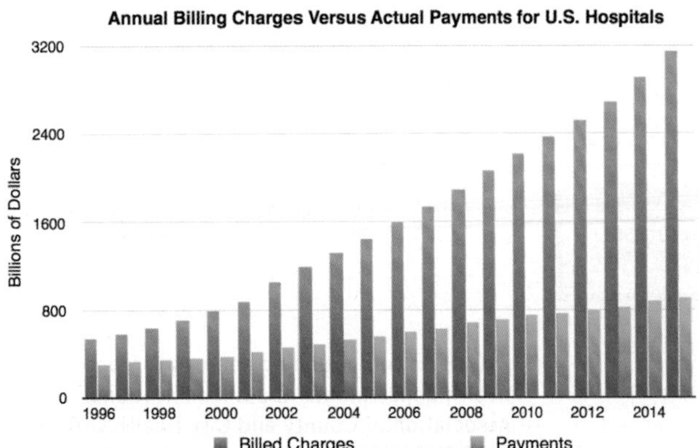

FIGURE 6-6 U.S. hospital overbilling, 1996 to 2014. (Reprinted with permission from Belk, D. (2019). *Hospital financial analysis: Print section. True Cost of Health-Care.* Retrieved from http://truecostofhealthcare.org/hospital_financial_analysis)

INTERNATIONAL HEALTH ORGANIZATIONS

International cooperation in health dates back to early concerns for epidemics. Besides important humanitarian and moral concerns, there are pragmatic reasons for addressing health issues at the international level. Today, health—along with politics and economics—has become a global issue, as the COVID-19 pandemic exemplifies. The modern era of collaboration truly began with the development of the World Health Organization, an agency of the United Nations. Formed in 1948, in the aftermath of World War II, the WHO currently has 194 member nations (WHO, 2020). International health agencies focus on issues of global concern, setting policy, developing standards, and monitoring health conditions and programs (see Chapter 16).

It may not seem possible that the health of a resident of a country 9,000 miles away can affect anyone in the United States or vice versa. However, the reality of international air travel means that illness in one part of the world can quickly move to another. Over one billion people traveled internationally during 2014, with 80 million international visitors to the United States in 2018, and travel/tourism accounted for 10.3% of global GDP in 2019 (World Travel & Tourism Council, 2020). Despite close scrutiny of airline passengers for passports, visas, customs regulations, weapons, drugs, and even symptoms such as cough and fever, how can anyone know if someone sitting next to them on a plane or in an airport is carrying a deadly, communicable disease on their journey? As described in Chapters 7 and 8, during early 2020, travelers did bring a novel coronavirus (COVID-19) to the United States and a pandemic ensued (CDC, 2020a; Gan, Xiong, & Mackintosh, 2020; Lovelace, 2020; Schuchat, 2020).

DEVELOPMENT OF TODAY'S HEALTH CARE SYSTEM

Many of the historical influences on health care, public health, and advancements in health and social systems were brought about through legislative efforts and influenced by market forces.

Significant Legislation

In comparison to earlier history, more recent history demonstrates an ever-widening sense of responsibility for citizen's health leading to the passage of expanded health-related legislation. This legislation was not always focused on providing care but eventually promoted disease prevention. For example, the Sheppard–Towner Maternity and Infancy Act in 1921 funded education about prenatal and infant care (Shi & Singh, 2019).

- During the Great Depression, the U.S. government enacted the first significant legislation that affected the health and well-being of a wide range of citizens, the Social Security Act of 1935 (Rosen, 2015; Social Security Administration, n.d.a).
  - This law ensured greater public health programs and provided retirement income to participating workers aged 65 years and older (SSA, n.d.a). The act included aid to dependent children, unemployment insurance, and supported educational programs similar to those in the Sheppard–Towner Act.
- Later legislation (e.g., Hill-Burton) provided federal support for expansion of hospitals; care for individuals with developmental delays; research and support for heart disease, cancer, and stroke; and training for health care personnel.
- The landmark Medicare and Medicaid legislation in 1965 moved the federal government deeper into the role of financing health care, especially for many older adults and people living in poverty, who, prior to this time, either could not get services or had to rely on charity care (CMS, 2019c).
- Health care legislation in the 1980s sought to contain health care spending, ensure the quality of health care, promote national health objectives, and facilitate data collection and research.
- President Bill Clinton made an unsuccessful attempt at universal health care during his first term in office. However, in 1997, the State Children's Health Insurance Program (SCHIP) was created to expand coverage to uninsured children at no or low cost, and this coverage was extended in 2009 under President Barak Obama (Brooks, 2018; CMS, n.d.a).
- The Medicare Modernization Act of 2003, signed into law by President George W. Bush, added prescription drug benefits and disease screening to Medicare and promoted health savings accounts.
- More recent laws have protected the confidentiality of health records and made it easier for workers to continue insurance coverage after being laid off. The ACA is the most recent legislation to impact health care financing in the United States (Knickman & Kovner, 2019), although efforts to repeal the act are ongoing as of 2020 (Frommer, 2018; Jost, 2019; Simmons-Duffin, 2019). (See http://thepoint.lww.com/Rector10e for a table of historical milestones.)

The ACA provided expanded health insurance for Americans, in an effort to bring the United States more in line with other high-income countries. See Chapter 13 for more information on legislation, policy, and advocacy.

Our Current Health Care System

Americans like to believe that ours is the best health care system in the world, but we have much to learn from other countries (Pross, Geissler, & Busse, 2017). Health care in the United States is very expensive.

- Health spending in 2018 was estimated at 17.7% of the U.S. gross domestic product (GDP)—the total amount of goods and services produced within a year (Centers for Medicare & Medicaid [CMS], 2019c). To put that in perspective, only 5.0% of GDP in 1960 was spent on health care (Catlin & Howard, 2015).
- CMS 2019b, (n.d.b) predicts that health care spending will grow 0.8% faster than the U.S. GDP and increase to 19.6% of U.S. GDP by 2027—meaning that almost one fifth of all goods and services produced in the United States will go toward health care.
- Total spending on health care services was $3.6 trillion in 2018 and is predicted to grow to more than $5 trillion in 2024. If viewed as a separate economy, the U.S. health care system would be the fifth largest economy in the world (CMS, 2019d, 2019f). The United States per person spending was $10,739 in 2017, about twice the average of comparable countries. This represented 17.1% of GDP, compared with an average of 10.6% in comparable countries (American Health Rankings, 2019).

Are we getting commensurate value in exchange for our expensive health care system? When overall U.S. health spending and outcomes are matched against comparable countries, the results are startling:

- The United States ranks 33rd out of 36 countries on infant mortality rates, with 5.9/1,000 live births compared to an average of 3.9 (America's Health Rankings, 2019).
- U.S. maternal death rate in 2015 was 26.4/100,000 live births, about 4 times the rates of 6.4 in Japan and 7.3 in Canada (Hoffer, 2019b).
- Average life expectancy in the United States is 78.6 years, compared to an average of 82.2 years, and this gap has been widening in recent years.
- Spurred by substance abuse and injuries, disease burden (a measurement of quality of life and longevity) is 31% higher in the United States, also demonstrating a widening gap.
- Rate of death responsive to health care is ranked on a scale from 0 to 100, and the United States falls behind at 88.7 compared to an average of 93.7.
- Preventable hospital admission rates are 143% higher for asthma, 55% higher for heart failure, and 38% higher for diabetes patients in the United States versus comparable countries (Kamal, Cox, McDermott, Ramirez, & Sawyer, 2019).
- In 2015, the United States had 7.9/1,000 practicing nurses versus a median of 9.9 when compared to other Organization for Economic Cooperation and Development (OECD) countries.
- The comparison for practicing physicians was 2.6 versus a median of 3.2 per 1,000 population (Anderson, Hussey, & Petrosyan, 2019).
- While high-quality new medications are often introduced in the United States, compared to four comparison countries, there is statistically significant evidence that "low-quality drugs diffuse more quickly" in the United States than those of higher quality (Kyle & Williams, 2017, p. 5).
- The United States ranks 11th out of 11 countries in health system effectiveness, a measure of access, equity, quality, efficiency, and healthy lives (Schneider, Sarnak, Squires, Shah, & Doty, 2017).

The U.S. health care system, in comparison to other countries, is often found lacking. In a study examining the quality of primary care coordination in 11 countries, the United States had the highest level of poor performance at 9.8% compared to the overall average of 5.2% (Penn, MacKinnon, Strakowski, Ying, & Doty, 2017).

The recent comprehensive evaluation of performance by Penn and colleagues (2017) examined five main indicators:

- Care process—including care coordination, preventive, and self-care, along with patient preference and engagement
- Access—encompassing promptness of care and affordability
- Administrative efficiency—effective use of time needed to complete administrative duties like processing insurance, prescriptions, mandated reports
- Equity—problems with care or prompt access related to lack of money/insurance, lack of providers
- Health care outcomes—measures of population health (e.g., life expectancy, infant mortality), mortality responsive to health care, health outcomes related to specific diseases (e.g., cancer survival rates, mortality 30 days after MI or stroke)

A Commonwealth Fund comparison of the United States and 10 other high-income countries (Box 6-2) noted that the United States ranked highest on health care spending (% of GDP) and last in overall performance, access, equity, and health outcomes (Schneider et al., 2017). This was also the case in an earlier study by the Commonwealth Fund in 2014. The United States was 10th in administrative efficiency and our highest ranking was 5th in care process (Fig. 6-7). You can examine the performance scores in more detail at https://interactives.commonwealthfund.org/2017/july/mirror-mirror/.

Out of 11 high-income countries in this analysis, only the United States is without universal health care. Even after increased access to care with the ACA, we remained last in access and equity. The highest-ranking countries overall were the United Kingdom, Australia, and The Netherlands.

- Statistical analysis of survey data comparing the United States with other high-income countries found that Americans are concerned about our current health care system, especially related to access to care and being able to receive preferred care. There are also profound concerns about health "insurance-related economic security" (Hero, Blendon, Zaslavsky, & Campbell, 2016, p. 507).
- A 2020 survey found that most Americans, regardless of their political views, want "substantial changes" to our health care system; goals include greater affordability, as well as coverage for preexisting conditions and long-term care (Public Agenda, 2020, para. 4).
  - Medicare for All, a public option plan, a market-based method, and a plan to give states wider health care responsibilities were offered as potential options; the market-based method and public option were the most widely accepted. Protection for those with preexisting conditions had the strongest support among all participants, despite political preference (Public Agenda, 2020).

Dissatisfaction with the U.S. health care system has resulted in various proposals for national health plans (e.g., universal coverage, Medicare for All) and closer examination of issues such as competition, managed care,

BOX 6-2 Comparison of Health Systems in the United Kingdom, Australia, and The Netherlands

United Kingdom

National Health Service (NHS) began in 1948, largely organized and care delivered by the national government, it is supported by taxes. Public hospitals and government staff employees are part of the NHS, but most primary care practices are independent and privately owned. Health care in the United Kingdom is more centrally managed, making accountability more governmentally driven than in the United States. About 10% of people purchase voluntary private health insurance, which excludes mental health, emergency care, and maternity care but does provide convenient and prompt access to care (Commonwealth Fund, n.d.; Schneider et al., 2017).

Australia

Medicare is the public insurance covering every citizen in Australia. It is paid for by taxes, and care is often available at private hospitals. About 50% of Australians also purchase private health insurance for access to care outside the Medicare system, but coverage is weighted higher among those with higher incomes. Coverage includes dental and vision care, along with other services. This system is similar to the U.S. Medicare system (Commonwealth Fund, n.d.; Schneider et al., 2017).

The Netherlands

Private health insurers cover the Dutch population. Funding is from payroll taxes and community-rated insurance premiums similar to the ACA insurance marketplaces. A standard benefit policy is available to everyone, with subsidies for low-income citizens, and those not enrolling in the plans being fined. The yearly deduction is around $500, and patients share some costs related to ambulance service and medical devices, for instance. Private providers are most common, and about 84% of people purchase additional voluntary insurance to cover dental, vision, and prescription drug copayments (Commonwealth Fund, n.d.; Schneider et al., 2017).

More comparisons of health care systems and statistics are available at https://international.commonwealthfund.org/countries/united_states/.

Source: Commonwealth Fund (n.d.); Schneider et al. (2017).

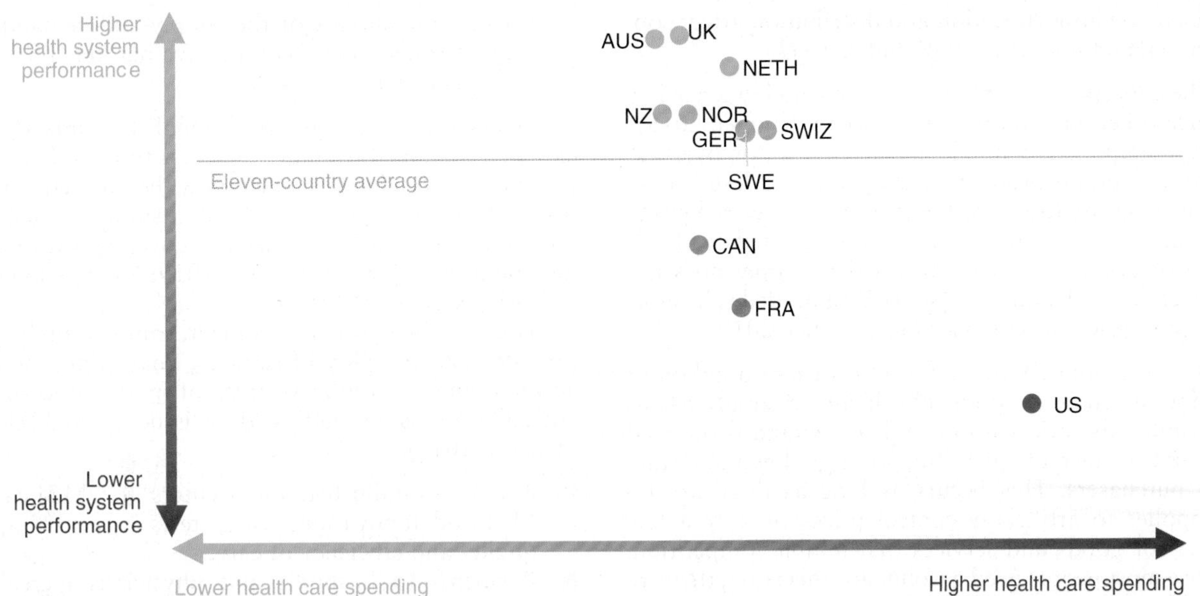

FIGURE 6-7 Health care system performance compared to spending, OECD countries. Note: Health care spending as a percent of GDP. Sources: Spending data are from OECD for the year 2014, and exclude spending on capital formation of health care providers; Commonwealth Fund analysis. (Reprinted with permission from Schneider, E. C., Sarnak, D. O., Squires, D., Shah, A., & Doty, M. M. (July, 2017). Mirror, mirror 2017: International comparison reflects flaws and opportunities for better U.S. health care. *Commonwealth Fund.* Retrieved from https://interactives.commonwealthfund.org/2017/july/mirror-mirror/assets/Schneider_mirror_mirror_2017.pdf (Exhibit 5).)

and health care rationing (Darvas, Moes, Myachenkova, & Pichler, 2018). To gain a deeper understanding, an examination of some basic economic concepts can provide a broader perspective on health care financing and issues with health care access and coverage.

THE ECONOMICS OF HEALTH CARE

- **Economics** is defined as the science of making decisions regarding scarce resources. It is concerned with the "production, distribution, and consumption of services" (Rambur, 2015, p. 8).

Economics permeates our social structure—it affects and is affected by policies. Consequently, health is closely tied to economic growth and development, in that a healthy population is necessary for adequate national productivity. A nation with a healthy population has better worker productivity; longer life expectancies provide an incentive for investment in education and innovation. These factors encourage income growth and higher GDP. For instance, an increased adult survival rate of 10% has been shown to increase labor productivity by over 9% (Bloom, Canning, Kotschy, Prettner, & Schunemann, 2018).

- Ample evidence exists for a **health–income gradient**, as personal income (specifically poverty) is linked to health status; people with lower incomes report poorer health and greater prevalence of diseases than those with higher incomes. They also live shorter lives (Urban Institute & Virginia Commonwealth University, 2015).
- Public health policies and programs that promote health and wellness can impact economic development by improving health outcomes, often on a more cost-effective basis than other interventions (APHA, 2020; Bloom et al., 2018).

Economic methods commonly employed by public health include analysis of (CDC, 2020b):

- Regulatory impact (How will this new law effect costs and behaviors?)
- Budget impact (How cost-effective is a new program or intervention?)
- Cost–benefit analysis (How much will a disease outbreak investigation cost, and how many lives will it benefit?)
- Decision modeling (How can mathematical models help determine cost-effectiveness of vaccine programs, pandemic spread, disease management, and injury prevention programs?)

Health economics can be better understood by examining the two basic theories underlying the science of economics: microeconomics and macroeconomics. In addition, concepts of health care payment must be understood.

Microeconomics

Microeconomic theory is concerned with supply and demand.

- Supply is the quantity of goods or services that providers are willing to sell at a particular price.
- Demand denotes the consumer's willingness to purchase goods or services at a specified price (Kramer, 2019).

In our free-market–driven economy, supply and demand is a key concept. Economists use **microeconomic theory** to study the supply of goods and services: how we, as consumers, allocate and distribute our resources, and how those marketing goods and services compete. They also examine how allocation and distribution affect consumer demand for these goods and services.

- The concepts of **supply and demand** are influenced by each other and, in turn, affect prices (Kramer, 2019).
- In a simplified example, an increase in, or oversupply of, certain products usually leads to less overall consumption (decreased demand) and lowered prices (Fig. 6-8). The opposite also is true. Limited availability of desired products means that supply does not meet demand, and when something needed is in short supply, prices usually increase (Kramer, 2019).

As an example, let's look at the price of a gallon of gasoline. When demand for oil is high and supply begins to dwindle, the prices go up. When demand drops and supplies become more plentiful, prices go down to attract more purchasers. This occurs as long as there are no monopolies to artificially control prices or only a few choices for goods and services that inhibit competition. Because most people need gasoline for their cars, they are more likely to continue to buy it even when the price is high. The same is true for health care.

- In health care economics, *demand-side policies* are enacted to reduce the demand for health care (e.g., raising insurance deductibles and copayments), and *supply-side policies* restrict the supply of resources (e.g., denial of coverage for specific services, utilization of preferred providers who practice within boundaries set by insurance companies, information overload for consumers) (Babaloa, 2017).
- Microeconomic theory is useful for understanding how prices are set and resources allocated. It comes into play when health care competition increases, because the success of the supply-and-demand concept depends upon a competitive market (Nicholson & Snyder, 2017).

Under the ACA, some traditional demand-side policies were removed to improve access to care. For example, preventive services must now be offered without deductibles or copayments, and insurance companies are limited in their ability to deny coverage for preexisting conditions (Healthcare.gov, 2019; Shaw, Asomugha, Conway, & Rein, 2014).

Issues such as cost containment, competition between providers, accessibility of services, quality, and need for accountability continue as areas of major concern. Several ACA provisions address these issues as well (Healthcare.gov, 2019):

- The law established the Centers for Medicare & Medicaid Innovation, which tests ways to improve quality and efficiency of care.
- Payments to hospitals and physicians increase or decrease based on the quality of care provided, and all hospitals must publicly report several indicators of quality.

Evaluation of how these provisions affect the supply and demand for health services is ongoing. Search for projects in your state at their Web site https://innovation.cms.gov.

Macroeconomics

Macroeconomic theory is concerned with the broad variables that affect the status of the economy as a whole, such as production, consumption, investment, international trade, inflation, recession, and unemployment on

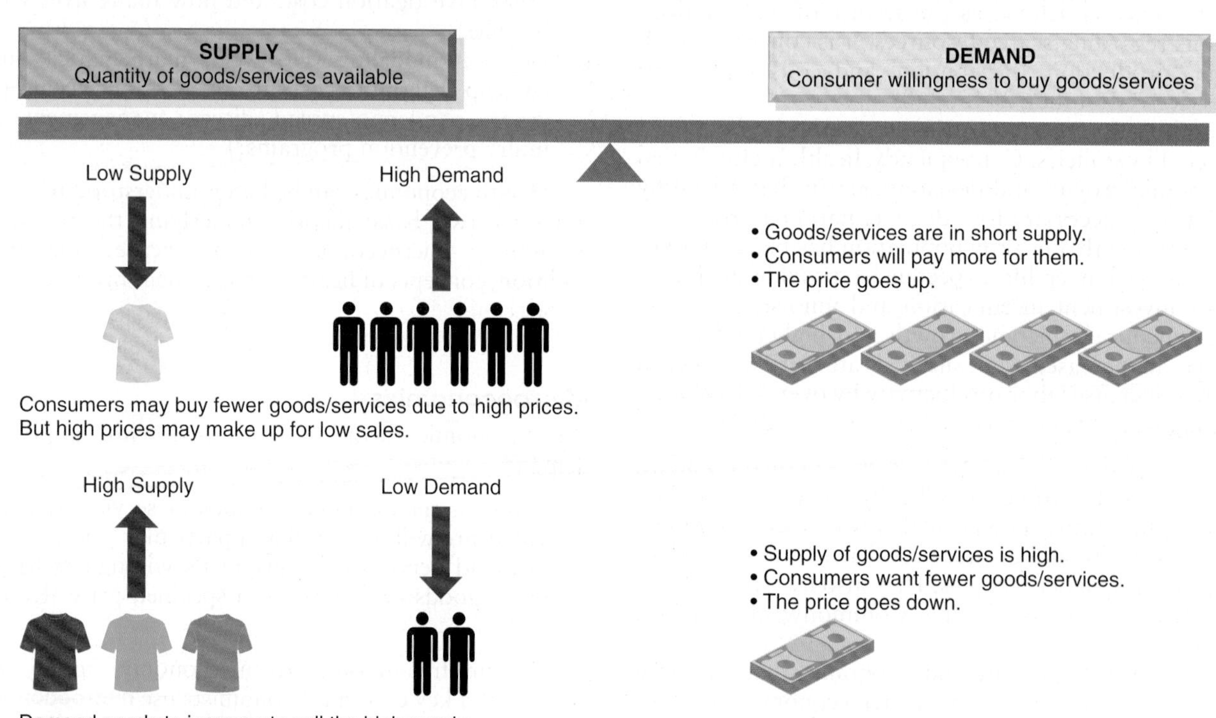

FIGURE 6-8 Supply and demand explained.

an aggregate level (Rice University, 2017). The focus is on the big picture, or larger view of economic stability and growth, and it is useful for providing a global or aggregate perspective of the variables affecting the total economic picture and subsequent economic policy development (Ross, 2018; Walsh, 2014).

The economics of health care encompasses both microeconomics and macroeconomics and an intricate and complex set of interacting variables. Health care economics is concerned with supply and demand, as well as the big picture: Are available resources sufficient to meet the demand by consumers and are the resources expended achieving the desired outcomes?

Supply and Demand in Health Care Economics

We have all learned first-hand about supply-and-demand economics. For instance, when you buy textbooks, you—as the purchaser—are able to determine the best value for your money (generally based on price, availability, and condition of the book) and you have choices of vendors (e.g., college bookstore, online bookseller, other students) and formats (e.g., print book, eBook). As a student, you know when you will need specific textbooks, but as a health care consumer, do you always know when you will need health care services? Is health care a competitive free market?

How does a patient determine what services are needed, where to buy them, and how to evaluate the quality of the goods and services? With health care, this is seldom the case; health care is typically unpredictable and often difficult to research (Hero et al., 2016). Even choosing a health insurance plan can be overwhelming considering the types of plans, the choices, the complexity, and one's level of health literacy (Taylor et al., 2016).

- With health insurance companies and managed care, different prices are often paid for the same service, and consumers have little information as to the costs. Hence, health care purchases are not easily understood.
- In a free-market system, competition is an important factor, but is competition truly possible with employer-based or government health insurance that limits the choice of plans and providers?

In 1963, economist Kenneth Arrow wrote an influential article about health care economics detailing the lack of information in the medical marketplace (reprinted as (Arrow, 2004). The main points of the article still apply; Arrow noted that risk and uncertainty prohibit a true market economy in health care because consumers:

- Do not know when or if they will become ill, but they know they will need and want medical treatment—thus the demand for health insurance.
- Do not know what services will be needed and what works best for their condition—thus the need for health care providers.
- Do not know about the quality of health care good and services—thus the need for government regulation (e.g., licensing, certification) and malpractice lawsuits.
- Are subject to an asymmetric level of information, compared to the insurer, about the likely demand for health care services. This can result in **adverse selection** (e.g., high-risk patients are denied insurance or care, smokers have higher health insurance premiums) and market failure (e.g., inefficiencies, lack of appropriate competition)—although this is less severe in large group insurance plans that spread out the risk (Mankiw, 2017).

Health care is an "opaque market" that keeps consumers in the dark about actual costs of services and medications due to confidential negotiations, discounts, and rebates (Walker, 2018, para. 3). For example, if you need an oil change for your car, the price is often clearly posted or advertised in advance, but are you aware of how much a chest x-ray or a vaccination will cost before you get one?

- Market consolidation (e.g., hospitals that monopolize a geographic area, buy up competitors) allows them to bargain for higher compensation from health insurance companies (Wolfe & Pope, 2020). A large study found that hospital billing for private insurance patients was 10.7% greater than those without coverage; Medicare patient billing was 8.9% higher (Woodworth et al., 2017).
- Consumers with health insurance are shielded from a typical business relationship with a provider or hospital. Costs have been the driver, not excess use of the health care system, and costs have risen faster than inflation since the mid-1960s.
- The multiple types of health insurance (variety of private companies and government plans like Medicare and Medicaid) in the United States lead to higher costs (Hoffer, 2019a).

For instance, the United States had the highest administrative costs when compared with seven peer countries; currently estimated costs are between 12% and 25% of national health care expenditures (Frakt, 2018; Hoffer, 2019a, 2019b).

- Health jobs grew faster than manufacturing jobs in 2008, and they surpassed retail sector jobs in 2017.
- Health care company revenues encompassed 16% of total revenues of firms on the S&P 500, increasing from just 4% in 1984.
- Since 1998, in an effort to sway policy decisions, twice as much money has been spent by health care companies on lobbying when compared to other businesses (Walker, 2018).

Waste is another factor in our high cost of health care. Cutler (2018, p. 494) estimated that as much as "one third of medical spending is wasteful," and 25% to 50% of our health care dollar "is not associated with improved health" outcomes. When interventions are not clinically sound, that wasteful spending makes it more difficult to sustain preventive measures.

As far as supply and demand are concerned, Indresano (2016) noted that these factors are at play:

- Higher demand due to an aging population. The number of people over 65 is roughly 52 million (with 85.6% having one or more chronic health conditions) and is projected to almost double by 2060.

- More people now have health insurance thanks to the ACA, estimated at about 20 million, and they have added to the demand.
- There is a projected physician shortage (about 90,000 doctors by 2025), just as demand for health care services skyrockets.
- Supply could be increased by hiring more nurse practitioners and increasing the number of medical residency slots available.
- Fully utilizing telemedicine would help extend care, especially into rural areas experiencing provider shortages (Mather, Scommegna, & Kilduff, 2019; National Center for Health Statistics, 2015).

Because traditional market forces of supply and demand work differently in health care, consumers are not solely responsible, as "government, insurers, employers, and providers themselves have a major role to play in controlling costs and ensuring access to care" (Meyer, 2016, para.15). Some governments and employers have taken action to control costs. Maryland's system of hospital rate setting is a broad-based approach to regulation, and Massachusetts has set spending growth targets on all health care spending, not just public plans. Target growth is in line with state GDP, and this program has helped them move from among the highest states in health care spending growth at the onset of the program in 2012 to one of the lowest states (Altman & Mechanic, 2018).

Consumers seek value and convenience in health care. An example of this is the case of urgent care clinics and retail clinics (Heath, 2017). These are now more prevalent than ever, with five times more retail clinics (i.e., low-cost, no appointment clinics in retail stores) in 2018 than in 2010. Younger people, generally in good health, are most often using them, even though 90% have health insurance and a **medical home** (coordinated care from a primary practice physician or nurse practitioner). The most common reasons for visits are minor illness or injury (40%) and vaccinations (30.9%). **High-deductible health plans** (deductible for individual $1,350 and family $2,700 or more) and convenience are drivers for this increased use; however, overutilization of retail clinics cancels out cost-savings and can boost health care costs (Bresnick, 2018; Heath, 2017).

There are, however, rare areas of health care where supply and demand works without any interference. These health care services are generally paid out-of-pocket, with direct interaction between the patient/consumer and the provider, as insurance does not cover them. Cosmetic procedures are a good example. Between 1998 and 2018, prices for overall U.S. medical care services increased by 109.8%, and costs for hospital and related services jumped 201.6%. Overall, consumer prices for health-related services increased 54%, following a steady pattern since 1998 of 3.8% per year for medical and 5.7% for hospital services, even though inflation averaged only 2.2% per year. Over almost 60 years, consumers actually paid fewer health-related costs out-of-pocket (47.6% in 1960 vs. 10.5% by 2017).

Elective cosmetic procedures are an area where prices are more transparent because costs are paid by the consumer and not usually by insurers. Therefore, consumers are cost conscious and providers operate in a competitive marketplace with more transparent pricing.

- Between 1998 and 2018, the average cost of 19 common cosmetic procedures and surgeries rose 34.3%, much less than the over 100% to 200% increases in medical and hospital services.
- Three of the most popular nonsurgical cosmetic procedures Botox injections, laser hair removal, and chemical peels actually dropped by 26.7%, 47.3%, and 15.6%, respectively (Perry, 2017).
- While elective procedures (e.g., cosmetic or LASIK surgery) demonstrate market influences, they are not typical of most health care expenditures. They also represent a select portion of the population—individuals who can afford them (Morelli, 2016).

Health Insurance Concepts

People are generally **risk averse**, meaning that they do not like uncertainty, and this is seen often in relation to health care. Conventional economic theories hold that people will pay small premiums monthly to offset the risk of large medical bills should they become seriously ill. This represents an *indemnity policy* (much like car or homeowners' insurance), and this was the type of health insurance first offered in the United States. In the past, patients could choose any doctor or hospital and submit the providers' bills to the insurance company for payment (Eeckhoudt, Fiori, & Gianin, 2018).

- **Moral hazard** is the term used by economists to explain how health insurance changes the behavior of people, resulting in more risk-taking and wasteful actions.
- They liken it to fire insurance without a deductible, noting that a person may be less careful about clearing brush from a house or may even resort to arson if it costs the owner nothing to have the home replaced.
- If a person has health insurance, many economists hypothesize, they are less likely to take good care of themselves, and if they do not pay for their health care (through premiums, copayments, and deductibles), they are more likely to overuse it, although empirical evidence of this is sparse (Nickitas, Middaugh, & Feeg, 2020).
- In other words, economists theorize that insurance has a paradoxical effect and may lead to wasteful or risk-taking behaviors. In this scenario, patients will demand expensive health care, even if it provides only the smallest benefit. The concept of moral hazard is a driver for larger deductibles and copayments; these are used to control waste and overuse.

A more recent viewpoint notes that consumers purchase health insurance not to avoid risk but to earn a claim for additional income (i.e., insurance paying for medical care) when they become ill and that copayments and managed care actually work against the system by reducing the amount of income transferred to ill persons or limiting their access to needed services. Think about what would happen if you or your loved one were to suddenly need an expensive heart surgery or lengthy cancer treatment—without health insurance. You would want health insurance to protect against this possibility—to be able to pay medical bills without losing your assets (e.g., home, car).

- For instance, Rose-Jacobs et al. (2019) found that families of children with special health care needs who were without government-sponsored insurance had significantly greater odds of missing rent or mortgage payments, moving frequently, and homelessness than did similar families who had this insurance.
- Families may face a genuine risk of financial disaster when confronted with a serious medical emergency or long-term illness, and this is why some economists argue that a focus on moral hazard in the health insurance industry is too limiting. Some suggest that it is also important to examine provider actions in forecasting health care costs (Einav & Finkelstein, 2018).

Moral hazard alone doesn't easily apply to health insurance because its effects may not be as predictable as in other instances of indemnity. Individuals who gain access to health insurance will use it, but there are still constraints (e.g., high deductibles, high copays) that moderate use and can be harmful to families who may have to choose between care for a sick child and rent or food (Einav & Finkelstein, 2018). The case can surely be made that even those with unlimited insurance coverage don't just "check into the hospital because it's free" as noted in a classic article by Gladwell (2005, para. 11). For example, most people do not seek infinite numbers of colonoscopies, root canals, or other invasive procedures or surgeries just because they are well insured.

- Adverse selection, however, is a concern for health insurance companies when sick individuals seek insurance because they have an urgent need for health care, while healthy people do not want to buy it because they have no pressing health concerns (Smith & Yip, 2016).
- This imbalance is not cost-effective, yet a key feature of the ACA is for insurers to provide coverage for people with preexisting conditions (without charging them outrageous prices), which was formerly a common practice. This was initially balanced out by requiring that everyone get insurance (Center on Budget & Policy Priorities, 2020a).

Cost sharing, which includes copayments and deductibles, divides the cost of health care services between insurance companies and patients. Insurance companies use cost sharing to prevent overuse of health services. The amount of a copayment or deductible may change for some types of care, such as a visit to the ED.

- In a systematic review of current "methodologically rigorous studies," Argawal, Mazurenko, and Menachemi (2017, p. 1762) found that newer **high-deductible health plans (HDHPs)** not only reduced costs but also led to a reduction in office visits and preventive care. The majority of studies reflected a decline in the use of preventive health care and medication compliance.
- A large study covering 42 states and the District of Columbia found that underinsured and uninsured adult women were significantly less likely to receive recommended screenings for colorectal, cervical, and breast cancer compared with those having adequate health insurance coverage (Zhao, Okoro, Li, & Town, 2018). Generally, the earlier a health problem is found, the less expensive the treatment and the better the patient outcomes.

Balancing the cost reduction against the lack of preventive care (that could eventually lead to more cost savings) is an important consideration. Also, the effect of cost sharing on use of services is not equal. Individuals with low incomes decrease their use of medications and services more than those with higher incomes. The ACA limited cost sharing for people with low or moderate incomes, in plans offered by employers and plans purchased through the marketplace (Healthcare.gov, 2019).

For some people, the cost-sharing component of their health insurance is so high that they are considered underinsured. To be **underinsured**, one must have a deductible that is 5% of income or out-of-pocket costs in excess of 10% of income (not including premium costs). Individuals and families often exhaust their savings, run up credit card debt, or else delay necessary medical care to avoid going into debt (Collins, Rasmussen, Beutel, & Doty, 2015). The numbers are rising:

- In 2018, 29% of American adults who reported having health insurance for the entire year were considered underinsured, compared to 23% in 2014 (Commonwealth Fund, 2019).
  - Of that group, 28% had employer-sponsored health insurance, up from 20% in 2014. But, 42% of those with individually purchased insurance were most likely to be inadequately covered.
  - Delayed care (41%) and problems paying medical bills (47%) were more common among underinsured than the insured population (23%, 25%).
  - A 2018 survey revealed that 55% of adults with employer-based health insurance reported being very confident that they could afford health care based on their coverage, while only 31% with individual market policies were very confident (Collins, Gunja, Doty, & Bhupal, 2018).

Employer-Sponsored Health Insurance

Employer-sponsored health insurance is the leading source of coverage for nonelderly U.S. citizens. A total of 49% of Americans had this type of insurance in 2017. Medicare, Medicaid, and other government plans provided coverage to 36%, while 7% purchased policies directly from insurers (Kaiser Family Foundation [KFF], 2019c).

The flaws in this system were blatantly exposed during the COVID-19 pandemic, as millions of Americans filed for unemployment when businesses shutdown, causing them to lose access to health care (Brown & Nanni, 2020). One example of the trickle-down effects of unemployment is the loss of reproductive health care for millions of women (Sonfield, Frost, Dawson, & Lindberg, 2020). About 56% of total jobs lost early on during the pandemic were among women, often those working in retail, education, and restaurant jobs. Black, Latina, and women with disabilities had the highest rates of unemployment. It is estimated that 40% of people losing employer-sponsored health insurance "will remain uninsured"; states without Medicaid expansion will be even harder hit (Sonfield et al., 2020, para. 6). Loss of access to contraceptive and preventive women's health care will place greater demands on publicly funded clinics that are continually underfunded and result in unplanned pregnancies or late diagnoses of cervical cancers and other health conditions.

How did the United States end up with this system of health insurance? Historically, employers became the leading source of coverage because of three policy decisions in the 1940s and 1950s.

1. During World War II, wage controls did not apply to health insurance, so employers used health insurance to lure workers from their competitors during wage freezes.
2. The U.S. government determined that health insurance could be part of collective bargaining.
3. In 1954, the IRS exempted health insurance premiums paid by employers from federal income tax (Rook, 2015).

A 2019 annual survey revealed that 57% of all U.S. employers offered health insurance to their workers and 99% of large companies offered coverage (KFF, 2019b). Small businesses may not offer employee health insurance because of the high cost and fewer employees (Fig. 6-9).

- The average annual costs for employees in 2019 were $7,188 for individual and $20,576 for family health insurance coverage (Fig. 6-10). This represents 4% and 5% increases, respectively, over 2018; however, family premiums are 22% higher than 5 years ago and 54% higher than 10 years ago. Wages increased only 1.4% above inflation from 2018 to 2019 (KFF, 2019b).
- Keep in mind that the median U.S. income in 2019 was just over $63,179; the employee cost for a family policy would represent almost one third of that year's wages (Rothbaum & Edwards, 2019).

The percent of employers offering health insurance decreased somewhat after the ACA went into effect but increased in 2017; the first time an increase was noted since 2008 (Joszt, 2018). However, employers are continuing to pass along some of the higher costs of health insurance to employees in the form of higher employee premiums, deductibles, copayments, and stricter enrollment requirements.

- The number of workers with insurance that includes an annual deductible has increased from 55% in 2006 and 70% in 2010 to 81% in 2015.
- Similarly, the percentage of covered workers enrolled in employer health plans with a deductible of $1,000 or more for single coverage increased from 10% in 2006 and 27% in 2010 to 46% in 2015 (KFF, 2019c).

Those people whose employers do not offer health insurance coverage or who are self-employed can purchase nongroup health insurance. However, premiums are greater than the worker's share of employer group coverage. The ACA has made purchasing a nongroup policy easier and subsidizes the premiums for eligible people. Even in states that did not expand Medicaid, a greater number of people with lower incomes purchased insurance on the federal marketplace (Blumenthal & Abrams, 2020; Sommers, Blendon, & Orav, 2016). Problematic changes in affordability and availability of ACA health plans, resulting in "churning and switching among enrollees," have been noted (McKillop et al., 2018, para. 4). Variation in costs has not been eliminated with the ACA's community rating, but the variation is geographical; specifically, costs vary by location, not within one location (Fehr & Cox, 2020; Gabel et al., 2016; Healthcare.gov, n.d.a).

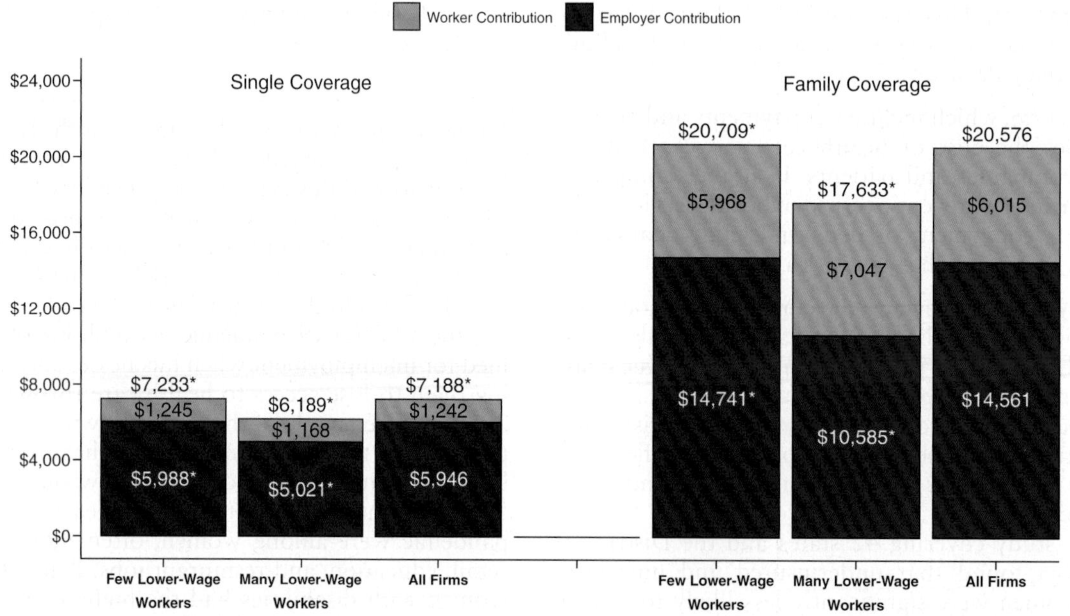

FIGURE 6-9 Average annual worker and employer contributions to premiums and total premiums for single and family coverage, by firm wage level, 2019. *Estimate is statistically different between All Small Firms and All Large Firms estimate ($p < .05$). (Reprinted with permission from Kaiser Family Foundation. (2019). *Employer health benefits 2019 annual survey*. Retrieved from http://files.kff.org/attachment/Report-Employer-Health-Benefits-Annual-Survey-2019)

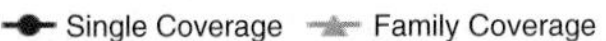

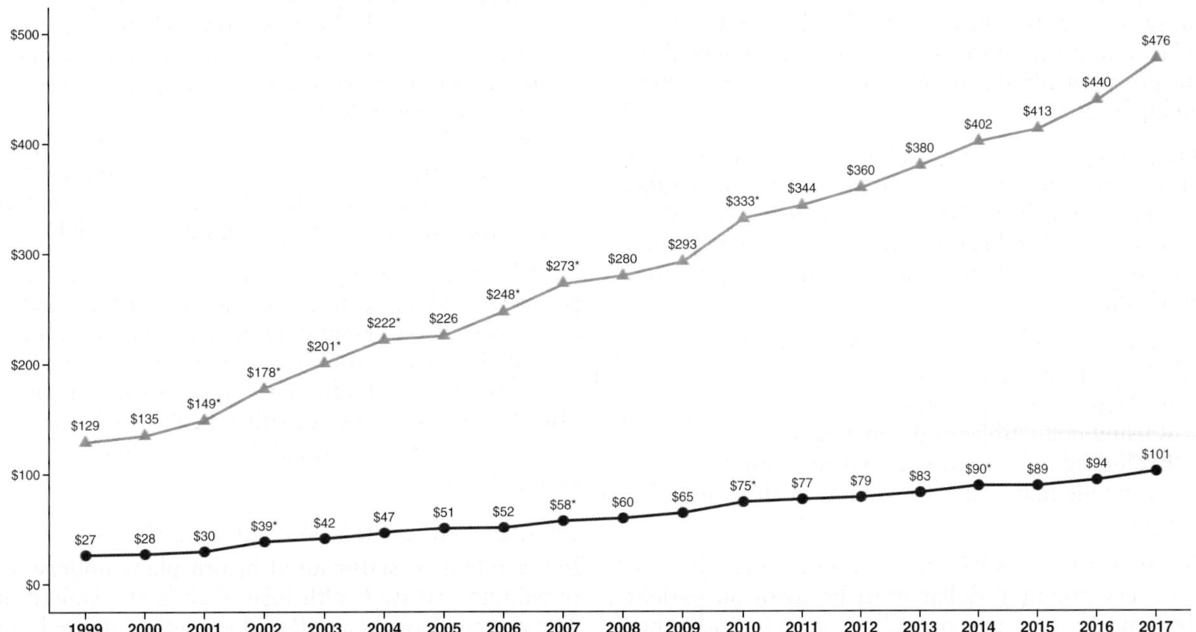

FIGURE 6-10 Average Worker Premium Contributions Paid by Covered Workers for Single and Family Coverage, 1999–2017. *Estimate is statistically different from estimate from the previous year (p <.05). (Reprinted with permission from Kaiser Family Foundation and Health Research & Educational Trust. (2017). *Employer health benefits: 2017 annual survey*. Retrieved from http://files.kff.org/attachment/Report-Employer-Health-Benefits-Annual-Survey-2017)

- For persons earning incomes "at or below 400% of the federal poverty level" ($103,000 per year for a family of four), premium subsidies are provided for those purchasing on the insurance "marketplaces." This keeps buyers from spending more than a "fixed percentage" of income (2.06% at the lowest level and 9.78% at the highest level) on health care premiums (Blumenthal, Collins, & Fowler, 2020, p. 964).
- Some "cost-sharing assistance" is available to subsidize private insurers, although it is only for those at lower income levels (100% to 250% of the federal poverty level, or $25,750 to $64,375).
- It is expected that about 94% of potential costs for a "moderately generous" plan will be covered for those receiving this benefit (Blumenthal et al., 2020, p. 964).

A study of coverage gains, from 2014 to 2015, found that about 40% was because of premium subsidies, and 60% was due to enrollment in Medicaid (Frean, Gruber, & Sommers, 2017).

- The cost of health insurance is a deterrent for many people. "In 2018, 45% of uninsured adults" stated that insurance costs were too high and that this was the reason they remained without it (Tolbert, Orgera, Singer, & Damico, 2019, para. 4).
- Prior to the ACA, only 4% to 11% of those at the lower-income levels purchased nongroup health coverage (Bernard, Banthin, & Encinosa, 2009). Although coverage levels generally increase as income rises, only 25% of those earning 10 times the poverty level purchased health insurance.

SOURCES OF HEALTH CARE FINANCING: PUBLIC AND PRIVATE

Financing of health care significantly affects community/public health nursing practice. It influences the type and quality of services offered, as well as the ways in which those services are used. Sources of payment may be grouped into three categories: third-party payments, direct consumer payment, and private or philanthropic support.

Third-Party Payments

Third-party payments are monetary reimbursements made to providers of health care by someone other than the consumer who received the care. The organizations that administer these funds are called *third-party payers* because they are a third party, or external, to the consumer–provider relationship. Included in this category are four types of payment sources: private insurance companies, independent or self-insured health plans, government health programs, and claims payment agents (California Department of Insurance, n.d.).

Private Insurance Companies

Payments from private companies make up approximately 34% of total health care spending (CMS, n.d.b). They market and underwrite policies aimed at decreasing consumer risk of economic loss because of a need to use health services.

- There are three types of private insurers—commercial stock companies that maintain profit margins for stockholders (e.g., Anthem, Cigna), mutual companies owned by policyholders (e.g., MassMutual), and nonprofit plans (e.g., American Postal Workers Union) that must be approved by states (Miller, 2018).

- Today, about one third of Americans are covered by a health plan offered by the Blues (Blue Cross Blue Shield, 2019).

Maintaining profits for stockholders means that insurance companies must control the *medical loss ratio* or the money paid for health services. If they can reduce the amount paid for health care services, then profits increase, and the stock is more attractive to potential buyers (CMS, 2018b).

- Four common ways to reduce the medical loss ratio include the following:
  - Reducing covered services
  - Raising deductibles and copayments
  - Excluding people with preexisting conditions
  - Targeting marketing to young, healthy populations

The ACA has an 80/20 rule requiring that at least 80% of every premium dollar must be spent on patient care, leaving 20% to pay for administrative and other costs of business. It was designed to protect both consumers and insurers (CMS, 2018b; Day, Himmelstein, Broder, & Woolhandler, 2015; Hall & McCue, 2019; Healthcare.gov, n.d.b).

- Previously, insurers also resorted to *rescission of coverage*—or canceling coverage for failure to disclose a preexisting condition (often unrelated to the person's current health care problem) or some other means of disqualifying coverage after large medical claims have been filed (Healthcare.gov, n.d.c). However, the ACA made this practice illegal, except in cases of consumer misrepresentation or fraud.
- A more recent trend in private insurance is the move to **high-deductible health plans with a savings option (HDHP/SOs)** such as **health savings accounts (HSAs)**—created and paid for by employees, or **health reimbursement accounts (HRAs)**—established and funded by employers (U.S. Office of Personnel Management [USOPM], n.d.b). About 28% of employers offered this type of plan (KFF, 2019f).
- Six times more common than HRAs, HSAs tied to HDHPs can be rolled over yearly and move with the employee. The high deductibles (minimum of $1,400 for an individual and $2,800 for a family) allow for lower premiums, but the attendant HSAs can only be used on medical expenses—nothing else—or tax-exempt status may be forfeited, and a penalty is incurred (KFF, 2019f; National Conference of State Legislation [NCSL], 2020).
- HRA funds are controlled by the employer and as the employee turns in medical bills; funds are released for payment. Generally, remaining HRA funds carry over to the following year but do not go with the employee when they leave the company (KFF, 2018a).
- Most plans require employees to pay coinsurance, a percentage of their total health costs (often 20% of charges)—rather than a fixed copayment per office visit or prescription as in many other plans.
- Most workers with employer-sponsored health insurance also have prescription drug coverage (more than 99%) with the most comprehensive health plan offered, and 83% of those covered have a plan with three or more tiers of cost sharing, such as copayment or coinsurance (KFF, 2018a).
  - For instance, the average prescription copayment with tier one medications is $11, and for the second tier, it is $31.Only about 3% of employers offer no cost sharing after deductible (KFF, 2018a).

While these copayments are used by insurance companies to reduce their costs, they can affect medication adherence. A systematic review of the literature concluded that lower (or no) copayments for medications not only improved adherence and patient outcomes but also decreased the use of other health care services and associated costs (Gourzoulidis et al., 2017; Kesselheim et al., 2015).

Independent or Self-insured Health Plans

Independent or self-insured health plans underwrite the remaining private health insurance in the United States. These plans have been offered through a limited number of organizations, such as large businesses, unions, school districts, consumer cooperatives, and medical groups. Employers with self-insured plans take on all or a major part of the risk for health care costs of their employees. These plans may be self-administered or utilize third-party claims administrators. Minimum premium plans are another form of self-insurance for which employers pay medical costs up to an agreed-upon limit, and insurers assume responsibility for the excess claims (Bureau of Labor Statistics, n.d.).

- About 61% of employees receiving employer health insurance benefits were covered in full or partly by self-insured plans in 2018 (remained the same in 2019), up from 51% in 1999. Employees of large firms are more likely to have self-funded plans than small firms (81% vs. 13%).
- Only 18% of large firms offering employee health benefits extend that benefit to retirees, significantly smaller than the 66% in 1988 or 34% in 2006 (KFF, 2018a, 2019b).

Government Health Programs

Government health programs make up the "largest single payer of health care in the United States" (Troy, 2015, p. 1).

- Federal sources comprised 28.3% of total payments from all sources in 2018. Spending for Medicaid rose by 3%, and growth in Medicare was 6.4% (CMS, 2020b).
- The U.S. government's four major health insurance programs are Medicare, Medicaid, the Federal Employees Health Benefits Plan, and the Civilian Health and Medical Program of the Uniformed Services.
- The VA (Veterans Administration) system is also part of the federal government, as are a few other specialized programs like Indian Health Services. The largest programs are Medicare and Medicaid.

Medicare. Medicare, known as Title XVIII of the Social Security Act Amendments of 1965, has provided mandatory federal health insurance since July 1, 1966, for adults aged 65 years and older who have paid into the Social Security system (CMS, 2019a). It also covers certain people with disabilities (regardless of age). Medicare is administered by the Centers for Medicare & Medicaid Services (CMS) of the USDHHS.

- In July 2019, Medicare covered more than 60.8 million people, the majority being aged 65 years or older (52.2 million), and paid health care costs of $618.7 billion (CMS, 2019e, f).
- In 2018, 21% of total federal spending was for Medicare ($750.2 billion), and it is expected to increase 7.6% per year between 2019 and 2028 (CMS, 2020b).
- Financing of Medicare is through general tax revenues (43%), payroll taxes (36%), premiums from beneficiaries (15%), and other sources (KFF, 2019a).
- Out-of-pocket spending for Medicare beneficiaries was $5,460 in 2016, almost equally divided between medical/long-term care and premiums (CMS, 2017; Cubanski, Neuman, & Freed, 2019).
- Individuals with multiple chronic diseases and poor health spent more than their healthier counterparts (Cubanski, Koma, Damico, & Neuman, 2019).

About 85% of beneficiaries were over the age of 65; the remaining beneficiaries qualified for Medicare 24 months after they became eligible for Social Security Disability Insurance (SSDI). These recipients are younger than age 65 and permanently disabled or chronically ill, including those with end-stage renal disease.

In 2017, almost 51 million Americans were aged 65 and older; by 2060, that number is expected to almost double, at 94.7 million (Administration for Community Living, 2018).

- Although there are financial challenges facing Medicare and Social Security, both program trust funds have sufficient resources to pay full costs and benefits, without any adjustments, through 2035. The disability insurance trust fund will be intact till 2052. Reforms enacted with the ACA, and other actions, extended the life of these trust funds (Zallman et al., 2016).
- Even after those funds have been spent, both programs can continue to pay 75% to about 90% of benefits using only their yearly tax revenues (Broaddus & Aron-Dine, 2019).

There are four parts to Medicare (Fig. 6-11):

Part A of Medicare, the hospital insurance program, covers inpatient hospitals, limited-skilled nursing facilities, home health, and hospice services to participants eligible for Social Security Disability Income (Medicare.gov, n.d.a).

- The 2020 deductible per benefit period for inpatient hospitalization, including inpatient mental health, is $1,408.
- Patients in a skilled nursing facility pay $176 per day after day 20 and assume all costs if care is needed longer than 100 days (Medicare.gov, n.d.c).

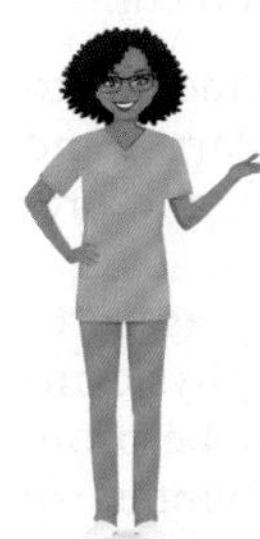
Medicare Made Simple
Provides **mandatory** federal health insurance for adults **age 65** years and older and people with **disabilities**.
Covers more than **60.8 million** people and pays health care costs of **$618.7 billion.**
About **15%** of the US population are age 65 and older; by 2060, that number is expected to **double**, increasing the need for Medicare.
What Medicare Covers...

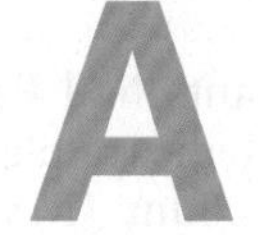
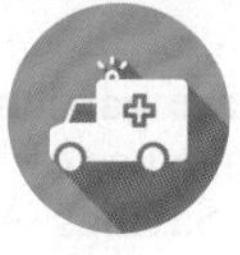
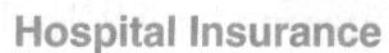
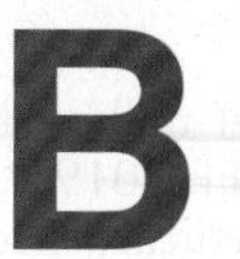
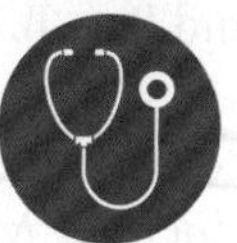

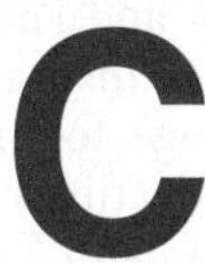

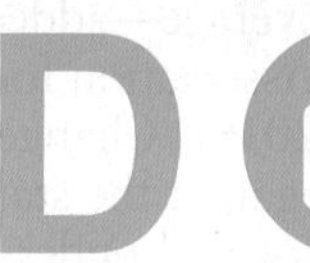
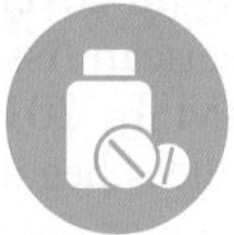
Medicare Advantage
• Deductible: depends on plan, averaging $468/year
• Private plan
• Replaces Medicare A and B
• Regional provider networks
• May cover dental, vision, and prescriptions
Drug Plan
• Monthly premium: $76.40 or less
• Prescription drugs
• Voluntary plan

FIGURE 6-11 Medicare coverage: Parts A to D. Figure concept by Claire Lindstrom; used with permission. (Data from www.medicare.gov (2020).)

- Information on hospice and home health can be found at https://www.medicare.gov/your-medicare-costs/medicare-costs-at-a-glance.

Part B of Medicare, the supplementary and voluntary medical insurance program, primarily covers necessary services to diagnosis or treat health issues and preventive services such as influenza vaccines (Medicare.gov, n.d.a).

- The 2020 annual deductible is $197, and recipients pay 20% of services once the deductible is met. No out-of-pocket charges are applied for annual wellness visits or preventive services that are rated "A" or "B" by the U.S. Preventive Services Task Force (USPSTF).
- Monthly premiums vary depending on yearly income ranging from $144.60 to $491.60 (Medicare.gov, n.d.c).

Part C Medicare plans, also called Medicare Advantage, are private plans subsidized by the federal government.

- Medicare Advantage plans are not supplemental to Part A and Part B—they take the place of Part A and Part B. Some may also cover vision, dental, and prescriptions (National Council on Aging, n.d.).
- Unlike traditional Medicare, Part C plans use provider networks, which limit the choice of physicians or hospitals. They are regional, which may be problematic for seniors who want to spend winters in Florida and summers in Montana, for instance.

Seniors can change their Part C plan during open enrollment periods or revert to traditional Medicare Part A and Part B.

- In 2018, 24 million Medicare participants had Part C plans (KFF, 2019a). Other types of Medicare plans include Medicare Medical Savings Account (MSA) plans, Medicare cost plans, Programs of All-Inclusive Care for the Elderly (PACE), and Medication Therapy Management (MTM) program; these are not available in all areas.

In 2018, over 14 million Medicare beneficiaries had supplemental coverage through a private company or employer retiree health insurance plans—known as *Medigap* coverage—added to Medicare Part A and Part B (American Association for Medicare Supplement Insurance [AAMSI], 2019). Changes in Medigap coverage for new enrollees began at the start of 2020. Part B deductibles are no longer covered under Medigap and Plans C and F are not allowed. However, these changes do not affect those enrolled prior to January 1, 2020 (Medicare.gov, n.d.g).

- People with Medigap coverage through their employers' retiree health plan generally pay lower premiums than people with coverage through a private company.
- With rising costs of health care coverage, companies are increasing premium costs for retirees, offering new options, such as Medicare Advantage to replace traditional health plans, or paying only a set amount for health coverage and leaving retirees to purchase their own insurance (AAMSI, 2020).

Part D is a volunteer prescription drug plan for those on Medicare or Medicare Advantage. The member can sign up for a Medicare Part D plan or an Advantage plan with medication coverage (KFF, 2019a: Medicare.gov n.d.b). Costs vary based on state of residence. Plans differ in coverage, so clients should be encouraged to research the plans to determine if their medications are included in the plan's formulary. See Box 6-3.

BOX 6-3 Deductibles, Copays, and the Donut Hole

Deductible Phase

- While plans vary, most have an annual deductible that must be met before the prescription drug plan takes effect. Medicare caps the deductible at $435, and some plans do not have a deductible (Medicare.gov, n.d.g; Social Security Administration [SAS], 2019).

Initial Coverage Phase

- When the deductible is met, members are responsible to pay a copayment (a set amount) or coinsurance (a percent of the price of the medication), with Medicare covering the rest of the cost (Medicare.gov, n.d.h; SSA, 2019).
- The monthly premium depends on the type of plan chosen and the income of an individual or family. Individuals may pay nothing over their plan premium up to a monthly fee of $76.40 plus plan premium. Costs vary based on state of residence as well (Medicare.gov, n.d.f).

Donut Hole

- The Bipartisan Budget Act of 2018 limits what members pay. Members pay no more than 25% of the brand name or generic cost, and the manufacturer pays 95% of the cost. When the combined paid amount is $4,020 out-of-pocket, the catastrophic coverage phase begins. Items that are included in the coverage gap are the deductibles, copayments and coinsurance, and what is paid in the gap (Medicare.gov, n.d.c; MedicareAdvantage.com, 2020; SSA, 2019).

Catastrophic Coverage Phase

- Between the initial coverage and the coverage gap, a total of $6,350 has been paid, at which time the member is only responsible for a small copay or coinsurance (Medicare.gov, n.d.d; SSA, 2019).

Source: Medicare.gov (n.d.c, n.d.d, n.d.e, n.d.f, n.d.g, n.d.h); Medicare Advantage.com (2020); SSA (2019).

Supplemental security income and social security disability insurance. Supplemental Security Income (SSI) and SSDI are federally funded programs to assist seniors and/or those with disabilities that have financial needs. Seniors and individuals with disabilities, regardless of age, with limited incomes can receive SSI. SSDI, however, is only available for those with disabilities that "have a qualifying work history" (Bauer, 2017, para. 3; SSA, 2019, 2020). Eligibility for health care benefits differs between the two programs as well (Fig. 6-12).

- Medicaid benefits are immediate for SSI recipients, whereas most individuals receiving SSDI can qualify for Medicare after 24 months (Bauer, 2017).
- To be eligible for SSI, an individual's income must be <$1,260 a month. In 2020, the highest amount individual SSI recipients receive is $783 a month (Social Security Administration, n.d.b).
- However, SSDI assistance is not based on income or severity of disability. Rather, the monthly amount is based on the person's income prior to the disability. The average monthly income from SSDI is $800 to $1,800 and a maximum monthly payment of $3,011 (Laurence, 2019).

Medicaid. Medicaid, known as Title XIX of the Social Security Amendments Act of 1965, provides medical assistance for children, pregnant women, parents with dependent children, seniors, and people with severe disabilities (Medicaid.gov, 2020).

Understanding SSI and SSDI

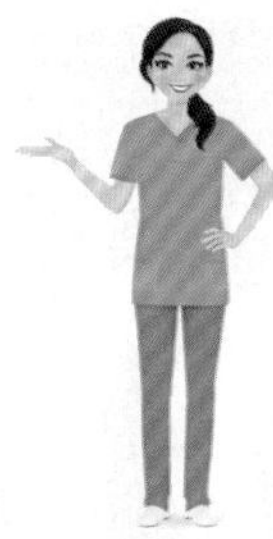

Social Security Income (SSI) and Social Security Disability Insurance (SSDI) are **federal programs to aid individuals with disabilities.**

What SSI and SSDI Cover...

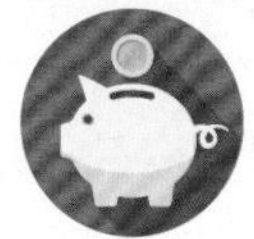

Supplemental Insurance Income (SSI)

- Supplemental income for disabled, blind, and aged with minimal or no income
- Receive immediate Medicaid benefits (Medicare after age 65)
- May qualify if individual monthly income is < $1,260
- Highest monthly SSI payment: $783

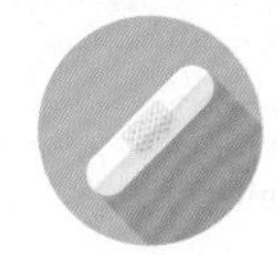

Social Security Disability Insurance (SSDI)

- Those under age 65 with sufficient work history and an eligible disability
- Can apply for Medicare after 24-month waiting period
- Monthly payment based on pre-disability income
- Average monthly payment: $800-$1,800; maximum payment: $3,011

FIGURE 6-12 Supplemental Security Income and Social Security Disability Insurance coverage. Figure concept by Claire Lindstrom; used with permission. (Data from www.ncoa.org (2017); www.disabilitysecrets.com (2019); https://www.ssa.gov/redbook/eng/overview-disability.htm (2020). For additional information and updates, see https://www.ssa.gov/benefits/disability/)

- About one in five Americans are covered by Medicaid (Rudowitz, Garfield, & Hinton, 2019). Medicaid is an optional program for states, but all states currently participate.
- Over time, the scope of Medicaid increased, and states opting to provide Medicaid were required to implement each increase—or lose their federal Medicaid funding (Cubanski et al., 2015).
- Medicaid covered over 70 million people in January 2020 (Medicaid.gov, 2020). Between October 1, 2017, and September 30, 2018, Medicaid spending was over $592 billion (KFF, 2018b).
- As the importance of social determinants of health gains wider acceptance, more states are requiring Medicaid managed care organizations (MCOs) to screen for determinants and provide social services, such as housing and nutrition assistance (Hinton, Rudowitz, Diaz, & Singer, 2019).
- Because Medicaid covers so many people, many of whom have complex health needs, it represents a significant proportion of health care spending in the United States (Rudowitz, Orgera, & Hinton, 2019).

In 2016, Medicaid covered 39% of all U.S. children and 77.9% of children living in households earning <$25,000 per year (Murphy, 2017). Medicare beneficiaries comprised 15% of Medicaid enrollment (Musumeci, 2017). Medicaid pays for 62% of individuals living in nursing homes, with the average yearly cost for nursing home care in 2016 topping $82,000 (KFF, 2017). About 33% of adults turning 65 will require nursing home care during the remainder of their lives (KFF, 2017).

- Prior to the ACA, childless adults without disabilities were not eligible for Medicaid. Under the ACA, Medicaid was expanded to all nonelderly adults with incomes up to 138% of the FPL, or $17,236 for an individual in 2019 (Garfield, Orgera, & Damico, 2020).
- Other changes made through the ACA were to extend Medicaid coverage for children in foster care until age 26—equal to the requirement that private plans allow dependent children to remain on a parent's plan until that age. States also needed to make the Medicaid application process easier (Congressional Research Service, 2018; Manatt, Phelps, & Phillips, 2019).

The ACA initially required all states to expand Medicaid. This was legally challenged by several states, leading to a Supreme Court case—*National Federation of Independent Business v. Sebelius* (KFF, 2012). The Medicaid expansion was ruled to be unconstitutional because it was highly coercive and the Medicaid expansion became optional for states.

- Currently, 37 states have expanded Medicaid coverage (KFF, 2020). However, a gap in coverage exists in states choosing not to expand Medicaid coverage (Fig. 6-13); Medicaid eligibility is 40% of the federal poverty level ($8,532 for a family of three in 2019).
- According to the Center on Budget and Policy Priorities (CPPB), since expanded Medicaid coverage was implemented, over 19,00 lives have been saved. Whereas, in states that have not expanded Medicaid, roughly 15,500 lives have been lost (Aron-Dine, 2019).
- The largest portion of Medicaid spending goes toward people with disabilities (40%) and older adults (21%), but these two groups comprise only 23% of Medicaid enrollees (Rudowitz, Orgera, et al., 2019).

Medicaid is jointly funded between federal and state governments to assist the states in providing adequate medical care to eligible persons. The federal government matches state Medicaid spending, and this is the largest source of federal funding for states. The federal government pays a portion of the costs, called the Federal Medical Assistance Percentage (FMAP), at 50% to 76%. Historically, the FMAP was around 62% (Schneider, 2019).

The funding model for Medicaid has both benefits and problems. There isn't a limit on federal spending, so as states expand their Medicaid programs, more federal funding flows to states (Paradise, Lyons, & Rowland, 2015). This allows Medicaid to expand during epidemics or pandemics (e.g., COVID-19), natural or man-made disasters, or short economic downturns. At the same time, when the economy contracts, as in the 2008 recession, many more people become eligible for Medicaid at a time when state and federal funds were decreasing (Cutler, 2018).

The states have some discretion in determining which population groups their Medicaid programs cover and the financial criteria for Medicaid eligibility, as well as the scope of services, rate of payment, and how the program will be administered, so long as they meet the minimum

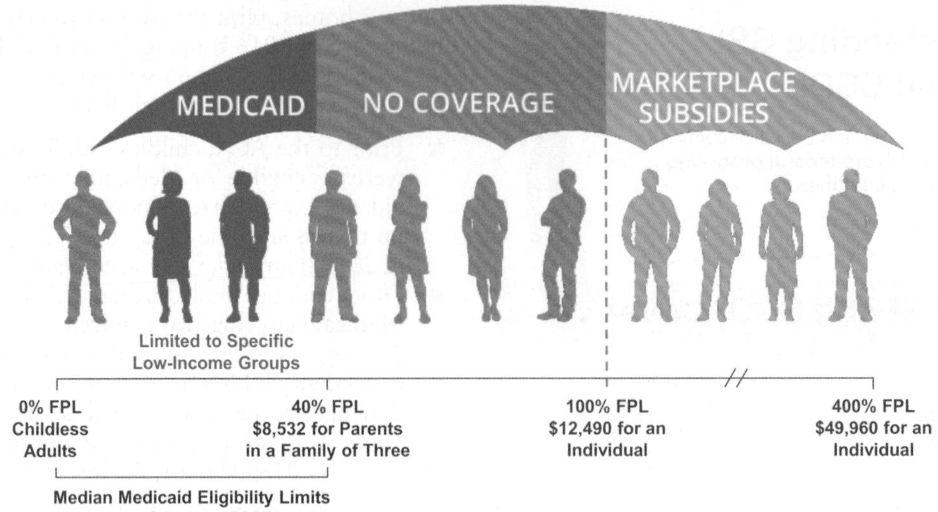

FIGURE 6-13 Gap in coverage for adults in states that do not expand Medicaid under the Patient Protection and Affordable Care Act. (Reprinted with permission from Garfield, R., Orgera, K., & Damico, A. (January 14, 2020). *The coverage gap: Uninsured poor adults in states that do not expand Medicaid.* Kaiser Family Foundation. Retrieved from https://www.kff.org/medicaid/issue-brief/the-coverage-gap-uninsured-poor-adults-in-states-that-do-not-expand-medicaid/)

requirements set by the federal government (Paradise et al., 2015).

Medicaid mandatory services include the following (Medicaid.gov, n.d.a):

- Outpatient and inpatient hospital services
- Early childhood screenings and well-child checkups (to age 21)
- Physician and nurse practitioner/certified nurse midwife services
- Lab and x-ray services
- Family planning services
- Tobacco cessation counseling for pregnant women
- Home health care and nursing home services for those over age 21 (including rehabilitation centers)
- Federally qualified health center and rural health clinic services
- Transportation to medical care

As with Medicare, Medicaid programs moved to a managed care concept following mandates within the Balanced Budget Act of 1997, in an attempt to restrain costs (Paradise et al., 2015).

- In July 2017, more than 66% of Medicaid beneficiaries were covered by managed care programs (Hinton et al., 2019), with nearly 50% of the Medicaid budget going to managed care programs (Rudowitz, Orgera, et al., 2019).
- In some states, a managed care plan is required. In states with lower per capita income, there are higher federal matches. Medicaid beneficiaries are economically disadvantaged, frequently reside in medically underserved areas, and often have more complex health and social needs than other adults with higher incomes do.
- They often must choose between multiple plans, fewer providers, and may need to drive long distances to see specialists. Some managed care plans lack sufficient oversight, leading to fragmented services and poor health outcomes (Rudowitz, Orgera, et al., 2019).

Medicaid is also a source of innovation in health care. States implemented medical homes, care coordination, integration of physical and mental health care, and other "new" services earlier than private health plans. The flexibility built into the federal requirements for Medicaid, Medicaid rule waivers to test ideas, and the new Innovation Center in CMS (part of the ACA) allow states to develop new models of health care delivery (CMS, 2019g; Paradise et al., 2015).

Patient advocates (e.g., physicians, nurses, community leaders) often express concerns that many Medicaid managed care plans (or state administrators) are more focused on keeping their costs down than on improving patient care. The system has wide variability in cost-effectiveness and quality (Paradise et al., 2015). Ensuring access and quality of care in a managed care environment will require fiscally solvent plans, established provider networks, and awareness of the unique needs of the Medicaid population (CMS, 2020a; National Conference of State Legislatures, 2017). Also, both providers and beneficiaries need more education about managed care.

- A key factor to Medicaid's future success is reimbursements to providers, both the amount of payments and administrative delays. Medicaid has historically reimbursed providers at a lower rate than Medicare, and other insurance programs and filing for reimbursement can be onerous.
- In 2016, Medicaid fees paid were an average of 72% of those paid by Medicare. In states where the fee ratio was above the median, physicians accepted Medicaid patients at higher rates than for those below the median (Holgash & Heberlein, 2019). This is problematic for C/PHNs who may have difficulty finding a health provider for clients.
- States may also take a long time to make the reimbursement payment. These issues create burdens for

clinics and private physician offices, leading to a lack of provider participation—and a lack of access to care for enrollees.

- When state resources are strained, provider reimbursement rates are often cut. This leads to fewer providers willing to take Medicaid patients—it is estimated that about 30% of physicians in the United States will not accept Medicaid patients (Cutler, 2018).
- Despite these issues, Medicaid provides societal benefits. Medicaid coverage is associated with reduced rates of infant mortality, especially in African American infants (Bhatt & Beck-Sagué, 2018).
- In addition, providing coverage to children early in life leads to higher educational achievement, higher income, and decreased use of public programs (Manatt, Phelps, & Phillips, 2019; Robert Wood Johnson Foundation, 2019).

Although there are access and quality problems with Medicaid, one large study examining differences between an uninsured population and those with Medicaid found that patients with Medicaid were more likely to see a physician at least once annually. Among low-income populations with high blood pressure, those with Medicaid had greater awareness and control of hypertension, although this was not the case for those with high cholesterol or diabetes (Christopher et al., 2016).

Children's Health Insurance Plan. Enacted as part of the Balanced Budget Act in 1997, the Children's Health Insurance Plan (CHIP) provides health coverage to uninsured children under age 19 for families caught in the gap between Medicaid and affordable health insurance (Healthcare.gov, n.d.d). Funding is provided from both federal and state budgets, and CHIP is a capped program; some states offer the program to pregnant women and their unborn child (Medicaid and CHIP Payment and Access Commission [MACPAC], 2018). In 2017, federal funding for this program lapsed, and it took 114 days to regain funding that is now good through 2023 (Mitchell, 2018).

- In 2018, 9.6 million children were enrolled or had been previously enrolled during the 2018 fiscal year (Medicaid.gov, n.d.b).
- While states differ on some services provided, all states must cover routine check-ups and doctor checks, dental and vision care, hospital services, immunizations, prescriptions, and emergency services.
- The program is free in many states, but premiums or enrollment fees vary by state; children up to the age of 19 are covered for families of four making up to $50,000 per year (InsureKidsNow.gov, n.d.).

Federal Reimbursements for Disproportionate Share Hospitals. In addition to payments from Medicare and Medicaid, the U.S. government reimburses safety net hospitals and other entities involved in care of the uninsured, known as designated Disproportionate Share Hospitals (DSH). The American Hospital Association (2018) reported a total of $38.3 billion in uncompensated care in 2016; this is an increase over 2015 figures of $35.7 billion. Although taxpayers help pay for uninsured patients, it does not fully cover costs of care.

- Camilleri (2018, p. 1562) examined national data on uncompensated care after the first year of ACA Medicaid expansion among hospitals with a "disproportionate share of low-income patients" and found significant reductions in the amount of uncompensated care for those participating in expansion.
  - DSH hospitals had greater reductions than non-DSH hospitals, and the differences in levels of uncompensated care for expansion and nonexpansion states were noticeably wider. The recent rash of hospital closures throughout the United States, mostly in rural and suburban areas and often safety net hospitals, has led to remaining hospitals being responsible for those patients (Khullar, Song, & Choski, 2018).
- In states with ACA-related Medicaid expansion, safety net hospitals had "improved operating margins" and those without expansion demonstrated declining operating margins (Dobson, DaVanzo, Haught, & Phap-Hoa, 2017, p. 1).
  - If Medicaid expansion were extended to those states, costs of uncompensated care are projected to drop by over $6 billion (Dranove, Gartwaite, & Ody, 2017).

Other Government Programs. In addition to third-party reimbursement, the government offers some direct health services to selected populations, including Native Americans, military personnel, veterans, merchant marines, and federal employees. Government support, largely through grants administered through the CDC, provides immunizations and well-child visits, as well as prenatal care and other programs at the state and local level.

Retrospective Payment

Reimbursement for health care services generally has been accomplished through one of two approaches: retrospective or prospective payment. A traditional form of reimbursement for any kind of service, including health care, is **retrospective payment**, which is reimbursement for a service after it has been rendered (Torrey, 2020). A fee may or may not be established in advance. However, payment of that fee occurs after the fact, or retrospectively, termed **fee-for-service (FFS)**.

In health care, limited accountability in the use of retrospective payment has created several problems (Hodgin, 2018).

- With third-party payers (e.g., insurance companies, the government) serving as intermediaries, neither consumers nor providers of health services were accountable for containing costs (Hodgin, 2018).
- As more advanced technology and new medications became available, costs increased. Third-party reimbursement also increased, along with other factors, to create an inflationary spiral of escalating costs.
- FFS promoted sickness care rather than wellness services. Providers were rewarded financially for treating illness and for providing additional tests and services. There were few incentives for prevention or health promotion (Hodgin, 2018).

Although retrospective payment worked well in other industries, from a cost-containment as well as a public health perspective, it has not worked well in health care and is now rarely used.

Surprise Medical Billing

"Surprise medical bills" occur when an individual is caught unaware that a provider is not in-network and receives a bill (Pollitz, 2016, para. 2). For instance, a visit to an emergency department is in-network hospital yet the ED physicians are contracted employees and out-of-network. A scheduled surgery at a hospital is covered under the plan yet the assistant surgeon, anesthesiologist or radiologist are not part of the plan.

- More than 42% of patients hospitalized or seen in emergency rooms at in-network hospitals received surprise bills in a recent study, with bills doubling or tripling between 2010 and 2016 (Kaiser Health News, 2019).
- Another study in New York found the average emergency care bill for out-of-network patients was $7,006. Despite efforts to address this common problem, it will most likely persist, especially with narrower networks of providers found with newer health insurance policies (Pollitz, 2016).

Prospective Payment

Prospective reimbursement, although not a new concept, was implemented for inpatient Medicare services in 1983, in response to the health care system's desperate need for cost containment (Rambur, 2015). It has since influenced the Medicaid program, as well as private health insurers. The prospective payment form of reimbursement has virtually eliminated the retrospective payment system (Nickitas et al., 2020). **Prospective payment** is a payment method based on rates derived from predictions of annual service costs that are set in advance of service delivery. Providers receive payment for services according to these fixed rates, set in advance. Payments may be in the form of premiums paid before receipt of service or in response to fixed-rate (not cost) charges. To correct unlimited reimbursement patterns and counteract disincentives to contain costs, prospective payment involves four classic steps (Dowling, 1979; Longest, 2016):

1. An external authority is empowered (by statute, market power, or voluntary compliance by providers) to set provider charges, third-party payment rates, or both.
2. Rates are set in advance of the prospective year during which they will apply and are considered fixed for the year (except for major, uncontrollable occurrences). The provider accepts the assignment of fees.
3. Patients, third-party payers, or both pay the prospective rates rather than the costs incurred by providers during the year (or charges adjusted to cover these costs).
4. Providers are at risk for losses or surpluses.

Prospective payment imposes constraints on spending and provides incentives for cutting costs. The federal government, as mentioned earlier, enacted a prospective payment plan (The Social Security Amendments Act of 1983; see Significant Legislation, above).

- The plan is a billing classification system known as **diagnosis-related groups (DRGs)**. The system is based on about 500 diagnosis and procedure groups. It provides fixed Medicare reimbursement to hospitals based on weighted formulas. Flat rates of payment are based on average national costs for a specific group, adjusted annually, with some regional variations accounting for higher wages and other costs (Longest, 2016).
- This system was enacted to curb Medicare spending in hospitals and to extend the program's solvency period. It was designed to create incentives for hospitals to be more efficient in delivering services.
- The prospective payment system reduced Medicare's rate of increase for inpatient hospital spending and increased hospital productivity by reducing hospital stays and unnecessary admissions, according to Clifton (2009) and Rambur (2015).
- The system, however, led to DRG creep or "upcoding" (i.e., classifying patients into more lucrative categories) and patient dumping (i.e., transferring patients whose reimbursement is expected to be lower than actual costs of services) in an effort to counteract the losses in revenue and in some circumstances make hefty profits.
  - The CEO of Prime Health Services and 14 of the company's hospitals settled a $65 million settlement for "upcoding," a practice in which patients are assigned a DRG requiring a higher level of care than what the patient needs (U.S. Department of Justice [USDOJ], 2018).

In a classic article, Kinney (2013) calculated that the three major concerns faced by Medicare (and the ACA) are "cost and volume inflation, quality assurance, and fraud and abuse" (p. 253).

- Cost inflation was addressed by DRGs and other measures; CMS has mechanisms in place to investigate fraud or abuse.
- Quality was addressed in October 2008, when Medicare began withholding payments to hospitals for preventable errors in an effort to provide an incentive to prevent avoidable mistakes and improve patient care. There are 29 preventable errors (often called "never events") grouped into 7 categories (Agency for Healthcare Research and Quality [AHRQ], 2019b).
- Appropriate mechanisms must be in place to provide accountability and take action when needed—as when billing and other fraud is prosecuted (Smith & Yip, 2016; USDOJ, 2018, 2019). Cutler (2018) estimated that overall health care fraud for public and private payers may be as high as 10% of total costs.

These changes were instituted at the request of Congress, and initially, many hospitals complained that their payments would be substantially reduced, especially for complicated patients.

"Never events" are medical errors or adverse events that never should happen and are largely preventable (Patient Safety Network 2019; AHRQ, 2019b). An expanded list of 24 never events for hospitals—serious incidents that could have been prevented—was approved for nonpayment by Medicaid beginning in July 2012 for all states. The goal was to reduce serious medical errors and preventable infections that should reduce costs and improve patient care (AHRQ, 2019a). Progress toward this goal of improved quality of care is evident by saving the lives of 8,000 people and saving close to $3 billion (CMS, 2018a). However, never events still occur. In 2017, there were 95 surgical events, 37 criminal events, and 89 patient protection events (Knowles, 2018). Medical errors account for 100,00 deaths and costs 20 billion a year. In addition, there are 4,000 surgical errors reported yearly (Rodziewicz & Hipskind, 2020). The ACA includes incentive payments to primary care providers who meet quality goals. Nursing instituted the QSEN initiative (QSEN Institute, 2020).

Debate continues about nonpayment outside of hospital settings and about which conditions should be included in the list of never events (Box 6-4).

Capitation

A more vigorous version of prospective payment is capitation. **Capitation** refers to a fixed fee per person that is paid to a MCO for a specified package of services. Fees remain in effect until renegotiated, regardless of the number of services provided. Because profit margins are very tight, utilization, quality, and costs are carefully monitored (Nickitas et al., 2020).

- The prospective payment concept has proved useful from a public health perspective. Prepaid services create incentives for providers to keep their enrollees healthy, thus reducing provider costs.
- A potential, indirect benefit from fixed rates and reduced costs is that prevention programs may capture a larger share of the health care dollar.

Claims Payment Agents

Claims payment agents administer the process for government third-party payments. That is, the government contracts with private fiscal agents to handle the claims payment process and function as an intermediary between them and the health care provider. As an example, Blue Cross Blue Shield, in addition to serving as a private insurance company, has also served as claims payment agent for Medicare since its inception (Blue Cross Blue Shield, 2019).

Direct Consumer Reimbursement or Out-of-Pocket Payment

Another source of health care financing comes from direct fees paid by consumers. This refers to individual out-of-pocket payments made for several different reasons, such as:

- Payments made by individuals who have no insurance coverage (fees must be paid directly for health and medical services)
- Payments for limited coverage, insurance caps, and exclusions (services for which the consumer must bear the entire expense)

For example, some individuals carry only major medical insurance and must pay directly for physician office visits, prescriptions, eyeglasses, and dental care. In other instances, deductibles and coinsurance leaves individuals and families with health care insurance out-of-pocket costs, with payments ranging from $360 to $1,500; the highest being $7,000 or more (Hayes, Collins, & Radley, 2019). Roughly, 30% of Americans are worried about health care insurance premiums, deductibles, and out-of-pocket expenses (Kirzinger, Muñana, Wu, & Brodie, 2019).

Two important factors to consider in health care costs are cost shifting and cross subsidization.

- **Cost shifting** consists of charging different prices for the same services, placing the burden of high cost of health care on others. The idea is that health care agencies and providers are able to make up for the lower reimbursements from Medicare and Medicaid by charging more to private payers (Feldhaus & Mathauer, 2018).
  - Over the past 20 years of research into cost shifting, it has been noted that, as Medicare and Medicaid decrease their payments to providers, this has not substantially increased costs to others. In fact, as government programs pay less, private insurance companies are charging less as well (Frakt, 2018).
- **Cross subsidization** is the practice of adjusting revenues from a central pool of funds to an area with higher health care needs to help cut site costs. The health risks of an area are calculated based on population's age, gender, poverty level, chronic diseases and disabilities (Mathauer, Vinyals Torres, Kutzin, Jakab, & Hanson, 2020).
  - Cross subsidization is used in many countries with decentralized health care such as Germany, Japan, Spain, and Switzerland (Mathauer et al., 2020).

Private and Philanthropic Support

Private or philanthropic support, a third funding source, contributes both directly and indirectly to health care financing. U.S. charities received $427.71 billion in

BOX **6-4** WHAT DO *YOU* THINK?

Nonpayment for Preventable Medical Errors

What if you were to hire a glass company to replace a broken windshield in your car, and while completing the repair, they accidentally broke off your rearview mirror. Would you expect them to pay for that mistake? Or would you just absorb the cost yourself?

In the past, we the taxpayers have been paying Medicare payments to hospitals and physicians who have made serious errors that have led to adverse events, spiraling costs, and resulted in poor patient outcomes. Congress and others feel that this is unfair and have enacted legislation to stop paying for these types of errors or preventable events.

Do you think this is fair? Can these conditions always be prevented? Are there extenuating circumstances that should be taken into account? Are there benefits to patients and taxpayers from holding health care providers accountable for errors and inadequate care?

donations in 2018. Many private agencies fund programs, underwrite research, and provide benefits for people who otherwise would go without services. Roughly, $9 billion was donated to help pay for medications by providing lower costs or medications at no charge to those who could not afford prescription drugs (Giving USA, 2019).

In addition, volunteerism, the efforts of numerous individuals and organizations that donate their time and services (e.g., hospital guild members), provides tremendous cost savings to health care institutions.

TRENDS AND ISSUES INFLUENCING HEALTH CARE ECONOMICS

The High Cost of Health Care in the United States

As described earlier, the United States pays the most for what are often some of the worst health outcomes. Mossialos, Wenzl, Osborn, and Sarnak (2016) reported health care comparisons across OECD countries and found that the United States ranked last on *amenable mortality levels* (deaths prior to age 75 that may be prevented through effective, timely health care). A study comparing mortality between the United States and seven European countries found that greater U.S. social and educational disparities "explain why U.S. adults have higher mortality" (van Hedel et al., 2015, p. e112). The United States was

- Among the lowest nations in the percentage of adults who smoke daily
- Among the lowest third of nations in cancer deaths
- In the lower half of countries on childhood vaccination rates but third highest on influenza vaccination rates
- Among the highest among nations on the percentage of adults who are obese
- Among the lower third of countries for life expectancy at birth (OECD, 2019)

Controlling Costs

The ACA has introduced many strategies to control the rise of health care costs, including increased funding for primary prevention strategies. A focus on primary prevention demands a paradigm shift in thinking about the practice and delivery of health care (see Chapter 1). It is one that fits more closely with the mission of public health. It expects that citizens are involved in their health care, are knowledgeable about their health status, can manage self-care practices, and can modify lifestyle behaviors to promote wellness. Our focus on illness and not health promotion or prevention has proven costly. Prevention should be at the forefront of a new era in health care. Trust for America's Health (TFAH, 2020) has developed 10 top priorities for a National Prevention Strategy:

1. Fighting the Obesity Epidemic
2. Thwarting the use or exposure to tobacco
3. Preventing/Controlling Infectious Diseases
4. Preparing for Possible Health Emergencies/Bioterrorism Attacks
5. Acknowledging the Connection Between Health and U.S. Economic Competitiveness
6. Safeguarding Our Food Supply
7. Planning for Adapting Senior Health Care Needs
8. Improving the Health and Wellbeing of Low-Income/Minority Communities
9. Diminishing Environmental Threats
10. Advancing Prevention of Diseases (para. 1)

Access to Health Services: The Uninsured and Underinsured

Many services, preventive or illness focused, are not available to a large portion of our population.

- The U.S. Census Bureau (2010) reported that 50.7 million people (16.7% of the population) were **uninsured** in 2009; the percentage of uninsured (those lacking health insurance) had been as high as 18% before passage of the ACA (Witters, 2019).
- The ACA (2010) improved access to care by making insurance available to people who were considered "uninsurable" due to preexisting health conditions. By 2014, the number of people who were uninsured decreased to 33 million or 10.4% of the population (U.S. Census Bureau, 2015).
  - The U.S. Census Bureau noted that 8.5%, approximately 27.5 million people, had no health insurance the entire year in 2018 (Berchik, Barnett, & Upton, 2019). The rate of those lacking health insurance varies by age group (Fig. 6-14).
  - The uninsured rate in 2018 is highest for those living below the poverty level (7.8%) and higher for Hispanics (8.7%) and Blacks (4.6%), and similar for Asians (4.1%) compared to non-Hispanic Whites (4.2%).
- The ACA expanded Medicaid in a number of states, extending coverage to low-income individuals and families. In addition, the ACA required insurance companies to cover preventative health care visits without a copay and to cover those with preexisting conditions.
- In recent years, political disagreements about the ACA have led to weakening of some protections. Despite this, federal surveys revealed a fairly stable national rate of uninsured between 2016 and 2017 at 8.8%. However, states that did not participate in Medicaid expansion had higher rates, averaging 12.2% (Keith, 2018).

At the end of 2018, a Gallup poll reported that the uninsured rate had increased to 13.7% (Witters, 2019). From 2016 to 2018, the number of uninsured Americans grew by 1.2 million. By the end of 20108, a Gallup poll reported that the uninsured rate had increased to 13.7% (KFF, 2019d; Witters, 2019).

Even those with Medicaid and Medicare can be underinsured or become uninsured.

- It is estimated that almost 25% (11.5 million) of Medicare participants are underinsured, with state data varying from a low of 16% to a high of 32% (Schoen & Solis-Roman, 2016).

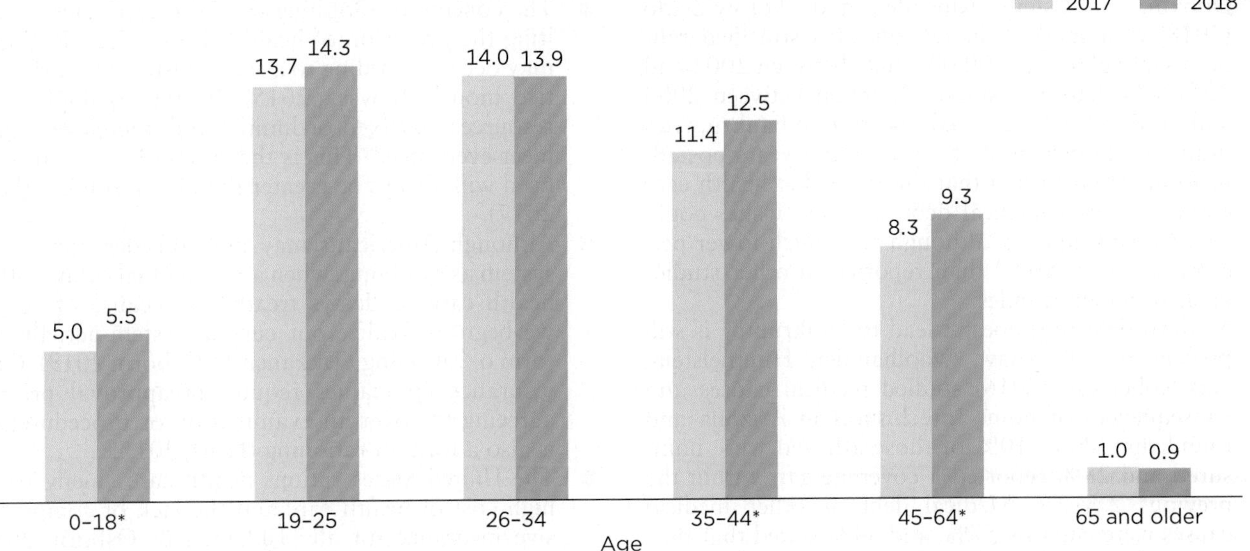

FIGURE 6-14 Percentage of people uninsured by age: 2017 and 2018. Note: population as of March of the following year. (From Berchik, E. R., Barnett, J. C., Upton, R. D., & for the U.S. Census Bureau. (November 2019). *Health insurance coverage in the United States: 2018.* Figure 4, p. 7. Retrieved from https://www.census.gov/content/dam/Census/library/publications/2019/demo/p60-267.pdf)

- The Kaiser Family Foundation estimated that between 1.4 and 4 million Medicaid recipients would lose their health care coverage in states where Medicaid work requirements are now being implemented (Fig. 6-15). Between 62% and 91% will be disenrolled for not correctly reporting work hours or exemptions and between 9% and 38% for not meeting the work requirements (Garfield, Rudowitz, & Musumeci, 2018).

Medical Bankruptcies

A wide variety of medical issues can lead to financial insecurity and bankruptcy. If you don't have health insurance and you undergo emergency surgery for appendicitis, it may take a great effort to pay off your medical debt (or you may turn to high-interest credit cards). Even if you have health insurance, long-term cancer treatments will likely mean large out-of-pocket costs—and your inability to work may lead to further financial problems. Bankruptcy has provided debt relief.

- Bankruptcy filings reached their peak in 2010; about 50% fewer filings were noted by 2017 (United States Courts, 2018). Experts credit that downturn to expanded health coverage with passage of the ACA, along with an improved economy and the 2005 legislation revising bankruptcy laws (St. John, 2017).
- Medical bankruptcies are uncommon in most developed countries, but GoFundMe efforts to help families with unexpected, crushing medical bills are commonplace in the United States, with over a quarter million requests for assistance annually, raising over $650 million annually (Hiltzik, 2019).

Medical debt is thought to be a major contributor to personal bankruptcy filings. In a classic study, Himmelstein, Thorne, Warren, and Woolhandler (2009) reported in a five-state study that 62% of bankruptcy filings were associated with medical expenses. This number has been widely cited—in academic journals, in the media, and in political speeches. However, more recent studies have not found the same patterns.

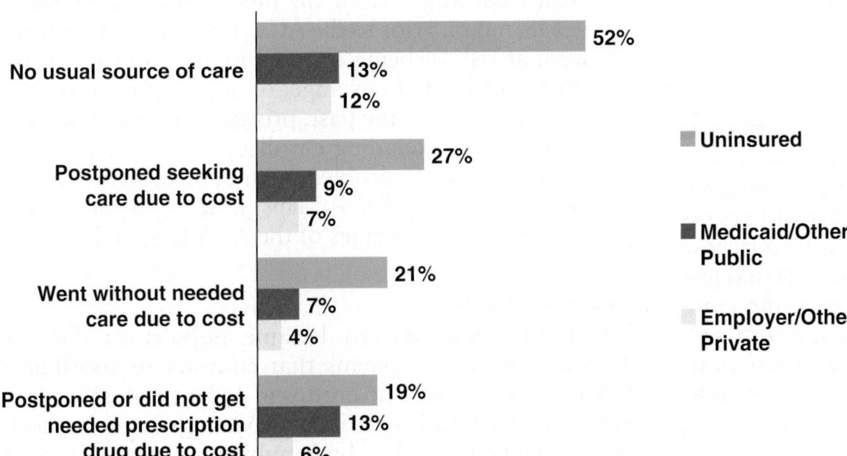

FIGURE 6-15 Barriers to health care among nonelderly adults by insurance status, 2018. (Reprinted with permission from the Kaiser Family Foundation. (December 13, 2019). *Key facts about the uninsured population.* Retrieved from https://www.kff.org/uninsured/fact-sheet/key-facts-about-the-uninsured-population/)

- Dobkin, Finkelstein, Kluender, and Notowidigdo (2018) examined credit records of a stratified random sample of over 500,00 adults between 2002 and 2011 who had a hospital admission between 2003 and 2007. They discovered that rate of bankruptcies dramatically increased at 1 year and 4 years postadmission. They posited that out-of-pocket health care costs, increased medical debt, and lost wages could lead to bankruptcies, although at a much lower percentage (under 10%) than reported in other studies using different samples.
- Medical debt that doesn't lead to bankruptcy is still problematic. Cutshaw, Woolhandler, Himmelstein, and Robertson (2016) studied medical causes and consequences of home foreclosures in Arizona and found that about 10% of those affected were uninsured and 28% reported a coverage gap within the previous 2 years. Medical debt or other medical causes were cited by 57%, and 54% stated that they incurred new debt in an effort to pay medical bills (10% had mortgaged homes). About 57% reported having a chronic condition, and over 50% had either delayed or missed medical visits. Five months after the first data collection, 33% reported that they could not afford food, and 63% had new medical debts. A few respondents were homeless.
- Medical debt redistributes income from the poor to wealthier individuals, and our health care system payment structure "exacerbates income inequality and impoverishes millions of Americans" (Christopher, Himmelstein, Woolhandler, & McCormick, 2018, p. 351).
- About 19% of people with employer-sponsored health insurance reported having been contacted by a collection agency within the last year because of unpaid health care expenses in a representative survey conducted by the Kaiser Family Foundation and the Los Angeles Times (Hamel, Munana, & Brodie, 2019). Over half of respondents reported skipping or postponing care.
- This is further evidence that the underinsured, along with those individuals without health insurance, are in danger of financial disaster when confronted with a serious medical emergency or long-term illness. Those with chronic health conditions, insured and uninsured, have even higher financial burdens from out-of-pocket health care expenses (Khera et al., 2018).

Health Care Rationing

In 2018, more than 30 million people, or 9.4% of the U.S. population, were uninsured (Cohen, Terlizzi, & Martinez, 2019). Health care in the United States is allocated based on price and the willingness and ability of patients to pay. In other words, patients are entitled to purchase a share of the medical services that they value. Social justice, in contrast, emphasizes the well-being of the community over the individual. Under this view, health care is regarded as a social good (as opposed to an economic good) that should be collectively financed and available to everyone regardless of ability to pay (APHA, 2020; Krau, 2015).

- The concept of rationing in health care refers to limiting the provision of health care services. Rationing may occur according to a social justice or market justice model (Bowser, 2015). Rationing implies that resources are fixed or limited and, therefore, cannot meet every need. This is the case in health care—the need will always be greater than the resources (Pearl, 2017).
- Although Americans may not consider our current system as rationing, when an individual cannot afford health care or delays treatment because of copays, we begin to realize our current system actually is a form of rationing (Tikkanen & Osborn, 2019). Often insurance companies require preapproval prior to agreeing to cover an examination or procedure; this is also a form of rationing (Pearl, 2017).
- The United States rations health care chiefly by the high cost of health care and the lack of comprehensive insurance for all (Tikkanen & Osborn, 2019). Rationing occurs by your zip code of residence, physicians rationing their time per patient, and hospitals' ratios of beds per unit (Khetpal, 2017).
- When rationing is based on social justice principles, it is considered a rational, fair and equal distribution of resources according to a clinical need or potential for effectiveness and is not based on income or where one lives. In this way, rationing focuses on the needs of the population more than the individual (Bowser, 2015).
- Rationing may occur by restricting people's choices, by denying access to services, or by limiting the supply of services or personnel. It may be overt, as in the oft-cited government health system of the United Kingdom, or more covert, as practiced by some U.S. health plans. When rationing is based on market justice principles, limited resources are distributed based on the ability to pay (Bowser, 2015).
- Rationing may jeopardize the well-being of groups of individuals (Bowser, 2015; Physicians for a National Health Program, 2020a). With limited resources for health services delivery, the government, insurers, and providers of health care services make rationing decisions to contain costs (Pearl, 2017). This has included strict eligibility levels or monitoring the use of resources to ensure the most equitable distribution.
- In 2014, companies were no longer allowed to deny health coverage based on preexisting health issues (CMS, n.d.c). Prior to the ACA, millions of Americans were at risk of being charged higher rates for insurance, had limited coverage, or were denied coverage (CMS, n.d.a.). In the past, private insurers engaged in rationing by excluding enrollees who were at greatest risk for health problems—and, thus, higher expenditures (Rosoff, 2014). This practice is no longer allowed under the rules of the ACA (Box 6-5).

Managed Care

The term **managed care** became popular in the late 1980s. It refers to systems that contract to coordinate medical care for specific groups in order to promote provider efficiency and control costs. Managed care is a cost-control strategy used in both public and private sectors

BOX **6-5** WHAT DO *YOU* THINK?

Rationing of Health Care Services

When several individuals need an organ transplant and only one organ is available, what criteria should be used to select the recipient? It is now commonly accepted that certain lifestyle behaviors, such as smoking, alcohol consumption, or driving without restraints, create health risks. Should people who engage in these activities pay a higher price for health care or be excluded from certain services? Should a younger person needing specialized surgery take priority over an older person needing similar care?

There are no easy answers. At the height of the COVID-19 pandemic, health care systems in several countries were stretched beyond their means, and a form of triaging evolved out of necessity. Was this form of rationing used in your area? Or was it used in other areas of our country? Which strategies do you feel are the most effective for the United States in controlling costs and improving health outcomes?

of health care. Care is *managed* by regulating the use of services and levels of provider payment. This approach is utilized in HMOs, ACOs, EPOs, and PPOs. Roughly 70 million Americans are enrolled in HMOs, compared to 90 million enrolled in PPOs (NCSL, 2017).

Managed care plans operate on a prospective payment basis and control costs by managing utilization and provider payments. Because costs are tight, preventive services are generally encouraged, so that more expensive tertiary care costs can be avoided if possible (NCSL, 2017).

Health Maintenance Organizations

Health maintenance organizations (HMOs) are systems in which participants prepay a fixed monthly premium to receive comprehensive health services delivered by a defined network of providers. In 2019, costs for employee health coverage were similar for HMO, PPO, and point-of-service plans with approximately a $500 difference for an individual and $2,000 for a family. Insurance premiums have continued to rise more than wage increases (KFF, 2019b).

HMOs are the oldest model of managed care. Several HMOs have existed for decades (e.g., Kaiser Permanente), but others have developed more recently. The unique set of properties of HMOs includes the following:

- A contract between the HMO and the beneficiaries (or their representative), the enrolled population.
- Absorption of prospective risk by the HMO.
- A regular (usually monthly) premium to cover specified (typically comprehensive) benefits paid by each enrollee of the HMO.
- An integrated delivery system with provider incentives for efficiency. The HMO contracts with professional providers to deliver the services due the enrollees, and the basis for reimbursing those providers varies among HMOs (Estes, Chapman, Dodd, Hollister, & Harrington, 2013).

Some HMOs follow the traditional model, employing health professionals (e.g., physicians, nurses), building their own hospital and clinic facilities, and serving only their own enrollees. Other HMOs provide some services while contracting for the rest (Shi & Singh, 2019).

- HMOs have a 20% higher rate of consumer complaints than customers with PPO plans (State of California, 2017).
- In response to concerns from managed care clients, a patient bill of rights stipulating the patient's right to timely emergency services, respect and nondiscrimination, as well as participation in treatment decisions and a more consumer-friendly appeals process was developed (California Department of Managed Care, 2020).

Preferred Provider Organizations

A **preferred provider organization (PPO)** is a network of physicians, hospitals, and other health-related services that contract with a third-party payer organization (health insurer) to provide health services to subscribers at a reduced rate. Employers with these plans offer medical services to their employees at discounted rates.

- In PPOs, consumer choice exists. Enrollees have a choice among providers within the plan and contracted providers out of the plan. PPOs practice utilization review and often use formal standards for selecting providers (KFF, 2019e).
- In 2016, PPOs were the most common form of health insurance offered by employers—with 48% of workers able to choose this type of policy; companies with over 200 employees have the highest rate of PPO usage at 52% (KFF, 2016).
- However, enrollment in PPOs began to decline, and increases were noted in HDHP/SO policies (KFF, 2016). In 2019, 44% of workers had PPOs, and 30% had HDHP/SOs. About 19% were enrolled in an HMO (KFF, 2019b).

Point-of-Service Plans

A variation on the plans described above is the **point-of-service (POS) plan**, which permits more freedom of choice than a standard HMO or PPO. Enrollees choose a primary physician from within the POS plan who monitors their care and makes outside referrals when necessary. At an extra cost, enrollees can go outside the HMO or PPO network of contracted providers unless their primary physician has made a specific referral (Downs, 2016). POS is a type of hybrid or combination of an HMO and PPO. In 2016, about 10% of employees were enrolled in POS plans and only 7% were in a POS plan in 2019 (KFF, 2016, 2019c). See Figure 6-16 for trends in types of health plan enrollment.

High-Deductible Health Plans

The **high-deductible health plan (HDHP)** is growing in popularity. Among employees in small and large size companies a **high-deductible health plan with a saving option (HDHP/SO)** is often favored over HMOs (Argawal et al., 2017). The plan has higher deductibles and out-of-pocket maximum limits. However, once these deductibles

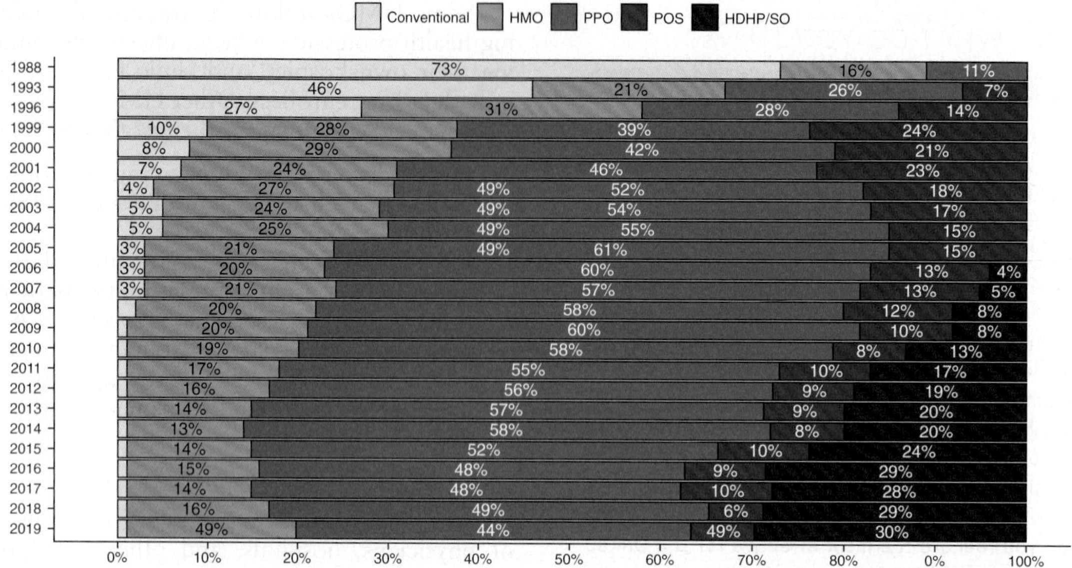

FIGURE 6-16 Distribution of health plan enrollment for covered workers, by plan type, 1988–2019. (Reprinted with permission from the Kaiser Family Foundation and Health Research & Educational Trust. (2019). *Employer health benefits: 2019 annual survey*. Retrieved from http://files.kff.org/attachment/Report-Employer-Health-Benefits-Annual-Survey-2019)

are met, the plan pays 100% of in-network health care. In addition, the HDHP plan is the only health plan that allows for money to be put aside pretaxed to be used to pay for deductibles and out-of-pocket expenses (USOPM, n.d.a.).

- The average annual out-of-pocket cost in 2018 for high-deductible, high-premium HDHP-HSA plans were not to exceed $6,650 for single and $13,300 for family coverage (KFF, 2018a). Similar saving plans tied to HDHP plans vary in maximum costs.
- Deductibles have risen 212% between 2008 and 2018, and over a quarter of covered employees have plans with $2,000 deductibles (or more). For employers with <200 employees, 42% of covered employees have at least $2,000 deductibles (Tozzi, 2018).
- In 2018, 29% of employers offering HDHPs also included a savings plan option, either HSA or HRA (Tozzi, 2018). HDHPs are more often available with large firms than with small ones, 58% versus 27% (KFF, 2018a).

Exclusive Provider Organizations

- Other than for medical emergencies, an **exclusive provider organization (EPO)** plan only covers services and providers within the network. Benefits of this type of plan are lower prices than an HMO and not needing a referral from a primary health care provider (Downs, 2016).
- However, if an individual goes out of network, 100% of the medical bill is owed by that person. A provider that was covered when you bought your policy may no longer be part of the plan the following year, and you will not necessarily know this until you are billed for the visit.

In 2016, there were projected to be about "60% more EPOs being sold through the federal insurance exchange" than the previous year (Zamosky, 2015, para. 13).

Competition and Regulation

Often, competition and regulation in health economics have been viewed as antagonistic and incompatible concepts.

- Competition describes a contest between rival health care organizations for resources and clients.
- Regulation refers to mandated procedures and practices affecting health services delivery that are enforced by law.

In a society in which there are long-held values of freedom of choice and individualism, competition provides opportunities for entrepreneurial endeavor, free enterprise, and scientific advancement. Yet, regulation also serves an important role in promoting the public good, overseeing equitable distribution of health services, and fostering community-wide participation (Smith & Yip, 2016).

Health care incorporates four major types of regulation—laws, regulations, programs, and policies (Longest, 2016; Young & Kroth, 2018).

Laws that regulate health care include any legislation that governs financing or delivery of health services (e.g., Medicare reimbursement to hospitals). Regulations guide and clarify implementation; they are issued under the authority of law and are part of most federal health care programs (e.g., CHIP eligibility requirements). Regulatory policies have a broader focus and involve decisions that shape the health care system by channeling the flow of resources into it and setting limits on key players' actions (e.g., state nurse practice acts, health manpower training, ACA rules on preexisting conditions) (Longest, 2016). Programs and policies are often developed in order to control costs and improve quality (e.g., HRRP, HIPAA). See Chapter 13.

- In the early 1980s, government cost-control measures were greatly diminished as the Reagan era ushered in deregulation (Young & Kroth, 2018). The passage of the Omnibus Budget Reconciliation Act caused dramatic changes affecting health care. The federal government, having failed to contain rising health care costs, shifted responsibility for the public's health and welfare back to state and local governments. From all this grew the competition-versus-regulation debate (KFF, n.d.; Young & Kroth, 2018).

- The 1990s were characterized by numerous hospital mergers and movement from nonprofit to for-profit status. More than 86% of the population in 1991 was covered by some form of prepaid health insurance, largely due to the effects of Medicare and Medicaid (Levit, Olin, & Letsch, 1992).
  - The Clinton health plan failed to gain support and many hospitals downsized and reduced the number of nurses on staff. Managed care became more popular, but by the late 1990s, fears were raised about MCOs withholding necessary care and a consumer "backlash" resulted (Melnick, Fonkych, & Zwanziger, 2018).
- Many states and the federal government enacted benefit laws between 1990 and 2008, in response to these concerns (KFF, n.d.). The ACA was passed into law in 2010 (KFF, n.d.). However, we still feel the results of decades of disjointed policies, and one of the most obvious consequences deals with competition in health care.
- Competition, its proponents say, offers wider consumer choice and positive incentives for cost containment and enhanced efficiency (Young & Kroth, 2018); that is, consumers are free to select among various health plans on the basis of cost, quality, and range of services.
- One downside is fragmentation of services, lack of coordination, and subsequent waste. Integrated delivery systems, such as Kaiser Permanente's fully integrated system, or more loosely organized public–private partnerships, could lead to improved quality, outcomes, and reduced costs (Enthoven & Baker, 2018).

Regulation advocates for almost 20 years have argued that there are at least four problems associated with the competition model: (1) consumers often do not make proper health care choices because they have limited knowledge of health services; (2) competition may discriminate against enrolling certain consumers, especially high-risk, high-cost patients, thus excluding those who may need services the most; (3) the competition model may not encourage enough teaching and research—expensive elements of our present system; and (4) quality may be sacrificed to keep costs down (Young & Kroth, 2018).

The following tenets often guide discussions on health care reform efforts (Fitzgerald & Yencha, 2019):

- Reduction in health care prices occurs when there is more competition among hospitals and among insurers.
- Reducing government regulations will lead to lower health care prices.
- Higher prices can reflect higher-quality care.
- Higher provider costs are reflected in higher prices.

A study by Fitzgerald and Yencha (2019) examining outcome measures for those tenets among seven million hospital and patient interactions found the following:

- Generally, the greater the competition among hospitals (more choice), the lower the prices.
- Depending upon the type of charge used (average total payment or "chargemaster" price), the price of average total payments is greater when there is more competition among insurers, and "chargemaster" prices (or the higher amount paid by those out of network or without insurance, like MSRP) increase when insurers are more concentrated, leading to fewer choices (p. 7).
- Regulation does not consistently affect health care prices; prices can increase or decrease depending upon the cost measure used.
- As hospitals gain in quality measures, their prices generally rise (both average and chargemaster); higher mortality rates were associated with lower prices. However, on two measures of quality, patient experiences and readmission rates, a negative relationship was found.
- Higher hospital costs are generally associated with higher prices.
- Regulation advocates conclude that standardization and controls are needed to guarantee quality and equal access (Longest, 2016). However, "regulation of prices and spending," as done in other health care systems, has not always been popular among U.S. policymakers (Altman & Mechanic, 2018, para. 5). Regulations are often viewed as excessively restrictive and costly. For instance, the American Hospital Association claims that $39 billion per year is spent by hospitals, health systems, and postacute care providers on administrative costs involved in meeting regulatory requirements (AHA, 2020). However, over 4,800 community hospitals reported increasing profits, rising 43% from 2011 to 2017, and reaching over $76 billion (Bannow, 2018).
  - From 2001 to 2016, hospital revenue rose dramatically (238% price increase), while experiencing a 10% drop in total care volume for privately insured patients (Melnick et al., 2018).
  - U.S. hospitals earned their highest level of profits post-ACA in 2016 (Altman & Mechanic, 2018).

California instituted a competitive model in an effort to control health care costs. This included promotion of competitive prices "through market-based, managed care policies" (Melnick et al., 2018, p. 1417). This model was successful until two emerging trends shattered competition: (1) hospitals were permitted by antitrust officials to merge into larger hospital systems (adding hospitals outside local markets) and (2) in order to adequately meet the demand for access to hospital emergency services, regulations were put in place that inadvertently gave hospitals new ability to gain an advantage in negotiations with health insurance companies. These actions led to a less competitive marketplace and the inability of health insurance companies to "leverage competition" to negotiate for lower costs and better benefits (Melnick et al., 2018, p. 1417).

- Our capitalist system is driven by profits, and the profit motive in health care can lead to excesses and higher costs for taxpayers and patients. In 2019, first quarter reporting more than half of all profits in the health care sector went to the top 10 companies, and 90% of those were large pharmaceutical companies like Pfizer ($3.9 billion), Eli Lilly ($4.2 billion), and Johnson & Johnson ($3.7 billion).
- These high profits are occurring at a time when drug prices are escalating, with almost half of the U.S. population reporting use of a prescription medication in the last month.
- Currently, 44 states have "joined an antitrust lawsuit accusing 20 drug manufacturers, including Pfizer and Teva Pharmaceuticals, of fixing prices for more than 100 generic drugs" (Jaggannathan, 2019, para. 5).
- The argument often made by pharmaceutical firms that more money is needed for research and development of new drugs was recently invalidated by examining the costs for 10 pharmaceutical companies introducing newly developed cancer drugs (cost = $9 billion) while their revenues reached over $67 billion (Anderson et al., 2019).

As the ACA was enacted, concerns arose about the continued financial stability of health insurers participating in the ACA marketplace exchanges, but the five largest health insurers have continued to be profitable. These five companies represent about 43% of the nation's insured population.

- Three of them have restricted or ended enrollment in ACA plans, but they have all benefited from growth in Medicare and Medicaid membership between 2010 and 2016, doubling from 12.8 million to 25.5 million.
- These companies now hold 52% of the Medicare Advantage market in 19 states. They have also moved to procuring more administrative service contracts, providing network and claims management for employers or entities who are converting from the usual health insurance policies to self-insurance plans.
- The five insurers report profit margins (some as high as 11% in 2017) and stock share prices have doubled or tripled from 2011 to 2016 (Schoen & Collins, 2017).

Leaders in the field have concluded that both competition and regulation are needed (Longest, 2016; Young & Kroth, 2018). With foresight, McNerney (1980) wrote, "It is rapidly becoming apparent that what we need is a proper balance between competition and regulation with more effective links [and] regulation [should be] used as a force to keep the market honest" (p. 1091).

Managed competition (market-based effort to provide wide access to health care while keeping costs down) and **universal coverage** (every person has health insurance), as well as **single-payer systems** (only one entity receives funds and pays for health care), have been part of the discussion around health care reform (Physicians for a National Health Program, 2020b). Two plans that are worth further review are managed competition and universal coverage, with and without a single-payer system. The benefits and drawbacks of each are discussed at http://thepoint.lww.com/Rector10e.

Drivers of Costs

- Drug spending is a "primary driver of higher cost" in the present U.S. health care system, and a continuing trend, with $1,011 per person spent on prescription drugs annually compared to $422 for other developed countries (Anderson et al., 2019, p. 12; Cox, Kamal, Jankiewicz, & Rousseau, 2016; NAHU, 2015).
  - While the U.S. Veterans Administration has a 30% discounted rate for prescription medications, the federal government is not allowed to negotiate drug prices for Medicare or Medicaid programs (Cai et al., 2020).
- Other drivers of health care costs include the following:
  - An aging population, new technologies, and biologics (e.g., biosimilars like synthetic insulin and monoclonal antibodies)
  - Lifestyle/behavioral choices (about 70% of health care costs may be related to smoking, abuse of alcohol, and obesity), inefficient systems (e.g., duplication of services/procedures, preventable medical errors, unwarranted prescriptions/visits/treatments, spotty quality improvement)
  - Medical malpractice costs, cost shifting, increased demand for health care, government regulations, and other market changes, like consolidations/monopolies (National Association of Health Underwriters, 2015)

We will need to decide how to move forward, either building on the ACA by offering a more meaningful public option and expanding markets while continuing to promote employer health insurance or making a significant shift to a single-payer system provided to all citizens.

With the lack of quality health outcomes in the United States, as described above, even if everyone received health insurance, how could quality be assured? Some believe that the overall performance of the health care system should improve as everyone gains access to care. However, some early evaluation of value-based incentive and penalty programs (e.g., Hospital Value-Based Purchasing Program, Hospital Readmission Reduction Program [HRRP]) reveal that they have not been "effectively calibrated" to achieve their expected results and need more fine tuning to produce better outcomes (Doran, Maurer, & Ryan, 2017, p. 464). A system that provides incentives to *both* providers and patients to use services efficiently and effectively may produce better results (Robinson, Brown, & Whaley, 2017). Another factor that may also improve outcomes is a means of providing health care consumers with pertinent, timely information so that they can be more active participants in their care. (See http://thepoint.lww.com/Rector10e for resources.)

Changing Our Health Care System

The cry for health care reform is not new. In a classic study, Perkins (1998) examined the work of the 1927 to 1932 Committee on the Costs of Medical Care. Almost 100 years ago, the committee defined *costs* as the major problem and *business models of organization* as the major solution.

An important health care reform element is a standard set of benefits, set by law and enjoyed by the entire population, regardless of age, health status, income level, and employment. Many countries have successfully implemented such a package under a plan called the *statutory model*. Various versions of this model have worked well in Austria, France, Belgium, Japan, Germany, Israel, Poland, The Netherlands, and Switzerland. In this model, health insurance falls under the rubric of social security and is funded through government-mandated payroll premiums or taxes. Payment is made to private sector health insurers, from a fund known in some countries as a *sickness fund* (Edwards & Dunn, 2019; IOM, 2013). Individuals can switch plans when desired. This statutory model eliminates the need for separate programs such as Medicaid and Medicare. It also provides uniform and comprehensive benefits (McClure, Enthoven, & McDonald, 2017).

- Health reform must focus on the central question: Is there coverage for the promotion of health and prevention of illness or simply payment for the diagnosis and treatment of those who are already ill?
- Research has shown that public health interventions are consistently more cost-effective than medical services, yet past health reform has often paid minimal attention to this critical issue (Owen, Pennington, Fischer, & Jeong, 2019; Smith et al., 2019; Tanner, 2015).
- In addition, our frequent emphasis on medical care cost containment does not take into account the social determinants of health that need to be addressed outside the health care system (Beckfield & Bambra, 2016). C/PHNs can play an influential role in emphasizing health promotion services as being central to future health reform efforts through political involvement and policy development.
- With the successful passage of HR 3590 (Public Law [PL] 111–148), *The Patient Protection and Affordable Care Act*, on March 23, 2010, and the March 25 passage of HR 4872 (PL 111–152), *Health Care and Education Affordability Reconciliation Act of 2010*, amending HR 3590, the long journey toward health care system reform crossed a threshold. Both pieces of legislation are referred to as the *Affordable Care Act* (ACA).
- Although by no means a grand vision for change with its incremental implementation, it has been noted to be a significantly consequential achievement in reducing the number of uninsured Americans (Gaffney & McCormick, 2017; Woolhandler & Himmelstein, 2017).
- The ACA has been described as "consumer friendly" with coordination and seamless transition between programs as the goal, with exchanges given to power to remove insurers who abuse the system or provide inadequate service. Coordination between insurance exchanges, Medicaid, and CHIP provides for better coverage (MACPAC, 2018).
- The ACA encourages comprehensive case management of chronic disease as one way to decrease hospitalizations and the cost of care. New methods of determining cost-effectiveness are being utilized to determine the realistic impact of population interventions (Arbel & Greenberg, 2016).

Another component of the ACA, the Patient-Centered Outcomes Research Institute (PCORI) provides additional information on effectiveness of treatments and interventions, and the Innovation Center at CMS develops, evaluates, and tests new programs and policies that reduce cost and enhance care for Medicaid and Medicare patients (CMS, 2020c; Hoagland & Parekh, 2019; PCORI, 2017). Improved value and quality outcomes are the proposed benefits of these programs. For a summary of the ACA, see http://kff.org/health-reform/fact-sheet/summary-of-the-affordable-care-act/.

EFFECTS OF HEALTH ECONOMICS ON COMMUNITY/PUBLIC HEALTH PRACTICE

Health economics has significantly affected community/public health practice by advancing disincentives for efficient use of resources, incentives for illness care, and conflicts with public health values.

Overcoming Disincentives for the Efficient Use of Resources

Public health has been affected in several ways. The trend of diminished federal and state allocations has had profound effects on community/public health programs, and severe budget cuts have affected even basic public health services, especially during the coronavirus pandemic.

Public health agencies and providers in Accountable Care Organizations are joining together for initiatives to improve quality along with cutting costs (e.g., Triple Aim, outcome accountable care). Public health professionals can offer their expertise in community assessment and design of population-based interventions. The 6/18 initiative follows the format of promoting population health by accelerating collaborative partnerships to implement 18 evidence-based interventions that target 6 high-cost, "high-burden, preventable conditions" in a community-integrated health care program (Hester et al., 2016, p. 4).

Managed Care and the Future of Public Health

Initially, managed care focused on event-driven cost avoidance (e.g., decreasing inpatient days and specialty physician use, using physician extenders). This evolved into a second stage, in which the principal objective was to control resource intensity and improve the delivery process. Now, emphasis has shifted to a focus on health promotion and population health. Community assessments are an important part of this approach, so that high-risk groups can be identified and provided early interventions. Case management of individuals with chronic illness is also a focus (Mendelson, 2019).

- Community health assessments could become standard quality tools for not only public health interventions but also health care in general. The ACA requires hospitals to conduct regular community assessments, and many have partnered with LHDs to do so.
- This provides an opportunity for collaborative partnerships or "cross-sector collaborations" needed to

improve population health and reach more community members. Health care reform legislation includes a requirement for community needs assessment every 3 years for state-licensed, tax-exempt health organizations such as hospitals and imposes a $50,000 annual penalty if this is not done. Prioritization of health needs and a description of community resources are to be included, as is input from those with expertise in public health (Adams, 2011; Erwin & Brownson, 2017a; Wahowiak, 2017, p. 1).

- While hospitals are required by the ACA to complete community health assessments, more research is needed to discover if intervention programs have been implemented to improve population health as a result (Cramer, Singh, Flaherty, & Young, 2017). See Chapter 15 for more on Community Assessment.

Improving the health status of a community mandates that health care agencies be actively involved in health teaching and health promotion, as well as developing community action plans to promote collaboration and focus on early intervention and treatment to improve health equity and health outcomes (National Academies of Sciences, Engineering, and Medicine, 2017). Are these not the proposals that public health advocates have been making for more than a century?

By partnering with hospitals on community assessment and research, these things, along with public health accreditation, may further improve the public health system (Wahowiak, 2017).

- Erwin and Brownson (2017a) described macro trends that will influence the future of public health. These include community health assessments in conjunction with hospitals, accreditation, and preparation for catastrophic weather events and other disasters related to climate change.
- The influences of Health in All Policies (HiAP, described in Chapters 13 and 16), informatics and social media, demographic trends (e.g., increased elderly and racial ethnic minority populations), and global travel will encourage C/PHNs to become more adept in these areas in order to meet the needs of their clients and communities. However, in some areas of the country, there is a decline in recruitment and retention of C/PHNs making it difficult to meet the coming challenges (Taylor, 2018).
- Public Health 3.0 is an initiative promoted by the U.S. Department of Health and Human Services (n.d.b) and amplified by leaders in the field of public health (Balio, Yeager, & Beitsch, 2019; DiSalvo et al., 2017).
    - Eight "strategic skill domains" were identified: "effective communication, data for decision-making, cultural competence, budget and financial management, change management, systems and strategic thinking, developing a vision for a healthy community, and cross-sector partnerships" (Resnick et al., 2019, p. 10).

Frieden (2015) called upon public health to join with clinical medicine, government agencies, health NGOs, private sector groups, and our communities to make our population healthier. He shared a powerful example from the United Kingdom.

- Knowing that decreasing sodium intake would have great benefits for health outcomes (reduced hypertension, stroke, heart attacks), but recognizing that individual efforts are difficult due to the use of processed foods, the government partnered with the food industry to cut sodium in breakfast cereals by 57% and bread by 20%, along with many other foods.
- This caused a drop in the population average for sodium intake by 15% over 8 years and a 40% reduction in heart attack deaths and 42% drop in strokes.

IMPLICATIONS FOR COMMUNITY/PUBLIC HEALTH NURSING

There are estimated to be over 47,000 public health nurses working in federal, state, and local public health agencies. A large number of nurses also work in educational community organizations. Together, they strive to promote and protect the health of individuals, families, and populations (Kub, Kulbok, Miner, & Merrill, 2017).

C/PHNs have had to adapt to a constantly changing system. They need the ability to assist their clients in accessing programs and services. Some of your clients may be able to access health care services through your LHD (e.g., immunizations, school physicals, women's health care), but others may need help in finding some type of health insurance to help pay for private health care services. Where do you begin? You will need the following information:

- What type of care is needed (e.g., primary provider, specialist)?
- Who needs the care (e.g., child, older adult, family)?
- Employment/finances (e.g., unemployed/laid off, intermittent or steady employment without health insurance/income level, sources of income)?

See Box 6-6 for online resources for accessing programs and services.

Nurses working within the public health system have developed innovative modes of service delivery (Nolte, 2018).

- One example of an innovative collaborative partnership is the inclusion of PHNs on case conference teams at Indianapolis health centers. The PHNs, with deep knowledge of their communities, help health center staff by following up on patients in their homes, and providing team members with information about available resources. In return, the public health department derives benefits from the health centers promoting population health (Vest et al., 2018).
- C/PHNs have recognized the importance of outcomes research to document the value of nursing interventions with at-risk populations (Christian, 2016; DiClemente, Nowara, Shelton, & Wingood, 2019; Hill, Penrod, & Milone-Nuzzo, 2014). An examination of 20 years of studies that focused on "health education, behavior change, and screening" demonstrated effective outcomes in almost 50%, but limitations included a need to "strengthen methods for documenting effectiveness of PHN practice" (Swider, Levin, & Reising, 2017, p. 324).

BOX 6-6 Online Resources for Accessing Programs and Services

Basic Information on Paying for Medical Care and Prescriptions

- https://www.usa.gov/paying-for-medical
- https://www.verywellhealth.com/how-to-get-help-paying-for-health-insurance-1738500
- https://www.thebalance.com/save-money-health-care-insurance-4124456
- https://www.livestrong.org/we-can-help/insurance-and-financial-assistance/health-care-assistance-for-uninsured

Information Based on Income Levels

- If incomes are low, check for Medicaid and CHIP eligibility at https://www.healthcare.gov/medicaid-chip/getting-medicaid-chip/.
- For those with higher-income levels, check your state's health insurance marketplace at:
  - https://www.healthcare.gov/apply-and-enroll/get-help-applying/
  - https://www.npr.org/sections/health-shots/2020/04/03/826316458/coronavirus-reset-how-to-get-health-insurance-now

Information for Older Adults

- https://www.nia.nih.gov/health/paying-care
- https://www.payingforseniorcare.com/homecare/paying-for-home-care
- https://www.caring.com/senior-living/nursing-homes/how-to-pay/

- The effectiveness of the PHN interventions in Nurse–Family Partnership research is well documented and extends over many years, taking place in many settings. See Chapter 4.

Utilizing collaborative skills and knowledge of their communities, they can work with partners to meet the challenges of Public Health 3.0 and provide services needed for the vulnerable populations in our future health care system (Kulbok, Kub, & Glick, 2017; Swider, Levin, & Kulbok, 2015; Swider et al., 2017).

SUMMARY

- Many factors and events have influenced the current structure, function, and financing of community/public health services. Understanding this background gives the C/PHN a stronger base for planning for population health.
- Historically, health care has progressed unevenly, marked by numerous influences. The Middle Ages saw a serious health decline in Europe, with raging epidemics leading to extensive 19th century reform efforts in England and, later, in the United States.
- Public health problems prompted the gradual development of official interventions. Quarantines to control the spread of communicable disease, sanitary reforms, and establishment of public health departments were discussed.
- By the early 1900s, the federal government had assumed a more active role in public health, with a proliferation of health, education, and welfare services.
- Efforts to address community/public health needs have been made by public agencies and private individuals. They work together to promote an emerging health care system.
  - The public arm includes all government, tax-supported health agencies and occurs at local, state, national, and international levels. A different structure and set of functions are found at each level.
    - Public health services include three core public health functions: assessment, policy development, and assurance.
    - Inadequate funding has been problematic for the public health system, especially during the recent pandemic.
  - Private health services are the unofficial arm. They include voluntary nonprofit agencies as well as privately owned (proprietary) and for-profit agencies. They often supplement and complement the work of official agencies.
- The delivery and financing of community/public health services have been significantly affected by various legislative acts.
  - These include such innovations as health insurance and assistance for people who are poor, elderly, or disabled; money to train health personnel and conduct health research; standards for health planning and delivery; health protection for workers on the job; and the financing of health services.
- Health care economics studies the production, distribution, and consumption of health care goods and services to maximize the use of scarce resources to benefit the most people.
  - The health care system is influenced by microeconomics (supply and demand) as well as macroeconomics.
- Health care is funded through public and private sources, which fall into three categories: third-party payers, direct consumer payment, and private support. Health care services have been reimbursed either retrospectively, typical of FFS plans, or prospectively, typical of most managed care plans.

- Several trends and issues have influenced community/public health care financing and delivery, including cost control, financial access, managed care, health care rationing, competition and regulation, managed competition, universal coverage, calls for a single-payer system, and health care reform.
- The changing nature of health care financing has adversely affected community/public health by promoting incentives to focus on illness care, and the competition model has generated a conflict with the basic public health values of health promotion and disease prevention for all persons.
- Health care reform has reduced the number of uninsured Americans, but access for many people is still difficult.
  - The United States remains the only industrialized nation without some type of universal health coverage.
  - It also ranks significantly lower than most other developed countries on health indicators, such as infant mortality and life expectancy, and we spend the highest percentage of GDP on health care.
- C/PHNs can lead the effort in making health care more accessible to all citizens and encourage policies and practices that promote health. C/PHNs should prepare for future changes in public health.

ACTIVE LEARNING EXERCISES

1. Explain how social, economic (e.g., Great Depression), political (e.g., WWII), and legislative actions have shaped our current health care system, public health system, policies, and practices. Give examples of legislation or policy that incorporates each of the three core public health functions (assessment, policy, and assurance) and identify which of the 10 essential public health services are implicated.
2. Describe an every-day life example of supply and demand. Summarize three exceptions to the law of supply and demand in health care economics. How can this promote rising health care costs? Form two teams and debate the advantages and disadvantages of managed competition as opposed to mandatory universal coverage.
3. Compare the United States with other similar countries. Where do we rank in spending on health care? Identify five measures (e.g., life expectancy) in which the United States has more negative outcomes. What health care system approach, that is common in all other high-income countries, does the U.S. lack? What are the advantages and disadvantages of a single-payer system? Debate with a classmate if further health care reform is feasible in the United States. What is the most efficient way of ensuring universal coverage, as evidenced by examples from other countries outlined in this chapter?
4. Debate the pros and cons of universal health care as outlined by Blumberg and Holahan (2019) at http://thepoint.lww.com/Rector10e. Describe three key potential benefits and the three most serious potential negative consequences. Talk with your classmates and other students at your university about their access to health care and if they have some type of health insurance. If they do not, explore the reasons for this. Does your campus have a student health center? What services are offered there? What are the average costs to students?
5. Interview two consumers about their perception of the problems and strengths of our health care system. What are their thoughts and feelings about our current health care system and availability of health insurance? Have they, or others they know, had problems with health care or health insurance coverage during the pandemic? Select people who represent distinctly different age groups and life situations, such as a single 25-year-old mother of three children making minimum wage and a 75-year-old widower; compare and contrast their responses.

thePoint: Everything You Need to Make the Grade!

thePoint® Visit http://thePoint.lww.com/Rector10e for NCLEX-style review questions, journal articles, supplemental materials, and more!

REFERENCES

Adams, A. (August 4, 2011). *Guidance issued on community health needs assessments for exempt hospitals*. Retrieved from http://www.healthcarereforminsights.com/2011/08/04/guidance-issued-on-community-health-needs-assessments-for-exempt-hospitals/

Administration for Community Living. (April, 2018). *2018 profile of older Americans*. Retrieved from https://acl.gov/sites/default/files/Aging%20and%20Disability%20in%20America/2018OlderAmericansProfile.pdf

Agency for Healthcare Research and Quality. (September, 2019a). *Health care-associated infections*. Retrieved from https://psnet.ahrq.gov/primers/primer/7/health-care-associated-infections

Agency for Healthcare Research and Quality. (2019b). *Patient safety primer: Never events*. Retrieved from https://psnet.ahrq.gov/primers/primer/3/never-events

Altman, S., & Mechanic, R. (July 13, 2018). Cost control: Where do we go from here? *Health Affairs Blog*. Retrieved from https://www.healthaffairs.org/do/10.1377/hblog20180705.24704/full/

America's Health Rankings. (2019). *2018 annual report*. Retrieved from https://www.americashealthrankings.org/learn/reports/2018-annual-report/findings-international-comparison

American Academy of Pediatrics (AAP). (2019). *Understanding the economics of the health care environment*. Retrieved from https://www.aap.org/en-us/

professional-resources/practice-transformation/economics/Pages/health-care-economics.aspx

American Association for Medicare Supplement Insurance. (2020). *Medicare supplement insurance statistics data—2019*. Retrieved from https://medicaresupp.org/medicare-supplement-statistics/

American Hospital Association. (January 4, 2018). *Hospital uncompensated care costs climb in 2016*. Retrieved from https://www.aha.org/news/headline/2018-01-04-hospital-uncompensated-care-costs-climb-2016

American Hospital Association. (2019). *Fast facts on US hospitals, 2019*. Retrieved from https://www.aha.org/statistics/fast-facts-us-hospitals

American Hospital Association (AHA). (2020). *Regulatory overload report: Assessing the regulatory burden on health systems, hospitals, and post-acute care providers*. Retrieved from https://www.aha.org/guidesreports/2017-11-03-regulatory-overload-report

American Public Health Association (APHA). (2019a). *Our history*. Retrieved from https://www.apha.org/about-apha/our-history

American Public Health Association (APHA). (March 11, 2019b). *President's budget would hinder public health programs, says APHA*. Retrieved from https://www.apha.org/news-and-media/news-releases/apha-news-releases/2019/president-budget-proposal

American Public Health Association (APHA). (2020). *Social justice and health*. Retrieved from https://apha.org/what-is-public-health/generation-public-health/our-work/social-justice

Anbazhagan, S. (2016). Role of non-governmental organizations in global health. *International Journal of Community Medicine & Public Health, 3*(1), 17–22.

Anderson, G. F., Hussey, P., & Petrosyan, V. (2019). It's still the prices, stupid: Why the US spends so much on health care, and a tribute to Uwe Reinhardt. *Health Affairs, 38*(1), 87–95.

Arbel, R., & Greenberg, D. (2016). Rethinking cost-effectiveness in the era of zero healthcare spending growth. *International Journal for Equity in Health, 15*, 33. doi: 10.1186/s12939-016-0326-8.

Argawal, R., Mazurenko, O., & Menachemi, N. (2017). High-deductible health plans reduce health care cost and utilization, including use of needed preventive services. *Health Affairs, 36*(10), 1762–1768.

Aron-Dine, A. (November 6, 2019). New research: Medicaid expansion saves lives. *Center on Budget and Policy Priorities*. Retrieved from https://www.cbpp.org/blog/new-research-medicaid-expansion-saves-lives

Arrow, K. (2004). Uncertainty and the welfare economics of medical care. *Bulletin of the World Health Organization, 82*(2), 141–149. Retrieved from http://www.who.int/bulletin/volume/82/2/PHCBP.pdf

Association of Public Health Nurses (APHN). (n.d.). *APHN's history*. Retrieved from http://www.phnurse.org/APHNs-Story

Association of State and Territorial Health Officials (ASTHO). (2017). *ASTHO profile of state public health: Volume four*. Retrieved from https://www.astho.org/Profile/Volume-Four/2016-ASTHO-Profile-of-State-and-Territorial-Public-Health/

Association of State and Territorial Health Officials (ASTHO). (2020). *Data brief: State public health resources and capacity*. Retrieved from https://www.astho.org/Research/Data-and-Analysis/Data-Brief-on-State-Public-Health-Resources-and-Capacity/

Babaloa, O. (2017). Consumers and their demand for healthcare. *Journal of Health & Medical Economics, 3*(1), 6. Retrieved from http://health-medical-economics.imedpub.com/consumers-and-their-demand-for-healthcare.php?aid=21061

Bai, G., & Anderson, G. F. (2016). A more detailed understanding of factors associated with hospital profitability. *Health Affairs, 35*(5), 889–897.

Balio, C., Yeager, V., & Beitsch, L. (2019). Perception of Public Health 3.0: Concordance between public health agency leaders and employees. *Journal of Public Health Management and Practice, 25*, S103–S112. Retrieved from https://journals.lww.com/jphmp/pages/articleviewer.aspx?year=2019&issue=03001&article=00015&type=Fulltext

Bannow, T. (January 6, 2018). Hospital profits, uncompensated care climb. *Modern Healthcare*. Retrieved from https://www.modernhealthcare.com/article/20180106/NEWS/180109940/hospital-profits-uncompensated-care-climb

Bauer, B. (April 6, 2017). SSI vs. SSDI: What are these benefits and how do they differ? *National Council on Aging*. Retrieved from https://www.ncoa.org/blog/ssi-vs-ssdi-what-are-these-benefits-how-they-differ/

Bekemeier, B., Walker Linderman, T., Kneipp, S., & Zahner, S. J. (2015). Updating the definition and role of public health nursing to advance and guide the specialty. *Public Health Nursing, 32*(1), 50–57.

Belk, D. (2019). *Hospital financial analysis: Print section*. Retrieved from http://truecostofhealthcare.org/hospital_financial_analysis/

Benedictow, O. J. (2005). The Black Death: The greatest catastrophe ever. *History Today, 55*(3). Retrieved from https://www.historytoday.com/archive/black-death-greatest-catastrophe-ever

Berchik, E. R., Barnett, J. C., & Upton, R. D. (November, 2019). Health insurance coverage in the United States: 2018. *U.S. Census Bureau*. Retrieved from https://www.census.gov/content/dam/Census/library/publications/2019/demo/p60-267.pdf

Bernard, D., Banthin, J., & Encinosa, W. (2009). Wealth, income, and the affordability of health insurance. *Health Affairs, 28*(3), 887–896.

Bernell, S. (2016). *Health economics: Core concepts and essential tools*. Chicago, IL: Health Administration Press.

Bhatt, C. B., & Beck-Sagué, C. M. (2018). Medicaid expansion and infant mortality in the United States. *American Journal of Public Health, 108*(4), 565–567. doi: 10.2105/AJPH.2017.304218.

Bivins, R. (2007). *Global health in historical perspective: The uses of history*. Retrieved from https://www.cugh.org/sites/default/files/29_Global_Health_In_Historical_Perspective_The_Uses_Of_History_FINAL.pptx__0.pdf

Bloom, D. E., Canning, D., Kotschy, R., Prettner, K., & Schunemann, J. (November, 2018). *Health and economic growth: Reconciling the micro and macro evidence*. IZA Institute of Labor Economics (Discussion Paper No. 11940). Retrieved from http://ftp.iza.org/dp11940.pdf

Blue Cross Blue Shield. (2019). *Leading the way in health insurance*. Retrieved from https://www.bcbs.com/about-us/industry-pioneer

Blumberg, A., & Davidson, A. (October 22, 2009). Accidents of history created U.S. health system. *NPR*. Retrieved from https://www.npr.org/templates/story/story.php?storyId=114045132

Blumenthal, D., & Abrams, M. K. (February 26, 2020). The Affordable Care Act at 10 years: What's changed in health care delivery and payment? *Commonwealth Fund*. Retrieved from https://www.commonwealthfund.org/publications/journal-article/2020/feb/aca-at-10-years-changed-health-care-delivery-payment

Blumenthal, D., Collins, S. R., & Fowler, E. J. (2020). The Affordable Care Act at 10 years—Its coverage and access provisions. *The New England Journal of Medicine, 382*(10), 963–969.

Bowser, R. (2015). Race and rationing. *Health Matrix, 25*(1), 87–107. Retrieved from https://scholarlycommons.law.case.edu/cgi/viewcontent.cgi?article=1019&context=healthmatrix

Bresnick, J. (November 5, 2018). Retail clinics, surprise bills changing healthcare purchasing patterns. *HealthpayerIntelligence*. Retrieved from https://healthpayerintelligence.com/news/retail-clinics-surprise-bills-changing-healthcare-purchasing-patterns

Broaddus, M., & Aron-Dine, A. (2019). Medicaid expansion has saved at least 19,000 lives, new research finds. *Center on Budget and Policy Priorities*. Retrieved from https://www.cbpp.org/research/health/medicaid-expansion-has-saved-at-least-19000-lives-new-research-findsCenter on Budget and policy priorities

Brooks, T. (January 30, 2018). CHIP funding has been extended, What's next for children's health coverage? *Health Affairs Blog*. Retrieved from https://www.healthaffairs.org/do/10.1377/hblog20180130.116879/full/

Brown, A. M., & Nanni, M. B. (2020). Risky business: Recognizing the flaws of employer-based health insurance during COVID-19. *Lerner Center for Public Health Promotion, Syracuse University*. Retrieved from https://lernercenter.syr.edu/2020/04/29/risky-business-recognizing-the-flaws-of-employer-based-health-insurance-during-covid-19/https://lernercenter.syr.edu/2020/04/29/risky-business-recognizing-the-flaws-of-employer-based-health-insurance-during-covid-19/

Bureau of Labor Statistics. (n.d.). *Definitions of health insurance terms*. Retrieved from http://www.bls.gov/ncs/ebs/sp/healthterms.pdf

Cai, C., Runte, J., Ostrer, I., Berry, K., Ponce, N., Rodriguez, M., ... Kahn, J. G. (2020). Projected costs of single-payer healthcare financing in the United States: A systematic review of economic analysis. *PLOS Medicine, 17*(1), e1003013. Retrieved from https://journals.plos.org/plosmedicine/article?id=10.1371/journal.pmed.1003013

California Department of Insurance. (n.d.). *Common health insurance terms*. Retrieved from http://www.insurance.ca.gov/01-consumers/110-health/10-basics/terms.cfm

California Department of Managed Care. (2020). *Your health care rights*. Retrieved from https://www.dmhc.ca.gov/HealthCareinCalifornia/YourHealthCareRights.aspx

Camilleri, S. (2018). The ACA Medicaid expansion, disproportionate share hospitals, and uncompensated care. *Health Services Research, 53*(3), 1562–1580. Retrieved from https://www.ncbi.nlm.nih.gov/pmc/articles/PMC5980407/pdf/HESR-53-1562.pdf

Catlin, C. A., & Howard, A. (November 19, 2015). *History of health spending in the United States: 1960–2013*. Retrieved from https://www.cms.gov/Research-Statistics-Data-and-Systems/Statistics-Trends-and-Reports/NationalHealthExpendData/Downloads/HistoricalNHEPaper.pdf

Center on Budget and Policy Priorities (CBPP). (February 7, 2020a). *Sabotage watch: Tracking efforts to undermine the ACA*. Retrieved from https://www.cbpp.org/sabotage-watch-tracking-efforts-to-undermine-the-aca

Centers for Disease Control and Prevention (CDC). (2013). *United States public health 101*. Retrieved from https://www.cdc.gov/publichealthgateway/docs/usph101.pdf

Centers for Disease Control and Prevention (CDC). (2019). *Resources organized by essential services*. Retrieved from https://www.cdc.gov/nceh/ehs/10-essential-services/resources.html

Centers for Disease Control and Prevention (CDC) (2020). 10 essential public health services. Retrieved from https://www.cdc.gov/publichealthgateway/publichealthservices/essentialhealthservices.html

Centers for Disease Control and Prevention (CDC). (January 17, 2020a). *Novel coronavirus in China*. Retrieved from https://wwwnc.cdc.gov/travel/notices/watch/novel-coronavirus-china

Centers for Disease Control and Prevention (CDC). (2020b). *Public health economics*. Retrieved from https://www.cdc.gov/publichealthgateway/pheconomics/index.html

Centers for Medicare & Medicaid Services (CMS). (2017). *Table of national health expenditures, aggregate and per capita amounts*. Retrieved from https://www.cms.gov/research-statistics-data-and-systems/statistics-trends-and-reports/nationalhealthexpenddata/nhe-fact-sheet.html

Centers for Medicare & Medicaid Services (CMS). (2018a). *Declines in hospital-acquired conditions save 8,000 lives and $2.9 billion in costs*. Retrieved from https://www.cms.gov/newsroom/press-releases/declines-hospital-acquired-conditions-save-8000-lives-and-29-billion-costs

Centers for Medicare & Medicaid Services (CMS). (2018b). *The Center for Consumer Information & Insurance Oversight: Medical loss ratio*. Retrieved from https://www.cms.gov/CCIIO/Programs-and-Initiatives/Health-Insurance-Market-Reforms/Medical-Loss-Ratio

Centers for Medicare & Medicaid Services (CMS). (2019a). *CMS fast facts*. Retrieved from https://www.cms.gov/research-statistics-data-and-systems/statistics-trends-and-reports/cms-fast-facts/index.html

Centers for Medicare & Medicaid Services (CMS). (August 15, 2019b). *CMS is bringing health plan quality ratings to all exchanges for the first time*. Retrieved from https://www.cms.gov/newsroom/press-releases/cms-bringing-health-plan-quality-ratings-all-exchanges-first-time

Centers for Medicare & Medicaid Services (CMS). (2019c). *History: Medicare and Medicaid*. Retrieved from https://www.cms.gov/About-CMS/Agency-information/History/

Centers for Medicare & Medicaid Services (CMS). (2019e). *National health expenditure data: Historical*. Retrieved from https://www.cms.gov/Research-Statistics-Data-and-Systems/Statistics-Trends-and-Reports/NationalHealthExpendData/NationalHealthAccountsHistorical

Centers for Medicare & Medicaid Services (CMS). (2019f). *National health expenditures 2018 highlights*. Retrieved from https://www.cms.gov/files/document/highlights.pdf

Centers for Medicare & Medicaid Services (CMS). (March 5, 2020a). *About the CMS Innovation Center*. Retrieved from https://innovation.cms.gov/about

Centers for Medicare & Medicaid Services (CMS). (2020b). *NHE fact sheet*. Retrieved from https://www.cms.gov/research-statistics-data-and-systems/statistics-trends-and-reports/nationalhealthexpenddata/nhe-fact-sheet

Centers for Medicare & Medicaid Services (CMS). (2020c). *The hospital value-based purchasing (VBP) program*. Retrieved from https://www.cms.gov/Medicare/Quality-Initiatives-Patient-Assessment-Instruments/Value-Based-Programs/HVBP/Hospital-Value-Based-Purchasing

Centers for Medicare and Medicaid Services (CMS). (n.d.a). *Children's health insurance program (CHIP)*. Retrieved from https://www.medicaid.gov/chip/index.html

Centers for Medicare and Medicaid Services (CMS). (n.d.b). *National Health Expenditures 2017 highlights*. Retrieved from https://www.cms.gov/Research-Statistics-Data-and-Systems/Statistics-Trends-and-Reports/NationalHealthExpendData/downloads/highlights.pdf

Centers for Medicare and Medicaid Services (CMS). (n.d.c). *Pre-existing conditions could affect 1 in 2 Americans*. The Center for Consumer Information & Insurance Oversight. Retrieved from https://www.cms.gov/CCIIO/Resources/Forms-Reports-and-Other-Resources/preexisting

Christian, B. J. (2016). Translational research—The value of family-centered care for improving the quality of care for children and their families. *Journal of Pediatric Nursing, 31*(3), 342–345.

Christopher, A. S., Himmelstein, D., Woolhandler, S., & McCormick, D. (2018). The effects of household medical expenditures on income inequality in the United States. *Public Health Policy, 108*(3), 351–354.

Christopher, A. S., McCormick, D., Woolhandler, S., Himmelstein, D. U., Bor, D. H., & Wilper, A. P. (2016). Access to care and chronic disease outcomes among Medicaid-insured persons versus the uninsured. *American Journal of Public Health, 106*(1), 63–69.

Clifton, G. L. (2009). *Flatlined: Resuscitating American medicine*. New Brunswick, NJ: Rutgers University Press.

Cohn, S. K. (2008). Epidemiology of the Black Death and successive waves of plague. *Medical History Supplement, 27*, 74–100.

Collins, S. R., Gunja, M., Doty, M. M., & Beutel, S. (May 20, 2018). Americans' confidence in their ability to pay for health care is falling. *Commonwealth Fund*. Retrieved from https://www.commonwealthfund.org/blog/2018/americans-confidence-their-ability-pay-health-care-falling

Collins, S. R., Rasmussen, P. W., Beutel, S., & Doty, M. M. (May 20, 2015). *The problem of underinsurance and how rising deductibles will make it worse: Findings from the Commonwealth fund biennial health insurance survey, 2014*. Retrieved from http://www.commonwealthfund.org/publications/issue-briefs/2015/may/problem-of-underinsurance

Commonwealth Fund. (2014). *U.S. health system ranks last among eleven countries on measures of access, equity, quality, efficiency, and healthy lives*. Retrieved from http://www.commonwealthfund.org/publications/press-releases/2014/jun/us-health-system-ranks-last

Commonwealth Fund. (February 7, 2019). *Underinsured rate rose from 2014–2018, with greatest growth among people in employer health plans*. Retrieved from https://www.commonwealthfund.org/press-release/2019/underinsured-rate-rose-2014-2018-greatest-growth-among-people-employer-health

Commonwealth Fund. (n.d.). *International health care systems profiles*. Retrieved from https://international.commonwealthfund.org/countries/united_states/

Congressional Research Service. (October 26, 2018). *Medicaid coverage for former foster youth up to age 26*. Retrieved from https://fas.org/sgp/crs/misc/IF11010.pdf

Congressional Research Service. (February 21, 2020). *Block grants: Perspectives and controversies*. Retrieved from https://fas.org/sgp/crs/misc/R40486.pdf

Cox, C., Kamal, R., Jankiewicz, A., & Rousseau, D. (2016). Recent trends in prescription drug costs. *Journal of the American Medical Association, 315*, 1326–1326. doi: 10.1001/jama.2016.2646.

Cramer, G. R., Singh, S. R., Flaherty, S., & Young, G. J. (2017). The progress of US hospitals in addressing community health needs. *American Journal of Public Health, 107*(2), 255–261.

Cubanski, J., Koma, W., Damico, A., & Neuman, T. (2019). *How much do Medicare beneficiaries spend out of pocket on health care*. Retrieved from https://www.kff.org/medicare/issue-brief/how-much-do-medicare-beneficiaries-spend-out-of-pocket-on-health-care/

Cubanski, J., Lyons, B., Neuman, T., Snyder, L., Jankiewicz, A., & Rousseau, D. (2015). Medicaid and Medicare trends and challenges. *Journal of the American Medical Association, 314*, 329–329. doi: 10.1001/jama.2015.8130.

Cubanski, J., Neuman, T., & Freed, M. (2019). The facts on Medicare spending and financing. *Kaiser Family Foundation*. Retrieved from https://www.kff.org/medicare/issue-brief/the-facts-on-medicare-spending-and-financing/

Cutler, D. M. (2018). What is the US health spending problem? *Health Affairs, 37*(3), 493–497.

Cutshaw, C. A., Woolhandler, S., Himmelstein, D. U., & Robertson, C. (2016). Medical causes and consequences of home foreclosures. *International Journal of Health Services, 45*(1), 36–47.

Darvas, Z., Moes, N., Myachenkova, Y., & Pichler, D. (August 23, 2018). *The macroeconomics implications of healthcare*. Retrieved from https://bruegel.org/2018/08/the-macroeconomic-implications-of-healthcare/

Day, B., Himmelstein, D., Broder, M., & Woolhandler, S. (2015). The Affordable Care Act and medical loss ratios: No impact first three years. *International Journal of Health Services, 45*(1), 127–131.

DiClemente, R., Nowara, A., Shelton, R., & Wingood, G. (2019). Need for innovation in public health research. *American Journal of Public Health, 109*(Suppl 2), S117–S120.

DiSalvo, K., Wang, Y. C., Harris, A., Auerbach, J., Koo, D., & Carroll, P. (September 7, 2017). Public health 3.0: A call to action for public health to meet the challenges of the 21st century. *Perspectives: Expert Voices in Health & Health Care. Discussion Paper*. Retrieved from https://nam.edu/wp-content/uploads/2017/09/Public-Health-3.0.pdf

Dobkin, C., Finkelstein, A., Kluender, R., & Notowidigdo, M. J. (2018). Myth and measurement: The case of medical bankruptcies. *New England Journal of Medicine, 378*(12), 1076–1078.

Dobson, A., DaVanzo, J. E., Haught, R., & Phap-Hoa, L. (November 1, 2017). Comparing the Affordable Care Act's financial impact on safety-net hospitals in states that expanded Medicaid and those that did not. *Issue Brief: The Commonwealth Fund*. Retrieved from https://www.commonwealthfund.org/publications/issue-briefs/2017/nov/comparing-affordable-care-acts-financial-impact-safety-net

Doran, T., Maurer, K. A., & Ryan, A. M. (2017). Impact of provider incentives on quality and value of health care. *Annual Review of Public Health, 38*, 449–465.

Dowling, W. L. (1979). Prospective rate setting: Concept and practice. *Topics in Health Care Financing, 3*(2), 35–42.

Downs, B. (2016). *Difference between PPO and POS health insurance*. Retrieved from https://www.bbgbroker.com/difference-between-ppo-pos-health-insurance/

Dranove, D., Gartwaite, C., & Ody, C. (May 3, 2017). Hospitals' uncompensated care burden and the potential effects of repeal. *Issue Brief: The Commonwealth Fund*. Retrieved from https://www.commonwealthfund.org/publications/issue-briefs/2017/may/impact-acas-medicaid-expansion-hospitals-uncompensated-care

Edwards, E., & Dunn, L. (June 30, 2019). Is Germany's health care system a model for the US? *NBC News*. Retrieved from https://www.nbcnews.com/health/health-news/germany-s-health-care-system-model-u-s-n1024491

Eeckhoudt, L., Fiori, A. M., & Gianin, E. R. (2018). Risk aversion, loss aversion, and the demand for insurance. *Risks, 6*, 60.

Einav, L., & Finkelstein, A. (2018). Moral hazard in health insurance: What we know and how we know it. *Journal of the European Economic Association, 16*(4), 957–982.

Enthoven, A. C. (2009a). *Building a health marketplace that works*. Retrieved from http://healthaffairs.org/blog/2009/07/31/building-a-health-marketplace-that-works/

Enthoven, A. C., & Baker, L. C. (2018). With roots in California, managed competition still aims to reform health care. *Health Affairs, 37*(9), 1425–1430.

Erwin, P. C., & Brownson, R. C. (2017a). Macro trends and the future of public health practice. *Annual Review of Public Health, 38*, 393–412. Retrieved from https://www.annualreviews.org/doi/full/10.1146/annurev-publhealth-031816-044224

Erwin, P. C., & Brownson, R. C. (Eds.). (2017b). *Scutchfield and Keck's Principles of public health practice* (4th ed.). Boston, MA: Cengage Learning.

Estes, C. L., Chapman, S. A., Dodd, C., Hollister, B., & Harrington, C. (2013). *Health policy: Crisis and reform* (6th ed.). Sudbury, MA: Jones & Bartlett Publishers.

Fehr, R., & Cox, C. (January 6, 2020). Individual insurance market performance in late 2019. *Kaiser Family Foundation*. Retrieved from https://www.kff.org/private-insurance/issue-brief/individual-insurance-market-performance-in-late-2019/

Feldaus, I., & Mathauer, I. (2018). Effects of mixed provider payment systems and aligned cost sharing practices on expenditure growth management, efficiency, and equity: A structured review of the literature. *BMC Health Services Research, 18*(1), 996.

Fitzgerald, M. P., & Yencha, C. (2019). A test of policy makers' formal and lay theories regarding health care prices. *Journal of Public Policy & Marketing, 38*(1), 3–18.

Frakt, A. B. (July 16, 2018). The astonishingly high administrative costs of US health care. *The New York Times*. Retrieved from https://www.nytimes.com/2018/07/16/upshot/costs-health-care-us.html

Frean, M., Gruber, J., & Sommers, B. D. (2017). Premium subsidies, the mandate, and Medicaid expansion: Coverage effects of the Affordable Care Act. *Journal of Health Economics, 53*, 72–86. doi: 10.1016/j.jhealeco.2017.02.004.

Frieden, T. R. (2015). The future of public health. *New England Journal of Medicine, 373*, 1748–1754. Retrieved from https://www.nejm.org/doi/pdf/10.1056/NEJMsa1511248?articleTools=true

Frommer, R. A. (2018). Efforts to repeal the Patient Protection and Affordable Care Act. *Columbia Medical Review, 2*(1). Retrieved from https://medicalreview.columbia.edu/article/affordable-care-act/

Gabel, J. R., Whitmore, H., Call, A., Green, M., Oran, R., & Stromberg, S. (January 28, 2016). *Modest changes in 2016 health insurance marketplace premiums and insurer participation*. Retrieved from http://www.commonwealthfund.org/publications/blog/2016/jan/2016-health-insurance-marketplace-premiums

Gaffney, A., & Mc Cormick, D. (2017). America: Equity and equality in health 2. The Affordable Care Act: Implications for health-care equity. *The Lancet, 389*, 1442–1452.

Gan, N., Xiong, Y., & Mackintosh, E. (January 20, 2020). China confirms new coronavirus can spread between humans. *CNN*. Retrieved from https://www.cnn.com/2020/01/19/asia/china-coronavirus-spike-intl-hnk/index.html

Garfield, R., Orgera, K., & Damico, A. (January 14, 2020). The coverage gap: Uninsured poor adults in states that do not expand Medicaid. *Kaiser Family Foundation*. Retrieved from https://www.kff.org/medicaid/issue-brief/the-coverage-gap-uninsured-poor-adults-in-states-that-do-not-expand-medicaid/

Garfield, R., Rudowitz, R., & Musumeci, M. (June 27, 2018). Implications of a Medicaid work requirement: National estimates of potential coverage losses. *Kaiser Family Foundation*. Retrieved from https://www.kff.org/medicaid/issue-brief/implications-of-a-medicaid-work-requirement-national-estimates-of-potential-coverage-losses/

Gee, E. (June 26, 2019). The high price of hospital care. *Center for American Progress*. Retrieved from https://www.americanprogress.org/issues/healthcare/reports/2019/06/26/471464/high-price-hospital-care/

Giving USA. (2019). *Giving USA 2019: Americans gave $427.71 billion to charity in 2018 amid complex year for charitable giving*. Retrieved from https://givingusa.org/giving-usa-2019-americans-gave-427-71-billion-to-charity-in-2018-amid-complex-year-for-charitable-giving/

Gladwell, M. (August 29, 2005). The moral-hazard myth. *The New Yorker*. Retrieved from http://www.newyorker.com/archive/2005/08/29/050829fa_fact

Goldsteen, R. L., Goldsteen, K., & Goldsteen, B. Z. (2017). *Jonas' introduction to the US health care system*. New York, NY: Springer Publishing.

Gourzoulidis, G., Kourlaba, G., Stafylas, P., Giamouzis, G., Parissis, J., & Maniadakis, N. (2017). Association between copayment, medication adherence and outcomes in the management of patients with diabetes and heart failure. *Health Policy, 121*(4), 363–377.

Hall, M. A., & McCue, M. J. (July 2, 2019). How the ACA's medical loss ratio rule protects consumers and insurers against ongoing uncertainty. *Commonwealth Fund*. Retrieved from https://www.commonwealthfund.org/publications/issue-briefs/2019/jul/how-aca-medical-loss-ratio-rule-protects-consumers-insurers

Hamel, L., Munana, C., & Brodie, M. (May, 2019). *Kaiser Family Foundation/L.A. Times survey of adults with employer-sponsored health insurance*. Retrieved from http://files.kff.org/attachment/Report-KFF-LA-Times-Survey-of-Adults-with-Employer-Sponsored-Health-Insurance

Hayes, S. L., Collins, S. R., & Radley, D. C. (2019). How much US households with employer insurance spend on premiums and out-of-pocket costs: A state-by-state look. *Commonwealth Fund*. Retrieved from https://www.commonwealthfund.org/publications/issue-briefs/2019/may/how-much-us-households-employer-insurance-spend-premiums-out-of-pocket

Healthcare.gov. (October 23, 2019). *About the affordable care act*. Retrieved from http://www.hhs.gov/healthcare/facts-and-features/key-features-of-aca/index.html

Healthcare.gov. (n.d.a). *Glossary: Community rating*. Retrieved from https://www.healthcare.gov/glossary/community-rating/

Healthcare.gov. (n.d.b). *Glossary: Medical loss ratio (MLR)*. Retrieved from https://www.healthcare.gov/glossary/medical-loss-ratio-mlr/

Healthcare.gov. (n.d.c). *Glossary: Recession*. Retrieved from https://www.healthcare.gov/glossary/rescission/

Healthcare.gov. (n.d.d). *The Children's Health Insurance program (CHIP)*. Retrieved from https://www.healthcare.gov/medicaid-chip/childrens-health-insurance-program/

Heath, S. (September 19, 2017). What is the difference between urgent care and retail health clinics? *Patient Engagement*. Retrieved from https://patientengagementhit.com/news/what-is-the-difference-between-urgent-care-retail-health-clinics

Hero, J. O., Blendon, R. J., Zaslavsky, A. M., & Campbell, A. L. (2016). Understanding what makes Americans dissatisfied with their health care system: An international comparison. *Health Affairs, 35*(3), 502–509.

Hester, J., Auerbach, J., Seeff, L., Wheaton, J., Brusuelas, K., & Singleton, C. (February 8, 2016). *CDC's 6/18 Initiative: Accelerating evidence into action*. Retrieved from https://nam.edu/wp-content/uploads/2016/05/CDCs-618-Initiative-Accelerating-Evidence-into-Action.pdf

Hill, N. L., Penrod, J., & Milone-Nuzzo, P. (2014). Merging person-centered care with translational research to improve the lives of older adults: Creating community-based nursing research networks. *Journal of Gerontological Nursing, 40*(10), 66–74.

Hiltzik, M. (September 4, 2019). Medical bankruptcy is an American scandal that's not debatable. *Los Angeles Times*. Retrieved from https://www.latimes.com/business/story/2019-09-04/hiltzik-medical-bankruptcy-american-scandal

Himmelstein, D. A., Thorne, D., Warren, E., & Woolhandler, S. (2009). Bankruptcy in the US, 2007: Results of a national study. *American Journal of Medicine, 122*(8), 741–746.

Himmelstein, D., & Woolhandler, S. (2016a). Public health's falling share of US health spending. *American Journal of Public Health, 106*(1), 56–57.

Himmelstein, D., & Woolhandler, S. (2016b). The current and projected taxpayer shares of US health costs. *American Journal of Public Health, 106*(3), 449–452.

Hinton, E., Rudowitz, R., Diaz, M., & Singer, N. (2019). 10 things to know about Medicaid managed care. *Kaiser Family Foundation*. Retrieved from https://www.kff.org/medicaid/issue-brief/10-things-to-know-about-medicaid-managed-care

Hoagland, G. W., & Parekh, A. (November 18, 2019). Patient-Centered Outcomes Research Institute: Healthcare's savior? *MedPage Today*. Retrieved from https://www.medpagetoday.com/publichealthpolicy/healthpolicy/83408

Hodgin, S. (July 30, 2018). *Capitation vs. fee-for-service*. Retrieved from http://www.insight-txcin.org/post/capitation-vs-fee-for-service

Hoffer, E. P. (2019a). America's health care system is broken: What went wrong and how we can fix it. Part 2: Health insurance. *The American Journal of Medicine, 132*(7), 791–794.

Hoffer, E. P. (2019b). America's health care system is broken: What went wrong and how we can fix it. Introduction to the series. *The American Journal of Medicine, 132*(7), 675–677.

Holgash, K., & Heberlein, M. (April 10, 2019). Physician acceptance of new Medicaid patients: What matters and what doesn't. *Health Affairs Blog*. Retrieved from https://www.healthaffairs.org/do/10.1377/hblog20190401.678690/full/

Indresano, R. (December 13, 2016). How to rebalance supply–demand scales in healthcare. *Becker's Hospital E-Weekly*. Retrieved from https://www.beckershospitalreview.com/patient-engagement/how-to-rebalance-the-supply–demand-scales-in-healthcare.html

Institute of Medicine (IOM). (2012). *For the public's health: Investing in a healthier future*. Washington, DC: National Academies Press.

Institute of Medicine (IOM). (2013). *U. S. health in international perspective: Shorter lives, poorer health*. Washington, DC: National Academies Press.

InsureKidsNow.gov. (n.d.). *Frequently asked questions*. Retrieved from https://www.insurekidsnow.gov/find-coverage-your-family/frequently-asked-questions/index.html#haveJob

Jaggannathan, M. (May 13, 2019). Most of the profit in health-care industry is going to drug companies: Here's why you should care. *MarketWatch*. Retrieved from https://www.marketwatch.com/story/most-of-the-profit-in-the-health-care-industry-is-going-to-drug-companies-heres-why-you-should-care-2019-05-13

Johnson, S. R. (2019). Report: Public health funding falls despite increasing threats. *Modern Healthcare*. Retrieved from https://www.modernhealthcare.com/government/report-public-health-funding-falls-despite-increasing-threats

Jost, T. S. (August 20, 2019). What do the courts have in store for the ACA? An update on health reform lawsuits. *The Commonwealth Fund*. Retrieved from https://www.commonwealthfund.org/blog/2019/what-do-courts-have-store-aca-update-health-reform-lawsuits

Joszt, L. (August 31, 2018). Percent of employers offering health coverage increases for first time since 2008. *American Journal of Managed Care, In Focus Blog*. Retrieved from https://www.ajmc.com/focus-of-the-week/percent-of-employers-offering-health-coverage-increases-for-first-time-since-2008

Kaiser Family Foundation (KFF). (January, 2012). *Explaining health care reform: How will the Affordable Care Act affect small businesses and their employees?* Retrieved from http://www.kff.org/healtHREForm/upload/8275.pdf

Kaiser Family Foundation (KFF). (2016). *2016 employer health benefits survey*. Retrieved from https://www.kff.org/report-section/ehbs-2016-section-five-market-shares-of-health-plans

Kaiser Family Foundation (KFF). (June 20, 2017). *Medicaid's role in nursing home care*. Retrieved from https://www.kff.org/infographic/medicaids-role-in-nursing-home-care/

Kaiser Family Foundation (KFF). (2018a). *Employer health benefits: 2018 summary of findings*. Retrieved from http://files.kff.org/attachment/Report-Employer-Health-Benefits-Annual-Survey-2018

Kaiser Family Foundation (KFF). (2018b). *Total Medicaid spending*. Retrieved from https://www.kff.org/medicaid/state-indicator/total-medicaid-spending/?currentTimeframe=0&sortModel=%7B%22colId%22:%22Location%22,%22sort%22:%22asc%22%7D

Kaiser Family Foundation (KFF). (2019a). *An overview of Medicare*. Retrieved from https://www.kff.org/medicare/issue-brief/an-overview-of-medicare/

Kaiser Family Foundation (KFF). (2019b). *Employer health benefits annual survey, 2019*. Retrieved from http://files.kff.org/attachment/Report-Employer-Health-Benefits-Annual-Survey-2019

Kaiser Family Foundation (KFF). (2019c). *Health coverage of the total population, 2017*. Retrieved from https://www.kff.org/other/state-indicator/total-population/?currentTimeframe=0&sortModel=%7B%22colId%22:%22Location%22,%22sort%22:%22asc%22%7D

Kaiser Family Foundation (KFF). (2019d). *Key facts about the uninsured population*. Retrieved from http://kff.org/uninsured/fact-sheet/key-facts-about-the-uninsured-population/

Kaiser Family Foundation (KFF). (2019e). *Percent of private sector establishments that offer health insurance to employees, 2018*. Retrieved from https://www.kff.org/other/state-indicator/percent-of-firms-offering-coverage/?currentTimeframe=0&selectedRows=%7B%22wrapups%22:%7B%22united-states%22:%7B%7D%7D%7D&sortModel=%7B%22colId%22:%22Percent%20of%20Firms%20Offering%20Coverage%22,%22sort%22:%22desc%22%7D

Kaiser Family Foundation (KFF). (2019f). *Section 8: High-deductible health plan with savings option. 2019 Employer Health Benefits Survey*. Retrieved from https://www.kff.org/report-section/ehbs-2019-section-8-high-deductible-health-plans-with-savings-option/

Kaiser Family Foundation (KFF). (April 27, 2020). *Status of state Medicaid expansion decisions: Interactive map*. Retrieved from https://www.kff.org/medicaid/issue-brief/status-of-state-medicaid-expansion-decisions-interactive-map/

Kaiser Family Foundation (KFF). (n.d.). *Timeline: History of health reform in the US*. Retrieved from https://www.kff.org/wp-content/uploads/2011/03/5-02-13-history-of-health-reform.pdf

Kaiser Health News. (August 13, 2019). *More patients are getting hit with surprise medical bills, and the price tags are going up, too*. Retrieved from https://khn.org/morning-breakout/more-patients-are-getting-hit-with-surprise-medical-bills-and-the-price-tags-are-going-up-too/

Kamal, R., Cox, C., McDermott, D., Ramirez, M., & Sawyer, B. (March 29, 2019). *US health system is performing better, though still lagging behind other countries*. Retrieved from https://www.healthsystemtracker.org/brief/u-s-health-system-is-performing-better-though-still-lagging-behind-other-countries/

Keith, K. (September 13, 2018). Two new federal surveys show stable uninsured rate. *Health Affairs Blog*. Retrieved from https://www.healthaffairs.org/do/10.1377/hblog20180913.896261/full/

Kesselheim, A. S., Huybrechts, K. F., Choudry, N. K., Fulchino, L. A., Isaman, D. L., Kowal, M. K., & Brennan, T. A. (2015). Prescription drug insurance coverage and patient health outcomes: A systematic review. *American Journal of Public Health, 105*(2), e17–e30.

Khera, R., Valero-Elizondo, J., Okunrintemi, V., Saxena, A., Das, S., de Lemos, J., … Nasir, K. (2018). Association of out-of-pocket annual health expenditures with financial hardship in low-income adults with atherosclerotic cardiovascular disease in the United States. *JAMA Cardiology, 2*(8), 729–738.

Khetpal, V. (October 13, 2017). *We have to ration health care: Medicare for all would be a much better plan if it acknowledged that simple reality*. Retrieved from https://slate.com/technology/2017/10/we-should-ration-health-care.html

Khullar, D., Song, Z., & Choski, D. A. (May 10, 2018). Safety-net health systems at risk: Who bears the burden of uncompensated care? *Health Affairs Blog*. Retrieved from https://www.healthaffairs.org/do/10.1377/hblog20180503.138516/full/

Kinney, E. D. (2013). The Affordable Care Act and the Medicare program: The engines of true health reform. *Yale Journal of Health Policy, Law & Ethics, 13*(2), 253–325.

Kirzinger, A., Muñana, C., Wu, B., & Brodie, M. (2019). Data note: Americans' challenges with health care costs. *Kaiser Family Foundation*. Retrieved from https://www.kff.org/health-costs/issue-brief/data-note-americans-challenges-health-care-costs/

Kisacky, J. (2019). An architectural history of US community hospitals. *AMA Journal of Ethics, 21*(3), e288–e296. Retrieved from https://journalofethics.ama-assn.org/article/architectural-history-us-community-hospitals/2019-03

Knickman, J. R., & Kovner, A. R. (Eds.). (2019). *Jonas & Kovner's health care delivery in the United States* (12th ed.). New York, NY: Springer.

Knowles, M. (2018). *13 statistics on never events*. Retrieved from https://www.beckershospitalreview.com/quality/13-statistics-on-never-events.html

Kramer, L. (June 25, 2019). *How does the law of supply and demand affect prices?* Retrieved from https://www.investopedia.com/ask/answers/033115/how-does-law-supply-and-demand-affect-prices.asp

Krau, S. D. (2015). Foreword. Social justice: A basis for health care delivery. *Nursing Clinics of North America, 50*, xiii-xv. Retrieved from https://www.nursing.theclinics.com/article/S0029-6465(15)00069-9/pdf

Kulbok, P. A., Kub, J., & Glick, D. F. (2017). Cornerstone documents and milestones: The changing landscape of public health nursing 1950–2015. *Online Journal of Issues in Nursing, 22*, 2. Retrieved from http://ojin.nursingworld.org/MainMenuCategories/ANAMarketplace/ANAPeriodicals/OJIN/TableofContents/Vol-22-2017/No2-May-2017/Articles-Previous-Topics/Cornerstone-Documents-Milestones-and-Policies.html

Kyle, M., & Williams, H. (2017). Is American health care uniquely inefficient? Evidence from prescription drugs. *American Economic Review, 107*(5), 486–490.

Laurence, B. K. (2019). *How much in Social Security Disability benefits can you get?* Retrieved from https://www.disabilitysecrets.com/how-much-in-ssd.html

Leider, J. P. (2016). The problem with estimating public health spending. *Journal of Public Health Management & Practice, 22*(2), e1–e11.

Leider, J. P., Castrucci, B. C., Hearne, S., & Russo, P. (2015). Organizational characteristics of large urban health departments. *Journal of Public Health Management & Practice, 221*(Suppl 1), S14–S19.

Leider, J. P., Resnick, B., Bishai, D., & Scutchfield, F. D. (2018). How much do we spend? Creating historical estimates of public health expenditures in the United States at the federal, state, and local levels. *Annual Review of Public Health, 39*, 471–487.

Levit, K. R., Olin, G. L., & Letsch, S. W. (1992). Americans' health insurance coverage, 1980–91. *Medicare & Medicaid Research Review, 14*(1), 31–57.

Lewis, R. A. (1952). *Edwin Chadwick and the public health movement, 1832–1854*. New York, NY: Longman's.

Longest, B. B. (2016). *Health policymaking in the United States* (6th ed.). Chicago, IL: Health Administration Press.

Lovelace, B. (February 28, 2020). WHO raises coronavirus threat assessment to its highest level: 'Wake up, get ready. This virus may be on its way'. *CNBC*. Retrieved from https://www.cnbc.com/2020/02/28/who-raises-risk-assessment-of-coronavirus-to-very-high-at-global-level.html

Manatt, Phelps & Phillips, LLP. (2019). Medicaid's role in children's health. *Robert Wood Johnson Foundation*. Retrieved from https://www.rwjf.org/en/library/research/2019/02/medicaid-s-role-in-children-s-health.html

Manchikanti, L., Helm, S., Benyamin, R. M., & Hirsch, J. A. (March/April, 2017). Evolution of US health care reform. *Pain Physician, 20*, 107–110.

Mankiw, N. G. (July 30, 2017). Why health care policy is so hard: Money and Business/Financial desk]. *New York Times*. Retrieved from https://search-proquest-com.falcon.lib.csub.edu/docview/1924309733?accountid=10345

Masterson, L. (May 25, 2017). *Nonprofit, for-profit hospitals play different roles but see similar financial struggles.* Retrieved from https://www.healthcaredive.com/news/nonprofit-for-profit-hospitals-play-different-roles-but-see-similar-financ/442425/

Mathauer, I., Vinyals Torres, L., Kutzin, J., Jakab, M., & Hanson, K. (2020). Pooling financial resources for universal health coverage: Options for reform. *Bulletin of the World Health Organization, 98*(2), 132–139. doi: 10.2471/BLT.19.234153.

Mather, M., Scommegna, P., & Kilduff, L. (July 15, 2019). Fact sheet: Aging in the United States. *Population Reference Bureau.* Retrieved from https://www.prb.org/aging-unitedstates-fact-sheet/

McClure, W., Enthoven, A. C., & McDonald, T. (July 25, 2017). Universal health coverage. Why? *Health Affairs Blog.* Retrieved from https://www.healthaffairs.org/do/10.1377/hblog20170725.061210/full/

McKillop, C., Waters, T., Kaplan, C. M., Kaplan, E. K., Thompson, M., & Graetz, I. (2018). Three years in—Changing plan features in the U.S. health insurance marketplace. *BMC Health Services Research, 18*, 450.

McNerney, W. J. (1980). Control of health care costs in the 1980s. *New England Journal of Medicine, 303*, 1088–1095.

Medicaid.gov. (2020). *Medicaid.* Retrieved from https://www.medicaid.gov/medicaid/index.html

Medicaid.gov. (n.d.a). *Mandatory & optional Medicaid benefits.* Retrieved from https://www.medicaid.gov/medicaid/benefits/mandatory-optional-medicaid-benefits/index.html

Medicaid.gov. (n.d.b). *Reports and evaluations.* Retrieved from https://www.medicaid.gov/sites/default/files/2019-12/fy-2018-childrens-enrollment-report.pdf

Medicaid and CHIP Payment and Access Commission (MACPAC). (2018). *State Children's Health Insurance Program: Fact sheet.* Retrieved from https://www.macpac.gov/wp-content/uploads/2015/03/State-Childrens-Health-Insurance-Program-Fact-Sheet.pdf

Medicare.gov. (n.d.a). *About Medicare health plans.* Retrieved from https://www.medicare.gov/sign-up-change-plans/medicare-health-plans/medicare-health-plans.html

Medicare.gov. (n.d.c). *Costs in the coverage gap.* Retrieved from https://www.medicare.gov/drug-coverage-part-d/costs-for-medicare-drug-coverage/costs-in-the-coverage-gap

Medicare.gov. (n.d.d). *Catastrophic coverage.* Retrieved from https://www.medicare.gov/drug-coverage-part-d/costs-for-medicare-drug-coverage/catastrophic-coverage

Medicare.gov. (n.d.e). *Medicare costs at a glance.* Retrieved from https://www.medicare.gov/your-medicare-costs/medicare-costs-at-a-glance

Medicare.gov. (n.d.f). *Monthly premium for drug plans.* Retrieved from https://www.medicare.gov/drug-coverage-part-d/costs-for-medicare-drug-coverage/monthly-premium-for-drug-plans

Medicare.gov. (n.d.g). *What's Medicare Supplement Insurance (Medigap)?* Retrieved from https://www.medicare.gov/supplements-other-insurance/whats-medicare-supplement-insurance-medigap

Medicare.gov. (n.d.h). *Yearly deductible for drug plans.* Retrieved from https://www.medicare.gov/drug-coverage-part-d/costs-for-medicare-drug-coverage/yearly-deductible-for-drug-plans

MedicareAdvantage.com. (2020). *Understanding the Medicare donut hole.* Retrieved from https://www.medicareadvantage.com/resources/medicare-donut-hole

Melnick, G. A., Shen, Y., & Wu, V. Y. (2011). The increased concentration of health plan markets can benefit consumers through lower hospital prices. *Health Affairs, 30*(9), 1728–1733.

Mendelson, D. (January 29, 2019). Are health plans the future of public health? *Forbes.* Retrieved from https://www.forbes.com/sites/danielmendelson/2019/01/29/are-health-plans-the-future-of-public-health/#38178938318c

Meyer, H. (March 12, 2016). Why consumer-based approaches are no panacea for US healthcare. *Modern Healthcare.* Retrieved from https://www.modernhealthcare.com/article/20160312/MAGAZINE/303129963/why-consumer-based-approaches-are-no-panacea-for-u-s-healthcare

Miller, M. (September 5, 2018). What are non-profit health insurance companies? *FirstQuote Health.* Retrieved from https://www.firstquotehealth.com/health-insurance-news/non-profit-health-insurance

Mitchell, A. (2018). Federal financing for the State Children's Health Insurance program (CHIP). *Congressional Research Service.* Retrieved from https://fas.org/sgp/crs/misc/R43949.pdf

Morelli, B. A. (August 16, 2016). Fact checker: Free market exposure would control health care costs. *The Gazette.* Retrieved from https://www.thegazette.com/subject/news/government/fact-check/fact-checker-free-market-exposure-would-control-health-care-costs-20160826

Mossialos, E., Wenzl, M., Osborn, R., & Sarnak, D. (2016). 2015 international profiles of health care systems. *Commonwealth Fund.* Retrieved from http://www.commonwealthfund.org/~/media/files/publications/fund-report/2016/jan/1857_mossialos_intl_profiles_2015_v7.pdf

Murphy, D. (May 12, 2017). Health insurance coverage improves child well-being. *Child Trends.* Retrieved from https://www.childtrends.org/publications/health-insurance-coverage-improves-child-well

Musumeci, M. (February 16, 2017). *Medicaid's role for Medicare beneficiaries.* Retrieved from https://www.kff.org/medicaid/issue-brief/medicaids-role-for-medicare-beneficiaries/

National Academies of Sciences, Engineering, and Medicine. (2017). *Communities in action: Pathways to health equity in the United States.* Washington, DC: National Academies Press.

National Academies Press. (2020). *Publications.* Retrieved from https://www.nap.edu/search/?rpp=20&ft=1&term=public+health+reports

National Association of County and City Health Officials (NACCHO). (2017). *2016 National profile of local health departments.* Retrieved from http://nacchoprofilestudy.org/wp-content/uploads/2017/10/ProfileReport_Aug2017_final.pdf

National Association of Health Underwriters (NAHU). (June, 2015). *Healthcare cost drivers: White paper.* Retrieved from https://nahu.org/media/1147/healthcarecost-driverswhitepaper.pdf

National Center for Health Statistics. (2015). *Percentage of U.S. adults 65 and over with one or more chronic conditions.* Retrieved from https://www.cdc.gov/nchs/health_policy/adult_chronic_conditions.htm

National Conference of State Legislatures (NCSL). (2020). *Health savings accounts.* Retrieved from https://www.ncsl.org/research/health/hsas-health-savings-accounts.aspx.

National Conference of State Legislatures. (2017). *Managed care, market reports and the States.* Retrieved from https://www.ncsl.org/research/health/managed-care-and-the-states.aspx

National Council on Aging. (n.d.). *What are Medicare Part C costs?* Retrieved from https://www.mymedicarematters.org/costs/part-c/

National Institutes of Health (NIH). (2017). *Office of History: Legislative chronology.* Retrieved from https://history.nih.gov/research/sources_legislative_chronology.html

National Institutes of Health (NIH). (2019). *Who we are.* Retrieved from https://www.nih.gov/about-nih/who-we-are

National Philanthropic Trust. (2018). *Leadership and mission.* Retrieved from https://www.nptrust.org/about-us/leadership/

Nicholson, W., & Snyder, C. (2017). *Microeconomic theory: Basic principles and extensions* (12th ed.). Boston, MA: Cengage Learning.

Nickitas, D. M., Middaugh, D. J., & Feeg, V. D. (Eds.). (2020). *Policy and politics for nurses and other health professionals: Advocacy and action* (3rd ed.). Burlington, MA: Jones & Bartlett Publishers.

Nolte, E. (2018). *How do we ensure that innovation in health service delivery and organization is implemented, sustained and spread?* World Health Organization. Policy Brief. Retrieved from http://www.euro.who.int/__data/assets/pdf_file/0004/380731/pb-tallinn-03-eng.pdf?ua=1

Nurse.org. (2019). *List of nursing organizations.* Retrieved from https://nurse.org/orgs.shtml

Office of Disease Prevention & Health Promotion (ODPHP). (2019). *Healthy People 2030 framework.* Retrieved from https://www.healthypeople.gov/2020/About-Healthy-People/Development-Healthy-People-2030/Framework

Organization for Economic Cooperation and Development (OECD). (2019). *Health for everyone? Social inequalities in health and health systems. Executive summary.* Retrieved from https://www.oecd-ilibrary.org/docserver/3c8385d0-en.pdf?expires=1588722920&id=id&accname=guest&checksum=4472A0DEAAF641AE601C47EB5C5B97BD

Owen, L., Pennington, B., Fischer, A., & Jeong, K. (2019). The cost-effectiveness of public health interventions examined by NICE from 2011 to 2016. *Journal of Public Health, 40*(3), 557–566.

Paradise, J., Lyons, B., & Rowland, D. (May 6, 2015). *Medicaid at 50.* Retrieved from http://kff.org/medicaid/report/medicaid-at-50/

Patient-Centered Outcomes Research Institute (PCORI). (March 29, 2017). *Our programs.* Retrieved from https://www.pcori.org/about-us/our-programs

Patient Safety Network. (2019). *Never events.* Retrieved from https://psnet.ahrq.gov/primer/never-events

Pearl, R. (February 2, 2017). Why healthcare rationing is a growing reality for Americans. *Forbes.* Retrieved from https://www.forbes.com/sites/robertpearl/2017/02/02/why-healthcare-rationing-is-a-growing-reality-for-americans/#546a2182dbad

Penn, J., MacKinnon, N. J., Strakowski, S. M., Ying, J., & Doty, M. M. (2017). Minding the gap: Factors associated with primary care coordination of adults in 11 countries. *Annals of Family Medicine, 15*(2), 113–119.

Perkins, B. B. (1998). Economic organization of medicine and the Committee on the Costs of Medical Care. *American Journal of Public Health, 88*(11), 1721–1726.

Perkins, B. B. (1998). Economic organization of medicine and the Committee on the Costs of Medical Care. *American Journal of Public Health, 88*(11), 1721–1726.

Perry, M. J. (March 16, 2017). What economic lessons about health care costs can we learn from the competitive market for cosmetic procedures? *Carpe Diem: American Enterprise Institute*. Retrieved from http://www.aei.org/publication/what-economic-lessons-about-health-care-costs-can-we-learn-from-the-competitive-market-for-cosmetic-procedures-2/

Physicians for a National Health Program. (2020a). *Does the U.S. ration health care?* Retrieved from https://pnhp.org/2016/08/01/does-the-u-s-ration-health-care/

Physicians for a National Health Program. (2020b). *Single payer vs. universal public coverage through managed competition*. Retrieved from https://pnhp.org/news/single-payer-vs-universal-public-coverage-through-managed-competition/

Pollitz, K. (2016). Surprise medical bills. *Kaiser Family Foundation*. Retrieved from https://www.kff.org/private-insurance/issue-brief/surprise-medical-bills/

Pross, C., Geissler, A., & Busse, R. (2017). Measuring, reporting, and rewarding quality of care in 5 nations: 5 policy levels to enhance hospital quality accountability. *Milbank Quarterly, 95*(1), 136–183.

Public Agenda. (February 5, 2020). *Taking the pulse: Where Americans agree on improving health care*. Retrieved from https://www.publicagenda.org/reports/taking-the-pulse-where-americans-agree-on-improving-health-care

Public Health Accreditation Board (PHAB). (2020). *Who is accredited?* Retrieved from https://phaboard.org/who-is-accredited/

Public Health Law Center. (n.d.). *State and local public health: An overview of regulatory authority*. Retrieved from https://www.publichealthlawcenter.org/sites/default/files/resources/phlc-fs-state-local-reg-authority-publichealth-2015_0.pdf

QSEN Institute. (2020). *Project overview: The evolution of the Quality and Safety Education for Nurses (QSEN) initiative*. Retrieved from https://qsen.org/about-qsen/project-overview/

Quad Council Coalition Competency Review Task Force. (2018). *Community/Public Health Nursing Competencies*. Retrieved from http://www.quadcouncilphn.org/wp-content/uploads/2018/05/QCC-C-PHN-COMPETENCIES-Approved_2018.05.04_Final-002.pdf

Rambur, B. (2015). *Health care finance, economics, and policy for nurses: A foundational guide*. New York, NY: Springer Publishing.

Resnick, B., Morlock, L., Diener-West, M., Stuart, E., Spencer, M., & Sharfstein, J. M. (2019). PH WINS and the future of public health education. *Journal of Public Health Management, 25*, S10–S12. Retrieved from https://journals.lww.com/jphmp/pages/articleviewer.aspx?year=2019&issue=03001&article=00004&type=Fulltext

Rice University. (2017). *How the AD/AS model incorporates growth, unemployment, and inflation*. Retrieved from http://cnx.org/contents/zJqU35Tm@5/How-the-ADAS-Model-Incorporate

Richardson, B. W. (1887). *The health of nations: A review of the works of Edwin Chadwick* (Vol. 2). London, UK: Longmans, Green.

Rook, D. (August 17, 2015). *How we got to now: A brief history of employer-sponsored healthcare*. Retrieved from http://www.griffinbenefits.com/employeebenefitsblog/history-of-employer-sponsored-healthcare

Rosen, G. (2015). *A history of public health* (rev. expanded ed.). Baltimore, MD: Johns Hopkins University Press.

Rose-Jacobs, R., Ettinger de Cuba, S., Bovell-Ammon, A., Black, M. M., Coleman, S. M., Cutts, D., ... Sandel, M. (2019). Housing instability among families with young children with special health care needs. *Pediatrics, 144*(2), e20181704. doi: 10.542/peds.2018-1704.

Rosoff, P. M. (2014). *Rationing is not a four-letter word: Setting limits on healthcare*. Cambridge, MA: The MIT Press.

Ross, S. (October 13, 2018). *Microeconomics vs. macroeconomics investments*. Retrieved from https://www.investopedia.com/articles/investing/052616/microeconomics-vs-macroeconomics-which-more-useful-investment.asp

Rothbaum, J., & Edwards, A. (September 10, 2019). U.S. median household income was $63,179 in 2018, not significantly different from 2017. *U.S. Census Bureau*. Retrieved from https://www.census.gov/library/stories/2019/09/us-median-household-income-not-significantly-different-from-2017.html

Rudowitz, R., Garfield, R., & Hinton, E. (2019). 10 things to know about Medicaid: Setting the facts straight. *Kaiser Family Foundation*. Retrieved from https://www.kff.org/medicaid/issue-brief/10-things-to-know-about-medicaid-setting-the-facts-straight/

Rudowitz, R., Orgera, K., & Hinton, E. (2019). Medicaid financing: The basics. *Kaiser Family Foundation*. Retrieved from https://www.kff.org/report-section/medicaid-financing-the-basics-issue-brief

Saving.org. (2020). *Value of $5 by year*. Retrieved from https://www.saving.org/inflation/inflation.php?amount=5

Schneider, A. (2019). Medicaid and state budgets: Checking the facts (yet again). *Georgetown University Health Policy Institute*. Retrieved from https://ccf.georgetown.edu/2019/02/28/medicaid-and-state-budgets-checking-the-facts-yet-again/

Schneider, E. C., Sarnak, D. O., Squires, D., Shah, A., & Doty, M. M. (July, 2017). Mirror, mirror 2017: International comparison reflects flaws and opportunities for better U.S. health care. *Commonwealth Fund*. Retrieved from https://interactives.commonwealthfund.org/2017/july/mirror-mirror/assets/Schneider_mirror_mirror_2017.pdf

Schoen, C., & Collins, S. (December 4, 2017). The big five health insurers' membership and revenue trends: Implications for public policy. *Commonwealth Fund*. Retrieved from https://www.commonwealthfund.org/publications/journal-article/2017/dec/big-five-health-insurers-membership-and-revenue-trends

Schoen, C., & Solis-Roman, C. (May 10, 2016). On Medicare but at risk: A state-level analysis of beneficiaries who are underinsured or facing high total cost burdens. *Commonwealth Fund*. Retrieved from https://www.commonwealthfund.org/publications/issue-briefs/2016/may/medicare-risk-state-level-analysis-beneficiaries-who-are

Schuchat, A. (May 1, 2020). *Public health response to the initiation and spread of pandemic COVID-19 in the United States, February 24-April 21, 2020*. Retrieved from https://www.cdc.gov/mmwr/volumes/69/wr/mm6918e2.htm

Shaw, F., Asomugha, C., Conway, P., & Rein, A. (2014). The patient protection and affordable care act: Opportunities for prevention and public health. *Lancet, 384*(9937), 75–82. Retrieved from https://www.thelancet.com/journals/lancet/article/PIIS0140-6736(14)60259-2/fulltext

Shi, L., & Singh, D. (2019). *Essentials of the U.S. health care system* (5th ed.). Burlington, MA: Jones & Bartlett.

Simmons-Duffin, S. (October 14, 2019). *Trump is trying hard to thwart Obamacare. How's that going?* Retrieved from https://www.npr.org/sections/health-shots/2019/10/14/768731628/trump-is-trying-hard-to-thwart-obamacare-hows-that-going

Smith, L., Atherly, A., Campbell, J., Flattery, N., Coronel, S., & Krantz, S. (2019). Cost-effectiveness of a statewide public health intervention to reduce cardiovascular disease risk. *BMC Public Health, 19*, 1234. Retrieved from https://bmcpublichealth.biomedcentral.com/track/pdf/10.1186/s12889-019-7573-8

Smith, P. C., & Yip, W. (2016). The economics of health system design. *Oxford Review of Economic Policy, 32*(1), 21–40.

Social Security Administration (SSA). (November, 2019). *Medicare*. Publication No. 095–10043. Retrieved from https://www.ssa.gov/pubs/EN-05-10043.pdf

Social Security Administration (SSA). (2020). *A guide to Supplemental Security Income (SSI) for groups and organizations*. Retrieved from https://www.ssa.gov/pubs/EN-05-11015.pdf

Social Security Administration (SSA). (n.d.a). *Historical background and development of Social Security*. Retrieved from http://www.ssa.gov/history/briefhistory3.html

Social Security Administration (SSA). (n.d.b). *SSI Federal payment amounts for 2020*. Retrieved from https://www.ssa.gov/oact/cola/SSI.html

Sommers, B. D., Blendon, R. J., & Orav, E. J. (2016). Both the 'private option' and traditional Medicaid expansions improved access to care for low-income adults. *Health Affairs, 35*, 96–105. doi: 10.1377/hlthaff.2015.0917.

Sonfield, A., Frost, J. J., Dawson, R., & Lindberg, L. D. (August 3, 2020). COVID-19 job losses threaten insurance coverage and access to reproductive health care for millions. *Health Affairs Blog*. Retrieved from https://www.healthaffairs.org/do/10.1377/hblog20200728.779022/full/

St. John, A. (May 2, 2017). How the Affordable Care Act drove down personal bankruptcy. *Consumer Reports*. Retrieved from https://www.consumerreports.org/personal-bankruptcy/how-the-aca-drove-down-personal-bankruptcy/

State of California. (2017). *Annual health care complaint data report to the legislature, measurement year 2017*. Retrieved from https://www.opa.ca.gov/ComplaintsReports/Documents/ComplaintDataReport-2017.pdf

Swider, S. M., Levin, P. F., & Kulbok, P. A. (2015). Creating the future of public health nursing: A call to action. *Public Health Nursing, 32*(2), 91–93.

Swider, S. M., Levin, P. F., & Reising, V. (2017). Evidence of public health nursing effectiveness: A realist review. *Public Health Nursing, 34*(4), 324–334.

Tanner, J. (December 9, 2015). *Reducing maternal and child mortality—What does the evidence show?* Retrieved from https://ieg.worldbankgroup.org/blog/reducing-maternal-and-child-mortality-what-does-evidence-show

Taylor, E. A., Carman, K. G., Lopez, A., Muchow, A., Roshan, P., & Eibner, C. (2016). Consumer decision making in the health care marketplace. *Rand Corporation*. Retrieved from https://www.rand.org/pubs/research_reports/RR1567.html

Taylor, S. (January 5, 2018). *Reversing the decline of public health nurse retention and recruitment in California, 2017*. Campaign for Action. Retrieved from https://campaignforaction.org/resource/reversing-decline-public-health-nurse-retention-recruitment-california-2017/

Tikkanen, R., & Osborn, R. (July 11, 2019). Does the United States ration health care? *Commonwealth Fund*. Retrieved from https://www.commonwealthfund.org/blog/2019/does-united-states-ration-health-care

Tolbert, J., Orgera, K., Singer, N., & Damico, A. (December, 2019). Key facts about the uninsured population. *Kaiser Family Foundation*. Retrieved from http://files.kff.org/attachment/Issue-Brief-Key-Facts-about-the-Uninsured-Population

Torrey, T. (2020). *Understanding healthcare reimbursement*. Retrieved from https://www.verywellhealth.com/reimbursement-2615205

Tozzi, J. (October 8, 2018). Employees' share of health costs continues rising faster than wages. *Insurance Journal*. Retrieved from https://www.insurancejournal.com/news/national/2018/10/08/503575.htm

Troy, T. D. (2015). How the government as a payer shapes the health care marketplace. *American Health Policy Institute*. Retrieved from http://www.americanhealthpolicy.org/Content/documents/resources/Government_as_Payer_12012015.pdf

Trust for America's Health (TFAH). (2019). *The impact of chronic underfunding on America's public health system: Trends, risks, and recommendations, 2019*. Washington, DC: Author.

Trust for America's Health (TFAH). (2020). *Ten top priorities for prevention*. Retrieved from https://www.tfah.org/report-details/ten-top-priorities-for-prevention/

Turnock, B. J. (2016a). *Essentials of public health* (3rd ed.). Sudbury, MA: Jones & Bartlett Learning.

Turnock, B. J. (2016b). *Public health: What it is and how it works* (6th ed.). Sudbury, MA: Jones & Bartlett Learning.

United States Courts. (March 7, 2018). Just the facts: Consumer bankruptcy filings, 2006–2017. *Administrative Office of the U.S. Courts*. Retrieved from https://www.uscourts.gov/news/2018/03/07/just-facts-consumer-bankruptcy-filings-2006-2017

Urban Institute & Virginia Commonwealth University. (April, 2015). *How are income and wealth linked to health and longevity?* Retrieved from https://www.urban.org/sites/default/files/publication/49116/2000178-How-are-Income-and-Wealth-Linked-to-Health-and-Longevity.pdf

U.S. Census Bureau. (2015). *Comparison of the prevalence of uninsured persons from the National Health Interview Survey and the Current Population Survey: January–April 2014*. Retrieved from https://www.cdc.gov/nchs/data/nhis/health_insurance/NCHS_CPS_Comparison092014.pdf

U.S. Census Bureau. (September 16, 2010). *Income, poverty and health insurance coverage in the United States: Summary of key findings*. Retrieved from http://www.census.gov/newsroom/releases/archives/income_wealth/cb10-144.html

U.S. Department of Health & Human Services (USDHHS). (2015). *HHS agencies and offices*. Retrieved from https://www.hhs.gov/about/agencies/hhs-agencies-and-offices/index.html

U.S. Department of Health & Human Services (USDHHS). (2020a). *About Healthy People*. Retrieved from http://www.healthypeople.gov/2020/about/default.aspx

U.S. Department of Health & Human Services (USDHHS). (2020b). *HHS Organizational Chart: HHS Agencies & Offices*. Retrieved from http://www.hhs.gov/about/agencies/hhs-agencies-and-offices/index.html

U.S. Department of Health & Human Services (USDHHS). (n.d.a). *Commissioned Corps of the U.S. Public Health Service: HHS offices and agencies*. Retrieved from https://www.usphs.gov/aboutus/agencies/hhs.aspx

U.S. Department of Health & Human Services (USDHHS). (n.d.b). *Public health 3.0: A call to action to create a 21st century public health infrastructure*. Retrieved from https://www.healthypeople.gov/sites/default/files/Public-Health-3.0-White-Paper.pdf?_ga=2.107795010.1356578261.1588809470-1969978574.1588809470

U.S. Department of Health & Human Services (USDHHS). (n.d.c). *HHS offices and agencies*. Retrieved from https://www.usphs.gov/aboutus/agencies/hhs.aspx

U.S. Department of Health & Human Services (USDHHS). (n.d.d). *Non-HHS agencies and programs*. Retrieved from https://www.usphs.gov/aboutus/agencies/non-hhs.aspx

U.S. Department of Justice. (2018). *Prime Healthcare Services and its CEO agree to pay $65 million to settle Medicare overbilling allegations at 14 California hospitals*. Retrieved from https://www.justice.gov/usao-cdca/pr/prime-healthcare-services-and-its-ceo-agree-pay-65-million-settle-medicare-overbilling

U.S. Department of Justice. (2019). *Federal health care fraud takedown in Northeastern U.S. results in charges against 48 individuals*. Retrieved from https://www.justice.gov/opa/pr/federal-health-care-fraud-takedown-northeastern-us-results-charges-against-48-individuals

U.S. Department of State. (n.d.). *Non-governmental organizations (NGOs) in the United States*. Retrieved from https://www.state.gov/non-governmental-organizations-ngos-in-the-united-states/

U.S. Office of Personal Management. (n.d.a). *Fast facts: High deductible health plans (HDHP)*. Retrieved from https://www.opm.gov/healthcare-insurance/fastfacts/high-deductible-health-plans.pdf

U.S. Office of Personal Management. (n.d.b). *Health savings accounts*. Retrieved from https://www.opm.gov/healthcare-insurance/healthcare/health-savings-accounts/

van Hedel, K., Avendano, M., Berkman, L., Bopp, M., Deboosere, P., Lundberg, O., ... Mackenbach, J. P. (2015). The contribution of national disparities to international differences in mortality between the United States and 7 European countries. *American Journal of Public Health, 105*(4), e112–e119.

Vest, J. R., Caine, V., Harris, L., Watson, D. P., Menachemi, N., & Halverson, P. (2018). Fostering local health department and health system collaboration through case conferences for at-risk and vulnerable populations. *American Journal of Public Health, 108*(5), 649–651.

Wahowiak, L. (2017). Community needs assessments leading to better outcomes: ACA requirement fortifying health. *The Nation's Health, 47*(4), 1–8. Retrieved from http://thenationshealth.aphapublications.org/content/47/4/1.4

Walsh, K. (2014). Medical education: Microeconomics or macroeconomics? *Pan African Medical Journal, 18*, 11.

Weber, L., Ungar, L., Smith, M. R., Recht, H., & Barry-Jester, A. M. (July 1, 2020). Hollowed-out public health system faces more cuts amid virus. *Kaiser Health News*. Retrieved from https://khn.org/news/us-public-health-system-underfunded-under-threat-faces-more-cuts-amid-covid-pandemic/

Witters, D. (January 23, 2019). *US uninsured rate rises to four-year high*. Retrieved from https://news.gallup.com/poll/246134/uninsured-rate-rises-four-year-high.aspx

Wolfe, I. D., & Pope, T. M. (2020). Hospital mergers and conscience-based objections—Growing threats to access and quality of care. *New England Journal of Medicine, 382*, 1388–1389. doi: 10.1056/NEJMp1917047.

Woodworth, L., Romano, P. S., & Holmes, J. F. (2017). Does insurance status influence a patient's hospital charge? *Applied Health Economics and Health Policy, 15*, 353–362.

Woolhandler, D., & Himmelstein, D. U. (2017). The Obama years: Tepid palliation for America's health scourges. *American Journal of Public Health, 107*(1), 22–24.

World Health Organization (WHO). (2020). *About WHO*. Retrieved from https://www.who.int/about

World Travel & Tourism Council. (2020). *Economic impact reports*. Retrieved from https://wttc.org/Research/Economic-Impact

Yale School of Public Health. (2019). *NGOs and nonprofits*. Retrieved from https://publichealth.yale.edu/career/toolkit/resources/ngos/

Young, K. M., & Kroth, P. J. (2018). *Sultz & Young's health care USA: Understanding its organization and delivery* (9th ed.). Burlington, MA: Jones & Bartlett Learning.

Zallman, L., Wilson, F. A., Stimpson, J. P., Bearse, A., Arsenault, L., Dube, B., ... Woolhandler, S. (2016). Unauthorized immigrants prolong the life of Medicare's Trust Fund. *Journal of General Internal Medicine, 31*(1), 122–127.

Zamosky, L. (November 20, 2015). Healthcare watch: EPO? Health plans tightly restrict doctors that patients can see. *Los Angeles Times*. Retrieved from https://www.latimes.com/business/la-fi-healthcare-watch-20151120-story.html

Zhao, G., Okoro, C. A., Li, J., & Town, M. (2018). Health insurance status and clinical cancer screenings among US adults. *American Journal of Preventive Medicine, 54*(1), e11–e19.

CHAPTER 7

Epidemiology in the Community

"Epidemiology dates back to the Age of Pericles in 5th Century B.C., but its standing as a 'true' science in 21st century is often questioned. This is unexpected, given that epidemiology directly impacts lives and our reliance on it will only increase in a changing world" (p. 1).

—Epidemiology is a science of high importance [Editorial]. (2018). *Nature Communications, 9*(1703), 1–2.

KEY TERMS

Association
Causal matrix
Causality
Chain of causation
Epidemic
Epidemiologic triangle
Epidemiology
Immunity
Incidence
Morbidity rate
Mortality rate
Natural history
Nosology
Pandemic
Prevalence
Reservoir
Risk
Vectors
Web of causation

LEARNING OBJECTIVES

Upon mastery of this chapter, you should be able to:

1. Discuss key highlights of the history of epidemiology.
2. Apply the epidemiologic triangle (host, agent, and environment model) to a common public health problem.
3. Describe theories of causality in health and illness.
4. Define immunity and compare and contrast passive, active, cross-, and herd immunity.
5. Explain how epidemiologists determine populations at risk.
6. Identify the four stages of a disease or health condition.
7. Describe sources of information for epidemiologic study, including existing data, informational observational studies, and scientific studies.
8. Discuss the types of epidemiologic studies that are useful for researching aggregate health and the process for conducting epidemiologic research.

INTRODUCTION

Epidemiology is the scientific discipline that seeks to describe, quantify, and determine how diseases occur in populations and aid in developing methods of controlling those diseases (Friis, 2018). The term is derived from the "Greek words *epi* (upon), *demos* (the people), and *logy* (study of)"; the knowledge or study of what happens to people (Friis, 2018, p. 6).

Purposes of epidemiology include the following:

- To examine determinants and distribution of diseases, disabilities, morbidity, and mortality, as well as health
- To provide a body of knowledge through research on which to base practice and methods for studying new and existing problems
- To provide C/PHNs with a methodology for assessing the health of aggregates
- To offer a frame of reference for investigating and improving clinical practice in any setting

Characteristics of epidemiology include the following:

- Is data driven
- Relies on an unbiased and systematic approach to collecting, analyzing, and interpreting data

- Draws on methods and principles from biostatistics, informatics, biology, and the social, economic, and behavioral sciences

Epidemiologists are considered "disease detectives" as they search for causes of illness and outbreak (Centers for Disease Control and Prevention [CDC], 2016, para. 1). Epidemiologists ask such questions as:

- What is the occurrence of health and disease in a population?
- Has there been an increase or decrease in a health state over the years?
- Does one geographic area have a higher frequency of disease than another?
- What characteristics of people with a particular condition distinguish them from those without the condition?
- What factors need to be present to cause disease or injury?
- Is one treatment or program more effective than another in changing the health of affected people?
- Why do some people recover from a disease and others do not?

As an example of epidemiology serving as a frame of reference, imagine that a county health department public health nurse's (PHN's) goal is to lower the incidence of sexually transmitted diseases (also referred to as sexually transmitted infections [STIs]) in a given community. Such a prevention plan would require information about population groups. The nurse would need to ask questions such as:

- How many STD cases have been reported in this community over the past year? What percentage of these are drug resistant (e.g., drug-resistant gonorrhea)?
- What is the expected number of STD cases (the morbidity rate)?
- Which members of the community are at highest risk of contracting STDs?

In fact, to be effective, any program of screening, treatment, or health promotion regarding STDs must be based on this kind of information about population groups.

Whether the PHN's goals are to improve a population's nutrition, control the spread of tuberculosis (TB), deal with health problems created by a flood, protect and promote the health of battered women, or reduce the number of automobile crash injuries and fatalities at a specific intersection, epidemiologic data are essential.

HOW EPIDEMIOLOGY SUPPORTS THE TEN ESSENTIALS OF PUBLIC HEALTH SERVICES

- Assessment
  - *Monitor Health:* by gathering vital and disease statistics, provides data necessary to define the scope of disease and health and visually trend disease spread
  - *Diagnose and Investigate:* by providing population health and disease data to determine whether new diseases are spreading into new segments of the population and providing the basis for launching epidemiologic investigations
- Policy Development
  - *Inform, Educate, and Empower:* by providing statistical reports of the status of disease spread, investigations, and their progress so policy makers can inform and educate the public about health factors and empower the public to address them
  - *Mobilize Community Partnerships:* by sharing community epidemiologic data so stakeholders can collaborate in addressing health issues that affect their constituents
  - *Develop Policies:* by providing health data to community planning agencies and organizations so policy makers can develop more informed strategies to address issues affecting the community
- Assurance
  - *Evaluate:* by providing population health data that can be used as objective measures to evaluate the effectiveness of health programs in reducing morbidity and mortality (CDC, 2020)

HISTORICAL ROOTS OF EPIDEMIOLOGY

Most of the early contributions to epidemiology were made by physicians who sought the cause of disease through methodical observation and conducting experiments to test their theories of new treatment methodologies. The work of these physicians formed the basic concepts that served as a foundation for the science of epidemiology.

Early Physician—Epidemiologists

The roots of epidemiology can be traced to Hippocrates (460 to 375 BC), a Greek physician who is sometimes referred to as the first epidemiologist.

Hippocrates:

- Explained disease occurrences from a rational, rather than a supernatural, viewpoint.
- In his essay, "On Airs, Waters, and Places," suggested that environmental and host factors (e.g., lifestyle behaviors) influence disease development (Bryant & Rhodes, 2018).
- Introduced observations of how diseases spread and affect populations.
- Considered diseases in relation to time and season, place, environmental conditions, and disease control.

Table 7-1 summarizes the contributions of the early physician–epidemiologists to the field of public health. Figure 7-1 shows an example of a spot map early epidemiologist John Snow used in tracking cholera cases.

Florence Nightingale: Nurse Epidemiologist

Nursing's epidemiologic roots can be traced to Florence Nightingale (1820 to 1910). Nightingale advocated training in science, strict discipline, attention to cleanliness, and the development of empathy for patients. She also established a nursing school at London's St. Thomas Hospital and is commonly referred to as "The Lady with the Lamp," a designation given to her by soldiers during the Crimean War as she ministered to them during the night. Queen Victoria recognized Nightingale's contributions to nursing and epidemiology. She was awarded the

TABLE 7-1 Physician–Epidemiologists and Their Contributions to Epidemiology

Physician–Epidemiologist	Contribution to Epidemiology
Thomas Sydenham (1624–1689)	Used empirical approaches and close observations of diseases to classification of London's fevers in 1660s and 1670s. Advocated for getting exercise and fresh air and eating a healthy diet as treatments and remedies when this was not the norm.
James Lind (1716–1794)	Used clinical observations and experimental design to identify the effect of diet on disease. Identified scurvy among British naval seamen that was effectively addressed by eating oranges and limes (why British sailors were called "limeys").
Edward Jenner (1749–1823)	Based on earlier observations and experiments by a farmer/dairyman (Benjamin Jesty), Jenner invented a vaccine for smallpox. Dairymaids never got smallpox but did get cowpox from the cows they milked. He theorized that vaccinating with cowpox would be a protection from smallpox. Thus, he is known as the "Father of Immunology."
Ignaz Semmelweis (1818–1865)	While director of a Viennese maternity hospital in the mid-1800s, he observed that many women died from childbed (puerperal) fever shortly after giving birth. He concluded these deaths were due to bacterial contamination from doctors who didn't wash their hands after performing autopsies of infected and decaying bodies and then performed pelvic examinations on postpartum women. Semmelweis instituted the use of chlorinated lime in hand washing between patient examinations, resulting in maternal deaths plunging to 1.3% in 1848 from a high of 12.1% in 1842.
John Snow (1813–1858)	In the 1800s, he conducted a descriptive epidemiologic investigation of a cholera outbreak in London's Soho district, and an analytic epidemiologic investigation of a cholera epidemic by comparing death rates of those getting their water from either the Lambeth Water Company or the Southward and Vauxhall Water Company. His spot (or dot) mapping of cholera cases, plotted where cholera deaths were occurring, helped to characterize when the epidemic started, peaked, and subsided. The removal of the handle from the Broad Street pump (so that water was unavailable) was the control measure that finally stopped the epidemic. Because of Snow's many contributions to epidemiology, he became known as the "Father of Epidemiology" (see Figs. 7-1 and 7-2).
William Farr (1807–1883)	Created the first national vital statistics system, compiling data on an annual basis (e.g., causes of death, mortality by occupation). Developed a **nosology** (classification of diseases) from which today's International Classification of Diseases (ICD) developed. Collaborated with Florence Nightingale in her British Army studies, publicizing the value of vital statistics. He supported Greenhow's systematic studies in occupational epidemiology and Seaton's analyses of the efficacy of smallpox vaccinations, forming the scientific basis for English public health policy that lasted for over 50 years. By careful analysis of mortality data and disease patterns among different geographical areas, he highlighted the association of disease with socioeconomic class (Lilienfeld, 2007; Merrill, 2017).

Source: Lilienfeld (2007); Merrill (2017).

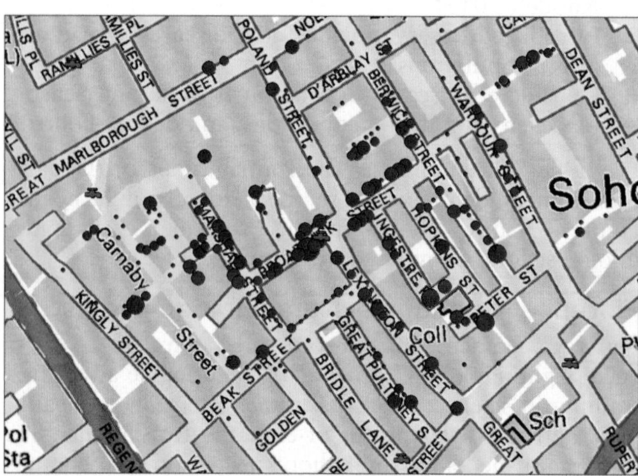

FIGURE 7-1 A spot map John Snow used to track cholera cases. Note the location of water wells/pumps (*blue*). (Reprinted with permission from Wilson, R. (2012). *John Snow's famous cholera analysis data in modern GIS formats. Robin's Blog.* Retrieved from http://blog.rtwilson.com/john-snows-famous-cholera-analysis-data-in-modern-gis-formats/)

highest civilian medal, the Order of Merit, and was the first woman to receive it (Florence Nightingale Museum, 2018). Her contributions include:

- Monitoring disease mortality rates to improve hospital sanitary methods that decreased death rates
- Using a research perspective to conducting systematic descriptive studies of the distribution and patterns of disease in a population (detailed records and descriptions of health conditions, morbidity [sickness] statistics)
- Using applied statistical methods to visualize data (shaded and colored wedge-shaped graphs) as a new way to improve medical and surgical practices
- Using published statistical reports to gain the attention of politicians and powerful people (i.e., William Farr) to bring about hospital and public health reforms that created changes in hygiene and overall treatment of patients (Schiotz, 2015)

Nightingale's contributions to nursing are further explored in Chapter 3.

TABLE 7-2 Eras in the Evolution of Modern Epidemiology

Era	Paradigm	Analytic Approach	Prevention Approach
Sanitary statistics (1800–1850)	Miasma: poisoning from foul emanations	Clustering of morbidity and mortality	Drainage, sewage, sanitation
Infectious disease epidemiology (1850–1950)	Germ theory: single agent related to specific disease	Laboratory isolation and culture from disease sites and experimental transmission/reproduction of lesions	Interrupt transmission (vaccines, isolation, and antibiotics)
Chronic disease epidemiology (1950–2000)	Exposure related to outcome	Risk ratio of exposure to outcome at individual level in populations	Control risk factors by modifying lifestyle (diet), agent (guns), or environment (pollution)
Eco-epidemiology (2000–present)	Ecological influences on human health: molecular, societal, and population based	Analysis using new information systems and biomedical techniques	Modifying molecular, societal, and population factors

Source: Susser and Susser (1996a, 1996b); Susser and Stein (2009).

Eras in the Evolution of Modern Epidemiology

Modern epidemiology can be described as having four distinct eras, each based on causal thinking: (1) sanitary statistics, (2) infectious disease epidemiology, (3) chronic disease epidemiology, and (4) eco-epidemiology. Table 7-2 summarizes these four eras in the evolution of modern epidemiology. Below, each is described in detail.

Sanitary Statistics

Early causal thinking was dominated by the *miasma theory*, which had its origins in the work of the Hippocratic School and was formally developed in the early 1700s. This theory held that a substance called *miasma* was composed of malodorous and poisonous particles generated by the decomposition of organic matter and was the cause of disease. Prevention based on this theory attempted to eliminate the sources of the miasma or polluted vapors.

Despite the faulty reasoning, this type of prevention had positive consequences because it made people aware that decaying organic matter can be a source of infectious diseases. This theory dominated until the first half of the 19th century, when environmental sources and the idea that sanitary conditions were linked to disease led John Snow to identify the source of cholera (Rosen, 2015; Schiotz, 2015).

Infectious-Disease Epidemiology

The era of *infectious-disease epidemiology* was dominated by the *contagion theory of disease*, which developed during the mid-19th century. Due to development of increasingly sophisticated microscopes, this theory attempted to identify the microorganisms that cause diseases as a first step in prevention. It inspired various theories of immunity, and even prompted some initial attempts at vaccination against smallpox.

Additionally, once an agent had been identified, measures were taken to contain its spread. Fumigating ships to kill rats, protecting wharf buildings and human habitations from rats, and removing rat food supplies from easy access were all measures taken to protect the public by further preventing the spread of plague bacilli. Based on the work of Louis Pasteur, Jakob Henle, and Robert Koch, the contagion theory was refined and became best known as the *germ theory of disease*, which was predominant from the late 19th century through the first half of the 20th century (McKenzie, Pinger, & Seabert, 2018; Merrill, 2017; Rosen, 2015).

In the era of *infectious disease epidemiology*, scientists viewed disease in terms of a simple cause-and-effect relationship. Finding a single cause (e.g., plague bacilli) and attacking it (e.g., eliminating rats) seemed to be the solution for preventing many diseases. In the case of bubonic plague, this approach appeared to be quite effective (Merrill, 2017).

However, scientific research eventually revealed that disease causation was much more complex than first suspected. For example, although most members of a group might be exposed to the plague, many did not contract it. With bubonic plague, as with many other infectious diseases, host characteristics can determine both the spread of the disease and its individual impact. Lessons learned from the bubonic plague include the following:

- Not everyone in a population is at equal risk; it is now known that untreated bubonic plague has a case fatality rate of 40% to 70%, meaning that about half of those who contract the disease and are not treated will eventually die.
- The agent and course of transmission can be quite complex. Although a flea carries the bacilli from rats to humans in bubonic plague, many infectious diseases spread directly from one human being to another.
- The environment must be considered as part of the cause of disease. Evidence suggests that the plague originated in the high plains of Asia and spread to other parts of the world. However, questions remain as to whether the bacillus spread from rats to ground squirrels or had always been part of the squirrels' ecology (CDC, 2015).

After World War II, the causative agents of major infectious diseases were identified, methods of prevention were recognized, and antibiotics were added to the arsenal to fight communicable diseases.

Chronic Disease Epidemiology

The focus then became understanding and controlling the new chronic disease epidemics, ushering in the era of *chronic disease epidemiology*. Researchers completed case–control and cohort studies, to be discussed more fully later, that linked the causative factors of cholesterol levels and smoking with coronary heart disease and associated smoking with lung cancer.

According to the CDC (2018a), noninfectious diseases are the major causes of mortality in the United States (Fig. 7-2). As you can see, infectious agents are not to blame for most of today's major health problems. See more in Chapters 21 and 22.

Eco-epidemiology

We are now in the new era of *eco-epidemiology*, distinguished by transforming global health patterns and technological advances. New and emerging global infections, such as the COVID-19 pandemic in 2020, are now a concern, as is the spread of medication-resistant diseases (see more in Chapters 8, 9, and 16). The West Nile virus (WNV), sudden acute respiratory syndrome (SARS), influenza A (H1N1), multidrug-resistant TB, HIV, Zika, and Ebola virus disease illustrate this transformation.

In most cases, causative organisms and critical risk factors are known, yet diseases occur, spread, and suddenly appear in countries or regions previously free of them (Abubakar, Stagg, Cohen, & Rodrigues, 2016; Bain & Awah, 2014). For example, we know how to prevent the transmission of HIV, yet 1.8 million new cases worldwide were reported in 2016 (HIV.gov, 2018). How can preventive practices be promoted among populations at risk for communicable diseases? The same situation is true for many current chronic diseases. For instance, how many nurses smoke? Do you exercise as often as you know you should? Do you know your cholesterol level and eat healthy foods? Do you regularly use sunscreen? What are we missing to effectively change social behaviors? See Chapter 11.

Technological developments drive research, primarily in biology and biomedical techniques and in information system capabilities. The science of *genetics* is useful in modern *epidemiology*. For example, *genetic influence* in some cases of insulin-dependent diabetes is linked to human leukocyte antigens, and particular combinations of this gene variant can predict risk of type 1 diabetes, whereas other combinations either cause no problems or may be protective (National Institute of Diabetes and Digestive and Kidney Diseases [NIDDKD], 2016). HIV, TB, and other infections can be tracked from person to person through identifying the molecular specificity of the organisms.

About 12% of women in the general population will develop breast cancer sometime during their lives, whereas about 72% of women who inherit a harmful *BRCA1* mutation and about 69% of women who inherit a harmful *BRCA2* mutation will develop breast cancer by the age of 80 years. About 1.3% of women in the general population will develop ovarian cancer sometime during their lives, whereas about 44% of women who inherit a harmful *BRCA1* mutation and about 17% of women who inherit a harmful *BRCA2* mutation will develop ovarian cancer by the age of 80 years (National Cancer Institute [NCI], 2018).

On a broader scale, using new technology, we can examine the *geographic distribution of* disease and correlate those data with other important health risks. For instance, using these geocoding systems, overweight and obesity in children can be correlated with other factors, such as after-school recreation opportunities, distribution of fast food restaurants, farmer's markets, or socioeconomic status. (See Chapter 10 for more on technology in public health). The possibilities of learning through technology have just begun in this current epidemiologic era.

Epidemics

An **epidemic** refers to a disease occurrence that clearly exceeds the normal or expected frequency in a community or region. When an epidemic, such as the bubonic plague (also called pneumonic plague or the Black Death) or HIV/AIDS, is worldwide in distribution, it is known as a **pandemic**. When a disease or infectious agent is continually found in a particular area or population, it is considered to be **endemic** (American Academy of Pediatrics, 2018).

Epidemic and pandemic diseases prompted the development of epidemiology as a science. Epidemiology became a distinct branch of medical science and provides public health with the tools to investigate disease outbreaks, as well as controlling disease to prevent future outbreaks. Despite hundreds of years of experience with disease outbreaks, new diseases arise all the time, such as COVID-19; see Box 7-1 for its epidemiology, and thePoint for information on its background, transmission, symptoms, and testing. New diseases challenge us to come up with new methods. Eradication would be ideal, but sometimes it may take a long time, or it may not happen at all. Read about smallpox eradication in Chapter 8.

Historically, as the threat of the great epidemic diseases declined, epidemiologists began to focus on other infectious diseases, such as diphtheria, infant diarrhea, typhoid, TB, and syphilis. They also studied diseases linked to occupations, such as scurvy among sailors and scrotal cancer among chimney sweeps (Remington & Brownson, 2011). In recent years, epidemiologists turned to the study of major causes of death and disability, such as cancer, cardiovascular disorders, AIDS, violence, mental illness, accidents, arthritis, and congenital defects (Meier, Sandler, Simonsick, & Parks, 2016).

Opioid Epidemic: A 21st Century Public Health Epidemic

The current, ongoing opioid epidemic is an example of how epidemiology has helped define the scope of the problem and how this knowledge impacts public health policies in addressing the epidemic. Public health

10 Leading Causes of Death by Age Group, United States—2018

Rank	<1	1–4	5–9	10–14	15–24	25–34	35–44	45–54	55–64	65+	Total
1	Congenital Anomalies 4,473	Unintentional Injury 1,226	Unintentional Injury 734	Unintentional Injury 692	Unintentional Injury 12,044	Unintentional Injury 24,614	Unintentional Injury 22,667	Malignant Neoplasms 37,301	Malignant Neoplasms 113,947	Heart Disease 526,509	Heart Disease 655,381
2	Short Gestation 3,679	Congenital Anomalies 384	Malignant Neoplasms 393	Suicide 596	Suicide 6,211	Suicide 8,020	Malignant Neoplasms 10,640	Heart Disease 32,220	Heart Disease 81,042	Malignant Neoplasms 431,102	Malignant Neoplasms 599,274
3	Maternal Pregnancy Comp. 1,358	Homicide 353	Congenital Anomalies 201	Malignant Neoplasms 450	Homicide 4,607	Homicide 5,234	Heart Disease 10,532	Unintentional Injury 23,056	Unintentional Injury 23,693	Chronic Low Respiratory Disease 135,560	Unintentional Injury 167,127
4	SIDS 1,334	Malignant Neoplasms 326	Homicide 121	Congenital Anomalies 172	Malignant Neoplasms 1,371	Malignant Neoplasms 3,684	Suicide 7,521	Suicide 8,345	Chronic Low Respiratory Disease 18,804	Cerebro-vascular 127,244	Chronic Low Respiratory Disease 159,486
5	Unintentional Injury 1,168	Influenza & Pneumonia 122	Influenza & Pneumonia 71	Homicide 168	Heart Disease 905	Heart Disease 3,561	Homicide 3,304	Liver Disease 8,157	Diabetes Mellitus 14,941	Alzheimer's Disease 120,658	Cerebro-vascular 147,810
6	Placenta Cord. Membranes 724	Heart Disease 115	Chronic Low. Respiratory Disease 68	Heart Disease 101	Congenital Anomalies 354	Liver Disease 1,008	Liver Disease 3,108	Diabetes Mellitus 6,414	Liver Disease 13,945	Diabetes Mellitus 60,182	Alzheimer's Disease 122,019
7	Bacterial Sepsis 579	Perinatal Period 62	Heart Disease 68	Chronic Low Respiratory Disease 64	Diabetes Mellitus 246	Diabetes Mellitus 837	Diabetes Mellitus 2,282	Cerebro-vascular 5,128	Cerebro-vascular 12,789	Unintentional Injury 57,213	Diabetes Mellitus 84,946
8	Circulatory System Disease 428	Septicemia 54	Cerebro-vascular 34	Cerebro-vascular 54	Influenza & Pneumonia 200	Cerebro-vascular 567	Cerebro-vascular 1,704	Chronic Low. Respiratory Disease 3,807	Suicide 8,540	Influenza & Pneumonia 48,888	Influenza & Pneumonia 59,120
9	Respiratory Distress 390	Chronic Low. Respiratory Disease 50	Septicemia 34	Influenza & Pneumonia 51	Chronic Low. Respiratory Disease 165	HIV 482	Influenza & Pneumonia 956	Septicemia 2,380	Septicemia 5,956	Nephritis 42,232	Nephritis 51,386
10	Neonatal Hemorrhage 375	Cerebro-vascular 43	Benign Neoplasms 19	Benign Neoplasms 30	Complicated Pregnancy 151	Influenza & Pneumonia 457	Septicemia 829	Influenza & Pneumonia 2,339	Influenza & Pneumonia 5,858	Parkinson's Disease 32,988	Suicide 48,344

Data Source: National Vital Statistics System, National Center for Health Statistics, CDC.
Produced by: National Center for Injury Prevention and Control, CDC using WISQARS™.

CDC Centers for Disease Control and Prevention National Center for Injury Prevention and Control

FIGURE 7-2 Ten leading causes of death by age group, United States: 2018. (Reprinted from National Vital Statistics System, National Center for Health Statistics. Retrieved from https://www.cdc.gov/injury/wisqars/pdf/leading_causes_of_death_by_age_group_2018-508.pdf)

BOX 7-1 Epidemiology and COVID-19

To control the spread of epidemics or pandemics, the following measures and terminology are useful to consider:

- **The S-I-R model**—This model is a mathematical model of spread that places the population into three categories: (1) "susceptibles"—those who do not have the disease yet; (2) "infectives"—those have contracted the disease; (3) "removed"—those who have had the disease and recovered and are now immune, or those who have died, and no longer spread the disease. The model supports the importance of social isolation of those infected to prevent the spread to those susceptible (Smith & Moore, 2020; Yates, 2020).
- **R_0 (pronounced "R-nought" or "R-zero")**—Whether an outbreak spreads or dies depends on the basic reproduction number. This is the average number of previously unexposed individuals infected by a single, freshly introduced disease. If a disease has an R_0 <1 (each infected person on average gives it to less than one other person), then the infection will die out quickly. The outbreak cannot sustain its own spread. If R_0 is larger than one, then the outbreak will grow exponentially (Yates, 2020).
  - The early estimates of the R_0 for COVID-19 was at least 2 (varying between 1.5 and 4). This means the first person with the disease spreads it to two others, who each, on average, is spreading the disease to two others and then to two others each, and so on.
  - The rate at which "susceptibles" become infected (the force of infection), and the rate of recovery or death from the disease can increase the R_0, while increasing recovery rate will reduce it.
  - The bigger the population and the faster the disease spreads between individuals, the larger the outbreak is likely to be. The quicker individuals recover, the less time they have to pass on the disease to others and, the easier it will be to bring an outbreak under control.
  - The "effective reproduction number" is the average number of secondary infections caused by an infectious individual at a given point in the outbreak's progression. If, by intervention, the effective reproduction number can be brought to below one, then the disease will die out (Yates, 2020, para. 19).
  - The fraction of the population that needs to be immune to protect the rest depends on how infectious the disease is. The basic reproduction number, R_0 can be used to determine the proportion of the population that will need to be immune. The higher the R_0, the higher the immune proportion of the population needs to be. If the Ro is 4, then three-quarters of the population must be immune. If R_0 is 1.5 then only one-third of the population must be immunized to protect the remaining two-thirds (Yates, 2020).
- **Case fatality rate**—R_0 does not capture the seriousness of the disease for an infected individual. The proportion of infected people who ultimately die from a disease is known as the case fatality rate. A high case fatality rate means that a high number of those who get the disease usually die from the disease. Diseases with high fatality rates are less infectious because those who are ill die quickly, thus reducing the chances of infecting others (Yates, 2020).
  - Early estimates indicate that the case fatality rate of COVID-19 is between 0.25% and 3.5%. This low fatality rate can end up killing more people because more people can become infected from those who are presymptomatic or have mild cases of the disease.
  - Case fatality rates for COVID-19 vary significantly with the age of the patient, with the elderly being worst affected. Older people are more likely to die from COVID-19 than the population as a whole (Yates, 2020).
  - Current estimates of the death rate of COVID-19 found that globally, the case fatality rate for those under age 60 was 1.4%. For those over age 60, it was 4.5%. For those 80 and over, the case fatality rate was 13.4% (Resnick, 2020).

Source: Resnick (2020); Smith and Moore (2020); Yates (2020).

surveillance of drug use has helped to better define who are most affected by the opioid epidemic by monitoring who is dying from drug overdoses. The latest compilation from the U.S. Department of Health and Human Services (USDHHS) about the opioid epidemic show the following (USDHHS, 2018a):

- 115 people die every day from opioid-related overdoses (Fig. 7-3)
- Opioid overdose deaths increased fivefold from 1999 to 2016
- New hepatitis C infections tripled from 2010 to 2016
- Hepatitis B and C and other infections associated with the injection of opioids increased in communities hardest hit

Mapping the statistically significant rise in overdose death rates shows how rapidly the opioid epidemic is spreading across various states (CDC, 2017a). This is why continuous monitoring over time is important to identifying trends (Fig. 7-4).

In 2016, drug overdose deaths totaled 63,632, increasing significantly from 2015 at a rate of 16.3 to 19.8 per 100,000. Opioids were involved in 66.4% of total deaths (CDC, 2017a). The most recent overdose death data indicate that different drugs are responsible for the rise in opioid deaths (Fig. 7-5). Between 2000 and 2016, deaths due to heroin steadily rose, to be overtaken by deaths from synthetic opioids (National Institute on Drug Abuse [NIDA], 2018a).

In August 2017, the CDC showed that opioid overdose deaths were occurring in three waves (CDC, 2017c; Fig. 7-6):

- Wave 1: Rise in prescription overdose deaths (1990s)
- Wave 2: Rise in heroin overdose deaths (2010 to now)
- Wave 3: Rise in synthetic overdose deaths (2013 to now)

THE OPIOID EPIDEMIC BY THE NUMBERS

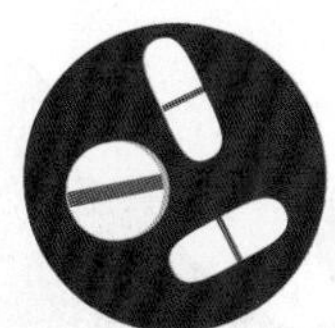

130+
People died every day from opioid-related drug overdoses[3] (estimated)

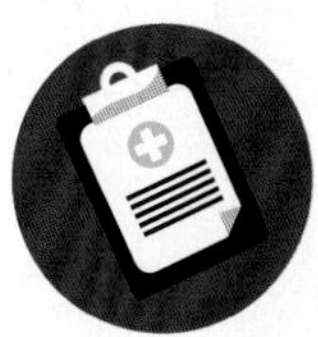

10.3 m
People misused prescription opioids in 2018[1]

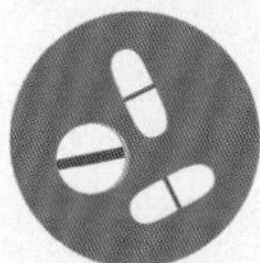

47,600
People died from overdosing on opioids[2]

2.0 million
People had an opioid use disorder in 2018[1]

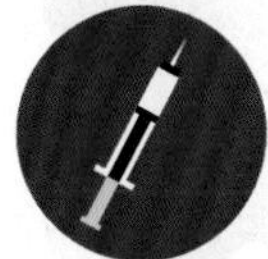

81,000
People used heroin for the first time[1]

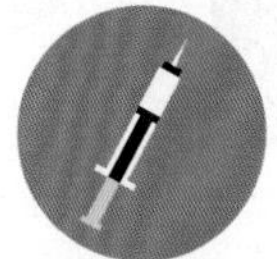

808,000
People used heroin in 2018[1]

2 million
People misused prescription opioids for the first time[1]

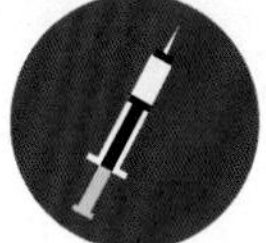

15,349
Deaths attributed to overdosing on heroin (in 12-month period ending February 2019)[2]

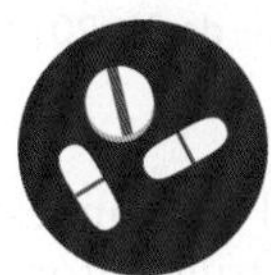

32,656
Deaths attributed to overdosing on synthetic opioids other than methadone (in 12-month period ending February 2019)[2]

SOURCES

1. 2019 National Survey on Drug Use and Health. Mortality in the United States, 2018
2. NCHS Data Brief No. 329, November 2018
3. NCHS, National Vital Statistics System. Estimates for 2018 and 2019 are based on provisional data.

Updated October 2019. For more information, visit:http://www.hhs.gov/opioids/

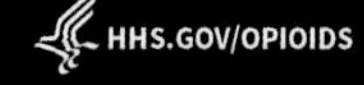

FIGURE 7-3 Opioid epidemic by the numbers. (Updated October 2019). Retrieved from https://www.hhs.gov/opioids/sites/default/files/2019-11/Opioids%20Infographic_letterSizePDF_10-02-19.pdf

Trends in opioid abuse include the following:

- Prescription opioid use is a risk factor for heroin use, with nearly 80% of heroin users in 2013 reporting using prescription opioids prior to heroin (NIDA, 2018b).
- Initiation into nonmedical use of opioids was through three main sources: family, friends, or personal prescriptions (NIDA, 2018b).
- Drug overdoses of cocaine, heroin, and OxyContin are occurring because popular illicit drugs are being laced with synthetic opioids (e.g., fentanyl; Fig. 7-7).
- Deaths due to fentanyl have not been well documented because they are usually mixed in with other drugs (Frankel, 2018).
- By July 2018, the CDC reported that drug deaths from fentanyl and fentanyl analogs were responsible for the growing opioid deaths seen in the United States (CDC, 2018b; Fig. 7-8).
- First responders are dying from accidental exposure to fentanyl, including nurses (Evans, 2017) and police dogs (Cima, 2018).

In July 2018, the CDC reported overdose deaths from fentanyl analogs in 10 states and viewed the rising

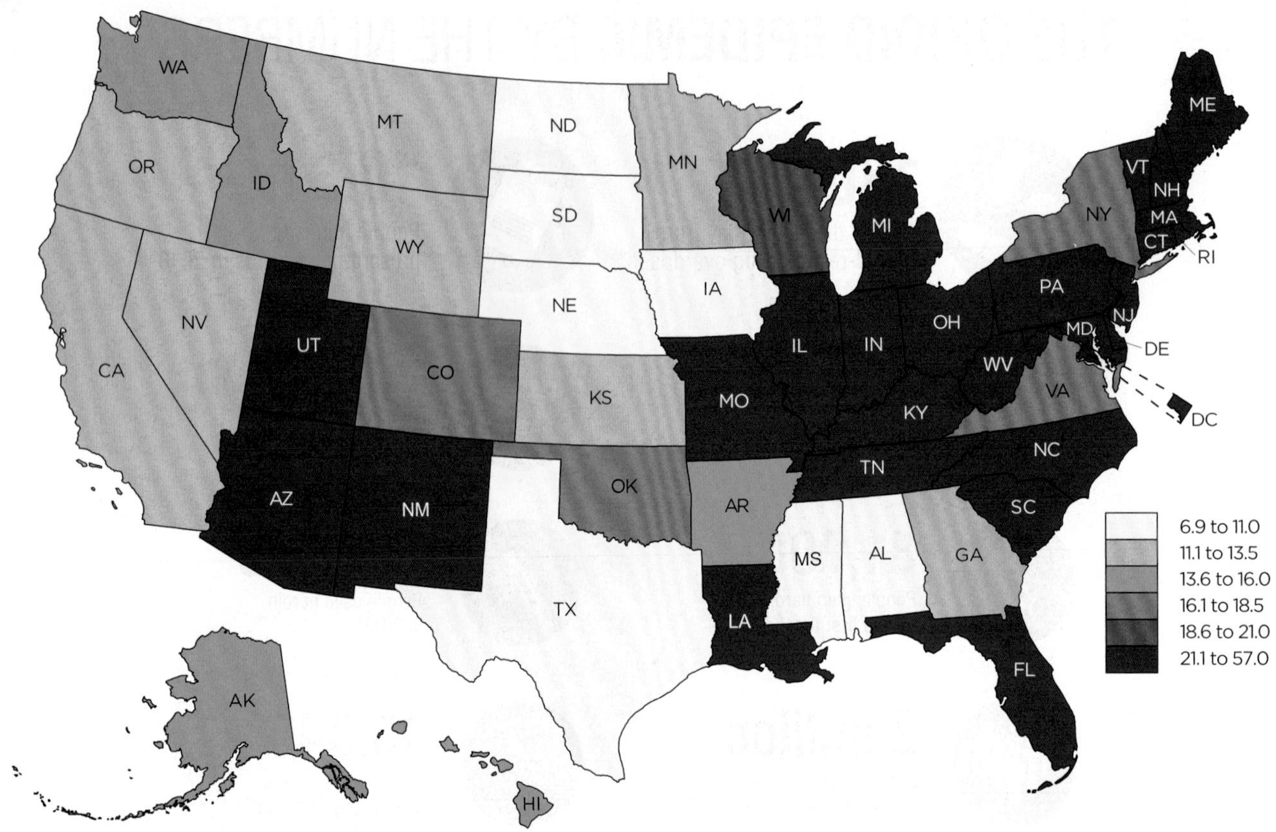

FIGURE 7-4 Age-adjusted rates of overdose deaths by state, US 2018. (Reprinted from CDC. (December 19, 2017). *Opioid overdose: Drug overdose death data.* Retrieved from https://www.cdc.gov/drugoverdose/data/statedeaths/drug-overdose-death-2018.html)

deaths to be alarming (CDC, 2018b; Fig. 7-9). Fentanyl analogs are illicitly manufactured forms of fentanyl (i.e., carfentanil, acetylfentanyl, furanylfentanyl, U-47700). The rise of fentanyl and its analogs in drug overdose deaths is the result of the high profit margin for drug traffickers (CDC, 2017b). One kilogram of fentanyl powder can yield hundreds of thousands of counterfeit pills that can be sold for millions of dollars in profit. Fentanyl is manufactured in clandestine labs found in Mexico and China (U.S. Drug Enforcement Administration, n.d.; EPR, 2018).

Trends in rates of serious infection and associated costs with opioid abuse/dependence were not investigated until 2016. At that time, research found hospitalizations related to opioid abuse/dependence both with and without associated serious infection significantly increased

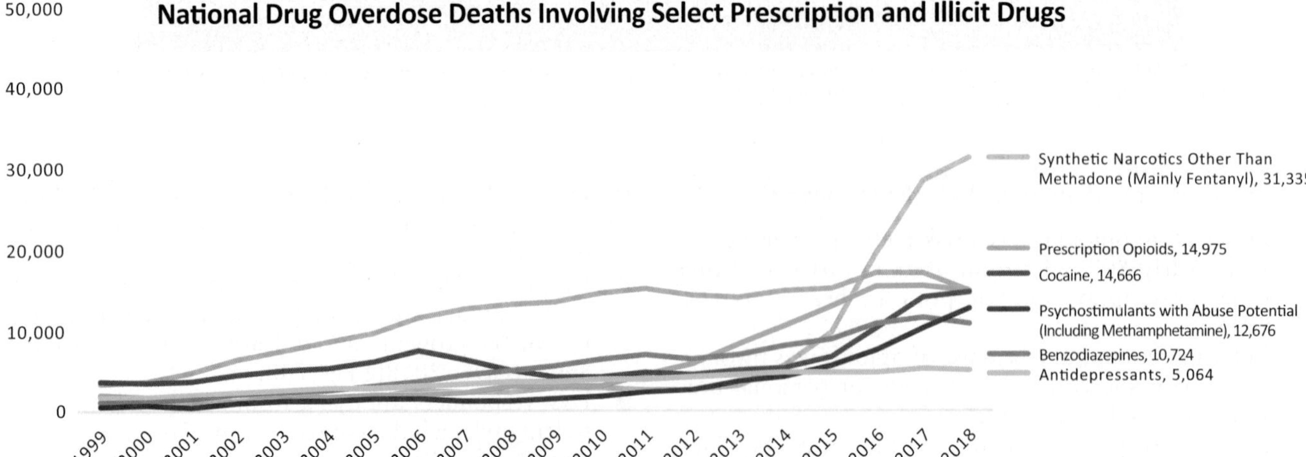

FIGURE 7-5 National drug overdose deaths by specific category—number among all ages, 1999–2018. (National Institute on Drug Abuse (NIDA). (2020). *Overdose death rates.* Retrieved from https://www.drugabuse.gov/drug-topics/trends-statistics/overdose-death-rates)

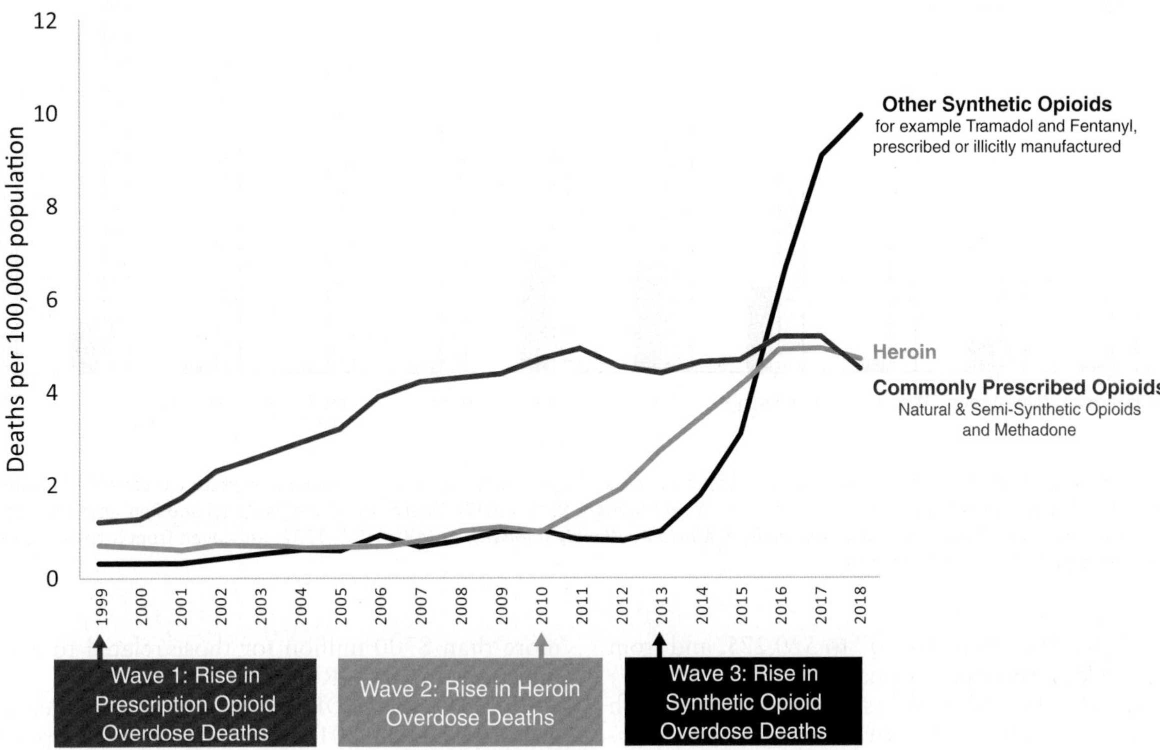

FIGURE 7-6 Three waves of opioid overdose deaths. (Reprinted from CDC. (2020). *Opioid overdose: Understanding the epidemic*. Retrieved from https://www.cdc.gov/drugoverdose/epidemic/index.html)

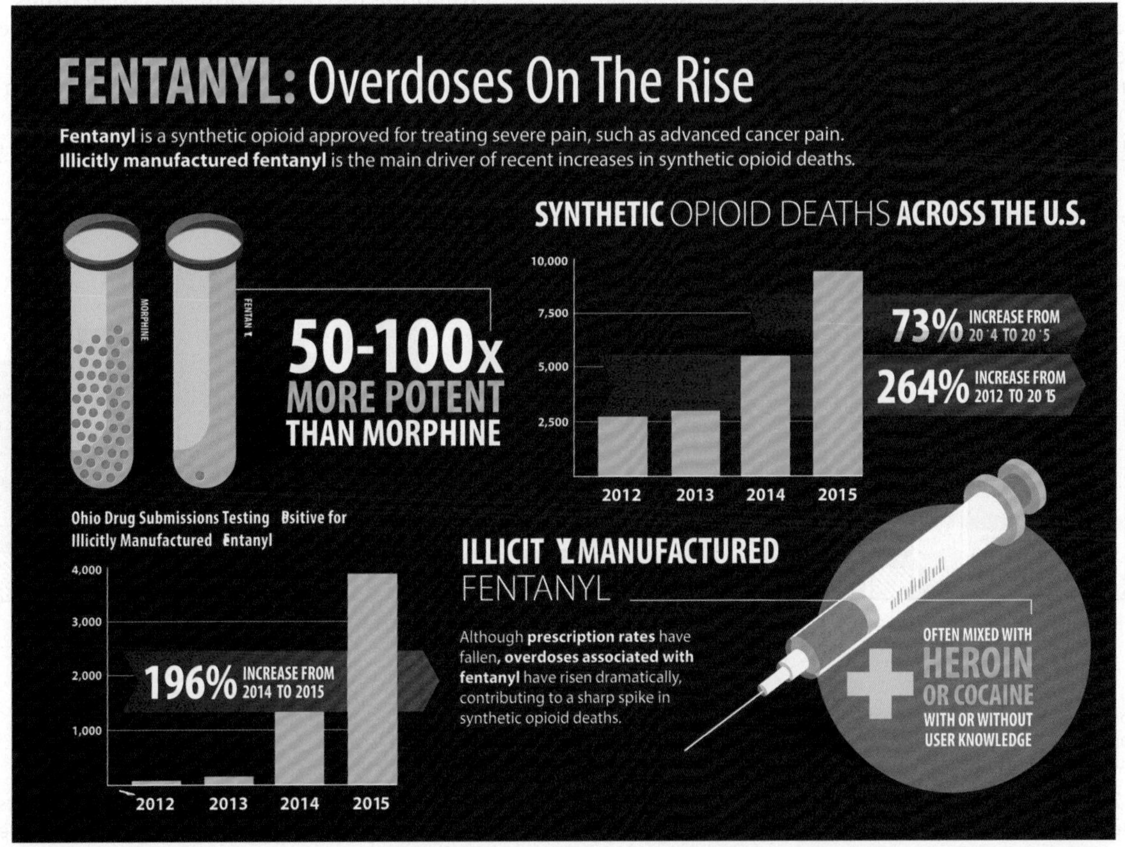

FIGURE 7-7 Fentanyl: Overdoses on the rise. (Reprinted from CDC. (2017). *Opioid overdose: Fentanyl*. Retrieved from https://www.cdc.gov/drugoverdose/opioids/fentanyl.html)

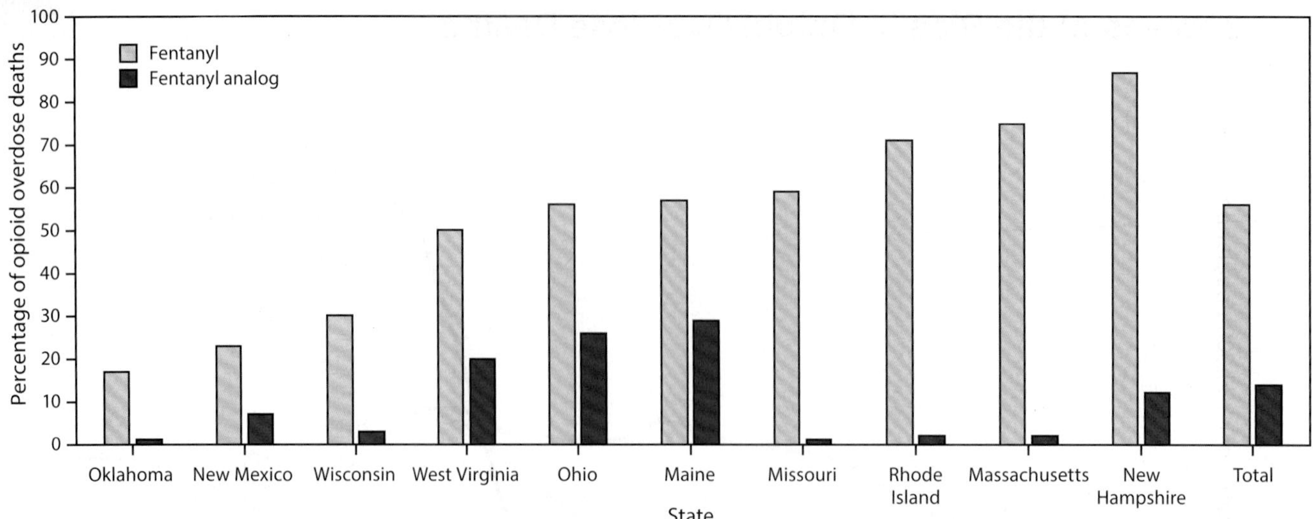

FIGURE 7-8 Percentage of opioid overdose deaths testing positive for fentanyl and fentanyl analogs, by state (10 states). (Reprinted from O'Donnell, J. K., Halpin, J., Mattson, C. L., Goldberger, B. A., & Gladden, R. M. (2017). Deaths involving Fentanyl and Fentanyl analogs, and U-47700—10 states, July-December 2016. *Morbidity & Mortality Weekly (MMWR), 66*(43), 1197–1202. Retrieved from https://www.cdc.gov/mmwr/volumes/66/wr/mm6643e1.htm)

from 2002 to 2012, from 301,707 to 520,275, and from 3,421 to 6,535, respectively (Ronan & Herzig, 2016).

The rise in HIV and hepatitis outbreaks, along with the dramatic increase in *Staphylococcus aureus* infections (often MRSA), have been linked to this epidemic. *S. aureus* can damage heart valves, and a North Carolina study found a 13-fold increase in endocarditis between 2007 and 2017 among those abusing drugs (Reardon, 2019; National Academies of Science, Engineering, and Medicine, 2018; USDHHS, 2018b). Inpatient charges for both types of hospitalizations quadrupled for the same time period. In all, almost $15 billion was paid for hospitalizations related to opioid abuse/dependence and more than $700 million for those related to associated infections in 2012 (Ronan & Herzig, 2016).

In 2017, the USDHHS declared a public health emergency (USDHHS, 2018a) and announced a 5-point strategy to combat the opioid crisis (USDHHS, 2017a):

1. Improving access to treatment and recovery services
2. Promoting use of overdose-reversing drugs
3. Strengthening our understanding of the epidemic through better public health surveillance
4. Providing support for cutting-edge research on pain and addiction
5. Advancing better practices for pain management

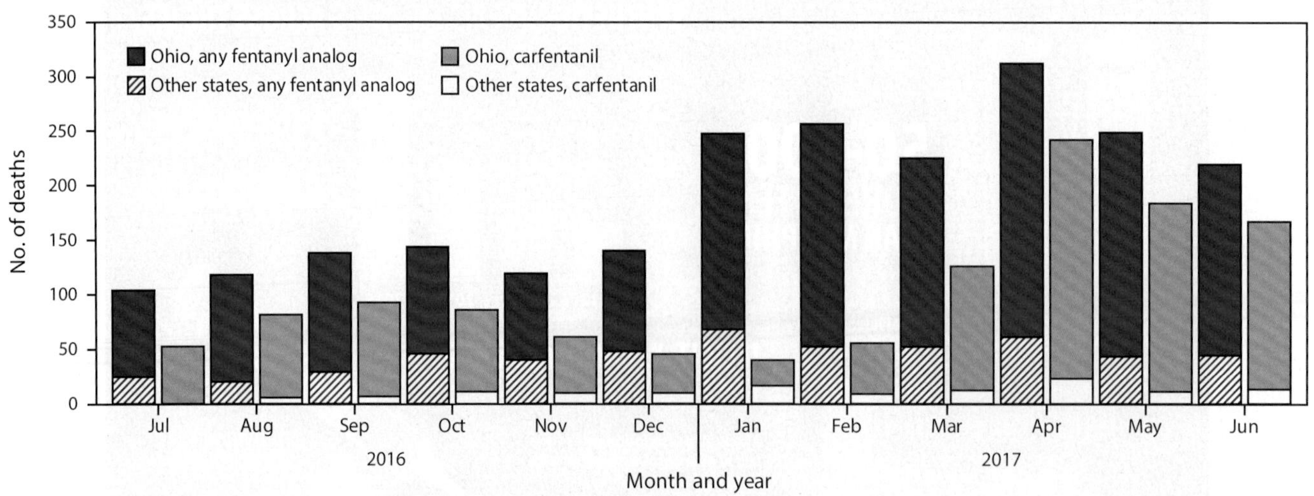

Abbreviation: SUDORS,State Unintentional Drug Overdose Reporting System.
* "Any fentanyl analog" includes carfentanil, so the categories are not mutually exclusive.
† Kentucky, Maine, Massachusetts, New Hampshire, New Mexico, Oklahoma, Rhode Island, West Virginia, and Wisconsin.

FIGURE 7-9 Number of overdose deaths with carfentanil and any fentanyl analog detected*—Ohio and nine other SUDORS states, July 2016–June 2017. (Reprinted from O'Donnell, J., Gladden, M., Mattson, C. L., & Kariisa, M. (2018). Notes from the field: Overdose deaths with Carfentanil and other Fentanyl analogs detected—10 states, July 2016-June 2017. *Morbidity and Mortality Weekly (MMWR), 67*(27), 767–768. Retrieved from https://www.cdc.gov/mmwr/volumes/67/wr/mm6727a4.htm)

Fortunately, epidemiological data were used to develop new guidelines for treating those who are brought in for treatment and provide data to drug enforcement agencies to develop strategies to reduce the trafficking of illegal drugs that will save lives in the long run.

CONCEPTS BASIC TO EPIDEMIOLOGY

The science of epidemiology draws on certain basic concepts and principles to analyze and understand patterns of occurrence among aggregate health conditions.

Disease Etiology

In 1856, John Stuart Mill formed three methods of hypothesis formulation for determining disease etiology. These methods include method of difference, method of agreement, and method of concomitant variation.

In 1965, Sir Austin Bradford Hill proposed expanding on Mill's postulates about causality by developing nine criteria to evaluate the relationship between environmental exposure and potential health outcomes. The criteria can be used with infectious disease as well as noninfectious disease. These elements are:

1. *Strength of Association*: The ratio of the rate of a disease in those with a suspected causal factor to the rate of the disease in those without it: a higher rate in the group with the factor than in the group without it indicates a strong association.
2. *Consistency of Association*: An association is demonstrated in varying types of studies among diverse study groups (i.e., replication).
3. *Specificity*: A cause leads to one effect (not always the case in noninfectious diseases).
4. *Temporality*: Exposure to the suspected factor must precede the onset of disease (i.e., time order or time sequence).
5. *Biological Gradient*: This relationship is demonstrated if, with increasing levels of exposure to the factor, there is a corresponding increase in occurrence of the disease (i.e., dose–response relationship).
6. *Biological Plausibility*: The hypothesized cause makes sense based on current biologic or social models (i.e., it is possible).
7. *Coherence of Explanation*: The hypothesized cause makes sense based on current knowledge about the natural history or biology of the disease (i.e., scientific knowledge).
8. *Analogy*: Similarities between the association of interest and others (e.g., potential links to birth defects from new drugs is a concern because we already recognize this potential from the use of the drug thalidomide during the 1950s and early 1960s).
9. *Experimental Evidence*: Experimental and nonexperimental studies support the association (e.g., reduced tobacco use in a population should lead to reduced lung cancer rates; Merrill, 2017).

The elements described by Hill are still used by epidemiologists and provide the fundamental principles C/PHNs can use to evaluate evidence of disease causation in all types of published reports, both scientific and lay.

In health education, these principles can be used to teach disease causation risk, especially when the evidence is not yet complete. For instance, a pregnant teen asks a nurse if she should drink diet soda while she is pregnant. The nurse can share with her that the evidence to date supports the safety of artificial sweeteners for most adults (experiment), but that it is probably not wise to drink diet soda while pregnant. When she asks why (because there isn't any reported risk), the nurse can respond that any chemical has the potential to cause harm (plausibility and analogy), and the effects on a growing fetus (biologic gradient) are often unknown until decades later (temporality and experiment).

Epidemiologic Triangle or Host, Agent, and Environment Model

Through their early study of infectious diseases, epidemiologists began to consider disease states in terms of the **epidemiologic triangle**, or the *host, agent, and environment model*, shown in Figure 7-10. Interactions among these three elements explained infectious and other disease patterns.

Host

The *host* is a susceptible human or animal who harbors and nourishes a disease-causing agent. Many physical, psychological, and lifestyle factors influence the host's susceptibility and response to an agent (Friis, 2018):

- Physical factors: age, sex, race, socioeconomic status, and genetic influences
- Psychological factors: outlook and response to stress
- Lifestyle factors: diet, exercise, and other healthy or unhealthy habits

The concept of resistance is important for community/public health nursing practice. People sometimes have an ability to resist pathogens, which is called *inherent resistance*. Typically, these people have inherited or acquired characteristics, such as the various factors mentioned ear-

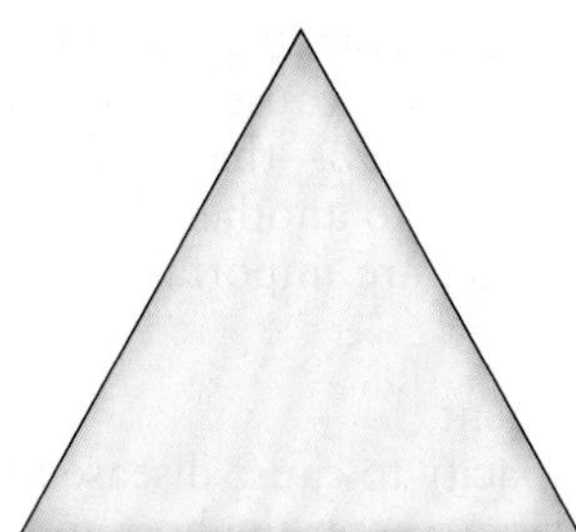

FIGURE 7-10 Epidemiologic triangle.

lier, that make them less vulnerable. For instance, people who maintain a healthful lifestyle may not contract influenza even if exposed to the flu virus. Resistance can be promoted through preventive interventions that improve one's immunity system and support a healthy lifestyle.

Such healthy habits include not smoking, eating more fruits and vegetables, exercising regularly, maintaining a healthy weight, drinking alcohol in moderation, getting adequate sleep, washing hands frequently, cooking meals thoroughly, and minimizing stress (Harvard Health Publishing [HHP], 2018).

Agent

An *agent* is a factor that causes or contributes to a health problem or condition (Friis, 2018). Causative agents can be factors that are present (e.g., bacteria that cause TB, rocks on a mountain road that contribute to an automobile crash) or factors that are lacking (e.g., a low serum iron level that causes anemia or the lack of seat belt use contributing to the extent of injury in an automobile crash).

Agents vary considerably and include five types: biologic, chemical, nutrient, physical, and psychological:

- *Biologic* agents include bacteria, viruses, fungi, protozoa, worms, and insects. Some biologic agents are infectious, such as influenza virus or HIV.
- *Chemical* agents may be in the form of liquids, solids, gases, dusts, or fumes. Examples are poisonous sprays used on garden pests and industrial chemical wastes. The degree of toxicity of the chemical agent influences its impact on health.
- *Nutrient* agents include essential dietary components that can produce illness conditions if they are deficient or are taken in excess. For example, a deficiency of niacin can cause pellagra, and too much vitamin A can be toxic.
- *Physical* agents include anything mechanical (e.g., chainsaw, automobile), material (e.g., rockslide), atmospheric (e.g., ultraviolet radiation), geologic (e.g., earthquake), or genetically transmitted that causes injury to humans. The shape, size, and force of physical agents influence the degree of harm to the host.
- *Psychological* agents are events that produce stress leading to health problems (e.g., war, terrorism).

Agents may also be classified as infectious or noninfectious. Infectious agents cause communicable diseases, such as influenza or TB—that is, the disease can be spread from one person to another. Certain characteristics of infectious agents are important for C/PHNs to understand:

- *Exposure* to the agent
- *Pathogenicity* (capacity to cause disease in the host)
- *Infectivity* (capacity to enter the host and multiply)
- *Virulence* (severity of disease)
- *Toxigenicity* (capacity to produce a toxin or poison)
- *Resistance* (ability of the agent to survive environmental conditions)
- *Antigenicity* (ability to induce an antibody response in the host)
- *Structure and chemical composition* (Friis, 2018)

Chapter 8 examines the subject of communicable disease in greater depth. Noninfectious agents have similar characteristics in that their relative abilities to harm the host vary with type of agent and intensity and duration of exposure (Szklo & Nieto, 2019).

Environment

The *environment* refers to all the external factors surrounding the host that might influence vulnerability or resistance and includes physical and psychosocial elements (Friis, 2018):

- The *physical environment* includes factors such as geography, climate and weather, safety of buildings, water and food supply, and presence of animals, plants, insects, and microorganisms that have the capacity to serve as reservoirs (storage sites for disease-causing agents) or **vectors** (carriers) for transmitting disease.
- The *psychosocial environment* refers to social, cultural, economic, and psychological influences and conditions that affect health, such as access to health care, cultural health practices, poverty, and work stressors, which can all contribute to disease or health (Szklo & Nieto, 2019).

Interaction of the Host, Agent, and Environment

Host, agent, and environment interact to cause a disease or health condition. For example, WNV is spread to people by mosquito bites and occurs during mosquito season (summer through fall). There are no vaccines to prevent or medications to treat WNV. Most people infected have no symptoms, but about 20% develop a fever and other symptoms. Around 1 out of 150 infected people develop a serious, sometimes fatal, illness. The risk of WNV can be reduced by using insect repellent and wearing long-sleeved shirts and long pants to prevent mosquito bites (CDC, 2018c). WNV, which was widespread in Africa and the Middle East, arrived in the United States in 1999 and spread throughout the continental United States. Mapping the distribution of infectious diseases (Fig. 7-11) helps authorities know where to make resources and aid available.

Another mosquito-borne viral illness, eastern equine encephalitis (EEE) virus, has recently gained attention. EEE cases are rare in humans, usually no more than 5 to 10 annually in the United States. However, about 30% of cases can be fatal; as of October 1, 2019, there have been 10 deaths reported from EEE virus, and patients are often left with neurological problems (Almasy, 2019; CDC, 2019a).

Causality

Causality refers to the relationship between a cause and its effect. As scientific knowledge of health and disease has expanded, epidemiology has changed its view of causality. The following section discusses some of those changes in thinking, which began in the 1960s and continue today.

Chain of Causation

As the scientific community is thinking about disease causation and the epidemiologic model (host–agent–environment) grew more complex, epidemiologists began to use the idea of a chain of causation (Fig. 7-12).

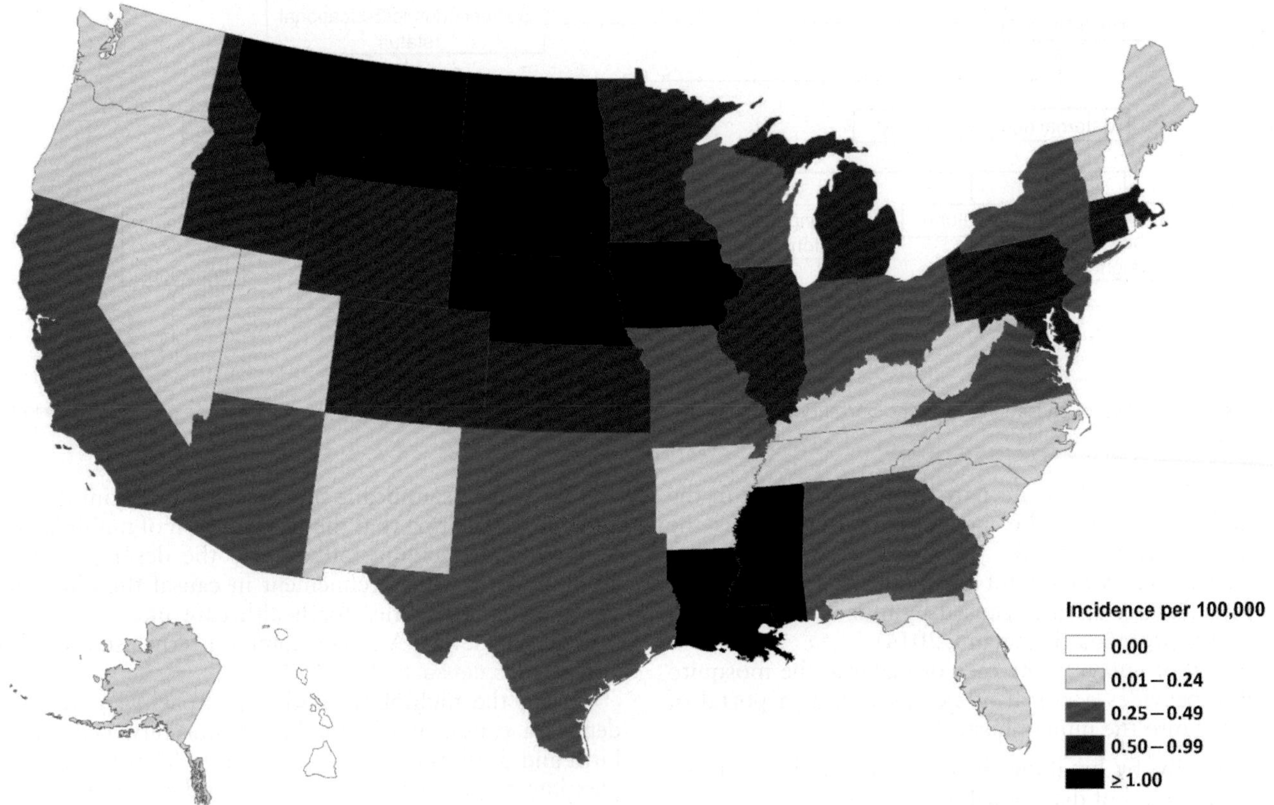

FIGURE 7-11 West Nile Virus incidence by State—United States. (Source: CDC. (2018). *West Nile virus neuroinvasive disease incidence reported to ArboNET, by state, United States, 2018*. Retrieved from https://www.cdc.gov/westnile/resources/pdfs/data/WNV-Neuro-Incidence-by-State-Map-2018-P.pdf)

The components of the **chain of causation** include:

- **Reservoir** (i.e., where the causal agent can live and multiply). With plague, that reservoir may be other humans, rats, squirrels, and a few other animals. With malaria, infected humans are the major reservoir for the parasitic agents, although certain nonhuman primates also act as reservoirs (Heymann, 2014).
- *Portal of exit* from the reservoir, which can be a mode of transmission. For example, the bite of an *Anopheles* mosquito provides a portal of exit for the malaria

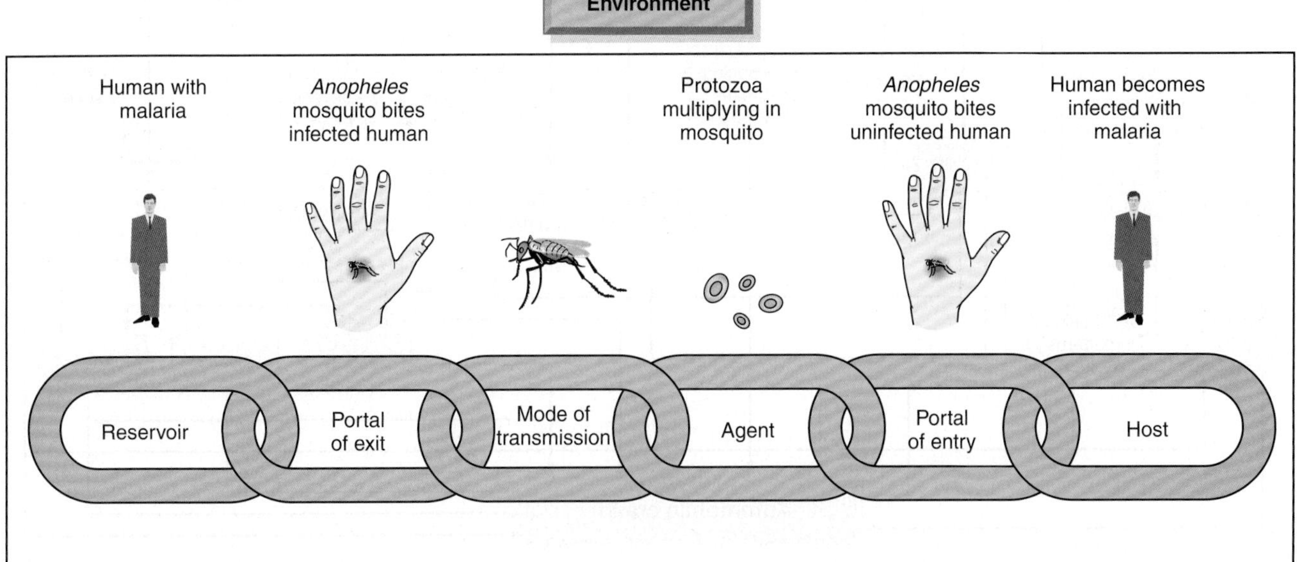

FIGURE 7-12 Chain of causation.

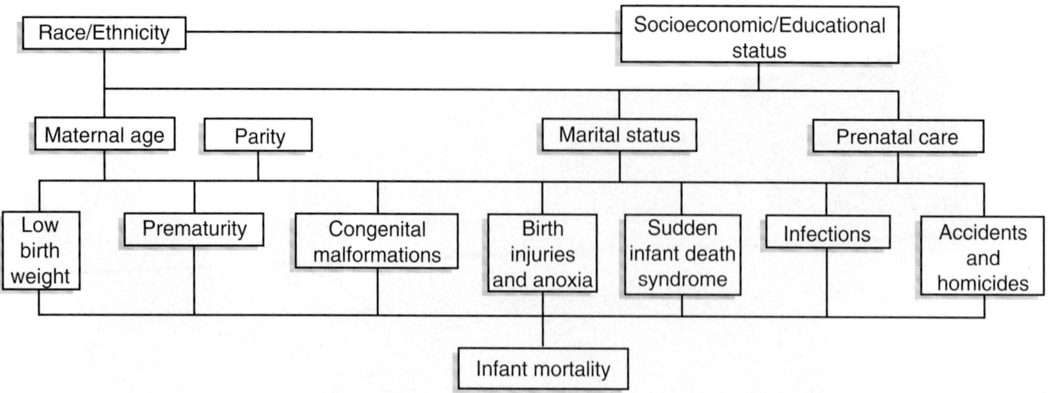

FIGURE 7-13 Web of causation for infant mortality.

parasites, which spend part of their life cycle in the mosquito's body; the mosquito in this case is the mode of transmission.

- *Agent* itself. Malaria, for example, actually consists of four distinct diseases caused by four kinds of microscopic protozoa (Heymann, 2014).
- *Portal of entry*. In the case of malaria, the mosquito bite provides a portal of exit as well as a portal of entry into the human host.

Basically, by breaking the chain of causation at any link, the spread of disease will be prevented.

Web of Causation

In the 1960s, the concept of multiple causation emerged to explain the existence of health and illness states and to provide guiding principles for epidemiologic practice. A causal paradigm that gained attention was referred to as the **web of causation**. The implication was that an intervention (or breaking of the web at any point nearest to the disease) could profoundly impact the development of that disease (Merrill, 2017; Szklo & Nieto, 2019).

This was a significant shift in thinking about disease and health, positing that the combination of multiple factors was the deciding influence in the development of poor outcomes. This refinement in causal thinking also provided opportunities for health care interventions at a variety of levels. Another common term used for this approach is **causal matrix**.

Using the multiple causation approach, Figure 7-13 depicts a causal matrix for infant mortality. Data from birth and death certificates were used to identify the complex interactions among multiple causal factors that produce a negative health condition leading to infant mortality. Another example (Fig. 7-14) shows a web of causation for automobile crashes. All of the numerous factors involved must be considered when diagramming a web of causation. Speed, faulty equipment, heavy traffic, confusing traffic patterns, road construction, poor visibility, weather conditions, driver inexperience, and drinking or drug use, in any combination, can cause an automobile crash.

All health conditions can be diagramed to depict a matrix of causation. A communicable disease that has

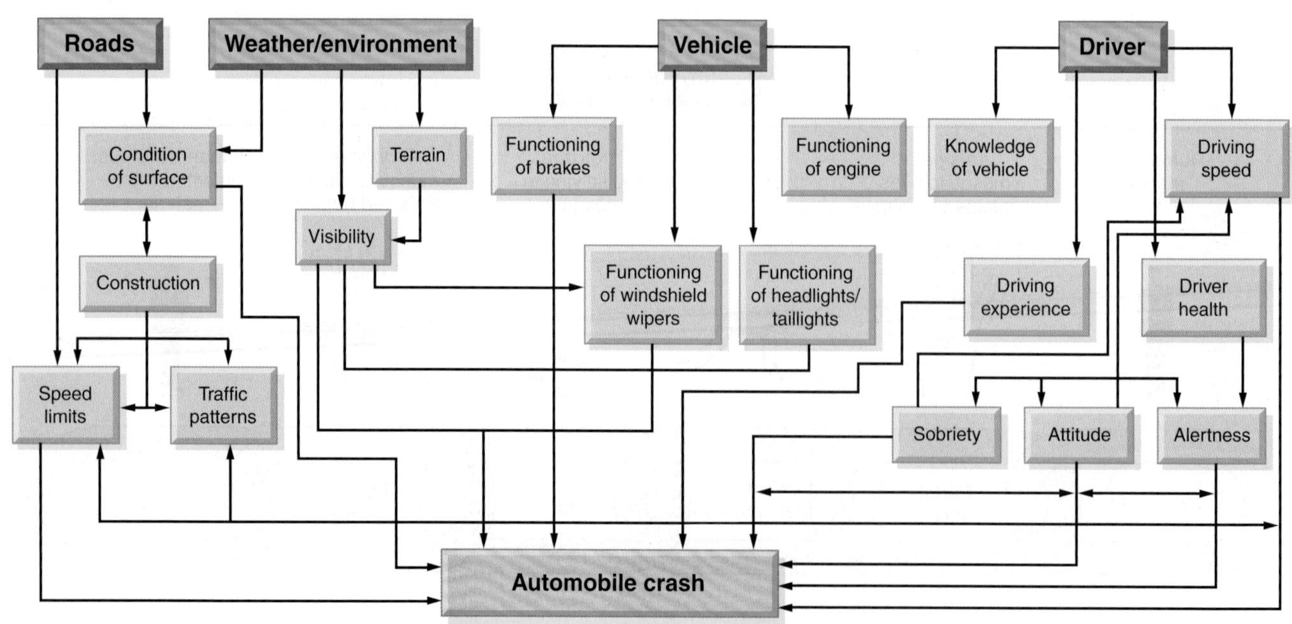

FIGURE 7-14 Web of causation for automobile crashes.

one clearly identified organism as the agent has the ability to be diagramed based on factors such as availability of emergency services (treatment), diagnostic skill of health professionals (early diagnosis), availability of medications and vaccines to treat the disease (reduced morbidity), and community communication networks (public awareness). Any of these factors could greatly influence the progression of disease within the community.

Association is a concept that is helpful in determining multiple causalities. Events are said to be associated if they appear together more often than would be the case by chance alone (see Box 7-10 later in this chapter). Such events may include risk factors or other characteristics affecting disease or health states. Examples are the frequent association of cigarette smoking with lung cancer, obesity with heart disease, and severe prematurity with infant mortality. The study of associated factors suggests possible causalities and points for intervention.

Contemporary epidemiologists continue to explore new and more comprehensive ways of viewing health and illness. The associations among lifestyle, behavior, environment, and stress of all kinds and the ways in which they affect health states are gaining importance in epidemiology (Szklo & Nieto, 2019).

Causation in Noninfectious (Noncommunicable) Disease

With the availability of vaccines and antibiotics by the mid-20th century to thwart most infectious diseases in the United States and the developed world, attention shifted to the causes of noninfectious diseases such as cancer and diabetes. A new causal paradigm was clearly needed. The linear thinking embodied in models such as the *chain of causation* was insufficient in understanding the causes of these emerging health threats.

The *web of causation* model, which previously was used to study infectious diseases and which encompasses multifactorial causes of health problems and issues, has therefore been adapted to study the causation of noninfectious (noncommunicable) diseases. One such adaptation of this model, proposed by Egger in 2012, explains the rise of chronic, noncommunicable diseases, for which there is no single underlying etiology, as the result of the body's reaction to its surrounding ecological environment. According to this model, the body develops systemic and chronic inflammation (*metaflammation*) at the molecular level to inducers (*anthropogens*) that are associated with lifestyles and modern built environments (Fig. 7-15).

Thus, preventive approaches to improving the health of those with chronic disease that are based on this model focus on reducing this inflammatory process through lifestyle changes (Straub & Schradin, 2016). Such preventive approaches are being taken today to address the top two leading causes of death—heart disease and cancer—and include modifying lifestyle and addressing environmental factors.

Examples of disease that can be studied using this model include:

- Air pollution, which has been identified as an independent risk factor for cardiovascular morbidity and mortality due to direct toxicity to the cardiovascular system or indirect injury by inducing systemic inflammation and oxidative stress in the peripheral circulation (Du, Xu, Chu, Guo, & Wang, 2016).
- Another example is how gene changes that alter cell function cause cancer. Genetic changes can occur naturally during the process of cell division, while others are the result of environmental exposures that damage the DNA. Such environmental exposures include tobacco smoke chemicals and ultraviolet radiation (NCI, 2020).

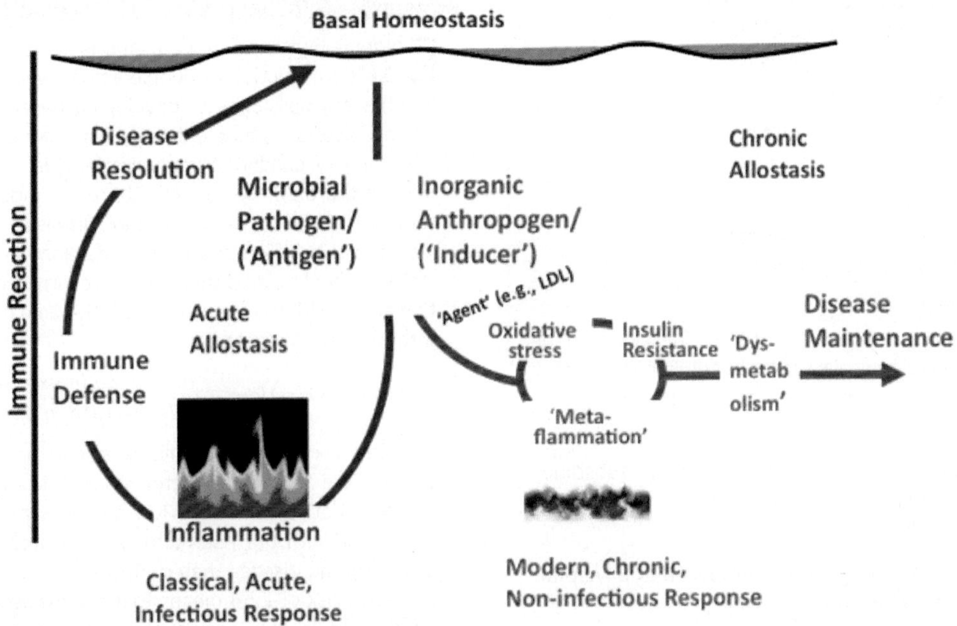

FIGURE 7-15 Anthropogen-induced metaflammation as the cause of chronic diseases. (Reprinted from Egger, G. (2012). In search of a germ theory equivalent for chronic disease. *Preventing Chronic Disease, 9*, e110301. Retrieved from https://www.cdc.gov/pcd/issues/2012/11_0301.htm)

Another aspect of this transition in focus from infectious to noninfectious disease is a shift from concern with individual susceptibility to the vulnerability of an entire population to chronic disease as a result of exposure to common environmental factors. Increasingly, public health workers came to realize the limitations imposed on individual control of health. After all, even individuals who are in the best of health may not withstand toxic agents in the workplace—for example, nuclear waste in the atmosphere from power plant accidents—or other debilitating conditions created by modern society. Therefore, more and more public health professionals are studying the environment and looking for methods to change conditions that contribute to illness in populations rather than just in individuals (see Chapter 9).

Immunity

Immunity refers to a host's ability to resist a particular infectious disease–causing agent. This occurs when the body forms antibodies and lymphocytes that react with the foreign antigenic molecules and render them harmless (Friis, 2018).

For community/public health nursing, this concept has significance in determining which individuals and groups are protected against disease and which may be vulnerable. Four types of immunity, seen in Box 7-2, are important in community health: passive, active, cross, and herd. Herd immunity is covered in greater detail in Chapter 8.

BOX 7-2 Basic Principles of Immunity

Immunity
Self versus nonself
Protection from infectious disease
Usually indicated by the presence of antibody
Generally specific to a single organism

Active Immunity
Protection produced by the person's own immune system
Often lifetime

Passive Immunity
Protection transferred from another animal or human
Effective protection that wanes with time

Cross Immunity
Immunity to one bacteria or virus is effective in protecting the person against an antigenically similar but different organism (e.g., cowpox vaccination protects against smallpox)

Antigen
A live (e.g., viruses and bacteria) or inactivated substance capable of producing an immune response

Antibody
Protein molecules (immunoglobulins) produced by B lymphocytes to help eliminate an antigen

Source: Centers for Disease Control & Prevention (CDC) (2018d); Merriam Webster Dictionary (n.d.).

Herd Immunity

Herd immunity or *community immunity* describes the immunity level that is present in a population group (USDHHS, 2017b). A population with low herd immunity is one with few immune members; consequently, it is more susceptible to a particular disease. Nonimmune people are more likely to contract the disease and spread it throughout the group, placing the entire population at greater risk.

Conversely, a population with high herd immunity is one in which the immune people in the group outnumber the susceptible people; consequently, the incidence of a particular disease is reduced. The level of herd immunity may vary with diseases. For instance, a level of community immunity of between 83% and 85% may be necessary for rubella, but for pertussis (whooping cough) 92% to 94% may be needed to be effective (Merrill, 2017). Mandatory preschool immunizations and required travel vaccinations are applications of the herd immunity concept. Figure 8-10 in Chapter 8 provides more information and a depiction of herd immunity.

Risk

Epidemiologists are concerned with **risk**, or the probability that a disease or other unfavorable health condition will develop. For any given group of people, the risk of developing a health problem is directly influenced, either positively or negatively, by such factors as their biology or inherited health capacity, living environment, lifestyle choices, and system of health care (McKenzie et al., 2018). When such factors are negative influences, they are called *risk factors*. The degree of risk is directly linked to susceptibility or vulnerability to a given health problem (Box 7-3).

BOX 7-3 Risk in Epidemiology

Epidemiologists study populations at risk. A *population at risk* is a collection of people among whom a health problem has the possibility of developing because certain influencing factors are present (e.g., exposure to HIV) or absent (e.g., lack of childhood immunizations, lack of specific vitamins in the diet), or because there are modifiable risk factors present (e.g., cardiovascular disease). Epidemiologists measure this difference using the *relative risk ratio*, which statistically compares the disease occurrence in the population at risk with the occurrence of the same disease in people without that risk factor.

$$\text{Relative risk ratio} = \frac{\text{Incidence in exposed group}}{\text{Incidence rate in unexposed group}}$$

If the risk of acquiring the disease is the same regardless of exposure to the risk factor studied, the ratio will be 1:1, and the relative risk will be 1.0. A relative risk >1.0 indicates that those with the risk factor have a greater likelihood of acquiring the disease than do those without it; for instance, a relative risk of 2.54 means that the exposed group is 2.54 times more likely to acquire the disease than the unexposed group (Merrill, 2017).

Natural History of a Disease or Health Condition

Any disease or health condition follows a progression known as its **natural history**, which refers to events that occur before its development, during its course, and during its conclusion. This process involves the interactions among a susceptible host, the causative agent, and the environment. The natural progression of a disease occurs in four stages in terms of how it affects a population: (1) susceptibility, (2) preclinical (subclinical) disease, (3) clinical disease, and (4) resolution (Fig. 7-16). The last stage, resolution, includes recovery, disability, or death (Friis, 2018). As shown in Fig 7-16, the stages may be grouped into two phases: phase I (prepathogenesis), which includes stages 1 and 2, and phase II (pathogenesis), which includes stages 3 and 4. Each stage is briefly described below.

1. *Susceptibility Stage*: The disease is not present, and individuals have not been exposed, but host and environmental factors influence their susceptibility. If a pathogen invades and the immune system's response is effective, then the infection is eliminated or contained and the disease does not occur (History of Vaccines, 2018).
2. *Subclinical Disease Stage*: Individuals have been exposed to a disease but are asymptomatic. In infectious diseases, it includes an *incubation period* of hours to months (or years, in the case of AIDS), during which the organism multiplies to sufficient numbers to produce a host reaction and clinical symptoms. In noninfectious disease, it includes an *induction* or *latency period*, which is the time from exposure to the onset of symptoms and is often years to decades (e.g., up to 40 years from exposure to asbestos and development of lung cancer).
3. *Clinical Disease Stage*: Signs and symptoms of the disease or condition develop, and diagnosis may occur. Early signs may be evident only through laboratory test findings (e.g., premalignant cervical changes evident on Papanicolaou smears), whereas later signs are more likely to be acute and clearly visible (e.g., enterocolitis in a salmonellosis outbreak; Heymann, 2014).
4. *Resolution or Advanced Disease Stage*: Depending on its severity, the disease may conclude with a return to health, a residual or chronic form of the disease with some disabling limitations, or death (Merrill, 2017).

C/PHNs can intervene at any point during these four stages to delay, arrest, or prevent the progression of the disease or condition. Primary, secondary, and tertiary prevention can be applied to each of the stages. However, primary prevention through health promotion and education strategies and health protection policies is the best and most cost-effective approach to ensuring population health (Box 7-4).

Epidemiology of Wellness

Epidemiology has moved from concentrating only on illness to examining how host, agent, and environment are involved in wellness at various levels. In response to an escalating need for improved methods of health planning and health policy analysis, epidemiology has developed more holistic models of health (Kiefer, 2017).

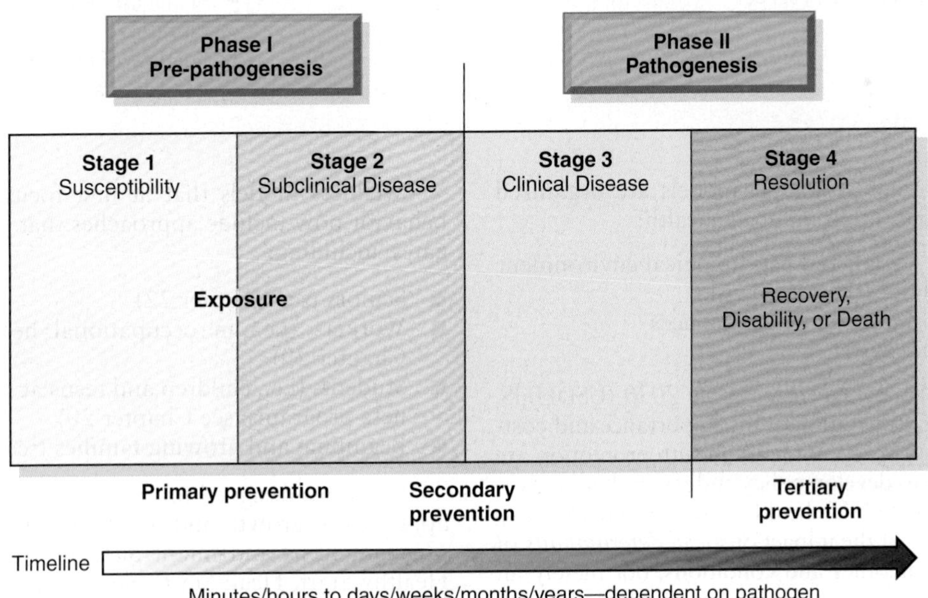

FIGURE 7-16 Natural history of stages of a disease. (Source: Centers for Disease Control and Prevention (CDC). (2012a). Lesson 1: Introduction to epidemiology. In *Principles of epidemiology in public health practice* (3rd ed.). Retrieved from https://www.cdc.gov/csels/dsepd/ss1978/lesson1/section9.html)

BOX 7-4 LEVELS OF PREVENTION PYRAMID

SITUATION: Apply the levels of prevention during the four stages of the natural history of a disease to eradicate or reduce risk factors (examples of potential conditions provided).

GOAL: Using the three levels of prevention, avoid or promptly diagnose and treat negative health conditions, and restore the fullest possible potential.

Tertiary Prevention

Rehabilitation	*Prevention*	
	Health Promotion and Education	***Health Protection***
■ Reduce the extent and severity of a health problem to minimize disability ■ Restore or preserve function	■ Training for employment—homeless population ■ Group treatment and rehabilitation—adolescent drug users ■ Food, shelter, rest/sleep, exercise	■ Health services ■ Immunizations as needed

Secondary Prevention

Early Diagnosis	*Prompt Treatment*
■ The third stage in the natural history of disease, the early pathogenesis or onset stage: ■ Screening programs—breast and testicular cancer, vision and hearing loss, hypertension, tuberculosis, diabetes	■ Initiate prompt treatment ■ Arrest progression ■ Prevent associated disability

Primary Prevention

Health Promotion & Education	*Health Protection*
■ May include ■ Nutrition counseling—diabetes ■ Sex education—pregnancy ■ Smoking cessation—lung cancer	■ May include ■ Improved housing and sanitation—waterborne diseases ■ Immunizations—communicable diseases ■ Removal of environmental hazards—accidents

These evolving epidemiologic models are organized around four attributes that influence health:

1. The physical, social, and psychological environment
2. Lifestyle, with its self-created risks
3. Human biology and genetic influences
4. The health care system

In the United States, *Healthy People 2030* (USDHHS, 2018c) and greater recognition of the importance and cost-effectiveness of illness prevention and health promotion are driving new efforts to develop policy and research initiatives that can improve the public's health (Box 7-5). There is also growing recognition of the impact of *social determinants of health* on health outcomes and conditions, not merely an individual role in one's health. Social determinants of health are "conditions in the environments in which people are born, live, play, worship, and age that affect a wide range of health, functioning, and quality of life outcomes and risks" (CDC, 2018h, para. 6). Population disparities result when these social determinants disproportionately impact individuals owing to race/ethnicity, socioeconomic status, gender, age, disability status, sexual orientation, and geographic location (USDHHS, 2018c). See Chapter 11 on health promotion and Chapters 15, 23, and 25 for more on this.

Wellness models that at first focused on individual behavior now include approaches that encompass aggregates, including:

- Seniors (see Chapter 22)
- Workers (i.e., in occupational health settings; see Chapter 29)
- Students (i.e., children and teens at schools with wellness programs; see Chapter 20)
- Beginning and growing families (see Chapter 19)

Programs designed for aggregates focus on a wellness approach to growth and development, such as those for pregnant teens and infant and child development (e.g., Healthy Start, Head Start). Societal changes, such as the aging population, the technological revolution, the global economy, environmental threats, health care reform with its focus on prevention, and the health and wellness movements, are driving these new approaches (see Chapter 6).

Another approach to wellness is applying the four stages of the natural history of disease to wellness states:

- *Susceptibility*: People are amenable ("vulnerable") to healthier practices and improved health system organization.

BOX 7-5 *SELECTED HEALTHY PEOPLE 2030 OBJECTIVES*

Core Objectives

PHI-01,02,03,07	Increase the proportion of state, local, tribal, and territorial public health agencies that are accredited
PHI-04,05,06	Increase the proportion of local, state, territorial jurisdictions, and tribal communities that have a health improvement plan

Developmental Objectives

PHI-D04	Increase the proportion of state public health labs that provide comprehensive lab services to support emerging public health issues
PHI-D05	Increase the proportion of state public health labs that use emerging technology to provide enhanced lab services

Research Objectives

PHI-R01	Explore and expand the use and impact of practice-based continuing education resources for public health professionals
PHI-R07	Explore the use and impact of quality improvement as a way to increase efficiency and/or effectiveness outcomes in health departments
PHI-R08	Explore financing of the public health infrastructure

Reprinted from U.S. Department of Health and Human Services (USDHHS). (2020). *Browse objectives: Public health infrastructure.* Retrieved from https://health.gov/healthypeople/objectives-and-data/browse-objectives/public-health-infrastructure

- *Subclinical*: A community is exposed to these health-promoting behaviors.
- *Clinical:* Signs of adoption of beneficial policies and activities are evident in the community.
- *Resolution:* The community fully adopts the beneficial policies and activities and achieves a higher level of well-being.

This approach has important implications for preventive and health-promotion practices in community/public health nursing as it can play a primary role in the investigation and identification of factors that not only prevent illness but also promote health. This means sharpening skills in epidemiologic research to uncover the factors that contribute to a full measure of healthful living. The time for an epidemiology of wellness has come (Merrill, 2017).

Causal Relationships

One of the main challenges to epidemiology is to identify causal relationships in disease and health conditions among populations. Causal inference is based on consistent results obtained from many studies. Frequently, the accumulation of evidence begins with a clinical observation or an educated guess that a certain factor may be causally related to a health problem (Friis, 2018). In epidemiological research, the types of studies to research causal relationships include:

- *Cross-sectional study:* Explores a health condition's relation to other variables in a specified population at a specific point in time and can show that the factor and the problem coexist (e.g., using the "broken window index" to correlate poor housing quality, public school deterioration, and the presence of abandoned cars, graffiti, and trash with crime and social isolation in neighborhoods [Aiyer, Zimmerman, Morrel-Samuels, & Reischl, 2015] and, by extension, perceived sexual partner risk level or other risk behaviors [Haley et al., 2018])
- *Retrospective study:* Looks backward in time to find a causal relationship, allowing a fairly quick assessment of whether an association exists. Such studies use existing data that have been recorded for reasons other than research and are generally less expensive and less labor intensive. One disadvantage is that the data may not be collected with a research outcome in mind. An example is a study of a giardia outbreak in a suburb of Boston caused by infection in a kiddy pool and then person-to-person spreading (Adam, Yoder, Gould, Hlavsa, & Gargano, 2016).
- *Prospective study:* Looks forward in time to find a causal relationship that is crucial to ensure that the presumed causal factor actually precedes the onset of the health problem (e.g., The Nurses' Health Study, with over 280,000 participants, related to women's health [NHS, 2018]).
- *Experimental study:* Controls or changes factors suspected of causing the condition and observes results, which are then used to confirm the associations obtained from observational studies (e.g., an experimental trial for a dengue virus vaccine in which 21 volunteers received the vaccine and 20 received a placebo injection; National Institutes of Health [NIH], 2016).

Epidemiologically, a causal relationship may be said to exist if two major conditions are met: (1) the factor of interest (causal agent) is shown to increase the probability of occurrence of the disease or condition as observed in many studies in different populations and (2) evidence suggests that a reduction in the factor decreases the frequency of the given disease.

The synthesis of data begins by selecting as many of the various types of epidemiologic studies of the problem as possible and reviewing those that are sound. The goal of any epidemiologic investigation is to identify causal mechanisms that meet Hill's nine criteria for disease causation and to develop measures for preventing illness and promoting health (Celentano & Szklo, 2019). The C/PHN may need to gather new data for this type of investigation but should thoroughly examine pertinent existing data first.

SOURCES OF INFORMATION FOR EPIDEMIOLOGIC STUDY

Epidemiologic investigators may draw data from any of three major sources: existing data, informal investigations, and scientific studies. The C/PHN will find all three sources useful in efforts to improve the health of aggregates. See Chapter 15 on community assessment for more on sources of data.

Existing Data

A variety of epidemiologic information is available nationally, by state, and by section (e.g., county, region, census tract, metropolitan statistical area). This information includes vital statistics, census data, and morbidity statistics on certain communicable or infectious diseases. Local health departments often can provide these data on request.

C/PHNs seeking information on communities may find local health agencies helpful. These agencies collect health information for groups of counties within states and interact with health planning authorities at the state level. They have access to many types of information and can give advice on specific problems. One newer source of data is social media (see Box 7-6).

Vital Statistics

Vital statistics refers to the information gathered from the ongoing registration of births, deaths, adoptions, divorces, and marriages. Certified births, deaths, and fetal deaths are the most useful vital statistics in epidemiologic studies.

The PHN can obtain blank copies of a state's birth and death certificates to become familiar with the information contained in each (for links to standard birth and death certificates, see thePoint). Death certificates report the fact and cause of death along with much more per-

BOX **7-6** POPULATION FOCUS

Epidemiology and Social Media

You probably use some form of social media. But, did you know that epidemiologists and C/PHNs have used Twitter and Yelp in foodborne illness investigations? Traditionally, most investigations begin with either a physician report to the local health department or a self-report called in by someone who became ill after eating out at a restaurant or a food truck. In most cases, people do not report when they have gotten ill when eating at restaurant, so food poisoning cases are underreported.

The Chicago Health Department used "FoodBorne Chicago" to track Twitter messages about food poisoning, leading to follow-up inspections of restaurants located within the city limits. Of the 133 Twitter-prompted health inspections, 20.3% identified at least one critical violation, compared with 16.4% of the 1,808 inspections initiated by usual methods. A total of 15.8% of restaurants failed inspection and were closed (Harris et al., 2014). Officials in St. Louis, Missouri, also instituted a Twitter message program of reporting foodborne illness and gathered 193 relevant tweets in 7 months. This method generated more reports than traditional mechanisms (Harris et al., 2017).

In New York City, health department staff noticed patron restaurant reviews often included reports of illness after eating at the same restaurant they were investigating for a recent gastrointestinal disease outbreak; most of these had not been reported to the health department. Thinking that this might be a reliable source for population-based investigation into foodborne illnesses, the New York City Department of Health and Mental Hygiene worked with Yelp in using data mining software to download weekly data that met the following criteria: (1) symptoms occurred after a meal, (2) symptoms occurred within 4 weeks of the posted review, and (3) two or more people became ill (or one person with symptoms of severe neurologic illness). An epidemiologist specializing in foodborne illness reviewed 893 potential postings and discovered three outbreaks causing 16 illnesses (Harrison et al., 2014). Officials in San Francisco worked with Yelp on a predictive model for health code violations, and their pilot study of 440 restaurant reviews, Yelp stars, and price ranges successfully predicted 78% of restaurants that would receive serious health code citations. When including specific key word analysis of reviews and expanding to 1,542 restaurants, the model was even more effective. They included New York City and found good predictive accuracy there, as well (Schomberg, Haimson, Hayes, & Anton-Culver, 2016).

The Web site iwaspoisoned.com is a consumer-led lead initiative, founded in 2009, that permits people to report online when they experience food poisoning symptoms. This real-time information collected from online reports is shared by consumers, food authorities, restaurants, and industry. There is also an app that informs consumers of whether a restaurant they were planning on eating at has had a food poisoning report. It was found that the site correctly identified several outbreaks before local officials became aware of problems (Neimark, 2017). These are examples of how collaborations of online sources with local health authorities have helped to reduce the incidence of food poisoning. Crowdsourcing such as this has been used in many areas of health care, especially during disasters and other emergencies (Wazny, 2018).

Source: Harris et al. (2014, 2017); Harrison et al. (2014); Neimark (2017); Schomberg et al. (2016); Wazny (2018).

tinent information. Birth certificates also can provide helpful information (e.g., weight of the infant, amount of prenatal care received by the mother), which can be used to identify high-risk mothers and infants.

However, nurses should note that the lack of standardization in collecting and reporting vital statistics data can lead to threats to reliability and validity. For example, if an agency changes the definitions for the categories used in grouping the data (reclassification), an inflation or deflation of the total of those affected can occur. Trending data over time would not be possible without including an explanation about the redefinitions used.

For example, according to the criteria of the *2017 AAP Clinical Practice Guideline*, about one in seven U.S. youths aged 12 to 19 years reported having hypertension during the period from 2013 to 2016. Prevalence of hypertension varied by weight status, ranging from 2% among healthy-weight youths to nearly 14% among those with severe obesity. The new guideline used a lower threshold of hypertension and new percentile references. Compared with the former guideline, the new guideline would reclassify 2.6% of U.S. youths (or nearly an additional 800,000) as having hypertension (CDC, 2018e).

Sources for vital statistical information include state Web sites, local and state health departments, city halls, and county halls of records (see list of Internet resources on thePoint®). Statistics regarding general aggregate morbidity and mortality for specific states are available from the CDC and, at the national level, from the National Center for Health Statistics (NCHS). State statistics are obtained from state health departments, and county information (regarding specific cities or census tracts) can be obtained from either the state or the county health department.

Census Data

Data from population censuses taken every 10 years in many countries are the main source of population statistics. This information can be a valuable assessment tool for the C/PHN who is taking part in health planning for aggregates. Population statistics can be analyzed by age, sex, race, ethnic background, type of occupation, income gradient, marital status, educational level, or other standards, such as housing quality.

Analysis of population statistics can provide the C/PHN with a better understanding of the community and help identify specific areas that may warrant further epidemiologic investigation. Data from the 2020 Census can be found on the U.S. Census Bureau Web site (https://www.census.gov/) and is an easily accessed source of population-level data.

Reportable Diseases

Each state has developed laws or regulations that require health organizations and practitioners to report to their local health authority cases of certain communicable and infectious diseases that can be spread through the community (Heymann, 2014). This reporting enables the health department to take the most appropriate and efficient action, for instance, in the case of foodborne illnesses. All states require that diseases subject to international quarantine regulations be reported immediately.

The World Health Organization (WHO, 2018a, 2018b) has numerous diseases under surveillance (e.g., TB, malaria, viral influenza) globally, and these must also be reported. Other reportable diseases (numbering between 20 and 40 in each state) are usually classified according to the speed with which the health department should be notified. Some should be reported by phone or e-mail, others weekly by regular mail. They vary in potential severity from varicella (chickenpox) to rabies and include AIDS, encephalitis, measles, meningitis, pertussis (whooping cough), syphilis, and toxic shock syndrome (MedlinePlus, 2017). The Laboratory Response Network (LRN) provides early response to biological and chemical agents involved in public health emergencies or bioterrorism (CDC, 2019b). See Chapter 16.

C/PHNs should obtain the list of reportable diseases from their local or state health department office. Following up on occurrences of these diseases is a task frequently assigned to PHNs working for local health departments. Chapter 8 includes more information on reporting and tracking communicable diseases at the local, regional, and national levels.

Disease Registries

Some areas or states have disease registries or rosters for conditions with major public health impact. TB and rheumatic fever registries were more common when these diseases occurred more frequently. Cancer registries provide useful incidence, prevalence, and survival data and assist the C/PHN in monitoring cancer patterns within a community. Nurses can access these registries through federal and state health department Web sites.

Federal registries include:

- Agency for Toxic Substances and Disease Registry (ATSDR, 2016) maintains three registries of major public concern:
    - *National Amyotrophic Lateral Sclerosis (ALS) Registry*: A congressionally mandated registry for persons in the United States with ALS (Lou Gehrig's Disease). It is the only population-based registry in the United States that collects information to help scientists learn more about who gets ALS and its causes.
    - *Rapid Response Registry*: A registry of persons who are exposed or potentially exposed to chemical and other harmful substances during catastrophic events to help local, state, and federal public health and disaster response agencies.
    - *World Trade Center Health Registry*: A comprehensive and confidential health survey of those directly exposed to fallout and debris on September 11, 2001.
- *Surveillance, Epidemiology, and End Results Program of the NCI:* An organization that collects and publishes cancer incidence and survival data from population-based cancer registries that cover a portion of the U.S. population (NCI, n.d.).

Surveillance Systems

The CDC maintains various surveillance systems to monitor diseases so it can develop and evaluate control strategies, including:

- The *Behavioral Risk Factor Surveillance System* conducts an ongoing state-based telephone survey of the civilian, noninstitutional adult population. Data collected provide the prevalence of high-risk behaviors, such as excessive alcohol consumption, cigarette smoking, physical inactivity and lack of preventive health care, such as screening for cancer. Results are published on a periodic basis in the *Morbidity and Mortality Weekly Report's* CDC Surveillance Summaries and are available online at https://www.cdc.gov/brfss/.

- The *Youth Risk Behavior Surveillance System* monitors unintentional injuries and violence, tobacco use, alcohol and other drug use, sexual behaviors that contribute to unintended pregnancy and STIs, unhealthy dietary behaviors, and physical inactivity, as well as the prevalence of obesity and asthma, in the national *Youth Risk Behavior Survey*. Results are available online at https://www.cdc.gov/healthyyouth/data/yrbs/index.htm (McKenzie et al., 2018).
- *Pregnancy Risk Assessment Monitoring System* (PRAMS) collects state-specific, population-based data on maternal attitudes and experiences before, during, and shortly after pregnancy. PRAMS surveillance currently covers about 83% of all U.S. births and the data can be used to identify groups of women and infants at high risk for health problems, to monitor changes in health status, and to measure progress toward goals in improving the health of mothers and infants (CDC, 2018f).
- *U.S. Zika Pregnancy and Infant Registry* was created in 2018 and is a collaborative system to learn about Zika virus infection during pregnancy and after birth. Information from the Registry is used to make recommendations for health care providers caring for families affected by Zika virus and plan for needed services (CDC, 2018g).

Environmental Monitoring

State governments, through health departments or other agencies, now monitor health hazards found in the environment. Pesticides, industrial wastes, radioactive or nuclear materials, chemical additives in foods, and medicinal drugs have joined the list of pollutants (see Chapter 9 for a detailed discussion). Concerned community members and leaders may view these as risk factors that affect health at both community and individual levels. C/PHNs can also obtain data from federal agencies such as the Food and Drug Administration, the Consumer Product Safety Commission, the Environmental Protection Agency (EPA), and, as previously mentioned, the ATSDR (USEPA, 2018). The CDC's *National Environmental Public Health Tracking Network* monitors the air, soil and water for potential threats to human health, as well as trends in chronic and other health conditions. The EPA has compiled a list of agencies and organizations addressing environmental asthma (USEPA, 2018).

National Center for Health Statistics Health Surveys

The NCHS furnishes valuable health prevalence data from surveys of Americans. Published data are also frequently available for regions. Examples are as follows:

- *The National Health Interview Survey* (formerly known as National Health Survey), established by Congress in 1956, provides a continual source of information about the health status and needs of the entire nation based on interviews from approximately 43,000 households each year (NCHS, 2018a, 2018b).
- *The National Nursing Home Survey*, which primarily samples institutional records of hospitals and nursing homes, provides information on those who are using these services, along with diagnoses and other characteristics (NCHS, 2018a, 2018b).
- *The National Health and Nutrition Examination Survey* reports physical measurements on smaller samples of the population and augments the information provided by interviews. It also provides prevalence information on injuries, diseases, and disabilities that appear frequently in the population (NCHS, 2018a).
- *The National Survey of Family Growth* focuses on fertility and family planning as well as other aspects of family health (NCHS, 2018a).

Other studies investigate vital statistics events and characteristics of ambulatory patients in physicians' community practices. Each of these nationally sponsored efforts suggests ways in which nurses can examine health problems or concerns affecting their communities (see Box 7-7). Interviews, physical examinations of subsets of community members, and surveillance of institutions, clinics, and private physicians' practices can be carried out locally after needs are identified and funds made available. Other sources may be found in data kept routinely, but not centrally, on the health problems of workers in local industries or the health problems of schoolchildren; a key issue for many C/PHNs. Existing epidemiologic data can be used to plan parent education programs, health promotion among students, and almost any other type of service.

BOX 7-7 STORIES FROM THE FIELD

How Public Health Nurses Make the Case

Public health nurses working for a local or county health department often find themselves more involved with program planning than direct patient care. Often, they are asked to help develop a health education program based on what is affecting the community the most, limited by budgetary constraints while still meeting reporting requirements of grant funders.

Let's say your health department has been given the opportunity to apply for funding from three sponsoring organizations. The choices are to develop public health education programs about alcohol consumption, smoking cessation, and community HIV testing. In an upcoming department meeting you are asked to make a case for and against applying for the funding of each of these programs.

1. *In preparing for this presentation, what specific types of data would you recommend to the department?*
2. *What would be the sources of these data? Are those sources from local, state, or national resources?*
3. *How could Healthy People 2030 help frame this presentation?*

Federal Public Health Agency Reports

The CDC issues the *Mortality and Morbidity Weekly Report*. This publication presents weekly summaries of disease and death data trends for the nation. It includes reports on outbreaks or occurrences of diseases in specific regions of the country and international trends in disease occurrences that may affect the U.S. population.

Most health departments subscribe to this publication, which provides important information both for epidemiologists and PHNs. It is also available free online from the CDC at https://www.cdc.gov/mmwr/index.html.

The Community Preventive Services Task Force (CPSTF) maintains the *Guide to Community Preventive Services* Web site. It houses the official collection of all the CPSTF findings, and the systematic reviews on which they are based are offered as a free resource to help C/PHNs and other public health professionals choose programs and policies to improve health and prevent disease within the communities with whom they work (CPSTF, n.d.).

Informal Observational Studies

In addition to perusing existing data, the C/PHN can also gain epidemiologic data by engaging in informal observation and description. The C/PHN can perform such study on almost any client group the nurse encounters.

If, for example, the nurse encounters an abused child at a clinic, a study of the clinic's records to screen for additional possible instances of child abuse and neglect could lead to more case finding. If several cases of diabetes come to the attention of a nurse serving on a Navajo reservation, a widespread problem might come to light through informal inquiries about the incidence and age at onset of the disease among this Native American population. Informal observational study often raises questions and suggests hypotheses that form the basis for designing larger-scale epidemiologic investigations.

Scientific Studies

A third source of information used in epidemiologic inquiry involves carefully designed scientific studies. The nursing profession has recognized the need to develop a systematic body of knowledge on which to base nursing practice. Systematic research is becoming an accepted part of the C/PHN's role.

Findings from epidemiologic studies conducted by or involving nurses are appearing more frequently in the literature. The Cochrane Database of Systematic Reviews is the most popular resource for systematic reviews in health care and includes a section on public health. Its Web site is searchable by topic or Cochrane Review Group. Additionally, the Web site includes reviews, methods studies, technology assessments, and economic evaluations (Wiley Online Library, 2018; see Chapter 4). Systematic reviews can routinely be found in many professional journals and the aforementioned Community Guide. These can provide the C/PHN with valuable information that can be used to positively affect aggregate health.

METHODS IN THE EPIDEMIOLOGIC INVESTIGATIVE PROCESS

The goals of an epidemiologic investigation are to identify the causal mechanisms of health and illness states and to develop measures for preventing illness and promoting health. Epidemiologists use an investigative process that involves a sequence of three approaches that build on one another: descriptive, analytic, and experimental studies. All three approaches have relevance for community/public health nursing (see Chapter 4 for a more detailed description).

Descriptive Epidemiology

Descriptive epidemiology includes investigations that seek to observe and describe patterns of health-related conditions that occur naturally in a population. At this stage in the epidemiologic investigation, the researcher seeks to establish the occurrence of a problem. Data from descriptive studies suggest hypotheses for further testing. Descriptive studies almost always involve some form of broad-based quantification and statistical analysis (Celentano & Szklo, 2019).

Descriptive studies can be *retrospective* (identify cases and controls, then go back to review existing data) or *prospective* (identify groups and exposure factors, and then follow them forward in time). In a descriptive study of child abuse, for example, the investigator would note the age, gender, race or ethnic group, and physical and emotional conditions of the children affected. In addition, the investigator would collect data that describe the economic status and occupation of parents, the location and setting of abusive behavior, and the time and season of the year when abuse occurred. In a retrospective study on reported varicella deaths, the investigators would describe the age, sex, ethnic background, and birthplace of victims and other information. Describing facets of these deaths provides information for further study and suggests avenues for intervention or prevention (Celentano & Szklo, 2019).

Counts

The simplest measure of description is a *count*. For example, an epidemiologic study to assess the impact of the routine 2-dose varicella vaccination program on death due to the disease used calculated rates to compare the prevaccine and mature 1-dose varicella vaccination program eras. Authors concluded that the new 2-dose varicella vaccination program significantly reduced varicella disease burden (Leung, Bialek, & Marin, 2015).

Obtaining a count of this type always depends on the definition of what is being counted and when it was counted. This particular count, for example, uses a large database that takes time to be made public and therefore may not provide a current picture of actual deaths. When using this type of data, the C/PHN should always consider the time delay involved. If a C/PHN needs more current information within a specific community or state, hospital records or death certificates may be another source.

Rates

Rates are statistical measures expressing the proportion of people with a given health problem among a population at risk. The total number of people in the group serves as the denominator for various types of rates. To express a count as a proportion, or rate, the population to be studied must first be identified. If those deaths are considered in relation to the total number of cases in the country, there will be one rate; if, however, those fatalities are considered in relation to the total population, there will be a quite different rate. It is important when reviewing rates that you understand which measures are being compared.

In epidemiology, the population represents the universe of people defined as the objects of a study. Because it is often difficult, if not impossible, to study an entire population, most epidemiologic studies draw a sample to represent that group.

Sometimes, it is important to seek a random sample (in which everyone in the population has an equal chance of selection for study and choice is made without bias). At other times, a sample of convenience (in which study subjects are selected because of their availability) is sufficient. In many small epidemiologic studies, it may be possible to study almost every person in the population, eliminating the need for a sample. Several rates have wide use in epidemiology (Merrill, 2017). Those most important for the C/PHN to understand are the incidence rate, the prevalence rate, and the period prevalence rate (see Box 7-8).

Computing Rates

To make comparisons between populations, epidemiologists often use a common base population in computing rates. For example, instead of merely saying that the rate of an illness is 13% in one city and 25% in another, the comparison is made per 100,000 people in the population. This population base can vary for different purposes from 100 to 100,000.

To describe the **morbidity rate**, which is the relative incidence of disease in a population, the ratio of the number of sick individuals to the total population is determined. The **mortality rate** refers to the relative death rate, or the sum of deaths in a given population at a given time (Celentano & Szklo, 2019). Table 7-3 includes formulas for morbidity rates, and Box 7-9 includes formulas for computing mortality and other rates used frequently in community/public health.

BOX 7-8 Incidence and Prevalence

Incidence

Not everyone in a population is at risk for developing a disease, incurring an injury, or having some other health-related characteristic. The *incidence rate* recognizes this fact. **Incidence** refers to *all new cases* of a disease or health condition appearing *during a given time*. Incidence rate describes a proportion in which the numerator is all new cases appearing during a given period of time and the denominator is the population at risk during the same period (Merrill, 2017).

$$\text{Incidence rate} = \frac{\text{Number of persons developing a disease}}{\text{Total number at risk per unit of time}}$$

Another rate that describes incidence is the attack rate. An *attack rate* describes the proportion of a group or population that develops a disease among all those exposed to a particular risk. This term is used frequently in investigations of outbreaks of infectious diseases such as influenza. If the attack rate changes, it may suggest an alteration in the population's immune status or that the disease-causing organism is present in a more or less virulent strain (Celentano & Szklo, 2019).

$$\text{Rate} = \frac{\text{Number of new cases in the population at risk}}{\text{Number of persons at risk in the population}}$$

Prevalence

Prevalence refers to all of the people with a particular health condition existing in a given population at a given point in time. The *prevalence rate* describes a situation at a specific point in time (McKenzie et al., 2018). If a nurse discovers 50 cases of measles in an elementary school, that is a simple count. When this number is divided by the total number of students in the school, the result is the prevalence of measles. For instance, if the school has 500 students, the prevalence of measles on that day would be 10% (50 measles/500 population).

$$\text{Prevalence rate} = \frac{\text{Number of persons with a characteristic}}{\text{Total number in population}}$$

The prevalence rate over a defined period of time is called a *period prevalence rate*:

$$\text{Period prevalence rate} = \frac{\text{Number of persons with a characteristic during a period of time}}{\text{Total number in population}}$$

Source: Celentano and Szklo (2019); Merrill (2017).

Analytic Epidemiology

A second type of investigation, *analytic epidemiology*, goes beyond simple description or observation and seeks to identify associations between a particular human disease or health problem and its possible causes. Analytic studies tend to be more specific than descriptive studies in their focus. They test hypotheses or seek to answer specific questions and can be retrospective or prospective in design (Merrill, 2017). Analytic studies fall into three types: prevalence studies, case–control studies, and cohort studies.

Prevalence Studies

When examining prevalence, it is helpful to remember that the health condition may be new or may have affected some people for many years. A *prevalence study* describes patterns of occurrence, as in the study of varicella-related deaths. It may examine causal factors, but a prevalence study always looks at factors from the same point in time and in the same population. Hypothesized causal factors are based on inferences from a single examination and most likely need further testing for validation. Intervening or confounding variables can lead to inaccurate assumptions about results, and studies must be carefully designed to avoid both falsely positive and falsely negative outcomes (Merrill, 2017). A recent international prevalence study found sociodemographic factors (e.g., education, gender) were moderators of the built environment (safety from crime) in meeting physical activity goals (Perez et al., 2018).

Case–Control Studies

A *case–control study* compares people who have a health or illness condition (number of cases with the condition) with those who lack this condition (controls). These

TABLE 7-3 Frequently Used Measures of Morbidity

Measure	Numerator	Denominator
Incidence* proportion (or attack rate or risk)	Number of new cases of disease during specified time interval	Population at start of time interval
Secondary attack rate	Number of new cases among contacts	Total number of contacts
Incidence* rate (or person-time rate)	Number of new cases of disease during specified time interval	Summed person-years of observation or average population during time interval
Point prevalence	Number of current cases (new and preexisting) at a specified point in time	Population at the same specified point in time
Period prevalence	Number of current cases (new and preexisting) over a specified period of time	Average or midinterval population

*Incidence refers to the occurrence of new cases of disease or injury in a population over a specified period of time. Although some epidemiologists use incidence to mean the number of new cases in a community, others use incidence to mean the number of new cases per unit of population.

Reprinted from CDC. (2012b). *Lesson 3: Measures of risk.* Retrieved from https://www.cdc.gov/csels/dsepd/ss1978/lesson3/section2.html

studies begin with the cases and look back over time (retrospectively) for presence or absence of the suspected causal factor in both cases and controls (Celentano & Szklo, 2019).

In a case–control study, Dabrera and colleagues (2015) explored whether maternal pertussis vaccination might prevent newborns younger than 8 weeks from being infected with pertussis. Cases included infants younger than 8 weeks who tested positive for pertussis infection with an onset of <8 weeks and healthy infants born subsequent to identified cases as controls. Mothers of 17% of the cases and 71% of the controls received pertussis vaccination during pregnancy. Vaccine effectiveness was 93%, and researchers concluded that maternal pertussis vaccine during pregnancy was effective in preventing infection of infants younger than 8 weeks (when they are too young to receive their own vaccination).

Cohort Studies

A *cohort* is a group of people who share a common experience in a specific time period. In epidemiology, a cohort of people often becomes a focus of study. Cohort studies, rather than measuring the relationship of variables in existing conditions, study the development of a condition over time.

A cohort study begins by selecting a group of people who display certain defined characteristics before the onset of the condition being investigated (Merrill, 2017). In studying a disease, the cohort might include individuals who are initially free of the disease but were known to have been exposed to a particular substance or risk factor. They would be observed over time to evaluate which variables were associated with the development or nondevelopment of the disease. These types of studies are often used with environmental hazard exposures, as with the Health Registry and the National Toxic Substance Incidents Program discussed earlier (ATSDR, 2016).

One workplace exposure study examined almost 48,000 employees who had contact with 11 toxins (e.g., dyes/inks, acids, paints, pesticides, metals, glues, petroleum products, soldering materials) and found that almost 2,000 cases of breast cancer were reported. They noted that premenopausal breast cancer was associated with exposure to soldering materials and that women with cumulative exposure to petroleum products at the highest level had 2.3 higher risk than those at the lowest level to for breast cancer and 2.5 higher risk for invasive breast cancer (Ekenga, Parks, & Sandler, 2015).

In 1993, the Women's Health Study, a 10-year national longitudinal, experimental, cohort study involving nearly 40,000 female health professionals was initiated (Harvard Medical School & Brigham and Women's Hospital, n.d.). Over the course of many years, significant findings regarding women's health issues were published (600+) and implemented to improve health outcomes.

In practice, the various types of studies just discussed are frequently mixed. A case–control study may include description and analysis with a retrospective focus; a cohort study may be conducted prospectively or retrospectively. The Women's Health Study is an example of a case–control study, a cohort study, and an experimental study. Flexibility is essential to allow the investigator as much freedom as possible in choosing the most useful methodology.

Experimental Epidemiology

Experimental epidemiology follows and builds on information gathered from descriptive and analytic approaches. In an experimental study, the investigator actually controls or changes the factors suspected of causing the health condition under study and then observe what happens to the health state (Merrill, 2017).

In human populations, experimental studies should focus on disease prevention or health promotion rather than testing the causes of disease, which is done primarily on animals. Experimental studies are carried out under carefully controlled conditions and must be approved by an Institutional Review Board. The investigator exposes an experimental group to some factor thought to cause disease, improve health, prevent disease, or influence

BOX 7-9 Common Epidemiologic Mortality Rates

A mortality rate is a measure of the frequency of occurrence of death in a defined population during a specified interval. Morbidity and mortality measures are often the same mathematically; it's just a matter of what you choose to measure, illness or death. The formula for the mortality of a defined population, over a specified period of time, is:

$$\frac{\textit{Deaths occurring during a given time period}}{\textit{Size of the population among which the deaths occurred} \times 10^n}$$

When mortality rates are based on vital statistics (e.g., counts of death certificates), the denominator most commonly used is the size of the population at the middle of the time period. In the United States, values of 1,000 and 100,000 are both used for 10^n for most types of mortality rates.

General Mortality Rates

$$\textit{Crude mortality rate} = \frac{\textit{Number of reported deaths during 1 year}}{\textit{Estimated population as of July 1 of same year}} \times 100{,}000$$

$$\textit{Cause-specific mortality rate} = \frac{\textit{Number of deaths from a specified cause during 1 year}}{\textit{Estimated population as of July 1 of same year}} \times 100{,}000$$

$$\textit{Case fatality rate} = \frac{\textit{Number of deaths from a particular disease}}{\textit{Total number with the same disease}} \times 100$$

$$\textit{Proportional mortality ratio} = \frac{\textit{Number of deaths from a specific cause within a given time period}}{\textit{Total deaths in the same time period}} \times 100$$

$$\textit{Age-specific mortality rate} = \frac{\textit{Number of persons in a specific age group dying during 1 year}}{\textit{Estimated population of the specific age group as of July 1 of same year}} \times 100{,}000$$

Specific Rates for Maternal and Infant Populations

$$\textit{Crude birth rate} = \frac{\textit{Number of live births during 1 year}}{\textit{Estimated population as of July of same year}} \times 1{,}000$$

$$\textit{General fertility rate} = \frac{\textit{Number of live births during 1 year}}{\textit{Number of females aged 15–44 as of July of same year}} \times 1{,}000$$

$$\textit{Maternal mortality rate} = \frac{\textit{Number of Deaths from puerperal causes during 1 year}}{\textit{Number of live births during same year}} \times 100{,}000$$

$$\textit{Infant mortality rate} = \frac{\textit{Number of deaths under 1 year of age for given year}}{\textit{Number of Live births reported for same year}} \times 1{,}000$$

$$\textit{Perinatal mortality rate} = \frac{\textit{Number of fetal deaths plus infant deaths under 7 days of age during 1 year}}{\textit{Number of Live births plus fetal deaths during same year}} \times 1{,}000$$

Source: Centers for Disease Control and Prevention (CDC) (2012b).

health in some way (as in the Women's Health Study). Simultaneously, the investigator observes a control group that is similar in characteristics to the experimental group but without the exposure factor. See Chapter 4 for more on experimental research studies.

The C/PHN should be alert for opportunities to conduct experimental studies in the course of working with groups. A study need not be elaborate to provide important data for future nursing practice. For example, a C/PHN can provide focused instruction to 20 new mothers encouraging them to breastfeed and then compare the health outcomes of their infants with infants of 20 mothers in the same service area who use formula.

An expanding area of experimental epidemiology involves the use of computers to simulate epidemics. With mathematical models, it is possible to determine the probabilities of various aspects of disease occurrence (Yang et al., 2015). This approach is making an increased contribution to epidemiologists' knowledge of etiology and prevention.

Occasionally, an experiment occurs naturally, thus affording the researcher a chance to make important discoveries. John Snow discovered such a "natural experiment" in London in 1854 (as discussed earlier in the chapter). In his seminal study of an epidemic of cholera, he observed one group that contracted the disease and another that did not. Closer inspection revealed that the major difference between these groups was their water supply. See Chapter 9 for a more current example from Flint, Michigan's lead-contaminated water.

A *community trial* is a type of experimental study done at the community level. Geographic communities are assigned to intervention (experimental) or nonintervention (control) groups and compared to determine whether the intervention produces a positive change in the community (Merrill, 2017).

Community trials can be extremely expensive and are not undertaken unless there is substantial evidence that the intervention will make a difference at the aggregate level. There are times when these community trials occur spontaneously, and it is important for the C/PHN to recognize these opportunities. For instance, one local public health department institutes an aggressive campaign to educate health care workers on the signs of elder abuse. Selecting a similar community where that level of training is not available, the PHN can then compare the rates of elder abuse reporting between these two communities. If you were conducting this research, what outcome would you expect in the community with the enhanced training? Where could you obtain this information? Think about what other measures you might also want to compare between these two communities.

CONDUCTING EPIDEMIOLOGIC RESEARCH

The C/PHN who engages in an epidemiologic investigation becomes a kind of detective. First, there is a problem to solve, a puzzle to unravel, or a question to answer. The nurse begins to search for basic information, for clues that might help answer the question.

Information is never self-explanatory, and, like a detective, the nurse must analyze and interpret every additional clue. Slowly, there is a narrowing of possible suspects until the causes of a particular disease, the consequences of a prevention plan, or the results of treatment are identified. On the basis of this investigation, the nurse can draw further conclusions and make new applications to improve health services.

Epidemiologic studies are a form of research. The steps outlined here are similar to those discussed in Chapter 4. Epidemiologic research involves seven steps (Table 7-4). Everything from an informal study in the course of nursing practice to the most comprehensive epidemiologic research project can be undertaken with these steps. An example of conducting an epidemiologic investigation can be found in Box 7-10 and will be used as examples for each step.

TABLE 7-4 Steps in Epidemiologic Research

Step	Description and Example from Box 7-10
Identify the problem	Any threat to the health of a group offers fertile ground for epidemiologic investigation. Issues can be identified by looking at local health statistics and trending data over time, defined by funding agencies, or unusual cases identified through screening and intervention activities. Box 7-10 example: Why did the woman have an elevated lead level?
Review the literature	Find out what has already been done to address the problem identified. Every epidemiologic investigation should begin with a review of the literature. Even discovering that little research has been done on the problem can be valuable information, a good source for conducting a literature review is the Community Guide Web site (see Internet resources on thePoint®). Conversely, if many studies have already been conducted in the area, this information can help narrow the study to areas that have not previously been investigated or allow researchers to replicate earlier studies to confirm findings in a different setting. A valuable source is the systematic review, which evaluates research studies done on specific topics. Box 7-10 example: Are the Koo Sar pills taken by the woman known to contain lead?
Design the study	The first step in designing a study is to formulate one or more specific questions to answer or hypotheses to test. Sometimes, the question or hypothesis emerges from the literature review or from the researcher's own analysis and hunches. Come up one or more hypotheses to test or questions to answer. Then plan what study type (descriptive, analytic, or experimental) or combination of study types, which best suits the goals of the research and how the study will be conducted. Will the data be collected retrospectively from existing records, or will new data be collected? Who will conduct interviews? What kinds of data will be needed to measure the outcomes of intervention? Box 7-10 example: Who else may be affected? The pills were bought at several locations. Did they also have lead?
Collect the data	Use available online sources (e.g., U.S. census demographic data; NCHS health-related data; CDC Behavioral Risk Factor Surveillance System risk factor data; geographic data from CDC's GIS, U.S. Geological Survey, and the Environmental Protection Agency), as well as data from state and local agencies and nongovernmental organizations. Data about a particular community may be available from the state, county, or local health departments, upon request. The Community Guide Web site may provide ideas about how to collect data for a particular purpose (e.g., assessment, evaluation, pilot testing), and what works and doesn't work. Development of data collection tools should start with why the data are being collected and what data are needed at the end of the study. This will help determine what kinds of data collection are most suited (e.g., mail surveys, telephone surveys, online surveys, face-to-face surveys, focus groups, etc.) in order to gather the data. There are many freely available data collection tools online. All methods of collection have pros and cons (DJS, 2015) that should be considered. Box 7-10 example: Gather samples of pills from cities she bought them at and test them for lead content.

TABLE 7-4 Steps in Epidemiologic Research *(Continued)*

Analyze the findings	In most epidemiologic studies, data analysis consists of summarizing the findings, computing rates and ratios, and displaying the findings in tables and graphs. At this stage, the data are used to address the original question or test the original hypothesis. Was the hypothesis supported or not supported by the data? Summarized data can also generate more questions or indicate areas that warrant further investigation. Box 7-10 example: Lead was found in three different sources, from three different cities, and each specimen contained different lead levels.
Develop conclusions and applications	Stating conclusions is an outcome of analysis and interpretation. The investigators summarize the results and their meaning for the purpose of making this information useful to the public and other public health and health service providers. Many times, research has direct practical application for improving health services, continuing or discontinuing services, or conducting future research. It is also important to describe mistakes made and lessons learned about study design and other aspects of the research and to propose further areas of study, to assist future investigators. Box 7-10 example: Laboratory findings indicated that lead was a contaminant during the manufacturing process.
Disseminate the finding	Finally, research findings should be shared. The audience for the reporting of findings should be considered during the development of the study to ensure that the concerns and questions of the audience will be addressed by the study. Of course, if the study is being sponsored, then the purpose for the study is clear, making the dissemination of the findings easier. Sponsorship, however, can affect how the findings are perceived. In medical research, financial conflicts of interest (e.g., pharmaceutical-funded studies) can negatively impact the value of the findings (Johnston, 2015). Nevertheless, information gained from epidemiologic studies must be disseminated throughout the professional community to strengthen the knowledge base for improved practice and to promote future research. Box 7-10 example: Findings from the 3-state investigation was reported to the CDC and published in the MMWR. As a result of the report, California and other environmental entities issued an alert that people can be poisoned by taking Koo Sar pills.

BOX 7-10 PERSPECTIVES: CONDUCTING AN EPIDEMIOLOGIC INVESTIGATION

Adult Lead Poisoning From the Use of an Asian Remedy for Menstrual Cramps—Example of an Epidemiologic Investigation

During a free lead-screening event, sponsored by a nursing school community health promotion center, a 33-year-old Cambodian woman who brought her two children to the center to be tested for lead poisoning also participated in being tested. She was found to have an elevated blood lead level (BLL) of 44 μg/dL, and a confirmatory BLL 1 month later of 42 μg/dL. Any level above 10 μg/dL is considered abnormal. The children and her husband were found to have normal BLLs. This woman was referred to the Connecticut Department of Public Health for follow-up.

As the Connecticut Adult Blood Lead Surveillance Program's Adult Lead Registry and Case Management Coordinator, I was responsible for compiling and analyzing BLL data from Connecticut laboratories performing these tests and following up on any reports of elevated lead levels, such as this woman who was identified through a community screening event sponsored by a nursing school.

After finding lead in the Koo Sar pills purchased in Connecticut, New York City and San Francisco and taken by the woman for menstrual cramps, public health department follow-up was conducted with the New York City and San Francisco health departments. Eventually it was determined that lead was not a listed ingredient of these pills but a contaminant during the manufacturing process. The investigation was considered significant and was reported in an issue of the CDC's *Morbidity and Mortality Weekly Report (CDC, 1999)*. As a result of this report, this case was further reported by various public health agencies to the public and their constituencies (Jung, 2018).

Lessons learned from this investigation:

- Collaboration between health care providers and public health entities allowed for a broader approach to addressing health and environmental issues, such as lead poisoning.
- Detailed follow-up at various points of an epidemiologic investigation allowed for cross-state efforts to identify new sources of exposure.
- Dissemination of findings by the CDC (via MMWR) provided scientific evidence that enabled the implementation of legislation in other states other than where the exposure initially occurred.
- Public health education regarding lead contamination of consumer products was expanded to include unusual sources of exposures.

Margie, case management coordinator

Source: Centers for Disease Control and Prevention (1999); Jung (2018); Poison Control (2018).

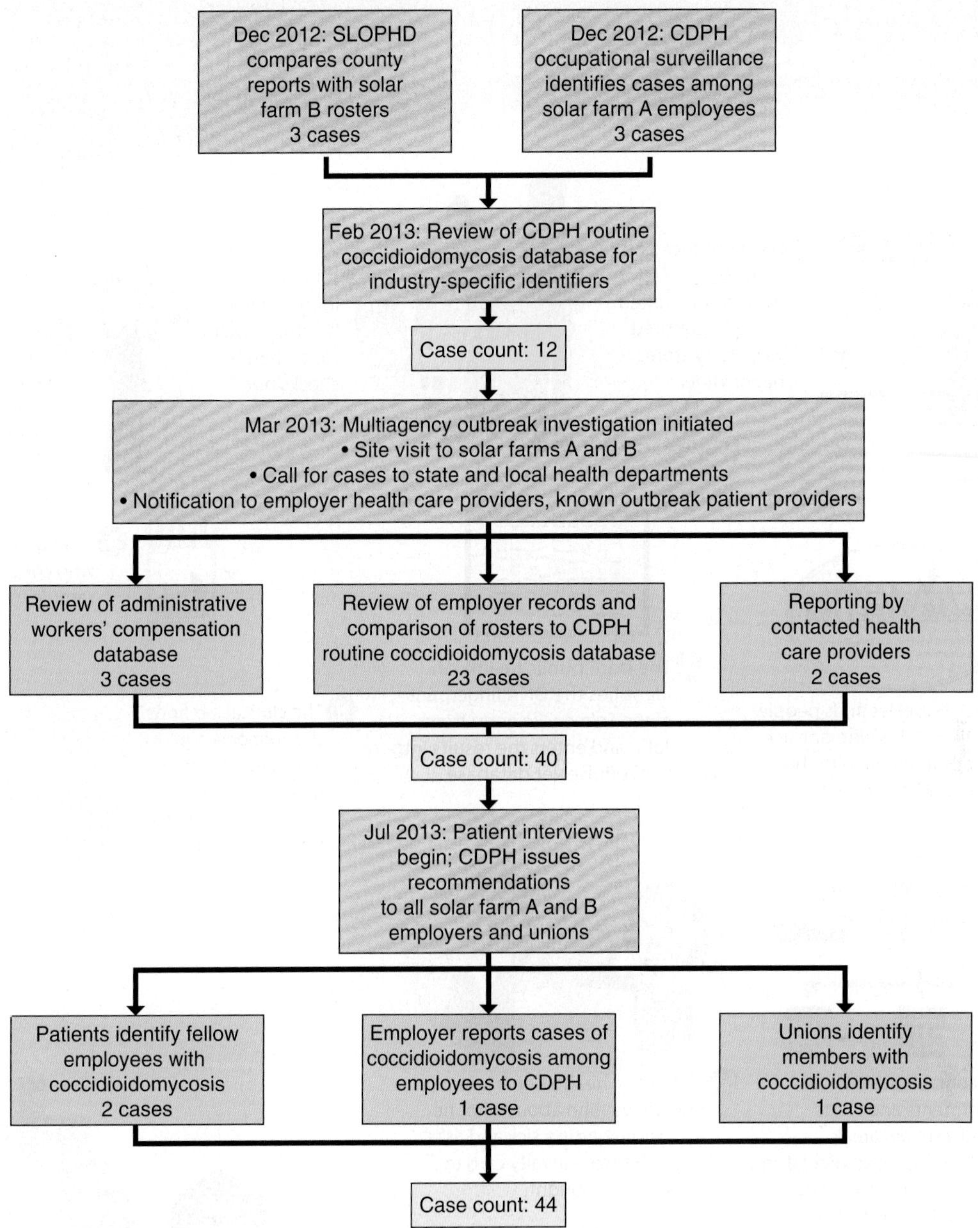

FIGURE 7-17 Flowchart of investigation of coccidioidomycosis among solar farm workers, San Luis Obispo County, CA, USA, October 2011 to April 2014. CDPH, California Department of Public Health; SLOPHD, County of San Luis Obispo Public Health Department. (Adapted from Wilkin, J. A., Sondermeyer, G., Shusterman, D., McNary, J., Vugia, D., McDowell, A., & ... Materna, B. L. (2015). Coccidioidomycosis among workers constructing solar power farms, California, USA, 2011=2014. *Emerging Infectious Diseases, 21*(11). doi: 10.3201/eid2111.150129. Retrieved from https://wwwnc.cdc.gov/eid/syn/en/article/21/11/15-0129.htm)

Findings from epidemiologic investigations should be disseminated in forms that are easily understood by the general public, such as the flow chart developed during an outbreak investigation of coccidioidomycosis among solar farm workers (Wilkin et al., 2015). See Figure 7-17 for a flowchart of the sequence of investigation that took place and how cases were identified, as well as what was done.

Figure 7-18 shows the impact of conducting investigations of multistate food outbreaks. Such outbreaks are becoming quite common because the manufacturing process of food products can affect people living in many states. It is vital that collaborative processes are in place in which all levels of public health agencies and health systems can communicate findings efficiently to prevent outbreaks as well as reduce morbidity and mortality.

Outbreak Investigations Help Everyone Make Food Safer

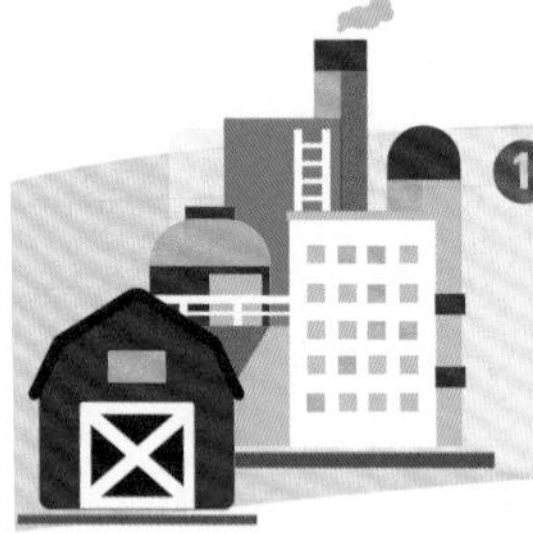

1 Food produced at company A's factory gets contaminated and is distributed to grocery stores nationwide.

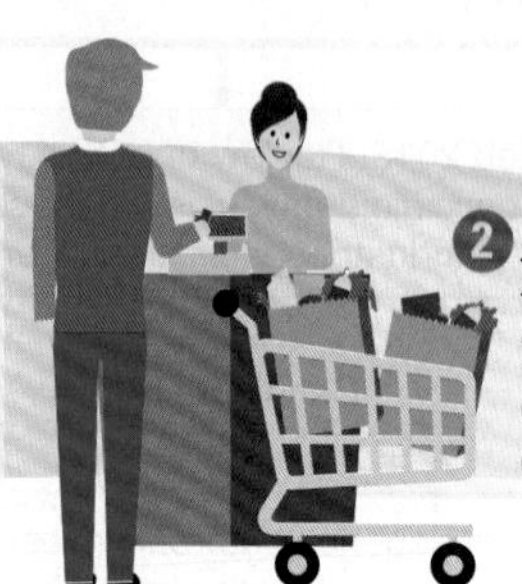

2 John buys the food and uses his store loyalty card when he checks out.

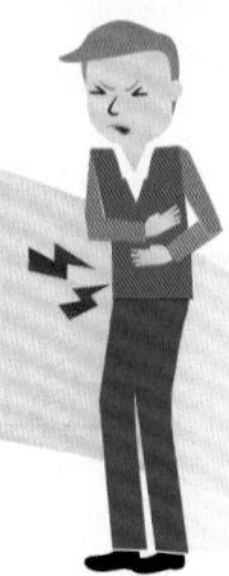

3 A few days after eating the food, John gets diarrhea, fever and stomach cramps.

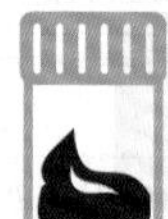

4 John goes to his doctor, who collects a stool sample to test for germs.

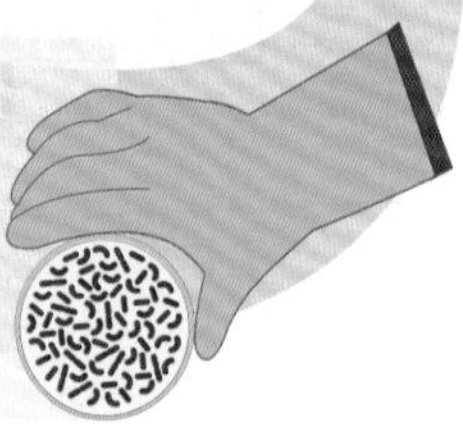

5 The clinical lab finds the *Salmonella* germ and sends a sample of it to the state public health lab for further testing.

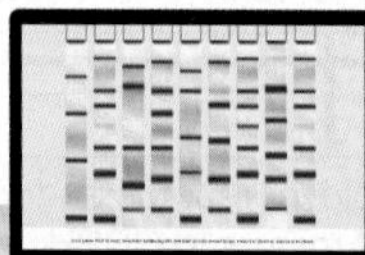

6 The state public health lab identifies the DNA fingerprint of the *Salmonella* germ from John and enters the results into CDC's PulseNet database.

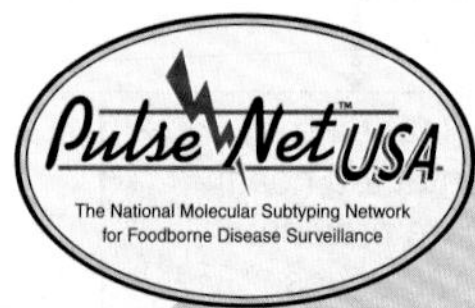

7 CDC's PulseNet finds people in other states who got sick from *Salmonella* with the same DNA fingerprint.

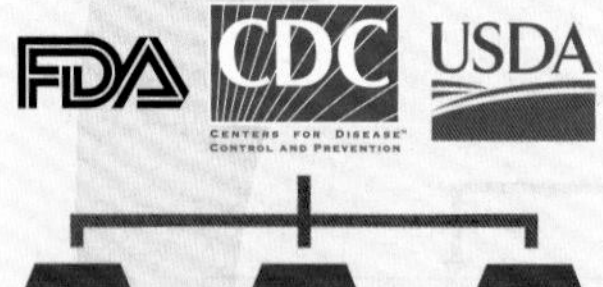

8a CDC contacts state health departments and starts a multistate outbreak investigation. Food regulators (FDA or USDA) trace suspect foods back to the source.

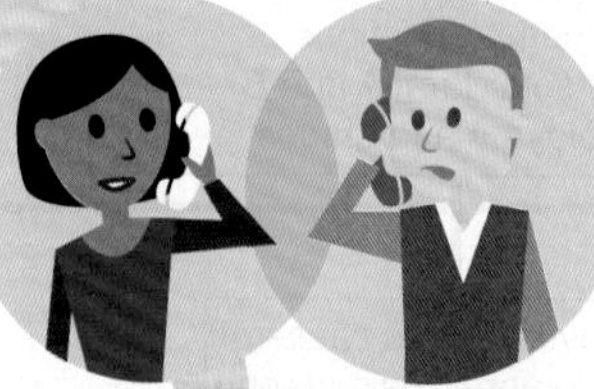

8b The public health department interviews John about what he ate before getting sick and asks to use his store loyalty card to see what he bought.

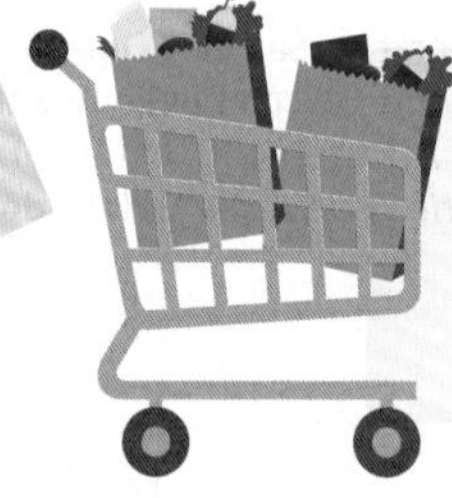

9 Interview results, store loyalty card data, source tracing and food tests show that many sick people ate a food from company A before getting sick.

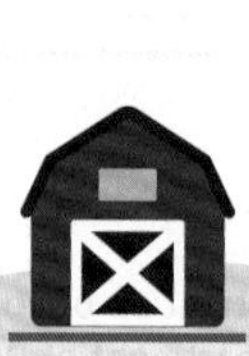
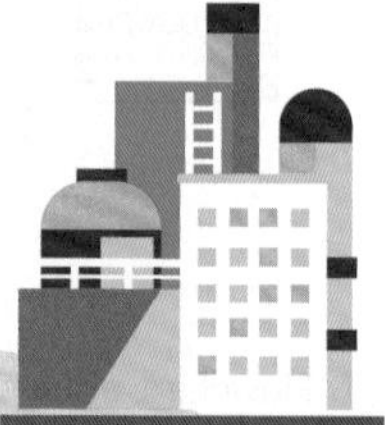

10 After discussing with public health officials and regulators, company A issues a recall and fixes the source of contamination.

11 Future illnesses and outbreaks are prevented when food regulators and companies that produce similar products improve practices based on company A's experience.

SOURCE: CDC Vital Signs, November 2015.

FIGURE 7-18 Outbreak investigations help everyone make food safer. (Reprinted from CDC. (2015). *Safer food saves lives*. Retrieved from https://www.cdc.gov/vitalsigns/foodsafety-2015/index.html)

SUMMARY

- Epidemiology is the study of the distribution and determinants of health, health conditions, and disease in human population groups.
- Epidemiology shares with community/public health nursing the common focus of the health of populations and provides a body of knowledge on which to base practice.
- Basic epidemiologic concepts the nurse should understand include:
  - The host, agent, and environment model
  - Causality
  - Immunity
  - Risk
  - The natural history of disease or health conditions
  - Wellness
  - Causal relationships
- C/PHNs can use three sources of information when conducting epidemiologic investigations:
  - Existing epidemiologic data
  - Informal investigations
  - Carefully designed scientific studies
- Epidemiology employs three investigative approaches:
  - Descriptive studies
  - Analytic studies
  - Experimental studies
- Epidemiologic research includes seven steps:
  1. Identifying the problem, which is usually a threat to the population's health
  2. Reviewing the literature to determine what other studies have found
  3. Carefully designing the study
  4. Collecting the data
  5. Analyzing the findings
  6. Developing conclusions and applications
  7. Disseminating the findings
- Thinking epidemiologically can significantly enhance community/public health nursing practice.

ACTIVE LEARNING EXERCISES

1. Identify an aggregate-level health problem in your community (e.g., hypertension, homelessness). Using the host, agent, and environment model, explain:
   a. Who the host is?
   b. What the causative agents are?
   c. What environmental factors have promoted or delayed the development of the problem?
   d. What vector control programs may be needed or enhanced?
2. Select an aggregate health (wellness) condition (e.g., preschoolers' normal growth and development, elders' healthy aging) and:
   a. List all the causal factors that might contribute to this healthy state.
   b. Plot these schematically in a diagram to show the web of causation model for this condition.
3. Using the same health condition that you selected in the previous exercise:
   a. Describe the natural history of this condition.
   b. Outline its four stages.
   c. Identify three preventive nursing interventions, one for each level of prevention that could apply to this condition.
4. Select an article that reports an epidemiologic study from a recent nursing or public health journal, and record your responses to the following questions:
   a. What prompted the study, and what was its purpose?
   b. Was it descriptive, analytic, or experimental research?
   c. Was the study design retrospective or prospective?
   d. Why did the investigators choose this design?
   e. What existing sources of epidemiologic data did this study use?
   f. List all sources specifically, such as *Morbidity and Mortality Weekly Report* or incomes by household in census data.
   g. What were the study findings? Identify the population group that will benefit from this research.
5. Interview one or more practicing C/PHNs in your community and identify an aggregate-level problem that needs epidemiologic investigation. Propose a rough draft study design to research this problem. How many of the 10 essential public health services would you need to employ? In relation to your identified problem, describe which three would be most useful.
6. Search for local or national news regarding a new disease threat (e.g., tick-borne diseases, Zika virus, COVID-19), an example of a foodborne illness outbreak (e.g., bacterial contamination of produce), or another example requiring epidemiological investigation. Work with a small group of classmates to develop a hypothetical case investigation and a potential epidemiological plan for action. Are there specific environmental factors that should be considered? If possible, watch for the resolution of the issue (e.g., conclusions of the investigation, public health recommendations).

REFERENCES

Abubakar, I., Stagg, H. R., Cohen, T., & Rodrigues, L. C. (Eds.). (2016). *Infectious disease epidemiology*. Oxford, UK: Oxford University Press.

Adam, E. A., Yoder, J. S., Gould, L. H., Hlavsa, M. C., & Gargano, J. W. (2016). Giardiasis outbreaks in the United States, 1971–2011. *Epidemiology & Infection, 144*(3), 2790–2801.

Agency for Toxic Substances and Disease Registry (ATSDR). (2016). *Exposure and health registries*. Retrieved from https://www.atsdr.cdc.gov/publications_health_registries.html

Aiyer, S. M., Zimmerman, M. A., Morrel-Samuels, S., & Reischl, T. M. (2015). From broken windows to busy streets: A community empowerment perspective. *Health Education & Behavior, 42*(2), 137–147.

Almasy, S. (October 1, 2019). *Eastern equine encephalitis death reported in Connecticut is 10th nationwide*. CNN Health. Retrieved from https://www.cnn.com/2019/10/01/health/eee-eastern-equine-encephalitis-connecticut-death/index.html

American Academy of Pediatrics. (2018). *Red book®*. Itasca, IL: Author.

Bain, L. E., & Awah, P. K. (2014). Eco-epidemiology: Challenges and opportunities for tomorrow's epidemiologists. *The Pan African Medical Journal, 17*, 317. doi: 10.11604/pamj.2014.17.317.4080.

Bryant, J. H., & Rhodes, P. (July 26, 2018). *Public health: Beginnings in antiquity*. Retrieved from https://www.britannica.com/topic/public-health#ref412417

Celentano, D. D., & Szklo, M. (2019). *Gordis epidemiology* (6th ed.). Philadelphia, PA: Saunders/Elsevier.

Centers for Disease Control and Prevention. (1999). Adult lead poisoning from an Asian remedy for menstrual cramps—Connecticut, 1997. *Morbidity and Mortality Weekly Report, 48*(20), 27–29. Retrieved from https://www.cdc.gov/mmwr/preview/mmwrhtml/00056277.htm

Centers for Disease Control and Prevention (CDC). (2012a). Lesson 1: Introduction to epidemiology. In *Principles of epidemiology in public health practice* (3rd ed.). Retrieved from https://www.cdc.gov/csels/dsepd/ss1978/lesson1/section9.html

Centers for Disease Control and Prevention (CDC). (2012b). *Principles of epidemiology in public health practice* (3rd ed.). Lesson 3: Measures of Risk. Retrieved from https://www.cdc.gov/csels/dsepd/ss1978/lesson3/section3.html

Centers for Disease Control and Prevention (CDC). (2015). *Plague: History*. Retrieved from https://www.cdc.gov/plague/history/

Centers for Disease Control and Prevention (CDC). (2016). *CDC disease detectives*. Retrieved from https://www.cdc.gov/about/facts/cdcfastfacts/disease.html

Centers for Disease Control and Prevention (CDC). (2017a). *Drug overdose data*. Retrieved from https://www.cdc.gov/drugoverdose/data/statedeaths.html

Centers for Disease Control and Prevention (CDC). (2017b). *Fentanyl*. Retrieved from https://www.cdc.gov/drugoverdose/opioids/fentanyl.html

Centers for Disease Control and Prevention (CDC). (2017c). *Understanding the epidemic*. Retrieved from https://www.cdc.gov/drugoverdose/epidemic/index.html

Centers for Disease Control and Prevention (CDC). (2018a). *What is the U.S. opioid epidemic?* Retrieved from https://www.hhs.gov/opioids/about-the-epidemic/index.html

Centers for Disease Control and Prevention (CDC). (2018b). *Notes from the field: Overdose deaths with Carfentanil and other Fentanyl Analogs Detected—10 States, July 2016–June 2017*. Retrieved from https://www.cdc.gov/mmwr/volumes/67/wr/mm6727a4.htm

Centers for Disease Control and Prevention (CDC). (2018c). *West Nile virus*. Retrieved from https://www.cdc.gov/westnile/index.html

Centers for Disease Control & Prevention (CDC). (2018d). *Immunology of vaccine-preventable diseases*. Retrieved from https://www.cdc.gov/vaccines/pubs/pinkbook/prinvac.html

Centers for Disease Control and Prevention (CDC). (2018e). *Hypertension among youths—United States, 2001–2016*. Retrieved from https://www.cdc.gov/mmwr/volumes/67/wr/mm6727a2.htm

Centers for Disease Control and Prevention (CDC). (2018f). *What is PRAMS?* Retrieved from https://www.cdc.gov/prams/

Centers for Disease control and Prevention (CDC). (2018g). *US Zika pregnancy and infant registry*. Retrieved from https://www.cdc.gov/pregnancy/zika/research/registry.html

Centers for Disease Control and Prevention (CDC). (2018h). *Social determinants of health: Know what affects health*. Retrieved from https://www.cdc.gov/socialdeterminants/

Centers for Disease Control and Prevention (CDC). (2019a). *Eastern equine encephalitis*. Retrieved from https://www.cdc.gov/easternequineencephalitis/index.html

Centers for Disease Control and Prevention (CDC). (2019b). *Frequently asked questions about the Laboratory Response Network (LRN)*. Retrieved from https://emergency.cdc.gov/lrn/faq.asp?CDC_AA_refVal=https%3A%2F%2Femergency.cdc.gov%2Flrn%2Ffactsheet.asp

Centers for Disease Control and Prevention (CDC). (2020). *10 essential public health services*. Retrieved from https://www.cdc.gov/publichealthgateway/publichealthservices/essentialhealthservices.html

Cima, G. (2018). *Synthetic opioids put police dogs at risk*. Retrieved from https://www.avma.org/News/JAVMANews/Pages/180201a.aspx

Community Preventive Services Task Force. (n.d.). *What is the community guide?* Retrieved from https://www.thecommunityguide.org/

Dabrera, G., Amirthalingam, G., Andrews, N., Campbell, H., Ribiero, S., Kara, E., ... Ramsay, M. (2015). A case–control study to estimate the effectiveness of maternal pertussis vaccination in protecting newborn infants in England and Wales, 2012–2013. *Clinical Infectious Diseases, 60*(3), 333–337.

DJS Research Ltd. (2015). *What are the pros and cons of data collection methods?* Retrieved from http://www.marketresearchworld.net/index.php?option=com_content&task=view&id=2118&Itemid=78

Du, Y., Xu, X., Chu, M., Guo, Y., & Wang, J. (2016). Air particulate matter and cardiovascular disease: the epidemiological, biomedical and clinical evidence. *Journal of Thoracic Disease, 8*(1), e8–e19. doi: 10.3978/j.issn.2072-1439.2015.11.37.

Egger, G. (2012). *In search of a germ theory equivalent for chronic disease*. Retrieved from https://www.cdc.gov/pcd/issues/2012/11_0301.htm

Ekenga, C. C., Parks, C. G., & Sandler, D. P. (2015). Chemical exposures in the workplace and breast cancer risk: A prospective cohort study. *International Journal of Cancer, 137*(7), 1765–1774.

Emergency Preparedness and Response (EPR). (2018). *Rising numbers of deaths involving fentanyl and fentanyl analogs, including carfentanil, and increased usage and mixing with non-opioids*. Retrieved from https://emergency.cdc.gov/han/han00413.asp

Evans, G. (2017). *Exposures to opioid patients endanger healthcare workers*. Retrieved from https://www.ahcmedia.com/articles/141390-exposures-to-opioid-patients-endanger-healthcare-workers

Florence Nightingale Museum. (2018). *Biography*. Retrieved from http://www.florence-nightingale.co.uk/resources/biography/?v=7516fd43adaa

Frankel, J. (May 2, 2018). *The hard-to-trace ingredient behind skyrocketing cocaine deaths*. The Atlantic. Retrieved from https://www.theatlantic.com/health/archive/2018/05/americas-opioid-crisis-is-now-a-fentanyl-crisis/559445/

Friis, R. H. (2018). *Epidemiology 101* (2nd ed.). Burlington, MA: Jones and Bartlett Learning.

Haley, D. F., Wingood, G. M., Kramer, M. R., Haardoirfer, R., Adimora, A. A., Rubtsova, A., &... Cooper, H. L. (2018). Associations between neighborhood characteristics, social cohesion, and perceived sex partner risk and non-monogamy among HIV-seropositive and HIV-seronegative women in the southern U.S. *Archives of Sexual Behavior, 47*(5), 1451–1463.

Harris, J. K., Hawkins, J. B., Nguyen, L., Nsoesie, E. O., Tuli, G., Mansour, R., & Brownstein, J. S. (2017). Using Twitter to identify and respond to food poisoning: The food safety STL project. *Journal of Public Health Management and Practice, 23*(6), 577–580.

Harris, J. K., Mansour, R., Choucair, B., Olson, J., Nissin, C., & Bhatt, J. (2014). Health department use of social media to identify foodborne illness: Chicago, Illinois, 2013–2014. *Morbidity and Mortality Weekly Report, 63*(32), 681–685. Retrieved from https://www.cdc.gov/mmwr/preview/mmwrhtml/mm6332a1.htm

Harrison, C., Jorder, M., Stern, H., Stravinsky, F., Reddy, V., Hanson, H., & ... Balter, S. (2014). Using online reviews by restaurant patrons to identify unreported cases of foodborne illness: New York City, 2012–2013. *Morbidity and Mortality Weekly Report, 63*(20), 441–446. Retrieved from https://www.cdc.gov/MMWr/preview/mmwrhtml/mm6320a1.htm

Harvard Health Publishing (HHP). (2018). *How to boost your immune system*. Retrieved from https://www.health.harvard.edu/staying-healthy/how-to-boost-your-immune-system

Harvard Medical School & Brigham and Women's Hospital. (n.d.). *Women's health study*. Retrieved from http://whs.bwh.harvard.edu

Heymann, D. L. (Ed.). (2014). *Control of communicable diseases manual* (20th ed.). Washington, DC: American Public Health Association.

History of Vaccines. (2018). *The human immune system and infectious disease*. Retrieved from https://www.historyofvaccines.org/content/articles/human-immune-system-and-infectious-disease

HIV.gov. (2018). *Global statistics: The global HIV/AIDS epidemic*. Retrieved from https://www.hiv.gov/hiv-basics/overview/data-and-trends/global-statistics

Johnston, J. (2015). *Conflict of interest in biomedical research*. Retrieved from https://www.thehastingscenter.org/briefingbook/conflict-of-interest-in-biomedical-research/

Jung, B. C. (2018). *Koo Sar pills epidemiological investigation*. Retrieved from https://www.bettycjung.net/Koosarnet.htm

Kiefer, D. (2017). *What is holistic medicine?* Retrieved from https://www.webmd.com/balance/guide/what-is-holistic-medicine#1

Leung, J., Bialek, S. R., & Marin, M. (2015). Trends in varicella mortality in the United States: Data from vital statistics and the national surveillance system. *Human Vaccines & Immunotherapeutics*, *11*(3), 662–668. Retrieved from https://www.tandfonline.com/doi/abs/10.1080/21645515.2015.1008880?src=recsys

Lilienfeld, D. E. (2007). Celebration: William Farr (1807–1883)—An appreciation on the 200th anniversary of his birth. *International Journal of Epidemiology*, *36*(5), 985–987. doi: 10.1093/ije/dym132.

McKenzie, J. F., Pinger, R. R., & Seabert, D. M. (2018). *An introduction to community & public health* (9th ed.). Burlington, MA: Jones & Bartlett Learning.

MedlinePlus. (2017). *Reportable diseases*. Retrieved from https://medlineplus.gov/ency/article/001929.htm

Meier, H. C., Sandler, D. P., Simonsick, E. M., & Parks, C. G. (2016). Association between vitamin D deficiency and antinuclear antibodies in middle-aged and older U.S. adults. *Cancer Epidemiology, Biomarkers & Prevention*, *25*(12), 1559–1563.

Merriam Webster Dictionary. (n.d.). Cross-immunity. Retrieved from https://www.merriam-webster.com/dictionary/cross-immunity

Merrill, R. M. (2017). *Introduction to epidemiology* (7th ed.). Burlington, MA: Jones & Bartlett Learning.

National Academies of Science, Engineering, and Medicine (NASEM). (2018). *Integrating responses at the intersection of opioid use disorder and infectious disease epidemics*. Proceedings of a Workshop. Retrieved from http://nationalacademies.org/hmd/reports/2018/integrating-responses-at-the-intersection-of-opioid-use-disorder-and-infectious-disease-epidemics-proceedings.aspx

National Cancer Institute (NCI). (2018). *BRCA1 and BRCA2: Cancer risk and genetic testing*. Retrieved from https://www.cancer.gov/about-cancer/causes-prevention/genetics/brca-fact-sheet#q1

National Cancer Institute (NCI). (2020). Cancer prevention overview (PDQ™)—health professional version. Retrieved from https://www.cancer.gov/about-cancer/causes-prevention/hp-prevention-overview-pdq#_92_toc

National Cancer Institute (NCI). (n.d.). *About the SEER registries*. Retrieved from https://seer.cancer.gov/registries/index.html

National Center for Health Statistics (NCHS). (2018a). *National Health Interview Survey*. About NHIS. Retrieved from https://www.cdc.gov/nchs/nhis/index.htm

National Center for Health Statistics (NCHS). (2018b). *Surveys and data collection systems*. Retrieved from https://www.cdc.gov/nchs/

National Institute of Diabetes and Digestive and Kidney Diseases (NIDDKD). (2016). *Symptoms and causes of diabetes*. Retrieved from https://www.niddk.nih.gov/health-information/diabetes/overview/symptoms-causes

National Institute on Drug Abuse (NIDA). (2018a). *Overdose death rates*. Retrieved from https://www.drugabuse.gov/related-topics/trends-statistics/overdose-death-rates

National Institute on Drug Abuse (NIDA). (2018b). *Prescription opioids and heroin: Prescription opioid use is a risk factor for heroin use*. Retrieved from https://www.drugabuse.gov/publications/research-reports/relationship-between-prescription-drug-heroin-abuse/prescription-opioid-use-risk-factor-heroin-use

National Institutes of Health (NIH). (March 16, 2016). *Experimental dengue vaccine protects all recipients in virus challenge study: Vaccine developed by NIH and FDA scientists*. Retrieved from https://www.nih.gov/news-events/news-releases/experimental-dengue-vaccine-protects-all-recipients-virus-challenge-study

Neimark, J. (2017). *"I was poisoned": Can crowdsourcing food illnesses help stop outbreaks?* Retrieved from https://www.npr.org/sections/thesalt/2017/11/30/565769194/i-was-poisoned-can-crowdsourcing-food-illnesses-help-stop-outbreaks

Nurses' Health Study (NHS). (2018). *Selected publications*. Retrieved from http://www.nurseshealthstudy.org/selected-publications

Perez, L. G., Conway, T. L., Bauman, A., Kerr, J., Elder, J., Arredondo, E. M., & Sallis, J. (2018). Sociodemographic moderators of environment-physical activity associations: Results from the International Prevalence Study. *Journal of Physical Activity and Health*, *15*(1), 22–29.

Poison Control. (2018). *Unusual sources of lead poisoning*. Retrieved from https://www.poison.org/articles/2011-dec/unusual-sources-of-lead-poisoning

Reardon, S. (June 28, 2019). The US opioid epidemic is driving a spike in infectious diseases. *Nature*, *571*(7763), 15–16.

Remington, P. L., & Brownson, R. C. (2011). Fifty years of progress in chronic disease epidemiology and control. *Morbidity and Mortality Weekly*, *60*(4), 70–77.

Resnick, B. (May 5, 2020). *Covid-19 is way, way worse than the flu. Vox.* Retrieved from https://www.vox.com/science-and-health/2020/5/5/21246567/coronavirus-flu-comparisons-fatality-rate-contagiousness

Ronan, M., & Herzig, S. (2016). Hospitalizations related to opioid abuse/dependence and associated serious infections increased sharply, 2002–2012. *Health Affairs*, *35*(5). doi: 10.1377/hlthaff.2015.1424.

Rosen, G. (2015). *A history of public health*. Baltimore, MD: Johns Hopkins University Press.

Schiotz, A. (2015). Medical statistics and epidemiology: The early history. *Norsk epidemiologi*, *25*(1–2), 3–9.

Schomberg, J. P., Haimson, O. L., Hayes, G. R., & Anton-Culver, H. (2016). Supplementing public health inspection via social media. *PLoS One*, *11*(3), e0152117.

Smith, D., & Moore, L. (2020). *The SIR Model for the spread of disease: The differential equation model*. Mathematical Association of America. Retrieved from https://www.maa.org/press/periodicals/loci/joma/the-sir-model-for-spread-of-disease-the-differential-equation-model

Straub, R. H., & Schradin, C. (2016). Chronic inflammatory systemic diseases: An evolutionary trade-off between acutely beneficial but chronically harmful programs. *Evolution, Medicine, & Public Health*, *1*(1), 37–51.

Susser, M., & Stein, Z. (2009). *Eras in epidemiology: The evolution of ideas*. New York, NY: Oxford University Press.

Susser, M., & Susser, E. (1996a). Choosing a future for epidemiology: I. Eras and paradigms. *American Journal of Public Health*, *86*(5), 668–673.

Susser, M., & Susser, E. (1996b). Choosing a future for epidemiology: II. From black box to Chinese boxes and eco-epidemiology. *American Journal of Public Health*, *86*(5), 674–677.

Szklo, M., & Nieto, J. (2019). *Epidemiology: Beyond the basics* (4th ed.). Burlington, MA: Bartlett & Jones Learning.

U.S. Department of Health and Human Services (USDHHS). (2017a). *Secretary Price announces HHS strategy for fighting opioid crisis*. Retrieved from https://www.hhs.gov/about/leadership/secretary/speeches/2017-speeches/secretary-price-announces-hhs-strategy-for-fighting-opioid-crisis/index.html

U.S. Department of Health and Human Services (USDHHS). (2017b). *Vaccines protect your community*. Retrieved from https://www.vaccines.gov/basics/work/protection/index.html

U.S. Department of Health and Human Services (USDHHS). (2018a). *What is the U.S. opioid epidemic?* Retrieved from https://www.hhs.gov/opioids/about-the-epidemic/index.html

U.S. Department of Health and Human Services (USDHHS). (2018b). *Integrating infectious disease prevention and treatment into the opioid response*. Retrieved from https://www.hhs.gov/blog/2018/07/17/integrating-infectious-disease-prevention-and-treatment-into-the-opioid-response.html

U.S. Department of Health and Human Services (USDHHS). (2018c). *Healthy people 2020: Public health infrastructure*. Retrieved from https://www.healthypeople.gov/2020/topics-objectives/topic/public-health-infrastructure/objectives?topicId=35

U.S. Drug Enforcement Administration (USDEA). (n.d.). *FAQ's-Fentanyl and Fentanyl-Related substances*. Retrieved from https://www.dea.gov/druginfo/fentanyl-faq.shtml

U.S. Environmental Protection Agency (USEPA). (2018). *Federal agencies and organizations addressing environmental asthma*. Retrieved from https://www.epa.gov/asthma/federal-agencies-and-organizations-addressing-environmental-asthma

Wazny, K. (2018). Applications of crowdsourcing in health: An overview. *Journal of Global Health*, *8*(1), e010502. doi: 10.7189/jogh.08.010502.

Wiley Online Library. (2018). *Cochrane database of systematic reviews*. Retrieved from http://www.cochranelibrary.com/cochrane-database-of-systematic-reviews/index.html

Wilkin, J. A., Sondermeyer, G., Shusterman, D., McNary, J., Vugia, D., McDowell, A., & ... Materna, B. L. (2015). Coccidioidomycosis among workers constructing solar power farms, California, USA, 2011–2014. *Emerging Infectious Diseases*, *21*(11). doi: 10.3201/eid2111.150129. Retrieved from https://wwwnc.cdc.gov/eid/syn/en/article/21/11/15-0129.htm

World Health Organization (WHO). (2018a). *Health topics: Epidemiology*. Retrieved from http://www.who.int/topics/epidemiology/en/

World Health Organization (WHO). (2018b). *International health regulations 2005*. Retrieved from http://www.who.int/ihr/en/

Yang, W., Zhang, W., Kargbo, D., Yang, R., Chen, Y., Chen, Z., & ... Shaman, J. (2015). Transmission network of the 2014–2015 Ebola epidemic in Sierra Leone. *Journal of the Royal Society Interface*, *12*(112). doi: 10.1098/rsif.2015.0536.

Yates, C. (April 1, 2020). *How to model a pandemic*. EarthSky. Retrieved from https://earthsky.org/human-world/how-to-model-a-pandemic

CHAPTER 8

Communicable Disease

"There are only two things a child will share willingly; communicable disease and its mother's age."

—Benjamin Spock (1903–1998), Pediatrician and Author

KEY TERMS

Active immunity
Antigenic drift
Antigenic shift
Cocooning
Communicable disease
Direct transmission
Disease control
Fomites
Herd immunity
Immunization
Incubation period
Indirect transmission
Infectious agent
Isolation
Novel
Pandemic
Passive immunity
Quarantine
Reservoir
Ring vaccination
Screening
Surveillance
Vaccine
Vaccine hesitancy
Vector

LEARNING OBJECTIVES

Upon mastery of this chapter, you should be able to:

1. Define the nurse's role in communicable disease control.
2. Describe the three modes of transmission for communicable diseases.
3. Identify four major communicable diseases in the United States.
4. Differentiate the strategies used for the three levels of prevention in communicable disease control.
5. Explain the significance of immunization as a communicable disease control measure.
6. Delineate the major concerns of parents who choose not to vaccinate their children.
7. Explain the importance of herd immunity in controlling vaccine-preventable diseases.
8. Discuss legal and ethical issues affecting communicable disease and infection control.

INTRODUCTION

In the United States, the highly contagious disease measles was eliminated in 2000. However, unvaccinated people and international travelers have been associated with outbreaks of this disease over the past few years. During 2019, there were 22 outbreaks and 1,249 confirmed measles cases, which is the highest annual number since 1992 (Patel et al., 2019). Imagine visiting Disneyland with your friends and family, only to learn that an infectious individual had been there on the same day. That occurred in 2019, and in 2014, "at least 131 California residents were infected with measles" in the state's most recent "large outbreak of measles" (California Department of Public Health, 2020, para. 3; Hassan, 2019). Communicable diseases pose a major threat to public health and are of significant concern to community/public health nurses. A **communicable disease** is caused by an **infectious agent**, such as a virus or bacteria, and can be transmitted from one source to another. Transmission to a susceptible host can occur directly either from person to person or animal to human, or transmission may occur indirectly through a **reservoir** such as contaminated water (Centers for Disease Control and Prevention [CDC], 2012; Heymann, 2015). Some noncommunicable diseases can also be caused by infectious agents, such as tetanus, but cannot be transmitted from one source to another (CDC, 2018a). Jurisdictional laws and regulations define the infectious and noninfectious diseases to be reported to local, state, and territorial public health departments. The National Notifiable Diseases Surveillance System allows sharing of notifiable disease information nationally and between jurisdictions for surveillance, control, and prevention purposes (CDC, 2018b).

Knowledge of communicable diseases is fundamental to the practice of community/public health nursing because these diseases typically spread through communities of people. It is essential for the nurse to understand the basic concepts of communicable **disease control**, which involves teaching important and effective preventive measures to community members, advocating for those affected, protecting the well-being of uninfected persons (including health care workers and nurses themselves), and controlling communicable disease in populations and groups (CDC, 2012).

In the last century, numerous changes occurred in the lives of people both nationally and globally related to issues of public health. Communicable disease control is recognized as one of the 10 great public health achievements of the 20th century (CDC, 2013). In the early 1900s, the top three causes of death were pneumonia, tuberculosis (TB), and diarrheal or enteric diseases. Then, control measures including improved sanitation and hygiene, vaccinations, and use of antibiotics and other antimicrobials, along with improved surveillance systems, have all contributed to a significant reduction of infant and child mortality and a nearly 30-year increase in life expectancy overall (Penn Wharton, 2016).

During the first decade of the 21st century, new vaccines reduced the number of serious illness and death due to pneumococcal infection and reduced rotavirus-related hospitalizations among children. Deaths related to other vaccine-preventable diseases (VPDs), including hepatitis A, hepatitis B, and varicella, were also reduced during this 10-year time period (Hinman, Orenstein, & Schuchat, 2011). In addition, improved public health infrastructure and changes in prevention strategies resulted in a 30% reduction in TB and a 58% reduction in bloodstream infections related to central lines. Improved testing has allowed more people with human immunodeficiency virus (HIV)/AIDS to be identified and receive lifesaving treatment earlier. Rabies control efforts have resulted in the elimination of canine rabies in the United States (CDC, 2018g). The CDC is charged to protect Americans against threats of disease, both in the United States and abroad (CDC, 2015a, 2019h). But, new challenges in communicable disease control have emerged:

- Human migration, modern transportation, and globalization leading to the spread of new pathogens and vectors such as the H1N1 influenza pandemic in 2009 and 2010 and Zika and Ebola virus outbreaks in West Africa in 2014 and 2017– 2018 (CDC, 2016e, 2019h, 2019p, 2020f; Heymann, 2015; Moreno-Madriñán & Turell, 2018; Porse, et al., 2018).
- Diseases with epidemic potential due to little or no countermeasures being in place, such as Zika virus, Ebola virus, and Middle East respiratory syndrome coronavirus (CDC, 2019p; WHO, 2016a). The COVID-19 (SARS-CoV-2) outbreak brought that reality to life, as the initial epidemic in China spread around the world as a pandemic, infecting millions (Johns Hopkins University of Medicine, 2020).
- Climate variability and increased rate of urbanization affecting the transmission patterns of vector-borne diseases such as dengue and Zika virus diseases (Otmani del Barrio, Simard, & Caprara, 2018).
- Development of antibiotic-resistant strains of the bacteria *Neisseria Meningitides*, groups A and B *Streptococcus*, TB, and gonorrhea that threaten the public's health and pose significant occupational health risk for health workers (CDC, 2015d, 2018i, 2019d; WHO, 2018c).
- The threat of bioterrorism, which involves the use of biologic agents with the intent to cause harm (Heymann, 2015); see Chapter 17 for more on emerging infections and bioterrorism.

This chapter provides information to help you better understand communicable diseases in communities and around the globe. It describes ways to plan and implement appropriate prevention interventions, including immunization of children and adults, environmental interventions, community education, screening programs, and disease investigation and case/contact finding. Ethical issues of communicable disease control are also discussed. A list of communicable disease information sources useful to you, the C/PHN, are also provided.

BASIC CONCEPTS REGARDING COMMUNICABLE DISEASES

Communicable diseases have challenged health care providers for centuries. Exposure to infectious agents can occur out in the community or within health care settings. The threat of these diseases has led to the development of important infection control measures over the last century (Heymann, 2015; Rosner, 2010):

- Hand washing
- Use of personal protective equipment
- Safe handling of contaminated sharp equipment
- Appropriate disposal of potentially infectious materials
- Community sanitation
- Pest control
- Vaccines
- Antimicrobial medications

Evolution of Communicable Disease Control

Although communicable diseases are no longer the leading cause of death in the world, they continue to pose a serious threat. Three of the top ten causes of death worldwide continue to be infectious illnesses. In 2016, lower respiratory infections, as a group, were the fourth-leading cause, responsible for 3.0 million global deaths. Even though the worldwide number of deaths attributed to diarrhea and TB have declined, these diseases are still responsible for the deaths of 1.4 million and 1.3 million people, respectively (WHO, 2020h).

Bubonic plague, caused by *Yersinia pestis*, is one example of how communicable diseases have changed the course of history. The first documented pandemic plague occurred in 541 AD. The next 200 years saw outbreaks in Africa, Egypt, Istanbul, Europe, and across the Middle East, with over 100 million deaths due to plague (CDC, 2019k; Frith, 2012). In 1347–1352, the great plague pandemic, known as "Black Death," killed 25% of the European population in the first plague and another 20% in the second one; it killed over 25 million people in Africa and Asia (Frith, 2012). Now, this deadly disease can be controlled through early identification and treatment with antibiotics. It may be transmitted when humans are bitten by infected fleas, when they come in contact with infected tissue or body fluids of an infected animal, or when droplets from a person infected with plague pneumonia are inhaled by another person. *Y. pestis* has been used as a weapon during wars over the centuries. Weaponization of *Y. pestis* remains a threat today (CDC, 2019k, 2019l).

Historically, as countries became industrialized, increased productivity, trade, and economic growth also brought on the four D's of disruption, deprivation, disease, and death. Industrialization brings large numbers of people close together in condensed living conditions. Trade brings populations together, exposing them to infectious agents they had not previously seen. These conditions, combined with poor sanitation leading to contaminated water supplies and infestation of disease-carrying insects or rodents, have all contributed to devastating epidemics in the past and continue to pose a threat today in developing countries (Boyce, Katz, & Standley, 2019).

To address this threat, the CDC is tasked with health promotion and disease prevention (see Chapter 6). It is recognized globally for its partnerships in disease surveillance, research, data collection, and analysis, as well as for responding nationally and globally with peer agencies to disease outbreaks (CDC, 2015a, 2020d). The World Health Organization (WHO) addresses communicable and noncommunicable diseases, working on emergency preparedness, surveillance, and response (WHO, 2018a, 2020a, WHO, 2020e). See more on global health in Chapter 16.

Smallpox, caused by the *variola* virus, is a classic example of a communicable disease control success story. The *variola* virus had been associated with devastating epidemics throughout the centuries. Smallpox became endemic in Europe in the 18th century and was responsible for 300 to 500 million deaths worldwide during the 20th century (Thèves, Biagini, & Crubezy, 2014). Smallpox first responded to a crude vaccine that was developed in the 18th century. The vaccine was studied and perfected and used globally for decades. A major worldwide eradication campaign began in 1967, under the direction of the WHO (Heymann, 2015). In 1980, the World Health Assembly declared the eradication of smallpox and made a call to cease smallpox vaccinations around the globe (WHO, 2014a). Outside of a small accidental laboratory-related outbreak in 1978, there have been no cases of smallpox since that time (Heymann, 2015).

Despite strides in controlling major disease outbreaks, nations and disease prevention organizations worldwide, such as the following, must continue to prepare for the future through collaboration, surveillance, and prevention (Heymann, 2015):

- Global Health Security Agenda (2018), an international partnership among nearly 50 participating nations and nongovernmental stakeholders, strives to make the world safe and secure from biological threats.
- The National Notifiable Diseases Surveillance System electronically collects, analyzes, and shares data on over 120 diseases provided by local, state, and territorial public health departments as per mandated jurisdictional laws and regulations (CDC, 2018b).
- Global Health Security is part of the CDC's prevention effort to stop the spread of disease through prevention, surveillance, and rapid response to outbreaks as a result of globalization (CDC, 2020d).

Community/Public Health Nurse's Role: Process of Investigating Reportable Communicable Diseases

Health care providers, veterinarians, and laboratories are required to report certain diseases in humans to the local health authority and, in some cases, to the CDC (Heymann, 2015). Each state has a State Health Department, and some states have local sites, such as a county or city health department. Such departments are typically staffed by a combination of nurses, epidemiologists, and communicable disease investigators (CDC, 2019h). See Chapter 6.

The local health department or agency is the initial point of notification of a communicable disease investigation. If a person is identified in one jurisdiction but was exposed in another, the health agency receiving the report should notify the health agency where the exposure occurred, so an investigation can be conducted in the originating region (Heymann, 2015). In most states, reporting known or suspected cases of a reportable disease is generally considered to be an obligation of:

- Physicians, dentists, nurses, veterinarians, pharmacists, and other health professionals
- Medical examiners
- Administrators of hospitals, clinics, nursing homes, schools, and nurseries

Some states also require or request reporting from:

- Laboratory directors
- Any individual who knows of or suspects the existence of a reportable disease (County of Los Angeles Department of Public Health, n.d.; Heymann, 2015).

Figure 8-1 outlines the Notifiable Disease Surveillance process. Each state has a disease report form (see example on thePoint), and the local health department or agency investigates a specific disease using a protocol set by the local, state, or federal public health official. Reportable diseases must be reported to the state health department. Notifiable diseases are voluntarily reported by the state to the CDC (CDC, 2020j). Individual citizens may also contact the CDC directly via mail, phone, or the Internet. You can reach them at:

Centers for Disease Control and Prevention
800-CDC-INFO (800-232-4636); TTY: (888) 232–6348, 24 hours/every day
E-mail: cdcinfo@cdc.gov; Website: https://www.cdc.gov/

Disease investigation requires a systematic approach. The nurse may be assigned to work on individual cases of a disease or several cases that make up a cluster or outbreak. Whether it is a single case of illness in a small town or a multijurisdictional outbreak, the nurse should follow similar steps (Heymann, 2015):

1. Identify additional people who might be infected (surveillance)
2. Determine the possible source of infection and means of transmission
3. Identify others who are at risk so screening and prevention measures can be implemented
4. Prevent further transmission
5. Monitor the response to these interventions

HOW WE DO
NOTIFIABLE DISEASE SURVEILLANCE

1 Patient

A person feels ill and goes to the doctor.

2 Healthcare Team

Doctor diagnoses or laboratory tests confirm a disease that is reportable by state law to the local or state public health department.

Doctor or lab sends information about this disease to the local or state public health department.

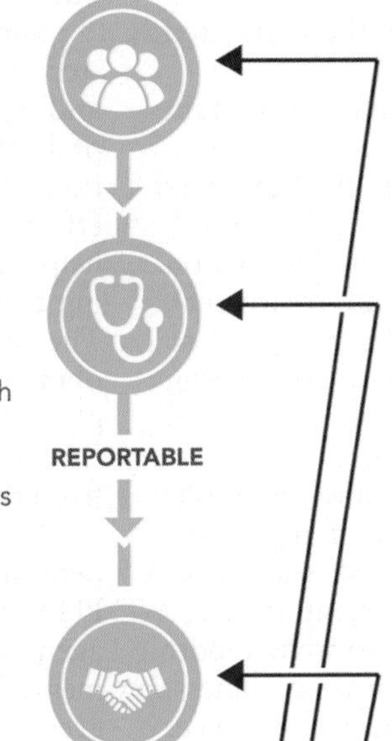

3 Public Health Department

The public health department receives disease data and uses them to:

- identify and control disease outbreaks
- ensure that the patient is effectively treated so disease is not spread
- provide testing and preventive care to those exposed to the disease
- control sources of exposure.

The state public health department sends information about national notifiable diseases to CDC.

NOTIFIABLE

4 CDC National Notifiable Diseases Surveillance System Team

NNDSS collects national notifiable disease data on behalf of CDC.

The NNDSS team receives, secures, processes, and provides these data to disease-specific programs across CDC.

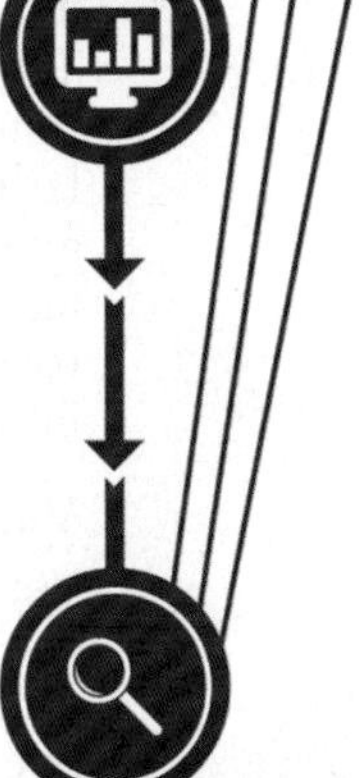

5 CDC Disease Program

CDC programs use disease-specific data to:

- support recognition of disease outbreaks
- monitor shifts in disease patterns
- evaluate and fund disease control activities.

CDC provides INFORMATION:

- ▶ Websites
- ▶ Fact sheets
- ▶ Toolkits
- ▶ Brochures and pamphlets

CDC provides GUIDANCE:

- ▶ Clinical guidance
- ▶ Research
- ▶ Publications
  - *Morbidity and Mortality Weekly Report*
  - Vital Signs
  - Community Guide

CDC provides SUPPORT:

- ▶ Guidance
- ▶ Data collection and reporting
- ▶ Alerts
  - Health Alert Network [HAN]
  - Epidemic Information Exchange [Epi-X] Network
- ▶ Large-scale outbreak assistance
- ▶ Small-scale outbreak assistance
- ▶ Funding

For more information about notifiable disease surveillance, please access the NNDSS website at **https://wwwn.cdc.gov/nndss/**

FIGURE 8-1 How we do notifiable disease surveillance. (Reprinted from Center for Disease Control and Prevention. (2018). *Defending America from Health Threats*. Retrieved from https://wwwn.cdc.gov/nndss/how-we-do.html)

In the event of an outbreak, the response should also include confirming the outbreak, establishing a task force to serve as the command-and-control center of the response, communicating with the public, managing care for those who are ill, and conducting an outbreak investigation (Heymann, 2015).

When investigating a disease outbreak, prior to contacting an individual for an interview:

- Review the information received from the mandated reporter for completeness.
- Clarify whether the disease is suspect (meeting certain clinical criteria) or lab confirmed.
- Review the case definition (criteria an individual must meet to be considered to have the disease).
- Review the disease information (reservoir, incubation and infectious periods, symptoms, and treatment), know the methods of control, and be prepared to provide education to the client while also conducting the investigation. See Chapter 7 to review the natural history of a disease or health condition.
- Review the disease-specific questionnaire, if applicable, to better understand the intent of the investigation and to identify questions to ask the client, allowing you to focus and putting the client at ease.
- If no questionnaire exists, write a narrative report including the information related to onset of illness, symptoms, medical evaluation, treatment if received, recovery state, and individuals the person has been in contact with, depending upon the nature of the disease. (See thePoint® for a sample disease investigation form.)

When conducting the interview:

- Maintain a neutral and nonjudgmental attitude to elicit information more readily, especially when discussing highly sensitive topics, such as a sexually transmitted infection (STI)
- Arrange to call or meet with the person (Fig. 8-2), depending on department protocol and/or disease being addressed
- Introduce yourself and explain the purpose of the confidential nature of the interview

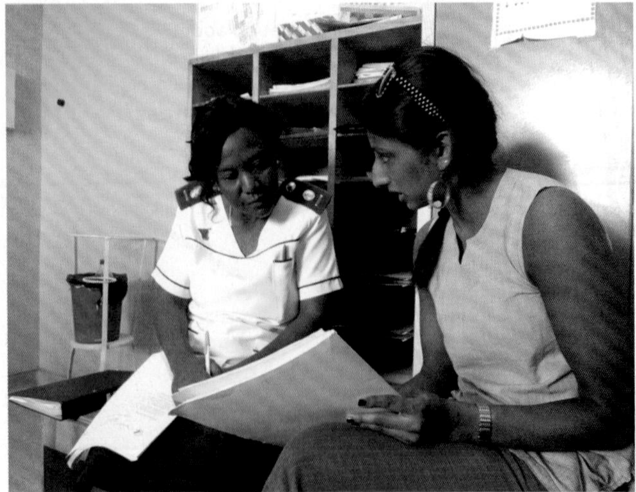

FIGURE 8-2 PHN interviews a health center nurse during TB/HIV investigation.

- Elicit what the individual knows about the disease to assess knowledge base and guide education
- Gather information using a disease-specific questionnaire, if available, and note any possible sources of the disease or additional infected contacts

After the interview, contact individuals identified as possibly infected, which may help establish whether an outbreak is occurring.

Surveillance of communicable diseases is the next step. The WHO has defined **surveillance** as the ongoing and systematic collection, analysis, and interpretation of health data. Surveillance allows for early identification of public health emergencies and evaluation of the effectiveness of public health interventions and is used to help inform policy changes (WHO, n.d). Contact tracing can identify additional people who are also affected. The nurse or other local investigator sends information obtained during the interview to the next higher level of government for analysis and interpretation. If an outbreak is occurring, properly addressing it may require assistance from the next level of government (Heymann, 2015).

Next is disease control. Disease control measures are determined by the characteristics specific to the disease. C/PHNs must understand the characteristics of the infectious agent so that appropriate control measures can be implemented. Prompt, appropriate action could minimize or even prevent an outbreak. Control measures may include testing, counseling, education, environmental modifications such as draining standing water, vaccination, treatment, or prophylaxis as appropriate (Heymann, 2015). Effective surveillance and control can lead to elimination and eradication of a disease in many cases. See Chapter 16 for more on global eradication of infectious diseases.

Modes of Transmission

Transmission of a communicable disease describes how disease is passed from person to person or from another source to a person. The spread can occur by **direct transmission** or **indirect transmission** methods (Heymann, 2015). Refer to Table 8-1, which summarizes the modes of infectious disease transmission. Two indirect modes of transmission particularly important for C/PHN, vector transmission and food and water transmission, are discussed in detail below. Chapter 9 describes both the government's role and the nurse's role in helping to prevent food and water contamination by infectious agents (Heymann, 2015).

Vector Transmission

Vectors are living organisms that can transmit infectious diseases to humans. Insects, a common type of vector, carry disease on their feet or expel it through their digestive tract. This *mechanical transmission* does not require the infectious organism to multiply. Insects can also transmit disease when the infectious agent has propagated within the insect, which is known as *biological transmission* (Heymann, 2015). This requires an incubation period for the infectious agent to be passed to the host. These modes of transmission, together known as vector-borne transmission, involve the bite of the infected insect (e.g., mosquito) or animal (e.g., rat) or some other form of exposure to the infected animal's body fluids, such as contact with the urine from the Hantavirus-infected rodent (CDC, 2020a; Heymann, 2015). Box 8-1 provides

TABLE 8-1 Modes of Infectious Disease Transmission

Routes	Method of Transmission	Examples
Direct: reservoir → host by direct contact or droplet spread		
▪ **Direct contact**	Sexual contact, kissing, skin-to-skin contact, bites, contact with soil or vegetation contaminated with infectious organisms	Gonorrhea, herpes, rabies, hookworm
▪ **Droplet spread**	Large, short-range aerosols produced by sneezing, coughing, or even talking	Pertussis, meningococcal infection
Indirect: reservoir → host by suspended air particles, inanimate objects (vehicles), or animate intermediaries (vector)		
▪ **Airborne**	Infectious agents are carried by dust or droplet nuclei and suspended in air	Measles virus, tuberculosis
▪ **Vehicles**	Indirect transmit an infectious agent include food, water, biologic products (blood), and fomites (inanimate objects such as handkerchiefs, bedding, surgical scalpels, or needles or	Hepatitis A virus
	The vehicle may provide an environment which the agent grows, multiplies, or produces toxin—improperly canned foods	Botulinum toxin by *Clostridium botulinum*

Source: CDC (2012).

an overview of vector-borne diseases that are a major public health concern and the most complex to prevent and control (CDC, 2018j, 2020a).

Food- and Water-Related Illness

Food- or water-related illness can be caused by bacteria (e.g., *Salmonella*, *Shigella*, *Escherichia coli* 0157, *Listeria monocytogenes*, and *Campylobacter*), viruses (e.g., norovirus, hepatitis A), or parasites (e.g., Cryptosporidium, *Giardia*; CDC, 2020c; Heymann, 2015). Toxins released in response to bacteria in the intestines can also result in severe illness. Ingestion of the pathogenic organism sets in motion the events of a food- or water-related intestinal illness or even death.

The contamination can occur:

- At the source (e.g., animal waste being introduced into the food or water chain)
- Through unsanitary food handling or practices (e.g., ingestion of fecal material, fecal–oral route)
- Due to food storage at improper temperatures, allowing microorganisms to grow (2016d)

Most commonly, exposure to contaminated food or water results in symptoms related to gastrointestinal function, including diarrhea, nausea, vomiting, stomach cramps, and bloating. Fever may accompany these infections, as well. Onset of symptoms may occur within a few hours after exposure or not until days or even weeks later, depending on the microorganism. This time interval between exposure and onset of symptoms is called the **incubation period**.

Microorganism contamination of food resulting in human illness occurs as a result of either infection or intoxication (Heymann, 2015):

- *Infection:* Ingestion of food contaminated with *Salmonella*, *Shigella*, *E. coli*, or other pathogen that has multiplied and grown in the food and that irritates the normal gastrointestinal mucosa

BOX 8-1 Vector-Borne Diseases

- Diseases from mosquito, tick, and flea bites have increased threefold between 2004 and 2016.
- The United States has had outbreaks of Zika and Chikungunya viruses.
- The U.S. population is at risk of infection from seven new tick-borne germs.
- Commerce and travelers spread mosquitos, ticks, and fleas around the world.
- Over 80% of vector control organizations report a need for improved performance in core competencies, including pesticide resistance testing.

Mosquito-Borne Diseases

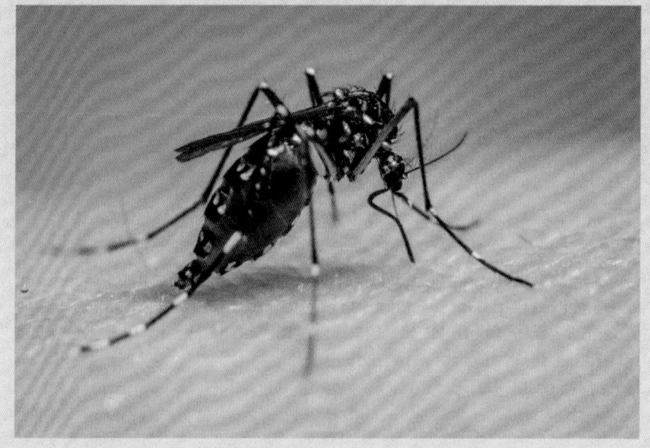

- California serogroup viruses
- Chikungunya virus
- Dengue viruses
- Eastern equine encephalitis virus
- Malaria plasmodium
- St. Louis encephalitis virus
- West Nile virus
- Yellow fever virus
- Zika virus

BOX 8-1 Vector-Borne Diseases (Continued)

Tick-Borne Diseases

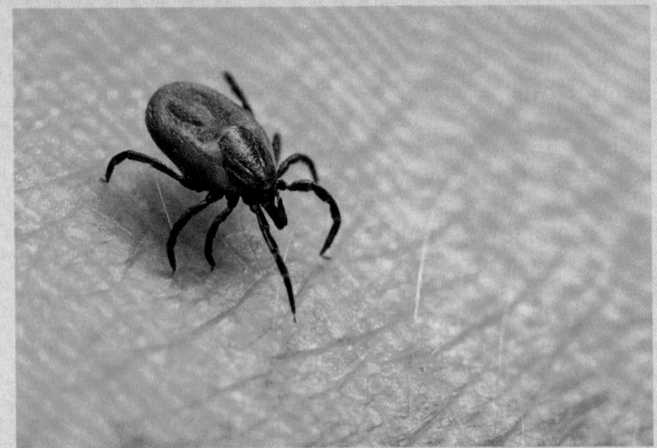

- Anaplasmosis/ehrlichiosis
- Babesiosis
- Lyme disease
- Powassan virus
- Spotted fever rickettsiosis
- Tularemia

Flea-Borne Disease

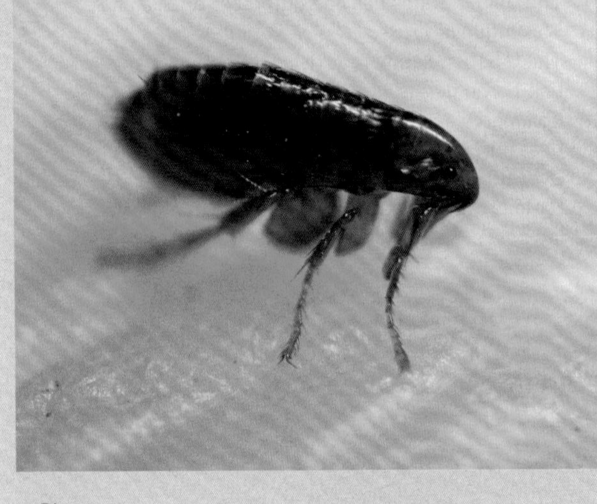

- Plague

Photo of mosquito reprinted from Centers for Disease control and Prevention. Public Health Image Library. Photo Image ID no. 23157—San Gabriel Valley Mosquito & Vector Control District (SGVMVCD), Pablo Cabrera. Retrieved from https://phil.cdc.gov/Details.aspx?pid=23157.
Adapted from CDC (2018c).

- *Intoxication:* Ingestion of food contaminated with a toxin, or by-product of the normal bacterial life cycle, rather than the microbe itself (e.g., heat-stable *Staphylococcus* toxin; the neurotoxin botulinum, produced by the bacterium *Clostridium botulinum*), which may be introduced to the food by bacteria in the food (e.g., cooked food left at room temperature) or living on the skin of a food preparer

This distinction is relevant because, compared with bacteria, toxins (Heymann, 2015):

- Are difficult to isolate and identify, causing some foodborne illnesses to go unidentified
- Are stable at normal cooking temperatures and therefore can occur in thoroughly cooked food
- Typically require only supportive care to address, rather than medical treatment

Food- and water-related outbreaks can impact large numbers of people. A famous historical example is Typhoid Mary. Mary Mallon was the "first identified healthy carrier of typhoid fever" who spread the bacteria (*Salmonella typhi*) in 10 outbreaks, resulting in 51 typhoid fever cases and three deaths (The College of Physicians of Philadelphia, 2019, para. 2). Such outbreaks serve to remind all C/PHP of the continuing need to teach and observe the most basic methods for preventing food and water contamination. Box 8-2 summarizes correct methods for maintaining the safety and cleanliness of food.

Investigating outbreaks involves three types of data:

1. Epidemiologic data:
   - Patterns in the geographic distribution, time of onset, and past incidents of illnesses
   - Associated exposures to foods, infected people, or other sources of disease
   - Clusters of unrelated sick people who share a common event (e.g., eating at the same restaurant, shopping at the same store, attending the same concert; CDC, 2019a)
2. Traceback data:
   - Common points of contamination in the distribution chain, identified by reviewing records collected from restaurants and stores where sick people ate or shopped
   - Findings of environmental assessment in food production facilities, farms, and restaurants identifying food safety risks (CDC, 2016d)
3. Food and environmental testing data:
   - Specimens collected from suspected food items and sent to the lab for processing and identification of the organism (CDC, 2016d)
   - Specimens processed through the CDC surveillance system, PulseNet, which is designed to identify organisms that may come from the same source, allowing outbreaks to be identified and sources to be eliminated (CDC, 2016h)

An example of one PulseNet success story occurred in 2014 when this system identified a rare fingerprint of *Salmonella* Newport in specimens from ill patients. This prompted multiple health departments to initiate an investigation (2016f). Chia powder used in people's smoothie drinks was determined to be the common source. Public health investigators included questions about Chia powder in their questionnaires and identified additional cases in the United States and in Canada. The product was pulled from shelves, eliminating the source from the food supply. A similar process occurred in 2019 with fresh basil from a company in Mexico when 132 lab confirmed *Cyclospora* infection cases were reported, and four people were hospitalized (CDC, 2019a, 2019i).

BOX 8-2 Correct Methods for Preserving the Safety and Cleanliness of Food

Before Handling Food

- Wash hands and all food preparation surfaces and utensils thoroughly with soap and water.

When Preparing Food

- Wash foods that are to be eaten raw and uncooked thoroughly in clean water. This includes foods that are to be peeled that grow on the ground or come in contact with soil.
- Cook all meat products thoroughly.
- Do not allow cooked meats to come in contact with dishes, utensils, or containers used when the foods were raw and uncooked.

When Storing Leftover Foods

- Cool cooked foods quickly; store under refrigeration in clean, covered containers.

When Reheating Leftover Foods

- Heat foods thoroughly. Bacteria contaminating food grow and multiply in a temperature range between 39°F and 140°F.

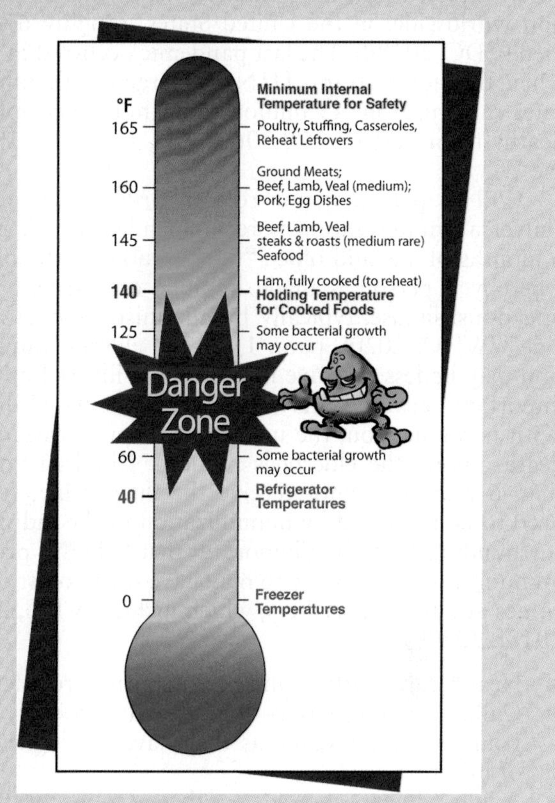

Source: U.S. Department of Agriculture (2015).

MAJOR COMMUNICABLE DISEASES IN THE UNITED STATES

C/PHN encounter many communicable diseases in their practice, some reportable, some not, though equally transmittable. These diseases are frequently diagnosed and treated in the community care setting rather than the hospital. The following sections discuss some of the more common communicable diseases, excluding many that are reportable. Diseases are presented in groups by similarity, rather than by virulence or prevalence.

Influenza (Seasonal or Novel) and Pandemic Preparedness

Influenza (flu) is an acute communicable viral disease of the respiratory tract. Symptoms include fever, headache, myalgia, prostration, coryza, sore throat, and cough. Influenza derives its importance from the rapidity with which epidemics evolve, the widespread morbidity, and the seriousness of complications, specifically pneumonias (Heymann, 2015). The antigenic types of influenza virus are as follows:

- Influenza A virus causes the most severe and widespread disease (**pandemic**) and undergoes minor genetic mutations from year to year, referred to as **antigenic drift**, and drastic transformations periodically, referred to as **antigenic shift**. Subtype description of proteins on the surface of the virus, hemagglutinin and neuraminidase antigens, are included in parentheses—A(H1N1), A(H3N2) (CDC, 2019o).
    - Most people around the world do not have antibodies to protect them from **novel** (new) strains, making them susceptible and increasing the risk of a pandemic. An explanation of differences between seasonal and pandemic flu is provided on thePoint.
- Influenza B virus causes milder disease outbreaks, and they change or mutate at a slower rate. They are not categorized by subtypes but do have two lineages: Victoria and Yamagata (CDC, 2019o; Heymann, 2015).
- Influenza C virus is connected with only sporadic cases of milder respiratory disease (Heymann, 2015).
- Influenza D viruses do not cause illness in people but do affect cattle (CDC, 2019o).

Influenza is usually seasonal in nature, occurring in the winter months, but may be found year-round if testing is done. Each year, a vaccine is developed to prepare for the upcoming flu season. The strains used in the vaccine are based on those the WHO identifies through ongoing surveillance as currently circulating around the globe (CDC, 2019o; Heymann, 2015).

Influenza, an Italian word that means *influence of the cold*, has been recognized since 412 BC and was first described by Hippocrates (Heymann, 2015). It existed throughout the early centuries, and about 30 probable pandemics have been documented in the past 400 years. Three have occurred in the 20th century: in 1918, 1957, and 1968. The 1918 "Spanish flu" pandemic was the most devastating, with 20% to 40% of the world population affected and an estimated death toll of 50 million worldwide; in the United States, roughly 675,000 died (CDC, 2018d). The last pandemic occurred in 2009, when the novel strain, H1N1, emerged with infection rates ranging from 43 million to 89 million people and deaths from 8,868 to 18,306 (CDC, 2018d, 2019n) in the US.

C/PHN play a major role in primary prevention. Universal immunization is recommended for all people 6 months of age and older. "**Immunization** is the process whereby a person is made immune or resistant to an infectious disease, typically by administration of a vaccine" (WHO, 2020f, para. 1). In the elderly, immunization may be less effective in preventing illness but is still important because it may reduce the severity of disease. With immunization, the incidence of complications and death among the elderly is reduced. Children younger than 6 months cannot receive the flu vaccine, so they need to be protected by immunization of the individuals surrounding them. It is important that C/PHNs promote immunization of those who may have the poorest of outcomes and their caretakers, which include (CDC, 2018e, 2018f, 2020b):

- Health care workers and personal care providers
- Children younger than 5 years, but especially those younger than 2 years, as they have the highest rate of infection
- Adults 65 years and older, as they account for 90% of deaths related to influenza and pneumonia
- Pregnant women
- Individuals with asthma
- Those with chronic disease of any organ system or on long-term medication for an illness

The injectable influenza vaccine is inactivated. The nasally inhaled version is a live attenuated vaccine and is licensed for use in people ages 2 to 49 years (Heymann, 2015). An adjuvanted and high-dose inactivated vaccine is recommended for those 65 years of age and older, whereas adults 18 to 64 years may receive a recombinant influenza (RIV) vaccine (CDC, 2019o; Fig. 8-3). The vaccine should be given every year *before* influenza is expected in the community. The season can begin as early as October, so vaccinating in September may be indicated, but usually it begins by the end of October in most of the United States. For those living or traveling outside the United States, timing of the immunization should be based on the seasonal patterns of influenza in the area to which they are traveling (Heymann, 2015). Influenza immunization clinics are frequently planned and organized by or with the local public health agency, with the injections usually administered by C/PHN. Flu shots are also available through major pharmacies.

The 2009 H1N1 pandemic provides an example of the emergency response to a pandemic event. On April 15, 2009, the first case of H1N1 strain influenza was diagnosed in the United States. Ongoing cases of this novel strain were being reported across the United States and around the world into the summer of 2010. There was a rapid response by the WHO and the CDC in investigating, typing the strain, and initiating the production of a vaccine. Vaccine production began by April 21, and on April 26, the federal government declared a public health emergency (CDC, 2019j). Within 6 months, a monovalent (single-strain) vaccine was available to the public. Eighty million doses were administered during that first season, which minimized the impact of this pandemic event (CDC, 2019j). The pandemic response to COVID-19 has been much slower with testing and vaccine development, because this is a novel coronavirus with community spread by asymptomatic as well as symptomatic individuals (Johns Hopkins University of Medicine, 2020).

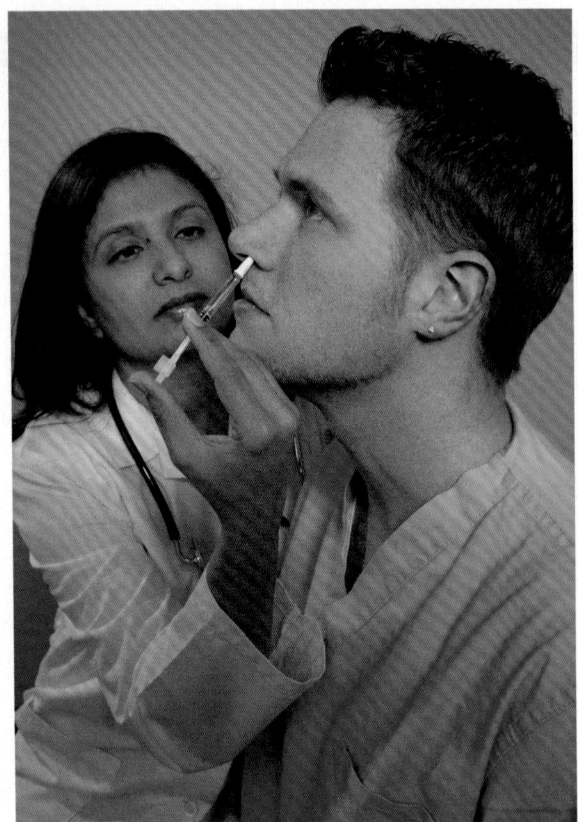

FIGURE 8-3 Administration of nasal spray flu vaccine. (Reprinted from Centers for Disease Control and Prevention. Public Health Image Library. Photo Image ID no. 11864—James Gathany.)

The WHO's Global Influenza Surveillance and Response System (GISRS) program began in 1952 and now involves 144 institutions from 114 WHO member states. The mission of GISRS is to protect the world from the threat of influenza (WHO, n.d.).

FluNet is an Internet-based tool for worldwide influenza surveillance. This program allows for the electronic submission of influenza data from participating global laboratories. Real-time data can be accessed through this resource. As new data arrive and are verified, the maps and tables are revised to give users an up-to-date overview of the influenza situation. Data are provided remotely through the GISRS, the WHO regional databases, and other designated laboratories. Only designated users can submit data, but the results—graphics, maps, and tables of influenza activity on a global scale—are available to the general public. FluNet has expedited the sharing of information on influenza patterns and virus strains and is becoming an essential tool in preparing for and preventing influenza pandemics. Collaborating national influenza centers in 112 countries have created a task force of influenza experts to develop a plan for the global management and control of influenza pandemics (WHO, 2020d). Real-time surveillance is provided by self-report on the app *Flu Near You*, in the United States, and *Flusurvey* in the United Kingdom (Heymann, 2017; Polansky, Outin-Blenman, & Moen, 2016). See more on global disease surveillance in Chapter 16.

Pneumonia

Pneumonia is a pulmonary infection that causes inflammation of the lobes of the lungs, bronchial tree, or interstitial space. People most susceptible to pneumonia are infants, the elderly, and people with a history of chronic diseases, a compromised immune system, or any condition affecting the anatomic or physiologic integrity of the lower respiratory tract. Malnutrition and smoking also increase risk (Heymann, 2015; MedlinePlus, 2020).

Key facts:

- Routes of transmission: droplet, direct oral contact, **fomites** (inanimate objects freshly soiled with respiratory discharges)
- Most common bacterial cause in the United States: *Streptococcus pneumoniae* (pneumococcus)
- Most common viral causes: influenza, parainfluenza, and respiratory syncytial viruses
- Symptoms: sudden onset with a shaking chill, fever, pleural pain, dyspnea, a productive cough of "rusty" sputum, and tachypnea
- Symptoms in older adults: less abrupt, including fever, shortness of breath, altered mental status
- Symptoms in infants and young children: initially, fever, vomiting, and convulsions
- Diagnosis: may require confirmation by radiographic studies (Heymann, 2015; MedlinePlus, 2020)

Community-acquired pneumonia is a significant cause of morbidity and mortality. The incidence of pneumonia is highest in winter. An increased incidence of pneumonia often accompanies epidemics of influenza. In the United States and Europe, morbidity rates range from 30 to 100 cases per 100,000 adults. Incidences are higher among people living in poverty or who have poor nutrition. Case fatality rates of pneumococcal pneumonia range from 5% to 35% and are 10% for children living in developing countries. Children under the age of 6 months who live in developing countries have a 60% fatality rate. Globally, pneumonia kills more than one and a half million children younger than 5 years of age each year. This is greater than the number of deaths from any other infectious disease, including AIDS, malaria, and TB (Heymann, 2015). Hospital admissions and mortality related to pneumonia are far more common among people older than age 65; the mortality rate is approximately 50%. Although this is not a reportable infectious disease, it can nevertheless have a great impact upon the community (Heymann, 2015).

Two vaccines are available to help protect against pneumonia. The pneumococcal protein–polysaccharide conjugate vaccine protects against 13 of the most common pneumonia serotypes and is included as part of the routine vaccination schedule for infants. The 23-valent pneumococcal polysaccharide vaccine is available for those in high-risk groups who are 2 years or older, with the following recommendations:

- High-risk groups: those with chronic diseases, immunosuppressing health conditions, or asplenia
- Reimmunization: recommended only for high-risk children or adults older than 65 years who received their first vaccine before age 65 and at least 5 years has passed since the previous vaccine
- Not effective in children younger than 2 years
- Not recommended for the healthy population between the ages of 2 and 65 years

For people who are not in a high-risk group, education about preventing pneumonia is a major part of the C/PHN role (Heymann, 2015).

Hepatitis

Of the five viral hepatitis infections that constitute serious liver disease, the three most commonly reported types are hepatitis A, B, and C. Infection with hepatitis is an ongoing global epidemic. Substantial progress is being made in the elimination of hepatitis viruses through the primary prevention practices of education and immunization with hepatitis A and B vaccines.

Hepatitis A

Hepatitis A is caused by infection with the hepatitis A virus (HAV). It occurs worldwide and is sporadic and epidemic, with cyclic recurrences affecting children and young adults most frequently. Case rates are highest in areas with poor sanitation, which include Central and South America, the Caribbean, Mexico, Asia (except Japan), Africa, and southern and eastern Europe (Heymann, 2015).

Key facts:

- Route of transmission: fecal–oral (person to person), with an incubation period of 28 days
- Risk factor: occupation as a food handlers or health care worker, due to increased risk of transmission (National Institutes of Health [NIH], 2019)
- Onset: 15 to 50 days after exposure to the virus
- Symptoms: abrupt, including fever, malaise, anorexia, nausea, abdominal discomfort, jaundice
- Symptoms in children: often asymptomatic
- Prognosis: self-limiting; does not result in chronic infection or chronic liver disease
- Duration: mild, 1 to 2 weeks; more severe, 1 month or longer
- Diagnosis: by the presence of immunoglobulin M antibodies against HAV in the serum of acutely or recently ill individuals
- Immunity: usually conferred by recovery from HAV
- Reporting: mandated for providers on diagnosis to the local health agency (Heymann, 2015; Mayo Clinic, 2020)

In areas of the world where environmental sanitation conditions are poor, endemic infection may exist and cause infection at an early age. In this setting, most adults have immunity due to previous exposure. In industrialized countries, cases tend to occur in the older population rather than children, in households of the infected, and among travelers returning from countries where the disease is endemic. At times, common-source outbreaks are related to contaminated water, food contaminated by infected food handlers, raw or undercooked shellfish harvested from contaminated water, or contaminated produce. Outbreaks of hepatitis A may warrant mass vaccination outreach with the hepatitis A vaccine or immunoglobulin (Heymann, 2015; USDA, 2015).

An inactivated hepatitis A vaccine has been available for use since 1995 (Hamborsky, Kroeger, & Wolfe, 2015; NIH, 2019). Administered in a two-dose series, these vaccines induce protective antibody levels in virtually all who are immunized. Ninety-five percent of immunized adults develop immunity after the first dose, and nearly 100% seroconvert after the second dose (CDC, 2015d). The vaccine is recommended as a routine vaccine for children and, as of 2005, was made available to children older than 12 months. C/PHN play an important role in the prevention and control of this disease. Vital to preventing and controlling this disease are offering hepatitis A vaccine to travelers, conducting case investigations, providing education, and identifying potential sources and exposed contacts who need referral or assistance in obtaining postexposure prophylaxis (PEP) and vaccination (CDC, 2016f; Hamborsky et al., 2015; NIH, 2019).

Hepatitis B

Hepatitis B is both an acute and chronic serious disease and is a global problem. Approximately 257 million people are living with hepatitis B virus (HBV). Approximately 800,000 people die each year due to complications related to HBV (WHO, 2018d). Rates are highest in China, Southeast Asia, most of Africa, most of the Pacific Islands, parts of the Middle East, and in the Amazon basin (CDC, 2020f; WHO, 2019a).

Key facts:

- Route of transmission: percutaneous or mucosal exposure to infected blood or body fluids (CDC, 2020f)
- Prognosis: a lifelong chronic infection (rarely resolving), possibly causing cirrhosis (scarring) of the liver, liver cancer, liver failure, and death (Heymann, 2015; NIH, 2017)
- Symptoms: range from unnoticeable to fulminating, including anorexia, fatigue, vague abdominal discomfort in the right upper quadrant, nausea and vomiting, light or gray stools, dark urine, fever, arthralgia, arthritis, and rash, often progressing to jaundice (Hamborsky et al., 2015; NIH, 2017)
- Symptoms in infants: rare
- Occurrence of jaundice: <10% of children and only 30% to 50% of adults (CDC, 2020f)
- Diagnosis: confirmed by the presence of specific antigens to HBV in serum (Heymann, 2015)

Immunization is the most effective way of preventing HBV transmission. The hepatitis B vaccine has been available in the United States since 1981. Since then, rates of HBV infection in the United States have declined by 75% (CDC, 2020f). Almost all infections would be prevented if hepatitis B vaccines were administered to all newborns and infants (Heymann, 2015). After receiving the recommended three doses of vaccine, 95% of infants and children develop immunity, whereas only 90% of adults become immune. By age 65 years, only 75% become immune (CDC, 2020f). Infants born to HBV carrier mothers are at an extremely high risk for developing hepatitis B. Receiving the hepatitis B vaccination and one dose of hepatitis B immunoglobulin within 24 hours after birth in combination with completing the three-dose series at 1 to 2 months and at 6 months of age is 85% to 95% effective (CDC, 2020f). C/PHN have an important role in the prevention and control of hepatitis B by encouraging immunization compliance, particularly following up on immunization of infants born to mothers with chronic HBV status, and consistent adherence to universal precautions, especially for people in high-risk lifestyles or occupations.

Hepatitis C

Hepatitis C virus (HCV) causes a complex infection of the liver and is one of the leading-known causes of liver disease in the United States. It was formerly known as hepatitis, non-A, non-B (NIH, 2016). Seventy-five to eighty-five percent of people with acute HCV develop chronic disease (Heymann, 2015). WHO estimates that in 2015, 71 million persons were living with chronic hepatitis C infection worldwide (WHO, 2018b). The Global Health Sector Strategy is to eliminate viral hepatitis as a public health threat by 2030, but funding is the "major hurdle" (Waheed, Siddiq, Jamil, & Najmi, 2018, p. 4959).

Key facts:

- Route of transmission (most common): direct contact with infected blood via shared intravenous needles, reuse or inadequate sterilization of medical equipment, or transfusion of unscreened blood or blood products (WHO, 2018b)
- Routes of transmission (less common): direct contact with infected blood via tattooing; sexual contact; and vertical (from infected mother to infant)
- Symptoms: similar to those of hepatitis A and B; 80% are asymptomatic after initial infection (WHO, 2018b)
- Diagnosis: confirmed by the presence of HCV antibody (WHO, 2018b)
- Treatment: may not be required if immune response clears infection or chronic infection does not result in liver damage (WHO, 2018b, 2019b)

Testing is recommended for those individuals at greater risk for HCV infection, as acute HCV infection is usually asymptomatic. These include:

- People who have injected drugs, even if only once
- People who received transfusions or organ transplants before 1992 or blood from a positive donor

- People who received clotting factors before 1987, are undergoing chronic hemodialysis, or have persistently elevated alanine aminotransferase levels
- People diagnosed with HIV/AIDS
- People with symptoms of liver disease
- People exposed to HCV-positive sources, such as through needle sticks, sharps, or mucosal exposures
- People who are HIV positive
- Children born to HCV-positive mothers; testing should be done after the child is 18 months old to avoid detecting the mother's antibodies (CDC, 2020g, 2020h)

There is currently no vaccine for HCV. When treatment for chronic hepatitis C is required, the goal is to cure, and the success rate depends on the strain of the virus and the type of treatment given. Treatment is rapidly changing with the introduction of direct-acting antivirals (DAA) like Vosevi® (sofosbuvir/velpatasvir/voxilaprevir) that can be administered to all regardless of genotyping, advancement of disease, or prior failed DAA treatment (WHO, 2018d). Another treatment drug, glecaprevir/pibrentasvir (Mavyrett™), is administered for 8 weeks, thus increasing the chance for compliance and decrease of overall cost of treatment. DAA medications have a >90% cure rate for most patients (Alkhouri, Lawitz, & Poordad, 2017). Protease and polymerase inhibitors, which are also effective, work by blocking the needed physiological processes the virus requires (Healthline, 2020).

The C/PHN's role is primarily supportive, encouraging testing for people who identified as having HCV infection risk factors, referring individuals for care and treatment and to support/educational groups, and encouraging adherence to standard precautions in the home (CDC, 2020g; WHO, 2018b).

HIV/AIDS

HIV is a retrovirus that attacks the body's immune system. HIV is a global health issue affecting 37.9 million people at the end of 2018, with more than half of new HIV infections among individuals and their sexual partners within the following groups: injection drug users, transgender, men having sex with men, sex workers and clients, and those living in prisons/closed facilities. About 95% of this increase is found in central Asian, eastern European, north African, and Middle Eastern countries (WHO, 2019c).

Key facts:

- Routes of transmission: direct contact with infected blood and body fluids via unprotected sex, sharing of needles, placental transmission from mother to fetus, or transfusion (WHO, 2019)
- Diagnosis: rapid diagnostic tests (RDTs), which can indicate the presence of HIV antibodies as early as 1 month after exposure (CDC, 2019e; WHO, 2019c)
- Symptoms (initial): none to flulike
- Symptoms (later): swollen lymph nodes, weight loss, diarrhea fever, and cough (WHO, 2019)
- Risk factors: having unprotected anal or vaginal sex; having another STI; sharing contaminated needles, syringes, or drug solution; using contaminated unsterile cutting or piercing equipment; and having an accidental needle stick injury, particularly among health workers. Transmission is through blood, semen/vaginal secretions, and breast milk/mother to baby (CDC, 2019e; WHO, 2019c).
- Prognosis: without treatment, AIDS can develop in 2 to 15 years after infection (WHO, 2019c)

Although there is no cure for HIV/AIDS, HIV infection is now treated with antiretroviral therapy (ART), which can reduce the viral load to the point that it is undetectable, thus reducing the risk of transmission of the virus by 96% (CDC, 2019f; WHO, 2019c). Antiretroviral (ARV) drugs are also being used for prevention of HIV. Preexposure prophylaxis (PrEP) drugs (e.g., ARVs) reduce the risk of infection by an HIV-negative partner when taken regularly. PEP is ART medication that is taken only in an emergency situation and within 72 hours after possible exposure to HIV (CDC, 2019f, 2019p; WHO, 2019c).

Acquired Immune Deficiency Syndrome (AIDS) is a severe, life-threatening condition, representing the late clinical stage of infection with HIV, in which there is progressive damage to the immune and other organ systems—particularly the central nervous system. AIDS has been delayed or deferred in many individuals by the use of medications during the HIV stage of the spectrum. AIDS reporting is obligatory in most countries (Heymann, 2015).

C/PHN interventions may include education about risk reduction behaviors for those who are at risk but not yet infected. For those who are infected, C/PHNs can provide education about treatment, noting that with early initiation of appropriate treatment, a person with HIV can expect to live almost as long as an uninfected person. Nurses can also play a role in promoting good health for those who are infected, helping them access care, and advising them on how to prevent transmitting the virus to others (CDC, 2019f).

Tuberculosis

TB is a disease primarily of the lungs and larynx, caused by the *Mycobacterium tuberculosis* (MTB) complex, *M. africanum*, *M. tuberculosis*, and *M. canettii*. These are all Gram-positive bacilli.

Key facts:

- Routes of transmission: airborne and spread of droplet nuclei (e.g., via coughing, sneezing, laughing, yelling, singing), in which one inhales the bacilli exhaled by a person with viable TB bacilli in the sputum
- Sites of infection: apex of the lung (most common), kidney, brain, bone, lymphatic channels (Parmer, Allen, & Walton, 2017)
- Process: two basic stages, latent and active; classification according to symptoms (Table 8-2)
- Communicability: depends on duration of the exposure with the infected person as well as the proximity or closeness and ventilation within the space where the exposure occurred
- Incubation period: approximately 10 to 12 weeks (Heymann, 2015)

Most individuals exposed to people with TB do not become infected. Of those who do, all but about 5% to 10% remain disease free. The remaining 90% harbor the organism in a latent stage; although not infectious, they represent a persistent pool of potential cases in a population (Heymann, 2015). Health factors such as poor nutri-

TABLE 8-2 Classification System for Tuberculosis

Class	Type	Description
0	No TB exposure ***Not*** infected	■ No history of TB exposure and no evidence of *M. tuberculosis* infection or disease ■ Negative reaction to tuberculin skin test (TST) or interferon gamma release assay (IGRA)
1	TB exposure No evidence of infection	■ History of exposure to *M. tuberculosis* ■ Negative reaction to TST or IGRA (given at least 8–10 weeks after exposure)
2	TB infection No TB disease (Latent)	■ Positive reaction to TST or IGRA ■ Negative bacteriological studies (smear and cultures) ■ No bacteriological or radiographic evidence of active TB disease
3	TB clinically active	■ Positive culture for *M. tuberculosis* ■ Positive reaction to TST or IGRA, plus clinical, bacteriological, or radiographic evidence of current active TB
4	Previous TB disease (***not*** clinically active)	■ May have past medical history of TB disease ■ Abnormal but stable radiographic findings ■ Positive reaction to the TST or IGRA ■ Negative bacteriologic studies (smear and cultures) ■ No clinical or radiographic evidence of current active TB disease
5	TB suspected	■ Signs and symptoms of active TB disease, but medical evaluation **not** complete

Reprinted from Centers for Disease Control and Prevention. (2013). *Core curriculum on tuberculosis: What the clinician should know* (6th ed.). Retrieved from http://www.cdc.gov/tb/education/corecurr/pdf/chapter2.pdf

tion or health status and chronic illness, such as diabetes, can inhibit the immune system's ability to prevent TB activation from the latent TB dormant state (Heymann, 2015). Figure 8-4 shows the geographic distribution of TB in the United States.

Once almost eradicated, TB has reemerged as a serious public health problem, with around one quarter of the world's population being infected with latent TB (WHO, 2020c). A total of 10 million cases of active TB were noted in 2018, and there were 1.5 billion deaths. TB is one of the ten leading causes of death globally (WHO, 2020h). The majority of new TB cases in 2018 (87%) were found in "high burden TB countries" (WHO, 2019d, para. 4). About 66% of these came from India, Pakistan, Bangladesh, China, Indonesia, the Philippines, South Africa, and Nigeria. The United States had a rate of 2.7 TB cases per 100,000 people in 2019. There are sharply disparate rates among racial/ethnic minority populations. In the United States, 87% of the reported TB cases in 2015 were among Hispanic, Black, and Asian

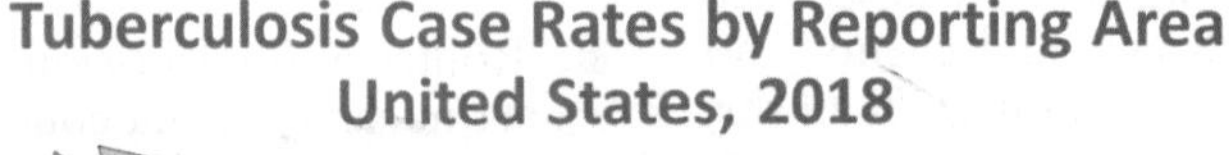

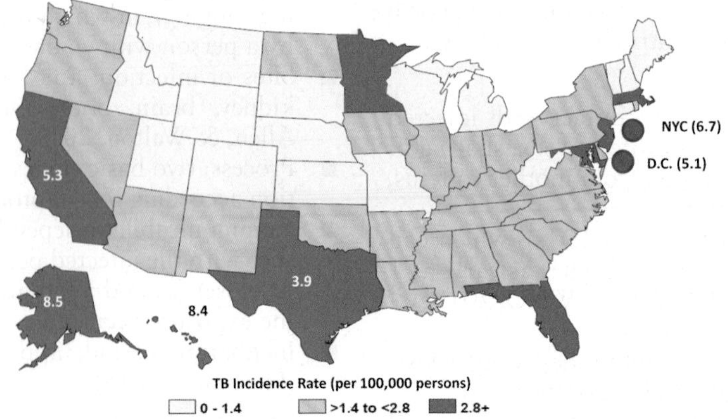

FIGURE 8-4 Reported tuberculosis (TB) case rates by states, United States, 2018. (Reprinted from Centers for Disease Control and Prevention [CDC]. (June 6, 2019). *Tuberculosis in the United States, 1993-2018. National Tuberculosis Surveillance System* (p. 5). Atlanta, GA: US Department of Health and Human Services. Retrieved from https://www.cdc.gov/tb/statistics/reports/2017/2017_Surveillance_FullReport.pdf)

individuals. In 2018, over 70% of reported TB cases were among individuals born outside the United States. Four states—California, Texas, New York, and Florida—reported 50.5% of the cases (CDC, 2019n).

The WHO describes global TB burden in three categories: TB, multidrug-resistant TB, and TB with HIV coinfection. HIV infection contributes dramatically to the development of active TB and is the leading killer of HIV-positive people (WHO, 2019d, 2020c). It is critical to rule out active disease before treating a person with HIV/AIDS for latent TB infection to reduce the risk of developing drug-resistant TB (CDC, 2014, 2020i; Heymann, 2015).

Screening

TB infection can be detected by screening through either a skin test or blood testing. The tests can only be used to identify a person who has been infected at some point; they do not differentiate between latent and active disease.

The Mantoux tuberculin skin test (TST) can detect whether a person is infected with *M. tuberculosis* 2 to 8 weeks after infection (CDC, 2014). Using the Mantoux technique, the nurse injects 0.1 mL of 5 TU of purified protein derivative (PPD) solution via the intradermal route. The nurse must conduct the reading within 48 to 72 hours after the test was administered. Interpretation of the results is based on measurement of induration and recorded in millimeters. Induration is described as the raised, hard area (redness is not considered part of the reaction). Results are considered positive based on various factors (CDC, 2016h). See Figure 8-5 and Table 8-3 for information on the correct administration, reading, and interpretation of TB skin tests.

Special considerations: Nurses should not administer the TST to individuals who report a previous positive TST. The bacille Calmette-Guerin (BCG) vaccine, used in TB-endemic countries to protect infants and young children from life-threatening TB illness, may cause a reaction to the TST. The effect of BCG often wanes over time; however, repeated TSTs may boost the reactivity in a BCG-vaccinated person. The results should be interpreted based on risk stratification regardless of BCG history.

Two-step TST testing may help to identify an infected person who might otherwise not be detected owing to a waning immune response because too much time had lapsed since a previous TST. The two-step approach allows the immune system to wake up and respond using a booster effect (CDC, 2014). The second test may be a blood test rather than another skin test (Lewinsohn et al., 2017).

Two different blood tests for interferon gamma release assays (IGRAs), the QuantiFERON test and the T-spot test, detect the immune response to TB proteins in the blood (CDC, 2016b).

Advantages of using an IGRA (CDC, 2016f, para. 5):

- Necessitates only one visit to be tested
- Allows a 24-hour turnaround time on results
- Does not boost responses measured by subsequent tests
- Is not affected by a health care provider's interpretation of the results
- Causes no false-positive results from past immunization with BCG vaccine

Disadvantages and limitations of using an IGRA (para. 6):

- Requires the blood sample to be processed within 8 to 30 hours after collection
- Can be less accurate due to errors in collecting or transporting the blood specimens or in running and interpreting the assay
- Lacks data supporting its use to predict who will progress to TB disease in the future
- Lacks data supporting its use for:
  - Children younger than 5 years
  - Persons who were recently exposed to *M. tuberculosis*
  - Immunocompromised persons
  - People requiring serial testing
- May be expensive

IGRAs are preferred for people who are not likely to return for reading of TST and people who have a history of receiving BCG vaccine. The TST is preferred for children under the age of 5 years (CDC, 2016b, 2020b).

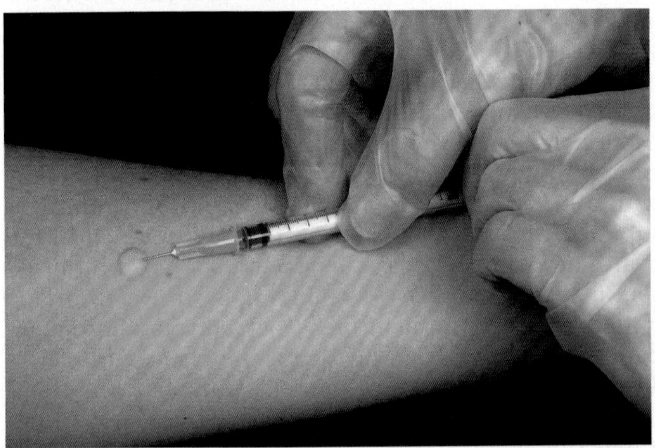

A

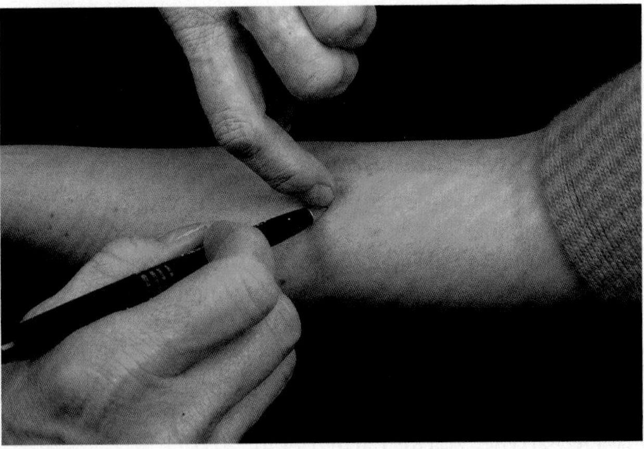

B

FIGURE 8-5 Mantoux tuberculin skin test. **A:** Inject 0.1 mL of purified protein derivative (5 tuberculin units) into the forearm between skin layers, producing a wheal (raised area) of 6 to 10 mm in diameter. **B:** After 48 to 72 hours, assess the reaction, measuring the diameter of the induration (not the area of redness surrounding the induration) across the forearm in millimeters.

TABLE 8-3 Interpreting the Mantoux Tuberculin Skin Test Reaction

 5 or More Millimeters	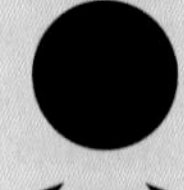 10 or More Millimeters	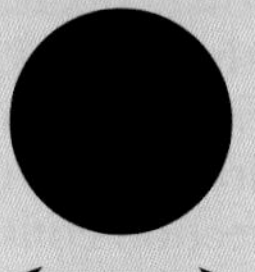 15 or More Millimeters
An induration of **5 or more millimeters** is considered positive for: ▪ HIV-infected persons ▪ Recent contacts of persons with infectious tuberculosis (TB) ▪ People who have fibrotic changes on a chest radiograph ▪ Patients with organ transplants and other immunosuppressed patients (including patients taking a prolonged course of oral or intravenous corticosteroids or TNF-α antagonists [tumor necrosis factor])	An induration of **10 or more millimeters** is considered positive for: ▪ People who have come to the United States within the last 5 years from areas of the world where TB is common (e.g., Asia, Africa, Eastern Europe, Russia, or Latin America) ▪ Injection drug users ▪ Mycobacteriology lab workers ▪ People who live or work in high-risk congregate settings ▪ People with certain medical conditions that place them at high risk for TB (silicosis, diabetes mellitus, severe kidney disease, certain types of cancer, and certain intestinal conditions) ▪ Children younger than 5 years of age ▪ Infants, children, and adolescents exposed to adults in high-risk categories	An induration of **15 or more millimeters** is considered positive for: ▪ People with no known risk factors for TB

Reprinted from Centers for Disease Control and Prevention. (2013). *Core curriculum on tuberculosis: What the clinician should know* (6th ed.). Retrieved from http://www.cdc.gov/tb/education/corecurr/pdf/chapter3.pdf

Diagnosis of Active TB

Diagnosis of suspected active TB disease is initially based on the presence of acid-fast bacilli in the sputum. Confirmation is determined by a culture that reveals MTB. The culture test also provides information about drug susceptibility that informs the decisions for treatment (CDC, 2016a, 2016h; Heymann, 2015). The nurse should conduct a full examination, including obtaining a chest x-ray and reviewing the person's history of risk factors and symptoms.

Prevention and Intervention

The C/PHN can apply all three levels of prevention when working with clients with TB. According to the CDC Division of TB Elimination (CDC, n.d., 2016d), a well-functioning TB control program must focus resources on those at risk for TB exposure and treating those with latent or active TB.

The U.S. Preventive Services Task Force (USPSTF) issued new recommended guidelines (the first since 1996) on offering testing and treatment for latent TB infection, as outlined in Table 8-4 (USPSTF, 2016). The recommendations for C/PHNs are to increase surveillance and take every opportunity to educate and encourage at-risk patients to get tested or seek treatment. Above all it is crucial for C/PHNs to work closely with local and state TB control programs to learn about at-risk populations in their community (CDC, 2016c, 2018i; Parmer et al., 2017).

Isoniazid therapy for individuals who are infected with TB but have no evidence of active disease has been shown to be highly effective in preventing progression to infectiousness and clinical symptoms. Isoniazid INH is a key component of the treatment for active disease (CDC, 2020i, 2020n; Heymann, 2015).

When candidates for drug therapy are identified, it is essential to provide program support to ensure that the maximum number of individuals comply with their medication regimen for the full duration of therapy. One of the most effective ways to achieve a high completion-of-therapy rate is through directly observed treatment (DOT). One variation of DOT is eDOT, which involves recording the patient taking the medication at home and review by trained staff. The eDOT method has a higher completion rate and is preferred over DOT as it costs 32% less than DOT (Garfein et al., 2018). eDOT and DOT are a public health strategy of delivering TB treatment and offer the benefits of timely completion of treatment, prevention of drug resistance, and prevention of further transmission (California Department of Public Health 2019). The DOT strategies have been demonstrated to work when they are implemented universally with all active TB patients within the county, and it is supported by the CDC and, in turn, by state and local health departments. It is not mandatory, but health officers may use the laws surrounding TB prevention and public protection to institute policy and statute to mandate its use. By using DOT with the client with active TB, providers can reduce ongoing potential sources of infection in the community (CDC, 2019; Zhang, Ehiri, Yang, Tan, & Li, 2016).

It is important to assess the patient to see what form of DOT therapy would work the best. The more difficult clients, such as alcohol and drug users, transient homeless people, and people stressed by socioeconomic problems,

TABLE 8-4 Screening for Latent Tuberculosis Infection in Adults

Population	Asymptomatic Adults at Increased Risk for Infection
Recommendation	**Screen for latent tuberculosis infection (LTBI)** **Grade: B**
Risk Assessment	Populations at increased risk for LTBI include persons who were born in, or are former residents of, countries with increased tuberculosis prevalence and persons who live in, or have lived in, high-risk congregate settings (e.g., homeless shelters and correctional facilities). Local demographic patterns may vary across the United States; clinicians can consult their local or state health departments for more information about populations at risk in their community.
Screening Tests	Screening tests include the Mantoux tuberculin skin test and interferon-gamma release assays; both are moderately sensitive and highly specific for the detection of LTBI.
Treatment and Interventions	The CDC provides recommendations for the treatment of LTBI at www.cdc.gov/tb/topic/treatment/ltbi.htm.
Balance of Benefits and Harms	The USPSTF concludes with moderate certainty that the net benefit of screening for LTBI in persons who are at increased risk for tuberculosis is moderate.

Recommendations made by the USPSTF are independent of the U.S. government. They should not be construed as an official position of the Agency for Healthcare Research and Quality or the U.S. Department of Health and Human Services.
For a summary of the evidence systematically reviewed in making this recommendation, the full recommendation statement, and supporting documents, please go to www.uspreventiveservicestaskforce.org.
CDC, Centers for Disease Control and Prevention; USPSTF, U.S. Preventive Services Task Force (September 6, 2016).
Reprinted from https://www.uspreventiveservicestaskforce.org/Page/Document/ClinicalSummaryFinal/latent-tuberculosis-infection-screening

may benefit from DOT therapy, as it ensures that patients are often met where they are located (school, shelter, bar, or job). Implementation of an eDOTS program requires input from information technology and legal representatives to ensure that it complies with both state and federal laws and that clients' HIPAA rights are protected (CDC, 2019).

Multidrug-Resistant TB

Epidemiologists and communicable disease specialists cite a number of factors that contribute to the development and spread of TB strains resistant to one or more of the standard TB drugs. Strains now exist that are resistant to almost all of the standard anti-TB drugs and according to the WHO, one in four persons contracting extensively drug-resistant TB (XDRTB) dies rapidly, within months from the disease. Chief among the factors contributing to drug resistance seems to be the political and social response to declining rates of TB over past decades, which has resulted in funding cuts for surveillance, treatment, and research and a premature sense that TB was defeated. On an individual case basis, the most common means by which resistant organisms are acquired is by noncompliance with therapy for the full, recommended period (WHO, 2018d, 2020c). Figure 8-6 compares MDRTB rates among people born in the United States and those born in other countries now living in the United States.

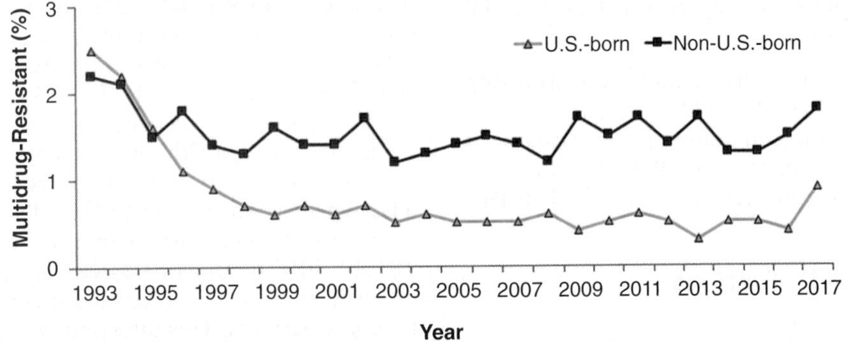

FIGURE 8-6 Multidrug-resistant tuberculosis patterns: comparison of U.S.-born and non–U.S.-born persons, 1993 to 2017. (Reprinted from Centers for Disease Control and Prevention (CDC). (2018). *Reported tuberculosis in the United States, 2017* (p. 119). Atlanta, GA: US Department of Health and Human Services, CDC. Retrieved from https://www.cdc.gov/tb/statistics/reports/2017/2017_Surveillance_FullReport.pdf)

Clients With HIV and TB

HIV infection is associated with an increased possibility of developing primary TB after exposure to a source. The person living with coinfection of latent TB infection and HIV infection has a 50% higher risk of developing active TB than the immunocompetent individual (Heymann, 2015).

The HIV-positive client may not have the ability to react to a skin test for TB because of a weakened immune system. Therefore, other methods to determine TB status are employed. People with HIV infection and TB infection should be counseled about the benefit of preventive treatment and possibility of TB activation without treatment. These clients must be monitored closely for effectiveness of the preventive therapy and for tolerance to isoniazid. This drug has the capacity to develop adverse reactions or negative side effects such as hepatitis or damage to the liver, and regular follow-ups are necessary to detect early symptoms such as nausea, vomiting, abdominal pain, fatigue, and dark urine signifying bleeding are sufficient to initiate liver function tests (CDC, 2020l; Heymann, 2015).

If it is determined that TB disease is present, HIV-infected clients should begin a regimen of drugs according to the accepted national and global medication schedule used in their country. The client should be closely monitored for response to treatment; if they do not seem to be responding, they should be reevaluated. Drug sensitivity is key to correct and successful treatment (USDHHS, 2019).

TB Case Management

The functional aspect of the program should ideally strive for (CDC, n.d.):

- Standardized public health practices for investigating, case and contact finding, as well as care and treatment.
- Case management of care and treatment of the individual with TB to ensure medication compliance and barriers to treatment completion are dealt with so treatment completion will occur.
- Close monitoring for sputum conversion in people with active disease, in order to adjust medication as necessary.
- A high completion-of-therapy rate within 1 year after diagnosis.
- Assurance of adequate funding and a dedicated TB control infrastructure.

C/PHNs have a responsibility to build a relationship of trust with individuals who have TB or latent TB infection which leads to seeking and adhering to treatment. It is also important to monitor for overall health and well-being, educating, and making referrals (CDC, 2016f; Parmer et al., 2017).

Sexually Transmitted Infections

Chlamydia

Chlamydia trachomatis (CT) infections are the most commonly reported notifiable STI in the United States (CDC, 2019b). In 2018, more than 1.8 million cases of *Chlamydia* were reported in the United States, with the highest proportion found in those ages 20 to 24. Disparities exist, resulting in infection rates among Black individuals that are 5.6 times higher than the rates of White individuals, even though between 2014 and 2018, there was a 17.6% increase in cases for Whites (CDC, 2019b).

Key Facts:

- Route of transmission: sexual contact and maternal transmission to a newborn (CDC, 2019b)
- Symptoms: often asymptomatic, resulting in a greater risk for going undetected, resulting in serious complications:
  - Pelvic inflammatory disease (PID)
  - Fallopian tube issues, including ectopic pregnancy and infertility
  - Chronic pain in the pelvis (CDC, 2019b)
  - Preterm delivery or complications for the newborn, including conjunctivitis or pneumonia (CDC, 2019b)
- Diagnosis: highly sensitive nucleic acid amplification urine tests (CDC, 2019b)
- Treatment: either a 7-day treatment with the antibiotics azithromycin, doxycycline, levofloxacin, ofloxacin, and erythromycin or a single dose of antibiotic followed by 7 days abstaining from sexual activity
- Barriers to successful treatment:
  - Noncompliance with the 7-day treatment with antibiotics or abstaining from sex
  - Stigma, costs of care, and treatment
  - Side effects of medication, such as gastric upset for erythromycin
  - Not treating infection of partner at the same time
  - Not following up with retesting if patient did not adhere to treatment guidelines (CDC, 2019b)
- Recommended screening guidelines:
  - Yearly for all women who are sexually active and 25 years or younger
  - For women older than 25 years who have a new sexual partner or multiple partners or a partner who has been diagnosed with an STI
  - All pregnant women at their first obstetrical visit
  - For men who have sex with men in settings with high rates of CT infection

Screening programs have been extremely effective in reducing the overall *Chlamydia* burden and reducing rates of PID in women (CDC, 2019b). As a result of increased screening efforts in many settings outside of the medical office, reported rates of *Chlamydia* continue to increase, especially in women aged 15 to 24 years (Fig. 8-7).

STI notification depends on the state health department, as some health departments use the Internet to anonymously notify partners of possible exposure to an STI, whereas others use patient-delivered partner treatment or expedited partner treatment (EPT; CDC, 2015d, 2019b). EPT treatment strategy is to give a prescription or medication to the infected patients to, in turn, give to their sex partners. This intervention has been shown to be more effective than encouraging the patient to notify the partner(s) to seek testing and treatment. Each state may have its own legal requirements related to this treatment option; nurses must review and understand their states'

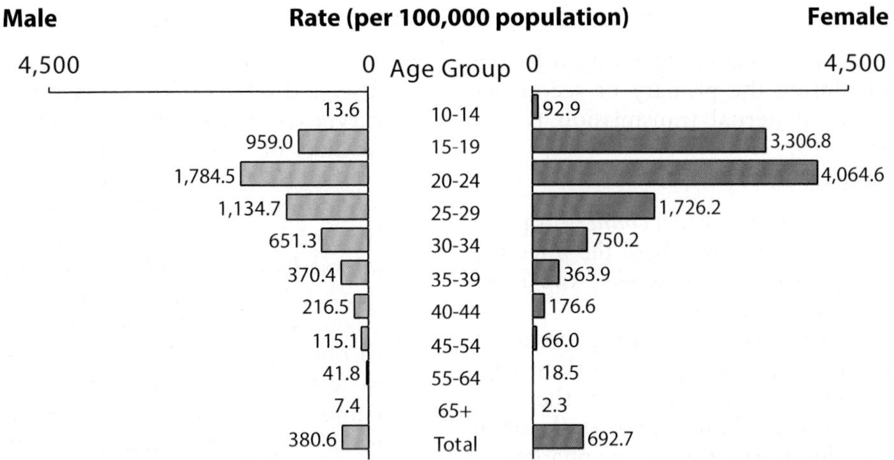

FIGURE 8-7 Chlamydia: rates of reported cases by age group and sex, United States, 2018. (Reprinted from Centers for Disease Control and Prevention. (September 30, 2019). *Sexually transmitted disease surveillance 2018: Chlamydia*. Retrieved from https://www.cdc.gov/std/stats17/figures/5.htm)

law (CDC, 2015d). With EPT, it is important to provide very specific written instructions that include self-administration of the medication, warnings about pregnancy and allergic reactions, when to seek medical care, and how to prevent reinfection. However, for men who have sex with men, this practice is not as customary, as there may be other coinfection issues needing evaluation and treatment, such as *Haemophilus influenzae* type b infection (CDC, 2015d).

Gonorrhea

The causative agent of gonorrhea is the gonococcus bacteria—*Neisseria gonorrhoeae*. Gonorrhea is the second-most commonly reported notifiable disease in the United States, with 583,405 cases reported in 2018, although it is estimated that there are 1.4 million new gonorrheal infections yearly (CDC, 2019d). About half of the cases each year are among people 15 to 44 years old. Compared with the rate of reported cases of gonorrhea among Whites, the rate was 7.7 times higher in Blacks, 4.6 times higher in American Indian/Alaska Natives, 2.6 times higher in Native Hawaiians and other Pacific Islanders, and 1.6 times higher in Hispanics (CDC, 2019d).

Key facts:

- Route of transmission: sexual contact and maternal transmission
- Symptoms (men): purulent drainage from the penis, accompanied by painful urination within 2 to 7 days after an infecting exposure
- Symptoms (women): asymptomatic; mild vaginal discharge or bleeding after intercourse (Heymann, 2015)
- Complications (women): if untreated, PID, infertility, or ectopic pregnancy
- Complications (dissemination): petechial or pustular lesions, requiring hospitalization for treatment and evaluation for complications such as endocarditis and meningitis
- Screening criteria: similar to those of *Chlamydia*; refer back to previous section on *Chlamydia* (CDC, 2015d, 2019b)

Antimicrobial resistance is a great concern when treating gonorrhea. In 2010, concerns over emerging resistant gonorrhea prompted the CDC to recommend dual therapy, combining cephalosporin with azithromycin or doxycycline. Resistance to cefixime, a third-generation cephalosporin, appeared in Asia, Europe, South Africa, and Canada, causing further changes in dual treatment guidelines advising the exclusive use of ceftriaxone and azithromycin (CDC, 2019b). Gonorrhea transmitted to neonates during delivery presents 2 to 5 days after delivery. This can result in ophthalmia neonatorum and sepsis. As a result, most states have a law that requires a prophylactic agent be given to all infants after delivery. Treatment during pregnancy is the best way to prevent gonorrhea infection in the newborn (CDC, 2019b).

Sex partners should be referred to a medical provider for testing and treatment, but if this is not possible, EPT can be used. This is not the preferred partner treatment course for men who have sex with other men owing to concerns of coexisting STD infection including HIV (CDC, 2015d). Once again, it is best to refer to your state's regulations regarding this method of treatment.

Syphilis

Syphilis is a systemic infection caused by the spirochete *Treponema pallidum*. Prior to 2014, the incidence rate of syphilis had been decreasing, but starting in 2014, the incidence rate has been increasing. In 2018, reported cases of all stages of syphilis increased by 13.3% from 2017 (CDC, 2019m). Increased incidence has been seen among men who have sex with men and women. The highest rates of primary and secondary syphilis infections in 2018 occurred in the age range of 25 to 29 years for both men and women, with 55.7 cases per 100,000 for men and 10 cases per 100,00 for women ages 20 to 24 (CDC, 2019m). The incidence rate of congenital syphilis also increased 39.7% from 2017 to 2018. Past historical data indicate a correlation between primary and secondary syphilis infectious rates of women in their reproductive years (CDC, 2019m).

Key facts:

- Routes of transmission: direct contact with a lesion; blood transfusion during the primary or secondary stage of the disease; maternal transmission (CDC, 2017g; Heymann, 2015)
- Process: Four distinct stages:
  1. Primary: A primary lesion called a *chancre* appears as a painless ulcer at the site where the infection entered the body, lasts 3 to 6 weeks, and heals regardless of medical treatment.
  2. Secondary: After 4 to 6 weeks, a more generalized secondary macular-to-papulosquamous skin eruption develops, classically appearing on the soles of the feet, palms of the hands, and trunk, often accompanied by fever, sore throat, lymphadenopathy, and fatigue. These secondary manifestations can resolve spontaneously within weeks or may persist up to 12 months.
  3. Latent: By this phase, the spirochete has invaded the central nervous system but there may not be any signs or symptoms of infection for weeks to years.
  4. Tertiary: One third of those infected who do not receive treatment progress to tertiary syphilis, associated with recurring lesions, severe systemic involvement, disability, abnormalities in the cerebral spinal fluid, deafness, meningitis, cranial nerve palsy, or even death (CDC, 2017g; Heymann, 2015).
- Complications (congenital syphilis): fetal death, premature birth, death of the newborn, failure to thrive, anemia, lesions, and central nervous system symptoms (CDC, 2017g; Heymann, 2015)

Penicillin is the treatment of choice for syphilis. The nurse should instruct patients to avoid sexual contact until the treatment is completed and the lesions have resolved and to encourage contacts to receive treatment. Contacts are defined as those with whom the patient had sex within the 3 months (for patients in the primary stage), 6 months (for patients in the secondary stage), or 1 year (for patients in the early latent stage) prior to the onset of symptoms or long-term sexual partners (for patients in the late latent stage (New York City Department of Health & STD Prevention Training Center, 2019). If an infant is diagnosed with congenital syphilis, all immediate family members should be treated. Anyone diagnosed with syphilis should also be evaluated for other STIs (Heymann, 2015).

Genital Herpes

Genital herpes is an STI caused by the herpes simplex virus types 1 (HSV-1) and 2 (HSV-2) and is one of the most common STIs in the United States. Most genital herpes infections are caused by HSV-2; however, rates of HSV-1 genital herpes are increasing among college students. HSV-1 is the virus that causes cold sores and spreads from the mouth to the genitals through oral sex. Most people with HSV-2 remain undiagnosed because of the symptoms being mild, causing the person to not recognize a need to seek medical care (CDC, 2017a).

Key facts:

- Symptoms (initial): systemic, including fever and malaise, and bilateral lesions lasting 2 to 3 weeks on the cervix (women), external genitalia (men or women), or anus or rectum (those who engage in anal intercourse) (CDC, 2017a; Heymann, 2015)
- Symptoms (subsequent outbreaks): lesions in areas beyond the initial exposure site, which usually are unilateral, less severe, and less frequent and resolve more quickly than the primary lesion (Heymann, 2015)
- Diagnosis: by isolation of the virus, DNA detection through polymerase chain reaction (PCR) testing, or tests that detect HSV antigens, with viral isolates being typed to determine whether the infection is due to HSV-1 or HSV-2 (Heymann, 2015)
- Prognosis: there is no cure for HSV, and the infection can remain in the body indefinitely; however, antiviral medications can prevent or reduce the duration of an outbreak and can reduce the risk of transmission to uninfected sexual partners (CDC, 2015b, 2015d).

If a pregnant woman becomes infected late in the pregnancy and has active lesions, delivery by cesarean section is often advised to reduce the risk of transmission to the neonate. Antiviral therapy can be given to the pregnant woman at 36 weeks of gestation to suppress the virus to help reduce the need for a cesarean section birth (Heymann, 2015).

Viral Warts

Condylomata acuminata, verruca vulgaris, papilloma venereum, and the common wart are all forms of a viral disease caused by the *human papillomavirus* (HPV). More than 120 HPV types have been identified, at least 40 of which are sexually transmitted. HPV is a common STD, with most sexually active persons becoming infected with it at least once during their lifetime (CDC, 2015c, 2019c). It is estimated that around 79 million people in the United States have been infected with HPV; between 340,000 to 360,000 have genital warts. Yearly, over 34,800 men and women are diagnosed with some type of cancer caused by HPV (e.g., cervical, anal, oropharyngeal), but these are preventable with the HPV vaccine (Cameron et al., 2016; CDC, 2019g).

Key facts:

- Routes of transmission: direct contact with fomites; sexual (skin-to-skin) contact; or transmission by a mother to a neonate during vaginal birth
- Process: incubation period of 2 to 3 months (Heymann, 2015)
- Symptoms: may include lesions on the skin or mucous membranes, including in the throat or respiratory tract (recurrent, respiratory papillomatosis) and in the genital region (condylomata acuminata, or genital warts); may include none (asymptomatic), with increased risk for lack of detection and diagnosis and ongoing transmission between or among sexual partners (CDC, 2019i; Heymann, 2015)
- Prevention: condoms are (not fully protective; CDC, 2019i)
- Prognosis: about 12,000 women are diagnosed with HPV-related cervical cancer each year, with oropharyngeal cancer being most common for men (CDC, 2019g)

- Vaccination: recommended for males and females against high-risk HPV (hrHPV) infection strains by the CDC, 2015e (Meites, Kempe, & Markowitz, 2016) as follows:
  - Routine vaccination is recommended for girls and boys at age 11 or 12 years.
    - Patients 9 to 14 years old: 2 doses, with 6 to 12 months between doses
  - Patients 15 to 26 years old: 3 doses, with at least 4 weeks between the first and second doses, 12 weeks between the second and third doses, and 5 months between the first and last doses
  - Extended use of Gardasil-9 to the age of 45 years for males and females (as approved by the U.S. Food and Drug Administration [FDA], 2018)

The vaccine works best if given prior to being sexually active but can still be given to individuals already sexually active to protect against any hrHPV (high risk) strains they have not yet acquired. The National Cancer Institute (NCI) stresses the importance of increasing the numbers of people vaccinated "to reduce the prevalence of the vaccine-targeted HPV types in the population, thereby providing some protection for individuals who are not vaccinated" (NCI, 2019, para. 15).

There is currently no routine recommended screening test for HPV-associated diseases other than cervical cancer. The USPSTF (2018, para. 6) has issued the following recommendations for women 21 to 65 years of age, "regardless of sexual history, who have a cervix and show no signs or symptoms of cervical cancer":

- Women aged 21 to 29 years: cervical cytology screening alone every 3 years
- Women aged 30 to 65 years: cervical cytology screening alone every 3 years or hrHPV testing alone every 5 years or hrHPV testing in combination with cervical cytology screening (cotesting) every 5 years
- Women younger than 21 years: no screening recommended (USPSTF, 2018)

Treatment may include curettage, trichloroacetic acid, cryotherapy with liquid nitrogen, or surgical debulking for larger lesions. Patient-applied treatment may include immunomodulator creams or ointments, but topical treatments may not be appropriate for pregnant women (Heymann, 2015).

Sexually Transmitted Infection Prevention and Control

Minority populations, the poor, the medically underserved, and women and children, in general, experience a disproportionate amount of the STI burden (see Chapters 5 and 23). Women also have a higher risk of serious complications from STIs, including PID, sterility, ectopic pregnancy, and cancer associated with HPV. Children can also be affected by exposure to maternal STIs, resulting in fetal and infant death, birth defects, blindness, and intellectual disability. Undiagnosed and untreated STIs may play a role in infertility (CDC, 2019m). Nurses need to be involved in accomplishing the *Healthy People 2030* goal of promoting healthy sexual behaviors, strengthening capacities within communities, and increasing access to quality services (ODPHP, 2020; see Chapter 21).

Infectious Diseases of Bioterrorism

The deliberate release of biological agents into the environment with the intent to cause harm is a real risk and can occur as an overt or covert event (Heymann, 2015). In the event of such a terrorist attack, C/PHNs can allay fears, provide the public with correct information, and promote and carry out immunization. Although many disease-causing organisms can be weaponized, only anthrax and smallpox, two biological agents that have a history of being used as terrorist weapons, are discussed here (see Chapter 17).

Anthrax

Shortly after the terrorist attacks of September 11, 2001, the U.S. population was further terrorized by a deliberate release of anthrax agent into the postal service system. As a result, 22 people were infected, five died, and 32,000 were identified as having been potentially exposed and were treated with antibiotics as a precaution (Heymann, 2015; NPR, 2011).

Anthrax spores are found in nature in the digestive tracks of herbivores and can be found in the soil. Infection in humans is infrequent and sporadic in most developed countries (Heymann, 2015). It is an occupational hazard among workers who process animal hides, hair, bone and bone products, and wool in some countries, leading to it being referred to as *woolsorter disease* and *ragpicker disease* (Heymann, 2015).

In humans, anthrax is an acute bacterial disease that affects mainly the skin or respiratory tract. The two main forms—cutaneous anthrax and inhalation anthrax—account for most human anthrax cases. Cutaneous anthrax, which has a case fatality rate of 5% to 20%, manifests as itchiness on the skin where exposed, a lesion that progresses from papular to vesicular, and, in 2 to 6 days after exposure, a depressed black eschar surrounded by extensive edema. The infection may spread to the lymph system and cause septicemia. Inhalation anthrax, which has a case fatality rate of 85% (although antimicrobial and supportive therapy can reduce this rate), manifests initially as mild symptoms—including fever, cough, chest pain, and malaise—but can then progress to respiratory distress, fever, and shock (Heymann, 2015).

The causative organism *Bacillus anthracis* is a Gram-positive, encapsulated, spore-forming agent found in livestock and wildlife as the main reservoirs. The incubation period for cutaneous infection is 5 to 7 days but for inhalational anthrax is 1 to 45 days. Person-to-person transmission is rare, but articles and soil contaminated with spores may remain infective for decades, so these items must be appropriately disposed of (Heymann, 2015).

A vaccine that protects against cutaneous and inhalational anthrax exists but is generally used only for those laboratory scientists handling anthrax specimens and some veterinarians who may have work-related exposure risk (Heymann, 2015).

Smallpox

The variola virus causes smallpox and is transmitted from person to person. Initial symptoms of infection include a febrile prodromal period, which includes a fever of 104°F, malaise, headache, abdominal pain, and vomiting

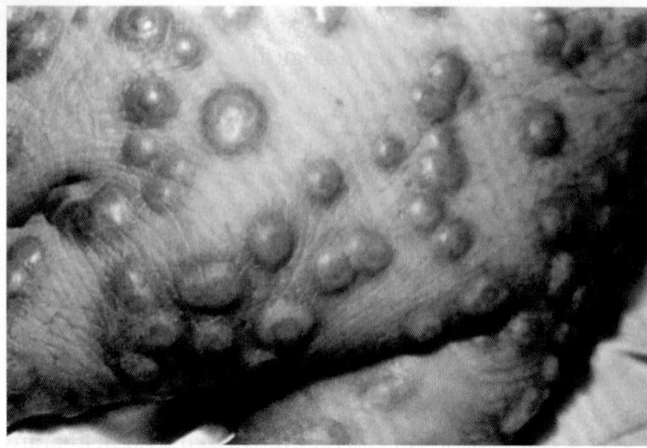

FIGURE 8-8 Maculopapular rash of smallpox. A smallpox patient in Cardiff, Wales during a 1962 epidemic. The lesions here upon his right hand were determined to be benign, semiconfluent focal variola eruptions. (Reprinted from Centers for Disease control and Prevention. Public Health Image Library. Photo Image ID no. 10375—Dr. Charles Farmer, Jr. Retrieved from https://phil.cdc.gov/Details.aspx?pid=10375)

followed by the eruption of a deep-seated rash that transitions from macular to papular to vesicular to pustular (Fig. 8-8). Eventually, these scab over and fall off approximately 3 to 4 weeks after onset. It is passed from person to person through respiratory droplets or skin inoculation, most easily by droplet during the first week after the rash has developed, but airborne and contact precautions (personal protective equipment-PPE) are recommended for health care workers (CDC, 2016g; Heymann, 2015).

Smallpox was declared globally eradicated in May of 1980. Officially, the smallpox virus presently exists at only two places: the CDC in Atlanta and the State Research Centre of Virology and Biotechnology in Koltsovo, Novosibirsk Region, Russian Federation. These samples remain available in the unlikely case of reemergence of smallpox disease (Heymann, 2015).

A vaccine made from the vaccinia virus exists. The vaccinia virus, also known as cowpox, is a similar organism that confers protection to smallpox. In 1798, Edward Jenner was able to demonstrate that the vaccinia virus could be used to protect people from smallpox (WHO, 2014a). Smallpox vaccination has risks as it is a live virus. To avoid spreading the vaccinia virus, vaccinated people should not touch or cover the vaccination site with a gauze bandage and should follow care instructions. Serious complications include eye infection or blindness if the vaccinated person has the vaccine virus on the hand and touches the eye, severe rash leading to scarring or even death, encephalitis, and preterm birth or fetal demise if the virus becomes transmitted to a fetus during pregnancy (CDC, 2017e). Reactions are rare, with only 14 to 52 per 1 million people experiencing a life-threatening reaction (CDC, 2017e). Less severe but more common side effects include the formation of satellite lesions, regional lymphadenopathy, fever, headache, nausea, muscle aches, fatigue, and chills. In addition, the vaccine is contraindicated for those who are immunosuppressed, those with eczema, and pregnant women (Heymann, 2015; Fig. 8-9).

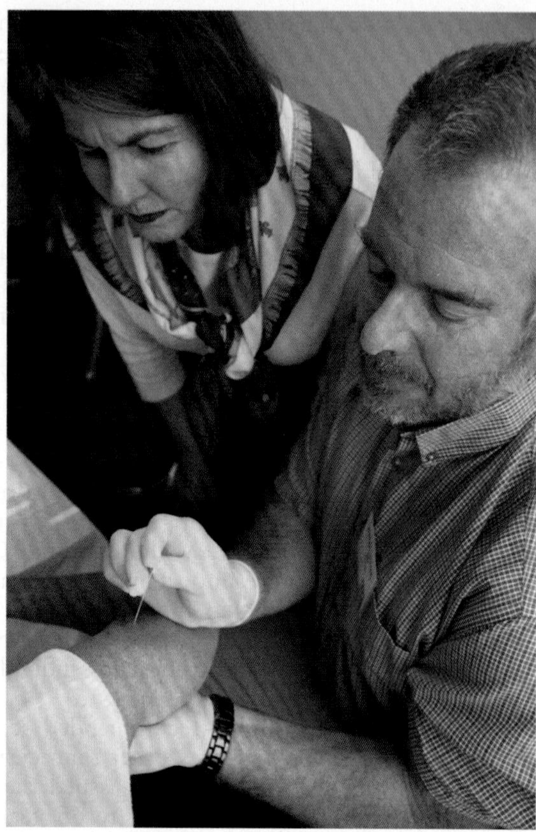

FIGURE 8-9 Smallpox inoculation of public health worker. (Reprinted from Centers for Disease Control and Prevention. Public Health Image Library. Photo Image ID no. 2825—James Gathany. Retrieved from https://phil.cdc.gov/Details.aspx?pid=2825)

Routine immunization against smallpox is no longer recommended for the general public because, at this time, the risk of harm from the vaccine is considered to be greater than the risk of contracting the disease. Laboratory workers who work in high-risk areas may still obtain the vaccine (Heymann, 2015).

The response plan for smallpox exposure may include the previously successful **ring vaccination** strategy—containing an outbreak by rapidly isolating and vaccinating people who have had close, face-to-face contact with the victim. This method refers to a ring of people around the exposed or ill person. Contacts would be monitored daily for fever and isolated if a fever develops (Heymann, 2015).

PRIMARY PREVENTION

In the context of communicable disease control, two approaches are useful in achieving primary prevention: (1) education using mass media with targeted health messages to aggregates and (2) immunizations.

Education

Health education in primary prevention is directed both at helping individuals understand their risk and at promoting healthy behaviors. Chapter 11 deals more extensively with the concepts of learning theory and the variety of health education approaches and materials available to C/PHN today.

Targeting Meaningful Health Messages to Aggregates

Marketing is based on the principles of exchange, paying a price for goods or services. The price may be money, effort, or time. The goods are the outcomes, such as good health. To effectively deliver a health promotion and disease prevention message, the following must be done (CDC, 2020e):

1. Identify the target (at-risk) market, a group of people who share common interests, needs, and behaviors.
2. Determine the target market's educational level, view of the salience of the issue, involvement with the issue, and access to media channels.
3. Consider the cultural, racial, and ethnic context of the target market and ensure that the message and educational materials are relevant to the needs and interests of the community and respect and reflect their values and traditions (Fig. 8-10).
4. Select or develop materials that relate to the delivery of health services that are available, accessible, and acceptable to the target population.
5. Pretest all materials and verify that they are attractive, comprehensible, acceptable, and persuasive to the target market and promote ownership.
6. Select or develop materials that are at the appropriate reading level for the intended audience.

Ways to Communicate

Social media, including Facebook, Instagram, YouTube, Snapchat, and Twitter, offers the ability to engage a large number of participants in an interactive, collaborative, and synchronous manner. It allows practitioners to reach populations that are diverse and that they might not easily arrange to meet face-to-face. It also makes sharing of information easier, through podcasts, YouTube, and blogs (CDC, 2020e); however, in using it, nurses must take care to maintain patients' privacy. This approach can also be integrated with other public health communication strategies. Public health organizations need to use social media engagement to its full potential (Andrade, Evans, Barrett, Edberg, & Cleary, 2018). Nurses can explore ways that social media can be used to augment current public health communication approaches. Chapters 10 and 12 have more information on social marketing and using technology to reach various populations.

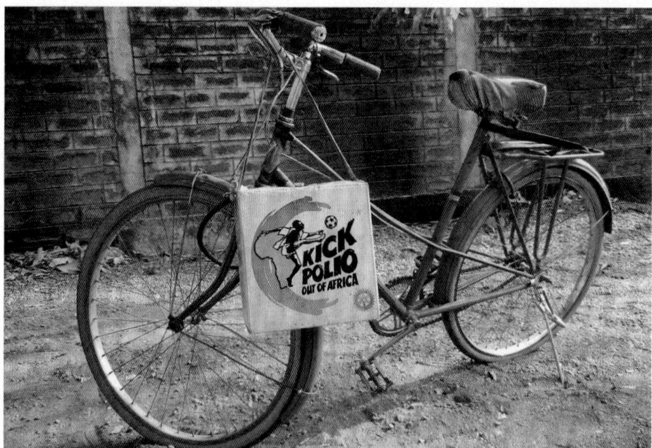

FIGURE 8-10 A targeted health message in Africa. A Stop Transmission of Polio (STOP) campaign volunteer's bicycle equipped with a vaccine-carrying satchel with the message "Kick Polio out of Africa." (From Centers for Disease control and Prevention. Public Health Image Library. Photo Image ID no. 19436—Molly Kurnit, MPH. Retrieved from https://phil.cdc.gov/Details.aspx?pid=19436)

Immunization

The extended life expectancy that has been enjoyed during the 20th century was largely due to the expansion of immunization programs that are provided to families. Immunizations are a cost-effective public health intervention that offers a high return on investment (see Fig. 8-11). Examples of the benefits gained through immunization programs include 92% to 100% drop in morbidity for ten communicable diseases including pertussis, polio, and smallpox, and preventing $14 million in lost income from disease while also saving $9.9 billion in health care costs and $33.4 billion in indirect costs (Ornstein & Ahmed, 2017; Vanderslott, Dadonaite, & Roser, 2019). Immunization and control of infectious diseases remain a national focus through *Healthy People 2030* (ODPHP, 2018). Box 8-3 highlights select objectives related to immunization and infectious diseases.

Challenges still exist. Over 3 million people, half of them children, die worldwide each year from VPDs. Pockets of communities with low vaccination rates among the children exist across the country. In addition, new and emerging diseases may develop (e.g., COVID-19) for which a vaccine has not yet been developed (Children's Hospital of Philadelphia, 2018; USDHHS, 2020).

The Advisory Committee on Immunization Practices (ACIP) reviews the schedule for administration of vaccines for various populations and age groups (CDC, 2020b). The ACIP provides vaccine recommendations based on research and scientific data related to vaccine safety and efficacy for adult and child vaccines. Recommendations include age when vaccines should be given, dosage, number of doses, time intervals between doses, and precautions and contraindications (CDC, 2020b). It also makes recommendations during times of disease outbreaks and vaccine shortages. An example is an outbreak of pertussis (whooping cough) in 2012. More than 14,000 people became infected and 14 babies died of pertussis. Given that young infants cannot receive the first dose of pertussis until they are 2 months old and their immunity would still be developing as they receive subsequent doses, ACIP recommends that pregnant women receive the vaccine to provide short-term protection, and the CDC encourages everyone close to the baby to receive an updated pertussis vaccine (CDC, 2017c, 2017f).

The majority of American society has accepted immunizations as a part of overall health care. However, some challenge the notion of immunizing their children for many reasons. Some oppose government mandates and the sheer number of vaccinations, whereas others want to veer from the recommended spacing schedule but plan to eventually complete the childhood series. Although

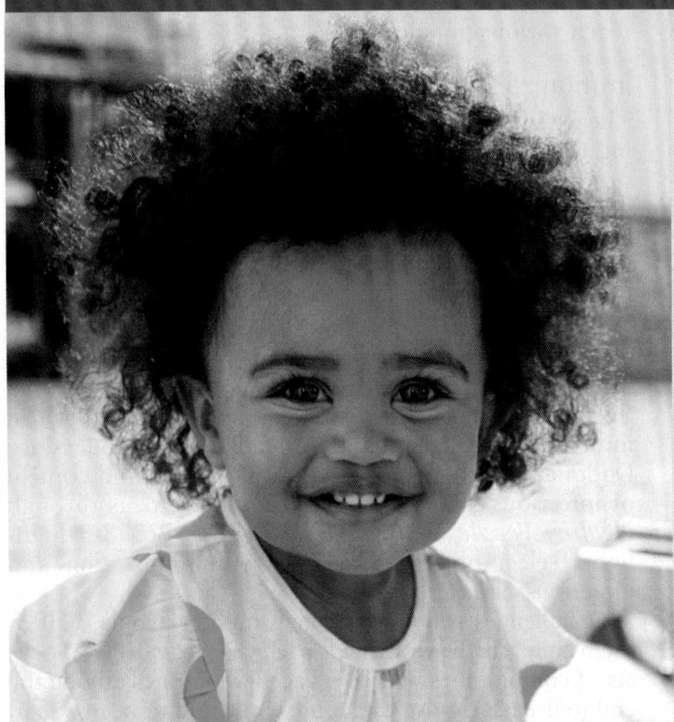

Vaccines for Children
Protecting America's children every day
The Vaccines for Children (VFC) program helps ensure that all children have a better chance of getting their recommended vaccines. VFC has helped prevent disease and save lives.
CDC estimates that vaccination of children born between 1994 and 2018 will:
prevent 419 million illnesses
(26.8 million hospitalizations)
help avoid 936,000 deaths
save nearly $1.9 trillion in total societal costs
(that includes $406 billion in direct costs)

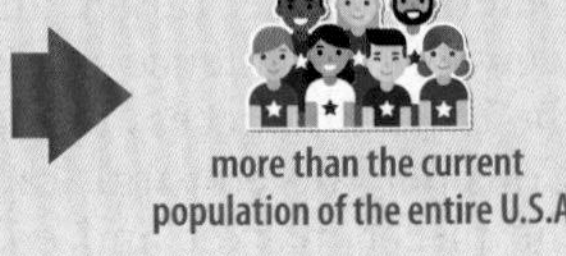

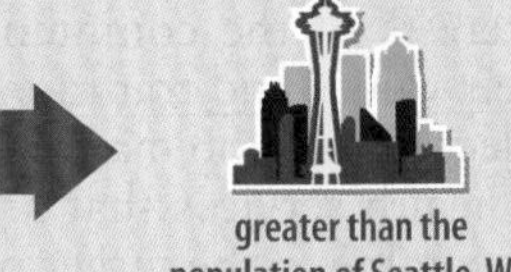
greater than the population of Seattle, WA
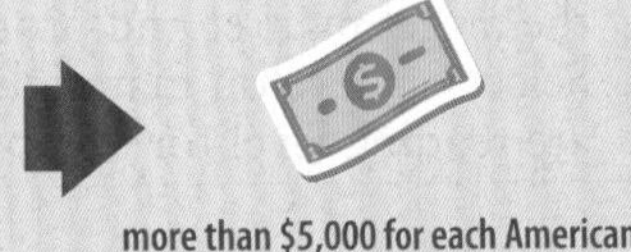
more than $5,000 for each American
Updated 2018 analysis using methods from "Benefits from Immunization during the Vaccines for Children Program Era—United States, 1994-2013"
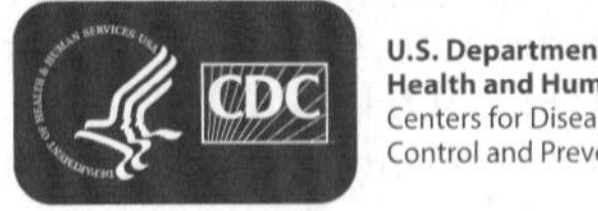
U.S. Department of Health and Human Services
Centers for Disease Control and Prevention
www.cdc.gov/features/vfcprogram
NCIRDig702 | 03/28/19

FIGURE 8-11 The Vaccines for Children (VCF) program ensures that children from all communities and income levels will be able to get recommended childhood vaccinations, preventing these infectious diseases and their sequelae. (Reprinted from Centers for Disease Control & Prevention (CDC). (2019). *Vaccines for Children Program (VCF)*. Retrieved from https://www.cdc.gov/vaccines/programs/vfc/protecting-children.html?CDC_AA_refVal=https%3A%2F%2Fwww.cdc.gov%2Fvaccines%2Fprograms%2Fvfc%2F20-year-infographic.html)

all states have established laws requiring immunizations in certain situations (such as for attendance in public schools and childcare facilities and employment in health care facilities), many allow for exempting immunizations for various reasons, whether religious, philosophical, or medical (Boxes 8-4 and 8-5). In 2019, 15 states allowed for personal, moral, or other beliefs exemption (National Conference of State Legislatures [NCSL], 2019). The C/PHN should look to immunization agency of the state of practice for the accepted exemption criteria (Immunization Action Coalition, 2020). This subject is further discussed under the section Barriers to Immunization Coverage.

At the time of this writing, data from the CDC's National Immunization Survey indicated the following (CDC, 2018c):

- Children's data for 2016 showed >80% compliance in vaccination for the diphtheria and tetanus toxoids and acellular pertussis (DTaP); measles, mumps, and rubella (MMR); polio; *Haemophilus influenzae* type b (HIB); hepatitis B; varicella; and pneumococcal conjugate vaccines.
- Of adolescents (boys and girls 13 to 17 years of age), 48.6% were up to date on the HPV vaccine, with higher HPV vaccine rates in Hispanic girls than in White girls and in girls living in poverty than those living at or above the poverty line.
- Adult immunization rates showed a modest increase of 1% to 3% from 2010 to 2015 but did not meet the Healthy People 2020 immunization goals, except for the herpes zoster rate, which was 30%.
- Racial and ethnic differences persisted, with Asians, Blacks, and Hispanics having lower rates for recommended immunizations, with the exception of influenza vaccination.
- Higher immunization rates could also be seen in U.S.-born adults when compared with foreign-born adults, with the exceptions of the influenza and hepatitis A vaccinations.

BOX **8-3** *HEALTHY PEOPLE 2030*

Immunization and Infectious Diseases: Selected 2030 Objectives

Core and Developmental Objectives	
IID-02	Reduce the proportion of children 2 doses of the MMR vaccine who get no recommended vaccines by age 2 years
IID-03	Maintain an effective vaccination coverage level of 1 dose of the MMR vaccine in children by age 2 years
IID-04	Maintain the vaccination coverage level of 1 dose of measles-mumps-rubella vaccine (MMR) for children in kindergarten
IID-05	Reduce cases of pertussis among infants
IID-06	Increase the vaccination coverage level of 4 doses of the DTaP vaccine in children by age 2 years
IID-08	Increase the percentage of adolescents aged 13 through 15 years who get recommended doses of the HPV vaccine
IID-09	Increase the proportion of people who get the flu vaccine every year
IID-10	Reduce the rate of hepatitis A
IID-11,12	Reduce the rate of acute hepatitis B and C
IID-17	Reduce tuberculosis cases
STI-01	Increase the proportion of sexually active females aged 16–24 years enrolled in Medicaid and commercial health plans who are screened for chlamydial infections
STI-02	Reduce gonorrhea rates in male adolescents and young men
STI-03	Reduce the incidence of primary and secondary syphilis in rate in females
STI-04	Reduce congenital syphilis
STI-05	Reduce the rate of syphilis in men who have sex with men
STI-06	Reduce the proportion of adolescents and young adults with genital herpes
STI-07	Reduce pelvic inflammatory disease in female adolescents and young women
IID-D01	Increase the proportion of women who get the Tdap vaccine during pregnancy

Reprinted from U.S. Department of Health and Human Services (USDHHS). (2020). *Browse 2030 objectives.* Retrieved from https://health.gov/healthypeople/objectives-and-data/browse-objectives

Adults who reported having a regular place to seek medical care, regardless of health insurance coverage, had higher vaccination rates than those who did not have a regular place to seek medical care (Williams et al., 2017).

Health care providers, C/PHN, and school nurses are in positions to review records, educate families, and provide opportunities for a child and adult to obtain immunizations. Nurses need to be aware that individuals now more often obtain their medial information from online sources than from medical professionals (Hussain, Ali, Ahmed, & Hussain, 2018). These online sources include Internet searches and social media platforms such as Facebook, Twitter, and Instagram. This change has allowed for users of social media to produce and disseminate their content directly, leading to widespread digital misinformation and "echo chambers," which has been listed as one of the main threats to our society (Schmidt, Zollo, Scala, Betsch, & Quattrociocchi, 2018, p. 3606). Researchers note that if parents are seeking information on the Internet about vaccination risks, they are likely to discover more Web sites perpetuating negative myths about and recommending against childhood vaccination than supporting it, according to a seminal systematic review by Kaufman et al. (2013). The

BOX 8-4 What Parents Should Know When Signing a Personal Beliefs Affidavit Exemption of Immunization

1. Please educate yourself to the symptoms and possible complications that can arise from a vaccine-preventable disease (VPD). Information for parents about these diseases may be found at the National Immunization Program site http://www.cdc.gov/nip/ or by calling *Insert Local County Public Health Department Name & Phone Number.*
2. Have a plan of care coordinated with your health care provider, to act upon the mildest to most severe symptoms of the disease.
3. It is the Parent/Guardian's responsibility to ensure an approved copy of the exemption is filed with the Child's school nurse.
4. An unimmunized child will be excluded from school by the County Health Officer when a VPD is identified in the school.
5. When a child is excluded from school, it is the responsibility of the parent/guardian to keep the child isolated[1] from the public at large to prevent spread of infection to the community.
6. VPDs are considered **reportable communicable diseases** under the Health and Safety Codes of *Insert Local County Public Health Department.* If your child contracts one of these diseases, a public health nurse will contact you. Be prepared to provide information about the illness to the investigator. **This information is confidential.**
7. The parent/guardian is also at risk of contracting any of these diseases when exposed to an ill child. If unimmunized, the parent or guardian will remain in isolation from the community through the incubation period.
8. The child who is exposed to the disease may be offered preventive medication or immunization to prevent the disease from occurring—either may keep the child from being excluded from school.

[1]The isolation time frame is determined by the county health officer. Isolation means that the exposed or ill child cannot leave home except for medical care. No social gatherings!

viewing of antivaccination Web sites cannot be underestimated, as studies have found that the perception of vaccine risk is evident 5 months after parents viewed the misinformation, resulting in parents choosing to not fully vaccinate their child (Hussain et al., 2018).

Common questions parents ask about vaccines and recommended responses by nurses are as follows:

- *Are the vaccines safe?* Nurses can provide information about the safety trials that the vaccines undergo prior to release to the public and advise parents of possible side effects and how to care for the child if side effects do arise.
- *I'm worried about giving so much at one time; how does that affect my child's immune system?* Nurses can assure parents that the small dose in the vaccine is not nearly as much as children are exposed to in everyday life (Donovan & Bedford, 2013; Kumar, Chandra, Mathur, Samdariya, & Kapoor, 2016). Nurses can explain that although incidences of diseases have declined, other than polio, they still exist

BOX 8-5 PERSPECTIVES

PHN: Personal Belief Exemption and Immunization

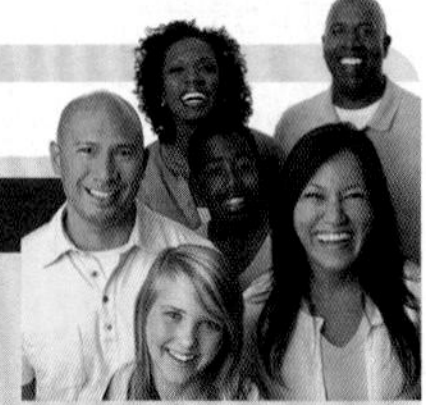

A whooping cough (pertussis) outbreak occurred in a small rural community. The outbreak of pertussis occurred in a small charter school, where the majority of the children were unvaccinated for reasons of parental personal belief objections. Unfortunately, with a large unvaccinated population and with many in the community against vaccinating children, 22 cases were reported among children and family members. The school closed early to stop the spread of the disease.

After meeting with parents, members in the community, and C/PHNs and school nurses, it was discovered that not all parents signed the personal belief exemption out of true conviction but instead signed them to stop the school staff from pestering them for not having the time to vaccinate their high-risk children.

The county's immunization coordinator, the community's immunization coalition, and the school nurses determined that the school secretaries were the most common point of entrance to school registration. It was discovered that these individuals needed an in-service on how to properly offer the exemption to a family and what information parents would need to make an informed decision before signing the exemption.

The immunization coordinator developed an education tool that explained to the parents their responsibility to the community at large if their child were to become ill with a vaccine-preventable illness. The Personal Beliefs Affidavit covered the points outlined in Box 8-4. The school secretaries were asked to give this document to parents who were interested in the exemption, as well as community resource information for families who may not have access to affordable immunizations.

The parents at the charter school were very accepting of the information on what to do for an ill child, and the school secretaries expressed relief regarding dealing with parents who may want to exempt out for convenience rather than conviction.

During the pertussis outbreak, as a C/PHN, what interventions would you direct to the parents who did not vaccinate their children due to true personal belief objections?

Ashley, PHN

in the natural setting and can easily resurface and be life-threatening.

- *Why are vaccines given at such a young age?* Nurses need to explain that vaccines are given as early as possible to provide the child with protection as early as possible and that declining an immunization at the time the child is eligible for it leaves the child vulnerable to the disease until the series is completed (CDC, 2018h; Donovan & Bedford, 2013).
- *Are preservatives or additives in the vaccine that will harm my baby?* The nurse could explain why the preservative is added to the vaccine. C/PHNs should be aware of any state law prohibiting the administration of a vaccine that contains thimerosal to a newborn (CDC, 2018h).

Vaccine-Preventable Diseases

Hepatitis A and B, *H. influenza* type b, measles, polio, diphtheria, pertussis, influenza, and chickenpox are examples of diseases that can be prevented through immunization, or VPDs. Immunization causes the body to become immune to an infectious agent by developing a defense against the invading infectious agent or antigen. The immunity allows the body to tolerate the presence of material that is foreign, such as a virus or bacterium (Hamborsky et al., 2015). Immunity may be either passive or active:

- **Passive immunity** is short-term resistance to a specific disease-causing organism; it may be acquired naturally (as with newborns through maternal antibody transfer) or artificially through inoculation with pooled human antibody (e.g., immunoglobulin) that gives temporary protection.
- **Active immunity** is long-term (sometimes lifelong) resistance to a specific disease-causing organism; it also can be acquired naturally or artificially. Naturally acquired active immunity occurs when a person contracts a disease, whereas artificial immunity occurs when a person receives an inoculation of an antigen through a vaccine.

Both prompt an immune response that stimulates the development of long-lasting antibodies that provide immunity against future exposure to that antigen (Hamborsky et al., 2015). See Chapter 7.

A **vaccine** is a preparation made from either a live organism or an inactivated form of the organism. Live attenuated vaccines are made from weakened wild virus organisms that are able to replicate but generally do not make the person ill. It only takes a small amount to initiate an immune response, and the organisms must replicate to be effective. Inactivated vaccines are made from a viral organism that has been inactivated by heat or chemicals. These vaccines cannot replicate in the recipient (Hamborsky et al., 2015). Currently, measles, mumps, rubella, vaccinia, yellow fever, rotavirus, and intranasal influenza are all live attenuated vaccines (Hamborsky et al., 2015).

Schedule of Recommended Immunizations

A schedule for the administration of childhood vaccinations, based on recommendations by the ACIP, the American Academy of Pediatrics, the American Academy of Family Physicians, and the CDC, is published annually (see https://www.cdc.gov/vaccines/schedules/hcp/imz/child-adolescent.html). The CDC also provides "catch-up" schedules for children not receiving their first immunizations at birth, according to the standard schedule. Current recommendations call for a child to receive 10 different vaccines or toxoids (many in combination form and all requiring more than one dose) in six or seven visits to a health care provider between birth and school entry, with boosters in the preteen to early teen years (Hamborsky et al., 2015).

Factors influencing the recommended age at which vaccines are administered include:

- Age-specific risks of the disease
- Age-specific risks of complications
- Ability of persons of a given age to produce an adequate and lasting immune response
- Potential for interference with the immune response acquired from passively transferred maternal antibodies

In general, vaccines are recommended for the youngest age group at risk whose members are known to develop an acceptable antibody response to the vaccination (Hamborsky et al., 2015).

Recommendations for vaccine administration may be revised in certain circumstances. For example, it is now recommended that infants receive hepatitis B vaccine at birth, whether or not their mothers have a positive or negative response to the hepatitis B surface antigen. This approach will catch any infant born to mothers who lack prenatal testing or who may live in households with individuals with unknown hepatitis B status (Heymann, 2015).

Herd Immunity

Herd immunity, or community immunity, is central to understanding immunization as a means of protecting community health. As described in Chapter 7, **Herd immunity** is the immunity level present in a particular group or community of people. If only a few immune persons exist within a community (i.e., if herd immunity is low), then the spread of disease is more likely (Fig. 8-12). However, if there are more individuals in the community who are immunized (i.e., if herd immunity is high), this helps minimize the chance that an unvaccinated person will become ill (Heymann, 2015).

The level of required herd immunity varies. For instance, a level of community immunity between 83% and 85% may be enough for rubella, but for pertussis (whooping cough), 92% to 94% may be needed to be effective (Merrill, 2017). Mandatory preschool immunizations and required travel vaccinations are applications of the herd immunity concept. An illustration of how herd immunity can cross all age groups is the Australian infant pneumococcal vaccination program, which created a herd immunity resulting in a 50% decline in hospitalization and deaths across all age groups over an 11-year period (Chen, 2018). See Box 8-6. An informative animation explaining herd immunity and how it varies depending on infectious agent can be found at: https://www.youtube.com/watch?v=XJFoOCmJsdg

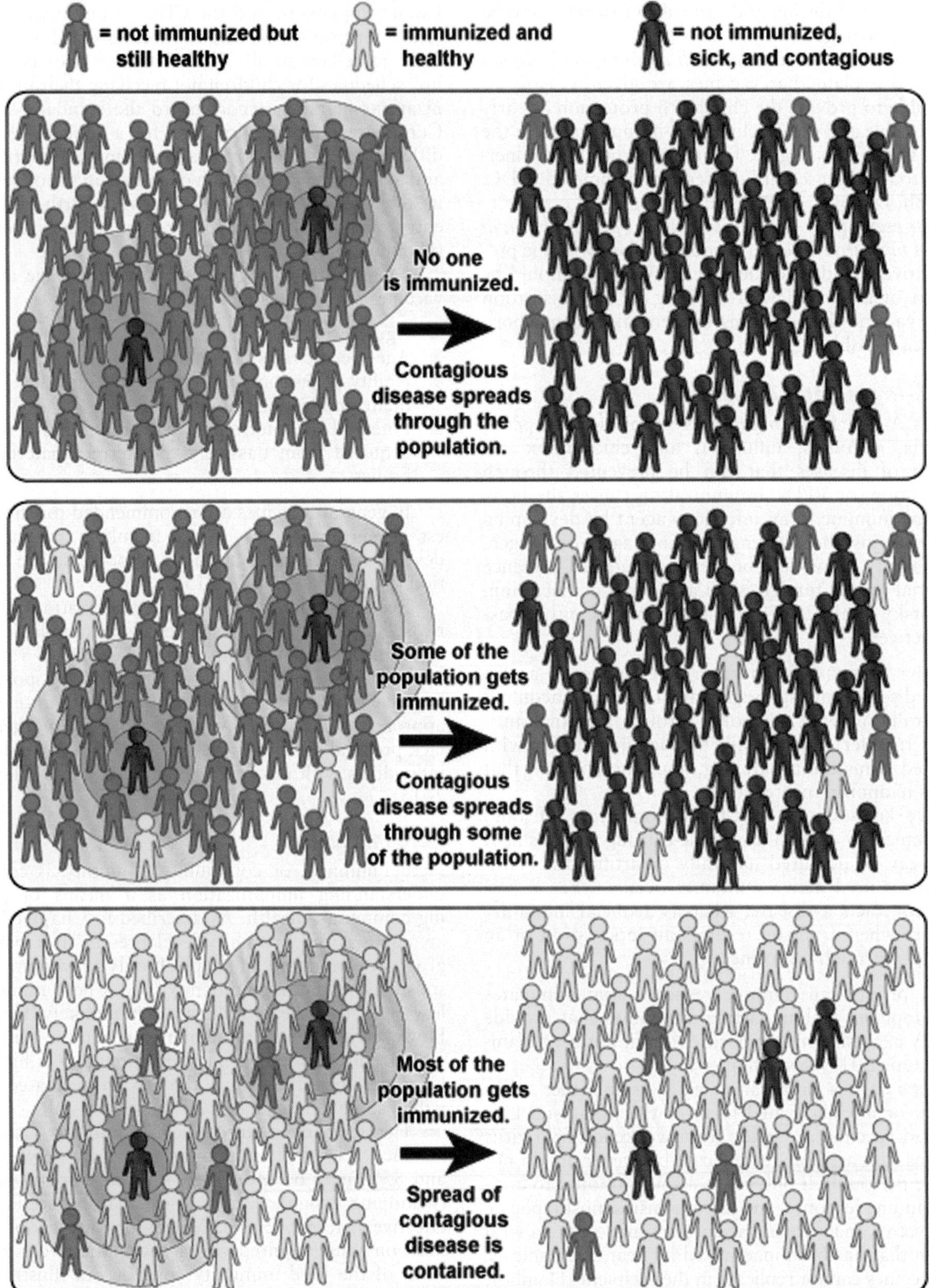

FIGURE 8-12 Community immunity/herd immunity. (From National Institute of Allergies and Infectious Diseases (NIAID). Retrieved from https://twitter.com/niaidnews/status/1105879923535867910?lang=en)

BOX **8-6** EVIDENCE-BASED PRACTICE

Pertussis: New Preventive Strategies for an Old Disease

In spite of high vaccination rates, pertussis outbreaks are occurring every 2 to 5 years in developed and developing countries. The population primarily being affected are infants <6 months of age followed by 10 to 14 years old who have yet to complete the vaccination series. The reasons may be due to the rising awareness of the disease, improved diagnostic tests, new strains of *Bordetella pertussis* not included in vaccine, asymptotic spread of *B. pertussis* in adolescents and adults or the decreased protection time of vaccine (Fernandes, Rodrigues, Sartori, De Soárez, & Novaes, 2018).

As a result, new strategies to protect against *B. pertussis* are under evaluation such as booster doses of vaccine to adolescents, adults, and pregnant women. Another method under evaluation is the practice known as **cocooning**. The goal is to immunize close family and friends or frequent contacts to reduce the risk of exposing the vulnerable person to these diseases (Di Mattia et al., 2018).

The C/PHN has an opportunity to evaluate the emerging research related to the booster doses, immunization of pregnant women, and cocoon approach and determine if their community could benefit from any of these strategies in reducing VPD outbreaks and poor outcomes for the infant at risk. A number of questions must be addressed in considering whether cocooning is a viable option in a community:

1. *Does the approach actually reduce infections in the target population and where is the evidence?*
2. *What is the risk to the persons being vaccinated?*
3. *What is the cost of this program?*
4. *Are there unintended consequences from this approach, such as delayed immunizations in the target population?*

Source: Di Mattia et al. (2018); Fernandes et al. (2018).

Herd immunity is not only important in relation to limiting exposure of infection but also in reducing risks for cancer. A 4-year study showed a connection between increased vaccination rates of HPV with decreased HPV-related cancers among nonvaccinated women, thereby confirming the potential benefits of herd immunity in reducing HPV-related cancers (Cameron et al., 2016).

Innovations are an important source of improved health-promoting practices and should not be discouraged, but, as always, solid research evidence is vital. With limited health care dollars, efforts must target the most cost-effective and proven methods possible. Only time and research will show which strategy will be an effective tool in the public health arsenal.

Assessing Immunization Status of the Community

Immunization rates still need to be improved. Nurses need to work to ensure that all those who need vaccines are receiving them. Laws have been implemented requiring students to receive vaccines prior to entering school. This section reviews approaches to address **vaccine hesitancy**, which is defined as a "delay in acceptance or refusal of vaccination despite availability of vaccination services" and listed as one of the top ten threats to global health (WHO, 2020g, para. 1). It is important to recognize that all clients who refuse vaccination are not all the same. They may have very different concerns. Refer to Figures 8-13 and 8-14 for the factors associated with vaccine hesitancy.

Vaccine hesitancy is closely connected with the Internet and social media such as Facebook, YouTube, Instagram, blogs, search engines, and Web sites (Schmidt et al., 2018), where much content on the subject decreases the confidence of the individual with regard to safety and need. Many Web sites are highly interactive and allow users to share their information without regard to validity. Antivaccination content ranks high in search engines as it is easy to read. Health institutions now understand the importance of spreading accurate information through the Internet, and the number of sites promoting vaccinations has grown (Mitra, Counts, & Pennebaker, 2016). As health professionals, it is important to understand the sources and quality of content on the Internet, and how to use tools such as Google Trends and HealthMap to monitor trends and help disseminate correct information (Bragazzi et al., 2018; Millard et al., 2018; Rosselli, Martini, & Bragazzi, 2016; Sampri, Mavragani, & Tsagarakis, 2016; Tustin et al., 2018).

Below are three different strategies that can be considered when dealing with vaccine hesitancy:

- Tell, don't ask: research has shown that a presumptive format, in which the health care provider leads the discussion (e.g., "well, we have to do some shots"), is associated with higher vaccination rates than a participatory format (e.g., "How do you feel about vaccines?"; Opel et al., 2018).
- Motivational interviewing (a brief intervention style developed by Miller and Rollnick): an empathetic, respectful approach in which the health care provider targets information based on the concerns of the parent only after permission has been given may be helpful (Gagneur, Gosselin, & Dube, 2018). See Chapter 10.
- "CASE" (Corroborate, About, Science, Explain):
  - *Corroborate* the concerns and have a respectful conversation with the parent.
  - Tell the parent *about* yourself and your level of expertise.
  - Refer to the evidence from *science*.
  - *Explain* and advise, following the ACIP guidelines (American Academy of Pediatrics, 2019; Domachowske & Suryadevara, 2013).

It is important to engage families who are hesitant about vaccines in open conversation. This may be a challenging task when a parent is confrontational with the health provider or perhaps even attempting to change the mind of the health care provider. Some who seemed adamant about refusing the vaccine may even decide to accept the vaccine after an honest discussion because they felt that they were heard, and their questions were answered (Attwell, Meyer, & Ward, 2018; MacDonald, 2015, WHO, 2014b).

Offering vaccines at home visits and in Women, Infants, and Children program offices has also been

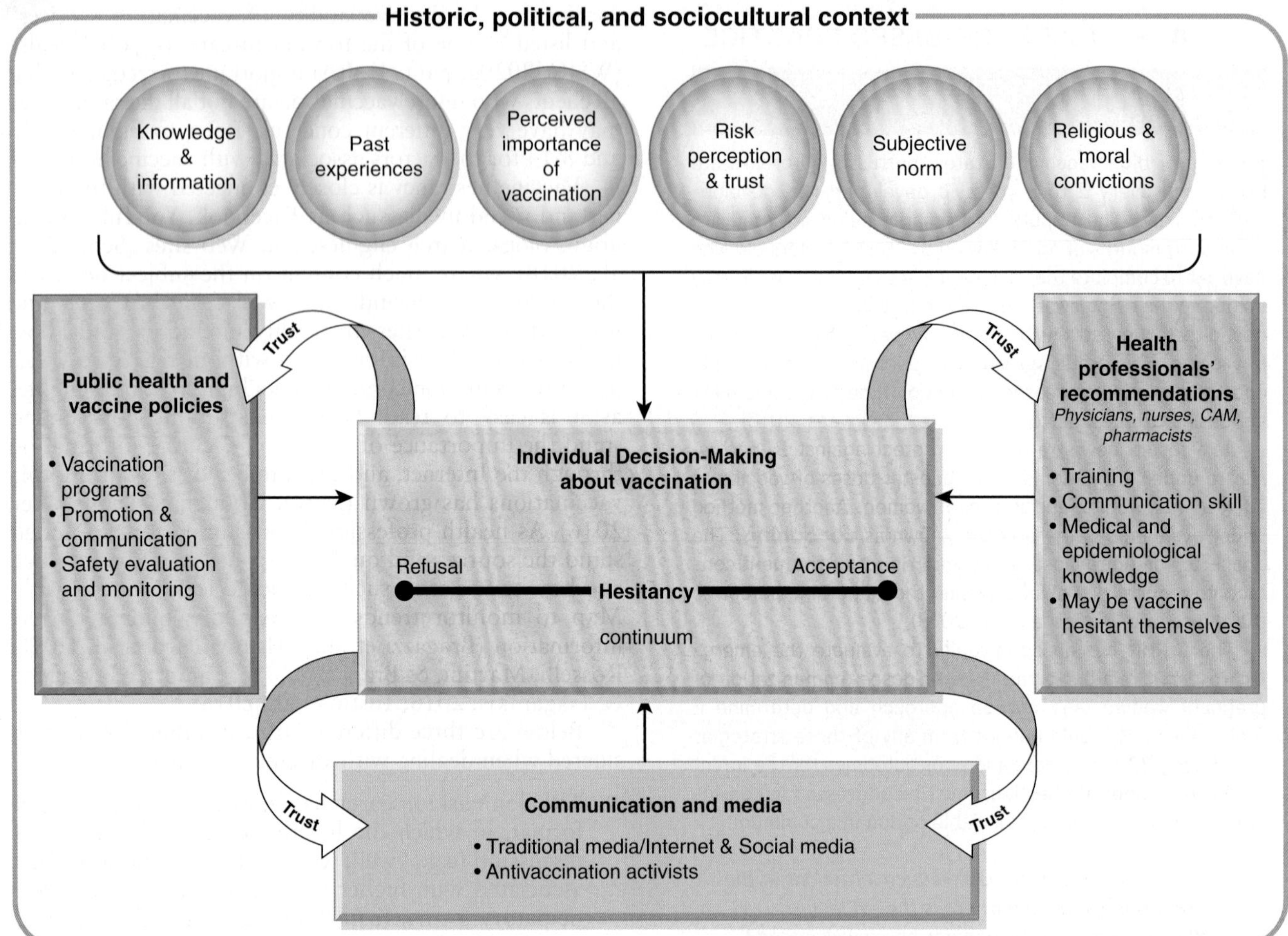

FIGURE 8-13 Conceptual Model of Vaccine Hesitancy. (Adapted with permission from Dubé, E., Laberge, C., Guay, M., Bramadat, P., Roy, R., & Bettinger, J. (2013). Vaccine hesitancy: an overview. *Human vaccines & immunotherapeutics, 9*(8), 1763–1773.)

found to be effective. Another strategy is to work with providers. The AFIX (assessment, feedback, incentives, and exchange) approach is designed to help providers recognize the problem:

- *Assess* the current immunization rates within the office to show the provider an accurate picture (computer applications from the CDC can help with this process).
- Give *feedback* to the provider about progress in increasing vaccination rates in a nonjudgmental way.
- Offer *incentives* to help motivate the provider to make the needed changes.
- Encourage an *exchange* of information with other providers about what has worked for them (Hamborsky et al., 2015).

Planning and Implementing an Immunization Campaign

Immunization campaigns targeting specific subgroups can be effective if they include the following:

- Community assessment for the target group(s)
- Assessment of and planning for the needs of the target group(s), such as:
  - Transportation
  - Language interpreters
  - Childcare
  - Literacy

Successful outreach efforts are motivated by the desire to reach the target population, even if specific or unusual accommodations must be made. An online presence, with information about the benefits of vaccines and clinic locations, is helpful. Clinics can be scheduled and held at times and places specifically intended to make the service more accessible and convenient to the target group. Materials in multilingual form can be obtained through the state's immunization agency or the CDC. The CDC and state immunization agencies have campaigns throughout the year for the C/PHN to participate in and provide to the public. Tool kits with the materials and tips for planning and implementation are available through the state immunization agency (Hamborsky et al., 2015). Box 8-7 outlines the process for administering an immunization campaign in a community setting. A 5-minute video on the importance of vaccines for older adults may be helpful for all age groups: https://www.youtube.com/watch?v=hodb65EkorM

CONTEXTUAL INFLUENCES Influences arising due to historic, socio-cultural, environmental, health system/institutional, economic or political factors	a. Communication and media environment b. Influential leaders, immunization program gatekeepers and anti- or pro-vaccination lobbies. c. Historical influences d. Religion/culture/ gender/socio-economic e. Politics/policies f. Geographic barriers g. Perception of the pharmaceutical industry
INDIVIDUAL AND GROUP INFLUENCES Influences arising from personal perception of the vaccine or influences of the social/peer environment	a. Personal, family and/or community members' experience with vaccination, including pain b. Beliefs, attitudes about health and prevention c. Knowledge/awareness d. Health system and providers-trust and personal experience. e. Risk/benefit (perceived, heuristic) f. Immunisation as a social norm vs. not needed/harmful
VACCINE/ VACCINATION–SPECIFIC ISSUES Directly related to vaccine or vaccination	a. Risk/ Benefit (epidemiological and scientific evidence) b. Introduction of a new vaccine or new formulation or a new recommendation for an existing vaccine c. Mode of administration d. Design of vaccination program/Mode of delivery (e.g., routine program or mass vaccination campaign) e. Reliability and/or source of supply of vaccine and/or vaccination equipment f. Vaccination schedule g. Costs h. The strength of the recommendation and/or knowledge base and/or attitude of healthcare professionals

FIGURE 8-14 Vaccine Hesitancy Matrix. (Reprinted with permission from WHO. (2014). *Report of the Sage Working Group on Vaccine Hesitancy* (p. 12). Retrieved from http://www.who.int/immunization/sage/meetings/2014/october/1_Report_WORKING_GROUP_vaccine_hesitancy_final.pdf)

Adult Immunization

Many people assume that vaccinations are for children only. Well-advertised influenza vaccination campaigns in recent years have, to some extent, helped to correct this notion.

Adults face risk for becoming infected with a VPD if they are unimmunized or underimmunized. Some of the immunizations that wane, meaning that the protection disappears over time, are tetanus, pertussis, influenza, and pneumococcal. Other vaccines are specific for adults, such as the varicella zoster, otherwise known as the shingles vaccine. The CDC (2020b) provides an adult immunization schedule of recommendations. See Chapter 21 for adult vaccination schedule and adult screenings.

Substantial numbers of VPDs still occur among adults despite the availability of safe and effective vaccines. C/PHN should be aware of factors that may contribute to low vaccination levels among adults:

1. Cost and reimbursement
2. Lack of a regular place to seek medical care
3. No reminder-recall system in place
4. Provider's lack of current knowledge of recommended immunizations or forgetting to ask about vaccinations at the time of the visit, leading to missed opportunities to vaccinate
5. Need for training of health care staff on recommended immunizations for adults
6. Patient's lack of awareness of adult vaccination standards

International Travelers, Immigrants, and Refugees

As Americans interact more and more with their neighbors in other parts of the world, the incidence of Americans with tropical or imported diseases also rises. Within about 36 hours of boarding an airplane, one can reach any destination in the world. An average flight can equal the incubation period of some infectious diseases, and before the onset of symptoms is realized, microbial agents could be spread around the globe.

Travelers can take steps to protect themselves prior to embarking on their journey to new and exotic places by:

BOX **8-7** C/PHN USE OF THE NURSING PROCESS

Administering an Immunization Campaign in a Community Setting

	Assessment	Planning	Implementation	Evaluation
Population Level	• Target community? • Are vaccines needed? • Identify and prioritize vaccine hesitant populations and subgroups? • Consider the political and social structure of the community. • Identify important leaders	• Engage community leaders to promote vaccination • Develop target message to reach specific population or subgroups and select appropriate method: e-mail, digital media (web pages, social media), places of worship, flyers, mail	• Inform target group of date, location, and times of immunization clinic • Provide information on reasons for and benefits (and contraindications to) immunization • Provide contact information for questions and concerns	• Evaluate and assess for gaps in communication system used. • Solicit feedback from community partners and leaders. • Assess if target group reached
Program Level	• Vaccine availability? • Medical staff knowledge of effective communication? • Availability of staff, vaccination sites and hours • Is there a reminder and follow-up system?	• Review budget • Determine goals and outcome measures • Estimate needs for vaccine and supplies • Plan immunization logistics: medical waste, anaphylaxis supplies, records, traffic control, and management of crowds. • Prepare staff with training and reinforcement of "herd immunity" message • Create or review reminder and follow-up system. • Plan on how to mitigate pain during immunization	• Designate a contact person(s) • Registration systems and records ready. • Register or assistant(s) ready for those not familiar with language of paperwork • System for call back, follow-up • System for dealing with other health issues and/or adverse events	• Assess numbers of immunizations given in relation to goals • Assess suitability of sites • Evaluate results in relation to expenditures • Solicit feedback from medical staff
Individual Level	• Complete assessment (physical, health history, environmental) • Surveillance of communicable diseases • Is the vaccine wanted? • What are the reasons behind vaccine hesitancy (barriers and enablers)?	• Educate and have evidence-informed responses • Have a consistent message: • Emphasize safety • Herd immunity • Remain free of signs and symptoms of disease • Complete vaccine (series)	• Education: informed consent, reporting of adverse reaction, and date next vaccine due. • Mitigate pain as much as possible • Reinforce message • Monitor for side effects • Provide opportunity for feedback	• Evaluate feedback • Evaluate the effectiveness of vaccine by confirming that the patient goals and expected outcomes have been met (see "Planning")

Source: MacDonald (2015); Martin (2018).

- Visiting the CDC Travelers Health Web site to access advise on staying healthy during and on return from a trip (CDC, 2020m)
- Making an appointment for a consultation with a tropical medicine or travel clinic to prepare for international travel
- Being immunized with the recommended vaccines for the particular area of the world
- Having the necessary chemical prophylaxis on hand (i.e., antimalarial medications as prescribed)
- Learning about food and water hygiene precautions and basic first aid for simple injuries (CDC, 2020m)

Traveling internationally has grown over the past decade, with 1.2 billion worldwide tourist arrivals in 2015. Promoting a traveler's health is important to safeguard not only the individual's health but also the health of the individual's community (CDC, 2017h).

Refugees and international travelers who arrive in the United States may be unfamiliar with U.S. health systems, health precautions, and practices. Refugees and immigrants must follow prescribed guidelines, including extensive health screening mandated by U.S. immigration laws, immunizations, and treatment, as appropriate (CDC, 2017i). More than ever before, C/PHNs have professional contact with these new Americans, whether close to their time of arrival or later, in schools, immunization clinics, or other locations. Visitors from other countries may also require the assistance of other C/PHP. For this reason, C/PHNs are encouraged to develop and maintain a global perspective on communicable diseases. See Chapter 16 for more information on global health.

SECONDARY PREVENTION

Two approaches to secondary prevention of communicable disease are possible: (a) screening and (b) disease case and contact investigation and notification (previously discussed).

Screening

Screening is a secondary prevention method because asymptomatic cases can be discovered and provided with prompt early treatment. Pregnant women can also be identified and treated to prevent infection to the neonate (Heymann, 2015).

The term **screening** is used in community/public health and disease prevention to describe programs that provide disease-testing opportunities to detect disease in groups of asymptomatic, apparently healthy individuals. Common screening measures can include prenatal hepatitis B screens, urine *Chlamydia* and gonorrhea screens, and Mantoux TSTs for TB infection (Heymann, 2015).

Remember that the screening test itself is not diagnostic but rather a method to identify those persons with positive or suspicious test findings who then require further medical evaluation or treatment. C/PHNs working with clients in a screening setting must be prepared to clearly and correctly explain to individuals that screening tests are not definitive and that positive findings require subsequent investigation before diagnostic conclusions can be drawn.

Criteria for Screening Tests

Some important criteria are used in deciding whether to carry out a screening intervention in a community. They include validity and reliability and predictive value and yield.

Validity and Reliability

The screening test must be valid and reliable. *Validity* refers to the test's ability to accurately identify those with the disease. *Reliability* refers to the test's ability to give consistent results when administered on different occasions by different technicians.

Predictive Value and Yield

The *predictive value* of a screening test is important for determining whether the screening intervention is justified. *Yield* refers to the number of positive results found per number tested. The predictive value and the yield of screening tests become important in planning screening programs for communicable disease detection and prevention because they can help planners locate screening efforts in areas or within population groups that are known to be at high risk for the disease. The predictive value of screening tests increases as the prevalence of the disease increases. For example, a screening test for TB among refugees would have a greater predictive value and yield than would TB screening in the population at large, owing to a higher endemicity of TB in many countries outside of the United States.

Epidemiologic criteria for screening interventions for the detection of health problems include the following (Trevethan, 2017):

- Is the disease an important public health problem?
- Is there a valid and reliable test?
- Is there an effective and tolerable treatment that favorably influences the early stages of the disease?
- After a positive screening result, are facilities for diagnosis and treatment available and accessible?
- Is there a recognizable early asymptomatic or latent stage in the disease?
- Do clear guidelines for referral and treatment exist?
- Is the total cost of the screening justifiable compared with the costs of treating the disease if left undiscovered?
- Is the screening test itself acceptable?
- Will screening be ongoing?

See Chapter 7 for more on epidemiology.

TERTIARY PREVENTION

The approaches to tertiary prevention of communicable disease include care and treatment of the infected person, isolation and quarantine of the infected person, and safe handling and control of infectious wastes.

Care and Treatment

Communicable diseases require care and treatment specific to the disease, and the nurse needs to:

- Understand the disease, the treatment, and follow-up requirements, and the educational component to discuss with the infected person
- Use information resources such as the CDC, state agency policies, and protocols provided by local public health agencies (Heymann, 2015)

Providing Services for Special High-Risk Populations

The LGBTQ community bears a disproportionate burden of STIs, particularly among men. Gay and bisexual men represent 83% of the cases of primary and secondary syphilis. Whereas men are generally at a lower risk for cancer due to HPV, men who have anal sex are 17 times more at risk for anal cancer (CDC, 2016e, 2020k).

C/PHNs can help alleviate the fear of bias that may be a barrier to accessing screening and treatment services by educating providers about LGBTQ-friendly practices such as nongender questions on patient history forms and nongender bathrooms. By educating medical staff, a more welcoming and supportive environment can be established encouraging LGBT people to seek out health care (Bristol, Kostelec, & MacDonald, 2018; CDC, 2020k).

Isolation and Quarantine

Communicable disease control includes two methods for keeping infected persons and noninfected persons apart to prevent the spread of a disease. **Isolation** refers to separation of the infected persons (or animals) from others for the period of communicability to limit the transmission of the infectious agent to susceptible persons. **Quarantine** refers to restrictions placed on healthy contacts of an infectious case for the duration of the incubation period to prevent disease transmission if infection should develop (Heymann, 2015). The CDC has quarantine stations located at land-border crossings and ports of entry, where public health officials determine if international travelers who are ill may be admitted into the United States or held to prevent spreading infectious disease (CDC, 2017d).

In 2020, some Americans who tested positive for a novel coronavirus (COVID-19) were quarantined, and travel bans were instituted in an effort to contain the spread of infection. The earliest reports of the new infection were made in the first week of January 2020, and as of February 29, 2020, there were 85,403 confirmed cases worldwide, with 79,394 reported cases in China, the suspected country of origin. Symptoms and potential spread of the novel virus are somewhat reminiscent of the SARS and MERS epidemics, although these were less widespread and had fewer total confirmed cases and deaths (but higher death rates). The WHO global risk assessment was raised to "very high" as the virus spread to 53 countries and 89 deaths were reported (Offord, 2020; WHO, 2020b). As of June 24, 2020, global cases reached 9,352,696 with 479,777 deaths. Despite statewide and area stay-at-home orders in most states in an effort to flatten the curve and reduce the burden on hospitals and health care workers, US cases reached 2,4224,168 and deaths totaled 123,473 (Mervosh, Lu, & Swales, 2020; Worldometer, 2020).

Safe Handling and Control of Infectious Wastes

The control of infection in C/PH also relies on the proper disposal of contaminated wastes. The CDC and the Occupational Safety and Health Administration (OSHA) support and encourage *standard precautions* that stress that health care workers think of all blood and body fluids and materials that they may come in contact with as potentially infectious (OSHA, n.d., 2011). Although universal precaution observance is primarily considered while the nurse is giving hands-on treatment or care to a patient, keeping these principles in mind while making community health visits in the primary and secondary setting is paramount to the safety of both the client and the nurse (Heymann, 2015).

Infectious waste is waste capable of producing an infectious disease provided it contains pathogens with sufficient virulence and quantity so that exposure to the waste by a susceptible host could result in an infectious disease (OSHA, n.d.). Requirements for medical waste disposal are for waste to be segregated into categories of:

- Used and unused sharps
- Cultures, specimens, and stocks of infectious agents
- Human blood and blood products
- Human pathologic, isolation, and animal waste

Although incineration has long been recognized as an efficient method for disposing safely of sharps and other contaminated medical waste, fewer incinerators are available now because of increasing regulation of emissions and particularly those regulations related to burning chemical wastes (Healthcare Environmental Resource Center, 2015; Heymann, 2015; OSHA, n.d., 2011).

Four key elements of an infectious waste management program are applicable to community practice:

1. Health professionals must be able to distinguish waste that poses a significant infection hazard from waste that does not.
2. The waste management program must have administrative support and authority to institute practice guidelines and provide the containers and other resources needed for safe disposal of infectious wastes.
3. Handling of the infectious wastes must be minimized. Containers should be rigid, leak-resistant (sealed), impervious to moisture, rupture-resistant, and, for sharps, puncture-resistant.
4. An enforcement or evaluation mechanism must be in place to ensure that the goal of reducing the potential for exposure to infectious waste in the community is met.

LEGAL AND ETHICAL ISSUES IN COMMUNICABLE DISEASE CONTROL

The threats presented by communicable diseases can bring public safety and ethical considerations to a crossroad. Public health interventions to protect the public often overlap individual rights (Gould, King, Wigglesworth, & Purssell, 2018). The communitarianism concept of what is good for the whole is good for the parts might be applied to public health practice. Considerations for ethical public health practice should include overall benefit to society, collective action, communitarianism, fairness in distribution of burden, harm principle, paternalism, liberty-limiting continua, social justice/fairness, and global justice. In addition, ethical issues of autonomy, beneficence, avoidance of maleficence, and justice also need to be taken into consideration (WHO, 2016b).

C/PHN must balance these ethical principles while working with the community to control the spread of infectious diseases. An example of this conflict might occur while conducting contact investigation for STI. The nurse must be mindful to conduct the investigation while maintaining confidentiality of the index case. Another example is mandating immunizations resulting in exclusion of unvaccinated children from a school setting (Gould et al., 2018). Public health practitioners walk a fine line to protect the rights of the individual while also protecting the health and safety of the community. Refer to Chapter 4 (ethical principles) for more details.

Enforced Compliance

Legally, the responsibilities of public health officials in communicable disease control include the police power to enforce compliance with treatment or restrict the activity of infectious people to protect the welfare of others (CDPH, 2020). Regulations that enforce compliance with disease prevention strategies are a justifiable restriction if the measures proposed are demonstrably effective and grounded in ethical principles (CDPH, 2020). However, during the recent Ebola epidemic, health care workers who treated Ebola victims in West Africa found themselves under 21-day quarantine once they returned to the United States even though they did not have symptoms, and some states took additional precautions not required by the CDC. As health care providers, it is important to be guided by scientific proof and not fear (Emrick, Gentry, & Morowit, 2016; Jones, 2020). Due process is crucial to protect individuals from government intrusion, particularly ensuring that fundamental fairness has been implemented in situations requiring imprisonment (CDPH, 2020).

Confidentiality, Privacy, and Discrimination

While carrying out communicable disease interventions, nurses and other health care professionals must ensure clients' confidentiality and privacy. The Health Insurance Portability and Accountability Act (HIPAA) Privacy Rule, last revised in 2003, seeks to protect patients' confidentiality and privacy by establishing laws that govern how health care providers, insurance companies, and other "covered entities" may use and disclose patients' personal health information. Health care providers may only disclose when necessary to provide care for the patient and then must provide only the minimum amount of information needed to provide that care (USDHHS, 2015). One exception is when disclosure of an individual's information is required to protect another person or people who are at risk of contracting an illness, but even then, the individual's identity is protected.

Human society has a long-standing aversion to infectious diseases. Ostracism, which in the past targeted people with leprosy and other contagious conditions, has shifted to discrimination against people with TB or AIDS (Jones, 2020). An example of this occurred in 2007 when an Atlanta attorney caused an international health scare and found his medical and personal information in the media as a result of flying to Europe after a recent diagnosis of drug-resistant TB (Night, 2007). People are protected from discrimination under the Americans with Disability Act but not with respect to posing a public health treat, such as with the contagious state of TB (U.S. Equal Employment Opportunity Commission, 2017).

SUMMARY

- Communicable diseases pose a major threat to the public's health and are transmitted globally as the result of mobile populations, increased urbanization, and international travel. They can be transmitted through direct contact from one person to another or indirectly through contaminated objects (air, water, food) or a vector (animal or insect; CDC, 2020a).
- Nurses concerned with communicable disease control must recognize who is at risk, where the potential reservoirs and sources of infectious disease agents are located, what environmental factors promote their spread, and what are the characteristics and vulnerability of community members and groups.
- Influenza is an evolving virus that is responsible for widespread outbreaks and pandemics as most of the world population do not have the antibodies to protect them from novel (new) strains.
- TB is one the biggest problems affecting our nation and is becoming more complicated to treat and manage with the introduction of MDR strains, the increasing number of people diagnosed with TB and HIV/AIDS, and the breaking down of international borders due to immigration, refugees, increased travel, poverty, and inadequate access to health care.
- STIs threaten the health and lives of millions of people. Control of STIs can be accomplished through effective screening, treatment, contact investigation, and aggressive public education.
- Primary prevention of communicable diseases includes methods such as using mass media education campaigns, one-on-one education, and immunization promotion and programs to reduce risk and help prevent diseases from occurring in the first place.
- Vaccine hesitancy is one of the ten leading causes of death worldwide. C/PHNs need to work with parents to learn about their concerns and provide education and strategies to assist them.
- Herd immunity, or community immunity, is central to understanding immunization as a means of protecting community health.
- Secondary prevention activities of screening and disease investigation are steps taken when primary prevention activities have failed.
- Tertiary prevention is needed to ensure additional people are not infected and those who are ill receive care and treatment. Ongoing disease transmission can be interrupted through treatment, isolation, or quarantine.
- Ethical issues in communicable disease control include enforced compliance, the justifiability of screening, preservation of confidentiality and privacy, and the avoidance of discrimination against infected people.

ACTIVE LEARNING EXERCISES

1. The antivaccine movement uses the Internet through social media, Web sites, and blogs to spread their antivaccine information. Find a Web site, social online group, or blog and summarize who they are targeting and why. Create a response to one argument against antivaccination using evidence-based research that could be easily understood by a non-medical person.
2. Find a case that was publicized in the media in which an individual was mandated to be quarantined due to a communicable disease. Identify how the case became public and whether it could have been prevented. As a C/PHN, what measures could be taken to prevent the enforced quarantine of this person? Explain how three of the 10 essential public health services (see Box 2-2) apply to this scenario.
3. In the United States, TB cases are highest among foreign-born individuals. Review your local health department Web site and identify the measures and services provided for the at-risk population. Create a diagram of the service(s) and how they address complacency, confidence, and convenience. What would you do differently, and why would that change be significant to the screening and treatment of latent TB?
4. Identify a WHO or CDC vaccination campaign/program and characterize the target audience. How can the nursing process can be used to plan, execute, and evaluate the success of the campaign/program?
5. How could social media be used by C/PHN in the prevention of vaccine preventable diseases? Provide two examples. What are the advantages and disadvantages of using social media for disease prevention?

REFERENCES

Alkhouri, N., Lawitz, E., & Poordad, F. (2017). Novel treatments for chronic hepatitis C: Closing the remaining gaps. *Current Opinion Pharmacology*, 6(37), 107–111. Retrieved from https://www.sciencedirect.com/science/article/pii/S0163725817302462

American Academy of Pediatrics. (2019). *Immunizations: Vaccine hesitant parents*. Retrieved from https://www.aap.org/en-us/advocacy-and-policy/aap-health-initiatives/immunizations/Pages/vaccine-hesitant-parents.aspx

Andrade, E. L., Evans, W. D., Barrett, N., Edberg, M. C., & Cleary, S. D. (2018). Strategies to increase Latino immigrant youth engagement in health promotion using social media: Mixed-methods study. *JMIR Public Health Surveillance, 4*(4), e71. doi: 10.2196/publichealth.9332.

Attwell, K., Meyer, S. B., & Ward, P. R. (2018). The social basis of vaccine questioning and refusal: A qualitative study employing Bourdieu's Concepts of "Capitals" and "Habitus". *International Journal of Environmental Research and Public Health, 15*(5). doi: 10.3390/ijerph15051044.

Boyce, M. R., Katz, R., & Standley, C. J. (2019). Risk factors for infectious diseases in urban environments of Sub-Saharan Africa: A systematic review and critical appraisal of evidence. *Tropical Medicine and Infectious Disease, 4*(4), 123.

Bragazzi, N. L., Gianfredi, V., Villarini, M., Rosselli, R., Nasr, A., Hussein, A., … Behzadifar, M. (2018). Vaccines meet big data: State-of-the-Art and future prospects. From the classical 3Is ("Isolate-Inactivate-Inject") vaccinology 1.0 to vaccinology 3.0, vaccinomics, and beyond: A historical overview. *Frontiers in Public Health*, 6, 62. doi: 10.3389/fpubh.2018.00062.

Bristol S., Kostelec T., & MacDonald, R. (2018). Improving emergency health care workers' knowledge, competency, and attitudes toward lesbian, gay bisexual, and transgender patients through interdisciplinary cultural competency training. *Journal of Emergency Nursing, 44*(6), 632–639. doi: 10.1016/j.jen.2018.03.013.

California Department of Public Health (CDPH). (2019). *Information for physicians regarding directly observed therapy (DOT) for active tuberculosis (TB)*. Retrieved from https://www.cdph.ca.gov/programs/tb/Documents/TBCB-PMD-DOT.pdf

California Department of Public Health (CDPH). (2020). *Health officer resources*. Retrieved from https://www.cdph.ca.gov/Programs/CCLHO/Pages/HealthOfficerResources.aspx

California Department of Public Health. (2020). *Measles: Outbreaks*. Retrieved from https://www.cdph.ca.gov/Programs/CID/DCDC/Pages/Immunization/measles.aspx

Cameron, R. L., Kavanagh, K., Pan, J., Love, J., Cuschieri, K., Robertson, C., … Pollock, K. (2016). Human Papillomavirus prevalence and herd Immunity after introduction of vaccination program, Scotland, 2009–2013. *Emerging Infectious Diseases, 22*(1), 56–64. doi: 10.3201/eid2201.150736.

Centers for Disease Control and Prevention. (n.d.). *TB 101 for health care workers: Lesson 6 treatment of TB disease*. Retrieved from https://www.cdc.gov/tb/webcourses/tb101/page3802.html

Centers for Disease Control and Prevention (CDC). (2012). *Lesson 1: Introduction to Epidemiology: Section 10: Chain of Infection*. Retrieved from https://www.cdc.gov/csels/dsepd/ss1978/lesson1/section10.html

Centers for Disease Control and Prevention (CDC). (2013). Ten great public health achievements, 1990–1999: Control of infectious diseases. *Morbidity and Mortality Weekly Report, 48*(29), 621–629.

Centers for Disease Control and Prevention (CDC). (2014). *Latent tuberculosis infection: A guide for primary health care providers*. Retrieved from https://www.cdc.gov/tb/publications/ltbi/diagnosis.htm#TST

Centers for Disease Control and Prevention (CDC). (2015a). *Epidemiology and prevention of vaccine preventable diseases: The Pink Book* (13th ed.). Washington, DC: Public Health Foundation.

Centers for Disease Control and Prevention (CDC). (2015b). *Genital HSV infections*. Retrieved from https://www.cdc.gov/std/tg2015/herpes.htm

Centers for Disease Control and Prevention (CDC). (2015c). *Human Papillomavirus (HPV) infection*. Retrieved from https://www.cdc.gov/std/tg2015/hpv.htm

Centers for Disease Control and Prevention (CDC). (2015d). *2015 Sexually transmitted diseases treatment guidelines: Clinical treatment guidance*. Retrieved from http://www.cdc.gov/std/tg2015/clinical.htm#partner

Centers for Disease Control and Prevention (CDC). (2015e). *2015 Sexually transmitted diseases treatment guidelines: Gonococcal infections*. Retrieved from http://www.cdc.gov/std/tg2015/gonorrhea.htm

Centers for Disease Control and Prevention (CDC). (2016a). *Fact sheets: A new tool to diagnose tuberculosis: The Xpert MT/RIF assay*. Retrieved from https://www.cdc.gov/tb/publications/factsheets/testing/xpert_mtb-rif.htm

Centers for Disease Control and Prevention (CDC). (2016b). *Fact sheets: Interferon-Gamma Release Assays (IGRAs)—blood tests for TB infection*. Retrieved from https://www.cdc.gov/tb/publications/factsheets/testing/igra.htm

Centers for Disease Control and Prevention (CDC). (2016c). *Fact sheets: Tuberculin skin testing*. Retrieved from https://www.cdc.gov/tb/publications/factsheets/testing/skintesting.htm

Centers for Disease Control and Prevention (CDC). (2016d). *Foodborne outbreaks: Investigating outbreaks*. Retrieved from https://www.cdc.gov/foodsafety/outbreaks/investigating-outbreaks/index.html

Centers for Disease Control and Prevention (CDC). (2016e). *Gay and bisexual men's health: Sexually transmitted diseases*. Retrieved from https://www.cdc.gov/msmhealth/STD.htm

Centers for Disease Control and Prevention (CDC). (2016f). *Lesson 6: Investigating an outbreak*. Retrieved from https://www.cdc.gov/csels/dsepd/ss1978/lesson6/section2.html

Centers for Disease Control and Prevention (CDC). (2016g). *Smallpox: Evaluating patients for smallpox. Acute, generalized vesicular or pustular rash illness protocol*. Retrieved from https://www.cdc.gov/smallpox/clinicians/algorithm-protocol.html

Centers for Disease Control and Prevention (CDC). (2016h). *TB guidelines: Infection control and health care personnel*. Retrieved from https://www.cdc.gov/tb/publications/guidelines/infectioncontrol.htm

Centers for Disease Control and Prevention (CDC). (2016i). *Twenty years of PulseNet*. Retrieved from https://www.cdc.gov/pulsenet/anniversary/index.html

Centers for Disease Control and Prevention (CDC). (2017a). *Genital Herpes-CDC fact sheet (Detailed)*. Retrieved from https://www.cdc.gov/std/herpes/stdfact-herpes-detailed.htm

Centers for Disease Control and Prevention (CDC). (2017b). *Implementing an electronic direct observed therapy (dDot) program: A toolkit for tuberculosis (TB) Programs*. Retrieved from https://www.cdc.gov/tb/publications/guidestoolkits/tbedottoolkit.htm

Centers for Disease Control and Prevention (CDC). (2017c). *Pregnancy and whooping cough*. Retrieved from https://www.cdc.gov/pertussis/pregnant/mom/get-vaccinated.html

Centers for Disease Control and Prevention (CDC). (2017d). *Quarantine stations*. Retrieved from https://www.cdc.gov/quarantine/quarantinestations.html

Centers for Disease Control and Prevention (CDC). (2017e). *Side effects of Smallpox vaccination*. Retrieved from https://www.cdc.gov/smallpox/vaccine-basics/vaccination-effects.html

Centers for Disease Control and Prevention (CDC). (2017f). Surround babies with protection (whooping cough). Retrieved from https://www.cdc.gov/pertussis/pregnant/mom/protection.html

Centers for Disease Control and Prevention (CDC). (2017g). *Syphilis-CDC fact sheet*. Retrieved from https://www.cdc.gov/std/syphilis/stdfact-syphilis.htm

Centers for Disease Control and Prevention (CDC). (2017h). *Yellow book: Homepage*. Retrieved from https://wwwnc.cdc.gov/travel/yellowbook/2018/introduction/introduction-to-travel-health-the-yellow-book#4924

Centers for Disease Control and Prevention (CDC). (2017i). *Yellow book: Newly arrived immigrants & refugees*. Retrieved from https://wwwnc.cdc.gov/travel/yellowbook/2020/posttravel-evaluation/newly-arrived-immigrants-and-refugees

Centers for Disease Control and Prevention (CDC). (2018a). *National Center for Emerging and Zoonotic Infectious Diseases*. Retrieved from https://www.cdc.gov/ncezid/dvbd/index.html

Centers for Disease Control and Prevention (CDC). (2018b). *National Notifiable Diseases Surveillance System (NNDSS)*. Retrieved from https://wwwn.cdc.gov/nndss/

Centers for Disease Control and Prevention (CDC). (2018c). *National, regional, state, and selected local area vaccination coverage among adolescents aged 13–17 years-United States, 2017*. Retrieved from https://www.cdc.gov/mmwr/volumes/67/wr/mm6733a1.htm

Centers for Disease Control and Prevention (CDC). (2018d). *Past pandemics*. Retrieved from https://www.cdc.gov/flu/pandemic-resources/basics/past-pandemics.html

Centers for Disease Control and Prevention (CDC). (2018e). *People at high risk of developing serious flu-related complications*. Retrieved from https://www.cdc.gov/flu/about/disease/high_risk.htm

Centers for Disease Control and Prevention (CDC). (2018f). *People 65 years and older & influenza*. Retrieved from https://www.cdc.gov/flu/about/disease/65over.htm

Centers for Disease Control and Prevention (CDC). (2018g). *Rabies*. Retrieved from https://www.cdc.gov/rabies/index.html

Centers for Disease Control and Prevention (CDC). (2018h). *Talking with parents about vaccines for infants*. Retrieved from https://www.cdc.gov/vaccines/hcp/conversations/talking-with-parents.html

Centers for Disease Control and Prevention (CDC). (2018i). *Tuberculosis (TB)*. Retrieved from https://www.cdc.gov/tb/default.htm

Centers for Disease Control and Prevention (CDC). (May 2018j). *VitalSigns: Illnesses on the rise from mosquito, tick, and flea bites*. Retrieved from https://www.cdc.gov/vitalsigns/pdf/vs-0518-vector-borne-H.pdf

Centers for Disease Control and Prevention (CDC). (2019a). *Asking the right questions quickly from the beginning*. Retrieved from http://www.cdc.gov/foodcore/successes/questions-from-beginning.html

Centers for Disease Control and Prevention (CDC). (2019b). *Chlamydia*. Retrieved from https://www.cdc.gov/std/stats18/chlamydia.htm

Centers for Disease Control and Prevention (CDC). (2019c). *Genital HPV infection—Fact sheet*. Retrieved from https://www.cdc.gov/std/hpv/stdfact-hpv.htm

Centers for Disease Control and Prevention (CDC). (2019d). *Gonorrhea-CDC fact sheet (Detailed)*. Retrieved from https://www.cdc.gov/std/gonorrhea/stdfact-gonorrhea-detailed.htm

Centers for Disease Control and Prevention (CDC). (2019e). *HIV basics*. Retrieved from https://www.cdc.gov/hiv/basics/

Centers for Disease Control and Prevention (CDC). (2019f). *HIV: Prevention*. Retrieved from https://www.cdc.gov/hiv/basics/prevention.html

Centers for Disease Control and Prevention (CDC). (2019g). *HPV cancers are preventable*. Retrieved from https://www.cdc.gov/hpv/hcp/protecting-patients.html

Centers for Disease Control and Prevention (CDC). (2019h). *Mission, role and pledge*. Retrieved from http://www.cdc.gov/about/organization/mission.htm

Centers for Disease Control and Prevention (CDC). (2019i). *Outbreak of Cyclospora infections linked to fresh basil from Siga Logisticsde de RL de CV of Morelos, Mexico*. Retrieved from https://www.cdc.gov/parasites/cyclosporiasis/outbreaks/2019/weekly/index.html

Centers for Disease Control and Prevention (CDC). (2019j). *Pandemic influenza*. Retrieved from https://www.cdc.gov/flu/pandemic-resources/

Centers for Disease Control and Prevention (CDC). (2019k). *Plague*. Retrieved from https://www.cdc.gov/plague/index.html?CDC_AA_refVal=https%3A%2F%2Fwww.cdc.gov%2Fplague%2Fhistory%2Findex.html

Centers for Disease Control and Prevention (CDC). (2019l). *Plague: Ecology and transmission*. Retrieved from https://www.cdc.gov/plague/transmission/index.html

Centers for Disease Control and Prevention (CDC). (2019m). *STD Surveillance 2018*. Retrieved from https://www.cdc.gov/std/stats18/default.htm

Centers for Disease Control and Prevention (CDC). (2019n). *Trends in tuberculosis, 2018*. Retrieved from https://www.cdc.gov/tb/publications/factsheets/statistics/tbtrends.htm

Centers for Disease Control and Prevention (CDC). (2019o). *Types of influenza viruses*. Retrieved from https://www.cdc.gov/flu/about/viruses/types.htm

Centers for Disease Control and Prevention (CDC). (2019p). *Years of Ebola virus disease outbreaks: 40 years of Ebola virus disease around the world*. Retrieved from https://www.cdc.gov/vhf/ebola/history/chronology.html

Centers for Disease Control and Prevention (CDC). (2020a). *About the Division of Vector-Borne Diseases*. Retrieved from https://www.cdc.gov/ncezid/dvbd/index.html

Centers for Disease Control and Prevention (CDC). (2020b). *Advisory Committee on Immunization Practices (ACIP)*. Retrieved from https://www.cdc.gov/vaccines/acip/index.html

Centers for Disease Control and Prevention (CDC). (2020c). *Foodborne germs and illnesses*. Retrieved from https://www.cdc.gov/foodsafety/foodborne-germs.html

Centers for Disease Control and Prevention (CDC). (2020d). *Global health: CDC and the Global Health Security Agenda*. Retrieved from https://www.cdc.gov/globalhealth/security/index.htm

Centers for Disease Control and Prevention (CDC). (2020e). *Health communication basics*. Retrieved from https://www.cdc.gov/healthcommunication/healthbasics/WhatIsHC.html

Centers for Disease Control and Prevention (CDC). (2020f). *Hepatitis B: For health professionals*. Retrieved from https://www.cdc.gov/hepatitis/hbv/index.htm

Centers for Disease Control and Prevention (CDC). (2020g). *Hepatitis C professional resource*. Retrieved from https://www.cdc.gov/knowmorehepatitis/HepCProfResources.htm

Centers for Disease Control and Prevention (CDC). (2020h). *Hepatitis C questions and answers*. Retrieved from https://www.cdc.gov/knowmorehepatitis/HepatitisC-FAQ.htm

Centers for Disease Control and Prevention (CDC). (April 2020i). *Latent TB infection testing and treatment: Summary of U.S. recommendations*. Retrieved from https://www.cdc.gov/tb/publications/ltbi/pdf/CDC-USP-STF-LTBI-Testing-Treatment-Recommendations-508.pdf

Centers for Disease Control and Prevention (CDC). (2020j). *Nationally notifiable infectious conditions, United States 2020*. Retrieved from http://wwwn.cdc.gov/nndss/conditions/notifiable/2020/

Centers for Disease Control and Prevention (CDC). (2020k). *STD health equity*. Retrieved from https://www.cdc.gov/std/health-disparities/default.htm

Centers for Disease Control and Prevention (CDC). (2020l). *TB and HIV coinfection*. Retrieved from https://www.cdc.gov/tb/topic/basics/tbhivcoinfection.htm

Centers for Disease Control and Prevention (CDC). (2020m). *Traveler advice*. Retrieved from https://wwwnc.cdc.gov/travel/page/traveler-information-center

Centers for Disease Control and Prevention (CDC). (2020n). *Treatment regimen for latent TB (LTBI) infection*. Retrieved from https://www.cdc.gov/tb/topic/treatment/ltbi.htm

Chen, C. (2018). Retrospective cost-effectiveness of the 23-valent pneumococcal polysaccharide vaccination program in Australia. *Vaccine, 36*(42), 6307–6313. Retrieved from https://www.clinicalkey.com/#!/content/playContent/1-s2.0-S0264410X18312349

Children's Hospital of Philadelphia. (2018). *Global immunization: Worldwide disease incidence.* Retrieved from https://www.chop.edu/centers-programs/vaccine-education-center/global-immunization/diseases-and-vaccines-world-view

County of Los Angeles Department of Public Health. (n.d.). *Communicable disease reporting system.* Retrieved from http://publichealth.lacounty.gov/acd/procs/ReportPage.htm

Di Mattia, G., Nicolai, A., Frassanito, A., Petrarca, L., Nenna, R., & Midulla, F. (2018). Pertussis: New preventive strategies for an old disease. *Paediatric Respiratory Reviews.* Retrieved from https://www.clinicalkey.com/#!/content/playContent/2-s2.0-29914744?returnurl=null&referrer=null

Domachowske, J. B., & Suryadevara, M. (2013). Practical approaches to vaccine hesitancy issues in the United States: 2013. *Human Vaccines & Immunotherapeutics, 9*(12), 2654–2657.

Donovan, H., & Bedford, H. (2013). Talking with parents about immunization. *Primary Health Care, 23*(4), 16–20.

Emrick, P. Gentry, C., & Morowit, L. (2016). Ebola virus disease: International perspective on enhanced health surveillance, disposition of the dead, and their effect on isolation and quarantine practices. *Disaster and Military Medicine, 2,* 13. doi: 10.1186/s40696-016-0023-6.

Fernandes, E. G., Rodrigues, C. C., Sartori, A. M., De Soárez, P. C., & Novaes, H. M. (2018). Economic evaluation of adolescents and adults' pertussis vaccination: A systematic review of current strategies. *Human Vaccines & Immunotherapeutics, 15*(35). doi: 10.1080/21645515.2018.1509646.

Frith, J. (2012). The history of plague—part 1. The three great pandemics. *Journal of Military and Veterans' Health, 20*(2), 11–16. Retrieved from https://jmvh.org/article/the-history-of-plague-part-1-the-three-great-pandemics/

Gagneur, A., Gosselin, V., & Dube, E. (2018). Motivational interviewing: a promising tool to address vaccine hesitancy. *Vaccine, 36,* 6553–6555. doi: 10.1016/j.vaccine.2017.10.049.

Garfein, R. S., Liu, L., Cuevas-Mota, J., Collins, K., Muñoz, F., Catanzaro, D. G., ... Raab, F. (2018). Tuberculosis treatment monitoring by video directly observed therapy in 5 health districts, California, USA. *Emerging Infectious Diseases, 24*(10), 1806–1815. doi: 10.3201/eid2410.180459.

Global Health Security Agenda. (February 2018). *Implementing the Global Health Security agenda: Progress and impact from U.S. Government investments.* Retrieved from https://www.cdc.gov/globalhealth/healthprotection/resources/pdf/GHSA-Report-_Feb-2018.pdf

Gould, D. J., King, M., Wigglesworth, N., & Purssell, E. (2018). Isolating infectious patients: Organizational, clinical, and ethical issues. *American Journal of Infection Control, 46*(8), e65–e69. Retrieved from https://core.ac.uk/reader/159067143

Hamborsky, J., Kroger, A., & Wolfe, C. (Eds.). (2015). *Epidemiology and prevention of vaccine-preventable diseases* (13th ed.). Washington, DC: Public Health Foundation. Retrieved from http://www.cdc.gov/vaccines/pubs/pinkbook/index.html

Hassan, A. (October 24, 2019). Disneyland visitor with measles may have exposed hundreds to infection. *New York Times.* Retrieved from https://www.nytimes.com/2019/10/23/us/disneyland-measles.html

Healthcare Environmental Resource Center. (2015). *OSHA standards for bloodborne pathogens.* Retrieved from http://www.hercenter.org/rmw/osha-bps.php

Healthline. (2020). *A full list of hepatitis C medications: Epclusa, Harvoni, Zepatier, and more.* Retrieved from https://www.healthline.com/health/hepatitis-c/full-medication-list

Heymann, D. L. (Ed.). (2015). *Control of communicable diseases manual* (20th ed.). Washington, DC: American Public Health Association.

Heymann, D. L. (2017). Public health surveillance for communicable diseases: From rigid and static to flexible and innovative. *American Journal of Public Health, 107*(6), 845–846.

Hinman, A. R., Orenstein, W. A., & Schuchat, A. (2011). Vaccine-preventable diseases, immunizations, and MMWR—1961–2011. *Morbidity and Mortality Weekly Report, 60*(4), 49–57.

Hussain, A., Ali, S., Ahmed, M., & Hussain, S. (2018). The anti-vaccination movement: A regression in modern medicine. *Cureus, 10*(7), e2919. doi: 10.7759/cureus.2919.

Immunization Action Coalition. (2020). *State laws and mandates by vaccine.* Retrieved from http://www.immunize.org/laws/

Johns Hopkins University of Medicine. (2020). *Coronavirus resource center.* Retrieved from https://coronavirus.jhu.edu

Jones, D. S. (March 12, 2020). History in a crisis: Lessons for COVID-19. *New England Journal of Medicine, 382*(18), 1681–1683. Retrieved from https://www.nejm.org/doi/pdf/10.1056/NEJMp2004361?articleTools=true

Kaufman, J., Synnot, A., Ryan, R., Hill, S., Horey, D., Willis, N., & Robinson, P. (2013). Face to face interventions for informing or educating parents about early childhood vaccines. *Cochrane Database of Systematic Reviews, 5,* CD010038. doi: 10.1002/14651858.CD010038.pub2.

Kumar, D., Chandra, R., Mathur, M., Samdariya, S., & Kapoor, N. (2016). Vaccine hesitancy: understanding better to address better. *Israel Journal of Health Policy Research, 5,* 2. doi: 10.1186/s13584-016-0062-y.

Lewinsohn, D., Loeffler, A., Mazurek, G., O'Brien, R., Pai, M., Richeldi, L., ... Woods, G. (2017). Official American Thoracic Society/Infectious Diseases Society of America/Centers for Disease Control and Prevention Clinical Practice Guidelines: Diagnosis of tuberculosis in adults and children. *Clinical Infectious Diseases, 64,* e1–e33. Retrieved from https://www.thoracic.org/statements/resources/tb-opi/diagnosis-of-tuberculosis-in-adults-and-children.PDF

MacDonald, N. (2015). Anti-vaccine movement: Strategies to address vaccine hesitancy presentation. *Canadian Centre for Vaccinology.* Retrieved from https://www.ammi.ca/Annual-Conference/2015/Presentations/2015-04-18.START%20-%20Noni%20MacDonald.pdf

Martin, B. (2018). Evidence-based campaigning. *Archives of Public Health, 76*(54). doi: 10.1186/s13690-018-0302-4.

Mayo Clinic. (2020). *Hepatitis A.* Retrieved from https://www.mayoclinic.org/diseases-conditions/hepatitis-a/symptoms-causes/syc-20367007

MedlinePlus. (2020). *Pneumonia.* Retrieved from https://medlineplus.gov/pneumonia.html

Merrill, R. M. (2017). *Introduction to epidemiology* (7th ed.). Burlington, MA: Jones & Bartlett Learning.

Meites, E., Kempe, A., & Markowitz, L. E. (2016). Use of a 2-dose schedule for Human papillomavirus vaccination-updated recommendations of the Advisory Committee on Immunization Practices. *Morbidity and Mortality Weekly Report, 65*(49), 1405–1408. Retrieved from https://www.cdc.gov/mmwr/volumes/65/wr/mm6549a5.htm

Mervosh, S., Lu, D., & Swales, V. (April 20, 2020). See which states and cities have told residents to stay at home. *New York Times.* Retrieved from https://www.nytimes.com/interactive/2020/us/coronavirus-stay-at-home-order.html

Millard, T., Dodson, S., McDonald, K., Klassen, K. M., Osborne, R. H., Battersby, M. W., ... Elliott, J. H. (2018). The systematic development of a complex intervention: HealthMap, an online self-management support program for people with HIV. *BMC Infectious Disease, 18*(1), 615. doi: 10.1186/s12879-018-3518-6.

Mitra, T., Counts, S., & Pennebaker, J. (2016). *Understanding anti-vaccination attitudes in social media.* International AAAI Conference on Web and Social Media, North America. Retrieved from https://www.aaai.org/ocs/index.php/ICWSM/ICWSM16/paper/view/13073/12747

Moreno-Madriñán, M. J., & Turell, M. (2018). History of mosquito borne diseases in the United States and implications for new pathogens. *Emerging Infectious Diseases, 24*(5), 821–826. doi: 10.3201/eid2405.171609.

National Institutes of Health (NIH). (2016). *Story of discovery: Hepatitis C from non-A, non-B hepatitis to a cure.* Retrieved from https://www.niddk.nih.gov/news/archive/2016/story-discovery-hepatitis-c-from-non-a-non-b-hepatitis-cure

National Institutes of Health (NIH). (2017). *Hepatitis B.* Retrieved from https://www.niddk.nih.gov/health-information/liver-disease/viral-hepatitis/hepatitis-b#diagnose

National Institutes of Health (NIH). (2019). *Hepatitis A.* Retrieved from https://www.niddk.nih.gov/health-information/liver-disease/viral-hepatitis/hepatitis-a

Night, S. S. (2007). Public health emergencies and HIPAA: When is the disclosure of individual health information lawful? *Houston Journal of Health Law & Policy.* Retrieved from https://www.law.uh.edu/healthlaw/perspectives/2007/(SN)SpeakerHIPAA.pdf

National Cancer Institute (NCI). (2019). *Human papillomavirus (HPV) vaccines.* Retrieved from https://www.cancer.gov/about-cancer/causes-prevention/risk/infectious-agents/hpv-vaccine-fact-sheet

National Conference of State Legislatures (NCSL). (2019). *States with religious and philosophical exemptions from school immunization requirements.* Retrieved from http://www.ncsl.org/research/health/school-immunization-exemption-state-laws.aspx

New York City Department of Health & the NYC STD Prevention Training Center. (March 2019). *The diagnosis, management, and prevention of syphilis: An update and review.* Retrieved from https://www.nycptc.org/x/Syphilis_Monograph_2019_NYC_PTC_NYC_DOHMH.pdf

NPR. (2011). *Timeline: How the anthrax terror unfolded.* Retrieved from https://www.npr.org/2011/02/15/93170200/timeline-how-the-anthrax-terror-unfolded

Occupational Safety & Health Administration (OSHA). (n.d.). *Workers protections against occupational exposure to infectious diseases.* Retrieved from https://www.osha.gov/SLTC/bloodbornepathogens/worker_protections.html

Occupational Safety & Health Administration (OSHA). (2011). OSHA's bloodborne pathogens standard. *OSHA FactSheet.* Retrieved from https://www.osha.gov/OshDoc/data_BloodborneFacts/bbfact01.pdf

Office of Disease Prevention and Health Promotion. (2018). *Proposed objectives for inclusion in Healthy People 2030.* Retrieved from https://www.healthypeople.gov/sites/default/files/ObjectivesPublicComment508_1.17.19.pdf

Office of Disease Prevention and Health Promotion. (2020). *Healthy People 2030 framework.* Retrieved from https://www.healthypeople.gov/2020/About-Healthy-People/Development-Healthy-People-2030/Framework

Offord, C. (February 21, 2020). How COVID-19 is spread. *The Scientist.* Retrieved from https://www.the-scientist.com/news-opinion/how-covid-19-is-spread-67143

Opel, D., Chuan, Z., Robinson, J. D., Henrikson, N., Lepere, K., Mangione-Smith, R., & Taylor, J. (2018). Impact of childhood vaccine discussion format over time on immunization status. *Academic Pediatrics, 18*(4), 430–436. doi: 10.1016/j.acap.2017.12.009.

Ornstein, W. A., & Ahmed, R. (2017). Simply put: Vaccinations save lives. *Proceedings of the National Academy of Sciences, 114*(16), 4031–4033.

Otmani del Barrio, M., Simard, F., & Caprara, A. (2018). Supporting and strengthening research on urban health interventions for the prevention and control of vector-borne and other infectious diseases of poverty: Scoping reviews and research gap analysis. *Infectious Diseases of Poverty, 7*, 94. doi: 10.1186/s40249-018-0462-z.

Parmer, J., Allen, L., & Walton, W. (2017). CE: Tuberculosis A new screening recommendation and on expanded approach to elimination in the United States. *American Journal of Nursing, 177*(8), 24–34. doi: 10.1097/01.NAJ.0000521946.45448.90.

Patel, M., Lee, A. D., Clemmons, N. S., Redd, S. B., Poser, S., Blog, D., ... Gastanaduy, P. A. (October 11, 2019). National update on measles cases and outbreaks—United States, January 1-October 1, 2019. *Morbidity and Mortality Weekly Report (MMWR), 68*(40), 893–896. Retrieved from https://www.cdc.gov/mmwr/volumes/68/wr/mm6840e2.htm

Polansky, L. S., Outin-Blenman, S., & Moen, A. C. (2016). Improved global capacity for influenza surveillance. *Emerging Infectious Diseases, 22*(6), 993–1001. Retrieved from https://wwwnc.cdc.gov/eid/article/22/6/15-1521_article

Penn Wharton. (June 27, 2016). *Mortality in the United States: Past, present and future*. Retrieved from https://budgetmodel.wharton.upenn.edu/issues/2016/1/25/mortality-in-the-united-states-past-present-and-future

Porse, C., Messenger, S., Vugia, D. J., Jilek, W., Salas, M., Watt, J., ... Kramer, V. (2018). Travel-associated Zika cases and threat of local transmission during global outbreak, California, USA. *Emerging Infectious Diseases, 24*(9), 1626–1632. doi: 10.3201/eid2409.180203.

Rosner, D. (2010). Public health in the early 20th century. *Public Health Reports, 125*(Suppl 3), 37–47.

Rosselli, R., Martini, M., & Bragazzi, N. L. (2016). The old and the new: vaccine hesitancy in the era of the Web 2.0. Challenges and opportunities. *Journal of Preventive Medicine and Hygiene, 57*(1), E47–E50. Retrieved from https://www.ncbi.nlm.nih.gov/pmc/articles/PMC4910443/pdf/2421-4248-57-E47.pdf

Sampri, A., Mavragani, A., & Tsagarakis, K. P. (2016). Evaluating Google Trends as a tool for integrating the 'Smart Health' concept in the Smart Cities' governance in USA. *Procedia Engineering, 162*, 585–592.

Schmidt, A. L., Zollo, F., Scala, A., Betsch, C., & Quattrociocchi, W. (2018). Polarization of the vaccination debate on Facebook. *Vaccine, 36*(25), 3606–3612.

The College of Physicians of Philadelphia. (2019). *Typhoid Mary. The history of vaccines*. Retrieved from https://www.historyofvaccines.org/content/typhoid-mary

Thèves, C., Biagini, P., & Crubezy, E. (2014). The rediscovery of smallpox. *Clinical Microbiology and Infection, 20*(3), 210–218. doi: 10.1111/1469.12536.

Trevethan, R. (2017). Sensitivity, specificity, and predictive values: Foundations, pliabilities and pitfalls in research and practice. *Frontiers in Public Health, 5*, 307. Retrieved from https://www.ncbi.nlm.nih.gov/pmc/articles/PMC5701930/pdf/fpubh-05-00307.pdf

Tustin, J. L., Crowcroft, N. S., Gesink, D., Johnson, I., Keelan, J., & Lachapelle, B. (2018). User-driven comments on a Facebook advertisement recruiting Canadian parents in a study on immunization: Content analysis. *JMIR Public Health Surveillance, 4*(3), e10090. doi: 10.2196/10090.

U.S. Department of Agriculture. (2015). *Kitchen companion: Your food safe handbook*. Retrieved from https://www.fsis.usda.gov/wps/wcm/connect/6c55c954-20a8-46fd-b617-ecffb4449062/Kitchen_Companion_Single.pdf?MOD=AJPERES

U.S. Department of Health and Human Services (USDHHS). (2015). *The HIPAA privacy rule*. Retrieved from https://www.hhs.gov/hipaa/for-professionals/privacy/index.html

U.S. Department of Health and Human Services (USDHHS). (2019). *Guidelines for the prevention and treatment of opportunistic infections in adults and adolescents with HIV*. Retrieved from https://aidsinfo.nih.gov/guidelines/html/4/adult-and-adolescent-oi-prevention-and-treatment-guidelines/325/tb

U.S. Department of Health and Human Services (USDHHS). (2020). *U.S. national vaccine plan*. Retrieved from https://www.hhs.gov/vaccines/national-vaccine-plan/index.html

U.S. Equal Employment Opportunity Commission. (2017). *Questions and answers about the association provision of the Americans with Disabilities Act*. Retrieved from http://www.eeoc.gov/facts/association_ada.html

U. S. Food & Drug Administration (FDA). (2018). *FDA approves expanded us of Gardasil 9 to include individuals 27 through 45 years old*. Retrieved from https://www.fda.gov/NewsEvents/Newsroom/PressAnnouncements/ucm622715.htm

U.S. Preventive Services Task Force (USPSTF). (2016). Screening for latent tuberculosis infection in adults: US Preventive Services Task Force recommendation statement. *JAMA, 316*(9), 962–969. doi: 10.1001/jama.2016.110.

U.S. Preventive Services Task Force (USPSTF). (2018). *Final recommendation statement: Cervical cancer screening*. Retrieved from https://www.uspreventiveservicestaskforce.org/Page/Document/RecommendationStatementFinal/cervical-cancer-screening2

Vanderslott, S., Dadonaite, B., & Roser, M. (December 2019). Vaccination. *Our World in Data*. Retrieved from https://ourworldindata.org/vaccination#progress-made-with-vaccination

Waheed, Y., Siddiq, M., Jamil, Z., & Najmi, M. H. (2018). Hepatitis elimination by 2030: Progress and challenges. *World Journal of Gastroenterology, 24*(44), 4959–4961. Retrieved from https://www.ncbi.nlm.nih.gov/pmc/articles/PMC6262254/

Williams, W. W., Lu, P. J., O'Halloran, A., Kim, D. K., Grohskopf, L. A., Pilishvili, T., ... Fiebelkorn, A. P. (2017). Surveillance of vaccination coverage among adult populations—United States, 2015. *MMWR Surveillance Summaries, 66*(11), 1–28. doi: 10.15585/mmwr.ss6611a1.

World Health Organization (WHO). (n.d.). *Global influenza surveillance and response system (GISRS)*. Retrieved from https://www.who.int/influenza/gisrs_laboratory/updates/GISRS_one_pager_2018_EN.pdf?ua=1

World Health Organization (WHO). (2014a). *Biologicals: Smallpox*. Retrieved http://www.who.int/biologicals/vaccines/smallpox/en/

World Health Organization (WHO). (2014b). *Report of the Sage Working Group on vaccine hesitancy*. Retrieved from http://www.who.int/immunization/sage/meetings/2014/october/1_Report_WORKING_GROUP_vaccine_hesitancy_final.pdf

World Health Organization (WHO). (2016a). *An R&D blueprint for action to prevent epidemics*. Retrieved from https://www.who.int/blueprint/about/r_d_blueprint_plan_of_action.pdf?ua=1

World Health Organization (WHO). (2016b). *Guidance for managing ethical issues in infectious disease outbreaks*. Retrieved from https://apps.who.int/iris/bitstream/handle/10665/250580/9789241549837-eng.pdf;jsessionid=417EFBAF79C31B363FB87714A933A35B?sequence=1

World Health Organization (WHO). (2018a). *2018 Annual review of diseases prioritized under the research and development blueprint*. Retrieved from http://www.who.int/emergencies/diseases/2018prioritization-report.pdf

World Health Organization (WHO). (2018b). *Guidelines for the care and treatment of persons diagnoses with chronic hepatitis C virus infection*. Retrieved from http://apps.who.int/iris/bitstream/han dle/10665/273174/9789241550345-eng.pdf?ua=1

World Health Organization (WHO). (2018c). *Monitoring global progress on addressing antimicrobial resistance: analysis report of the second round of results of AMR country self-assessment survey 2018*. Retrieved from http://apps.who.int/iris/bitstream/handle/10665/273128/9789241514422-eng.pdf?ua=1

World Health Organization (WHO). (January 16, 2018d). *Newsroom: What is multidrug-resistant tuberculosis (MDR-TB) and how do we control it?* Retrieved from https://www.who.int/news-room/q-a-detail/what-is-multi-drug-resistant-tuberculosis-(mdr-tb)-and-how-do-we-control-it

World Health Organization (WHO). (2019a). *Fact Sheets: Hepatitis B*. Retrieved from http://www.who.int/news-room/fact-sheets/detail/hepatitis-b

World Health Organization (WHO). (2019b). *Fact Sheets: Hepatitis C*. Retrieved from http://www.who.int/news-room/fact-sheets/detail/hepatitis-c

World Health Organization (WHO). (2019c). *Fact Sheets: HIV/AIDS*. Retrieved from http://www.who.int/en/news-room/fact-sheets/detail/hiv-aids

World Health Organization (WHO). (2019d). *Global tuberculosis report 2019*. Retrieved from https://apps.who.int/iris/bitstream/han dle/10665/329368/9789241565714-eng.pdf?ua=1

World Health Organization (WHO). (2020a). *About WHO: What we do*. Retrieved from http://www.who.int/about/what-we-do/en/

World Health Organization (WHO). (February 29, 2020b). *Coronavirus disease 2019 (COVID-19): Situation report 40*. Retrieved from https://www.who.int/docs/default-source/coronaviruse/situation-reports/20200229-sitrep-40-covid-19.pdf?sfvrsn=849d0665_2

World Health Organization (WHO). (2020c). *Fact Sheet: Tuberculosis*. Retrieved from http://www.who.int/en/news-room/fact-sheets/detail/tuberculosis

World Health Organization (WHO). (2020d). *FluNet*. Retrieved from www.who.int/influenza/gisrs_laboratory/flunet/en/

World Health Organization (WHO). (2020e). *History of WHO*. Retrieved from http://www.who.int/about/history/en/

World Health Organization (WHO). (2020f). *Immunization*. Retrieved from http://www.who.int/topics/immunization/en/

World Health Organization (WHO). (2020g). *Ten threats to global health in 2019*. Retrieved from stories/ten-threats-to-global-health-in-2019

World Health Organization (WHO). (2020h). *The top 10 causes of death*. Retrieved from http://www.who.int/news-room/fact-sheets/detail/the-top-10-causes-of-death

Worldometer. (June 24, 2020). *COVID-19 coronavirus pandemic: Reported cases and deaths*. Retrieved from https://www.worldometers.info/coronavirus/

Zhang, H., Ehiri, J., Yang, H., Tang, S., & Li, Y. (2016). Impact of community-based DOT on Tuberculosis treatment outcomes: A systematic review and meta-analysis. *PLoS One, 11*(2), e0147744. Retrieved from https://www.ncbi.nlm.nih.gov/pmc/articles/PMC4744041/

CHAPTER 9

Environmental Health and Safety

"When we try to pick out anything by itself, we find it hitched to everything else in the Universe."

—John Muir (1838–1914), Naturalist

KEY TERMS

Bioaccumulation
Biomonitoring
Brownfields
Built environment
Climate change
Ecosystems
Endocrine-disrupting chemicals
Environmental epidemiology
Environmental justice
Epigenetics
Exposure pathways
Health risk assessment
Integrated pest management (IPM)
One Health
Planetary health
Precautionary principle
Risk management
Social determinants of health
Superfund
Sustainability
Sustainable Development Goals (SDGs)
Toxicology

LEARNING OBJECTIVES

Upon mastery of this chapter, you should be able to:

1. **Apply the ecological perspective to human and environmental relationships.**
2. **Discuss concepts of prevention and upstream approaches to health impact and environmental health.**
3. **Discuss the community/public health nurse's role in reducing and managing environmental risk.**
4. **Discuss guiding documents for public health nursing that pertain to environmental health.**
5. **Discuss how the core functions of public health can be applied to environmental health.**
6. **Describe how nurses can collaborate with other professionals, government agencies, and communities to reduce environmental threats to health.**

INTRODUCTION

Recent events such as lead contamination in the drinking water in Flint, Michigan; growing piles of plastics in our oceans; wildfires in the western United States and in northern Europe; and hurricanes and severe flooding in the southeast United States remind us of the impact of the built and natural environments on the health of local and global communities, as well as the impact on patients in our care in clinics and hospitals.

The effect on health of environmental factors has been noted in nursing and by national and international agencies. In nursing, the concern for the environment dates back to Florence Nightingale (1960/1969), who reminds us that health depends on clean air, clean water, safe food, control of noise, and exposure to light. More recently, the World Health Organization defined health as "a complete state of physical, mental, and social wellbeing" and environment, as it relates to health, as "all the physical, chemical, and biological factors external to a person, and all the related factors impacting behaviors" (WHO, 2020b, para. 1). In its definition, the WHO was careful to identify environmental factors that could be modified.

The ability to live in a healthy environment increases not only the number of years of a healthy life but also one's quality of life. Thus, nurses, as the largest group of health care professionals globally, can play a key role in supporting environments that sustain health.

In 2015, the United Nations implemented a new set of global goals called the **Sustainable Development Goals (SDGs)**. The SDGs identify the need to care for the natural and built environments that support the health of our planet and its inhabitants (UN, 2020). See Chapter 16 on global health for more on SDGs.

Increasingly, a number of environmental factors have been recognized as detrimental to health, including:

- Exposures to hazardous materials in air, water, food, and soil
- The rise in development and deforestation
- The use of synthetic chemicals not well tested for safety

- The adverse effects of natural and human-caused disasters, the built environment, and climate change

The framework for the nation's health in the United States is *Healthy People 2030*. It addresses the social, economic, and physical factors, as well as behaviors, that can influence exposure to physical, chemical, and biological environmental risks (Office of Disease Prevention and Health Promotion, 2019). Our national framework for health is therefore in line with global goals and the WHO definition of health.

ENVIRONMENTAL HEALTH AND NURSING

Historically, public health and occupational health nurses (OHNs) have been leaders in addressing the impact of the physical and natural environments through their work in homes, in communities, and with governmental organizations. As evidence of environmental impact on our health continues to grow, it is important for nurses in all practice settings to be knowledgeable of environmental risks, the relationship of exposures to disease and illness, prevention measures, and growing scientific evidence to best protect and promote the health of the populations in the nurse's care. Professionally, nurses must be aware of the guiding documents that call for nurses to incorporate environmental health into all areas of practice.

The documents are:

- Public health nursing: *Environmental Principles for Public Health Nursing* in 2005
- The American Nurses Association (ANA): *ANA's Principles of Environmental Health for Nursing Practice and Implementation Strategies* in 2007 (http://ojin.nursingworld.org/MainMenuCategories/WorkplaceSafety/Healthy-Nurse/ANAsPrinciplesofEnvironmentalHealthforNursingPractice.pd)
- The ANA: *Nursing: Scope and Standards of Practice*, Standard 17 Environmental Health (American Nurses Association, 2015b; Box 9-1)

BOX 9-1 American Nurses Association, Public Health Nursing: Scope and Standards of Practice

Standard 17. Environmental Health: "The registered nurse practices in an environmentally safe and healthy manner" (p. 84).

The registered nurse:

1. In nursing practice and the workplace, fosters health and safety.
2. Incorporates concepts of environmental health in nursing practice.
3. Evaluates the health risk factors present in the environment.
4. Works to decrease environmental health risks for self, nursing counterparts, and patients.
5. Shares knowledge of environmental risk factors and strategies to reduce risk of exposure.
6. Acts as an advocate for product safety, as well as proper use and disposal.
7. Utilizes new technologies to ensure safe environments for nursing practice.
8. Applies evidence-based practice principles in the use of products or therapies to decrease environmental risks.
9. Actively works to develop interventions that promote healthier environments in workplace and community environments.

Adapted from American Nurses Association (ANA) (2015b)

Brief History of the Occupational and Environmental Health Movement in Nursing

Florence Nightingale's (1969) work in identifying the relationship between the patient environment and health highlighted the importance of incorporating environmental health into nursing practice. As a result, nurses consider the environment of the home, hospital, or community as a factor to promote and restore health.

However, the specific role of nurses in occupational and environmental health first occurred in the workplace. Initially called industrial nurses, OHNs assess workers' health status and strive to ensure worker safety and prevent adverse health effects from workplace hazards. The American Association of Occupational Health Nurses (2020) cites the need for specific education and training in toxicology, epidemiology, workplace hazards, regulations, and prevention strategies. OHNs can be certified through the American Board of Occupational Health Nurses (see Chapter 29). Public health has included environmental health as a central aspect of health promotion and disease prevention. More recently, the nursing profession has responded to the call for nurses to establish environmental health competencies for nursing practice.

Significant historical milestones in environmental health nursing are:

- 1995: The Institute of Medicine report *Nursing, Health, and the Environment* (Pope, Snyder, & Mood, 1995) identified the need for nursing environmental health knowledge, research, and interventions.
- 1995 to 2008: Many nursing programs incorporated environmental health into the curriculum. Nurses incorporated environmental health into their practice settings to reduce hazardous exposures to both health professionals and patients. Environmental health nursing advanced, and nurses became involved in a number of policy and advocacy efforts (Leffers, McDermott-Levy, Smith, & Sattler, 2014).
- 2005: *Environmental Health Principles for Public Health Nursing* was published (APHA, 2005).
- 2007: *ANA Principles of Environmental Health for Nursing Practice* was published (ANA, 2007).
- 2008: The Alliance of Nurses for Healthy Environments (ANHE) was formed—the first professional nursing organization solely focused on environmental health (ANHE, 2019).

- 2010: ANA, Standard 16: Environmental Health was included in the second edition of *Nursing: Scope and Standards of Practice* (ANA, 2010) and revised for the 2015 edition (ANA, 2015b). Since the publication of the 2010 Standard 16: Environmental Health, all nurses must incorporate environmental health principles into nursing practice.

Healthy People 2030 Initiatives

In addition to guidelines for environmental health in nursing, there are federal guidelines from the Surgeon General Report on Healthy People and the core functions of public health (Centers for Disease Control and Prevention [CDC], 2018a) to support environmental health in nursing practice.

First released in 1990 as *Healthy People 2000*, *Healthy People* is the federal document produced every decade to set health goals to promote the health of Americans (Box 9-2). This document provides guidance for nurses to identify targets for health and is used for many public health nursing interventions. The most current version of this document, *Healthy People 2030*, identifies overarching goals that support environmental health and policies to promote a healthier population. These goals can be found in Chapter 1, Box 1-4. (Office of Disease Prevention and Health Promotion, (2020, para. 13).

BOX **9-2** *HEALTHY PEOPLE 2030*

Objectives for Environmental Health

Core Objectives

EH-01	Reduce the number of days people are exposed to unhealthy air
EH-02	Increase trips to work made by mass transit
EH-03	Increase the proportion of people whose water supply meets Sage Drinking Water Act regulations
EH-04	Reduce blood lead level in children aged 1–5 years
EH-05	Reduce health and environmental risks from hazardous sites
EH-06	Reduce the amount of toxic pollutants released into the environment
EH-07,08,10,11	Reduce exposure to arsenic, lead, bisphenol A, and perchlorate in the population, as measured by blood or urine concentrations of the substance or its metabolites
EH-09	Reduce exposure to mercury in children
D02-13, 14, 15	Reduce diseases and deaths related to heat

Reprinted from U.S. Department of Health and Human Services (USDHHS). (2020). *Browse 2030 objectives.* Retrieved from https://health.gov/healthypeople/objectives-and-data/browse-objectives

Importance of Environmental Health for Nursing

Nurses are essential to improve environmental health through nursing research, education, advocacy, and practice. We work with diverse populations in homes, workplaces, and communities and are the largest group of health care providers in the United States, with almost 3 million registered nurses.

In addition, we are in one of the most trusted professions, are able to communicate complex information to our patients and communities, interact with many other health care organizations, and serve in policy setting roles (Brenan, 2018). Therefore, nurses are ideally situated to assess for and address environmental health risk.

CONCEPTS AND FRAMEWORKS FOR ENVIRONMENTAL HEALTH

Ecosystems

Ecosystems are dynamic communities of plants, animals, microorganisms, and the nonliving environments in which they live. No organism, including humans, can live removed from its ecosystem or other species. Ecosystems help regulate water, gases, waste recycling, nutrient cycling, pollination, infectious disease, climate, and biology, as well as provide recreational and cultural opportunities for human use (Frumkin, 2016).

The synergistic relationship between humans and the environment has been highlighted through the multidisciplinary approach of **One Health**. One Health relies on an ecological approach to monitor and control diseases spread through the environment, animals, and humans (CDC, 2018b; Rabinowitz, 2018). Through One Health, botanists, microbiologists, nurses, physicians, and veterinarians have worked closely to understand and address the impact of ecosystem on public health (see Chapter 16).

Community/public health nurses (C/PHNs) find that the science of ecology has been applied to social ecological perspectives that identify not only the physical environment but also the social, political, economic, and cultural factors that exist for populations.

In public health, the ecological model of population health (Fig. 9-1) is used to illustrate that determinants of health (biological, behavioral, and environmental) interact to affect health (Friis, 2019). In addition, the framework of **planetary health** relies on an ecological perspective to attain health, well-being, and equity through stewardship of the political, economic, and social systems

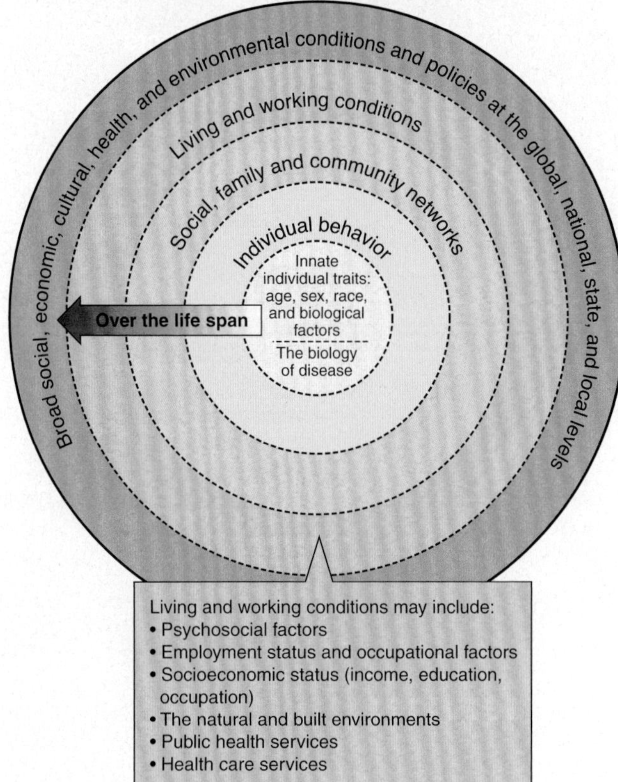

FIGURE 9-1 Ecological model for public health.

as well as natural ecosystems (Haines, 2016; Whitmee et al., 2015). Using the ecological perspective of planetary health, nurses are able to collaborate to address social, political, economic, cultural, and natural environmental factors that influence human health within their practice setting (Kurth, 2017).

Sustainability

Sustainability is based on the principle that human beings and the natural environment must coexist harmoniously for survival (U.S. Environmental Protection Agency [EPA], 2020b). When the concept of sustainability is applied to human systems, it is evident that the public must protect the environment and promote healthy characteristics in the population and in their communities.

Currently, much of human/environment interactions are not sustainable. For example, our food production and energy use create pollution that threatens human life and ecosystems. Solutions to improve sustainability for humans and the environment include strategies that are socially desirable, economically feasible, and ecologically viable (Wright & Boorse, 2016).

One example of how our energy use impacts sustainability is the increased use of fossil fuels for home heating and cooling. Our increased use of natural gas, for example, increases air pollution from the toxic emissions released from gas extraction and distribution. Many of these emissions lead to increases in ground-level ozone, particulates, and greenhouse gases that contribute to climate change. Current estimates indicate that the global need for oil has exceeded available resources that are not sustainable, according to a seminal article by Howarth (2014). Concerns about the depletion of natural resources, disruption of nutrient cycles, widening economic disparities between the rich and poor, and climate change are key issues addressed in the EPA's *Framework for Sustainability Indicators at EPA* (2012).

Sustainability is an important concept in relationship to nursing practice and the health care setting. The U.S. health care industry is a $2.5 trillion enterprise that contributes to 8% of all greenhouse gases and 7% of all carbon dioxide emissions. Hospitals generate as much as 5 million tons of solid waste annually, much of which is hazardous materials (EPA, 2017c).

Nurses were instrumental in the formation of Health Care Without Harm, a leading organization that promotes environmentally responsible health care (Health Care Without Harm, 2018). The ANA (2015a) has long supported efforts to address medical and pharmaceutical waste. For example, Beth Schenk, PhD, MHI, RN, serves as the Nurse Scientist and Sustainability Coordinator with Providence St. Patrick Hospital in Montana. In this role and in her shared appointment at Washington State University, Dr. Schenk seeks to advance environmental stewardship in health care and promote research for sustainability.

Although this example highlights the work of a nurse leader for a large health care system, nurses who work in community settings must comply with best practices for waste disposal as well as greening their practice environments. Pharmaceutical waste is a serious concern for nurses who work in home and school settings. This topic is more fully addressed in the section about water contaminants.

Upstream Focus

C/PHNs incorporate an "upstream" focus into their work with populations. This approach emerged from the seminal publication by John McKinley in 1979, *A Case for Focusing Upstream*, which identified root causes of disease and the multiple factors that lead to illness. The C/PHN approach to prevention and health promotion relies on an upstream approach to address the root causes that influence health at the institutional and system level rather than looking solely at healthy lifestyle issues; in other words, C/PHN direct their care "upstream" from the identified problem or issue (Butterfield, 2017).

For example, a C/PHN is taking an upstream approach to asthma prevention by working with legislators to strengthen ambient air quality polices. Thus, the nurse is moving up along the system to address a leading factor, outdoor air pollution that causes asthma (Fig. 9-2).

Two related concepts for environmental health nursing associated with upstream focus are health disparities

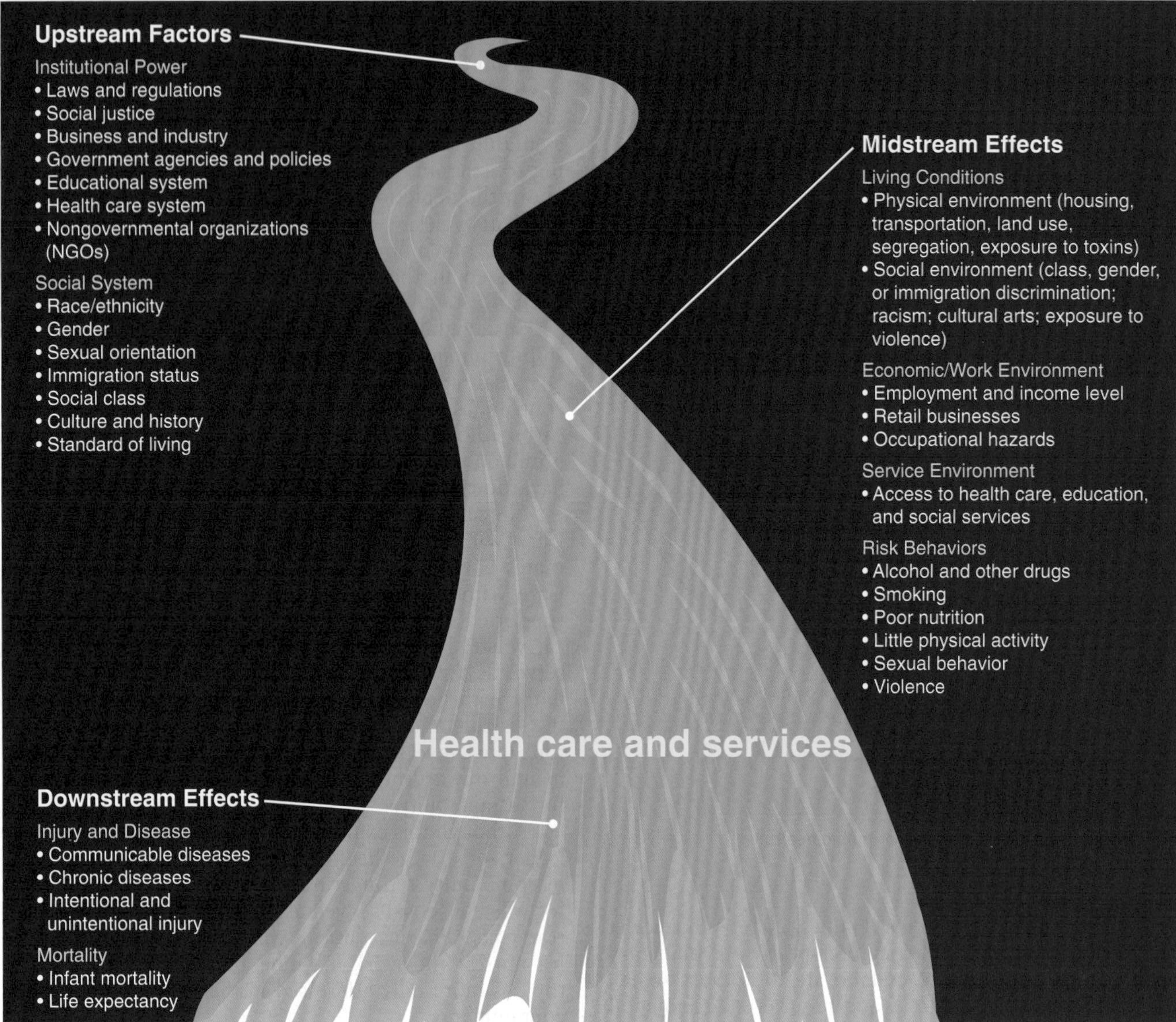

FIGURE 9-2 The influence of upstream factors on midstream and downstream effects. (Source: City of Richmond CA. (n.d.). *Health in all policies (HIAP) report.* Retrieved from http://www.ci.richmond.ca.us/2575/Health-in-All-Policies-HiAP; RAND Health. (2015). *Understanding the upstream social determinants of health.* Retrieved from https://www.rand.org/content/dam/rand/pubs/working_papers/WR1000/WR1096/RAND_WR1096.pdf)

and the social determinants of health. This focus for public health and environmental health nursing was introduced in a classic article by Butterfield (1990), who reminds the nursing profession that nurses, particularly C/PHNs, serve to reduce risks. C/PHNs are often the "sentinels of surveillance" (Butterfield, 2002, p. 33), who detect unusual illness patterns and respond to environmental emergencies in work and community settings.

With emphasis on data it is estimated that as much as 33% of disease occurrence is attributable to environmental exposures and that the prevalence of environmentally linked health problems such as asthma, neurological problems, certain cancers, and birth defects are all on the rise, a case can be made for nurses to use an upstream framework to assess, monitor, educate, advocate, and create policies to reduce environmental health risks (Frumkin, 2016). See Chapter 1, Figure 1-2.

Dr. Butterfield's original work, the Butterfield Upstream Model for Population Health (BUMP), applies an upstream public health nursing approach to environmental risks by giving nurses the framework to address the determinants of health and health inequities that influence health outcomes across the life course of a population (Butterfield, 2017).

Specific points that are part of the BUMP framework are:

- Assessing and analyzing the environmental exposures for the community or population
- Establishing health goals that include a multisector approach
- Determining where interventions will have the greatest impact
- Aligning with community partners to carry out the interventions

- Measuring effectiveness of interventions by process, outcome, and impact evaluations

The BUMP needs to be further tested by communiiy/public health nursing research. However, by using an upstream approach, C/PHNs can impact the prevalence of disease within a population by intervening where the root causes exist (Butterfield, 2017).

Health Disparities

Health disparities are a serious concern for overall health in the United States and globally. As noted in the discussion of upstream approaches to health, environmental factors are basic determinants of health and well-being. However, great inequities occur between the environments of people with higher incomes and those of low-income communities, people of color, and tribal and indigenous populations.

There are complex relationships between genes and environment that are related to social determinants of health (National Institute of Environmental Health Sciences [NIEHS], 2019; World Health Organization, 2020a). Disparities that are directly correlated with environmental exposures include rates of asthma among children, elevated blood lead levels (EBLLs), cancers that are linked to environmental exposures, and lung diseases among adults. Social and economic factors have created disproportionate exposures to pesticides, toxic chemicals in the workplace, poor indoor air quality in schools, and lead in housing.

At the federal level, the U.S. government responds to health disparities related to children's health through the President's Task Force for Environmental Health and Safety Risks to Children. This interagency effort includes 18 federal departments and White House Offices, including the EPA and Departments of Agriculture, Health and Human Services, Education, Energy, Housing and Urban Development, Justice, Labor, Transportation, and Homeland Security (National Institutes of Health [NIH], 2016). Issues that are being addressed include lead exposure, asthma disparities, healthy settings, and chemical exposures.

Social Determinants of Health

According to the WHO, **social determinants of health** are defined as "the conditions in which people are born, grow, live, work, and age. These circumstances are shaped by the distribution of money, power, and resources at global, national, and local levels" (WHO, 2020a, para. 1).

Social determinants of health include a number of social factors that affect families and communities, such as education, housing conditions, options for safe and active transportation, access to health care services, access to healthy food, employment and income, neighborhood environment and safety, and the quality of the built environment, such as parks, buildings, and green spaces (see Chapter 23). These social factors and non-chemical stressors contribute to the inequities in health outcomes, burden of disease, and quality of life (Fig. 9-3).

Environmental Justice

Closely related to social determinants of health and health disparities is the issue of environmental justice.

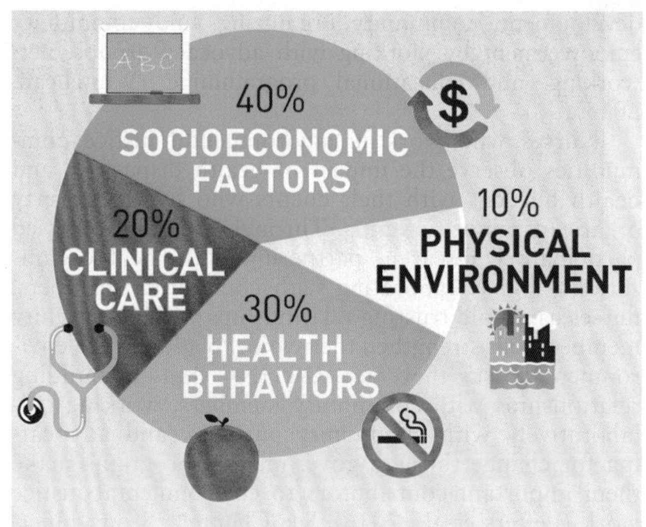

FIGURE 9-3 Infographic "What Affects Health." (Reprinted from https://www.cdc.gov/chinav/docs/chi_nav_infographic.pdf; data from www.countyhealthrankings.org.)

The EPA defines **environmental justice** as "the fair treatment and meaningful involvement of all people regardless of race, color, national origin, or income with respect to the development, implementation, and enforcement of environmental laws, regulations, and policies" (EPA, 2020a, para. 1). The key difference between social determinants and environmental justice is that the former addresses social factors that contribute to health disparities, whereas environmental justice is responsive to the inequities in the distribution of environmental hazards and exposure risks. The federal government took action to address environmental injustice though President Clinton's Executive Order 12898 in 1994 (EPA, 2020a, 2020b).

In communities across the United States, people of color, minorities, people with low income, and tribal communities bear a higher burden of exposures to environmental risks where they live (Brugge, 2016; EPA, 2020a). Children are at particular risk in such disadvantaged communities, where they have cumulative risk from exposures in homes, schools, and neighborhoods. Developmental and behavioral factors make children more vulnerable to environmental contaminants, and they have little control over where they live, what they eat, or the socioeconomic factors of their lives (Chakraborty, Collins, & Grineski, 2016).

Poor and minority children, who are more likely to live in neighborhoods with incinerators, industrial plants, toxic waste sites, and poor-quality housing, show higher rates of asthma, learning disabilities, and EBLLs than do nonminority children and those who come from more affluent families (Leffers, Smith, Huffling, McDermott-Levy, & Sattler, 2016). Cumulative environmental exposures, unique exposure pathways, and chronic psychosocial stress contribute to the environmental health disparities of those living in environmental justice communities (McPartland, Dantzker, & Portier, 2017).

Communities can promote healthier environments through a multifaceted approach to community development, community organizing, and community empowerment by working with advocacy groups, networking, and educational programming (Whitehead, 2015).

Nurses who work in environmental justice communities observe the impact of health disparities and health burdens with their clients who live in poverty or are of minority status. Through community-based participatory research, partnering with local organizations, and collaborating with community members, nurses can build trusting relationships with community members that strengthen their voice to address the environmental risks they face. C/PHNs' skills in building relationships with community members, working collaboratively with community partners, and advocating for change through governmental programs make them important contributors to environmental justice work (Leffers et al., 2016). See Chapter 23 on vulnerable populations and Box 9-3 for further sources of environmental health information and thePoint for more in-depth resources.

BOX 9-3 Environmental Health Regulatory Agencies

Environmental Protection Agency (EPA)

This federal agency was established in December 1970 for the purpose of standard setting, monitoring, and enforcement of environmental protection in order to work for a cleaner and healthier environment for America. EPA is tasked with setting regulations based on scientific evidence that addresses environmental risks in homes, schools, workplaces, and natural environments. https://www.epa.gov/history

Food and Drug Administration (FDA or USFDA)

This is an agency of the USDHHS that regulates food safety, dietary supplements, prescription and over-the-counter pharmaceuticals, veterinary medications, cosmetics, biopharmaceuticals, blood transfusions, medical devices, tobacco products, and products that emit radiation (www.fda.gov/aboutfda/whatwedo/and tobacco products. www.fda.gov/aboutfda/whatwedo/).

Consumer Product Safety Commission (CPSC)

CPSC was created in 1972 as an agency of the U.S. government to protect the public from risks of injury or death from consumer products. Commonly reported products are cribs, toys, household chemicals, and power tools but include any commercially traded product. As an independent agency, the CPSC does not report to any other agency of the U.S. government (https://www.cpsc.gov/About-CPSC/).

Occupational Safety and Health Administration (OSHA)

This agency was created in 1970 as a regulatory federal agency of the United States to assure safe working conditions. OSHA sets and enforces standards for health and safety in work environments (https://www.osha.gov/about.html).

Determining Risk

Merriam-Webster dictionary defines risk as "something that creates or suggests a hazard" (2019, para. 2). In the case of environmental health risks, exposure to a toxic substance within the environment creates a hazard to human health and thus increases risk of illness or disease. C/PHN must rely on the existing science to assess and determine environmental risk to communities. Nurses determine risk by relying on risk identification frameworks.

One such framework is the **precautionary principle**, which states, "When an activity raises threats of harm to human health or the environment, precautionary measures should be taken if some cause and effect relationships are not fully established scientifically. In this context the proponent of an activity, rather than the public, should bear the burden of proof" (Science and Environmental Health Network [SEHN], 2018, para. 6). The precautionary principle relies on credible evidence to determine an action to protect the population from a potential environmental health risk and is rooted in precaution, scientific uncertainly, and human rights.

The ANA and the American Public Health Association adopted the precautionary principle in 2006 as a measure to protect public health, as noted in a classic article by Chaudry (2008). It is used when there is limited evidence to determine risk, but there are concerns of threats to human health. As scientific methods have advanced, public health practitioners, including nurses and policy makers, have sought to better understand the impact of the environment on the health of communities.

Recently, health risk assessments and health impact assessments (HIA) have gained greater use in the United States. These assessments provided a more comprehensive and systematic examination of a potential environmental health risk and thus addressed limitations of the evidence that result in the need to rely on the precautionary principle.

The **health risk assessment** is a systematic evaluation of risk of a specific exposure. It involves four steps: (1) identification of the hazard; (2) exposure assessment (determining how are people exposed, who is at risk, and who is most vulnerable); (3) characterization of the health risk (determining whether the risk exists, how the exposure presents in humans, and what the toxic levels of exposure are); and (4) **risk management**: if there is a health risk, identifying how it can be managed and reduced (Finland National Institute for Health and Welfare, 2018).

An HIA is a systematic method of evaluating a planned change to a community *before* the change occurs. The purpose of a HIA is to inform decision-makers of the impacts of a proposed change on the health of the population. An HIA has six steps: (1) screening, (2) scoping, (3) assessment, (4) recommendations, (5) reporting, and (6) monitoring and evaluation (Quattrone, Callahan, Brown, Lin, & Pina, 2018).

Public health nurse Cynthia Stone, DrPH, RN, has identified the HIA as a valuable tool to address the health risks of communities. She has taken leadership in HIAs and developed HIA courses at Indiana University. Dr. Stone is also the editor-in-chief of *Chronicles of Health Impact*

Assessment. An example of the application of HIA (support of a full service grocery store in a food desert neighborhood) can be found at https://pdfs.semanticscholar.org/7d28/bef26232f0ee8796abb1bb788480674e4c4c.pdf .

Specific Vulnerabilities

Some groups are at more risk during specific periods of physical development or due to existing health issues or from social or environmental exposures related to where they live, work, or attend school. Exposures for pregnant women create a number of risks to both the mother and fetus and can produce lifelong or intergenerational adverse outcomes. Some of these effects include fetal loss, low-birth-weight infants, menstrual abnormalities, recurrent miscarriage, malformations of the reproductive system, reduced fertility, hormonal changes, intrauterine growth restriction, altered semen quality, neurodevelopmental performance, and alterations in onset of puberty (Chan, Chalupka, & Barrett, 2015; Kim et al., 2018; St. Cyr & McGowan, 2018).

Infants and children are at risk due to their stage of physical development, behavioral factors, and specific environments, such as neonatal intensive care units, schools, and homes. Children's exposures begin in utero, when many pollutants reach the developing fetus.

Although breastfeeding is the best source of infant nutrition, many chemicals, such as polychlorinated biphenyls (PCBs), dichlorodiphenyltrichloroethane (DDT), dioxin, and benzene, have been identified in breast milk. The stage of physical development of the respiratory, neurological, and excretory systems can also lead to increased risk of exposure and decreased ability to metabolize toxins.

Childhood behaviors such as hand-to-mouth exploration, crawling and playing on or near the ground, and use of toys all contribute to vulnerability to environmental hazards. Toxic materials on floors, in soil where children play, and in playthings (e.g., pressure-treated wood, toys, and paints) can increase risk for childhood exposures. Exposures to lead, mercury, and PCBs increase the risk for developmental disabilities. Studies suggest that the rise in attention deficit hyperactivity disorder, as well as antisocial and aggressive behavior diagnoses and possibly autism, can be attributed to the harmful effects of neurotoxic agents in the environment (Kalkbrenner, Schmidt, & Penlesky, 2014; Kim et al., 2018; Schmidt et al., 2017).

One specific type of vulnerability involves a chronic disease arising from complex interactions between the environment and the genes. **Epigenetics** is the field of study that examines the gene–environment interaction to study the processes in which genes are expressed differently as a result of environmental influences (EPA, 2016). **Endocrine-disrupting chemicals (EDCs)** mimic or block natural hormones in the human body and are linked to changes in genes inherited by offspring (English, Healy, Jagais, & Sly, 2015).

One example of epigenetic change was the use of diethylstilbestrol (DES) to treat women at risk of miscarriage. Female offspring of mothers who took DES showed increased rates of vaginal adenocarcinoma. Other cancers (breast, pancreatic) may now linked to the estrogen taken by their mothers during pregnancy (Troisi et al., 2019).

In addition, a landmark long-term follow-up study of 4,653 women who were exposed to DES in utero (comparison group of 1,927 women not exposed) found that those women exposed to DES while in utero were 1.42 to 3.77 times more likely to experience reproductive problems such as infertility, spontaneous abortion, preterm delivery, loss of second-trimester pregnancy, ectopic pregnancy, preeclampsia, stillbirth, gynecological conditions such as early menopause, grade 2 or higher cervical intraepithelial neoplasia, and breast cancer at 40 years of age or older (Hoover et al., 2011). Current perspectives on DES show that some of these effects occur in DES-exposed daughters and potentially future generations, as DES is considered a "biological time bomb" that requires continued study (Al Jishi & Sergi, 2017, p. 71).

Experts argue that the genetic changes that result from epigenetic processes because of developmental exposure to environmental stressors create negative effects on the health of future generations and contribute to rising rates of neurological conditions, alterations in reproductive organ development, and cancer (Grandjean et al., 2015).

Sciences for Environmental Health

Environmental health sciences include environmental epidemiology, toxicology, risk assessment, and risk management. In Chapter 7, you learned about the principles of epidemiology. **Environmental epidemiology** is a particular branch of epidemiology that focuses on environmental exposures and the risks that contribute to adverse health effects such as cancer, developmental disabilities, neurological problems, reproductive health issues, or death. Environmental epidemiology seeks to understand the specific vulnerabilities of population groups, to understand how toxic exposures adversely affect health, and to contribute to public health policies that address risk and risk management (National Cancer Institute, 2018).

Toxicology is the study of the adverse effects of chemical, physical, or biological agents on living organisms and the ecosystem, including the prevention and amelioration of such adverse effects" (Society of Toxicology, 2020, para. 1). Toxicants are those substances that are harmful and made by humans or result from human activities, in contrast to toxins that are naturally produced. By studying the physical properties of chemicals, scientists are able to examine the toxicity of chemicals as manifested by enzyme inhibition, cytotoxicity, inflammation, necrosis, immune hypersensitivity or immune suppression, neoplasia, and mutagenic reactions.

These processes should be familiar to nurses, because they parallel the effects and adverse effects of pharmacotherapeutic chemicals. Chemicals are classified as alcohols, solvents, heavy metals, oxidants, and acids and may be found as industrial wastes, agricultural chemicals, waterborne toxicants, air pollutants, or food additives. Factors such as dose level and timing can make a difference in efficacy or toxicity of a drug; dose and timing can also affect the toxicity of chemicals. Toxicity is affected by factors such as gender, age, lifestyle, diet, genetics, and disease states.

Furthermore, **exposure pathways**, or the routes by which a chemical enters the body, can affect toxicity, absorption, and metabolism. For example, children have less well-developed metabolic processes and are less able to detoxify chemical exposures. Likewise, older adults have reduced defense mechanisms in their lungs, skin, and other systems that make them more prone to adverse health effects (Gangemi et al., 2016). Nurses can learn more about toxicology and risk of specific toxicants through the National Library of Medicine (2020) TOXNET site, available at http://toxnet.nlm.nih.gov/.

Although health care screening does not test for most hazardous chemicals, some studies highlight the importance of biomonitoring. **Biomonitoring** refers to the body's burden of toxic chemicals or, more precisely, the "standard for assessing people's exposure to chemicals that may be toxic, and for responding to serious environmental public health problems" (CDC, 2017b , para. 1). Nurses can learn more about the CDC National Biomonitoring Program on their Web site: https://www.cdc.gov/biomonitoring/index.html.

Scientists identify health risks from epidemiology and toxicology, which provide information for government agencies to regulate hazards to human health (EPA, 2018b). For example, the EPA uses risk assessments to "characterize the nature and magnitude of health risks to humans (e.g., residents, workers, recreational visitors) and ecological receptors (e.g., birds, fish, wildlife) from chemical contaminants and other stressors that may be present in the environment" (EPA, 2018a, para. 4).

CORE FUNCTIONS OF PUBLIC HEALTH

The U.S. Department of Health and Human Services has identified 10 essential public health services, which are divided into 3 core functions: assessment, policy development, and assurance (see Chapter 2). These services have become the national Environmental Health Performance Standards (CDC, 2017a). They are used to guide community-level environmental health interventions (CDC, 2016, 2018a).

- Assessment: investigation of health hazards, surveillance of health issues, examining causes, and assessing needs. Activities include
  - Monitoring community environmental health status
  - Diagnosing and investigating community environmental health hazards
- Policy development: science-based decision-making and education of the community to create involvement to develop polices:
  - Informing, educating, and empowering community members regarding environmental health
  - Mobilizing community partnerships and activities to recognize and address environmental health problems
  - Developing policies and efforts that support individual and community environmental health
- Assurance: seeks innovative solutions to health issues, guarantees necessary services, and provides oversight to policy implementation:
  - Enforcement of laws and regulations that protect environmental health and ensure safety
  - Connect people to environmental health services and assure that the services are provided
  - Assure a competent environmental health workforce
  - Evaluate effectiveness, accessibility, and quality of individual and community environmental health services
  - Research to develop new knowledge and solutions to address environmental health problems

C/PHN fulfill these functions but extend them by emphasizing education for health promotion, disease prevention, and integrating nursing knowledge and practice into these functions to advocate for communities (Box 9-4). Additionally, C/PHN work collaboratively with others in the community to promote health. Some of the most common areas of public health nursing practice to address environmental impacts on health are schools, homes, and the broader community.

School nurses have been leaders in addressing indoor air quality in schools, particularly as rates of asthma in children rise (EPA, 2018h, 2018i), and serving as advocates for **integrated pest management (IPM)** programs for pest prevention without increasing exposure to harmful toxins.

IPM uses data on life cycles of pests and their environmental impact, along with environmentally friendly, economical methods of pest control, to effectively manage damage done by pests with the least hazardous effects to humans and the environment (EPA, 2017b, 2019f).

At the community level, C/PHN are involved with efforts to reduce pediatric obesity by participation in efforts to improve the built environment by advocating for safe walking paths, parks, and recreational areas and reducing exposure to pesticides in playgrounds (National Association of School Nurses, 2018).

Assessment

The breadth of environmental health information available exceeds the scope of this chapter. Our discussion is organized around the settings where people live, work, and go to school, the routes of exposure, the types of hazards, and the health effects of environmental toxins (Box 9-5). It is important for nurses working in the community to identify priority environmental concerns where people spend the majority of their time (home, work, school). Although community assessment and epidemiology are essential skills for public health nursing, the ability to perform critical assessments for environmental health requires background in the environmental health sciences.

Community/Public Health Nursing Assessments

In community/public health nursing practice, nurses routinely complete assessments for individuals, families, groups, and communities. There are many assessment tools available to help guide both C/PHN and the people they serve to assess environmental health risks.

Individual Assessments

The *ecological model of public health* offers a framework to consider where to target public health nursing interventions (Fig. 9-1). The framework offers spheres of influence at individual, social sphere or family, community, and national levels. The nurse must first identify the needs of the targeted sphere by assessing the environmental risk.

BOX 9-4 LEVELS OF PREVENTION PYRAMID

Pesticides Exposures

SITUATION: Provide education, resources, and support to prevent and treat pesticide exposures and poisoning.
GOAL: Using the three levels of prevention, avoid or promptly diagnose and treat negative health conditions, and restore the fullest possible potential.

Tertiary Prevention	
Rehabilitation	***Prevention***
Call Poison Control Center at 1-800-222-1222 HAZMAT teams Disaster preparedness	Health education: Continue to educate employers and workers about common risks in their businesses and specific hazardous chemicals. Health protection: Advocate for safe use and storage of pesticides and how to proceed during emergencies.

Secondary Prevention	
Early Diagnosis	***Prompt Treatment***
Recognition of early signs or pesticide poisoning. Laboratory screening for pesticide toxicity (blood or urine samples)	Poisoning signs can be seen, for example, vomiting, sweating, or pinpoint pupils. Symptoms can also include functional changes in normal condition that can be described by the victim of poisoning (e.g., nausea, headache, weakness, dizziness, others). National Pesticide Information Center http://npic.orst.edu/ingred/specchem.html

Primary Prevention	
Health Promotion and Education	***Health Protection***
Educate community members to reduce exposures to pesticides in their homes and outdoor areas. Educate employers and workers about Safety Data Sheets to understand hazardous chemicals	Advocate for: ▪ Clear product labeling with a package insert of warnings in multiple languages ▪ Community-level policy to restrict exposures to hazardous chemicals in pesticides in public places and use integrated pest management (IPM) for schools and playgrounds ▪ Safe use of pesticides and prepare for emergencies Teach parents, teachers, and caregivers pesticide risk, exposure routes, and methods of pesticide exposure prevention

BOX 9-5 STORIES FROM THE FIELD

Chemical Exposure Risks in the Clinical Setting

How many chemicals do you come in contact with on a daily basis in your nursing practice? Of particular interest to nurses is the survey conducted by the National Institute for Occupational Safety and Health (NIOSH) that found that American nurses and other health care professionals are at risk of exposure to chemicals in the clinical setting. These chemicals are used to sterilize and disinfect equipment and are the medications, such as chemotherapeutic agents, that are used to treat patients. Exposure to these chemicals can place nurses, their patients, and others in the health care setting at risk of asthma, reproductive problems, and cancer (NIOSH, 2017). Another finding of the NIOSH survey was that health care workers do not know nor do they always follow the proper procedures to reduce the risk of chemical exposures in the workplace. These are important environmental health factors for the nurse practicing in the clinical setting to consider. A large-scale study of nurse workplace exposure during pregnancy to sterilizing agents, dangerous drugs, anesthetic gases, and chemicals used in housekeeping found an increase in birth defects among their offspring (Environmental Working Group, 2019). Higher incidences of asthma, contact dermatitis, cancer, and miscarriages were also noted in nurses who reported high exposure rates.

1. *How are decisions made about the products used in your facility?*
2. *Who determines policies and procedures for use of chemicals and medications that can affect the health of staff and patients?*
3. *Where would you find information about the cleaning chemicals used in your place of practice?*
4. *Where would you find information to reduce the risk of exposure to chemotherapeutic agents?*
5. *Develop a plan to share the information you found with other nurses within a health care setting.*

At the individual level, individuals should complete a personal environmental health exposure assessment. Ideally, this should be part of every health visit, workplace assessment, or other health history. Though there are some shared characteristics for environmental exposures, individual risks from work, home, school, and recreation all contribute to an individual's overall risk.

The Agency for Toxic Substances and Disease Registry provides continuing education trainings to learn about a variety of environmental risks and how to take an exposure history; see their Web site (https://www.atsdr.cdc.gov/csem/exphistory/docs/exposure_history.pdf; this document includes information on continuing education trainings and, as appendices, an exposure history form and a material safety data sheet).

In addition, they created an environmental exposure history card using the mnemonic "I PREPARE" to aid nurses and other health professionals in adding environmental health exposure questions to patient assessment (Table 9-1). This tool that is both brief and easy to remember can be incorporated into any health assessment easily.

TABLE 9-1 Environmental Health Assessment "I PREPARE"

Mnemonic Cue	Examples of Questions
I Investigate potential exposures	Have you ever felt sick after coming in contact with a chemical, pesticide, or other substance? Do you have any symptoms that improve when you are away from your usual location (e.g., home or work)?
P Present work	Are you exposed to solvents, dusts, fumes, radiation, loud noise, pesticides, or other chemicals? Do you know where to find Safety Data Sheets on chemicals that you work with? Do you wear personal protective equipment? Are work clothes worn home? Do coworkers have similar health problems?
R Residence	When was your residence built? What type of heating do you have? Have you recently remodeled your home? What chemicals are stored on your property? Where does your drinking water come from?
E Environmental concerns	Are there environmental concerns in your neighborhood (i.e., air, water, soil)? What types of industries or farms are near your home? Do you live near a hazardous waste site or landfill?
P Past work	What are your past work experiences? What is the longest job held? Have you ever been in the military, worked on a farm, or done volunteer or seasonal work?
A Activities	In what type of activities and hobbies do you and your family engage in? Do you burn, solder, or melt any products? Do you garden, fish, or hunt? Do you eat what you catch or grow? Do you use pesticides? Do you engage in any alternative healing or cultural practices?
R Referrals and resources	Use these key referrals and resources: Agency for Toxic Substances and Disease Registry www.atsdr.cdc.gov Association of Occupational and Environmental Clinics www.aoec.org Environmental Protection Agency www.epa.gov Safety Data Sheets https://www.osha.gov/Publications/HazComm_QuickCard_SafetyData.html Occupational Safety and Health Administration www.osha.gov Local Health Department, Environmental Agency, Poison Control Center
E Educate	Are materials available to educate the patient? Are alternatives available to minimize the risk of exposure? Have prevention strategies been discussed? What is the plan for follow-up?

Reprinted from Agency for Toxic Substances and Disease Registry. (n.d.). *Environmental exposure history*. Retrieved from http://www.atsdr.cdc.gov/asbestos/site-kit/docs/IPrepareCard.pdf

While completing an individual assessment, it is important to consider those exposures specific to the workplace, school, or neighborhood. Workplace exposures are often addressed by OHNs and include not only physical hazards such as injuries from machinery, burns, falls, and crushing injuries but also hazardous exposure to toxic chemicals, particulate matter in the form of dust, volatile organic compounds (VOCs) and aerosols, heavy metals, and other chemicals that can contribute to poor indoor air quality (EPA, 2020d). See Chapter 29.

School nurses often address students' exposures in school settings, but it is very important for C/PHNs to identify potential risks to educate parents about environmental hazards in schools. Similar to the workplace, many schools have issues of poor indoor air quality with the increased use of synthetics in building materials and reduced access to outdoor air (EPA, 2020d). Neighborhood exposures affect individual health and are discussed in the community assessment section of this chapter. It is especially important to assess for hazards among school-aged children and the routes taken to school and playgrounds. See Chapter 28.

Home Assessments

C/PHNs frequently conduct home assessments for case finding, follow-up, screening, or other public health services. Home assessments often involve looking for safety hazards in the home, but do not always include potential environmental exposures. During the home visit, C/PHNs must assess the home for environmental tobacco smoke; the possibility of asbestos, the presence of a carbon monoxide detector and heating sources; lead paint risk; the water source and the possibility of lead pipes (EPA, 2018g); and other potential or actual hazardous materials (Table 9-2). Depending on the region of the country, C/PHNs should ensure that the family has their home tested for radon (EPA, 2019e).

Likewise, family members should be reminded to safely dispose of unused medication and old mercury thermometers. Cleaning products, paints, varnishes, strippers and other home remodeling materials, gardening fertilizers and pesticides (which can be carried into the home on shoes or pets; see Chapter 27), pest management insecticides and other materials, air fresheners, and mold and moisture can all be sources of exposure in the

TABLE 9-2 Common Hazards in the Home Setting

Hazard	Source	Exposure Pathway	Risk Groups	Health Effects
Asbestos	Asbestos is a fiber that has been used for insulation and as a fire retardant Used in shipbuilding and other occupational exposures to metal work	Inhalation	Children of metal workers Home residents	Lung cancer (mesothelioma) and lung disease
Arsenic	Used in pressure-treated wood, was formerly used in industrial sites, can be present in soil and water	Drinking water Inhalation from indoor or outdoor air	Children playing in playgrounds with pressure-treated wood, those with contaminated water supply	High levels are lethal Exposure can cause decreased red and white blood cells
Carbon monoxide	Colorless and odorless gas that is a by-product of combustion from home heating sources as well as automobiles housed in attached garage	Inhalation	Persons with respiratory and cardiovascular disease	Unconsciousness and death due to hypoxia
Environmental tobacco smoke	Cigarette smoking	Inhalation	Those people in area where smoking occurs in indoor space/home	Lung disease; lung cancer; cardiovascular problems
Formaldehyde	Carpeting, particle board, glues, adhesives used in home construction, or decorating Also some personal care products	Inhalation		Cancer
Lead	Paint used prior to 1978; leaded gasoline prior to ban in 1970s; ceramics, pottery, pipes, soil; some alternative medical therapies	Ingestion from dust in home or soil	Children	Nervous system

TABLE 9-2 Common Hazards in the Home Setting (*Continued*)

Hazard	Source	Exposure Pathway	Risk Groups	Health Effects
Mold	Normal growth of fungi in and outside of home Can produce VOCs	Spores travel in the air Inhalation	Those people most sensitive to molds	Respiratory symptoms
Pests	Mites, cockroaches	Inhalation, physical contact with droppings	Children and those with asthma	Exacerbation of asthma
Pesticides	Used in homes and outside lawns and gardens to protect plants from pests, home from insects	Indoor or outdoor air; inhalation Dermal absorption	Children All people exposed	Specific types of pesticides have been linked to neurological problems, others to cancer, and many as EDCs
Pharmaceutical Waste	Unused, out-of-date prescriptions	If discarded by waste or water systems, may seep into aquifers	All people exposed	Possible health concerns (hormone disruption, antibiotic resistance) to humans
Radon	Naturally occurring radioactive gas	Seeps into homes through cracks in foundation of home; inhalation	Residents of home	Lung damage particularly lung cancer
Solvents such as paint thinners, varnishes, and resins (ethers)	Dry cleaning, home improvements	Inhalation Percutaneous absorption	Home residents	Neurological problems renal, liver, and reproductive effects
Personal care products	Shampoo, soaps, cosmetics	Percutaneous	Individuals using them, children, adolescents	Varied EDCs, cancer, and neurological effects
Volatile organic compounds (VOCs)	Alcohols, ketones, and esters that are present in thousands of products such as paint thinners, cleaning supplies, pesticides, building materials, office equipment, copiers, printers, glues, adhesives	Inhalation	Those exposed in indoor settings	Eye, nose, and throat irritation, headaches, kidney damage, and central nervous system disorders

home and land around the home. C/PHN must be well versed in identifying hazardous materials and assess for them in their routine home visits, as noted in a classic, large, two-state study by Butterfield, Hill, Postma, Butterfield, and Odom-Maryon (2011).

Identify everyday products in clients' homes that contain hazardous materials and communicate to them the risk they pose to health and the importance of eliminating them or securing them to minimize risk of exposure (Oneal, Eide, Hamilton, Butterfield, & Vandermause, 2015).

Finally, a home assessment should address nearby environmental hazards or potential hazards such as coal-fired power plants, farms, industries, **brownfields** (properties where pollutants, contaminants, or hazardous substances may be present), toxic waste sites, highways, and contaminated waterways (EPA, 2018c, 2019g). Frequently, these hazards are visible in the neighborhood, but often, there are hidden routes of exposure from contaminated groundwater, ambient air, and contaminated soil. It is important that the C/PHNs is aware of local industry and potential contaminations that can place families at risk in their home.

Below is a list of useful home environmental assessment tools:

- *A Healthy Home Checklist* from the U.S. Surgeon General: https://www.surgeongeneral.gov/library/calls/checklist.pdf
- *Home Environmental Health and Safety Assessment Tool*, which is easy to use and addresses key exposure topics (Davis, 2007): https://envirn.org/wp-content/uploads/2017/03/davis-home-environmental-health-and-safety-assessment-tool.pdf
- *Healthy Home Checklist* from the Environmental Working Group: https://secure.ewg.org/images/EWG_HealthyHomeChecklist_201710.pdf

Community Assessments

A comprehensive community health assessment considers environmental factors in a number of ways. In Chapter 15, community health assessment is introduced with a focus on aspects of the community that promote health or provide risks to health. Environmental assessment refers to the natural and built environments.

Community assessment is central to public health nursing practice and to the core functions of public health. Typically, a *windshield* or walking survey is useful for observation of environmental hazards (see Chapter 15). By knowing likely hazards in the community, C/PHNs can identify many possible environmental risks simply by observation.

Various tools have been developed to help nurses assess for environmental risks. Though most community assessment tools address environment, C/PHNs must also consider specific threats that may not be covered by general community assessments. To assess air quality, for instance, nurses should look for visible sources of air pollution from smokestacks, identify exhaust from vehicular traffic, and learn of significant industries, power sources, and incinerators in the community.

To assess water quality, C/PHNs must identify the source of drinking water as public or private, understand water treatment and quality, recognize evidence of pollution and whether there are fish alerts for local waterways, examine stagnant water and possible waterborne risks, and identify issues related to sewer function and possible contamination, as well as the likelihood of floods and other water emergencies (USGS, 2018b).

To assess land, nurses must consider both current and former land use. **Superfund** refers to funding made possible by the Comprehensive Environmental Response, Compensation, and Liability Act of 1980 to address those contaminated areas of the United States that needed to be remediated; the EPA administers the funding. Well-known examples of Superfund sites in which land contamination caused public health disasters are Love Canal in New York State and Times Beach, Missouri. Nurses must be aware of such sites in their communities, which are listed on the National Priorities List and can be located by searching on the EPA Web site: https://www.epa.gov/superfund/superfund-national-priorities-list-npl (EPA).

Brownfield sites refer to real "property, the expansion, redevelopment, or reuse of which may be complicated by the presence or potential presence of a hazardous substance, pollutant, or contaminant" (EPA, 2018c, para. 1). In 2018, the Brownfields Utilization, Investment, and Local Development (BUILD) Act was ratified to bring more opportunities for sustainable local development and to redevelop brownfield sites that still required remediation (EPA, 2018c, 2019d). Nurses should monitor the impact of the BUILD Act of 2018 and advocate that the goals of this act serve their communities.

Built Environment. The **built environment** refers to all aspects of our environment that are not naturally occurring and includes not only the physical structures (e.g., homes, schools, workplaces, dams, roadways, buildings, energy sources) but also the features that contribute to social cohesiveness or disruption (Fig. 9-4). The impact of the built environment includes indoor and outdoor physical environments, which in turn affect the social environments where people live, work, and engage with others. Considering that Americans spend upwards of 90% of their time indoors, our built environment can have significant impact on our health (Robert Wood Johnson Foundation, 2018).

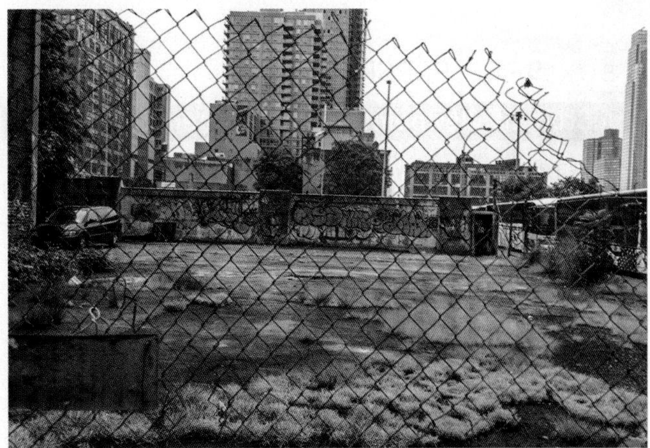

FIGURE 9-4 Neighborhoods, or the built environment, can contribute to population health or illness.

In recent years, there has been a shift in community development to consider the influence of the built environment on community health and cohesion. Evidence suggests that many physical and mental health problems are related to the built environment, such as asthma, cardiovascular disease, lung conditions, obesity, and cancer (Ying, Ning, & Xin, 2015). Increasingly, communities are promoting social engagement and human health in the built environment by improving public transportation, promoting areas for walking and biking, enhancing green spaces, and addressing sustainable energy sources (Koehler et al., 2018).

Many U.S. cities are addressing issues related to community/public health and the built environment by implementing the UN SDGs. The UN Sustainable Development Solutions Network ranks U.S. cities in meeting the SDGs, which serves as an indication of impacts of the built environment on community health http://unsdsn.org/resources/publications/leaving-no-u-s-city-behind-the-2018-u-s-cities-sdgs-index/.

Another C/PHN role is to assess the quality of the housing. Buildings that were constructed prior to 1978 are likely to have lead-based paint, and homes built before 1987 may have lead soldering in the plumbing that delivers household drinking water (Hanna-Attisha, LaChance, Sadler, & Schnepp, 2016). Homes or buildings constructed between 1930 and 1950 are likely to have asbestos in the insulation, as well as in the hot water and steam pipes (U.S. Consumer Product Safety Commission, 2018).

The overall condition of the community indicates sanitation factors, safe waste disposal, and potential sources of contamination. The location of schools, playgrounds, and public transportation and access to green spaces should be part of the community assessment. Examination of the overall community environment provides C/PHNs with essential information about how the environment is likely to impact the residents' health (Box 9-6).

BOX 9-6 PERSPECTIVES

A Student Viewpoint on Environmental Health in Health Systems

As a nursing student, I was bothered by the amount of waste I saw in the hospital during my clinical rotations. When we covered environmental health in class, I learned that while healing patients, health systems also contribute to greenhouse gases, use toxic materials to maintain the patient care units, and generate 29 lb of waste per patient bed per day (Slutzman, 2018). I did not want to be part of a health system that was contributing to pollution and illness.

I spoke to my nursing professor, and we both agreed that education is the way to make the change. With the support of my professor and the simulation lab staff, I developed a waste reduction program for the students within my nursing school's simulation lab. I started with the urinary catheterization lab and taught the sophomore students about hospital waste and what items can be recycled, reused, and must be discarded. By weighing the reusable, recycled, and discarded items from the urinary catheterization lab, I demonstrated the impact that education and end-use product management can have. The faculty, simulation lab staff, and students were excited to see that they could make a difference in the environment by being aware of end-use product management.

As I prepared for the educational session for my fellow nursing students, I learned where to find information about products that are used in the hospital. I looked first at the USDHHS Household Products Database (http://householdproducts.nlm.nih.gov/) to learn more about the types of exposures that the staff and patients might have in the hospital setting. Through my research, I also learned about hospital Green Teams or Sustainability Teams that support institutional sustainability in purchasing, foods for dietary services, energy use, waste management, and product safety. Nurses can serve on these important hospital teams and support green practices on their units. I also learned about two organizations that support this important work:

- Practice Greenhealth (https://practicegreenhealth.org/) and Health Care Without Harm (https://noharm.org/)
- Health Care Without Harm (2020b) (https://noharm.org)

When I look for my first staff nurse position, I am going to seek employment at a hospital where I can serve on the Green Team so I can continue to have an environmental health focus in my nursing career.

Marina, senior nursing student

Source: Slutzman, 2018.

Climate Change. Climate change is our greatest global public health threat (Costello, Montgomery, & Watts, 2013; Costello et al., 2009; Desmond, 2016). **Climate change** "refers to significant changes in global temperature, precipitation, wind patterns and other measures of climate that occur over several decades or longer" (Fig. 9-5; UC Davis, n.d., para. 1).

Unfortunately, in the United States, instead of addressing the realities of climate change, it has become politicized, leading to inaction and avoidance of our very serious reality. For example, the U.S. EPA has removed most of the documents concerning climate change and its impact on human health from its Web site, and, in 2017, President Trump withdrew the United States from the Paris Climate Agreement.

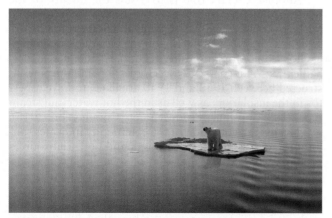

FIGURE 9-5 Climate change is related to melting ice caps, warming oceans, and increased volatile weather patterns.

- The Paris Agreement is an international agreement of signatory countries to limit greenhouse gas emissions in an effort to keep temperature rise below 2°C of preindustrial temperatures and to target temperature reduction to 1.5°C. The target of 1.5°C preindustrial temperatures has been further supported by a sobering report from the Intergovernmental Panel on Climate Change (IPCC, 2018), in which the world's leading climate scientist stated that to avoid severe impacts of climate change, the world must reduce carbon emissions by 45% now.
- In 2018, the National Oceanic and Atmospheric Administration found the average temperature (all land and ocean surfaces) to be 1.42°F higher than the average 20th century temperature. This was the fourth hottest year ever recorded (Lindsey & Dahlman, 2019; EPA, 2020e).
- Temperature changes affect weather patterns that can result in more frequent extreme weather events, disease outbreaks, food and water shortages, and changing migration patterns (see Boxes 9-7 and 9-8).

Nurses are in a position to take a lead in addressing climate change through individual, professional, local, and national mitigation, adaptation, and resilience strategies. When assessing communities, the nurse should note vulnerable groups such as pregnant women, infants, children, older adults, people with disabilities, non-English speakers, and the poor. In addition, communities may experience risks related to food and water

BOX **9-7** WHAT DO *YOU* THINK?

Climate Refugees

In addition to those already affected, it is estimated that by 2050, 143 million people around the globe will be climate refugees. In 2017, between 22.5 and 25 million people were displaced due to sudden severe weather events such as forest fires and flooding. More climate migration will occur as slow-onset changes like rising sea levels and air pollution increase. Eight western Pacific islands have already submerged, with a projected 48 being under water by 2100 (Podesta, 2019).

One example in Louisiana highlights the dire circumstances. Isle de Jean Charles, about 50 miles southwest of New Orleans, was first settled by a Frenchman who described it not as an island, but as a ridge covered with live oak trees and encircled by swampy marshlands. Native American tribes later settled there, hunting, trapping, fishing, raising domestic animals, and growing rice. In 1953, the marshland was linked to the mainland by a 2-mile causeway. Now the island is 98% submerged into the Gulf of Mexico and is only a quarter-mile wide and two miles long. From a high of 300, now there are only 40 residents remaining. Over the last 20 years, six hurricanes have pummeled the island. Although residents are conflicted about being relocated to the mainland, they will eventually become climate refugees (Jarvie, 2019).

1. *Is climate change a driver for the increase in Central Americans requesting asylum at the U.S. southern border?*
2. *How many Puerto Ricans left their island country to resettle to the U.S. mainland? What percentage have returned?*

Source: Jarvie, 2019; Podesta, 2019.

quality and availability, heat stress for those most vulnerable, increased air pollution, and severe weather-related events. Severe weather events such as flooding, droughts, hurricanes, and tornados require emergency preparedness and disaster response from the public health sector (EPA, 2020e; U.S. Global Change Research Program, 2016, 2018).

BOX **9-8** WHAT DO *YOU* THINK?

Pandemics and Pollution

Italy is considered a leader in lowering greenhouse gases, having reduced greenhouse gases 30% between 2004 and 2018. In mid-March 2020, satellite readings revealed a rapid drop in nitrogen dioxide levels since January. Because of the COVID-19 outbreak and isolation measures enacted in the northern part of Italy, fewer diesel-powered cars were being used as people remained in their homes. Time-lapse maps showed striking results, similar to even more dramatic results noted earlier in China, where the disease outbreak began (Mooney, Muyskens, Dennis, & Freedman, 2020). Although these changes are temporary, they demonstrate how humans have an impact on their environment. What other changes might occur if the trend continued?

Specifically, C/PHNs must be prepared for surge events by developing skills such as the ability to (1) be personally prepared, (2) comprehend state and local disaster plans, (3) conduct a rapid needs assessment, (4) investigate outbreaks, (5) perform public health triages, (6) communicate risk effectively, (7) participate effectively in mass dispensing interventions, and (8) respond after the event to the debriefing and public health impact of the event, as outlined in a seminal article by Polivka et al. (2008, 2012). Nurses need to be prepared for inadequate resources and infrastructure, as well as the lack of electricity and technology (Ruskie, 2016).

Nurse leaders are disseminating timely and accurate information for nursing practice through resources and collaboration with national organizations. All nurses must understand the implications of climate change on health.

Together with nine other organizations, including the National Student Nurses' Association and the Public Health Nursing Section of the American Public Health Association, the ANHE (2019) established the Nursing Collaborative for Climate Change and Health to bring leaders and institutions together to advance climate solutions to protect the health of Americans.

In addition, ANHE has cooperated with Health Care Without Harm to offer the Nurses Climate Challenge. This project educates practicing nurses about the health impacts of climate change so that they, in turn, can educate their nurse colleagues about climate health. This program can be accessed at https://nursesclimatechallenge.org. Another valuable resource for nurses is the U.S. Global Change Research Program report, *Forth National Climate Assessment* (2018). See Box 9-9 for what you need to know about climate change.

Land Use. Topics that must be considered when conducting community health assessment to address land use include zoning regulations and enforcement, industries and their toxic releases, types of transportation, sidewalks, bikeways, public transportation, recreational space including green space, what fertilizers or pesticides are applied to the fields, safe play areas for children, and information regarding a tree ordinance to promote health environments (EPA, 2020b).

School locations should be examined for accessibility by foot or bicycle, the safety of the surrounding area, and the use of pesticides on school fields. The community should be assessed for commercial lots, their safety and use, and vacant lots or unused property. Specific commercial businesses such as gas stations, auto repair shops, and dry cleaners are often common sources of toxic exposures (Leffers et al., 2016).

If the community has agricultural areas, these must be assessed for irrigation practices, use of pesticides, runoff, and land use practices. In addition, waste can be a source of environmental hazards. C/PHNs must assess for the presence of landfills or municipal waste incinerators, medical waste incinerators, and municipal trash collection or dumpsters throughout the community (Leffers et al., 2016).

Land use and transportation patterns and plans can influence the health of the community. The design of a

BOX **9-9** PERSPECTIVES

A C/PHN Viewpoint on Climate Change

In June 2017, President Trump announced that the United States would withdraw from the Paris Agreement to reduce greenhouse gas emissions (Dalton, 2017). However, the United States did sign on to the Paris Agreement rules that were established during COP24, or the Conference of the Parties to the U.N. Framework Convention on Climate Change, in December 2018 in Katowice, Poland. This may have been in response to the Intergovernmental Panel on Climate Change (IPCC, 2018) scientific report that the world must come together to keep temperature rise below preindustrial temperature increase of 1.5°C.

The WHO has noted that health professionals globally must be knowledgeable and prepared to respond to the health impacts of climate change. The political volleying of climate change in the national and international arenas can be challenging, especially when trying to maintain a nonpolitical stand and advocate for public health.

As a C/PHN, I feel the best response is to focus on the scientific evidence related to climate change and health. C/PHNs should be aware that the world's leading climate scientists from the IPCC have made recommendations after vetting and reviewing the global scientific evidence. Furthermore, when addressing climate change, a local response makes it easier to avoid the politicization of climate change. Communities in the United States and globally have been affected by unprecedented hurricanes, drought, and wildfires. These events have a direct impact on human health. Other health impacts include poor birth outcomes, malnutrition, water quality and disease, vector-borne diseases, respiratory diseases, and psychological impacts (U.S. Global Change Research Program, 2016). Certain vulnerable populations such as infants, children, and older adults are at higher risk for adverse health outcomes as well at those living in poverty.

This is a global health issue for all nurses. C/PHNs must be prepared to address the health impacts of climate change for the populations they serve (Leffers & Butterfield, 2018). This includes mitigation of climate risk, adaptation to climate health impacts, and building resilient communities and health systems (Leffers, McDermott-Levy, Nicholes & Sweeney, 2017). Communicating climate risk to gain community action can be a challenge. You can find current research and weather trends at the National Oceanic and Atmospheric Administration website (https://www.noaa.gov/categories/climate-change), and EcoAmerica has a climate communication resource that can support a C/PHNs climate work with communities: https://ecoamerica.org/wp-content/uploads/2017/03/5_ea_15_steps.pdf

Source: Dalton (2017); IPCC (2018); Leffers & Butterfield (2018); Leffers et al. (2017); U.S. Global Change Research Program (2016).

city, community, or neighborhood affects physical activity, automobile dependence, ability of those of older age and those with physical disabilities to navigate the community, and opportunities for children to walk to school. Community design also highlights concerns for environmental justice when those who live in areas of low accessibility and high exposure to pollution are more likely to be of minority status or living in poverty (Leffers et al., 2016).

There is need for further research that includes assessing (Leffers et al., 2016):

- Walking as an indicator of community health
- Physical activity levels and contributory factors
- The public health consequences of public safety design choices
- The types and determinants of travel to school
- The influence of community design on risk of injury
- The influence of community design on emissions of overall and specific pollutants
- Physical activity, mobility, and social integration in persons with disabilities
- Social equity and health outcomes in relation to community design
- The influence of physical setting characteristics on mental health
- The impact of community engagement on environmental health

For example, studies of air quality exposures of bicyclists in urban settings have shown that they are exposed to higher levels of air pollution while biking in areas of heavy vehicular traffic (Cole, 2018; Hofman, Samson, Joosen, Blust, & Lenaerts, 2018). As communities transition to sustainable practices with more walking and biking areas, considerations should be made to reduce environmental risks for walkers and bikers in areas of high vehicular traffic.

Types of Toxic Exposures.

Air. Air quality is a major variable in the health of populations. People living in areas that have poor air quality experience higher rates of disease and adverse health effects. Climate change contributes to air pollution and adversely affects health.

Ambient air, or outdoor air, can be affected by a number of air pollutants. Air pollution is composed of a variety of materials such as aerosols, criteria air pollutants (carbon monoxide, lead, ground-level ozone, nitrogen dioxide, sulfur dioxide, particulate matter), VOCs, and hydrofluorocarbons, as well as radon and other gases that contain harmful toxins (EPA, 2018d, 2020h).

In response to the Clean Air Act of 1970, air quality is monitored by the EPA. In an effort to inform citizens about the air quality in their own communities, the EPA created the Air Quality Index (AQI) (see thePoint®), which is often reported in media sources on a daily basis. The AQI is calculated for four of the six criteria air pollutants (ground-level ozone, particle pollution, carbon monoxide, and sulfur dioxide) to see if they exceed the national air quality standard set by the EPA, with an emphasis on their effect on health (EPA, n.d., 2018f, 2020h).

The EPA's Web site presents a guide for citizens to understand the importance of monitoring the ambient air, what the six criteria air pollutants are and how they affect health, and efforts to monitor air quality to provide public health advisories (EPA, n.d., 2018d, 2020h). Additionally, the EPA offers the AirNow app, which can be used to monitor regional AQI readings.

The EPA publishes a *Plain English Guide to the Clean Air Act* available on their Web site for the public to learn more about air quality (EPA, 2018f, 2019c).

Reports from the EPA monitoring of air pollution indicate that from 2010 to 2017, the overall levels of the six major pollutants measured by the federal government (carbon monoxide, ozone, sulfur dioxide, nitrogen dioxide, lead, and particulate matter) declined by a high of 80% for lead and a low of 5% for ozone because of cleaner cars, industries, and consumer products. However, millions of people live in areas that exceeded the national ambient air quality standard (NAAQS) set by the EPA (2019c).

Our health is influenced by the air we breathe both indoors and outdoors. Ambient air is composed of gases such as nitrogen, oxygen, argon, carbon dioxide, hydrogen, neon, helium, and other gases, which are part of the atmosphere. It also contains moisture and particulate matter. The amount of hazardous material that is contained in ambient air is the reason that the Clean Air Act of 1970 was created (U.S. Environmental Protection Agency [EPA], 2020h).

C/PHNs must understand the adverse effects of ambient air pollution to assess, monitor, and advocate for those most vulnerable, which includes children, people with lung disease, older adults, and even healthy individuals who are active outdoors (EPA, 2020f).

Health effects include irritation of the respiratory system with inflammation of the cell lining. This makes the lungs more susceptible to infection. Air pollution can also exacerbate asthma and cause chronic lung disease, reduced lung function, and lead to permanent lung damage. In addition, air pollution causes increased risk of cardiac disease, in particular acute myocardial infarctions and arrhythmias (EPA, 2019c).

Indoor air quality is particularly important for home, school, and workplace assessments. When the AQI for outside air is high, in order to avoid pollutants, people are instructed to stay inside. However, indoor air quality may be poor and expose people to pollutants, microbials, and particulates that may also lead to adverse health conditions.

Air pollution in homes occurs from exposure to heating or combustion sources such as oil, coal, kerosene or wood, radon gas, secondhand smoke from cigarettes, building materials and furniture that contains pressed wood products, carpeting and adhesives that emit VOCs, asbestos in insulation, cleaning products, paints, varnishes, and paint removers, personal care products, and other sources used around the home such as pesticides (EPA, 2020d).

Mild health effects might be headaches and nausea; the more serious health effects include damage to the liver, kidneys, and central nervous system, as well as cancer. In addition, molds, dust, and known asthma triggers in the home can not only exacerbate asthma symptoms but also cause irritation to those with heart and lung conditions.

BOX 9-10 Indoor Air Quality in Schools

School environments can influence a child's health. This has been demonstrated in research studies. For example, environmental triggers have been shown to worsen asthma symptoms in children and effect student and staff absentee rates.

The U.S. EPA offers a program, Healthy Schools, Healthy Kids. This program offers tools for schools regarding school air quality, building structure, transportation, and chemicals used in the building. The EPA AirNow.gov (n.d.) also offers webinars to address school indoor air quality.

In addition, the EPA offers the "Air Quality Flag Program" that uses the flag colors that respond to the current local AQI to alert parents and the school community about ambient air quality. This supports parents, children, and the school community to take proper precautions to reduce asthma symptoms in the student population. Nurse scientist Laura Anderko, PhD, RN, has worked with Washington, DC, school nurses on the flag program, and school officials have observed the parents respond to the air quality flags and take appropriate action to reduce asthmatic episodes for their children (Tomkins, Anderko, & Patten, 2016).

Source: Tomkins et al. (2016); AirNow.gov (n.d.).

Air quality in school buildings is very important for staff, teachers, and students (Box 9-10). More than 56 million children and adults spend up to 6 to 8 hours in elementary and secondary school each day. In particular, children are at increased risk for a variety of reasons. Young children are more likely to spend time on or near the floor where toxins are likely to settle; they use more hand-to-mouth behavior, and they take in more air per size than adults. Although exposures can be the same as in the home, those who attend or work in schools are in the same air environment for 6 to 8 hours or more where they are exposed to the toxins for long periods of time (EPA, 2018h).

Nurses who work in the school setting can access information through the EPA Web site to aid in assessments and interventions to improve air quality in schools. A comprehensive guide to healthier school environments is available on their Web site (EPA, 2018h).

Water. The human body is composed of 50% to 60% water, which illustrates how necessary water is for our survival. In public health, the concern is for safe water consumption; safe lakes, rivers, and streams for recreation; and safe waterways to support animal and plant life necessary for transport of nutrients and ecology of the environment. The availability of clean water is becoming a very serious threat to human survival (U.S. Geological Survey [USGS], 2018a).

Globally, 2.1 billion people lack access to safe water, and in 2017, approximately 4.5 billion did not have access to an improved sanitation facility creating threats to safe water (United Nations, 2018).

Poverty is linked with lack of access to clean water and sanitation. Every day, approximately 1,000 children die from a water and sanitation-related diarrheal disease (United Nations, 2018). The critical importance of this issue is born out by the UN including water and sanitation as one of its SDGs. See Chapter 16.

Drinking water is available in two forms: surface water and groundwater. Both are potential sources of contamination or pollution. Surface water sources include lakes, streams, and municipal reservoirs for water use. Underground sources, or groundwater, include aquifers that run beneath the ground level and are reached via wells and springs.

Many municipalities use reservoirs and other surface sources for their water supply, whereas in many areas, people must rely upon wells to provide their source of water. Safe drinking water is essential for human health. Public water systems provide water for community members. More than 90% of Americans are served by public water systems. Public water systems are monitored and regulated through the EPA. These regulations require that public water suppliers protect consumers from microorganisms and contaminants that are harmful to health (Box 9-11; EPA, 2018g).

The EPA does not regulate private sources of water from private wells. The individual users must be responsible for monitoring their own wells. Private well owners should test their water annually and anytime there is a risk of contamination such as flooding, repair to the well system, changes in water quality, or local construction (EPA, 2018g).

Water can become contaminated from a number of sources, including point and nonpoint sources.

- *Point sources* are those that can be traced to one source, such as a wastewater facility release into municipal water or discharge from an industrial site.
- *Nonpoint sources* are runoff from agricultural areas, gasoline stations, and other contaminants carried by rain and waterways. Some common water contaminants are microbial (frequently *Cryptosporidium* and *Giardia*).

To rid public water systems of microorganisms, disinfection processes are used. Disinfectants that are chlorine based can produce by-products that can also be hazardous to health. Additionally, other inorganic (such as nitrogen derivatives, arsenic, lead, fluoride, cadmium, and mercury) and organic chemicals (commonly organophosphates, phthalates), as well as radionuclides, are frequent water contaminants (EPA, 2018b, 2018e, 2018g).

More recently, there is a global concern about pharmaceutical waste in water. During 1999 to 2000, the U.S. Geological Survey (USGS, 2018b) found chemicals such as medications for humans and animals, natural and synthetic hormones, metabolites, pesticides, insecticides, plasticizers, and fire retardants in 80% of the streams sampled (Health Care Without Harm, 2020a).

Not only are pharmaceuticals used by humans, excreted in their urine, and discarded into locations where they can reach water supplies but also animals are fed with hormones and antibiotics in animal feeding operations that can leach into water supplies (Diaz-Sanchez, D'Souza, Biswas, & Hanning, 2015).

C/PHNs must be aware of sources of water contamination that puts vulnerable population groups such as the growing fetus, infants and children, older adults, and those with compromised immunity at great risk (Marcoux & Vogenberg, 2015). Organizations such as Health Care Without Harm seek to address the pharmaceutical waste issue through measures that address production, use, discharge, and disposal, treatment in wastewater facilities, and collection of unused medications (Health Care Without Harm, 2020a).

The Right to Know legislation and use of Safety Data Sheets provide some assurance and can be helpful in teaching our clients how to better protect themselves as well. C/PHNs can direct community members to consult the EPA Web site to learn about their right to know. To locate local information, nurses and community members can visit the EPA Web site at www.epa.gov. One link connects to "your own community" and leads to *MyEnvironment*, where consumers can learn more about the risks for one's own community, how to address specific pollution, and ensure safe drinking water. Nurses can teach their community partners how to access a consumer confidence report. Every public water system is required to provide information to consumers that identify any detected contaminants or factors that affect the water quality for those customers that they serve. This responsibility to provide the public with information about public water systems is mandated through the SDWA enacted in 1974 that established standards for safe drinking water. Individuals can access information from their own water supplier or can visit the EPA Web site (EPA, 2020j). In September of 2019, the Trump administration announced plans to repeal the 2015 rules related to the 1972 Clean Water Act and to roll back protections on wetlands and tributaries (Eliperin & Dennis, 2019).

Finally, a risk to community water supplies occurs in the communities where unconventional natural gas or oil extraction, also known as fracking, occurs. This is a process to extract natural gas or oil from deep underground for public use. Fracking has the potential to contaminate air and water from chemical sources such as methane, benzene, and other hydrocarbons, and it poses health risks to community members as well as the workers involved in extraction operations.

Fracking is occurring throughout the United States. In fact, 21 states permit fracking, including Arkansas, California, Colorado, Pennsylvania, Texas, and Wyoming. Methane, benzene, and other chemicals have been found in the groundwater in communities where fracking takes place. Health concerns, such as respiratory and nervous system problems, along with blood disorders, cancers, and birth defects, have been noted (McDermott-Levy, Katkins & Sattler, 2013; Wilke & Freeman, 2017).

It is important to remember that process of fracking and health risk is not only related to exposures from the well sites but the entire process from well preparation to delivering the fuel to the marketplace, sometimes across

BOX **9-11** STORIES FROM THE FIELD

Flint, Michigan

The public health of citizens in Flint, Michigan, was compromised in April 2014 when, in an attempt to save money, the city changed its water supply from Lake Huron water supplied by Detroit to the Flint River. Flint was once a booming automotive manufacturing area and the site of early labor strikes and conflicts. Now, the plants are closed, and jobs are scarce. Flint has some of the highest levels of violent crime, preterm birth/infant mortality, domestic violence, and illicit drug use in the state, as well as some of the poorest health outcomes (Hanna-Attisha et al, 2016). It is also marred by the effects of largely unrestrained industrial pollution from the industries that dominated the area for 80 years, as "huge amounts of lead and other toxins were pumped into the air, water, streams, and ground" (Rosner, 2016, p. 200).

After the water supply switch, residents noted changes in the taste, odor, and color of their drinking water. Flint's water system was old (with estimates of 10% to 80% of it with lead plumbing), and the city has struggled to maintain basic services in the face of declining tax revenues and high unemployment. City officials claimed that the water was fine. By August 2015, researchers had found high levels of lead in the Flint water supply, noting that the water was likely corroding the plumbing lines (Edwards, 2015). In October 2015, the Flint water supply was switched back to Detroit water from Lake Huron, but by then, Flint residents had been drinking and bathing in the tainted water for over a year. In January 2016, President Obama declared federal emergency status to help resolve the water issues (EPA, 2017a).

In the meantime, researchers from Flint's Hurley Children's Hospital conducted a spatial analysis of risk and pre–/post–water system change blood lead levels for over 700 Flint children tested in their facility. They found statistically significant changes in elevated blood lead level (EBLL) in blood collected between the months of January to September 2014, compared to blood drawn from January to September 2015. Before the water system change, 2.4% of Flint children had EBLL, but after the change, the proportion increased to 4.9%; those children living outside Flint with no change in water source had no significant changes and low levels of lead in both samples. There were also statistically significant changes noted on demographic data, with higher proportions of African American children and greater levels for those with socioeconomic disadvantages. The "preexisting disparity in lead poisoning" broadened for those children living in Flint, especially for those with high levels of lead in their home water supply (Hanna-Attisha et al., 2016, p. 286). High blood lead levels can cause learning problems, lower IQ, behavioral issues, attention problems, aggression, and poor academic achievement, and the damage is irreversible (Keuhn, 2016 & Wood, 2019).

By July 2018, the EPA had filed a report of the Flint water crisis and acknowledged lapses in EPA's, Michigan's, and Flint's oversight of water regulations (EPA, 2018e). The EPA agreed to improve the agency's oversight of the Safe Drinking Water Act and revise the Lead and Copper Rule to improve the effectiveness of drinking water monitoring requirements. Although this revision reduced the amount of lead required to trigger action from 15 to 10 parts per billion, critics note that enforcement requirements still appear weak and do not mandate removal of underground lead pipes (Dennis, 2019; EPA, 2018e, 2020h). Studies following the water crisis found that there was a 26% increase in White mothers delivering low-birth-weight babies (there was no statistical significance for Black mothers) during that time (Abouk & Adams, 2018). Additionally, 40% of parents surveyed reported changes in their child's health and 65% reported changes in their own health (Heard-Garris et al., 2017). In 2016, criminal charges were filed against nine city and state officials for tampering with evidence, conspiracy, willful neglect of duty, and misconduct; these were dismissed but may be refiled (Kennedy, 2016). Residents are angry and no longer trust officials at any level of government to provide them with clean water (Wood, 2019).

Other communities will be affected by this issue. In 2019, the city of Newark, New Jersey, finally admitted that the city's water had problems with lead levels and distributed water filters on a limited basis. The filters were ineffective; residents needed bottled water because of "ineffective corrosion treatment" at the water treatment plant that permitted lead to leach into the water supply (Fitzsimmons, 2019, para. 9).

It may be decades until we realize the full health impact of this crisis, as more cities with older buildings and infrastructure discover problems with their water. C/PHNs are among those who continue to be concerned about the current situation as well as the long-term consequences of lead exposure for the citizens of Flint, Michigan. Given the recent findings of the potential for multigenerational epigenetic changes in grandchildren linked to lead exposure in pregnant women, this environmental exposure has exponential potential for harm (Sen et al., 2015).

1. *What is the role of the community/public health nurse in addressing this issue? Which primary, secondary, and tertiary interventions could be applied?*
2. *Describe ethical issues, and potential health and social repercussions, related to this case.*
3. *List issues related to environmental justice in this case and describe how to address them.*

Source: Abouk & Adams (2018); Dennis (2019); Edwards (2015); Fitzsimmons (2019); Hanna-Attisha et al. (2016); Heard-Garris et al., 2017; Kennedy (2016); Keuhn (2016); Rosner (2016); Sen et al. (2015); U.S. Environmental Protection Agency (2017a, 2018e); EPA (2020h); Sen et al. (2015); Wood (2019).

state lines where gas or oil extraction is not permitted. An example of this is discussed in Box 9-12.

Food. Food quality, quantity, and safety are essential to human health. Food quality refers to the relative nutritional value, cost, and variety of food available. The CDC estimates that each year more than 3,000 people die from foodborne illness and 1 in 6 Americans becomes ill from food consumption (CDC, 2020).

C/PHNs frequently work closely with environmental sanitarians in state and local health departments who routinely monitor food establishments for their safety to prevent exposure to microbial agents that cause foodborne illness (CDC, 2014).

BOX 9-12 STORIES FROM THE FIELD

Fracking

Laurel is a small community in rural northeastern Pennsylvania where the local citizens have become concerned about their drinking water as a result of fracking activities. In your work in the local community hospital, you have noted more pediatric hospital admissions for asthma exacerbations, and a recent study pointed out that children exposed to Pennsylvania's newly drilled gas wells were 1.25 (OR 95% CI: 1.07, 1.47) times more likely to be hospitalized for an asthma-related diagnosis compared with children who did not live near gas wells (Willis, Jusko, Halterman, & Hill, 2018).

Community members also reported feeling powerless as they noted health problems and were concerned about the quality of their air and water; yet, the elected officials and government agencies were not responding to their concerns (McDermott-Levy & Garcia, 2016). Meanwhile, nurses and other health professionals in New York state, to the north of Laurel, were attending town halls and meeting with state and federal policy makers to prevent Pennsylvania's natural gas from coming through their communities via the new proposed pipeline. The New York health professionals cited air quality, water quality, and safety concerns related to the required infrastructure to transport the gas through their region and on to New England.

In 2012, the ANA passed a resolution, "Nurses' Role in Recognizing, Educating, and Advocating for Healthy Energy Choices," that states nurses must be knowledgeable about the health risks involved with fossil fuel energy, such as fracking (McDermott-Levy et al., 2013). Because the local community shows great trust in nurses and seeks advice from nurses in hospitals, schools, and community settings, it is important for all nurses to understand and provide education for community members about this health concern.

1. *How might you learn more about hydraulic fracturing and the associated health risks?*
2. *Describe the role of the nurse working in communities where hydraulic fracturing occurs.*
3. *Describe how an interdisciplinary approach might be used to address the health issues of Laurel, PA, and in the state of New York.*
4. *How might you identify issues related to environmental justice in this scenario?*

Source: McDermott-Levy et al. (2013); McDermott-Levy & Garcia (2016); Willis et al. (2018).

Environmental issues that affect food quality extend beyond the microbial exposures and include the availability of adequate nutritious food, chemical exposures through food additives and from agrichemicals and antibiotics, contaminated food from diseased animals, and improper food handling. Pesticides are ubiquitous in the environment and are transmitted to humans through foods (EPA, 2020). Fresh fruits and vegetables must be thoroughly washed to remove pesticide residue. In addition, antibiotics fed to animals in animal feeding operations are transmitted through this food (EPA, 2017b).

After production, many foods are processed for market. Food additives such as dyes and flavors provide the color and often improve flavor of foods. Leavening and thickening agents improve consistency, while preservatives keep food from spoiling on the shelf. Many of these additives can be harmful to health with examples being linked to cancer and endocrine disruption. Recently, there is a concern about genetically modified foods being marketed. These concerns not only address the safety of the food for human consumption but also raise questions about the ecological impact and sustainability.

Microbial outbreaks are common from a variety of bacteria (*Shigella*, *Salmonella*, *Campylobacter*, *Escherichia coli*) and parasites (*Cryptosporidium parvum*, *Amoeba*; CDC, 2020). In 2018, for example, there were two national recalls of romaine lettuce as the result of *E. coli* O157:H7 contamination. FDC, state and local authorities, and CDC joined to investigate food contamination outbreaks, isolate the cause, and inform health professionals and the public (CDC, 2020).

Although the public often hears about these outbreaks through the media, they may not be as aware of the risks from chemical contaminants. A great resource for families and community members is the Partnership for Food Safety Education (2018) that promotes safe food handling and education for both children and adults.

The U.S. Food and Drug Administration (FDA) is charged with the responsibility to ensure the safety of food produced, shipped, imported, and sold in the United States. This includes the monitoring of microbial toxins and chemicals such as lead and cadmium, pesticides, food additives, and packaging (EPA, 2020; Johnson, 2016; Maffini, Neltner, & Vogel, 2017).

Although the FDA operates to ensure that the genetically modified foods meet the same safety standards as other foods, the technology used to modify or engineer new food varieties from plant and animal breeding techniques is expanding rapidly (FDA, 2020).

Fish and other seafood are an important part of food safety. Nurses should be aware and instruct communities to monitor fish advisories (EPA, 2019a). The advisories warn consumers of contaminants (mercury, PCBs, chlordane, dioxins, and DDT). These contaminants persist in the environment, particularly in river and lake sediments where fish consume them from bottom-feeding organisms (Fig. 9-6).

Bioaccumulation refers to the process where toxins accumulate in greater concentration in an organism than the rate of elimination. Toxins can accumulate from direct exposure or from eating contaminated food products. Through biomagnification, the toxins present at lower levels of the food chain are in greater concentration in those species further up the chain.

Therefore, humans who eat contaminated fish are exposed to toxins at all levels across the food chain. Public health nurse and Georgetown University faculty member, Dr. Laura Anderko (2015), has been involved with fish advisories for many years. In collaboration with the EPA, she prepared the educational set of four modules on this topic: *Fish Facts for Health Professionals: Methylmercury Exposure, Fish Consumption, and Health Risks/Benefits*. This is available through the Web site (www.fishfacts.org).

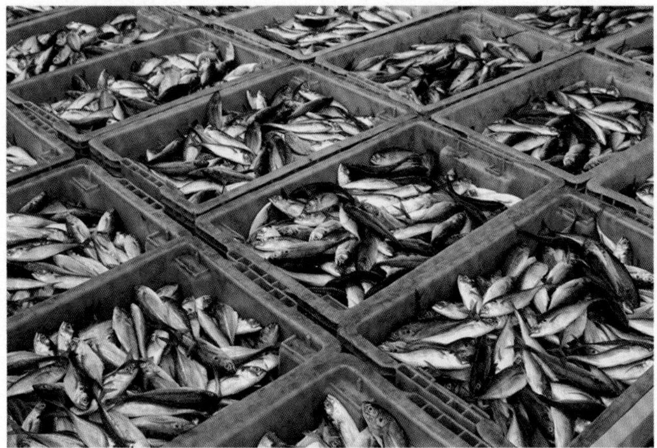

FIGURE 9-6 Fish contain valuable nutrients, but contaminated waterways can make fish a health risk.

Vulnerable Groups. C/PHNs must also be aware of the increased vulnerability of certain groups. For example, pregnant women are likely to transmit their exposure to chemicals, pesticides, and toxins to the unborn fetus, children are more susceptible to hazards from food because of their immature gastrointestinal systems and increased food intake per size compared to adults, and those with altered immunity due to cancer, diabetes, and other health conditions are more likely to be affected by food exposures.

Nurses can be a resource to ensure that community members learn about the specific local risks and identify ways to decrease their risk. The EPA produces a booklet entitled *Citizen's Guide to Pesticides and Pesticide Safety* that is available from their Web site (EPA, 2005). The booklet is written to help nonprofessionals understand pesticides. Although it is not directly focused upon food, it helps community members understand the hazards present in pesticides and strategies to reduce their use and to ensure safety when using pesticides.

The Pesticide Action Network (2018) uses data from the USDA Pesticide Program to identify commonly applied pesticides for many foods. Consumers can consult their Web site to be informed of foods that pose the most serious threats to health, particularly for the most vulnerable groups.

In addition, the effect of climate change on weather extremes (droughts, foods, and storms), changes in rainfall and water supply for soil, rising atmospheric greenhouse gases, and the ecology of microbial growth will have negative impacts upon the food supply. Extreme weather events increase the likelihood of chemical contaminants and pesticide exposures from runoff that occurs with flooding.

Agriculture and fisheries industries are sensitive to specific climate conditions related to changes in temperature and levels of CO_2 in the atmosphere (EPA, 2019b; Smith & Fazil, 2019). Additionally, our changing climate has led to loss of nutritional content (Zhu et al., 2018) and impact on water resources and crop production (Blanc, Caron, Fant, & Monier, 2017).

Globally, these changes can also affect human health. Scientists report the risks for waterborne and foodborne pathogens in drinking water, seafood, and fresh produce from climate variability and the potential for ecological changes that can affect watershed and drainage (EPA, 2019a).

Toxic Waste. Individuals, families, schools, governmental agencies, health care facilities, and industries all create waste that must be managed to minimize environmental impact and to protect human health. The EPA reports that in 2017, Americans generated about 267 million tons of municipal solid waste. This comes to 4.51 lb of waste per person, per day (EPA, 2020c).

In an effort to minimize waste and environmental impact, local, state, and federal agencies have begun supporting sustainable practices that highlight the environmental value of reducing and reusing products. The EPA offers a waste management hierarchy that highlights (this image would be good to include) the value of reducing and reusing materials as a priority and recycling is the second level, when the items are not able to be reused (EPA, 2020c).

In particular, our use of plastics and its ecological impact on sea life highlights the importance of reducing and reusing products. The waste management hierarchy offers an upstream approach of reducing waste at the source of waste generation. For health care facilities, this can mean environmentally preferred purchasing of products that are less toxic, contain recycled materials, more energy efficient, and are safer and healthier for patients, health care workers, and the environment (Health Care Without Harm, 2020a).

Although efforts are made to reduce health risk, hazardous wastes continue to be produced. These wastes include solvent wastes, dioxins, and wastes from electroplating and other metal finishing operations, wastes from oil refineries, organic chemicals, pesticides, explosives, lead processing materials, and wood preservatives. We are exposed to these chemicals if they are aerosolized into the ambient air, leach into ground or wells, and reach the soil where children play, or crops are produced. What is particularly dangerous for human exposure is the fact that most community members are unaware of the hazards in their communities.

Communities may be burdened with many brownfield sites, as well as those listed on the National Priorities List of hazardous sites as Superfund sites (EPA, 2018j). Popular media such as books, films, newspapers, television, and social media may be the first place that nurses become aware of communities affected by toxic waste. The Flint water crisis was played out in the news and chronicled in Dr. Mona Hanna-Attisha's book, *What the Eyes Don't See.* Nurses should be knowledgeable about the toxic hazards in their own communities and those where the patients and families they care for reside. Through the EPA Superfund Web site (EPA, 2018j), nurses can assist community members in learning about Superfund sites that impact their communities. Further, on the EPA Brownfields Web site, nurses and community members can learn about *Brownfields Near You* (EPA, 2019g). It is important for the nurse to be alert for reports of toxic exposure risk, evaluate the science and toxicological risk, and advocate for community/public health.

Radiation. Humans are exposed to radiation in a variety of forms. Risks and forms of radiation are generally categorized as ionizing and nonionizing radiation. Ionization refers to the process where the atomic particle (ion) breaks away from the nucleus of the atom. Ionizing radiation occurs in natural forms as radon gas and cosmic radiation from the atmosphere. Nonionizing radiation refers to radiation from sources such as infrared, microwave, and radio wave radiation (EPA, 2020i).

Radon is an odorless, ionizing, radioactive gas. Radon can seep into the foundation of homes from the ground and expose residents to the radiation effects. Radon exposure is a leading cause of lung cancer.

Nurses must be aware of areas with high radon risk and should be sure that community members are educated about the risks of radon. Community members can access the EPA's *A Citizen's Guide to Radon: The Guide to Protecting Yourself and Your Family from Radon* from their Web site (EPA, 2020i). EPA map of radon zones is available at https://www.epa.gov/sites/production/files/2015-07/documents/zonemapcolor.pdf

Policy Development

Community/public health nurses participate in the other core functions of public health for environmental health nursing. Policy development is the core function that addresses the need for legislation to protect human health. In addition, policy development also provides opportunities for nurses to engage with communities in addressing policies specific to their needs (CDC, 2018c).

To advocate for change, C/PHN must be informed about the community hazards, existing legislation, and governmental and nongovernmental groups that can be partners in the efforts to protect health (Leffers & Butterfield, 2018).

Nurses can begin their environmental advocacy by writing letters to their legislators in support of health-protective laws such as sustainable energy choices, improved air quality, or ecological agricultural practices. Important nursing actions related to environmental policy are to advocate for health-protective policies and to inform community members about the health risks related to the specific issue (Moyer, 2016).

Additionally, letters to local newspapers and periodicals can remind community members of safe practices in the home and personal environment. Nurses can also present testimony at public forums or hearings (Waddell, Audette, DeLong, & Brostoff, 2016). As knowledgeable and trusted members of the community, C/PHN help to educate and empower community members; nurses in many other settings are also realizing the benefits of population-based advocacy (Christopher, Duhl, Rosati, & Sheehan, 2015); (Waddell et al., 2016).

C/PHN serve on local and national committees and boards to advocate for change. Examples of agencies where nurses play an advocacy role are the Children's Environmental Health Network, Just Green Partnership, local and country environmental groups, state nurses association environmental affairs committees, and Health Care Without Harm, to name just a few. Nurses engaged in environmental health research can share the findings of successful environmental health nursing interventions to promote policy change (Snell, 2015).

For nurses to function effectively as advocates for safer environments, it is essential to be aware of important legislation for environmental health. Nurses can also use the *EnviRN* Web site to follow current advocacy efforts in nursing practice (ANHE, 2019). For more on policy development and advocacy, see Chapter 13. See thePoint for a list of important legislation related to environmental protection.

Assurance

The regulatory function for policy ensures that appropriate services are provided. This public health function demands that C/PHNs must incorporate environmental health principles into practice (ANA, 2015b; Leffers & Butterfield, 2018).

For example, a nurse can educate families to reduce their risks from environmental hazards in the home, an OHN will ensure that safety regulations are followed in the work settings, or a school nurse can ensure that indoor air quality is monitored for the school setting. Assurance guarantees that policy and regulatory functions are followed through the provision of public health essential services. The following examples illustrate how community nurses fulfill the assurance function.

Home

People spend 90% of their time in their homes. To assure that nurses are prepared to address environmental risks to health in home settings, competencies for nursing education include home assessment strategies (Leffers et al., 2017). Nurses working with families and in communities participate in research programs and collaborative projects that impact home environments.

To address some of those health issues, particularly for children, the U.S. Department of Housing and Urban Development (USHUD, 2018) created the Healthy Home Intuitive (HHI) to protect children and their families from health and safety hazards in their homes (Ashley, 2015). The program targets multiple childhood diseases and injuries in the home by using a comprehensive approach. Some of the environmental health concerns addressed include lead, carbon monoxide, pesticides, radon, mold, home safety, and asthma.

In New York, the Erie County Health Department took an upstream approach and addressed lead exposure, carbon monoxide, falls, and burn risks for low-income families before they moved into their homes (USHUD, 2018). In Ohio, C/PHN collaborated with other professionals (program manager, health educator, sanitarians, community outreach worker) through a Healthy Homes Program Grant to perform housing control assessments, education, and interventions in housing units. The interventions included home visits and education, and they were found to reduce asthma symptoms, school days missed, workdays missed, and the number of emergency room visits for asthma events. Results continued 6 months postintervention (Sweet, Polivka, Chaudry, & Bouton, 2014).

Severe Weather Events

A second area for nurses to assure that essential services are provided to community members is in response to severe weather events (Fig. 9-7). Although studies indicate

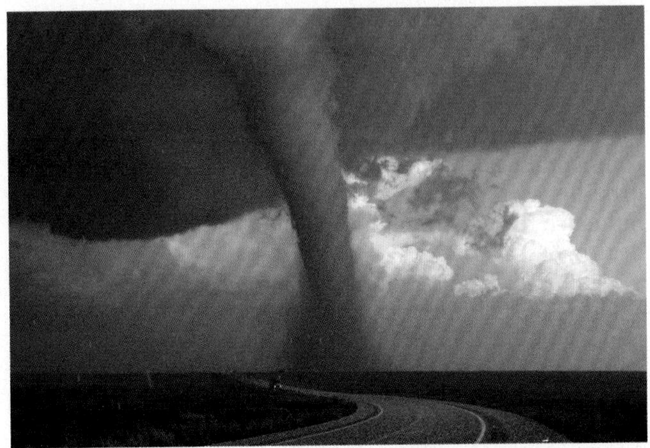
A

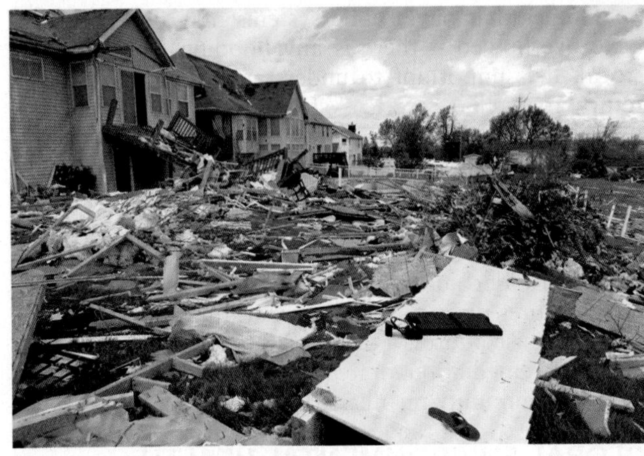
B

FIGURE 9-7 Severe weather, like tornadoes, can have a serious impact on the environment and population health.

that nurses are involved in disaster response, results indicate that nurses are not always prepared for their role in emergency response situations (Usher et al., 2015; Yan, Turale, Stone, & Petrini, 2015).

The United States is experiencing more frequent and severe weather events. In 2018, extreme weather events caused damage and destruction across the United States. Colorado, Maryland, Michigan, North Carolina, South Carolina, and Wisconsin all experienced 1,000-year rainfall events with severe flooding. A 1,000-year event means that there is a 0.1% chance of such rainfall occurring in any given year (The Weather Chanel, 2018).

In addition, California experienced devastating wildfires (Box 9-13), Alaska had a 7.0-magnitude earthquake, and EF3 tornadoes were reported in Montana, South Dakota, and Virginia. Loss of power and homes, and disruption of services from flooding, fires, earthquakes, tornados, and hurricanes, put many people at risk from natural disasters. Category 5 hurricanes ravaged the Bahamas and Puerto Rico (Korten, 2019).

Whereas Chapter 17 discusses disasters and the role for public health, this chapter covers some specific issues related to environmental risks that occur after severe weather events or disasters that are important for C/PHNs. These include power outages, safe water and food supply, wastewater, mold, toxic exposures, and poor air quality (EPA, 2012, 2020g).

For example, when there is a power outage, many families depend upon generators to supply electricity. These can be a source of carbon monoxide poisoning if not effectively functioning or not well ventilated. During cold weather, families may use wood or kerosene for heat that can pose danger of fire, explosion, and asphyxiation from carbon monoxide, but kerosene heaters can also emit other pollutants including carbon dioxide, nitrogen dioxide, and sulfur dioxide.

In particular, pregnant women, asthmatics, individuals with cardiovascular disease, older adults, and young children are at particular risk from these toxic emissions. Nurses must inform community members of safety in the home when using alternate sources of heat or power (Wisconsin Department of Health Services, n.d.).

If a home is without power, there is a risk for food storage and safety. If the home has a well and water pump, there may not be access to potable water during the power outage. Community members should be informed of issues related to safe storage of food and the need to dispose of improperly refrigerated foods.

BOX **9-13** PERSPECTIVES

A Nurse's Viewpoint on a California Wildfire

In November 2018, California experienced the worst wildfire in its history to date. Eighty-eight people lost their lives and 12,000 homes were destroyed. The town of Paradise, California, was engulfed in flames, and nurse manager, Allyn Pierce, was among the last to evacuate patients from the town's hospital. As they traveled through the evacuation route with heavy traffic and smoke fires burned on both sides of the road, Mr. Pierce knew that his family had already been evacuated to safety days earlier. After a harrowing evacuation, he returned to the hospital to assist first responders, physicians, and other nurses help smoke inhalation victims and those with more serious injuries. Afterwards, Mr. Pierce reported that although he was frightened for his own safety, he did what nurses are trained to do, remain calm, work within the team, and address the situation. He also reported that following the wildfires, he has had unsettling moments where he sees fires in his sleep.

In addition to the loss of life and property, the air quality in the surrounding area had reached the "dangerously unhealthy" range for 10 consecutive days requiring San Francisco bay area (roughly 170 miles away) to close schools and issue warnings to limit outdoor activity.

Source: Santiago (2018).

Homes that have septic systems may find that they have overflowed if there is any flooding from a severe storm. It is important to understand when it is safe to return to well or septic system use after ground-level flooding.

Floods also pose a problem to residents who have water enter their homes. Standing water can cause mold and mildew, possibly harm home furnaces, pose a risk of fire, and release toxins into the water and air. Small children and older adults are at more risk of environmental exposures during and after a natural disaster, and the C/PHN must address not only emergency planning but also safe remediation strategies to avoid toxic exposures among community members (EPA, 2020g).

GLOBAL ENVIRONMENTAL HEALTH

Nurses must engage in strategies to protect human health in their communities through the core functions of public health: assessment, policy development, and assurance. To effectively do this, nurses must think globally in order to be effective locally. This means adopting an ecological perspective related to impacts on human health.

By broadening our perspectives, consideration of foods imported from countries around the world, toys made in other countries and used in the United States, and the manufacture of products in locations where the regulations for safety are not as stringent (or in some cases more stringent) as in the United States is helpful for nurses in addressing environmental health knowledge and advocacy. See Chapter 7 for an example.

Nurses who endorse “green nursing” by promoting more ecological and environmentally safe practices in their workplace are making an impact upon global environmental health. The UN SDGs call on us to think more broadly as global citizens of the multiple factors that influence thriving communities and thus enhance human health. See Chapter 16.

Climate change reinforces that we are one ecosystem. What is placed in the environment, in the form of greenhouse gases affects the entire planet and the human family. Although it is now illegal in most countries to dump waste into the ocean or to ship waste to less developed countries that have less stringent laws to protect their citizens from toxins, large quantities of toxic industrial waste, medical waste, toxic ash from incinerators, as well as the growing issue of e-waste from computers and other electronic products, have found their way to ocean waters and poorer countries. In order to fully promote the health of populations, nurses must take personal action to reduce their use of products (particularly those with toxic chemicals), reuse as much as possible, and recycle (in safe processes) to decrease their personal environmental footprint (ANA, 2015a; EPA, 2020c). Nurses must also incorporate the environmental health knowledge and skills mandated by the ANA *Scope and Standards of Nursing Practice* into their nursing practice (ANA, 2015b). See Chapter 16 for more on global health issues.

SUMMARY

- Environmental health is a discipline encompassing all of the elements of the environment that influence the health and well-being of its inhabitants.
- C/PHNs include environmental health in their practice by:
  - Accessing environmental information from reliable resources
  - Relying on environmental frameworks such as HIA and the precautionary principle to determine and address risk
  - Utilizing an upstream approach to reduce environmental risk
  - Monitoring for causal links between people and their environments
  - Including an ecologic perspective by linking the human–environment relationship and how the health of one affects the health of the other
  - Addressing specific needs of groups that are vulnerable to environmental risk
  - Understanding that what is done today may affect the health of future generations
- Both public and private sectors are involved in regulating, monitoring, and preventing environmental health problems.
- Utilizing the core functions for public health, the C/PHN recognizes the key role of assessment, assurance, and policy development to influence change in the health of individuals, families, communities, and the environment.
- The C/PHN should be a leader of the team of health professionals who promote and protect the reciprocal relationship between the environment and the public’s health.

ACTIVE LEARNING EXERCISES

1. How important is engaging in climate mitigation and adaptation? This effort has met with resistance from a variety of people. There are several organizations that have examined messaging climate and health risk.
   a. Examine the Yale Climate Opinion Map at http://climatecommunication.yale.edu/visualizations-data/ycom-us-2018/?est=personal&type=value&geo=county&id=42029.
   b. Select your state and county or a state and county of interest.
   c. Choice five topics in the select topic response for the selected state and county. Look at the county level response to the topic you selected. Were you surprised by the response? Why or why not? How can you address this as a C/PHN?

2. Review EcoAmerica's *15 Steps to Create Effective Climate Communications* found at https://ecoamerica.org/wp-content/uploads/2017/03/5_ea_15_steps.pdf
   a. Given what you learned about the county you examined in question 1, how would you communicate climate risk with the selected county?
   b. Would you change the message between your selected group and your family? Why is there or is there not a difference in your communication?
3. Have you heard alerts on TV or radio or seen Internet reports about unhealthy air quality? Do you know what toxic substances are in your community's air? How do these may impact you and sensitive groups such as children and older adults?
   a. You can find out by examining the EPA's MyEnvironment and AirNow Web sites (http://www.airnow.gov/). Other helpful sites may be found through the CDC, the EPA, and local air resources board or agencies. Go on a computer scavenger hunt and see what you can find.
   b. Look around your city or neighborhood. What are the most common environmental hazards? Visit the EPA "MyEnvironment" site. Look at the AQI and air facilities on the map on this site. Be sure to read about radon too. How might these impact the air you breathe?
   c. Find the AirNow Web site and enter your zip code. For your city or area, which three companies have the highest amounts of emissions? Are there any VOCs, metals, or polycyclic aromatic hydrocarbons listed for the top company?
   d. If you were an OHN, what safety measures would you want in place to respond to accidental exposures to these chemicals? What could you do for emergency first aid until assistance arrives?
   e. If you were a school nurse, what would be your concerns for the children's exposures to air pollution?
   f. If you were a home care nurse, what would be your concerns for the elderly patients you care for?
4. To explore personal care and cleaning products in the hospital setting, on the ToxTown site (https://toxtown.nlm.nih.gov), next to Sources of Exposure, click on "Explore," scroll down to Health Care Services, and then click on the "Hospitals" link.
   a. Select one possible chemical exposure in the hospital setting. Read the information about exposure risk including the ASTDR Web site source offered at the bottom of the web page.
   b. Select a personal care product that you use (shampoo, conditioner, moisturizer, deodorant, etc.). Visit the EWG Web site Skin Deep database https://www.ewg.org/skindeep/ of commonly used products. Search for the item you selected and identify the risks posed to your personal health and that of your patients.
   c. Visit the DHHS Web site for the Household Products Database (https://householdproducts.nlm.nih.gov), and examine other a common product that you use at home (cleanser, pet care products, pesticide). Review the information for health risks.
   d. Finally, consider a population group (neonates, adolescents, older adults) in the community that might be at risk when using any of the products you reviewed, and consider how you might educate that group about their exposures.
5. As a nursing student, it is important to know about common community hazards in order to educate community members. Visit the EPA's MyEnvironment Web site, and enter you home zip code or that of the community where you work. The link for this site is http://www3.epa.gov/enviro/myenviro/.
   There you will find headings for MyMaps, MyAir, MyWater, MyEnergy, MyHealth, MyClimate, MyLand, MyEnvironmentReports, and MyCommunity.
   a. Look through these headings to identify the hazards in your community. What is the air quality? Are there particular industries, power plants, or high areas for auto emissions that affect health? What about water quality? Are there significant toxic waste sites? What types of exposures are there in the community?
   b. Can you identify possible risks from climate change and severe weather events? What might be ways to assure emergency preparedness for those most at risk?
   c. Using the framework for this chapter, the core public health functions, select a strategy that is most appropriate for your community for each area: assessment, policy development, and assurance.
6. Conduct a walking tour of a community. Consider housing stock, industry, the built environment, and open space.
   a. What do you observe that could be an environmental risk for this community?
   b. Do you observe specific vulnerable populations in the community?
   c. Use the resources at the EPA Web site, including MyEnvironment, and develop a list of five recommendations to reduce environmental health risk in the community you observed. Identify why these are an environmental health risk for this community.
   d. Describe which of the 10 essential public health services applies here.

REFERENCES

Abouk, R., & Adams, S. (2018). Birth outcomes in Flint in the early stages of the water crisis. *Journal of Public Health Policy, 38*(1), 68–85.

AirNow.gov. (n.d.). *Air quality flag program*. Retrieved from https://www.airnow.gov/air-quality-flag-program/

Al Jishi, T., & Sergi, C. (2017). Current perspectives of diethylstilbestrol (DES) exposure in mothers and offspring. *Reproductive Toxicology, 71*, 71–77.

Alliance of Nurses for Healthy Environments (ANHE). (2019). *History of AHNE*. Retrieved from https://envirn.org/about/

American Association of Occupational Health Nurses. (2020). *What is occupational & environmental health nursing?* Retrieved from http://aaohn.org/page/profession-of-occupational-and-environmental-health-nursing

American Nurses Association (ANA). (2007). *ANA's principles of environmental health for nursing practice with implementation strategies*. Silver Spring, MD: Author.

American Nurses Association (ANA). (2015a). *Medical waste*. Retrieved from http://www.nursingworld.org/MainMenuCategories/WorkplaceSafety/Healthy-Work-Environment/Environmental-Health/Issues/Facility/MedicalWaste

American Nurses Association (ANA). (2015b). *Nursing: Scope and standards of practice* (3rd ed.). Silver Spring, MD: Author.

American Nurses Association (ANA). (2010). Nursing: *Scope and standards of practice* (2nd ed.). Silver Spring, MD: Author.

American Public Health Association (APHA). (2005). *Environmental health principles for public health nursing*. Washington, DC: Author.

Anderko, L. (2015). *Fish facts for health professionals: Methylmercury exposure, fish consumption, and health risks/benefits*. Retrieved from http://www.fish-facts.org/fishfactsworkbook.pdf

Ashley, P. J. (2015). HUD's healthy homes program: Progress and future directions. *Journal of Environmental Health, 78*(2), 50–53.

Blanc, E., Caron, J., Fant, C., & Monier, E. (2017). Is current irrigation sustainable in the United States? An integrated assessment of climate change impact on water resources and irrigated crop yields. *Earth's Future, 5*(8), 877–892.

Brenan, M. (2018). *Nurses again outpace other professions for honesty, ethics*. Gallup, Inc. Retrieved from https://news.gallup.com/poll/245597/nurses-again-outpace-professions-honesty-ethics.aspx

Brugge, D.D. (2016). Why has it taken so long to address the problems created by uranium mining in the Navajo Nation? *New Solutions, 25*(4), 436–439.

Butterfield, P. G. (1990). Thinking upstream: Nurturing a conceptual understanding of the societal context of health behavior. *Advances in Nursing Science, 12*(2), 1–8.

Butterfield, P. G. (2002). Upstream reflections on environmental health: An abbreviated history and framework for action. *Advances in Nursing Science, 25*(1), 32–49.

Butterfield, P. G. (2017). Thinking upstream: A 25-year retrospective and conceptual model aimed at reducing health inequities. *Advances in Nursing Science, 40*(1), 2–11.

Butterfield, P. G., Hill, W., Postma, J., Butterfield, P. W., & Odom-Maryon, T. (2011). Effectiveness of a household environmental health intervention delivered by rural public health nurses. *American Journal of Public Health, 101*(S1), S262–S270.

Centers for Disease Control and Prevention (CDC). (2014). *Environmental public health performance standards (Version 2.0)*. Retrieved from https://www.cdc.gov/nceh/ehs/envphps/docs/EnvPHPSv2.pdf

Centers for Disease Control and Prevention (CDC). (2016). *10 essential environmental public health services*. Retrieved from https://www.cdc.gov/nceh/ehs/10-essential-services/index.html

Centers for Disease Control and Prevention (CDC). (2017a). *Environmental public health performance standards (Env)PHPS*. Retrieved from https://www.cdc.gov/nceh/ehs/envphps/default.htm

Centers for Disease Control and Prevention (CDC). (2017b). *National biomonitoring program*. Retrieved from https://www.cdc.gov/biomonitoring/index.html

Centers for Disease Control and Prevention (CDC). (2018a). *Multistate Outbreak of E. coli O157:H7 Infections linked to romaine lettuce (Final Update)*. Retrieved from https://www.cdc.gov/ecoli/2018/o157h7-04-18/index.html

Centers for Disease Control and Prevention (CDC). (2018b). *One Health Basics*. Retrieved from https://www.cdc.gov/onehealth/basics/index.html

Centers for Disease Control and Prevention (CDC). (2018c). *The public health system & the 10 essential public health services*. Retrieved from https://www.cdc.gov/publichealthgateway/publichealthservices/essentialhealthservices.html

Centers for Disease Control and Prevention (CDC). (2020). *Foodborne germs and illnesses*. Retrieved from http://www.cdc.gov/foodsafety/foodborne-germs.html

Chakraborty, J., Collins, T. W., & Grineski, S. E. (2016). Environmental justice research: Contemporary issues and emerging topics. *International Journal of Research and Public Health, 13*(11), 1072. Retrieved from https://www.ncbi.nlm.nih.gov/pmc/articles/PMC5129282/

Chan, L. M., Chalupka, S. M., & Barrett, R. (2015). Female college student awareness of exposures to environmental toxins in personal care products and their effect on preconception health. *Workplace Health & Safety, 63*(2), 64–70.

Chaudry, R. V. (2008). The precautionary principle, public health, and public health nursing. *Public Health Nursing, 25*(3), 261–268.

Christopher, A., Duhl, J., Rosati, R., & Sheehan, K. (2015). Advocacy for vulnerable patients: How grassroots organizations can influence health care policy. *American Journal of Nursing, 115*(3), 66–69.

City of Richmond CA. (n.d.). *Health in all policies (HIAP) report*. Retrieved from http://www.ci.richmond.ca.us/2575/Health-in-All-Policies-HiAP

Cole, C. (2018). Particulate matter exposure and health impacts of urban cyclists: a randomized crossover study. *Environmental Health, 17*(1), 78.

Costello A, Abbas M, Allen A, Ball S, Bell, S, Bellamy R., ... Patterson C. (2009). Managing the health effects of climate change: Lancet and University College London Institute for Global Health Commission. *Lancet*, 33, 1693–1733.

Costello, A., Montgomery, H., & Watts, N. (2013). Climate change: The challenge for healthcare professionals. *British Medical Journal, 347*, f6060. https://doi.org/10.1126/bmj.f6060

Dalton, M. (2017). U.S. withdrawal from climate deal draws rebuke, resolve from leaders. *The Wall Street Journal*, June 1. Retrieved from **https://www.wsj.com/articles/u-s-withdrawal-leaves-paris-accord-in-limbo-1496346071**

Davis, A. (2007). Home environmental health risks. *OJIN*: The Online Journal of Issues in Nursing, 12(4), 4. Retrieved from http://ojin.nursingworld.org/MainMenuCategories/ANAMarketplace/ANAPeriodicals/OJIN/TableofContents/Volume122007/No2May07/HomeEnvironmentalHealthRisks.html

Dennis, B. (October 10, 2019). For the first time in decades, EPA is overhauling how communities must test for lead in water. *The Washington Post*. Retrieved from https://www.washingtonpost.com/climate-environment/2019/10/10/first-time-decades-epa-is-overhauling-how-communities-must-test-lead-water/

Desmond, S. (2016). Implementing climate change mitigation in health services: The importance of context. *Journal of Health Services Research & Policy, 21*(4), 257–262.

Diaz-Sanchez, S., D'Souza, D., Biswas, D., & Hanning, I. (2015). Botanical alternatives to antibiotics for use in organic poultry production. *Poultry Science, 94*(6), 1419–1430.

Edwards, M. (September 8, 2015). *Our sampling of 252 homes demonstrates a high lead in water risk: Flint should be failing to meet the EPA Lead and Copper Rule*. Retrieved from http://flintwaterstudy.org/2015/09/our-sampling-of-252-homes-demonstrates-a-high-lead-in-water-risk-flint-should-be-failing-to-meet-the-epa-lead-and-copper-rule/

Eliperin, J., & Dennis, B. (2019). Administration finalizes repeal of 2015 water rule Trump called 'destructive and horrible'. *The Washington Post*. Retrieved from https://www.washingtonpost.com/climate-environment/administration-finalizes-repeal-of-2015-water-rule-trump-called-destructive-and-horrible/2019/09/11/fddfa49a-d4aa-11e9-9343-40db57cf6abd_story.html

English, K., Healy, B., Jagais, P., & Sly, P. D. (2015). Assessing exposure of young children to common endocrine disrupting chemicals in the home environment: A review and commentary of the questionnaire approach. *Reviews on Environmental Health, 30*(1), 25–49.

Environmental Working Group. (2019). *Nurses' health: A survey on health and chemical exposures*. Retrieved from https://www.ewg.org/research/nurses-health

Finland National Institute for Health and Welfare (2018). *Human Impact Assessment*. Retrieved from https://thl.fi/en/web/health-promotion/human-impact-assessment

Fitzsimmons, E. G. (August 12, 2019). In echo of Flint lead crisis, Newark offers bottled water after long denial. *The New York Times (Late Edition; East Coast), A17*.

Friis, R. H. (2019). *Essentials of environmental health* (3rd ed.). Burlington, MA: Jones & Bartlett Learning.

Frumkin, H. (2016). *Environmental health: From global to local* (3rd ed.). San Francisco, CA: John Wiley.

Gangemi, S., Gofita, E., Costa, C., Teodoro, M., Briguglio, G., Nikitovic, D., ... Fenga, C. (2016). Occupational and environmental exposure to pesticides and cytokine pathways in chronic diseases (review). *International Journal of Molecular Medicine*, 38(4), 1012–1020.

Grandjean, P., Barouki, R., Bellinger, D. C., Castelevn, L., Chadiwck, L. H., Cordier, S., ... Paige, L. B. (2015). Life-long implications of developmental exposure to environmental stressors: New perspectives. *Endocrinology, 156*(10), 3408–3415. doi: 10.1210/EN.2015-1350.

Haines, A. (2016). Addressing challenges to human health in the Anthropocene epoch—an overview of the findings of the Rockefeller/Lancet Commission on Planetary Health. *Public Health Reviews, 37*, 14. Retrieved from https://www.ncbi.nlm.nih.gov/pmc/articles/PMC5810099/pdf/40985_2016_Article_29.pdf

Hanna-Attisha, M., LaChance, J., Sadler, R. C., & Schnepp, A. C. (2016). Elevated blood lead levels in children associated with the Flint drinking water crisis: A spatial analysis of risk and public health response. *American Journal of Public Health, 106*(2), 283–290.

Health Care Without Harm. (2018). *Leading the global movement for environmentally responsible healthcare*. Retrieved from https://noharm.org/

Health Care Without Harm. (2020a). *Pharmaceutical pollution*. Retrieved from https://noharm-europe.org/content/europe/pharmaceutical-pollution-faqs

Health Care Without Harm. (2020b). *Sustainable procurement*. Retrieved from https://noharm-uscanada.org/issues/us-canada/environmentally-preferable-purchasing

Heard-Garris, N. J., Roche, J., Carter, P., Abir, M., Walton, M., Zimmerman, M., & Cunningham, R. (2017). Voices from Flint: Community perceptions of the Flint water crisis. *Journal of Urban Health, 94*(6), 776–779.

Hofman, H., Samson, R., Joosen, S. Blust, R. & Lenaerts, S. (2018). Cyclist exposure to black carbon, ultrafine particles and heavy metals: An experimental study along two commuting routes near Antwerp, Belgium. *Environmental Research, 164*, 530–538.

Hoover, R. N., Hyer, M., Pfeiffer, R., Adam, E., Bond, B., Cheville, A. L., … Troisi, R. (2011). Adverse health outcomes in women exposed in utero to diethylstilbestrol. *New England Journal of Medicine, 365*, 1304–1314. Retrieved from https://www.nejm.org/doi/full/10.1056/NEJMoa1013961

Howarth, R. (2014). A bridge to nowhere: methane emissions and the greenhouse gas footprint of natural gas. *Energy Science & Engineering, 2*(2): 47–60.

Intergovernmental Panel on Climate Change (IPCC). (2018). *Special Report: Global Warming of 1.5° Celsius*. Retrieved from https://www.ipcc.ch/sr15/

Jarvie, J. (April 23, 2019). On a sinking Louisiana island, many aren't ready to leave. *Los Angeles Times*. Retrieved from https://www.latimes.com/nation/la-na-jean-charles-sinking-louisiana-island-20190423-htmlstory.html

Johnson, R. (December 16, 2016). The federal food safety system: A primer. *Congressional Research Service*. Retrieved from https://fas.org/sgp/crs/misc/RS22600.pdf

Kalkbrenner, A. E., Schmidt, R. J., & Penlesky, A. C. (2014). Environmental chemical exposures and autism spectrum disorders: A review of epidemiological evidence. *Current Problems in Pediatric and Adolescent Health Care, 10*, 277–318. Retrieved from http://www.ncbi.nlm.nih.gov/pubmed/25199954

Kennedy, M. (April 20, 2016). *Lead-laced water in Flint: A step-by-step look at the makings of a crisis*. Retrieved from https://www.npr.org/sections/thetwo-way/2016/04/20/465545378/lead-laced-water-in-flint-a-step-by-step-look-at-the-makings-of-a-crisis

Keuhn, B. M. (2016). Pediatrician sees long road ahead for Flint after lead poisoning crisis. *JAMA, 315*(10), 967–969.

Kim, S. Eom, S., Kim, H. J., Lee, J. J., Choi, G., Choi, S., … Eun, S. H. (2018). Association between maternal exposure to major phthalates, heavy metals, and persistent organic pollutants, and the neurodevelopmental performances of their children at 1 to 2 years of age—CHECK cohort study. *Science of the Total Environment, 15*, 377–384.

Koehler, K., Latshaw, M., Matte, T., Kass, D., Frumkin, H., Fox, M., … Burke, T. A. (2018). Building healthy community environments: A public health approach. *Public Health Reports, 133*(Suppl 1), 35s–43s.

Korten, T. (2019). The Bahamas and the Caribbean have withstood hurricanes for centuries. *Smithsonian Magazine*. Retrieved from https://www.smithsonianmag.com/history/bahamas-and-caribbean-have-withstood-hurricanes-centuries-180973157/

Kurth, A. E. (2017). Planetary health and the role of nursing: A call to action. *Journal of Nursing Scholarship, 49*(6), 598–605. doi: 10.1111/jnu.12343

Leffers, J., & Butterfield, P. (2018). Nurses play essential roles in reducing health problems due to climate change. *Nursing Outlook, 66*(2), 210–213.

Leffers, J., McDermott-Levy, R., Nicholas, P., & Sweeney, C. (2017). Mandate for the nursing profession to address climate change through nursing education. *Journal of Nursing Scholarship, 49* (6), 679–687.

Leffers, J., McDermott-Levy, R., Smith, C. M., & Sattler, B. (2014). Nursing education's response to the 1995 Institute of Medicine report: Nursing, health, and the environment. *Nursing Forum*, 49(44), 214–224. doi: 10.1111/nuf.12072.

Leffers, J., Smith, C., Huffling, K., McDermott-Levy, R., & Sattler, B. (Eds.). (2016). *Environmental health in nursing. ANHE e-book*. Retrieved from https://envirn.org/e-textbook/

Lindsey, R., & Dahlman, L. (September 19, 2019). *Climate change: Global temperature*. Retrieved from https://www.climate.gov/news-features/understanding-climate/climate-change-global-temperature

Maffini, M. V., Neltner, T. G., & Vogel, S. (2017). We are what we eat: Regulatory gaps in the United States that put our health at risk. *PLoS Biology, 15*(12), e2003578. Retrieved from https://www.ncbi.nlm.nih.gov/pmc/articles/PMC5737876/

Marcoux, R. M., & Vogenberg, F. R. (2015). Hazardous waste compliance in health care settings. *Pharmacy and Therapeutics, 40*(2), 115–118.

McDermott-Levy, R. & Garcia, V. (2016). Health concerns of Northeastern Pennsylvania residents living in an unconventional oil and gas development county. *Public Health Nursing, 33*(6), 502–510.

McDermott-Levy, R., Katkins, N., & Sattler, B. (2013). Fracking, the environment, and health: New energy practices may threaten public health. *American Journal of Nursing, 133*(6), 45–51.

McKinley, J. (June, 1979). *A case for focusing upstream: The political economy of illness*. Proceedings of the American Heart Association Conference: Applying Behavioral Science to Cardiovascular Risk, Seattle, WA.

McPartland, J., Dantzker, H., & Portier, C. (2017). Elucidating environmental dimensions of neurological disorders and disease: Understanding new tools from federal chemical testing programs. *Science of the Total Environment, 593–594*, 634–640. Retrieved from https://www.sciencedirect.com/science/article/pii/S0048969717305296?via%3Dihub

Merriam Webster On-Line Dictionary. (2019). *Risk*. Retrieved from https://www.merriam-webster.com/dictionary/risk

Mooney, C., Muyskens, J., Dennis, B., & Freedman, A. (2020). Pollution is plummeting in Italy in the wake of coronavirus, emissions data show. *New York Times*. Retrieved from https://www.washingtonpost.com/climate-environment/2020/03/13/italy-emissions-coronavirus/?arc404=true

Moyer, A. (2016). Using nursing process to guide advocacy for environmental health. In Leffers, J., Smith, C., Huffling, K., McDermott-Levy, R., & Sattler, B. (Eds.), *Environmental Health in Nursing. Alliance of Nurses for Healthy Environments*. Retrieved from https://envirn.org/e-textbook/

National Association of School Nurses (NASN). (2018). *The role of the 21st century school nurse*. Retrieved from https://www.nasn.org/advocacy/professional-practice-documents/position-statements/ps-role

National Cancer Institute. (2018). *Environmental epidemiology*. Retrieved from https://dceg.cancer.gov/about/organization/programs-ebp/oeeb

National Institute of Environmental Health Sciences (NIEHS). (2018). *Environmental health disparities and environmental justice*. Retrieved from https://www.niehs.nih.gov/research/supported/translational/justice/index.cfm

National Institutes of Health (NIH). (2016). *President's Task Force on Environmental Health Risk and Safety to Children*. Retrieved from https://ptfceh.niehs.nih.gov/about/assets/files/health_safty_risks_to_children_508.pdf

National Institute for Occupational Safety and Health (NIOSH). (2017). *Health and Safety Practices. Survey of Healthcare Workers*. Retrieved from **https://www.cdc.gov/niosh/topics/healthcarehsps/default.html**

National Library of Medicine. (2020). *How to access TOXNET information*. Retrieved from https://www.nlm.nih.gov/toxnet/index.html

Nightingale, F. (1969). *Notes on nursing: What it is and what it is not*. New York, NY: Dover Publications, Inc. (Original work published 1860).

Office of Disease Prevention and Health Promotion. (2018). *Proposed objectives for inclusion in Healthy People 2030*. Retrieved from https://www.healthypeople.gov/sites/default/files/ObjectivesPublicComment508_1.17.19.pdf

Office of Disease Prevention and Health Promotion. (2019). *Healthy People*. Retrieved from https://health.gov/our-work/healthy-people/

Office of Disease Prevention and Health Promotion. (2020). *Healthy people 2030 framework*. Retrieved from https://www.healthypeople.gov/2020/About-Healthy-People/Development-Healthy-People-2030/Framework

Oneal, G. A., Eide, P., Hamilton, R., Butterfield, P., & Vandermause, R. (2015). Rural families' process of re-forming environmental health risk messages. *Journal of Nursing Scholarship, 47*(4), 354–362.

Partnership for Food Safety Education. (2018). *Food safety*. Retrieved from http://www.fightbac.org/

Pesticide Action Network. (2018). *What's on my food?* Retrieved from http://whatsinmyfood.org/index.jsp

Podesta, J. (July 25, 2019). The climate crisis, migration, and refugees. *Brookings*. Retrieved from https://www.brookings.edu/research/the-climate-crisis-migration-and-refugees/

Polivka, B., Chaudry, R., & Crawford, J. (2012). Public health nurses' knowledge and attitudes regarding climate change. *Environmental Health Perspectives, 120*(3), 321–325.

Polivka, B. J., Stanley, S. A., Gordon, D., Taulbee, K., Kieffer, G., & McCorkle, S. M. (2008). Public health nursing competencies for public health surge events. *Public Health Nursing, 25*(2), 159–165.

Pope, A. M., Snyder, M. A., & Mood, L. H. (1995). *Nursing, health and the environment: Strengthening the relationship to improve the public's health*. Washington, DC: National Academy Press.

Quattrone, W., Callahan, M., Brown, S., Lin, T., & Pina, J. (2018). Health impact assessment: An information needs analysis of HIA practitioners across sectors. *Chronicles of Health Impact Assessment, 3*(2). 1–13. Retrieved from https://journals.iupui.edu/index.php/chia/article/view/22536/22164

Rabinowitz, P. M. (2018). A planetary vision for one health. *BMJ Global Health, 3*(5), 1–6.

RAND Health. (2015). *Understanding the upstream social determinants of health*. Retrieved from https://www.rand.org/content/dam/rand/pubs/working_papers/WR1000/WR1096/RAND_WR1096.pdf

Robert Wood Johnson Foundation. (2018). *Built environment and health*. Retrieved from https://www.rwjf.org/en/our-focus-areas/topics/built-environment-and-health.html

Rosner, D. (2016). Flint, Michigan: A century of environmental injustice. *American Journal of Public Health, 106*(2), 200–201.

Ruskie, S. E. (2016). All the resources was gone: The environmental context of disaster nursing. *Nursing Clinics of North America, 51*(4), 569–584.

Santiago, E. (November 14, 2018). *Allyn Pierce, Camp Fire hero: 5 fast facts you need to know*. Retrieved from https://heavy.com/news/2018/11/allyn-pierce-camp-fire-hero-toyota/

Schmidt, R. J., Kogan, V., Shelton, J. F., Delwiche, L., Hansen, R. L., Ozonoff, S., … Volk, H. E. (2017). Combined prenatal pesticide exposure and folic acid intake in relation to autism spectrum disorder. *Environmental Health Perspectives, 125*(9), 097007, doi: 10.1289/EHP604

Science and Environmental Health Network (SEHN). (2018). *Precautionary principle*. Retrieved from https://www.sehn.org

Sen, A., Heredia, N., Senut, M. C., Land, S., Hollocher, K., Lu, X., … Ruden, D. M. (2015). Multigenerational epigenetic inheritance in humans: DNA methylation changes associated with maternal exposure to lead can be transmitted to the grandchildren. *Scientific Reports, 5*, 14466.

Slutzman, J. E. (2018). The hidden harm of health care: Air, water, and other pollution. *STAT*. Retrieved from https://www.statnews.com/2018/09/25/pollution-health-care-harm/

Smith, B. A., & Fazil, A. (2019). How will climate change impact microbial foodborne disease in Canada? *Canada Communicable Disease Report, 45*(4), 108–113. Retrieved from https://www.ncbi.nlm.nih.gov/pmc/articles/PMC6587690/

Snell, D. (2015). Leading the way: Implementing a domestic violence assessment pilot project by public health nurses. *Nursing Leadership, 28*(1), 65–72.

Society of Toxicology. (2020). *What is toxicology?* Retrieved from https://www.toxicology.org/about/relevance.asp

St. Cyr, S., & McGowan, P. O. (2018). Adaptation or pathology? The role of prenatal stressor type and intensity in the developmental programing of adult phenotype. *Neurotoxicology and Teratology, 66*, 113–124.

Sweet, L., Polivka, B. J., Chaudry, R. V., & Bouton, P. (2014). Impact of an urban home-based intervention program on asthma outcomes. *Journal of Environmental Health, 73*(9), 16–20.

The Weather Chanel. (2018). *American's "One-in-1000-year" rainfall events*. Retrieved from https://weather.com/safety/floods/news/2018-09-27-1000-year-rainfall-events-lower-48

Tomkins, C.M., Anderko, L., & Patten, M. (2016). *Air quality flag program influences behavioral change on poor air quality days. Mid Atlantic Center for Children's Health and the Environment*. Retrieved from http://www.enviro.center/epas-air-quality-flag-program-influences-behavioral-change-poor-outdoor-air-quality-days-d-c-elementary-school-2/

Troisi, R., Hatch, E., Titus, L., Strohsnitter, W., Gail, M. H., Huo, D., … Palmer, J. R. (2019). Prenatal diethylstilbestrol exposure and cancer risk in women. *Environmental and Molecular Mutagenesis, 60*(5), 395–403. doi: 10.1002/em.22155.

UC Davis. (n.d.). *Science & climate: Climate change terms & definitions*. Retrieved from https://climatechange.ucdavis.edu/science/climate-change-definitions/

United Nations. (2018). *Water*. Retrieved from http://www.un.org/en/sections/issues-depth/water/index.html

United Nations (UN). (2020). *About the Sustainable Development Goals*. Retrieved from https://www.un.org/sustainabledevelopment/sustainable-development-goals/

U.S. Consumer Product Safety Commission. (2018). *Asbestos in the home*. Retrieved from http://www.cpsc.gov/safety-education/safety-guides/home/asbestos-in-the-home/

U.S. Department of Housing and Urban Development (USHUD). (2018). *Healthy homes program*. Retrieved from https://www.hud.gov/program_offices/healthy_homes/hhi

U.S. Environmental Protection Agency (EPA). (n.d.). *Air quality flag program*. Retrieved from https://cfpub.epa.gov/airnow/index.cfm?action=flag_program.index

U.S. Environmental Protection Agency (EPA). (March, 2005). *Citizen's guide to pest control and pesticide safety*. Retrieved from https://www.epa.gov/sites/production/files/2017-08/documents/citizens_guide_to_pest_control_and_pesticide_safety.pdf

U.S. Environmental Protection Agency (EPA). (2012). *Framework for sustainability indicators at EPA*. Retrieved from http://www2.epa.gov/sites/production/files/2014-10/documents/framework-for-sustainability-indicators-at-epa.pdf

U.S. Environmental Protection Agency (EPA). (2016). *EPA workshop on epigenetics and cumulative risk assessment*. Retrieved from http://cfpub.epa.gov/ncea/risk/recordisplay.cfm?deid=308271&CFID=51323330&CFTOKEN=62079592

U.S. Environmental Protection Agency (EPA). (March 17, 2017a). *News releases from headquarters: EPA awards $100 million to Michigan for Flint water infrastructure upgrades*. Retrieved from https://archive.epa.gov/epa/newsreleases/epa-awards-100-million-michigan-flint-water-infrastructure-upgrades.html

U.S. Environmental Protection Agency (EPA). (2017b). *Pesticides and food: What you and your family need to know*. Retrieved from https://nepis.epa.gov/Exe/ZyNET.exe/94X00NFN.txt?ZyActionD=ZyDocument&Client=EPA&Index=1995%20Thru%201999&Docs=&Query=&Time=&EndTime=&SearchMethod=1&TocRestrict=n&Toc=&TocEntry=&QField=&QFieldYear=&QFieldMonth=&QFieldDay=&UseQField=&IntQFieldOp=0&ExtQFieldOp=0&XmlQuery=&File=D%3A%5CZYFILES%5CINDEX%20DATA%5C95THRU99%5CTXT%5C00000038%5C94X00NFN.txt&User=ANONYMOUS&Password=anonymous&SortMethod=h%7C-&MaximumDocuments=1&FuzzyDegree=0&ImageQuality=r75g8/r75g8/x150y150g16/i425&Display=hpfr&DefSeekPage=x&SearchBack=ZyActionL&Back=ZyActionS&BackDesc=Results%20page&MaximumPages=1&ZyEntry=1

U.S. Environmental Protection Agency (EPA). (2017c). *Sustainable materials management: Non-Hazardous materials and waste management hierarchy*. Retrieved from https://www.epa.gov/smm/sustainable-materials-management-non-hazardous-materials-and-waste-management-hierarchy

U.S. Environmental Protection Agency (EPA). (2018a). *About risk assessment*. Retrieved from http://www2.epa.gov/risk/about-risk-assessment#whatisrisk

U.S. Environmental Protection Agency (EPA). (2018b). *Assessing human health risk from pesticides*. Retrieved from http://www2.epa.gov/pesticide-science-and-assessing-pesticide-risks/assessing-human-health-risk-pesticides

U.S. Environmental Protection Agency (EPA). (2018c). *Brownfields Utilization, Investment and Local Development Act (BUILD)*. Retrieved from https://www.epa.gov/sites/production/files/2018-08/documents/1-pg_build_summary_handout_508_0818.pdf

U.S. Environmental Protection Agency (EPA). (2018d). *Criteria air pollutants*. Retrieved from https://www.epa.gov/criteria-air-pollutants

U.S. Environmental Protection Agency (EPA). (July 19, 2018e). *Management weaknesses delayed response to Flint water crisis*, Report 18-P0221. Retrieved from https://www.epa.gov/sites/production/files/2018-07/documents/_epaoig_20180719-18-p-0221.pdf

U.S. Environmental Protection Agency (EPA). (2018f). *Plain English guide to the Clean Air Act*. Retrieved from http://www2.epa.gov/clean-air-act-overview/plain-english-guide-clean-air-act

U.S. Environmental Protection Agency (EPA). (2018g). *Protect your home's water*. Retrieved from https://www.epa.gov/privatewells/protect-your-homes-water#welltestanchor

U.S. Environmental Protection Agency (EPA). (2018h). *Report on the Environment: Indoor Air Quality*. Retrieved from https://www.epa.gov/report-environment/indoor-air-quality

U.S. Environmental Protection Agency (EPA). (2018i). *Schools*. Retrieved from http://www.epa.gov/schools/

U.S. Environmental Protection Agency (EPA). (2018j). *What is Superfund?* Retrieved from https://www.epa.gov/superfund/what-superfund

U.S. Environmental Protection Agency (EPA). (2019a). *Advisories and technical resources for fish and shellfish consumption*. Retrieved from http://www2.epa.gov/fish-tech

U.S. Environmental Protection Agency (EPA). (2019b). *Agricultural crops*. Retrieved from https://www.epa.gov/agriculture/agricultural-crops

U.S. Environmental Protection Agency (EPA). (2019c). *Air Quality: National Summary*. Retrieved from https://www.epa.gov/air-trends/air-quality-national-summary

U.S. Environmental Protection Agency (EPA). (2019d). *Brownfields and land revitalization activities near you*. Retrieved from https://www.epa.gov/brownfields/brownfields-and-land-revitalization-activities-near-you

U.S. Environmental Protection Agency (EPA). (2019e). *Health risks of radon*. Retrieved from http://www2.epa.gov/radon/health-risk-radon

U.S. Environmental Protection Agency (EPA). (2019f). *Integrated pest management (IPM) principles*. Retrieved from https://www.epa.gov/safepestcontrol/integrated-pest-management-ipm-principles

U.S. Environmental Protection Agency (EPA). (2019g). *Overview of EPA's Brownfields Program*. Retrieved from https://www.epa.gov/brownfields/overview-epas-brownfields-program

U.S. Environmental Protection Agency (EPA). (2020a). *Environmental justice*. Retrieved from http://www.epa.gov/environmentaljustice/

U.S. Environmental Protection Agency (EPA). (2020b). *Environmental justice equals healthy, sustainable, and equitable communities*. Retrieved from http://www3.epa.gov/environmentaljustice/sustainability/index.html

U.S. Environmental Protection Agency (EPA). (2020c). *Facts and figures about materials, waste, and recycling*. Retrieved from https://www.epa.gov/facts-and-figures-about-materials-waste-and-recycling/advancing-sustainable-materials-management-0

U.S. Environmental Protection Agency (EPA). (2020d). *Indoor air quality*. Retrieved from http://www2.epa.gov/indoor-air-quality-iaq

U.S. Environmental Protection Agency (EPA). (2020e). *Learn about sustainability*. Retrieved from http://www2.epa.gov/sustainability/learn-about-sustainability#what

U.S. Environmental Protection Agency (EPA). (2020f). *National overview: Facts and figures on materials, wastes and recycling*. Retrieved from https://www.epa.gov/facts-and-figures-about-materials-waste-and-recycling/national-overview-facts-and-figures-materials

U.S. Environmental Protection Agency (EPA). (2020g). *Natural disasters and weather emergencies*. Retrieved from http://www2.epa.gov/natural-disasters

U.S. Environmental Protection Agency (EPA). (2020h). *Overview of the Clean Air Act and air pollution*. Retrieved from https://www.epa.gov/clean-air-act-overview

U.S. Environmental Protection Agency (EPA). (2020i). *Radon*. Retrieved from http://www2.epa.gov/radon

U.S. Environmental Protection Agency (EPA). (2020j). *Safe Drinking Water Act*. Retrieved from https://www.epa.gov/sdwa

U.S. Food and Drug Administration (FDA). (2020). *New plant variety regulatory information*. Retrieved from https://www.fda.gov/food/food-new-plant-varieties/new-plant-variety-regulatory-information

U.S. Geological Survey (USGS). (2018a). *The water in you*. Retrieved from https://water.usgs.gov/edu/propertyyou.html

U.S. Geological Survey (USGS). (2018b). *Water quality data for pharmaceuticals, hormones and other organic wastewater contaminants in streams, 1999–2000*. Retrieved from http://toxics.usgs.gov/pubs/OFR-02-94/index.html

U.S. Global Change Research Program. (2016). *The impacts of climate change upon human health in the United States: A scientific assessment*. Washington, DC: Author. Retrieved from https://health2016.globalchange.gov

U.S. Global Change Research Program. (2018). *Impacts, risks, and adaptation in the United States: Fourth national climate assessment, 2018*. Retrieved from https://nca2018.globalchange.gov

Usher, K., Mills, J., West, C., Casella, E., Dorji, P., Guo, A., ... Woods, C. (2015). Cross-sectional survey of the nurses across the Asia-Pacific region. *Nursing & Health Sciences, 17*(4), 434–443.

Waddell, A., Audette, K., DeLong, A., & Brostoff, M. (2016). A hospital-based interdisciplinary model for increasing nurses' engagement in legislative advocacy. *Policy, Politics & Nursing Practice, 17*(1), 15–23.

Whitehead, L. (2015). The road towards environmental justice from a multifaceted lens. *Journal of Environmental Health, 77*(6), 106–108.

Whitmee, S., Haines, A., Beyrer, C., Boltz, F., Capon, A. G., de Souza Dias, B. H., ... Yack, D. (2015). Safeguarding human health in the Anthropocene epoch: Report of The Rockefeller Foundation-Lancet Commission on planetary health. *The Lancet, 386*(10007), 1973–2028. Retrieved from https://www.thelancet.com/journals/lancet/article/PIIS0140-6736(15)60901-1/fulltext

Wilke, R. A., & Freeman, J. W. (2017). Potential health implications related to fracking. *JAMA, 318*(7), 1645–1646.

Willis, M. D., Jusko, T. A., Halterman, J. S., & Hill, L. (2018). Unconventional natural gas development and pediatric asthma hospitalizations in Pennsylvania. *Environmental Research, 166*, 401–408.

Wisconsin Department of Health Services. (n.d.). *Portable generator hazards*. Retrieved from https://www.dhs.wisconsin.gov/publications/p4/p45106.pdf

Wood, M. R. (July 2, 2019). How the Flint water crisis set students back: Lead-poisoned children struggle to keep up with their peers academically and socially. *Pittsburgh Post-Gazette*, A-9.

World Health Organization (WHO). (2020a). *Social determinants of health*. Retrieved from http://www.who.int/social_determinants/sdh_definition/en/

World Health Organization (WHO). (2020b). *WHO constitution*. Retrieved from https://www.who.int/about/who-we-are/constitution

Wright, R. T., & Boorse, D. F. (2016). *Environmental science: Toward a sustainable future* (13th ed.). Boston: Pearson.

Yan, Y. E., Turale, S., Stone, T., & Petrini, M. (2015). Nursing skills, knowledge, and attitudes required in earthquake relief: implications for nursing education. *International Nursing Review, 62*, 351–359.

Ying, Z., Ning, L. D., & Xin, L. (2015). Relationship between built environment, physical activity, adiposity, and health in adults aged 46–80 in Shanghai, China. *Journal of Physical Activity & Health, 12*(4), 569–578.

Zhu, C., Kobayashi, K., Loladze, I., Zhu, J., Jiang, Q., Xy, X., ... Ziska, L. (2018). Carbon dioxide (CO_2) levels this century will alter the protein, micronutrients, and vitamin content of rice grains with potential health consequences for the poorest rice-dependent countries. *Science Advances, 4*(5), eaaq 1012.

UNIT 3

Community/Public Health Nursing Toolbox

CHAPTER 10

Communication, Collaboration, and Technology

"Think like a wise man but communicate in the language of the people."

—William Butler Yeats (1865–1939)

KEY TERMS

Active listening
Asset-based community development (ABCD)
Big data
Brainstorming
Community-based participatory research (CBPR)
Critical pathway
Electronic health records (EHRs)
Emotional intelligence (EI)
Feedback loop
Geographic information system (GIS)
Group process
Health literacy
Health technology
Integrative strategies
Interpersonal skills
Mobile health (mHealth)
Nominal group technique
Telehealth

LEARNING OBJECTIVES

Upon mastery of this chapter, you should be able to:

1. Describe five barriers to effective communication in community/public health nursing and how to deal with them.
2. Summarize the key issues related to health literacy.
3. Explain the stages of group development.
4. Discuss the value of contracting to both clients and community/public health nurses.
5. Design a contract useful in community/public health nursing.
6. Debate the pros and the cons of using electronic health records.
7. Describe the unique features of big data and areas of public health where it is most helpful.
8. Explain the main trends in mobile health and give a public health–related example of each.
9. Identify a current example of the combination of data and geographic information system applications in public health.

INTRODUCTION

Although you have learned how to effectively communicate with your patients in acute care settings, communication with community/public health nursing (C/PHN) clients entails additional skills and techniques. Communication, collaboration, and contracting are primary tools for community health nurses. They form the basis for effective relationships that contribute both to the prevention of illness and to the protection and promotion of population health. Health literacy is a concept that is important because of its relationship to health promotion and disease prevention and management. For the nurse accustomed to communicating one-on-one with clients, communicating with community groups requires new skills, because the effective application of group process skills facilitates collaboration with both task and support groups. Unlike ordinary social relationships, collaborative relationships

- Are based on a team approach, with shared responsibilities and mutual participation in establishing and achieving goals
- Involve working creatively across sectors and disciplines
- Lead to improved health outcomes
- Foster organizational commitment

Health technology serves as a powerful equalizer for improving health education and access to care among vulnerable and minority populations by reaching people where they are and in whatever environment they live. This chapter examines these tools and discusses their integration into C/PHN practice.

COMMUNICATION IN COMMUNITY/PUBLIC HEALTH NURSING

Effective communication is vital to all areas of nursing but is considered to be a fundamental core competency needed in C/PHN practice. The Quad Council Community/Public Health Nursing Competencies (Quad Council Coalition Competency Review Task Force, 2018) include communication skills as one of the eight competency domains (see the appendix). Nurses working in community/public health must be skilled in effective communication to be able to maintain relationships with individual clients, families, the community, members of the health care team, and community partners (Joyce et al., 2018). The lack of effective communication can lead to misunderstanding, poor performance, interpersonal conflict, ineffective program development, and medical mistakes, all resulting in poorer health outcomes. Whereas ineffective communication is one of the major causes of preventable adverse events in acute care settings (Robertson & Long, 2018), effective communication skills empower community/public health nurses to (Hansson et al., 2017)

- Provide quality health care and health education that improves patient outcomes
- Advocate effectively for clients, families, and populations
- Enhance professional collaboration and organizational commitment
- Initiate public health policy
- Implement programs designed to meet the needs of clients despite societal, organizational, and individual obstacles

Successful nurses must use both sound clinical skills and good communication skills (Arnold & Boggs, 2016). Necessary communication skills include soliciting input from others and listening to others in a nonjudgmental way.

Communication provides a two-way flow of information that nourishes nurse–client and nurse–professional relationships. For communication to take place, client and professional messages are sent and received. As participants in the communication process, community/public health nurses play both roles: sender and receiver. The nurse must be able to elicit ideas as well as contribute to the planning process by speaking and acting in ways that promote information sharing.

The Communication Process

Communication in its simplest form is the sending and receiving of a message, a process by which one assigns and conveys meaning to create shared understanding. This process incorporates the conventional aspects of communication: sender, receiver, message, channel (e.g., verbal, nonverbal, social networking), encoding, decoding, and feedback (e.g., checking the message meaning, revising for clarity) (El-Shafy et al., 2017). Effective communication is seen only when the message sent is received and interpreted by the receiver as intended (Borkowski, 2016 and Slade et al., 2018). This process forms a communication loop, which is shown in Figure 10-1.

Strategies to Overcome Communication Barriers

Community/public health nurses should be aware of the barriers that block effective communication (Box 10-1).

Overcoming barriers to effective communication requires the development of sound communication skills, including sending, receiving, and **interpersonal skills**.

Establish Trust and Rapport

Nurses are considered to be knowledgeable professionals who have standing within the community. Those working

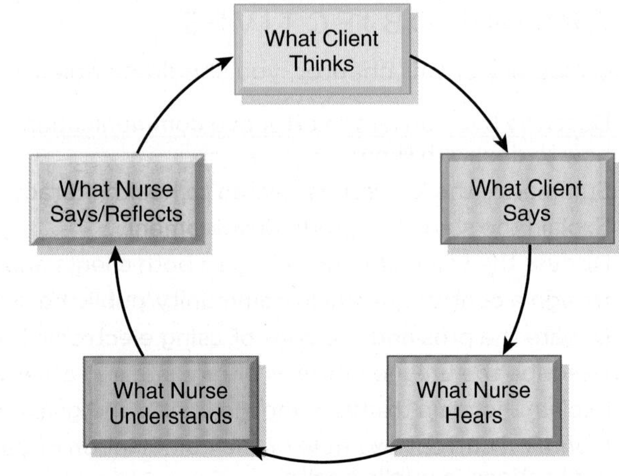

FIGURE 10-1 The communication process.

for public health agencies have power and authority as representatives of a government agency. Clients may feel apprehensive about C/PHNs entering their homes. Therefore, it is essential for the nurse to demonstrate respect for the client, especially for those clients who lack self-respect. Having an appreciation for the dignity and worth of all individuals, being nonjudgmental, and demonstrating empathy (acceptance and acknowledgement of the client's situation and feelings) are prerequisites for successful communication with clients in the community setting (Townsend & Morgan, 2018). To establish trust and rapport with clients, nurses must

- Develop a relationship with the client, not just around the public health issues of interest to the nurse but concerning the client's life and challenges
- Over time, by being consistently trustworthy, reliable, sincere, and truthful with clients

To promote trust, nurses can

- Commit to develop knowledge and experience of the client and their situation
- Clarify expectations, anticipated behaviors, and boundaries of the nurse–client relationship
- Be aware of attitudes and behaviors that do not promote trust (Springer & Skolarus, 2019)

Many factors that are often shaped by clients' cultural background and upbringing influence trust and rapport. For many, the societal norm is to agree with someone in a position of authority, such as a community/public health nurse, even if they do not fully understand what that person is communicating. This can lead to mistrust and poor client outcomes. Establishing a trusting relationship can empower clients to accomplish important lifestyle changes (Box 10-2). However, it is important to keep in

BOX 10-1 Barriers to Effective Communication in Community/Public Health Nursing

Selective Perception

Individuals interpret a message through their own perceptions, which are influenced by their own experience, interests, values, motivations, and expectations. This perceptual screen leads to possible distortion or misinterpretation of the meaning from the sender's original intent. Nurses can overcome this barrier by using the **feedback loop** to ask clients to voice their understanding of the message they just received from the nurse. This enhances clarification and correction of misunderstandings, which is an essential step in the communication process.

Filtering

Filtering is described as manipulation of information by the sender in order to make it seem more favorable to the receiver (Cain, Surbone, Elk, & Kagawa-Singer, 2018).

Clients sometimes use filtering during the assessment process, giving only partial or distorted information because they think this is what health professionals want to hear. Filtering can also affect community/public health nurses. Cole (1990), in a classic work, notes that we have "filters" through which we view others—often influenced by culture, ethnicity, and socioeconomic class or even gender—and these can lead to miscommunication. Cole's premise is that people from different backgrounds actually view the world differently, thus confounding communication and leading to prejudice and stereotyping. Community/public health nurses should consider their communication style and those of the people with whom they come in contact (Cain et al., 2018).

Emotional Influence

How a person feels at the time a message is sent or received influences the meaning. Emotions can interfere with rational and objective reasoning, thus blocking communication. Nurses need to be aware of their own emotions and the emotional status of clients or health professionals with whom they are communicating. For example, it is important for community/public health nurses to remain calm and unruffled when dealing with families in crisis. Family communication may be angry, blaming, and confrontational because of a child's serious health crisis, for instance. A calm, firm, reassuring presence can go far in diffusing the situation and promoting clearer and more constructive communication. You may say, "I sense that you are feeling upset about Joey's diagnosis. Are there any questions I can answer for you? How can I be of help to you?"

Language Barriers

People interpret the meaning of words differently, depending on many variables, such as age, education, cultural background, and primary spoken language. For example, an adolescent might understand the term "lit" to mean that something is good or exciting, whereas an 80-year-old person might understand the word refers to lighting. In the community, nurses work with a wide range of clients and professionals whose disparate ages, education levels, and cultural backgrounds lead to different communication patterns.

Language of Nursing

The context of health care provides nurses with a unique vocabulary that may not be understood by clients, family, and community members. The use of scientific terminology or jargon by some health professionals can be confusing to clients. Communication techniques would be different when educating a new mother on proper breast-feeding techniques than when discussing community health needs with the director of a public health department (Cain et al., 2018).

Source: Cain et al. (2018); Cole (1990).

BOX 10-2 EVIDENCE-BASED PRACTICE

Community/public Health Nurse—Client Communication

Evidence-based research has verified the importance of establishing rapport and trust, understanding clients, and the complex communication skills used by nurses with their clients. For trust to occur, the nurse must be accessible and available, be competent, and have a good bedside manner, and the client's past experiences with the health care system must be positive (Ozaras & Abaan, 2018). A trusting relationship is developed over time and is dynamic and changing; it is a reciprocal relationship, and the nurse earns continued trust by meeting patient expectations. Characteristics of the nurse that facilitate trust include being honest, sensitive, authentic, respectful, caring, accepting of the patient, encouraging, and committed to giving good care. Barriers include the use of professional jargon, not listening for understanding, being neglectful, being incompetent, and having power struggles. The trust relationship is negotiated over time and becomes more stable as the patient feels respected and accepted and values the ethical and moral practice of the nurse.

Talk with your instructor and community/public health nurses about these findings. Do they concur? How can you use this information to promote more effective trusting relationships with your clients? What experiences can you draw upon that may promote an understanding of how trust affects the relationship of the client and community health nurse?

Source: Ozaras and Abaan (2018).

mind that although nurses have a good deal of knowledge and education, to be effective they must appreciate the knowledge gained by clients through life experiences and the environments in which they live (Strandas & Bondas, 2018). An "analogy about shoes" is helpful in understanding this; it involves a shoemaker and a shoe customer in a classic story by Clement and Roberts (1983, p. 192): The shoemaker is an expert in making shoes, but the shoe wearer can tell if the shoe made by the shoemaker is uncomfortable and can give the shoemaker important information (e.g., exactly where it pinches). If both appreciate the knowledge that each one possesses and can work together, a comfortable shoe can be the outcome.

Showing respect is a fundamental behavior that conveys the attitude that clients and others have knowledge, importance, dignity, and worth (Sabatino, Rocco, Stievano, & Alvaro, 2015). C/PHNs can work with clients in many ways to change their lives for the better, but just like acute care nurses need to "know the patient" in the hospital setting in order to pick up subtle cues that may indicate serious problems, we must begin with what is important to the client rather than our own agenda (Johansson & Martensson, 2019, p. 120). A new nurse making a home visit to a mother who has missed several immunization clinic appointments for her infant may think that the mother needs only information on why immunizations are important for her baby. However, the mother may be dealing with an abusive husband who has drug and alcohol problems. If the nurse begins the visit with a reminder about the missed appointments and the potential consequences involved, it may end abruptly. It is best to begin by asking about the client's concerns so the nurse can gain a deeper understanding of the client's experiences, fears, and perspectives while communicating a demeanor of understanding and the intention to help (Gholamzadeh, Khastavaneh, Khademian, & Ghadakpour, 2018).

Actively Listen

An essential skill is **active listening**, also referred to as reflective listening (Hardavella, Aamli-Gaagnat, Saad, Rousalova, & Sreter, 2017). Active listening is the skill of assuming responsibility for and striving to understand the feelings and thoughts in a sender's message, thus giving importance to the person speaking (Karp, 2015). Skills that promote active listening (see Fig. 10-2) include the following:

- **Being attentive and mindful:** Being focused and engaged in conversation with your client gives insight into the client's frame of mind, reactions, and body language (Raphael-Grimm, 2015).
- **Conveying a nonjudgmental attitude**: Keeping an open mind, having interest in what your client is saying, and not arguing help build client self-confidence.
- **Using reflection:** Mirroring the client's message by occasionally paraphrasing key points demonstrates empathy and shows the client you can view the world through the client's eyes.
- **Asking for clarification:** By asking probing questions to clear up ambiguity or to expand on the client's ideas, you check your interpretation of their message, closing the loop and preventing communication breakdowns.

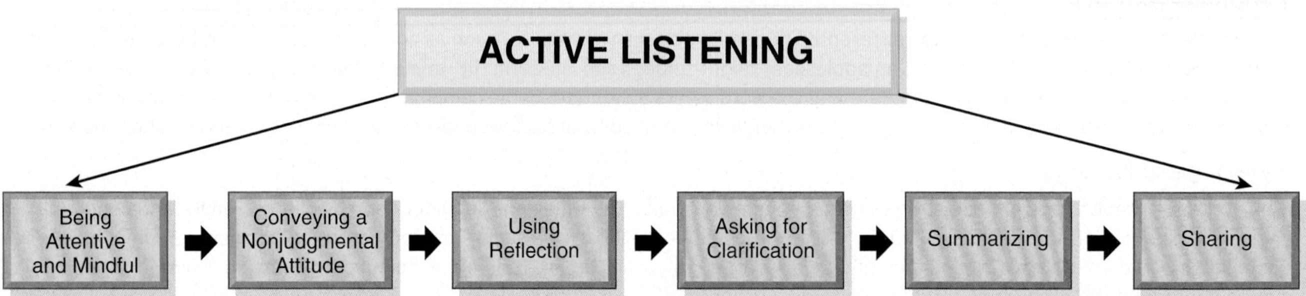

FIGURE 10-2 Six key skills for active listening. (Source: Center for Creative Leadership. (2019). *Active listening: Improve your ability to listen and lead.* Greensboro, NC: Author.)

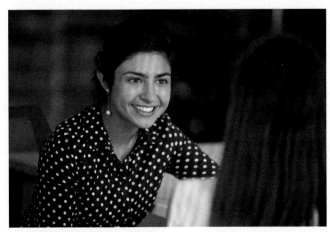

FIGURE 10-3 An example of active listening.

- **Summarizing:** By restating key themes of your conversation, you ensure that you understand the true nature of the message and help the client reflect and focus on issues raised (Schumacher & Madson, 2015).
- **Sharing:** Explain your ideas, feelings, or messages only after client indicates readiness and you have first fully understood the other person's views (Center for Creative Leadership, 2019; Harmon, 2016; Schumacher & Madson, 2015).

Active listening with nonjudgmental empathy (see Fig. 10-3) helps to communicate acceptance and increase trust (Heslip, 2015). It also allows for an accurate understanding of another person's viewpoint and helps to bring issues and concerns into the open, where they can be more easily resolved (Canpolat, Kuzu, Yildirim, & Canpolat, 2015). However, our own personal beliefs and values may confuse the message. A critical response to the client's message by the nurse can cut off communication and cause the client to disengage; therefore, a nonjudgmental approach better supports a therapeutic relationship (Karp, 2015). Students interested in learning more about active listening skills can listen to a podcast developed by the Centers for Creative Leadership (2019), which may be found at https://www.ccl.org/multimedia/podcast/the-big-6-an-active-listening-skill-set/.

Communicate Clearly

The CDC hosts a site that provides valuable resources to augment clear communication, including a clear communication index use guide, index widget, example material, and everyday words for public health communication found at https://www.cdc.gov/ccindex/. The basic rules for effective verbal or written communication can be summarized in this manner:

1. Use everyday words.
2. Use as few words as possible.
3. Use active voice.
4. Ask for feedback to make certain that the message is understood (CDC, 2019d).

Promoting Effective Communication and Change: Motivational Interviewing and OARS

Many techniques promote effective communication. One of the most successful is using motivational interviewing

BOX 10-3 Characteristics of a Helping Relationship

In a helping relationship, it is important to promote

- Openness, genuineness, trustworthiness, and self-awareness (ability to reflect on one's strengths and weaknesses)
- Sensitivity, acceptance, and concern for the client
- Respect for the client as an individual, which includes
  - Encouraging client to take an active role in health care and to be included in all decisions and choices
  - Considering ethnic and cultural backgrounds
  - Considering family background, beliefs, and values
- Knowledge, self-confidence, creativity, compassion, and empathy
- Ability to problem solve and to confront or direct when necessary (Ozaras & Abaan, 2018)

Source: Ozaras and Abaan (2018).

(MI) to join with clients to help them change behaviors. MI was first developed as a method of counseling to break through ambivalence and motivate clients to change problem behaviors such as excessive drinking (Miller & Rollnick, 2013). It involves having a conversation that establishes a "collaborative partnership" with the client about change and is focused on client feelings of ambivalence regarding the need for change. The nurse elicits client motivations and ideas about change (Schumacher & Madson, 2015, p. 2). This technique can be used in conjunction with the Transtheoretical or Stages of Change Model to determine the client's stage from his or her statements (see Chapter 11). Listen carefully to what the client is saying about the issue (e.g., smoking, hypertension, dietary changes), and determine if the client is amenable to making changes (see Box 11-3). Clients in the last three stages are most amenable to change, and MI can then be most helpful (Haque & D'Souza, 2019; Schumacher & Madson, 2015).

OARS is an acronym encompassing the skills needed in MI:

Open-ended questions: Rather than closed-ended questions that often result in only Yes or No answers, these questions open up conversation and help clients talk about thoughts and feelings, as well as behaviors and motivations for change. An example follows:
Nurse: "What are your concerns for your baby (Rose)?"

Affirmations of client strengths: These are genuine and congruent statements about clients' positive behaviors, skills, and accomplishments. An example follows:
Nurse: "You were very caring in comforting Rose while she was getting her shots."

Reflective listening: Similar to active listening, discussed earlier. It helps discern what the client is saying and if the nurse is hearing and understanding the client's meaning. Reflective comments demonstrate empathy and understanding and can move conversations to deeper levels. An example follows:
Nurse: "So it sounds like you would like some information on how to sign up for WIC."

Summaries: Statements used to move the conversation into different areas or to review final highlights of a conversation; can also be helpful in adding information about resources or future planning. Two examples follow:

Nurse: "Let me see if I understand what you said so far…."

Nurse: "We talked about x, y, z; let me know if I understood you correctly or missed anything."

Through MI conversations, client statements may reflect indecision or motivation to change. If motivated to change, clients may discuss their desire, ability, or reasons for change along with importance and urgency. The nurse can help them mobilize these feelings by asking open-ended questions about their commitment to change, how they could begin to plan for change, and other steps they need to take to move toward their goal (Dobber et al., 2019; Palmer, 2018; Schumacher & Madson, 2015). See thePoint for a list of Web sites that offer more information on MI and OARS, including suggestions for open-ended questions and shared decision making.

Research demonstrates the effectiveness of MI and OARS delivered by counselors (including lay counselors), physicians, nurses, and nurse practitioners working with a variety of clients:

- Heart failure patients with depression (Navidian, Mobaraki, & Shakiba, 2017)
- Patients with inflammatory arthritis (Palmer, 2018)
- Coronary artery disease patients (promoting a healthy lifestyle; Dobber et al., 2019)
- Individuals with HIV (Dillard, Zuniga, & Holstad, 2017)
- Intimate violence partner treatment clients (Soleymani, Britt, & Wallace-Bell, 2018)
- Appalachian women (supporting breast-feeding; Addicks & McNeil, 2019)

Emotional Intelligence

The concept of **emotional intelligence (EI)** is central to nursing practice. EI is the ability to recognize and understand one's own emotions and those of others as well as to manage one's own emotions so as to be able to adjust appropriately to a wide range of situations (Goleman, 1995; Park & Oh, 2019; Raghubir, 2018).

Studies have shown that nurses who possess a high level of EI have increased job performance and job satisfaction, both of which lead to improved health outcomes (Park & Oh, 2019; Raghubir, 2018).

Recently, EI has further been defined as an eclectic mix of traits or attributes. The five most widely recognized attributes are self-awareness, self-management, social skills, motivation, and empathy (Raghubir, 2018; Goleman, 1995). People who demonstrate high levels of EI

- Consider other people's feelings
- Examine their own feelings and how they react to stressful situations
- Practice empathy for others and relate to them in conversation
- Operate on trust, by communicating honestly and building trust through verbal and nonverbal cues
- Recognize, identify, and resolve ambiguity or misunderstandings
- Take responsibility for their own actions
- Consider how their actions affect others (Ackerman, 2019)

TABLE 10-1 Online Sites Offering Free Emotional Intelligence Testing

Name of Test and Source	Web Link
Emotional Intelligence Test (Psychology Today)	https://www.psychologytoday.com/us/tests/personality/emotional-intelligence-test
MindTools Test for How EI Are you? (MindTools)	https://www.mindtools.com/pages/article/ei-quiz.htm
Test your Emotional Intelligence (The Institute of Health and Human Potential)	http://www.ihhp.com/free-eq-quiz/

Table 10-1 details online sites that offer free testing to assess your level of EI.

A person can increase EI attributes through training and practice. Practice focuses on making a conscious effort to display the positive behaviors indicated above. MindTools has a number of online resources at https://www.mindtools.com/search?search_term=Emotional+Intelligence. Formal training is also available through a variety of programs found online.

In a helping relationship, it is important for the community/public health nurse to demonstrate effective communication. Box 10-3 lists key components that assist in promoting a helping relationship.

Cultivating Cultural Awareness

Effective communication is also strongly influenced by previous experiences and the culture of both the nurse and the client. For example, adolescents who are having difficulty with authority may hear the nurse's suggestion to "learn more about sexually transmitted diseases" as an authoritarian command or an effort to exert control. Differences in culture, ethnicity, and linguistics pose even greater challenges in establishing a helping relationship (Box 10-4).

Community/public health nurses often find themselves communicating cross-culturally and sometimes through an interpreter. This requires patience and constant effort to ensure accurate and inoffensive messages. For example, silence in Native American cultures may indicate patience and thoughtfulness, but someone not familiar with these cultures may interpret it as weakness or indifference. Culture is dynamic, and community/public health nurses cannot make assumptions about a client's cultural background, but it has been shown that knowledge of someone's cultural background can aid in providing quality care within the cultural context of the client (Crawford, Candlin, & Roger, 2015; Henderson, Horne, Hills, & Kendall, 2018). See Chapter 5.

BOX **10-4** PERSPECTIVES

Mr. Sanchez Needs an Interpreter

I am a student in community/public health nursing now, but I work as an extern at our small, local county hospital helping in the emergency department (ED). A man came in one Saturday a month or so ago with a bad cut to his right hand from a manual push lawnmower. The ED doc asked him if he had received a tetanus shot recently, and he quickly nodded "yes." He spoke little English, and none of us spoke Spanish. The interpreter was not available. We cleaned his wound, closed it with stitches, bandaged it, and told him to keep it clean. He was given a prescription for an antibiotic medication, but a tetanus shot was not administered.

A short time later, Mr. Sanchez was back in the hospital because his wound had gotten infected; he used a needle to drain some pus from his hand and developed tetanus. He ended up in the ICU on a ventilator. Mr. Sanchez spent 30 agonizing days in the ICU because of miscommunication about the tetanus booster. We should have used an interpreter, and I truly understand the importance of a translator now. I have some Spanish-speaking clients in my community/public health nursing rotation. I do my best to speak with them, and they are usually very welcoming and patient, but when I need to be sure that something is fully understood, I request that an interpreter accompany me on my home visits. I always remember Mr. Sanchez and what can happen when you don't use an interpreter, and communication is not clearly understood.

Amy, age 24

1. *What first comes to mind when you think of this scenario?*
2. *Can you imagine an incident like this occurring in your facility?*
3. *What barriers exist in using an interpreter? How can communication and understanding be validated in a situation where language is a barrier?*

Health Literacy and Health Outcomes

Health literacy is essential to client autonomy and good client outcomes. Any client in need of health services or information needs health literacy skills to:

- Access services and information.
- Communicate individual needs and preferences.
- Internalize the meaning of health information and services available.
- Grasp the context, options, and resulting consequences in health settings.
- Make choices that are aligned with their preferences and needs (CDC, 2019c).

Health literacy is critical to health promotion, and disease prevention encompasses cultural, scientific, media, and technological literacy (Feinberg, Tighe, Greenberg, & Mavreles, 2018). Vulnerable groups such as older adults, recent immigrants, migrants, ethnic minorities, and clients with low levels of education and dominant language proficiency are most affected by low health literacy (Johnson, 2015).

Presenting information in a manner that matches the clients' health literacy level can help address health disparities and empower clients to effectively manage their health by

- Understanding and complying with self-care instructions, including complex daily medical regimens
- Planning and attaining necessary lifestyle adjustments to improve their health
- Making positive, informed health-related decisions
- Knowing when and how to access necessary health care
- Addressing health issues in their community and society by sharing health-promoting activities with others (Feinberg et al., 2018)

Health information is disseminated in person, in print, and online, so health literacy is relevant to all of these processes (Rowlands, Berry, Protheroe, & Rudd, 2015). Clear communication is important to outcomes; one example is the link between the level of health literacy among rural heart failure patients and morbidity and mortality rates (CDC, 2019d; Moser et al., 2015; Nouri & Rudd, 2015). In addition, adequate health literacy among the nursing population is imperative in addressing the problem. A study by Erunal, Ozkaya, Mert, and Kucukguclu (2019) revealed that approximately 50% of nursing students failed to demonstrate adequate health literacy skill levels. Hence, it is vital that nursing students (and nurses) improve health literacy skills to communicate effectively with clients and fellow health care personnel (Erunal et al., 2019).

- Low health literacy skills are associated with poorer health status, increased health care costs, and use of emergency care, because patients with low health literacy levels are less knowledgeable about their health conditions and are less likely to seek preventative care, especially in older adults (≥65 years of age; Fabbri et al., 2018; Mantwill & Schulz, 2015).
- Children with caregivers who have low literacy skills have poor health outcomes, because the caregivers are less knowledgeable about their child's condition and less likely to engage in behaviors to help improve it (Kakarmath, Denis, Encinas-Martin, Borgonovi, & Subramanian, 2018).

The federal government has set standards to encourage health professionals to consider clients' health literacy when communicating with them. Table 10-2 details the most relevant acts, guidelines, and standards addressing our nation's health literacy goal.

The U.S. Department of Health and Human Services (USDHHS) developed the National Action Plan to Improve Health Literacy based on the vision and principles that "(1) everyone has the right to health information

TABLE 10-2 Acts, Guidelines, and Standards on Health Literacy

Resource	Web site Link
National Standards for Culturally and Linguistically Appropriate Services	https://minorityhealth.hhs.gov/omh/browse.aspx?lvl=2&lvlid=53
National Action Plan to Improve Health Literacy	https://health.gov/communication/initiatives/health-literacy-action-plan.asp
National Health Education Standards 2018	https://www.cdc.gov/healthyschools/sher/standards/index.htm
Federal Plan Language Guidelines	https://www.plainlanguage.gov/
Federal Plan Writing Act	https://www.plainlanguage.gov/law/
Health Literacy Training	https://www.cdc.gov/healthliteracy/gettraining.html

that helps them make informed decisions and (2) health services are delivered in ways that are understandable and beneficial to health, longevity, and quality of life" (USDHHS, 2010, p. 16). Online health literacy suggestions are found in Box 10-5.

BOX 10-5 Health Literacy Online: Helpful Suggestions for Digital Access

People often search the web for answers to a specific question or problem or to gain knowledge of a particular subject. They want to

- Have a better understanding of the health problem or behavior
- Learn about actions they can take to change the behavior or deal with the problem
- Find information that is concise, focused, engaging, and actionable
    - Checklists, conversation tools, or interactive features improve engagement

Individuals with limited health literacy may get easily distracted; they decide within the first few words or sentences if they can understand the content and want to keep reading.

- Start with the most important information to pique their interest.
- Briefly describe the health behavior or problem to hold their interest.
- Describe the benefits of changing a behavior or addressing a problem to motivate them.
- List specific steps or actions to take. Break the information into small steps, and use bulleted points.
- Use plain language, including short, simple sentences and paragraphs, no jargon (only common language used by clients), and active voice. (An example is "You need to have a yearly mammogram.")
- Use simple sans serif (e.g., Verdana, Arial, Calibri) fonts in 12- or 14-point sizes.
- Identify links with color or underlining so users can easily click on them.
- Use images or graphics to reinforce your message and to ensure your meaning is clear.
- Check the accuracy of your content.

Source: DeSalvo (2016).

To be sure that these goals are being met, the improvement of health literacy and health communication for our population continues to be a priority in the *Healthy People 2030* goals (Box 10-6).

Health communication includes health literacy, but it also incorporates health messages and campaigns targeted to populations. Population health promotion is best achieved by health communication that uses multiple communication channels to reach stakeholders, including television, radio, newspapers, Web sites, social media, smartphones/applications, text messaging, educational pamphlets, and nutrition and medication labels. To manage disease and promote health, we must make sure our patients can understand the health information they see, hear, and read from multiple sources (Feinberg et al., 2018). More information on these topics can be found in Chapter 11.

COMMUNICATING WITH GROUPS

An important aspect of communication in C/PHN involves working with groups of people. C/PHNs are regularly involved in committees, task forces, support groups, and other work-related groups (Fig. 10-4). Group communication patterns can be complex, and interaction requires skill on the nurse's part to elicit feedback from all members to generate a common understanding among the group's members. C/PHNs need to understand how to organize groups and how groups function and develop over time as well as techniques for facilitating group support and decision making.

Group Development

In 1977, Tuckman and Jenson identified five stages of group development:

1. *Forming*

- Members: feel awkward and hesitant and depend on the group leader to help them develop mutual trust and give them structure and guidance (Carter & Mossholder, 2015)
- Group leader: helps members become oriented to each other and to the work
- "Ice-breaker" activities at the first group meeting
- Setting of ground rules (e.g., confidentiality)

BOX **10-6** *HEALTHY PEOPLE 2030*

Selected Objectives Related to Health Literacy or Health Communication

Core Objectives

HC/HIT-01	Increase the proportion of adults whose health care provider checked their understanding
HC/HIT-02	Decrease the proportion of adults who report poor communication with their health care provider
HC/HIT-03	Increase the proportion of adults whose health care providers always involved them in decisions about their health care as much as they wanted
HC/HIT-04	Increase the proportion of adults who talk to friends or family about their health
HC/HIT-05	Increase the proportion of adults with broadband internet
HC/HIT-06	Increase the proportion of adults offered online access to their medical record
HC/HIT-07	Increase the proportion of adults who use IT to track health care data or communicate with providers

Developmental Objectives

HC/HIT-D01	Increase the number of state health departments that use social marketing in health promotion programs
HC/HIT-D02	Increase the proportion of emergency messages in news stories that give complete information
HC/HIT-D07	Increase the proportion of doctors with electronic access to information they need
HC/HIT-D08	Increase the proportion of doctors who exchange and use outside electronic health information
HC/HIT-D09	Increase the proportion of people who can view, download, and send their electronic health information

Reprinted from U.S. Department of Health and Human Services (USDHHS). (2020a). *Browse 2030 objectives.* Retrieved from https://health.gov/healthypeople/objectives-and-data/browse-objectives

- Defining scope of work and timeline for completion (Box 10-7)

2. *Storming*

- Group begins to work together
- Conflict and competition over different agendas, ideas, and approaches
- Group leader: guides group in problem-solving and setting goals, models maintenance roles (e.g., encouraging all to participate), and summarizes group feelings

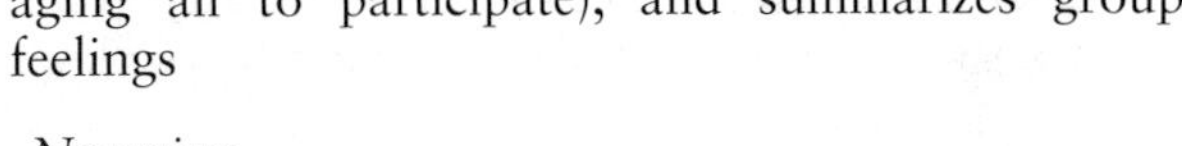

3. *Norming*

- Group shows signs of cohesiveness, trust, openness, shared sense of "belonging"
- Work begins to progress
- Creativity and shared ideas and opinions
- Group leader: continues to role model good maintenance behaviors

4. *Performing*

- May not occur with all groups
- Members: can work as a total group, in subgroups, or independently
- Most productive stage, as group members are motivated and able to handle the decision-making process in a competent and autonomous manner
- High level of team satisfaction

5. *Adjourning*

- Emphasis is on wrapping up the project
- Withdrawal from both task and relationship or maintenance activities
- Members: often feel happy to have accomplished goal but sad about the loss or disbanding of the group (Betts & Healy, 2015)

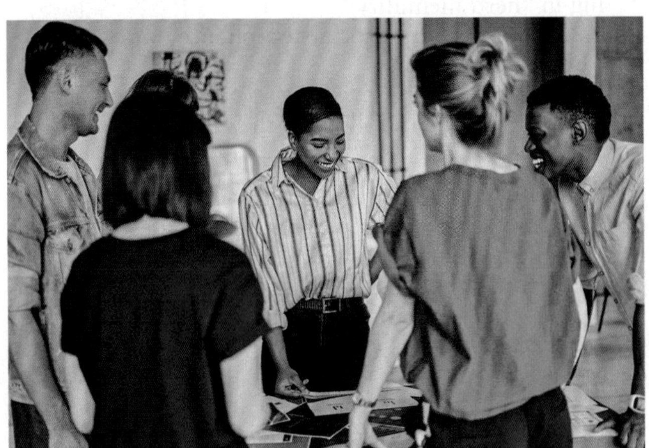

FIGURE 10-4 An example of a functioning group.

BOX 10-7 Task, Maintenance, and Nonfunctional Roles in Groups

Task Role Behaviors

Behaviors required in selecting and carrying out group tasks include the following:

- **Initiates Activity:** Proposes solutions; suggests new ideas and new approaches to the problem
- **Seeks Information:** Asks for clarification and requests additional information
- **Seeks Opinions:** Looks for input from members; seeks clarification of values, suggestions, or ideas
- **Gives Information:** Offers facts or observations; relates one's own experiences to the group problem
- **Gives Opinions:** States an opinion or belief related to concerning a suggestion; generally based on value rather than its factual basis
- **Elaborates:** Envisions how a proposal might work if adopted; gives examples and clarifies meaning
- **Coordinates:** Shows relationships among various ideas or suggestions; draws together activities of various subgroups or members
- **Summarizes:** Restates a summary of suggestions after the group has discussed them

Maintenance Role Behaviors

Behaviors required in maintaining group relationships and activities include the following:

- **Encourages:** Praises others and their ideas accepts contributions of others; maintains a warm and friendly manner
- **Gatekeeps:** Ensures that all have a chance to be heard; suggests limited talking time for everyone
- **Sets Standards:** Suggests standards for the group to use in choosing its content or procedures or in evaluating its decisions
- **Follows:** Goes along with decisions of the group, thoughtfully accepting ideas of others, and serving as audience during group discussion
- **Expresses Group Feelings:** Summarizing what group feeling is sensed to be and describing reactions of the group to ideas or solutions

Both Task and Maintenance Role Behaviors

The following behaviors are true of both task roles and maintenance roles:

- **Evaluates:** Compares group decisions or accomplishments with group standards and goals
- **Diagnoses:** Determines sources of difficulties, appropriate steps to take next, and analyzes the main block to progress
- **Tests for Consensus:** Asks for group opinions in order to find out whether the group is nearing consensus on a decision
- **Mediates:** Harmonizes differences in points of view and suggests compromise solutions
- **Relieves Tension:** Balances negative feelings by putting a tense situation in a wider context

Nonfunctional Roles

Roles that harm the group and its work include the following:

- **Being Aggressive:** Strives for status by criticizing or blaming others, showing hostility toward the group or some individual, and deflating egos or status of others
- **Blocking:** Interferes with the progress of the group by arguing too much on a point and rejecting ideas without consideration
- **Self-confessing:** Uses the group as a sounding board to express personal, non–group-oriented feelings or points of view
- **Competing:** Vies with others to produce the best idea; talks the most
- **Seeking Sympathy:** Tries to induce other group members to be sympathetic to one's problems or disparaging one's own ideas to gain support
- **Special Pleading:** Persistently lobbies in support of one's own opinion, concern, or philosophy
- **Horsing Around:** Clowns, jokes and disrupts the work of the group
- **Seeking Recognition:** Calls attention to one's self by loud or excessive talking, extreme ideas, and unusual behavior
- **Withdrawal:** Acts indifferent or passive, using excessive formality, daydreaming, doodling, and whispering to others

Source: Boyd (2018); Schneider Corey et al. (2018).

Group Functions in Decision Making

Groups are often called on to make important decisions. It is widely accepted that decisions made by groups are stronger than those made by individuals (Bang & Frith, 2017). However, group decision making can go astray when group members

- Lack independent knowledge, which results in "groupthink"
- Bring background and experiences that are too similar, resulting in similar biases to the problem being addressed
- Adapt to each other's knowledge too quickly, resulting in "herd mentality"
- Fall into the trap of social compliance out of a desire to fit into the group
- Believe that others have better knowledge and ignore their own instincts, following the others instead (Bang & Frith, 2017)

One way to avoid these pitfalls is to ensure strong diversity among group members. This is best achieved by recruiting members with diverse identities (age, gender, ethnicity), cognitive styles, and even goals. Although this sometimes invites conflict, working through the conflict is often how groups reach the best decisions. Harnessing the group diversity draws on vastly different experiences and expertise allows for a wider range of potential solutions and minimizes individual biases (Bang & Frith, 2017).

Techniques for Enhancing Group Decision Making

As a member of many decision-making groups in the community, the community/public health nurse can facilitate the process through certain techniques such as brainstorming, multivoting, and nominal group technique.

Brainstorming. Brainstorming is an idea-generating process that encourages group members to freely offer suggestions. Group members are asked to present creative ideas without criticism or discussion. This technique is helpful for generating creative possibilities and is most useful in the early stages of decision making. Research has shown that brainstorming is considered to be the most widely used method of generating creative ideas (Oztop, Katsikopoulos, & Gummerum, 2018).

Multivoting. Multivoting is a decision-making tool that enables members to prioritize a long list of ideas with minimal discussion and difficulty. Multivoting often follows brainstorming to narrow the list to a few items worthy of immediate attention. All of the ideas are listed on a flip chart and members are allowed to vote on one third of the total number of items (Minnesota Department of Health, 2016).

Nominal Group Technique. Nominal group technique is a group decision-making method in which group members are asked to not speak to each other but instead are asked to write down their ideas, along with the advantages and disadvantages of the issue being addressed. After everyone has completed the task, the members' ideas are presented to the group, and discussion takes place so that the information can be categorized and prioritized (Gorman & McDowell, 2018).

Advances in technology have resulted in the availability of a number of online tools and apps that can help facilitate group decision making, whether the groups are sitting together in a room or working virtually. A Web site that provides links to 14 free online applications that support various forms of group decision making can be found at https://tallyfy.com/brainstorming-tools/.

Other Group Communication Settings

Not all C/PHN work with groups involves group process and group decision making. Often, nurses are called on to incorporate group-teaching methods to change behaviors (see Chapter 11 for more on health teaching). Group teaching can be an effective tool for many health care challenges, such as for diabetes teaching and education (Aeyoung, De Gagne, Sunah, & Young-Oak, 2015; Kewming, D'Amore, & Mitchell, 2016).

Community/public health nurses are also called on to share best practices and research findings. Public speaking is an important community/public health nurse skill. This involves developing public speaking and presentation skills that engage and draw in audiences, ultimately influencing improvements in health outcomes for individuals and populations (Sherman, 2016).

CONTRACTING IN COMMUNITY/PUBLIC HEALTH NURSING

Contracting means negotiating a working agreement between two or more parties in which they come to a shared understanding and mutually consent to the purposes and terms of the transaction. Contracts are common and include legal and nonbinding agreements. Legal contracts, such as signing a contract for a loan, are legally binding, and the terms are clearly provided.

Contracts in C/PHN can be either verbal or written, and clients can make them with themselves, family members, or health care practitioners. Such contracts commit clients to a set of behaviors, with the goal to improve adherence to a health promotion program or plan.

Box 10-8 shows a contract used by C/PHNs when counseling clients who desire to stop smoking. Contracts in a collaborative relationship or a nurse–client alliance are flexible and changing and are based on mutual understanding and trust, making this a valuable tool for community/public health nurses (Ackley, Ladwig, Makic, Martinez-Kratz, & Zanotti, 2020). The same format is followed with clients who are receiving home health care services called a critical pathway. It consists of the written plans for client care with a timetable. This is a more formal type of contracting that is typically a fiscally driven and agency-required tool designed to document standards and quality of care while reducing costs (see Chapter 30 for additional information).

Value of Contracting

C/PHN has used the concept of contracting for many years, developing partnerships with clients to address issues such as weight loss, exercise, and substance abuse. Without always labeling it contracting, these techniques are used with clients who want to lose weight, for instance. In this case, the contract involves mutual agreement on certain exercise and eating patterns for clients and teaching and support responsibilities for the nurse. Contracts set time limits (e.g., 6 months) within which to achieve the intended goal (e.g., weight loss). Nurses can help take a complex behavior and break it into manageable steps, such as by contracting to walk at a moderate pace for 30 minutes three times a week, which may seem more feasible than beginning by jogging 2 miles a day. Success in meeting the contract may encourage future efforts to increase exercise activities. Nurses and clients are, in effect, contracting even though they may see it simply as setting goals with clients (Ackley et al., 2020).

Community/public health nurses may use contracting when implementing health promotion programs. Contracting may be appropriate when planning to stop or reduce substance use, change eating habits, or increase physical activity. Contracting can also be done with groups or agencies (e.g., schools, businesses). For instance, a school district may want to contract with a public health agency to provide C/PHNs and health educators to address pregnancy prevention, and the nurse may informally contract with the students about sharing aggregate information gleaned in the small-group

BOX 10-8 Client Service Plan With Contract

Madera County Public Health Department
Public Health Nursing: Client Individual Service Plan

Client Name: Angelica Luz-Smith
RN Case Manager: M. Stanley, PHN

Client's Signature:____________
Start Date: 3/1/2022

Date: 3/1/2022	Client Goal:	Case Manager: Teaching/Counseling/Referral Case Manager will:	Follow-up/ Reassessment Date: 5/2022
Strengths Identified: Angelica desires to improve the length and quality of life to be healthier to spend time with grandchildren Problems/Risks: Has smoked 1–2 packs per day for 20 years	ANGELICA will decrease to fewer than 10 cigarettes per day within the next 2 months. Contract agreement: Angelica will avoid temptations or situations associated with pleasurable aspects of smoking by the following: ■ Instead of smoking after meals, brush teeth or take a walk. ■ Limit social activities to where smoking is prohibited. ■ Find new activities that make smoking difficult such as swimming or bicycle riding. ■ Identify a new activity to spend time on during work breaks (reading, crosswords, etc.). ■ Avoid alcoholic drinks. ■ Keep oral substitutes such as carrots, pickles, and sugarless gum handy. ■ Take a yoga class to learn relaxation techniques. Angelica will explore community resources: ■ American Lung Association Program: Freedom from Smoking ■ California Smokers' Helpline: 1-800-NO-BUTTS	■ Promote positive expectations for success; encourage self-efficacy. ■ Prepare Angelica for relapse. ■ Assist in developing timeframe with goal ultimately to be that Angelica will stop smoking completely. ■ Partner with Angelica for evaluation, feedback, and revision of health plan as needed. ■ Provide resources for Freedom from Smoking and California Smoker's Helpline.	Outcome/Evaluation Angelica will be smoking fewer than 10 cigarettes (1/2 pack) per day by 5/2022.

Source: Gulanik and Myers (2017).

teaching exercises with their parents to encourage adolescent–parent communication.

Common benefits of contracting in C/PHN include that it

- Involves clients in promoting their own health
- Motivates clients to perform necessary tasks
- Focuses on clients' unique needs, regardless of aggregate size
- Increases the possibility of achieving the health goals identified by collaborating team members
- Enhances all team members' problem-solving skills
- Fosters client participation in the decision-making process
- Promotes clients' autonomy and self-esteem as they learn self-care
- Makes nursing service more efficient and cost-effective (Duiveman & Bonner, 2012)

Characteristics of Contracting

The concept of contracting, as used in the collaborative relationship, incorporates four distinctive characteristics: partnership and mutuality, commitment, format, and negotiation. Box 10-9 displays the concept and process of contracting.

Partnership and Mutuality

All aspects of contracting involve shared participation and agreement between team members; they become partners in the relationship (Westefeld, 2019). In a mutual partnership, the nurse and partner come to an agreement on what the partner needs and what the nurse can provide. Together, they develop goals, outline methods to meet those goals, explore resources to help achieve them, define the time limits for the contract, and outline their separate responsibilities (Fig. 10-5). The contract involves reciprocal negotiation and shared evaluation.

BOX 10-9 Concept and Process of Contracting

Contracting is based on four distinctive features, shown here as spokes of a wheel, that form the basis of a nurse–client collaboration. This relationship is a dynamic process that moves through phases, represented here as the outer rim of the wheel, and is focused on meeting client needs and aiding in the achievement of their goals.

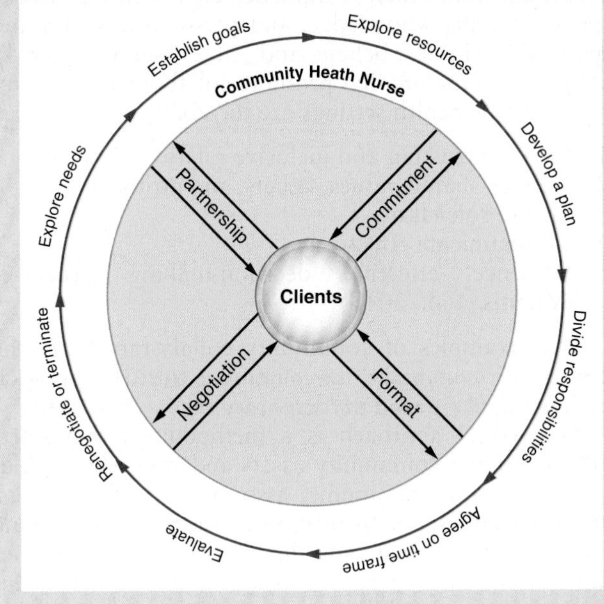

Commitment

Second, every contract implies a commitment. The involved parties make a decision that binds them to fulfilling the purpose of the contract (Westefeld, 2019). In community/public health collaboration, there is a pledge of trust and dedication to see the contract through to completion. All parties feel responsible for keeping promises; all want to achieve the intended outcomes. When the nurse and the partners identify their tasks, they commit to success.

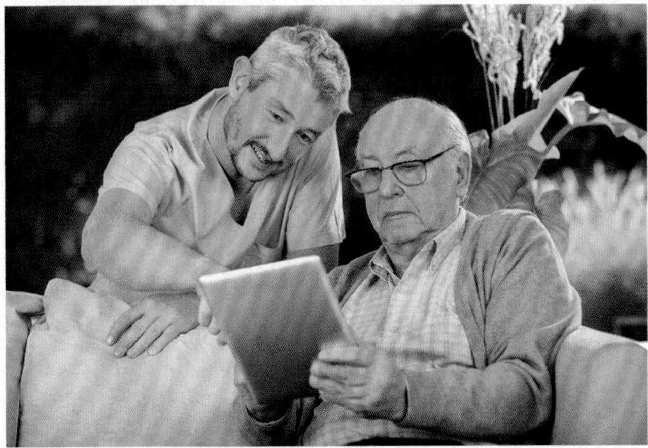

FIGURE 10-5 Contracting is an important aspect of client care.

Format

Format, the third distinctive feature of contracting, involves outlining the specific terms of the relationship. Clients and professionals gain a clear idea of the purpose of the relationship, their respective responsibilities, and the specific limits to their work. Expectations are clarified for all parties involved. The format of contracting provides the framework for collaboration to clearly articulate the logistics, avoid the difficulty of terminating long-term relationships, and shift health care responsibilities from the professionals to the client.

Negotiation

Finally, contracting always involves negotiation (Westefeld, 2019). The nurse and other team members propose certain responsibilities and then ask whether the clients agree. A period of give-and-take then occurs in which ideas are discussed and conclusions and consensus are reached without coercion. Team members may find over time that terms or goals on which they had agreed need modification. Negotiation is dynamic and allows for changes that facilitate the ultimate achievement of goals and encourages ongoing communication among all team members. Although C/PHNs are experts in nursing care, our clients know more about their life own circumstances and how health and illness impact them. Think of the shoemaker and shoe wearer, described earlier.

Principles of Contracting

Contracting applies the basic principles of adult education: self-direction, mutual negotiation, and mutual evaluation. Contracting may be formal or informal, written or verbal, simple or detailed, and signed or unsigned by client and nurse. It should be adapted to the particular client's abilities and may vary greatly from situation to situation. The nurse should date initial interventions as well as follow-up and reassessment visits. Like all nursing tools, contracting enhances a client's health only if it is adapted to each particular client.

The Nursing Process and Contracting

Contracting follows a sequence of steps that are aligned with the nursing process. As a working agreement, it depends on knowing what clients want, agreeing on goals, identifying methods to achieve these goals, knowing the resources that collaborating members bring to the relationship, using appropriate outside resources, setting limits, deciding on responsibilities, and providing for periodic reviews. The tasks are incorporated into the contracting process and can be described in eight phases that follow the nursing process.

Assessment

1. *Explore needs*: Assess the clients' health and needs, with the involvement of the clients and other relevant persons.

Nursing Diagnosis/Goal Setting

2. *Establish goals*: Discuss goals and objectives with contracting members and come to an agreement.

Plan/Intervention

3. *Explore resources*: Define what each member has to offer (clarifying the C/PHN role, client's role) and can expect from the others; identify appropriate resources and agencies.
4. *Develop a plan*: Identify methods, activities, and a timeline for achieving the stated goals.
5. *Divide responsibilities*: Negotiate the activities for which each member will be responsible.
6. *Agree on time frame*: Set limits for the contract in terms of length of time or number of meetings.

Evaluation

7. *Evaluation*: Conduct formative and summative assessments of progress toward goals at agreed-on intervals.
8. *Renegotiation or termination*: Agree to modify, renegotiate, or terminate the contract.

As community/public health nurses use this process to negotiate a contract, they must adapt it to each situation. Nevertheless, the basic elements remain important considerations for successful contracting.

Levels of Contracting

Community/public health nurses use contracts at levels ranging from formal to informal, based on the situation. To fund a community health program for preventing child abuse, for example, a formal contract in the form of a written grant proposal may be needed. To conduct a wide-scale needs assessment of a homeless population, the services of an epidemiologist and statistician may require a formal contract to clarify roles and expectations as well as fees. *Formal contracting* involves all parties negotiating a written contract by mutual agreement, signing the agreement, and sometimes having it witnessed or notarized.

Informal contracting involves some form of verbal agreement about relatively clear-cut purposes and tasks. A client group may agree to prioritize their list of needs, the nurse may agree to conduct health teaching sessions, the social worker may agree to obtain informational materials, and so on. Sometimes, nurses use contracting informally without realizing it. They conclude a session with clients by agreeing with them about the purpose and time of the next meeting. Clients often find it helpful if the nurse gives them a written list or reminder of tasks or goals.

The level of contracting also may change during the development of communication and collaboration. Clients often need education about their options. Initially, they may have difficulty in identifying needs and making choices. The professional team can work to promote clients' self-confidence and help them assume increasing responsibility for their own health.

COLLABORATION AND PARTNERSHIPS IN COMMUNITY/PUBLIC HEALTH NURSING

Effective interdisciplinary and interprofessional collaboration is essential in the health care system to achieve quality health care and assure successful outcomes (Morgan, Pullon, & McKinlay, 2015). Collaboration is a purposeful interaction among nurses, clients, other professionals, and community members to develop strategies for improving the health of individuals, families, and communities (Hudson & Croker, 2017; Mitchell et al., 2013).

Although collaboration is a complex, dynamic process, it has two basic components: (1) a goal and (2) two or more parties assisting one another to achieve that goal. The overriding purpose of collaboration in community/public health practice is to benefit the health of the public.

According to a study done by Valaitis et al. (2018), two *intrapersonal factors* influence collaborative efforts: a person's skills, knowledge, and personal qualities and a person's attitudes, beliefs, and values (see Chapter 4). *Interpersonal factors* that promote collaboration in community/public health settings are the ability to

1. Develop trusting and inclusive relationships
2. Identify shared values, beliefs, and attitudes
3. Ensure role clarity
4. Communicate effectively
5. Influence effective decision-making processes (Valaitis et al., 2018)

Two examples of community collaboration are the **asset-based community development (ABCD)** approach and **community-based participatory research (CBPR)**.

The ABCD approach is a methodology that starts with identifying community assets and strengths, including local persons, community associations and networks, natural resources, and institutions, as a means of working with residents to create sustainable communities. Rather than a needs-focused approach, ABCD starts with identifying the types of skills and resources already available in the community and then involves consulting with the community members on improvements they would like to make (Nel, 2015; 2018). If you are interested in learning more about how to apply the ABCD methodology, you can access a free, easy-to-complete training at http://www.uniteforsight.org/community-development/abcd/. You will learn more about community assessment in Chapter 15.

Similarly, CBPR involves community members in the entire research process, from identifying a topic of importance to the community to implementing the research and disseminating the results (Springer & Skolarus, 2019). See more on CBPR in Chapter 4. Involving stakeholders in planning and implementing programs and research increases their buy-in and the likelihood of success as well as the quality of research findings.

Key principles for establishing partnerships and collaboration with communities and interprofessional team members include the following:

- Think "outside the box" when looking for partners or collaborators.
- View plans as guides toward a goal, staying flexible.
- Incorporate partners as part of the planning process; continuously expand participants, being prepared to replan.
- Maintain different levels of collaboration.
- Use consensus-building techniques that are creative and visual.
- Establish a shared vision; then share the plans and leadership (Nel, 2015; Suarez-Balcazar, Mirza, & Garcia-Ramirez, 2018).

To meet the needs of clients, C/PHN practice draws on the expertise and assistance of numerous individuals. The list of team members can include many different interdisciplinary health care professionals, as well as the population being reached. All partners should be encouraged and allowed to use their skills and knowledge to optimize outcomes (Springer & Skolarus, 2019; Suarez-Balcazar et al., 2018).

Depending on the need to be addressed, C/PHNs may work with many people on a single project or on multiple endeavors. Remember to involve the most important team players, members from the client population, which facilitates addressing potential barriers. Refer to the CoursePoint+ case study on community health improvement partnerships for an in-depth look at this process.

Culture and Collaborative Services

Culture is a set of shared understandings related to knowledge, attitudes, and behaviors that give meaning to an experience. In C/PHN, clients and providers are often separated by their own distinct cultures. Therefore, clients' cultural background, experience in collaboration and partnership building, perspectives, and expressions of need provide important information for the planning and delivery of services. By being aware of one's own culture and the difference between one's culture and the client's, a nurse can participate in cultural exchanges with clients that promote stronger alliances (Dyches, Haynes-Ferere, & Haynes, 2019). See Chapter 5 for more on culture in C/PHN.

Characteristics of Collaborative Partnerships in Community/Public Health Nursing

To explore the meaning of collaboration in the context of C/PHN, this section examines five characteristics that distinguish collaboration from other types of interaction: shared goals, mutual participation, maximized resources, clear responsibilities, and set boundaries.

Shared Goals

First, collaboration in C/PHN is goal directed. The nurse, clients, and others involved in the collaborative effort or partnership recognize specific reasons for entering into the relationship (Kraaijenbrink, 2019). For example, a lumber company with 150 employees seeks to develop a wellness program. The interdisciplinary health team will work together to develop specific physical and mental health goals. The team enters into the collaborative relationship with broad needs or purposes to be met and specific objectives to accomplish.

Mutual Participation

Second, in C/PHN, collaboration involves mutual participation; all team members contribute and are mutually benefited (Ma, Park, & Shang, 2018). Collaboration involves a reciprocal exchange, in which individual team players discuss their intended involvement and contribution, and all members of a team should feel equally valued—no hierarchies should exist (Davis & Travers Gustafson, 2015). In interdisciplinary teams, physicians, nurses, lay community health workers, clients, outside agency personnel, and others must be able to effectively share ideas and frustrations on an equal, reciprocal basis.

Maximized Use of Resources

A third characteristic of collaboration is that it maximizes the use of community assets (Majee, Goodman, Vetter-Smith, & Canfield, 2016). That is, the collaborative partnership is designed to draw on the expertise of those who are most knowledgeable and in the best positions to influence a favorable outcome. In this age of dwindling resources, it is now common for public health agencies to seek additional funding assistance from other agencies to support new community/public health programs or to provide educational information or interventions. Being able to demonstrate fiscal responsibility and evidence-based outcomes will assist nurses in sustaining health promotion efforts on a long-term basis through collaborative partnerships.

Clear Responsibilities

Fourth, the collaborating team members work in partnership and assume clearly defined responsibilities. Each member in the partnership plays a specific role with related tasks. Effective collaboration clearly designates what each member will do to accomplish the identified goals. Each member of the team develops an understanding of individual responsibilities based on realistic and honest expectations. This understanding comes through effective communication. The collaborating partners explore necessary resources, assess their capabilities, and determine their willingness to assume tasks.

Boundaries

Fifth, collaboration in community/public health practice has set boundaries, with a beginning and an end, that fall within the goals of the partnership. An important part of defining collaboration is determining the conditions under which it occurs and when it will be terminated. The temporal boundaries sometimes are determined by progress toward the goal, sometimes by the number of team member contacts, and often by setting a time limit (Browning, Torain, & Patterson, 2016). Once the purpose for the collaboration has been accomplished, the group as a formal entity can be terminated.

In some settings, the partnership may desire to continue to work on other, mutually agreed-on activities. Some partnerships are ongoing. For example, a university department of nursing might use a neighborhood community center for clinical experiences for their students. When people collaborate and work together in partnership, many possibilities exist.

Levels of Prevention

In Box 10-10, the levels of prevention are used to provide a framework for the collaborative process in C/PHN. One objective in *Healthy People 2030* is the Environmental Health objective EH-04: Reduce blood lead levels in children aged 1 to 5 years (USDHHS, 2020). To achieve this objective, community/public health nurses need to be able to collaborate effectively with community partners in the design and implementation of health programs that address this very significant issue.

The importance of effective collaboration to address lead contamination (Fig. 10-6) was highlighted when the United States witnessed the tragic contamination of

BOX **10-10** LEVELS OF PREVENTION PYRAMID

Children's Health and the Environment

SITUATION: High lead blood levels were identified in a community
GOAL: Using the three levels of prevention:

- Develop programs and policies to prevent childhood lead poisoning.
- Screen children for elevated blood levels.
- Ensure that lead-poisoned infants and children receive appropriate medical care and environmental follow-up.

Tertiary Prevention*

Prevent Death and Further Disability	*Interventions*
■ Restore child to healthful state. ■ Restore the environment to a healthful state.	■ Medical treatment as indicated ■ Removal of child from environment ■ Aggressive environmental remediation

Secondary Prevention*

Early Diagnosis	*Prompt Treatment*
■ Surveillance and screening activities for early detection, treatment, and referral for management of lead exposure	■ Identification of children with elevated blood lead levels ■ Routine maintenance and repair of homes in high-risk communities

Primary Prevention*

Health Promotion and Education	*Health Protection*
■ Identify populations at high-risk for housing-based lead exposure. ■ Develop strategies to ensure lead-safe housing. ■ Collaborative partnerships to provide educational programs increasing knowledge of lead safety ■ Evaluate and redesign current prevention programs to achieve primary prevention.	■ Identify high-risk geographic areas using surveillance data ■ Identify high-risk families who could benefit from immediate assessment ■ Educate community partners on the cost of inaction; highlight risk disparities. ■ Incorporate lead hazard screening into home visits by community health nurses.

*The goal of Tertiary Prevention is to reduce morbidity from lead exposure. The goal of Secondary Prevention is to minimize absorption of lead and eliminate chronic exposure. The goal of Primary Prevention is to remove lead from the environment to eliminate exposure.
Source: CDC (2019a).

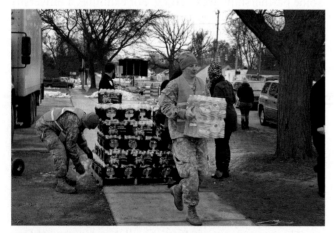

FIGURE 10-6 Emergency water distribution following the discovery of lead contamination of water supplied in Flint, Michigan in 2014.

publicly supplied drinking water in Flint, Michigan. The contamination occurred in 2014 when the community's water source was switched to the Flint River as a cost-saving measure (Zahran, McElmury, & Sadler, 2017). Signs and symptoms of lead poisoning are primarily neurologic, especially in children, and include seizures, stupor, delirium, behavioral changes, and headaches (Craft-Blacksheare, 2017). For more on this, see Chapters 7 and 9.

Nurses played a major role in the public health response to the contamination in Flint, including assessing clients for lead exposure and offering health education aimed at primary, secondary, and tertiary prevention. Nurses also offered emotional support, particularly to those most vulnerable and marginalized (Craft-Blacksheare, 2017). This modern-day example of a major public health response involved nurses working in collaboration with the U.S. Public Health Service; the

Centers for Disease Control and Prevention; the U.S. Surgeon General; county and state health departments; the Environmental Protection Agency; federally qualified health centers; the Red Cross; free medical clinics; local, state, and national political leaders; and a wide array of other community agencies.

Effective public health responses are possible only when interdisciplinary, cross-sectoral bodies collaborate efficiently and effectively. The Public Health Leadership Forum (2018) and the Health Care Transformation Task Force developed a framework aimed to support and improve collaboration between health care and public health bodies. Five primary elements of collaboration include establishing a governance structure, creating a financing plan, utilizing cross-sector prevention models, developing a data-sharing strategy, and ensuring that performance is measured and evaluated.

Fostering Client Participation

This chapter has stressed that communication and collaboration are based on mutual participation. The extent of clients' participation varies, however, depending on their readiness and ability to participate (Biswas, Faulkner, Oh, & Alter, 2017). The client's level of wellness at the time of the initial nurse–client encounter directly influences participation. In this case, the nurse may have to take a stronger initial leadership role; however, the nurse should not abandon the goals of collaboration. Gradually, as the client's wellness level improves or the client's family becomes more involved, the nurse can encourage more active participation. Clients with developmental disabilities or cognitive impairment may not have the capacity for true collaboration at any point in the process.

Engaging clients in a collaborative process may be difficult at times. Clients with low literacy, with low income, or from different cultural backgrounds may need extensive encouragement to actively participate in a collaborative relationship. Sometimes, a client's previous experience with health personnel limits participation in collaboration. For example, clients who were not previously encouraged to participate in decision making by health care providers or team members may take a passive role and not feel that they can truly collaborate. Unless the nurse persists in efforts to empower clients, the relationship can fall short of therapeutic goals (Dawson-Rose et al., 2016).

The nurse's own view of collaboration also influences the degree of client participation. Nurses who see their position as more informed and the client's position as one of complete ignorance and need may find that a paternalistic relationship develops. All clients have resources on which to build, and the community/public health nurse should help clients to discover these resources and empower clients to use them to enhance collaboration and attain health goals.

Barriers to Effective Collaboration

Communication barriers and miscommunication can inhibit effective collaboration. This is sometimes caused by misconceptions on the part of team members regarding the professional knowledge and motives of other team members. Stereotypes and the perception of unequal power and authority can sabotage the effectiveness of communication and collaboration. Organizational or structural factors, such as ineffective coordination and lack of agency support, are also cited as barriers to effective collaboration (Hanson et al., 2018).

Conflict is inevitable when dealing with groups of diverse individuals, but how potential anger, resentment, and mistrust are handled is the key to getting beyond conflict (Gerardi, 2015). Agreeing on how conflict will be handled prior to any incidents sets a positive stage for resolution. One strategy is to agree to handle conflict by using the **carefronting** model, which is described as a method of addressing and resolving conflict by confronting others in a caring, responsible, yet self-asserting manner (Sherman, 2016). Using "I" messages ensures that all parties in the conflict matter and that you care enough to negotiate differences so that common goals can be met. Key principles in the carefronting model are presented in Table 10-3.

HEALTH TECHNOLOGY

Health technology/informatics incorporates processes, procedures, theories, and concepts from information and computer science, health sciences, and social sciences. Nurses use the tools of information technology to support delivery of care and improve the health status of all. Health data, information, wisdom, and knowledge can be collected, stored, processed, and communicated. Nurses and other health professionals, administrators, policy and decision makers, consumers, and clients or patients can use information technology, hardware, and software (Veazie et al., 2018).

Electronic Health Records

Electronic health records (EHRs) are, at their simplest, digital (computerized) versions of patients' paper charts. The contemporary EHR is a complex piece of software with multiple functions and capabilities that enables a health care provider to record patient progress in free text, place prescription orders, receive decision-support alerts and reminders, order laboratory tests, receive and review results electronically, message patients or fellow providers, and perform a variety of other documentation and clinical tasks. It may contain lab and x-ray results and medications and medical history, along with administrative and billing information (Office of the National Coordinator for Health Information Technology [ONC], 2019).

The use of EHRs in community/public health has followed a slower progression than in hospitals. Reporting (e.g., communicable disease, immunizations) has moved from paper to unidirectional electronic reporting in many areas. In public health, EHRs have been shown to improve efficiency, productivity, quality of care, cost reduction, and data management, although drawbacks include missing data, complex technology, and the learning curve (Kruse, Stein, Thomas, & Kaur, 2018; Pyron & Carter-Templeton, 2019). Agencies may find EHRs helpful in areas such as epidemiology, large-scale planning, budgets, and grant writing. For example, an agency may search for specific characteristics and

TABLE 10-3 Key Principles for Carefronting: Facing Client Aggression

Principle	Action
Seeking truth	■ Active listening with empathy to understand viewpoints ■ Speak honestly about one's own feelings and attitudes ■ Use simple, nonjudgmental speech
Owning your anger	■ Acknowledge anger in a constructive way that affirms emotion and self-worth ■ Take responsibility for your own anger
Inviting change	■ Gently invite change in a caring manner; do not force or demand change ■ Focus on change in behavior, not the person
Demonstrating trust	■ Approach all conflict trusting that the other person is being honest and frank while being committed to finding a solution ■ When trust is broken, work to restore trust
Stopping blame	■ Avoid blaming ■ Ask where we go from here
Getting unstuck	■ Own responsibility for one's role in the conflict
Making peace	■ Appreciate multiple viewpoints ■ Risk being present to resolve conflict and make piece

Source: Lamont & Brunero (2018); Sherman (2016).

target vulnerable populations to best determine more effective planning and targeted interventions (e.g., clients with specific chronic diseases, current smokers). Individuals may also gain access to their own health information, and this is especially helpful in the case of immunization records (Birkhead, Klompas, & Shah, 2015; Kruse et al., 2018).

Big Data

We live in a digitized world. Massive amounts of data are captured daily as we browse the Internet, swipe our credit cards, visit a clinic for a flu vaccine, or use social media sites. Other sources include biological or genomic data, geospatial analyses (statistical analysis of geographic mapping) data sets, readings from personal monitoring devices people wear (e.g., GPS, FitBit), payer and EHRs, or "effluent data" constantly flowing from computer searches, online records, cell phone accounts, or social media (Mooney & Pejaver, 2017, p. 96).

- **Big data** represent "largescale data collections..." from a wide variety of sources and includes the unique methods of data processing, analyses, and storage (e.g., cloud servers, distributed data warehouses) needed to accommodate massive data sets (Zhu, Han, Su, Zhang, & Duan, 2019, p. 229).
- The four V's of big data include
  - Volume: Denotes the massive amount of data (2.5 quintillion bytes of data every day)
  - Velocity: Refers to the speed of data generation, collection, analysis, and transmission
  - Variety: Means the different types of data (often unstructured) that are collected that require sophisticated technology to overcome data inconsistencies
  - Veracity: Refers to assuring accuracy and trustworthiness of massive data sets that may be used for secondary analysis, have missing items, or need statistical cleaning to assure validity (Massachusetts Medical Society, 2018; Zhu et al., 2019)

Nurses in all settings add to big data through sharable and comparable documentation in the EHR. The use of big data makes it easier to drill down (or view more detailed information), drill up (or see data in an aggregate view), as well as combine different data variables than when using more traditional forms of data collection and analysis (Garcia, 2015).

A goal of EHR documentation is capturing health and nursing care data in structured ways that help build a foundation for accurate, reliable, clinically meaningful measurement across systems and settings of care (ONC, 2019). Big data are the core of that documentation, but the lack of standardized data and a common data structure are barriers to nursing research that highlights the outcomes of nursing care linked to assigned patients. The consistent and reliable use of data elements will allow information to be collected once and reused for multiple purposes (Sensmeier, 2015). If EHR systems are not integrated (e.g., if they do not work together and talk to each other), the task is much more challenging.

- The National Patient-Centered Clinical Research Network (PCORnet) is a central source of data from EHRs and provider billing that is currently used for health care research. Providers can be linked to patients, and nursing researchers are "working on a structure to make the location of care and nurse characteristics visible to researchers" (Garcia, Harper, & Welton, 2019, p. 100).
- The Nursing Value Data Model (NVDM) is a framework to guide big data use in nursing research, and

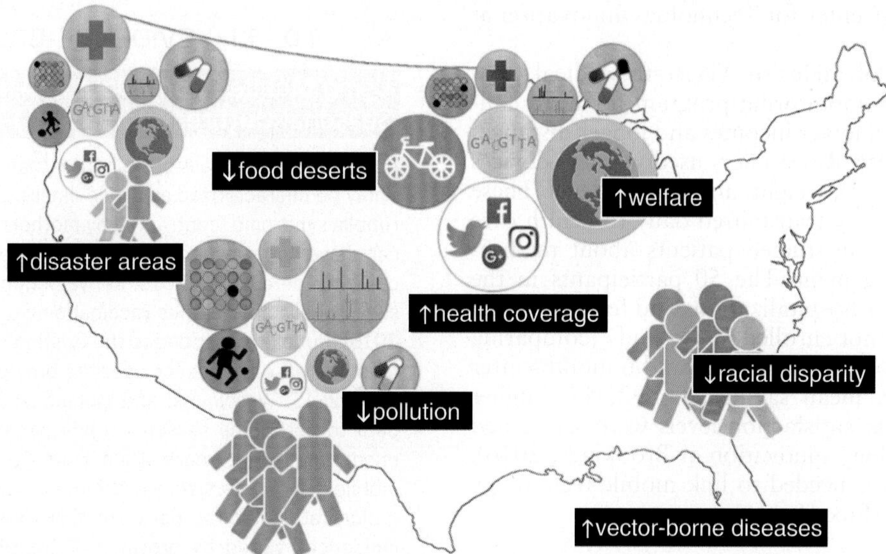

FIGURE 10-7 Precision public health infographic. (Reprinted from Prosperi, M., Min, J. S., Bian, J., Bian, J., & Mopdave, F. (2018). Big data hurdles in precision medicine and precision public health. *BMC Medical Informatics and Decision Making, 18*(1), 139. doi: 10.1186/s12911-018-0719-2. Reprinted under the Creative Commons License http://creativecommons.org/licenses/by/4.0)

the National Database of Nursing Quality Indicators (NDNQI) provides a means of consistent coding for various populations receiving nursing care (Garcia et al., 2019). Because nursing is a process-oriented profession, to effectively demonstrate nursing interventions and patient outcomes, data specific to nursing must be collected (Hersh, 2019).

Precision medicine (Fig. 10-7), using genomic and other big data, can provide more individualized care and treatments, along with more personally tailored medication regimens. It is also useful in disease prediction and differential diagnosis (Prosperi, Min, Bian, & Modave, 2018). In the future, even vaccines may be tailored for "homogeneous subpopulations" rather than a single vaccine given to everyone (Dolley, 2018, p. 4). Big data are used in precision public health to promote population health through epidemiology, disease surveillance, risk prediction, research, and preventive care. Big data have also been used to identify treatment and intervention in public health research on childhood obesity and asthma, HIV, misuse of opioid medications, use of smokeless tobacco and with HIV and the Zika virus (Dolley, 2018) (Fig. 10-7).

Mobile Health (mHealth)

The rapid expansion of mobile technology provides an opportunity for nurses and other clinicians to improve health and health care through forms of interactive **mobile health (mHealth)**, referred to as mHealth services. mHealth includes the use of wireless technologies, such as smartphones, tablets, and notebooks for improving health. mHealth offers great opportunities for improving global health, safety, and preparedness. The potential of mobile technology's impact on sharing health information and collecting disease/health data is tremendous due to its portability, affordability, and availability; it also has the potential to save billions of dollars in health care costs (Naqvi & Shah, 2018). The potential of mHealth will be further established as patients' experiences with technology and clinical/psychosocial outcomes are evaluated (Marcolino et al., 2018).

Three current mHealth trends have been identified by USDHHS (2014). The trends include mHealth technology that is interactive, integrated, and multimedia.

- Interactive strategies enable "two-way flow of information that engages patients more actively" in their health management.
- **Integrative strategies** use multiple "self-management applications to share health information between patients and providers through text messages, centralized web-based" tracking and management programs, and mobile monitoring (such as glucose monitoring).
- Multimedia use "games and quizzes" to communicate preventive messages and motivate behavior change (USDHHS, 2014, p. 5).

mHealth is extending health care to underserved and hard to reach areas. Technology puts health care providers in a position to change how health care is delivered, the quality of the patient experience, and the cost of health care. Advantages include management of chronic disease, empowering the elderly and expectant mothers, reminding people to take medication, serving underserved areas, and improving health outcomes and medical system efficiency. However, big differentials in the number of mobile devices exist among nations. In 2020, China and India (1.65 billion and 1.2 billion, respectively), followed by the United States (422 million), had the highest number of mobile devices, whereas several island nations (e.g., Falkland Islands, Marshall Islands, Cook Islands) had the lowest number—between 5000 and 14,000 (Central Intelligence Agency, 2020). A report cited common uses for mHealth globally that included call centers, reminders, and telemedicine. Mobile medical applications and wearable medical devices were projected to be growth areas for mHealth (Center for Technology Innovation at Brookings, 2016).

As an example of mHealth, Flagstaff Medical Center piloted a remote monitoring program for heart failure patients who had lower incomes and longer distances to drive to the facility. Researchers used wireless devices to track blood pressure, weight, and activity level. These data were electronically transmitted daily to health care providers, who then instructed patients about medication and diet management. The 50 participants in the pilot study had fewer hospitalizations and fewer hospital days than did those not enrolled in the study (comparing baseline 6 months before enrollment and 6 months after enrollment), with a mean savings of $92,317. Higher patient and caregiver satisfaction levels were also noted (Center for Technology Innovation at Brookings, 2016). Continued research is needed to link mobile technology to health outcomes (Box 10-11).

Mobile Phones

Approximately 96% of Americans own a cell phone, and 81% of those are smartphones (Pew Research Center, 2019). And 67% of cell owners find themselves checking their phone for messages, alerts, or calls—even when they don't notice their phone ringing or vibrating. Konok, Gigler, Bereczky, and Miklósi (2016) reported that people are extremely attached to their mobile phones; most were kept within arm's reach. Mobile phone use is highest among individuals who use a cell phone as their primary method of communication.

Text messaging and the use of applications and other mHealth interventions can reduce geographic and economic barriers to health information and services. These interventions have the potential to reduce health disparities and leverage a profound effect on health (USDHHS, 2020b). A recent study found Black and Hispanic participants used mobile digital devices to access patient portals more often than White participants, who relied more on computers (Chang, Blondon, Courtney, Lyles, Jordan, & Ralston, 2018). Another study found that "racial/ethnic minorities and patients living in poorer neighborhoods" most often checked personal health records exclusively by means of a mobile device (Graetz et al., 2018, para. 1). Optimizing Web sites for mobile devices could be helpful in reaching diverse populations and would enable a wide audience to test and review apps in development. Mobile phone technologies offer promising opportunities for nurses working in the community setting (Brayboy, McCoy, Thamotharan, Zhu, Gil, & Houck, 2018).

Connected health offers the patient the opportunity to feel constantly connected to the health delivery system and offers the system a just-in-time messaging opportunity that can be motivating, educational, and caring (Health Information and Management Systems Society, 2019). A disadvantage is that mobile or cellular phones are less reliable than landlines, with users sometimes citing spotty service, dropped calls, and text messages delayed or lost in cyberspace.

Text messages are the initial, simplest, and most common type of mobile data service and are becoming a vital tool for the delivery of health information and engaging users to improve their health (CDC, 2019e; Kazemi et al., 2017). Text messaging is a way of connecting quickly with a large population (Benetoli, Chen, & Aslani, 2018). The use of text messaging has been advocated in HIV testing as a means of improving health quality and preventing complications (Brown, Tan, Guerra, Naidoo, & Nardone, 2018). Marcolino et al. (2018) conducted a systematic review of text messaging and the implications in health care and noted that this is growing in use and popularity. Given the widespread use of mobile phone text message reminders among different patient groups, it may have the potential to improve adherence to medication and attendance at clinical appointments globally.

BOX **10-11** EVIDENCE-BASED PRACTICE

Using Mobile Phone Data to Assess Drivers of Seasonal Outbreaks of Rubella in Kenya

Incidence of rubella is often higher than reported because it may be characterized as a mild illness. However, congenital rubella syndrome, contracted by mothers in early pregnancy, can have long-lasting repercussions (e.g., stillbirth, serious birth defects). In 2016, Kenya began a large-scale measles—rubella and tetanus vaccination campaign (WHO Africa, 2016). Rubella was added to the existing measles vaccine due to an increased incidence over the previous few years.

In 2015, Wesolowski and colleagues used mobile phone data to determine seasonal travel patterns that may influence rubella outbreaks. Data from 15 million anonymous mobile phone users revealed higher movement and aggregation rates at three peak times of rubella incidence. Peak incidences varied by province. Rates of rubella and other communicable diseases often rise during the school year, when children are gathered in classrooms. However, in the western area of Kenya, the risk of rubella transmission was highest during school breaks. Researchers statistically controlled for rainfall and school terms and used maps to examine spatial and temporal patterns of risk based on the mobile phone data of population movements. They were able to identify high-risk areas and variations over the 1-year period of the study. They found that all regions except Nairobi varied in areas of high risk for rubella during the year.

The Wesolowski et al. study verified a new tool in the fight against communicable diseases, as "patterns of population fluxes inferred from mobile phone data are predictive of disease transmission ....showing .... that mobile phone data capture epidemiologically relevant patterns of movement" (Wesolowski et al., 2015, p. 11114).

1. *How could public health departments use mobile phone data to track communicable diseases in your area? Which data would be most critical?*
2. *In what other instances would knowledge of population mobile phone use in your area be helpful (e.g., disaster notification, health promotion, immunization reminders)? Are these being utilized in your area?*
3. *Find other research about digital technology in public health. Are the findings significant, valid, and helpful to your population?*

Source: Wesolowski et al. (2015); WHO Africa (2016).

Text messaging is simple, low cost, and ubiquitous. It continues to increase as a form of communication. Text messaging is considered more private and less intrusive than a phone call. Pictures, video, and text reminders can also be sent. Text messaging allows for automatic contact with groups of clients without the sender having to send an individual message to each intended recipient (Griffiths et al., 2017). Response may be real time or at the leisure of the recipient. Text messages are less expensive than phone calls and less prone to spam than e-mail. Texts may be stored and revisited, and all languages are supported. The benefits of text messages and social media are numerous (Eckert et al., 2018). However, health literacy and cultural appropriateness for diverse populations must be considered when using text messages (USDHHS, 2014).

Reminder and educational text messages have the ability to be disseminated widely and broadly, reaching mass number of recipients quickly and inexpensively (Arya et al., 2018). Tailored, user-friendly interventions delivered by mobile phone may be a better fit with many individuals' lifestyles than traditional treatment and an attractive option for both clinicians and patients or clients. Mobile phones have a broad range of uses, diverse functions, and the ability to intercede in "real time." Text messaging can overcome barriers of time and access to reach even high-risk populations (Arya et al., 2018).

Much research in public health has found that it is possible to use text messages to help deliver health-related information and to aid people in disease management (e.g., diabetes) and make better health decisions such as smoking less and exercising more. Text message interventions promote healthy lifestyle behaviors, have become widely integrated into routine daily life, and are simple, low cost, and nonlabor intensive. Use of text messaging to deliver information about more sensitive topics, such as sexual health and reducing risky behaviors, seems promising. Opt-in features, which allow choice for the recipient, can also be used (Arya et al., 2018). These are helpful for immunization reminders, encouraging healthy behaviors, and more. Text messages may be used for simple reminders to have blood pressure checked, to notify individuals about an upcoming appointment, or to pick up prescriptions (Benetoli et al., 2018). Box 10-12 provides selected examples of how text messaging has been used to implement interventions as well as supporting research.

BOX 10-12 Selected Examples of Text Messaging Interventions and Research

- PHNs providing case management to low-income women with chronic conditions results in improved mental health and functional status.
- A series of automated text messages to predominantly low-income, Hispanic parents about influenza and the importance of flu shots results in a small but meaningful increase in child vaccinations.
- Sexual health clinics communicate most test results via text message, leading to quicker diagnoses and treatment and improved clinic capacity for processing new cases.
- Weekly text messaging service for teens and young adults improves access to sexual health information/services and engenders positive changes in behavior and knowledge.
- Low-income, African American, rural HIV patients receive regular text message reminders that encourage them to regularly access HIV/AIDS primary care, leading to improved retention in care and quality of life.
- Daily, automated text messages combined with nurse follow-up improved diabetic patient self-management behaviors and led to better glycemic control, fewer doctor visits, and higher patient satisfaction.
- A statewide text messaging service targeting minority youth and young adults in Illinois provides accurate information on HIV/AIDS and how to access free HIV testing and related services.
- A Medicaid managed care organization uses cell phone text messaging to remind members with type 2 diabetes to get blood glucose testing, resulting in a significant increase in members being tested on a regular basis.
- Regular reminders via text message increase adherence to medication regimens and reduce risk of organ rejection in pediatric liver transplant patients.
- SexInfo provided free basic information and referrals for in-person health consultations to at-risk youth in San Francisco via an opt-in text messaging service.
- Weekly text messaging service for teens and young adults improves access to sexual health information and services and produces positive changes in behavior and knowledge.

Source: Agency for Health Care Quality & Research (AHRQ) (2018).

Loescher, Rains, Kramer, Akers, and Mossa (2016) conducted a systematic review of research studies on adult physical activity and a text messaging intervention. They concluded that text messaging as a method to promote health activities shows improvement in healthy behaviors and health outcomes.

Text messaging is used globally to communicate and to motivate individuals to engage in healthy or healthier behaviors, deliver public health messages, and alert populations about available resources or disasters. In some cases, other digital solutions may be more effective. A systematic review of research studies using texting, video-observed therapy (VOT), or medication monitors in tuberculosis care found that text messaging did not significantly affect completion of treatment, whereas VOT rates of treatment completion were comparable to the much more expensive directly observed treatment (DOT) option. Groups using medication monitors demonstrated statistically significant reductions in missed doses over those using standard care measures (Ngwatu et al., 2018).

Nurses and other clinicians may use texting to assist patients and caregivers with management of chronic conditions and disease prevention. Text messaging provides a venue to deliver information to hard-to-reach populations and the opportunity to have a positive influence on health knowledge and behaviors, as evidenced by clinical outcomes in a recent study among college students (Glowacki et al., 2018; USDHHS, 2014). See Box 10-13 for best practices in using text messages.

BOX 10-13 Text Messaging Best Practices

1. *Keep messages short.* Text messages should be short and concise. The entire message should be <160 characters, including spaces and punctuation and any branding or links to additional information (p. 25).
2. *Make messages engaging:* Write relevant, timely, clear, and actionable messages.
3. *Make content readable:* Content should be at or below an 8th grade reading level.
4. *Use abbreviations sparingly:* Only use those that are easily understood and don't change meaning.
5. *Limit foreign language characters:* Accented letters do not work well in texts.
6. *Provide access to additional information:* Include a way for users to follow up or respond to the message (e.g., URL, phone number, mobile Web site).
7. *Include opt-out options:* Include information on how to opt-out of the text message program.
8. *Evaluate your efforts.* Evaluation can be accomplished with surveys and metrics reviews.

Source: Centers for Disease Control and Prevention (CDC) (2016).

Applications

An application, or app for short, may be defined as a software program developed to help the user perform specific tasks (Greenie, Morgan, Sayani, & Meghani, 2018). Apps are self-contained programs, used to enhance existing functionality, in a simple and user-friendly way. Today's modern smartphones come with powerful web browsers, meaning nearly anything that can be done on a desktop computer can be done with a smartphone's browser. The portability of the app that allows the user to remain connected is very appealing to both nurses and clients. Many new mobile apps are targeted to assist individuals in their own health and wellness management. Other mobile apps are targeted to health care providers as tools to improve and facilitate the delivery of patient care (Greenie et al., 2018).

Application developers have noticed the potential of health care apps. Health professionals are necessary in app development to peer-review the reliability, usability, and usefulness of medical apps. Zweig, Shen, & Jug (2019) conducted a national survey of 4000 adults about digital health adoption that revealed an upward trend from 2015 to 2017 in the use of digital tools like online health information, online health provider reviews, wearables, and telemedicine. The most common reasons for wearable use were to lose weight and increase physical activity. Those keeping track of their blood pressure rarely utilized digital tracking. Almost a quarter of respondents owned a wearable device (Fig. 10-8), but about a quarter of users discontinued use either due to reaching their goals or due to inability to reach goals. Data security was important to participants; although 87% reported willingness to share health data with their providers, they were less confident in the security of their data in the hands of health insurance companies, pharmacies, government organizations, and tech companies and were therefore less willing to share data with these entities. Although older adults could reap greater benefits from the use of health tools, they were less likely to use them than young, high-income adults. There is a significant market for these technologies to promote health (Brayboy et al., 2018).

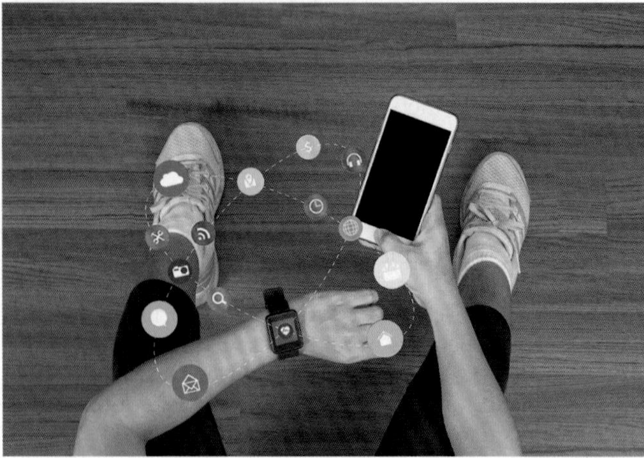

FIGURE 10-8 Social media and technology have the capacity to reach and influence the health behaviors of a wide audience.

The Food and Drug Administration (FDA) is responsible for the protection of public health by assuring the safety, effectiveness, quality, and security of human and veterinary drugs, vaccines and other biological products, and medical devices (FDA, 2019). The FDA intends to apply regulatory oversight to medical mobile apps and identifies apps as medical devices whose functionality could pose a risk to an individual's safety if the mobile app did not function as intended (Shuren, Patel, & Gottlieb, 2018).

FastStats and Mobile Apps

The CDC offers a Web site called FastStats, which provides quick access to statistics on topics of public health importance and is organized alphabetically. Links are provided to publications that include the statistics presented, sources of more data, and related web pages (CDC, 2019b). The site can be accessed at https://www.cdc.gov/nchs/fastats/default.htm.

In addition, CDC offers a free "CDC Mobile App" where you can access important public health information at any time. The app automatically updates when your device in online, so you are sure to receive the most up-to-date health news and information. The app also provides direct links to social media, text, and email, enabling you to share information with clients and colleagues. In addition, you can gain access to CDC's *Morbidity and Mortality Weekly Report (MMRW)* and their Disease of the Week articles (CDC, 2018). The following link will take you to CDC's site where you can download the free CDC Mobile App: https://www.cdc.gov/mobile/applications/cdcgeneral/promos/cdcmobileapp.html.

Twitter

Twitter is a micro-messaging/microblogging technology and an online social networking service that enables users to send and read short 140-character messages called "tweets." Posts are delineated by a hashtag (#) symbol to organize topics (Benetoli et al., 2018). Microblogging began with the advent of Twitter in 2006 and is a method of mass communication. "Followers" or users sign up to follow the microblog (Benetoli et al., 2018). Twitter is real time and designed for mobility. E-registered users can read and post tweets by computer or smartphone, and anyone on Twitter (not just followers) can see tweets on a public account. Twitter provides important insight related to health and is a useful tool to promote health behaviors (Baumann, 2016; Grover, Kar, & Davies, 2018).

Grover et al. (2018) found that Twitter was a helpful tool to engage patients. Nurses/clinicians and health care systems can use Twitter to communicate timely information, both within the medical community and to patients as well as the general public. Short messages, or tweets, are delivered to a group of recipients simultaneously, providing an easy and quick method to reach large groups in limited time. There are obvious advantages for sharing time-critical information such as disaster alerts and drug safety warnings, tracking disease outbreaks, or disseminating health care information. Twitter applications can deliver information about clinical trials, for example, or link brief news alerts from the CDC to reliable Web sites that provide more detailed information (Vijaykumar, Nowak, Himelboim, & Jin, 2018). Clinicians can tweet from the operating room or a disaster site allowing live updates (Eckert et al., 2018).

The CDC also encourages the use of Twitter as an effective vehicle to disseminate health information and engage communities and partners. Box 10-14 offers CDC's best practices for using Twitter to improve health (CDC, 2019e).

BOX 10-14 Twitter Best Practices

1. *Clearly Define Your Objectives:* Do you want to highlight content, spark action, or encourage awareness of an issue?
2. *Know Your Target Audience(s):* Knowing your target audience informs how you develop and communicate messages that resonate with your audience.
3. *Determine Resource Needs:* Who will manage the Twitter profile? Who will be the point of contact and monitor the posts on a regular basis?
4. *Keep Your Content Short and Simple:* Use not more than 120 characters (including URL, punctuation and spaces) to make it easy for followers to retweet the message without having to edit it.
5. *Determine Schedule and Frequency of Twitter Posts:* Set a posting schedule that defines a frequency for posts per week.
6. *Conduct Promotion Activities:* Promote your Twitter profile to the extent possible to expand your reach.
7. *Determine Approach for Engaging with Twitter Followers:* Develop a strategy for identifying and retweeting or replying to posts from partners and followers.
8. *Evaluate:* Regularly monitor your Twitter account to review the number of followers, updates, retweets and mentions in Twitter; also consider monitoring the increases in traffic to your Web site.
9. *Establish a Records Management System:* Set-up a system to keep track of your Twitter posts, @replies, retweets, and mentions to comply with Federal guidelines for records management and archiving.

Source: Centers for Disease Control and Prevention (CDC) (2019e); Christofferson et al. (2015).

Blogging and Online Support Communities

Blogs or weblogs are web-based chronological journals (Thomas, Allison, & Latour, 2018). They are free or low cost and easy to use. Blogs typically include date-stamped, multiple entries in chronological order and are updated frequently. Blogs usually focus on a particular subject or topic. One type of blog, referred to as a simple blog, is a form of online personal diaries. Other blogs relate to group causes such as political or social concerns, and some may ask for contributions. Blogs may contain reflections, commentaries, comments, images, videos, and often hyperlinks to other information of interest to the blogger or that she/he feels will be of interest to their readers. The ability for readers to leave comments on a blog post depends on the settings that the blog administrator uses (Thomas et al., 2018).

- The popularity or success of a blog is judged by its ability to draw individuals together who are interested in a specialized topic. Many journals, health care systems, nursing and other professional organizations, health care provider networks, and educational institutions create blogs to provide the latest information and promote discussion (Thomas et al., 2018).
- Many people create personal blogs when faced with an illness or are a family member/support for someone facing health challenges. Participating in the creation of health information through blogging and social networking contributions influences experiences and supports an individual's understanding of their role in health care management and ability to copy with their disease process (Tsai, Crawford, & Strong, 2018).

Traditional forms of contact and support groups are limited to certain hours of the day, week, or month. Some face-to-face support groups meet weekly or monthly and may require considerable travel and effort. Telephone help lines may be available only during office hours. Conversely, online blogs allow for contact and support that are available at any hour of the day or night via the Internet. Individuals who have joined an online support group benefit from venting their feelings and from the support they receive as well as feeling connected by helping and supporting others (CDC, 2015; Partridge, Gallagher, Freeman, & Gallagher, 2018). Online supportive relationships generally provide a safe environment. Others' experiences can induce feelings of compassion, and one becomes less self-absorbed and may gain a better perspective (Wagner, 2018). Finding a safe place to share can be very empowering, and the value of first-person accounts, the appeal and memorability of stories, and the need to make contact with peers all strongly suggest that reading and hearing others' accounts of their own experiences of health and illness will remain an important component of health management/care. For example, PatientsLikeMe (https://www.patientslikeme.com/) is a great example of a free Internet-based tool for sharing and learning.

Video Games and Virtual Reality Games

As of 2018, 67% of American adults have played video games (Electronic Entertainment Design and Research, 2019). Public attitudes toward video games and the people who play them are complex and often mixed. Video games are typically thought of as entertainment. However, there is a growing interest in video games as a means to facilitate healthy behaviors. Exercise programs based on video game activities provide an alternative to motivate and increase adherence to activity and exercise (Taylor, Kerse, Frakking, & Maddison, 2018).

Games can serve as a means to engage patients behaviorally in order to improve their health outcomes. Behaviors, often necessary to maintain and improve health, are reinforced.

- A recent 9-month study examined the use of an augmented reality game, Pokémon Go (Fig. 10-9), and discovered that it provided opportunities for increased exercise levels and suggested further research in public health (Wong, Turner, MacIntyre, & Yee, 2017).
- A systematic review of virtual reality rehabilitation found some evidence of improvement in motor skills and balance for children and adolescents with cerebral palsy (Ravi, Kuman, & Singhi, 2017).
- Researchers developed a game to help individuals with Parkinson's disease improve coordination, gross and fine dexterity, and strength of upper limb muscle grip. Results showed significant improvement in the experimental group (Fernandez-Gonzalez et al., 2019).

With game play, tension and fears are released in a safe setting, and aversive or shameful aspects of an illness may be managed. The focus of attention on an engaging distraction (the game) may explain how individuals manage aversive symptoms through video game play. An example of distractive use of a virtual reality game is SnowWorld (see Table 10-4 for description) that is used to distract patients during burn care.

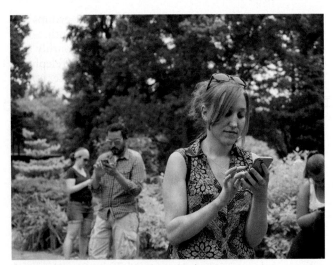

FIGURE 10-9 Individuals playing Pokémon Go.

Telehealth

Telehealth is the "use of technology to deliver health care, health information, or health education at a distance" (Association of State and Territorial Health Officials, 2017, p. 4). Telehealth Nursing: A Position Statement from the Telehealth Special Interest Group of the American Telemedicine Association states: Telehealth is "remote healthcare.....via electronic communications to improve patients' health status" using "different types of programs and services" (2019, p. 8). Telehealth gives the community/public health nurse an opportunity to see and speak with clients located at remote sites as well as provide education and counseling. Telehealth consists of delivery, management, and coordination of health services, integrating telecommunication and electronic technologies, to increase client access to health care and improve outcomes while lowering costs (Smith, Watts, & Moss, 2018).

Telehealth provides access to care and the ability to export clinical expertise to individuals who require care, regardless or geographic location of the patient or the clinician (Donelan et al., 2019). The boundaries of telehealth are limited only by the technology available, and new applications are being developed and tested every day. Telehealth can be divided into two general types of applications: real-time or synchronous communication and store-and-forward or asynchronous communication.

- Real-time communication scenarios include a patient and clinician consulting with a specialist via a live audio/video link, a clinician and a patient in an exam room communicating through an interpreter connected by phone or webcam, or a patient at home communicating with a C/PHN via a live audio/video link (Fig. 10-10).
- Asynchronous telehealth applications do not require members to be present at the same time but share the same information at the time most convenient to each one (Siwicki, 2019).

Telehealth has been growing rapidly because it offers four fundamental benefits:

- Improved access: Can reach patients in distant locations
- Cost efficiencies: Reduces the cost of health care
- Improved quality: Similar to traditional in-person care
- Patient convenience/satisfaction: Reduces travel time and related stresses

Telehealth shows great potential for advancing preventative medicine and the treatment of chronic conditions. The first year of reimbursement for telehealth services delivered outside of care settings occurred in 2015 (Wicklund, 2015). Between 2016 and 2017, telehealth

TABLE 10-4 Selected Health-Related Video Games and Virtual Reality Games

Name of Game if Specifically Named	Medical Condition Targeted	Game Description
Snow World Common Ground VR	Burn pain Vision	This game was created to minimize body motion during wound debridement by gameplay through the use of a joystick. Simulates visual disabilities (e.g., glaucoma, macular degeneration) to promote understanding and accommodation needs.
Packy and Marlon, (Super Nintendo system)	Diabetes for children	The game was designed to better understand how to maintain stable glucose levels and manage their insulin.
Bronkie the Bronchiasaurus (Super Nintendo)	Asthma for children	Players help the characters keep their asthma in control by avoiding dust, smoke, and other triggers while on their quest.
reSET & reSET-O	Individuals with substance abuse	Mobile app for tracking substance abuse, triggers, and cravings to promote abstinence.
Nonspecifically titled games that use biofeedback to control gameplay	Bladder and bowel dysfunction Pediatric voiding dysfunction in children	The child's compliance and motivation influence the success of biofeedback. Children are often not interested in dealing with embarrassing topics and may have difficulty staying focused on a biofeedback-training task. When combined with a game interface, interest and motivation in biofeedback are increased. The games helped improve symptoms and treatment compliance.
Nonspecifically titled games that employee biofeedback to control gameplay	Irritable bowel syndrome in adults	A computer biofeedback game designed for patients with IBS. The game teaches deep relaxation and stress management. The patients had more control of the animated gut movement when they were more relaxed.
Re-Mission2	Cancer in adolescents and young adults	A collection of six games. The goal of the games is to improve treatment, with players controlling a nanobot named Roxxi, who flies through tumors with chemotherapy and radiation. Animations and direct interactions with environments provide information. Studies revealed greater knowledge, self-efficacy, and treatment compliance.

Source: Cigna (2019); Coravos (2018); Lee (2017).

use grew 53%, outpacing growth in urgent care clinics (14%) and retail clinics (7%). Injuries, respiratory infections, and digestive problems were most commonly seen, along with mental health and joint/soft tissue issues. The growth in telehealth services demonstrates continued demand for this service (FAIR Health, 2019).

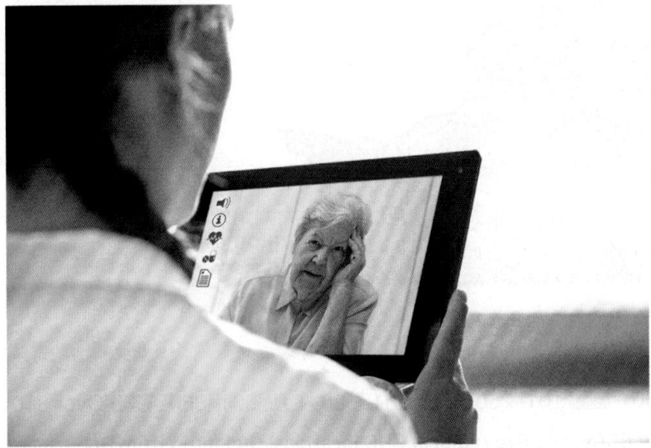

FIGURE 10-10 Telehealth gives the community/public health nurse an opportunity to see and speak with clients located at remote sites, as well as provide education and counseling.

In a survey of state health departments, ASTHO (Kearly & Oputa, 2019) found that over 51% used telehealth services to provide patient and professional health education. Other uses included behavioral health (42.4%), specialty care (40.2%), chronic disease (23.9%), and infectious disease (23.9%). Increased access was the greatest achievement (33.8%), whereas securing funding (22.4%) was the greatest challenge.

There are nursing licensure barriers, as nurses working in telehealth must be licensed in the state where patients are located at the time services are provided. Licensure compact regulations provide for multistate nursing licenses through the Enhanced National Licensure Compact (eNLC), which requires criminal background checks and licenses within states and reporting between states participating in the compact (Mataxen, 2019). As of January 2020, there were 38 member states of eNLC, either enacted or pending (Gaines, 2020).

Telehealth can be a lifeline during disasters and pandemics, such as the Covid-19 pandemic in 2020. In March 2020, because a national emergency declaration was issued, a waiver was made for the requirement that physicians or other health care professionals hold licenses in the state in which they provide services, as long as they have an equivalent license from another state. In addition, the Medicare telehealth waiver expanded chronic care management, interprofessional consultations, and digital evaluations (e-visits) and lifted geographical limitations as well as the requirement for a prior health care relationship to exist between the client and the health care provider. Other constraints were relaxed for the duration of the public health emergency, including restrictions on prescribing controlled substances and HIPAA-related limitations on the use of Facebook or Skype for telehealth (Center for Connected Health Policy, 2020).

Geographic Information Systems

A **geographic information system (GIS)** is a computer-based information system designed to capture, store, manipulate, analyze, manage, and present all types of spatial (relating to space) or geographical data (Fig. 10-11). GIS allows the user to visualize, question, analyze, and interpret data to understand relationships, patterns, and trends. Spatial or mappable data are integrated with conventional data. GIS can be thought of as a two-dimensional Google earth map. Google earth allows you to zoom in and out and pan around, and GIS additionally allows users to select a feature on the map and, in return, will be provided with any information in the database associated with that feature (University of Mary Washington, 2016). Much of community/public health is spatially related, so the use of GIS can provide information about demographic, epidemiological, and logistical issues and emerging trends. GIS output is location-based information. GIS can provide

- Better understanding of a current situation
- Planning/targeting of appropriate interventions
- Monitoring and revision of interventions as needed
- An opportunity for cooperation with other organizations and government departments through a culture of data sharing and working together

Sharing, comparing, and integrating GIS data will eliminate silos and result in better outcomes providing additional information to identify health disparities (Mohammadi et al., 2018). There is great potential for GIS to inform C/PHN. Nurses can play an important role in demonstrating how various data sources come together to enable informed decisions for populations and individuals (Kolifarhood, Khorasani-Zavareh, Salarilak, Shoghli, & Khosravi, 2015). Understanding of GIS may be considered an essential skill for the evolution of nursing practice (Mohammadi et al., 2018).

The tremendous potential of GIS to benefit health care delivery is being realized. Both public and private organizations are developing innovative ways to use GIS, from public health departments and public health policy and research organizations to hospitals, medical centers, and health insurance organizations. Public health uses of GIS include tracking child immunizations, evaluating the spread and clustering of diseases, conducting health policy research, and establishing service areas and districts (ArcUser Online, n.d.).

An example of how GIS has been used to benefit health care delivery is the research by DeGuzman et al. (2018). The purpose of their study was to use GIS and other mapping to identify local and regional access gaps of children with special health care needs (CSHCN), with the aim of pinpointing and reducing disparities. This collaborative group of academic and practice researchers recognized that access to necessary services for families of CSHCN is less convenient for rural populations due to distance and travel required. Public health departments often serve as safety net providers in these areas but sometimes need to refer clients to specialized programs at child development centers (CDCs). In the state of Virginia, there were only five CDCs helping children with motor/physical disorders, speech/developmental delays, attention-deficit hyperactivity disorder, or autism spectrum disorder. Researchers "layered individual-level data over county-level socioeconomic data" to bring the sociodemographic environment into focus (p. 2). A chloropeth map (i.e., color progression from lighter to darker areas) indicated the number of uninsured CSHCN children at the county level. As

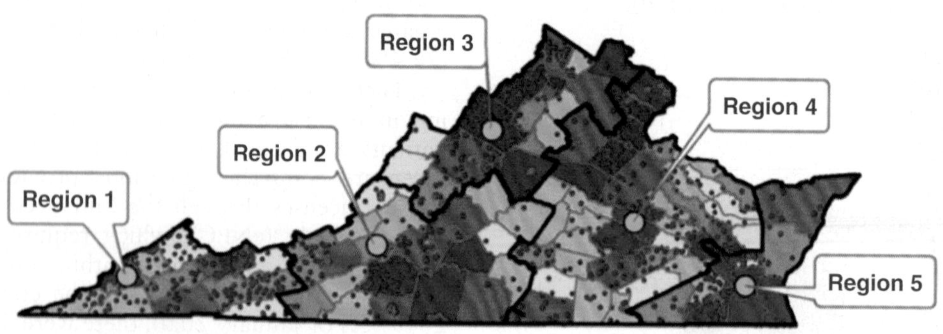

FIGURE 10-11 Map of Virginia indicating uninsured, children accessing CDCs, and five regional CDC locations.. (Adapted from DeGuzman, P., Altrui, P., Doede, A. L., Allen, M., Deagle, C., & Keim-Malpassa, J. (2017). Using geospatial analysis to determine access gaps among children with special healthcare needs. *Health Equity, 2*(1), 1–4. doi: 10.1089/heq.2017.0050. Copyright © Pamela DeGuzman et al. Reprinted under the Creative Commons License http://creativecommons.org/licenses/by/4.0)

Figures 10-11 depict, darker red and orange areas have a greater number of uninsured children. You can easily discern larger cities (groupings of dots) and rural areas (scattered dots) as well as the distance of the child from the nearest CDC. At a quick glance, it is evident that many children live in rural areas, and many of them are uninsured. One of the significant limitations of this chloropeth map is that it cannot include the unknown number of unserved children who never made contact with a CDC.

Electronic Health Literacy and the Digital Divide

The rapid development of communication technology affects every aspect of society as information is instantly available. Health communication and health information technology competencies are identified as vital skills of an informed consumer and essential for improving population health outcomes and health care quality. Electronic health literacy was first defined by Norman and Skinner (2006, para. 1) as the "ability to seek, find, understand, and appraise health information from electronic sources and apply the knowledge gained to addressing or solving a health problem."

Computer literacy and knowledge of the use of current technologies are part of health literacy. Increasingly, individuals must be able to use technology and navigate through a vast array of information, tools, and sources to acquire and critically analyze the information necessary to make appropriate and informed decisions (Vajan & Baban, 2015). The same is true for community/public health nurses, as noted in the Quad Council C/PHN competencies (2018) (see the appendix).

A digital divide exists between those who have easy access to computers, broadband Internet, and smartphones/tablets and those who do not. Often this affects those living in rural areas (Perrin, 2019). Recent technological developments have elevated the importance of assessing how electronic health tools have empowered patients and improved health, especially among the most vulnerable populations. There is potential for electronic health technologies to aid in reducing communication inequalities and disparities in health. The need exists to educate at-risk and needy groups (e.g., chronically ill) and design technology in a way that works for them. Addressing these areas may not diminish the digital divide, but it may ameliorate its consequences (Griebel et al., 2018).

SUMMARY

- Communication and collaboration are important tools for community/public health nurses to promote aggregate health. Communication involves the transfer and understanding of meaning between individuals. Motivational interviewing and OARS are means of joining with clients to effect change or meet needs. There are many barriers, skills, factors, and core skills essential to effective communication in community health nursing.
- In community/public health, nurses frequently need to promote group communication and in-group decision making. Decisions made by groups have many advantages, including sharing of members' experience and expertise, diversity of opinions, potential for broadening members' perspectives, and a focus on arriving at consensus solutions. There are several methods of enhancing group decision making.
- Collaboration and partnership building are purposeful interactions among the nurse, clients, community members, and other professionals based on mutual participation and joint effort. It is characterized by shared goals, mutual participation, maximized use of resources, clear responsibilities, set boundaries, and collaborative relationships.
- Contracting is a helpful tool in promoting clients' participation, independence, and motivation. It is used at all levels of community/public health nursing to promote partnership in the collaborative process, to encourage commitment to health goals, and to ensure a format and a means for negotiation among the collaborating parties. Contracts may be formal or informal, written or verbal, and simple or complex.
- EHRs are becoming more prevalent in public health and are commonplace in hospital and outpatient settings. There are both advantages and disadvantages to using electronic records.
- Big data include very large and complex data sets that are analyzed to uncover trends, associations, and patterns. This is very helpful in public health agencies in the areas of disease surveillance, population health management, and immunization trends.
- mHealth involves the use of mobile devices (e.g., smartphones, tablets, notebooks) for communication between clients and community/public health nurses and can be useful in promoting health. Trends in mHealth include interactive (two-way communication), integrative (patient/provider and tracking systems), and multimedia uses (games/quizzes to promote health).
- Technology applications are used for computers, tablets, and smartphones, and more health-related apps are available every year. C/PHNs must be aware of reliable applications to assist in health promotion.
- Blogging and online support communities have proven to be helpful to those with chronic diseases or others needing emotional support.
- Video games and virtual reality games, such as exercise programs, are being used for health applications, in addition to their usual entertainment value.
- Telehealth provides health information or health care to many individuals and groups who may otherwise not be able to access it, and its popularity is increasing.
- Electronic health literacy and the digital divide often prevent full use of technology among vulnerable and rural populations.

ACTIVE LEARNING EXERCISES

1. Pick a classmate and take turns practicing motivational interviewing (using OARS). Role play working with a client who has a problematic behavior (e.g., needs to eat healthier, exercise more). How will you approach them? Describe how you can demonstrate active listening and effective communication skills. List three effective communication skills and practice them.
2. Think of a patient you have worked with who may have low health literacy. Give three examples of how to help them better communicate with their physician and other health professionals. Debate with a classmate if health literacy is important, not only for the patient as an individual but for the community and society as a whole. Which of the 10 essential public health services (see Box 2-2) is being utilized here?
3. Discuss with a community/public health nurse or supervisor collaboration and the importance of collaborative skills. Ask about examples of types of collaborative projects or interventions. What facilitates effective collaboration in the community? What inhibits effective collaboration, and how can you overcome this? Describe how collaboration is essential in mobilizing community partnerships (see number 4 of the 10 essential public health services listed in Box 2-2).
4. Search the literature for research examples of the use of big data in assessing public health problems and designing interventions. Were the findings significant and applicable to your community? Explain ways in which these data are more helpful than traditional data. How is this most useful in public health?
5. Consider the various types of technology available (e.g., mHealth, mobile health applications, video games, telehealth, GIS). Which would you find most effective as you design public health interventions for various age groups and populations (e.g., low-income, Spanish-speaking Latino women needing nutritional information; adolescents seeking information on STDs and sexual health; addressing an outbreak of foodborne illness in a large metropolitan area; 10- to 14-year-olds with asthma)?

thePoint: Everything You Need to Make the Grade!

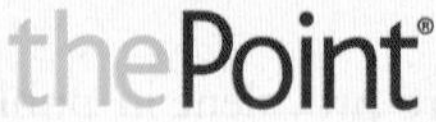

Visit http://thePoint.lww.com/Rector10e for NCLEX-style review questions, journal articles, supplemental materials, and more!

REFERENCES

Ackerman, C. (2019). *What is emotional intelligence? +18 ways to improve it*. Retrieved from https://positivepsychologyprogram.com/emotional-intelligence-eq/#references

Ackley, B. J., Ladwig, G. B., Makic, M. B., Martinez-Kratz, M., & Zanotti, M. (2020). *Nursing diagnosis handbook: An evidence-based guide to planning care* (12th ed.). St. Louis, MO: Elsevier.

Addicks, S. H., & McNeil, D. W. (2019). Randomized controlled trial of motivational interviewing to support breastfeeding among Appalachian women. Journal of Obstetric, *Gynecologic and Neonatal Nursing, 48*(4), 418–432.

Aeyoung, S., De Gagne, J. C., Park, S., & Young-Oak, K. (2015). The effect of a workshop on a urinary incontinence self-management teaching program for community health nurses. *Journal of Korean Academy of Community Health Nursing*, 26(3), 260–267. doi: 10.12799/jkachn.2015.26.3.260.

Agency for Health Care Quality & Research (AHRQ). (2018). *Building rapport with patients: OARS communication skills*. Retrieved from https://www.ahrq.gov/evidencenow/tools/oars-model.html

Agency for Health Care Quality & Research (AHRQ). (n.d.). *Innovations exchange: Search innovations*. Retrieved from https://innovations.ahrq.gov/search/innovations/Text%20Messaging?page=1

American Telemedicine Association. (2019). *Telehealth nursing: A position statement from the Telehealth Special Interest Group of the American Telemedicine Association*. Retrieved from https://www.americantelemed.org/?s=Telehealth+Nursing%3A+A+position+statement

ArcUser Online. (n.d.). *GIS for healthcare: Using GIS for public health*. Retrieved from https://www.esri.com/news/arcuser/0499/umbrella.html

Arnold, E. C., & Boggs, K. U. (2016). *Interpersonal relationships: Professional communication skills for nurses* (7th ed.). St. Louis, MO: Elsevier.

Arya, M., Huang, A., Kumar, D., Hemmige, V., Street, R., & Giordano, T. P. (2018). The promise of patient-centered text messages for encouraging HIV testing in an underserved population. *Journal of the Association of Nurses in AIDS Care*, 29(1), 101–106. doi: 10.1016.j.jana.2017.07.002.

Association of State and Territorial Health Officials (ASTHO). (2017). *Telehealth resource guide*. Retrieved from http://www.astho.org/Health-Systems-Transformation/Medicaid-and-Public-Health-Partnerships/2017-Telehealth-Resource-Guide/

Bang, D., & Frith, C. D. (2017). Making better decisions in groups. *Royal Society Open Science*, 4(8). doi: 10.1098/rsos.170193.

Baumann, P. (2016). *140 health care uses for Twitter*. Retrieved from http://philbaumann.com/140-health-care-uses-for-twitter/

Benetoli, A., Chen, T. F., & Aslani, P. (2018). How patients' use of social media impacts their interactions with healthcare professionals. *Patient Education and Counseling*, *101*(3), 439–444. doi: 10.1016/j.pec.2017.08.015.

Betts, S., & Healy, W. (2015). Having a ball catching on to teamwork: An experiential learning approach to teaching the phases of group development. *Academy of Educational Leadership Journal*, *19*(2), 1–9.

Birkhead, G. S., Klompas, M., & Shah, N. R. (2015). Uses of electronic health records for public health surveillance to advance public health. *Annual Review of Public Health*, *36*, 345–359.

Biswas, A., Faulkner, G. E., Oh, P. I., & Alter, D. A. (2017). Patient and practitioner perspectives on reducing sedentary behavior at an exercise-based cardiac rehabilitation program. *Disability and Rehabilitation*, *40*(19), 2267–2274. doi: 10.1080/09638288.2017.1334232.

Borkowski, N. (2016). *Organizational behavior in health care* (3rd ed.). Burlington, MA: Jones and Bartlett.

Boyd, M. A. (2018). *Psychiatric nursing: Contemporary practice* (6th ed.). Philadelphia, PA: Wolters Kluwer.

Brayboy, L. M., McCoy, K., Thamotharan, S., Zhu, E., Gil, G., & Houck, C. (2018). The use of technology in the sexual health education especially among minority adolescent girls in the United States. *Current Opinion in Obstetrics and Gynecology*, *30*(5), 305–309. doi: 10.1097/GCO.0000000000000485.

Brown, L. J., Tan, K. S., Guerra, L. E., Naidoo, C. J., & Nardone, A. (2018). Using behavioral insights to increase HIV self-sampling kit returns: A randomized controlled text message trial to improve England's HIV self-sampling service. *HIV Medicine*, *19*(9), 585–596. doi: 10.1111/hiv.12634.

Browning, H. W., Torain, D. J., & Patterson, T. E. (2016). *Collaborative healthcare leadership: A six-part model for adapting and thriving during a time of transformative change*. Retrieved from http://insights.ccl.org/wp-content/uploads/2015/04/CollaborativeHealthcareLeadership.pdf

Cain, C. L., Surbone, A., Elk, R., & Kagawa-Singer, M. (2018). Culture and palliative care: Preferences, communication, meaning, and mutual decision making. *Journal of Pain and Symptom Management*, *55*(5), 1408–1491. doi: 10.1016/j.jpainsymman.2018.01.007.

Canpolat, M., Kuzu, S., Yildirim, B., & Canpolat, S. (2015). Active listening strategies of academically successful university students. *Eurasian Journal of Educational Research*, *60*, 163–180. doi: 10.14689/ejer.2015.60.10.

Carter, M. Z., & Mossholder, K. W. (2015). Are we on the same page? The performance effects of congruence between supervisor and group trust. *Journal of Applied Psychology, 100*(5), 1349–1363. doi: 10.1037/a0038798.

Center for Connected Health Policy. (March 19, 2020). *Telehealth coverage policies in the time of Covid-19 to date.* The National Telehealth Policy Resource Center. Retrieved from https://www.cchpca.org/sites/default/files/2020-04/CORONAVIRUS%20TELEHEALTH%20POLICY%20FACT%20SHEET%20APRIL%206%202020.pdf

Center for Creative Leadership. (2019). *The big 6: An active listening skill set.* Retrieved from https://www.ccl.org/multimedia/podcast/the-big-6-an-active-listening-skill-set/

Center for Technology Innovation at Brookings. (2016). *mHealth in China and the United States: How mobile technology is transforming healthcare in the world's two largest economies.* Retrieved from https://www.brookings.edu/wp-content/uploads/2016/06/mHealth_finalx.pdf

Centers for Disease Control and Prevention (CDC). (2015). *The health communicator's social media toolkit.* Retrieved from http://www.cdc.gov/socialmedia/Tools/guidelines/pdf/SocialMediaToolkit_BM.pdf

Centers for Disease Control and Prevention (CDC). (2016). *The health communicator's social media toolkit.* Retrieved from https://www.cdc.gov/socialmedia/tools/guidelines/guideforwriting.html

Centers for Disease Control and Prevention (CDC). (2018). *CDC mobile app.* Retrieved from https://www.cdc.gov/mobile/applications/cdcgeneral/promos/cdcmobileapp.html

Centers for Disease Control and Prevention (CDC). (2019a) *CDC's childhood lead poisoning prevention program.* Retrieved from http://www.cdc.gov/nceh/lead/about/program.htm

Centers for Disease Control and Prevention (CDC). (2019b). *FastStats.* Retrieved from https://www.cdc.gov/nchs/fastats/default.htm

Centers for Disease Control and Prevention (CDC). (2019c). *Health literacy.* Retrieved from https://www.cdc.gov/healthliteracy/learn/index.html

Centers for Disease Control and Prevention (CDC). (2019d). *The CDC clear communication index.* Retrieved from https://www.cdc.gov/ccindex/

Centers for Disease Control and Prevention (CDC). (2019e). *Twitter guidelines and best practices.* Retrieved from https://www.cdc.gov/socialmedia/tools/guidelines/twitter.htm

Central Intelligence Agency (CIA). (2020). *The world factbook: Mobile cellular telephone subscribers.* Retrieved from https://www.cia.gov/library/publications/resources/the-world-factbook/fields/197rank.html

Chang, E., Blondon, K., Lyles, C. R., Jordan, L., & Ralston, J. D. (2018). Racial/ethnic variation in devices used to access patient portals. *The American Journal of Managed Care, 24*(1), e1–e8.

Christofferson, D. E., Hamlett-Berry, K., & Augustson, E. (2015). Suicide prevention referrals in a mobile health smoking cessation intervention. *American Journal of Public Health, 105*(8), e7–e9.

Cigna. (2019). *Download Hopelab's Re-Mission2™.* Retrieved from https://www.cigna.com/about-us/corporate-responsibility/remission/

Clement, I. W., & Roberts, F. B. (Eds.). (1983). *Family health: A theoretical approach to nursing care.* New York, NY: John Wiley & Sons.

Cole, J. (1990). *Filtering people: Understanding and confronting our prejudice.* Philadelphia, PA: New Society Publishers.

Coravos, A. (November 28, 2018). *The doctor prescribes video games and virtual reality rehab.* Wired. Retrieved from https://www.wired.com/story/prescription-video-games-and-vr-rehab/

Craft-Blacksheare, M. G. (2017). Lessons Learned from the crisis in Flint, Michigan regarding the effects of contaminated water on maternal and child health. *Journal of Obstetric, Gynecologic & Neonatal Nursing, 46*, 258–266. doi: 10.1016/j.jogn.2016.10.012.

Crawford, T., Candlin, S., & Roger, P. (2015). New perspectives on understanding cultural diversity in nurse–patient communication. *Collegian, 24*(1), 63–69. doi: 10.1016/j.colegn.2015.09.00.

Davis, R. A., & Travers Gustafson, D. (2015). Academic-practice partnership in public health nursing: Working with families in a village-based collaboration. *Public Health Nursing, 32*(4), 327–338. doi: 10.1111/phn.12135.

Dawson-Rose, C., Cuca, Y. P., Webel, A. R., Solis Báez, S. S., Holzemer, W. L., Rivero-Méndez, M., ... Lindgren, T. (2016). Building trust and relationships between patients and providers: An essential complement to health literacy in HIV care. *Journal of the Association of Nurses in AIDS Care, 27*(5), 574–584.

DeGuzman, P., Altrui, P., Doede, A., Allen, M., Deagle, C., & Keim-Malpass, J. (2018). Using geospatial analysis to determine access gaps among children with special healthcare needs. *Health Equity, 2*(1), 1–4. doi: 10.1089/heq.2017.0050.

DeSalvo, K. B. (2016). *Health literacy online: A guide for simplifying the user experience* (2nd ed.). USDHHS Office of Disease Prevention and Health Promotion. Retrieved from https://health.gov/healthliteracyonline/

Dillard, P. K., Zuniga, J. A., & Holstad, M. M. (2017). An integrative review of the efficacy of motivational interviewing in HIV management. *Patient Education and Counseling, 100*(4), 636–646. doi: 10.1016/j.pec.2016.10.029.

Dobber, J., Latoour, C., Snaterse, M., van Meijel, B., Ter Riet, G., Reimer, W. S., & Peters, R. (2019). Developing nurses' skills in motivational interviewing to promote a healthy lifestyle in patients with coronary artery disease. *European Journal of Cardiovascular Nursing, 18*(1), 38–37. doi: 10.1177/1474515118784102.

Dolley, S. (2018). Big data's role in precision public health. *Frontiers in Public Health, 6*, 68.

Donelan, K., Barreto, E. A., Sossong, S., Michael, C., Estrada, J. J., Cohen, A. B., ... Schwamm, L. H. (2019). Patient and clinician experiences with telehealth for patient follow-up care. *American Journal of Managed Care, 25*(1), 40–44.

Duiveman, T., & Bonner, A. (2012). Negotiating: Experiences of community nurses when contracting with clients. *Contemporary Nurse, 41*(1), 120–125.

Dyches, C., Haynes-Ferere, A., & Haynes, T. (2019). Fostering cultural competence in nursing students through international service immersion experiences. *Journal of Christian Nursing, 36*(2), E29–E35. doi: 10.1097/CNJ.0000000000000602.

Eckert, S., Sopory, P., Day, A., Wilkins, L., Padgett, D., Novak, J., ... Gamhewage, G. (2018). Health related disaster communication and social media: Mixed-method systematic review. *Health Communication, 33*(12), 1389–1400. doi: 10.1080/10410236/2017.1351278.

Electronic Entertainment Design and Research. (2019). *Gamer segmentation syndicated report 2018.* Retrieved from https://www.eedar.com/post/introducing-the-2018-gamer-segmentation-syndicated-report

El-Shafy, I. A., Delgado, J., Akerman, M., Bullaro, F., Christopherson, N. A. M., & Prince, J. M. (2017). Closed-loop communication improves task completion in pediatric trauma resuscitation. *Journal of Surgical Education, 75*(1), 58–64. doi: 10.1016/j.jsurg.2017.06.025.

Erunal, M., Ozkaya, B., Mert, H., & Kucukguclu, O. (2019). Investigation of health literacy levels of nursing students and affecting factors. *International Journal of Caring Sciences, 12*(1), 270–277.

Fabbri, M., Yost, K., Rutten, L. J. F., Manemann, S. M., Boyd, C. M., Jensen, D., ... Roger, V. L. (2018). Health literacy and outcomes in patients with heart failure: A prospective community study, *Mayo Clinic Proceedings, 93*(1), 9–15. doi: 10.1016/j.mayocp.2017.09.018.

FAIR Health. (2019). *FH healthcare indicators and FH medical price index 2019: An annual review of place of service trends and medical pricing.* FAIR Health White Paper. Retrieved from https://s3.amazonaws.com/media2.fairhealth.org/whitepaper/asset/FH%20Healthcare%20Indicators%20and%20FH%20Medical%20Price%20Index%202019%20-%20A%20FAIR%20Health%20White%20Paper.pdf

Feinberg, I., Tighe, E. L., Greenberg, D., & Mavreles, M. (2018). Health literacy and adults with low basic skills. *Adult Education Quarterly, 68*(4), 297–315. doi: 10.1177/0741713618783487.

Fernandez-Gonzalez, M., Monge-Pereira, E., Collado-Vazquez, S., Baeza, P., Cuesta-Gomez, A., Ona-Simbana, E. D., ... Cano-dela Cuerda, R. (2019). Leap motional controlled video game-based therapy for upper limb rehabilitation in patients with Parkinson's disease: A feasibility study. *Journal of NeuroEngineering and Rehabilitation, 16*(1), 133.

Food and Drug Administration (FDA). (2019). *Device software functions including mobile medical applications.* Retrieved from https://www.fda.gov/medical-devices/digital-health/device-software-functions-including-mobile-medical-applications

Gaines, K. (2020). *Updated map: Enhanced Nursing Licensure Compact (eNLC), July 2019.* Retrieved from https://nurse.org/articles/enhanced-compact-multi-state-license-eNLC/

Garcia, A. L. (2015). How big data can improve health care. *American Nurse Today, 10*(7), 53–55.

Garcia, A. L., Harper, E. M., & Welton, J. M. (2019). National clinical research networks: Where is the nurse? *Nursing Economic$, 37*(2), 100–102.

Gerardi, D. (2015). Conflict engagement: Creating connection and cultivating curiosity. *American Journal of Nursing, 115*(9), 60–65.

Gholamzadeh, S., Khastavaneh, M., Khademian, Z., & Ghadakpour, S. (2018). The effects of empathy skills training on nursing students' empathy and attitudes toward elderly people. *BMC Medical Education, 18*(1), doi: 10.1186/s12909-018-1297-9.

Glowacki, E. M., Kirtz, S., Hughes Wagner, J., Cance, J. D., Barrera, D., & Bernhardt, J. M. (2018). HealthyhornsTXT: A text-messaging program to promote college student health and wellness. *Health Promotion Practice, 19*(6), 844–855. doi: 10.1177/1524839917754089.

Goleman, D. (1995). *Emotional intelligence.* New York, NY: Banton Books.

Gorman, L. L., & McDowell, J. R. S. (2018). Identifying the needs of critical and acute cardiac care nurses within the first two years of practice in Egypt using a nominal group technique. *Nurse Education in Practice, 28*, 127–134. doi: 10.1016/j.nepr.2017.10.005.

Graetz, I., Huang, J., Brand, R., Hsu, J., Yamin, C., & Reed, M. (January 2018). Bridging the digital divide: Mobile access to personal health records among patients with diabetes. *The American Journal of Managed Care, 24*(1), 43–48.

Greenie, M. M., Morgan, B., Sayani, S., & Meghani, S. H. (2018). Identifying mobile apps targeting palliative care patients and family members. *Journal of Palliative Medicine, 21*(10). doi: 10.1089/jpm.2018.0157.

Griebel, L., Enwald, H., Gilstad, H., Pohl, A. L., Moreland, J., & Sedlmayr, M. (2018). eHealth literacy research—Quo vadis? *Informatics for Health and Social Care, 43*(4),427–442. doi: 10.1080/17538157.2017.1364247.

Griffiths, F., Bryce, C., Cave, J., Dritsaki, M., Fraser, J., Hamilton, K., ... Sturt, J. (2017). Timely digital patient-clinician communication in specialist clinical services for young people: A mixed-methods study. *Journal of Medical Internet Research, 19*(4), e102. doi: 10.2196/jmir.7154.

Grover, P., Kar, A. K., & Davies, G. (2018). "Technology enabled Health"—Insights from Twitter analytics with a socio-technical perspective. *International Journal of Information Management, 43*, 85–97. doi: 10.1016/j.ijinfomgt.2018.07.003.

Gulanik, M., & Myers, J. (2017). *Nursing care plans: Diagnosis, interventions, and outcomes* (9th ed.). St. Louis, MO: Elsevier.

Hanson, R. F., Saunders, B. D., Peer, S. O., Ralston, E., Moreland, A. D., Schoenwald, S., & Chapman, J. (2018). Community-based learning collaboratives and participant reports of interprofessional collaboration, barriers to, and utilization of child trauma services. *Children and Youth Services Review, 94*, 306–314. doi: 10.1016/j.childyouth.2018.09.038.

Hansson, A., Svensson, A., Ahlstrom, B. H., Larsson, L. G., Forsman, B., & Alsen, P. (2017). Flawed communications: Health professionals' experience of collaboration in the care of frail elderly patients. *Scandinavian Journal of Public Health, 46*(7), 680–689. doi: 10.1177/1403494817716001.

Haque, S. F., & D'Souza, A. (2019). Motivational interviewing: The RULES, ACE, and OARS. *Current Psychiatry, 18*(1), 27–28. Retrieved from https://pdfs.semanticscholar.org/0c3f/2fa823056bcae014ae01f51078a23b4737a6.pdf?_ga=2.126197065.555666267.1594673694-1371952598.1594673694

Hardavella, G., Aamli-Gaagnat, A., Saad, N., Rousalova, I., & Sreter, K. B. (2017). How to give and receive feedback effectively. *Breathe (Sheffield, England), 13*(4), 327–333.

Harmon, J. (2016). The top 4 communication skills of effective student leaders. *Campus Activities Programming, 48*(7), 30–34.

Health Information and Management Systems Society. (2019). *Connected health: It's personal*. Retrieved from https://www.himss.org/resources/connected-health-its-personal

Henderson, S., Horne, M., Hills, R., & Kendall, E. (2018). Cultural competence in healthcare in the community: A concept analysis. *Health and Social Care in the Community, 26*(4), 590–603. doi: 10.1111/hsc.12556.

Hersh, E. (2019). *Improving patient experience and reducing cost by measuring outcomes*. Harvard T. H. Chan School of Public Health. Retrieved from https://www.hsph.harvard.edu/ecpe/improving-patient-experience-and-reducing-cost-by-measuring-outcomes/

Heslip, N. (2015). Active listening: An important audit skill. *New Perspectives on Healthcare Risk Management, Control, and Governance, 34*(1), 14–15.

Hudson, J. N., & Croker, A. (2017). Rural multidisciplinary training: Opportunity to focus on interprofessional rapport-building. *Rural and Remote Health, 17*(3), 4180. Retrieved from https://www.rrh.org.au/journal/article/4180

Johansson, B., & Martensson, L. B. (2019). Ways of strategies to knowing the patient described by nursing students. *Nurse Education in Practice, 38*, 120–125.

Johnson, A. (2015). Health literacy: How nurses can make a difference. *Australian Journal of Advanced Nursing, 33*(2), 20–27.

Joyce, B. L., Harmon, M., Johnson, R. H., Hicks, V., Brown-Shott, N., Pilling, L., & Brownrigg, V. (2018). Community/public health nursing faculty's knowledge, skills and attitudes of the Quad Council Competencies for Public Health Nurses. *Public Health Nursing, 35*(5), 427–439. doi: 10.1111/phn.12409.

Kakarmath, S., Denis, V., Encinas-Martin, M., Borgonovi, F., & Subramanian, S. V. (2018). Association between literacy and self-rated poor health in 33 high- and upper middle-income countries. *International Journal of Public Health, 63*(2), 213–222. doi: 10.1007/s00038-017-1037-7.

Karp, L. (2015). Can empathy be taught? Reflections from a medical student active-listening workshop. *Rhode Island Medical Journal, 98*(6), 14–15.

Kazemi, D. M., Borsari, B., Levine, M. J., Li, S., Lamberson, K. A., & Matta, L. A. (2017). A systematic review of the mHealth interventions to prevent alcohol and substance abuse. *Journal of Health Communication, 22*(5), 413–432. doi: 10.1080/10810730.2017.1303556.

Kearly, A., & Oputa, J. (November 5, 2019). *Telehealth state capacity survey*. Association of State and Territorial Health Officials (ASTHO). Retrieved from http://www.astho.org/Programs/Clinical-to-Community-Connections/Documents/ASTHO-Telehealth-Capacity-Survey_2019-APHA-Presentation/

Kewming, S., D'Amore, A., & Mitchell, E. L. (2016). Conversation maps and diabetes education groups: An evaluation at an Australian rural health service. *Diabetes Spectrum, 29*(1), 32–36. doi: 10.2337/diaspect.29.1.32.

Kolifarhood, G., Khorasani-Zavareh, D., Salarilak, S., Shoghli, A., & Khosravi, N. (2015). Spatial and non-spatial determinants of successful tuberculosis treatment outcomes: An implication of Geographical Information Systems in health policymaking in a developing country. *Journal of Epidemiology and Global Health, 5*, 221–230. doi: 10.1016/j.jegh.2014.11.001.

Konok, V., Gigler, D., Bereczky, B. M., & Miklósi, Á. (2016). Full length article: Humans' attachment to their mobile phones and its relationship with interpersonal attachment style. *Computers in Human Behavior, 61*, 537–547. doi: 10.1016/j.chb.2016.03.062.

Kraaijenbrink, J. (April 9, 2019). *Seven tips for developing goal-directed collaborations and ecosystems*. Forbes. Retrieved from https://www.forbes.com/sites/jeroenkraaijenbrink/2019/04/09/seven-tips-for-developing-goal-directed-collaborations-and-ecosystems/#31135bff5a2e

Kruse, C. S., Stein, A., Thomas, H., & Kaur, H. (2018). The use of electronic health records to support population health: A systematic review. *Journal of Medical Systems, 42*(11), 214.

Lamont, S., & Brunero, S. (2018). The effect of a workplace violence training program for generalist nurses in the acute hospital setting: A quasi-experimental study. *Nurse Education Today, 68*, 45–52.

Lee, B. Y. (August 28, 2017). *Virtual reality is a growing reality in health care*. Forbes. Retrieved from https://www.forbes.com/sites/brucelee/2017/08/28/virtual-reality-vr-is-a-growing-reality-in-health-care/#18af6eac4838

Loescher, L. J., Rains, S. A., Kramer, S. S., Akers, C., & Moussa, R. (2016). A systematic review of interventions to enhance healthy lifestyle behaviors in adolescents delivered via mobile phone text messaging. *American Journal of Health Promotion, 32*(4), 865–879. doi: 10.1177/0890117116675785.

Ma, C., Park, S. H., & Shang, J. (2018). Inter- and intra-disciplinary collaboration and patient safety outcomes in U.S. acute care hospital units: A cross-sectional study. *International Journal of Nursing Studies, 85*, 1–6. doi: 10.1016/j.ijnurstu.2018.05.001.

Majee, W., Goodman, L., Vetter-Smith, M., & Canfield, S. (2016). Healthy Communities initiative: A preliminary assessment of the University of Missouri-Sedalia health promotion partnership. *Community Development, 47*(1), 91. doi: 10.1080/15575330.2015. 1100643.

Mantwill, S., & Schulz, P. J. (2015). Low health literacy associated with higher medication costs in patients with type 2 diabetes mellitus: Evidence from matched survey and health insurance data. *Patient Education and Counseling, 98*, 1625–1630. doi: 10.1016/j.pec.2015.07.006.

Marcolino, M. S., Oliveira, J. A. Q., D'Agostino, M., Ribeiro, A. L., Alkmim, M. B. M., & Novillo-Ortiz, D. (2018). The impact of mHealth interventions: Systematic review of systematic reviews. *JMIR mHealth and uHealth, 6*(1). doi: 10.2196/mhealth.8873.

Massachusetts Medical Society. (January 1, 2018). *Healthcare big data and the promise of value-based care*. NEJM Catalyst. Retrieved from https://catalyst.nejm.org/big-data-healthcare/

Mataxen, P. A. (2019). Licensure barriers to telehealth nursing practice. *Nursing2020, 49*(11), 67–68.

Miller, W. R., & Rollnick, S. (2013). *Motivational interviewing: Helping people change*. New York, NY: The Guilford Press.

Minnesota Department of Health. (2016). *Multivoting*. Retrieved from http://www.health.state.mn.us/divs/opi/qi/toolbox/nominalgroup.html

Mitchell, R., Paliadelis, P., McNeil, K., Parker, V., Giles, M., Higgins, I., ... Ahrens, Y. (2013). Effective interprofessional collaboration in rural contexts: A research protocol. *Journal of Advanced Nursing, 69*(10), 2317–2326. doi: 10.1111/jan.12083.

Mohammadi, A., Valinejadi, A., Sakipour, S., Hemmat, M., Zarei, J., & Majdabadi, H. A. (2018). Improving the distribution of rural health houses using elicitation and GIS in Khuzestan Province (the Southwest of Iran). *International Journal of Health Policy and Management, 7*(4), 336–344. doi: 10.15711/ijhpm.2017.101.

Mooney, S. J., & Pejaver, V. (2017). Big data in public health: Terminology, machine learning, and privacy. *Annual Review of Public Health, 39*, 95–112.

Morgan, S., Pullon, S., & McKinlay, E. (2015). Observation of interprofessional collaborative practice in primary care teams: An integrative literature review. *International Journal of Nursing Studies, 52*(7), 1217–1230. doi: 10.1016/j.ijnurstu.2015.03.008.

Moser, D. K., Robinson, S., Biddle, M. J., Pelter, M. M., Nesbitt, T. S., Southard, J., ... Dracup, K. (2015). Clinical investigation: Health literacy predicts morbidity and mortality in rural patients with heart failure. *Journal of Cardiac Failure, 21*, 612–618. doi: 10.1016/j.cardfail.2015.04.004.

Naqvi, S. B. & Shah, A. A. (2018). Modeling historically mHealth care environments. *International Journal of Reliable and Quality E-Healthcare (IJRQEH), 7*(3). doi: 10.4018/IJRQEH.2018070104.

Navidian, A., Mobaraki, H., & Shakiba, M. (2017). The effect of education through motivational interviewing compared with conventional education on self-care behaviors in heart failure patients with depression. *Patient Education and Counseling, 100*(8), 1499–1504. doi: 10.1016/j.pec.2017.02.023.

Nel, H. (2015). An integration of the livelihoods and asset-based community development approaches: A South African case study. *Development Southern Africa, 32*(4), 511–525. doi: 10.1080/0376 835X.2015.1039706.

Nel, H. (2018). A Comparison between the asset-oriented and needs-based community development approaches in terms of systems changes. *Practice, 30*(1), 33–52.

Ngwatu, B. K., Nsengiyumva, N. P., Oxlade, O., Mappin-Kasirer, B., Nguyen, N. L., Jaramillo, E., ... Schwartzman, K. (2018). The impact of digital health technologies on tuberculosis treatment: A systematic review. *European Respiratory Journal, 51*(1), 1701596.

Norman, C. D., & Skinner, H. A. (2006). eHealth literacy: Essential skills for consumer health in a networked world. *Journal of Medical Internet Research*, *8*(2), e9.

Nouri, S. S., & Rudd, R. E. (2015). Health literacy in the "oral exchange": An important element of patient-provider communication. *Patient Education and Counseling*, *98*, 565–571.

Office of the National Coordinator for Health Information Technology (ONC). (2019). *What is an electronic health record (EHR)?* Retrieved from https://www.healthit.gov/faq/what-electronic-health-record-ehr

Ozaras, G., & Abaan, S. (2018). Investigation of the trust status of the nurse-patient relationship. *Nursing Ethics*, *25*(5), 628–639. doi: 10.1177/0969733016664971.

Oztop, P., Katsikopoulos, K., Gummerum, M. (2018). Creativity through connectedness: The role of closeness and perspective taking in group creativity. *Creativity Research Journal*, *30*(3), 266–275. doi: 10.1080/10400419.2018.1488347.

Palmer, D., & El Miedany, Y. (2018). Incorporating motivational interviewing into rheumatology care. *British Journal of Nursing (BSN)*, *27*(7), 370–376. doi: 10.12968/bjon.2018.27.7.370.

Park, J., & Oh, J. (2019). Influence of perceptions of death, end-of-life care, stress, and emotional intelligence on attitudes towards end-of-life care among nurses in the neonatal intensive care unit. *Child Health Nursing Research*, *25*, 38–47. doi: 10.4094/chnr.2019.25.1.38.

Partridge, S. R., Gallagher, P., Freeman, B., & Gallagher, R. (2018). Facebook groups for the management of chronic diseases. *Journal of Medical Internet Research*, *20*(1). doi: 10.2196/jmir.7558.

Perrin, A. (2019). *Digital gap between rural and nonrural America persists*. Pew Research Center. Retrieved from https://www.pewresearch.org/fact-tank/2019/05/31/digital-gap-between-rural-and-nonrural-america-persists/

Pew Research Center. (June 12, 2019). *Mobile fact sheet*. Retrieved from https://www.pewresearch.org/internet/fact-sheet/mobile/

Prosperi, M., Min, J. S., Bian, J., & Modave, F. (2018). Big data hurdles in precision medicine and precision public health. *BMC Medical Informatics and Decision Making*, *18*(1), 139. doi: 10.1186/s12911-018-0719-2.

Public Health Leadership Forum. (2018). *Partnering to catalyze comprehensive community wellness: An actionable framework for health care and public health collaboration*. Retrieved from https://hcttf.org/wp-content/uploads/2018/06/Comprehensive-Community-Wellness-Report.pdf

Pyron, L., & Carter-Templeton, H. (2019). Improved patient flow and provider efficiency after the implementation of an electronic health record. *Computers, Informatics, Nursing*, *17*(10), 513–521.

Quad Council Coalition Competency Review Task Force. (2018). *Community/Public Health Nursing Competencies*. Retrieved from http://www.quadcouncilphn.org/documents-3/2018-qcc-competencies/

Raghubir, A. E. (2018). Emotional intelligence in nursing practice: A concept review using Rodger's evolutionary analysis approach. *International Journal of Nursing*, *5*, 126–130.

Raphael-Grimm, T. (2015). *The art of communication in nursing and health care: An interdisciplinary approach*. New York: Springer Publishing.

Ravi, D. K., Kuman, N., & Singhi, P. (2017). Effectiveness of virtual reality rehabilitation for children and adolescents with cerebral palsy: An updated evidence-based systematic review. *Physiotherapy*, *103*(3), 245–258.

Robertson, J. J. & Long, B. (2018). Suffering in silence: Medical error and its impact on health care providers. *The Journal of Emergency Medicine*, *54*(4), 402–409. doi: 10.1016/j.jemermed.2017.12.001.

Rowlands, G., Berry, J., Protheroe, J., & Rudd, R. E. (2015). Building on research evidence to change health literacy policy and practice in England. *Journal of Communication in Healthcare*, *8*(1), 22–31.

Sabatino, L., Rocco, G., Stievano, A., & Alvaro, R. (2015). Learning and teaching in clinical practice: Perceptions of Italian student nurses of the concept of professional respect during their clinical practice learning experience. *Nurse Education in Practice*, *15*, 314–320. doi: 10.1016/j.nepr.2014.09.002.

Schneider Corey, M., Corey, G., & Corey, C. (2018). *Groups: Process and practice* (10th ed.). Boston, MA: Cengage Learning.

Schumacher, J. A., & Madson, M. B. (2015). *Fundamentals of motivational interviewing: Tips and strategies for addressing common clinical challenges*. New York: Oxford University Press.

Sensmeier, J. (2015). Big data and the future of nursing knowledge: How can we use these technologies to improve care quality, optimize outcomes, and reduce healthcare costs? *Nursing Management*, *46*(4), 22–27.

Sherman, R. (2016). *Managing conflict*. Retrieved from https://www.emergingrnleader.com/9180-2/

Shuren, J., Patel, B., Gottlieb, S. (2018). FDA regulation of mobile medical apps. *Journal of the American Medical Association*, *320*(4), 337–338. doi: 10.1001/jama.2018.8832.

Siwicki, B. (September 9, 2019). *How asynchronous telemedicine saved SSM Health 18 minutes per visit*. Healthcare IT News. Retrieved from https://www.healthcareitnews.com/news/how-asynchronous-telemedicine-saved-ssm-health-18-minutes-visit

Slade, D., Pun, J., Murray, K. A., Eggins, S. (2018). Benefits of health care communication training for nurses conducting bedside handovers: An Australian hospital case study. *The Journal of Continuing Education in Nursing*, *49*(7), 329–336. doi: 10.3928/00220124-20180613-09.

Smith, T. S., Watts, P., & Moss, J. A. (2018). Using simulation to teach telehealth nursing competencies. *Journal of Nursing Education*, *57*(10), 624–627. doi: 10.3928/01484834-20180921010.

Soleymani, S., Britt, E., & Wallace-Bell, M. (2018). Motivational interviewing in intimate partner violence (IVP) treatment: A review of the literature. *Aggression and Violent Behavior*, *40*, 119–127. doi: 10.1016/j.avb.2018.05.005.

Springer, M. V., & Skolarus, L. E. (2019). Community-based participatory research: Partnering with communities. *Stroke*, *50*(3), e48–e50. doi: 10.1161/STROKEAHA.118.024241.

Strandas, M., & Bondas, T. (2018). The nurse-patient relationship as a story of health enhancement in community care: A meta-ethnography. *Journal of Advanced Nursing*, *74*(1), 11–22. doi: 10.1111/jan/13389.

Suarez-Balcazar, Y., Mirza, P., & Garcia-Ramirez, M. (2018). Health disparities: Understanding and promoting healthy communities. *Journal of Prevention & Intervention in the Community*, *46*(1), 1–6. doi: 10.1080/10852352.2018.1386761.

Taylor, L. M., Kerse, N., Frakking, T., & Maddison, R. (2018). Active video games for improving physical performance measures in older people: A meta-analysis. *Journal of Geriatric Physical Therapy*, *41*(2), 108–123. doi: 10.1519/JPT.0000000000000078.

Thomas, C. M., Allison, R., & Latour, J. M. (2018). Using blogs to explore the lived experience of life after stroke: "A journey of discovery I never wanted to take". *Journal of Advanced Nursing*, *74*(3), 579–590. doi: 10.1111/jan.13457.

Townsend, M. C., & Morgan, K. I. (2018). *Psychiatric mental health nursing: Concepts of care in evidence-based practice* (9th ed.). Philadelphia, PA: F.A. Davis Company.

Tsai, S., Crawford, E., & Strong, J. (2018). Seeking virtual social support through blogging: A content analysis of published blog posts written by people with chronic pain. *Digital Health*, *4*, 1–10. doi: 10.1177/2055207618772669.

U.S. Department of Health and Human Services (USDHHS). (2020a). *Browse 2030 objectives*. Retrieved from https://health.gov/healthypeople/objectives-and-data/browse-objectives

U.S. Department of Health & Human Services (USDHHS). (2020b). *2020 Topics and objectives: Health communication and health information technology*. Retrieved from http://www.healthypeople.gov/2020/topicsobjectives2020/overview.aspx?topicId=18

U.S. Department of Health and Human Services (USDHHS). (2014). *Using health text messages to improve consumer health knowledge, behaviors, and outcomes: An environmental scan*. Retrieved from https://www.hrsa.gov/sites/default/files/archive/healthit/txt4tots/environmentalscan.pdf

U.S. Department of Health and Human Services: Office of Disease Prevention & Promotion. (2010). *National action plan to improve health literacy*. Retrieved from http://www.health.gov/communication/HLActionPlan/pdf/Health_Literacy_Action_Plan.pdf

University of Mary Washington. (2016). *Geographic information science: What is GIS*? Retrieved from http://cas.umw.edu/gis/what-is-gis/

Vajan, C. C., & Baban, A. (2015). Emotional and behavioral consequences of online health information-seeking: The role of eHealth literacy. *Cognition, Brain, Behavior: An Interdisciplinary Journal*, *19*(4), 327–345.

Valaitis, R., O'Mara, L., Wong, S., MacDonald, M., Murray, N., Martin-Misener, R., & Meagher-Stewart, D. (2018). Strengthening primary health care through primary care and public health collaboration: The influence of intrapersonal and interpersonal factors. *Primary Health Care Research & Development*, *19*(4), 378–391. doi: 10.1017/S1463423617000895.

Veazie, S., Winchell, K., Gilbert, J., Paynter, R., Ivlev, I., Eden, K., ... Helfand, M. (2018). *Mobile applications for self-management of diabetes* (Technical brief No. 31). Agency for Healthcare Research and Quality. Retrieved from https://www.ncbi.nlm.nih.gov/books/NBK518944/

Vijaykumar, S., Nowak, G., Himelboim, I., & Jin, Y. (2018). Virtual Zika transmission after the first U.S. case: Who said what and how it spread on Twitter. *American Journal of Infection Control*, *46*(5), 549–557. doi: 10/1016/j.ajic.2017.10.015.

Wagner, B. (2018). Coping with bereavement online? An overview of web-based interventions for the bereaved. *Grief Matters: The Australian Journal of Grief and Bereavement*, *21*(1), 10–14.

Wesolowski, A., Metcalf, C., Eagle, N., Kombich, J., Grenfell, B., Bjornstad, O., ... Buckee, C. (2015). Quantifying seasonal population fluxes driving rubella transmission dynamics using mobile phone data. *Proceedings of the National Academy of Sciences*, *112*(35), 11114–11119.

Westefeld, J. S. (2019). Suicide prevention and psychology: A call to action. *Professional Psychology: Research and Practice*, *50*(1), 1–10. doi: 10.1037/pro0000209.

Wicklund, E. (October 9, 2015). *AMA workgroup targets telemedicine and CPT codes*. mhealth News: The Voice of Mobile Care. Retrieved from http://www.mhealthnews.com/news/cms-boosts-telehealth-2015-physician-pay-schedule

Wong, M. C., Turner, P., MacIntyre, K., & Yee, K. C. (2017). Pokémon Go: Why augmented reality games offer insights for enhancing public health interventions on obesity-related diseases. *Studies in Health Technology and Informatics*, *241*, 128–133.

World Health Organization (WHO) Africa. (2016). *Kenya rolls out massive measles-rubella and tetanus campaign*. Retrieved from https://www.afro.who.int/news/kenya-rolls-out-massive-measles-rubella-and-tetanus-campaign

Zahran, S., McElmurry, S. P., & Sadler, R. C. (2017). Four phases of the Flint water crises: Evidence from blood lead levels in children. *Environmental Research*, *157*. 160–172. doi: 10.1016/j.envres.2017.05.028.

Zhu, R., Han, S., Su, Y., Zhang, C., & Duan, Z. (2019). The application of big data and the development of nursing science: A discussion paper. *International Journal of Nursing Science, 6*(2), 229–234.

Zweig, M., Shen, J., & Jug, L. (2019). *Healthcare consumers in a digital transition: Results from our third national consumer survey (2017 data) on digital health adoption and sentiments*. Rock Health. Retrieved from https://rockhealth.com/reports/healthcare-consumers-in-a-digital-transition/

CHAPTER 11

Health Promotion Through Education

"It is health that is real wealth and not pieces of gold or silver."

—Mahatma Gandhi

KEY TERMS

Affective domain
Anticipatory guidance
Change
Cognitive domain
Evolutionary change
Health literacy
Health promotion
Learning theory
Planned change
Psychomotor domain
Revolutionary change
Social determinants of health
Social marketing
Socioeconomic gradient
Stages of change

LEARNING OBJECTIVES

Upon mastery of this chapter, you should be able to:

1. Describe social determinants of health and how each relates to health inequities and change through education.
2. Explain the three stages of change and planned change strategies.
3. Describe the C/PHN role as an educator in promoting health and improving quality of life.
4. Identify educational activities for the nurse to use that are appropriate for each of the three domains of learning.
5. Identify health teaching models for use when planning health education activities.
6. Develop teaching plans focusing on primary, secondary, and tertiary levels of prevention for clients of all ages and learning needs.

INTRODUCTION

Think about one of your favorite teachers from nursing school, high school, or earlier. How did the teacher get and hold your interest? How can you apply that in your work with public health nursing clients? Teaching has been a critical role of the community/public health nurse (C/PHN) since the origins of the profession, and frequently it is the primary role or function. C/PHNs develop partnerships with clients to achieve behavior changes that promote, maintain, or restore health. This partnership focuses on self-care—the ability to effectively advocate and manage a person's own health. The rationale for health teaching is to equip people with the knowledge, attitudes, and practices that will allow them to live the fullest possible life for the greatest length of time.

This chapter begins by discussing the *Healthy People 2030* goals and objectives, as well as key concepts related to health promotion. It then covers the nature and stages of change and the process and principles of planned change. Next, we consider some foundational concepts related to learning and teaching, including the domains of learning, learning theories, health teaching models, and teaching at the three levels of prevention. Finally, the chapter concludes by providing guidance on effective client teaching, including some principles of learning and teaching, steps in the teaching process, teaching methods and materials, and teaching clients with special learning needs.

HEALTHY PEOPLE 2030 AND KEY CONCEPTS RELATED TO HEALTH PROMOTION

To understand the goals of health promotion and the C/PHN's role in meeting them, we must explore relevant aspects of the *Healthy People 2030* initiative and some key concepts, including the social determinants of health, the socioeconomic gradient in health, health disparities, access to care, and quality of care.

Healthy People 2030

The vision of *Healthy People 2030* is for "a society in which all people can achieve their full potential for health and well-being of all people" (U.S. Department of Health and Human Services [USDHHS], 2020, para. 6). The *Healthy People 2030* objectives address social determinants of health and health equity (USDHHS, 2019). *Healthy People 2030* objectives for Educational and Community-Based Programs are listed in Box 11-1

BOX **11-1** *HEALTHY PEOPLE 2030*

Objectives for Educational and Community-Based Programs

Core Objectives	
ECBP-01	Increase the proportion of adolescents who participate in daily school physical education
ECBP-02	Increase the proportion of schools that don't sell less healthy foods and drinks
Developmental Objectives	
ECBP-D01	Increase the proportion of middle and high schools that provide case management for chronic conditions
ECBP-D03	Increase the proportion of worksites that offer employee health promotion program(s)
ECBP-D04	Increase the proportion of worksites that offer an employee physical activity program
ECBP-D05	Increase the proportion of worksites that offer an employee nutrition program
ECBP-D06	Increase the proportion of worksites with policies that ban indoor smoking
ECBP-D07	Increase the number of community organizations that provide prevention services
ECBP-D08	Increase the interprofessional prevention education in health professions training programs
ECBP-D09, D10, D11, D12, D13	Increase core clinical prevention and population health education in medical, nursing schools, dental, and pharmacy schools and physician assistant training programs

Reprinted from U. S. Department of Health and Human Services (USDHHS). (2020). *Educational and community-based programs objectives.* Retrieved from https://health.gov/healthypeople/search?query=ECBP

(USDHHS, 2020). These objectives, when viewed in the broader context, can be used to identify client needs and align educational efforts that will advance this national initiative.

Social Determinants of Health

The World Health Organization has defined the **social determinants of health** as "the conditions in which people are born, grow, live, work, and age" (World Health Organization, 2018, para. 1). Economic stability, education, health and health care, neighborhood and built environment, and social and community context are five key domains associated with social determinants of health (Centers for Disease Control and Prevention [CDC], 2017). The unequal distribution of these factors among certain groups contributes to health disparities that are persistent and pervasive. Recognizing and reducing health inequities is a priority of *Healthy People 2030*.

- Understanding social determinants of health requires examination of numerous factors, beyond individual behavior, that contribute to our state of health.
- Factors that influence an individual's ability to maintain good health include social, economic, and physical factors such as access to social and economic opportunities; safe housing; quality education; clean water, food, and air; safe workplaces; equitable social interactions (class, race, and gender); and adequate community resources (USDHHS, 2018).
- Addressing these factors in a manner that has a positive impact on social, economic, and physical conditions and supports positive health behavior change can improve the health of communities over time.

Social determinants of health influence both morbidity and mortality. Singh et al. (2017) examined the health inequalities among different populations in the United States from 1935 to 2016 and found that although life expectancy increased during this time, gender and racial/ethnicity disparities were present. Life expectancy was lowest in African American populations and rural populations. Additionally, infant mortality rates were greater in Black infants and rural, poor communities (Singh et al., 2017).

In an effort to improve the health of disadvantaged groups, early public health efforts addressed determinants of health such as sanitation and poverty, along with living conditions and other environmental issues, as noted in Chapters 3 and 7. It is now widely acknowledged that to truly have an impact on the health of the population, there is a need to improve social conditions (Bharmal, Derose, Felician, & Weden, 2015). Political action and participatory action research are vital tools in reducing the effects of these conditions, as are methods of community empowerment (Lee et al., 2018). See Chapters 4 and 13. See Box 23-5 for the *Healthy People 2030* social determinants of public health.

Socioeconomic Gradient in Health

Socioeconomic gradient in health refers to the improvement in health outcomes as socioeconomic position improves (CDC, 2014). A series of large-scale, longitudinal studies in England, the now-classic Whitehall studies, divided British civil servants into socioeconomic groups based upon their occupational status (e.g., from executives to unskilled workers). What the investigators discovered was an improvement in mortality and morbidity rates as the level of occupation and pay increased. Those at the lowest levels had the poorest health, but as they moved up the salary scale and occupational level, their health improved. What makes this so interesting is that all of the workers had basic health insurance coverage and free medical care—no real problems with access to health care existed. Although less pronounced, even when the researchers adjusted for diet, exercise, and smoking, the gradient persisted (Center for Social Epidemiology, 2018). Researchers have found higher rates of mortality in all causes and cardiometabolic disorders among those with lower socioeconomic position (Petrovic et al., 2018).

Globally, socioeconomic gradients in health are noted. For example, the infant mortality rate is 2 per 1,000 live births in Iceland compared with more than 120 per 1,000 live births in Mozambique. The life expectancy for men is 54 years in Calton (a neighborhood in Glasgow, Scotland) compared with 81 years in Lenzie (a neighborhood just a few miles away; Marmot, 2015). The socioeconomic gradient has also been noted in behaviors, such as smoking, that are highest among those who are from the working class and who have low income and low educational levels (Petrovic et al., 2018).

As noted above, the social determinants of health involve the conditions in which we live, work, and exist, which include socioeconomic factors such as income, education, and social status. Our health is determined to a great extent by these upstream social determinants, such as "education, labor, criminal justice, transportation, economics, and social welfare" (Adler et al., 2016, p. 2). Social determinants of health affect both morbidity and mortality, and targeted programs such as the Nurse-Family Partnership and the Supplemental Nutrition Assistance Program (SNAP) address some of health disparities resulting from these factors (Adler et al., 2016). See Chapter 23 for more on the social determinants of health.

Health Disparities

Health disparities are differences among populations in the quantity of disease, burden of disease, age and rate of mortality due to disease, health behaviors and outcomes, and other health conditions (Duran & Pérez-Stable, 2019). Put another way, health disparities can be objectively viewed as a disproportionate burden of morbidity, disability, and mortality found in a specific portion of the population in contrast to another. Although health disparities can result from poor choices by an individual despite health education and counseling efforts, most are thought to be due to social inequities that can be corrected (CDC, 2018). A long-held belief about health inequities, adopted by the World Health Organization, is that health differences that are avoidable and unnecessary are patently unfair and unjust (World Health Organization, 2020).

The topic of social determinants of health was added to *Healthy People 2020* and continues to be a focus of *Healthy People 2030* (Office of Disease Prevention & Health Promotion, 2020). Reported disparities exist in the areas of quality of health care, access to care, levels and types of care, and care settings; they exist within subpopulations (e.g., older adults, women, children, rural residents, those with disabilities) and across clinical conditions. Thus, to continue the work on eliminating health disparities, one overarching goal for *Healthy People 2030* is to "eliminate health disparities, achieve health equity, and attain health literacy to improve the health and well-being of all" (USDHHS, 2020, para. 10).

- Poor access to quality care and overt discrimination are examples of disparities.
- Discrimination can occur during service delivery if health care providers are biased against a specific group or hold stereotypical beliefs about that group.
- Providers may also not be confident about providing care for a racial or ethnic group with whom they are unfamiliar.
- Language barriers can be a problem, as can cultural values and norms that are unfamiliar to providers. Patients can also react to providers in a way that promotes disparities; patients may not trust the information given to them and may not follow it as explained, leading to inadequate care (Kaiser Family Foundation, 2018).

Access to Health Care

The Institute of Medicine's (2003) classic report *Unequal Treatment: Confronting Racial and Ethnic Disparities in Health Care* noted a large body of research highlighting the higher morbidity and mortality rates among all racial and ethnic minority groups when compared with Whites. This report drew attention to an issue that continues today and remains relevant. Differences in health care access were also explained, be it in the form of inadequate or no health insurance, problems getting health care, the quality of care, fewer choices in where to go for care, or the lack of a regular health care provider.

- Residential segregation, although illegal, still exists and can play a role in health disparities.
- Historically, vulnerable populations, especially racial and ethnic minority groups and low-income populations, have found access to health care difficult. Recent data showed that the Patient Protection and Affordable Care Act is improving access to health care for Hispanic and African American young adults (Lipton, Decker, & Sommers, 2017). However, it is estimated that approximately 55% of all uninsured who are not older adults are people of color (Kaiser Family Foundation, 2016).
- Other geographic factors can affect access to health care services. For example, the opioid epidemic has impacted low-income, low-employment areas harder than other geographic areas. Additionally, there remains a lack of access to drug treatment programs for minority groups (Santoro & Santoro, 2018).

Health care access is also problematic for other vulnerable groups. For example, services and resources for the mentally ill and those with substance use disorders are often fragmented and inadequate, as are those for victims of abuse and homeless persons. Refugees and immigrants may have difficulty finding affordable and easily accessible health care, largely because of their lack of health insurance and the need to find care at free clinics or emergency rooms (McNeely & Morland, 2016). When vulnerable individuals cannot get appropriate health care or treatment for illness or disease, for whatever reason, they are more likely to have health deficits.

Quality of Health Care

Quality of care is essential for positive health outcomes. The World Health Organization states that "health care must be safe, effective, timely, efficient, equitable, and people centered" (2019, para. 4). To receive quality care, people must be able to access it. Research confirms that minority groups have more barriers to access health care when compared with White populations and use less care (Kaiser Family Foundation, 2016). One factor contributing to the lower use of care could be the lack of diversity that exists in the U.S. health care system. Research indicates that racial and ethnic minority clients feel more comfortable and satisfied with care from a health care provider who comes from the same racial and/or ethnic group (Fig. 11-1; Duke & Stanik, 2016). The USDHHS reports that all minority groups, except Asians, were underrepresented in health diagnosis and treating occupations. These occupations include nursing, occupational therapy, physical therapy, dietetics, physicians, pharmacists, dentists, speech language pathology, respiratory therapy, and optometrists (USDHHS, 2017).

Lack of access to quality health care services is common among racial and ethnic minority groups. Significant disparities in the quality of care were found in a study examining diabetes quality of care. The study was a cross-sectional study examining adults diagnosed with type 2 diabetes. Study findings revealed that when compared with White adults, Hispanic adults had fewer HbA1c lab tests, eye exams, cholesterol lab tests, foot exams, and flu vaccinations; Black adults had fewer flu vaccinations; and Asian adults had fewer HbA1c tests, foot exams, and flu vaccinations (Canedo, Miller, Schlundt, Fadden, & Sanderson, 2018). Other studies have similar findings. A review of 25 studies examining

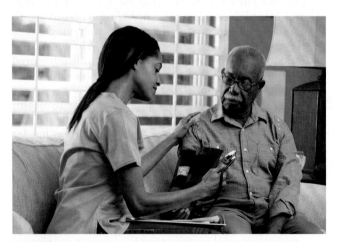

FIGURE 11-1 Racial and ethnic minority clients often prefer health care providers from the same racial and ethnic background.

quality of care in cardiovascular disease revealed racial disparities. The use of statins for treatment of peripheral artery disease, prescription for ischemic vascular disease, hyperlipidemia behavioral counseling, and clinical measures for coronary artery disease and congestive heart failure were lower for Black and Hispanic populations when compared with non-Hispanic White populations (Dong, Fakeye, Graham, & Gaskin, 2017).

Communication can be a factor in poor quality of care. Marginalized vulnerable populations are at a greater risk for experiencing communication problems in health care. Vulnerable populations include those who are uninsured, low-income, low-education, or low health literacy; those with cultural barriers (social, cultural, or linguistic); and those with environmental challenges (lack of housing or instability, environmental exposures, limited physical activity opportunities). Poor health outcomes may result as effectiveness of health care for vulnerable populations is not often considered or even well defined (Bhatt & Bathija, 2018).

- The C/PHN can play a significant role in addressing social determinants of health by first being aware and educated about factors that influence health beyond an individual's choices, looking at root causes of disease.
- C/PHNs can educate their client base on the social determinants of health, facilitate community action that supports positive change, and advocate for policies that address the root causes of disease and health inequities (USDHHS, 2018).

The Robert Wood Johnson Foundation conducted seminal research to determine the most effective messages on social determinants of health that are meaningful and understandable to Americans (Robert Wood Johnson Foundation, 2010). The C/PHN educator can use these messages to communicate concepts about social determinants of health to clients and communities (see Boxes 11-1 and 11-2). See Chapters 14, 15, and 23 for additional information.

One example of an effective intervention using social determinants of health is the Kaiser Permanente's Healthy Eating Active Living program. There were a series of several implementation programs that were conducted over a period of 10 years that touched 60 communities and over 700,000 individuals from five states. These programs included nutrition patient education programs, physical activity programs, healthy school lunch programs, programs to reduce food insecurity, and improved physical education school programs. Over 60% of the 143 obesity-prevention strategies revealed improvements in behavior change (Heath, 2018).

For health education to be effective, awareness of the underlying principles of behavior change is vital. The C/PHN should consider what motivates individuals and groups to adopt new behaviors and what factors may inhibit or prevent that change. By understanding the principles of teaching and behavior change, the C/PHN can work toward the ultimate goal of health promotion for individuals, families, groups, and communities.

BOX **11-2** *HEALTHY PEOPLE 2030*

Key Factors for Social Determinants of Health (Selected Objectives)

Core Objectives

SDOH-01	Reduce the proportion of people living in poverty
SDOH-02	Increase employment in working-age people
SDOH-03	Increase the proportion of children aged 0 to 17 years living with at least one parent who works full time
SDOH-04	Reduce the proportion of families that spend more than 30% of income on housing
SDOH-05	Reduce the proportion of children with a parent who has served time in jail
SDOH-06	Increase the proportion of high school graduates in college the October after graduating.

Research Objectives

SDOH-R01	Increase the proportion of federal data sources that collect country of birth as a variable

Reprinted from U.S. Department of Health and and Human Services (USDHHS). (2020). *Browse objectives.* Retrieved from https://health.gov/healthypeople/objectives-and-data/browse-objectives

HEALTH PROMOTION THROUGH CHANGE

Health promotion has been defined as health behaviors that improve well-being and lead to a desire to meet one's human potential (Pender, Murdaugh, & Parsons, 2015). Another term often confused with health promotion is *disease prevention* (or *health protection*), which is "behavior motivated by a desire to actively avoid illness, detect it early, or maintain functioning within the constraints of illness" (Pender et al., 2015, p. 17).

These two terms, so often used interchangeably, are clearly both important aspects of health education efforts, yet they imply a decidedly different motivation. For the C/PHN, both terms relate to practice at the primary level of prevention. Box 11-3 later in this chapter describes educational activities within both of these approaches in relation to primary prevention. For instance, a C/PHN may plan an educational program for community-dwelling older adults to learn about the need for a balanced diet, rich in fruits and vegetables. This would be an example of a health promotion focus, because there is no clear disease or condition at issue. As the nurse continues to work with these individuals, the nurse learns that several clients have had recent falls. Fortunately, none of the falls were serious, yet the nurse recognizes the need to discuss foods that will help reduce bone loss and promote healthy bone growth. To protect the clients' health,

BOX **11-3** **Theoretical Propositions of the Health Promotion Model**

1. Inherited and acquired characteristics along with prior behavior influence beliefs, affect, and health-promoting behavior.
2. People engage in behaviors from which they anticipate deriving personally valued benefits.
3. Perceived barriers can constrain action to change behavior and the behavior itself.
4. Perceived self-efficacy to embrace a given behavior increases the likelihood to commit to action and implementing the behavior.
5. Greater perceived self-efficacy results in fewer perceived barriers.
6. Positive affect toward a behavior results in greater perceived self-efficacy, which can result in increased positive affect.
7. When positive affect is associated with a behavior, commitment, and action are increased.
8. People are more likely to commit to and participate in health-promoting behaviors when significant others model the behavior, expect it, and provide assistance and support for the behavior.
9. Others—family members, peers, and health care providers—are important sources of influence that can positively or negatively influence commitment to and implementation of health-promoting behavior.
10. Situational influences can positively or negatively influence commitment to and implementation of health-promoting behavior.
11. The greater the commitment to a behavior change, the more likely the change will be maintained over time.
12. Distracting demands over which the person has little control may affect commitment to a behavior change.
13. Commitment to a behavior change is less likely to be maintained when other actions are more attractive and preferred.
14. People can modify the interpersonal and physical environments to create incentives for behavior changes.

Source: Murdaugh et al. (2019).

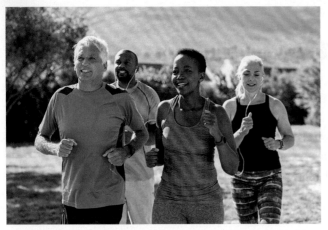

FIGURE 11-2 A goal of health promotion is to encourage clients to develop healthy behaviors.

the nurse provides information on a variety of foods rich in calcium and explains the need for adequate vitamin D, a safe home environment, weight-bearing exercise (Fig. 11-2), and medication review. This effort would be still primary prevention, but with the purpose of health protection.

For the C/PHN, teaching is the primary means to influence health at all levels, primary, secondary, and tertiary. But consider the educational program just described: The C/PHN has provided a well-developed educational program that was well received by the participants. They listened attentively, took the nurse's well-prepared handouts home, and even promised to add more fruits, vegetables, and calcium-rich foods to their diet. A few weeks later, in another educational program, the nurse learns from the participants that they have not altered their dietary patterns in the slightest. This is an example of how understanding the principles of behavior change may provide guidance to this C/PHN in planning a more effective program, with a greater chance for success.

The Nature of Change

To be a C/PHN is to be a health educator with the goal of effecting change in people's behaviors. When nurses suggest that families adopt healthier communication patterns, they are asking them to change. Teaching parenting skills to teenagers is introducing a change. Promoting a community's self-determination in choosing a safer environment requires that the individuals involved must change. Therefore, it becomes imperative for C/PHNs to understand the nature of change, how people respond to it, and how to effect change for improved community health.

Definitions and Types of Change

Change is "any planned or unplanned alteration of the status quo in an organism, situation, or process," per Lippitt's (1973, p. 37) classic definition. This definition explains that change may occur either by design or by default. From a systems perspective, change means that things are out of balance or the system's equilibrium is upset (Roussel, Harris, & Thomas, 2016). For instance, when a community is ravaged by floodwaters, its normal functioning is thrown off balance. Adjustments are required; new patterns of behavior become necessary. The change process can also be described as sudden or drastic (revolutionary) or gradual over time (evolutionary).

Evolutionary change is change that is gradual and requires adjustment on an incremental basis. It modifies rather than replaces a current way of operating. Some examples of evolutionary change include becoming parents, gradually cutting back on the number of cigarettes smoked each day, and losing weight by eliminating desserts and snacks. Gradual change may "ease the pain" that change brings to some individuals. Sometimes, this type of change may be viewed as *reform*.

Revolutionary change, in contrast, is a more rapid, drastic, and threatening type of change. It involves different goals and perhaps radically new patterns of behavior. Sudden unemployment, stopping smoking overnight, losing the town's football team in a plane accident, removing children from abusive parents, or rapidly replacing human workers with computers are examples of revolutionary changes. In each instance, the people affected have little or no advance warning and little or no time to prepare. High levels of emotional, mental, and sometimes physical energy and rapid behavior change are required to adapt to revolutionary change. If the demands are too great, some may experience defense mechanisms such as incapacitation, resistance, or denial of the new situation.

The impact of a proposed change on a system clearly depends on the degree of the change's evolutionary or revolutionary qualities, a factor to be considered in planning for change. Some situations lend themselves better to one kind of change than to another. A community in need of improved facilities for the handicapped (e.g., ramps, wider doors) can introduce this change on an evolutionary, incremental basis, whereas a community that is involved in an unsafe, intolerable, or life-threatening situation, such as a hurricane or serious influenza epidemic, may require revolutionary change.

Two powerful examples of social and public health change occurred during the last decades of the 20th century—dramatic decreases in both motor vehicle crashes and tobacco consumption. These changes did not come about simply through education alone. Rather, "multilevel and multicomponent" approaches were used, and social norms were changed by the use of epidemiology and surveillance as a basis for **social marketing** in bringing the problems to the attention of the American public; with the social influence of individuals, along with supportive legislation and policies, changes in health behaviors occurred (Gielen & Green, 2015, p. 21). Because of research, surveillance, monitoring of risk factors, and subsequent interventions related to these two problems, more people became aware of the significance of them. Although cigarettes had been proclaimed a health risk in 1964, many people still smoked. It was not until smoking cessation research began to show promise and new over-the-counter treatments and medications became available that more people attempted to stop smoking. In 1992, secondhand smoke was declared to be a carcinogen. Mass media was used to educate the public on the risks and the benefits of quitting; this also began to change public opinion. At the same time, legislation to control the advertising of tobacco products and tighten sales to minors gained momentum. Smoke-free policies were enacted, and higher cigarette taxes made it more difficult for some to smoke. Counseling and education strategies were increasingly empowering individuals and communities to change health behaviors, and multiple attempts at quitting were accepted. Cigarette sales began to drop, and stroke and heart attack death rates quickly improved after smoke-free zones were established. Child asthma admissions to hospitals and premature births also significantly declined within a year after the United States enacted bans on smoking in public places. Researchers point to the synergistic effect of the interventions (Gielen & Green, 2015).

Stages of Change

The phrase **stages of change** refer to the three sequential steps leading to change:

- Unfreezing (when desire for change develops)
- Changing (when new ideas are accepted and tried out)
- Refreezing (when the change is integrated and stabilized in practice)

Kurt Lewin first described these stages in the 1940s and early 1950s, and they have become a cornerstone for understanding the change process (Kaminski, 2011; Lewin, 1947, 1951; Lippitt, Watson, & Westley, 1958):

- Unfreezing: The first stage, unfreezing, occurs when a developing need for change causes disequilibrium in the system. A system in disequilibrium is more vulnerable to change. People are motivated to change either intrinsically or by some external force. The unfreezing stage involves initiating the change.
- Changing/moving: The second stage of the change process, changing or moving, occurs when people examine, accept, and try the innovation (Kaminski, 2011). This is the period when participants in a prenatal class are learning exercises or when elderly clients in a senior citizens' center are discussing and trying ways to make their apartments safe from accidents. During the changing stage, people experience a series of attitude transformations, ranging from early questioning of the innovation's worth to full acceptance and commitment and then to accomplishing the change. The change agent's role during this moving stage is to help clients see the value of the change, encourage them to try it out, and assist them in adopting it.
- Refreezing: The third and final stage in the change process, refreezing, occurs when change is established as an accepted and permanent part of the system (Kaminski, 2011). The rest of the system has adapted to it. People no longer feel resistant to it, because it is no longer viewed as disruptive, threatening, or new. As the change is integrated, the system becomes refrozen and stabilized. Refreezing involves integrating or internalizing the change into the system and then maintaining it.

Planned Change

Leaders in community health nursing have been change agents for decades. They have planned and managed change in a variety of systems. **Planned change** is a purposeful, designed effort to effect improvement in a system with the assistance of a change agent per Spradley's classic definition (1980). Planned change, also known as managed change, is crucial to the development of successful community health nursing programs, and various models of change have been proposed over the years (Table 11-1; Roussel et al., 2016). Regardless of the specific model used, the following characteristics of planned change are a key to its success:

- *The change is purposeful and intentional:* There are specific reasons or goals prompting the change. These goals give the change effort a unifying focus and a specific target. Unplanned change occurs haphazardly, and its outcomes are unpredictable.
- *The change is by design, not by default:* Thorough, systematic planning provides structure for the change process and a map to follow toward a planned destination.
- *Planned change in community health aims at improvement:* That is, it seeks to better the current situation, to promote a higher level of efficiency, safety, or health enhancement. Planned change aims to facilitate growth and positive improvements. Plans to provide shelter and health care for a homeless population, for example, are designed to improve this group's well-being.
- *Planned change is accomplished through an influencing agent:* The change agent is a catalyst in developing and carrying out the design; the change agent's role is a leadership role, often as an educator.

Planned Change Process

The planned change process involves a systematic sequence of activities that follows the nursing process. The eight basic steps lead to the successful management of change. These steps include (1) recognize symptoms; (2) diagnose need; (3) analyze alternative solutions; (4) select a change; (5) plan the change; (6) implement the change; (7) evaluate the change; and (8) stabilize the change (Table 11-1; Spradley, 1980).

Applying Planned Change to Larger Aggregates

C/PHNs use the change process when managing change at organization, population group, community, and larger aggregate levels. For example, as a result of information gleaned from parents, C/PHNs, other community health partners, and other data that track health outcomes, a nurse may suspect that there is a widespread lack of confidence among young parents (Fig. 11-3). This hypothesis could be tested through a social media survey to determine parenting needs among the entire community's population of young parents. If symptoms are present (step 1), the nurse, in collaboration with health department personnel or other appropriate professionals, could analyze the symptoms and reach a diagnosis (step 2) that many young parents in the community are lacking

TABLE 11-1 Change Models

Change Model	Steps in the Model	Example of Application
Six phases of planned change (Havelock & Havelock, 1973)	1. Develop the relationship 2. Diagnose the problem 3. Acquire resources for change 4. Select a pathway for the solution 5. Establish and accept change 6. Maintain the change (maintenance and separation)	A new family planning client is requesting birth control but is unsure of the method. Developing rapport and trust (relationship) is essential to allow the C/PHN to be able to identify the young woman's needs (diagnose). Several birth control methods are discussed (resources), and the young woman feels a long-acting birth control would be ideal (pathway). After education, a progesterone intrauterine device is inserted (maintenance).
Seven phases of planned change (Lippitt et al., 1958)	1. Diagnose the problem 2. Assess motivation and capacity for change 3. Assess the change agent's motivation and resources 4. Select progressive change objectives 5. Choose an appropriate change agent role 6. Maintain the change 7. Terminate the helping relationships	A young woman is in for a well woman's exam. Her body mass index is 30 (diagnose). The C/PHN asks if the woman has any health concerns, and the woman reports she is concerned with her weight (assess motivation). The woman is interested in working with the nurse to identify resources and a weight loss plan (assess change agent's motivation). A nutrition and physical activity plan is developed along with a return appointment (choose appropriate change agent). Upon the first return visit, the client has lost 4 lb in a 4-week period, and at the next visit in 4 weeks, the client has lost a total of 7 lb (maintain). Once weight loss goals have been accomplished, the visits end (terminate).
Innovation-decision process (Rogers, 2003)	1. Knowledge 2. Persuasion 3. Decision 4. Implementation 5. Confirmation	A client wants to stop tobacco use. She has tried several times but has been unsuccessful. The client seeks assistance from the C/PHN. The nurse provides information regarding the risks of tobacco use and tobacco cessation options (knowledge), and the need to set a stop date (persuasion). The client determines a stop date (decision) with consultation of a primary care provider a tobacco cessation medication is prescribed (implementation). A follow-up appointment is scheduled in 2 weeks and the client is tobacco free. Additional follow-up is set up to track the client's progress (confirmation).
Kotter's 8-step model of change (Kotter, 2012)	1. Create a sense of urgency 2. Build a guiding coalition 3. Form a strategic vision and initiative 4. Enlist a volunteer army 5. Enable action by removing barriers 6. Generate short-term wins 7. Sustain acceleration 8. Institute change	Data reveal an increase in teen suicide (urgency). Several agencies, including the school system, the public health department, mental health providers, parents, students, etc., schedule a meeting (coalition). The meeting consists of developing a vision to reduce teen suicide in the community (vision/initiative). Additional resources and support for the coalition are established (volunteer army). Focus groups with teens are conducted to determine concerns (remove barriers). Information from the focus groups is used to implement change (short-term wins). Interventions and evaluation continue (sustain acceleration and institute change).

Source: Havelock and Havelock (1973); Kotter (2012); Lippitt, Watson, and Westley (1958); Rogers (2003).

in confidence and knowledge of parenting skills. Several approaches to meeting this need could be considered, such as instituting a parenting center in the community with satellite clinics, organizing churches or clubs to sponsor parenting support groups, or working through the community college system to hold workshops and classes on parenting skills (step 3). The most feasible and useful alternative could be selected (step 4), and a parenting program for the community could be planned (step 5) and implemented (step 6). The nurse, with parents and other professionals involved, would then evaluate the outcomes (step 7) and make necessary adjustments in the parenting program before finally stabilizing it (step 8), making certain that this change, undertaken to meet a population group need, remains an established and effectively functioning service (Table 11-1).

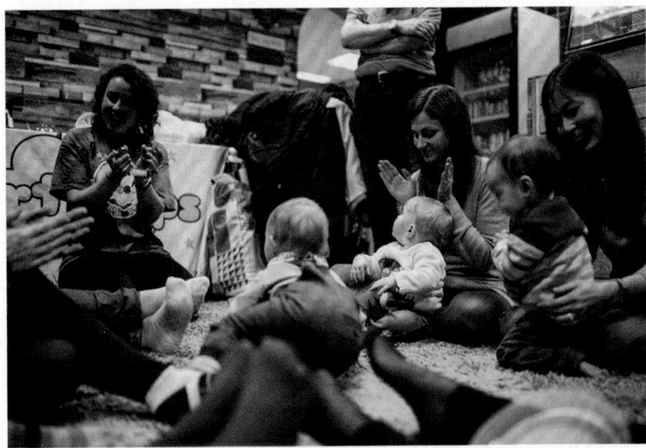

FIGURE 11-3 Parents and their young children in a play group.

Change and Health Promotion Within Communities/Populations

Changes in behavior and health promotion can also be directed to even larger audiences—communities and larger populations. Similar approaches can be used but may be varied depending upon age, most pertinent issues, and how to best reach targeted audiences. For instance, in an effort to address cardiovascular health by encouraging prevention and health promotion, researchers stratified their approaches based upon what they determined were the most beneficial age ranges.

- They began with 3- to 5-year-olds and a family-centered educational strategy about hearts and how to keep them healthy by reducing obesity and other risk factors.
- Then, between 25 and 50 years of age, the focus changes to education about screening and early detection of potential problems.
- Over age 50, the approach is directed more toward education about discovering cardiovascular disease and early treatment.
- Physical activity programs for all age groups are important to reduce cardiovascular disease. Additionally, cardiovascular risk factors, physical activity, and exercise assessments should be completed on all individuals. Health care professionals should refer those with risk factors to specialists for and exercise prescription (Fletcher et al., 2018).

Change and health promotion in communities begin with understanding the basics of health communication and social marketing. The CDC provides information regarding these areas (CDC, 2019b).

It involves six phases in health communication basics:

1. Problem definition and description (e.g., health problem of concern, who this affects, how you can address it)
2. Problem analysis/market research (e.g., analyze data on problem, target audience's values, behaviors, beliefs, attitudes, and barriers/facilitators to changing behavior)
3. Planning communication/market strategy (e.g., determine target audience, what behaviors that you wish to address, benefits offered [such as better health] with interventions to support change)
4. Program planning/interventions (e.g., methods you will use to influence change [for instance, a Web site to promote better nutrition/physical activity for adolescents], plan, objectives)
5. Program evaluation (e.g., is your program useful, feasible, accurate, ethical)
6. Implementation (e.g., plan for launching program, publicity, threats/opportunities)

This method has been used with many health problems and issues (e.g., arthritis, breast-feeding, drug abuse prevention, smoking cessation, HIV/AIDS, colorectal cancer screening, chronic fatigue syndrome, immunizations, influenza) and is a helpful means of reaching targeted populations (CDC, 2019b). See Chapters 10, 12, and 15 for more on health promotion, communication, and use of technology in assessing communities and developing programs for health promotion.

Principles for Effecting Positive Change

C/PHNs introduce change every day that they practice. Every effort to solve a problem, prevent another problem from occurring, meet a potential community need, or promote people's optimal health requires changes. For these changes to be truly successful, so that desired outcomes are reached, they must be well thought out and managed. The following six principles provide guidelines for effecting positive change: (1) participation; (2) resistance to change; (3) proper timing; (4) interdependence; (5) flexibility; and (6) self-understanding (Table 11-1).

Principle of Participation

- Persons affected by a proposed change should participate as much as possible in every step of the planned change process, including group meetings to discuss the proposed change (Fig. 11-4).
- This involvement is important for several reasons. Collaboration with those who have a vested interest in the change can produce a wealth of ideas and insights that can greatly improve the change plan.
- Furthermore, such participation can help remove obstacles and reduce resistance.

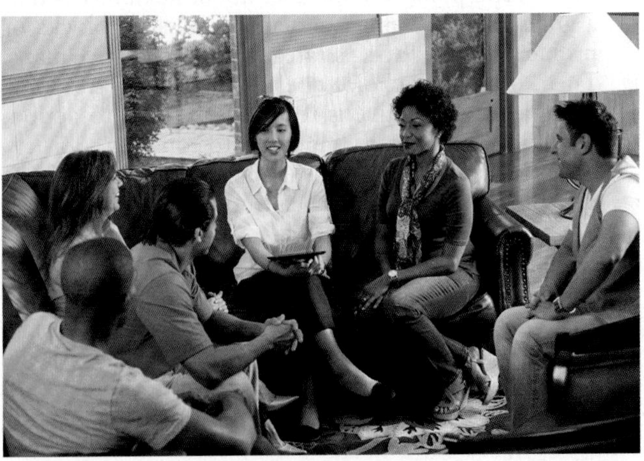

FIGURE 11-4 A C/PHN leading a group.

Principle of Resistance to Change

- Because all systems instinctively preserve the status quo, the change agent can expect people to resist change.
- The homeostatic mechanism operating in any system seeks to maintain equilibrium; change poses a threat to that stability and security.
- Furthermore, all systems experience inertia, that is, they resist beginning movement. People do not undertake a change until they are convinced of its worth.
- Resistance may also come from a conflict over goals and methods or from misunderstanding about what the change will mean and require. Involving people in the planned change process, as discussed in the previous section, is one way to overcome resistance.

Principle of Proper Timing

- Proper timing is as important to a planned change as well-timed seed planting is to a good harvest.
- The change idea must be appropriate, the change recipient prepared, the climate right, and the resources available before the change can be fostered to grow into full maturity and usefulness.

Principle of Interdependence

- This principle of interdependence reminds the nurse that change does not take place in a vacuum.
- Every system has many subsystems that are intricately related to and interdependent on one another. When workers learn new health and safety practices associated with their jobs, their relationships with one another, and their bosses, their overall productivity in the organization may easily be affected.
- One must anticipate and prepare for the impact of the proposed change on the clients involved, other persons, departments, organizations, or even geographic areas.

Principle of Flexibility. Unexpected events can occur in every situation. This fifth principle—flexibility—emphasizes two points.

- First, the nurse needs to be able to adapt to unexpected events and make the most of them.
- The second point to remember about flexibility is that a good change planner anticipates possible blocks or problems by preparing strategies and alternative plans.
- Then, if the first choice does not work out for some reason, an alternative is ready to be put into action. Flexibility involves a willingness to consider a variety of options and suggestions from many sources, and it is the hallmark of public health professionals.

Principle of Self-Understanding

- Self-understanding is essential for an effective change agent (Michigan State University, 2019). The community nurse (as change agent) should be able to clearly define his or her role and seek to understand how others define it.
- It is important to understand your own values and motives in relation to each change that you are asking people to make. Nurses should also understand their own personality traits, so that they can capitalize on or adjust them in order to be more effective change agents. Understanding yourself is crucial to learning to make use of your best qualities and skills in order to effect change (Jerome & Powell, 2016).

Change is inevitable. Understanding the principles of planned change can assist the C/PHN in guiding individuals, families, and communities toward achieving the highest level of health.

CHANGE THROUGH HEALTH EDUCATION

For the C/PHN, health education is a foundation of practice. Whether the nurse is providing one-on-one education to a new mother about the benefits of breast-feeding, briefing county officials on the need to maintain breast-feeding support centers, or working with community partners and grant funders to develop a Web-based social marketing campaign to promote breast-feeding among adolescent mothers, educational techniques are being used to promote health in the community. Knowledge of educational theories and teaching methods can assist the nurse to frame these "health messages" for the greatest impact and chance of success.

- *Teaching* is a specialized communication process in which desired behavior changes are achieved. The goal of all teaching is learning.
- *Learning* is a process of assimilating new information that promotes a permanent change in behavior. Learning is gaining knowledge, comprehension, or mastery.

After learning, clients are capable of doing something that they could not do before learning took place. Effective teaching is the cause; learning becomes the effect. To teach effectively, especially in the community where teaching is the focus of care, nurses need to understand the various domains of learning and related learning theories.

Domains of Learning

Learning occurs in several realms or domains: cognitive, affective, and psychomotor. Understanding of the differences among the domains and of the related roles of the nurse provides the background necessary to teach effectively.

Cognitive Domain

The **cognitive domain** of learning involves the mind and thinking processes. When the meaning and relationship of a series of facts is grasped, cognitive learning has occurred. The cognitive domain deals with the recall or recognition of knowledge and the development of intellectual abilities and skills (Bloom, 1956), as follows:

- Remember.
  - Recall basic facts.
  - Example: A school nurse asks adolescents in a weight loss group to list foods high in fat.

- Understand.
    - Comprehend concepts when they are explained.
    - Example: A school nurse asks adolescents in a weight loss group to identify ways to lose weight.
- Apply.
    - Transfer understanding into practice.
    - Example: A school nurse asks adolescents in a weight loss group to keep a food and physical activity record for a week, draw up a diet, and share this plan with the group at the next meeting.
- Analyze.
    - Break down concepts into parts; establish the relationship among the parts.
    - Example: A school nurse asks adolescents in a weight loss group to distinguish the fat content in a variety of packaged foods.
- Evaluate.
    - Validate information.
    - Example: A school nurse asks adolescents in a weight loss group to select a menu that is low in fat.
- Create.
    - Produce new or original work.
    - Example: A school nurse asks adolescents in a weight loss group to develop a menu that is low in fat.

(Vanderbilt University Center for Teaching, 2019).

How to Measure Cognitive Learning. Cognitive learning at any of the levels described can be measured easily in terms of learner behaviors. Nurses know, for instance, that clients have achieved teaching objectives for the application of knowledge if their behavior demonstrates actual use of the information taught. Client roles in cognitive learning range from relatively passive (at the knowledge level) to a more active role (at the evaluation level). Conversely, as clients become more active, the nurse's role becomes less overtly directive. Not all clients need to be brought through all levels of cognitive learning, and not every client needs to reach the evaluation level for each aspect of care. For some clients and situations, comprehension is an adequate and effective level; for others, the nurse should focus on the application level. Table 11-2 illustrates client and nurse behaviors for each cognitive level (Iowa State University Center for Excellence in Learning and Theory, 2019).

Affective Domain

The **affective domain** involves learning that occurs through emotion, feeling, or *affect*. This kind of learning deals with changes in interest, attitudes, and values (Bloom, 1956; Miller, Linn, & Gronlund, 2012). Here, nurses face the task of trying to influence what their clients may value and feel. Nurses want clients to develop an ability to accept ideas that promote healthier behaviors, even if those ideas conflict with the clients' own values.

TABLE **11-2** Domains of Learning

Level	Illustrative Client Behavior	Illustrative Nurse Behavior
A. Cognitive Learning: A Case Study in Controlling Diabetes		
Remember (recalls, knows)	States that insulin, if taken, will control own diabetes	Provides information
Understand (describes)	Describes insulin action and purpose	Explains information
Apply (uses learning)	Adjusts insulin dosage daily to maintain proper blood sugar level	Suggests how to use learning
Analyze (draws a connection)	Compares relationships between insulin, diet, activity, and diabetic control	Demonstrates and encourages analysis
Evaluate (judges according to a standard)	Selects a plan, incorporating above learning, for controlling own diabetes	Facilitates evaluation
Create (generates new ideas)	Designs a plan of diabetic control	Formulates own plan
B. Affective Learning: A Case Study in Family Planning		
Receptive (listens, pays attention)	Is attentive to family planning instruction	Directs client's attention
Responsive (participates, reacts)	Discusses pros and cons of various methods	Encourages client involvement
Valuing (accepts, appreciates, commits)	Selects a method for use	Respects client's right to decide
Internal consistency (organizes values to fit together)	Understands and accepts responsibility for planning for desired number of children	Brings client into contact with role models
Adoption (incorporates new values into lifestyle)	Consistently practices birth control	Positively reinforces healthy behaviors

Attitudes and values are learned. They develop gradually, as family, peers, experiences, and culture influence the way a person feels and responds. These feelings and responses are the result of imitation and conditioning. In this way, clients acquire their health-related beliefs and practices. Because attitudes and values become part of the person, they are difficult to change unless the nurse is aware of how they develop.

Affective learning occurs on several levels as learners respond with varying degrees of involvement and commitment:

- At the first level, learners are simply receptive; they are willing to listen, to show awareness, and to be attentive. The nurse aims at acquiring and focusing learners' attention (Miller & Stoeckel, 2016; Miller et al., 2012). This limited goal may be all that clients can achieve during the early stages of the nurse–client relationship.
- At the second level, learners become active participants by responding to the information in some way. Examples are a willingness to read educational material, to participate in discussions, to complete assignments (e.g., keeping a diet record), or to voluntarily seek out more information (Miller & Stoeckel, 2016; Miller et al., 2012).
- At the third level, learners attach value to the information. Valuing ranges from simple acceptance through appreciation to commitment (Miller & Stoeckel, 2016; Miller et al., 2012).
- The final level of affective learning occurs when learners internalize an idea or value. The value system now controls learner behavior. Consistent practice is a crucial test at this level (Miller & Stoeckel, 2016; Miller et al., 2012).

Affective learning often is difficult to measure and is often attempted through self-report surveys or tools (Miller & Stoeckel, 2016; Miller et al., 2012). This elusiveness may influence C/PHNs to concentrate their efforts on cognitive learning goals instead. Yet, client attitudes and values have a major effect on the outcome of cognitive learning—which is desired behavioral changes. Therefore, both cognitive and affective domains must be linked when teaching clients about health-related topics; otherwise, results may quickly fade (Hales, 2016).

Psychomotor Domain

The **psychomotor domain** includes visible, demonstrable performance skills that require some kind of neuromuscular coordination (Miller & Stoeckel, 2016; Miller et al., 2012). Clients in the community need to learn skills such as infant bathing, temperature taking, breast or testicular self-examination, prenatal breathing exercises, range-of-motion exercises, catheter irrigation, walking with crutches, changing dressings, and performing cardiopulmonary resuscitation (Fig. 11-5).

For psychomotor learning to take place, three conditions must be met: (1) learners must be capable of the skill; (2) learners must have a sensory image of how to perform the skill; and (3) learners must practice the skill.

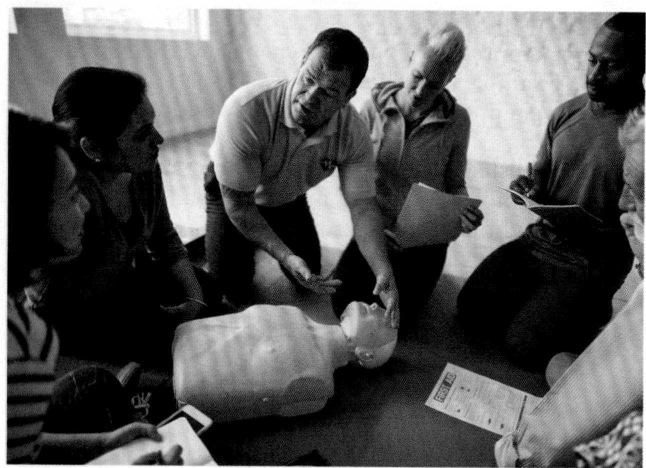

FIGURE 11-5 A C/PHN demonstrates cardiopulmonary resuscitation to clients before having them return the demonstration to show that they can put this learning into practice.

- C/PHNs must be certain that the client is physically, intellectually, and emotionally capable of performing the skill. It may be difficult for an elderly diabetic man with tremulous hands and fading vision to give his own insulin injections; it could frustrate and harm him. He may need some assistance or accommodations.
- Clients' intellectual and emotional capabilities also influence their capacity to learn motor skills. It may be inappropriate to expect persons with significant developmental delays to learn complex skills. The degree of complexity should match the learners' level of functioning. However, educational level should not be equated with intelligence.
  - Developmental stage is another point to consider in determining whether it is appropriate to teach a particular skill. For example, most children can put on some article of clothing at 2 years of age but are not ready to learn to fasten buttons until they are past their third birthday.
- Learners also must have a sensory image of how to perform the skill through sight, hearing, touch, and sometimes taste or smell. This sensory image is gained by demonstration. To teach clients motor skills effectively, the C/PHN has to provide them with an adequate sensory image. It is best to demonstrate and explain slowly, one point at a time, and sometimes repeatedly, until clients understand the proper sequence or combination of actions necessary to carry out the skill.
- Another condition for psychomotor learning is practice. After acquiring a sensory image, clients can start to perform the skill. Mastery comes over time as clients repeat the task until it is smooth, coordinated, and unhesitating (Miller & Stoeckel, 2016; Miller et al., 2012).
  - During this process, the C/PHN should be available to provide guidance and encouragement. In the early stages of practice, you may need to use hands-on guidance to give clients a sense of how the performance should feel.

- When clients give return demonstrations, you can make suggestions, give encouragement, and thereby maximize the learning.
- For example, a C/PHN demonstrates passive range-of-motion exercises on a client's wife to show her how the exercises should feel (giving her a sensory image). The wife then learns to perform the exercises on her husband. During practice, feedback from the nurse enables the wife to know whether the skill is being performed correctly.
- At this guided response stage, objectives may include action verbs such as *fastens*, *manipulates*, *measures*, *organizes*, and *calibrates*.

The psychomotor domain, like the cognitive and affective domains, ranges from simple to complex levels of functioning. It is necessary to exercise judgment in assessing a client's ability to perform a skill. Even clients with limited ability often can move to higher levels once they have mastered simple skills. Nursing tasks that facilitate psychomotor learning in the client include the following:

- Determine the client's capability for learning by assessing the client's physical, intellectual, and emotional ability.
- Physically demonstrate and explain the skill, providing the client with a sensory image.
- Encourage practice by providing guidance and positive reinforcement.

Learning Theories

A **learning theory** is a systematic and integrated look into the nature of the process whereby people relate to their surroundings in such ways as to enhance their ability to use both themselves and their surroundings more effectively (Schunk, 2020). Each nurse has and uses a particular theory of learning, whether consciously or unconsciously, and that theory, in turn, dictates the way the C/PHN teaches clients. It is useful to discover what each nurse's learning theory is and how it affects the role of health educator. A brief examination of these learning theories can be viewed in Table 11-3.

Health Teaching Models

Theories on learning provide a general understanding of how people learn. In addition, various health teaching models specifically focus on explaining individual health experiences, behaviors, and actions. These models fit with the learning theories to give nurses a more accurate picture of the client and the clients' learning needs. Four useful models are described here: the health belief model (HBM), Pender's health promotion model (revised) (HPM), the transtheoretical or stages of change model, and the PRECEDE and PROCEED models.

Health Belief Model

The HBM, which was developed by social psychologists and brought to the attention of health care professionals by Rosenstock (1966), is useful for explaining the behaviors and actions taken by people to prevent illness and injury. It postulates that readiness to act on behalf of a person's own health is predicated on the following (Skinner, Tiro, & Champion, 2015):

- Perceived susceptibility to the condition in question
- Perceived seriousness of the condition in question
- Perceived benefits to taking action
- Barriers to taking action
- Cues to action, such as knowledge that someone else has the condition or attention from the media
- Self-efficacy—the ability to take action to achieve the desired outcome

Using the HBM, parental intention to participate in parenting classes was examined. Researchers found that high intentions to participate was related to low barriers to attend the program (Salari & Filus, 2017). C/PHNs may find the use of the HBM (and variations) to be helpful in assessing the health behaviors and beliefs of culturally diverse populations.

Pender's Health Promotion Model

First published in the 1980s by nurse Nola Pender, the HPM was envisioned as a framework for exploring health-related behaviors within a nursing and behavioral science context (Murdaugh, Parsons, & Pender, 2019). Reflecting the growing body of literature relevant to the HPM, Pender revised the model to reflect a number of major theoretical changes. The revised HPM includes three general areas of concern to health-promoting behavior: *Individual characteristics and experiences* are seen to interact with *behavior-specific cognitions and affect* to influence specific *behavioral outcomes* (Murdaugh et al., 2019). The revised HPM focuses on predicting behaviors that influence health promotion. In addition, the HPM includes the variable of interpersonal influence of others, including family and health professionals.

Being able to predict health promotion behaviors enhances the C/PHN's ability to work with clients. Awareness of their characteristics, experiences, comprehension of their health-related issues, perceived barriers, self-efficacy, support (or lack of it) from significant others, and commitment provides the nurse with a picture that clarifies the client–nurse role and gives direction for action taking. The HPM (Fig. 11-6) is based on the theoretical propositions found in Box 11-3.

Using these propositions, researchers explored clients' health behaviors in many studies conducted in the 1980s, 1990s, and into the 21st century. Research using the model includes a study determining factors influencing breakfast consumption in female high school students in the Yazd Province of Iran. Results revealed that by including family and friends in breakfast and being positive about breakfast reduces barriers and increases self-efficacy; thus, improving female high school students' participation in breakfast (Mehrabbeik, Mahmoodabad, Khosravi, & Fallahzadeh, 2017).

Transtheoretical or Stages of Change Model

The transtheoretical model (TTM) addresses change by anticipating relapses and recognizing those as opportunities to better plan for how to sustain the needed change in future attempts (Bartholomew, Markham, Mullen, & Fernandez, 2015; Prochaska, Norcross, & DiClemente, 2007). The model, sometimes called stages of change, is not linear but is depicted as a spiral, with plateaus, relapses, and false starts. It can be used with individuals, groups, and populations. The stages include the following (Prochaska et al., 2007, p. 39):

TABLE **11-3** Learning Theories

Theory Type and Name	Theorists and Dates of Landmark Publications	Theory Description	Example of Theory in Practice
Behavioral			
Stimulus–response "bond" theory	Ivan Pavlov (1957)	With conditioning, certain causes (stimuli) evoke certain effects (responses).	C/PHN teaches a family client to take her birth control pill each morning after she brushes her teeth.
No-reinforcement approach	Edward Thorndike (1932, 1969)	The learner has an innate reflexive drive to accomplish the desired response after conditioning.	C/PHN repeatedly emphasizes to a group of pregnant women that their prenatal classes promote a positive delivery experience and healthy newborns.
Conditioning through reinforcement	B. F. Skinner (1974, 1987)	Reinforcement through successive, systematic changes in the learner's environment enhances the probability of desired responses.	A school nurse gives rewards (e.g., stickers, activity books) to children who attend each class on safety.
Cognitive			
Theory of cognitive development	Jean Piaget (1966, 1970)	Each stage signifies a transformation from the previous one, and a child must move through each stage sequentially. Three abilities are used to make the transformation: 1. *Assimilation*: reacting to new situations by using skills already possessed 2. *Accommodation*: being sufficiently mature so that previously unsolved problems can now be solved 3. *Adaptation*: the ability to cope with the demands of the environment	The nurse uses puppets with 3-year-olds in a presentation on safety but group discussion with young teens with diabetes on the benefits and consequences of taking or not taking their insulin.
Insight theory		1. Learning is a process in which the learner develops new insights or changes old ones. 2. Learners intuitively and intelligently sense their way through problems. 3. However, the "insight" is useful only if the learner understands its significance.	The C/PHN provides a career planning class and Amy, a high school dropout, realizes that she has limited job skills and that if she learned more about computer skills, she could get a better job.
Goal-insight theory		The learner goes beyond intuitive hunches to tested insights.	Amy takes a beginning and then an advanced computer class and is offered a higher-paying job. The C/PHN discusses Amy's successes with her and asks Amy whether she ever thought about going to college. Amy begins to think about completing the requirements to go to community college, because if she had an associate degree she could be promoted to a supervisory position and make more money.
Cognitive-field theory		The learner is purposive and problem centered.	Amy confers with the C/PHN about her choices and has changed her thinking about herself so much that she is planning to get an apartment in a neighborhood that is better for her child and she may continue taking classes.

TABLE 11-3 Learning Theories *(Continued)*

Theory Type and Name	Theorists and Dates of Landmark Publications	Theory Description	Example of Theory in Practice
Social Learning			
Overview of theory	Bandura (1977, 1986)	1. Relationships often are dysfunctional and produce undesirable or inappropriate behavior. 2. The learner, influenced by role models, builds self-confidence, persuasion, and personal mastery. 3. Self-efficacy can lead to the desired behaviors and outcomes.	N/A
Coincidental association		Outcomes typically are preceded by numerous events, and the client selects the wrong events as predictors of an outcome.	Juanita had a negative experience with a man who wore a hearing aid. Afterward, all of her experiences with men who wore hearing aids were negative. Juanita may begin to separate her negative experiences with men from their hearing disabilities after attending a class on building self-esteem suggested by the C/PHN.
Inappropriate generalization		One negative experience provokes negative feelings for future experiences.	Three-year-old Ryan accidentally drank some spoiled milk. He generalized that milk tastes bad and now refuses to drink it. The nurse can suggest to Ryan's mother that she might have Ryan try chocolate milk. She then can slowly reintroduce plain milk.
Perceived self-inefficacy		"Persons who judge themselves as lacking coping capabilities, whether the self-appraisal is objectively warranted or not, will perceive all kinds of dangers in situations and exaggerate their potential harmfulness" (Bandura, 1986, p. 220).	An older client, William, tells the C/PHN about two missing Social Security checks but refuses to take a bus to the post office. He states that he does not know what to say to the postal clerk and has read about senior citizens getting mugged on buses. He refuses to follow up on his lost income. The C/PHN introduces him to another gentleman in the apartment complex who feels confident in the neighborhood and improves William's self-confidence.
Humanistic			
Hierarchy of human needs	Abraham Maslow (1970)	A person's needs must be met in order of priority, with more basic needs having to be met before others. In order from most basic to least, needs are: 1. Physiologic (air, food, water) 2. Safety and security 3. Love and belonging 4. Self-esteem (positive feelings of self-worth) 5. Self-actualization	It would be difficult for a group of young mothers to concentrate on learning about proper infant nutrition if they are worried about their babies crying in the next room. Their need to care for their children (need for love and belonging) would be greater than the need to learn about future health considerations (self-esteem and self-actualization).

(Continued)

TABLE 11-3 Learning Theories *(Continued)*

Theory Type and Name	Theorists and Dates of Landmark Publications	Theory Description	Example of Theory in Practice
Client-centered counseling approach	Carl Rogers (1969, 1989)	1. The learning environment is to be learner centered so that students become more self-directed and guide their own learning. 2. The learner is the person most capable of deciding how to find the solutions to problems. The client identifies the problem and, given time and space, can find a way through the problem to a solution. 3. The C/PHN acts as a facilitator in this learning process.	A 55-year-old man wants to quit smoking after a prolonged upper respiratory tract infection that is aggravated by his habit and comes to a stop-smoking class led by the C/PHN at the county health department.
Adult Learning			
Adult learning theory	Knowles (1984, 1989, 1990) Knowles, Holton, and Swanson (2015)	Adult learners: 1. Are self-directed in their learning 2. Have a lifetime of experience to draw on when learning 3. Are more ready to learn when the learning is focused on helping them meet requirements for their personal and occupational roles 4. Have a problem-centered time perspective, in that they need to apply and try out their learning quickly	Susan, a 65-year-old retired librarian, was open to learning more about her type 2 diabetes after a recent discharge from the hospital. When the C/PHN arrived at her house, Susan was asked what she already knew about diabetes and included Susan in goal-setting regarding her health. Susan appreciated that the C/PHN provided information that built on her previous understanding of the disease and worked with Susan to find manageable solutions to improve her health.

Source: Bandura (1977, 1986); Knowles (1984, 1989, 1990); Knowles et al. (2015); Maslow (1970); Pavlov (1957); Piaget (1966, 1970); Rogers (1969, 1989); Skinner (1974, 1987); Thorndike (1932, 1969).

- Precontemplation—This is usually the normal state of denial or the problem may not be perceived (either don't know about it or don't want to think acknowledge it). Clients may say, "I don't really smoke that many cigarettes, so I don't have to worry about lung cancer or the other health problems."
- Contemplation—At this stage, the client is more realistic and may be more open to discussing the problem of smoking. However, the client may not be able to seriously consider behavior change or feel able to confront the issue. The client may say, "I know I should probably try to quit smoking, but I am really stressed right now and can't think about it."
- Preparation—During this stage, the client is moving away from contemplation toward action. The client may be trying to gather information and may be talking to others about how they quit smoking. They may be concerned that it may take more than one try in order to accomplish their goal. A client may talk to the physician about medications that are helpful, tell friends and family that they are planning to quit smoking, and may even begin to cut back on the number of cigarettes smoked each day.
- Action—This stage is the beginning of the behavioral change. The client sets a date to quit smoking, begins using a nicotine patch or medication, and finds replacement behaviors for smoking (e.g., using breath mints, exercising during usual smoking breaks). The client knows that this attempt may not be successful the first time and should be encouraged to acknowledge and plan for this.
- Maintenance—In this stage, the behavior has been changed. The smoker has stopped smoking, but now needs to be vigilant in avoiding a relapse. The client needs a support system and rewards to encourage maintenance. If the client relapses, the C/PHN and others can help the client learn from this and begin their preparation and action stages again until longer periods of maintenance are achieved.
- Termination—This occurs when the former behavior is no longer appealing. The smoker no longer has an interest in cigarettes and does not have to exert the constant vigilance needed in the maintenance stage. Prochaska et al. (2007) note that not everyone can truly reach this stage, and therefore, it is not always included in health promotion programs or research.

Researchers have used this model with many topics related to health promotion and prevention (e.g., substance abuse, smoking cessation, weight loss, physical activity). One research study found that this model could help determine physical activity behavior in

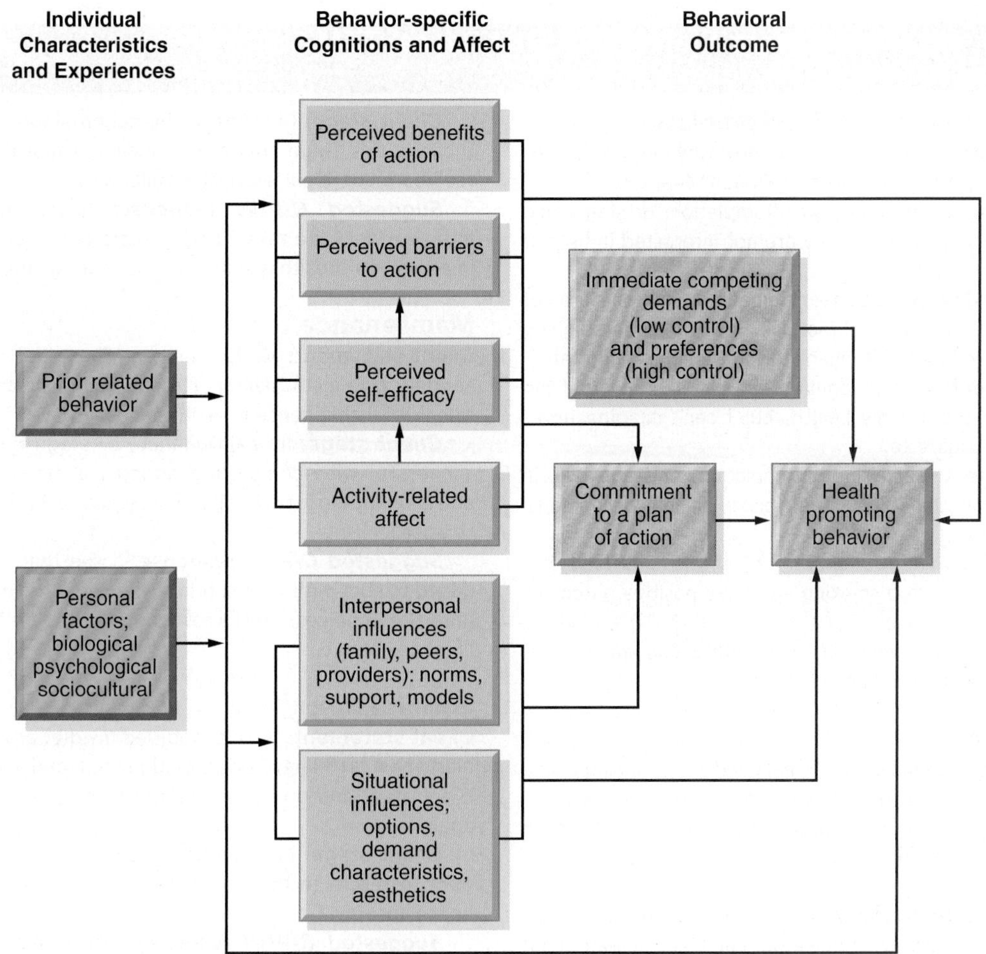

FIGURE 11-6 Health promotion model. (Reprinted with permission from Pender, N. L., Murdaugh, C.L., Parsons, M.A. (2015). *Health promotion in nursing practice* (7th ed.). Upper Saddle River, NJ: Prentice Hall. © 2015. Reprinted by permission of Pearson Education, Inc., New York, NY.)

women. Results found that stages of change were significantly correlated with self-efficacy, processes of change, and decisional balance (Pirzadeh, Mostafavi, Ghofarniphour, & Mansorian, 2017). Often, the nurse can determine the stage the client is in from the client's statements; see Box 11-4 for some example statement and suggested nurse responses.

The PRECEDE and PROCEED Models

First published by Green in 1974, the PRECEDE model was developed for educational diagnosis (Glanz, Rimer, & Viswanath, 2015). The acronym PRECEDE has been slightly revised from the original to stand for *p*redisposing, *r*einforcing, and *e*nabling *c*onstructs in *e*ducational/ecological *d*iagnosis and *e*valuation (Bartholomew et al., 2015; Green & Kreuter, 2005).

- The PROCEED model (Green, Cross, Woodal, & Tones, 2019) works in tandem with the PRECEDE model as the C/PHN proceeds to plan, implement, and evaluate health education programs.
- This acronym stands for *p*olicy, *r*egulatory, and *o*rganizational *c*onstructs for *e*ducational and *e*nvironmental *d*evelopment (Bartholomew et al., 2015). The entire PRECEDE–PROCEED model includes eight phases in the formulation and evaluation of health educational programs.
- The first five of these phases are included in the PRECEDE portion of the model and include (1) social, (2) epidemiologic, and (3) education/ecological assessments, followed by (4) administrative and policy assessment and intervention alignment, and (5) implementation.
- The PROCEED model is emphasized in the last three phases: (1) process evaluation, (2) impact evaluation, and (3) outcome evaluation.

A hallmark of the PRECEDE–PROCEED model is the emphasis on the desired outcome. The model both begins and ends with *quality of life*, which includes "subjectively defined problems and priorities of individuals and communities" (Green et al., 2019). The emphasis on what the individual or community perceives as the problem, not what the professional believes it to be, is crucial. Outcome evaluation is logically linked back to that same individual or community in assessing achievement of the desired change.

The steps in this model are similar to those of the nursing process. Because of this familiarity, the model has become a useful tool for nurses teaching in the community.

BOX 11-4 Example Clients' Statements That Reveal TTM Stage and Suggested Nurse Responses

Precontemplation and Contemplation

Client statement: Jeff says: "I don't know why my wife is concerned about my high blood pressure, I don't feel sick."

Client stage: Client is in precontemplation, or stage one, in which clients demonstrate they are not interested in help or thinking about change.

Suggested C/PHN response: "Sometime symptoms are not always present, so you may not feel sick. However, understanding your diagnosis and what this means to your health is important."

Client statement: Jessica comments, "I can see how quitting smoking could improve my health, but I can't imagine never having another cigarette."

Client stage: Client is in contemplation, or stage two, in which clients may think about their behavior and the personal consequences of it.

Suggested C/PHN response: "I know this is difficult, but taking steps now to stop smoking can have positive outcomes for your health."

Neither client is committed to making a change; each is unaware or thinking of pros/cons.

Preparation

Client statement: Jamie states, "I feel good about setting a date to go into rehab, but I wonder if I can really go through with it."

Client stage: Client is in preparation, or stage three, in which clients think about change and take small steps like gathering information.

Suggested C/PHN response: "I'm glad you are taking steps to improve your health. What questions can I help answer about rehab?"

Action

Client statement: Kevin reports, "I have been on my low salt, low fat diet for a month now, and my blood pressure is better, but I'd really like to be able to eat fast food more often."

Client stage: Client is in the action stage, or stage four; those in this stage are actually moving toward their goal and feel more confident exercising willpower.

Suggested C/PHN response: "Incorporating change into your daily life takes time. You are taking positive steps to improve your health and modify your eating choices."

Maintenance

Client statement: Maria remarks, "These last few months of sobriety give me a feeling of accomplishment, but I still question if total abstinence is really mandatory."

Client stage: In maintenance, or stage five, people are successful with completing actions, avoiding temptations, and developing new habits. There is awareness of potential relapse.

Suggested C/PHN response: "I see that you are determined to stick with your sobriety. It is often too easy to slip into unhealthy choices, but I know you can stay on track with this lifestyle change."

Termination

Client statement: "I have modified my diet and exercise regularly now, and I have decreased my BMI and lowered my A1C. I feel great and do not want to go back to feeling unhealthy again."

Client stage: In termination, or stage six, people do not want to return to their previous unhealthy behaviors and will not relapse.

Suggested C/PHN response: "Your decision to include healthy behaviors in your life has made a difference in how you now manage your diabetes. These positive choices might also influence other family members."

The nurse builds on the assessment formulated from the PRECEDE model, determines the best interventions, and then proceeds to evaluate the outcome of those interventions. The emphasis on the perceived needs of the individual or community as the starting point for all community efforts is consistent with public health nursing practice. The model reminds us of the importance of an organized approach to health educational programs, one that begins and ends with the "experts"—the individuals, families, and communities we hope to help through our efforts. The PRECEDE–PROCEED model can be seen in Figure 11-7.

This model has been used to address many public health problems. Over 1,000 examples of published applications of PRECEDE–PROCEED may be found at www.lgreen.net, including studies on health care workers' hand hygiene behaviors, follow-up with multicultural women with abnormal mammograms, implementation of church-based heart health promotion programs for older adults, developing a healthy-eating curriculum for schools, evaluation of a physical activity and nutrition program for senior citizens, and determining health promotion motivators in Asian populations. Other models used in community assessment and intervention may be found in Chapter 15.

Teaching at Three Levels of Prevention

C/PHNs should develop teaching programs that coincide with the level of prevention needed by the client. The three levels of primary, secondary, and tertiary prevention are demonstrated in the levels of prevention pyramid for nurses who teach clients, families, aggregates, or populations (Box 11-5).

Ideally, the C/PHN focuses teaching at the primary level. If nurses were able to reach more people at this level, it would help to diminish years of morbidity and limit subsequent incapacity. Many people experience disabilities that could have been prevented if primary prevention behaviors had been incorporated into their daily activities.

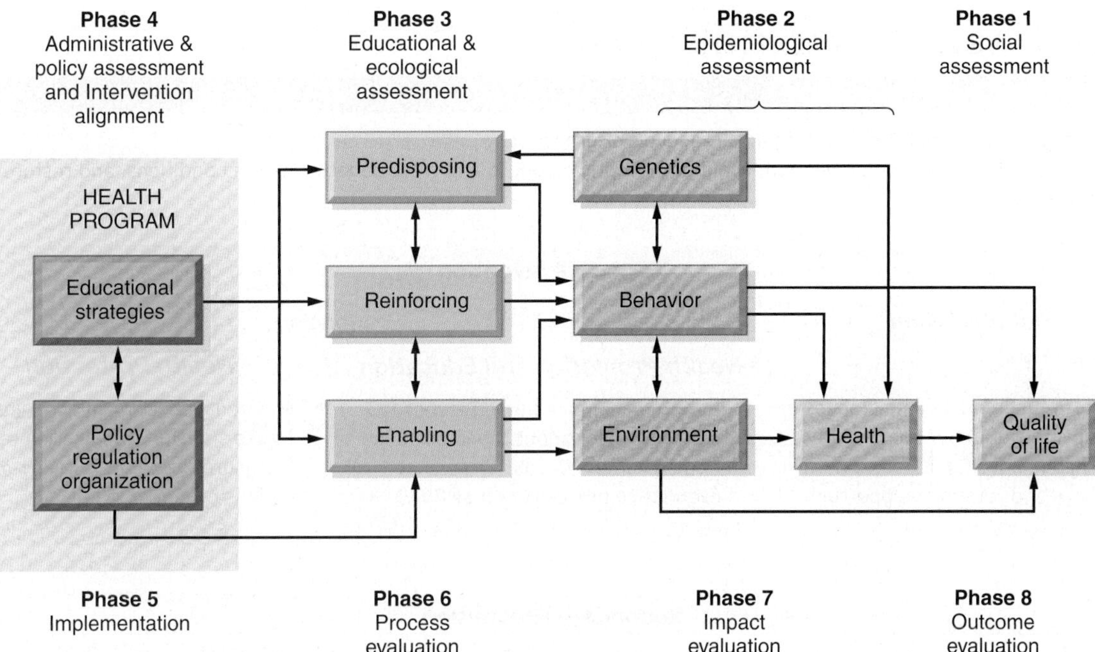

FIGURE 11-7 The PRECEDE–PROCEED model. (Reprinted with permission from Green, J., Cross, R., Woodall, J., & Tones, K. (2019). *Health promotion: Planning and strategies* (4th ed.). Los Angeles, CA: Sage.)

Effective Teaching

Teaching is an art. It can be performed with such skill and grace that the client becomes part of a well-orchestrated event, with learning as the natural outcome. Instead of relying on prescribed teaching methods, the skillful C/PHN can make judgments based largely on client qualities, situations, and needs that guide the experience. The desired changes emerge in the course of the interaction rather than at a level conceived before the teaching. Before the C/PHN can reach this level of artistry, there is much to learn about being an effective teacher.

Teaching–Learning Principles

- Teaching lies at one end of a continuum. At the other end is learning. Without learning, teaching becomes useless in the same way that communication does not occur unless a message is both sent and received.
- Both the teacher and the learner have responsibilities on that continuum.
- Learners must take responsibility for their own learning.
- Teachers obstruct that process if they assume complete responsibility for bringing about changed behavior.
- Clients can be directed toward health knowledge, but they will not acquire knowledge unless they have the desire to learn.

Teaching, then, becomes a matter of facilitating both the desire and the best conditions for satisfying it (Gilbert, Sawyer, & McNeill, 2015). Teaching in community health nursing means to influence, motivate, and act as a catalyst in the learning process. To do this, the C/PHN needs to understand the basic principles underlying the art and science of the teaching–learning process and the use of appropriate materials to influence learning.

Client Readiness. The client's readiness to learn influences the C/PHN's teaching effectiveness. Four facets of client readiness have been identified (Kitchie, 2019):

1. Physical readiness, which deals with their ability, task complexity, environment, health status, and gender
2. Emotional readiness, which deals with the state of receptivity to learning (e.g., motivation, anxiety, developmental stage, risk-taking behavior)
3. Experiential readiness, which reflects the learner's past experiences with learning (cultural background, orientation, locus of control, coping mechanisms used)
4. Knowledge readiness, which encompasses the learner's knowledge and understanding (e.g., learning disabilities, learning style, current knowledge base)

For instance, one C/PHN found that a young primipara was not ready for prenatal teaching on fetal growth and development. She had strong fears that she would be unable to lose her baby weight and that this would make her sexually unattractive to her partner. Until these anxieties were addressed, the teaching would remain ineffective. Clients' needs, interests, motivation, stress, and concerns determine their readiness for learning.

Another factor that influences readiness is educational background. If a group of women who never completed grade school meet to learn how to care for a sick person in the home, material should be presented in a factual and easily accessible manner and in terms that they understand. To discuss complex concepts of health, illness, and scientific research would be above their level of readiness. However, you can begin to introduce more complex concepts as you work with the women and assess their readiness for additional knowledge.

BOX 11-5 LEVELS OF PREVENTION PYRAMID

Application to Client Teaching

SITUATION: Several examples of teaching at three levels of prevention.

GOAL: Using the three levels of prevention, avoid or promptly diagnose and treat negative health conditions, and restore the fullest possible potential.

Tertiary Prevention		
Rehabilitation	*Prevention*	
	Health Promotion and Education	*Health Protection*
▪ Restore function: a nurse teaches a stroke survivor about home safety, alternative housing options, physical therapy, and retraining opportunities	▪ Health teaching: a nurse teaches the stroke survivor about the importance of medication use, diet, rest, and exercise to prevent another CVA	▪ Maintenance: a nurse observes the stroke survivor's medication regime to ensure the client is taking medications properly

Secondary Prevention	
Early Diagnosis	*Prompt Treatment*
▪ Screening and case finding: a nurse takes blood pressure measurements from all family members at each home visit and teaches them the importance of maintaining a healthy blood pressure reading	▪ Treatment: a nurse teaches clients how to navigate through the complexities of the health care delivery system to receive prompt treatment

Primary Prevention	
Health Promotion and Education	*Health Protection*
▪ Health education: a nurse teaches a class on sensible weight control for teenagers	▪ Immunizations: a nurse teaches about the importance of pneumonia and flu vaccines for seniors, followed by an immunization clinic

Maturational level also affects readiness. An adolescent mother who is still working on the normal developmental tasks of her age group, such as seeking independence or selecting a career path, may not be ready to learn parenting skills. Readiness of the client determines the amount of material presented in each teaching session. The pace or speed with which information is presented must be manageable. A small amount of anxiety often increases client receptivity to learning; however, high levels of anxiety can have the opposite effect.

Client Perceptions. Clients' perceptions also affect their learning, serving as a screening device or filter through which all new information must pass. Individual perceptions help people interpret and attach meaning to things.

Frequently, clients use selective perception. They screen out some statements and pay attention to those that fit their values or personal desires. For example, a C/PHN is teaching a client about the various risk factors in coronary disease; the individual screens out the need to quit smoking and lose weight, paying attention only to factors that would not require a drastic change in lifestyle. Nurses must know their clients, understand their backgrounds and values, and learn about their perceptions before health teaching can influence their behavior (Kitchie, 2019).

Educational Environment. The setting in which the educational experience takes place has a significant impact on learning (Kitchie, 2019). Students probably have had the experience of sitting in a cold room and trying to concentrate during a lecture or of being distracted by noise, heat, or uncomfortable seating. Physical conditions such as ventilation, lighting, room temperature, view of the speaker, and noise level should be controlled to provide an environment that is conducive to learning.

Equally important for learning is an atmosphere of mutual respect and trust. The nurse needs to convey this attitude both verbally and nonverbally. The way the C/PHN addresses clients, shows concern, and gives recognition makes a considerable difference in establishing clients' rapport and trust.

- Both nurse and clients need to be mutually helpful and considerate of one another's needs and interests.
- All participants in the educational experience should feel free to express ideas, should know that their views will be heard, and should feel accepted despite differences of opinion and perspective.

- According to the adult learning theorist Knowles, this requires that the nurse refrain from seeming judgmental or inducing competitiveness among learners. Knowles (1980, p. 58) adds that teachers should share their own feelings and knowledge "as a co-learner in the spirit of inquiry."

Client Participation. The degree of participation in the educational process directly influences the amount of learning (Moffett, Berezowski, Spencer, & Lanning, 2014). One nurse discovered this principle while working with a group of clients who were nearing retirement. After talking to them about the changes they would face and receiving little response, the nurse shifted to a different method of teaching. Handouts on Social Security benefits were distributed, and everyone was asked to read them during the week and come the next week with questions generated by the pamphlets. The C/PHN began the next session with a story about an older couple unprepared for retirement and the problems that they incurred. He then asked the group to share questions and concerns they had about retirement. This strategy prompted the group to slowly begin to participate in their own learning (Fig. 11-8).

- Learning is facilitated when the student is engaged and fully participates in the learning process. C/PHNs should begin from the client's place of interest.
- When the client chooses own directions, helps to discover own learning resources, formulates own problems, decides own course of action, and lives with consequences of each of these choices, then the client has significantly maximized his or her learning.
- Contracting is a tool that allow the client to participate in the process as a partner to determine goals, content, and time for learning. This can contribute to client learning and active participation (see Chapter 10).

The amount of learning is directly proportional to the learner's involvement. In another example, a group of senior citizens attended a class on nutrition and aging yet made few changes in eating patterns. It was not until the members became actively involved in the class, encouraged by the nurse to present problems and solutions for food purchasing, understanding how to read nutrition labels, and preparation of meals on limited budgets, that any significant behavioral changes occurred.

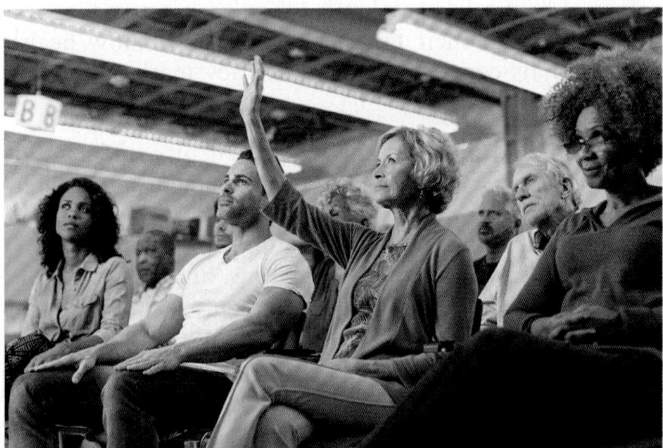

FIGURE 11-8 Client engagement is a key to successful health promotion programs.

Subject Relevance. Subject matter that is relevant to the client is learned more readily and retained longer than information that is not meaningful. Learners gain the most from subject matter that is immediately useful to their own purposes. This is particularly true for adult learners, who have more life experiences that can be related to learning and who tend to see the immediate relevance of the material taught (Bastable, Gramet, Sopczyk, Jacobs, & Braungort, 2020; Knowles, 1980). When clients see the relevance in learning, they accomplish it more promptly. When the subject matter is relevant to the learner, more knowledge is retained.

Client Satisfaction. To maintain motivation and increase self-direction, clients must derive satisfaction from learning. Learners need to feel a sense of steady progress in the learning process. Realistic goals contribute to learner satisfaction. Objectives should be set within the learner's ability, thereby avoiding the frustration resulting from a task that is too difficult and the loss of interest resulting from one that is too easy. Once objectives are met, it is important to provide recognition or reward for the accomplishment. Setting objectives requires agreement on goals, periodic reviews, and revision of goals if they become too easy or too difficult (Bastable et al., 2020). Obstacles, frustrations, and failures along the way discourage and impede learning. Many clients who have had strokes and have potential for rehabilitation often give up trying to regain speech or move paralyzed limbs because they become frustrated and discouraged. On the other hand, clients who experience satisfaction and progress in their speech and muscle retraining maintain their motivation and may work on exercises without prompting. C/PHNs can promote client satisfaction through support and encouragement.

Client Application. Learning is reinforced through application (Bastable et al., 2020). Learners need as many opportunities as possible to apply the knowledge in daily life. If such opportunities arise during the teaching–learning process, clients can try out new knowledge and skills under supervision. Learners are given an opportunity to begin integrating the learning into their daily lives at a time when the teacher is there to help reinforce that pattern.

Teaching Process

The process of teaching in community health nursing follows steps similar to those of the nursing process:

1. *Interaction:* Establish basic communication patterns between clients and nurse.
2. *Assessment and diagnosis*: Determine client's present status and identify client's need for teaching through surveys, interviews, open forums, or task forces that include representative clients as members (keeping in mind that clients should determine their own needs).

3. *Setting goals and objectives*: Analyze needed changes, establish the goal (a broad statement of outcome), and prepare objectives that describe the desired learning outcomes. Objectives should be stated in measurable behavioral terms, using a grammatical structure that contains a subject, verb, condition/criterion, and time frame. That is, each objective should include a single idea that describes an outcome that can be measured within a certain time frame (see the example that follows these steps).
4. *Planning:* Design a plan for the learning experience that meets the mutually developed objectives; include content to be covered, sequence of topics, best conditions for learning (place, type of environment), methods, and materials (e.g., visual aids, exercises). A written plan is best; it may be part of the written nursing care plan.
5. *Teaching*: Implement the learning experience by carrying out the planned activities.
6. *Evaluation:* Determine whether learning objectives were met, and if not, why not. Evaluation measures progress toward goals, effectiveness of chosen teaching methods, or future learning needs.

Here is an example of a short-term goal, a long-term goal, and a set of objectives related to a specific client need:

Need: A group of smokers wish to end their addiction to nicotine.

Short-term goal: Within 1 month, all members of the group will reduce the number of cigarettes smoked.

Long-term goal: Ninety percent of group members will remain tobacco-free for 6 months.

Objectives: At the end of the program, all clients should be able to do the following:

- *List* three reasons why smoking is unhealthy.
- *Identify* at least two factors that influence their smoking habit.
- *Apply* a series of action steps leading to smoking cessation within 1 month.
- *Examine* the steps as they work to live tobacco-free in the first 3 months.
- *Design* a way to live a fulfilled, tobacco-free life.
- *Evaluate* successful strategies to remain tobacco-free for 6 months.

Teaching Methods and Materials

Teaching occurs on many levels and incorporates various types of activities.

- It can be formal or informal, planned or unplanned. Formal presentations, such as group lectures, usually are planned and fairly structured.
- Lecturers tend to create a passive learning environment for the audience unless strategies are devised to involve the learners.
- Many individuals are visual rather than auditory learners. To capture their attention, computer-generated slide programs or video presentations can supplement the lecture.
- Allowing time for questions and discussion after a lecture also actively involves learners. This method is best used with adults, but even they have a limited attention span, and breaks should be given every 30 to 60 minutes.
- Distributing printed material that highlights and summarizes, or supplements, the shared content also reinforces important points.

Some teaching is less formal but still planned and relatively structured, as in group discussions in which questions stimulate the exploration of ideas and guide thinking. Informal levels of teaching, such as counseling or **anticipatory guidance** (in which the client is assisted in preparing for a future role or developmental stage), require the teacher to be prepared, but there is no defined presentation plan. The C/PHN may use a handout or agency protocol steps as a guide. C/PHNs use one or a combination of methods, along with a variety of materials, to facilitate the teaching–learning process. Two-way communication is an important feature of the learning process. Learners need an opportunity to raise questions, make comments, reason out loud, and receive feedback to develop deeper understanding. When discussion is used in conjunction with other teaching methods, such as demonstration and role playing, it improves their effectiveness.

Effective education also includes an understanding and awareness of health literacy and the need to evaluate patient understanding of medical information. **Health literacy** is defined as, "The degree to which individuals have the capacity to obtain, process, and understand basic health information needed to make appropriate health decisions" (HRSA, 2019, para. 1). Health literacy can be prevalent among older adults, minority populations, underserved populations, and those with low socioeconomic status (SES) (HRSA, 2019). The populations C/PHNs serve may be poor and underserved. Risk factors such as SES have been shown to have a casual relationship with health literacy, which can then influence clinical and behavioral choices, thereby affecting heath care use and outcomes (Knighton, Brunisholz, & Savitz, 2017). Low literacy may be due to limited English proficiency (LEP), cultural barriers, medical terms that patients may not understand, or low educational skills, which can affect their understanding of medication directions, their management of health conditions, or their ability to fill out forms (HRSA, 2019). C/PHN must be aware of health literacy levels when providing education to patients and their families. Examples of how health professionals can mitigate low literacy may include the following:

- Assume all patients may have difficulty understanding medical information, and implement health literacy universal precautions.
- Supplement instruction with appropriate materials.
- Ask open-ended questions (how and what) rather than closed-ended questions (yes and no).
- Have patients "teach back" or demonstrate a procedure.
- Teach so that age, culture, and ethnic diversity are considered.
- Provide information in the primary language for LEP patients (HRSA, 2019).

- Use health literacy tools (such as those found on thePoint® to provide information that patients can understand (AHRQ, 2016, 2019; CDC, 2019b; Readability Formulas, 2020).

Demonstration. The demonstration method often is used for teaching psychomotor skills and is best accompanied by explanation and discussion, with time set aside for return demonstration by the client or caregiver. It gives clients a clear sensory image of how to perform the skill. Because a demonstration should be within easy visual and auditory range of learners, it is best to demonstrate in front of small groups or a single client. Use the same kind of equipment that clients will use, show exactly how the skill should be performed, and provide learners with ample opportunities to practice until the skill is perfected.

Role Playing. At times, having clients assume and act out roles maximizes learning. A parenting group, for example, found it helpful to place themselves in the role of their children. In doing so, their feelings about various ways to respond became more apparent. Reversing roles can effectively teach conflicting couple's better ways to communicate. To prevent role playing from becoming a game with little learning, it should be planned with clear objectives in mind.

- What behavioral outcomes should be achieved?
- Define the context (the "stage") clearly, so that everyone shares in the situation. Then define each role ahead of time, making sure that participants understand their performance roles.
- Emphasize that no wrong or right performance exists and that participants should behave the way people behave in everyday life.
- Avoid having people play themselves, because it can embarrass them and make it difficult for them to achieve objectivity.
- After the drama has concluded, begin discussion with carefully prepared questions.

This technique can be used with staff, coworkers, young children, teenagers, and adults. However, it can be a risk-taking experience for some people, and they may be reluctant to participate. The nurse should use judgment, begin with volunteers, and avoid pushing this technique on unwilling or nonreceptive people. It is best to build up to full participation.

Teaching Materials. Many different kinds of teaching materials are available to the nurse (Fig. 11-9). They often are employed in combination and are useful during the teaching process. Visual images—such as PowerPoint presentations (using graphics, photos), pictures, posters, chalkboards, flannel boards, DVDs, online videos, bulletin boards, flash cards, pamphlets, flyers, charts, and gestures—can enhance most learning. Americans readily learn from television and the Web, as there is visual and auditory appeal. Other tools, such as anatomic models and improvised or purchased equipment, provide clients with both visual and tactile learning experiences. Still others, such as interactive computer games or instruction, actively involve the learners.

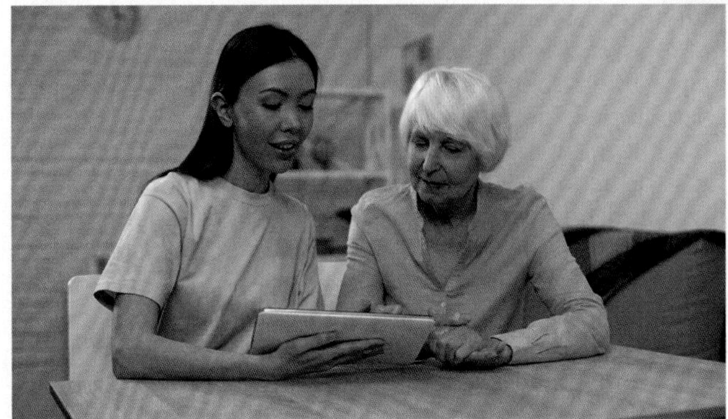

FIGURE 11-9 Teaching materials help to make your point.

The choice of teaching materials varies with the client's interests and abilities and the resources available. Teaching often occurs in casual conversations, spontaneously in situations when clients raise unexpected questions, or when a crisis arises. In these instances, C/PHNs draw on their background of knowledge and exercise professional judgment in their selection of content, methods, and materials.

Printed educational support materials are available, such as pamphlets, brochures, booklets, flyers, and informational sheets. Each should be evaluated for appropriateness and effectiveness with particular individuals, families, or groups. Many come from state and local public health sources. Nurses can create their own handouts, customizing them to the needs of individual clients. The nurse can get educational information from state, federal, and international health agencies. Example include state health departments, the U.S. Food and Drug Administration (FDA), the Centers for Disease Control and Prevention (CDC), the National Institutes of Health (NIH), and the World Health Organization (WHO). Other materials come from nonprofit national agencies such as the American Diabetes Association (ADA), the March of Dimes, the American Association for Retired Persons (AARP), and the American Heart Association (AHA).

Factors to be considered with all educational literature include the material's content, complexity, and reading level. There are several ways to assess the readability of the printed word. One easy way is to use the Fry Readability Graph or the Gunning-Fog formula. These tools are rough way of determining the years of schooling needed to understand printed material. It works by analyzing words and sentence length; the higher the number, the more difficult the reading level. A Gunning-Fog Index of 6 is a sixth grade reading level, and a score of 11 is at the junior year in high school. Fortunately, most word processing programs now include a feature to allow assessment of the reading level in text. Another very common tool is the Flesch Reading Ease program, available in Microsoft Word grammar checker, which evaluates reading material. Similar to the Fry Graph, the Flesch-Kincaid Grade Level readability score rates the material in terms of typical grade level; however, it may not be as accurate and you may need to adjust results downward (Medline Plus, 2019). The nurse should always consider the population when selecting a reading level, as many individuals cannot understand materials at even the 6th grade level. Also, clients, including those speaking a language other than English, may not be able to read and write in their dominant language.

Culturally appropriate health education materials must be acquired or developed for the predominant cultural and linguistic minority populations taught by the nurse. Developing printed materials is an important first step, but the development of video, audio, and public service announcements in community-appropriate languages is also necessary. When translating printed materials from English into another language, it is strongly suggested that a separate translator "back-translate" the materials. This added step helps assure that the meaning from the original has not been distorted or lost in the translation. Essentially one person or group translates the material, and another individual or group translates it back into English. This can add time and cost to the project, but it may prevent inaccuracies in the final material (Huff, Klein, & Peterson, 2015).

Finally, nurses teach by example. Actions speak louder than words. If a nurse teaches the importance of washing hands to reduce disease transmission and then begins a newborn assessment without hand washing, the message of observed actions carries more impact than the words. Nurses who exhibit healthy practices use themselves as teaching tools and serve as role models as well as health teachers.

Clients With Special Learning Needs

At times, the nurse experiences a challenging teaching situation with an individual, family, or group. These challenges may involve clients who have cultural or language differences, hearing impairments, developmental delays, memory losses, visual perception distortions, and problems with fine or gross motor skills, distracting personality characteristics, or demonstrations of stress or emotions. Culture can play a role in communication because it influences belief systems, communication styles, and understanding and response to health information (National Network of Libraries of Medicine, n.d.). The inability to see, hear, and understand health information places those with disabilities at a greater disadvantage impacting their health and health outcomes. Regardless of the situation, C/PHNs will feel most comfortable and confident if they are prepared to deal with these situations before they are experienced.

Before beginning to teach a client, family, or aggregate, thorough preparation is important for successful learning to occur. This includes finding out whether it is possible to teach in English or whether other modifications are needed as the teaching plan is being developed. C/PHNs should never assume anything, including the primary language spoken by clients, their visual or hearing ability, or their capacity to understand. When teaching unfamiliar groups, the nurse can obtain information regarding the interests and abilities of the members from a center manager, caretaker, or program director. These human resources are invaluable in planning any teaching when English may be a second language or when other barriers exist that may impede success if they are not known by the nurse. Interpreters may be needed, and the C/PHN should work closely with the interpreter to assure that the intended message is sent and received by the clients (Huff et al., 2015). The phases of the nursing process continue to guide the nurse as a teacher.

Another difficulty that can arise is unexpected behavior from a client who disrupts the group process. The client may monopolize the discussion, answer questions asked of others, burst out with personal experiences that have no relevance to the topic, become irate at the comments of others, or sit silently and never speak. This can be unnerving to even the most experienced nurse. The C/PHN must tactfully diffuse any behavior that has the potential to distract the other learners. This is accomplished by considerately giving the recognition sought by the person while also setting limits.

SUMMARY

- *Healthy People 2030* objectives recognize the health and well-being of all people and communities, which is an essential component of a thriving, equitable society.
- The purpose of health education is to effect change, which alters the equilibrium in a system.
- Change occurs in three stages: *unfreezing* when the system is ready for change, *changing* when the innovation is implemented, and *refreezing* when the change is stabilized.
- The cognitive domain refers to learning that takes place intellectually. It ranges in levels of learner functioning from simple recall to complex evaluation. As learners move up the scale of cognitive learning, they become more self-directed; the nurse then assumes a more facilitative role.
- Affective learning involves the changing of attitudes and values. Learners may experience several levels of affective involvement, from simple listening to adopting the new value. Again, as the client increases involvement, the nurse uses a less directive approach.
- Psychomotor learning involves the acquisition of motor skills. Clients who learn psychomotor skills must meet three conditions: they must be capable of the skill, they must develop a sensory image of the skill, and they must practice the skill.
- Learning theories can be grouped into four broad categories:
  - Behaviorist theories, which view learning as a behavioral change accomplished through stimulus–response or conditioning;
  - Cognitive learning theories, which seek to influence learners' understanding of problems and situations through promoting their insights;
  - Social learning theories, which explain dysfunctional behavior and facilitate learning; and
  - Humanistic theories, which assume that people have a natural tendency to learn and that learning flourishes in an encouraging environment. Knowles' adult learning theory provides a framework for understanding adult characteristics and appropriate teaching interventions.

- Health teaching models work together with the learning theories to give nurses a more accurate picture of the client and the client's learning needs.
  - The health belief model is useful in explaining the behaviors that are triggered by people with an interest in preventing diseases.
  - The health promotion model helps to predict behaviors that lead to health promotion and includes concepts about the interpersonal influence of others, such as health professionals, friends, and family.
  - The transtheoretical or stages of change model is not a linear model but recognizes that behavior change occurs more like a spiral, with plateaus, relapses, and false starts.
  - The PRECEDE–PROCEED model is designed to guide health educational program development. The model has a strong focus on the perceived problems and priorities of a particular individual or group as they impact quality of life.
- The teaching process in community health nursing is similar to the nursing process, including steps of interaction, assessment and diagnosis, goal setting, planning, teaching, and evaluation.
- The teaching may be formal or informal, planned or unplanned, and methods may range from structured lecture presentations and discussions to demonstration and role playing.

ACTIVE LEARNING EXERCISES

1. Using "Assess and Monitor Population Health" (1 of the 10 essential public health services; see Box 2-2), identify the leading cause of adult mortality in your community. Discuss the social determinants of health that may influence this mortality statistic.
2. As a staff C/PHN, you have been asked to develop a sexual health educational program for group of students aged 14 to 16. Explain your educational plan (include the domain of learning and the learning theory along with the need, goal, objectives, implementation, and evaluation methods).
3. Using behavioral objectives that match the learning level desired, develop a flyer or program for an educational presentation for clients.
4. Select a patient educational handout from CDC: https://www.cdc.gov/hepatitis/resources/patientedmaterials.htm
5. Determine the readability level of the handout and discuss the implications for a nurse using this handout in an educational program. Explain how it best meets the educational needs of your target population.
6. Select a current research article that demonstrates application of one of the health teaching models. How do the results compare with the constructs of the model?

REFERENCES

Adler, N. E., Cutler, D. M., Fielding, J. E., Galea, S., Glymour, M. M., Koh, H. K., & Satcher, D. (2016). Addressing social determinants of health and health disparities: A vital direction for health and health care. *Perspectives: Expert voices in health care*. Retrieved from https://nam.edu/wp-content/uploads/2016/09/Addressing-Social-Determinants-of-Health-and-Health-Disparities.pdf

Agency for Healthcare Research and Quality (AHRQ). (2016). *Health literacy measurement tools (revised)*. Retrieved from https://www.ahrq.gov/health-literacy/quality-resources/tools/literacy/index.html#short

Agency for Healthcare Research and Quality (AHRQ). (2019). *AHRQ health literacy universal precautions toolkit*. Retrieved from https://www.ahrq.gov/health-literacy/quality-resources/tools/literacy-toolkit/index.html

Bandura, A. (1977). *Social learning theory*. Englewood Cliffs, NJ: Prentice-Hall.

Bandura, A. (1986). *Social foundations of thought and action: A social cognitive theory*. Englewood Cliffs, NJ: Prentice-Hall.

Bartholomew, L. K., Markham, C., Mullen, P., & Fernandez, M. E. (2015). Planning models for theory-based health promotion interventions. In K. Glanz, B. K. Rimer, & K. Viswanath (Eds.), *Health behavior: Theory, research, and practice* (5th ed., pp. 359–388). San Francisco, CA: Jossey-Bass.

Bastable, S. B., Gramet, P., Sopczyk, D. L., Jacobs, K., & Braungort, M. M. (2020). *Health professional as educator: Principles of teaching and learning* (2nd ed.). Sudbury, MA: Jones & Bartlett Learning.

Bharmal, K., Derose, K. P., Felician, M., & Weden, M. (2015). *Understanding the upstream social determinants of health*. Rand Corporation. Retrieved from https://www.rand.org/pubs/working_papers/WR1096.html

Bhatt, J., & Bathija, P. (2018). Ensuring access to quality health care in vulnerable populations. *Academic Medicine, 93*(9), 1271–1275.

Bloom, B. (Ed.). (1956). *Taxonomy of educational objectives: The classification of educational goals. Handbook I: Cognitive domain*. New York, NY: Longman.

Canedo, J. R., Miller, S. T., Schlundt, D., Fadden, M. K., & Sanderson, M. K. (2018). Racial and ethnic disparities in diabetes quality of care: The role of healthcare access and sociodemographic status. *Racial and Ethnic Health Disparities, 5*(1), 7–14. Retrieved from https://doi.org/10.1007/s40615-016-0335-8

Centers for Disease Control and Prevention (CDC). (2014). *NCHHSTP social determinants of health*. Retrieved from https://www.cdc.gov/nchhstp/socialdeterminants/definitions.html

Centers for Disease Control and Prevention (CDC). (2017). *Social determinants of health*. Retrieved from https://www.cdc.gov/nchs/data/hpdata2020/HP2020MCR-C39-SDOH.pdf

Centers for Disease Control and Prevention (CDC). (2018). *Adolescent and school health*. Retrieved from https://www.cdc.gov/healthyyouth/disparities/index.htm

Centers for Disease Control and Prevention (CDC). (2019a). *Health communication basics*. Retrieved from https://www.cdc.gov/healthcommunication/healthbasics/WhatIsHC.html

Centers for Disease Control and Prevention (CDC). (2019b). *Health literacy*. Retrieved from https://www.cdc.gov/healthliteracy/developmaterials/guidancestandards.html

Center of Social Epidemiology. (2018). *Unhealthy work*. Retrieved from https://unhealthywork.org/classic-studies/the-whitehall-study/

Dong, L., Fakeye, O. A., Graham, G., & Gaskin, D. J. (2017). Racial/ethnic disparities in quality of care for cardiovascular disease in ambulatory settings: A review. *Medical Care and Research Review, 75*(3), 263–291.

Duke, C. C., & Stanik, C. (2016). *Overcoming lower-income patients' concerns about trust and respect from providers*. Retrieved from https://www.healthaffairs.org/do/10.1377/hblog20160811.056138/full/

Duran, D. G., & Pérez-Stable, E. J. (2019). Novel approaches to advance minority health and health disparities research. *American Journal of Public Health, 109*, S8–S10, Retrieved from https://doi.org/10.2105/AJPH.2018.304931

Fletcher, G. F., Landolfo, C., Niebauer, J., Ozemek, C., Arena R., & Lavine, C. J. (2018). Promoting physical activity and exercise: JACC health promotion series. *Journal of the American College of Cardiology, 72*(4), 1622–1639. doi: 10.1016/j.jacc.2018.08.2141.

Gielen, A. C., & Green, L. W. (2015). The impact of policy, environmental, and educational interventions: A synthesis of the evidence from two public health success stories. *Health Education & Behavior, 42*(Suppl. 1), 20s–34s.

Gilbert, G. G., Sawyer, R. G., & McNeill, E. B. (2015). *Health education: Creating strategies for school and community health* (4th ed.). Burlington, MA: Jones & Bartlett.

Glanz, K., Rimer, B. K., & Viswanath, K. (Eds.). (2015). *Health behavior: Theory, research, and practice*. San Francisco, CA: Jossey-Bass.

Green, J., Cross, R., Woodall, J., & Tones, K. (2019). *Health promotion: Planning and strategies* (4th ed.). Los Angeles, CA: Sage.

Green, L. W., & Kreuter, M. W. (2005). *Health program planning: An educational and ecological approach* (4th ed.). New York, NY: McGraw Hill.

Hales, D. (2016). *An invitation to health: Build your future* (9th ed.). Belmont, CA: Wadsworth, Cengage Learning.

Havelock, R. G., & Havelock, M. C. (1973). *Training for change agents: A guide to the design of training programs in education and other fields*. Inst for Social Research the Univ.

Heath, S. (2018). *Programs targeting social determinants of health improve wellness*. Retrieved from https://patientengagementhit.com/news/programs-targeting-social-determinants-of-health-improve-wellness

Health Resources & Service Administration (HRSA). (2019). *Health literacy*. Retrieved from https://www.hrsa.gov/about/organization/bureaus/ohe/health-literacy/index.html

Huff, R. M., Kline, M. V., & Peterson, D. V. (Eds.). (2015). *Health promotion in multicultural populations: A handbook for practitioners and students*. Thousand Oaks, CA: Sage.

Institute of Medicine. (2003). *Unequal treatment: Confronting racial and ethnic disparities in healthcare*. Washington, DC: The National Academies Press.

Iowa State University Center for Excellence in Learning and Theory. 2019. *Revised Bloom's taxonomy*. Retrieved from http://www.celt.iastate.edu/teaching/effective-teaching-practices/revised-blooms-taxonomy/

Jerome, B., & Powell, C. (2016). *The disposable visionary: A survival guide for change agents*. Santa Barbara, CA: ABC-CLIO, LLC.

Kaiser Family Foundation. (2016). *Key facts on health and health care by race and ethnicity*. Retrieved from https://www.kff.org/disparities-policy/report/key-facts-on-health-and-health-care-by-race-and-ethnicity/

Kaiser Family Foundation. (2018). *Disparities in health and health care: Five key questions and answers*. Retrieved from https://www.kff.org/disparities-policy/issue-brief/disparities-in-health-and-health-care-five-key-questions-and-answers/

Kaminski, J. (2011). Theory applied to informatics: Lewin's change theory. *Canadian Journal of Nursing Informatics, 6*(1). Retrieved from http://cjni.net/journal/?p=1210

Kitchie, S. (2019). Determinants of learning. In S. B. Bastable, P. Gramet, K. Jacobs, & D. L. Sopczyk (Eds.), *Health professional as educator: Principles of teaching and learning* (5th ed., pp. 119–168). Sudbury, MA: Jones & Bartlett Learning.

Knighton, A., Brunisholz, K., & Savitz, S. (2017). Detecting risk of low health literacy in disadvantaged populations using area-based measures. *Journal for Electronic Health Data and Methods, 5*(3), 1–10. Retrieved from https://doi.org/10.5334/egems.191

Knowles, M. (1980). *The modern practice of adult education: Andragogy versus pedagogy* (2nd ed.). Chicago, IL: Follett.

Knowles, M. (1984). *The adult learner: A neglected species* (3rd ed.). Houston, TX: Gulf.

Knowles, M. (1989). *The making of an adult educator: An autobiographical journey*. San Francisco, CA: Jossey-Bass.

Knowles, M. (1990). *The adult learner: A neglected species* (4th ed.). Houston, TX: Gulf Publishing.

Knowles, M. S., Holton, E. F., & Swanson, R. A. (2015). *The adult learner: The definitive classic in adult education and human resource development* (8th ed.). New York, NY: Routledge.

Kotter, J. P. (2012). *Leading change*. Boston, MA: Harvard Business Review Press.

Lee, J., Schram, A. Riley, E., Harris, P., Baum, F., et al. (2018). Addressing health equity through action on the social determinants of health: A global review of policy outcome evaluation methods. *International Journal of Health Policy Management, 7*(7), 581–592.

Lewin, K. (1947). Frontiers in group dynamics: Concept, method, and reality in social science; social equilibria and social change. *Human Relations, 1*(1), 5–41.

Lewin, K. (1951). *Field theory in social science: Selected theoretical papers*. New York, NY: Harper & Row.

Lippitt, G. L. (1973). *Visualizing change: Model building and the change process*. La Jolla, CA: University Associates.

Lippitt, R., Watson, J., & Westley, B. (1958). *The dynamics of planned change*. New York, NY: Harcourt.

Lipton, B. J., Decker, S. L., & Sommers, B. D. (2017). The Affordable Care Act appears to have narrowed racial and ethnic disparities in insurance coverage and access to care among young adults. *Medical Care and Research Review, 76*(1), 32–55.

Marmot, M. (2015). The health gap: The challenge of an unequal world. *Lancet, 386*(10011), 2442–2444.

Maslow, A. H. (1970). *Motivation and personality* (2nd ed.). New York, NY: Harper and Row.

McNeely, C. A., & Morland, L. (2016). The health of the newest Americans: How U.S. Public Health Systems can support Syrian refugees. *American Journal of Public Health, 106*(1), 13–15.

Medline Plus. (2019). *How to write easy-to-read health materials*. Retrieved from https://medlineplus.gov/etr.html

Mehrabbeik, A., Mahmoodabad, S., Khosravi, H. M., & Fallahzadeh, H. (2017). Breakfast consumption determinants among female high school students of Yazd Province based on Pender's Health Promotion Model. *Electronic Physician, 9*(8), 5061–5067.

Michigan State University. (2019). *Qualities of effective change agents*. Retrieved from https://www.michiganstateuniversityonline.com/resources/leadership/qualities-of-effective-change-agents/

Miller, D. M., Linn, R., & Gronlund, N. E. (2012). *Measurement and assessment in teaching* (11th ed.). Upper Saddle River, NJ: Pearson.

Miller, M. A., & Stoeckel, P. R. (2016). *Client education: theory and practice*. Burlington, MA: Jones & Bartlett.

Moffett, J., Berezowski, J., Spencer, D., & Lanning, S. (2014). An investigation into the factors that encourage learner participation in a large group medical classroom. *Advances in Medical Education and Practice, 5*, 66–71.

Murdaugh, C. L., Parsons, M. A., & Pender, N. J. (2019). *Health promotion in nursing practice* (8th ed.). Upper Saddle River, NJ: Prentice Hall.

National Network of Libraries of Medicine. (n.d.). *Health literacy*. Retrieved from https://nnlm.gov/initiatives/topics/health-literacy

Office of Disease Prevention & Health Promotion. (2020). *Browse Healthy People 2030 objectives*. Retrieved from https://health.gov/healthypeople/objectives-and-data/browse-objectives

Pavlov, I. P. (1957). *Experimental psychology and other essays*. New York, NY: Philosophical Library.

Pender, N. L., Murdaugh, C. L., & Parsons, M. A. (2015). *Health promotion in nursing practice* (7th ed.). Upper Saddle River, NJ: Prentice Hall.

Petrovic, D., de Mestral, C. Bochud, M., Bartley, M., & Kivimäki, M. (2018). The contribution of health behaviors to socioeconomic inequalities in health: A systematic review. *Preventive Medicine, 113*, 15–31.

Piaget, J. (1966). *The origin of intelligence in children*. New York, NY: Norton.

Piaget, J. (1970). *Child's conception of movement and speed*. Abingdon, UK: Routledge.

Pirzadeh, A., Mostafavi, F., Ghofarnipour, F., & Mansourian, M. (2017). The application of the Transtheoretical Model to identify physical activity behavior in women. *Iranian Journal of Nursing and Midwifery Research, 22*(4), 299–302.

Prochaska, J. O., Norcross, J. C., & DiClemente, C. C. (2007). *Changing for good: A revolutionary six-stage program for overcoming bad habits and moving your life positively forward* (reprint ed.). New York, NY: William Morrow Paperbacks.

Readability Formulas. (2020). *The SMOG readability formula, a simple measure of gobbledygook*. Retrieved from https://readabilityformulas.com/smog-readability-formula.php

Robert Wood Johnson Foundation. (2010). *A new way to talk about social determinants of health*. Retrieved from http://www.rwjf.org/en/library/research/2010/01/a-new-way-to-talk-about-the-social-determinants-of-health.html

Rogers, C. (1969). *Freedom to learn*. Columbus, OH: Merrill.

Rogers, C. (1989). *Freedom to learn for the eighties*. Columbus, OH: Merrill.

Rogers, E. M. (2003). *Diffusion of innovations* (5th ed.). New York, NY: Simon & Schuster.

Rosenstock, I. M. (1966). Why people use health services. *Milbank Memorial Fund Quarterly, 44*, 94–127.

Roussel, L. A., Harris, J. L., & Thomas, T. (2016). *Management and leadership for nurse administrators* (7th ed.). Sudbury, MA: Jones & Bartlett.

Salari, R., & Filus, A. (2017). Using the Health Belief Model to explain mothers' and fathers' intention to participate in university parenting programs. *Prevention Science, 18*(1), 83–94.

Santoro, T. N., & Santoro, J. D. (2018). Racial bias in the US opioid epidemic: A review of the history of systemic bias and implications for care. *Cureus, 10*(12), e3733. doi: 10.7759/cureus.3733.

Schunk, D. H. (2020). *Learning theories: An educational perspective*. Hoboken, NJ: Pearson.

Singh, G. K., Daus, G. P., Allender, M., Ramey, C. T., Martin, E. K., et al. (2017). Social determinants of health in the United States: Addressing major health inequality trends for the nation, 1935–2016. *International Journal of MCH and AIDS, 6*(2), 139–164.

Skinner, B. F. (1974). *About behaviorism*. New York, NY: Knopf.

Skinner, B. F. (1987). *Upon further reflection*. Englewood Cliffs, NJ: Prentice-Hall.

Skinner, C. S., Tiro, J., & Champion, V. L. (2015). The health belief model. In K. Glanz, B. K. Rimer, & K. Viswanath (Eds.), *Health behavior: Theory, research, and practice* (5th ed., pp. 75–94). San Francisco, CA: Jossey-Bass.

Spradley, B. W. (1980). Managing change creatively. *Journal of Nursing Administration, 10*(5), 32–37.

Thorndike, E. L. (1932). *The fundamentals of learning*. New York, NY: Teachers College Press.

Thorndike, E. L. (1969). *Educational psychology*. New York, NY: Arno Press.

U.S. Department of Health and Human Services (USDHHS). (2017). *Sex, race, and ethnic diversity of U.S. health occupations (2011-2015)*. Retrieved from https://bhw.hrsa.gov/sites/default/files/bhw/nchwa/diversityushealthoccupations.pdf

U.S. Department of Health and Human Services (USDHHS). (2018). *Healthy People 2020: Social determinants of health*. Retrieved from http://www.healthypeople.gov/2020/topicsobjectives2020/overview.aspx?topicid=39

U.S. Department of Health and Human Services (USDHHS). (2019). *Secretary's advisory committee on national health promotion and disease prevention objectives for 2030 report #7*. Retrieved from https://www.healthypeople.gov/sites/default/files/Report%207_Reviewing%20Assessing%20Set%20of%20HP2030%20Objectives_Formatted%20EO_508_05.21.pdf

U.S. Department of Health and Human Services (USDHHS). (2020). *Healthy People 2030 framework*. Retrieved from https://www.healthypeople.gov/2020/About-Healthy-People/Development-Healthy-People-2030/Framework

Vanderbilt University Center for Teaching. (2019). *Bloom's taxonomy*. Retrieved from https://cft.vanderbilt.edu/guides-sub-pages/blooms-taxonomy/

World Health Organization. (2018). *Social determinants of health*. Retrieved from http://www.who.int/gender-equity-rights/understanding/sdh-definition/en/

World Health Organization. (2019). *What is quality of care and why is it important?* Retrieved from https://www.who.int/maternal_child_adolescent/topics/quality-of-care/definition/en/

World Health Organization. (2020). *Social determinants of health*. Retrieved from https://www.who.int/social_determinants/sdh_definition/en/

CHAPTER 12

Planning, Implementing, and Evaluating Community/Public Health Programs

"True genius resides in the capacity for evaluation of uncertain, hazardous, and conflicting information."

—Winston Churchill (1874–1965), British Prime Minister (1940–1945; 1951–1955)

KEY TERMS

Advisory group
Authoritative knowledge
Benchmarking
Community action model
Enabling factors
Grant
Grant writing
Letter of inquiry
Predisposing factors
Quality indicators
Reinforcing factors
Request for proposal (RFP)
Social marketing
Target population

LEARNING OBJECTIVES

Upon mastery of this chapter, you should be able to:

1. List sources of information that can be used to identify group and community health problems.
2. Describe methods to gain input from target populations to define the scope of a health problem.
3. Identify change strategies that maximize cooperation of target populations.
4. Identify quality of care models that are useful in program evaluation.
5. Describe the role of social marketing and potential uses of social media in health promotion programs.
6. Locate appropriate grant funding sources for select health promotion programs.

INTRODUCTION

In the early 20th century, after suffering several personal tragedies, Mary Breckinridge committed herself to a noble cause—bringing effective health care to one of the poorest, most remote regions of the United States. A trained nurse and daughter of a politician, she used her skills and influence to establish a public health program, the Frontier Nursing Service (FNS) in rural Appalachia (Fig. 12-1). During the humble beginnings of the FNS, Breckinridge and her team of nurse–midwives rode through the hills of Leslie County, Kentucky, on horseback, providing primary care and midwifery services to the impoverished residents. Breckinridge dedicated the rest of her life to the effort, ultimately developing a network of clinics, a hospital, and a school to train midwives, as well as becoming an advocate for the region's economic development (Goan, 2015). Thanks to the FNS, the maternal mortality rate in Appalachia dropped from among the highest in the country to well below the national average. The school Breckinridge founded continues to operate today as Frontier Nursing University, which trains some of the nation's most influential nurse–midwives and nurse practitioners (see Chapter 3).

In the early 21st century, the emerging role of the community/public health nurse (C/PHN) offers opportunities to plan and implement programs that not only improve the health of individuals but of entire communities. Due to shrinking health department budgets and high demand for services, C/PHNs now provide health promotion and educational programs to larger and larger constituencies. Nurses must develop unfamiliar skills such as writing grants, creating social marketing campaigns, and collaborating with a variety of organizations to effectively address new challenges that are just as significant in our generation as those faced by the FNS. These activities and challenges might include the following:

- Writing a grant proposal to fund a naloxone distribution program for a community struggling with widespread opioid misuse and overdose deaths.
- Collaborating with local school districts to reduce the use of e-cigarettes and vaping among school children.

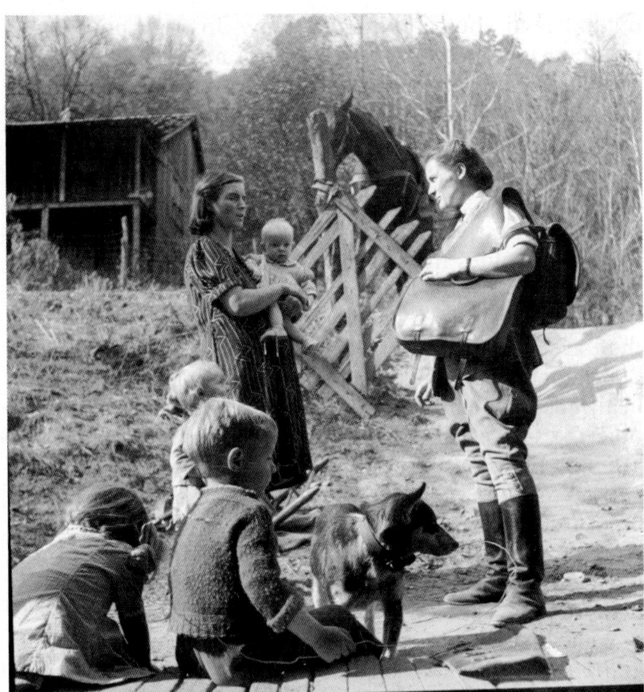

FIGURE 12-1 The Frontier Nursing Service used a public health program approach in improving the health of poor families in rural Kentucky. (Photo Courtesy of Frontier Nursing University Archives. Used with permission. Retrieved from https://frontier.edu/about-frontier/history-of-fnu/)

- As a global health specialist, assisting a nongovernmental organization in India to create a social marketing campaign aimed at discouraging violence against women and girls.

Communities are rarely in a position to fund all needed health programs, so they must carefully prioritize those that are important and feasible and then turn to a variety of agencies for financial support through grants or contracts. The C/PHN frequently assumes responsibility for locating, securing, and maintaining grant funding.

Evaluation of program outcomes is a requirement of most funding sources, whether public or private. A nurse who receives $500 to start an emergency preparedness program for low-income families may not be expected to provide the level of evaluation data that a million-dollar effort to address postdischarge care of hospitalized homeless patients would require. Nevertheless, the nurse will need to provide evidence that demonstrates the impact of the program.

The populations served may also want to know whether the programs were successful and why. For instance, a mother who enrolls her daughter in an after-school program to increase self-esteem may want to know the results of the first 6-week session before granting permission for a second session, particularly if her daughter is interested in attending a dance class that conflicts with the program session. With competing alternatives, the mother may want details about what was accomplished in the first session and what will be the future results. With this information, the mother and daughter can weigh the options. For future planning, funders, consumers, and nurses should all be aware of the demonstrated program outcomes.

You were previously introduced to theories and models that are commonly used in the community setting. In this chapter, we'll build on concepts discussed in prior chapters and describe the resources, knowledge, skills, and actions that help nurses plan and develop effective community health programs. These include the following:

- National, state, and local health objectives, initiatives, and resources that will help you identify high-priority health issues
- How to recognize community problems that lead to poor health
- How to partner with community members, organizations, and leaders to better understand the community, determine priorities for improving community health, and develop successful programs
- Factors that influence the changes in individual behavior that are necessary to improve the health of communities as a whole
- Tools and models that can organize your thinking about health program aims and development
- How to set measurable goals and objectives
- Quality assurance and improvement tools and models that will help you evaluate community health programs
- Social marketing for community health and program promotion
- How to obtain and manage grants to fund health programs

PLANNING COMMUNITY HEALTH PROGRAMS: THE BASICS

In the classic writings of Ottoson and Green (2008, p. 590), public health education programs are defined as interventions "designed to inform, elicit, facilitate, and maintain positive health practices in large numbers of people." Likewise, the American Nurses Association's *Public Health Nursing: Scope and Standards of Practice* (2013) focuses on the role of the nurse in planning, implementing, and evaluating population-focused health promotion/health education programs (Fig. 12-2).

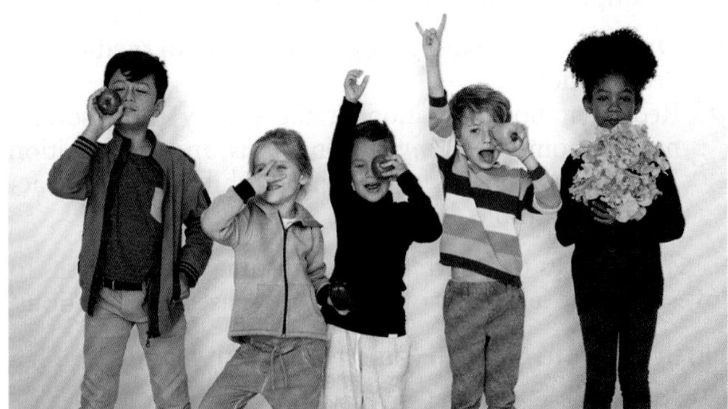

FIGURE 12-2 Contemporary public health nurses plan public health programs that improve the health of entire communities.

- Standard 5B calls on the PHN to "employ multiple strategies to promote health, and a safe environment" (p. 37), through programs and services that include appropriate teaching–learning methods, that are culturally and age appropriate, and that also include an evaluation component.
- Advanced PHNs plan "evidence-based health promotion programs and services" and engage with consumers and advocacy groups in promoting health and modifying programs (p. 38).

With so much emphasis on planning and developing health education/health promotion programs, the process can seem overwhelming to the new C/PHN or even to the acute care nurse who is involved in some aspect of health initiative development. The first part of this chapter is designed to take some of the mystery out of the process. You will be guided through the complex problem of teen vaping, which poses significant health risks for school children and young adults. The principles applicable to this example can be used in other situations and programs, even those that are very broad in scope and involve many practice partners.

In your nursing program, you may have been tasked with developing a health program, working on an existing community program, or simulating the process in a written assignment. Whatever your experience level, the essential elements are the same. As you begin this next section, think about your past experiences, such as taking blood pressures at a local health fair or developing a pamphlet on the need for prostate screening for non–English-speaking residents. Did these actions have the impact you hoped for? Successful health promotion programs do not occur by accident; they take skill, time, patience, and most of all listening to and understanding the needs and opinions of the individuals who are the focus of your program (the **target population**).

IDENTIFYING GROUP OR COMMUNITY HEALTH PROBLEMS

Student nurses are educated in the care of individuals, families, *and* communities, yet nurses most often practice at the individual and family levels. When is it appropriate for a nurse to expand his or her practice to the community level? Perhaps the most natural time is when a nurse identifies an ongoing issue that does not change with traditional interventions.

Examples include the following:

- Overuse of the emergency room for pain medication prescriptions
- Recurrent hospitalization of the elderly from several nursing homes for dehydration, sepsis, and malnutrition
- Hospitalization of unvaccinated children with vaccine-preventable diseases

These types of recurrent problems might lead nurses to investigate the feasibility of community-based interventions.

National and State Health Objectives and Initiatives

Individually or in a group, identify a possible issue to explore—one you believe is leading to poor health outcomes in your community. How do you know if this problem is widespread or if others also find it to be a problem? Several methods can be used to validate the importance of the issue. One method would be to consider *Healthy People 2030* objectives for the nation (Office of Disease Prevention and Health Promotion [ODPHP], 2019).

What are the major areas of concern for improving health outcomes in the United States? What are the priorities of the state in which you live? Take some time to review federal agency Web sites to identify programs that are being developed to meet the *Healthy People 2030* goals and objectives (Box 12-1). Your state or local health department may also publish *Healthy People 2030* objectives on its Web site, highlighting those issues that are high priorities in your region. You can monitor progress on meeting the *Healthy People 2020* objective targets by searching for current results for national- and state-level data on the *Healthy People 2020* widget (https://www.healthypeople.gov/2020/data-search/Search-the-Data#hdisp=1).

The overarching national goals of *Healthy People 2030* are found in Box 1-4 in Chapter 1.

Local Health Priorities and Initiatives

Community agencies and organizations frequently network to establish community-wide goals, with the local health department spearheading the effort. It may also be organized by community-based health agencies and volunteer organizations. Improved outcomes for individuals who have diabetes or asthma is an example of a goal a local community might want to set. Another topic of concern may be adolescent suicide. Nurses can work collaboratively with these special interest groups to find solutions for affected individuals and families.

As a specific problem is identified, it is crucial to analyze the scope of the problem within the community. It is a poor use of resources to set up a program if the condition or situation is rare. For example, it would be a waste of resources to establish a program on diabetes and pregnancy for a local homeless shelter that only serves 35 women a year. Of those 35 women, none may be pregnant, and only 5.6% of pregnant women develop gestational diabetes (Deputy, Kim, Conrey, & Bullard, 2018), so it may be several years before an eligible client is found. A better use of resources would be to target a community with a high proportion of individuals at risk for diabetes during pregnancy, such as a community with a large population of non-Hispanic Asian mothers, among whom the prevalence of gestational diabetes is higher (11.1%) than other racial/ethnic groups. Another target group may be pregnant women age 40 years or older, who are also at increased risk of gestational diabetes (Deputy et al., 2018).

Using Data to Confirm Needs

There are many ways a nurse can determine whether a problem affects enough of the population to warrant intervention. The best way to start is to review the local, state, and national data available through government repositories. This can be done by going to a university library for assistance, asking for specific data from local

BOX **12-1** *HEALTHY PEOPLE 2030*

Recommended Leading Health Indicators and Objectives

Life Expectancy	■ Increase life expectancy (at birth)
Child Health	MICH-02 Reduce the rate of all infant deaths IVP-D03 Reduce the number of young adults who report three or more adverse childhood experiences
Self-Rated Health	■ Increase the mean healthy days (CDC-HRQOL-14 Healthy Days)
Well-Being	■ Increase proportion thriving on Cantril's Self-Anchored Striving scales
Disability	■ Reduce the percentage of adults ages 65 years and over with limitations in daily activities
Mental Disability	■ Reduce the rate of mental disability
Substance Use	SU-03 Reduce drug overdose deaths
Unintentional Injury Deaths	IVP-03 Reduce unintentional injury deaths
All Cancer Deaths	C-01 Reduce the overall cancer death rate
Suicide	MHMD-01 Reduce the suicide rate
Firearm-Related Mortality	IVP-12 Reduce firearm-related deaths
Mental Health	■ Reduce percentage of adults who reported their mental health was not good in 14 or more days in the past 30 days (i.e., frequent mental distress)
Oral Health Access	OH-08 Increase use of the oral health care system
Reproductive Health Care Services	FP-11 Increase the proportion of adolescent females at risk for unintended pregnancy who use effective birth control
HIV Incidence	HIV-03 Reduce the number of new HIV diagnoses
Tobacco	TU-04 Reduce current tobacco use in adolescents
Obesity	NWS-04 Reduce the proportion of children and adolescents with obesity
Alcohol Use	SU-13 Reduce the proportion of people with alcohol use disorder in the past year
Immunization	■ Increase the proportion of children 19- to 35-month-old children up to date on DTaP, MMR, polio, Hib, HepB, varicella, and pneumococcal conjugate vaccines
Hypertension Rate	HDS-04 Reduce the proportion of adults with high blood pressure
Ambulatory Sensitive Conditions/ Avoidable Hospitalization	■ Reduce discharges for ambulatory care-sensitive conditions per 1,000 Medicare enrollees (CMS-2[a])
Medical Insurance Coverage	AHS-01 Increase the proportion of persons with medical insurance
Affordable Housing	SDOH-04 Reduce the proportion of families that spend more than 30% of income on housing
Environment	■ Improve the Environmental Quality Index ■ Lower the Heat Vulnerability Index
Education	AH-04 Increase the proportion of 4th graders with reading skills at or above the proficient level
Poverty	SDOH-03 Reduce the proportion of people living in poverty
Food Security	NWS-01 Reduce household food insecurity and hunger
Civic Engagement	■ Increase the proportion of voting eligible population who vote
Social Environment	■ Lower the Neighborhood Disinvestment Index ■ Reduce the level of residential segregation captured by the Index of Dissimilarity ■ Reduce the level of residential segregation captured by the Isolation Index

[a]CMS-2 is a chronic conditions composite measure developed by the Centers for Medicare & Medicaid Services.

Reprinted with permission from National Academies of Sciences, Engineering, and Medicine. (2020). *Leading health indicators 2030: Advancing health, equity, and well-being.* Washington, DC: The National Academies Press. Retrieved from https://www.nap.edu/catalog/25682/leading-health-indicators-2030-advancing-health-equity-and-well-being health and social service agencies, police and judicial departments, and local school districts, or by searching the Internet. The National Center for Health Statistics (NCHS) offers public-use data files through the file server of the Centers for Disease Control and Prevention (CDC). The NCHS data collection systems include (CDC, 2019a) the following:

- Population surveys, such as the National Health and Nutrition Examination Survey and National Survey of Family Growth
- Vital records, such as the National Death Index
- Provider surveys, such as the National Hospital Care Survey and other national health care surveys
- Historical surveys, which provide an overview of surveys and programs administered by the NCHS that have been completed

The U.S. Department of Health and Human Services (USDHHS) makes high-value health data accessible to the public via HealthData.gov. The data are collected from agencies within the USDHHS as well as its state partners and include U.S. data on (USDHHS, 2019b):

- Environmental health
- Medical devices
- Social services
- Community health
- Mental health
- Substance abuse
- Medicare and Medicaid

Hospital discharge data are also reported to state agencies, and this information is sometimes available at the local level (Lane et al., 2017). For more information on data collection systems, see thePoint®.

Target Groups and Neighborhoods

As nurses and community groups narrow their focus, they can identify target groups and neighborhoods by using geographic information system (GIS) technology. Many organizations use GIS to identify target groups by race, age, and family status. GIS data can be found through a variety of federal sources (see Chapter 10), including the CDC, the National Cancer Institute, the Center for Mental Health Services, the National Library of Medicine, the Environmental Protection Agency, and, as previously mentioned, the NCHS, which maintains GIS maps on the major causes of mortality in the United States (USDHHS, 2019a). GIS mapping can depict deaths by regions or in clusters, such as one depicting drug overdose mortality that can be found at https://www.cdc.gov/pcd/issues/2019/18_0405.htm.

Earthquake seismic hazard maps may be helpful in disaster planning. National and state maps are available (https://earthquake.usgs.gov/hazards/hazmaps/), and Figure 12-3 displays a map highlighting major populations exposed to potentially damaging earthquakes.

Collaborating With Other Health Care Professionals

Talking about the problems you have identified in your community with other nurses and health care professionals may help you identify resources and solutions as you brainstorm ideas about the problem and what should be done to alleviate it. Find out what has been tried in the past and why those interventions may have failed. A very helpful source of information is the Community Preventive Services Task Force (CPSTF) Web site, thecommunityguide.org

The CPSTF developed a federally sponsored resource, the *Guide to Community Preventive Services: What Works to Promote Health*—now known as *The Community Guide.* Originally published in 2005, *The Community Guide* is an online collection of evidence-based findings and other resources that C/PHNs can use to select and implement interventions to improve health and prevent disease within communities or at state and national levels (CPSTF, 2019).

The interventions with limited evidence may be very effective but need to be confirmed by further research; perhaps your idea is among those listed. For example, as a means of increasing community demand for vaccinations, client reminder and recall systems are recommended, yet there is not enough evidence to support client or family incentives, or the use of patient-held medical records. If a C/PHN develops a program to implement these interventions, the additional step of publishing the program results would add to the body of evidence that determines the value of such a program.

Engaging the Target Population

The next step is the most important of all, as it will determine whether your interventions succeed or fail. A nurse may think, "I know what the problem is—now I will think up an intervention to alleviate it!" This is a well-intentioned, but doomed, approach. At this point, only part of the assessment is complete; the most important component of the assessment is to find out the views of the target population about the identified problem. What do they think are the causes? What ideas do they have about solving it? Which approaches do they think will work?

It is crucial to hear and respect the views of the target population (Fig. 12-4). Anthropologists talk about a concept called **authoritative knowledge**. This is based not on whose knowledge may be right but rather on what is accepted as substantial and legitimate because it comes from authoritative sources, such as health care providers (Anderson, Mah, & Sellen, 2015; Henley, 2015). Nurses may think they know more about a topic (e.g., diabetes) than their target population and therefore conclude that their solutions must also be superior. Members of the target population may hold just as strongly to their own beliefs. If nurses don't learn about the target population's beliefs and only consider their own, they will not be able to work out an acceptable and appropriate solution. Interventions that fail to engage the target population will likely be unsuccessful. It is imperative that positive working relationships be established with high-risk target communities and that chosen interventions involve effective use of health resources (see the story of the shoemaker and shoe customer in Chapter 10).

Understanding the Target Population

When working with target groups, it's important to get as much information about the population as possible.

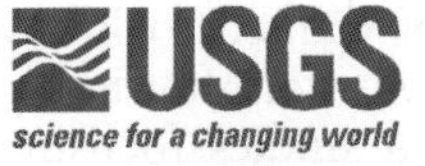

FIGURE 12-3 Population exposed to potentially damaging earthquake ground shaking. (Reprinted from U.S. Geological Survey. (October 11, 2016). *Population exposed to potentially damaging earthquake ground shaking*. Retrieved from https://www.usgs.gov/media/images/population-exposed-potentially-damaging-earthquake-groundshaking)

Start by asking those you know, as colleagues and as patients/clients, about their local community (Gordon, 2018). What are their thoughts about the problem of interest? What do they think about the quality of services currently available? What do they see as barriers to services? What about barriers to adherence to treatment and other health care recommendations? In Chapter 15, you will learn that nurse interaction with the community is an essential first consideration in promoting community health.

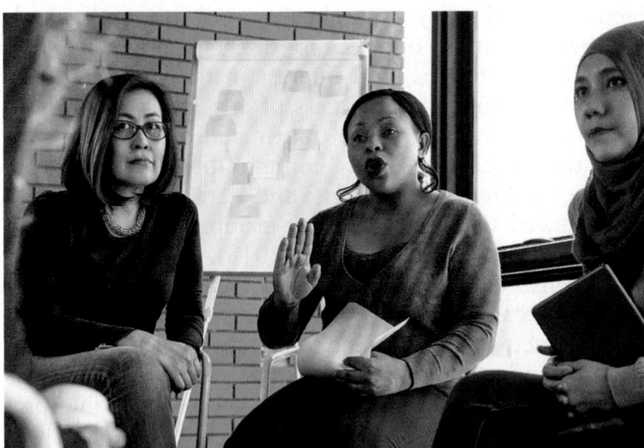

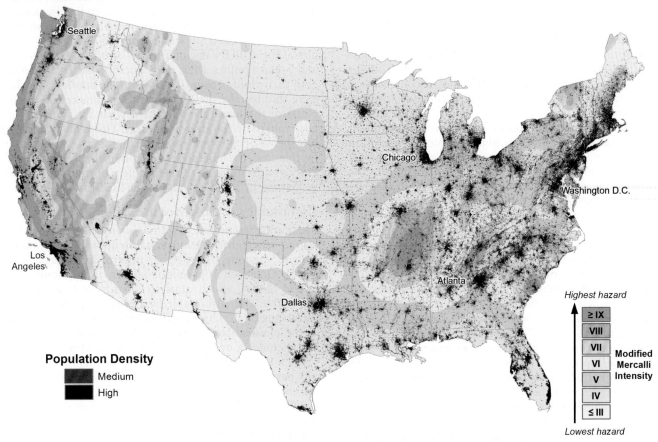

FIGURE 12-4 It is crucial to hear and respect the views of the target population.

Additional issues to explore include the following:

- Who else can provide insights about this problem?
- Who are key people with whom you should build relationships?
- What are their customs regarding health care?
- Who are the leaders within families?
- What is the best way to form collaborations and linkages within this community?
- Who are their *formal* and *informal leaders*?
- What types of events bring them together?
- What are the roles of family, church, and health care providers within their community?
- Should you approach church groups, school groups, or other organizations?
- What radio stations do they listen to, and what television stations are they most likely to watch?

Which Web sites do they visit when seeking health information? The answers to these questions will provide insight into factors influencing the health problem and will also help you understand how to reach out to the target population (Community Tool Box, 2019a). Mobilizing Action through Planning and Partnerships (MAPP) is one of many tools that begin with this community mobilization step; it can be found at the Community Tool Box Web site: https://ctb.ku.edu/en/table-of-contents/overview/models-for-community-health-and-development/mapp/main.

As you gain insight into relevant environmental and social factors, you are also building interest among the community members about the issue. As you participate in discussions with others, be open to their input. Your original ideas will likely change in response to feedback from members of the target and service communities. For example, an experienced C/PHN was involved in a project developed to serve Hispanic women with gestational diabetes. When interviewed, the Spanish-speaking women expressed concern that they were told to go on a diabetic "diet" and were then chastised for not eating enough. To these women, going on a "diet" meant they should eat less. They were also told that if they followed the diabetic diet, they wouldn't have such "big babies." They thought a "big" baby was a healthy baby and couldn't understand why they were being told to avoid having a larger baby. These were simple issues to fix but required knowledge of how the "diabetic teaching plan" was interpreted by the target audience. Another key factor was that the clinic was a family event; thus, all of the children were brought along. The clinic staff had been irritated by the presence of large groups of children but learned they should alter the clinic setup and resources to accommodate their clients' expectations. Modifications were made based on dialogue with members of the target population that contributed to the eventual success of the clinic's program.

This example demonstrates how use of *local knowledge* can increase the effectiveness of a community-based intervention. Working with community partners is a technique that has been used in providing services within developing countries. This type of approach ensures community *buy-in* for an intervention. It also builds networks that increase the capacity of communities to resolve other health care issues, both current and emerging (Bolton, Moore, Ferreira, Day, & Bolton, 2016; Piltch-Loeb, Abramson, & Merdjanoff, 2017; Worthman, Tomlinson, & Rotheram-Borus, 2016).

Using Evidence to Guide Interventions

The search for evidence-based guidelines and interventions is important to program success. It is essential to review literature regarding health problems, factors influencing the outcomes of interventions, and the role of families and communities in adhering to interventions. The literature review can offer insights that may shape interviews with community members (Leadbeater, Gladstone, & Sukhawathanakul, 2015). How does the target group compare to other target groups? Are there issues that should be addressed that are not found in the literature?

Consider this situation: A C/PHN wanted to know why parents were using emergency rooms for after-hours urgent care. A literature review found studies focusing heavily on the "misuse" of emergency rooms by parents to treat urgent ambulatory care health problems, such as otitis media. Based on input from an emergency room nurse, the C/PHN decided to go directly to the source and asked families what their doctors had told them to do if their child became ill at night. The families said they were told to take their children to the emergency room! None of the literature addressed what the families had been told to do for after-hours care. This is an example of how being open to information from a variety of sources (in this case, the emergency room nurse) enhanced the C/PHN's understanding of the problem beyond what could be learned by solely relying on the literature.

Community Action Model

Facilitating community action is most effective when using participatory action research approaches (Cusack, Cohen, Mignone, Chartier, & Lutfiyya, 2018; deChesnay, 2015). One such approach is known as the **Community Action Model**, which aims to identify actions that are achievable and sustainable and propels changes for the well-being of all. This model builds on concepts presented in the planned-change process described in Chapter 11 and includes a cyclical five-step process (Fig. 12-5). The C/PHN educator can use this model to facilitate community participation and ownership of change that improves the community's health.

An example of a successful application of the Community Action Model is Pennsylvania's School Nutrition Policy Initiative, targeted to combat obesity in 4th to 6th graders. About 48 hours of interactive nutrition lessons are presented in classrooms yearly, with participation from families and local community partners. Incentives are offered to students who choose healthier snacks. Program evaluation revealed a 50% reduction in the number of students who were overweight (The Food Trust, 2012). Other successful programs incorporate farm-fresh foods into school lunches and snacks or aim to reduce consumption of soda (Duggan, 2017).

Advisory Groups

As nurses work with community members to identify factors contributing to a health problem, individuals will begin to stand out because of their knowledge, networking capabilities, and interest in the subject. A key factor for ensuring the success of any intervention is to appoint an **advisory group** that includes representatives from the target and service communities. Findings from interviews, literature reviews, and data analyses should be reviewed with this advisory group (Sharma, Huang, Knox, Willard-Grace, & Potter, 2018).

To ensure success of the advisory group, all meetings should be carefully planned, so that they are well organized, punctual, and efficient. Strategies to encourage input from the advisory group should be employed; meetings should focus on getting the advisory group to interpret findings and community feedback and to develop possible solutions. Contributions from each member should be sought and valued equally (Chapter 10). Depending

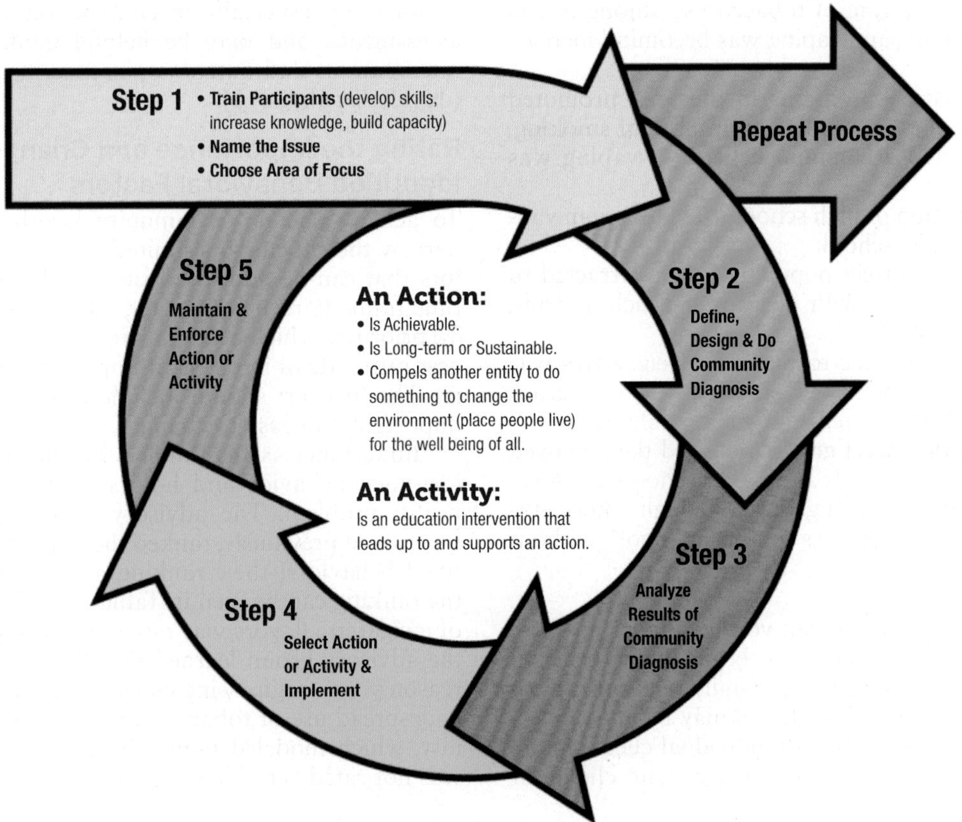

FIGURE 12-5 Community action model: Creating change by building community capacity. (Reprinted with permission from San Francisco Department of Public Health, Tobacco Free Project, and Bright Research Group. (September 2016). *Community action in public health policy*. Retrieved from https://sanfranciscotobaccofreeproject.org/wp-content/uploads/CAM-Case-Study-Final-9.12.16-to-TFP.pdf)

on the size of the group, it may be most effective to hold breakout sessions as well as larger group sessions. Every member should do an evaluation at the conclusion of each meeting, so that any problems can be addressed before the next meeting. Maintaining a record of these meetings—in the form of minutes or a brief written overview—is also very helpful. Be certain to also keep a record of attendees. Maintaining a *paper trail* is always important.

Delineating the Problem(s)

With the help of the advisory group, it's important to define the problem or problems to be addressed. The process of determining the real or perceived needs of a defined community is called community assessment. There are a variety of assessment tools and methods that help nurses delineate community health problems by collecting, analyzing, and interpreting information—these are discussed in detail in Chapter 15. The following is a case example.

A group of school nurses identified teenage use of e-cigarettes ("vaping" or "JUULing") as a problem (Fig. 12-6). Input from community members, as well as a review of data, demonstrated a high rate of teen vaping in a local high school. Although the original plan made by the school nurses was to establish a special educational presentation for all high school students, input from members of the service and target community indicated significant problems with this approach:

1. Many of the high school students began using e-cigarettes in middle school.
2. There was a widespread belief in the community that vaping was a safer alternative to tobacco use.
3. The e-cigarette users were predominantly male, and the nurses did not understand the association between gender and vaping within the targeted community.

The use of an advisory group helped the nurses first identify what behavioral factors contributed to vaping in the target population. These behavioral factors included the following:

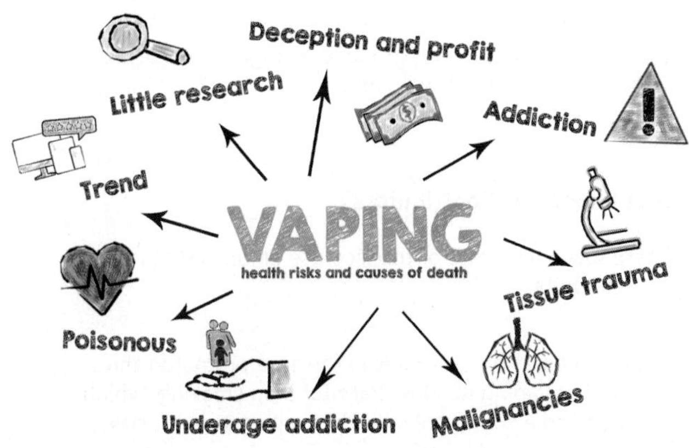

FIGURE 12-6 There are risks associated with e-cigarette use.

- There was a high rate of tobacco use among adults in the community, and vaping was becoming increasingly popular.
- Smoking cessation programs in the area promoted the idea that vaping was less harmful than smoking, which supported a common belief that vaping was not risky.
- A high proportion of high school students began vaping during middle school.
- Teenagers in the target population were attracted to the flavors available with e-cigarettes, such as fruit, mint, and chocolate.
- Although the legal age to purchase e-cigarettes was 18, local vendors were lax in enforcing the restrictions and vaping products were easily accessible online.
- Teenagers in the target group indicated they enjoyed vaping with their friends as an after-school activity.
- Many males in the target group were high school athletes who used e-cigarettes to appear "cool" without the risks of smoking.

What nursing diagnoses can you identify from these behavioral factors? Would you begin with deficient knowledge or risk for injury? Are family relationships or self-concept involved? Although you may be most familiar using nursing diagnoses with individual clients, nursing diagnoses can be advanced for aggregate clients or populations, especially in conjunction with community assessments, and may be helpful guides in proposing interventions and outcomes, as described in Chapter 15 (da Silva et al., 2018).

Rating the Importance and Changeability of Identified Behavioral Factors

To achieve success, community health programs must narrow their focus to a limited number of health behaviors that can be addressed successfully within a specific time frame (Green & Kreuter, 2005; Green et al., 2014). To prioritize which behaviors to address, the authors suggest rating them in terms of importance and changeability. The final list should include problems that are both important and easy to change.

Importance is determined by the frequency of the identified behavior and how strongly it is linked to a health problem. The advisory group for teen vaping, mentioned previously, ranked the importance of the identified behaviors; their ranking and rationale (basis) for the ranking can be seen in Table 12-1. The attractiveness of e-cigarette flavors was rated highly important because the advisory group learned that flavors are the primary reason youth begin using e-cigarettes (CDC, 2019b). The widespread use of tobacco among adults in the community, which modeled unhealthy practices for the youth, was not rated very highly by the advisory group because

TABLE 12-1 Importance Ratings of Behaviors Contributing to Teen Vaping at a Local High School

Behavior/Data	Basis for Rating
More Important Contributors	
A high proportion of high school students began vaping during middle school.	Long-established habits are more difficult to change than those which have been more recently adopted (Green & Kreuter, 2005).
Teenagers in the target population were attracted to the flavors available with e-cigarettes, such as fruit, mint, and chocolate.	Adolescents usually begin vaping with flavored e-cigarettes. Many teens are curious about the products, and flavors are the most common reason they begin using them (CDC, 2019b).
Although the legal age to purchase e-cigarettes was 18, local vendors were lax in enforcing the restrictions and vaping products were easily accessible online.	Unrestricted access to e-cigarettes supports widespread use and research showing early vaping is related to a greater chance of switching to cigarettes (Fairchild, Bayer, & Lee, 2019).
Teenagers in the target group indicated that they enjoyed vaping with their friends as an after-school activity.	Peer smoking behaviors are very influential and are more strongly associated with e-cigarette use during teenage years than smoking by adult family members (Wang, Cap, & Hu, 2019).
Many males in the target group were high school athletes that used e-cigarettes to appear "cool" without the risks of smoking.	The perceived high status of the athletes may increase the influence of their conduct among fellow athletes as well as other students. There are significant risks associated with vaping, especially among children, teens, and young adults (CDC, 2019b).
Less Important Contributors	
There was a high rate of tobacco use among adults in the community.	Adult smoking is associated with uptake of smoking by young family members; nevertheless, sibling and peer smoking behavior more strongly influences teen vaping (Wang et al., 2019).
Smoking cessation programs in the area promoted the idea that vaping was less harmful than smoking, which supported a common belief that vaping was not risky.	Recognition of the risks of e-cigarettes may be undermined by the perceived support for vaping in the smoking cessation program (Fairchild et al., 2019). However, most of the teens in the community were not directly involved in the program.

the members felt the influence of peers was a more important factor.

The advisory group was then asked to rate the changeability of the behaviors. In their classic book, Green and Kreuter (2005) indicate that behaviors that are easiest to change:

- Are usually still developing
- Are more recently adopted
- Do not have deep roots in culture or lifestyle
- Have been attempted before with some success

In this round of assessments, the advisory group believed that the smoking cessation programs' promotion of inaccurate information about vaping could potentially be changed. This rating was based on the fact that the smoking cessation program leaders were well-intentioned, but misinformed, and could easily change the program content. The program leaders could, in fact, become valuable allies in disseminating accurate information about the risks of vaping. The advisory group also determined that it may be more effective to target middle school rather than, or in addition to, high school students, because they had not yet begun using e-cigarettes or had vaping habits that were not yet deeply ingrained (Fig. 12-7).

After rating the identified problems based on changeability and importance, the nurses and advisory group sought to narrow their focus to specific goals. Ranking the behaviors in a simple table, as seen in Table 12-2, is suggested (Community Tool Box, 2019b; Green & Kreuter, 2005; Green et al., 2014). This effort yielded a table with the problems categorized in four groups: more important/more changeable, less important/more changeable, more important/less changeable, and less important/less changeable (Table 12-2). One issue seen as most important and changeable was the use of e-cigarettes among male athletes, who represented the subpopulation most likely to vape (high school males) and who were influential among other male teens. This had support from coaches, so there was greater motivation to abandon unhealthy behaviors.

The use of this grid enabled the advisory group to focus on more changeable and important issues. They wrote behavioral objectives for each identified factor they hoped to change. These objectives identified *who* was targeted, *what* they hoped would change or what action would be taken, *how* the change would be measured, and what the *time frame* was for achieving the expected outcome. The following are their behavioral objectives:

1. By the end of the fall semester, all local smoking cessation programs will discontinue the promotion of vaping as a safer alternative to tobacco.
2. By the end of the fall semester, 90% of all high school athletes will sign a "no-vaping" contract as a condition of participation in high school sports.
3. By the end of the school year, 90% of 6th through 12th grade students will attend a presentation aimed at preventing or discontinuing participation in vaping.

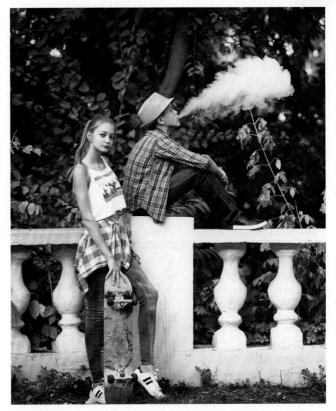

FIGURE 12-7 Vaping is increasingly popular among school-age children and is associated with significant health risks.

TABLE 12-2 Changeability Ratings of Behaviors Contributing to Teen Vaping at a Local High School

Changeability of Behavior	More Important Behaviors	Less Important Behaviors
More changeable	A high proportion of teenagers began vaping during middle school.	Smoking cessation programs promoted the idea that vaping was less harmful than smoking.
	Teenagers in the target group enjoyed vaping with friends.	—
	Male high school athletes used e-cigarettes to appear "cool" without the risks of smoking.	—
Less changeable	Teenagers in the target population liked the flavors available with e-cigarettes.	High rate of tobacco and e-cigarette use among adults in the community.
	Local vendors were lax in enforcing the restrictions and vaping products were easily accessible online.	—

Factors That Influence Behavior Change: Predisposing, Reinforcing, and Enabling Factors

Three categories of factors affecting individual behavior can contribute or create barriers to successful behavioral change (Green & Kreuter, 2005; Green et al., 2014). Per the PRECEDE–PROCEED model, discussed in Chapter 11, these factors are as follows (Fig. 12-8):

- **Predisposing factors** provide the rationale or *motivation* for subsequent behavior.
- **Reinforcing factors** provide a continued motivation to repeat or persist in the behavior.
- **Enabling factors** promote or facilitate the behavior based upon availability.

The advisory group followed the PRECEDE–PROCEED model and identified the predisposing, enabling, and reinforcing factors that affected each behavioral objective. For the behavioral objective:

- By the end of the fall semester, 90% of high school athletes will sign a "no-vaping" contract as a condition of participation in sports.
- A *predisposing factor* seemed to be the athletes' belief that vaping would help them look "cool" among their peers.
- *Reinforcing factors* included the common use of tobacco and e-cigarettes among adults in the community, as well as the belief that e-cigarettes were a relatively safe alternative to tobacco.
- An *enabling factor* that promoted the change was the support of high school athletics coaches who agreed to monitor the conduct of the athletes while at school and enforce the no-vaping contract.
- On the other hand, the apathy of local vendors in enforcing restrictions on the sale of vaping products to children under the age of 18 was seen as inhibiting change.

In addition to the vaping education presentations, the advisory group decided to establish a peer-mentoring program, in which student leaders would work with the advisory group and provide mentoring and support to students who wanted to quit vaping (Fig. 12-9). The advisory group had teachers nominate students for this intervention. The principal allowed the nominated students to attend educational classes conducted by the nurses to increase their knowledge about vaping cessation. The nurses worked collaboratively with the students to ensure that their mentoring and support approaches were effective. Student peer mentors suggested rewards that the students could work for that would encourage them to persist. One of the rewards that students felt should be offered is sports equipment for student use during recess and lunch periods. One local community-based organization offered to sponsor a fund-raising event that would allow them to purchase sports equipment for the school.

Working with the advisory group, the nurses developed a program that outlined activities for each objective, as well as the individual responsible for the activity, the date by which the activities were to be accomplished,

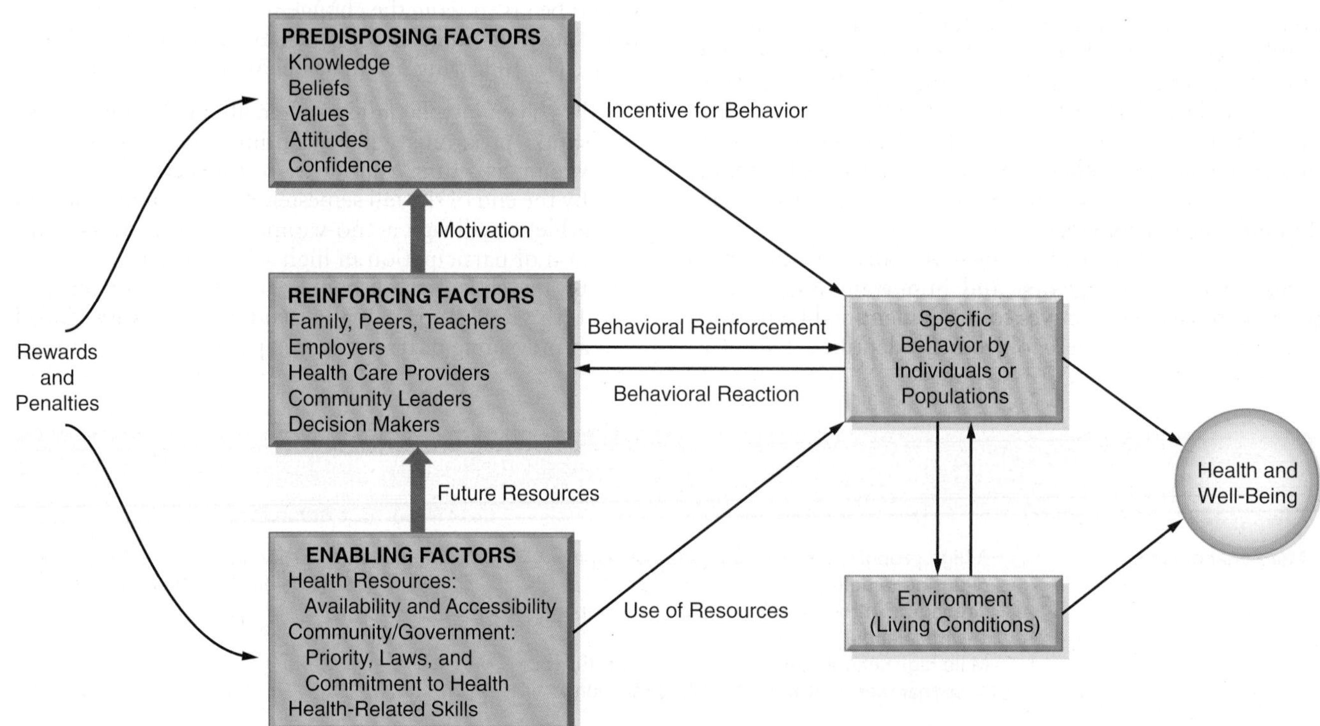

FIGURE 12-8 Predisposing, enabling, and reinforcing factors that categorize various behavioral influences. (Source: Hood, S., Linnan, L., Jolly, D., Muqueeth, S., Hall, M. B., Dixon, C., & Robinson, S. (2015). Using the PRECEDE planning approach to develop a physical activity intervention for African American men who visit barbershops: Results from the FITShop study. *American Journal of Men's Health, 9*(4), 262–273. doi: 10.1177/1557988314539501.)

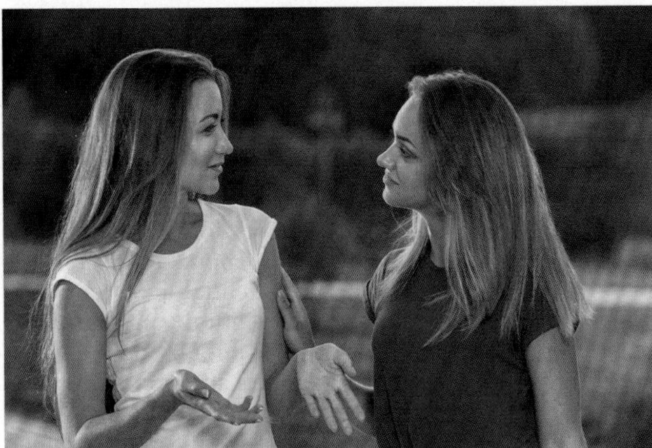

FIGURE 12-9 Peer mentoring can aid individuals in changing unhealthy behaviors.

and how outcomes would be documented. This allowed the group to stay focused, share responsibilities, and monitor outcomes. For instance, student mentors were asked to meet with their assigned students to evaluate their progress and provide support at least once a week. The nurses were tasked with meeting each week with the student leaders to provide peer-mentoring training.

Working with the advisory group allowed the nurses to contextualize the problem of teen vaping within the target community. The advisory group ensured that the nurses identified solutions that were culturally acceptable, appropriate, and ultimately effective. This process also helped them develop outcome measures that were consistent with the concerns of the community. As data were gathered, findings could be interpreted with input from the advisory group. This approach grounded the findings and ensured that interpretations were culturally consistent with the target population. Evaluation was facilitated by clearly defined goals that could be measured against actual results.

EVALUATING OUTCOMES

The previous section of this chapter discussed the issues of program planning, implementation, and evaluation as they related to a small health program. This section focuses on programs and services provided by agencies. Although the scope of the effort to address outcome evaluation is understandably broader, the concepts are essentially the same (Kidder & Chapel, 2018). According to the CDC (2017, para. 1), "Effective program evaluation is a systematic way to improve and account for public health actions by involving procedures that are useful, feasible, ethical, and accurate." The CDC proposes a framework and standards for program evaluation in public health, which includes six steps, usually taken in order (Fig. 12-10). There are several approaches and tools for evaluating health care agencies, programs, and outcomes, a few of which will be discussed in this section.

Accreditation

The Institute of Medicine (IOM) report, *The Future of the Public's Health in the 21st Century* (IOM, 2002), called for examining the benefits that accreditation of governmental public health departments might bring. The benefits of and requirements for accreditation are discussed in Chapter 6 (IOM, 2004).

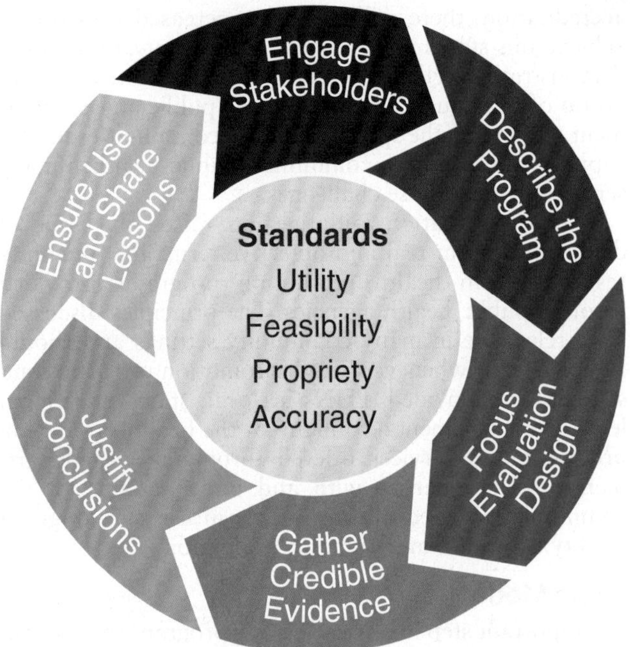

FIGURE 12-10 The framework of the Centers for Disease Control and Prevention for program evaluation in public health. (Reprinted from Centers for Disease Control and Prevention. (1999). Framework for program evaluation in public health. *Morbidity and Mortality Weekly Report, 48*(RR-11), 4. Retrieved from https://www.cdc.gov/eval/framework/index.htm)

The Public Health Accreditation Board (PHAB) is a nonprofit entity that is the independent accrediting body. With support from the CDC, Office for State, Tribal, Local, and Territorial Support (2018), and the Robert Wood Johnson Foundation, the PHAB was launched in 2011. By August of 2019, PHAB accredited or re-accredited a total of 275 U.S. health departments, which included 36 state, 3 tribal, and 236 local health departments. Eighty percent of the U.S. population is now served by a PHAB-accredited health department (PHAB, 2019). The National Association of County and City Health Officials (2020) and PHAB offer resources that assist health departments to assess the feasibility of becoming accredited and tools to further support a successful accreditation process if departments choose to seek accreditation. Of the 12 domains in Standards and Measures version 1.5 for accreditation, 3 are particularly applicable to program development and outcome measurement (PHAB, 2014, p. 3):

- Domain 4: Engage with the community to identify and address health problems.
- Domain 9: Evaluate and continually improve health department processes, programs, and interventions.
- Domain 10: Contribute to and apply the evidence base of public health.

A review of the impact of the accreditation process suggests that one of the leading benefits is strengthening health departments' quality improvement efforts (Kronstadt, Bender, & Beitsch, 2018). As more agencies seek accreditation, there will likely be increased pressure to achieve this status at all levels (local, county, or state) to demonstrate excellence. Accreditation promotes the provision of high-quality services to the public and commitment to meeting the specific needs of communities. It also supports the need for community/public health nursing services to meet those challenges.

The accreditation initiative has raised the issue of demonstrating in real and objective terms the outcomes resulting from health promotion programs provided through public health agencies. The principles discussed have relevance in many community settings and should be considered whenever health promotion programs and services are provided. PHNs at local, state, and global levels are instrumental to many of the health promotion programs and services offered through health departments; their expertise with and understanding of the communities served are invaluable in assuring ongoing quality assurance and outcome evaluation.

Logic Models

An important step in evaluating any program entails constructing a clear model of what the program is meant to achieve (Cornell University, 2016). Logic models, or pathway logic models, are often used to articulate the causal relationship between planned program activities and the expected outcome. While community problems may be easy to recognize, it is harder to determine which strategies offer the highest likelihood for successful change and, more importantly, what evidence will indicate progress or success. It is important to develop a framework for change and use it as a road map in planning and implementing individual and community change (Community Tool Box, 2019c). Based on change theory, logic models offer a clear picture of the desired outcome, the changes that must be realized in order to achieve the outcome, the activities and outputs that will affect the change, and the inputs necessary to carry out the planned activities. In other words, logic models provide a process for planning backward in order to implement forward (Ball et al., 2017).

In developing a causal framework or pathway, you are able to map out what will be done to produce a desired effect. It demonstrates how inputs (e.g., community resources), outputs (e.g., potential interventions), impact (e.g., initial results of intervention), and outcomes (e.g., improvement in behaviors or population statistics) are interrelated. A visual roadmap can be examined by starting with intended outcomes and "walking back" through the steps that are needed to produce the intended result. A logic model is a type of flow chart and usually takes up one page or less. The left side deals with process and the right side with outcomes. To be effective, a logic model should (Community Tool Box, 2019c):

- Logically link activities and effects
- Demonstrate appropriate level of detail about the program (enough to clearly understand but not too much to overwhelm)
- Be thought-provoking and visually engaging
- Include the known forces needed to promote program outcomes

See Figures 12-11 and 12-12 for more on developing program logic models and evaluating program outcomes.

Setting Measurable Goals and Objectives

Using the logic model as a guide, planned programs should have specific goals to help identify who the program is supposed to serve, what services are provided, the length of time the services are to be provided, and the resources that

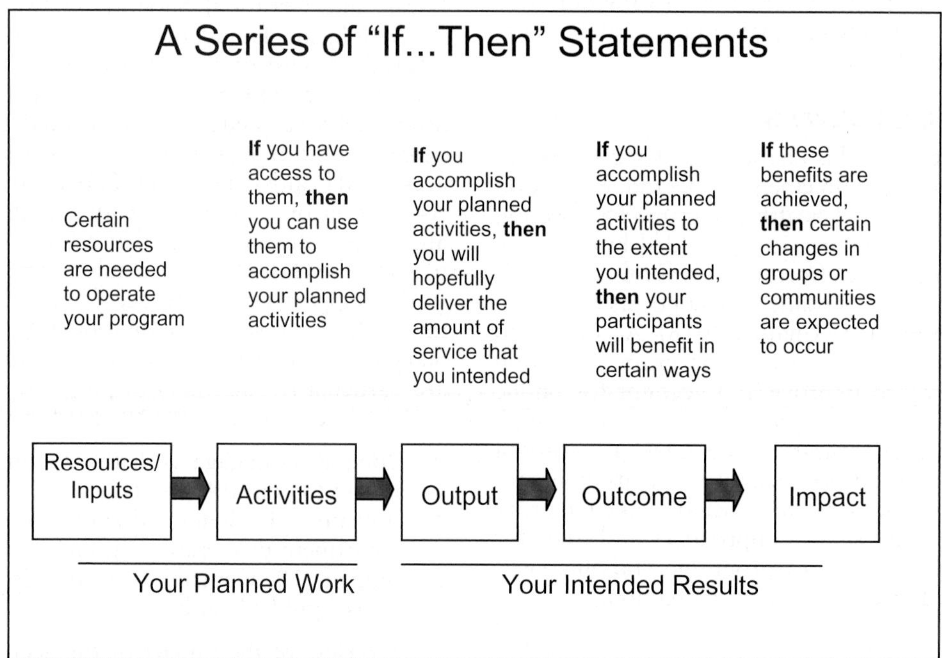

FIGURE 12-11 A series of "If...Then" statements to develop the program logic model by connecting inputs to interventions and outcomes to impacts. (From the Centers for Disease Control and Prevention, Division for Heart Disease and Stroke Prevention. (n.d.). *Evaluation guide: Developing and using a logic model.* Retrieved from https://www.cdc.gov/dhdsp/docs/logic_model.pdf)

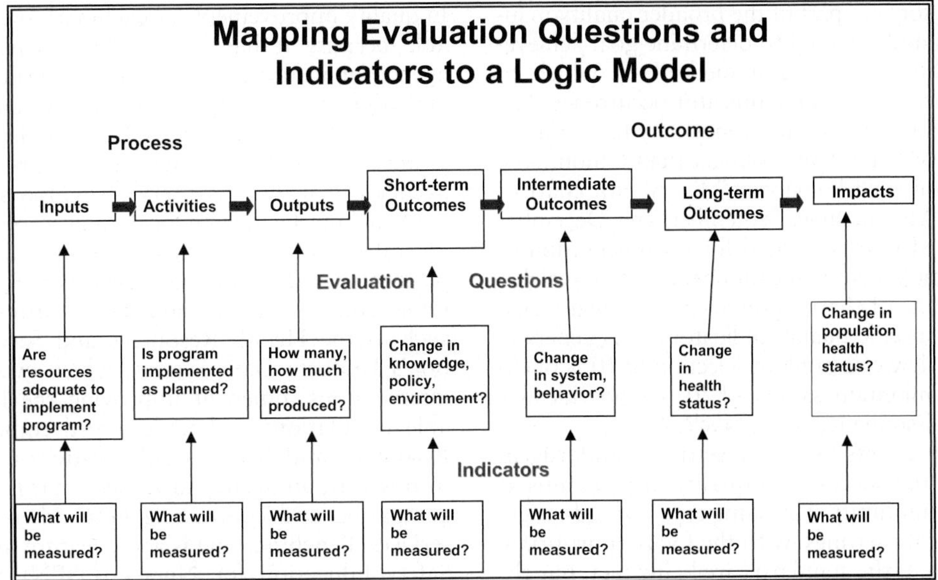

FIGURE 12-12 Mapping evaluation questions and indicators to a logic model to determine the effectiveness of a program. (From the Centers for Disease Control and Prevention, Division for Heart Disease and Stroke Prevention. (n.d.). *Evaluation guide: Developing and using a logic model.* Retrieved from https://www.cdc.gov/dhdsp/docs/logic_model.pdf)

are needed. Then, measurable objectives are developed that describe the expected outcomes. Use of selected verbs indicates the expected level of achievement, such as "clients will be able to demonstrate safe administration of insulin after three home visits" or "parents will have their infants' recommended immunizations up to date by 24 months of age." Goal setting is imperative when developing an educational program for an entire health program or service (see Chapter 11). These statements of measurable goals are then examined during the program evaluation. Without such statements, accurate evaluations cannot be conducted. Consider the overarching goal of your program, what you plan to accomplish, as well as why this program is important. The timeline and personnel resources must be considered, along with which actions must be taken to achieve your intended results (CDC, n.d.).

One helpful acronym, SMART is frequently used in developing outcome measures. The general consensus is that SMART stands for *S*pecific, *M*easurable, *A*ttainable, *R*elevant, and *T*ime Bound, and may include *E*valuate and *R*eevaluate—SMARTER when added (CDC, 2018).

Box 12-2 describes specific questions that must be asked and answered at each step of the SMART process.

In evaluating programs and care, outcomes must be measured against certain standards. *Standards* are generic guidelines of expected functioning. They can focus on the client, the caregiver, or the organization (finances). All care and services must also be measured against these guidelines. The core standards of care, practice, and finance must be integrated and compatible if they are to ensure quality care.

Quality Indicators and Benchmarks

Quality indicators of client outcomes are the quantitative measures of a client's response to care (Gordon, 2016). Defining and quantifying client outcomes from these indicators are worthwhile processes that enable the nursing staff to evaluate the results of the care they provide. The goal of care in the community is successful client outcomes. By starting with measurable indicators, successful outcomes can be demonstrated in quantifiable terms. When client care meets the standards set, client satisfaction—another quality outcome indicator—is greater.

BOX 12-2 Developing SMART Objectives

Specific

- What: What do we want to accomplish?
- Why: Specific reasons, purpose, or benefits of accomplishing the goal.
- Who: Who is involved?
- Where: Identify a location.
- Which: Identify requirements and constraints.

Measurable

- How much?
- How many?
- How will we know when it is accomplished?

Attainable

- How can the goal be accomplished?

Relevant

- Does this seem worthwhile?
- Is this the right time?
- Does this match our other efforts/needs?
- Are we the right group or agency?

Time-Bound or Timely

- When?
- What can we do 6 months from now?
- What can we do 6 weeks from now?
- What can we do today?

Source: Doran (1981).

Quality indicators are part of the broader quality management program and are used to determine goal achievement. Chart auditing is a useful method by which to measure the frequency of quality indicator occurrence (Bissonnette, 2016). For example, an agency may have a quality indicator such as "all infants younger than 6 months of age are weighed on each home visit." Every fifth chart of infants visited in March, June, September, and December during a designated year is audited for documentation of the number of home visits and the number of infant weights recorded. A sampling of charts is sufficient to measure goal achievement and specific quality indicators. It is generally accepted that a review of a random selection of 10% of eligible cases, with a minimum sample of 20, will provide useful information (Bissonnette, 2016; Nock, 2016).

Indicators are necessary when setting standards in order to measure the success and quality of programs at home or in the community. The same types of indicators are used in acute care settings, with the focus appropriate to that population. If the standards are being met, but client outcomes are unacceptable, the process indicators are explored for possible areas of weakness. Such areas may need further study to identify the cause of the poor client outcomes. For example, a process such as the catheter-care protocol used by an agency, or the communication between hospital and health department or home health nurses, may be examined to determine why there is a high incidence of catheter-associated urinary tract infections among home care patients. In addition, Medicaid and Medicare regulations in some states mandate that a percentage of records be audited each year.

While striving for excellence and best practices, agencies may use the **benchmarking** process. Benchmarking compares the performance of an individual practice, department, or agency with an external standard (Fig. 12-13).

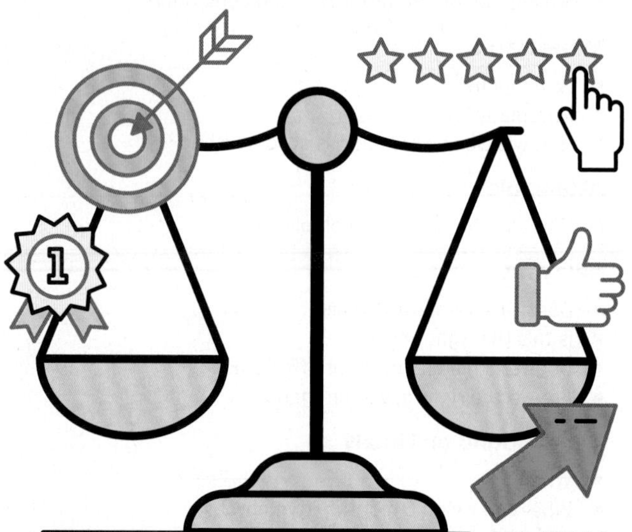

FIGURE 12-13 Benchmarking compares the performance of one entity against that of another entity or standard.

In quality improvement, a benchmark is considered achievable because it has already been achieved by another agency or institution (Agency for Health Care Research and Quality [AHRQ], 2016). Internal benchmarking occurs within organizations, between departments or programs. External benchmarking occurs between similar agencies providing like services. Good sources for external benchmarks include local quality collaboratives where several practices or agencies collect and compare similar performance data among themselves (Seow et al., 2018). Other sources include data reports from federal agencies such as the Health Resources and Services Administration's Uniform Data System, which evaluate services or interventions aimed at improving the health of vulnerable populations and underserved communities (Health Resources and Services Administration [HRSA], 2019). In this way, an agency identifies what is achievable while comparing and contrasting how others provide quality services. Benchmarking is a key feature of the Quality and Safety Education for Nurses (QSEN) project discussed later in this chapter and throughout this book.

The Nurse's Role in Quality Assurance and Improvement

Some quality improvement activities for C/PHNs include daily prioritizing of care needs for a caseload of clients, seeking supervision or skills development for a difficult case, systematizing charting so that needed documentation is efficiently completed, proposing better ways to organize care of chronically ill clients, and establishing new agency procedures. Staff meetings, peer review, and case conferences are common settings for nurses to bring the lessons of their practices to the larger group for examination and potential adoption. In particular, nursing peer review shows promise as a means to improve quality and safety in health care (Herrington & Hand, 2019).

It is the role of nursing administration to develop a formalized quality management program that includes a three-pronged focus, based on a classic approach to quality management: (1) review organizational *structure*, personnel, and environment; (2) focus on nursing care standards and delivery methods (*process*); and (3) focus on the *outcomes* of that care (Donabedian, 2003; Pelletier & Beaudin, 2018). In its essential competencies for health care quality professionals, the National Association for Healthcare Quality (NAHQ) identifies six key components of a robust quality management program, which are as follows:

- Performance and process improvement
- Population health and care transitions
- Health data analytics
- Patient safety
- Regulatory and accreditation
- Quality review and accountability (NAHQ, n.d., para. 2)

The issue of quality and safety has more recently been addressed through the QSEN project (QSEN, 2019). The QSEN competencies are consistent with the Donabedian approach to quality improvement and provide a framework for nursing education. They also form a sound basis for community health program evaluation, especially as it relates to quality. More details about the QSEN project follow.

Nurses should recognize the value of quality improvement efforts and the importance of their role in ensuring that quality care is delivered. Direct service providers are the best judges of care problems and potential solutions. For this reason, it is critical that quality assurance reviews and other quality improvement activities focus on issues relevant to staff and client concerns and are structured to be accomplished quickly and with minimal effort. When these activities are clear, concise, and well-integrated into daily routines, they become less time-consuming, and staff members may recognize the positive client outcomes as rewards for their efforts. Moreover, when health care providers have the opportunity to systematically examine the care they provide, they can identify problems and generate potential solutions sooner.

Program Evaluation: Concepts and Tools

Studies of community health programs suggest that they are often successful in changing community policies and individual behavior but may not have a significant impact on health outcomes over time (Fry, Nikpay, Leslie, & Buntin, 2018). This may have more to do with the complex causes of health-related issues, involving both "proximal risk factors as well as upstream determinants of health" (Andermann, Pang, Newton, Davis, & Panisset, 2016, p. 3). Whether small or large, health care agencies are complex organizations with many interrelated components. Assuring they provide services that protect or promote health can be an equally complex task. Avedis Donabedian, a physician credentialed in public health, offered a conceptual framework for evaluating health care, which is foundational to 21st century quality initiatives (Backer, 2019). The concepts of structure, process, and outcome offer the basis for his own and related models of care evaluation.

Structure, Process, and Outcomes

The organizational *structure* should:

- Fulfill its mission statement or philosophy (Dunham-Taylor, 2015)
- Be client-focused, with enough resources to maintain present services and introduce additional services as needed
- Operate efficiently and within budget, maintaining financial stability and promoting trust and confidence among stakeholders
- Have a well-developed system of acquiring additional funding for new services through grants and contract expansion if needed
- Attract and retain clients and qualified, highly motivated staff

The agency should integrate *processes* which:

- Provide client services in a manner that is safe, effective, client-centered, timely, efficient, and equitable (Agency for Healthcare Research and Quality [AHRQ], 2018)
- Maintain standards set by the professional staff that comply with or surpass those recommended by relevant accrediting bodies (Sills, 2015)
- Encourage staff to contribute to the evaluation and revision of standards
- Assure that staff members maintain current skills and knowledge pertinent to their job requirements
- Foster a collaborative work environment in which quality of care is continuously monitored and improved using a variety of participative management tools (e.g., audit instruments, peer review, incident reporting systems)
- Minimize staff turnover by providing a supportive work environment in which administration and staff have compatible working relationships
- Assure that employee values are compatible with the goals of the agency and that the conduct of all employees is consistent with organizational values
- Maintain effective feedback mechanisms for clients to share their perceptions about the care and services received (e.g., questionnaires, surveys, interviews)
- Act upon suggestions and opportunities for improvement that are identified by clients

The client health *outcomes* reflect the impact of the services provided by the agency (AHRQ, 2015). Outcomes are the result of numerous factors, including structure and processes, and others that are often beyond the agency's control. Examples include the following:

- Review the charts of hospitalized clients to identify any opportunities for improvement in the agency's teaching or care that could have prevented hospitalization.
- Review clinic or home visit records when poor client outcomes are reported to determine whether any aspect of the clinic's or home visit care might have prevented these occurrences.
- Focus on outcomes among commonly served high-risk populations in order to optimize care delivery as well as to benefit high-risk clients.
- Review national, state, and local health care initiatives and objectives (discussed earlier in this chapter) to identify priority health indicators or outcomes in the agency's client population.
- Develop SMART goals (discussed earlier in this chapter) focusing on the priority health indicators and outcomes in the client population.
- Develop aim statements—the tactics to achieve the SMART goals—which are outcome-focused (Institute for Healthcare Improvement [IHI], 2019).
- Enlist individuals with health care analytics skills, within or outside the agency, who can offer expertise in measuring and analyzing outcomes.
- Identify the metrics, or measures, that will show the agency has achieved its goals for client outcomes.
- Develop and implement strategies to improve and monitor client outcomes.
- Modify and improve structure and/or processes when client outcome targets are not met.

Models Useful in Program Evaluation

Donabedian Model. As previously mentioned, Donabedian (2003) was the original proponent of using the concepts of structure, process, and outcome in evaluating quality of care (Fig. 12-14). The Donabedian model is:

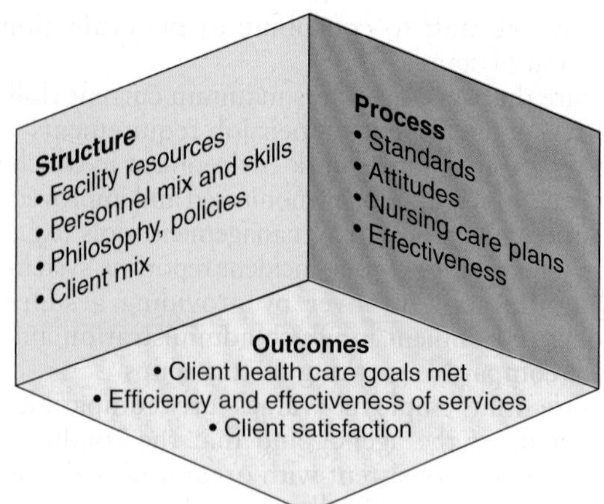

FIGURE 12-14 Structure, process, and outcome of quality model.

- Essentially linear in form, suggesting that structure influences processes which, in turn, produce outcomes
- Recognized as a simplistic and basic method of measuring quality
- Widely used as the framework for more elaborate models
- Relevant to common domains of nursing

Omaha System. Also discussed and graphically displayed in Chapter 15, the Omaha System includes measurement approaches that make it a useful model for evaluating the quality of nursing care provided to individuals, families, and communities (Box 12-3).

- Evaluation focuses on process indicators, client outcome measures, and satisfaction with care (Martin, 2005; The Omaha System, 2019).

The model is currently used in "home care, public health, and school health practice settings, nurse-managed center staff, hospital-based and managed care case managers, educators and students, occupational health nurses, faith community staff, acute care and rehabilitation hospital/long-term care staff, researchers, members of various disciplines, and computer software vendors" (The Omaha System, 2019, para. 10). The evaluation components of the Omaha System include the following:

- Outcomes that are rated in terms of *knowledge* (what the client knows), *behavior* (what the client does), and *status* (how the client is)
- Quantification of outcomes in a range of severity, as well as on a continuum toward or away from optimal health
- Ongoing monitoring of individual, family, or community health to assess the quality of nursing interventions

Quality and Safety Education for Nurses. The QSEN project, which is frequently referenced in this book, arose from the groundbreaking IOM (1999) report on medical errors and the subsequent 2004 report focusing on nursing quality and safety. This recognition prompted funding from the Robert Wood Johnson Foundation for what would become known as the QSEN project. The purpose of the project is "preparing future nurses who will have the QSEN competencies (knowledge, skills, and attitudes, or 'KSAs') necessary to continuously improve the quality and safety of the health care systems within which they work" (QSEN, 2020, para. 1). See Figure 12-15. Some have called for these competencies to move beyond the individual to systems of care, bringing it more in line with the population-based focus of public health (Dolansky & Moore, 2013; Dolansky, Schexnayder, & Patrician, 2017).

- The KSAs can be used across all settings where a nurse may be employed, whether hospital, outpatient center, home care, hospice, or community/public health nursing services.
- The KSAs are similar to the Omaha System outcome measures of knowledge, behavior, and status.
- The QSEN competencies are significant in community/public health nursing because they provide a method of evaluating both individual nurse performance and the use of aggregated data to assess programmatic outcomes.

The CDC's model for continuous program improvement cycle or its National Public Health Improvement Initiative is other example of quality improvement methods for public health. Additional information on program evaluation and related resources can be found at: https://www.cdc.gov/eval/index.htm.

MARKETING AND COMMUNITY HEALTH PROGRAMS

Each of the program evaluation models presented provide a mechanism to plan, implement, and evaluate community-based programs and services. Demonstrating quality through measurable outcomes is a crucial aspect of community health. Health promotion and health education programs must demonstrate achievement of stated goals to justify continuation. Community health services are also challenged to provide programs in ways that reach and engage their target populations. In this section, the roles of social marketing and social media are explored as additional tools for influencing health behaviors and lifestyle choices. These methods must be selected carefully and evaluated against the same standards as previously presented, perhaps more so, because of the potentially higher costs of this type of intervention.

The Value of Marketing

During the 2019 Super Bowl broadcast, television networks charged between $5.1 million and $5.3 million for a 30-second commercial spot (Calfas, 2019). Businesses have long recognized the value of "catchy," memorable advertisements. Marketing can literally make or break an enterprise. If the message is effective, the business often thrives; if not, it may dwindle.

Children as young as 3 years have been found to be "branded" with current fast-food items and beverages, meaning that they recognize and prefer one particular brand or logo over another (Enax et al., 2015; Kelly et al., 2019; Tatlow-Golden, Hennessy, Dean, & Hollywood, 2014). The techniques used by some corporations have contributed to health issues we currently face

BOX **12-3** STORIES FROM THE FIELD

Application of the Omaha System in Reducing Community Transmission During an Influenza Outbreak

During the holiday season, a metropolitan county of 120,000 people in Minnesota experienced concern and panic after a local store clerk at a regional mall contracted influenza and died 5 days later. The local health department quickly used their supply of vaccine, and the next week received enough vaccine for all residents from the CDC. Public health clinics were flooded with worried residents, and security became a concern. Cough and fever are early symptoms of flu and other less serious illnesses. It was difficult to determine if someone needed to be quarantined in order to thwart the spread of influenza.

In conjunction with the state health department and other partners, the local health department launched a vigorous media campaign about prevention and treatment of the flu and how to get the flu vaccine. Information was also given about the limitations of the vaccine and the importance of reducing contact with others (e.g., avoiding public places, using the ER). However, residents were hesitant to cancel holiday events and were continuing to visit the ER. PHNs completed contact investigations and "attempted to quarantine exposed family members" (para. 5). As the influenza outbreak ended, there were over 200 confirmed cases and 31 deaths.

DOMAIN: PHYSIOLOGICAL

Problem: Communicable/infectious condition (high priority)

Problem Classification Scheme (Community and Actual):

- Signs/Symptoms (Actual): infection, fever, positive screening/labs, inadequate policies to prevent transmission, refusal to follow infection control regimen, inadequate immunity.

Intervention Scheme:

- Teaching, Guidance, and Counseling (Targets/Client-Specific Information): anatomy/physiology (transmission), communication (media campaign), education (reduce risk of transmission), infection precautions (voluntary quarantine, MD not ER), medical/dental care (correct use of MD vs. ER).
- Treatments and Procedures (Targets/Client-specific Information): medication administration (antiviral medication for those with the flu).
- Case Management (Targets/Client-specific Information): communication (media campaign/many partners), infection precautions (enforced quarantine for those exposed).
- Surveillance (Targets/Client-specific Information): Infection precautions (contact investigations, monitoring of adherence, tracking reported cases and deaths).

Problem Rating Scale for Outcomes:

Knowledge: 2—minimal knowledge (residents aware of outbreak, residents with the flu knew they needed antiviral medication but not aware of other precautions; some residents were "overly concerned") (para. 10).

Behavior: 3—inconsistently appropriate behavior (most of the ill residents were given antiviral medication; many residents refused to restrict their activities/follow voluntary quarantine advice).

Status: 2—severe signs/symptoms (extensive flu infections, many cases and deaths, statistics monitored).

1. *How could compliance with voluntary quarantines be improved?*
2. *How could the Omaha System help PHNs evaluate the effectiveness of the media campaign and other interventions?*
3. *How could a PHN use Omaha System measures (i.e., Knowledge, Behavior, and Status) to evaluate the impact of the interventions to reduce teen vaping (discussed earlier in this chapter)?*

Adapted with permission from Olson Keller, L., & Minnesota Omaha System Users Group. (2019). Solving the clinical information puzzle: Influenza outbreak. *Omaha Systems.* Retrieved from www.omahasystem.org/casestudies.html

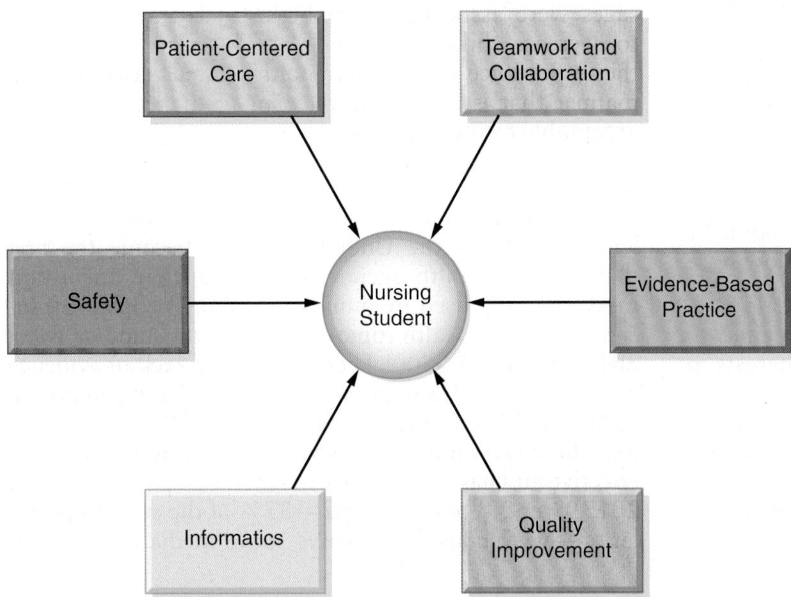

FIGURE 12-15 The knowledge, skills, and attitudes associated with the QSEN competencies facilitate learning and competence of the nursing student. (Source: QSEN. (2019). *QSEN competencies: Overview.* Retrieved from https://qsen.org/competencies/pre-licensure-ksas/)

as a nation (e.g., obesity in children, teen vaping). For instance, research examining awareness among 3- to 6-year-old children of products high in salt, fat, and sugar found that brand knowledge was a significant predictor of the child's BMI. After controlling for gender, age, and amount of television viewing, the researchers concluded that the link between brand knowledge, consumption of the products, and higher BMI had policy implications (Cornwell, McAlister, & Polmear-Swendris, 2014). In another study, products with cartoon characters were chosen by 8- to 10-year-olds when comparing the taste of yogurt–cereal–fruit snacks with plain labels, health-focused labels, or labels with unknown cartoon characters (Enax et al., 2015). An analysis of e-cigarette brand Web sites found marketing claims of being healthier, having fewer restrictions for public use, and being less expensive than cigarettes. E-cigarettes were also touted as helpful in smoking cessation (Eysenbach, 2018).

The health care sector has also recognized the power of marketing. Although health message marketing has been used in some capacity since the 1960s, it was not recognized as a potential health promotion tool until the 1990s, when federal agencies, such as the CDC, spearheaded efforts to utilize it (Lee & Kotler, 2020).

Social Marketing of Community Health Programs

The term **social marketing** refers to using marketing principles to influence or advance "the voluntary behavior of target audiences" (Leuking et al., 2017, p. 1426). You may have seen brief examples on television (or in print) of the CDC's *Tips from Former Smokers* campaign (Howard, 2019). An example of a very successful social marketing campaign was the ALS Association's "Ice Bucket Challenge," which raised over $115 million during an 8-week period in 2014 for amyotrophic lateral sclerosis (ALS) research (ALS Association, 2019). The objective of social marketing in public health is to improve society's health by influencing changes in individual health behaviors (e.g., healthy eating) and implementing policies that improve health behaviors of populations (e.g., seat belt laws). The integration of marketing with public health is seen as a means to enhance the effectiveness of public health practitioners (Leuking et al., 2017; Resnick & Siegel, 2013); nevertheless, this has yet to be confirmed by substantial research (Giustin, Ali, Fraser, & Boulos, 2018).

Key Social Marketing Concepts

Concepts that are important in marketing are also applicable to social marketing as noted in a seminal book by Resnick and Siegel (2013). These include the following:

- Exchange: Individuals give something to get something; they weigh the costs and perceived benefits.
- Self-interest: People act in their own best interests in most cases.
- Behavior change: Change in behavior is the focus; thoughts and ideas may also need to change but are not the ultimate goal.
- Competition: Selecting one option (or action) inherently involves giving up another option (or action).
- Consumer orientation: Problem-solving process is directed at the target—the consumer (this could be an individual, group, or organization).
- Four Ps (product, price, place, and promotion): Also called the marketing mix; each can be altered to increase market share.
- Partners and policy: Organizations with similar interests may form partnerships to achieve mutual objectives; identification of policy changes necessary for behavioral change, those supportive of the change, and those that the organization could help influence.

These principles seem rather straightforward, yet public health practitioners are often at a disadvantage when attempting to implement social marketing campaigns (Resnick & Siegel, 2013). They may lack training in the necessary skills, be outspent by the competition (e.g., the fast-food industry), or have limited options for distributing their message (e.g., public service announcements). Another example of a very successful social marketing campaign is the *Go Red for Women* initiative begun in 2004 by the American Heart Association (2020). Using a red dress as the symbol of the program, the initiative seeks to raise awareness of heart disease among women. Both of these health issues are equally important (heart disease, ALS), but one has a more broadly recognized campaign; the other was humorous but not necessarily educational. Ultimately, the issues are whether public health practitioners will take full advantage of social marketing to promote community or population health and whether behaviors and health outcomes will improve as a result.

Zahid and Reicks (2018) reported on a quantitative study of messaging that promotes healthy beverage intake among children. The study evaluated the effectiveness of gain-framed messaging (outcomes framed in positive light), on parenting practices that affect child intake of sugar-sweetened beverages (SSBs). Gain-framed messaging aimed to support parental motivation for reducing child SSB intake, as opposed to loss-framed messaging (outcomes framed in negative terms), which aimed to undermine it. Parents completed a survey after viewing gain- and loss-framed messages. The gain-framed messages were associated with higher parental motivation to decrease child intake of SSBs. This study exemplifies the importance of framing health-related messages in a manner that is appealing, relevant to the situation, and acceptable to the audience.

Social Media

In 2017, the National Institute for Health and Care Excellence (NICE) in the United Kingdom became the first major public health agency to use Snapchat, an instant messaging app used by millions of young people, to educate them on a health topic—antibiotic resistance (Owen, 2017). The cost? $500! There is, as yet, a lack of evidence confirming the effectiveness of social media in promoting public health programs (Giustin et al., 2018); nevertheless, there is no doubt that social media can be very cost-effective and has the capacity to reach vast populations. In 2017, over 2.7 billion people—37% of the world's population—were considered active social media users (Hart,

Stetten, Islam, & Pizarro, 2017). In 2019, approximately 72% of Americans used social networking tools, such as Facebook, Snapchat, Instagram, Twitter, and YouTube (Pew Research Center, 2019).

The capacity of social media to reach individuals with strategic and effective health messages is immense (CDC, 2019c) and must be harnessed (Fig. 12-16). A thematic analysis of research on the use of social media in public health and medicine suggests that patients, health care professionals, and the general public are already using social media for a variety of health-related purposes including behavioral change support and disease surveillance, prevention, and management (Giustin et al., 2018). The example below, in Box 12-4, demonstrates how social marketing principles can be utilized when you have a limited budget, limited time, and limited creativity. What role can social media play in these efforts?

When planning and beginning development of a social marketing approach, there are many resources available to the C/PHN and other public health professionals.

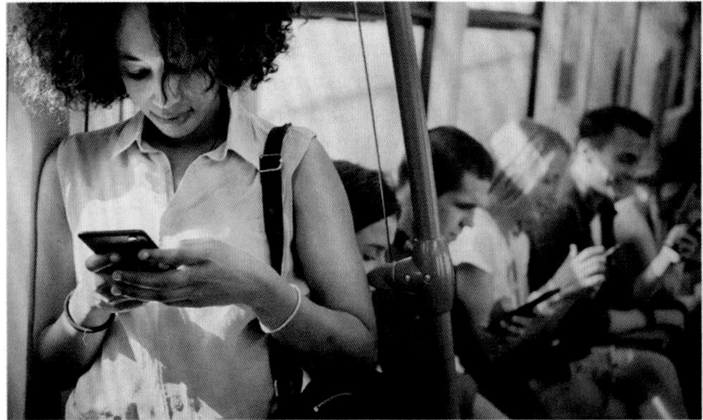

FIGURE 12-16 Social media and technology have the capacity to reach and influence the health behaviors of a wide audience.

- The CDC offers an excellent Web site, *Gateway to Health Communications and Social Marketing* (CDC, 2019d), that includes links to a wide variety of resources. For instance, one of the social marketing resources, *Social Media at CDC*, offers guidelines and best practices, including a social media toolkit and a guide to writing for social media (CDC, 2019a, 2019d).
- The European Centers for Disease Prevention and Control (2014) offers a comprehensive *Social Mar-*

BOX **12-4** STORIES FROM THE FIELD

Nursing Students and a Social Marketing Campaign

University campuses hold a wealth of often-untapped expertise. For nursing students working on a health promotion program, the substance of the effort (the health issue) is often pretty straightforward, but the presentation is more challenging. Many schools of nursing are providing collaborative experiences for students, supporting partnerships with nonnursing students and faculty in addressing health education needs. The following is one example of how collaboration can be effective:

In conversation with an instructor, two nursing students learned that university administration was concerned about a surge in measles cases statewide. The university recommended students be current on all standard immunizations prior to admission; nevertheless, it was not a requirement. After further discussion with their instructor, the nursing students sought input from several student organizations. From those discussions, they identified a low level of knowledge and concern about the issue among the students.

Recognizing that college students are not prone to worrying about measles, the nursing students sought help from the university's student health center. The health center administration agreed this was an important issue and collaborated with the public health department to offer free measles, mumps, and rubella (MMR) immunizations at the student health center. The student health center posted information about the free immunizations on its Web site, but there was very little response from students.

The nursing students realized they needed to spread the word about the importance of the issue and the availability of the free immunizations. Based on input from the student groups, they decided to develop social media messaging that was informative, engaging, and brief. In conjunction with their instructor, they contacted the university's animation department and found an instructor who was willing to assign his or her students to develop an animated video promoting MMR vaccination. The nursing students provided information about the current measles outbreak, educational materials about the MMR vaccine, and details about its availability at the student health center. The animation students then developed brief videos within those parameters. In the end, several outstanding videos were submitted.

The animation student's videos were posted on several of the university's social media outlets, including Facebook and Instagram. The campus newspaper also published an article about the MMR campaign and the collaborative efforts of the health center and students from different colleges. In response, there was a surge in students visiting the health center for free MMR vaccination. The campaign also reached parents who saw the videos on the webpages and social media. Many messages were sent to the university by the parents regarding the campaign, and the responses were handled by the nursing students.

The campaign was not expensive, it engaged the most skilled individuals for each task, and it provided much-needed information to the university students and their parents. Even though they had targeted the college students, the nursing students found that the parents were just as interested in the campaign.

1. *In what ways has social marketing influenced your actions or behaviors?*
2. *Can you think of an issue on your university campus that could benefit from social marketing?*
3. *Do you recognize any social marketing efforts sponsored by your university or your school of nursing?*

keting Guide for Public Health Programme Managers and Practitioners. Another very helpful publication *What Works: Health Communication and Social Marketing—Evidence-Based Interventions for Your Community* (CPSTF, 2014).

- *Social Media Toolkit: A Primer for Local Health Department PIOs and Communications Professionals* (National Association of County and City Health Officials (NACCHO) (2019) provides information on the importance of social media tools to "reinforce and personalize messages, reach new audiences, and build a communication infrastructure based on open information exchange" (p. 2). However, there are also downsides to this approach.

Ethical Issues in Social Marketing

The plethora of social marketing campaigns have raised a spotlight on ethical issues that must be carefully considered when designing, implementing, and evaluating social marketing programs for good causes (Olson, 2018). The International Union for Health Promotion and Education (2016) is dedicated to seeing optimum health and well-being globally. Their values highlight the importance of ethics in this arena:

- Respect—for the innate dignity of all people, for cultural identity, for cultural diversity, and for natural resources and the environment
- Inclusion and involvement of people in making the decisions that shape their lives and impact upon their health and well-being
- Equity in health, social, and economic outcomes for all people
- Accountability and transparency—within governments, organizations, and communities
- Sustainability
- Social justice for all people
- Compassion and empowerment (International Union for Health Promotion and Education, 2016, para. 3)

Social media platforms, which are potent social marketing tools, are powerful but often unreliable sources of information. It may be difficult for consumers to discern truth from fiction in social media posts about health and wellness, many (or perhaps, most) of which may originate from sources that are not authoritative or credible. Social media platforms are also vulnerable to nefarious uses such as hacking and fraud, which also makes them potent sources of misinformation. In 2019, Facebook and Twitter took action against China for using hundreds of fake accounts to sow political discord during protests in Hong Kong. As Olson (2018) points out, social marketers should resist the temptation to use questionable tactics, even when it might seem justified from their perspective about "the greater good."

Social marketing is not a panacea, but it does provide techniques that can support health education and promotion programs. The method can be very expensive and elaborate, or it can provide simple, straightforward messages. The point is that well-presented marketing can prompt behavior change. Media messages are not a replacement for a sound health promotion program; but they are a tool that can be used for great impact.

SECURING GRANTS TO FUND COMMUNITY HEALTH PROGRAMS

Public health departments and other community agencies often require outside funding to develop new health intervention programs. A common practice is to seek grant funding. What is a grant? A **grant** is, very simply, one individual or group providing another individual or group with the support (i.e., money) for a specified purpose. Some basic knowledge about grants can demystify the topic.

In health promotion and education, grants offer a source of funding for program development or project support. These types of grants fall into the following common categories:

- Planning grants (i.e., initial project development)
- Start-up grants (i.e., seed money)
- Management or technical assistance grants (e.g., for fund raising or marketing)
- Research grants
- Facilities or equipment grants (National Institutes of Health, 2019)

Grants are a reality in public health efforts, similar to a new program or research proposal. They are not easy to locate, secure, or manage (once you have one), but they are vital in providing a wide range of programs and services to a community. Grants are available from government sources, private philanthropic sources, and corporations. Private organizations often have sections on their Web sites with information on available grant funding. Grant money is not typically paid back; however, it is a contractual agreement, and the terms and conditions are usually clearly delineated.

Federal Grants

Federal grants award government funds to implement projects that provide public service and stimulate the economy (Grants.gov, n.d.) and are available from 26 grant-making agencies. The funding categories most applicable to community health include the following:

- Community development
- Disaster preparation and relief
- Food and nutrition
- Health

Federal grants are available to a wide variety of groups, but typically, health-related grants are available to state or local governments, which include public health departments, public housing organizations, educational organizations, and nonprofit organizations (Grants.gov, n.d.). Nonprofit means the organization was not established to earn a profit. This does not mean it doesn't generate income, but only that there are restrictions on how its funds can be used. Federal grants can be found on the Web site www.grants.gov or on individual federal agency Web sites.

Of particular importance to the discussion of grants is the term *501c3*. This is a designation that refers to the Internal Revenue Service (IRS) tax-exempt status granted to certain nonprofit organizations. To be granted this designation, an entity must be organized and operated exclusively for specific purposes, which include charity, science, education, or the prevention of cruelty to children or animals (IRS, Department of the Treasury, 2020). Some grants are only available to 501c3 organizations, and the funders will request proof of this in the grant application. Only corporations, community chests, funds, or foundations can receive this designation; individuals or partnerships do not qualify (IRS, Department of the Treasury, 2020). Essentially, the 501c3 organization can be the provider of the grant funding or the organization seeking the funding.

The Grant Process

The grant process, although arduous, provides the opportunity to focus clearly on what you intend to accomplish, why it is needed, and what part you will play in the successful outcome of the project. Here are some of the steps involved:

- Select a funder that is a good match for your organization and your program/project. For instance, applying to a faith-based organization that supports abstinence-only educational programs would not be a good fit for your program that seeks to provide contraceptive information in an after-school program for teens.
- Be prepared to provide proof of interdisciplinary or community involvement; many grant funders favor or require grant applications that show collaboration with others.
- Submit a **letter of inquiry**; this may be by invitation-only or be part of the original advertisement of the grant funding. This letter is brief, yet clearly lays out your plan.
- Read the **request for proposal (RFP)** carefully and write a clear, well-prepared grant proposal that carefully follows the guidelines; failure to submit all required items prior to the deadline means your grant application is unlikely to be reviewed or funded.
- If your grant is not selected, contact the funder to request a review of your submission; this is common with government-sponsored grants. Understanding what hampered your selection puts you in a better position to be successful in future submissions to this or other funding sources.

It is wise to seek the help of an experienced mentor—someone who has been successful in **grant writing**—as they can critique your proposal and offer suggestions prior to submission. In grant funding, experience counts! A proven record in securing grants and completing the requirements, means you or your organization will have an easier time securing additional funding (Jaykus, 2017). For the new grant seeker, this can be discouraging.

So, where to begin? Don't start with complicated grants. Begin building your reputation with small local grants. Work with partners. A school of nursing could partner with a home health agency to write a grant to provide worksite wellness programs for uninsured agricultural workers. Or several faith-community groups could partner in a grant application to provide free health screenings for uninsured adults in their area.

Finally, be certain that the grant will allow you to meet the mission and goals of your program. With limited funds available, funders are looking for proof of the sustainability of your program after their support ends. For instance, a breast-feeding support program sought funding in a high-risk area where there was a clear need. Although the need was demonstrated, the agency had no plan for continuing the program after the funding ended, so they did not receive funding. Grant support is often seen as funding to get programs started—not to provide for long-term operations (Jaykus, 2017; Karsh & Fox, 2019).

Many courses are available on how to successfully locate and write grants. A wide variety of information is available online. Helpful Web sites are included in the Internet resources found on *thePoint*.

The Nurse's Role in Grant Applications and Management

Many health departments see grants as an integral part of their service delivery, even hiring grant writers and managers in some cases. For the small nonprofit organization seeking funding, one effective approach is to partner with a local university, which allows for more access to grant-locating programs, as well as the expertise offered on the campuses (e.g., content area experts, experienced researchers, statisticians, business plan experts).

For most health agencies, the task of locating grant funds, writing the grant application, and doing the work stipulated by the grant falls on the nurses and other professionals within those agencies. On the positive side, it provides an opportunity for C/PHNs to explain to others what they can provide in terms of services and programs targeting the community's health.

The following tips may be helpful as you begin the process of seeking grant funding (Federal Grants Wire, 2020):

- Gain a sound understanding of the grant and specific criteria required, ensuring your interests and intentions are in line with the grantor agency.
- Seek input from the community the services are intended to benefit.
- Compile all required documents, such as articles of information, tax exemption certification, etc.
- Conform the proposal to the RFP requirements. The order of contents may vary but usually include a proposal summary, problem statement, project goal and objectives, project methods or design, project evaluation, and budget.
- Review, proofread, and ensure all requirements are met prior to submitting your proposal.
- Submit the proposal prior to the deadline.

Even if you are never required to write a grant, you will likely be involved in some part of a programmatic grant at some point in your career, either in the delivery of services stipulated by the grant (product) or in evaluating the outcomes of the services provided (e.g., satisfaction surveys). You may even be asked to provide ideas for services to be included in the grant application. Take advantage of these opportunities. The experience you gain will enhance your knowledge of the process and prepare you for future opportunities.

SUMMARY

- The first step in developing effective community health programs is identifying the problems which should be addressed.
- National health objectives and initiatives, such as Healthy People 2030, as well as state and local priorities and programs, offer ideas for community health aims.
- There are a variety of tools for identifying local health needs, including federal resources.
- Establishing partnerships with other health care professionals and community organizations, leaders, and members is a crucial element in planning community health programs.
- Nurses must integrate their own "authoritative knowledge" with the target population's "local knowledge" into the community health program.
- The Community Action Model is a form of participatory action research that identifies actions that are achievable and sustainable.
- A key factor in ensuring the success of an intervention is to appoint an advisory group, including representatives from the target community.
- The changeability and importance of health behaviors should be considered when developing community health programs.
- Successful community health programs require that the nurse listen to the target population and not determine the problem and solution without their assistance.
- Outcome measures should be consistent with the concerns of the community, and evaluation can be facilitated by clearly defined goals that can be measured against actual results.
- The PRECEDE–PROCEED model offers a framework for understanding the predisposing, reinforcing, and enabling factors that influence behavior.
- Accreditation is an evaluation process that promotes high-quality services among health departments.
- Quality indicators are measures of a client's response to care. The goal of community health programs is successful client outcomes.
- Benchmarking compares the performance of an individual entity with an external standard. Good sources for external benchmarks include local quality collaboratives.
- The concepts of structure, process, and outcome offer the basis for Donabedian's and other related models of health care evaluation (e.g., QSEN). The Omaha System provides standardized language for classifying problems, interventions, and outcomes.
- Social marketing in public health can promote changes in individual health behaviors and/or policies that improve health behaviors of populations.
- Social media has immense potential for reaching individuals with public health messages; however, there is a lack of evidence confirming its effectiveness.
- Grants offer a source of funding for program development or project support. Nurses play a key role in grant writing and management.

ACTIVE LEARNING EXERCISES

1. With the information provided in the teen vaping example, work with a group of students to complete the planning of a viable program that meets the stated goals. List nursing diagnoses and develop measurable objectives (SMART objectives). Use Figure 12-10 as a guide to develop predisposing, reinforcing, and enabling factors related to teen vaping. Use the logic model diagrams in Figures 12-13 and 12-14, and other information on evaluation, to determine resources and activities, as well as available data that could be used to evaluate short-term and long-term outcomes.
2. Inquire about past and present public health programs targeted to specific populations in your area (or at the state level). How was the need discovered? What steps did they take to understand community concerns about this issue? Was a model or framework used to develop an intervention (if so, which one)? How were the outcomes measured? Did program evaluation determine if the intervention was effective? Describe how 4 of the 10 essential public health services (see Box 2-2) were used in this process.
3. Compare common quality improvement measures found in acute care (hospital) settings and potential areas for quality improvement in public health (e.g., CDC's continuous program improvement cycle or National Public Health Improvement Initiative). Is your local public health agency accredited? If so, ask an administrator how this has changed PHN practice and client outcomes. If not, ask for examples of public health quality improvement measures or benchmarks.
4. Identify a health-related social marketing campaign that you viewed recently on television, social media sites, or in print (e.g., the National Institute for Health and Care Excellence [NICE] Snapchat campaign about antibiotic resistance). Alternately, find a research article on the use of social marketing in public health. Who is the target audience? What is the main message it is sending? What is the target behavior or problem? Does it reach the target audience? What works? What doesn't seem to be effective? How could you improve on methods to reach the target audience?
5. Talk with PHNs or PHN supervisors at your local or state public health department or other community health agency. How many and what types of grants do they have? What programs do they fund exclusively from grant writing? How are they involved in grant writing? How do they manage grant funding and data gathering to justify outcomes for grant funders?

REFERENCES

Agency for Healthcare Research and Quality (AHRQ). (2015). *Types of health care quality measures*. Retrieved from https://www.ahrq.gov/talkingquality/measures/types.html

Agency for Healthcare Research and Quality (AHRQ). (2016). *Comparing quality scores to a benchmark*. Retrieved from https://www.ahrq.gov/talkingquality/translate/compare/choose/benchmark.html

Agency for Healthcare Research and Quality (AHRQ). (2018). *Six domains of health care quality*. Retrieved from https://www.ahrq.gov/talkingquality/measures/six-domains.html

ALS Association. (2019). *Every drop adds up*. Retrieved from http://www.alsa.org/fight-als/ice-bucket-challenge.html

American Heart Association. (2020). *Go red for women*. Retrieved from https://www.goredforwomen.org/

American Nurses Association. (2013). *Public health nursing: Scope and standards of practice* (2nd ed.). Silver Spring, MD: Nursesbooks.org.

Andermann, A., Pang, T., Newton, J. N., Davis, A., & Panisset, U. (2016). Evidence for health I: Producing evidence for improving health and reducing inequities. *Health Research Policy and Systems, 14*, 18. Retrieved from https://www.ncbi.nlm.nih.gov/pmc/articles/PMC4791875/pdf/12961_2016_Article_87.pdf

Anderson, L. C., Mah, C. L., & Sellen, D. W. (2015). Eating well with Canada's food guide? Authoritative knowledge about food and health among newcomer mothers. *Appetite, 91*, 357–365. doi: 10.1016/j.appet.2015.04.063.

Backer, L. A. (2019). Rediscovering the secret of quality: It's probably not what you think. *Family Practice Management, 26*(2), 4.

Ball, L., Ball, C., Leveritt, M., Ray, S., Collins, C., Patterson, E., ... Chaboyer, W. (2017). Using logic models to enhance the methodological quality of primary health-care interventions: Guidance from an intervention to promote nutrition care by general practitioners and practice nurses. *Australian Journal of Primary Health, 23*(1), 53–60. doi: 10.1071/PY16038.

Bissonnette, J. (October, 2016). *Chart audits: Pros and cons as a research/QI and data collection methodology*. Retrieved from http://www.ohri.ca/clinicalresearchtraining/documents/0820%20Chart%20Audits.pdf

Bolton, M., Moore, I., Ferreira, A., Day, C., & Bolton, D. (2016). Community organizing and community health: Piloting an innovative approach to community engagement applied to an early intervention project in south London. *Journal of Public Health, 38*(1), 115–121. doi: 10.1093/pubmed/fdv017.

Calfas, J. (2019). Here's how much it costs to buy a commercial during Super Bowl 2019. *Money*. Retrieved from http://money.com/money/5633822/super-bowl-2019-commercial-ad-costs/

Centers for Disease Control and Prevention (CDC). (n.d.). *State heart disease and stroke prevention program. Evaluation guide writing SMART objectives*. Retrieved from https://www.cdc.gov/dhdsp/docs/smart_objectives.pdf

Centers for Disease Control and Prevention (CDC). (2017). *A framework for program evaluation*. Retrieved from https://www.cdc.gov/eval/framework/index.htm

Centers for Disease Control and Prevention (CDC). (2018). *Writing SMART objectives*. Retrieved from https://www.cdc.gov/healthyyouth/evaluation/pdf/brief3b.pdf

Centers for Disease Control and Prevention (CDC). (2019a). *National Center for Health Statistics*. Retrieved from https://www.cdc.gov/nchs/index.htm

Centers for Disease Control and Prevention (CDC). (2019b). *Quick facts on the risks of e-cigarettes for kids, teens and young adults*. Retrieved from https://www.cdc.gov/tobacco/basic_information/e-cigarettes/Quick-Facts-on-the-Risks-of-E-cigarettes-for-Kids-Teens-and-Young-Adults.html

Centers for Disease Control and Prevention (CDC). (2019c). *Social media at CDC*. Retrieved from https://www.cdc.gov/socialmedia/tools/guidelines/index.html

Centers for Disease Control and Prevention (CDC). (2019d). *Gateway to health communication*. Retrieved from https://www.cdc.gov/healthcommunication/index.html

Centers for Disease Control and Prevention, Office for State, Tribal, Local, and Territorial Support. (2018). *National voluntary accreditation for public health departments*. Retrieved from https://www.cdc.gov/publichealthgateway/accreditation/docs/AccreditationFactsheet.pdf

Community Preventive Services Task Force (CPSTF). (2014). *What works: Health communication and social marketing—Evidence-based interventions for your community*. Retrieved from https://www.thecommunityguide.org/sites/default/files/assets/Health-Communication-Mass-Media.pdf

Community Preventive Services Task Force (CPSTF). (2019). *About the community guide*. Retrieved from https://www.thecommunityguide.org/about/about-community-guide

Community Tool Box. (2019a). *Developing a plan for assessing local needs*. Retrieved from https://ctb.ku.edu/en/table-of-contents/assessment/assessing-community-needs-and-resources/develop-a-plan/main

Community Tool Box. (2019b). *Increasing participation and membership*. Retrieved from https://ctb.ku.edu/en/increasing-participation-and-membership

Community Tool Box. (2019c). *Developing a framework or model of change*. Retrieved from https://ctb.ku.edu/en/best-change-processes/developing-a-framework-or-model-of-change/overview

Cornell University. (2016). *Modeling the program: Conceptualization, logic models, & pathway models*. Retrieved from https://core.human.cornell.edu/resources/modeling.cfm

Cornwell, T. B., McAlister, A. R., & Polmear-Swendris, N. (2014). Children's knowledge of packaged and fast food brands and their BMI. Why the relationship matters for policy makers. *Appetite, 81*(1), 277–283. doi: 10.1016/j.appet.2014.06.017.

Cusack, C., Cohen, B., Mignone, J., Chartier, M. J., & Lutfiyya, Z. (2018). Participatory action as a research method with public health nurses. *Journal of Advanced Nursing, 74*(7), 1544–1553. doi: 10.1111/jan.13555.

da Silva, F., Paiva, F., Guedes, C., Frazao, I., Vasconcelos, S., & da Costa Lima, M. (2018). Nursing diagnoses of the homeless population in light of self-care theory. *Archives of Psychiatric Nursing, 32*(3), 425–431. doi: 10.1016/j.apnu.2017.12.009.

deChesnay, M. (Ed.). (2015). *Nursing research using participatory action research: Qualitative designs and methods in nursing*. New York, NY: Springer Publishing.

Deputy, N. P., Kim, S. Y., Conrey, E. J., & Bullard, K. M. (2018). Prevalence and changes in preexisting diabetes and gestational diabetes among women who had a live birth—United States, 2012–2016. *Morbidity and Mortality Weekly Report, 67*, 1201–1207. doi: 10.15585/mmwr.mm6743a2.

Dolansky, M. A., & Moore, S. M. (2013). Quality and Safety Education for Nurses (QSEN): The key is systems thinking. *Online Journal of Issues in Nursing, 18*(3), 1. Retrieved from http://ojin.nursingworld.org/quality-and-safety-education-for-nurses.html

Dolansky, M. A., Schexnayder, J., & Patrician, P. A. (2017). New approaches to integrating Quality and Safety Education for Nurses competencies in nursing education. *Nurse Educator, 42*(5 Suppl), S12–S17. doi: 10.1097/NNE.0000000000000422.

Donabedian, A. (2003). *An introduction to quality assurance in health care*. New York, NY: Oxford University Press.

Doran, G. T. (1981). There's a S.M.A.R.T. way to write management's goals and objectives. *Management Review (American Management Association Forum), 70*(11), 35–36.

Duggan, T. (May 18, 2017). Fresh approach with farm-to-school meals in Oakland. *San Francisco Chronicle*. Retrieved from https://goodfoodpurchasing.org/fresh-approach-with-farm-to-school-meals-in-oakland/

Dunham-Taylor, J. (2015). Organizations: Surviving within a chaotic, complex, value-based environment. In J. Dunham-Taylor & J. Z. Pinczuk (Eds.), *Financial management for nurse managers: Merging the heart with the dollar* (3rd ed., pp. 81–165). Burlington, MA: Jones and Bartlett.

Enax, L., Weber, B., Ahlers, M., Kaiser, U., Diethelm, K., Holtkamp, D., ... Kersting, M. (2015). Food packaging cues influence taste perception and increase effort provision for a recommended snack product in children. *Frontiers in Psychology, 6*, 882. Retrieved from https://www.frontiersin.org/articles/10.3389/fpsyg.2015.00882/full

European Centre for Disease Prevention and Control. (2014). *Social marking guide for public health programme managers and practitioners*. Retrieved from https://www.ecdc.europa.eu/sites/default/files/media/en/publications/Publications/social-marketing-guide-public-health.pdf

Eysenbach, G. (2018). Evolution of electronic cigarette brands from 2013–2014 to 2016–2017: Analysis of brand websites. *Journal of Medical*

Internet Research, 20(3), e80. Retrieved from https://www.ncbi.nlm.nih.gov/pmc/articles/PMC5869180/

Fairchild, A. L., Bayer, R., & Lee, J. S. (2019). The e-cigarette debate: What counts as evidence? *American Journal of Public Health, 109*(7), 1000–1006. Retrieved from https://ajph.aphapublications.org/doi/10.2105/AJPH.2019.305107

Federal Grants Wire. (2020). *How to write a federal grant proposal.* Retrieved from http://www.federalgrantswire.com/writing-a-federal-grant-proposal.html#.Vr2CePkrL3Q

Fry, E., Nikpay, S. S., Leslie, E., & Buntin, M. B. (2018). Evaluating community-based health improvement programs. *Health Affairs, 37*(1), 22–29. doi: 10.1377/hlthaff.2017.1125.

Giustin, D., Ali, S. M., Fraser, M., & Boulos, M. N. K. (2018). Effective uses of social media in public health and medicine: A systematic review of systematic reviews. *Online Journal of Public Health Informatics, 10*(2), e215. doi: 10.5210/ojphi.v10i2.8270.

Goan, M. B. (2015). *Mary Breckenridge: The frontier nursing service and rural health in Appalachia.* Chapel Hill, NC: The University of North Carolina Press.

Gordon, M. (2016). *Manual of nursing diagnosis* (13th ed.). Burlington, MA: Jones & Bartlett Learning.

Gordon, L. (2018). The community as patient: Assessing needs for public health program planning and intervention. *Journal of the Academy of Nutrition and Dietetics, 118*(10), A157. Retrieved from https://jandonline.org/article/S2212-2672(18)31778-7/fulltext

Grants.gov. (n.d.). *Grants 101: A short summary of federal grants.* Retrieved from http://www.grants.gov/web/grants/learn-grants/grants-101.html

Green, L. W., & Kreuter, M. W. (2005). *Health program planning: An educational and ecological approach* (4th ed.). New York, NY: McGraw-Hill.

Green, L. W., Ottoson, J. M., & Roditis, M. L. (2014). Public health education and health promotion. In L. Shi & J. A. Johnson (Eds.), *Novick & Morrow's public health administration: Principles for population-based management* (3rd ed., pp. 477–504). Burlington, MA: Jones & Bartlett Learning.

Hart, M., Stetten, N. E., Islam, S., & Pizarro, K. (2017). Twitter and public health (part 1): How individual public health professionals use Twitter for professional development. *JMIR Public Health and Surveillance, 3*(3), e60. doi: 10.2196/publichealth.6795.

Health Resources & Services Administration. (2019). *Uniform data system (UDS) resources.* Retrieved from https://bphc.hrsa.gov/datareporting/reporting/index.html

Henley, M. M. (2015). Alternative and authoritative knowledge: The role of certification for defining expertise among Doulas. *Social Currents, 2*(3), 260–279. doi: 10.1177%2F2329496515589851.

Herrington, C. R., & Hand, M. W. (2019). Impact of nurse peer review on a culture of safety. *Journal of Nursing Care Quality, 34*(2), 158–162. doi: 10.1097/NCQ.0000000000000361.i.

Howard, A. (2019). 10 effective public health social media campaigns. *Strategic Social Media Lab.* Retrieved from https://strategicsocialmedialab.com/10-effective-public-health-social-media-campaigns/

Institute for Healthcare Improvement. (2019). *Science of improvement: Setting aims.* Retrieved from http://www.ihi.org/resources/Pages/HowtoImprove/ScienceofImprovementSettingAims.aspx

Institute of Medicine (IOM). (1999). *To err is human: Building a safer health system.* Washington, DC: National Academies Press. Retrieved from https://www.nap.edu/resource/9728/To-Err-is-Human-1999-report-brief.pdf

Institute of Medicine (IOM). (2002). *The future of the public's health in the 21st century.* Washington, DC: National Academies Press. Retrieved from https://www.ncbi.nlm.nih.gov/books/NBK221239/

Institute of Medicine (IOM). (2004). *Keep patients safe: Transforming the work environment of nurses.* Washington, DC: National Academies Press. doi: 10.17226/10851.

Internal Revenue Service, Department of the Treasury. (2020). *Tax-exempt status for your organization.* Retrieved from http://www.irs.gov/publications/p557/index.html

International Union for Health Promotion and Education. (2016). *Mission and values.* Retrieved from http://www.iuhpe.org/index.php/en/

Jaykus, L. A. (2017). Keys to successful grant writing. *Journal of Food Science, 82*(7), 1511–1512. doi: 10.1111/1750-3841.13457.

Karsh, E., & Fox, A. S. (2019). *The only grant-writing book you will ever need* (5th ed.). New York, NY: Basic Books.

Kelly, B., Boylan, E., King, L., Bauman, A., Chapman, K., & Hughes, C. (2019). Children's exposure to television food advertising contributes to strong brand attachments. *International Journal of Environmental Research and Public Health, 16*(13), 2358. Retrieved from https://www.ncbi.nlm.nih.gov/pmc/articles/PMC6651128/pdf/ijerph-16-02358.pdf

Kidder, D. P., & Chapel, T. J. (2018). CDC's program evaluation journey: 1999 to present. *Public Health Reports, 133*(4), 356–359. Retrieved from https://doi.org/10.1177/0033354918778034

Kronstadt, J., Bender, K., & Beitsch, L. (2018). The impact of public health department accreditation: 10 years of lessons learned. *Journal of Public Health Management & Practice, 24*(Suppl 3), S1–S2. doi: 10.1097/PHH.0000000000000769.

Lane, S. D., Cashman, D. M., Keefe, R. H., Narine, L., Ducre, B., Chesna, S., … Oliver, D. (2017). Community health agency administrators' access to public health data for program planning, evaluation, and grant preparation. *Social Work in Health Care, 56*(2), 65–77. doi: 10.1080/00981389.2016.1268661.

Leadbeater, B., Gladstone, E., & Sukhawathanakul, P. (2015). Planning for sustainability of an evidence-based mental health promotion program in Canadian elementary schools. *American Journal of Community Psychology, 56*(1), 120–133. doi: 10.1007/s10464-015-9737-8.

Lee, N. R., & Kotler, P. (2020). *Social marketing: Changing behaviors for good* (6th ed.). Thousand Oaks, CA: Sage Publications, Inc.

Leuking, C., Hennink-Kaminski, H., Ihekweazu, C., Vaughn, A., Mazzucca, S., & Ward, D. S. (2017). Social marketing approaches to nutrition and physical activity interventions in early care and education centers: A systematic review. *Obesity Reviews, 18*(12), 1425–1438. doi: 10.1111/obr.12596.

Martin, K. S. (2005). *The Omaha System: A key to practice, documentation, and information management* (2nd ed.). Omaha, NE: Health Connections Press.

National Association for Healthcare Quality. (n.d.). *HQ essentials: Competencies for the healthcare quality professional.* Chicago, IL: Author. Retrieved from https://nahq.org/education/hq-essentials

National Association of County & City Health Officials. (2019). *Social media toolkit: A primer for local health department PIOs and communications professionals.* Retrieved from https://www.naccho.org/uploads/downloadable-resources/Social-Media-Toolkit-for-LHDs-2019.pdf

National Association of County & City Health Officials. (2020). *Accreditation readiness.* Retrieved from https://www.naccho.org/programs/public-health-infrastructure/performance-improvement/accreditation-preparation

National Institutes of Health (NIH). (2019). *Grants & funding: Types of grant programs.* Retrieved from https://grants.nih.gov/grants/funding/funding_program.htm

Nock, B. (August 2, 2016). *Auditing medical records in 8 easy steps.* Ease the Way Blog. Retrieved from https://www.gebauer.com/blog/auditing-medical-records

Office of Disease Prevention and Health Promotion. (2019). *Healthy people 2030 framework.* Retrieved from https://www.healthypeople.gov/2020/About-Healthy-People/Development-Healthy-People-2030/Framework

Olson, E. (2018). The Fakegate scandal: Social marketing ethics in promoting a difficult-to-sell good cause. *Journal of Social Marketing, 8*(3), 297–313. doi: 10.1108/JSOCM-04-2017-0030.

Ottoson, J. M., & Green, L. W. (2008). Public health education and health promotion. In L. F. Novick, C. B. Morrow, & G. P. Mays (Eds.), *Public health administration: Principles for population-based management* (2nd ed., pp. 589–619). Sudbury, MA: Jones & Bartlett Publishers.

Owen, J. (2017). NICE turns to Snapchat to connect with young people. *PR Week.* Retrieved from https://www.prweek.com/article/1423560/nice-turns-snapchat-connect-young-people

Pelletier, L. C., & Beaudin, C. L. (2018). *HQ solutions: Resource for the healthcare quality professional* (4th ed.). Philadelphia, PA: Wolters Kluwer.

Pew Research Center. (2019). *Social media fact sheet.* Retrieved from https://www.pewinternet.org/fact-sheet/social-media/

Piltch-Loeb, R., Abramson, D., & Merdjanoff, A. (2017). Risk salience of a novel virus: US population risk perception, knowledge, and receptivity to public health interventions regarding the Zika virus prior to local transmission. *PLoS One, 12*(12), e0188666. doi: 10.1371/journal.pone.0188666.

Public Health Accreditation Board. (2014). *Standards and measures: Summary of version 1.5 revisions and clarifications.* Retrieved from http://www.phaboard.org/wp-content/uploads/Version-1.5-changes-and-clarifications-FINAL1.pdf

Public Health Accreditation Board. (2019). *National voluntary accreditation for public health departments.* Retrieved from https://phaboard.org/who-is-accredited/

Quality and Safety Education for Nurses (QSEN). (2019). *Project overview: The evolution of the Quality and Safety Education for Nurses (QSEN) project.* Retrieved from https://qsen.org/about-qsen/project-overview/

Quality and Safety Education for Nurses (QSEN). (2020). *QSEN competencies: Overview.* Retrieved from https://qsen.org/competencies/pre-licensure-ksas/

Resnick, E. A., & Siegel, M. (2013). *Marketing public health: Strategies to promote social change.* Burlington, MA: Jones & Bartlett Learning.

Seow, H., Qureshi, D., Barbera, L., McGrail, K., Lawson, B., Burge, F., & Sutradhar, R. (2018). Benchmarking time to initiation of end-of-life homecare nursing: A population-based cancer cohort study in regions across Canada. *BMC Palliative Care, 17,* 70. Retrieved from https://www.ncbi.nlm.nih.gov/pmc/articles/PMC5936018/pdf/12904_2018_Article_321.pdf

Sharma, A. E., Huang, B., Knox, M., Willard-Grace, R., & Potter, M. B. (2018). Patient engagement in community health center leadership: How does it happen? *Journal of Community Health, 43*(6), 1069–1074. doi: 10.1007/s10900-018-0523-z.

Sills, F. W. (2015). Contemporary legal issues for the nurse administrator. In J. Dunham-Taylor & J. Z. Pinczuk (Eds.), *Financial management for nurse managers: Merging the heart with the dollar* (3rd ed., pp. 347–378). Burlington, MA: Jones and Bartlett.

Tatlow-Golden, M., Hennessy, E., Dean, M., & Hollywood, L. (2014). Young children's food brand knowledge. Early development and associations with television viewing and parent's diet. *Appetite, 80,* 197–203. doi: 10.1016/j.appet.2014.05.015.

The Food Trust. (2012). *What we do: Nutrition education*. Retrieved from http://thefoodtrust.org/what-we-do/schools/nutrition-education

The Omaha System. (2019). *Omaha system overview*. Retrieved from http://www.omahasystem.org/overview.html

U.S. Department of Health and Human Services. (2019a). *Geospatial data resources*. Retrieved from https://www.cdc.gov/gis/geo-spatial-data.html

U.S. Department of Health and Human Services. (2019b). *HealthData.gov*. Retrieved from https://healthdata.gov/node/1

Wang, J. W., Cap, S. S., & Hu, R. Y. (2019). Smoking by family members and friends and electronic-cigarette use in adolescence: A systematic review and meta-analysis. *Tobacco Induced Diseases, 16*, 5. doi: 10.18332/tid/84864.

Worthman, C. M., Tomlinson, M., & Rotheram-Borus, M. J. (2016). When can parents most influence their child's development? Expert knowledge and perceived local realities. *Social Science & Medicine, 154*, 62–69. doi: 10.1016/j.socscimed.2016.02.040.

Zahid, A., & Reicks, M. (2018). Gain-framed messages were related to higher motivation scores for sugar-sweetened beverage parenting practices than loss-framed messages. *Nutrients, 10*(5), 625. doi: 10.3390/nu10050625.

CHAPTER 13

Policy Making and Advocacy

"Never doubt that a small group of thoughtful citizens can change the world. Indeed, it is the only thing that ever has."

—Margaret Mead

KEY TERMS

Advocacy
Community empowerment
Health policy
Lobbying
Polarization
Policy
Policy analysis
Policy competence
Political action committee (PAC)
Politics
Power
Public policy
Special interest groups

LEARNING OBJECTIVES

Upon mastery of this chapter, you should be able to:

1. Describe the relationship between social policy and health outcomes.
2. Define health policy and explain how it is established.
3. Provide one health-relevant example of policy in each jurisdiction: local, state, and federal.
4. Describe how a bill becomes a law on the federal level.
5. Discuss policy examples for legislation, regulation, and policy modification.
6. Contrast the rational framework with Kingdon's framework for policy analysis and identify when each would be most useful for public health nurses (PHNs).
7. Identify three ways a PHN can engage in policy activism.
8. Identify the difference between advocacy and lobbying, as well as the influence of both on policy.
9. Describe three components of the Patient Protection and Affordable Care Act that impact the health of the public.
10. Discuss power and empowerment and the roles these concepts play in policy development.

INTRODUCTION

Public health policy consists of the rules, regulations, legislation, and funding that we, as members of the public, choose to establish to govern the provision, regulation, and research of health care for our fellow Americans. All legislation and health care regulation decision making include discussions over priorities and how they will be addressed. In all legislative activities and reforms, social and political factions are at work—special interest groups, business, and industry each bring their influence into play (Payne, 2017).

Because the outcomes determine the availability and quality of all health and social services, nurses need to develop a working knowledge of health policy formation and the political process in order to advocate for and protect the individuals, families, and communities they serve, as well as support their own nursing practice. For community/public health nurses (C/PHNs), policy outcomes impact the communities in which we practice, our personal health, and the health of our neighborhoods and country. The C/PHN needs to understand how to provide input to policy through advocacy and leadership in decision making.

In this chapter, we will discuss the current state of the health of people in the United States, how policy impacts health, how policy is developed, and how C/PHNs can be involved in health policy formation. We will discuss specific examples of C/PHN policy involvement and potential action, given the current health care policy environment in the United States.

HEALTH IN THESE UNITED STATES: HOW HEALTHY ARE WE?

The US health care system is recognized worldwide for medical achievements such as the mapping of the human genome, advances in biomedical technologies, and increasing numbers of pharmaceuticals that hold promise for addressing the myriad chronic and acute illnesses that affect the world's populations. The US health care system is also known to be expensive. Current data indicate that the United States spends 17.8% of its gross domestic product on health care costs; this is twice as much as the average health care expenditures from countries with similar levels of economic development (Rapaport, 2018). High expenditures are not necessarily problematic as long as the nation can afford them and they result in positive health outcomes. However, for the amount the United States spends on health care, are we achieving the results we desire (Box 13-1)?

The United States performs better than comparable countries in some areas and grossly underperforms in others. According to the Organization for Economic Co-operation and Development (OECD, 2017) the United States performs poorer than peer countries in the areas of

- Infant mortality and low birth weight
- Injuries and homicides
- Adolescent pregnancy and sexually transmitted infections (STIs)
- HIV and AIDS
- Drug-related deaths (Box 13-2)
- Obesity and diabetes
- Cardiovascular disease
- Chronic lung disease
- Disability

The OECD report (2017) also documents areas where the Unites States compares favorably to peer countries. These areas include

- Cancer mortality
- Stroke mortality
- Control of blood pressure and cholesterol levels
- Suicide
- Elderly survival
- Self-rated health

Areas of strength for the United States include cancer and stroke mortality and control of blood pressure and cholesterol (OECD, 2017). These are a result of advances in early diagnosis and development of new, more effective pharmaceutical treatments. Elderly survival is also likely related to medication therapy and technological advances in old age. For those who live to age 75 years, their odds of living longer are greatly increased. Self-rated health is high in the United States, possibly because our technological developments provide consumers with the perception of great medical advances from which it is logical to conclude that one's health outcomes are positive. Lastly, although the United States compares favorably in the area of suicide, the US population does not compare favorably in the category of gun-assisted suicide, for which our numbers far exceed those in our peer countries.

More recent data indicate similar trends. The Peterson-Kaiser Health System Tracker shows that although mortality rates have fallen for all developed countries, they remain slightly higher in the United States than in similar countries. In addition, measures of potential years of life lost (PYLL) (Fig. 13-1), disease burden, and hospitalizations for preventable conditions are all higher in the United States than in comparable countries (Sawyer & Gonzales, 2017). The Commonwealth Fund presents data on health care system performance across 11 developed countries. The United States ranks last among the countries in this study. Five aspects are ranked, including access, equity, administrative efficiency, care process, and health care outcomes. Among these, the United States ranks last in access, equity, and health care outcomes and next to last in administrative efficiency, as reported by patients and providers (Schneider, Sarnak, Squires, Shah, & Doty, 2017).

These rankings all highlight outcomes related to problems with the health care system in the United States. The authors present a variety of explanations for these

BOX 13-1 WHAT DO *YOU* THINK?

Access to Health Care

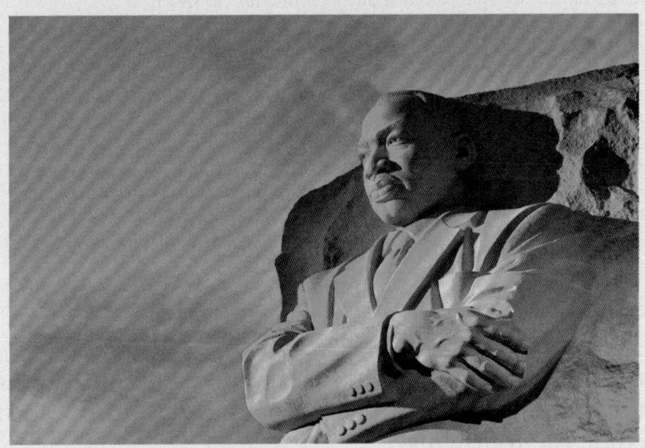

Martin Luther King, Jr. Memorial.

"Of all the forms of inequality, injustice in health is the most shocking and the most inhuman because it often results in physical death."

—Dr. Martin Luther King

In the decade or so leading up to President Clinton's attempt at health care reform in the 1990s, the debate about access to health care centered on whether health care was a right or a privilege. What do you think? Should there be some basic rights regarding access to services as found in most other developed nations (e.g., a safety net)? Or is this a privilege that is accessed as a primary good that people budget for out of their personal resources? With the Patient Protection and Affordable Care Act (ACA), those with preexisting conditions were protected, but this and other provisions of the law are being challenged. What changes have happened in the ACA since it was enacted? Have these new changes affected you or someone you know?

BOX **13-2** STORIES FROM THE FIELD

Opioids in America

In the United States, from 1999 to 2017, more than 700,000 people died as a result of a drug overdose. In 2017, 68% of overdose-related deaths involved an opioid (including prescription and illegal opioids), making this six times higher than in 1999. On average, 130 Americans die each day as a result of an opioid overdose (CDC, n.d.).

The causes of this epidemic are complex. One contributor was the increase in prescription of opioid medications, which lead to misuse, before it was known that these medications are highly addictive (DHHS, 2019; NAM, 2017). Established addiction leads many prescription opioid users to seek nonprescription opioids (NAM, 2017). In fact, 80% of heroin users started with prescription opioid use (Muhuri, Gfroerer, & Davies, 2017). There is a complex interaction between obesity, disability, chronic pain, depression, and substance use that has not been fully explored in relation to opioid misuse (Dasgupta, Beletsky, & Ciccarone, 2018). Further, the communities in which people live are influential factors in the opioid epidemic. Risk is compounded by overall poor health, poverty, lack of opportunity, and inadequate living and working conditions. The contributors to the opioid epidemic are public health policy issues.

Taylor is a 35-year-old who visits her primary care provider (PCP) for a chronic pain follow-up visit. During this visit, the PCP notes that the patient was prescribed an opioid for pain management 6 months ago. The patient has requested refills 4 to 7 days early each month. The patient reports limited pain relief and becomes agitated when the PCP offers alternative, nonopioid pain management options. By using motivational interviewing techniques, the PCP engages the patient in a discussion about her medication use. During this discussion, the patient shares that she has been misusing her opioid prescription for the past 5 months and has resorted to using nonprescription opioids when her prescriptions run out. After much discussion, the patient acknowledges her misuse of opioids and asks for assistance in seeking treatment. Together, the PCP and patient develop a plan for next steps of care.

The health care system, in this case, functioned well in that Taylor had access to care and her care provider provided high-quality, evidence-based care to assist her in seeking treatment.

However, when Taylor leaves the clinic, there are additional resources necessary to help her reach her goals.

1. *Does she have access to transportation necessary to seek treatment? Such access could be related to where she lives, or her income level.*
2. *Will her health insurance cover necessary follow-up and treatment options?*
3. *What community factors influence her opioid use? Does she live in poverty, with few opportunities for safe work and housing?*

The ability of Taylor to carry out a plan for treating her opioid misuse is related to policies that impact adequate housing, safe working conditions, social and economic stability, health insurance coverage, and access to illegal opioids.

1. *How does the health care system use its knowledge to influence such policies in ways that combat the opioid epidemic?*
2. *How can and should health professionals be involved in the development or implementation of policies to promote healthy lifestyles?*

Source: CDC (n.d.); Dasgupta et al. (2018); DHHS (2019); Muhuri et al. (2017); NAM (2017).

health inequities, including a lack of attention within the current health care system to the social determinants of health, the challenges to access to health care, and public policies that do not address the nonclinical causes of poor health.

PYLL is a measure of premature death and provides a method to measure deaths that occur at a younger age and that may be preventable. PYLL is calculated by multiplying the number of deaths that occur at each age by the number of years left to live, up to a specific age limit. The age used by the OECD is 70 years old. This measure is used across countries to compare preventable mortality (OECD, 2017; see https://data.oecd.org/healthstat/potential-years-of-life-lost.htm).

This raises the question: what is health policy and how it is relevant to community/public health nursing? If C/PHNs are to promote and protect the health of populations (American Public Health Association [APHA], PHN Section, 2013), they need to understand health policy as it relates to the health of the public. Policies affect our daily lives, regardless of whether they are related to health or work. Thus, C/PHNs need an understanding of health policy to better address the issues affecting the health of the communities they serve and improve health outcomes. Relevant questions include the following:

- How does health policy impact the health of the population?
- How is policy important in addressing both issues of access to care and of creating and supporting the social conditions that support health?
- What is the relationship between politics and health policy?
- What do C/PHNs need to understand about health policy and its formation?
- How can nurses become involved in the political process and in promoting effective health policies?

In the remainder of the chapter, we will discuss policy, how it is formed, how C/PHNs can gain policy competence to impact policy in their practice, and the policy changes resulting from the Patient Protection and Affordable Care Act (ACA) and its implementation over time (U.S. Department of Health and Human Services [USDHHS], 2015). We will also discuss the relationship of politics and health policy.

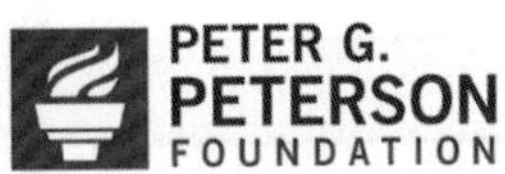

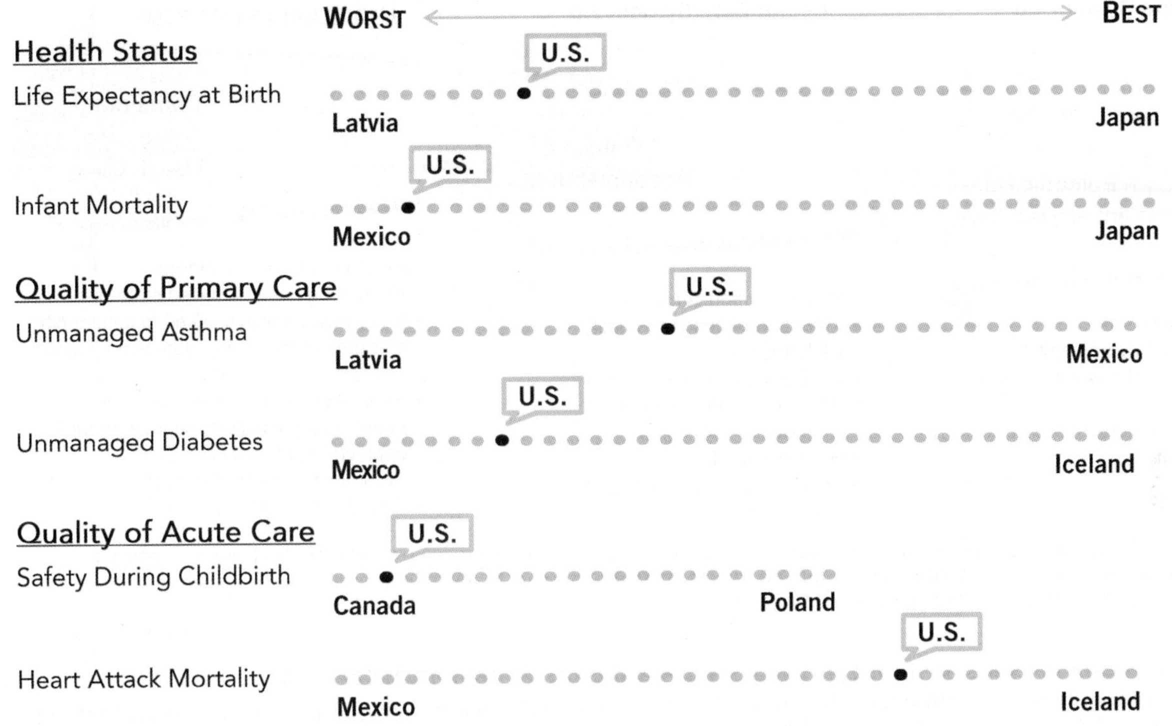

FIGURE 13-1 Global health outcomes rankings. (© 2019 Peterson G. Peterson Foundation. Used with permission. Retrieved from https://www.pgpf.org/sites/default/files/0011_health-outcomes.pdf)

HEALTH POLICY ANALYSIS

What Is Policy?

To effect changes in the health care system requires changes in health care policies. What does that mean? Policy analysts define **policy** as

- A relatively stable, purposive course of action taken over time to deal with a problem or matter of concern
- Actions that emerge in response to needs or demands; can be negative or positive; authoritative
- Actions that relate to government action, not stated intention; based on law/regulation (Anderson, 2015)

Policies lead to laws, regulations, or administrative rulings. When issued by national, state, or local governments, they are called **public policy**. **Health policy** refers to specific policies involving health and health care. There are also different types of policies:

- *Substantive policy:* This refers to policy that involves an action or activity, such as funding for a health program or health-related agency. One example would be federal funding for the Indian Health Service and its activities.
- *Procedural policy:* These involve the procedure by which an outcome is sought. An example of this would be voting rights policies, which stipulate the process for voting eligibility.
- *Distributive policy:* These include policies that allocate services or benefits to specific groups of people. Medicare, for example, distributes resources to people who meet age and/or physical condition criteria.
- *Regulatory policy:* These put limitations on the activities or behaviors of certain groups or individuals, such as age limits for purchase of alcohol or health professional licensing regulations (Birkland, 2019).

Nancy Milio, a well-known PHN, wrote extensively on policy and public health nursing practice, coining the term *healthy public policy*. In her classic work on health policy, Milio (1981) defined policy as option setting:

> To bring about the largest improvement in health requires the development of policies that will change the options that organizations and individuals face today… It would provide new, easier opportunities, or reduce the cost of current options, in areas that now lack health-promoting resources. (p. 76)

Neal Halfon illustrated how the US health care system has evolved over time in its policy options, moving

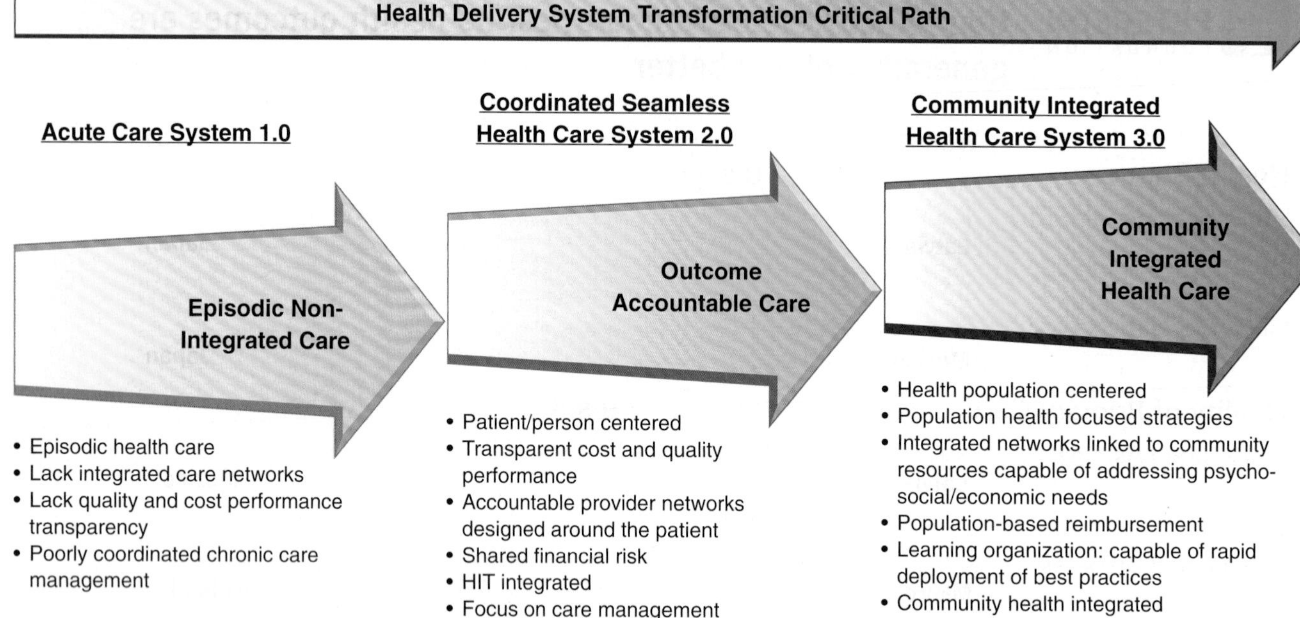

FIGURE 13-2 Health delivery system transformation critical path. (Adapted with permission from Halfon, N., Long, P., Chang, D. I., Hester, J., Inkelas, M., & Rogers, A. (2014). Applying A 3.0 transformation framework to guide large-scale health system reform. *Health Affairs, 33*(11), 2003–2011. doi: 10.1377/hlthaff.2014.0485.)

from a focus on short-term system of episodic nonintegrated care to a system of community integrated care—with an increased focus on population health strategies that address the social determinants of health (2014; see Fig. 13-2).

What Is Politics?

While defining policy is important, understanding policy also requires attending to policy formation, implementation, and evaluation. An essential aspect of this is knowing the role politics plays in the policy process.

Politics is defined as the process by which society determines who gets what, when they get it, and how they get it (Birkland, 2019). It is often discussed as the art of using influence to bring about change, which includes the efforts in which groups or individuals engage to influence, gain power, or get their way.

- The legislative and regulatory process may start with lofty goals, but the final product is usually the result of compromise often encouraged by special interest groups, coalition groups, political realities, or the current economic environment.
- Politics includes discussions related to the values or ethics of a society, such as the conflict between individual needs and the needs of a community. Examples include the debate around assisted suicide or the continuing dispute regarding universal health care.
- The classic understanding of politics was stated by the late Massachusetts Congressman and former Speaker of the House, Tip O'Neill, in his book, "*All Politics Is Local*" (1993). No matter the definition of politics or the topic of debate, the role of C/PHNs is to be responsive to the needs of the community they serve.

Local, State, and National Level Policy

One of the first policy questions to address is that of jurisdiction. Public policy is decided and impacts health and well-being at local, state, and national levels (Box 13-3). Because of this, it is essential to know whether the key decision makers are local, state, or national policymakers.

Local Policy

Many policies that impact health care are developed and implemented at the local level. Although local policies may also be subject to guidelines from other jurisdictions (e.g., state, federal), a hallmark of the US governmental system has been to have robust local policy authority (National League of Cities, 2016). While the U.S. Constitution specifically details state authority, each state also gives powers to local governments. This means the policy-competent C/PHN needs to know what jurisdiction governs any relevant issue.

- Public policies such as tobacco use in public places, requirements for gun ownership, or speed limits on public roads are often made by local-level governing bodies.
- At the local level, these policies are very open to public involvement, because often the legislative and regulatory bodies are easily accessed and composed of community residents. The C/PHN is often able to collect or interpret data relevant to the health impact of local policies and can talk directly to decision makers about local policy concerns.

State Policy

There is a limit to municipal powers and some policies are developed and regulated at the state level. Longest (2016) notes that the role of states in health policy includes being public health guardians (e.g., protect public health and

BOX 13-3 POLICY IMPACTS AT THE LOCAL, STATE, AND NATIONAL LEVELS

Local Policy

In January 2016, the mayor of the city of Chicago called for legislation to increase the minimum age for purchasing of tobacco from 18 to 21 years. Teenagers are the largest group of new smokers, and research suggests that increasing the legal age to purchase tobacco is part of an overall strategy to discourage teens from using tobacco products (Rhodes, 2016).

State Policy

As of 2017, two states have signed into law new regulations about prescription drug pricing. California enacted legislation to require advance notice and justification to public and private health plans about significant prescription drug price increases—those of 16 percent or more over 2 years. Maryland passed a law allowing the state's attorney general to sue generic drug manufacturers who engage in price gouging and rveturn that money to consumers and others who pay for the drugs or make the drug available at its previous price (Families USA Blog, 2017).

National Policy

Data indicate that climate change can have detrimental health effects on populations including increased respiratory and cardiovascular disease, injuries and premature deaths related to extreme weather events, changes in the prevalence and geographical distribution of food- and water-borne illnesses and other infectious diseases, and threats to mental health (NIEHS, 2018). National policy efforts, implemented by the Environmental Protection Agency (2019), included voluntary business participation resulting in cost savings of $37 billion and avoided emissions of 470 million tons carbon dioxide equivalent.

Source: Environmental Protection Agency (2019); Families USA (2017); NIEHS (2018); Rhodes (2016).

welfare through laws and regulations), health care service purchasers (often in conjunction with the federal level; safety-net providers), and providers of education and public health laboratory services.

- Health and related policies such as Medicaid eligibility and services, health professional license regulation and scope of practice, and public health codes, including immunization regulations, are some of the functions that fall within state powers.
- With the passage of the ACA in 2010, participation in the marketplace of insurance plans and expanded federal funding for Medicaid were decisions made by some state legislatures and had significant impacts on access to care (Kaiser Family Foundation, 2019).

National Policy

- Public health policies are also developed and implemented at the national level. Funding for the health insurance plan, Medicare, the ACA, parts of Medicaid, and health research are all national-level policies.
- This level of policy has the advantage of being broadly applicable across the country, with the potential for significant impact on population health.
- It can be challenging to work at this level because there are a large number of stakeholders and an enormous political and policy bureaucracy for creation implementation and evaluation of legislation. However, federal funding and regulatory requirements impact the role and practice of C/PHNs, and C/PHN practice includes being aware of, and in compliance with, federal policies.

Legislative Process at the National Level

The federal model for how an idea becomes a bill and how a bill is passed into legislation is relevant across the country. States each have their own mechanism.

- The first step in becoming policy competent on any issue is to know under which jurisdiction the issue falls (local, state, or federal) and then know how policy is developed and regulated at that level. There are a wide variety of Web sites and descriptions of the legislative process, but the definitive version can be found on the House of Representatives Web site: http://www.house.gov/content/learn/legislative_process/.
- It is estimated that 5% or less of bills introduced into any session of Congress actually become laws (Govtrack, 2019). The two session of Congress between 2013 and 2017 only enacted 3% of bills into law (Civic Impulse, 2018).

How a Bill Becomes a Law

This section will review the process for how a bill becomes a law at the federal level, but the process is very similar at the state level. See Figures 13-3 and 13-4 for state and federal examples.

Ideas for legislation can originate anywhere and be introduced as legislation at the state and federal levels. For federal legislation, the bill is introduced in either the House of Representatives or the Senate. Only budget bills must originate in the House of Representatives. This was done to keep the budget process closest to the "people's house," the body of the legislature where members represent relatively small numbers of constituents for 2-year terms and thus are thought to be more responsive to their constituents (Longest, 2016).

- When a bill is introduced to either house, it is assigned to a committee based upon the general area of focus (e.g., appropriations, agriculture). The committee structure is designed to allow members of each house to focus on a smaller number of issues in depth and then vote, as a whole, on issues that are deemed worthy of going before the whole legislature (i.e., going to the "floor") for a vote.
- Often, bills never leave the committee, stalling there because of lack of interest from the majority party, whose members chair committees and thus set the committee's agenda in both houses.

Some bills have hearings, where experts are brought in to testify to facets of the bill and answer questions from the committee members. For bills where there is

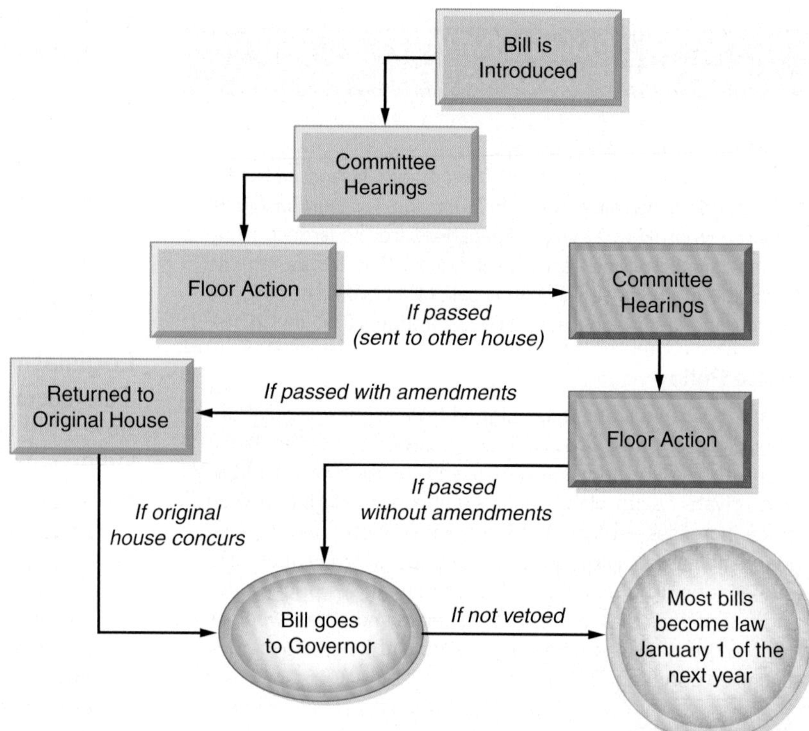

FIGURE 13-3 How a bill becomes a law—state process. The process may vary by state, but generally the schematic shows how the process unfolds. (Source: California Legislative Counsel.)

sufficient interest or political will, the bill will be discussed, amended as needed, and voted upon in the committee. If the bill passes in committee, it is sent to the full house for further discussion, possible amendments, and an ultimate vote (Longest, 2016).

- If the bill passes the full house, it is sent to the other chamber, and the process begins again. Sometimes, bills are introduced simultaneously to both houses, which can speed the process, as each committee and house reviews and votes on the bill during the same time period.
- If the bill is passed in each house, but in a slightly different version, a conference committee, composed of members of both houses, is convened to discuss, amend, and vote on the bill.
    - The bill can stall in the conference committee until the session of Congress ends, and then it would need to be reintroduced in the next session, as bills do not carry over from one session to the next.
    - Alternatively, the bill may be passed by the conference committee and then be returned to each chamber for a final vote. At this point, amendments would not be added or the bill would be stalled again and have to go back through the process once again (Longest, 2016; U.S. House of Representatives, n.d.).
- After both chambers of Congress pass the same version of a bill, it goes to the president for signature.
    - The president can sign the bill, in which case it becomes law and is sent to the appropriate administrative agency for rulemaking.
    - The president can actively or passively veto the legislation, in which case the bill needs to be sent back to each chamber for a 2/3 vote to override the president's veto, or the bill stalls again, and the process begins anew.

In summary, passing legislation is a complex process, designed for maximum debate and representation to avoid frivolous, dangerous, or unnecessary legislation (U.S. House of Representatives, n.d.).

There are other important aspects of the legislative process of which the C/PHN needs to be aware. These include the rulemaking process, implementation, evaluation, policy modification, and judicial action.

Rulemaking and Implementation

- After a bill is passed and signed into law, it is sent to the appropriate administrative agency to develop rules and processes for implementation.
- After these rules are developed, they are published in the Federal Register with a designated time period for public comment. Comments are reviewed and used to revise and edit the rules as needed.
- The rules are then published, along with an effective date for implementation, and are used to guide organizations and individuals in implementing the policy; rules provide the "who, what, where, when, how, and why" of the law.

These rules can be critical to the actual impact of legislation, as they guide how the policy intent will be carried out (Office of the Federal Register, n.d.). Subtle changes to one or two words can significantly alter the legislature's intent.

Evaluation and Judicial Action

Evaluation of policy is sometimes written into the law and sometimes requested as part of the rulemaking process as a step in implementation. These evaluation data can be used for policy modifications or for modifications of the rules for implementation. Policy evaluation is designed to help the legislature know whether a policy is

HOW DOES A BILL BECOME A LAW?

1 EVERY LAW STARTS WITH AN IDEA

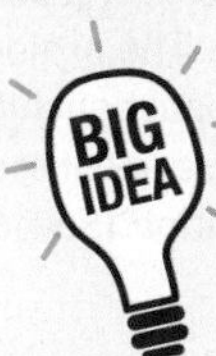

That idea can come from anyone, even you! Contact your elected officials to share your idea. If they want to try to make it a law, they will write a bill.

2 THE BILL IS INTRODUCED

A bill can start in either house of Congress when it's introduced by its primary sponsor, a Senator or a Representative. In the House of Representatives, bills are placed in a wooden box called "the hopper."

the HOPPER

Here, the bill is assigned a legislative number before the Speaker of the House sends it to a committee.

3 THE BILL GOES TO COMMITTEE

Representatives or Senators meet in a small group to research, talk about, and make changes to the bill. They vote to accept or reject the bill and its changes before sending it to:

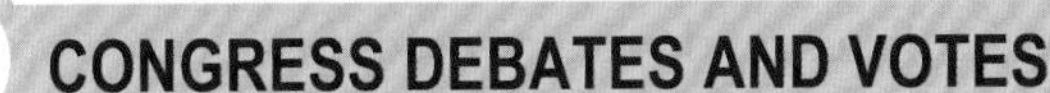

the House or Senate floor for debate or to a subcommittee for further research.

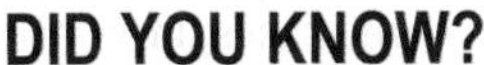

4 CONGRESS DEBATES AND VOTES

Members of the House or Senate can now debate the bill and propose changes or amendments before voting. If the majority vote for and pass the bill, it moves to the other house to go through a similar process of committees, debate, and voting. Both houses have to agree on the same version of the final bill before it goes to the President.

DID YOU KNOW?

The House uses an electronic voting system while the Senate typically votes by voice, saying "yay" or "nay."

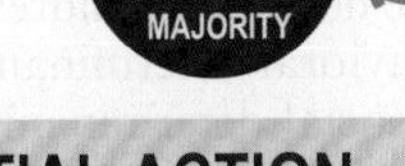
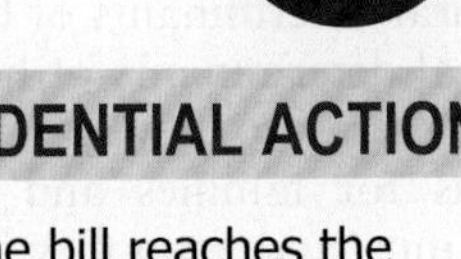

5 PRESIDENTIAL ACTION

When the bill reaches the President, he or she can:

✓ APPROVE and PASS

The President signs and approves the bill. The bill is law.

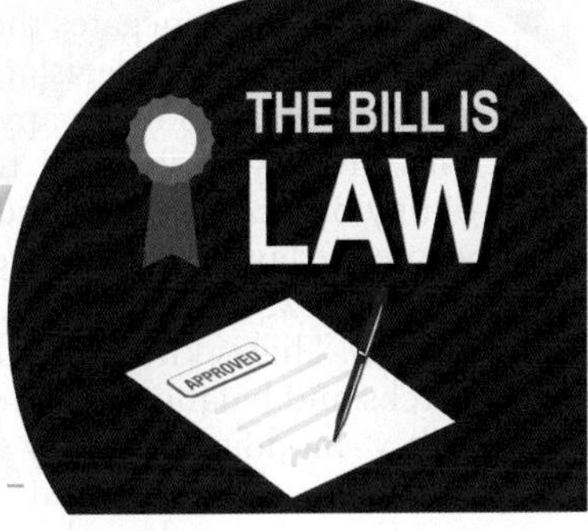

The President can also:

Veto

The President rejects the bill and returns it to Congress with the reasons for the veto. Congress can override the veto with 2/3 vote of those present in both the House and the Senate and the bill will become law.

Choose no action

The President can decide to do nothing. If Congress is in session, after 10 days of no answer from the President, the bill then automatically becomes law.

Pocket veto

If Congress adjourns (goes out of session) within the 10 day period after giving the President the bill, the President can choose not to sign it and the bill will not become law.

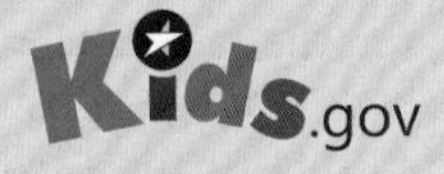

Brought to you by usa gov

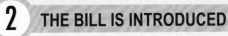

FIGURE 13-4 How does a bill become a law?—federal level. (Reprinted from *How laws are made and how to research them.* (2020). Retrieved from https://www.usa.gov/how-laws-are-made)

BOX 13-4 An Example of Evaluating Policy Changes: Paying for Performance

In the past, injury or illness related to hospital stays were often recognized as inevitable consequences. However, the Patient Protection and Affordable Care Act created a Hospital-Acquired Condition (HAC) Reduction Program. The goal of this program is to reduce the number of HAC and improve overall patient outcomes (CMS, 2019). This is encouraged through reduced Medicaid payments for hospitals that do not meet benchmarks for HAC (CMS, 2019). The promise of reduced reimbursement has led to a number of nurse-led interventions to reduce HAC and improve patient outcomes. A nurse-led effort to combat a common HAC is explored below.

Central line–associated bloodstream infections (CLABSIs) are defined as "a laboratory-confirmed bloodstream infection not related to an infection at another site that develops within 48 hours of a central line placement." CLASBIs increase patient mortality and health care costs. In fact, they are the most expensive of all hospital-acquired infections, costing approximately $46,000 per case (Haddadin & Regunath, 2019).

Nursing leadership at a Tennessee pediatric medical facility developed, implemented, and evaluated an intervention to prevent CLASBIs in their pediatric and neonatal intensive care units. Nurses created an evidence-based CLASBI prevention bundle that included a variety of insertion, maintenance, and prevention strategies. After the implementation of this nurse-led intervention, the hospitals CLASBI rate decrease from 3.80 out of 1,000 lines day to 0.45 ($p < 0.001$). The project resulted in decreases across all units to below national benchmarks. This project demonstrates the success of a nurse-led intervention to decrease CLASBIs for a vulnerable population (Savage, Hodge, Pickard, Myers, & Powell, 2018).

1. *Do you think nurses are generally aware of legislation that affects their workplace, practice, and patient outcomes? Why? Why not?*
2. *How could nurses become involved in the implementation of new laws/regulations and policy evaluation?*

Source: CMS (2019); Haddadin and Regunath (2019); Savage et al. (2018).

having the intended impact on the problem or condition it was designed to address. See Box 13-4 for an example of policy evaluation.

- The judicial branch of government is designed to interpret laws and ensure they align with the constitution. In some cases, laws are challenged, and the challenge works its way through various levels of judicial decision making.
- Courts can void a law or require that it be changed in some way to comply with the constitution. If this involves omitting part of the law, this can be done while implementation continues.
    - If such a change negates the intent or desired outcome of the law, the legislative process would have to begin again to make any substantive changes.
    - This process is designed to minimize the power of any branch of government: the legislators who wrote the law, the executive branch who administers the law, or the judicial branch who interprets the law. This is known as the American system of checks and balances (White House, 2016).
    - Policy modification may occur, such as those related to the ACA, and may involve adjusting regulations to reflect changes in political climate or cost impacts (Commonwealth Fund, 2018). See Box 13-5 for an example of policy modification.

Policy and Public Health Nursing Practice

Now that we have some basic definitions of policy and politics, we can explore how policy is relevant to public health nursing practice. The definition of PHN practice developed and disseminated by the PHN Section of the APHA in 1996 and reaffirmed in 2013 is as follows:

> Public health nursing is the practice of promoting and protecting the health of populations using knowledge from nursing, social, and public health sciences. (APHA, PHN Section, 2013, para. 5)

The definition, and its background statements, includes several key elements:

- A focus on the health needs of an entire population
- Assessment of population health using a comprehensive, systematic approach
- Attention to multiple determinants of health
- An emphasis on primary prevention
- Application of interventions at all levels—individuals, families, communities, and the systems that impact their health

Therefore PHNs, by definition, are interested in health policy broadly, including both health care services and also policy as it relates to creating conditions in which people can be healthy by addressing the social, physiological, and behavioral determinants of health. Assessing and treating the social determinants of health includes working with communities to develop policies that impact living conditions for families and communities. Thus, C/PHN practice must address policy implications of health needs and conversely look at creating policies to promote and maintain health for communities and populations.

The term *public health nursing* was coined in 1893 by Lillian Wald, who described PHNs as nurses who worked outside the hospital "to provide decent health care" to those people living in poor communities and tenements (Jewish Women's Archive, 2016, para. 2). See Chapter 3 for more information on PHN nursing history. These nurses specialized in both preserving health and implementing prevention measures as they responded to referrals from patients and physicians; they were only paid for their services if the patient was able to afford payment. In 1893, Lillian Wald and Mary Brewster established the Visiting Nurse Service, and a year later, the famed Henry Street Settlement House was established. Wald's exposure to the plight of newly arrived immigrants to the Lower East Side and the appalling living conditions there spurred her to action. She was determined that these immigrants

BOX 13-5 A History of Tobacco Legislation in the United States

The tobacco industry has been regulated through state and national legislation since the early 1900s, with several policies and policy modifications. Policies have been created and modified as a result of new scientific discoveries about the negative impact of tobacco use and in an effort to protect the health of the public. With the recent advent of electronic cigarettes, many tobacco policies have been created or modified to include new methods of tobacco use.

1906 The Food and Drugs Act of 1906 did not include mention of tobacco. However, a 1914 advisor groups recommended that tobacco be included in modified legislation but only when used to prevent or treat disease.

1914 The Federal Trade Commission (FTC) Act of 1914 empowers the FTC to take action preventing people or organizations from using "unfair or deceptive acts or practices in commerce." This is important legislation as it allowed the FTC to regulate advertising of tobacco products. The FTC completed seven formal cease-and-desist order proceedings for medical or health claims of cigarettes between 1945 and 1960.

1938 The 1906 legislation was superseded by the Federal Food, Drug, and Cosmetic Act (FFDCA) of 1938, which allowed the government to regulate tobacco products used to prevent or treat disease. For example, in 1959, the FDA asserted jurisdiction over Trim Reducing-Aid Cigarettes that claimed to aid in weight reduction due to the additive tartaric acid.

1965 Federal Cigarette Labeling and Advertising Act of 1965 required cigarette packages to include a warning label stating, "Caution: Cigarette Smoking May Be Hazardous to Your Health" but did not require this warning to be included on advertisements.

1969 The Public Health Cigarette Smoking Act of 1969 required the following to be place on all cigarette packing and print advertising: "Warning: The Surgeon General Has Determined that Cigarette Smoking Is Dangerous to Your Health." This Act also prohibited radio and television advertising.

1984 The Comprehensive Smoking Education Act of 1984 requires four rotating warning labels on cigarettes about lung cancer, heart disease, pregnancy, and carbon monoxide. The Act also requires cigarette companies to provide a confidential list of ingredients to the government.

1986 The Comprehensive Smokeless Tobacco Health Education Act of 1986 required warning labels and prohibited radio and television advertising for smokeless tobacco products.

1987 Public Law 100–202 bans smoking on domestic airline flights 2 hours or less.

1992 The Synar Amendment to the Alcohol, Drug Abuse, and Mental Health Administration (ADAMHA) Reorganization Act of 1992 requires that all states adopt and enforce restrictions the sale and distribution of tobacco to minors.

2009 The Family Smoking Prevention and Tobacco Control Act of 2009 gives the Food and Drug Administration (FDA) the authority to regulate cigarettes, smokeless, and roll-your-own tobacco.

2016 The "Deeming Rule": Tobacco Products Deemed to be Subject to the Federal Food, Drug, and Cosmetic Act extended the reach of the FDA to regulate "hookah, e-cigarettes, dissolvables, smokeless tobacco, cigarettes, all cigars, roll-your-own tobacco, pipe tobacco, and future tobacco products that meet the statutory definition of a tobacco product" (USFDA, 2016, para 2).

The history of tobacco legislation in the United States is an example of how policies are created and/or modified in response to science to protect the nation's health.

1. *Can you think of an example of a current policy that requires modification based on new or emerging science?*
2. *What modifications would you suggest?*

Source: Centers for Disease Control and Prevention (CDC) (2017); Public Health Law Center (2019); U.S. Federal Drug Administration (FDA) (2016).

and other poor people, regardless of ethnicity or religious affiliation, would have access to health care and adequate housing. Wald went on to encourage the establishment of the Department of Nursing and Health at Columbia University's Teachers College through a series of lectures she presented starting in 1910. She was also instrumental in creating the U.S. Children's Bureau in 1912, an agency that oversaw fair child labor laws (see Chapter 3). Her work exemplifies how public health nursing and policy go hand-in-hand.

A recent movement in public health of interest to nurses is that of *Health in All Policies* (California Dept. of Public Health, 2018). The APHA presents this as embedding health considerations into decision-making processes across all sectors. An example of a *Health in All Policies* approach is a city planning policy that determines zoning for a new retirement community for seniors. In the planning phase for the project, a health impact assessment would be done.

- A health impact assessment (HIA) is a process that accesses potential health impacts of a plan, project, or policy prior to implementation.
- Results of a HIA are used by including public health impact in the decision-making process for projects and policies that fall outside of traditional public health arenas. Conducting a HIA reveals possible positive and negative health impacts (California Department of Public Health, 2018; CDC, 2016).

In this case, the HIA would look at health implications of different site options. For example, what are the health implications for the residents if the facility is built just off a major highway? Is the population being served particularly vulnerable to noise or auto exhaust? What about building the facility on the outskirts of a town? Does this population have unique transportation needs? *Health in all Policies* as an approach helps guide decision making across sectors to maximize health-enhancing options and minimize options that increase health risks for the populations involved.

For C/PHNs to be effective in the policy process, they need to be aware of policy implications on health planning and health-promoting interventions and be prepared to provide data to support policy recommendations that enhance the health opportunities for a target group or community. This is called being *policy competent* (Longest, 2016). **Policy competence** means being able to:

- Assess the impact of public policies on one's domain of interest/responsibility
- Understand policy and the policy process sufficiently to be able to exert influence on the process and impact policy
- Exert influence on the policymaking process

For Community/public health nursing practice, this means that the C/PHN is able to assess relevant policies and determine where the policy is in the policymaking process. The C/PHN must also be able to determine where action is needed to influence the policy process: data support, lobbying, development/testing of potential policy solutions, stakeholder convening, etc. The C/PHN might not be able to lobby due to his/her position (for instance, working for a government agency), but there are many other policy process activities that are relevant in planning and implementing health policy. There are few studies documenting the impact of C/PHN involvement in policy efforts, but those that exist demonstrate the importance of policy efforts in PHN practice.

- A study of African nurse leaders found that having knowledge of policy and practicing health policy development enhanced nursing's image, whereas a lack of policy involvement promoted a more negative nursing image and promoted processes and structures that excluded nurses (Shariff, 2014).
- Another study of Canadian PHNs in a rural community presented perspectives from the PHNs on how much of their role involved interpreting health policy to be able to meet the needs of rural women (Leipert, Regan, & Plunkett, 2015).

As we shall see later in the chapter, there are many activities relevant to the policy process in addition to lobbying for legislation.

POLICY ANALYSIS FOR THE PHN

Once C/PHNs understand how an idea becomes law, and how that law is implemented, they can begin to analyze the policy process to determine where they might become involved to create "healthy public policy." **Policy analysis** is the technique of understanding a policy from a variety of perspectives. Such analysis can provide results for better understanding policy, finding ways to impact policy development, understanding the values behind policy, tracking the history of policy in specific areas, and other policy-relevant research and practice questions. Policy analysis can be done using a variety of approaches and methods. Here, we will present policy analysis for practicing C/PHNs to help them develop policy competence.

Developing Policy Competence

- Policy competence means understanding policy and the policy process sufficiently to be able to exert influence on the process and impact policy (Longest, 2016).
- This can be done at a variety of levels. Because policy sets the context for much of C/PHN practice, policy competence is particularly important for C/PHNs, but all nurses should have some concept of how policy affects nurses, patients, and population health.
- For example, changes in Medicaid funding, at either the national or state level, might directly impact which clients the C/PHN is allowed to include in certain health promotion/disease prevention programs. Therefore, the C/PHN should understand this impact, the reasons for the Medicaid changes, and where useful input might be provided.
- This might be as straightforward as explaining to agency administrators what the impact of these changes will be on individuals in the community, or it may be more complicated and involve policy evaluation mechanisms or development of alternative policy solutions to meet the health goals of the community.

Frameworks for Policy Analysis

For the purposes of policy competence in C/PHN practice, we will discuss two frameworks for policy analysis, the rational framework and John Kingdon's framework. These frameworks provide two interrelated mechanisms for looking at the policy process and are combined into a useful diagram by Longest (2016) (Fig. 13-5).

The Rational Framework

- The rational framework is commonly found in policy texts as a straightforward way to comprehend the intent and effect of a particular policy.
- The framework involves defining the policy problem to be addressed. The more clear and measurable this problem definition is, the more specific any policy response can be.
- The second step in this framework is to understand possible solutions to this policy problem and compare and contrast them to each other in order to determine which is optimal in terms of being politically feasible, easily implemented, and likely to result in the desired outcome.
- The third step, based on comparing and contrasting the possible policy alternatives, is to select an alternative, implement it, and evaluate for its effectiveness (Kingdon, 2011).
- This logical analytic framework is very similar to the nursing process, in its structure and components, and as such is easily understood by C/PHNs (ANA, 2016b).

Policy researchers use policy analysis frameworks to guide research on policy impacts and outcomes. One classic example of Longest's framework in practice is as follows:

An example from Sri Lanka involves achieving a consensus on the public health problem of high rates of suicide (47 overall and 80 for males per 100,000—the highest in the world at that time). A presidential committee of experts was convened to examine and make recommendations about the problem, using the rational framework approach. A large proportion of suicides were

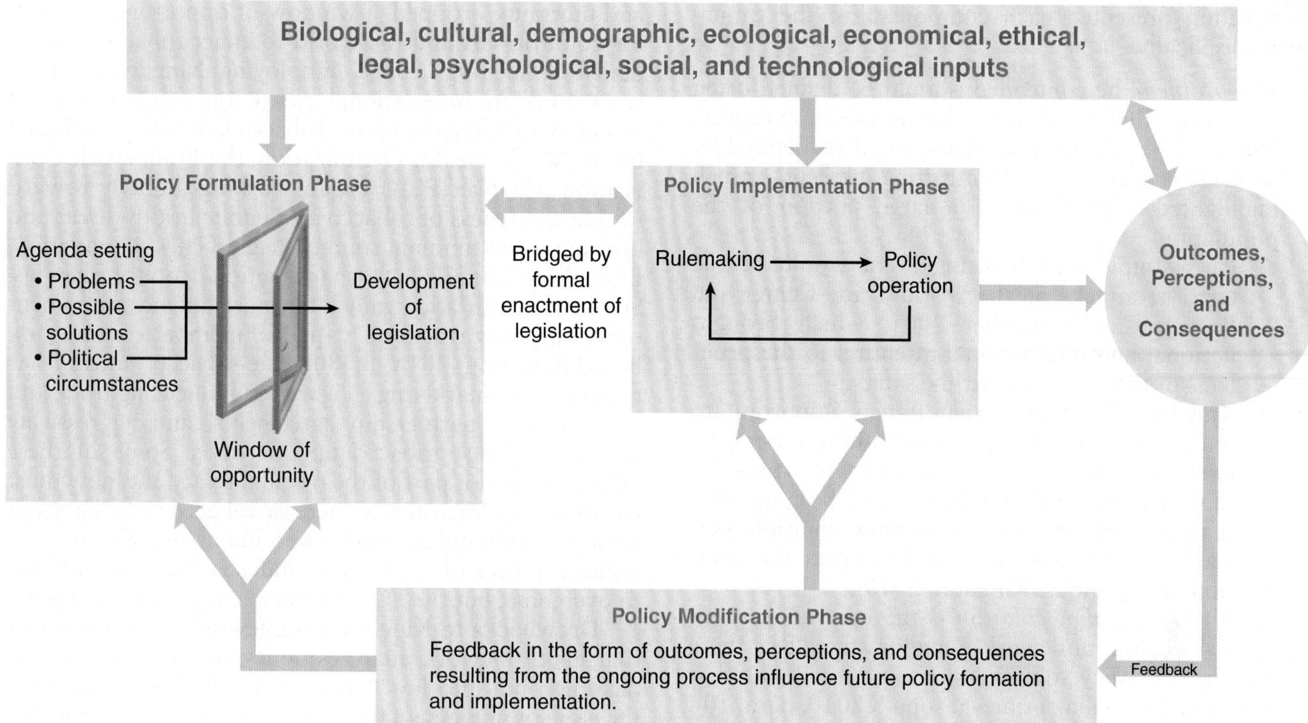

FIGURE 13-5 Longest's model. (Adapted with permission from Longest, B. B. (2016). *Health policymaking in the United States* (5th ed., p. 82). Chicago, IL: Health Administration Press.)

deemed self-poisoning, and suggestions ranged from reducing access to lethal pesticides, research to decrease the lethality level of pesticides, changing the culture to discourage suicides, repackaging pesticides into nonlethal doses, and increasing access to care to improve survival rates after suicidal poisoning. Once the data and the potential interventions were discussed, policy analysis was used to determine weaknesses, strengths, and costs of options. Interventions that required further political actions, such as taxation, new programs, or private sector self-interest, were weighed. The influence of expert evidence and data are not sufficient to change policies—political action is needed with an understanding of "context, networks, knowledge, implementation, and impact" (Pearson, Anthony, & Buckley, 2010, para. 37). Understanding of technical feasibility, budgets, marketability, and dominant cultural values is necessary, along with evidence and data, in order to exert political influence and change cultural practices.

There are several challenges to using this framework. Much like the nursing process, it examines policy as a structured, linear process, and that is often not the case. Challenges in defining the problem or in comparing viable solutions might often influence policy to be formed with insufficient data or based on the power and influence of specific stakeholders, meaning that all elements may not be considered carefully and in the order presented in the framework (Kingdon, 2011), Additionally, this framework doesn't assist the C/PHN in addressing the politics involved or in determining why one issue might be addressed when another—equally important to the community—might languish with no policy activity taking place.

Kingdon's Framework

The second framework to be discussed here is that developed by John Kingdon (2011) in his classic book (Fig. 13-6). Kingdon set out in his research to address the question of why some issues came to the forefront in policy development and others did not.

- Kingdon argued, based on his research results, that policy was enacted when a *window of opportunity* was opened. During the period of this open window, bills could be voted on and new legislation made.
- The window of opportunity opened when there was a confluence of a *policy problem*, a *viable solution* or solutions, and *political will* on this issue. This confluence opened a window of opportunity for the issue to be acted upon (however briefly).

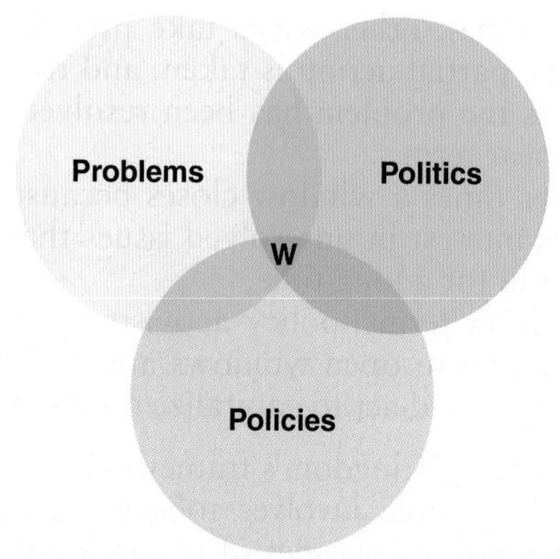

FIGURE 13-6 Kingdon's model of the policy process.

Kingdon presented each component of the framework specifically.

- The *problem*, he contended, should be defined using *indicators*, that is, data to document its existence. However, he also said problems could be defined by *focusing events*, or attention-getting incidents, which highlighted a problem for a large portion of the population.
  - An example of a focusing event would be the terrorist attacks on the World Trade Center and Pentagon in September 2001, which brought national and international attention to the problems of terrorism and airline safety.
  - Kingdon also argued that it was important to understand the problem from multiple perspectives, recognizing how others can interpret the same problem and data. In this way, he contended that the analyst could understand multiple perspectives and how they might impact the solutions and politics (Kingdon, 2010).
- Identifying a *policy solution* is the next component of the Kingdon framework. Kingdon stated that there are always policy solutions floating around in what he called the "policy primeval soup" (2010, para. 10).
  - He provided some parameters for assessing solutions: technical feasibility, acceptability in terms of public values, acceptable costs, alignment with the current size and role of government, fairness, and equity. He used these parameters to compare solutions for those most likely to align with problems and politics (Kingdon, 2011).
- When analyzing the *politics* of an issue, Kingdon had several facets to consider. First, being the political climate at the current time.
  - For example, immediately after the 9/11 terrorist attacks, the US political climate was focused almost entirely on safety and security, and very few other issues were being seriously addressed.
  - Kingdon (2010) also advised looking at stakeholders on both sides of an issue and assessing relative power and influence. This can be done by looking at the numbers of people they represent, resources available for lobbying, and political reputation and past achievements.
- When a *window of opportunity* does open, Kingdon (2010, 2011) cautioned that it does not remain open forever.
  - Sometimes, other issues take precedence. Sometimes, partial action is taken, and the public perceives the problem has been resolved, at least in the near term.
  - Other times a window closes because the public loses interest in unresolved issues that have been around for a long time.
- In Kingdon's terms, policy activists should look for opportunities to open windows and, when windows are open, should act to capitalize on the opportunity.

An example of Kingdom's framework in practice:

A global example involves tobacco control. As the United States utilized decades of research and began legislating no-smoking ordinances and tax increases on tobacco products and rates of tobacco-related morbidity and mortality dropped, a window of opportunity opened for countries around the world to enact tobacco control policies (Gneiting, 2016). Employing Kingdon's framework and an international treaty on tobacco control (Framework Convention on Tobacco Control) established by the World Health Organization, the Framework Convention Alliance (FCA) began working globally toward raising awareness of tobacco as a public health threat and utilizing new funding sources (e.g., Gates Foundation, Bloomberg Initiative) to shape national policy agendas. Smoke-free legislation gained the most "advocacy momentum and policy traction," with 120 member countries on board (Gneiting, 2016, p. i80). The tobacco industry has responded by marketing e-cigarettes, influencing trade and governmental partnership agreements, and aggressively lobbying against tobacco tax increases. Some of these measures are not part of the original treaty and now must be addressed. Measures to increase tobacco taxes have not been as successful as smoke-free initiatives. The relative political power of the tobacco industry has been difficult to overcome, but the FCA members continue their work.

Drawbacks to Kingdon's framework include the fact that his framework analyzes policy only to the point of passing a bill into law. His framework does not address the issue of implementation, evaluation, or policy modification. As mentioned earlier, Longest combined the rational framework and Kingdon's framework into a figure encompassing all facets of policymaking (Fig. 13-5).

For the policy analyst, both frameworks present important components of understanding an issue. The rational framework allows the analyst to look post hoc at an issue and learn from the process as it unfolded. For policy activists, or C/PHNs who want to use policy effectively in practice (policy competence), the Kingdon framework allows you to examine a current issue in real time and determine if a window of opportunity exists or if one could be created. This helps the C/PHN, or a public health organization, to prioritize its time and resources and focus policy efforts where they can be most effective.

Policy Analysis for Activism

Now, we will put this altogether to demonstrate how a C/PHN can use this information to be policy active in practice.

- The first step is to select a policy issue to address. Consider what health concern in your community has policy implications or is being impacted by current health policy or the lack thereof.
  - Perhaps there are water quality concerns in the community, or the most recent community assessment has identified an increase in STIs among adolescents and young adults. These are public policy issues; that is, they are issues that involve public decisions about laws and regulations related to funding, services, or rights and behaviors.
- The second step, once the C/PHN has determined that the issue is indeed one of public policy, is to conduct a brief policy analysis using Kingdon's framework initially: What is the *problem*? Are there *solutions*, and are they adequate and appropriate? What are the *politics*—or who are the stakeholders and what is their level of influence?

- This preliminary analysis will inform the C/PHN whether this is a new issue on the agenda or whether it is an issue of *implementation* or *evaluation* of existing legislation or regulations.
- Given this analysis, the C/PHN can determine the next steps. First, the C/PHN needs to know under what jurisdiction the policy falls (local, state, federal) and who key stakeholders and the target audiences are for any action. Perhaps, the key concern is the problem; it may not be well defined, the definition may need to be expanded, or more data may be needed.
- The goal may be to get the issue on the policy agenda via outreach to policymakers. Action may be necessary to develop and test solutions based on practice standards and population needs.
    - Developing policy solutions is a fundamental role for nurses—for the welfare of patients and communities, as well as the profession (Mason, Gardner, Outlaw, & O'Grady, 2016).
    - Perhaps, the issue is the way a regulation is being implemented, and thus, change could be made by working with legislators to identify the problem and develop implementation modifications. The policy evaluation may lack clarity.

Once the C/PHN considers all of these factors, then the level of involvement necessary can be determined. Given constraints on time, lobbying, access to data, and the priority of the issue, the level of engagement can be established. A number of avenues for activism are available, based on the above criteria. Table 13-1 demonstrates how the analysis framework relates to concerns of the C/PHN and possible actions in response.

POLITICAL ACTION AND ADVOCACY FOR C/PHNS

The definition of C/PHN practice describes efforts to promote and protect the public's health. When looking at *Healthy Public Policy*, C/PHN efforts to do so can take many forms from active participation as an informed citizen to actions taken as part of C/PHN practice to promote *Healthy Public Policy.* The Association of Public Health Nurses (APHN) put out a booklet for their C/PHN members to help understand advocacy and policy in their practice (APHN, 2016).

The C/PHN as an informed citizen, who has valuable knowledge and experience in health and health promotion, can be involved at a basic level by being aware of health policy and using this awareness for informed voting in elections across levels of jurisdiction.

- Individual C/PHNs might choose to increase their involvement by serving in a campaign to support a legislator that espouses public policies promoting health and preventing disease.

TABLE 13-1 C/PHN Practice Mechanisms to Address Policy Issues

Component of Analysis Framework	Action Needed	Mechanisms of Action
Problem	Data to define	▪ Collect or analyze evaluation data; assessment data ▪ Collaborate with researchers on problem definition
	Expand definition	▪ Collaborate with researchers on problem definition
Policies/solutions	Develop/pilot possible solutions	▪ Develop and implement model projects
	Change context to increase solution viability	▪ Evaluate/collect outcome data on projects to evaluate process of implementation
Politics	Educate public or other stakeholders	▪ Letters, phone call, e-mails, office visits to key stakeholders ▪ Communicate via letters to the editor or social media ▪ Present program results or assessment results in public forum ▪ Disseminate reports on service outcomes or new conditions to key stakeholders
Implementation	Revise regulations to improve implementation	▪ Work with regulators to revise regulations and rules
	Expand implementation to others affected	▪ Work with legislators and/or regulators to expand eligible populations for interventions
Evaluation	Data needed to measure impact	▪ Evaluate services provided
	Disseminate evaluation results	▪ Present program results or assessment results in public forum ▪ Disseminate reports on service outcomes or new conditions to key stakeholders
	Policy modification needed (see Problem)	▪ Collaborate to collect data for problem definition

- Additionally, the C/PHN might choose to share their expertise with others, as a means to inform their voting and citizen involvement.
- The C/PHN could also choose to be involved in professional organizations or citizen organizations to advocate for *Healthy Public Policies* and the legislators who promote them.

C/PHN practice, looking broadly at health and the social determinants of health, can provide background that is valuable in any number of professional and civic organizations. For example:

- At the state level, the C/PHN can ensure that the state nursing organizations maintain a broad-based focus on the health of the public.
- Locally, C/PHNs can serve on health boards but can also provide valuable input into health and education by serving on school boards or parent–teacher organizations. Working toward eliminating health inequities, healthier built environments, HIAs, and sharing knowledge are all worthwhile endeavors for nurses who want to affect population through health policy work (Kostas-Polston, et al., 2015).
- C/PHN researchers can influence policy by focusing on research questions related to the social determinants of health or health in all policies and sharing results in a clear and persuasive manner with policymakers and legislators. C/PHN research might include assessing the impact of public policies on community health outcomes or on evaluating public health promotion efforts in the community (Williams, Phillips, & Koyama, 2018).
- Lastly, C/PHNs can provide input by serving on policymaking bodies. A C/PHN serving on a hospital board could be critical in helping the hospital better understand population health and the role of the hospital in enhancing it.
- Alternatively, the C/PHN could serve on state or national advisory groups such as MedPAC (www.medpac.gov) or the Community Preventive Services Task Force (https://www.thecommunityguide.org/task-force/what-task-force). The organization, Nurses on Boards, is campaigning to put 10,000 nurses on various boards at all levels by 2020. Types of boards may include advisory, elected, appointed, constituency, and regulatory. The organization provides a wide variety of examples across each state, along with guidance on how to prepare to serve on a board (http://nursesonboardscoalition.org/).

Public Health and Social Justice

The concept of social justice is seen as the very foundation of community/public health and C/PHN (deChesnay & Anderson, 2016). The American Association of Colleges of Nursing (2017) emphasizes that the guiding values of nursing include social justice at all levels of educational preparation, and the ANA *Code of Ethics with Interpretive Statements* (2015, preface) states that nurses should "act to change those aspects of society that detract from health and wellbeing." The ANA's *Public Health Nursing: Scope and Standards of Practice* document also highlights the basic value of social justice in community health nursing (2013). The many definitions of social justice depend on the discipline involved; for purposes of this chapter, social justice is focused on health equity, which is ensuring that individuals have an equal opportunity to maximize their health (deChesnay & Anderson, 2016). See Chapter 23 for more information on social justice.

- As a C/PHN, you are expected to give voice to the health and social inequities found in the communities you serve (e.g., substandard housing, high rates of unemployment, death, and disability).
  - These are disparities that often could be prevented or alleviated at early stages. In order to promote and protect the health of populations, your nursing interventions will need to address not only health issues but also the educational, social, and economic issues that give rise to these disparities (deChesnay & Anderson, 2016).
  - The nexus between social justice, advocacy, and policy is interrelated, complex, and one that will affect every aspect of your community health nursing career.

History of Public Health Nursing Advocacy

Nurses have a long history of action in social justice and **advocacy**, which can be defined as pleading the case of another or championing a cause (see Chapter 3). To advocate is to try to influence outcomes that affect people, communities, and systems. Additionally, advocacy is a process, not an outcome, one that includes identifying an issue, collecting information, identifying who can be influenced to make the decision sought, building support, and taking action. Advocacy also includes litigation and public education campaigns. Advocacy can present itself in a variety of ways:

- Self-advocacy: advocating for oneself
- Individual advocacy: pleading the case of others
- Community/public health advocacy: creating awareness of, and generating support for meeting, the community's health needs
- Legislative advocacy: changing or modifying local, state or federal laws

Advocacy is also the process of empowering those less able to present their views or needs, with the goal of giving them a voice and/or achieving their objectives. Nurses have long been advocates for their patients, and advocacy can and does affect the larger systems of care (deChesnay & Anderson, 2016). Both nurses and communities have a common goal—the best possible health outcomes for all.

The importance of early nurse advocates such as Lillian Wald, Sojourner Truth, Margaret Sanger, Clara Barton, Mary Seacole, Susie King Taylor, Mary Mahoney, and others is that they wielded influence even at a time when women were not allowed to vote (see Chapter 3). In fact, many women in the 1800s, regardless of socioeconomic status, did not attend school. Women during these times rarely, if ever, voiced their opinions about issues affecting their lives, the lives of their children, their families, or their communities; it was neither expected nor accepted. African American women in the early 20th century were legally forbidden to learn to read and write (Nickitas, Middaugh, & Aries, 2016). For these women to influence policy during the 19th century is a tribute to their ability to take on the system in which they lived and to triumph over it.

The early pioneers are seen as feminists, and the entrance of these women into the political arena opened the way for others, such as Nancy Pelosi, first-ever female Speaker of the U.S. House of Representatives, and the four women Supreme Court justices (including one retired). The numbers of women in elected office continues to grow, and after the 2018 midterm elections, 24% of members of the senate and 23% of House members were female. In state legislatures, those numbers were 22.9% and 26.4%, respectively (Rutgers Center for American Women and Politics, 2018).

Professional Advocacy

One of the chief ways in which nurses have been successful in advocating is through membership in their professional organizations. The late 19th century may be seen as the beginning of nurse activism. The Nurses Associated Alumnae of the United States and Canada and the American Society of Superintendents of Training Schools of the United States and Canada were formed in the 1890s (ANA, n.d.a.; National League for Nursing, 2016). Out of these groups came the ANA and the National League for Nursing (see Chapter 3). However, in the 1980s, with the stratification of nursing into various specialties and organizations, representing an assortment of specialty groups, came the realization that the many nursing groups needed to coordinate efforts in order to be more successful, per a seminal article by Cohen et al. (1996). Throughout the next few decades, the nursing organizations realized, regardless of internal differences and competition, that to be politically successful, they must join together to work toward their common political goals. The formation of the following coalitions occurred:

- *Tri-Council for Nursing*—comprising the American Nurses Association (ANA), the American Association of Colleges of Nursing (AACN), the National League for Nursing (NLN), and the American Organization of Nurse Executives (AONE)
- *American Association of Nurse Practitioners (NPs)*—state and national NP groups initially met for a national forum and eventually to influence health policy
- *Nursing Organizations Alliance (The Alliance)*—an alliance of National Federation for Specialty Nursing Organizations and Nursing Organizations Liaison Forum

These and other coalitions permitted the organizations to lobby for common nursing issues (e.g., maintenance of federal funding for nursing education and research) and ultimately the establishment of the National Institute of Nursing Research within the National Institutes of Health (Milstead, 2016). Many of the current state nurse practice acts and expanded responsibilities for NPs are the result of these new coalitions. But more significantly, the profession worked together to demonstrate that there is a difference between "self-interest" and "selfishness" (Milstead, 2016).

- One of the most significant outcomes of this era was the development of *Nursing's Agenda for Health Care Reform* (ANA, 1994), which exemplified the maturing of nursing as a special interest group and demonstrated consensus building and collaboration among the more than 60 nursing and various health care provider organizations.
- Despite nursing's early history of political activism and the fact that nurses are the largest group of health care providers in the United States, widespread political involvement has not been fully realized (Nickitas et al., 2016).
    - Nursing has the potential to be a major player in Washington when discussing health care policy. For a recent example of successful professional advocacy, see Box 13-6.

Nurses must take advantage of how the public views the profession. For more than a decade, nurses have ranked highest in a Gallup poll for honesty and ethical standards (Gallup, 2018). Clearly, there is favorable impression of nursing as a profession among the general public. Despite criticism about special interest and professional organizations "protecting their turf," professional nursing organizations demonstrate how a critical mass can be influential and successful in moving the discussion forward on health care and the public's perception of nursing. Large professional organizations have the resources, relationships with policymakers, success at coalition building, and reputation for the ability to compromise needs to assure viable outcomes. It is the professional nursing organizations that have elevated nursing professionalism, given voice to the inequities that affect our society, and developed the paradigms that influence and affect public health at the institutional, state, and national level in the 21st century. A united voice on public policy is more powerful than individual nurses pleading with their legislators (Taylor, 2016). Being a part of your professional organization demonstrates your professionalism, promotes your organization's viability, and demonstrates your social responsibility to advocate for the needs of your patients.

The pursuit of personal agendas over the common good results in a piecemeal approach to problems and promotes polarization. **Polarization** is the process by which a group is severely split into two or more factions over a political issue. Polarization can be so intense that people perceive one another as good or wicked, depending on their ideological opinions. One of the primary goals of a professional nursing association is to build a collective voice for nurses. A strong professional association limits polarization by developing the political skills of its members and ensures that its structure and processes equitably meet the needs of its constituencies. This is the essence of politics: people must listen to each other, learn from others' viewpoints, and compromise to ensure the most positive outcomes from their endeavors (Nickitas et al., 2016).

Nurses are increasingly becoming shapers of policy on both the local and federal level; this is occurring because of our experience, perspective, and expertise in health care (Box 13-7). The realization that improving conditions for nursing also improves conditions for the communities we serve and the larger society in which we live and work has enhanced our ability to organize. This increases our visibility, access to policymakers, and, more importantly, our capacity to influence the political process (Kostas-Polston et al., 2015).

BOX 13-6 Expanding Practice Opportunities for Nurse Practitioners as a Result of Professional Advocacy

The Patient Protection and ACA is estimated to have decreased the numbers of uninsured in the United States by 5% to 7% by 2028 from 2010 levels. Thus, an estimated 15 million more Americans will have access to primary health care (Inserro, 2018). The demand for nurse practitioners (NPs) or advanced practice nurses (APNs) is increasing; nationally, it is expected to reach an increase of 30% between 2016 and 2020 (Xue & Intrator, 2016). NPs are often thought by patients to provide quality care, excellent communication with patients, and clear education about self-management of chronic conditions (e.g., diabetes). Given this increased demand for services—and specifically those provided by APNs, there are several provisions in the ACA that promote APN practice including the following:

- Five years of funds for demonstration projects to expand NP education programs.
- Increased funds for hiring NPs into the National Health Service Corps.
- Increased support for Federally Qualified Health Centers (FQHC) and Nurse-Managed Health Clinics (NMHCs), as safety-net providers, to hire APNs to care for their often vulnerable, high-risk clients.
- Medicare beneficiaries with functional limitations and chronic illnesses are able to receive home-based primary care from NPs through a 3-year project, Independence at Home Demonstration (Carthon, Barnes, & Sarik, 2015).

Although these gains have been the hard won result of consistent lobbying and advocacy efforts on the part of professional nursing organizations and individuals, the bright future on the horizon for APNs is at risk because of inconsistent scope of practice laws at the state level (Poghosyan, Boyd, & Clarke, 2016). In 2015, only 21 states and the District of Columbia had full autonomy rules for NPs (e.g., NPs could evaluate/treat patients, order/interpret diagnostic tests, and prescribe medications). That leaves 29 states with laws for NPs that restrict or reduce their scope of practice; often, this involves requiring physician oversight or collaboration (Xue & Intrator, 2016). Some states prohibit NPs from certifying home health or long-term care and limit their admitting privileges to hospitals. This practice leads to barriers to practice and uneven distribution of primary health care providers, with per capita rates for NPs ranging from 1.7 to 8 per 10,000 people in rural areas of the country. Most are working in large cities and urban areas (Xue & Intrator, 2016).

Another important consideration is the fact that NPs often work with the most vulnerable populations in areas where other health care providers are scarce, and "their active participation in advocating for both health and social policies" for their clients is helpful in promoting health equity in access and quality (Xue & Intrator, 2016, p. 5). Although NPs are achieving success in the area of policymaking and expanded practice opportunities, it is still vitally important for them to advocate and politically support health policies that benefit the clients they serve.

1. *What are the APN laws in your state?*
2. *How could allowing for APN full practice authority change how health care is provided in your community?*

Source: Carthon et al. (2015); Inserro (2018); Poghosyan et al. (2016); Xue and Intrator (2016).

BOX 13-7 QSEN: FOCUS ON QUALITY

Safety

Safety: Minimizes risk of harm to patients and providers through both system effectiveness and individual performance (p. 128).

(See https://qsen.org/competencies/pre-licensure-ksas/#quality_improvement for the knowledge, skills, and attitudes associated with this QSEN competency.)

Do not underestimate the power of nurses in action! On May 1, 2018, over 400 nurses from California visited the state capitol to push for important legislation that could impact them and the patients and populations they serve. They lobbied in support of A.B. 2874, which would require hospital systems to give the public 180-day notice before closing facilities or cutting specific services and would give the state attorney general the authority to approve or deny hospital closures. As a result, this bill was amended but became inactive. The nurses also advocated against A.B. 1795 and S.B. 944; these bills would allow paramedics to make clinical decisions about whether patients should be transported to emergency rooms or taken to other treatment sites, which the California Nurse Association worried could threaten patient safety and intrude on the RN scope of practice. Further, if passed, these policies could increase disparities in health care quality and access by providing a mechanism for vulnerable populations to be transported to subpar treatment facilities (National Nurses United, 2018). Both bills died in the Senate Assembly.

1. *Do you know about "lobby days at your local state capitol?" Do nurses participate?*
2. *Which nursing organizations or groups have lobbyists working with your state legislators?*

At https://leginfo.legislature.ca.gov/faces/billCompareClient.xhtml?bill_id=201720180AB2874&showamends=false, look up A.B. 2874 and analyze how this legislation might improve nursing care and patient outcomes.

Source: Cronenwett et al. (2007); National Nurses United (2018).

Nursing's Role in Health Care Reform

Since the 1950s, the ANA has advocated for reforms in health care that will benefit both nurses and their patients. Their involvement in federal health care reform began in the 1960s with the passage of Medicaid and Medicare. In the 1970s, the ANA formed a **political action committee (PAC)**. PACs are organizations that raise money to contribute to political parties or candidates, with the understanding that those receiving financial and political support will be sympathetic toward issues of interest to members of the PAC.

In 1991, the ANA released Nursing's Agenda for Health Care Reform: A Call to Action—a plan so ambitious and forward-looking that Senator Edward Kennedy referenced this document when introducing his legislation on health care reform. Even though this legislation failed to pass, the ANA and other nursing organizations gained wide recognition for their policy acumen and leadership abilities. During the Clinton-era health care debate, the ANA continued to play a key role in the policy and political discussions on health care reform. As research and experience continued to show the need for health care reform, the ANA remained steadfast in its advocacy and updated the policy agenda on health care reform and progress toward a more balanced approach incorporating primary care, community-based care, and preventive services. The ANA supported the development of a single-payer system. Understanding the time was ripe for health care reform, the ANA-PAC identified those legislators supportive of ANA's legislative and regulatory agenda. They provided financial and political support and increased their grassroots organizing. RNs nationwide responded and through multiple activities (e.g., contacting members of Congress, testifying at hearings, sharing personal stories, participating in high-profile press conferences, attending rallies and events) lobbied for action. The frontline nurses also joined ANA's health care reform team, and through these concentrated efforts and collaborations, health care reform became a reality in March 2010 (Lewenson, 2015).

Since the enactment of the ACA, ANA has worked to support implementation and to identify and disseminate the impact of any efforts to repeal the ACA (ANA, n.d.b.). The strongest efforts to repeal the ACA came at the end of 2016. The ANA carefully analyzed all proposals, compared them against the ANA's Principles for Health System Transformation (see Box 13-8), and made decisions regarding which proposals the organization would support. As a result of these efforts, in 2017, the ANA was crucial in stopping the passage of legislation that would repeal aspects of the ACA important to nursing practice and patient outcomes. Further, in May 2017, the ANA followed this same process and was vocal in opposition to the American Health Care Act, which the organization believed would threaten the health of the public and compromise the quality of health care delivery in the United States. See Box 13-8.

Nurses represent the largest number of health care practitioners in America—more than 3 million—and are poised at the frontline in patient care to play a major role in the evolving health care system. However, to change the existing system, the barriers to competent, quality care (e.g., nursing shortages, faculty shortages, a lack of proper education and training) that prevent nursing from taking its rightful place among the cadre of providers must be addressed. To that end, the Robert Wood Johnson Foundation (2010) in collaboration with the IOM sponsored a report, *The Future of Nursing: Leading Change, Advancing Health* (IOM, 2011). *The Future of Nursing* is a seminal document that addressed the need to reform the health care and public health system of the 21st century and outlined nursing's pivotal role in this. Four key messages from *The Future of Nursing: Leading Change, Advancing Health* (IOM, 2011, p. 4) include the following:

Nurses should:

1. Practice to the full extent of their education and training
2. Achieve higher levels of education and training that promote seamless academic progression
3. Be full partners in redesigning health care
4. Be part of health care policy and planning using data collection and an improved information infrastructure to inform decision making

The resulting seven recommendations and indicators of progress as of August 2019 are as follows:

1. *By 2020, increase the number of nurses with a baccalaureate degree to 80%.* As of 2018, 56% of nurses have baccalaureate or higher degrees (Campaign for Action, 2019).
2. *By 2020, the number of nurses with a doctorate should be doubled.* This recommendation has been achieved with over 23,800 employed nurses with doctoral degrees (Campaign for Action, 2019).
3. *Allow for advanced practice nurses to practice to the full extent of their education and training.* Nine states have achieved full access to care provided by

BOX 13-8 American Nurses Association's Principles for Health System Transformation

The system must:

- Provide to everyone universal access for essential health care services including mental health services, preexisting condition coverage, expansion of safety net through Medicaid, cost-effective practices, primary care that works in partnership with the patient, and coordination of care with all team members
- Address economics of health care costs through government and private partnerships, payment systems that include quality and resource use; address how lifetime caps/coverage limits/deductibles/copayments may be barriers to care and use an income-based sliding scale for insurance coverage purchase
- Ensure a skilled workforce that provides high-quality health care services through RN education, increased support for nursing faculty, and health care work force development and diversity funding

Source: American Nurses Association (2016a).

APNs since the campaign began, resulting in a total of 22 states with full practice authority for APNs (Campaign for Action, 2019).

4. *Provide opportunities for nurses to participate in collaborative improvement efforts. The number of required clinical courses and/or activities at top nursing* schools that include both RN students and graduate students of other health professions has increased by 183% over the last 6 years (Campaign for Action, 2019).
5. *Allow leadership opportunities in health care for nurses.* As of July 2019, over 6,300 nurses serve on boards across the nation (Campaign for Action, 2019).
6. *Collect and analyze interprofessional health care workforce data.* To date, almost all states collect nursing workforce data related to the supply of nurses, with smaller but increasing numbers of states collecting data on nursing education and demand for nursing services (Campaign for Action, 2019).
7. *Prioritize diversity in the nursing workforce.* As of 2016, 30% of all nursing students across levels of education are members of racial and ethnic minority groups and 14% of nursing students are male (Campaign for Action, 2019).

Nurses are an important force in health care and should be at the table with other stakeholders when important decisions are being made. The IOM report on nursing is a clear hallmark of our growth in the area of health policy and health reform. A new National Academy of Sciences report on nursing, scheduled for completion in 2020, will focus on nurses' value added to health outcomes for all Americans. "Nurses' regular, close proximity to patients and scientific understanding of care processes ... give them a unique ability to act as partners with other health professionals and to lead in the improvement and redesign of the health care system and its many practice environments..." (IOM, 2011, p. S-3). This is a mandate for community health nurses to be actively involved in advocacy and influencing the future development of our health care system.

CURRENT US HEALTH POLICY OPTIONS

What does the current health care system look like for C/PHNs? Earlier in this chapter, we discussed current health outcomes and the need for an increased focus on disease prevention and addressing the social determinants of health. The ACA has changed the policy options for health care on a national level; concerns persist regarding whether this is the best solution to ensuring access and controlling costs of care. However, in the past decade, policy and public health researchers have begun to examine seriously the health outcomes that have derived from the US health care system as configured, with access to care largely through employer-based insurance and a focus on medical treatment. Although the system has spawned innovations in pharmaceuticals and technological innovations, these services have often been effective for a small number of people, in acute need and at a large cost. Thus, the system has developed to be expensive and largely ineffective for the overall population health, disease prevention, and chronic disease management needs. The health care system has been very successful as measured in terms of education of health care professionals, pharmacological treatments for many illnesses, surgical innovations, and diagnostic technologies. As discussed earlier, however, these achievements have not led to overall positive health outcomes for the population as a whole. The passage of the ACA (Medicaid.gov, n.d.) has led to policy changes designed to address these concerns (see Chapter 6 for more information on the ACA).

The ACA and C/PHN Practice

The ACA provided a dramatic change in US policy options. Recognizing that the US health care system was not addressing all the factors necessary to improve the health of the public, and that it was costing US taxpayers an ever-increasing and sustainable proportion of the national budget, the Obama administration moved to pass health care reform legislation in 2010. The focus of the ACA, in the minds of the public, was to mandate health insurance coverage for all US citizens. This would be done through a required employer minimal health insurance package, a mandate on employer provision of health insurance or employer contribution to a marketplace of insurance options for individuals to access, and government provision of subsidies for low-income people without employer insurance coverage. Indeed, data indicate that the ACA was initially successful at insuring those previously uninsured. The percentage of uninsured adults (ages 19 to 64) dropped from 20% in 2010 to 12% in 2018, but more people are underinsured (Collins, Bhupal, & Doty, 2019). In the current administration, however, there have been efforts to repeal the ACA, and related efforts to curtail ACA expansion have led to projections of numbers of uninsured beginning to rise again, with projections of 13% of Americans uninsured by 2028 (Isarra, 2018). See Chapter 6.

Lesser known but equally critical aspects of the ACA include a focus on health promotion and disease prevention, strengthened requirements for nonprofit hospitals to demonstrate their community value, and a restructuring of governmental payment plans to move toward value-based payments. These aspects are important for C/PHN practice and are not expected to be impacted dramatically by efforts to repeal or weaken the ACA (Kacic & Castellucci, 2018).

As part of the ACA efforts to move to a culture of disease prevention, the ACA mandated formation of a National Prevention Council, composed of cabinet officials representing the social determinants of health, chaired by the Surgeon General of the United States. The council developed a National Prevention Strategy Assocaition of State and Territorial Health Offficals (2011), which addressed core strategic directions and priorities for an increased focus on public health and well-being, including recommendations for evidence-based interventions in each area (Fig. 13-7).

Subsequent work by the National Prevention Council and the federal advisory group appointed to advise and guide these efforts included work to disseminate the interventions and strategies, document successes and lessons learned, and promote model and exemplary interventions and policies to promote health and prevent disease across all levels of government (Surgeon General, n.d.).

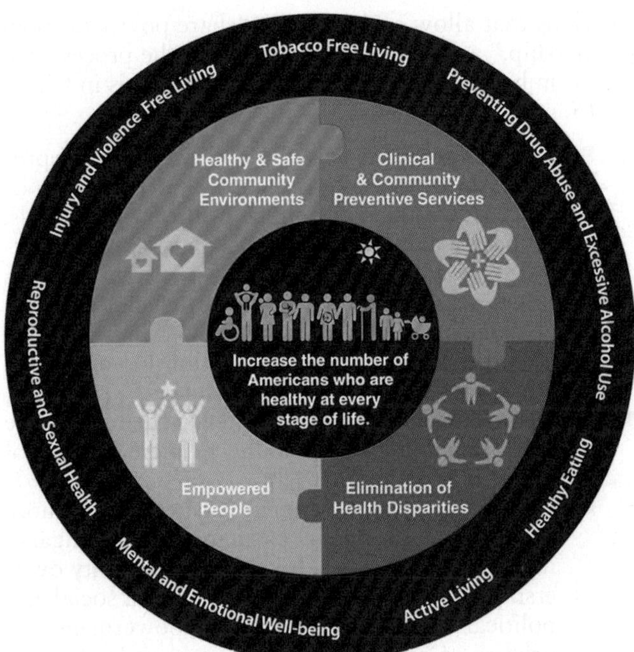

FIGURE 13-7 National prevention strategy model. (Reprinted from *National Prevention Strategy*. Washington, DC: U.S. Department of Health and Human Services, Office of the Surgeon General. Retrieved from https://www.hhs.gov/sites/default/files/disease-prevention-wellness-report.pdf)

The federal advisory group, appointed by the president, included two nurses, who worked to disseminate the NPS to C/PHNs across the country so that it may be incorporated as part of their practice initiatives (Surgeon General, n.d.). Successes of the NPS implementation included efforts in violence prevention in Minnesota; the Healthy Chicago 2.0 health blueprint adopted by Chicago; and efforts to work with American Indians in Maine to assess and plan community health improvements (Advisory Group, 2016). Although the NPS is not being actively used in this administration, much of the strategy has been adopted around the country and appears in Healthy People 2030.

Additional components of the ACA that have the potential for great changes in health and health policy at the community level include value-based purchasing and accountable care organizations (ACOs), along with the expanded Internal Revenue Service (IRS) requirement for nonprofit hospitals to conduct regular community health needs assessments and develop implementation plans based on these data for improving the health of their communities (Kacic & Castellucci, 2018).

Value-Based Purchasing and Accountable Care Organizations

The ACA began a movement away from the traditional fee-for-service care where health providers diagnose and treat individuals and are paid for each service provided (e.g., office visits, lab fees, prescriptions, follow-up visits) and that has thought to have led to increasing health care costs (Kacic & Castellucci, 2018). This style of reimbursement for care has had the problem of indirectly encouraging additional care, as each service is reimbursed separately. National health policy has begun to reverse this by mandating no reimbursement for specific services required because of medical error. See Chapter 6.

- The ACA expands this with a move toward *value-based purchasing* or reimbursing a specific amount based on achieving the likely outcome for clients within specific diagnostic categories.

Instead of fees for office visits, lab fees, and prescriptions, the federal government is proposing paying for achievable health outcomes in a bundled manner based on the client's demographics and diagnosis. A diabetic would not have each service reimbursed, but rather a lump sum reimbursement would be provided upon the client achieving a level of stability in the disease (e.g., lab values for hemoglobin A1c within normal limits). This reimbursement would cover whatever services were required to achieve this outcome, which might be lab tests and medications, but might also include C/PHN-provided chronic disease self-management training or clinical nutrition counseling.

- Such a change in reimbursement mechanisms would have a large impact on health care services, as clinical agencies would need to begin looking at what services and providers were most effective at achieving the desired outcomes, with a focus on addressing the social determinants of health. This would provide an opportunity for C/PHNs to demonstrate the effectiveness of their practice interventions in improving health outcomes for individuals and populations (LaPointe, 2019; Swider, Levin, & Reising, 2017).

When a national sample of C/PHNs was asked about their involvement with components of the ACA, over 65% responded that they were actively involved with integration of public and primary health care, and nearly as many were working in clinical preventive services. Almost 60% noted activity with patient navigation, care coordination, and establishing public/private collaborations. Slightly fewer mentioned involvement with population health strategies and data, along with community health assessments (Edmonds, Campbell, & Gilder, 2015).

- *Accountable Care Organizations* (ACOs) are another feature of health care reform that is intended to emphasize quality over quantity. Physicians and other health care providers are forming groups, sometimes in conjunction with hospitals, and will be paid based on patient's treatment outcomes (not the number of visits or tests).
  - Thus, duplicative tests or procedures should be avoided, as a more coordinated form of treatment is available.
  - One goal of ACA is to provide 30% of Medicare services to alternative payment models, such as ACOs, and away from fee-for-service models.
  - In addition to cost savings, quality is also a focus. In 2014, Medicare ACOs demonstrated $411 million in cost savings, while 27 out of 33 quality measures were improved between 2013 and 2014 (USDHHS, 2016).
  - Newer types of ACOs not only pay based on quality outcomes but also penalize for negative outcomes, shifting risk to providers and away from the government. The number of ACOs is

growing, with 923 public and private ACO's identified in 2017 (Muhlstein et al., 2017). ACO case study examples can be found at the Center for Medicare and Medicaid Services (CMS) website: https://innovation.cms.gov/initiatives/ACO/

Policy Competence as an Integral Part of C/PHN Practice

The US health care system is undergoing significant changes to improve the health of the public and contain costs. These changes are impacting health care across the system but are particularly critical for those who work in communities with the increased emphasis on population health and disease prevention. The C/PHN can lead the way in addressing the social determinants of health and focusing efforts on prevention and long-term health promotion for families and communities. Along with other public health professionals, C/PHNs need to do this by understanding the policy process and then determining where their efforts would be most effective in improving overall population health (Kub, Kulbok, Miner, & Merrill, 2017). This is a critical time for nursing in general, and C/PHN specifically, as the health care system focuses attention on what has always been at the core of C/PHN concern—health where people live, work, play, and pray.

POWER AND EMPOWERMENT

Collaborating with underserved populations to elicit change can be a difficult task. Citizen participation is never particularly easy in communities that are excluded from political or economic resources. Sherry Arnstein, in her classic (1969) treatise *A Ladder of Citizen Participation*, stated that "citizen participation is citizen power," and without access to information about how the system functions, these populations cannot obtain the resources they need to make their communities livable and nurturing (p. 217). Arnstein goes on to point out that those in power often work to prevent those in need from accessing the process (Fig. 13-8).

Although Arnstein writes about the anger that disenfranchised populations feel, she does offer possible solutions that allow each party to "share power through partnership," as outlined by engaging in the process discussed in her treatise (p. 217). See more on this in Chapter 15.

- **Power** can be defined as the ability to act or produce an effect, possession of control, or authority or influence over others. As public health professionals, nurses have a commitment to social justice and working with disadvantaged communities. This means that nurses have a responsibility to ensure community participation in issues affecting them, and they must continually examine the relationship and position they hold within these communities.
- The term **community empowerment** is defined as the process of enabling communities to increase control over their lives (WHO, 2019).
  - Community empowerment, therefore, is more than the involvement, participation, or engagement of communities. It implies community ownership and action that explicitly aims at social and political change. Community empowerment is a process of renegotiating power in order to gain more control, and power is a central concept of this process.
  - Community empowerment necessarily addresses the social, cultural, political, and economic determinants that underpin health and seeks to build partnerships with other sectors in finding solutions (WHO, 2019).

An empowered community is one in which members effectively use resources (human and fiscal) and collaborate to meet identified needs (Fig. 13-9). Individuals and organizations within empowered communities support each other, work together for conflict resolution, and increasingly have the ability to facilitate social change, gaining power over the quality of life in their community. This demonstrates how empowerment of communities is linked to empowerment at the individual and organizational level.

How does the C/PHN make sure that preconceived ideas about certain communities are not forced on the community in order to meet the goals and objectives of

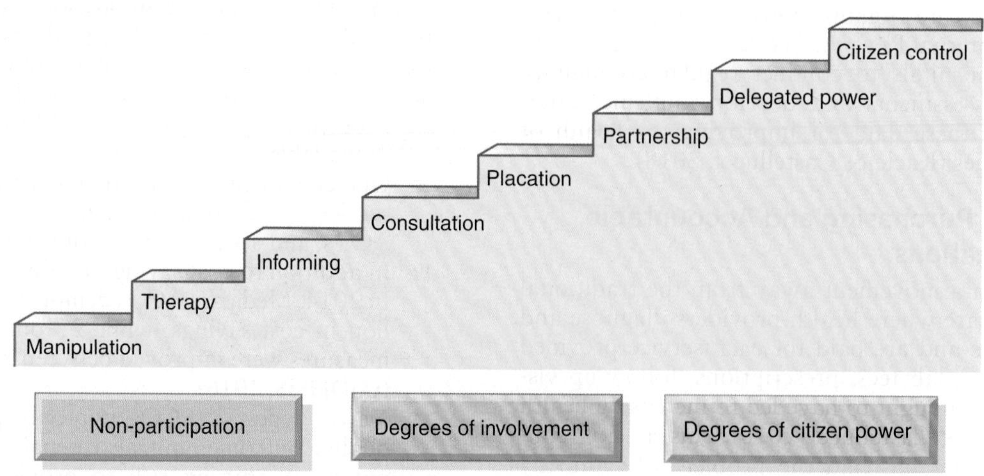

FIGURE 13-8 Arnstein's ladder: Eight steps of citizen participation. (Adapted from Arnstein, S. R. (July 1969). A ladder of citizen participation. *Journal of the American Institute of Planners, 35*(4), 217–224.)

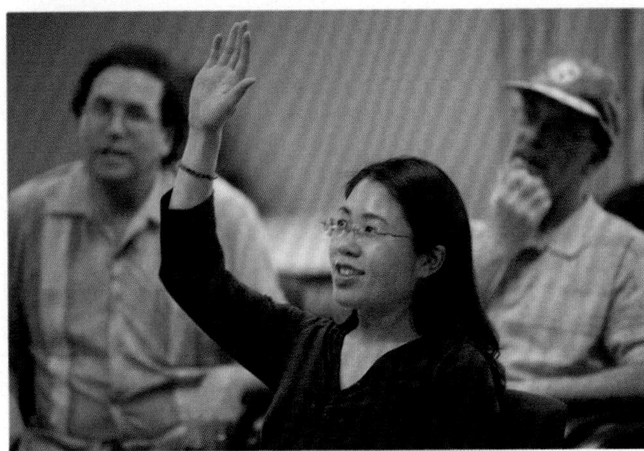

FIGURE 13-9 Town hall meetings promote community participation in public policy. (Photo courtesy of CDC Photo Image Library.)

the public health agency? In the past, community health promotion practice often only met the bottom rung of Arnstein's ladder by using the rhetoric of community participation, while the professionals working with the community actually set the agenda. Health promotion may best be facilitated by the use of empowerment and assisting individuals and communities in articulating their problems and solutions. This suggests a change in the relationship between professionals and communities—a change from the customary hierarchical patient–provider relationship to one of a partnership. Discovering what is most important to the community and providing access to that information while supporting leadership from within the community and encouraging them to overcome bureaucratic hurdles to action are important parts of community empowerment. Real stories about clients having problems, such as gaining access to services or resources, not receiving adequate or timely treatment, or about the need for more school nurses who are currently spread so thin that they cannot adequately perform their assigned roles and functions. First-hand knowledge of how our health care system works (or does not work) can be very persuasive when a nurse shares personal examples in a way that demonstrates a passion for clients and communities.

So, how can C/PHNs influence policies that affect the clients and communities they serve? And, how do we influence policymakers to hear our concerns and act on them? Using persuasion, through either written or oral methods, to influence government is known as **lobbying**. While personal stories may call attention to your issue, effective lobbying requires more substance. Seasoned advocates developed ground rules by which to be effective. Some call them the "ten commandments of lobbying." However these steps are named, advocates adhere to the basic ideas inherent in the following:

- **Honesty is the best policy**. Being known as someone who has integrity is a lasting virtue. Never mislead a legislator about the importance of an issue or the position of the opposition as it is difficult to regain credibility once lost. Do not speak beyond your level of expertise. If you do not know the answer, say so. If you promise to get the answer, then do so. Do not promise what you cannot deliver.
- **Start early**. Planning always takes longer than you think it will. Your interests are not everyone's interests, and convincing others they should be involved always involves time. If you are planning policy change at the state or federal level, it is vital to know the legislative process and the critical time lines.
- **Know what you want and be prepared.** Understand the role politics plays in getting what you want and how policymakers may respond to your issue. Targeting your story to the goals, emotions, and interests of the legislator is important and may result in a positive outcome. It is crucial to understand the role funding may have on your policy issue.
- **KISS** (Keep it simple, stupid). Be able to articulate your issues in a clear and concise manner. Do not confuse possible supporters with complicated arguments. Key issues should be concise and clear and on one page, no more than two.
- **No permanent enemies, no permanent friends.** Political affiliation does not always determine what interests a person has or whether they are likely to support your issue. It behooves you to speak with everyone. Respectful disagreement keeps the door open for future agreement and compromise. Remember, an opponent on one issue may be an ally on another. Always be polite and professional.
- **Know your opponents**. Understand all sides of the issue prior to approaching a policymaker. Be prepared to answer questions and provide data on both sides of the issue.
- **Make an "ask":** Be *clear* about what you are asking the legislator for—to carry legislation or to vote no or yes on specific legislation. Asking your legislator to vote a certain way is perfectly legitimate, and if you don't ask, the opposition will. Ask for much more than you think you can get. When negotiating, this allows you to give up something without hurting your priorities or your bottom line. In politics, rarely does anyone get all they want, but priority setting is a key.
- **There is strength in numbers**. The more groups involved, the more likely you are to be successful. Any opportunity for networking is an opportunity to enlarge your coalition. Including disparate groups means you may have accessed conflicting political persuasions. Additionally, it is useful to have groups who can speak with those who are not viewed as "friends." Cross-fertilization of groups is politically expedient but understands that next time you or they may be in opposition.
- **Know your legislators and work at the local level.** Legislators are interested in their constituents—these are the people who elected them to office and who will keep them in office. To be noticed by policymakers, sharing information with them about their constituents is the surest way to capture their attention. Information sharing should occur on issues both in the community where you live and in the one where you work.
- **Thank you.** Everyone loves to be told, "Job well done." To maintain your coalitions, always recognize the work of others. Spreading the credit is like sowing seeds: the wider the spread, the more bountiful the crop.

Common methods of making contact with legislators are by e-mail, over phone, or in person. Often, your first contact will be a staff member. This person is the gatekeeper and your interaction may determine the level of communication you have with your legislator. It is important to organize your thoughts and carefully craft a pitch that ends with an "Ask" or how you want the legislator to take action (Kostas-Polston et al., 2015, p. 12).

- If you plan to make contact in person, prepare a "one-pager," with your contact information and credentials listed, along with brief bulleted points on the subject of interest that includes current statistics and research (p. 13).
- If you meet with a legislator, it is important to remember that they are not allowed to discuss campaign contributions in their legislative offices. Finally, it is important for those new to advocacy to understand that the thing with the most critical influence on policy is *money*.

Nurses, even with the passage of the recent health care reform legislation, must become even more actively involved in the process of influencing policy. How many nurses understand that the nurse practice acts, or portions thereof, under which they work are developed by legislators or special interest groups who don't have a background in health care? How many nurses know who their legislators are at either the state or federal level? How many nurses have written their legislators about pending health care legislation or legislation that affects nursing?

Political Action Committees

- Financial resources are essential to effective advocacy. One reason why nurses are less politically active can be tied to a lack of money.
  - As mentioned earlier, the ANA has a PAC that supports federal candidates on a nonpartisan basis. Candidates must demonstrate an interest in and willingness to vote for nursing issues or issues that nurses support.
  - To participate in the PAC, you must be a member of the ANA (this also allows your family to contribute to the PAC). By contributing to the ANA-PAC, one maximizes his/her contribution by joining with other nurses. Power in numbers increases our influence with those candidates we choose to endorse.

During the 2016 election cycle, the ANA-PAC contributed just over $200,000 to federal candidates who supported nurses and nursing issues. While this is a large amount of money, it is significantly less than the $1.2 million that the American Medical Association's PAC contributed during the same time frame (U.S. FEC, n.d.). Because nursing organizations do not have as much money as other health care groups (e.g., hospitals, physicians, insurance companies, and health care plans), there is less opportunity to employ lobbyists and contribute to supportive candidates. This often means nurses have less influence than other groups.

- Another way to influence policy is to make contributions to your personal legislator. This will keep you on his/her mailing list and may lead to invitations to local legislative activities. It also lets your legislator know you are interested in whether he/she remains in office. Being in regular contact with your legislators provides an avenue for introducing legislation that impacts nursing or important community issues, and when you call to ask for a vote "for" or "against" an issue, the legislator may be more likely to entertain your request.
- Lobbyists may work for PACs or independently represent various special interests or groups. Professional organizations or other **special interest groups** (individuals who share a common interest and work politically to make their goals a reality) may retain paid lobbyists.

Lobbyists are professionals who know the rules governing the state or federal political process, have or develop relationships with policymakers, provide guidance for members of the organizations employing them on how to impact public policy decisions, and work behind the scenes to influence policy discussions and outcomes. States and the federal government have laws and regulations that determine the legal actions of lobbyists as well as the organizations that employ those (Mason et al., 2016; Milstead, 2016). However, some lobbyists are former legislators or staff members who "take lucrative jobs representing the very industries" they formerly regulated, and this "revolving door" lobbying is disconcerting to most citizens as they are often seen as selling their access to current key legislators (LaPira & Thomas, 2014, p. 4).

Volunteering

Money is *not* the only way to build a relationship with your legislator. Being involved in local and state elections can take many forms. Volunteering your time can be just as important (Box 13-9). Candidates develop position papers to tell their constituents where they stand on key campaign concerns. Nurses have the expertise to assist legislators in developing position papers and setting policy agendas for health care issues, including the social determinants of health. Legislators and legislative candidates also need people to assist in everyday tasks such as phone banking, stuffing mailers, answering phones, putting up flyers and campaign posters, and walking door to door to spread support.

- *Relationships* are critical in policy development and in affecting public policy. As demonstrated earlier, being a friend can reap huge benefits when health care policy is on the line. Voting, for instance, is vital—RNs represent a substantial block of potential voters (Nickitas et al., 2016).
- Joining your local and state professional organizations is imperative to having the voice of nursing heard at all levels.

You can become more actively involved by writing legislators about the health care issues that impact the communities, both where you live and work. It is also vital to understand the importance of critically timing those communications. Effective communications with

BOX 13-9 PERSPECTIVES

A Volunteer's Viewpoint on Campaigning for an RN

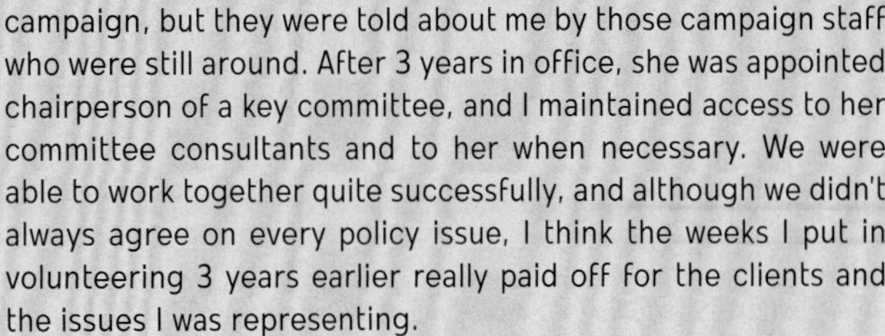

A registered nurse (RN) who had been through what I called the women's legislative career ladder—School Board, City Council, and the County Board of Supervisors—was now poised to run for the state legislature. Because we had had numerous contacts and I believed she would make a good state legislator and a voice for nursing and health care, I volunteered to work in her campaign office. I primarily answered the phones on the evenings I worked, but I met the office staff—many of them were much younger than me. And, even once, she came in while I was there. I talked with the staff about some of my experiences as a lobbyist, and they shared their experiences; many of them were fresh out of college.

She was successful in her run for office, and whenever I needed to meet with her or her staff, I was shown right in. I was also asked my opinion about the hiring of certain staff. Her staff knew me by name—many of them did not work on her campaign, but they were told about me by those campaign staff who were still around. After 3 years in office, she was appointed chairperson of a key committee, and I maintained access to her committee consultants and to her when necessary. We were able to work together quite successfully, and although we didn't always agree on every policy issue, I think the weeks I put in volunteering 3 years earlier really paid off for the clients and the issues I was representing.

Lydia, professional lobbyist

legislators should be tied to times when the issues are being heard in policy committee—thus, you must know when your issue is scheduled to be discussed in committee. For example, it is prudent to send letters on your issue—via fax or regular mail—close to the time of the committee hearing. Holding a press conference or getting other media coverage when the bill is introduced, or on the day it will be heard in committee, is quite effective in drawing attention to your issue. Writing letters to the editor of your local newspaper on health issues and writing articles for various publications are also effective methods of persuading others to back your issue.

- Other methods for influencing health policy or nursing issues include applying for positions on boards and commissions; each local area has advisory committees for their locally elected officials at the city and county level.
  - The state board of RNs needs nurses willing to sit on their board or to serve on various advisory committees and task forces.
  - At your state capitols, there are usually vacancies on policy committees, or legislators may be looking for new staff. And, who better to serve in this capacity than a nurse! Serve your patients and communities by *running for office*!

SUMMARY

This chapter briefly reviewed health outcomes in the United States.

- Health outcomes for Americans do not compare well with peer countries, particularly considering the high cost of the US health care system; this is largely due to system issues and not addressing the SDOH.
- Health policy guides health care and governmental actions related to the SDOH; C/PHNs can use policy in their practice to improve the health of the communities with which they work.
- Policy competence as it relates to local, state, and federal health policy—and how nurses are impacted by these policies—is an essential skill for C/PHNs.
- An understanding of how a bill becomes a law helps inform policy process, implementation, and evaluation.
- Frameworks such as the rational and Kingdon provide guidance in health policy analysis.
- Policy analysis as a call for activism can be used to support social justice in public health, professional advocacy, and the C/PHN's role in health care reform, PACs, and volunteerism.
- Current US health policy includes the ACA within community and public health practice, value-based purchasing, and accountable care organizations.

ACTIVE LEARNING EXERCISES

1. Using "Utilize Legal and Regulatory Actions" (1 of the 10 essential public health services; see Box 2-2), describe a legislative bill related to health at either your state or the federal level and where the bill is in the legislative process. Identify who is sponsoring the bill, who is opposing it, and why. Determine the population that will be affected most by the bill if it passes and in what ways they will be affected. Discuss what you, as a C/PHN, could do to be involved in this bill and then develop a political action plan to support or oppose the bill. E-mail your legislator regarding your position.
2. Who are your state legislators? What are the critical health issues in your state, and how have your legislators responded to the issues? How have your state legislators voted on policies to advance the nursing profession?
3. Attend a meeting of a professional organization, board of directors, government agency, or council when a health policy or health care issue is on the

agenda. Analyze the positions of the major interest groups involved and describe to what extent economics comes into the discussion. Describe who controls the discussion and why. Compare your findings with classmates.

4. Are nurses the most qualified group to articulate national health care issues? If so, why? If not, why not?
5. Pick a policy issue and take a position related to political action and advocacy. What stance does your nursing professional organization have on this issue?

REFERENCES

Advisory Group on Prevention, Health Promotion, and Integrative and Public Health. (2016). *Fulfilling the legacy report*. Washington, DC: U.S. Department of Health and Human.

American Association of Colleges of Nursing (AACN). (2017). *Diversity, inclusion, and equity in academic nursing*.

American Nurses Association. (1994). *Nursing's agenda for health care reform*. Retrieved from http://ojin.nursingworld.org/MainMenuCategories/ANAMarketplace/ANAPeriodicals/OJIN/TableofContents/Vol31998/No1June1998/References.html

American Nurses Association (ANA). (2015). *Code of ethics for nurses with interpretive statements (revised)*. Silver Spring, MD: Author.

American Nurses Assocation. (2016a). ANA's prinicples for health system transformation 2016. Retrieved from https://www.nursingworld.org/~4afd6b/globalassets/practiceandpolicy/health-policy/principles-healthsystemtransformation.pdf

American Nurses Association (ANA). (2016b). *The nursing process*. Retrieved from https://www.nursingworld.org/practice-policy/workforce/what-is-nursing/the-nursing-process/

American Nurses Association (ANA). (n.d.a). *ANA historical review*. Retrieved from http://www.nursingworld.org/history

American Nurses' Association (ANA). (n.d.b). *Health system reform resources*. Retrieved from https://www.nursingworld.org/practice-policy/health-policy/health-system-reform/resources/

American Public Health Association (APHA). (2013). *Health in all policies: A guide for state and local governments*. Retrieved from http://www.apha.org/~/media/files/pdf/factsheets/health_inall_policies_guide_169pages.ashx

American Public Health Association, PHN Section. (2013). *Definition of public health nursing*. Retrieved from https://www.nursingworld.org/practice-policy/workforce/public-health-nursing/

Anderson, J. E. (2015). *Public policymaking: An introduction* (8th ed.). Stamford, CT: Cengage Learning.

Arnstein, S. (1969). A ladder of citizen participation. *Journal of American Planning Association*, *35*(4), 216–224.

Association of Public Health Nurses (APHN). (2016). *Public health policy advocacy guide book and tool kit*. Retrieved from https://www.phnurse.org/assets/docs/APHN%20Public%20Health%20Policy%20Advocacy%20Guide%20Book%20and%20Tool%20Kit%202016.pdf

Birkland, T. (2019). *An introduction to the policy process* (5th ed.). Abingdon, UK: Routledge.

California Department of Public Health. (2018). *Health in all policies (HIAP)*. Retrieved from https://www.cdph.ca.gov/Programs/OHE/Pages/HIAP.aspx

Campaign for Action. (2019). *Dashboard indicators*. Retrieved from https://campaignforaction.org/resource/dashboard-indicators/

Carthon, J. M. B., Barnes, H., & Sarik, D. A. (2015). Federal policies influence access to primary care and nurse practitioner workforce. *Journal for Nurse Practitioners*, *11*(5), 526–531.

Center for Medicare and Medicaid Services (CMS). (2019). *Hospital acquired condition (HAC) reduction program*. Retrieved from https://www.cms.gov/Medicare/Quality-Initiatives-Patient-Assessment-Instruments/Value-Based-Programs/HAC/Hospital-Acquired-Conditions.html

Centers for Disease Control and Prevention (CDC). (2016). *Disability and obesity*. Retrieved from http://www.cdc.gov/ncbddd/disabilityandhealth/obesity.html

Centers for Disease Control and Prevention (CDC). (2017). *Smoking and tobacco use: Legislation*. Retrieved from https://www.cdc.gov/tobacco/data_statistics/by_topic/policy/legislation/index.htm

Centers for Disease Control and Prevention (CDC). (n.d.). *Opioid overdose*. Retrieved from https://www.cdc.gov/drugoverdose/index.html

Civic Impulse. (2018). *Statistics and historical comparison: Bills by final status*. Retrieved from https://www.govtrack.us/congress/bills/statistics

Cohen, S. S., Mason, D. J., Kovner, C., Leavitt, J. K., Pulcine, J., & Sochalshi, J. (1996). Stages of nursing's political development: Where we've been and where we ought to go. *Nursing Outlook*, *44*(6), 259–266.

Collins, S., Bhupal, H., & Dhoty, M. (2019). *Health insurance coverage eight years after the ACA*. Retrieved from https://www.commonwealthfund.org/publications/issue-briefs/2019/feb/health-insurance-coverage-eight-years-after-aca

Commonwealth Fund. (2018). *The Affordable Care Act under the Trump administration*. Retrieved from https://www.commonwealthfund.org/blog/2018/affordable-care-act-under-trump-administration

Cronenwett, L., Sherwood, G., Marnsteiner, J., Disch, J., Johnson, J., Mitchell, P., ... Warren, J. (2007). Quality and safety in education for nurses. *Nursing Outlook*, *55*, 122–131. doi: 10.1016/j.outlook.2007.02.006.

Dasgupta, N., Beletsky, L., & Ciccarone, D. (2018). Opioid crisis: No easy fix to its social and economic determinants. *American Journal of Public Health*, *108*, 182–186. doi: 10.2105/AJPH.2017.304187.

deChesnay, M., & Anderson, B. A. (2016). *Caring for the vulnerable: Perspectives in nursing theory, practice, and research* (4th ed.). Burlington, MA: Jones & Bartlett Learning.

Department of Health and Human Services (DHHS). (January 22, 2019). *What is the U.S. opioid epidemic?* Retrieved from https://www.hhs.gov/opioids/about-the-epidemic/index.html

Edmonds, J. K., Campbell, L. A., & Gilder, R. E. (2015). Public health nursing and the Affordable Care Act: Survey results. Presented at the 143rd meeting of the American Public Health Association, 3393.0. Health Systems and Practice Reform Round Table, Chicago, IL.

Environmental Protection Agency. (August 8, 2019). *Greenhouse gas emissions*. Retrieved from https://www.epa.gov/ghgemissions

Families USA. (November 14, 2017). *Health and health care in the 2017 State Legislatures: Opportunities, threats, and what to expect in 2018*. Retrieved from https://familiesusa.org/resources/health-and-health-care-in-the-2017-state-legislatures-opportunities-threats-and-what-to-expect-in-2018/

Gallup. (2018). *Nurses again outpace other professions for honesty, ethics*. Retrieved from https://news.gallup.com/poll/245597/nurses-again-outpace-professions-honesty-ethics.aspx

Gneiting, U. (2016). From global agenda-setting to domestic implementation: Successes and challenges of the global health network on tobacco control. *Health Policy and Planning*, *31*, i74–i86.

Govtrack. (2019). *Statistics and historical comparison*. Retrieved from https://www.govtrack.us/congress/bills/statistics

Haddadin, Y., & Regunath, H. (2019). *Central Line Associated Blood Stream Infections (CLABSI)*. Retrieved from https://www.ncbi.nlm.nih.gov/books/NBK430891/

Halfon, N., et al. (2014). Applying A 3.0 transformation framework to guide large-scale health system reform. *Health Affairs*, *33*(11). doi: 10.1377/hlthaff.2014.0485.

Inserro, A. (2018). *CBO projects additional uninsured through 2028 after ACA changes*. Retrieved from https://www.ajmc.com/newsroom/cbo-projects-additional-uninsured-through-2028-after-aca-changes

Institute of Medicine (IOM). (2011). *The future of nursing: Leading change, advancing health*. Washington, DC: National Academies Press.

Isarra, A. (2018). *CBO Projects additional uninsured through 2028 after ACA changes*. AJMC Managed Markets Network. Retrieved from https://www.ajmc.com/newsroom/cbo-projects-additional-uninsured-through-2028-after-aca-changes

Jewish Women's Archive. (2016). *Women of valor: Lillian Wald*. Retrieved from http://jwa.org/womenofvalor/wald

Kacic, A., & Castellucci. (December 18, 2018). ACA repeal wouldn't stop transition to value based payment, efforts to lower drug spending. *Modern HealthCare*. Retrieved from https://www.modernhealthcare.com/article/20181219/NEWS/181219885/aca-repeal-wouldn-t-stop-transition-to-value-based-payment-efforts-to-lower-drug-spending

Kaiser Family Foundation. (August 1, 2019). *Status of state medicaid expansion decisions: An interactive map*. Retrieved from https://www.kff.org/medicaid/issue-brief/status-of-state-medicaid-expansion-decisions-interactive-map/

Kingdon, J. W. (2010). *Agendas, alternatives and public policies*. Retrieved from http://marieljohn.blogspot.com/2010/02/agendas-alternatives-and-public.html

Kingdon, J. W. (2011). *Agendas, alternatives and public policies* (2nd ed.). Boston, MA: Pearson/Longman.

Kostas-Polston, E. A., Thanavaro, J., Arvidson, C., & Taub, L. M. (2015). Advanced practice nursing: Shaping health through policy. *Journal of the American Association of Nurse Practitioners*, *27*, 11–20.

Kub, J., Kulbok, P., Miner, S., & Merrill, J. (2017). Increasing the capacity of public health nursing to strengthen the public health infrastructure and to promote and protect the health of communities and populations. *Nursing Outlook*, *65*(5), 661–664.

LaPira, T. M., & Thomas, H. F. (2014). Revolving door lobbyists and interest representation. *Interest Groups & Advocacy*, *3*(1), 4–29.

LaPointe, J. (2019). *Social determinants of health key to value based purchasing success*. Retrieved from https://revcycleintelligence.com/news/social-determinants-of-health-key-to-value-based-purchasing-success

Leipert, B. D., Regan, S., & Plunkett, R. (May 6, 2015). Working through and around: exploring rural public health nursing practices and policies to promote rural women's health. *Online Journal of Rural Nursing and Health*, *15*(1). doi: 10.14574/ojrnhc.v15i1.342.

Lewenson, S. B. (2015). Overview and summary: Cornerstone documents in healthcare: Our history, our future. *Online Journal of Issues in Nursing*, *20*(2). Retrieved from http://www.nursingworld.org/MainMenuCategories/ANAMarketplace/ANAPeriodicals/OJIN/TableofContents/Vol-20-2015/No2-May-2015/OS-Cornerstone-Documents.html

Longest, B. B. (2016). *Health policymaking in the United States* (6th ed.). Chicago, IL: Health Administration Press.

Mason, D. J., Gardner, D. B., Outlaw, F. H., & O'Grady, E. T., (Eds.). (2016). *Policy and politics in nursing and health care* (7th ed.). St. Louis, MO: Elsevier.

Medicaid.gov. (n.d.). *Affordable Care Act*. Retrieved from https://www.medicaid.gov/about-us/program-history/index.html

Milio, N. (1981). *Promoting health through public policy*. Philadelphia, PA: F. A. Davis.

Milstead, J. A. (Ed.). (2016). *Health policy and politics: A nurse's guide* (5th ed.). Burlington, MA: Jones & Bartlett Learning.

Muhlstein, D., Saunders, R., & McClellan, M. (June 28, 2017). Growth of ACOs and alternative payment models in 2017. In *Health Affairs Blog*. Retrieved from https://www.healthaffairs.org/do/10.1377/hblog20170628.060719/full/

Muhuri, P., Gfroerer, J., Davies, M. C. (2017). *Associations of nonmedical pain reliever use and initiation of heroin use in the United States. CBHSQ Data Review 2013*. Retrieved from https://www.samhsa.gov/data/sites/default/files/DR006/DR006/nonmedical-pain-reliever-use-2013.htm

National Academy of Medicine. (2017). *Pain management and the opioid epidemic: Balancing societal and individual benefits and risks of prescription opioid use*. Retrieved from https://www.ncbi.nlm.nih.gov/books/NBK458661/

National Institute of Environmental Health Sciences (NIEHS). (2018). *Health impacts: Climate and human health*. Retrieved from https://www.niehs.nih.gov/research/programs/geh/climatechange/health_impacts/index.cfm

National League for Nursing. (2016). *Overview*. Retrieved from http://www.nln.org/about

National League of Cities. (2016). *Cities 101-delegation of power*. Retrieved from https://www.nlc.org/resource/cities-101-delegation-of-power

National Prevention Strategy Assocaition of State and Territorial Health Officals. (2011). *National Prevention Strategy*. Retrieved from https://www.astho.org/NPS/

National Nurses United. (2018). *Your Handy Guide to CAN Lobby Day 2018*. Retrieved from https://www.nationalnursesunited.org/blog/your-handy-guide-cna-lobby-day-2018

Nickitas, D. M., Middaugh, D. J., & Aries, N. (2016). *Policy and politics for nurses and other health professionals* (2nd ed.). Burlington, MA: Jones & Bartlett Learning.

Office of the Federal Register. (n.d.). *A guide to the rulemaking process*. Retrieved from https://www.federalregister.gov/uploads/2011/01/the_rulemaking_process.pdf

O'Neill, T. (1993). *All politics is local*. New York, NY: Crown Publishing.

Organization for Economic Cooperation & Development (OECD). (2017). *Health at a Glance 2017: OECD Indicators*. Paris: OECD Publishing. Retrieved from https://doi.org/10.1787/health_glance-2017-en

Payne, K. (2017). *The broken ladder: How inequality affects the way we think, live, and die*. New York, NY: Viking.

Pearson, M., Anthony, Z. B., & Buckley, N. A. (2010). Prospective policy analysis: How an epistemic community informed policymaking on intentional self poisoning in Sri Lanka. *Health Research Policy and Systems*, *8*, 19. doi: 10.1186/1478-4505-8-19.

Poghosyan, L., Boyd, D. R., & Clarke, S. P. (2016). Optimizing full scope of practice for nurse practitioners in primary care: A proposed conceptual model. *Nursing Outlook*, *64*(2), 146–155.

Public Health Law Center. (2019). *U.S. E-Cigarette Regulations—50 State Review*. Retrieved from https://www.publichealthlawcenter.org/resources/us-e-cigarette-regulations-50-state-review

Rapaport, L. (March 13, 2018). *U.S. Health spending twice other countries with worse results*. Retrieved from https://www.reuters.com/article/us-health-spending/u-s-health-spending-twice-other-countries-with-worse-results-idUSKCN1GP2YN

Rhodes, D. (January 17, 2016). Raising cigarette-buying age to 21 a new strategy in fighting addiction. *Chicago Tribune*. Retrieved from http://www.chicagotribune.com/news/ct-minimum-tobacco-age-emanuel-met-20160117-story.html

Robert Wood Johnson Foundation. (November 30, 2010). *Robert Wood Johnson Foundation launches national campaign to advance health through nursing*. Retrieved from https://www.rwjf.org/en/library/articles-and-news/2010/11/robert-wood-johnson-foundation-launches-national-campaign-to-adv.html

Rutgers Cetner for American Women and Politics. (2020). Current numbers. Retrieved from https://cawp.rutgers.edu/search?fulltext=current+numbers

Savage, T., Hodge, D., Pickard, K., Myers, P., & Powell, K. (2018). Sustained reduction and prevention of neonatal and pediatric central line-associated bloodstream infection following a nurse-driven quality improvement initiative in a pediatric facility. *Journal of the Association for Vascular Access*, *23*(1), 30–41.

Sawyer, B., & Gonzalez, S. (2017). *How does the quality of the US health care system compare to other countries?* Kaiser Family Foundation. Retrieved from https://www.healthsystemtracker.org/chart-collection/quality-u-s-healthcare-system-compare-countries/#item-mortality-rate-cancers-falling-u-s-across-comparable-countries

Schneider, E., Sarnak, D., Squires, D., Shah, A., & Doty, M. (2017). *Mirror, Mirror 2017: International Comparison Reflects Flaws and Opportunities for Better U.S. Health Care*. Commonwealth Fund. Retrieved from https://interactives.commonwealthfund.org/2017/july/mirror-mirror/

Shariff, N. (2014). Factors that act as facilitators and barriers to nurse leaders' participation in health policy development. *BMC Nursing*, *13*, 20.

Surgeon General. (2011). *National prevention strategy*. Washington, DC: U.S. Department of Health and Human Services, Office of the Surgeon General. Retrieved from https://www.hhs.gov/sites/default/files/disease-prevention-wellness-report.pdf

Swider, S. M., Levin, P. F., & Reising, V. (2017). Evidence of public health nursing effectiveness: A realist review. *Public Health Nursing*, *34*(4). doi: 10.1111/phn.12320.

Taylor, M. R. (2016). Impact of advocacy initiatives on nurses' motivation to sustain momentum in public policy advocacy. *Journal of Professional Nursing*, *32*(3), 235–245.

U.S. Department of Health and Human Services. (2015). *About the Affordable Care Act*. Retrieved from http://www.hhs.gov/healthcare/about-the-law/read-the-law/index.html

U.S. Department of Health and Human Services. (January 11, 2016). *New hospitals and health care providers join successful, cost-cutting federal initiative that cuts costs and puts patients at the center of their care*. Retrieved from https://www.prnewswire.com/news-releases/new-hospitals-and-health-care-providers-join-successful-cutting-edge-federal-initiative-that-cuts-costs-and-puts-patients-at-the-center-of-their-care-300215344.html

U.S. Federal Drug Administration (FDA). (2016). *The Facts on the FDA's New Tobacco Rule*. Retrieved from https://www.fda.gov/consumers/consumer-updates/facts-fdas-new-tobacco-rule

U. S. Federal Election Commission. (n.d.). *Committees*. Retrieved from https://www.fec.gov/data/advanced/?tab=committees

U.S. House of Representatives. (n.d.). *The legislative process*. Retrieved from http://www.house.gov/content/learn/legislative_process/

White House. (2016). *The judicial branch*. Retrieved from https://www.whitehouse.gov/1600/judicial-branch

Williams, S., Phillips, J., & Koyama, K. (2018). Nurse advocacy: Adopting a health in all policies approach. *Online Journal of Issues in Nursing*, *23*(3). doi: 10.3912/OJIN.Vol23No03Man01.

World health Organization (WHO). (2019). *Community empowerment*. Retrieved from https://www.who.int/healthpromotion/conferences/7gchp/track1/en/

Xue, Y., & Intrator, O. (2016). Cultivating the role of nurse practitioners in providing primary care to vulnerable populations in an era of health-care reform. *Policy, Politics & Nursing Practice*, *17*(1), 24–31.

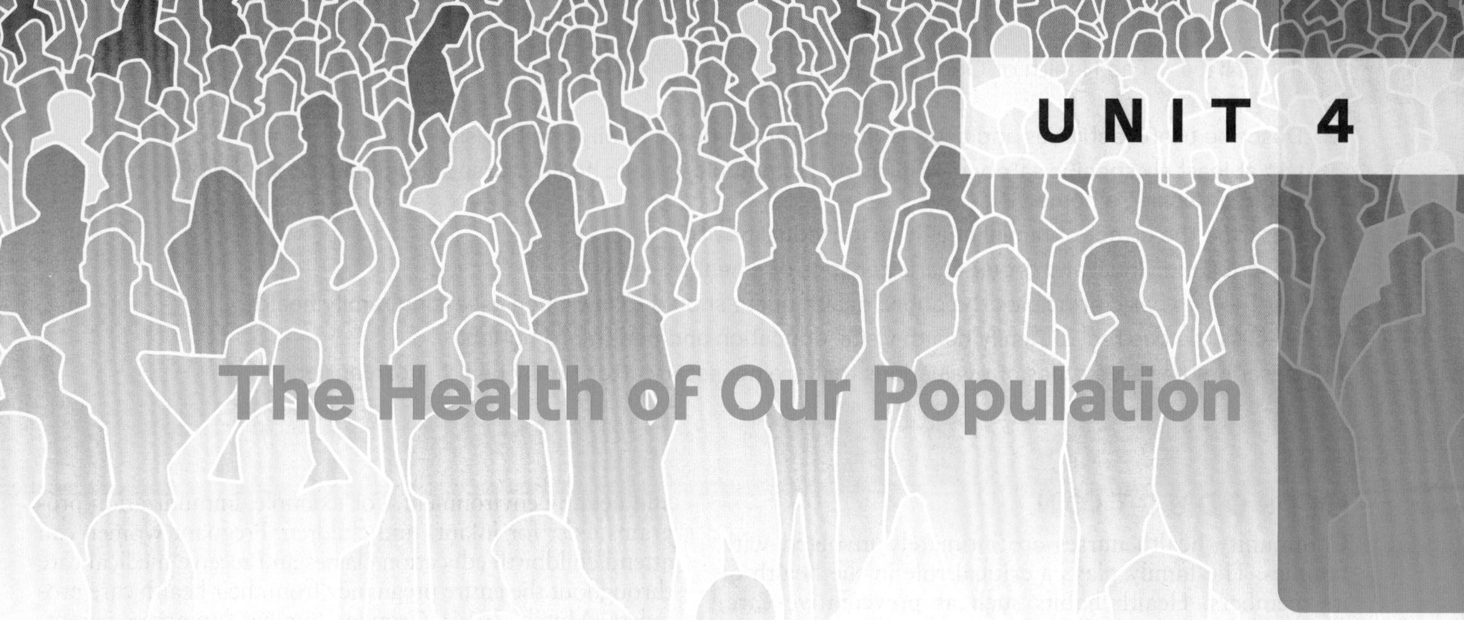

CHAPTER 14

Family as Client

"I yearn to enter the 'Promised Land'—a land of ideal health care where family nursing is 'usual care,' where families are included and welcomed, where family preferences are invited, and where family illness suffering is softened."

—Janice Bell (2014, p. 8), Family Nurse Theorist

KEY TERMS

- Asset-based approach
- Conceptual framework
- Developmental framework
- Eco-map
- Family
- Family health
- Family health nursing
- Family life cycle
- Genogram
- Home
- Interactional framework
- Outcome evaluation
- Population
- Referral
- Resource directory
- Roles
- Strengthening
- Structural–functional framework

LEARNING OBJECTIVES

Upon mastery of this chapter, you should be able to:

1. Discuss characteristics all families have in common.
2. Identify the stages of the family life cycle and the developmental tasks of a family.
3. Discuss how a family's culture influences its values, behaviors, and roles.
4. Describe the functions of a family.
5. Analyze the role of the community health nurse in promoting the health of the family.
6. Describe the components of the nursing process as they apply to enhancing family health.
7. Identify the steps in a successful family health intervention.

8. Describe useful activities and actions when intervening on family health visits.
9. List at least six specific safety measures the community/public health nurse should take when traveling to a home or making a home visit.
10. Describe the effect of family health on individual health.
11. Describe individual and group characteristics of a healthy family.
12. List the five basic principles the public health nurse should follow when assessing family health.
13. Discuss the two foci of family health visits: education and health promotion.
14. Describe the three types of evaluations that are necessary after family health interventions.

INTRODUCTION

Community health nurses are intimately involved with families. The family plays a critical role in the health of its members. Health habits such as preventative care, diet, exercise, and physical activity are developed through your experiences in a family. Health beliefs, genetic influences, and care of the ill family member all take place within the family environment. The community/public health nurse (C/PHN) is in a unique position to influence and promote **family health**. Families should be considered at every point of nursing care.

The definition of family varies by organization, discipline, and individual. Family theorists suggest that a family consists of two or more individuals who share a residence or live near one another; possess some common emotional bond; engage in interrelated social positions, roles, and tasks; and share cultural ties and a sense of affection and belonging (Kaakinen, Coehlo, Steele, Tabacco, & Robinson, 2018).

Today's C/PHN needs to understand and work with many types of families, each of which has unique health needs. For example, a young, single mother seeks help in caring for her infant. A 67-year-old provides care for his mother, who was recently discharged from the hospital after a stroke. A family from Haiti needs instruction on the purchase and preparation of food for the kidney dialysis diet their father has been given. The effectiveness of C/PHN depends on knowing how to work with all kinds of families.

This chapter draws from various theories to strengthen the student's understanding and appreciation of families as clients. This information will promote the effectiveness of interventions with families at the primary, secondary, and tertiary levels of prevention (Box 14-1).

The family is the basic element of a community and a population. A **family** refers to a group of individuals whose behaviors, actions, health conditions, and interrelationships impact the health of the group and the individuals (Kaakinen et al., 2018). As discussed in Chapter 1, a community is a set of people in families that share a common purpose with a sense of belonging and place (Kaakinen et al., 2018). A **population** encompasses the total number of persons in families within communities at a specific geographic location (Kaakinen et al., 2018). Based on the above definitions, the family's positive experience when accessing health services improves the health for the community that leads to a healthier population.

Families need to have equal access to optimal health care, social services, and community resources in a supportive and healthy environment. For example, immunization programs exist for infants and children. Pregnant women can attend childbirth education classes and receive medical care throughout the entire pregnancy from their health care providers (Mutch, 2016). Growing families can access parenting classes and support groups for help with developmental crises and in the management of chronic illness (Lee et al., 2017). Older adults have senior centers for a myriad of social and recreational activities as well as numerous services and activities offered at senior discounts (Frost, Beattie, Bhanu, Walters, & Ben-Shlomo, 2019). All these clients have one point in common—they are members of families. Clearly, the health of the family influences the health and wellness of the population.

Within the family, the interactions are unique because a family member can knowingly or unknowingly influence another. The health of one family member can influence other members' perspective(s) about health or their social value system. The emotional state of a family member can be the deciding factor in another family member's choice for a career or the schools you attended. The impact can be as mundane as the type of meals eaten. Will the meal include chicken if the dinner guests include vegetarian parents? Family members clearly influence each other and the entire family. This makes for a unique unit of service.

Just as each family is unique, so too are their homes. A public health nurse may feel comfort in some families' homes and not in others. A **home** is a structure or building where families live (e.g., mobile homes, high-rise inner-city apartments, rural cabins, cardboard boxes, farm labor camps). It can be daunting for students to enter a home that is a small and cluttered apartment, a sparsely furnished single room, or a makeshift structure in disrepair. Each home brings its own set of unique challenges and strengths that can influence the way the public health nurse perceives and interacts with the community to promote health, prevent illnesses, and reduce risk.

Public health nurses rely on the nursing process when working with families, the "core unit of service," to promote health and wellness, prevent illness, and improve the overall health of the population. The delivery of care occurs in various community settings (i.e., homes, work settings, classrooms, clinics and outpatient departments, neighborhood centers, and homeless shelters). Although caring for the family, as a unit of service, is an effective way to treat the population in the communities, practice does not always match a family nursing theory. The problem,

BOX **14-1** LEVELS OF PREVENTION PYRAMID

A Home Visit to an Infant With Gastroesophageal Reflux

SITUATION: A young single mother with a new infant (Patrick) asks for help with her baby at a well-baby visit as the baby is spitting up after feeding. The baby is diagnosed with gastroesophageal reflux. The mother was referred to a PHN for a home visit.
GOAL: Using the three levels of prevention, avoid negative health conditions, and promptly diagnose, treat, and/or restore the fullest possible potential.

Tertiary Prevention

Rehabilitation	*Health Promotion and Education*	*Health Protection*
▪ Monitor infant's reflux. ▪ Work closely with the provider to ensure follow-up for concerns. ▪ Be alert for any complication.	▪ The family continues to see provider for well visits. ▪ Encourage more frequent feedings (feed Patrick half as much, twice as often). ▪ Keep baby upright for 30 minutes after feeding.	▪ Educate and follow up to assure that infant immunization schedule begins on time and continues through childhood. ▪ Baby maintains weight and developmental milestones.

Secondary Prevention

Early Diagnosis	*Prompt Treatment*
▪ Parents discuss feeding with provider and when to introduce solids. ▪ Baby has irritability after eating and refuses to eat. ▪ Baby has not gained weight.	▪ The child has projectile vomiting; yellow, green, or coffee ground spit; blood in spit. ▪ Parents use feeding techniques to minimize infant reflux.

Primary Prevention

Health Promotion and Education	*Health Protection*
▪ Address infant feeding. ▪ Discuss anticipatory guidance.	▪ Baby continues to gain weight. ▪ Milestones for development are obtained. ▪ Review immunization schedule.

in part, is that health care services are often tailored to an individual and not a family and/or a community. Third-party payer and reimbursement policies impose limits to the kinds of services funded. Public health agencies often organize services around individuals. The government requires that public health agencies structure disease statistics or service categories on an individual instead of aggregated data on a family.

Family-level problem-solving techniques are used to deal with health issues including health promotion, pregnancy and childbirth, acute life-threatening illness, chronic illness, substance abuse, domestic violence, and terminal illness (Beck, Le, Henry-Okafor, & Shah, 2017; Coker, Martin, Simpson, & Lafortune, 2019; De Grubb, Levine, & Zoorob, 2017; Dyess-Nugent, 2018). The first step is a detailed family assessment that emphasizes internal and external influences (Salmond & Echevarria, 2017; Shajani & Snell, 2019). This creates a database from which a family diagnosis is generated, an essential step before planning, implementation, and evaluation of services.

The novice public health nurse must be able to practice within the nursing process. Moreover, when public health nurses address the health needs of the core unit of service, the family, the nurses are treating the health needs of the communities and the population (Association of Public Health Nurses [APHN], 2016a, 2016b). Public health nurses are legally the leaders in using the accessible health care services to prevent illnesses and promote health in families (APHN, 2016a, 2016b; Salmond & Echevarria, 2017). Family health is the cornerstone for community and population health, making the family the focus of health care and related services. Therefore, the health of the *family* is addressed through the nursing process that involves assessing, diagnosing, planning, implementing, and evaluating the family.

FAMILY HEALTH AND FAMILY HEALTH NURSING

Throughout history, the family has been the most basic unit. One of the first steps for nurses is to explore how a family influences the care that they provide and how they interact with the family. Most of us were raised in families and spent a good portion of our lives within families. Our first experiences with others are influenced by our families of origin. Feetham (2018) asserts that the way we interact with families actually comes from how we define family. So we come to our nursing practice with ideas about families based on our own experiences.

- The United States Census Bureau (Pemberton, 2015) views family as people living together and related by birth, adoption, or marriage.
- Kaakinen et al. (2018, p. 5) define family as "two or more individuals who depend on one another for emotional, physical, and economical support."
- Kaakinen et al. (2018, p. 5) define family health as a "dynamic changing state of wellbeing, which includes the biological, psychological, spiritual, sociological, and culture factors of individual members and the whole family system."

Family health is concerned with how well the family functions together as a unit. It involves not only the health of the members and how they relate to other members but also how well they relate to and cope with the community, outside the family. In fact, family health, like individual health, ranges along a continuum from wellness to illness. A family may be at one point on that continuum now and at a much different point 6 months from now. Family health refers to the health status of a given family at a given point in time (Kaakinen et al., 2018).

Family health nursing is how public health nurses care for individuals within the family or for the family as the client (family as context) or for the family as a system (Fig. 14-1). There are multiple ways that community health nurses can approach families. Some nurses view family nursing as part of other specialties such as public health nursing, maternal child nursing, or behavioral health nursing. However, some nurses view family nursing as its own distinct specialty, rich with its own body of literature and research. Each of these approaches with families has its own distinct set of beliefs.

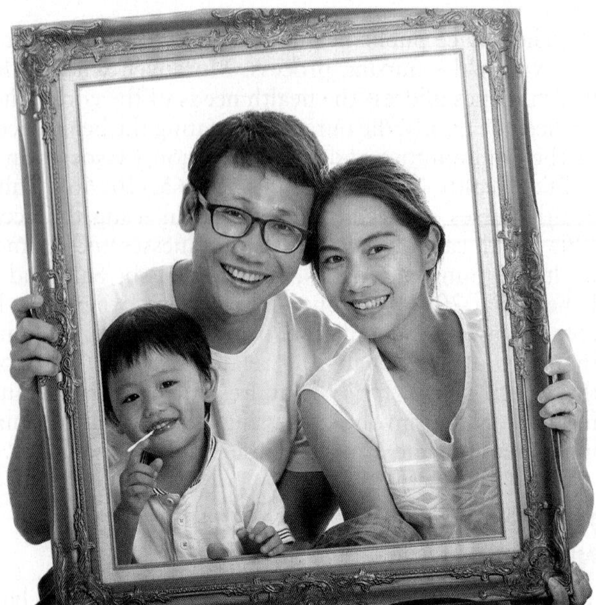

FIGURE 14-1 Community health nurses work with families and individual family members.

Nurses work with individuals within families every day. Most often, the individual is the recipient of care. While assessing the needs of the individual, the nurse needs to include the family in the assessment, as the family is the pivotal provider of care. How does the family assist the individual family member or hinder his or her progress? What are their available resources (physically, emotionally, and spiritually)?

Nurses working with families as a system view the family as part of a larger suprasystem that includes many subsystems. The family becomes greater than the sum of all of its parts. Any change within the family system affects all of the family members (Shajani & Snell, 2019).

When visualizing a family as a system, it may help to compare it to a mobile. Think of all the pieces suspended freely by a string. If you pull lightly on one piece, all the pieces move, just as a change in one member's health affects the entire family. Can you think of some examples of this in your own family?

FAMILY CHARACTERISTICS AND DYNAMICS

Several observations can be made about families. First, each family is unique, with its own distinct set of strengths. As a nurse you want to look first at the family's strengths. When you approach the door of a house to begin your visit with a family, you cannot be sure of what they will be like. You will have to gather information about the family in order to provide the best nursing care possible. Starting with their strengths will assure your success.

Families share universal characteristics with every other family (Box 14-2). For instance, families in every culture throughout history have engaged in similar functions: families have produced children, physically cared for their members, protected their health, encouraged their education or training, given emotional support and acceptance, and provided supportive and nurturing care during illness. These characteristics provide an important key to understanding each family's uniqueness. No matter how many families a nurse may visit over the course of a year, each one will have universal features; it is important for PHNs to know each family's unique set of characteristics and their effects on family health.

Family Stage of Development

Many of the characteristics and defined developmental stages of individual growth also apply to families. For example, families change continuously. Families grow and develop as the individuals within them mature and adapt to changes. A family's composition, set of roles, and interpersonal relationships change with time. Families vary with each stage of the **Family life cycle**. See Box 14-3 for some questions to ask yourself about your own family.

As Duvall and Miller (1985) first pointed out, no two children come to precisely the same family. Consider the following example of how families change over time. The

BOX 14-2 Universal Characteristics of Family Life

- Every family is a small social system.
    - Families are interdependent.
    - Families maintain boundaries.
    - Families exchange energy with their environments.
    - Families adapt.
    - Families are goal oriented (providing love, security, and a sense of belonging).
- Every family moves through stages in its life cycle.
- Every family has its own cultural values and rules.
- Family members share certain values that affect their behavior.
- Certain roles are defined for family members.
- A family's culture influences its distribution and use of power.
- Every family has certain basic functions:
    - Providing affection
    - Providing security
    - Instilling identity
    - Promoting affiliation
    - Providing socialization
    - Establishing controls
- Every family has structure.

Source: Duvall and Miller (1985).

Garcia family, a young married couple, begins their family by getting to know each other, learning more about their new roles, and developing a satisfying marriage. They have difficulty getting pregnant, so they decide to adopt a baby. Their baby, Rosa, changes the family and their roles as parents. Thus new roles are added (father, mother, and daughter). Within 2 years they become pregnant and Luis is born. This once again changes the family. Both family size and a reorganization of family occurred. The children entered school; Mrs. Garcia went back to work, and soon, Rosa was leaving for college. The Garcia family, like every family, is moving through a predictable and sequential pattern of stages known as the family life cycle.

PHNs who are knowledgeable about this cycle can provide anticipatory guidance to families. For instance, nurses can help prepare the family for having children. The nurse can help the soon-to-be parents to anticipate the responsibility and costs of raising her child by helping them calculate child care needs. The nurse can assist the family in figuring out the monthly costs of breastfeeding versus buying formula, disposable versus cloth diapers, and the clothing, equipment, and medical costs of infant care.

BOX 14-3 WHAT DO *YOU* THINK?

Questions for Self-Evaluation

1. What are your first memories of family?
2. What is your definition of family?
3. How would you describe your own family?
4. Who do you now include as family members?

To progress through the stages of the life cycle, a family must carry out its basic functions and the developmental tasks associated with those functions. Often, how we define family will determine how the family functions are filled. Unlike developmental tasks, which are specific to each age level, family developmental tasks are ongoing throughout the life cycle. The manner and degree to which each function is carried out varies depending on how well members accomplish individual developmental tasks and meet the demand of a particular stage (Kaakinen et al., 2018).

Some functions require greater emphasis at certain stages. Socialization, for example, consumes much of a family's time during the early years of child development. Duvall and Miller (1985) described these activities as "stage critical" family developmental tasks that must be completed before moving onto the next stage. Sample community health nursing actions with the family at different stages are presented in Table 14-1.

Family Values and Their Effect on Behavior

Every family has its own set of values and rules for operation (McGoldrick, Garcia-Preto, & Carter, 2016). Like all cultural values, many family values remain outside the conscious awareness of family members. These values, often not verbalized, become powerful determinants of what the family believes, feels, thinks, and does. Family values include those beliefs transmitted by previous generations, religious influences, immediate social pressures, and the larger society. Values become an integral part of a family's life and are difficult to change (Box 14-4).

Family Roles

Roles, the assigned or assumed parts that members play during day-to-day family living, are bestowed and defined by the family (Kaakinen et al., 2018). Families distribute among their members all the responsibilities and tasks necessary to conduct family living.

Family members may play several roles at the same time. This can be taxing. A single parent often takes on the role of both father and mother but may distribute responsibilities and tasks more widely. A grandmother or a child may assume responsibility for some chores and thereby relieve some of the demands on the single parent. Among families, there is great variation in expectations for each role and in the degree of flexibility in divisions of roles. An example may be specific tasks given to girls versus boys within the family. Girls may be given child care or kitchen responsibilities and boys given yard tasks.

Many families enjoy the fellowship of organized religious or cultural groups. This fellowship can be a source of support or comfort, as well as an additional role function for the family members. Family members can also participate in roles outside the family. These may involve local or regional politics, community improvement, volunteerism for nonprofit groups, or other groups outside the home that the community may offer. These diverse role relationships should enrich and energize the participants. The community health nurse may work with families to help them achieve a balance of activities that promote family health.

TABLE 14-1 Critical Family Developmental Tasks

Stage of the Family Life Cycle	Developmental Tasks	Role of the Community Health Nurse
Forming a partnership	Establishing a mutually satisfying relationship	Interact with family where they are at
Childbearing	Adjusting to pregnancy and the promise of parenthood Fitting into the kin network Having and adjusting to infants and encouraging their development Establishing a satisfying home for both parents and infant(s)	Assist them in developing strong relationships
Preschool-age children	Adapting to the critical needs and interests of preschool children in stimulating, growth-promoting ways Coping with energy depletion and lack of privacy as parents	Assist in preparing for family expansion through education and anticipatory guidance
School-age children	Fitting into the community of school-age families in constructive ways Encouraging children's educational achievement	Encourage time for each other as adults in a relationship separate from parenting role
Teenage children	Balancing freedom with responsibility as teenagers mature and emancipate themselves Establishing outside interests and careers as growing parents	Provide anticipatory guidance for the school-aged children as they grow into adulthood
Launching children	Releasing young adults into work, military service, college, marriage, etc., with appropriate rituals and assistance Maintaining a supportive home base	Provide anticipatory guidance for the contracting family as children leave home
Middle-aged parents	Rebuilding the relationship Maintaining kin ties with older and younger generations	Prepare adults for grandparenting role
Aging family members	Adjusting to retirement Coping with bereavement and living alone Closing the family home or adapting it to aging	Assist aging adults with emotional and financial security, as they approach retirement Prepare the aging adults with ways to cope with the losses of old age, including changes in space, work, health, status, and loss of friends and family members

Source: Duvall and Miller (1985).

Power is the possession of control, authority, or influence over others—assuming patterns in each family. In some families, power is concentrated primarily in one member; in other families, it is distributed on a more egalitarian basis (McGoldrick et al., 2016).

The traditional patriarchal family, in which the father holds absolute authority over the other members, is rare in American society. However, the pattern of husband as head of the household and dominant member of the family is still frequently seen. The dominant power, whether male or female, holds the majority of the decision-making power, particularly over more important family matters such as employment, finances, and health care. With changing societal influences, however, the present trend among American families is toward egalitarian power distribution.

BOX 14-4 Cultural Values

Cultural values such as the following shape most decisions and choices in our lives:

- Education
- Sex roles
- Health care
- Courtship/marriage
- Lifestyle
- Childrearing

Family Social Class and Economic Status

As a community health nurse, it is important for your assessment to include social class of families you are visiting. Social class often shapes a family's access and choices to work, educational, and health care opportunities (McGoldrick et al., 2016). Their overall health is often determined by their class position. The biggest predictor of health is your level of wealth (Penman-Aguilar et al., 2016). How healthy we are and how long we live are often related to our social standing. The neighborhoods families choose to live in, and the schools their children attend, are often determined by social class. These decisions/choices have lifelong implications and shape the history of families. See Chapter 23 for more on social determinants of health and the socioeconomic gradient.

Most people who experience homelessness are single adults. In 2017:

- 184,661 people in families were homeless.
- 57,971 families with children were homeless.
- This represents one third (33%) of the total homeless population.
- 16,938 people in families with children who were counted in unsheltered locations (living on the streets, in cars, or in another place not meant for human habitation) (National Alliance to End Homelessness, 2018).

Families who are homeless are not necessarily incomeless. They may include working parents who just are not making enough money to pay for housing. On average, a homeless family household consisted of three people. Homeless families present the C/PHN with unique challenges. Primarily, the family is in crisis and often not able to provide for their most basic needs. When families are unable to meet these needs, they are unable to address other concerns such as medical appointments, healthy eating and exercise, and other preventative actions that nurses typically recommend.

Children who experience homelessness have higher risks of emotional and behavioral problems, serious health problems, school mobility, repeating a grade, and being expelled or dropping out of school and have lower academic performance (National Alliance to End Homelessness, 2018).

Community health nurses should be aware of this and focus on first assisting the family in getting their essential needs met. They should also acknowledge that the behaviors seen in children may be the direct result of the situation that the family finds itself in. A C/PHN's knowledge of the resources available in the community is an important first step in providing the family with the help to deal with the crisis and assisting in the provision of ongoing shelter, food, health, employment, and schooling needs. See Chapter 26 for more on homeless populations. You can check your state rates at https://endhomelessness.org/homelessness-in-america/homelessness-statistics/state-of-homelessness-2020/

Family Composition

Globally, families—in all varied forms—are the basic social unit (Shajani & Snell, 2019). The meaning of family among the Hmong of northern Laos may include hundreds of people who make up a clan. In Mexico, families remain close, are large, and extend into multiple generations. In Germany and Japan, families are small and tend to the needs of their elders at home.

In the United States, where families come from many cultural groups, many variations coexist within communities. Families come in many shapes and sizes (Fig. 14-2).

It is a privilege to gain entry into a family's home. This is a uniquely private space belonging to the family. The people who are members of this household interact, care for one another, and bond in ways that may never be fully understood by anyone outside the family. Therefore, being granted entrance into this system gives the community health nurse an opportunity to work with the family that few other professionals experience. Each type of household requires recognition and acceptance by community health nurses, who must help families achieve optimal health.

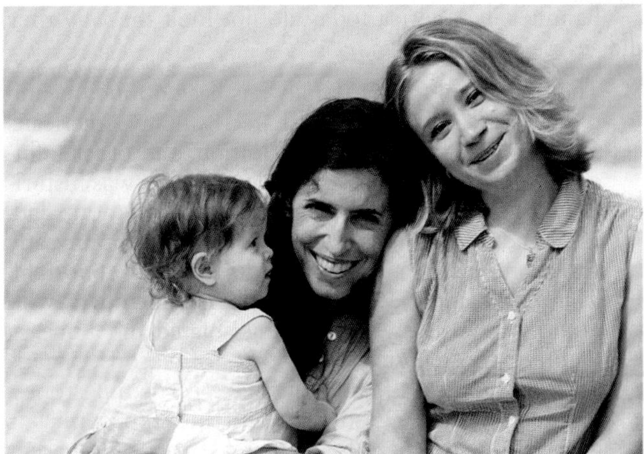

FIGURE 14-2 Families exist in many forms.

Traditional Versus Contemporary Families

Traditional families are those that are likely most familiar to us:

- The nuclear family—husband, wife, and children living together in the same household. In nuclear families, the workload distribution between the two adults can vary. Both adults may work outside the home; one adult may work outside the home, whereas the other stays at home and assumes primary responsibilities for the household; or partners may alternate, constantly renegotiating work and domestic responsibilities.
- A nuclear dyad family consists of two adults living together who have no children or who have grown children living outside the home.
- A single adult family is one in which one adult is living alone by choice or because of separation from a spouse or children or both. Separation may be the result of divorce, death, or distance from children.

Half of American adults are married today, which is drastically different than 72% in 1960 (Pew Research Center, 2017). Couples are putting off marriage as they get their careers started and begin working on their futures. In 2016, the median age for marriage among men was 29.5 and for women 27.4, which is roughly 7 years more than in 1960 (Pew Research Center, 2017). In 2017, 65% of children under the age of 17 years old lived with two-parent families which is up slightly from 64% in 2014 (ChildStats.gov, 2019).

Sometimes, in close-knit ethnic communities, families form a kin network, in which several nuclear families live in the same household or near one another and share goods and services. They may own and operate a family business, sharing work and child care responsibilities, income and expenses, and even meals. Variations of this trend are increasing among all groups as children postpone leaving home because of economic conditions, educational plans, or student loans. This is the most popular living arrangement for young adults today (Vespa, 2017).

The number of young adults who continue to live with their parents is on the rise. A third of young adults aged 18 to 34 lived with their parents, and more young adults lived in their parents' home than with a spouse in 2016 (Vespa, 2017).

Families in America today do not look the way they did several years ago.

- The traditional nuclear family has been a fundamental part of our cultural heritage shared by many Americans and reinforced by religion, education, and other influential social institutions. The "ideal" family was historically considered a nuclear family including a mom, dad, and children. By thinking of this as the ideal family, any variation was often treated as deviant and abnormal. This view can leave families and family members, who do not fit this description, feeling isolated and alone.
- Families are changing for a variety of reasons; Americans are putting off previously expected milestones, families are getting smaller, and life expectancy is getting longer. There is an increase in single-parent adoptions; an increase in lesbian, gay, bisexual, transgender, or queer (LGBTQ) couples and families; and high divorce and remarriage rates.
- The role of women in the family is changing, they are marrying at older ages, and children are being born outside of marriage. Families should no longer be defined as "what" they are but rather "who" they are (Feetham, 2018).
- McGoldrick et al. (2016) fosters the importance of putting a positive spin on the families that make up our world. The nurse is in a unique position to assess families in a strength-based model rather than viewing certain families as deviant.

As society struggles with what they consider to be the ideal family, the media portrays them in various forms, showing that society is beginning to accept more contemporary definitions of family.

- Television shows such as Gilmore Girls, Blackish, Modern Family, and The Fosters are all examples of the ways that television is changing along with family structures. The days of Leave it to Beaver type shows are becoming less common. People want to see characters like themselves, going through similar experiences, on the shows that they watch.
- Another way that families are impacted by media is through social media. It can be a positive or negative influence on the family and its members. In a study done by Valdermorose-San-Emeterio, Sanz-Arazu, & Ponce-de-Leon-Elizondo (2017), it was discovered that children who report more digital leisure time as one of their favorite leisurely practices had less family cohesion. Digital leisure time can be considered playing video games, social networking, and scanning the Internet. Since these activities are becoming more commonplace, the public health nurse should consider these factors when working with families. See Chapter 10.
- One of the positive aspects of social media is its use in promoting health care resources to families. Nurses can use messaging and other platforms to reach patients who otherwise may be limited by distance or transportation issues. Families turn to online resources for many reasons and health care questions are no exception. With the high usage of social media, families and its members are likely to use it for health access and information (Schroeder, 2017). Nurses can play a role in using them to communicate and teach families with current and evidence-based information.

Families Experiencing Divorce, Remarriage, and Blending

Divorce, remarriage, and blending of families can result in distinct emotional responses and developmental issues among family members, as shown in Table 14-2.

Divorce. Divorce does not just affect the involved couple; it changes the entire family structure and each family member's life course. Demographics play a role in divorce with those who are less educated and earning a lower income. Approximately 850,000 marriages in the United States end in divorce and even more parents who are never married break up, which also greatly impacts the family (Dissing, Dich, Nybo-Andersen, Lund, & Rod, 2017). As divorce becomes more acceptable, couples are making this choice for a variety of reasons. These can vary from marital dissatisfaction, infidelity, finances, and many other factors. Something new to consider in this day and age is the effect of social media on couples. It is now easier than ever to form emotional relationships online. Through various online platforms, couples are able to reconnect with old friends and even make new ones. Social media boundaries are important for couples to discuss and agree on. These virtual relationships can become part of a family's daily lives and can lead to infidelity and even divorce (Abassi & Alghamdi, 2017).

Divorce affects all members of the family in a different way, since each is at a different stage in life. Each member is going through unique adjustments and transitions as they cope with their new normal.

- For children, it may require coping with a new geographic location and a new school, as well as adjusting to changes in the mental and physical health of family members.
- In addition to the normal growth and developmental changes, children from divorced families may face an absent father or mother, interparental conflict, economic distress, parental adjustment, multiple life stressors, and short-term crises.
- New schools mean that children must find new friends and social groups, proving themselves once again and trying to gain acceptance in a completely new social setting. Their previous sense of security and comfort at home is forever changed. These adjustments take time and C/PHN can provide support for the children involved (Table 14-2).
- The frequency of divorce does appear to be stabilizing in America today; the number of children living with unmarried parents has remained unchanged in the 21st century (Kaakinen et al., 2018).

Remarriage and Blending. The United States Census Bureau uses the term "blended families" to describe families who bring nonbiological children into a new marriage. In this structure, single parents marry and raise the children from each of the previous relationships together. If this is the result of divorce or death, this can be an especially painful transition (Table 14-2).

TABLE 14-2 Phases of the Divorce–Remarriage–Blending Cycle and Expected Family Member Responses

Phase	Emotional Responses	Developmental Issues
Divorce	■ Continue working on emotional recovery by overcoming hurt, anger, or guilt	■ Giving up fantasies of reunion ■ Staying connected with extended families ■ Rebuild and strengthen own social network
Postdivorce	■ Separate feelings about ex-spouse from parenting role ■ Prepare self for possibility of changes in custody as child(ren) get older; be open to their needs ■ Risk developing a new intimate relationship	■ Make flexible and generous visitation arrangements for child(ren) and noncustodial parent and extended family members ■ Deal with possibilities of changing custody arrangements as child(ren) get older ■ Deal with child(ren)'s reaction to parents establishing relationships with new partners
Meeting new people	■ Allowing for the possibility of developing a new intimate relationship	■ Dealing with child(ren)'s and ex-family members' reactions to a parent "dating"
Entering a new relationship	■ Completing an "emotional recovery" from past divorce ■ Accepting one's fears about developing a new relationship ■ Working on feeling good about what the future may bring	■ Recovery from loss of marriage is adequate ■ Discovering what you want from a new relationship ■ Working on openness in a new relationship
Planning a new marriage	■ Accepting one's fears about the ambiguity and complexity of entering a new relationship such as: ■ New roles and responsibilities ■ Boundaries: space, time, and authority ■ Affective issues: guilt, loyalty, conflicts, and unresolvable past hurts	■ Recommitment to marriage and forming a new family unit ■ Dealing with stepchild(ren) as custodial or noncustodial parent ■ Planning to help child(ren) deal with fears, loyalty conflicts, and memberships in two systems ■ Realignment of relationships with ex-family to include new spouse and child(ren)
Remarriage and blending families	■ Final resolution of attachment to previous spouse ■ Acceptance of new family unit with different boundaries	■ Restructuring family boundaries to allow for new spouse of stepparent ■ Realignment of relationships to allow intermingling of systems ■ Expanding relationships to include all new family members ■ Sharing family memories and histories to enrich members' lives

Source: McGoldrick et al. (2016).

- They may be custodial parents who have the children except during planned visits with the noncustodial parent, or they may share custody, so that the children live in the blended arrangement only part time or possibly live in two separate blended homes.
- The family may include children from the couple, in addition to the children brought into the relationship. Not all divorced adults stay single; most remarry or cohabitate with another adult, who may or may not have children. This new couple may have children from their union, or adopt, creating an even more complex family.
- Merged or blended families require considerable adjustment and relearning of roles, tasks, communication patterns, and relationships.
- Traditional nuclear families have well-established roles and stages that members go through, but this is not true for blended families, which leads to the complexity of the family dynamics and structure (Kaakinen et al., 2018).
- We all come to new relationships with our own history from the past.

Since this emerging family pattern is becoming more prominent, it is very possible that the C/PHN is familiar with this pattern or lives in such a family. In the blended family, there isn't a definitive and common definition of who makes up the family among its members (Kaakinen et al., 2018). This is something for the nurse to keep in mind as the family is assessed. The data on blended families can be challenging to track since the United States Census information is done only every 10 years. The American Community Survey done in 2017 found that 3,927,266 households included stepchildren (U.S. Census, 2017).

Some of the challenges that blended families face are merging traditions, adjustment to change, sibling rivalry, change in discipline styles, and managing age differences (Guzzo, Hemez, Anderson, Manning, & Brown, 2019). This adds to the complexity of the dynamics and health of families.

Nursing skills that are needed when working with divorced or blended families include the ability to listen and be empathetic, as well as a nonjudgmental attitude. The nurse should meet the family where they are at and provide resources that the family may need. Resources may include support groups, reading materials, or interventions available in the community. Communication among all parents and family members should be encouraged. Peer support groups for children and adolescents and support from within the schools should be used, if available, or started if they do not exist. The school nurse could be a rich resource for families also. The community health nurse can have a significant role in community-wide planning if services are needed but unavailable.

Single-Parent Families

One of the most common contemporary family structures is the single-parent family, mostly headed by women. These families are created in several ways. Sometimes single women choose to adopt or have children without being married, and some become single parents through divorce. Depending on how single-parent families come about, there can be loss and grief to deal with. Family strength and security is important for the family members regardless of the situation.

- In 2016, the birth rate for unmarried women was 42.4 births per 1,000 aged 15 to 44, which is down 2% from 2015 (Martin, Hamilton, Osterman, Driscoll, & Drake, 2018).
- The percentage of all births to unmarried women was 39.8% in 2016, a 1% decline from 2015 and the lowest level since 2007 (Martin et al., 2018).

Nonmarital birth rates declined from 2015 to 2016 for women in age groups under 35, with the rate for teenagers ages 15 to 19 dropping 8% (to 18.5 per 1,000 in 2016).

- The rate for females aged 15 to 17 was at an all-time low (8.6).
- Conversely, rates rose for all age groups aged 35 and over, reaching historic peaks for women aged 35 to 39 (35.6) and 40 to 44 (10.0) (Martin, Hailton, Osterman, & Driscoll, 2019).

This is thought to be the result of two trends; the increased financial independence of women and the tightening of the job market for men. Although Kaakinen et al. (2018) mentions that the wage gap between men and women still exists, women are better able to support themselves than in the past.

Over time, this form of family has become more accepted by society. It is important for C/PHNs to view the strengths of single-parent families. Building on their current strengths can be most helpful in terms of meeting the challenges that they may face. These challenges will typically result from one parent being solely responsible for the financial income, caregiving, and support for the family. The needs of the family will depend on their stage in the family cycle and experiences that brought them into the single-parent family. Nurses with their connections in the community can assist these families through advocacy and collaboration.

Families Headed by an Adolescent Parent or Parents

Statistics indicate that teenagers are increasingly the heads of single-parent families; some of these teen heads of households become pregnant in junior high or high school. The birth rate among teens 15 to 19 years old has continued a steady decline, but teen birth rates in the United States remain the highest among those in developed countries (Guttmacher Institute, 2015).

- The birth rate for women aged 15 to 19 in the United States in 2016 was 20.3 births per 1,000 women, down 9% from 2015 (22.3) and another record low.
- The number of births to teenagers aged 15 to 19 was 209,809 in 2016, also down 9% from 229,715 in 2015.
- The 2016 birth rates for teenagers aged 15 to 17 and 18 to 19 were 8.8 and 37.5 births per 1,000 women, respectively, down 11% and 8% from 2015 to record lows for both groups (Martin et al., 2018).

Teenagers are still developing physically, mentally, and emotionally and are not prepared to take on parenthood without help. Consideration should be given to helping the mother on her life course as well as the baby. The mother needs support and structure so that she may support her child. Home visitation programs such as the Nurse Family Partnership are able to provide this stability for both mom and baby if available in the community.

Specific factors related to teen birth rates are low education and low-income levels of a teen's family, few opportunities in a teen's community for positive youth involvement, neighborhood racial segregation, neighborhood physical disorder (e.g., graffiti, abandoned vehicles, litter, alcohol containers, cigarette butts, glass on the ground), and neighborhood-level income inequality, and teens in child welfare systems are at increased risk of teen pregnancy and birth than other groups. For example, young women living in foster care are more than twice as likely to become pregnant than those not in foster care (CDC, 2019). Teenagers also lack availability to contraceptives and the education to use them properly. They may be afraid to ask for resources and fear judgment which adds to risk of pregnancy and unsafe sex practices.

Housing is another significant issue that affects teen mothers. A study conducted by SmithBattle (2018a), which started in 1988 and continues today, found that housing is a concern that needs to be addressed when assessing teen moms. Housing was especially a concern for black moms who grew up in poverty. Compared to their white counterparts, they lived in various situations that increased toxic stress associated with discriminatory housing policies (SmithBattle, 2018a). Children raised without safe and secure housing struggle in other aspects of their lives. It is also difficult for teen moms to become productive members of society if they do not have a home to call their own.

Teen fathers are often left out of the loop for services that communities provide for the teen mother and infants, and there is a lack of research in the literature on the experiences and roles of teen fathers (Ngweso, Peterson, & Quenlivan, 2017). However, it has been established that partner involvement contributes positively to the outcomes in pregnancy (SmithBattle, Phengnum, Shagavah, & Okawa, 2019).

- A father who is emotionally supportive of the mother and provides child care and financial support directly and indirectly affects the well-being of his child.
- Children with absent fathers are at increased risk for behavioral difficulties and poor academic performance. Longitudinal research found lower birth weights and lower cognitive and behavioral scores at age 2 and poorer health for children of adolescent fathers when compared with those of adult fathers.
- Ngweso et al. (2017) found that teen fathers feel unprepared and unincluded in the birth and decision-making process. It would benefit teen moms, babies, fathers, and the community if we were to involve teen fathers in the preparation and education of birth and early parenting.
- There are home visiting programs that include the father in the visits and activities (Nurse Family Partnership, 2019). This encourages a sense of inclusion and promotes healthy family relationships. Teens often feel misunderstood; and this is even more true in the case of teen pregnancy. See Chapter 4 for research demonstrating the effectiveness of NFP.

The implications for the role of the C/PHN are greatest with the adolescent parent population. For example, nurses work with young teens through schools, clinics, or home visiting programs to ensure healthy pregnancies and teach parenting skills to the parents and grandparents.

- Nurses can also ensure that the infant receives immunizations and primary care health services, reaches age-appropriate milestones, and can provide family planning information to the new parents.
- Teen mothers experience high levels of psychological distress, and one of the recommendations given by SmithBattle and Freed (2016) is to be proactive and screen for distress in pregnant and parenting teens.
- Teens may have trauma in their backgrounds that may not have been addressed. They may feel stigmatized and this can prevent them from reaching out for help. If C/PHNs focus on the teen mothers' strengths and aspirations to prevent childhood trauma, which they themselves may have experienced, they will be in a unique position to help these families (SmithBattle, 2018b).
- On a broader scale, C/PHNs should collaborate with other professionals to make sure that the community has resources for all levels of prevention, with a focus on primary prevention.

Families Headed by a Cohabitating Couple

Cohabitating couples' ages can range from young adults to elderly couples. The couples may be heterosexual or LGBTQ; they may or may not share a sexual relationship. In some instances, these couples have their own biologic or adopted children. Cohabitation has increased for all race groups of unmarried mothers in America over the last decade (Pew Research, 2018). There is a wide class gap in marriage in America. Marriage is more prevalent and more durable among better educated, higher-income Americans. It should come as no surprise, then, to find an education gap between married and cohabiting parents. Married mothers and fathers are over four times more likely to hold a bachelor's or advanced degree than cohabiting biological parents (Reeves & Krause, 2017).

Young adults may put off marriage to complete their education, work on their careers, or simply experiment with different living experiences. Since many have delayed marriage, it has become more likely that couples will live together prior to marriage. Living together does not necessarily mean that marriage is imminent though. Raley (2016) explains that nearly two thirds of married couples lived together prior to marriage and that couples who cohabitate are less likely to marry and are more likely to break up within the first 3 years (Raley, 2016). Elderly couples may choose to cohabitate after losing a spouse or experiencing loneliness but not wanting to go through a legal marriage. Similar to the other families mentioned in this chapter, cohabiting couples have become an accepted family structure in America.

LGBTQ Families

Although the exact number of LGBTQ families is not known, this emerging family type is increasing. The United States Census estimates close to 900,000 same-sex households. Romero (2017) states that 1.1 million LGBTQ individuals are married to a same-sex partner. There are over 10.7 million American adults identifying themselves as LGBTQ, and 2 to 3.7 million children report having a LGBTQ parent. Almost one half of LGBTQ women and about one fifth of LGBTQ men are raising a child. Foster and adopted children are often being raised by LGBTQ couples, and over 25% of same-sex couples are raising siblings, grandchildren, or other related/nonrelated children (Jones, 2015).

Healthy People 2030 addresses lesbian, gay, bisexual, and transgender Health. This speaks to the importance of understanding the discrimination and oppression that LGBTQ families have faced. Although much progress has been made in accepting people with values and beliefs different from those of the mainstream, LGBTQ still face health-related challenges and disparities (U.S. Department of Health and Human Services, 2020).

These families have many of the same hopes regarding parenting that any family may have. In addition, they experience the stress that accompanies being stigmatized by much of a society.

- Lack of acceptance from their families and communities may have negative implications on their own family.
- Out and Equal: Workplace Advocates (2019) reports that one in four of LGBTQ participants surveyed has experienced workplace discrimination. Other markers of discrimination (e.g., rejected by family/

friend; been a subject of jokes/slurs; threatened or physically attacked; poor service at business, hotel, restaurant) have shown decreases from the past year to current year; this indicates that some progress has occurred. Healthy People 2030 addresses reduction in bullying as an objective for this population (USDHHS, 2020).
- Annual family income is lower (39% vs. 38% earning <$30,000; 20% vs. 34% earning <$75,000) for LGBTQ families than for the overall US population.

The nurse can become a valued resource for the family. Through education and anticipatory guidance, the nurse can assist the family to successfully navigate the developmental stages of their children as well as the varied issues faced by families. The nurse can work with parents to anticipate what questions to expect from their children about their family.

Families With Older Adults

Aging is something that begins the day we are born; however, it is not focused on until a person turns 65 or older or begins to experience declining health. It is often thought of as something negative rather than a normal process. Elderly individuals are the fastest-growing segment of the population and their value is often overlooked. Since Americans are getting older and families are getting smaller, there is an increase in elderly and a decrease in adult children to care for them. However, family relationships remain strong and last longer than ever due to the increase in life expectancy (Kaakinen et al., 2018).

- In 2010, 40 million people in the United States were over the age of 65 years or 11% of the total population. This is projected to double by 2030 (AgingStats.gov, 2015).
- Many older adults live independently well into their eighties and maintain healthy contacts with family and friends.
- Others feel isolated because of chronic health problems that limit mobility, thereby reducing or eliminating the ability to interact or contribute meaningfully in society. Relationships in later life are affected by several factors: retirement status, health, mental health, and caregiving roles (Eliopoulos, 2018).
- The way that individual members of the family react to these factors will affect how the rest of the family copes. This is where the nurse can help.

The community health nurse needs to understand the complex dynamics of such situations and offer support and encouragement as family members work through chronic health problems. Adult children may become caregivers as their parents become older which is a change in the family dynamic for nurses to keep in mind. Often, a nurse serves an entire community of elders in a senior apartment complex, an assisted living center, or a mobile home community, for whom maintaining wellness is the focus. Keeping physically active, eating healthy meals, receiving appropriate medical care and immunizations, and establishing and maintaining social contacts are some of the tasks elders should focus on to stay healthy well into old age. The community health nurse can intervene by advocating for the individual medical and social needs for the elderly.

Foster Families

Many children are removed from their families because of maltreatment due to abuse, violence, or neglect. When this occurs, children are often placed with foster families. On September 30, 2016, there were an estimated 437,465 children in foster care, more than a quarter (32%) were in relative homes, and nearly half (45%) were in nonrelative foster family homes (childwelfare.gov, 2018).

- Foster families take a variety of forms, but all foster families have formal training to accept unrelated children into their homes on a temporary basis, while the children's parents receive the help necessary to reunify the original family.
- Although this arrangement is not ideal, most foster families provide safe and loving homes for these children in transition.
- Roughly half (55%) had a case goal of reunification with their parents or primary caretakers, and a little over half (51%) of the children who left foster care in 2016 were discharged to be reunited with their parents or primary caretakers.
- Close to half of the children (45% who left foster care in 2016 were in care for <1 year. (childwelfare.gov, 2018).

Often, foster children have emotional and physical health problems, and they may never have experienced the positive structure that foster families provide. Consideration should be given to the loss that typically present in foster situations. The losses may include biological parents losing their children, foster parents unable to have biological children, and foster children losing biological parents (Turney &Wildeman, 2016). These problems, which can cause stress and grief for everyone involved, are typically ones that the community health nurse may help to alleviate.

Implications of Family Composition Diversity for Community/public Health Nurses

The variety of family structures raises three important issues for consideration:

- First, C/PHNs can no longer hold to a myth that idealizes the traditional nuclear family. They must be prepared to work with and accept all types of families. Unless the C/PHN can accept the full array of family lifestyles and address the special needs of each, it is questionable that they will be able to fully help the family and may even create additional difficulties.
- Second, the structure of an individual's family may change several times over a lifetime. A girl may be born into a nuclear family and then become part of a single-parent family when her parents are divorced. As she matures, she may become a single adult living alone and then become a part of a cohabitating couple. Still later, she may marry and have children in a nuclear family. After the death of her husband as a senior citizen, she may have a relationship outside of marriage and choose not to remarry. For the

BOX 14-5 Questions the Nurse May Ask the Family

1. What are your strengths as a family?
2. If you had to tell me your three most favorite things about your family, what would they be?
3. Name one quality about your mother that you really respect. About your father? Your partner? Your child?
4. What is your best memory of your family?

individual, each family form involves changes in roles, interaction patterns, socialization processes, and links with external resources. The community health nurse must learn to address clients' needs throughout these life changes equipping people with the skills needed to deal with the inevitability of changing structures.

- Finally, each type of family structure creates different issues and problems that, in turn, influence a family's ability to perform basic functions. Shajani and Snell (2019) discuss the need for nurses to identify and develop strengths with families in planning nursing care. This should be a community health nurse's starting point. What are the family strengths? How does the family see their strengths? All families have strengths, although sometimes these are not easily recognized. It is important for the nurse to identify these with the family's collaboration (Box 14-5).

The family is the basic unit of a community and a population. Maintaining the health of family transitions into the health of both the community and the population. Caring for family impacts the health of the community, which in turn affects the health of the population (APHN, 2016a, 2016b; Kub, Kulbok, Miner, & Merrill, 2017). This interdependence is evident even within the family because one family member can positively or negatively impact other family members and the family unit itself. As a result, public health nurses must first understand what constitutes a "healthy family" so that they can use the nursing process with family-level problem-solving techniques for health prevention and promotion within the family and subsequently the community and the population.

Traits Associated With Healthy Family Functioning

A family is a health aggregate from the interrelationships of the family members. The health of the family is affected by each family member and all family members collectively. A healthy family promotes each family member's growth and resistance to illnesses so that the family's health can sustain members during times of crisis such as serious illness, emotional dilemmas, divorce, or death of a family member (Gladding, 2019; Kaakinen, et al., 2018). Conversely, a family with underdeveloped coping skills or a limited capacity for problem-solving, self-management, or self-care is often unable to promote the potential of its members or assist them in times of need.

Adherence to cultural practices and family standards for family health can influence each member's health. Many families comply with cultural norms when deciding about utilizing preventative health care, adhering to immunization recommendations, completing routine health assessments, or investing in family planning (Spector, 2017). In turn, these cultural norms dictate how family members will participate in their health care. This interlacing can either obstruct or facilitate the health of the family and the family members.

The description of "normal" family health is challenging given the heterogeneity and subjectivity of the data related to family health. However, there are some standards that characterize a healthy family. Major family strengths have emerged for family functioning and coping with crisis— family pride, family support, cohesion, adaptability, communication, religious orientation, and social support (Nichols & Davis, 2019). Specific topics have been used to characterize a healthy family (Kaakinen, et al., 2018):

- Communicates and listens
- Has a balance of interaction among members
- Exhibits a sense of shared responsibilities
- Teaches a sense of right and wrong
- Abounds in rituals and traditions
- Respects the privacy of each member
- Admits to problems and seeks help

From this information, six signs have persisted about a healthy family—maintaining a spiritual foundation, making the family a top priority, asking for and giving respect, communicating and listening, valuing service to others, and expecting and offering acceptance (Clark-Jones, 2018; Parachin, 1997). While using these signs to guide and understand family-oriented interventions (Clark-Jones, 2018), six important characteristics have consistently emerged (Kaakinen et al., 2018):

1. A facilitative process of interaction exists among family members.
2. Individual member development is enhanced.
3. Role relationships are structured effectively.
4. Active attempts are made to cope with problems.
5. There is a healthy home environment and lifestyle.
6. Regular links are established with the broader community.

Healthy Communication Among Family Members

- Healthy families communicate in patterns that are regular, varied, and supportive (Fig. 14-3). Adults talk and engage with adults, children with children, and adults with children; it is through communications that families find ways to adapt to changes as they seek family stability (Denham, Eggenberger, Young, & Krumwiede, 2016).

Healthy families discuss problems, confront each other when angry, share ideas and concerns, and write or call each other when separated. They communicate through nonverbal means. This level of family communication sensitizes family members to one another. They watch for cues and verify messages to ensure understanding, which intensifies the family's recognition and dealing

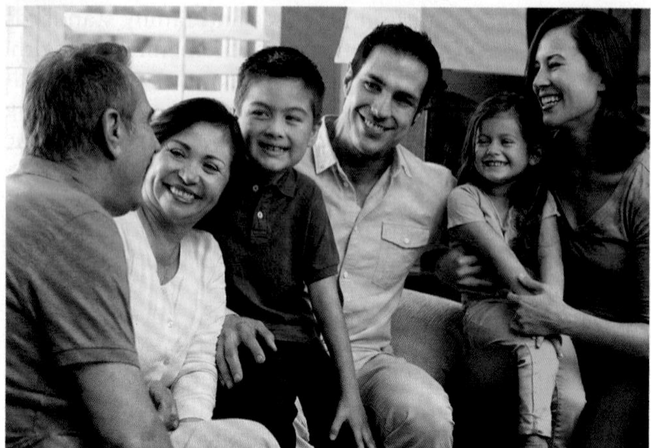

FIGURE 14-3 Good communication promotes healthy families.

with conflict. Thus, a communicative family knows to share and collaborate with each other.

Furthermore, family members use communication to demonstrate affection and acceptance, to promote identity and fellowship, and to guide behavior through socialization and social ethics. Importantly, effective communication patterns are associated with a family that promotes the health and development of each family member.

Enhancement of Family Members' Development

Healthy families respond to the needs of family members and provide the freedom and support necessary to promote each member's growth. This family tolerates differences of opinion or lifestyle because each member has the right to be an individual, and the family respects this right. A healthy family encourages freedom and autonomy for each of its members because it contributes to the family's stability (Kaakinen et al., 2018).

Freedom and autonomy are supported even if the patterns of promoting family members' development vary from family to family. As a result, family members will experience increased competence, self-reliance, social skills, intellectual growth, and overall capacity for self-management among family members (Kaakinen et al., 2018; Salem et al., 2017; Shajani & Snell, 2019).

Effective Structuring of Family Role Relationships

In healthy families, role relationships are structured to meet the family's changing needs over time (Kaakinen et al., 2018). In a stable society, families establish members' roles and tasks to maintain workable patterns throughout the life of the family. There is high role consistency because family members experience little to no external pressure or the need to change their role(s).

In a technologically advanced society, most families establish roles for the changing family needs that are created by external forces. The degree of role consistency is highly influenced by the permanency of the external forces on the family members' roles and expected tasks. Finally, changing life cycle stages require alterations in the structure of relationships. With each stage, family members change in their developmental needs so that the family must adapt their roles, tasks, and controls in a healthy family (Kaakinen et al., 2018; Salem et al., 2017).

Active Coping Effort

Healthy families actively attempt to cope with life's problems and issues. When faced with a challenge, the family assumes responsibility for coping and seeks to meet the demands of the situation (Gladding, 2019; Kaakinen et al., 2018; Nichols & Davis, 2019).

Family members may pursue treatment opportunities for other family members in order to maintain the health of the family. The collective support of family members may be essential for a family member to acquire any type of assistance outside the family. Clearly, the healthy family recognizes the need for assistance, accepts help, and pursues opportunities to eliminate or decrease the stressors that affect it (Gladding, 2019; Salem et al., 2017).

Even if most healthy families are dealing with less dramatic, day-to-day changes, the healthy families remain receptive to innovation, new ideas, and creative and energetic ways to solve problems. Moreover, healthy families actively seek and use a variety of resources to solve problems, which may be internal or external within the family.

Healthy Environment and Lifestyle

Another sign of a healthy family is a healthy home environment and lifestyle. Healthy families maintain safe and hygienic living conditions for their members. Steps are taken to minimize the risk of damage to any family member while maximizing the potential for health within the family.

A healthy family lifestyle encourages family members to find balance or harmony in their lives so that the family will have sufficient energies for daily living. A balanced and varied family diet is nutritious and appealing. Adequate physical activity helps to maintain a healthy weight while promoting cardiac health. Family members seek out and use health care services and demonstrate adherence to recommended regimens. The emotional climate of a healthy family is positive and supportive of growth. Contributing to this healthful emotional climate is a strong sense of shared values, often combined with a strong moral ethical orientation. When the home environment makes family members feel welcomed, they express their individuality in simple ways (Gladding, 2019).

Regular Links With the Broader Community

Healthy families maintain dynamic ties with the broader community. They participate regularly in external groups and activities. They use external resources suited to family needs.

Healthy families also show an interest in current events and attempt to understand significant social, economic, and political issues. The families are exposed to a wider range of alternatives and a variety of contacts, which can increase options for finding resources and strengthen coping skills. Public health nurses need to assess and encourage family's involvement within the broader community as it facilitates a relationship between the family and the community (Kaakinen et al., 2018).

FAMILY HEALTH NURSING: PREPARING FOR THE HOME VISIT

Because the nurse encounters most family members in their homes and neighborhoods, the focus of this section

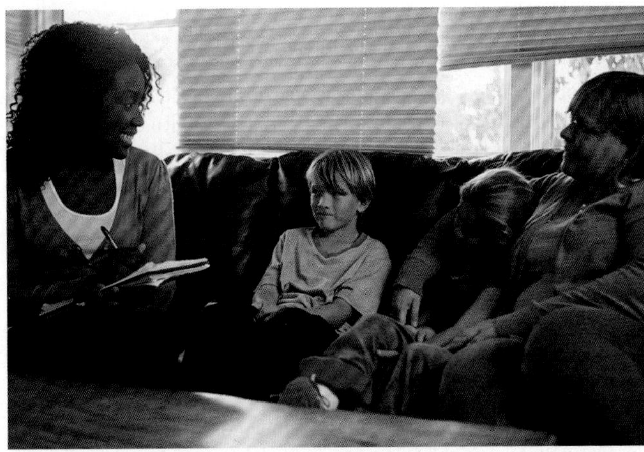

FIGURE 14-4 Family health assessments are foundational to the community/public health nurse's work with families.

is on the home visit (Fig. 14-4). However, some nurses encounter families in other settings in the community, including on the streets, in homeless shelters, and in the homes of relatives or friends. For more on family health nursing in nonhome community settings, see Box 14-6. Regardless of the family's location, the family is the client; the family is the unit of service in public health nursing (Kaakinen et al., 2018).

In the unique setting of the patient's home, the nurse is permitted into the most intimate of spaces that human beings have. The key to this privilege is trust. Family members must have a certain amount of trust to let a stranger and representative of a governmental agency into their home. Family members believe that you are there to help enhance their ability to function as a healthy family with internal and external resources. In the same manner, the nurse must have a certain amount of trust to enter the family's home. Once the door closes, the nurse enters the client's world where they are the experts, and the nurse is the guest, a stranger. Nevertheless, you are trusting that the family welcomes your visit and is ready to work with you for healthier outcomes.

To be best prepared to enter a client's home, you must have an understanding of the skills of observation and communication, the components of the home visit, the various purposes for the home visit, and how to maintain your own personal safety while making the home visit. These topics are covered below. For general guidelines on public health nursing practice when the family is the client, see Box 14-7.

BOX 14-6 Working With Families in Nonhome Community Settings

There is a variety of nonhome settings or public places for visits to accommodate the family's schedules and routines provided the family member is comfortable with the nonhome setting. A visit may occur during a lunch break, after work/school, in a day care or senior center, or public setting. Be mindful of maintaining a confidential atmosphere.

Visiting a family member in public places can enhance the family assessment. The nurse can assess an individual's ability to function outside the home setting. It decreases the potential of issues in the home impacting the individual's response(s) to the questions. The family member may feel comfortable talking about problems and issues related to the home environment from other family members such as parents.

Skills Used During the Home Visit

Many skills are needed when assessing, diagnosing, planning, implementing, and evaluating families in their home at a variety of functional levels. Expert interviewing skills and effective communication techniques are essential for effective family intervention (see Chapter 10). It is equally important to enhance these established techniques with your relational skills (e.g., intuition, openness, nurturing, and compassion) (Stastny, Keens, & Alkon, 2016). A trusting relationship is the key to a productive home health visit and effective use of nursing skills (Healthy Families America, 2019). Through home visits nurses can assist families in promoting nurturing relationships leading to stronger family-centered healthy development (Healthy Families America, 2019). The following paragraphs describe special skills required when making home visits.

Acute Observational Skills

You will be using your acute observational skills to assess both the family and the environment, which are equally important for a detailed assessment. This refers to the ability to take note of every detail (physical and nonphysical) that is directly and indirectly related to the family, the environment, the visit, and the entire process. Throughout the visit, the nurse focuses on the family members' concerns and the purpose of the visit, while being observant about the neighborhood, travel safety, home environmental conditions, number of household members, client demeanor, and body language, as well as other nonverbal cues. All this information contributes to understanding the family, identifying patterns, and recognizing how to navigate the neighborhood. Addresses on referrals may be incorrect, incomplete, or generally dubious. Confirm with the referring agency to identify any anomalies and environmental conditions of the neighborhood.

Observation of Home and Neighborhood Environmental Conditions. Conditions in the neighborhood and home environments reveal important information that can guide diagnosing, planning, and intervention with families. While traveling to and arriving at the family home, you have been gathering information about the neighborhood conditions and the physical appearance of the apartment or house. Observing the home environment conditions provides an assessment about the resources and barriers encountered by the family. The external environment may contradict the family's values, resources, and goals. They may have little control over the neighborhood or the building in which they live, especially if they are renting. While these external factors may influence the behavior of the family, they may not define the behavior.

Observation of Body Language and Other Nonverbal Cues. You gather data as soon as you knock on the door

BOX 14-7 Public Health Nursing Practice Guidelines for Working With Families

The family is the unit of service in public health nursing (Kaakinen et al., 2018). The nurse assesses the family to determine what services are needed to move the family to a state of health, which can be determined by using five guidelines for practice.

Work With the Family Collectively

The family is a group of several persons living together with a collective personality, collective interests, and a collective set of needs. The family functions collectively as a single entity with common attributes and activities so that all family members are involved in the nurse–client interactions (Gladding, 2019; Shajani & Snell, 2019).

Start at the Family's Present Level of Functioning

The C/PHN begins by conducting a detailed family assessment to ascertain the needs and health level of each family member. The nurse can also recognize patterns of behaviors to determine collective interests, concerns, problems, risks, and priorities.

Adapt the Nursing Intervention to the Family's Stage of Development

Every family engages in the same basic functioning but not the same approaches to accomplish these functions within the family's development. A young family meets the family members' affiliation needs by establishing mutually satisfying relationships and meaningful communication patterns. The bonds of a family in the later stages of development change due to some family members becoming part of another family unit or family member(s) dying (Box 14-8). With this assessment, the nurse recognizes the family's appropriate level of functioning, determines the problems/risks, and implements the tailored interventions needed to move the family to a state of health (Kaakinen et al., 2018; Shajani & Snell, 2019).

Recognize the Validity of Family Structure Variations

C/PHNs work with families from communities with varying family structures and individualized patterns of family functioning. The nurse must learn to understand and accept variations in family structure to address the needs of the families. Two principles guide this acceptance and understanding (Kaakinen et al., 2018; Sperry, 2019; Shajani & Snell, 2019):

1. Principle One—Each family is unique in its combination of structures, composition, roles, and behaviors. This uniqueness is valid, while family functions effectively and demonstrates the characteristics of a healthy family.
2. Principle Two—Families are constantly changing throughout the life cycle, which leads to a family to adapt to its circumstances.

There may be a change in the family structure and the family members' roles due to internal and external environmental issues from the addition, loss, or alteration of persons related to the family. It is the C/PHN's responsibility to help the family to cope with these changes with a nonjudgmental and acceptance manner about the family structure. A nurse personally may find it difficult to work with same-sex couples or respect same-sex marriages because this lifestyle conflicts with the nurse's personal set of values. As a professional, however, it is the nurse's responsibility to help promote the collective health of that family because all families are unique groups, each with its own set of needs that are best served through unbiased care.

Empower Families

Throughout the family visit, the public health nurse realizes that the ultimate goal is to assist the family in becoming independent of services (Kaakinen et al., 2018; Salem et al., 2017; Sperry, 2019). This positive outcome is accomplished via the working nurse–family relationship, which can be guided by four suggestions:

- The current functioning of the family has worked for the family before meeting you.
- Before doing "something" for a family, consider who did this "something" before you.
- Find family strengths even in the most challenging and compromised family situation.
- Think about your ability to manage, cope, or function as well as the family members if you were in a similar situation.

With an **asset-based approach**, the nurse collaborates with the family to discern the family's strengths and positive potentiality embedded in the family weaknesses so that independence from the agency's services reflects a positive outcome (Marshall & Easton, 2018). Regrettably, too often, C/PHNs perceive family weaknesses as *needs* or *problems*, which can undermine any hope of a therapeutic relationship between nurse and family as well as the use of an asset-based approach. It is the nurse's job to recognize the strengths in families and to help families recognize them and understand their potential for self-efficacy (Kaakinen et al., 2018; Shajani & Snell, 2019). The asset-based approach fosters a positive self-image, promotes self-confidence and self-efficacy, and often helps a family feel better able to address other problems as they arise (Marshall & Easton, 2018). Furthermore, C/PHNs need to ensure that whatever assistance they offer/provide to a family will promote the family's independence and self-efficacy.

The C/PHN should be able to say, at the least, that the family is managing as best as possible so that the assessment can explore all aspects of family functioning, positive and negative. It also emphasizes the positive outcomes, indicating to the family that they are important to the nurse—creating a collaborative relationship.

One helpful communication technique is **strengthening**, which involves verbally listing the positive aspects of an otherwise negative situation in a natural and conversational manner (Gladding, 2019). This strengthening technique empowers the family through positivism instead of negativity that may be viewed by the family as condescending or punitive. Strengthening also facilitates the use of the nurse as a resource and guide (Shajani & Snell, 2019).

Through empowerment, the family can meet the needs of each family member and the demands made by systems outside the family unit. Of course, all behaviors must first be assessed in terms of promoting the family functioning before deemed a strength. Some behaviors that are considered as strengths are related to basic family functions, family developmental tasks, and characteristics of family health. Thus, it is the context in which the behavior exists that makes it a strength, not the behavior alone.

BOX 14-8 STORIES FROM THE FIELD

Factoring in the Ravina Family's Stage of Development

The Ravinas, a couple in their early 70s, recently moved to a retirement complex. They had received nursing visits after Mrs. Ravina's stroke 3 years earlier but requested service now because Mr. Ravina was feeling "poorly" all the time. He thought that perhaps his diet and lack of activity might be the cause and hoped the nurse might have some helpful suggestions. The couple had eagerly awaited Mr. Ravina's retirement from teaching, with plans to be lazy, travel, visit all their children, and do all those things they never had time to do when they were young. Now, neither of them seemed to have enough energy or the capacity to enjoy their new life. The move from their home of 28 years had been difficult: they were still trying to find space in the tiny apartment for their cherished books and mementos, although they had given many items away.

Ronald Bell, a C/PHN, recognized that the Ravinas were experiencing a situational crisis (leaving their home of 28 years) and a developmental crisis (aging and entering retirement) and may perhaps have some underlying health problems. Many of the Ravinas' expectations for this new life stage were unrealistic; they had not adequately prepared themselves for the adjustments that the loss of their home and retirement would demand. Through discussion, Ronald was able to help the Ravina family understand their situation and express their feelings. He completed physical assessments on the Ravinas and encouraged regular follow-up with their health care provider. He also helped them join a support group of retired persons who were experiencing some of the same difficulties. Because this nurse was able to help the Ravina family through their crisis in a supportive and nonjudgmental manner, he found them receptive later to discussing preparation for the inevitable loss and bereavement that would occur when one of them died. He was adapting his nursing intervention to this family's stage of development.

1. *What concerns might the C/PHN have in this situation?*
2. *What strategies might the C/PHN employ for this situation?*

BOX 14-9 STORIES FROM THE FIELD

A Home Visit to James Cutler and Brian Hoag

James Cutler and Brian Hoag have a 6-year monogamous relationship. A same-sex couple, they worked with an attorney to privately adopt a child. The arrangements were completed and their 2-week-old son, Adrian, arrived in their home last week. Helen Jeffers, a public health nurse, receives a referral from the county hospital where Adrian was born. The request is for an assessment of the home situation and parenting skills. At the hospital, the baby tested positive for cocaine with APGAR scores of 6 and 8 and had some initial difficulty sucking. Birth weight was 2,900 g. Discharge weight, at 3 days, was 2,850 g. At her first home visit, Helen finds a neat and orderly two-bedroom condominium that is well equipped with baby supplies. The infant has gained 200 g and is being well cared for by two fatigued parents whose previous contact with infants was limited. James and Brian have many questions and are anxious learners. Helen plans with the couple to make weekly home visits to assess infant growth and development, provide support, and answer questions. She suggests a neighborhood parenting class and finding a reliable babysitter. She also helps James and Brian develop an infant care work schedule. After 6 weeks of intervention, Adrian is thriving. Helen closes the case to home visits, feeling confident that the parents' goal of becoming knowledgeable and confident has been achieved.

1. *As the C/PHN, identify the family life cycle and developmental tasks of this family.*
2. *How can the C/PHN support this family in health promotion and education?*

or ring the doorbell, greet the people in the doorway, and enter the home (Box 14-9). Observations of previsit nonverbal cues and body language contribute to your initial opinions and perceptions about the family. Also, *all* family members (present or absent) are doing the same with you (Box 14-10). Thus, you need to be aware of all family members; acknowledge and greet them. Inquire about those who are absent. Make this a habit on all visits. Each family member has opinions and health care needs, even if you only see certain members of the family on each visit.

Be observant of the family's nonverbal cues such as body language and demeanor because they provide information that must not be overlooked. Opening statements such as "You seem anxious today," or "Did I come at a bad time? You seem distracted," will encourage family members to express what is on their minds, which otherwise might not be indicated or addressed. Through their facial expressions, hand gestures, subtle glances, eye movement, and body language, detailed information will be generated to address both direct and indirect concerns of the family. Overlooking the body language makes it easy to continue with *your* agenda instead of the *family member's* agenda, although the family is distracted by another, more pressing issue.

Nonverbal Communication

It is equally important to be aware of your body language that can tell the family a great deal about how you feel being in their home, dealing with the family members, and completing the home visit. Suggestive behaviors like fidgeting with car keys during the entire visit or appearing to be in a hurry or rushed can be perceived as nervousness, anxious, or not wanting to be in the current situation. Minimal eye contact or continuously looking at your paperwork may be viewed as rudeness, unprofessionalism, and unknowledgeable about the family and/or the purpose of the visit. Your "fear" can be implied from the refusal to sit on any of the furniture or a shocked expression from a roach or mouse scampering across the floor. Your behavior impacts the family's trust in you, subsequent visits, and interventions.

BOX **14-10** PERSPECTIVES

A C/PHN Nursing Instructor's Viewpoint on Home Visits—How Your Knock Helps Families Open the Door

This question may seem trite, but how do you knock on the door when you visit a family? Do you use the "I don't want to be here, and if they don't hear the knock I can quickly and quietly leave" type of knock that even Superman can't hear? Or do you knock like, "I'm a bill collector and ***you better*** open this door!" During this knock, the entire family may be running out the back door or through a window! The preferred knock is loud enough to be heard, yet friendly and nonthreatening. If necessary, practice "your knock" until you can create this beneficial combination.

With some families, it is helpful to call toward the door as you knock or ring the bell with, "Mrs. Smith, this is Jenny from the Health Department—remember I was coming by today," or "Ms. Jiminez, it's the student public health nurse, Terry De Leon, and I brought some pamphlets for you," or "Hello, it's James from the neighborhood clinic; we planned to meet today." Using such a greeting allows the family to know who is at the door and choose to open the door if they want. It will get you into more homes than the "quiet-as-a-mouse" or "bill-collector" knocks.

—*Alice K., PHN*

Components of the Family Health Visit

The components of the family health visits align with the nursing process. Previsit preparation steps encompass assessment, diagnosing, and planning, which are necessary for implementation or completion of the actual family health visit. The documentation and planning for the next visit (or evaluation) terminates one visit and prepares the nurse for the next action needed.

Previsit Preparation

Public health nurses identify preliminary family diagnoses and design a plan for the initial family health visit based on a referral to the agency. A **referral** is a request for service from another agency or person. They are the source of new cases and need timely responses. This request can be a form letter or the transferal of information from the originating agency to the receiving agency. Referrals may be formal (from physicians or complementary agencies) or informal (verbal or telephone referrals from friends or relatives who believe that someone needs help). Some examples include:

- Labor and delivery hospital units request service for low-birth-weight babies and teen mothers.
- Social service agencies request a home assessment for a child being returned to parents after previous removal.
- A homeless shelter might be seeking services for homeless or transient persons showing signs of uncontrolled diabetes.
- A battered woman's shelter needs services to treat emotional issues of a mother and her children who are running from an abusive husband and father.
- A woman in a city 500 miles away requests that a nurse check on an elderly relative who lives alone in the community and has recently exhibited slurred speech and/or has been homebound.

Follow-up visits are based on the family's needs and agency protocol. Public health nurses must be equipped with the appropriate tools to establish a physical place to work:

- Access to a telephone, the Internet, and other necessary resources
  - Educational material (pamphlets, brochures, and related Web information)
  - Charting tools
  - Any other supplies required for home visits
- **Resource directory**, which is a list of resources for the broader community, or a nurse-made directory of resources created over years of working with people in the community
- A nursing bag or carryall tote (issued by agency or devised by the nurse) for medical supplies
  - Specialized supplies depending on the visit (a tote for each type of visit)
  - Basic supplies to treat basic needs of a new mother and her infant or an elderly man with hypertension

Once the nurse is prepared, the family is contacted to schedule a visit. The referral ideally contains a correct telephone number for the family, a relative, or a neighbor. The nurse needs to extract as much information as possible from the referral so that the preparation can be exact and specific for the health visit. This sets the stage for a detailed assessment, appropriate family diagnosing, and family-oriented care planning (Arbaje et al., 2018). If the referral does not contain this information, an unannounced visit is scheduled. During this visit, it is important to get a contact number for the family. When calling for the first time, you, the C/PHN, will:

1. Introduce yourself
2. Explain the reason for the call
3. Give the reason why the family was referred
4. Indicate what the visit consists of
5. Determine when a visit would be convenient for the family and you
6. Get explicit directions to where the family is staying (the referral may have a different address, or the family did not mention that they are staying elsewhere)
7. Repeat the date and time of the scheduled visit

The nurse's intention(s) may be questioned with some people becoming defensive or suspicious. A new young mother may wonder, "Why is this nurse visiting me so close to my time in the hospital? Did I say or do something wrong with my baby when I was in the hospital?" The C/PHN will explain that:

- The visit is a follow-up one to see if the move from the hospital to home is okay.
- The visit is an opportunity for her to ask questions that she might have about her new baby since her return home. It is also a chance to learn more about handling her baby in the home if needed.
- The visit is a service provided by the agency to all mothers.
- The visit is paid for by taxes or donations, or by the client's health maintenance organization (if applicable). There is no direct cost to her or the family.

Following logical steps in the previsit preparation enhances the nurse's confidence in her or his ability to intuitively recognize patterns and/or trends from the referral information for preliminary diagnoses to guide preliminary care planning.

Making the Visit

It is recommended to call the family to remind them of the scheduled meeting and your arrival time prior to the scheduled visit. State the purpose of the visit and the anticipated length of time needed. Once you arrive, the following guidelines for initial contact should be used (Kaakinen et al., 2018):

1. Engage the family in a manner to build a supportive and trusting relationship (Box 14-11).
   a. Introduce yourself to the family.
   b. Explain the value of the nursing services provided by the agency.
   c. Spend the first few minutes of the visit establishing cordiality and getting acquainted (a mutual discovery or "feeling out" time).
   d. Become acquainted with all family and household members if you are making a home visit.
   e. Encourage each person to speak for himself.
2. Use acute observational skills.
   a. Use your "sixth sense" or intuition as a guide regarding family responses, questions they ask, and your personal safety (trust your feelings).
   b. Be sensitive to verbal and nonverbal cues.
   c. Be accepting and listen carefully.
   d. Be cognizant of possible internal and external stressors and effect on mental status of family.
   e. Be aware of your own personality—balance talking and listening—and be aware of your nonverbal behaviors.
3. Help the family focus on issues and move toward the desired goals.
   a. Be adaptable and flexible (you may be planning a prenatal visit, but the woman delivered her baby the day after you made the appointment, and now there is a newborn).
   b. Be aware that most clients are not extremely ill and have higher levels of wellness than are generally seen in acute care settings.
   c. Be prepared to develop a sustained continuity of care by actively collaborating with the family in addressing their issues.
4. Near the end of the visit, review the important points and emphasize the family strengths.
5. Plan with the family for the next visit.

BOX 14-11 Developing a Trusting Relationship with the Stevenson Family

The public health nurse, David Dow, made an initial home visit after referral by an outpatient physician who was concerned about possible child abuse. The physician suspected abuse after seeing bruises on the arm of a baby boy (Eugene) who was in the emergency room for treatment of a laceration on the forehead. Alice Stevenson, the mother, claimed that the laceration resulted from Eugene falling off a table when she was changing him. She also explained that the bruise happened when Phillip (Eugene's older brother) was playing too rough. David began the visit by stating that he was simply following up on the emergency room visit and wanted to see how Eugene was progressing. David made no mention of child abuse. He simply observed Alice and the children closely to learn more about the family's background and used the strengthening technique to create a trusting relationship interaction. Due to David's supportive demeanor, Alice agreed to further visits, and at one of the visits, Alice confessed that her ring cut Eugene's forehead when she slapped him. "I could not get him to stop crying, no matter what I did," she whimpered. "I just could not endure it any longer." She also confessed that the bruises happened when she, not Phillip, grabbed Eugene roughly to stop him from pulling and touching things he should not. David learned that Alice's husband abandoned her while she was still pregnant with Eugene. David realized that Alice would be particularly vulnerable to any criticism, so he concentrated on her strengths such as managing the home, dressing the children, and reading to little Eugene. During subsequent visits, Alice and David were able to discuss her feelings frankly and work toward improving the health of the Stevenson family. Alice started counseling and attended a support group for single parents counseling.

The length of the visit varies depending on its purpose and can influence the C/PHN–family relationship.

Less than a 20-minute visit

- Not enough time for a thorough assessment, but ideal for
  - Dropping off supplies
  - Relaying information about a referral
  - Stopping by at the family's request, for instance

More than a 60-minute visit

- Avoid; not a productive way to provide nursing services.
- Any lengthy assessments should be conducted over two visits.
- Disruptive to the family with the potential for unwanted outcomes.
  - Families have routines that are important to them.
  - The family may feel that nothing of value occurred during a visit.
  - The family may not continue to make themselves available for future visits. This becomes a balancing act for the family and the nurse, and you may want to work at picking up on nonverbal cues.

- May reflect the nurse's hesitation in trusting the family to understand and/or follow the instructions and feedback.
- Limits the family's ability to seek out community resources for community-based health care.

Remember, the outcome of better health for family members must be demonstrated in order to support and validate the value, as well as justify the cost of public health nursing services.

Concluding and Documenting the Visit

The current home visit concludes after planning for the follow-up visit with the family. You will say goodbye and pack up any paperwork, materials, and supplies used for this visit in your car. Before leaving this community, you need to get ready for the next home visit on your schedule. By arriving prepared at the next home, you demonstrate respect for the family's time, efficiency, and professionalism (Arbaje et al., 2018).

Documentation or charting of each home visit used to be typically completed as soon as the nurse returned to the agency. Today, it is recommended that charting happens *immediately* at the end of the home visit (not upon arrival at the next one) on an agency-provided device (laptop, smartphone, or tablet) linked to electronic charting forms and records (Arbaje et al., 2018). For the most part, most agencies expect the charting to be completed as soon as practically possible in that workday.

Agencies use a variety of forms that assist the nurse to document fully and succinctly. Some forms use a checklist format that contains code numbers, letters, or checkmarks on developmental or disease-specific care plans. A four-paged postpartum visit and newborn assessment may consist of two narrative forms to chart the expectations for the mother and baby plus two forms for the head-to-toe assessment of the newborn. There is a place to document parent teaching within the expected parameters and for listing other professionals' involvement with the family. Other forms may focus on chronic illness common in the agency's clientele (e.g., alcoholism, chronic obstructive pulmonary disease, communicable diseases diabetes, HIV/AIDS, hypertension).

Focus of the Family Health Visit

The focus of family health visits depends on the agency's mission and resources or services and the needs of the families. Some agencies provide education, recreational activities, and support groups for families of persons with Alzheimer's disease, asthma, or diabetes. Other agencies provide services to address issues related to immigration, poverty, and/or homelessness (Beck et al., 2017; de Grubb et al., 2017; Lee et al., 2017). In general, family health visits are designed to educate, provide anticipatory guidance, and focus on health promotion or prevention.

Family Education and Anticipatory Guidance

Local health departments distribute their services based on the broader community's needs. The health department may contract with health care providers to treat a community with a high rate of teen pregnancies and high-risk infants through home or clinic visits to all teens and women with high-risk pregnancies and their newborns after delivery (Tachibana et al., 2019). The treatment involves teaching prenatal, postpartum, and newborn care and providing anticipatory guidance to promote regular health care provider visits for the infant, immunizations, and safety awareness. The health department may address the needs of another community with a significant number of older adults or migrant workers who need to learn how to manage a chronic illness, enhance their nutrition, and practice safety measures to prevent injuries and falls (Coker et al., 2019; Frost et al., 2019).

Family Promotion and Illness Prevention

Family members can be taught health promotion activities for healthy living even within the limitations of chronic illnesses. These activities may include screening for hypertension and elevated cholesterol, performing a physical assessment, teaching about nutrition and safety, and promoting immunization.

Immunizations protect the health of all individuals and the larger community. Although such services are not brought into the home, it remains the C/PHN's responsibility to provide information about immunizations, teach the importance of following an immunization schedule, and follow up with the family during home visits. A focus on population health shifts care to the needs of the community and strengthens the focus on aggregate health promotion strategies that optimize personal health (APHN, 2016a, 2016b). Adding social determinants of health also contributes to the ultimate goal of creating "social, physical, and economic environments that promote attaining the full potential for health and well-being for all" (USDHHS, 2020, para. 4; see Box 14-12).

C/PHNs provide health promotion services during a family health visit in any setting. During prenatal classes, the C/PHN teaches couples about the expected changes during pregnancy and provides anticipatory guidance for safe infant care and postpartum care (Mutch, 2016). The C/PHN screens older adults for hypertension or elevated cholesterol at the senior center, educates family members attending Alcoholics Anonymous, or provides mental and health assessments for homeless persons in shelters.

Personal Safety During the Home Visit

Being streetwise is essential when interacting and traveling throughout communities. Continuation of personal safety must be considered while maintaining respect for the families, a trusting relationship, and professionalism.

Traveling to and in the Neighborhood

When leaving your "base of operation," make sure you have all the necessary supplies, materials, and paperwork for the scheduled home visits. To ensure safety and promote coordination with your agency, always inform your agency about your planned itinerary and all contact information (your mobile phone number and telephone numbers of families scheduled to visit) so that the agency can promptly reach you (Arbaje et al., 2018). Traveling safely in a community can mean different things to different people.

BOX 14-12 *HEALTHY PEOPLE 2030*

Selected Goals and Objectives Related to Family Health

Family Planning

Core Objectives

FP-01	Reduce the proportion of unintended pregnancies
FP-02	Reduce the proportion of pregnancies conceived within 18 months of a previous birth
FP-03	Reduce pregnancies in adolescents
FP-04	Increase the proportion of adolescents who have never had sex
FP-05	Increase the proportion of adolescent females who used effective birth control the last time they had sex
FP-06	Increase the proportion of adolescent males who used a condom the last time they had sex
FP-07	Increase the proportion of adolescents who use birth control the first time they have sex
FP-08	Increase the proportion of adolescents who get formal sex education before age 18 years
FP-09	Increase the proportion of women who get needed publicly funded birth control services and support
FP-10	Increase the proportion of women at risk for unintended pregnancy who use effective birth control
FP-11	Increase the proportion of adolescent females at risk for unintended pregnancy who use birth control

Developmental Objectives

FP-D01	Increase the proportion of publicly funded clinics that offer the full range of reversible birth control

Adolescent Health

Core Objectives

AH-01	Increase the proportion of adolescents who had a preventative health care visit in the past year
AH-02	Increase the proportion of adolescents who speak privately with a provider at a preventive medical visit
AH-03	Increase the proportion of adolescents who have an adult they can talk to about serious problems
AH-04	Increase the proportion of students participating in the School Breakfast Program
AH-05	Increase the proportion of 4th-graders with reading skills at or above the proficient level
AD-06	Increase the proportion of 4th-graders with math skills at or above the proficient level
AH-07	Reduce chronic school absence among early adolescent
AH-08	Increase the proportion of high school students who graduate in 4 years

Developmental Objectives

IVP-D03	Reduce the number of young adults who report 3 or more adverse childhood experiences
EH-D01	Increase the proportion of schools with policies and practices that promote health and safety

Maternal, Infant, and Child Health

Core Objectives

Morbidity and Mortality

MICH-01	Reduce the rate of fetal deaths at 20 or more weeks of gestation
MICH-02	reduce the rate of infant deaths

Infant Care

MICH-14	Increase the proportion of infants who are put to sleep on their backs
MICH-15	Increase the proportion of infants who are breastfeed exclusively through age 6 months

(Continued)

BOX **14-12** *HEALTHY PEOPLE 2030 (Continued)*

Health Services

MICH-08	Increase the proportion of pregnant women who receive early and adequate prenatal care
MICH-19	Increase the proportion of children and adolescents who receive care in a medical home
MICH-20	Increase the proportion of children and adolescents with special health care needs who have a system of care

Developmental Objectives

MICH-D01	Increase the proportion of women who get screened for postpartum depression

Reprinted from U.S. Department of Health & Human Services (USDHHS). (2020). *Healthy People 2030: Browse objectives.* Retrieved from https://health.gov/healthypeople/objectives-and-data/browse-objectives

Traveling in an agency or private car requires

- A full gas tank
- Addresses for families you are visiting, city/county map, or GPS
- A cell phone

Using public transportation requires

- Change/bus card or smartphone app for each bus trip
- A current bus schedule
- Knowledge of the exit at the bus stop closest to your family's home
- Knowledge of the bus stop for the return trip to agency or to the next home visit
- A cell phone

You should *always* call ahead to the family and give them an estimated time of your arrival. Be "streetwise" when walking in neighborhoods. A C/PHN understands the value of safety measures used by expert nurses, following these measures for personal safety, and not challenging them. Another focus of concern is the perceived risk to self when making a home visit. Feeling and being safe can relate to the nurse's perception of a situation, views on risk-taking, awareness of the traveling conditions (e.g., the time and/or the setting), and coping process. What one person sees as a risk, another sees as a challenge or an opportunity, and another may see nothing. We each perceive risks differently based on knowledge, experience, and personality.

Arriving at the Home

Make sure you are at the right house. Do not go into the home until you are assured that the family you are intending to visit does live there and is home. You are scheduled to visit 16-year-old Jennifer and her 5-day-old infant, Marcus. A 50-year-old man answers the door when you knock. Give your name and ask if Jennifer can come to the door because you are here to see her. Do not enter the house even if he invites you in to wait for Jennifer. Smile and let him know that you are comfortable waiting for Jennifer at the door. Remain outside the house and go inside *only after* you talk to Jennifer at the door. This precaution ensures that the family members you want to visit are in the house and that this is the right address.

Dealing With Challenging Situations

Due to the nature of the home setting, you may encounter unexpected and challenging situations, including family conflict, family members under the influence, and the presence of strangers.

Friction Between Family Members. During a home visit, two or more family members may begin to argue or physically fight. You should immediately terminate the visit and inform the family what will take place regarding the home visit. Follow these steps:

1. Inform the family that the visit is now terminated.
2. Calmly let the family know that such distraction takes away from the purpose of the visit.
3. Inform the family that you will return at another convenient time.
4. Calmly and quickly remove yourself from the home.

When two or more family members are physically fighting, never intervene, try to stop the fight, serve as a referee, or assist an adult family member. You may be the next victim. Once you are out of the house, call 911, if necessary, from your cell phone. Once you are safe, rely on your acute observation skills to recall the altercation. This data may provide significant information about the family's structure, process, and health. Depending on your assessment and processing of the information, it may be appropriate to discuss the altercation and the friction in the family at a later visit.

Family Members Under the Influence. If the focus of the visit is on two family members, but a third member's behavior suggests the use of drugs or alcohol, use your judgment as to the best action to take. It is important for you to assess the situation and proceed accordingly within the parameters of guidelines provided by your agency or your school. If the intoxicated or high person goes to another room and remains quiet/calm, it might be appropriate to continue the visit. You might want to discuss your observations with the two family members. If the intoxicated or high person remains in another room but interrupts the visit by being abusive or distractive, it is best to terminate the visit. Let the two family members know that you want to reschedule when the intoxicated or high family member is not under the influence or is not present. Never put yourself in the middle of a situation that could deteriorate rapidly and compromise your safety.

The Presence of Strangers. In some families, it is common to have extended family members, neighbors, and friends present in the home. This may be the norm for the family but not for the nurse because it is a different setting from her or his experience. The nurse may have to weave your way past five teenage boys sitting on the front stoop in order to enter the home and step over three men sleeping on the living room floor in the small apartment of a teenage mother and her infant. Children may be riding their tricycles inside the house during a teaching visit to two young parents who do not seem fazed by the commotion. These situations may not be indicative of danger, but they can make you feel vulnerable and uncomfortable, while distracting you from the purpose of the visit. Always rely on your observation skills; inquire about the people you observe in the periphery of the home visit; ask about their relationship to the family and if they should be included in the visit. The family may suggest that you ignore these people or say they are transient family members. It may be important to learn who they are, if they have unmet health care needs, or if their presence influences the health of the family you are visiting.

APPLYING THE NURSING PROCESS TO FAMILY HEALTH

The nursing process (assessing, diagnosing, planning, implementing, and evaluating nursing care) includes steps used to deliver care to families and aggregates in community health settings. These steps are, interestingly, the same ones used to care for clients in acute care settings and in the extensive clinic system. The difference in implementing this process in family health nursing is the context (the home), the client focus (the family), and the consideration of external variables not typically encountered in other contexts. In public health nursing, addressing the health needs of the core unit of service (in this case, the family) should always transition to addressing the health needs of the community and the population. The context and application of each step are tailored to the needs of the population by focusing on the core unit of service (APHN, 2016a, 2016b).

The nursing process commences on the first visit when the public health nurse performs an initial assessment (Box 14-13). Subsequent visits entail the nurse and the family working collectively to reach the targeted goals.

Preliminary Considerations

Before implementing the nursing process, the nurse must establish (1) a conceptual framework, (2) a clearly defined set of data collection categories, and (3) a method of measuring a family's functional level.

Conceptual Frameworks

A **conceptual framework** is a set of concepts integrated into a meaningful explanation (Hosseini Shokouh et al., 2017). Three conceptual frameworks are used in public health nursing: the interactional, structural–functional, and developmental (Hill & Hansen, 1960; Raingruber, 2017; Shajani & Snell, 2019).

Theories structured on the **interactional framework** focuses on the family's internal environment, their relationships. The family is a unit of interacting personalities with emphasis on communication, roles, conflict, coping patterns, and decision-making processes (Raingruber, 2017; Shajani & Snell, 2019).

The **structural–functional framework** creates a structure that focuses on the family's internal and external environments. The family is a social system with a specific

BOX **14-13** C/PHN USE OF THE NURSING PROCESS

Family Health

- Family assessment refers to a detailed collection of information from the C/PHN's observations about the family and external environment that includes verbal cues, nonverbal cues, and what is observed as well as what is not observed (certain barriers to health care may be invisible, camouflaged as another issue, or understated).
- During the family diagnosis process, the C/PHN recognizes patterns, behaviors, constraints of health (positive and negative), and/or seen/unseen routines from the collected information during the assessment (Swartz, 2018). This step involves identifying issues, risks, concerns, and problems that can negatively and positively alter the health of the family. During the family planning of care step, targeted outcomes and goals are identified based on the patterns of unhealthy/healthy behavior and relationships.
- A plan of care is created. It includes interventions, strategies, and interactions, which involves family resources and external services to promote the health of the family.
- Implementation of family care plan involves the C/PHN collaborating with the family, community resources, and external services to organize and complete the plan of care. The family is educated about the resources and how to use them to address the health problems and promote the family health. It is equally important to include seen/unseen cultural and social issues in completing the interventions and strategies.

Finally, the evaluation step is where the entire nursing process is reviewed to determine if (1) the targeted outcomes and goals were achieved, (2) the process was a positive experience for the family, (3) new and current relationships with internal and external resources will maintain and strengthen the efforts for the family health, and (4) the family feels comfortable in participating in their care. With this understanding of the nursing process, the novice public health nurse is ready to prepare to work with families in the community (Swartz, 2018).

structure that exists in an external environment defined by interactions with other social systems (e.g., other families, church, work, and the health care system). The family structure is used to process, analyze, and understand how the family functions in the external environment (Raingruber, 2017; Shajani & Snell, 2019).

The theories based on the **developmental framework** incorporate elements from both interactional and structural–functional frameworks. For a life cycle perspective, one examines the changing roles and tasks as family members progress through life cycle stages within the environment. Internal relationships elucidate the development of the family. External environmental influences highlight how the family is structured, functions as a social system, and interacts with other social systems. This framework gives context to the family development within the environment (2018; Raingruber, 2017; Shajani & Snell, 2019).

Even though these three core frameworks are the basis for theories and conceptual models used by C/PHNs, these frameworks are the foundations for various methods of family assessment. Their concepts have been combined to design family assessments, diagnosing process, and intervention models.

Data Collection Categories

The conceptual framework gives the nurse a format to group the data about the family into specific categories in order to organize the collected data. This data may be useful for assessing, diagnosing, care planning, and serving as a guide for subsequent visits in which to obtain additional information. For an example of a data collection tool that lists 12 assessment categories in which data are grouped for three data sets (family strengths and self-care capabilities, family stresses and problems, and family resources), see thePoint (Edelman & Kudzma, 2017).

Methods of Measuring a Family's Functioning

Family function includes the relationships, interactions, and structural properties within the family system in which communication, conflict, cohesion, adaptability, and organization are assessed. The C/PHN will evaluate the strengths, resources, and protective factors of a family including any underlying behaviors that might create unsafe conditions.

Family Health Assessment

A thorough family health assessment relies on the public health nurse's commitment to understand the family, to determine the value of the referred information, and to process any prior opinions about the family in order to promote family health. See Box 14-14 for guidelines that can help the C/PHN conduct a detailed family assessment and organize data. See Box 14-15 for an application-oriented exercise in conducting a family assessment.

Assessment Methods

Assessment methods generate information about selected aspects of family structure and function, while matching the purpose for assessment. An informal approach consists of the nurse's acute observational skills and occasional questioning to confirm the observations and determine the next direction to take. A formal approach entails the use of specific questions and assessment tools to assess each family member in terms of health data, family history, physical data, family's development, or potential health problems not detected by family members.

The **genogram** (Fig. 14-5) diagrams the family's genealogy, relationships, and complex family patterns. The PHN can formulate hypotheses about a family over a significant period of time and across generations (de Souza, Bellato, de Araujo, & de Almeida, 2016). Completing the genogram with the family encourages family expression, which can reveal family behavior and problems. The genogram has been useful in linking health outcomes to preventive strategies based on potential health risks and guiding clinical and public health interventions (Centers for Disease Control and Prevention [CDC], 2018).

The **eco-map** (Fig. 14-6) shows the connections between a family and the other systems in the ecologic environment. It visually depicts dynamic family–environment interactions (de Souza et al., 2016). A central circle represents the family or family member with smaller peripheral circles indicative of people and systems significantly relating to the central circle. Connecting lines

BOX 14-14 STORIES FROM THE FIELD

Assessing the Beck Family's Nutritional Status

A public health nurse had an initial contact with Mr. and Mrs. Beck and their youngest child at the well-baby clinic. The 9-month-old child was over the 95th percentile for weight and at the 40th percentile for height. The nurse also noted that both parents were obese. The nurse asked about the family's eating patterns, the baby in particular, and suggested a home visit to determine whether the Becks were interested in family nursing. The nurse explained the purpose of home visits (to assess all family members, coping patterns, eating patterns, and food purchasing choices) and the importance of including all family members and asked for a time that would be good for the family as a whole. The nurse explained that each person should be involved and committed to the agreed-upon goals and that, like a team of oarsmen, the family has to pull together to accomplish the purpose of the visits. To help the Beck family improve its nutritional status, the nurse might suggest a session of brainstorming to uncover many causes of poor nutrition. More brainstorming might also lead to more solutions and plans for action. On each visit, the nurse views the Becks as a group so that group responses and actions would be expected. Evaluation of outcomes will be based on what the family did collectively. The Becks were interested, and a home visit date was made.

1. *What developmental stages appear to have been achieved?*
2. *What is your plan of action for this family over the next three visits?*
3. *What are the goals for this family (immediate, midrange, and long-term)?*

BOX **14-15** STORIES FROM THE FIELD

A Family Assessment for Lorenzo

You are a C/PHN assigned to a small surburb in Chicago. Your new client is Lorenzo, a 103-year-old White American male. He is being released from the geriatric ICU of Uptown Hospital after being treated for severe pneumonia, three episodes of delirium, and 2-degree bedsores. He resides in his own house in the center of Othertrackside. The local hospital is the only medical facility with a geriatric unit in a 75-mile radius that will accept Medicare clients.

His respiratory complications started 4 weeks ago. He experienced SOB and pain with breathing after working in his garden 3+ hours at 43°F temperature while it was raining. The frequency and severity of the respiratory problems resulted in Lorenzo significantly decreasing his activities while increasing his time in the bed. When he was rushed to the hospital, due to severe chest pains and arrhythmia, his neighbor Adam, a 97-year-old African American male, expressed to the admitted nurse, "Please fix him Ms. Nurse. He has just been lying in bed staring at the ceiling for a while now. Even at bedtime, it was like sleeping next to a dead person; he didn't even roll around or sit up. He even didn't speak to his sister and brother when they made their occasional visit or any of the neighbors who stopped by to check on us." The nurse later discovered that Lorenzo and Adam are in a 50+ year intimate relationship.

Your job is to facilitate Lorenzo's return to his home from Uptown Hospital, assist him in regaining his preillness level of activity, and address issues affecting his mental health. The teaching over your scheduled visits will include but not limited to the following:

- Signs and symptoms warranting follow-up
- Medication and administration
- Nutrition and fluid consumption
- Bladder, bowel, skin, and mental health care
- ADLs and IADLs
- Physical activity/endurance
- Safety/injury prevention
- Altered significant other/family/neighbor processes
- Community resources

Consider the following questions:

1. *How will you empower the family to avoid Lorenzo's isolation (self-imposed and socially constructed), risky behavior, and potential for noncompliance with his treatment?*
2. *How would you prioritize Lorenzo's issues, both medical and psychosocial?*
3. *As the public health nurse, what interventions can you utilize to achieve the indicated goals without offending, embarrassing, alienating, and/or "outing" the core family system?*

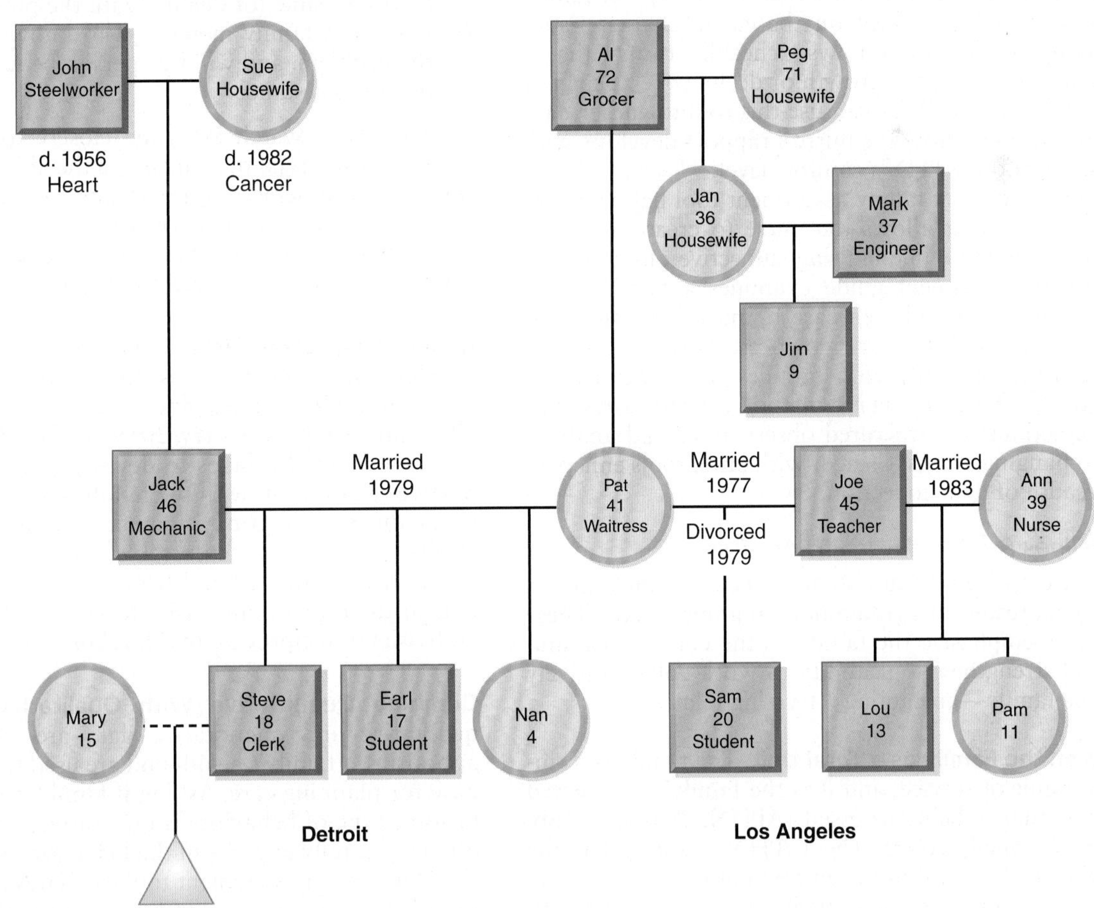

FIGURE 14-5 A genogram.

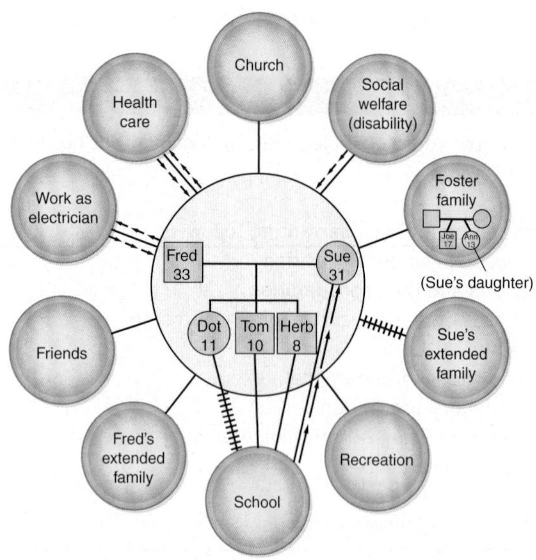

FIGURE 14-6 An eco-map of a family's relationship to its environment.

between the central circle and smaller ones depict the strength of relationships.

For consistency and ease of documentation, public health nursing agencies usually develop their own tools, often in the form of questionnaires, checklists, flow sheets, or interview guides (Chapman et al., 2017; Pontin et al., 2019) to fit organizational needs (for examples of family assessment tools, visit thePoint). One type of family assessment tool uses questions based on characteristics of healthy families and follows a checklist format that is useful to observe family growth or decline over a span of time. The novice C/PHN can use this tool to gather data and to document how the nurse's rapport develops with the family and the PHN's comfort level.

Another type of family assessment tool has an open-ended format that allows the nurse to create an informative document while limiting subjective observations. A self-care assessment guide examines a family member's ability to provide self-care by measuring the family's stressors and self-care practices. This tool is used adjunctively, especially with families from various cultural groups. Videotaping is a method used to assess family interactions for structured observations and analyses of life-changing events. Using it with other tools enhances the breadth of data collection.

Guidelines for Family Health Assessment

There are five guidelines to use since a family health assessment results in a voluminous amount of data. These guidelines emphasize the family as the core service unit and will strengthen your ability to work collaboratively with the family—promoting a trusting relationship.

Focus on the Family as a Total Unit. The family is a single core unit of service, and it is the family's aggregated behavior that is being assessed (APHN, 2016a, 2016b; Shajani & Snell, 2019). The C/PHN ensures that the information is typical of the entire family.

Getting families to share their stories can be a health promotion tool by creating meaning for individuals and the family. The story can tell nurses what is important to the family to help develop interventions. Nurses can begin by asking the family who are you from rather than where are you from? Practice telling and listening to family stories with someone (Driessnack, 2017).

When assessing the communication patterns of two family members, the nurse is also thinking about how other family members communicate among themselves and with the two being assessed. After analyzing the data, the nurse may decide that the family, as a whole, communicates well and supportively even if one family member does not. The nurse documents this deviation and considers it in the care planning.

Ask Goal-Directed Questions. Goal-directed questions are the cornerstone of a detailed assessment (Sperry, 2019; Shajani & Snell, 2019). They facilitate the C/PHN in determining a family's level of health, making family diagnoses, and crafting a care plan. These relevant questions yield relevant and comprehensive data that goes beyond the family dynamics at the moment (Sperry, 2019). Examples of goal-directed questions include the following:

- Does this family recognize when a change needs to be made?
- How does the family react when a change is forced on the family?
- If a problem arises from the change, such as the baby having diarrhea or constantly crying, will the family be responsible for dealing with the problem?
- Is there a family member who knows how to solve the problem, and will this person be willing to accept outside assistance?

Thus, you watch everyone closely for signs of the family's response(s) to change and the ability to problem-solve any problems resulting from the change. Another more open-ended format or approach is to use assessment categories to stimulate questions to explore family support systems for a specific category.

Collect Data Over Time. You want to take your time to accumulate observations, make notes, identify both major and minor issues, and observe the interactions of all family members (Sperry, 2019; Shajani & Snell, 2019).

Timeliness also helps to develop a trusting and supportive relationship with the family since assessment can occur during any family activity such as mealtime. The family needs to feel comfortable with you, the observing nurse. Even if the C/PHN feels welcomed and comfortable at the initial home visit, it may take the family several visits to reciprocate that level of comfort.

Combine Quantitative With Qualitative Data. Both qualitative and quantitative data are collected when appraising a family's health and are used to create a database for planning care. Asking if family members engage in some type of behaviors is qualitative, and asking how often the family engages in the behaviors is quantitative.

One type of assessment tool evaluates a family's ability to enhance individuality by rating the family's behavior on a scale of 0 (never) to 4 (most of the time), which provides a way to compare the family's development over several home visits. The difference between the present and previous scores assists the C/PHN in executing the intervention(s). For this reason, it is useful to conduct periodic assessments when a case is reopened or every 3 to 6 months if it is kept open for an extended period.

Exercise Professional Judgment. The content of a family assessment is driven by the nurse's professional judgment with the assessment tools guiding the nurse's observations and quantifying the nurse's decisions (McDowell & Boyd, 2018; Sperry, 2019).

The nurse may observe that a family makes good use of a community agency, but the decision that using this external resource contributes to the family's health results from a professional judgment. An assessment tool is only a tool, and its value should never be interpreted as an absolute and irrevocable statement about a family's health status.

As a professional, the C/PHN knows that the completion of an assessment tool should occur at the end of the home visit(s). The C/PHN may review the assessment tool before entering a family's home or keep it in a folder for easy reference or note during the visit. However, the assessment tool is not completed in the presence of the family. Even with an eco-map or genogram, the C/PHN uses professional judgment to determine when the family is ready.

Family Health Diagnosis

The family diagnosing process moves the data from assessment to care planning, implementation, and evaluation. This process is an expected standard of practice for public health nurses (APHN, 2016a, 2016b). The C/PHN uses observational skills and clinical reasoning to understand the patterns in the data.

Specifically, the C/PHN identifies patterns of behavior, barriers preventing the family from being healthy, and internal relationships with the external environment (APHN, 2016a, 2016b). Next, the nurse prioritizes the information while taking the best action(s) for the desired outcome or goal (Kaakinen et al., 2018). The diagnosing process can occur as follows (Kaakinen, et al., 2018):

1. Identify the family health problems.
   a. Determine what family members are directly and indirectly related to the problem.
   b. Determine what factors from the external environment are related to the problem.
   c. Describe the problem as it impacts the identified family members and external environment.
   d. Indicate the risks that are associated with the problem(s).
   e. Prioritize the problems along with their risks with an emphasis on the problems that are overlapping and/or have overlapping risks.
2. Indicate the factors from the family (family unit and family members) and the external environment that are associated with the health problems.
3. Determine the measurements (quantitative and qualitative data) that confirm or verify the health problems.

The diagnosing process is an ongoing one with two major goals: improve the family health and give them the tools for health promotion. It should be completed several times, especially with a lot of assessment data so that the nurse can craft a plan of care to move the family toward a state of health.

Family Health Planning and Implementation

A formal care plan occurs after identifying the main concerns, problems, and risks. The nurse and the family collaborate to identify the problem(s), to suggest interventions, and to discuss the plan of action (Fiese, Celano, Deater-Deckard, Jouriles, & Whisman, 2018; Stastny et al., 2016; Shajani & Snell, 2019).

If there is no agreement, the data should be reviewed and discussed with family members to reach a mutual understanding about the best interventions and how to put them into action. The family needs to believe in the plan of action or the nurse will be limited in her or his efforts to prevent identified problems and/or risks while promoting the family's health (Shajani & Snell, 2019). Once family members are ready to learn ways to improve their health status, then the nurse determines the best teaching approach to use and tailors interventions to the specific family needs and functional capability (Sperry, 2019; Shajani & Snell, 2019). If the family's level of functioning does not enable them to use anticipatory guidance and teaching, then the nurse can serve as a counselor.

Planning for subsequent visits assures that the nurse is totally prepared for the next encounter with the family, assuring a successful family visit. This planning ensures that the family transitions toward a healthy outcome in the visit. Planning commences during the first home visit as the nurse collects data so that subsequent visits can be individualized and tailored to meet the family's needs, especially since this information is not available from a paper referral. Consequently, planning for the next visit will affect the nurse's continued success with the family.

Implementation includes making referrals and contacting appropriate resources.

Making Referrals

The nurse makes a referral so that the family can have access to services that might be beyond the agency's resources. The referral reflects the nurse's knowledge of resources within the community, which includes the eligibility requirements and availability of services, provided by official, voluntary, religious, and neighborhood organizations (Kaakinen et al., 2018; McDowell & Boyd, 2018). The nurse must also be aware of any updates or changes to the information about these organizations. Therefore, C/PHNs need to network with colleagues on a regular basis in order to remain up-to-date with community services for family referrals (APHN, 2016a, 2016b; Kaakinen et al., 2018).

Contacting Resources

Public health nurses know how to access key personnel in agencies, which can eliminate some of the red tapes involved in obtaining services, while giving family members pointers on procuring needed services. When C/PHNs seek informal services for families, the nurse establishes a relationship with the agency's staff that can help nurses secure services for the family over time. This rapport can also be used to connect with other agencies, which increases the nurse's database of services.

Family Health Evaluation

Evaluation represents the final step in the nursing process and involves appraising the work with the family and preparing for the next visit. A formal evaluation concludes with the documenting of the outcomes, which facilitates the nurse in making appropriate referrals and contacting key resources to meet the needs of family.

The components of the evaluation are the structure–process, the outcome, and the nurse's self-evaluation. Each one contributes to determining what made the visit a success and what made it less than successful by evaluating if the outcomes were achieved and if they can be advanced to the next level of family health. The nurse must be prepared to determine if a change is needed in the structure–process, the nurse's level of preparedness, or the nurse's behavior in order to promote health in the family, the community, and eventually the population.

Structure–Process Evaluation

The structure–process evaluation should be completed first as it refers to the organization of the visit and how it proceeded (see Chapter 12). The nurse identifies where the organization or the flow of the assessment needs to be changed or modified in order to avoid distractions in the next visit.

Specifically, the nurse will analyze the available resources, number of persons present, timing of home visit(s), environmental factors, or materials/supplies used as well as the use of observational skills, people's attitudes, and reliance on standards of assessment and analysis. Every aspect must be used in the evaluation in order to effectively and thoroughly modify subsequent visits.

Outcome Evaluation

The outcome evaluation facilitates the nurse in deciding if the anticipated outcomes were achieved and what made them possible. This **outcome evaluation**, a formal appraisal process, happens with documentation of the home visits. The effectiveness of any achieved outcomes is determined with standards and/or agency-driven criteria.

The standards are the Nursing Outcomes Classification (NOC) System, the Nursing Intervention Classification (NIC) System, and the Omaha System (see Chapter 15). The agency-driven criteria may be the successful achievement of the indicated expectations for each client category or visit type. Evaluating the outcomes with the agency-driven criteria may be more exact if the effectiveness is demonstrated by small changes over time in the family dynamics as noted on a visit-by-visit basis instead of cumulatively as represented in the standards. Therefore, the nurse must use professional judgment to determine the success or failure of the family to achieve certain outcomes at the conclusion of agency services, with the family included in the decision process.

Self-Evaluation

The self-evaluation encompasses the nurse appraising the ability to facilitate the desired outcome during the home visit(s), the level of being prepared, the thoroughness in data collection, the degree of preparedness for subsequent home visits, and the pros and cons of completed home visits. In other words, this self-evaluation affords the community/public health nurse the opportunity to recognize her or his strengths and failings with internal measures to improve practice (Edelman & Kudzma, 2017).

In some agencies, routine peer evaluations are conducted to recognize strengths and/or weaknesses not indicated in a self-evaluation. The peer evaluation can be completed by an agency staff nurse who makes a family visit with the community/public health nurse and provides feedback based on her or his observations. This might be helpful when working with a family that has not made progress toward the desired outcomes or to a family you have not been able to reach (Sperry, 2019). Peer consultation can also assist the C/PHN in becoming better prepared or more focused in order to improve the interaction(s) with families from different cultures or in difficult situations (Spector, 2017).

SUMMARY

- Because today the family is recognized as an important unit of service, an effective C/PHN must understand family theory and characteristics. Family health and individual health strongly influence each other, and family health affects community health.
- Although every family on the globe is unique in terms of its needs and strengths, each family is at the same time alike because of certain shared universal characteristics: every family is a small social system, has its own cultural values and rules, has structure, has certain basic functions, and moves through stages in its life cycle.
- The C/PHN needs to understand the different needs of various family patterns. Whereas the single adolescent parent needs the community health nurse's knowledge of family developmental theory, more complex interaction patterns and living arrangements are created by divorce, remarriage, the blending of families, and the unique relationships these arrangements create. Gay and lesbian families with children may also have special needs, calling for a sensitive understanding of society's reaction to their family.
- The essential starting point in the community health nurse's work is to accept the family's definition of who their family is and listen to the family's ideas. The nurse and the family become partners in providing health care, with the nurse beginning the work assessing the family's strengths, which will begin to build a positive relationship between the nurse and the family. The family unit remains the focus of service in public health nursing because each family member strongly influences the other, which affects the community health.
- Healthy families demonstrate six important characteristics. The characteristics of a healthy family provide one assessment framework that public health nurses can use.

- Making family health visits is a unique role for nurses and is one of the activities common to most public health nurses.
- The nurse's preparation for the visit facilitates (1) an orderly and organized flow for the visit and (2) the nurse becoming acquainted with the family, which is indispensable for the comprehensive execution of the nursing process and development of a trusting relationship.
- For a comprehensive assessment, C/PHNs employ acute observational skills, good verbal and nonverbal communication, assessment skills, and intuition to guide them safely in the community and with the families they visit.
- The family is a total unit or single entity, and the nurse must consciously recall this point through the home visits and every stage of the nursing process, especially during assessment.
- To systematically assess a family's health, the nurse needs a conceptual framework, categories for data collection, and a measure of the family's level of functioning.
- The main broad categories of a family health visit are previsit preparation, conduct of the visit, postvisit documentation, and preparation or planning for the next visit. Each step contributes to the success of the subsequent one.
- There are specific precautions for safety that a nurse must follow if using a personal or agency car or public transportation or walking to visit families. Safety must be considered in a family's home even if it means terminating the visit and rescheduling.
- The nurse empowers the family by establishing a verbal or written contract with the family so that the family members (1) understand their personal roles and responsibilities in the relationship and (2) feel confidence in making independent decisions about their own health.
- The C/PHN makes referrals to other agencies on behalf of the family in order to provide all the services that a family needs; therefore, the C/PHN needs to know how and where to locate official and voluntary services within their community.

ACTIVE LEARNING EXERCISES

1. Analyze two families you know well (other than your own) and answer the following questions:
   If the major breadwinner in this family was unable to work or lost his or her job, how would the family most likely respond immediately and in the long term?
   What are the strengths of the family?
   How could a nurse most effectively intervene in this situation?
2. Talk with members of a blended family, and discuss with each member his or her relationships with stepchildren, stepparents, or siblings. What strengths can they identify in their family? How has this helped them adapt to their blended family?
3. Listen to two to three stories on Story Corp https://storycorps.org/. What did you learn? Are there themes that you recognize among the stories?
4. Construct an eco-map of your family and ask a peer to do the same, which can be completed face-to-face or online (i.e., Google Docs). Compare the eco-maps. Assess the balance between your family and the resources in its environment. How does your eco-map compare with that of your peer? What changes are needed in each family system? Are you able to influence the changes that are needed?
5. Using "Build a Diverse and Skilled Workforce" (1 of the 10 essential public health services; see Box 2-2), watch one of the two YouTube videos, A Day in the Life of a Public Health Nurse (https://www.youtube.com/watch?v=n8FvhaMvcDQ) or A Day in the Life-Mary (Public Health Nursing) https://www.youtube.com/watch?v=fGj5wncmuX0, with one or two classmates. Evaluate the public health nurse in terms of structure–process and outcomes as well as a peer evaluation of the PHN. With your classmates, discuss the PHN's strengths and weaknesses, and identify what actions you would emulate, change, or leave as is. Identify five instances in the video that made you feel uncomfortable, discuss with your classmates why these occurrences affected you, and discuss ways to process these feelings.

REFERENCES

Abassi, I. S., & Alghamdi, N. G. (2017). When flirting turns into infidelity: The Facebook dilemma. *The American Journal of Family Therapy*, *45*(1), 1–14.

AgingStats.gov. (2015). *Population*. Retrieved from http://www.agingstats.gov/agingstatsdotnet/Main_Site/Data/2015_Documents/Population.aspx

American Academy of Pediatrics. (2015). *Promoting the wellbeing of children whose parents are gay*. Retrieved from https://pediatrics.aappublications.org/content/131/4/827

Arbaje, A. I., Hughes, A., Werner, N., Carl, K., Hohl, D., Jones, K., … Gurses, A. P. (2018). Information management goals and process failures during home visits for middle-aged and older adults receiving skilled home healthcare services after hospital discharge: A multisite, qualitative study. *BMJ Quality & Safety*, *28*(2), 111–120. doi: 10.1136/bmjqs-2018-008163.

Association of Public Health Nurses (2016a). *Definition of public health nurses*. Retrieved from http://phnurse.org/Mission-and-Vision

Association of Public Health Nurses. (2016b). *The public health nurse: Necessary partner for the future of healthy communities. A position paper of the Association of Public Health Nurses*. Retrieved from http://www.quadcouncilphn.org/wp-content/uploads/2016/08/APHN-PHN-Value-Position-P_APPROVED-5.30.2016.pdf

Beck, T. L., Le, T. K., Henry-Okafor, Q., & Shah, M. K. (2017). Medical care for undocumented immigrants: National and international issues. *Primary Care, 44*(1), 127–140. doi: 10.1016/j.pop.2016.09.014.

Centers for Disease Control and Prevention. (2018). *My family health portrait: A tool from the surgeon general.* Retrieved from https://phgkb.cdc.gov/FHH/html/index.html

Centers for Disease Control and Prevention. (2019). *Social determinants and eliminating disparities in teen pregnancy. Reproductive Health: Teen Pregnancy.* Retrieved from https://www.cdc.gov/teenpregnancy/about/social-determinants-disparities-teen-pregnancy.htm

Chapman, H., Kilner, M., Matthews, R., White, A., Thompson, A., Fowler-Davis, S., & Farndon, L. (2017). Developing a caseload classification tool for community nursing. *British Journal of Community Nursing, 22*(4), 192–196. doi: 10.12968/bjcn.2017.22.4.192.

ChildStats.gov. (2019). *America's children: Key national indicators of well-being, 2019.* Retrieved from https://www.childstats.gov/americaschildren/

Childwelfare.gov. (2018). *Foster care statistics 2016.* Retrieved from https://www.childwelfare.gov/pubs/factsheets/foster/

Clark-Jones, T. (2018). *Qualities of a healthy family.* Retrieved from https://www.canr.msu.edu/news/traits_of_a_healthy_family

Coker, J. F., Martin, M. E., Simpson, R. M., & Lafortune, L. (2019). Frailty: An in-depth qualitative study exploring the views of community care staff. *BMC Geriatrics, 19*(1), 1–12. doi: 10.1186/s12877-019-1069-3.

de Grubb, M. C., Levine, R. S., & Zoorob, R. J. (2017). Diet and obesity issues in the underserved. *Primary Care, 44*(1), 127–140. doi: 10.1016/j.pop.2016.09.014.

de Souza, I. P., Bellato, R., de Araujo, L. F. S., & de Almeida, K. B. B. (2016). Genogram and eco-map as tools for understanding family care in chronic illness of the young. *Texto & Contexto-Enfermagem, 25*(4), e1530015 doi: 10.1590/0104-07072016001530015.

Denham, S., Eggenberger, S., Young, P., & Krumwiede, N. (2016). *Family focused nursing care.* Philadelphia, PA: Wolters Kluwer.

Dissing, A. S., Dich, N., Nybo-Andersen, A. M. N., Lund, R., & Rod, N. H. (2017). Parental break-ups and stress: Roles of age and family structure in 44 509 pre-adolescent children. *European Journal of Public Health, 27*(5), 829–834.

Driessnack, M. (2017). "Who are you from?": The importance of family stories. *Journal of Family Nursing, 23*(4), 434–449

Duvall, E. M., & Miller, B. (1985). *Marriage and family development* (6th ed.). Philadelphia, PA: Lippincott Williams & Wilkins.

Dyess-Nugent, P. (2018). Nurses' unique opportunity to promote patient engagement in prenatal care. *Nursing Forum, 53*(1), 1–68. doi: 10.1111/nuf.12210.

Edelman, C. L., & Kudzma, E. E. (Eds.). (2017). *Health promotion throughout the life span* (9th ed.). St. Louis, MO: Mosby.

Eliopoulos, C. (2018). *Gerontological Nursing* (9th ed.). Philadelphia, PA: Wolters Kluwer.

Feetham, S. (2018). Revisiting Feetham's criteria for research of families to advance science and inform policy for the health and well-being of families. *Journal of Family Nursing, 24*(2), 115–127.

Fiese, B. H., Celano, M., Deater-Deckard, K., Jouriles, E. N., & Whisman, M. A. (2018). *APA handbook of contemporary family psychology (Volumes 1–3). APA handbooks in psychology.* Washington, DC: American Psychological Association.

Frost, R., Beattie, A., Bhanu, C., Walters, K., & Ben-Shlomo, Y. (2019). Management of depression and referral of older people to psychological therapies: A systematic review of qualitative studies. *The British Journal of General Practice, 69*(680), e171–e181. doi: 10.3399/bjgp19X701297.

Gladding, S. T. (2019). *Family therapy: History, theory, and practice* (7th ed.). New York, NY: Pearson.

Guttmacher Institute. (2015). *Teen pregnancy rates declined in many countries between the mid-1990s and 2011.* Retrieved from https://www.guttmacher.org/news-release/2015/teen-pregnancy-rates-declined-many-countries-between-mid-1990s-and-2011

Guzzo, K., Hemez, O., Anderson, L., Manning, W., & Brown, S. (2019). Is variation in biological and residential ties to children linked to mothers' parental stress and perceptions of co-parenting? *Journal of Family Issues, 40*(4), 488–517.

Healthy Families America. (2019). *Our approach; home visiting.* Retrieved from https://www.healthyfamiliesamerica.org/our-approach/

Hill, R., & Hansen, D. (1960). The identification of conceptual frameworks utilized in family study. *Marriage and Family Living, 22*, 299–311.

Hosseini Shokouh, S. M., Arab, M., Emamgholipour, S., Rashidian, A., Montazeri, A., & Zaboli, R. (2017) Conceptual models of social determinants of health: A narrative review. *Iranian Journal of Public Health, 46*(4), 435–446.

Jones, S. (2015). Implications of case managers' perceptions and attitude on safety of home-delivered care. *British Journal of Community Nursing, 20*(12), 602–607.

Kaakinen, J. R., Coehlo, D. P., Steele, R., Tabacco, A., & Robinson, M. (2018). *Family health care nursing: Theory, practice, and research* (6th ed.). Philadelphia, PA: F. A. Davis.

Kub, J. E., Kulbok, P. A., Miner, S., & Merrill, J. A. (2017). Increasing the capacity of public health nursing to strengthen the public health infrastructure and to promote and protect the health of communities and populations. *Nursing Outlook, 65*, 661–664.

Lee, L. H., Jun, J. S., Kim, Y. J., Roh, S., Moon, S. S., Bukonda, N., & Hines, L. (2017). Mental health, substance abuse, and suicide among homeless adults. *Journal of Evidence-Informed Social Work, 14*(4), 229–242. doi: 10.1080/23761407.2017.1316221.

Marshall, K., & Easton, C. (2018). The role of asset-based approaches in community nursing. *Primary Health Care, 28*(5). doi: 10.7748/phc.2018.e1339.

Martin, J., Hailton, B., Osterman, M., & Driscoll, A. (2019). *National vital statistics report.* Births: Final data for 2018. Retrieved from https://www.cdc.gov/nchs/data/nvsr/nvsr68/nvsr68_13-508.pdf

Martin, J. A., Hamilton, B. E., Osterman, M. J. K., Driscoll, A. K., & Drake, P. (2018). Births: final data for 2016. *National Vital Statistics Report, 67*(1). Retrieved from https://www.cdc.gov/nchs/data/nvsr/nvsr67/nvsr67_01.pdf

McDowell, J., & Boyd, E. (2018). Community diabetes nurse specialists: Service evaluation to describe their professional role. *British Journal of Community Nursing, 23*(9), 426–434.

McGoldrick, M., Garcia-Preto, N., & Carter, B. (2016). *The expanding family life cycle: Individual, family, and social perspectives* (5th ed.). Upper Saddle River, NJ: Prentice Hall.

Mutch, L. (2016). *Public health nursing prenatal services: Clinical practice guideline (working document). Evidence informed practice tools. Population and public health prenatal and postpartum working group.* Winnipeg, Manitoba, Canada: Winnipeg Regional Health Authority.

National Alliance to End Homelessness. (2018). *Who experiences homelessness?* Retrieved from https://endhomelessness.org/homelessness-in-america/who-experiences-homelessness/

Ngweso, S., Petersen, R. W., & Quinlivan, J. A. (2017). Birth experience of fathers in the setting of teenage pregnancy: Are they prepared? *World Journal of Obstetrics and Gynecology, 6*(1), 1–7.

Nichols, M. P., & Davis, S. D. (2019). *The essentials of family therapy, 7th edition. The Merrill Social work and human services series.* New York, NY: Pearson

Nurse Family Partnership. (2019). *Dads need help, too: Your personal nurse can help him be a great dad.* Retrieved from https://www.nursefamilypartnership.org/first-time-moms/expectant-fathers/

Out and Equal: Workplace Advocates. (2019). *Workplace equality factsheet 2019.* Retrieved from https://www.readkong.com/page/equality-factsheet-workplace-2019-6813772

Parachin, V. M. (March/April, 1997). Six signs of a healthy family. *Vibrant Life, 13*, 5–6.

Pemberton, D. (2015). *Statistical definition of 'family' unchanged since 1930.* Retrieved from https://www.census.gov/newsroom/blogs/random-samplings/2015/01/statistical-definition-of-family-unchanged-since-1930.html

Penman-Aguilar, A., Talih, M., Huang, H., Moonsinghe, R., Bouye, K., & Beckles, G. (2016). Measurement of health disparities, health inequities, and social determinants of health to support the advancement of health equity. *Journal of Health Managment PRactice,* 22(Suppl 1), S33–S42. doi: 10.1097/PHH.0000000000000373.

Pew Research. (2018). *The changing profile of unmarried parents.* Retrieved from https://www.pewsocialtrends.org/2018/04/25/the-changing-profile-of-unmarried-parents/

Pew Research Center. (September 14, 2017). *As U.S. marriage rate hovers at 50%, education gap in marital status widens.* Retrieved from http://www.pewresearch.org/fact-tank/2017/09/14/as-u-s-marriage-rate-hovers-at-50-education-gap-in-marital-status-widens/

Pontin, D., Thomas, M., Jones, G., O'Kane, J., Wilson, L., Dale, F., ... Wallace, C. (2019). Developing a family resilience assessment tool for health visiting/public health nursing practice using virtual commissioning, high-fidelity simulation and focus groups. *Journal of Child Health Care, 24*(2), 195–206. doi: 10.1177/13674935198664743.

Raingruber, B. (2017). Health promotion theories. In B. Raingruber (Ed.), *Contemporary health promotion in nursing practice* (pp. 53–94). Sudbury, MA: Jones & Bartlett Learning.

Raley, K. (2016). Cohabitating couples with lower education levels marry less: Is this because they do not want to? *PRC Research Brief Series, 1*(3).

Reeves, R. V., & Krause, E. (2017). *Cohabiting parents differ from married ones in three big ways. Brookings Report.* Retrieved from https://www.brookings.edu/research/cohabiting-parents-differ-from-married-ones-in-three-big-ways/.

Romero, A, (2017). *Estimates of marriages of same-sex couples at the two-year anniversary of Obergefell v. Hodges.* Retrieved from https://williamsinstitute.law.ucla.edu/wp-content/uploads/Obergefell-2-Year-Marriages-Jun-2017.pdf

Salem, H., Johansen, C., Schmiegelow, K., Winther, J. F., Wehner, P. S., Hasle, H., ... Bidstrup, P. E. (2017). FAMily-oriented support (FAMOS): Development and feasibility of a psychosocial intervention for families of childhood cancer survivors. *Acta Oncologica*, *56*(2), 367–374. doi: 10.1080/0284186X.2016.1269194.

Salmond, S. W., & Echevarria, M. (2017). Healthcare transformation and changing roles for nursing. *Orthopaedic Nursing*, *36*(1), 12–25.

Schroeder, W. K. (2017). Leveraging social media in family nursing practice. *Journal of Family Nursing*, *23*(1), 55–72.

Shajani, Z., & Snell, D. (2019). *Nurses and families: A guide to family assessment and intervention* (7th ed.). Philadelphia, PA: F.A. Davis.

SmithBattle, L. (2018a). Housing trajectories of teen mothers and their families over 28 years. *American Journal of Orthopsychiatry*, *89*(2), 258–267.

SmithBattle, L. (2018b). The past is prologue? The long arc of childhood trauma in a multigenerational study of teen mothering. *Social Science & Medicine*, *216*, 1–9.

SmithBattle, L., & Freed, P. (2016). Teen mothers' mental health. *The American Journal of Maternal/Child Nursing*, *41*(1), 31–36.

SmithBattle, L., Phengnum, W., Shagavah, A. W., & Okawa, S. (2019). Fathering on tenuous ground: A meta-synthesis on teen fathering. *MCN: The American Journal of Maternal/Child Nursing*, *44*(4), 186–194.

Spector, R. E. (2017). *Cultural diversity in health and illness* (9th ed.). New York, NY: Pearson.

Sperry, L. (2019). *Couple and family assessment: Contemporary and cutting-edge strategies. The family therapy and counseling series*. New York, NY: Routledge

Stastny, P. F., Keens, T. G., & Alkon, A. (2016). Supporting SIDS families: The public health nurse SIDS home visit. *Public Health Nursing*, *33*(3), 242–248. doi: 10.1111/phn.12251.

Swartz, G. (2018). 2018 insights, drivers and constraints of community-based primary care practices. *Remington Report*, *26*(4), 1–2. Retrieved from https://remingtonreport.com/intelligence-resources/marketwatch/insights-drivers-and-constraints-of-community-based-primary-care-practices/attachment/businessman-hand-drawing-light-bulb-with-design-word-knowledge/constraints-of-community-based-primary-care-practices.html

Tachibana, Y., Koizumi, N., Akanuma, C., Tarui, H., Ishii, E., Hoshina, T., … Ito, H. (2019). Integrated mental health care in a multidisciplinary maternal and child health service in the community: The findings from the Suzaka trial. *BMC Pregnancy and Childbirth*, *19*(1), 1–11. doi: 10.1186/s12884-019-2179-9.

Turney, K., &Wildeman, C. (2016). Mental and physical health of children in foster care. *Pediatrics*, *38*(5), e20161118.

U.S. Census. (2017). *2017 data release new and notable*. Retrieved from https://www.census.gov/programs-surveys/acs/news/data-releases/2017/release.html

U.S. Department of Health & Human Services (USDHHS). (2020). *Healthy People 2030: Browse objectives*. Retrieved from https://health.gov/healthypeople/objectives-and-data/browse-objectives

Valdermorose-San-Emeterio, M. A., Sanz-Arazu, E., & Ponce-de-Leon-Elizondo, A. (2017). Digital leisure and perceived family functioning in youth of upper secondary education. *Media Education Research Journal*, 99–107.

Vespa, J. (2017). *Jobs, marriage and kids come later in life*. Retrieved from https://www.census.gov/library/stories/2017/08/young-adults.html

CHAPTER 15

Community as Client

"The health of the public is another shared value. Not only does each individual have an interest in staying healthy, but all of us together share an interest in having a healthy population."

—Dan E. Beauchamp & Bonnie Steinbock, New Ethics for the Public's Health

KEY TERMS

Assets assessment
Community as client
Community development
Community diagnosis
Community-oriented, population-focused care
Community subsystem assessment
Conceptual model
Descriptive epidemiologic study
Key informants
Outcome criteria
Partnerships
Priority setting
Problem-oriented assessment
Social determinants of health
Windshield survey

LEARNING OBJECTIVES

Upon mastery of this chapter, you should be able to:

1. Discuss three essential characteristics of nursing service when a community is the client.
2. Describe the contributions of two models of nursing practice to community/public health nursing practice.
3. Describe the characteristics of a healthy community.
4. Describe the meaning of community as client.
5. Articulate three specific considerations of each of the three dimensions of the community as client.
6. Discuss methods of community health assessment.
7. Delineate five sources of community data.
8. Describe the role of the community health nurse as a catalyst for community development.

INTRODUCTION

When you open the door of a senior center where you will be promoting cardiovascular fitness, advocating for exercise equipment, and suggesting changes in the on-site meal program, how might theories of public health nursing contribute to your success? When you approach your city council about the need to increase staffing for public health services, what models of public health nursing practice might support your argument? What are *theories, models*, and *principles*, and what is their relevance to day-to-day public health nursing practice? These are the key issues explored in the first three sections of this chapter.

The remainder of the chapter explores the definition of a healthy community, dimensions of the community as client, and application of the nursing process to the community as client. Included in this discussion are the types of community needs assessment, methods of collecting and sources of community data, data analysis and diagnosis, and making, implementing, and evaluating plans for community health promotion.

WHEN THE CLIENT IS A COMMUNITY: CHARACTERISTICS OF COMMUNITY/PUBLIC HEALTH NURSING PRACTICE

Nursing exists to address people's health care needs, and nurses fulfill this purpose through their work in various specialty areas. Specialties are characterized by the unit of care for which the specialty is responsible and by the goal of the specialty. Each specialty requires a particular area of knowledge and a set of skills for excellence in practice.

Public health nursing is a specialty in which the unit of care is a specific community or aggregate, and the nurse has responsibility to promote group health. The goal of this specialty is health improvement of the community. Some of the skills required for excellence in public health nursing practice include epidemiology, research, teaching, community organizing, and managing programs and outcomes related to interpersonal relational care.

Public health nursing is characterized by **community-oriented, population-focused care** and is based on interpersonal relationships. In the following sections, each of these characteristics is examined in more depth.

A community is a collection of people interacting with one another because of geography, common interests, characteristics, or goals. These interactions include social institutions, such as schools, government agencies, and social services. The concept of community as client refers to a group or population of people as the focus of nursing service (Anderson & McFarlane, 2019).

As described in Chapters 1 and 2, understanding the concept of the community as client is a prerequisite for effective service at every level of community nursing practice. Population-focused practice distinguishes community health nursing from other nursing specialties (American Nurses Association [ANA], 2018; American Public Health Association, Public Health Nursing Section, 2013).

Community orientation is a process that is actively shaped by the unique experiences, knowledge, concerns, values, beliefs, and culture of a given community. For example, when an outbreak of hepatitis occurs, the public health nurse (PHN) does more than simply treat infection in individuals. The nurse also

- Uses disease investigation skills to locate possible sources of infection (see Chapter 7)
- Determines how the community's knowledge, values, beliefs, and prior experiences with infectious disease may influence its interpretation of the disease, response to the outbreak, and treatment preferences
- Uses knowledge and suggestions gathered from the community to develop, in collaboration with other health professionals, a community-specific program to prevent future outbreaks

A community-oriented nurse who provides education about sexually transmitted diseases to a group of students at a Catholic university includes consideration of community values regarding sexual behavior. Similarly, a community-oriented nurse who provides nutritional counseling to a community of Hispanic older adults considers the meaning of food in their culture, the types of food most commonly consumed, and the cooking methods most commonly used.

A *population* refers to all people occupying an area, such as a city, county, or state. Parts of populations may be subpopulations or aggregates. Smokers and refugees are two subpopulations. The nurse's place of employment commonly limits the population that the nurse serves. For example, a nurse who works for a county health department is limited professionally to caring for the population residing in that county.

A *population focus* requires that a nurse use population-based knowledge and skills such as epidemiology, community assessment, and community organizing as bases for interventions. For example, a population-focused nurse employed by an autoworkers' union may study all cases of repetitive use injury occurring in the auto industry in the United States in the past 5 years, develop a program for reducing repetitive use injury, and lobby industry executives for adoption of the program.

Community-oriented, population-focused care employs population-based knowledge and skills and is shaped by the characteristics and needs of a given aggregate, community, or population. C/PHNs provide community-oriented, population-focused care when they count and interview homeless people sleeping in a park and, based on these data, help develop a program to provide food, clothing, shelter, health care, and job training for this population.

THEORIES AND MODELS FOR COMMUNITY/PUBLIC HEALTH NURSING PRACTICE

Nursing is a theory- and evidence-based profession. "Theory-guided, evidence-informed practice is the hallmark of any professional discipline" (Smith, 2019, p. 3). As a nursing specialty, community/public health nursing is not only guided by theories and evidence that pertain to the nursing profession, but also theories and evidence that have been specifically developed and tested for the specialty. Borrowed and shared theories are also major parts of the practice of community and public health nursing. Examples of shared theories are health behavior, learning theory, and diffusion of innovations.

In the classical definition, a theory is "a set of interrelated constructs, definitions, and propositions that present a systematic view of phenomena by specifying relations among variables, with the purpose of explaining and predicting the phenomena" (Kerlinger, 1973, p. 9). A theory is based either explicitly or philosophically on a conceptual model (also referred to as a conceptual framework, a conceptual system, or a paradigm). A **conceptual model**, as originally defined, is a set of concepts and the propositions that integrate them into a meaningful configuration (Lippitt, 1973). These concepts are presented in a framework format used to explain the relationships among variables. A conceptual model cannot be used directly in research or clinical practice. Linking a conceptual model with one or more theories to form the conceptual-theoretical systems of knowledge is needed for action (Fawcett, 2017).

Having been exposed to nursing theories throughout your nursing program, you will recall that nursing theories are usually classified as grand theories, middle-range theories, and situation-specific theories (Smith & Liehr, 2018).

Grand theories are frameworks composed of concepts and relational statements that explain abstract phenomena (Smith, 2019). These theories have a high level of abstraction and are not directly applicable to nursing practice. An example of a grand theory is Rogers' Model of the Science of Unitary Human Beings. This model emphasized that the individual and environment should be viewed as one unit; that is, focusing on the individual without examining her or his environment or examining parts of a community, such as its health care or housing, does not provide an adequate picture of its totality in relation to the person (Johnson & Webber, 2015). Rogers also incorporated developmental theory into her model by describing the development of "unitary" persons or systems according to three principles: (1) life proceeds in one direction along a rhythmic spiral, (2) energy fields follow a certain wave pattern and organization, and (3) human and environmental energy fields interact simultaneously and mutually, leading to completeness and unity (Rogers, 1990).

Middle-range theories have more limited scope and are less abstract than grand theories. These theories are intended to be used for practice as well as research. An example of a middle-range theory is self-care of chronic illness (Riegel, Jaarsman, & Stromberg, 2012). The core elements of this theory are self-care maintenance, self-care monitoring, and self-care management. Self-care management is a process of recognizing changes in signs and symptoms, making decisions about self-care actions, and evaluating outcomes of that action. Several factors influence whether a patient is successful in performing self-care, such as confidence, motivation, and support from others. Community/public health nurses provide care to many individuals who use self-care to manage their chronic illnesses. This theory would be helpful to care for these individuals.

Situation-specific theories focus on specific nursing phenomena that reflect clinical practice and are limited to specific populations or to particular fields of practice. "They are theories that are more clinically specific, that reflect a particular context, and that may include blueprints for action" (Im & Meleis, 1999, p. 13). An example of a situation-specific theory is depression in Black single mothers (Atkins, 2016). The investigator hypothesized and tested a model of the relationships of perceived stress, perceived racism, and self-esteem to depression. Although further study is needed, this model of situation-specific theory of depression can be used to improve care to single Black mothers (Atkins, 2016).

Betty Neuman's Systems Model provides a comprehensive holistic and system-based approach to nursing that contains an element of flexibility (Fig. 15-1). The theory focuses on the patient's response to actual or potential environmental stressors and the use of primary, secondary, and tertiary nursing prevention intervention for retention, attainment, and maintenance of patient system wellness. Table 15-1 shows an example of applying Neuman's model to the prevention of cardiovascular disease (CVD) in an ethnic minority population (Neuman, 1980).

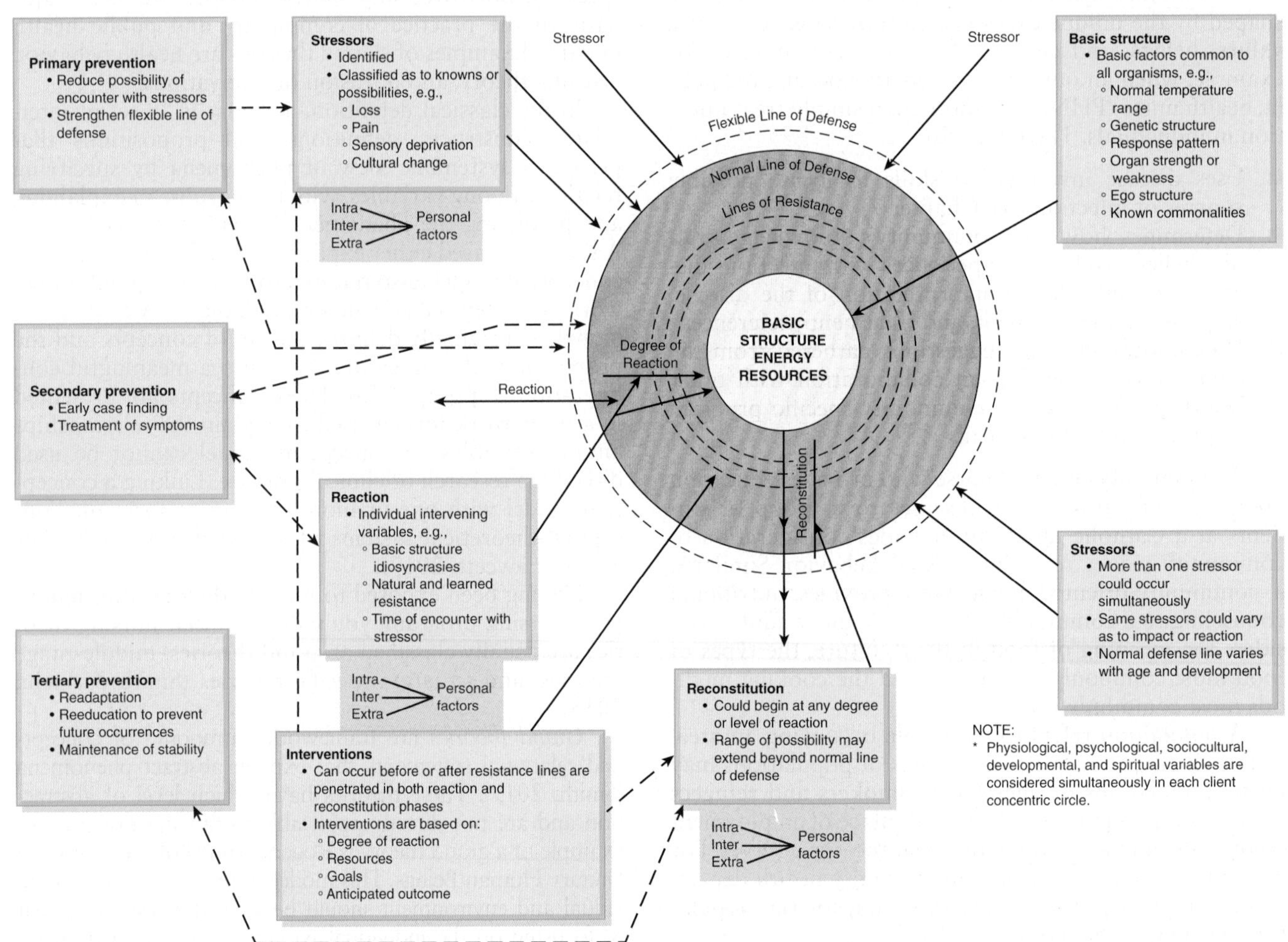

FIGURE 15-1 Neuman's health care systems model. (Adapted with permission from Neuman, B., & Fawcett, J. (2011). *The Neuman systems model* (5th ed., Fig. 1-3, p. 13). Upper Saddle River, NJ: Pearson. Original diagram copyright © 1970 by Betty Neuman.)

TABLE 15-1 Applying Neuman's Model to Prevention of Cardiovascular Disease (CVD) in an Ethnic Minority Population

Part of Model	Description	Application to CVD Prevention
Flexible line of defense	Buffer that expands and contracts to protect normal line of defense from stressors.	Primary prevention efforts include culturally competent education on risk factors for CVD (hypertension, diabetes, obesity, high cholesterol, smoking) and promoting health through regular exercise, healthy eating, and not smoking.
Normal line of defense	Typical responses to stressors; changes over time. Behaviors strengthen or weaken this line in response to stressors.	Promotion of regular medical care and limitation of sodium, sugar, and fat intake. Screening and monitoring cholesterol, blood sugar, B/P.
Lines of resistance	These lines are final protection for the central core.	Providing culturally competent smoking cessation, healthy eating, and exercise programs. Encouraging referrals to cardiologists/other specialists for continued follow-up of early signs/symptoms. Education on importance of continuing medications, self-checks of B/P, food/sodium intake, and weight.
Central core	This component is the basic client system structure common to all people.	CVD may be influenced by genetic factors as well as strength and weaknesses of the system parts.
Stressors	These can originate in the external or internal environment.	Stressors include: ■ Intrapersonal (within the self—e.g., how one deals with stress) ■ Interpersonal (a result of how one copes with others/family/work) ■ Extra-personal (from outside the self—e.g., discrimination, financial crisis, no health insurance, limited health care providers)

Source: Angosta, A.D., Ceria-Ulep, C.D., & Tse, A.M. (2014). Care delivery for Filipino Americans Using the Neuman Systems Model. *Nursing Science Quarterly*, 27(2), 142-148.

Salmon's Construct for Public Health Nursing

Although not a theory, Salmon proposed a model to specifically guide community health nursing practice. Salmon (1982, 1993) described public health as an organized societal effort to protect, promote, and restore the health of people and public health nursing as focused on achieving and maintaining public health.

The model describes three practice priorities:

- Prevention of disease and poor health
- Protection against disease and external agents
- Promotion of health

The three general categories of nursing intervention are:

- Education that is directed toward voluntary change in the attitudes and behavior of the subjects
- Engineering that is directed at managing risk-related variables
- Enforcement that is directed at mandatory regulation to achieve better health

The scope of practice spans individual, family, community, and global care. Interventions target determinants in four categories: human/biologic, environmental, medical/technologic/organizational, and social.

Using Salmon's approach, a C/PHN attempting, for example, to reduce the transmission of tuberculosis, would use education, engineering, and enforcement in working with the population of affected individuals and families. Strategies could include collaboration with the client community on a variety of interventions, from mandating isolation precautions to providing education about medications and connecting the client and his or her family to social support, in an effort to prevent further disease in the community and to promote global health.

Minnesota Wheel: The Public Health Interventions Model

The Minnesota Department of Health, Division of Community Health Services, Public Health Nursing Section, developed a model that depicts public health interventions and applications for public health practice. In the form of a wheel (Fig. 15-2), the model contains 17 different interventions for population-based interventions within three levels of public health practice: community-focused practice, systems-focused practice, and individual-focused practice (Minnesota Department of Health, 2019).

The Wheel can be applied in a variety of activities, including public health practice, nursing education, and management. Keller and colleagues emphasized that the "use of the Wheel has empowered nurses to explain in a better way how their practice contributes to the improvement of population health" (Keller, Strohschein, Lia-Hoagberg, & Schoffer, 2004, p. 454). The wheel is useful

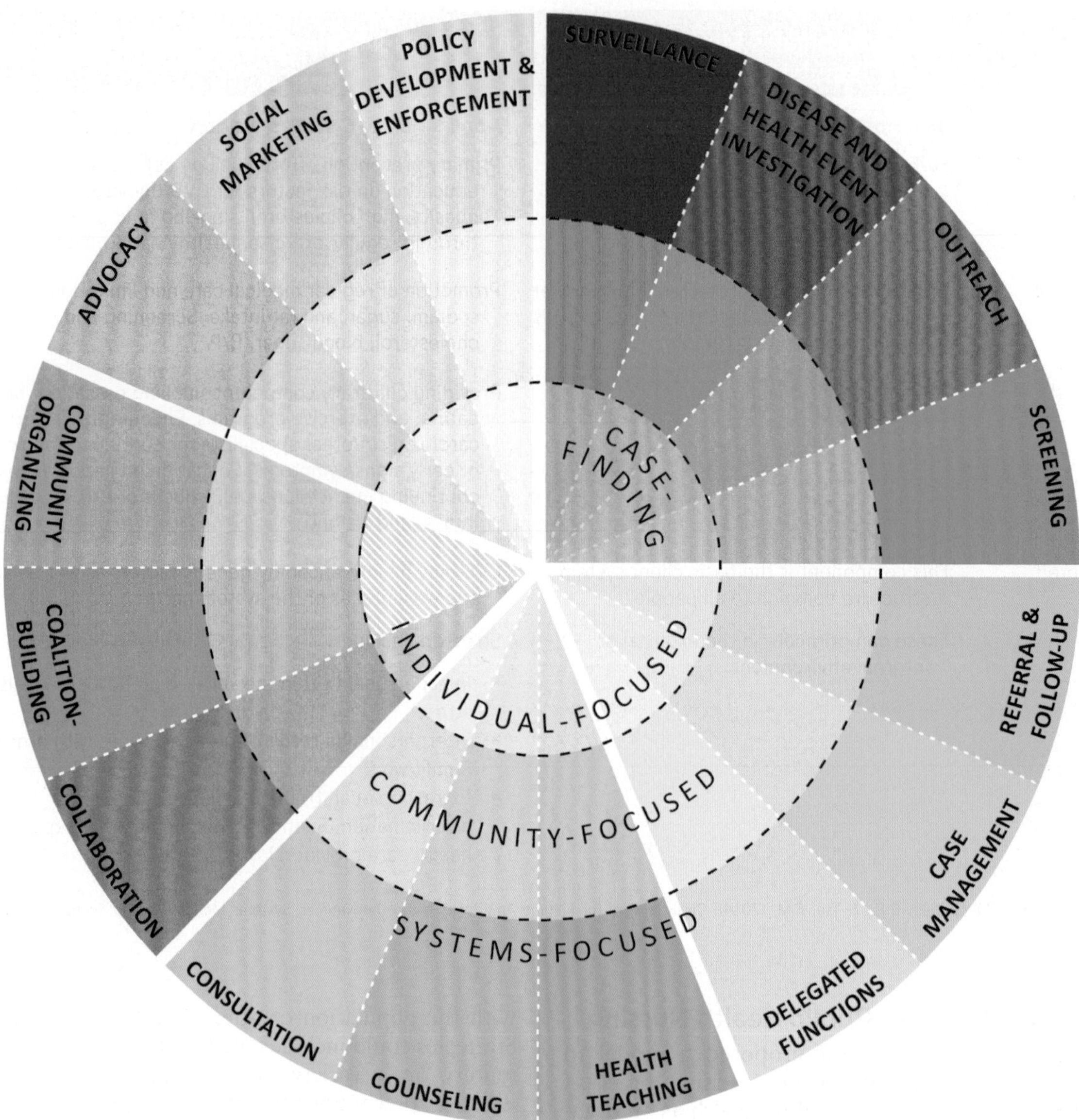

FIGURE 15-2 The Minnesota wheel. (Reprinted with permission from Minnesota Department of Health, Division of Community Health Services, Public Health Nursing Section. Retrieved from https://www.health.state.mn.us/communities/practice/research/phncouncil/docs/PHInterventions.pdf)

for C/PHNs because it visually depicts the comprehensive list of interventions nurses must consider in the scope of practice. Schaffer, Anderson, and Rising (2016) described how school nurses used the model interventions in their day-to-day work.

Public Health Nursing Practice Model

The Los Angeles County Public Health Nursing (LAC PHN) Practice Model was developed in response to an identified need for a model that could blend public health nursing practice and the principles of public health, which could be applicable to both the generalist nurse and nurses working in specific programs (Smith & Bazini-Barakat, 2003). The LAC PHN Practice Model (Public Health Nursing, Los Angeles County Department of Health Services [PHN, LAC-DHS], 2013) integrates foundational nursing and public health guiding documents, including the Public Health Nursing Standards of Practice, the 10 essential public health services, the *Healthy People* health indicators, and the Public Health Nursing Practice Model (Fig. 15-3). The LAC PHN Practice Model provides a "conceptual framework that assists in clarifying the role of the C/PHN and presents a guide for public health practice applicable to all public health disciplines" (Smith & Bazini-Barakat, 2003, p. 42).

The principles of population-based practice are included in the LAC PHN Practice Model (PHN, LAC-DHS, 2013; Smith & Bazini-Barakat, 2003). C/PHNs integrate assessment, policy development, and assurance into their work. The three levels of population-based practice—individuals and families, community, and systems—are addressed, with the nursing process applied throughout the model. The 17 interventions, as first presented in the Minnesota Public Health Nursing

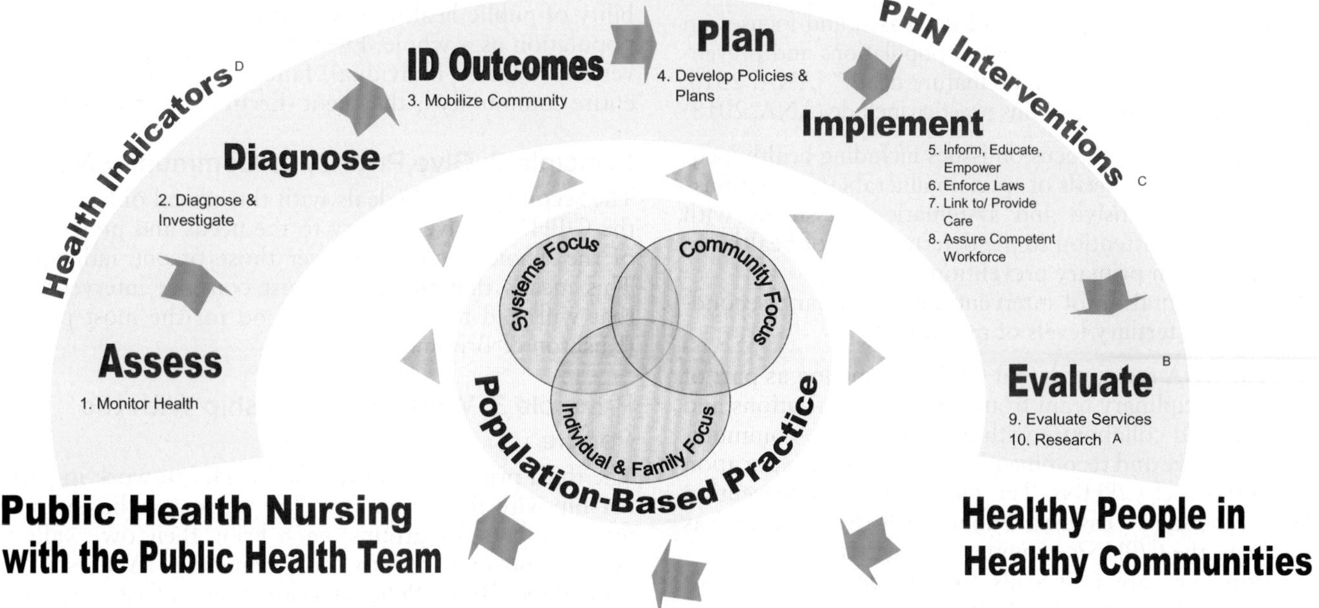

FIGURE 15-3 Public health nursing practice model. (Reprinted from the Los Angeles County Department of Public Health, Public Health Nursing. Retrieved from http://publichealth.lacounty.gov/phn/docs/PracticeModelfinal2.pdf)

Model described above, are also incorporated into the LAC PHN Practice Model. This model promotes the concepts of an interdisciplinary public health team working together with an emphasis on primary prevention. The model also recognizes the importance of active participation of the individual, family, and community (PHN, LAC-DHS, 2013; Smith & Bazini-Barakat, 2003).

Omaha System

The Omaha System (Fig. 15-4) is a multidisciplinary standardized interface that incorporates documentation of nursing assessment and interventions (Thompson, Monsen, Wanamaker, Augustyniak, & Thompson, 2012). It is a comprehensive system, with the following components (Martin, 2005):

- *The problem classification scheme* is a holistic, comprehensive method for identifying clients' health-related concerns. Included are domains, problems, modifiers, and signs/symptoms. Problems can be identified at the individual, family, or community level.
- *The intervention scheme* provides a framework for documenting plans and interventions in the client record in the areas of health teaching, guidance, and counseling; treatments and procedures; case management; and surveillance.
- *The problem rating scale* for outcomes consists of a Likert-type scale that is a systematic and recurring method to document the progress of clients in the record and in case conferences during their time of service in the agency. It is used in conjunction with any problem in the problem classification scheme. Central to problem rating is quantifying outcomes in three dimensions: knowledge (what the client knows), behavior (what the client does), and status (how the client is).

The model is applicable to individuals, families, and communities and provides a mechanism to evaluate both individual and group change over time. With ongoing pressure for public health program funding, outcome data are vital and can be captured through the application of the Omaha System.

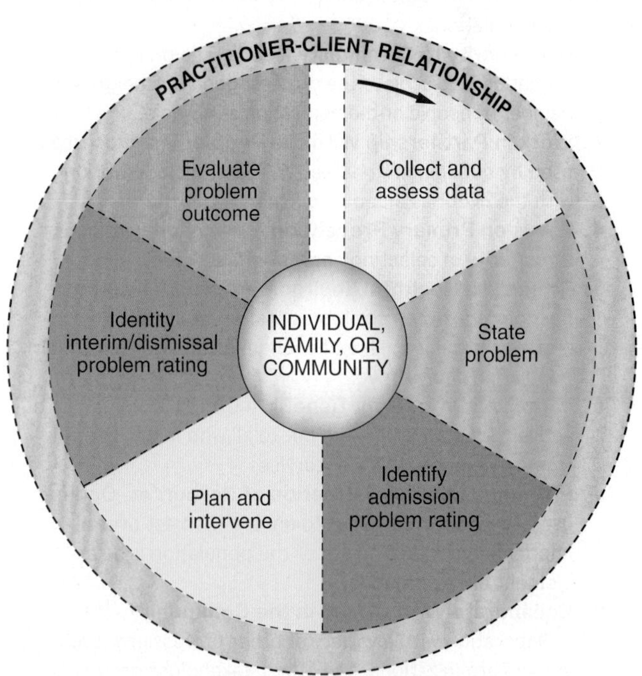

FIGURE 15-4 Omaha system model of the problem-solving process. (Reprinted with permission from Martin, K. S. (2005). *The Omaha System: A key to practice, documentation, and information management* (2nd ed.). Omaha, NE: Health Connections Press.)

PRINCIPLES OF COMMUNITY/PUBLIC HEALTH NURSING

Public health nursing is "…evidence-based and focuses on promotion of the health of entire populations and prevention of disease, injury, and premature death" (ANA, 2013, p. 3). The key elements of this practice include (ANA, 2018)

- Population-level focus on issues including health inequities and the needs of special vulnerable populations
- A comprehensive and systematic assessment with particular attention to the determinants of health
- A focus on primary prevention
- Implementation of interventions of primary, secondary, and tertiary levels of prevention

The ANA recognizes that C/PHNs function as part of an interdisciplinary team from various organizations and agencies and collaborate with members of the communities they serve and recommends a baccalaureate education for entry-level C/PHNs. The Public Health Intervention Wheel and the 10 Essential Public Health Services serve as guides to the C/PHN's activities (ANA, 2018).

Principles are universals to help achieve the most beneficial outcomes. The goals of public health nursing, to promote and protect the health of communities, are facilitated by adhering to eight principles identified by the ANA (2018) for public health nursing practice. These principles are summarized in Box 15-1 and discussed in depth below (ANA, 2018).

BOX 15-1 Principles of Public Health Nursing

1. **Focus on the Community.** The client or unit of care is the population.
2. **Give Priority to Community Needs.** The primary obligation is to achieve the greatest good for the greatest number of people or the population as a whole.
3. **Work in Partnership With the People.** The processes used by public health nurses (C/PHNs) include working with the client as an equal partner.
4. **Focus on Primary Prevention.** Primary prevention is the priority in selecting appropriate activities.
5. **Promote a Healthful Environment.** Public health nursing focuses on strategies that create healthy environmental, social, and economic conditions in which populations may thrive.
6. **Target All Who Might Benefit.** A C/PHN is obligated to actively identify and reach out to all who might benefit from a specific activity or service.
7. **Promote Optimum Allocation of Resources.** Optimal use of available resources to ensure the best overall improvement in the health of the population is a key element of the practice.
8. **Collaborate With Others in the Community.** Collaboration with a variety of other professions, populations, organizations, and other stakeholder groups is the most effective way to promote and protect the health of the people.

Adapted from American Nurses Association (2018, pp. 8–9).

Principle 1: Focus on the Community

The first principle reminds us that the ultimate responsibility of public health nursing is to direct services to the population as a whole. Even though C/PHNs may intervene to address individual, family, or group needs, the entire community is the client (Ervin & Kulbok, 2018).

Principle 2: Give Priority to Community Needs

The second principle deals with the ethical obligation of the C/PHN to give priority to the needs and preferences of the whole community over those of one individual. This means that the nurse must consider interventions that will lead to the greatest good for the most people (Rushton & Broome, 2015).

Principle 3: Work in Partnership With the People

The third principle requires the C/PHN to work in partnership with the community. The nurse and the community members (or groups) each bring their own values, beliefs, and expertise to the partnership (Anderson & McFarlane, 2019). Policy development and assurance are more likely to be accepted and applied if there is mutual consideration of and respect for these elements. Developed policies need to be communicated in language that reflects an understanding of the community

Principle 4: Focus on Primary Prevention

The fourth principle of public health nursing underscores the importance of primary prevention in promoting the health of people. Public health nursing has an obligation to prevent health problems and injuries and to promote a higher level of wellness (Anderson & McFarlane, 2019).

Principle 5: Promote a Healthful Environment

The fifth principle highlights the importance of ensuring that people live in conditions conducive to health. C/PHNs, along with other public health professionals, understand the effects of social determinants of health and work to improve those (O'Brien, 2019).

Principle 6: Target All Who Might Benefit

The sixth principle involves outreach strategies to meet the obligation to serve all people who might benefit from an intervention. This tenet requires that the nurse examine policies or programs to determine whether they are accessible and acceptable to the entire population in need and advocate for change if necessary (Ervin & Kulbok, 2018).

Principle 7: Promote Optimum Allocation of Resources

The seventh principle addresses resource allocation decisions. In most communities, the available resources are not sufficient to meet all needs of all people. The nurse must ensure that the community is using limited resources in ways that lead to the greatest improvement in health (Swider, Berkowitz, Valentine-Maher, Zenk, & Bekemeier, 2017). To promote optimum allocation of resources, the nurse must

- Know the latest research on the effectiveness of various programs in addressing needs
- Collect information about the short- and long-term costs of programs
- Evaluate existing programs and policies for ways to improve or discontinue them
- Communicate this information to community decision makers, so that they can make resource allocation decisions that are most likely to improve the community's health

C/PHNs should continue to work on all levels to promote greater funding for public health programs and more effective allocation of resources.

Principle 8: Collaborate With Others in the Community

The eighth principle underscores the importance of collaboration with other nurses, health care providers, social workers, educators, spiritual leaders, business leaders, and government officials within the community. This interdisciplinary collaboration is essential to execute effective programs and improve health outcomes. Programs that are planned and implemented in isolation can lead to fragmentation, gaps, and overlaps in health services (Ervin & Kulbok, 2018).

WHAT IS A HEALTHY COMMUNITY?

Just as health for an individual is relative and will change, all communities exist in a relative state of health. A community's health can be viewed within the context of health being more than just the absence of disease and including things that promote the maintenance of a high quality of life and productivity. A key vision for healthy communities is presented in *Healthy People 2030* the national agenda for health and well-being published by the U.S. Department of Health and Human Services (USDHHS, 2020). See Chapter 1. The five overarching goals for the health of the nation are to:

- Attain healthy, thriving lives and well-being free of preventable disease, disability, injury, and premature death.
- Eliminate health disparities, achieve health equity, and attain health literacy to improve the health and well-being of all.
- Create social, physical, and economic environments that promote attaining the full potential for health and well-being for all.
- Promote healthy development, healthy behaviors, and well-being across all life stages.
- Engage leadership, key constituents, and the public across multiple sectors to take action and design policies that improve the health and well-being of all (USDHHS, 2020).

Healthy People 2030 objectives and targets provide guidelines for communities to follow to promote the health of their members. By encouraging collaboration across communities, empowering individuals to make better choices, and measuring progress toward set benchmarks, *Healthy People 2030* can be used as a road map for achieving longer and healthier lives for all Americans.

The National Prevention Strategy (NPS), largely based on *Healthy People* priorities, was developed in 2011 to further national health improvement efforts. The NPS aims to guide national efforts in the most effective and achievable means for improving health and well-being. The strategy prioritizes prevention by integrating recommendations and actions across multiple settings to improve health and save lives. To realize this vision and achieve this goal, the strategy identifies four strategic directions and seven targeted priorities (Association of State and Territorial Health Officials, 2019).

The *strategic directions* provide a strong foundation for all of our nation's prevention efforts and include core recommendations necessary to build a prevention-oriented society. They include

- Healthy and safe community environments: Create, sustain, and recognize communities that promote health and wellness through prevention.
- Clinical and community preventive services: Ensure that prevention-focused health care and community prevention efforts are available, integrated, and mutually reinforcing.
- Empowered people: Support people in making healthy choices.
- Elimination of health disparities: Eliminate disparities, improving the quality of life for all Americans.

Within this framework, the *priorities* provide evidence-based recommendations that are most likely to reduce the burden of the leading causes of preventable death and major illness and include

- Tobacco-free living
- Preventing drug abuse and excessive alcohol use
- Healthy eating
- Active living
- Injury- and violence-free living
- Reproductive and sexual health
- Mental and emotional well-being

The NPS serves as a road map for community health nurses collaborating with stakeholders and community partners, to address priority areas such as healthy eating, active living, and tobacco control through the prioritization of prevention and integration of recommendations and actions across multiple settings. By working on shared priorities, community health nurses can serve as a valuable partner in identifying community health needs and connecting communities with available resources. Nurses can also serve as community educators, empowering people with information to make healthy choices while working to create environments where healthy choices are more accessible and affordable, which is the ultimate intent of the strategy (Lushniak, Alley, Ulin, & Graffunder, 2015).

DIMENSIONS OF THE COMMUNITY AS CLIENT

The health of a community can be characterized through a number of perspectives. Donabedian's classic theory of structure, process, and outcomes provides unique insight into the health status of the community (Donabedian, 2005).

- *Status/people* is the most common measure of the health of a community. It typically comprises morbidity and mortality data identifying the physical, emotional, and social determinants of health.

- *Structure* of a community refers to its services and resources. Community associations, groups, and organizations provide a means for accessing needed services. Adequacy and appropriateness of health services can be determined by examining patterns of use, number and types of health and social services, and quality measures. These measures provide key information and correlate to health status.
- *Process* reflects the community's ability to function effectively. It includes processes within the community and between the community and the state or national levels to maintain health and improve outcomes.

These characteristics are discussed in more detail later in this chapter under the discussion on "Planning to Meet the Health Needs of the Community." See Chapter 1 for more information on healthy communities.

Addressing community health by examining the process, in addition to the structure and status dimensions, provides a broader view into the complexities of community health and community actions for change. It is a key not only to examine health outcomes but also to consider how the interactions between processes and structure impact health outcomes (Public Health Accreditation Board, 2019). These are detailed in Tables 15-2 and 15-3.

Location

The health of a community is affected by location, because placement of health services, geographic features, climate, plants, animals, and the human-made environment are intrinsic to geographic location. The location of a community places it in an environment that offers resources and also poses threats.

TABLE 15-2 Community Profile Inventory: Location Perspective

Location Variables	Community Health Implications	Community Assessment Questions	Information Sources (For All—Various Internet Sites)
Boundary of community	These serve as basis for measuring incidence of wellness and illness and for determining spread of disease.	Where is the community located? Is it a part of a larger community? Smaller communities included?	Google Maps State maps County maps City maps City directory Public library
Location of health services	Use of health services depends on availability and accessibility.	Where are the major health institutions located in the community? Outside the community?	www.Healthfinder.gov Chamber of commerce State health department County or local health departments Maps
Geographic features	Injury, death, and destruction may be caused by floods, earthquakes, volcanoes, or hurricanes. Recreational opportunities at lakes, seashore, and mountains promote health and fitness.	What major landforms are in or near the community? Which features pose possible threats? Which offer opportunities for healthful activities?	Atlas Chamber of commerce Maps State health department Public library www.NGMDB.USGS.gov
Climate	Extremes of heat and cold affect health and illness. Extremes of temperature and precipitation may tax community's coping ability.	What are the average temperature and precipitation? What climatic features affect health and fitness? Is the community prepared to cope with emergencies?	www.CLIMATE.gov Chamber of commerce State health department Maps Local government Weather bureau Public library
Flora and fauna	Poisonous plants and disease-carrying animals can affect community health. Plants and animals offer resources as well as dangers.	What plants and animals pose possible threats to health?	State health department Poison control center Police department Emergency rooms Encyclopedia Public library
Human-made environment	All human influences on environment (housing, dams, farming, type of industry, chemical waste) can influence levels of community wellness.	What are the major industries? Are there air, land, and water pollution concerns? What is the quality of housing?	Chamber of commerce Local government City directory State health department University research reports Public library

TABLE **15-3** Community Profile Inventory: Population Perspective

Population Variables	Community Health Implications	Community Assessment Questions	Information Sources (For All—Various Internet Sites)
Size	The number of people influences number and size of health care institutions.	What is the population? Is it an urban, suburban, or rural community?	State health department Census data Chamber of commerce
Density	High and low density often affects the availability of health services.	What is the density of the population per square mile?	Census data State health department
Composition	Composition of the population often determines types of health needs.	What are the population's demographic?	Census data State health department U.S. Department of Labor Statistics
Rate of growth or decline	Rapidly growing communities may place excessive demands on health services. Marked decline in population may signal a poorly functioning community.	How has population size changed over the past two decades? What are the health implications of this change?	Census data State health department
Cultural differences	Health needs vary among subcultural and ethnic populations. Utilization of health services varies with culture. Health practices and extent of knowledge are affected by culture.	What is the ethnic breakdown of population? What racial groups are represented? What subcultural populations exist? Are different ethnic and cultural groups included in health planning?	Census data State health department Social and cultural research reports City government Health planning boards
Mobility	Mobility of the population affects continuity of care. Mobility affects availability of service to highly mobile populations.	How frequently do members move into and out of the community? Are there any specific populations that are highly mobile? Is the community organized to meet the health needs of mobile groups?	State health department Census data Health agencies serving migrant workers Program serving transients and the homeless
Income level	Economic disparities may lead to health disparities.	What percentage of the population is below federal poverty levels? How many children qualify for free or reduced cost school lunch?	Census data State data Local data (schools)
Education level	Education disparities may lead to health disparities.	What is the literacy rate?	State data Local data (schools)
Unemployment rate	Health insurance is often tied to employment. Lack of regular income can be a family stressor. Both can lead to health disparities.	What is the rate of unemployment? How variable is this rate?	U.S. Department of Labor State data Local data
Population by age	A high proportion of children and elderly can overburden health care and social systems.	What is the dependency ratio? Has this rate changed dramatically? What is the trend?	Census data State data Local data
Health status	Community members' status relative to the 10 Leading Health Indicators can impact overall community health.	What is the rate of obesity/overweight? What are the rates of tobacco use and substance abuse? What is the immunization rate? What are rates of injury and violence? What are the STD and HIV/AIDS rates?	State data Local data Centers for Disease Control and Prevention (CDC) data Vital statistics—numbers of births, deaths, marriages, and infant mortality rate (Compare local to state data; state to national data)
Environmental health status	Poor environmental health (e.g., presence of coliform bacteria in well water, toxic chemicals, or poor air quality) can lead to increased incidence of communicable or chronic diseases.	What are rates of communicable or chronic diseases (e.g., *Escherichia coli* infections, asthma)?	CDC data State data Local data

The healthy community is one that makes wise use of its resources and is prepared to meet threats and dangers. In assessing the health of any community, it is necessary to collect information not only about variables specific to location but also about relationships between the community and its location. Do groups cooperate to identify threats? Do health agencies cooperate to prepare for an emergency such as a flood, tornado, or earthquake? Does the community make certain that its members are given available information about resources and dangers?

Table 15-2 describes the location perspective of the Community Profile Inventory, including the six location variables: community boundaries, location of health services, geographic features, climate, flora and fauna, and the human-made environment.

Community Boundaries

To talk about the community in any sense, one must first describe its boundaries. Measurement of health within a community must be preceded by definition of geographic and informal boundaries around the target population. Nurses need to be clear, for example, that a target community of older adults includes a description of age and location (e.g., all persons 65 years and older in a given city or county). Some communities are distinctly separate, such as an isolated rural town, whereas others are closely situated to one another, such as the suburbs of a large metropolis. Therefore, it is important for the nurse to know the nature of each location and clearly define its boundaries.

Location of Health Services

If the members of a town must travel 200 miles to the nearest clinic or dental office, the health of the community will be affected. When assessing a community, the community health nurse needs to identify the major health centers and know where they are located. For example, an alcoholism treatment center for indigent alcoholics was located 30 miles outside of one city. This location presented transportation problems and profoundly affected the length of time they remained at the center and the willingness of clients to voluntarily seek treatment there. If a well-baby clinic is located on the edge of a high-crime district, parents may be deterred from using it. It is often helpful to plot the major health institutions, both inside and outside the community, on a map that shows their proximity and relationship to the community as a whole.

Geographic Features

Communities have been constructed in every conceivable physical environment, and environment certainly can affect the health of a community (see Chapter 9). A healthy community is one that takes into consideration the geography of its location, identifies possible problems and likely resources, and responds in an adaptive fashion. For example, Anchorage, Alaska, and San Francisco, California, are both located on a geologic fault line and are subject to major earthquakes. In such places, the health of the community is determined, in part, by its preparedness for an earthquake and its ability to cope and respond quickly when such a crisis occurs.

Climate

Winter weather patterns are expected to become more variable as average global temperatures continually increase. Research findings indicate that there is a relationship between temperature variability and health outcomes, including cardiovascular, respiratory, cerebrovascular events, and all-cause morbidity and mortality. Populations most vulnerable to global changes are older adults, residents of rural areas, children living in poor countries, and those with preexisting medical conditions (World Health Organization, 2019a, 2019b, 2019c).

Flora and Fauna

Plant and animal populations in a community are often determined by location. The way a community responds to these populations, whether wild or domesticated, can affect the health of the community.

Public health officials note chronic environmental factors as a possible cause for increased asthma cases: pollution from high-traffic areas, secondhand smoke in homes, and poor living conditions characterized by dust mites, mold, industrial air pollution, mouse and cockroach droppings, and animal dander.

C/PHNs need to know about the major sources of danger from plants and animals affecting the community under study. Are there community agencies that provide educational information about these dangers? Does the populace understand their significance? Are emergency services, such as a poison control center, available to community members?

The Built Environment

Every community is located in the midst of an environment created and transformed by human ingenuity. People build houses and factories, dump wastes into streams or vacant lots, fill the air with gases, and build dams to control streams. All of these human alterations of the environment have important implications for community health. A C/PHN might improve the health of a community by working with community members, legislators, and stakeholders to improve the design of the built environment to promote health and well-being.

Population Characteristics

When one considers the community as the client, examining the health status of the total population in a given community is a critical component. Table 15-3 presents the population perspective section of the Community Profile Inventory.

Size

Knowing a community's size provides community health nurses with important information for planning. For example, when conducting emergency preparedness planning, knowledge of the population size will ensure that an adequate number of resources can be made available in the event of an emergency. See Chapter 27 for issues related to rural and urban population health.

Density

In some communities, thousands of people are crowded into high-rise apartment buildings. In others, such as farm communities, people live great distances from one another. Population density, or the number of people residing within a square mile area, is used to describe how many people live within a community. Living in high-density, crowded communities affects individual and community health by increasing community members' exposure to pollution and an urbanized diet (The Healthy City, 2018). A low-density community, however, may also pose problems. When people are spread out, provision of health care services can become difficult.

A healthy community takes into consideration the density of its population. It organizes to meet the differing needs created by its density levels (e.g., it recognizes differences in density between the inner city and the suburbs and allocates services accordingly). See Chapter 27 for more on health risks specific to rural and urban areas.

Composition/Demographics

Communities differ in the types of people who live within their boundaries. Age, sex, educational level, occupation, and many other demographic variables affect health concerns (CDC, 2019a). Understanding a community's composition is an important early step in determining its level of health. For example, when planning a cost-free vaccination program, knowledge of community demographics allows nurses to identify those who are eligible and those who would benefit most from the program.

Rate of Growth or Decline

Community populations change over time. Some grow rapidly. As people leave to find new employment or better living conditions, consumption of goods and services drops. Community morale may suffer, and community leadership may decline. Even a stable community can have problems (e.g., members may resist needed change because they notice little fluctuation in their population; commercial and residential properties may be abandoned or left vacant). This trend is widely observed across the country, as the United States has progressed from being a manufacturing society to a postindustrial and technologically focused one.

Cultural Characteristics

A healthy community is aware of the diversity and the needs of the cultural subgroups (McElfish et al., 2017). See Chapter 5 for more about transcultural nursing in the community.

Social Class and Educational Level

Social determinants of health impact a wide range of health, functioning, and quality of life outcomes (Fig. 15-5; National Academies of Sciences, Engineering, and Medicine, 2019; USDHH, 2020). They reflect social factors and the physical conditions in the environment in which people are born, live, learn, play, work, and age. They are shaped by the distribution of money, power, and resources at global, national, and local levels and contribute to health inequities among different groups of people based on social and economic class, gender, and ethnicity. For these reasons, social determinants of health are an underlying cause of today's major societal health dilemmas (National Academies of Science, Engineering, and Medicine, 2019). See Chapter 23.

It is generally known that different groups have different health problems, as well as a variety of resources for coping with illness and diverse ways of using health services. A healthy community recognizes these

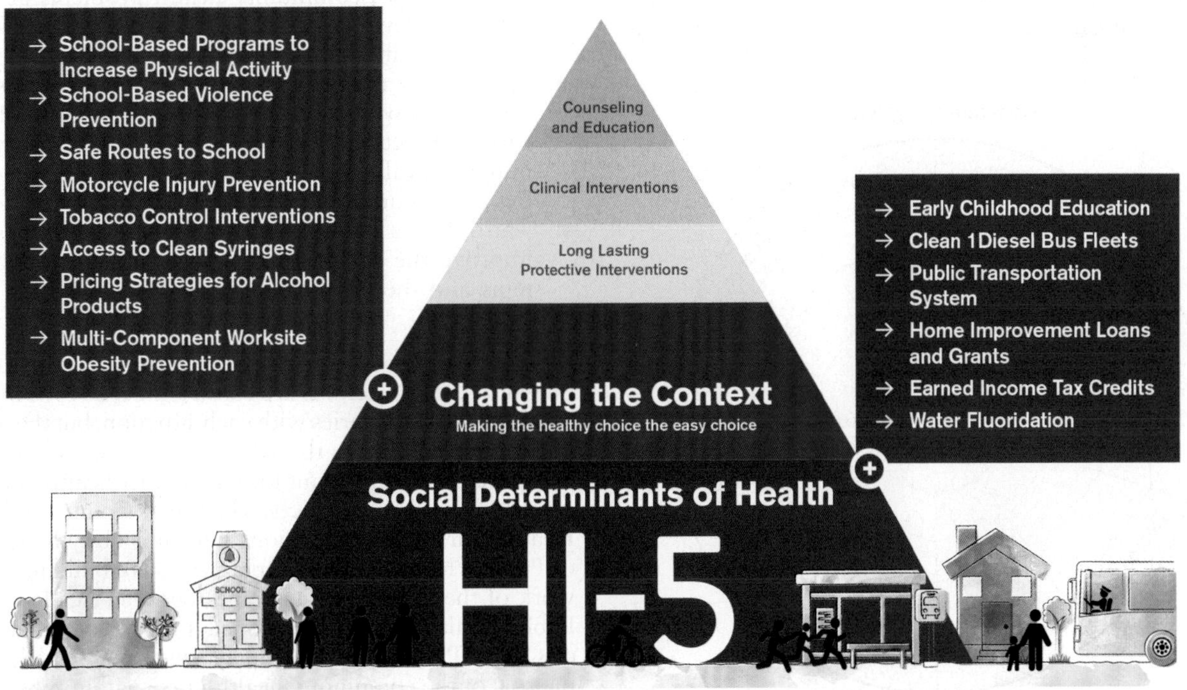

FIGURE 15-5 Health impact pyramid. (Reprinted from CDC. (2018). *Health Impact in 5 years.* Retrieved from https://www.cdc.gov/policy/hst/hi5/)

differences and creates health care services to meet these varied needs.

Mobility

Americans are a mobile population. Outcomes from the 2017 American Community Survey indicate that approximately 40 million people moved annually within their region, 3.8 million moved between regions, and nearly another 2 million moved to the United States from abroad between 2013 and 2017. Oftentimes these fluctuations are linked to social and economic factors (U.S. Census Bureau, 2019). If the population turnover is extensive, continuity of services may suffer. Leadership for improving the health of the community may change so frequently that concerted action becomes difficult. High turnover may necessitate special attention to health education about local conditions.

Population groups may arrive and depart in seasonal swings; fluctuations in the number of migrant farm workers, tourists, or college students can affect a community. Immigrants and refugees may represent a significant population subgroup in many areas of a country, and public health officials must recognize their unique health needs and barriers (Philbin, Flake, Hatzenbuehler, & Hirsch, 2018). A healthy community neither ignores nor overreacts to this kind of mobility. Rather, its members work collaboratively to recognize and address their unique needs and barriers to health.

Social System

In addition to location and population, every community has a third feature—a social system. The various parts of a community's social system that interact and influence the health of a community are called social system variables. These variables include health, family, economy, education, religion, welfare, politics, recreation, law, and communication (Fig. 15-6). Whether assessing a community's health, developing new services for the mentally ill within the community, or promoting the health of older adults, the community health nurse needs to understand the community as a social system. A community health nurse working in a tiny village in Alaska needs to understand and work with the social system of that village no less than a nurse practicing in New York City. When a group of organizations are linked and have similar functions, such as all those providing social services, they form a community system or subsystem. The various community systems have a profound influence on one another. Because this interaction among parts determines the health of the whole, it is the total social system that concerns community health nurses. Table 15-4 guides the nurse in assessing a community's social system variables.

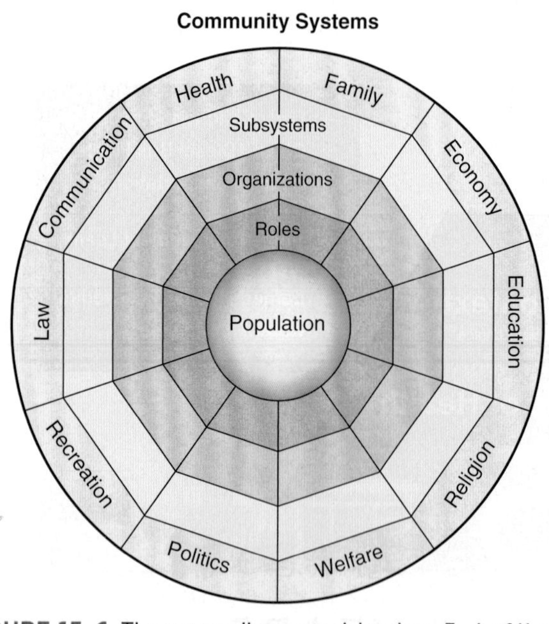

FIGURE 15-6 The community as a social system. Each of the 10 major systems of a community includes a number of subsystems that are made up of organizations. Members of the community occupy roles in these organizations.

THE NURSING PROCESS APPLIED TO THE COMMUNITY AS CLIENT

Consisting of a systematic, purposeful set of interpersonal actions, the nursing process provides a structure for change that remains a viable tool employed by the community health nurse. This chapter examines the use of the nursing process as applied at the aggregate or community level. Five components—assessment, diagnosis, planning, implementation, and evaluation—give direction to the dynamics for solving problems, managing nursing actions, and improving the health of communities and community health nursing practice. Three characteristics support the use of the nursing process in community health nursing.

- First, the nursing process is a problem-solving process that addresses community health problems at every aggregate level with the goals of preventing illness and promoting public health.
- Second, it is a management process that requires situational analysis, decision-making, planning, organization, direction, and control of services, as well as outcome evaluation. As a management tool, the nursing process addresses all aggregate levels.
- Third, it is a process for implementing changes that improve the function of various health-related systems and the ways that people behave within those systems.

The nursing process provides a framework or structure on which C/PHN actions are based (ANA, 2013). Application of the process varies with each situation, but the nature of the process remains the same. Certain characteristics of that process are important for community health nurses to emphasize in their practices. The Quad Council of Public Health Nursing Organizations (which is now the Council of Public Health Nursing Organizations), building on the work of the Council on Linkages Between Academia and Public Health Practice, developed a list of core competencies for C/PHNs. These competencies have helped clarify the role of the community health nurse within the context of community as client (see the appendix and http://www.quadcouncilphn.org/wp-content/uploads/2018/05/QCC-C-PHN-COMPETENCIES-Approved_2018.05.04_Final-002.pdf; Quad Council, 2018).

TABLE 15-4 Community Profile Inventory: Social System Perspective

Social System Variables	Community Health Implications	Community Assessment Questions	Information Sources (For All—Various Internet Sites)
Health system Family system Economic system Educational system Religious system Welfare system Political system Recreational system Legal system Communication system	Each system must fulfill its functions for a healthy community. Collaboration among the systems to identify goals and problems affects health of community. Undue influence of one system on another may lower the health of the community. Agreement on the means to achieve community goals affects community health. Communication among organizations in each system affects community health.	What are the functions of each major system? What are the major subsystems of each system? What are the major organizations in each subsystem? How well do the various organizations function? Are the subsystems in each major system in conflict? Is there adequate communication among the major systems? Is there agreement on community goals? Are there mechanisms for resolving conflict? Do any parts of the total system dominate the others? What community needs are not being met?	Chamber of Commerce Telephone book City directory Organizational literature Officials in organizations Community self-study Community survey Local library Key informants

Deliberative

The nursing process, like the research process in evidence-based practice, is deliberative—purposefully, rationally, and carefully thought out. It requires the use of sound judgment that is based on adequate information. C/PHNs often practice in situations that demand the ability to think independently and make difficult decisions. Furthermore, thoughtful, deliberative problem solving is a necessary skill for working with the community health team to address the needs and problems of aggregates in the community. The nursing process is a decision-making tool to facilitate these determinations (ANA, 2018).

Adaptable

The dynamic nature of the nursing process enables the community health nurse to adapt it appropriately to each situation and apply it to meeting aggregate health needs. Furthermore, its flexibility is a reminder to the nurse that each client group and each community situation is unique. The nursing process must be applied specifically to the individual situation and group of people. Based on assessment and sound planning, the nurse adapts services to meet the identified needs of each community client group.

Cyclical

The nursing process is cyclical and in constant progression. Steps are repeated over and over in the nurse–aggregate client relationship. The nurse engages in continual interaction, data collection, analysis, intervention, and evaluation. As interactions between nurse and client group continue, various steps in the process overlap with one another and are used simultaneously. The cyclic nature of the nursing process enables the nurse to engage in a constant information feedback loop: the information gathered and lessons learned at each step of the process promote greater understanding of the group being served, the most effective way to provide quality services, and the best methods of raising this group's level of health.

Client Focused

The nursing process is used for and with clients. Community health nurses use the nursing process for the express purpose of addressing the health of populations. They are helping aggregate clients, directly or indirectly, to achieve and maintain health. Clients as total systems—whether groups, populations, or communities—are the targets of the C/PHN's nursing process (ANA, 2018).

Interactive

The nurse and clients are engaged in a process of ongoing interpersonal communication. Giving and receiving accurate information is necessary to promote understanding between nurse and clients and to foster effective use of the nursing process. Furthermore, because of the movement toward informed use of health care, demands for clients' rights and the concept of self-care have gained emphasis. Client groups and community health nurses have increasingly joined forces to assume responsibility for promoting community health. The nurse–aggregate client relationship can and should be a partnership, a shared experience by professionals (nurses and others) and client groups (Tucker, Arthur, Roncoroni, Wall, & Sanchez, 2015).

Need Oriented

A long association with problem solving has tended to limit the focus of the nursing process to the correction of existing problems. Although problem solving is certainly an appropriate use of the nursing process, the community health nurse can also use the nursing process to anticipate client needs and prevent problems. The nurse should think of nursing diagnoses as ranging from health problem identification to primary prevention and health promotion opportunities. This focus is needed if the goals of community health—to protect, promote, and restore the people's health—are to be realized.

Interacting With the Community

All steps of the nursing process depend on interaction, reciprocal exchange, and influence among people. Although nurse–client interaction is often an implied or assumed element in the process, it is an essential first consideration for community health nursing. This type of engagement was observed during the Flint water crisis, where C/PHNs established relationships with community members and were thereby able to identify and directly aid in addressing their needs. These relationships also facilitated communication between community members and service providers (see Chapter 10 for more details). Listening to a group of older people, teaching a class of expectant mothers, lobbying in the legislature for the poor, working with parents to set up a dental screening program for children—all of these involve relationships, and relationships require interaction. Mutual give and take between nurse, clients, and community stakeholders—whether a family, a group of mothers on a Native American reservation, or representatives from resource agencies within the community—is an expected and much needed skill that should be integrated throughout the nursing process.

Need for Communication

C/PHNs can serve as effective liaisons—facilitating communication between stakeholders and clients to ensure that health needs are both identified and adequately addressed.

Interaction and Effective Communication. Through open and honest sharing, the nurse (and others on the health team) can begin to develop trust and establish lines of effective communication. For instance, the nurse explains the nurse's role and purpose for being there. The nurse encourages the group members to talk about themselves. The nurse and group members together discuss their relationship and clarify the desired nature of that alliance. Does the group want help to identify and work on its health needs? Would its members like this nurse to continue regular contacts? What will their respective roles be? Effective communication, as a part of interaction, is essential to develop understanding and facilitate a free exchange of information between nurse and client.

Interaction Is Reciprocal. Sharing of information, ideas, feelings, concerns, and self goes both ways. The community health nurse (and other collaborating health professionals) represents one system and the client group represents the other. Health care professionals tend to prioritize based on their own perspective and many times neglect to take the clients' wishes into account. Whether the client is a parent group, a homeless population, or an entire community, this exchange involves a two-way sharing between the nurse and client group. The key elements of interaction are mutuality and cooperation.

Consider the following example: After several weeks of meeting with a community member focus group to discuss disease management and physical activity, a C/PHN noticed that community violence was a recurring theme during group discussions. Community residents described conditions in the neighborhood as unsafe and many indicted that they were afraid to adopt the nurse's recommendations to increase physical activity because of ongoing violence near their homes. The nurse initially felt unprepared to address this issue but, after consulting with other support agencies within the community, realized that resources were available. After meeting and coordinating with community members and support agencies, the nurse was able to develop a feasible and safe physical activity plan for residents. Engagement with community members and communication were the first step in reapplying the nursing process and allowed goals for the group to be accomplished.

Interaction Paves the Way for a Helping Relationship. As nurse and client interact, each learns about the other. A test period occurs before trust can be fully established (Summach, 2011). For a female school nurse working with middle school students about health education and human sexuality, establishing interaction was more difficult at the time of the initial contact with the boys than with the girls. They had been reluctant to talk and felt embarrassed to discuss personal subjects with an adult they did not know. Nonetheless, their interests in bodybuilding and personal appearance were strong enough to bring them to these optional sessions. Interaction began with a friendly exchange on nonthreatening topics and gradually deepened, as the boys seemed ready to discuss personal subjects. Eventually, it was relatively simple to talk about a new "problem" (and start the nursing process over again), because a helping relationship had already been developed. The nurse had a track record. The boys trusted, respected, and liked the nurse, so they were happy to interact around a newly stated need.

Aggregate Application

As noted in earlier chapters, community health practice focuses largely on the health of population groups; therefore, interaction goes beyond the one-on-one with individual patients. The challenge that the community health nurse faces is a one-to-aggregate approach. A group of parents concerned about teenage alcohol abuse, people with physical disabilities needing access ramps, and a neighborhood's older adult population frightened by muggings and thefts are all aggregates or clients with different concerns and opinions. As defined in Chapter 1, an aggregate refers to a mass or grouping of distinct individuals who are considered as a whole and who are loosely associated with one another. Each person in an aggregate is influenced by the thoughts and behavior of other group members. Nursing interaction with an aggregate client demands an understanding of group behavior, group dynamics, and group-level decision-making. It requires interpersonal communication skills applied at the group level. Interaction is more complex and challenging with an aggregate than with an individual but also can be rewarding. Once community health nurses acquire an understanding of aggregate behavior, they can capitalize on the potential of group influence to make a far-reaching impact on the health of the total community. Chapter 10 more closely examines communication and interaction with groups.

Forming Partnerships and Building Coalitions

Community-level nursing practice also requires teamwork. The job of planning for the health of an entire community or a community subsystem requires that the nurse collaborate with other professionals. Usually, the nurse is part of an organized team, separate from the agency that employs the nurse. The team is brought together with the goal of improving the health of the community. Each group member brings expertise and a particular view of the problem. These interprofessional work groups are often formed as either partnerships or coalitions (Wyer, Umscheid, Wright, Silva, & Lang, 2015).

The Maryland Collaborative is an example of a collaborative practice approach to reduce college drinking and related problems (Arria & Jernigan, 2018). A priority for the Maryland Department of Health and Hygiene was to reduce excessive drinking among college students. A collaboration was formed with the state health department, the Chancellor of the UC System, and other university presidents in the state to address excessive drinking on college campuses through the lens of individual, interpersonal networks, and organizational and environmental factors. Using assessment techniques, hot spot areas on campuses were identified, and campus teams worked with local community members to develop strategies to reduce excessive drinking and related problems. An evidence-based and community partnership approach can address serious health issues at the individual and community, level thereby providing a "...positive academic and social experience for students, quality of life for the campus community, and viability of the surrounding neighborhoods" (Arria & Jernigan, 2018, p. 311).

Partnerships are agreements between people (and agencies) that support a joint purpose. A partnership can be large (e.g., a multinational corporation and several high schools; a city government and the county jail system), or it can be a more modest endeavor (e.g., a group of older adult citizens and a preschool program; a Girl Scout troop and a community recycling program).

To enhance the outcomes of a program for the homeless while improving the health needs of homeless individuals and families, the Shelter Nurse Program and public health nursing service, along with community members, worked in partnership to develop a plan to demonstrate population outcomes formalizing goals and objectives for the agency (Minnich & Shirley, 2017). By collaborating on this project, the partnership identified program needs, developed goals and objectives, and created a comprehensive evaluation plan to meet the needs of the local homeless population. Working together to develop areas for improvement to meet the needs of homeless clients, both the agency and the shelter nurses learned the value of a program development model and the importance of front-line workers' participation in the process (Minnich & Shirley, 2017).

Community-wide partnerships require more planning and coordination than do small partnerships. For example, because of increased student enrollment, a college may need two additional temporary and part-time faculty members who can teach the C/PHN course. The county public health department is interested in more new graduate nurses coming to work in the agency. The nursing program and the health department form a partnership and design a plan to solve both problems. The health department selects two staff nurses who have master's degrees and are qualified to teach undergraduate clinical courses in C/PHN one day a week for two semesters. The benefits for everyone are numerous. The nursing program solves a temporary staffing problem; the nurses from the health department share their expertise with students, enhancing their practice and the students' learning experience; and the health department successfully introduces a pool of students, who may be potential staff members, to the agency and the services that it provides for the community.

A coalition is an alliance of individuals or groups that work together to influence the outcomes of a specific problem. Coalitions are an effective means to achieve a collaborative and coordinated approach to solving community problems. Steps to coalition building include (CDC, 2015b)

- Defining goals and objectives
- Conducting a community assessment
- Identifying key players or leaders
- Identifying potential coalition members

Staying in touch with the coalition members, running effective meetings, and keeping every participant involved are means of keeping the coalition active.

Sound public health practice depends on pooling resources—including people—in ways that will best serve the public. In planning for a community's health, the community (represented by appropriate individuals and agencies) must be involved. Community health nurses cannot lose sight of the need for client involvement at all levels and in all stages of community health practice (Box 15-2).

TYPES OF COMMUNITY NEEDS ASSESSMENT

Assessment is the key initial step of the nursing process; it involves collecting and evaluating information about a community's health status to discover existing or potential needs and assets as a basis for planning future action (Anderson & McFarlane, 2019). Assessments are also a critical requirement for public health department accreditation (Public Health Accreditation Board, 2019).

Several models or frameworks can be used for assessment. Three such models are

- Mobilizing for Action through Planning and Partnerships
- Protocol for Assessing Community Excellence in Environmental Health
- Planned Approach to Community Health

These models have been developed through partnership with the Centers for Disease Control and Prevention (CDC) to improve community assessment in relation to healthy people goals (CDC, 2015a) and to assist communities in assessing health promotion and chronic disease prevention programs. The *Healthy People* Web site also provides planning tools and toolkits to assist local communities

BOX **15-2** PERSPECTIVES

A Public Health Nurse's Viewpoint on Addressing Adolescent Pregnancy

I am a public health nurse and my health department serves a community with a large proportion of adolescents and young adults aged 18 to 24. After reviewing data from a recent community health status assessment, members of our community council observed a significant increase in the number of unplanned pregnancies among members of this age group. We proceeded to convene a group of community stakeholders with the intention of partnering with them to identify and implement solutions to address these issues. Several meetings were held, and key members of the community were invited to participate, including a local church pastor, youth group leaders, and administrators representing nonprofit organizations targeting this same issue. Further analysis of this issue, the group agreed to develop a plan to address unplanned pregnancy and to also target resources toward secondary prevention in order to support those who had experienced unplanned pregnancies and were now raising their children as single parents.

An assessment of community resources was conducted to identify available programs and resources. We searched the literature for best practices on this topic and collaborated with program planners to develop an implementation plan for our target population. The group engaged local leaders to request funding for areas where gaps in services were identified. After 2 months of planning, community resources were identified and coordination was conducted to begin marketing and outreach efforts. Referral mechanisms in local clinics were used to link potential clients to our program, and we received several word-of-mouth recommendations for participants. The program consists of birth control education, counseling, participation in group informational sessions, and the assignment of a primary care manager in our community-based clinic.

A 6- and 9-month outcome evaluation is planned to monitor the effect of our program. Anecdotal feedback has been resoundingly positive. The commitment of our partners is evident as our efforts have been embraced and supported by a wide range of leaders and community members. This commitment appears to have yielded a great response from program participants. Participants have remarked about the quality of services received, and many have commented on the quality of care they received in our program.

Tara, public health nurse

(see internet resources on thePoint). These are all valuable resources that provide specific guidelines focusing on local-level strategies to improve the health of communities.

Assessment involves two major activities:

- Collection of pertinent data
- Analysis and interpretation of data

These actions overlap and are repeated constantly throughout the assessment phase of the nursing process. While assessing a community's ability to enhance its health, the nurse may simultaneously collect data on community lifestyle behaviors and interpret previously collected data on morbidity and mortality.

Community health assessment is the process of determining the real or perceived needs of a defined community. In some situations, an extensive community study may be the first priority; in others, all that is needed is a study of one system or even one organization. At other times, community health nurses may need to perform a cursory examination or **windshield survey** to familiarize them with an entire community without going into any depth (Anderson & McFarlane, 2019).

Familiarization or Windshield Survey

A familiarization assessment is a common starting place in evaluation of a community. Familiarization assessment involves studying data already available on a community and then gathering a certain amount of firsthand data in order to gain a working knowledge of the community. Such an approach may use a windshield survey—an activity often used by nursing students in public health courses and by new staff members in community health agencies. Nurses drive (or walk) around the community of interest; find health, social, and governmental services; obtain literature; introduce themselves and explain that they are working in the area; and generally become familiar with the community and its residents. This type of assessment is needed whenever the community health nurse works with families, groups, organizations, or populations.

The windshield survey provides knowledge of the context in which these aggregates live and may enable the nurse to better connect clients with community resources (Box 15-3). See an example in Box 15-4.

Problem-Oriented Assessment

A second type of community assessment, problem-oriented assessment, begins with a single problem and assesses the community in terms of that problem. Instead of working to gather information about the larger community, the nurse would identify resources, programs, and support networks of potential benefit to the family. Steps taken to complete this assessment would include collecting data on local prevalence and incidence, interviewing officials to obtain information on processes and policies, and identifying local programs and services.

The problem-oriented assessment can be used when familiarization is not sufficient, and a comprehensive assessment is not feasible. This type of assessment is responsive to a particular need and should also seek to describe contextual issues associated with the need. The data collected can support community efforts to address specific problems. Data should address the magnitude of the problem to be studied (e.g., prevalence, incidence), the precursors of the problem, and information about population characteristics (e.g., community resources, strengths, and weaknesses), along with the attitudes and behaviors of the population being studied (Kirst-Ashman, 2014).

BOX 15-3 Community Familiarization (Windshield) Survey

A windshield survey is often done to help you become familiar with a new community or public health service area. Walking/driving around neighborhoods and interacting with community members can provide a context for further community assessment. You might begin at the local Chamber of Commerce or government building to determine history, current statistics, and demographics and to access maps and further resources for data you might use for a more formal community health assessment.

Physical

- Look at the age and conditions of the buildings, the density (apartments, houses on large lots) and materials used (bricks, plywood), and the zoning and maintenance of yards/empty lots. What clues does that give you about the community as a whole?
- How similar are the houses (are some neighborhoods very rich, others very poor)? Are there abandoned vehicles, piles of excess trash, large numbers of stray animals/for sale signs, or vacant houses?
- Are there open spaces (parks, agricultural areas, public/private areas like golf courses) and are they being used; by whom?
- Are there boundaries separating the community (e.g., natural boundaries like rivers, economic boundaries, commercial/residential boundaries)?
- What about air/water quality, signs of pollution?

Economic

- Does the area look like it is a thriving community?
- Are there areas where homeless gather? Soup kitchens?
- Is there adequate shopping (e.g., grocery stores, shopping centers)?
- Does it appear that food stamps are accepted/welcomed?
- Are there businesses, industries, manufacturing, and adequate places for employment? What is the unemployment rate?

Services

- Are there schools (how many, in what condition)? School nurses? What are the main concerns or problems with the educational system here (e.g., dropout rates)?
- Are there libraries? Do they provide additional services (e.g., internet)? Are they well used?
- Are there recreational facilities (e.g., gyms, playgrounds, soccer fields, baseball diamonds)? Are these being used and by whom?
- How many churches do you see? What denominations?
- Is there adequate health care? Does the community have a hospital? Are there adequate health care services (e.g., physicians, clinics, nurses, mental health/substance abuse facilities, PH department services, nursing homes, traditional health care providers)? Is it a medically underserved area or a health professions shortage area?
- What types of social services are available (e.g., welfare/social workers, shelters, mental health counseling)? Do you see one main location for social services (e.g., government center) or are they dispersed around the community?
- What types of public/private transportation are available? Are highways and roads crowded with traffic? Accident rate? Are there bike paths/trails and adequate sidewalks? How is transportation access for the disabled?
- Does the community "feel" safe to you? Is there adequate fire and police protection? What is the crime rate? What are the most common types of crimes?
- Are there signs of political activity (e.g., posters, notices of meetings, predominant party affiliations)? Do people feel that they can be involved in decisions made by their local government?

Social

- Are there common "hangouts" (e.g., teen gathering spots, chess playing for older adults)? What about local newspapers, radio, and TV (e.g., satellite dishes)?
- Who do you see on the streets? Are there indications of homogeneity or diversity of ethnicities, languages spoken, SES (socioeconomic status), and occupations? How are people dressed?
- How do people feel about living in this community? What problems or concerns do they express? What strengths do they note? How "healthy" is their community?
- What are your impressions of this community?

Source: Anderson and McFarlane (2019).

BOX 15-4 STORIES FROM THE FIELD

Working With the Community on a Safety Assessment

Consider the following example: After several weeks of meeting with a community-member focus group to discuss disease management and physical activity, a public health nurse (C/PHN) noticed that community violence was a recurring theme during group discussions. Community residents described conditions in the neighborhood as unsafe and many indicted that they were afraid to adopt the nurse's recommendations to increase physical activity due because of ongoing violence near their homes. The nurse initially felt unprepared to address this issue but after consulting with other support agencies within the community, she realized that resources were available. After meeting and coordinating with community members and support agencies, she was able to develop a feasible and safe physical activity plan for residents. Engagement with community members and communication were the first step in reapplying the nursing process and allowed goals for the group to be accomplished.

1. *What should the C/PHN know about location, population, and social system to be better prepared to work with this group?*
2. *How can the C/PHN use the nursing process to direct the plan of care with this community?*

Community Subsystem Assessment

In **community subsystem assessment**, the C/PHN focuses on a single dimension of community life. For example, the nurse might decide to survey churches and religious organizations to discover their roles in the community. What kinds of needs do the leaders in these organizations believe exist? What services do these organizations offer? To what extent are services coordinated within the religious system and between it and other systems in the community?

In one situation, churches and other cultural leaders were instrumental in providing information to address the local public health department's concerns. A small county health department worked with the nearby university C/PHN clinical instructor and the instructor's students to determine why two specific racial/ethnic groups did not use free women's health clinics. Students from the university conducted focus groups with local clergy and representatives from the racial groups to better understand the group's health seeking behaviors. Health department officials reviewed transcripts from the focus groups and discovered that most members of the groups were unaware of the services provided through the county health department. The students then conducted additional interviews with families within the groups and found that, as part of their cultural practice, husbands generally accompany their wives when getting prenatal care or family planning services. They also learned that members of the group felt more comfortable with health care personnel of their own race and that there was a provider from their ethnic group practicing in a neighboring county. As a result of these subsystem engagements, health department staff were able to tailor their service offerings to better meet the needs to these groups and a partnership for health was established with local clergy and group members.

Community subsystem assessment can be a useful way for a team to conduct a more thorough community assessment. If five members of a nursing agency divide up the 10 systems in the community and each person does an assessment of two systems, they could then share their findings to create a more comprehensive picture of the community and its needs.

Comprehensive Assessment

Comprehensive assessment seeks to discover all relevant community health information. It begins with a review of existing studies and all the data presently available on the community. A survey compiles all the demographic information on the population, such as its size, density, and composition.

Key informants are interviewed in every major system—education, health, religious, economic, and others. **Key informants** are experts in one particular area of the community, or they may know the community as a whole. Examples of key informants would be a school nurse, a religious leader, key cultural leaders, the local police chief or fire captain, a mail carrier, or a local city council person. Then, more detailed surveys and intensive interviews are performed to yield information on organizations and the various roles in each organization.

A comprehensive assessment describes the systems of a community and also how power is distributed throughout the system, how decisions are made, and how change occurs (Anderson & McFarlane, 2019).

Because comprehensive assessment is an expensive, time-consuming process, it is not often undertaken. Performing a more focused study, based on prior knowledge of needs, is often a better and less costly strategy. Nevertheless, knowing how to conduct a comprehensive assessment is an important skill when designing smaller more focused assessments (Box 15-5).

Community Assets Assessment

Assets mapping focuses on the strengths and capacities of a community rather than its problems (Jakes,

BOX 15-5 PERSPECTIVES

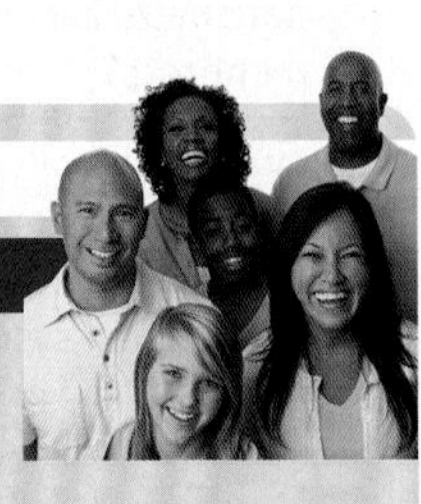

A Public Health Nursing Student Viewpoint on Addressing Adolescent Pregnancy

After completing my Med-Surg courses, I was excited to begin my Community Health rotation. I looked forward to stepping outside of the clinical environment to engage community members but I absolutely I dreaded the thought of having to complete the perfunctory comprehensive community health assessment. To my delight, the assessment process had recently been revamped and, instead of repeating the task of collecting the same data that the previous classes had collected, my class was able select from a list of community health projects for which data were needed. These projects were directly related to grants currently being written by staff and state-directed program evaluations that the department was working on. The fact that these were real-time projects made the assignment feel less like a task and more like a meaningful opportunity to contribute to the health of community members served by the department. My class voted to collect data for a grant-funded project to address teen pregnancy, and we set about creating our own survey tools drawing from standardized assessment products. We were excited about our work and tackled the project bunch of detectives chasing down leads! We divided into subgroups, gathered data, problem-solved and worked together to achieve our goals. We also worked with other agencies and NGOs, and spoke with local health care providers and members of the community. Toward the end of our project, we collaborated with the program director for a teen pregnancy program to distribute questionnaires to local teens so that we could gather information on sexual activity and attitudes. At that time, the conservative county that we worked in had the highest rate of teen pregnancies in the state and many parents opposed *Sex Ed*. However, we were able to gather information and statistics on teen pregnancies in this county and compared it with state and national data. After investigating best practices for teen pregnancy prevention programs, we formed into smaller work groups, some met with school officials, high school students, teachers, and parents to educate them about this project. In the end, everyone in my class felt that by working on this project, they made a meaningful contribution to the community and the health department and the university heartily agreed!

Mikinsey, nursing student

Hardison-Moody, Bowen, & Blevins, 2015) and evaluates variables such as the needs that exist, the goals to be achieved, and the resources available for carrying out the study.

Although it is difficult to determine the type of assessment needed in advance, understanding the various types of community assessment in advance helps to facilitate your decision. Based on a classic model developed by McKnight and Kretzmann in the 1980s (Kretzman & McKnight, 1993), the **assets assessment** provides a framework for conducting a complete functional community assessment and serves as a guide to the community for the nurse, as well as the foundation for community development.

The previously mentioned methods are needs oriented and deficit based—in other words, they are *pathology* models, in which the assessment is performed in response to needs, barriers, weaknesses, problems, or perceived scarcity in the community. This may result in a fragmented approach to solutions for the community's problems rather than an approach focused on the community's possibilities, strengths, and assets. The assets assessment also provides the community the ability to "identify a variety and richness of skills, talents, knowledge, and experience of people" and "provides a base upon which to build new approaches and enterprises" (p. 4).

Assets assessment begins with what is present in the community (Jakes et al., 2015). The capacities and skills of community members are identified, with a focus on creating or rebuilding relationships among local residents, associations, and institutions to multiply power and effectiveness. This approach requires that the assessor look for the positive or see the glass as half full. The nurse can then become a partner in community intervention efforts, rather than merely a provider of services. Assets assessment includes three levels (Kramer, Seedat, Lazarus, & Suffla, 2011):

1. Specific skills, talents, interests, and experiences of individual community members such as individual businesses, cultural groups, and professionals living in the community.
2. Local citizen associations, organizations, and institutions controlled largely by the community such as libraries, social service agencies, voluntary agencies, schools, and police.
3. Local institutions originating outside the community controlled largely outside the community such as welfare and public capital expenditures (p. 14).

The key, however, is linking these assets together to enhance the community from within. The community health nurse's role is to assist with those linkages.

METHODS FOR COLLECTING COMMUNITY DATA

The health status of the community may be assessed using a variety of methods. Regardless of the assessment method used, data must be collected. The Community Health Assessment and Group Evaluation (CHANGE) Tool (https://www.cdc.gov/nccdphp/dch/programs/healthycommunitiesprogram/tools/change/downloads.htm) is an example of a current process to prioritize community needs for community-based improvements (CDC, 2019d). The tool assists C/PHNs and community members through the community change process (commitment, assessment, planning, implementation, and evaluation). Once a CHANGE team is assembled, data must be gathered to fully assess the community's need. Data collection in community health requires the exercise of sound professional judgment, effective communication techniques, and special investigative skills. Four important methods are discussed here: surveys, descriptive epidemiologic studies, community forums or town meetings, and focus groups.

Surveys

A survey is an assessment method in which a series of questions is used to collect data for analysis of a specific group or area. Surveys are commonly used to provide a broad range of data that will be helpful when used with other sources or if other sources are not available.

To plan and conduct community health surveys, the goal should be to determine the variables (selected environmental, socioeconomic, and behavioral conditions or needs) that affect a community's ability to control disease and promote wellness. The nurse may choose to conduct a survey to determine such things as health care use patterns and needs, immunization levels, demographic characteristics, or health beliefs and practices.

The survey method involves self-report, or response to predetermined questions, and can include questionnaires, telephone, or in person interviews (Polit & Beck, 2017).

Survey findings can be combined with other health data in order to better understand the health status of the community and the determinants of health. These data include reports of health risks and outcomes by zip code (Agarwal, Menon, & Jaber, 2015; Wang, Ponce, Wang, Opsomer, & Yu, 2015) and CDC Environmental Health Tracking Network reports of local environmental health exposures (Charleston, Wilson, Edwards, David, & Dewitt, 2015). Consideration of these data along with survey results allows for a more comprehensive understanding of the community's health status and the conditions impacting health.

Descriptive Epidemiologic Studies

A second assessment method is a descriptive epidemiologic study, which examines the amount and distribution of a disease or health condition in a population by person (Who is affected?), by place (Where does the condition occur?), and by time (When do the cases occur?). In addition to their value in assessing the health status of a population, **descriptive epidemiologic studies** are useful for suggesting which individuals are at greatest risk and where and when the condition might occur. They have also long been known to be useful for health planning purposes and for suggesting hypotheses concerning disease etiology (Merrill, 2017). Their design and use are detailed in Chapter 7.

Geographic Information System Analysis

In Chapter 10, the concept of GIS was introduced as a health information technology. GIS technology is an integration of research methods and analytic techniques from both medical geography and spatial epidemiology. It has been well documented as a tool that can collect, organize, and display public health data, and it is widely used in assessment and research of health disparities, resource availability, and health-related behaviors (WHO, 2019a).

Harvard's T.H. Chan School of Public Health offers a Web site designated to the use of GIS in public health, including particular research studies. For instance, one line of research examines effects of air pollution on MI rates within the community of Worchester and spatial mapping of incidence and levels of pollution. Researchers are also working on developing a predictive model for pollution's effect on death rates in Eastern Massachusetts. A prospective study of normative aging began with data collected from healthy cohort of 2,500 individuals in the 1970s; and GIS data on exposure are used to estimate cumulative exposure to pollution and its association with COPD, MI, and death (Harvard University, 2019). The WHO has been using GIS for leprosy elimination (WHO, 2019a).

Community Forums and Social Media

The community forum or town hall meeting is a qualitative assessment method designed to obtain community opinions. It takes place in the neighborhood of the people involved, perhaps in a school gymnasium or an auditorium. The participants are selected to participate by invitation from the group organizing the forum.

Members come from within the community and represent all segments of the community that are involved with the issue. For instance, if a community is contemplating building a swimming pool, the people invited to the community forum might include potential users of the pool (residents of the community who do not have pools and special groups such as the Girl Scouts, elders, and disabled citizens), community planners, health and safety personnel, and other key people with vested interests. They are asked to give their views on the pool: Where should it be located? Who will use it? How will the cost of building and maintaining it be assumed? What are the drawbacks to having the pool? Any other pertinent issues the participants may raise are included. This method is relatively inexpensive, and results are quickly obtained.

A drawback of this method is that only the most vocal community members, or those with the greatest vested interests in the issue, may be heard. This format does not provide a representative voice to others in the community who also may be affected by the proposed decision.

Town halls are used to elicit public opinion on a variety of issues, including health care concerns, political views, and feelings about issues in the public eye, such as school safety.

Frequently, local news may stream important city government or school board meetings. Other methods of opinion gathering include e-mailing to support a particular view, Web-based survey sites, and text messaging a Yes or No vote on an issue. Social media sites, like Facebook and Twitter, are also popular forums for opinion sharing. Digital media is often used to elicit grassroots opinions from local community members. See more ideas on the use of social media in Chapter 10.

Focus Groups

Focus groups are similar to the community forum or town hall meeting in that it is designed to obtain grassroots opinion with a small group of participants, usually 5 to 15 people.

The members chosen for the group are homogeneous with respect to specific demographic variables. For example, a focus group may consist of female community health nurses, young women in their first pregnancy, or retired businessmen. Leadership and facilitation skills are used in conjunction with the small group process to promote a supportive atmosphere and to accomplish set goals. The interviewer guides the discussion according to a predetermined set of questions or topics. A focus group can be organized to be representative of an aggregate, to capture community interest groups, or to sample for diversity among different population groups. Whatever the purpose, however, some people may be uncomfortable expressing their views in a group situation.

The choice of assessment method varies depending on the reasons for data collection, the goals and objectives of the study, and the available resources. It also varies according to the theoretical framework or philosophical approach through which the nurse views the community. In other words, the community health nurse's theoretical basis for approaching community assessment influences the purposes for conducting the assessment and the selection of methodology. For example, Neuman's health care systems model forms the basis for the "community-as-partner" assessment model developed by (Anderson & McFarlane, 2019). Additional resources on methodologies for assessing community health (e.g., list of internet resources) are available on thePoint.

SOURCES OF COMMUNITY DATA

The community health nurse can look in many places for data to enhance and complete a community assessment. Data sources can be primary or secondary, and they can be from international, national, state, or local sources. Web sites for many primary and secondary data sources are included in internet resources on thePoint.

Primary and Secondary Sources

C/PHNs make use of many sources in data collection. Community members, including formal leaders, informal leaders, and community members, can frequently offer the most accurate insights and comprehensive information.

Information gathered by talking to people provides primary data, because the data are obtained directly from the community. Specific examples are health team members, client records, community health (vital) statistics, census bureau data, reference books, research reports, HEDIS measures, and community health nurses.

Secondary sources of data include people who know the community well and the records such people create in the performance of their jobs. Because secondary data may not totally describe the community and do not necessarily reflect community self-perceptions, they may need augmentation or further validation through focus groups, surveys, and other primary data collection methods.

International Sources

International data are collected by several agencies, including the World Health Organization (WHO) and its six regional offices and health organizations, such as the Pan-American Health Organization. The WHO publishes health statistics by country and information about specific diseases and health measures in their annual Global Health Observatory. Information from these official sources can give the nurse in the local community information about immigrant and refugee populations he serves. More information on international health agencies can be found in Chapter 16.

National Sources

C/PHNs can access a wealth of official and nonofficial sources of national data (see Chapter 6 for more information). Official sources develop documents based on data compiled by the government. The following are the major official agencies:

USDHHS. This is the main agency from which data can be retrieved, and the National Center for Health Statistics (NCHS) at the **Centers for Disease Control and Prevention (CDC)** was specifically established under its auspices for the collection and dissemination of health-related data. This agency is the nation's principal health statistics agency, compiling data from many sources. These data provide information for many functions, including health status for various populations and subgroups, identification of disparities, monitoring trends, identifying health problems, and supporting research.

USDHHS also developed *Healthy People 2030* (USDHHS, 2020), designed to focus America's attention on the major national health problems, including realistic goals for national, state, and local agencies to work toward over one decade. Other data sources are also available through the CDC (2019b).

U.S. Census Bureau. This agency undertakes a major survey of American families every 10 years, gathering data on health, socioeconomic, and environmental conditions. This information is available on the Web or on a CD-ROM, allowing numerous variables to be viewed in combination, for easier development of a community profile (U.S. Census Bureau, 2019).

National Institutes of Health (NIH). This system focuses on improving the health of the nation. An emphasis is placed on discovery of new cures or treatments and preventing disease. Employees of these agencies prevent, diagnose, and treat diseases and conduct research and disseminate research findings (NIH, 2019).

Nongovernmental organizations (NGOs) have data sources generated from research they conduct that focuses on the population, disease, or condition they were developed to serve. Each agency collects data at the national level; however, the more accessible arm for services functions at state, county, and local levels. Examples of these agencies are the American Cancer Society (ACS), American Heart Association (AHA), the American Association of Retired Persons (AARP), Mothers Against Drunk Drivers (MADD), and Students Against Drunk Drivers (SADD). The Public Health Foundation (2020) offers information on many areas of interest to C/PHNs: teams toolbox, critical thinking tools, population heath driver diagrams, and other quality improvement tools for public health. The Kaiser Family Foundation and the RAND Corporation have a variety of fact sheets and compilations of data from various sources. The Gallup Poll provides national survey information on various topics, including health. Information from such national sources allows community health assessment teams to compare local data with national and state statistics and trends—a very valuable function. The Robert Wood Johnson Foundation's (2019) County Health Rankings and Roadmaps is based on a model of population health that emphasizes the many factors that, if improved, can help make communities healthier places to live, learn, work, and play. Proprietary data sources include the American Hospital Association, the American Medical Association, or various health insurance companies. See Chapter 6 for a list of data collection systems.

State and Local Sources

For nurses, the most significant state source of assessment data comes from the state health department. This official agency is responsible for collecting state vital statistics and morbidity data.

The Behavioral Health Surveillance System (BRFSS) is the world's largest telephone health survey that monitors health risk at the state level (CDC, 2019c). Supported by the CDC, the information is used at various levels to identify risk and prevent disease. As a resource to local health departments, the state health department provides invaluable support services, and it is the main source of health-related data on the state level.

Nonofficial agencies have state chapters or headquarters and compile their information at the state level. Local nonofficial agency chapters have documents of compiled state and national data on the population, disease, or condition they address.

State and county budgets or public health agency Web sites may also provide helpful information. All states collect vital statistics (e.g., births, deaths), and many collect information on hospitalization and morbidities related to infectious diseases, cancer, or cardiovascular disease. State departments of education may have school-based data on immunizations and overall school health. Information on traffic accidents, mental health, and environmental hazards is often available at the state level. States may also organize their statistics by county level, making it easier to compare your county's data with others.

Many sources of information may be obtained at the local level. Some key sources are the local visitor's bureau, city chamber of commerce, city planner's office, health department, hospitals, social service agencies, county extension office, school districts, universities or colleges, libraries, clergy, business and service organizations, and community leaders and key informants. Some of these sources compile their own statistics, but all have views of the community particular to their discipline, interest, or knowledge base. Some agencies at the local level develop city or county directories. These are updated periodically and are valuable resources for community health assessment teams and community health nurses. More detailed information on national, state, and local health agencies, and information available from them, can be found in Chapter 6.

DATA ANALYSIS AND DIAGNOSIS

This stage of assessment requires analysis of the information gathered, so that inferences or conclusions may be made about its meaning. Such inferences must be validated to determine their accuracy, after which a nursing diagnosis can be formed.

The Analysis Process

First, the data must be validated: Are they accurate, complete, representative of the population, and current? Several validation procedures may be used (Northwest Center for Public Health Practice, n.d.):

- Data can be rechecked by the community assessment team.
- Data can be rechecked by others.
- Subjective and objective data can be compared.
- Community members can consider the findings and verify them.

Validated data are then separated into categories such as physical, social, and environmental data. In many instances, data spreadsheets are used to provide a structure for data organization. Next, each category is examined to determine its significance. At this point, there may be a need to search for additional information to clarify the meaning of the data. Only then can inferences be made and a tentative conclusion about the meaning of the data be reached (Anderson & McFarlane, 2019).

Big data have increasingly become a go-to source for clinical and community health professionals seeking to learn more about the health status of communities. Defined as large volumes of data that is amassed, managed, and analyzed from multiple sources, big data provide the level of detail necessary predict and understand public health risks and to develop interventions for specific groups within a larger population. These data are used in disease surveillance, predicting health risk, targeting interventions, and understanding disease (Zhu et al., 2019). It can be found in clinical information systems (i.e., electronic health records), public payer data claims (i.e., Medicare), and research databases.

Some computer programs are designed to analyze community assessment data. For large, complex, or ongoing community assessment plans, this may be the best method. For smaller, one-time assessments, the paper-and-pencil method may be sufficient and less unwieldy. Some communities may hire an outside professional assessment service. These teams often use the latest technology when analyzing data. Not all communities can afford such a service, and if key leaders become familiar with assessment, analysis, and diagnostic processes, an investment in a computer program may be worthwhile. Regardless of the analysis method used, data interpretation remains a critical phase of the process.

In data interpretation, the ever-present danger exists of making inaccurate assumptions and diagnoses. The importance of validation cannot be overemphasized. Before making a diagnosis, all assumptions must be validated: Are they sound? Community members should participate actively in validation efforts by clarifying perceptions, explaining the circumstances surrounding the situation, and acting as sounding boards for testing assumptions. Other resources, such as the health team members and community leaders, are used to explore and confirm inferences. Data collection, data interpretation, and nursing diagnosis are sequential activities, with validation serving as the bridges between them. When performed thoroughly, these steps lead to accurate diagnoses.

Community Diagnosis Formation

The next step of the nursing process, after analysis, is the development of the community diagnosis. **Community diagnosis** stems from analysis of assessment data.

The diagnosis "describes a situation" and "implies a reason" or etiology focusing on a specific community (Anderson & McFarlane, 2019).

Various taxonomies and classification systems are used in nursing to describe specific nursing problems, and each one has its limitations when dealing with community-level diagnoses. The North American Nursing Diagnosis Association (NANDA) is much more oriented to nursing diagnoses of individuals and families than to community-level problems. Nursing Outcomes Classification (NOC) is also generally individual oriented. The Omaha System, originally designed by the Omaha Visiting Nurse Association and described earlier in this chapter, is again primarily used in nursing diagnoses of individuals, families, and small groups, and some community health applications have been developed (Omaha System, 2017).

An example of a research study that used the Omaha System was one in which researchers evaluated the following behaviors of Syrian refugees living in urban areas of Turkey (Ardic, Esion, Koc, Bayraktar, & Sunal, 2018):

- In the environmental domain: income, sanitation, and residence
- In the psychosocial domain: communication with community resources, social contact, interpersonal relationships, mental health, neglect, and caretaking/parenting
- In the physiological domain (communicable/infectious conditions)
- Health-related behaviors (nutrition, personal care, substance use, health care supervision, and medication regimen)

A sociodemographic questionnaire provided individual and housing characteristics, and the Omaha System-Problem Classification List was used to identify issues and plan for intervention based on the specified nurse-identified domains and behaviors of concern. Due to language issues and limited time with an interpreter, there was no detailed evaluation of outcomes. However, The Omaha System components can be used by the local health departments to support the diagnosis and planning of further initiatives for the refugee population (Ardic et al., 2018).

This chapter discusses nursing diagnosis as characterized by Neufeld and Harrison (1996), based on the classic work of Mundinger and Jauron (1975). These authors proposed the use of nursing diagnoses in the community by substituting the term *client, family, group*, or *aggregate* for the word *patient*.

Neufeld and Harrison (1996) described a nursing diagnosis as the statement of a [client's] response which nursing intervention can help to change in the direction of health and which also identifies essential factors related to the unhealthful response.

Nursing diagnosis was used by Neufeld and Harrison as the foundation for development of wellness diagnosis (Neufeld & Harrison, 1996): "…the statement of a client's [or community's] healthful response which nursing intervention can support or strengthen. It should also identify the essential factors related to the healthful response."

In 1996, Stolte developed a manual dedicated solely to nursing wellness diagnosis which were later incorporated with community diagnosis by Carpenito (2017) in her well-known handbook of nursing diagnosis application.

By substituting the term community for client, family, group, or aggregate, the nursing or wellness diagnosis can be applied to the community as a whole. These diagnoses identify the conclusion the nurse draws from interpretation of collected data and describe a community's healthy or unhealthy responses that can be influenced or changed by nursing interventions. These findings allow the nurse to collaborate with community and health team members to affect positive changes in outcomes.

In community health, nurses do not limit their focus to problems; they consider the community as a total system and look for evidence of all kinds of responses that may influence the community's level of wellness. Responses encompass the whole health–illness continuum, from specific deficits, such as a lack of senior centers or day care programs, to opportunities for maximizing a community's health, such as promoting farmer's markets for better access to fresh fruits and vegetables or improving the safety of the roadways. The statement of community response—the diagnosis—can focus on a wide range of topics.

Community Diagnoses

Data have been gathered from a variety of sources and have been validated by several means. The data have been recorded, tabulated, analyzed, and synthesized, so that patterns and trends can be seen. The use of charts, graphs, and tables assists in visualizing the synthesized data. The community assessment team should present their findings to peers and colleagues and use their expertise to assist in the formulation of the community diagnoses.

Inferences are drawn from the data, and these statements refer to *actual* or *potential* problems. Additional statements involve *etiology*, by stating that this condition is *related to* certain conditions or problems. There may be a number of these statements, involving several subsystems, for every one diagnosis. Signs and symptoms of the diagnosis relate to the *magnitude* or *duration* of the problem, usually documented "as manifested by" (Anderson & McFarlane, 2019).

Continuing with the nursing process format, nursing diagnoses for the community are developed. Community diagnoses refer to nursing diagnoses about a community's ineffective coping ability and potential for enhanced coping. The statements about the community should include the strengths of the community and possible sources for community solutions, as well as the community's weaknesses or problem areas.

Community-level diagnoses can be developed (Carpenito, 2017). These diagnoses are used as tools as the community begins to plan, intervene, and evaluate outcomes. Diagnostic categories for individuals (e.g., knowledge deficit of senior services, high risk for injury or falls) can often be applied at the community level.

Community-level nursing diagnoses should portray a community focus, include the community response, and identify any related factors that have potential for change through community health nursing. These may also include wellness diagnoses, which indicate maintenance or potential change responses (due to growth and development), when no deficit is present.

Community nursing diagnoses must also include statements that are narrow enough to guide interventions, have logical linkages between community responses and related factors, and include factors within the domain of community health nursing intervention.

Examples of wellness and deficit community nursing diagnoses and several diagnoses for a specific community follow:

1. *Wellness nursing diagnosis for an assisted living community of elders*. The senior residents of an assisted living center (*community focus*) have the potential for achieving optimal functioning related to (*host factors*) their expressed interest in exercise, diet, and meaningful activities and to (*environmental factors*) their access to exercise opportunities, nutritional information, and social outlets.
2. *Deficit community nursing diagnosis for a rural farmworker community*. The inhabitants of (*name of the town*) in (*name of the state*) are at risk for illness and injury related to (*host factors*) exposure to pesticides, lack of motivation to add or use safety devices on farm machinery, lack of safety knowledge, choice to take unnecessary risks (*environmental factors*), lack of family income to purchase newer equipment, and long hours of work that lead to stress and exhaustion.
3. *Community diagnoses for Anytown, Kansas*. Anytown, Kansas, is experiencing an increase in crime, a problem compounded by the small size of the police force and an influx of many new community members. The community has worked together constructively in the past, communicates well, and has strong recreational outlets for community members. The community:
   - Has expressed vulnerability and feels overwhelmed related to threats to community safety
   - Has failed to meet its own expectations related to inadequate law enforcement services
   - Has expressed difficulty in meeting the demands of change related to an influx of new community members
   - Has a successful history of coping with a previous crisis of teenage pregnancy

- Has positive communication among community members
- Has a well-developed program for recreation and relaxation

Such diagnoses can guide communities toward maximizing or improving their health as they plan, implement, and evaluate changes to be measured by established outcome criteria. Broad goals can form the basis for planning interventions. From these goals, more specific activities, interventions, and targeted programs can be designed. Measurable objectives can be written and evaluated (Anderson & McFarlane, 2019). **Outcome criteria** are measurable standards that community members use to measure success as they work toward improving the health of their community. Outcome-based or evidence-based nursing practice applies to aggregates in the community as well as to patients in acute care settings.

Nursing diagnoses change over time because they reflect changes in the health status of the community; therefore, diagnoses need to be periodically reevaluated and redefined. The changing diagnosis can be a useful means of moving a community toward improved health because it gives community members a clear standard against which to measure progress.

PLANNING TO MEET THE HEALTH NEEDS OF THE COMMUNITY

Planning is the logical decision-making process used to design an orderly, detailed series of actions for accomplishing specific goals and objectives. Planning for community health is based on assessment of the community and the nursing diagnoses formulated, but assessment and diagnosis alone do not prescribe the specific actions necessary to meet clients' needs (Anderson & McFarlane, 2019; Minnesota Department of Health, n.d.a). See Chapter 12 for more on program planning.

Knowing that a group of mothers at the well-child clinic need emotional support does not tell the nurse what further action is indicated. A diagnosis of culture shock (adjustment deficit to a contrasting culture) for a family newly arrived from Cuba does not reveal what action to take. The nurse must systematically develop an appropriate plan (Box 15-6). See Chapter 12 for more

BOX 15-6 LEVELS OF PREVENTION PYRAMID

The Problem of Child Abuse

SITUATION: Desire to reduce the incidence of child abuse in a given community by 50% within 2 years.
GOAL: Using the three levels of prevention, avoid or promptly diagnose and treat negative health conditions, and restore the fullest possible potential.

Tertiary Prevention

Rehabilitation	*Prevention*	
	Health Promotion and Education	***Health Protection***
▪ Establish rehabilitation programs for abused children, including safe home placement, physical and emotional treatment, and self-esteem building ▪ Rebuild the family unit if appropriate or possible	▪ Provide family life education programs for families ▪ Develop resources to support health promotion programs	▪ If unable or inappropriate to rehabilitate the abuser or family, keep abuser away from victim through incarceration or court order

Secondary Prevention

Early Diagnosis	*Prompt Treatment*
▪ Develop early detection programs through schools, clinics, and physicians' offices ▪ Promote enforcement of child protection laws	▪ Establish programs to provide prompt treatment for abused children and abusing parents

Primary Prevention

Health Promotion and Education	*Health Protection*
▪ Assess factors contributing to child abuse ▪ Institute family life education programs through schools and community groups ▪ Develop community resources to support health protection programs	▪ Identify families in the community who are at greatest risk (e.g., parents with history of child abuse, families under great stress) ▪ Develop community resources to support health promotion programs

on planning, implementing, and evaluating community health.

Tools to Assist With Planning

- A wide variety of tools are available to enhance community health improvement planning; these include activity descriptions, templates, and models (Minnesota Department of Health, n.d.a; NACCHO, 2015).
- Such tools help prioritize health issues, develop goals and objectives, specify interventions, and anticipate client outcomes.
- Tools that assist with planning also enable the nurse to test ideas and adjust solutions before actual implementation. Finally, the use of standardized tools enhances the planning process and promotes effectiveness of services, as well as professional standards of practice.

In addition to using tools, a systematic approach guides the community health nurse in the development of a feasible plan that adequately and appropriately addresses the needs of the community (Anderson & McFarlane, 2019). As they do in the rest of the nursing process, community health nurses collaborate with clients and other appropriate professionals throughout each of these planning activities.

The Health Planning Process

The health planning process is a four-stage system used to design new health-related programs or services in the community and includes

- Priority setting
- Establishing goals and objectives
- Implementing health promotion plans
- Evaluating implemented programs

The process is often used by health educators when designing educational programs or by administrators in community health agencies when initiating new services. The nursing process is similar to the health planning process. Each model helps to promote service effectiveness in addition to maintaining standards of practice. Community health nurses familiar with both the health planning process and the nursing process should be able to work collaboratively with community health professionals using either model.

Setting Priorities

Priority setting involves assigning rank or importance to the identified needs to determine the order in which goals should be addressed.

There are numerous ways to set priorities in the planning process. Many have identified useful criteria that can guide ranking problems for order of action (National Association of County & City Health Officials, n.d.; Office of the Assistant Secretary for Planning and Evaluation, n.d.; Public Health Institute, 2012). They are presented here as a combination of criteria:

1. Significance of the problem or the number of people affected in the community
2. Level of community awareness of the problem
3. Community motivation to act on the problem (or, Is this important to the community?)
4. Nurse and partnership's ability to reduce risk and/or influence the solution
5. Cost of risk reduction in terms of financial, social, and ethical capital
6. Ability to identify a specific target population for an intervention
7. Availability of expertise to solve the problem within the partnership, coalition, or community
8. Severity of the outcome if left unresolved or the consequences of inaction
9. Speed with which the problem can be resolved

A common test for priority setting is called PEARL, an acronym for "propriety, economics, acceptability, resources, and legality" (Public Health Institute, 2012, p. 50). A priority matrix may also be developed, but decisions must not be unilateral and should include input from all stakeholders, including community members. For example, a community assessment not only revealed that a group of elderly residents living within a specific zip code were fearful of crime but also identified the lack of public transportation as issues to be addressed. Using the above criteria, the community health nurse working in this community identified that 85% of residents of the community had fears about crime but did not see transportation as an issue. The residents saw crime as an important concern and were also motivated to act on the crime issue but were not willing to explore the transportation issue at the current time. The nurse, along with the community coalition partners, would be better able to influence the crime problem by helping to form town watch groups and getting the local police district to provide increased patrols during evening hours when robberies were more likely to occur. However, the partners had little influence to extend the hours of operation on buses or influence the creation of new bus routes. Members of the coalition included the local police chief and chamber of commerce director. If the crime problem was left unchecked, more people could be adversely affected, including businesses, because people would not be willing to leave their homes to shop or might even be forced to move away. Finally, these initiatives could be put in place rather quickly and inexpensively after the formation and training of volunteer town watch groups. There certainly are no adverse social, economic, or ethical consequences attached to addressing this problem. Therefore, it would seem that the crime issue would take priority over the transportation issue. It is important to remember that each community diagnosis is examined separately and then compared. Priorities for action are discussed, ranked, and then prioritized for action (Hauck & Smith, 2015).

Establishing Goals and Objectives

Goals and objectives are crucial to planning and should be feasible, specific, and measurable (Anderson & McFarlane, 2019). The diagnosis that identifies needs must be translated into goals to give focus and meaning to the nursing plan.

- Goals are broad statements of desired outcomes.
- Objectives are specific statements of desired outcomes, phrased in behavioral terms that can be measured.

Target dates for expected completion of each objective are also stated. Objectives are the stepping-stones to help one reach the end results of the larger goal. For the elderly group concerned about crime in the neighborhood, the need, the goal, and the objectives were defined as follows:

- *Need*: The group of elderly people has altered coping ability related to their fear of crime.
- *Goal*: Within 6 months, this group of elderly people will feel comfortable to walk the streets of their neighborhood without experiencing any incidents of criminal assault.
- *Objectives:*
    1. By the end of the 1st month, a safety committee (composed of senior citizens, nurses, police, and other appropriate community members) will be established to study the crime patterns in the neighborhood.
    2. The safety committee will develop strategies for crime reduction and elder protection, which will be presented to the city council for approval by the end of the 3rd month.
    3. Safety strategies, such as increased police surveillance, town watch patrols, and escort services, will be implemented by the end of the 5th month.
    4. By the end of the 6th month, nursing assessment will determine that senior citizens feel free to walk about the neighborhood.
    5. By the 6th month, there will be fewer reported incidents of criminal assault.

Development of objectives depends on a careful analysis of all the ways in which one could accomplish the larger goal. C/PHNs should first select the course of action that is best suited to meet the goal and then build objectives. For the group of elderly people, other alternatives, such as staying indoors or always walking in pairs, were considered and rejected. The ultimate choice was to find a way to make their environment safe and enjoyable.

Some rules of thumb are helpful when writing objectives.

- First, each objective should state a single idea. When more than one idea is expressed—as in an objective to both obtain equipment and learn procedures—it is more difficult to measure the completion of the objective.
- Second, each objective should describe one specific behavior that can be measured. For instance, the fourth objective from the list states that the seniors will report feeling free to walk outdoors within 6 months. It describes a behavior that can be measured at some point in time. One can more readily evaluate objectives that include specifics—such as what will be done, who will do it, and when it will be accomplished. Then it is clear to everyone involved exactly what has to be done and within what time frame.
- Writing measurable objectives makes a tremendous difference in the success of planning. See Chapter 11 for more information on writing behavioral objectives.

The acronym SMART is another useful guideline when writing objectives (Minnesota Department of Health, n.d.b). SMART objectives are

- **Specific:** Concrete, detailed, and well defined so that you know where you are going and what to expect when you arrive.
- **Measurable:** Numbers and quantities provide means of measurement and comparison.
- **Achievable:** Feasible and easy to put into action.
- **Realistic:** Considers constraints such as resources, personnel, cost, and time frame.
- **Time bound:** A time frame helps to set boundaries around the objective.
- Planning means thinking ahead. The nurse looks ahead toward the desired end and then decides what intermediate actions are necessary to meet that goal.
- Sometimes, an objective itself describes the intermediate actions. At other times, an objective may be further broken down into several activities. For example, the second objective states that the safety committee will be charged with developing strategies, presenting them to the city council, and gaining their approval. Good planning requires this kind of detail.
- Making decisions is an important part of planning. Decisions must be made during the process of establishing priorities. Decisions are necessary for selecting goals and for choosing the best course of action from many possible courses. Further decision-making is involved in selecting objectives and taking action to accomplish the objectives.
- To facilitate planning and decision-making, the community health nurse involves other people. Clients must be included at every step because they are the ones for whom the planning is being done. Without their insight and cooperation, the plan may not succeed. Additionally, the involvement of other nurses may be important.
- Team meetings, nurse–supervisor conferences, and nurse–expert consultant sessions are all useful resources for planning. In addition, it is essential that you confer with members of other health and professional disciplines (e.g., teachers, social workers, mental health professionals, hospital representatives, city planners). Interdisciplinary team conferences are valuable for gaining a broader perspective and enlisting wider support for the evolving plan.

IMPLEMENTING HEALTH PROMOTION PLANS FOR THE COMMUNITY

Implementation is putting the plan into action. The nurse, other professionals, or clients carry out the activities of the plan.

Implementation is often referred to as the action phase of the nursing process. In community health nursing, implementation includes not just nursing action or nursing intervention, but collaboration with clients, stakeholders, and other professionals. An example of this process can be seen in the community action plan of the CHANGE tool (CDC, 2019d). After community data are assessed and analyzed, the final step is to create an action plan using SMART objectives. The action plan should include big-picture outcomes as well as incremental progress (CDC, 2019d).

When bringing about change in a community organization, implementation involves the greatest commitment of time and planning. This often includes an implementation timetable, as well as funding or organizing physical/informational/staff/management resources, collaboration with outside agencies, training staff and working with community volunteers as needed for program implementation, and actually putting into action those interventions created during the planning phase (Anderson & McFarlane, 2019; Public Health Institute, 2012).

Certainly, the nurse's professional expertise and judgment provide a necessary resource to the client group. The nurse is also a catalyst and facilitator in planning and activating the action plan. However, a primary goal in community health is to help people learn to help themselves in achieving their optimal level of health. To realize this goal, the nurse must constantly involve clients in the deliberative process and encourage their sense of responsibility and autonomy. Other health team members may also participate in carrying out the plan. All are partners in implementation.

Preparation

The actual course of implementation, outlined in the plan, should be fairly easy to follow if goals, expected outcomes, and planned actions have been designed carefully. Professionals and clients should have a clear idea of *who*, *what*, *why*, *when*, *where*, and *how*. Who will be involved in carrying out the plan? What are each person's responsibilities? Do all understand why and how to do their parts? Do they know when and where activities will occur? As implementation begins, nurses should review these questions for themselves, as well as for clients. This is the time to clarify any doubtful areas, thereby facilitating a smooth implementation phase. An operations manual may be needed, as well as organizational charts, clear budgets, and social marketing plans (Anderson & McFarlane, 2019).

Even the best planning may require adjustments. For example, some nurses who planned a health fair for seniors discovered that the target group would not have transportation to the site because the volunteering bus company had withdrawn its offer. To smoothly implement the plan, the nurses arranged for volunteers from local churches to pick up the seniors, bring them to the health fair, and deliver them afterward to their homes. Implementation requires flexibility and adaptation to unanticipated events.

Activities or Actions

The process of implementation requires a series of nursing actions or activities:

- The nurse applies appropriate theories, such as systems theory or change theory, to the actions being performed.
- The nurse helps to facilitate an environment that is conducive to carrying out the plan (e.g., a quiet room in which to hold a group teaching session or solicitation of support from local officials for an environmental cleanup project).
- The nurse and other health team members prepare clients to receive services by assessing their knowledge, understanding, and attitudes and by carefully interpreting the plan to clients. This interaction nurtures open communication and trust between nurse and clients. Professionals and clients (or representatives if the aggregate is large) form a contractual agreement about the content of the plan and how it is to be carried out.
- The plan is carried out, or modified and then carried out, by professionals and clients. Modification requires constant observation and interchange during implementation, because these actions determine the success of the plan and the nature of needed changes.
- The nurse and the team monitor and document the progress of the implementation phase by process evaluation, which measures the ongoing achievement of planned actions (Anderson & McFarlane, 2019).

EVALUATION OF IMPLEMENTED COMMUNITY HEALTH IMPROVEMENT PLANS

Evaluation is usually seen as the final step, but because the nursing process is cyclic in nature, the nurse is constantly evaluating throughout the entire process. For instance, in the assessment phase, the nurse must evaluate whether the collected data are sufficient and appropriate to beginning planning.

- Evaluation methods must be addressed during the planning phase as goals and objectives as well as interventions are identified (Anderson & McFarlane, 2019).
- Evaluation refers to measuring and judging the effectiveness of goal or outcome attainment. Too often, emphasis is placed primarily on assessing client needs and on planning and implementing service. The nursing process is not complete until evaluation takes place.
- Ideally, the nursing process should be observed as cyclical instead of linear, and when this occurs, it is obvious that evaluation guides the next assessment.
- The Community Toolbox (2019) provides suggestions for participatory evaluation that includes examination of the process (e.g., how the assessment was conducted), implementation (e.g., how the program was designed and executed), and outcomes (e.g., if desired results were accomplished). Appropriate questions include the following: Was all potential information assessed? How effective was the service provided? Were client needs truly met? How has health status changed? Professional practitioners owe it to their clients, themselves, and other health service providers to fully and effectively evaluate a program (Box 15-7).

Evaluation is woven throughout the Community Change Process and the CHANGE tool. The evaluation process should assist in determining if the team is creating the measurable impact envisioned (CDC, 2019d). An example of evaluation to improve program plans includes the Health in Action Project (Nieves et al., 2019). In conjunction with the East Neighborhood Health Action

Center, this project implemented a participatory grant-making process to fund projects that improved the community's health. The project engaged stakeholders in decision-making by including local residents in the decision-making process for allocation of grant funds. Evaluation findings showed that inclusion of residents as part of the process for decision-making was a strength of the project. Participants learned about the local organizations and services, and they felt included in a process that affected them and their neighborhood. Reciprocally, the funded organizations expanded their work and piloted new programs, forming new partnerships and building community networks (Nieves et al., 2019).

As stated earlier, evaluation is an act of appraisal in which one judges value in relation to a standard and a set of criteria. Evaluation requires a stated purpose, specific standards, and criteria by which to judge and judgment skills.

Types of Evaluations

To determine the success of their planning and intervention, community health nurses use two main types of evaluation: formative and summative evaluation.

The focus of *formative* evaluation is on process during the actual interventions. In formative evaluation, performance standards are developed and used to determine what is and is not working throughout the process. These could include the physical and organizational structure of the agency, as well as resources that provide a foundation for any interventions. Formative evaluation essentially looks at the step-by-step process of program implementation. Could I do anything better or differently to increase

BOX **15-7** **STORIES FROM THE FIELD**

Community Assessment of a Rural County in a West Coast State

Our group completed a community assessment of a rural county in a west coast state. We found data from many sources (e.g., census, health department reports), including key informants and a community survey completed by community members. Many resources were available on the CDC Web site for Mobilizing for Action through Planning and Partnerships (MAPP) (https://www.naccho.org/programs/public-health-infrastructure/performance-improvement/community-health-assessment/mapp/phase-3-the-four-assessments).

Windshield Survey

The windshield survey had the following findings.

Physical

In touring the area, it is noted that there are many older homes in need of repair. Some homes are vacant and boarded up on the SW part of town. Sidewalks are broken up, making them unsafe to walk on. Few playgrounds are noted on this side of town. The NE area has new home subdivisions and a new park. the NW area of town has apartment buildings, while the SE side has a large tomato processing plant. Most of the county is open land or is used for agriculture. Two state prisons are at opposite ends of the county. There is a community swimming pool in the largest town. The downtown areas of the larger towns have different types of businesses, but some areas are vacant. In the more rural areas, there are acres of land in production (e.g., dairies, cotton, cattle, pistachios, almonds, tomatoes, walnuts, corn), and some abandoned old farmhouses or dilapidated buildings can be found.

Economic

There are two large supermarkets in the largest town, and most of the smaller towns have at least one local market. Convenience/liquor stores are found in every community and some rural crossroads areas. There are a bulk warehouse store and two pharmacies in the largest city and a small local pharmacy in a smaller community at the far southern edge of the county. Food stamps are accepted in many places. The largest town has a farmer's market and a flea market weekly. There is a shopping mall, and smaller towns have second-hand and antique stores. Most jobs are agriculture related. People gather in the parking lot of the local home improvement store looking for day work. There is a small military base on the outskirts of the county with medical services and a store. There is an American Indian reservation with housing, a casino, and a small health clinic.

Services

For transportation, there is a county bus, but times/days are limited; there is an Amtrak station that includes intercity bus service. Medical transport services and cabs are available. A freeway runs through the middle of the county. Most people drive their own cars, but bus ridership has increased over the past few years. A community hospital is located in the largest city, and there are two small hospitals in the most distant small towns (now closed or used as clinic). The county is a Health Professional Shortage Area (HPSA) for primary care, dental care, and mental health. There is a county public health department in the largest town, with satellite clinics or rotating C/PHN access in every smaller town. There are two dialysis clinics in the largest town and one in the adjoining town, and several rural health clinics. The nearest Planned Parenthood clinics are in two adjoining counties. There are churches in every community (some in poor repair). There is a county library, with some service to smaller towns. Fire, police, and sheriff department offices are found in several areas throughout the county, along with eight post offices. There are high schools in three larger towns, and K-8 schools are found in local communities throughout the county. There is also a community college satellite center.

Social

There is a local newspaper. Most people have access to TV/radio, and there are Spanish language stations available. There are political bumper stickers on some cars and also billboards in populated areas. People can be seen smoking and occasionally vaping outside of stores or when walking downtown. Homeless individuals gather in several areas of the county. High school students gather after school at local fast food restaurants and arcades. People shopping at grocery stores are overheard speaking English, Spanish, and Portuguese.

BOX 15-7 STORIES FROM THE FIELD

Community Assessment of a Rural County in a West Coast State (*Continued*)

Data Collection

The data collected are shown in the following table.

	County	State
Population	150,467	30.5 million
Mortality Rates		
Average adjusted death rate	696.2 per 100,000	610.3 per 100,000
Diabetes death rate	30.3	20.4
Lung cancer death rate	38.4	27.5
Motor vehicle accidents death rate	15.5	9.5
Firearm death rate	10.5	7.9
Morbidity Rates		
Smoking (adults)	14.5%	11.3%
Hypertension on discharge	30.3%	28.4%
Adolescent mothers	30.4 per 1,000 live births	15.7 per 1,000 live births
Infant mortality rate	6.8	4.4
Prenatal care, 1st trimester	71.1	83.5
% Births late/no prenatal care	8%	2.9%
% Births ≤ 24 mo prior birth	16.8%	13.1%
Socioeconomic Data		
Ethnicity (majority)	53.5% Hispanic/Latino	39.3% Hispanic/Latino
Median household income	$49,742	$67,169
Children < poverty level	35.3%	22.8%
No high school diploma	30.1%	17.5%
Bachelor's degree or higher	10.2%	30.6%
Have health insurance	87.3%	91%
Unemployment	12%	5.3%
Of working population		
Worked 50–52 wk/y	40%	57%
Did not work/past year	32%	25%
Worked part of year/seasonal	28%	18%
Violent crime rate	4.6 per 1,000	3.96 per 1,000
Property crime rate	23.0	24.4

1. *List the strengths and weaknesses of this community.*
2. *What diagnoses would you apply, and why?*
3. *What interventions might be done to address these issues? Identify one that your student group might be able to complete during this clinical experience.*
   a. *Who would be involved (what collaboration would be needed)?*
   b. *What level of prevention (primary, secondary, tertiary) does the intervention represent?*
   c. *What outcomes could you measure to show improvement?*
   d. *How can your plan best be evaluated?*

my desired outcome? An example would occur when looking at the poor attendance at two sessions of an evening health promotion class for senior citizens. The nurse identifies the reason for poor attendance as being seniors' reluctance to attend an evening class because they either don't drive at night, have low vision at night, or fear coming out in the dark. The class is rescheduled for midmorning, and the attendance dramatically increases.

Summative evaluation focuses on the outcome of the interventions: Did you meet your goals? Summative evaluation examines outcomes of the interventions. The *effect*, or degree to which an outcome objective has been met, informs the agency or program leader of the program's impact on clients' health. As an example, one manufacturing company had an 80% adherence rate for employees who were supposed to wear proper protective devices (goggles, safety shoes, and hard hats) in the plant. Noncompliance on the part of some workers was a concern to union representatives, the health and safety team, and the company management. They were concerned that 20% of their employees were at risk for injury that would cause pain, suffering, loss of work time, disruption to the manufacturing process, and reduced profitability. The occupational health nurse along with the safety officer began a month-long safety campaign that included safety mini-classes, posters, and incentives for departments with 100% safety equipment adherence. Three months after the program, 95% of the employees were adhering to the safety regulations. This 15% increase was attributed to the effect of the safety program.

The *impact* of a program determines how close it comes to attaining its goals. In the earlier example, the objective of the safety campaign was to increase safety equipment use, and use was significantly increased as a result of the program. However, if the goal of the program had been to decrease accidents and save the company money, the result could be determined only with additional information. Were there fewer injuries caused by accidents? Were there fewer days lost to injuries? Did the company save money as the direct result of employee safety adherence? What was the cost–benefit ratio? Depending on the answers to these questions, the overall goal of the program may or may not have been met, even though the objective of the program was met. The full impact of the program cannot be determined without additional data. See Chapter 12 for more on program evaluation.

Community Development Theory

An outcome of effective community-level nursing practice is community development. **Community development** is the process of collaborating with community members to assess their collective needs and desires for positive change and to address these needs through problem solving, collaboration with community stakeholders, and resource development (Leigh & Blakely, 2013). A community development perspective assumes that community members participate in all aspects of change—assessment, planning, development, delivery of services, and evaluation. With this approach, the focus is on healthful community changes generated from within the community, as a partnership between health care providers and inhabitants, rather than a commodity dispensed by health care providers.

Houghtaling, Banks, Ahmed, and Rink (2018) addressed breastfeeding in American Indian culture by looking at the role of American Indian grandmothers to inform breastfeeding practices in a rural community in the United States. Interviews with American Indian grandmothers identified the following: the importance of breastfeeding for healthy maternal–infant bonding, the passing of knowledge for family support for breastfeeding including attachment and bonding, and an overburdened health care system as a barrier to maternal–child health. Outcomes of the study were that breastfeeding practices need to be grounded in tribal resources and that American Indian grandmothers and health care professionals need to use a collaborative community approach (Houghtaling et al., 2018). The community as partner model exemplifies this approach (Anderson & McFarlane, 2019). Chapter 11 details community change theory.

- The outcomes are more positive when community members have a sense of ownership in the health programs and services that address their needs. This enhances empowerment among members of the community and enables them to more effectively control and participate in transforming their environment and their personal circumstances.
- This implies that health care agency infrastructures are appropriate additions to services that are planned and delivered in an acceptable manner to the community. This empowerment leads to greater resilience and ultimately, wellness (RAND Corporation, 2015).

When applying community development theory, the agent of change (often the C/PHN) is considered a partner rather than an authority figure responsible for the community's health. To achieve acceptance as a partner, the nurse must listen and learn from the community members, because they are the experts with respect to their health care needs, culture, and values. They have mastered adaptation to the community, and they have firsthand knowledge of prevention methods and interventions that are appropriate to their lifestyles. Members of the community are engaged as coresearchers, and time is spent building trust and developing collaborative relationships with community members, stakeholders, and neighborhood health care providers. The expertise of community members is valued and can be useful in designing recruitment strategies, as well as in data analysis. This experience can enrich the community as a whole, as well as the actual participants.

The outcomes of the services provided by any organization can be benchmarked against those of other groups. *Benchmarking* involves comparing an organization's outcomes against those of a similar organization or an organization that is known for its excellence in a particular area of client care (Haustein et al., 2011). Information from this comparison can be used to identify an organization's areas of weakness and to focus attention on specific outcomes. The establishment of *best practice* activities entails constant comparisons between high- and low-performance programs and interventions (Ettorchi-Tardy, Levif, & Michel, 2012).

From a global perspective, the Conference on Primary Health Care held at Alma-Ata in 1978 concluded that people have little control over their own health care services and that the emphasis should be on health problems identified by the members of the community in their attempts to attain a state of wellness (WHO, 2019b). Leadership in the use of community development methods to improve global health includes

- Promote active, representative participation to influence decisions affecting community members' daily lives.
- Engage community members in economic, social, political, environmental, psychological, and other issues that impact them.
- Interest them in learning more about alternative courses of action.
- Incorporate diverse cultures, ethnic and racial groups, and varied interests in the process of community development.
- Refrain from supporting efforts that are likely to adversely affect disadvantaged members of the community.
- Actively work to build leadership capacity of community leaders and groups, and individuals.
- Work toward long-term sustainability and community well-being.

SUMMARY

- Public health nursing is a community-oriented, population-focused nursing specialty that is based on interpersonal relationships.
- The unit of care is the community or population rather than the individual, and the goal is to promote healthy communities.
- Theories and models of community/public health nursing practice aid the nurse in understanding the rationale behind community-oriented care.
- Salmon's construct for public health nursing prescribes education, engineering, and enforcement with individuals, families, communities, and nations.
- Models used in public health nursing practice, the Minnesota Intervention "Wheel," the LAC PHN Practice Model, and the Omaha System Model of the Problem-Solving Process provide guidance for C/PHNs to assess, plan, intervene, and evaluate the care they provide to communities.
- The eight principles of public health nursing provide a framework within which the nurse works to promote and protect the health of populations.
- Characteristics of healthy communities include those elements that enable people to maintain a high quality of life and productivity by increasing health and decreasing disease and disparities in health and health care delivery. The effectiveness of community health nursing practice depends on how well the nursing process is used as a tool to enhance aggregate or population health. The nursing process involves appropriate application of a systematic series of actions with the goal of helping clients achieve their optimal level of health. The components of this process are assessment, diagnosis, planning, implementation, and evaluation.
- The concept of **community as client** refers to a group or population of people as the focus of nursing service. The community's health is reflected in its status (e.g., morbidity and mortality rates, crime rates, educational and economic levels), structure (availability, use, and quality of services and resources), and processes (how well it functions in regard to its strengths and limitations). The dimensions of a community's health may be seen in regard to its location (e.g., climate, vegetation, boundaries), population (e.g., diversity or homogeneity, old, young, pregnant, addicted, or academic members), and social systems (e.g., schools, businesses, communications, health care, and religious organizations, among others).
- Assessment for community health nurses means collecting and evaluating information about a community's health status to discover existing or potential needs and assets as a basis for planning future action. Assessment involves two major activities. The first is collection of pertinent data, and the second is analysis and interpretation of that data.
- Community health nurses may use various assessment methods to determine a community's needs. They include *familiarization assessments*, such as windshield surveys, which involves studying data already available on a community; **problem-oriented assessment**, which focuses on a single problem and looks at the community in terms of that problem; *community subsystem assessment*, by which the community health nurse focuses on a single dimension of community life; a complicated and often time-consuming *comprehensive assessment*, to discover *all* relevant community health information; or an *assets assessment* that focuses on the strengths of a community as opposed to its deficits. Combinations may also prove useful (e.g., problem oriented and assets assessments).
- Community data may be provided by many means—surveys, descriptive epidemiologic studies, community forums, and town meetings. Focus groups as well as primary and secondary sources (e.g., people who are familiar with the community and its character and history) are also common sources of data, along with Web sites, and government departments and agencies that compile statistics (e.g., U.S. Census Bureau, state or county health departments). Sources can include national, international, state, county, and local agencies, as well as business and social organizations.
- Using the nursing process in the community would not be complete without looking at the role of the C/PHN as a catalyst for community health improvement. Community development theory is the foundation that supports citizen empowerment and use of key players in the community to plan for the health and safety of that community.

ACTIVE LEARNING EXERCISES

1. Using "Enable Equitable Access" (1 of the 10 essential public health services; see Box 2-2), search your local public health agency's Web site to determine what population-focused programs are offered in your locality. How do you know if the programs are population-focused?
2. Talk with a public health nursing director or a program manager to explore nursing's role in the assessment, development, implementation, and evaluation of population-focused programs offered by the local health department.
3. Discuss with a public health nursing director or supervisor how public health nurses might expand their population-focused interventions.
4. Describe a situation in community/public health nursing practice in which the use of an educational intervention would be most appropriate. Do the same with engineering (Salmon) and enforcement interventions. Discuss your rationale for matching each situation with that intervention.
5. What populations define your community? What are the needs and deficits for specific groups? Use the nursing process to assess potential or actual problems. Using data and your assessment, determine a community diagnosis. As the community/public health nurse, what are next steps in addressing your community's issues?

thePoint: Everything You Need to Make the Grade!

thePoint® Visit http://thePoint.lww.com/Rector10e for NCLEX-style review questions, journal articles, supplemental materials, and more!

REFERENCES

Agarwal, S., Menon, V., & Jaber, W. A. (2015). Outcomes after acute ischemic stroke in the United States: Does residential ZIP code matter? *Journal of the American Heart Association*, *4*(3), e001629.

American Nurses Association (ANA). (2013). *Public health nursing: Scope and standards of practice* (2nd ed.). Silver Spring, MD: Nursesbooks.org.

American Nurses Association (ANA). (2018). *Public health nursing: Scope and standards of practice* (3rd ed.). Silver Spring, MD: Nursesbooks.org.

American Public Health Association, Public Health Nursing Section. (2013). *The definition and practice of public health nursing: A statement of the public health nursing section*. Washington, DC: American Public Health Association.

Anderson, E. T., & McFarlane, J. (2019). *Community as partner: Theory and practice* (8th ed.). Philadelphia, PA: Lippincott Williams & Wilkins.

Angosta, A. D., Ceria-Ulep, C. D., & Tse, A. M. (2014). *Care delivery for Filipino Americans Using the Neuman Systems Model*. Nursing Science Quarterly, 27(2), 142–148.

Ardic, A., Esion, M., Koc, S., Bayraktar, B., & Sunal, N. (2018). Using the Omaha system to determine health problems of urban Syrian immigrants. *Public Health Nursing*, *36*, 126–133. doi: 10.111/phn.12563.

Arria, A., & Jernigan, D. (2018). Addressing college drinking as a statewide public health problem: Key findings from the Maryland collaborative. *Health Promotion Practice*, *19*(2), 303–313.

Association of State and Territorial Health Officials. (2019). *Implementing the national prevention strategy*. Retrieved form http://www.astho.org/NPS/

Atkins, R. (2016). Coping with depression in single black mothers. *Issues in Mental Health Nursing*, *37*(3), 172–181.

Carpenito, L. J. (2017). *Nursing diagnosis: Application to clinical practice* (14th ed.). Philadelphia, PA: Lippincott Williams & Wilkins.

Centers for Disease Control and Prevention (CDC). (2015a). *Assessment & planning models, frameworks & tools*. Retrieved from http://www.cdc.gov/stltpublichealth/cha/assessment.html

Centers for Disease Control and Prevention (CDC). (2015b). *Developing program goals and measurable objectives*. Retrieved from http://www.cdc.gov/std/Program/pupestd/Developing%20Program%20Goals%20and%20Objectives.pdf

Centers for Disease Control and Prevention (CDC). (2019a). *Populations and vulnerabilities*. Retrieved form https://ephtracking.cdc.gov/showPcMain

Centers for Disease Control and Prevention (CDC). (2019b). *Data & statistics*. Retrieved from https://www.cdc.gov/datastatistics/index.html

Centers for Disease Control and Prevention (CDC). (2019c). *Behavioral risk factor surveillance system*. Retrieved from https://www.cdc.gov/brfss/index.html

Centers for Disease Control and Prevention (CDC). (2019d). *Download the community health assessment and group evaluation (change) action guide*. Retrieved from https://www.cdc.gov/nccdphp/dch/programs/healthycommunitiesprogram/tools/change/downloads.htm

Charleston, A. E., Wilson, H. R., Edwards, P. O., David, F., & Dewitt, S. (2015). Environmental public health tracking: Driving environmental health information. *Journal of Public health Management and Practice: JPHMP*, *21*, S4–S11.

Community Toolbox. (2019). *Section 6: Participatory evaluation*. Retrieved from http://ctb.ku.edu/en/table-of-contents/evaluate/evaluation/participatory-evaluation/main

Donabedian, A. (2005). Evaluating the quality of medical care. *Milbank Quarterly*, *83*(4), 691–729.

Ervin, N. E., & Kulbok, P. A. (2018). *Advanced public and community health nursing practice: Population assessment, program planning, and evaluation* (2nd ed.). New York, NY: Springer Publishing Company.

Ettorchi-Tardy, A., Levif, M., & Michel, P. (2012). Benchmarking: A method for continuous quality improvement in health. *Healthcare Policy*, 7(4), e101.

Fawcett, J. (2017). *Applying conceptual models of nursing: Quality improvement, research, and practice*. New York, NY: Springer Publishing Company, LLC.

Harvard University. (2019). *Center for Geographic analysis*. Retrieved from https://gis.harvard.edu/gis-institute

Hauck, K., & Smith, P. C. (2015). *The politics of priority setting in health: A political economy perspective—working paper 414*. Retrieved from http://www.cgdev.org/publication/politics-priority-setting-health-political-economy-perspective-working-paper-414

Haustein, T., Gastmeier, P., Holmes, A., Lucet, J., Shannon, R. P., Pittet, D., & Harbarth, S. (2011). Use of benchmarking and public reporting for infection control in four high-income countries. *The Lancet Infectious Diseases*, *11*(6), 471–481.

Houghtaling, B., Shanks, C., Ahmed, S., & Rink, E. (2018). Grandmother and health care professional breastfeeding perspectives provide opportunities for health promotion in an American Indian community. *Social Science and Medicine*, *208*, 80–88.

Im, E. O., & Meleis, A. I. (1999). Situation-specific theories: Philosophical roots, properties, and approach. *Advances in Nursing Science*, *22*(2), 11–24.

Jakes, S., Hardison-Moody, A., Bowen, S., & Blevins, J. (2015). Engaging community change: The critical role of values in asset mapping. *Community Development*, *46*(4), 392–406.

Johnson, B., & Webber, P. (2015). *An introduction to theory and reasoning in nursing* (4th ed). Philadelphia, PA: Wolters Kluwer.

Keller, L., Strohschein, S., Lia-Hoagberg, B., & Schoffer, M. (2004). Population-based public health intervention: Practice-based and evidence-supported. Part 1. *Public health Nursing*, *21*, 453–468.

Kerlinger, E. N. (1973). *Foundations of behavioral research* (2nd ed.). New York, NY: Holt, Rinehart & Winston.

Kirst-Ashman, K. (2014). *Human behavior in the macro social environment* (4th ed.). Belmont, CA: Brooks/Cole–Cengage Learning.

Kramer, S., Seedat, M., Lazarus, S., & Suffla, S. (2011). A critical review of instruments assessing characteristics of community. *South African Journal of Psychology*, *41*(4), 503–516.

Kretzman, J., & McKnight, J. (1993). *Building communities from the inside out: A path toward finding and mobilizing a community's assets*. Chicago, IL: ACTA Publications.

Leigh, N. G., & Blakely, E. J. (2013). *Planning local economic development: Theory and practice* (5th ed.). Thousand Oaks, CA: Sage Publications, Inc.

Lippitt, G. L. (1973). *Visualizing change. Model building and the change process*. Fairfax, VA: NTL Learning Resources.

Lushniak, B. D., Alley, D. E., Ulin, B., & Graffunder, C. (2015). The National Prevention Strategy: Leveraging multiple sectors to improve population health. *American Journal of Public Health*, *105*(2), 229–231.

Martin, K. S. (2005). *The Omaha system: A key to practice, documentation, and information management* (2nd ed.). Omaha, NE: Health Connections Press.

McElfish, P., Long, C., Rowland, B., Moore, S., Wilmoth, R., & Ayers, B. (2017). Improving culturally appropriate care using a community-based participatory research approach: Evaluation of a multicomponent cultural competency training program, Arkansas 2015-2016. *Preventing Chronic Disease*, *14*, 170014. doi: 10.5888/pcd14.170014.

Merrill, R. M. (2017). *Introduction to epidemiology* (6th ed.). Sudbury, MA: Jones & Bartlett Learning.

Minnesota Department of Health. (2019). *Public health interventions: Applications for public health nursing practice* (2nd ed.). Retrieved from https://www.health.state.mn.us/communities/practice/research/phncouncil/wheel.html

Minnesota Department of Health. (n.d.aaaaaa). *Local public health assessment and planning*. Retrieved from https://www.health.state.mn.us/communities/practice/assessplan/index.html

Minnesota Department of Health. (n.d.bbbbbb). *SMART and meaningful objectives*. Retrieved from http://www.health.state.mn.us/divs/opi/qi/toolbox/objectives.html

Minnich, M., & Shirley, N. (2017). Enhancing a public health nursing shelter program. *Public Health Nursing*, *34*(6), 585–591.

Mundinger, M. O., & Jauron, G. D. (1975). Developing a nursing diagnosis. *Nursing Outlook*, *23*(2), 94–98.

National Academies of Sciences, Engineering, and Medicine. (2019). *Investing in Interventions That Address Non-Medical, Health-Related Social Needs: Proceedings of a Workshop*. Washington, DC: The National Academies Press. Retrieved from https://doi.org/10.17226/25544.

National Association of County & City Health Officials (NACCHO). (2015). *Developing a community health improvement plan*. Retrieved from http://www.naccho.org/topics/infrastructure/CHAIP/chip.cfm

National Association of County & City Health Officials (NACCHO). (n.d.). *Guide to prioritization techniques*. Retrieved from https://www.naccho.org/uploads/downloadable-resources/Gudie-to-Prioritization-Techniques.pdf

National Institutes of Health (NIH). (2019). *National institute of health*. Retrieved from https://www.nih.gov/

Neufeld, A., & Harrison, M. J. (1996). Educational issues in preparing community health nurses to use nursing diagnosis with population groups. *Nurse Education Today*, *16*, 221–226.

Neuman, B. (1980). The Betty Neuman health-care system model: a total person approach to patient problems. In J. P. Riehl & C. Roy (Eds.), *Conceptual Models for Nursing Practice* (pp. 119–134). Norwalk, OH: Appleton-Century-Crofts.

Nieves, C., Chan, J., Dannefer, R., De La Rosa, C., Diaz-Malvido, C., Realmuto, L., ... Manyindo, N. (2019). Health in action: Evaluation of a participatory grant-making project in east harlem. *Health Promotion Practice*, March 7, Online. doi: 10.1177/1524839919834271.

Northwest Center for Public Health Practice. (n.d.). *Module one: An overview of public health data*. Retrieved from http://www.nwcphp.org/docs/bcda_series/data_analysis_mod1_transcript.pdf

O'Brien, K. H. (2019). Social determinants of health: The how, who, and where screenings are occurring; a systematic review. *Social Work in Health Care*, *58*(8), 719–745.

Office of the Assistant Secretary for Planning and Evaluation. (n.d.). *Strategic planning*. Retrieved from https://aspe.hhs.gov/strategic-planning

Omaha System. (2017). *The Omaha System: Solving the clinical data-information puzzle*. Retrieved from http://www.omahasystem.org/overview.html

Philbin, M. M., Flake, M., Hatzenbuehler, M. L., & Hirsch, J. S. (2018). State-level immigration and immigrant-focused policies as drivers of Latino health disparities in the United States. *Social Science & Medicine*, *199*, 29–38.

Polit, D. F., & Beck, C. T. (2017). *Essentials of nursing research: Appraising evidence for nursing practice* (8th ed.). Philadelphia, PA: Lippincott Williams & Wilkins.

Public Health Accreditation Board. (2019). *Standards & measures, version 1.5. 2013*. Retrieved from http://www.phaboard.org/wp-content/uploads/SM-Version-1.5-Board-adopted-FINAL-01-24-2014.docx.pdf

Public Health Foundation. (2020). *Programs*. Retrieved from http://www.phf.org/Pages/default.aspx

Public Health Institute. (2012). *Best practices for community health needs assessment and implementation strategy development: A review of scientific methods, current practices, and future potential*. Retrieved from http://www.phi.org/uploads/application/files/dz9vh55o3bb2x56lcrzyel83fw-fu3mvu24oqqvn5z6qaeiw2u4.pdf

Public Health Nursing, Los Angeles County Department of Health Services (PHN, LAC-DHS). (2013). *Public health nursing practice model*. Retrieved from http://publichealth.lacounty.gov/phn/docs/Narrative%20of%20Revised%20PHN%20Practice%20Model%202013.pdf

Quad Council. (2018). *Community/public health nursing competencies*. Retrieved from http://www.quadcouncilphn.org/wp-content/uploads/2018/05/QCC-C-PHN-COMPETENCIES-Approved_2018.05.04_Final-002.pdf

RAND Corporation. (2015). *County health and well-being*. Retrieved from https://www.rand.org/topics/community-health-and-well-being.html

Riegel, B., Jaarsma, T., & Stromberg, A. (2012). A middle-range theory of self-care of chronic illness. *Advances in Nursing Science*, *35*, 194–204.

Robert Wood Johnson Foundation. (2019). *2019 County health rankings key findings report*. Retrieved from https://www.countyhealthrankings.org/

Rogers, M. (1990). Nursing: Science of unitary, irreducible human beings: Update 1990. In E. A. M. Barrett (Ed.), *Visions of Rogers' science-based nursing* (pp. 5–11). New York, NY: National League for Nursing.

Rushton, C. H., & Broome, M. E. (2015). Safeguarding the public's health: Ethical nursing. *Hastings Center Report*, *45*(1). doi: 10.1002/hast.410.

Salmon, M. E. (1982). Construct for public health: Where is it practiced, in whose behalf, and with what desired outcome. *Nursing Outlook*, *30*(9), 527–530. (Originally published under the author name Marla Salmon White.)

Salmon, M. E. (1993). Public health nursing: The opportunity of a century. *American Journal of Public Health*, *83*(12), 1674–1675.

Schaffer, M., Anderson, L., & Rising, S. (2016). Public health intervention for school nurse practice. *Journal of School Nursing*, *32*(3), 195–208. doi: 10.1177/1059840515605361

Smith, M. C. (2019). Regenerating nursing's disciplinary perspective. *Advances in Nursing Science*, *42*(1), 3–16.

Smith, K., & Bazini-Barakat, N. (2003). A public health nursing practice model: Melding public health principles with the nursing process. *Public Health Nursing*, *20*, 42–48.

Smith, M. J., & Liehr, P. R. (Eds.). (2018). *Middle range theory for nursing* (4th ed.). New York, NY: Springer Publishing Company.

Summach, A. H. (2011). Facilitating trust engenderment in secondary school nurse interactions with students. *The Journal of School Nursing*, *27*(2), 129–138.

Swider, S. M., Berkowitz, B., Valentine-Maher, S., Zenk, S. N., & Bekemeier, B. (2017). Engaging communities in creating health: Leveraging community benefit, *Nursing Outlook*, *65*(5), 657–660.

The Healthy City. (2018). *The effects of urbanization on human's physical health*. Retrieved from https://medium.com/the-healthy-city/the-effects-of-urbanization-on-humans-physical-health-e2cd73c91001

Thompson, C. W., Monsen, K. A., Wanamaker, K., Augustyniak, K., & Thompson, S. L. (2012). Using the Omaha system as a framework to demonstrate the value of nurse managed wellness center services for vulnerable populations. *Journal of Community Health Nursing*, *29*(1), 1–11.

Tucker, C. M., Arthur, T. M., Roncoroni, J., Wall, W., & Sanchez, J. (2015). Patient-centered, culturally sensitive health care. *American Journal of Lifestyle Medicine*, *9*(1), 63–77.

U.S. Census Bureau. (2019). *Data*. Retrieved from http://www.census.gov/data.html

U.S. Department of Health and Human Services (USDHHS). (2020). *Healthy People 2030 framework- overarching goals*. Retrieved from https://health.gov/healthypeople/about/healthy-people-2030-framework

Wang, Y., Ponce, N. A., Wang, P., Opsomer, J. D., & Yu, H. (2015). Generating health estimates by zip code: A semiparametric small area estimation approach using the California health interview survey. *American Journal of Public Health*, *105*(12), 2534–2540.

World Health Organization. (2019a). *Climate change and health*. Retrieved from https://www.who.int/news-room/fact-sheets/detail/climate-change-and-health

World Health Organization. (2019b). *Geographic information system*. Retrieved from https://www.who.int/lep/monitor/gis/en/

World Health Organization. (2019c). *WHO called to return to the declaration of alma-alta*. Retrieved from https://www.who.int/social_determinants/tools/multimedia/alma_ata/en/

Wyer, P. C., Umscheid, C. A., Wright, S., Silva, S. A., & Lang, E. (2015). Teaching evidence assimilation for collaborative health care (TEACH) 2009–2014: Building evidence-based capacity within health care provider organizations. *eGEMs*, *3*(2).

Zhu, R., Han, S., Su, Y., Zhang, C., Yu, Q., & Zhiguang, D. (2019). The application of big data and the development of nursing science: A discussion paper. *International Journal of Nursing Sciences*, *3*, 229–234.

CHAPTER 16

Global Health Nursing

"When it comes to global health, there is no 'them'... only 'us'."

—Global Health Council (2010)

KEY TERMS

Community health worker (CHW)
Demographics
Disability-adjusted life year (DALY)
Era of Chronic, Long-Term Health Conditions
Era of Infectious Diseases
Era of Social Health Conditions
Global health
Global burden of disease (GBD)
Primary health care (PHC)
Sustainable Developmental Goals (SDGs)
Years lived with disability (YLD)
Years of life lost (YLL)
World Health Organization (WHO)

LEARNING OBJECTIVES

Upon mastery of this chapter, you should be able to:

1. Describe a framework for delivering community-based nursing care within the context of global health.
2. Explain how epidemiologic and demographic transition theories assist in understanding the impact of disease patterns on the health of a community, country, or region.
3. Define the global burden of disease according to common social determinants of health.
4. Describe the major health care trends currently affecting the world's populations.
5. Explain how a focus on primary health care provides the basis for health promotion and disease prevention.
6. Describe issues of global health conduct and regulation, including ethical concerns.

INTRODUCTION

The world has come to us; we encounter the world every day where we live. In the Los Angeles Unified School District, second largest K-12 district in the nation, students speak 92 languages other than English at home (Los Angeles Regional Adult Education Consortium, 2018). Even Montana, a sparsely populated state, has identified 22 world languages spoken in their homes (City-Data, 2020). Local health has become global health.

What do you think of when you hear the phrase "global health?" Would you first think about the survival rates of women and children? Or basic nutrition as a foundation for health worldwide? More likely, you might think about the news of respiratory pandemics spreading from one country to another. What would you do if an international traveler from a pandemic area is admitted to your unit for care? Knowledge about global health could guide you to find targeted resources when you write a nursing care plan for your traveler patient. What are the special health needs of refugees fleeing conflict or extreme weather, or of immigrants simply looking for better opportunities? These questions all point to the importance of understanding the concept of global health, or the "world as client," which is the focus of this chapter. How can the whole world be our client as the recipient of nursing care? Even if you think you will never practice nursing overseas, it is important to realize that global events affect nursing actions locally and the health of others globally.

This chapter describes the intersection of global health and community/public health nursing. It introduces basic global health concepts and how global events can impact the health and health care of a community, country, region, or the world.

- We begin with a quick review of the context for global health and some key events over the years that show the evolution of global health. **Global health** includes health within the borders of each nation, within population groups with unique cultures and languages, and across international borders and cultures.

- We briefly examine selected global health trends and examine the influence of global political initiatives. Usually when we think of global health trends, we think of data describing epidemiology and contagious diseases. Other trends are equally important, such as management of noncommunicable diseases and increased access to primary health care (PHC). One important initiative is *Health in All Policies* (HiAP), which aims to address the health impact of every program or initiative.
- We also consider how these trends influence global health goals. We know health promotion and disease prevention are important goals, but do some strategies work better than others? Smaller nations with emerging economies have figured out how to deliver quality health care despite limited resources and challenging infrastructure. How do these countries achieve success? Sometimes they partner with a nongovernmental agency (NGO), which is a nonprofit or voluntary citizens' group formed to address a social issue. Which agencies achieve the best results? Could we adapt their successes for our local communities? Good ideas anywhere can improve good health everywhere and make the world a better place for all.

This chapter ends with a brief discussion of global health ethics. You are already familiar with the primary ethical concept in nursing of nonmalfeasance, "first do no harm" (see Chapter 4). This is also a key principle in global health ethics. Someday you might have the opportunity to participate in an overseas internship or perhaps volunteer as a nurse following a disaster in another country. Being aware of the special ethical concerns unique to global health will help you be successful wherever you practice nursing. Ultimately, we want the nursing care we provide to be ethical and positive with lasting benefits, whether we care for patients down the street or across the world.

A FRAMEWORK FOR GLOBAL HEALTH NURSING ASSESSMENT

The slogan, *think globally and act locally*, captures the essence of caring for our interconnected world. When community/public health nurses (C/PHNs) partner with the community client to assess health status, one useful guide is the universal imperatives of care. For instance, determining how many nurses a community needs depends in part on knowing the characteristics of the community, the people, and the predominant state of health. These universal imperatives are reflected in the elements of the following community assessment framework:

- Patterns of care
- Demographic transitions
- Epidemiologic transitions

After completing a community assessment, C/PHNs determine which services to provide by referring to the core functions and 10 essential public health services to guide their care (CDC, 2017c). See Chapter 2 and examples throughout this book.

Patterns of Care

As with any assignment in nursing, our first task is to assess the client. When the client is an entire population, the assessment can be quite substantial. In this case, we can use a framework to guide our review. Certain social conditions of living are known to influence and even determine health among all populations. When the social determinants of health are reviewed together, we quickly learn about the client population and their knowledge, behavior, and values. We also assess the health infrastructure within their country or region. Data describing these patterns have proven to be good predictors of the overall health of a population. Patterns allow us to design culturally appropriate care solutions affecting health, wellness, and illness of populations, both within and between countries and communities. These patterns of **demographics** are recognizable and measured across populations. What other aspects can you think of to add to the categories shown in Box 16-1?

Demographic Transitions

The next type of assessment is to determine the demographics of a population group by evaluating whether they are increasing or decreasing in number based on the balance between births and deaths and whether there are any migrations, such as rural-to-urban (Slogett, 2015). Demographic transition theory explains that population demographics in high-income countries changed slowly over several centuries. As low- and middle-income countries began to evolve in the 20th century, populations changed more rapidly over a few decades. Below is a summary of both demographic transition trends (Colburn & Seymour, 2018). Where do you see opportunities for nursing care?

- "Long life, small family": Starting in the 18th century, high-income Western European and English-speaking countries followed four stages in population change at a fairly slow rate. The final result for such populations today is a demographic with low fertility rates, an aging population, and decline in total numbers. Reasons for decline in mortality are thought to be from advances in public health, nutrition, medical care, and management of infectious disease.
- "Short life, large family": During the 20th century, low-income countries experienced a rapid growth in the total population, primarily from a rapid decline in deaths while birth rates remained high resulting in a very young population. Socioeconomic development in low-income countries also resulted in the movement of populations from rural to urban settings in search of employment while also gaining improved access to health. The availability of family planning has also had a stabilizing influence on population size (Colburn & Seymour, 2018).

Epidemiologic Transitions

The third concept in our framework of population assessment is to evaluate epidemiologic transitions. These are grouped according to the predominant health outcomes,

BOX 16-1 Patterns of Care

- Patterns of place or the lived environment
  - Rural
  - Urban
  - Climate influence
- Patterns of perceptions of health care
  - Influence of culture
  - Influence views and acceptance of healing treatments
  - Influence acceptance of nurses and other health care providers
  - Affected by attitudes toward women
- Patterns of privilege or inequality
  - Living conditions, including access to nutritional food and clean water
  - Daily functioning including physical safety
  - Quantity and quality of education for children, especially girls and women
  - Level of health literacy
  - Preference of learning style
  - Access to employment
  - Access to affordable health care resources
  - Informed health care decisions, including who lives or dies
- Patterns of population health differences (demographics)
  - Birth rates (fertility)
  - Infant and child survival rates
  - Life expectancy rates
  - Rates of infectious and communicable diseases
  - Rates of noncommunicable diseases and chronic illnesses (morbidity)
  - Death rates (mortality)
- Patterns of providers
  - Traditional healers
  - Trained community health workers
  - Community health nurses
  - Midwives and physician extenders
  - Physicians
  - Differing education levels and requirements for licensure
- Patterns of procedures and interventions
  - Sustainable and culturally appropriate
  - Primary care
  - Health promotion
  - Primary prevention
- Patterns of partnerships
  - Peripheral health unit and health station
  - District hospitals
  - Public health and governmental health care agencies
  - Nonprofit and nongovernmental organizations (NGOs)
  - Universities
- Patterns of politics and policies
  - Universal health care
  - Access to treatment and pharmaceuticals
  - Payment to providers
  - Local health care policies
  - Municipal governments
  - National governments
  - International collaboration
  - Cooperation versus conflict or violence
- Patterns of personal insight of health care workers
  - Personal health and physical well-being
  - Personal values and cultural beliefs, including religious beliefs and attitudes
  - Personal knowledge of community health nursing theory and practice

or levels of public health, experienced by a society. There are three eras of epidemiologic transitions of public health, named according to historical trends of health and health conditions as described in a classic articles by Breslow (2006) and Omran (2005). In high-income nations, these eras progressed sequentially. However, in our world today, some countries may experience two or all three eras in different regions of their nation at the same time.

- The **Era of Infectious Diseases**: Throughout most of history, populations died from infectious diseases such as the plague, tuberculosis, puerperal fever, measles, and others. The death rate was high, and life expectancy was not very long. During this era, the birth rate was also high. Families had many children because they knew that most children would die before adulthood and yet as adults aged, they depended on their children for care.
- The **Era of Chronic, Long-Term Health Conditions**: With the advent of antibiotics, people survived common infections and started to live longer. Because children survived into adulthood, the birth rate dropped. As people survived infections and aged, they developed chronic, long-term illnesses such as heart disease, cancer, and arthritis.
- The **Era of Social Health Conditions**: More recently, a new array of health conditions are affecting world populations. These new problems are anchored in social issues, as reflected in the slogan, *where you live determines your health* (Colburn & Seymour, 2018).
  - The wealth or poverty of your neighborhood reflects whether the streets are safe, housing is adequate, healthy food options are available, and schools and municipal services are adequate.
  - Personal lifestyle behaviors contribute to social health conditions, such as addictions and obesity, while social behaviors contribute to others, such as gang membership, prostitution, sexual abuse, and deviant behavior. The popular press has exposed many of these conditions.
  - Documentaries and reports have helped raise awareness about the effects of methamphetamine on entire communities, the abuse of opioid prescription painkillers, the obesity epidemic growing throughout the world, and the exploitation of children through human trafficking (Brundage & Levine, 2019; Bureau of Justice Assistance, 2019; Colburn & Seymour, 2018).

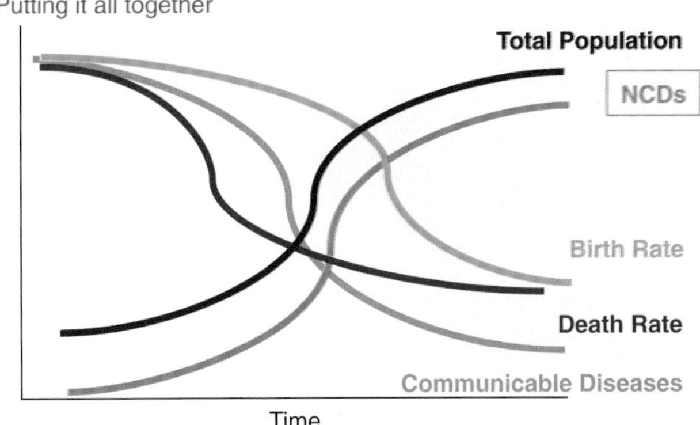

FIGURE 16-1 Demographic and epidemiologic transition theories combined. (Reprinted with permission from Seymour, B., & Colburn, C. (2018). Module 1: Global trends. In: B. Seymour, J. Cho & J. Barrow (Eds.), *Toward competency-based best practices for global health in dental education: A global health starter kit* (p. 18). A project of the Consortium of Universities for Global Health Global Oral Health Interest Group. Retrieved from https://hsdm.harvard.edu/global-health-starter-kit; Data from: Omran, A. R. (2005). The epidemiologic transition: A theory of the epidemiology of population change. *Milbank Quarterly, 83*(4), 731–757.)

Bringing Together the Framework Components

Review each component in the community assessment framework. What examples from your own experience explain longevity in your community? Consider the combination of patterns of care, the demographic transition theory, and the epidemiology transition theory together. What is the impact of communicable diseases and noncommunicable diseases? See Figure 16-1.

Explore differences between the development of countries through the concept of "we" in the Western world and "them" in the third world. In his Ted Talk, Hans Rosling debunks myths about the "developing world" in *The best stats you've ever seen* (19:46): https://www.ted.com/talks/hans_rosling_the_best_stats_you_ve_ever_seen?utm_campaign=tedspread&utm_medium=referral&utm_source=tedcomshare

GLOBAL HEALTH CONCEPTS

Key global health concepts, discussed below, include global burden of disease (GBD), the Health for All and HiAP initiatives, primary health care (PHC) achievements, sustainable development goals (SDGs), telehealth, and women's health.

Global Burden of Disease

Data collection and data analysis are an important part of the C/PHN toolkit. In addition to morbidity and mortality rates, one data tool used in global health helps to measure what it costs society when not everyone is healthy and helps answer the following questions.

- If a member of your family dies, what is the impact to your family?
- What does it cost if you miss a month of work or school because of an illness?
- What does it cost a country when adults have high rates of diabetes or depression, or when the greatest cause of disability in children age 5 to 14 years is from iron deficiency?

When populations or societies experience disadvantages socially, economically, or environmentally, these differences are called health disparities. The calculation of health disparities is the goal of a series of studies known as the **global burden of disease (GBD)**.

The first GBD study was commissioned by the World Bank in 1990. It was unique for its time because it brought together economists and health experts to evaluate health as an economic investment. That same year, the World Health Organization (WHO) assumed responsibility for the GBD study which emphasized the impact of disability (morbidity) and death (mortality) rates (Institute for Health Metrics and Evaluation (IHME), 2019a, 2019b; WHO, 2020f). Since 2010, the IHME has repeated the study at regular intervals. Because the GBD studies attempt to assess all health conditions using the same methodology, comparison of one condition to another is now possible. We can also compare disease rates and trends over time and by location.

The 2017 GBD report published by the independent IMHE provided data for 195 countries and territories around the globe. Updated mortality and morbidity estimates covered 359 diseases and injuries and 80 new risk-outcome data pairs were added (IMHE, 2019a). GBD data were also used to generate projections of health into the future (WHO, 2020b, 2020f). Review the report and other GBD resources at the IHME Web site (http://www.healthdata.org/gbd/gbd-2017-resources).

How is the GBD calculated? GBD is the measure for a population of **disability-adjusted life years (DALY)**, which is an equation that adds the total **years of life lost (YLL)** due to diseases and premature mortality to the **years lived with disability (YLD)** (Population Services International [PSI], 2014; WHO, 2014). The impact of public health interventions is calculated the same way, but using presumed years saved. See Figure 16-2.

For example, let's say one community has a high rate of death from measles for children under 5 years of age, but after a measles vaccine campaign the next year, there are no deaths from measles. When the DALYs are calculated from the year with measles, they are able to demonstrate the burden of measles on that community related to the lost lifetime productivity of the children who died. Comparing DALYs to the year without measles demonstrates the impact of the vaccine. Children who might have died did not die and are now counted among those in the community who are healthy. Children who received the vaccine can become productive adults. The GBD on the community is lessened with the vaccine.

The information obtained from calculating the GBD informs decisions related to investments in health, research, human resource development, and physical infrastructure. Assessment of global and regional information on diseases and injuries can be reviewed directly online using the *GBD Compare* interactive tool at http://www.healthdata.org/data-visualization/gbd-compare.

Compare the global disease trends by DALYs for 1990 and 2017 in Figure 16-3. Notice that 1990 had a greater area for burden of communicable disease. By 2017, there was a shift, showing a greater burden of

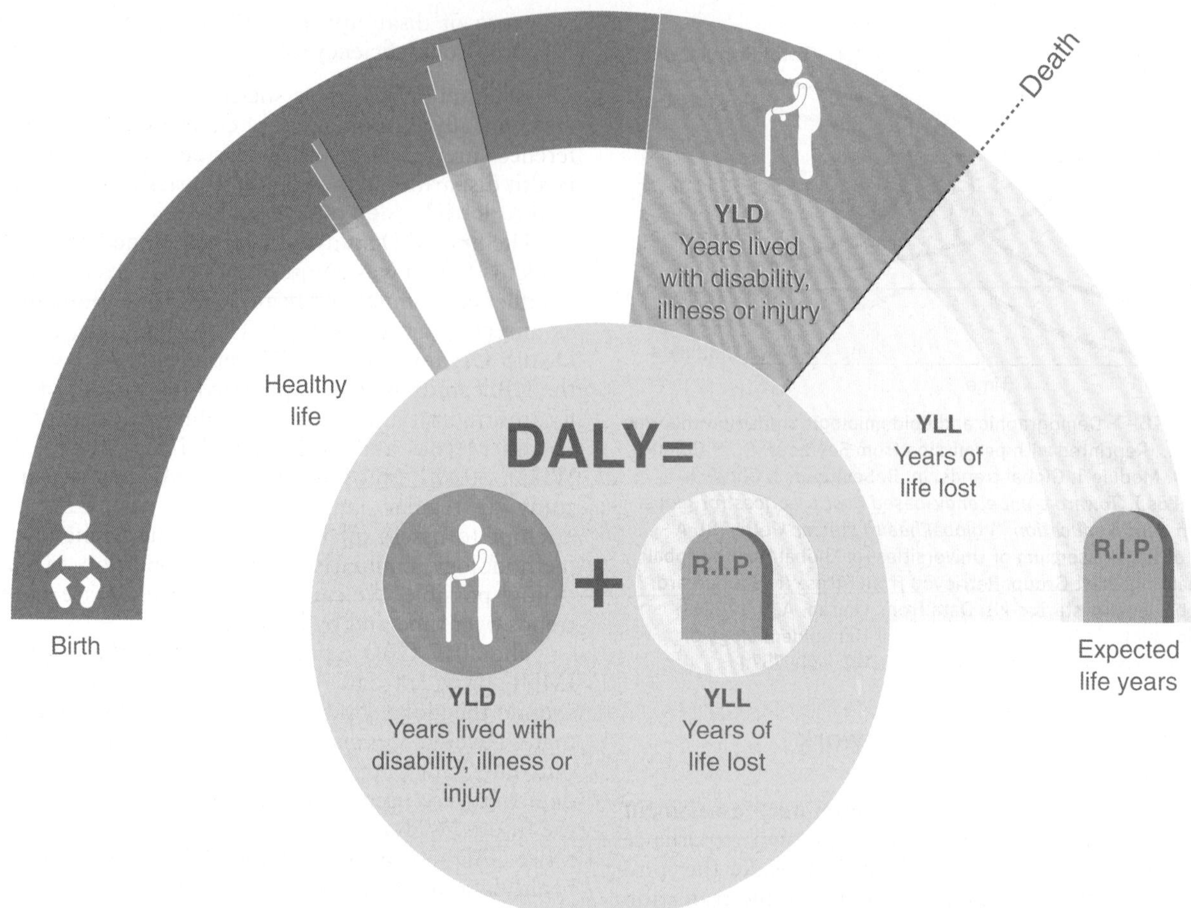

FIGURE 16-2 Calculating the global burden of disease by DALYs. (Reprinted from Newton, J. (September 15, 2015). *The burden of disease and what it means in England. Public Health Matters Blog.* Retrieved from https://publichealthmatters.blog.gov.uk/2015/09/15/the-burden-of-disease-and-what-it-means-in-england/)

noncommunicable disease. How might changing demographics account for that?

Health for All: A Primary Health Care Initiative

In its earlier years after World War II, the focus of the WHO was on building hospitals and costly health establishments throughout the world. The thinking was that hospitals brought health to a region. However, many countries could not afford to build health care centers, nor could they afford to train large numbers of health professionals. Because of those emerging trends and, believing that a major change in thinking and practice was needed, many health leaders from throughout the world met in Alma-Ata, Kazakhstan, in 1978 at the International Conference on Primary Health Care. They created a sweeping set of recommendations emphasizing the importance of PHC that became the *Declaration of Alma-Ata* (see Chapter 1) or *Health for All*. Section VI in the Declaration (International Conference on Primary Health Care, 1978) states that **primary health care (PHC)** "is essential health care based on practical, scientifically sound and socially acceptable methods and technology made universally accessible to individuals and families in the community through their full participation and at a cost that the community and country can afford to maintain… spirit (underscoring) self-reliance and self-determination" (p. 1–2).

It was a lofty goal to implement PHC for all by the year 2000. Each country was encouraged to develop goals for their specific population needs (WHO, 2019c). The United States responded by launching *Healthy People* in 1979 with the specific goal to reduce preventable death and injury. Updated every decade since the first report, *Healthy People 2030* represents the nation's current health goals and objectives for the next decade. *Healthy People 2030* covers many objectives for health attainment while still including objectives for the prevention of death and injury. Global health objectives can be found at https://health.gov/healthypeople/objectives-and-data/browse-objectives/global-health Compared to the initial goals from 40 years ago, one can see the evolution in our understanding of how to best achieve health for all (Haskins, 2017; USDHHS, 2020).

Health for All emphasized PHC that is affordable, culturally acceptable, appropriate, accessible, and delivered through partnerships between national health services and local communities. Communities assumed responsibility for identifying their own priority health concerns, with planning and implementing PHC services that match their unique needs. Common PHC services include health promotion, disease prevention, treatment, and rehabilitative care provided by health care workers who live in the same community (Fig. 16-4) (WHO, 2020a).

A

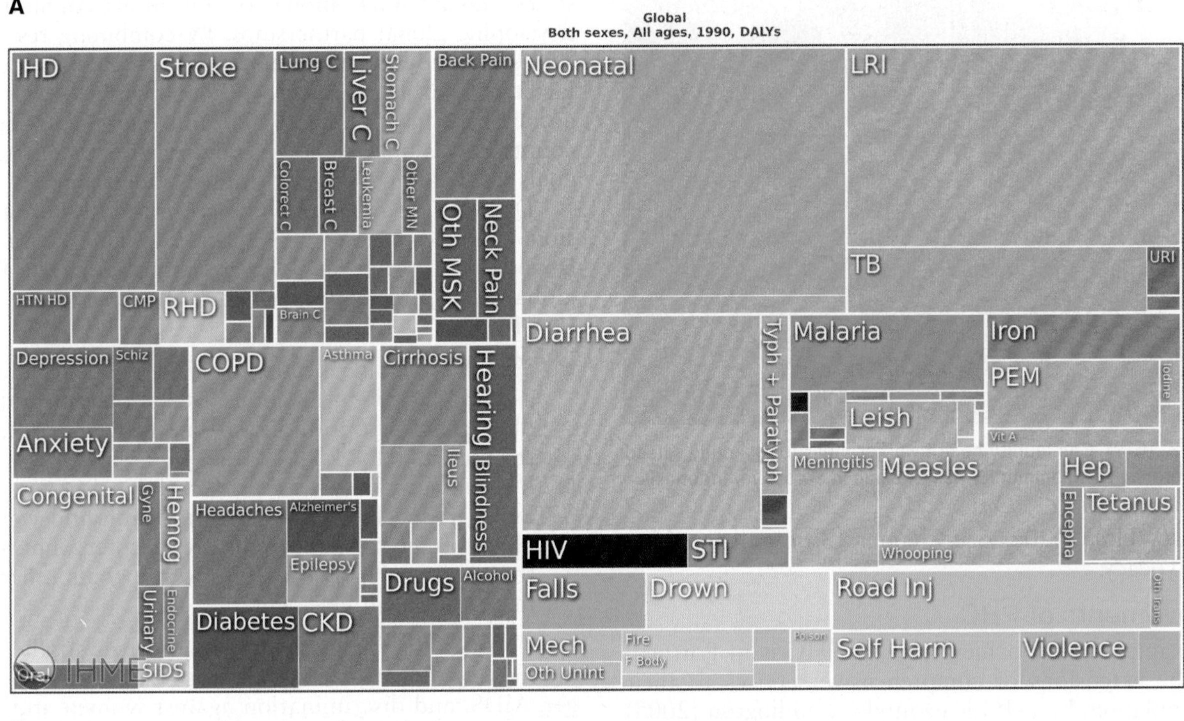

B

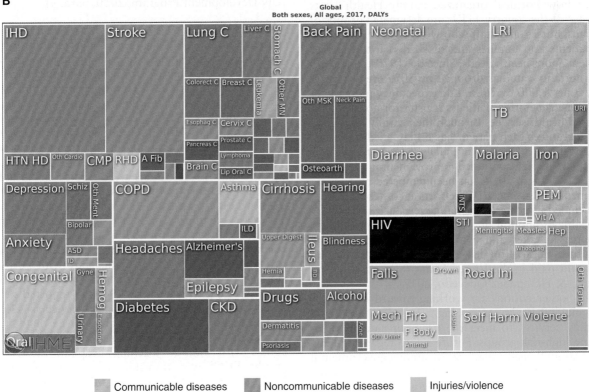

Communicable diseases Noncommunicable diseases Injuries/violence

FIGURE 16-3 Global disease trends in DALYs by cause, 1990 **(A)** and 2017 **(B)**. (Reprinted with permission from Institute for Health Metrics and Evaluation. (2020). *GBD Compare DALYs (global, by cause, all ages, both sexes)*. Retrieved from https://vizhub.healthdata.org/gbd-compare/)

Health in All Policies

In 2006, *Health for All* was expanded to *HiAP* as an essential component of PHC. The idea of HiAP is that good health in any society requires policies across all sectors to actively support health. This expanded approach requires policymakers to incorporate consideration of the health impact in policies for transportation, housing, employment, nutrition, water and sanitation, and education. By acknowledging the impact that any policy has on health, optimal health is maintained for the community's

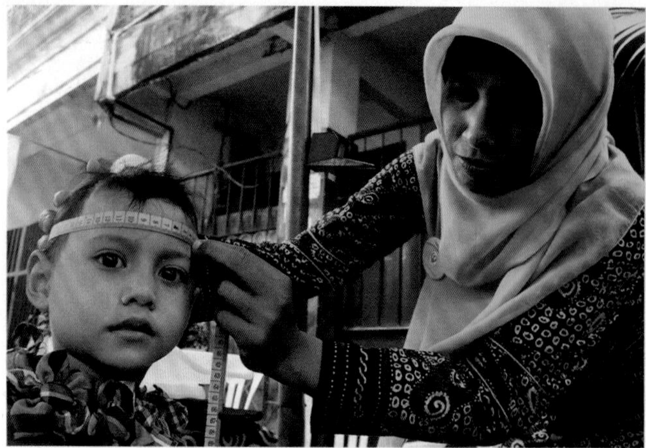

FIGURE 16-4 Community health worker measuring a child's head circumference at a community health clinic in Surabaya, Indonesia.

benefit (WHO, 2020e). See Chapter 13 on policymaking and advocacy.

Achievements of PHC

One example in the achievement of PHC is in Portugal with the extensions of comprehensive services to their full population. In a classic example, Waddington (2008) reported how Portugal organized Family Health Units (FHU) across the country. FHUs are designated groups of physicians, nurses, and staff who work to provide care to local patients and families and make decisions together with them about health needs. Since the 1970s, Portugal's infant mortality rate has dropped by 50% every 8 years to only 3 per 1,000 by 2006. Life expectancy jumped 9.2 years in one generation. Patients register for government-sponsored health services through their family physician, which guarantees each patient has a PHC medical home. MD/RN salaries are based on FHU productivity and performance. However, continued improvement in life expectancy (81.3 years in 2014) has been tempered by ongoing health inequalities. Since 2011, efforts at cost containment have included a greater focus on governance and regulation, health promotion, more reliance on generic drugs, and increased taxes and cost-sharing. The total health expenditures in 2014 totaled 9.5% of GDP, or about half the amount paid in the United States (Simoes, Augusto, Frontiera, & Hernandez-Quevedo, 2017).

Many other nations are working toward *Health for All* by making health care a right for all citizens and expanding services to meet the needs of rural populations and high-risk groups. Future action regarding PHC calls for strengthened collaboration among governmental agencies and NGOs in public and private sectors. Only when PHC is accessible to all people will the world have a realistic chance of achieving all the goals set out in the Declaration of Alma-Ata (WHO, 2020l).

Sustainable Development Goals

In 2000, during the Millennium Summit, the United Nations (UN) approved eight international health goals for the year 2015. These goals were named the Millennium Development Goals (MDGs), targeting health improvement, eradication of poverty and hunger, and achievement of universal education and gender equality. All UN member states and 22 international organizations committed to developing global partnerships. By combining resources, skills, and knowledge, these partnerships were assumed to facilitate goal achievement. Although some MDGs were accomplished before the 2015 deadline, progress between countries was uneven. Some countries found some of the goals were not appropriate for their populations.

Drawing on the experience from the MDGs, a revision and expansion was approved. The **Sustainable Development Goals (SDGs)** were launched as the future global development framework to be achieved by 2030 (Fig 16-5).

- The SDGs are a collection of 17 global goals and "are a call for action by all countries—poor, rich, and middle-income—to promote prosperity while protecting the planet" (UN, 2020, para. 1).
- Interestingly, only goal 3, Good Health and Well-Being, is specifically devoted to health and wellness. However, because the goals are all interconnected in the spirit of HiAP, each one of the goals reflects an important health element.

Through the pledge to leave no one behind, the SDGs are looking for "life-changing zeros": zero "poverty, hunger, AIDS, and discrimination against women and girls" (UN Development Program, 2020, para. 3).

Telehealth

Achieving these goals has been facilitated by the expansion of broadband and the Internet throughout the world. Ministries of health are training community care workers in communication, observation, and technical skills for telehealth systems that link remote areas to academic health centers (Fig. 16-6). For example, in Brazil's Minas Gerais state, PHC centers in 608 municipalities, some in remote areas, are now connected through the country's Telehealth Network (TN). In the first 5 years of the TN, 6,000 health professionals were trained in its use. The system was shown to be cost-effective and simple to use. With access to specialist teleconsultations, users of the TN were able to prevent 81% of case referrals from leaving the local community (Alkmim et al., 2012). A 2016 evaluation study found that the network had expanded to include 88% of Minas Gerais state with 40 teleconsults occurring each day. User satisfaction with the services provided through the TN was reported at 95%, demonstrating that this telehealth service is successful and sustainable (Marcolino et al., 2016).

A feasibility study in India networked five rural health clinics with a large teaching hospital. Electrocardiographs (EKGs) were transmitted from portable EKG tablet devices using WiFi hotspots at the clinics. The 12-lead EKGs were transmitted as secure PDF files for cardiologists to read (Shetty, Samant, Nayak, Maiya, & Reddy, 2017). Individuals and their local primary care providers now receive support and information from distant providers without traveling or being away from home. See Chapter 10 for more on technology and telehealth.

Women's Health

The WHO estimates that almost 295,000 women died in 2017 from complications of pregnancy and childbirth.

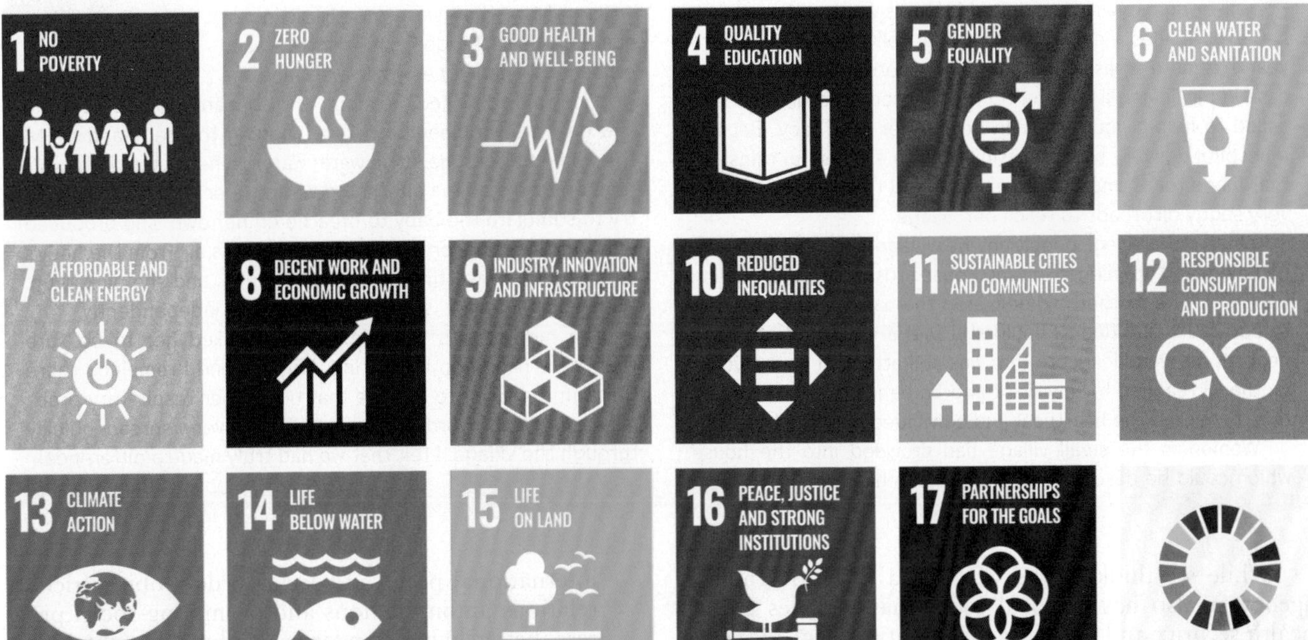
SUSTAINABLE DEVELOPMENT GOALS
1 NO POVERTY
2 ZERO HUNGER
3 GOOD HEALTH AND WELL-BEING
4 QUALITY EDUCATION
5 GENDER EQUALITY
6 CLEAN WATER AND SANITATION
7 AFFORDABLE AND CLEAN ENERGY
8 DECENT WORK AND ECONOMIC GROWTH
9 INDUSTRY, INNOVATION AND INFRASTRUCTURE
10 REDUCED INEQUALITIES
11 SUSTAINABLE CITIES AND COMMUNITIES
12 RESPONSIBLE CONSUMPTION AND PRODUCTION
13 CLIMATE ACTION
14 LIFE BELOW WATER
15 LIFE ON LAND
16 PEACE, JUSTICE AND STRONG INSTITUTIONS
17 PARTNERSHIPS FOR THE GOALS

FIGURE 16-5 Sustainable development goals. Reprinted with permission from United Nations Sustainable Development Goals. Retrieved from https://www.un.org/sustainabledevelopment/. The content of this publication has not been approved by the United Nations and does not reflect the views of the United Nations or its officials or Member States.

Ninety-four percent of these deaths are in economically poor countries. Nigeria and India had an estimated 35% of all maternal deaths in 2017. Pregnant women living in rural areas and adolescent mothers face higher mortality rates. The death of a mother profoundly impacts the well-being of the entire family. Between 2000 and 2017, due to efforts to improve prenatal and delivery care, global rates of maternal mortality dropped by 38% (Box 16-2; WHO, 2019a, 2019b). Women's health continues to be a major emphasis in Health for All. See Chapters 19 and 21.

FIGURE 16-6 Mother and child sleeping in a hammock near the Amazon River in Peru.

All populations we serve deserve respect for their personal choices, including our health care colleagues. See Box 16-3.

GLOBAL HEALTH TRENDS

The overarching perspective of global health nursing is one planet of interdependent nations. What happens in one country affects others in important ways. For example, air travel can transport health problems from any remote village halfway around the world to any major city within 36 hours. Detecting disease quickly has become more urgent for everyone's health since the outbreak of SARS in 2003 and more recently the COVID-19 pandemic, caused by the novel coronavirus SARS-CoV2. By February 16, 2020 China had 51,174 cases and 1,666 deaths, but there were only 683 cases and 3 deaths outside of China (WHO, 2020b). By October 2, 2020, the United States had 7,260,425 total cases and 207,302 deaths, with 302,093 new cases in the last 7 days (CDC, 2020a). Other global issues with an impact on population health include ongoing efforts to eradicate old diseases such as TB or malaria while maintaining ongoing efforts to improve basic health care services. See Box 16-4.

BOX 16-2 PERSPECTIVES

Volunteering as a Nurse-Midwife in Africa

Delivering babies in the United States is vastly different from experiences I encountered while delivering babies for 1 year in remote areas near the Ethiopian border. I remember one case in particular. It was during the monsoon season, and I was called to help a young woman having her first baby. Because a hospital delivery was impossible due to a powerful rainstorm that made roads impassable, my aide and I walked for miles on very soggy dirt roads to reach her village.

When we arrived, people in the village said that the baby had died, and upon entering the house I rushed toward the limp baby girl. The mother had delivered the baby on the mat used to cover the dirt floor. I could still feel a very muffled heartbeat on the umbilical cord that was still attached to the young mother. I reached for my mask and bag and started resuscitation. I checked the heartbeat and continued bagging the baby.

Women in the small village had crowded into the house, which could be described as a hut; some had been crying and wailing. Now, they were quietly sitting or standing near the door, speaking to each other in hushed tones while watching me work. My aide checked the mom, who appeared to be stable and had only a little bleeding. I kept bagging the baby and asked the women to get me some warm water to help keep the baby's temperature stable. I alternated warm water with cold water to try to stimulate the baby to breathe on her own; she produced only an occasional breath. I removed excess air from the baby's stomach after inserting a nasogastric tube, and she pinked up. Within a short while, she began to breathe independently.

The mother was relieved, and I checked her to be sure that there had been no tearing. My aide and I remained there through the night to be sure that no further respiratory problems returned. Word of the baby's recovery spread quickly through the village. I felt that we had truly made a difference!

Robin, nurse—midwife

While we think of the CDC as a U.S. government agency, it also has a global focus that includes global health security and outbreak investigation (Fig. 16-7).

UN and WHO

- At the end of World War II after earlier attempts to form international agreements, the United Nations (UN) Charter was signed and ratified in 1945 by 50 countries who were "committed to maintaining international peace and security, developing friendly relations among nations and promoting social progress, better living standards and human rights" (UN Systems Chief Executives Board for Coordination [UNSCEB], 2016, para. 1). The UN today supports and manages several international funds, programs, and specialized agencies that focus on health. Some of these existed before World War I, some were part of the League of Nations, and some were established

BOX 16-3 PERSPECTIVES

A Nurse Volunteer's Viewpoint on Personal Challenges While Serving Overseas

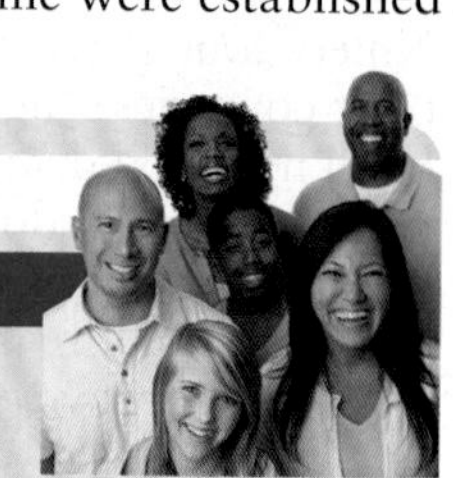

From an early age, I was exposed to nursing. My mother was a nurse, and I saw firsthand how she cared for us as a family and how she cared for her friends when they were in need. I also listened intently when she talked about the patients she helped over the years. Furthermore, I witnessed how she integrated her own faith with her nursing practice in the simplest of forms: genuine service to others. After I became a nurse, I also felt a deep calling to use my nursing skills in volunteer ways to serve others.

My first volunteer experience was in the rural mountains of Guatemala where I worked with indigenous women to improve birth practices. I thought I was going there to teach them how to safely deliver babies. But after spending 2 months caring for women during pregnancy and childbirth, they actually taught me more about the miracle of birth than I ever learned in my hospital-based experiences. We shared our knowledge with each other and I came away from the experience with a deeper understanding of what it means to become a mother.

Later in life, I met a nurse with the same deep passion for service to others. She was preparing to move to West Africa to serve women with childbirth injuries. She and I had both been raised within the same Christian faith and we both felt our nursing practice was very integrated into our values and beliefs. Then, we fell in love with each other. This was a challenging time for us, as we navigated the minority of being in a same-sex relationship within the Christian community. We struggled as some of our friends and family made it clear they did not approve of our relationship. But we also found new friends and family in the journey as well who were willing to see the greater value of who we were together.

In addition to navigating our home-front challenges, we also had to negotiate our relationship abroad. My wife was working for a faith-based organization in a predominately Muslim country, both of which do not condone same-sex relationships. In order for me to visit with her, to spend time together, and to also offer myself for service when I was there, we had to be silent about the depth of our relationship. We acted only as friends, with no public displays of affection. This was a compromise we both felt committed to in order to make a difference in the lives of the nurses and the women we cared for. Although some might find this compromise too costly, we continue to be grateful for the opportunities we had to serve and would do it again in a heartbeat.

Posted anonymously in order to protect future service opportunities.

BOX 16-4 STORIES FROM THE FIELD

Addressing Malaria in the Community

The Kenya Strategy for Community Health 2014 to 2019 included an objective to "enhance community access to health care in order to improve productivity and thus reduce poverty, hunger, and child and maternal deaths, as well as improve education performance across all stages of life" (Kenya Ministry of Health, 2014, para. 1). The goal was to empower Kenyan communities to take charge of improving their own health. One community strategy was to develop the capacity of the community health extension workers (CHEWs) and community-owned resource persons (CORPs) to recognize and respond to emerging health trends in the community.

Atieno is a community nurse working as a CHEW in Siaya County. Over a period of 3 months, she noted a rise in the number of malaria cases involving children in one particular community. Though the county is a malaria endemic area, Atieno was concerned about the new trend and began to have conversations with the mothers.

The steady increase in the number of children under 5 years of age with fever-related symptoms coincided with the start of the rainy season. Some of the mothers thought the fever was from children playing in the stagnant ponds and catching cold.

On her return to her health unit, she proposed a visit by the extension team. The visit was arranged with the community elders. During the visit, the team learned that the community had recently started making clay bricks as an income-generating venture. Almost every home was participating and had built furnace-like structures. These were surrounded by freshly dug clay pits that quickly became small ponds of stagnant rainwater which attracted mosquitoes. The team sought permission to check sleeping areas and noticed that most did not have mosquito bed nets.

A "*baraza*" (public meeting) with the brick works managers, the community elders, and CHEWs was arranged to discuss the situation. The team shared the connection between their findings and the new cases of malaria. The community acknowledged that the brick-making venture had contributed to the increase in stagnant water that became breeding pools for malaria-transmitting mosquitoes. Together, they developed a plan to reduce and treat the cases of malaria without compromising the community's new business venture:

- Drain stagnant water around the homesteads.
- Use treated bed nets, especially with pregnant women and young children.
- Monitor malarial symptoms. When fever develops, seek immediate medical attention.

Collaborative roles and shared responsibilities were also approved:

- All households were encouraged to purchase and use locally available bed nets treated with approved insecticides. The community leader negotiated for free insecticide-treated bed nets for the most vulnerable households.
- Workers committed to relocating their brick works away from homes.
- The local brick works leader coordinated with health dispensary officials for fumigation of existing mosquito breeding grounds.
- The CHEW enhanced existing community-based health services for malaria with additional health education, outreach services, and community–facility referrals.
- Community nurses provided information directly to residents of the community on the causes, symptoms, and the importance of early treatment of malaria. They also demonstrated the proper treatment and use of bed nets.

Once the plan was put into action, malaria cases decreased in the community overall while encouraging their new business venture. The community leaders and local population had the tools and knowledge to manage their own environment and take preventative steps against future cases of malaria. This account demonstrates highly effective PHC and community-owned action, all spurred by one community nurse's observations and follow-up.

1. *What steps of the nursing process are demonstrated in this global health nursing story where the community is client?*
2. *Which of the 10 essential public health services are pertinent to this situation?*
3. *What was the role of the community meeting (the "baraza") in reducing the number of malaria cases?*
4. *What would happen if the solution for malaria prevention and treatment were not managed by the community, but by health experts coming from outside the local area?*

Missie Oindo, BA, MCHD, and Serah Malaba-Kambale, BSc, MPH, PRINCE2 Practitioner, Kenya

Source: Kenya Ministry of Health (2014).

more recently to meet emerging needs such as the Joint UN Programme on HIV/AIDS (UNSCEB, 2016).

- Located in Geneva, Switzerland, the **World Health Organization (WHO)** is a specialized agency under the UN with the objective for "the attainment by all peoples of the highest possible level of health" (WHO, 2006, p. 2). As of 2020, there are 194 member states in the WHO divided into 6 geographical regions for the purposes of reporting, analysis, and administration (WHO, 2020m).

Other organizations are also active in promoting health internationally but are not necessarily sponsored by governments. Nongovernment organizations (NGOs) are often philanthropic and some are for profit. See Table 16-1 for a list of selected global health organizations and their areas of focus.

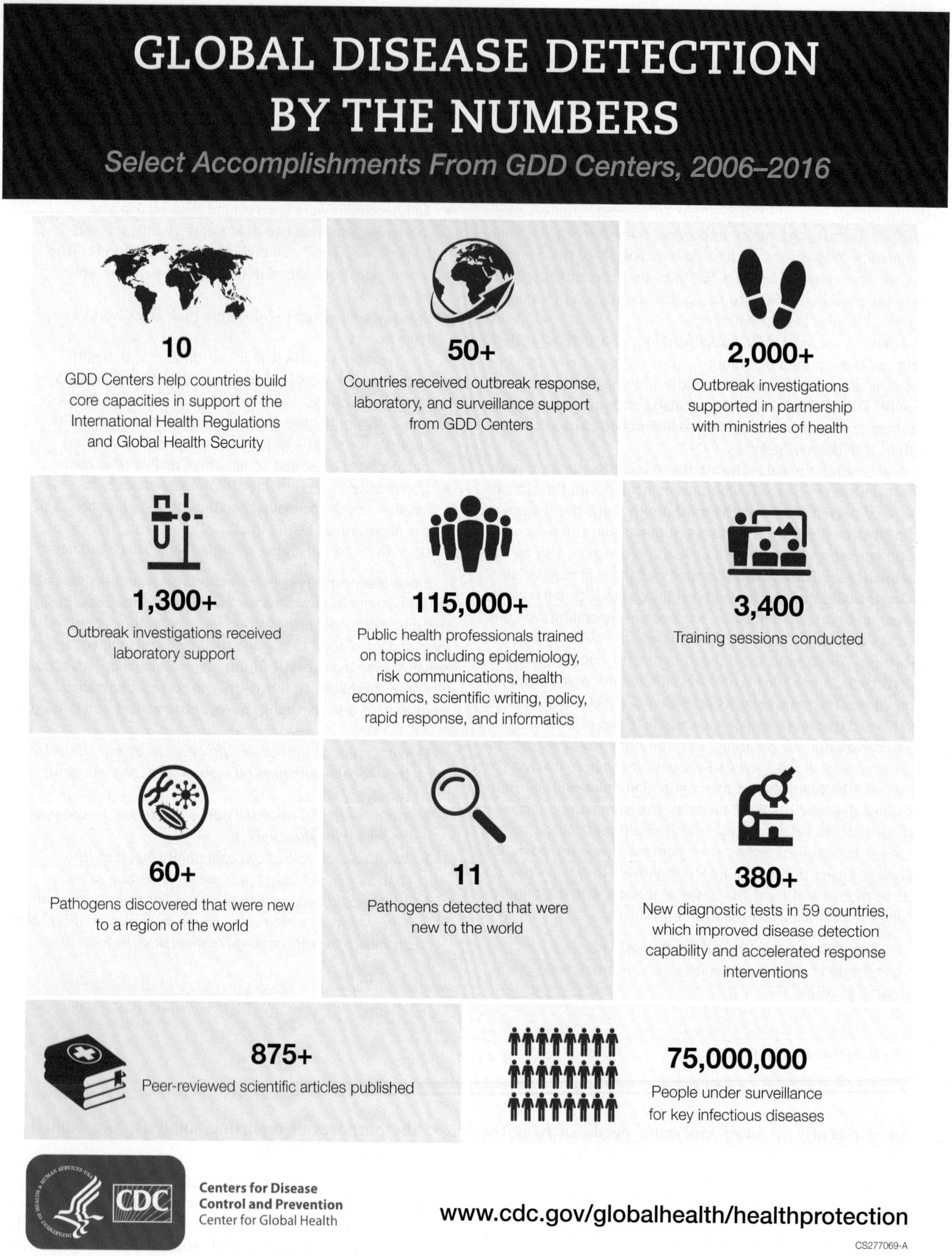

GLOBAL DISEASE DETECTION BY THE NUMBERS

Select Accomplishments From GDD Centers, 2006–2016

10

GDD Centers help countries build core capacities in support of the International Health Regulations and Global Health Security

50+

Countries received outbreak response, laboratory, and surveillance support from GDD Centers

2,000+

Outbreak investigations supported in partnership with ministries of health

1,300+

Outbreak investigations received laboratory support

115,000+

Public health professionals trained on topics including epidemiology, risk communications, health economics, scientific writing, policy, rapid response, and informatics

3,400

Training sessions conducted

60+

Pathogens discovered that were new to a region of the world

11

Pathogens detected that were new to the world

380+

New diagnostic tests in 59 countries, which improved disease detection capability and accelerated response interventions

875+

Peer-reviewed scientific articles published

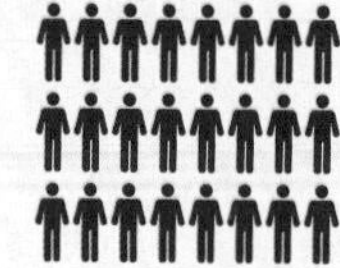

75,000,000

People under surveillance for key infectious diseases

Centers for Disease Control and Prevention
Center for Global Health

www.cdc.gov/globalhealth/healthprotection

CS277069-A

FIGURE 16-7 Global disease detection accomplishments. (Reprinted from Centers for Disease Control and Prevention (CDC). (2017). *Global disease detection by the numbers: Select accomplishments from GDD centers, 2006-2016 [Infographic]*. Retrieved from https://www.cdc.gov/globalhealth/infographics/uncategorized/global_disease_detection.htm)

TABLE **16-1** Global Health Organizations

Organization	Type	Funding Source	Purpose/Audience
World Health Organization (WHO)	Intergovernmental agency related to UN	Dues of member countries Donations (governments, private)	Directing, coordinating authority on international health Improves global health
United Nations International Children's Emergency Fund (UNICEF)	UN agency	Voluntary contributions of governments (70%) and private sources (30%): NGOs, foundations, corporations, and individuals	Promotes maternal and child health and welfare across the globe
United Nations Educational, Scientific, & Cultural Organization (UNESCO)	UN agency	Voluntary contributions of governments, NGOs, foundations, corporations, and individuals	Assists people in forming peaceful and inclusive societies Preserves the heritage of countries (World Heritage Centre)
The World Bank (WB)	Intergovernmental agency related to the UN	Primarily financed by selling AAA-rated bonds in the world's financial markets, from reserves paid in by 188-member country shareholders	Not a bank in the ordinary sense but a unique partnership of five institutions to reduce poverty and support development with financial and technical assistance to developing countries
Pan American Health Organization (PAHO)	Intergovernmental agency	Member country (52) assessments Funds from WHO, UN, private donations	Coordinating agency for public health in Western hemisphere Provides technical and epidemiologic assistance
U.S. Agency for International Development (USAID)	Independent, bilateral agency of the U.S. executive branch, under the Secretary of State	Congressional justifications, annual appropriations bill, budget for the State Department	Strategic global health priorities for developing countries: (1) preventing child and maternal deaths; (2) controlling the HIV/AIDS epidemic; and (3) combating infectious diseases Advances U.S. foreign policy
Centers for Disease Control and Prevention (CDC; including the Center for Global Health)	U.S. federal agency within the U.S. Department of Health and Human Services	Congressional justifications, annual appropriations bill	Works 24/7 to protect America from health, safety, and security threats, both foreign and domestic
Partners in Health	501(c)(3) nonprofit corporation	Corporate and government donations, academic and public sector partners	To provide a preferential option for the poor in health care, strives to achieve two overarching goals: to bring the benefits of modern medical science to those most in need of them and to serve as an antidote to despair
Medecins Sans Frontieres (Doctors Without Borders)	NGO	International agencies and governments, along with private donors	International, neutral organization sending emergency medical assistance in times of war, epidemics, disasters, or denial of care
Bill and Melinda Gates Foundation	Private foundation	Endowment fund from the Bill and Melinda Gates Foundation Trust	Provides grants to U.S. tax-exempt organizations that are independently identified for partnership on global health, development, growth and opportunity, policy and advocacy, and U.S. educational improvement
International Council of Nurses (ICN)	Professional federation	Membership dues, limited to one nursing organization per nation (The American Nurses Association is the organization representing U.S. nurses.)	Represents the global interests and concerns of the nursing profession. Maintains the role of nursing in health care through its global voice Includes nursing organizations from 130 countries, representing 20 million nurses

NGO, nongovernmental organization; UN, United Nations.
Source: Bill and Melinda Gates Foundation (2019); Doctors Without Borders USA (n.d.); International Council of Nurses (2020); Kaiser Family Foundation (January 24, 2019); Partners in Health (2020); PAHO (n.d.); UNICEF (2016); World Bank Group (2020).

Managing Global Diseases During Epidemics and Pandemics

An example of the interdependency of all nations is the cooperation needed when epidemics or pandemics occur. The WHO has led the way with developing an approach to respond to, coordinate, and assist all nations during such outbreaks.

- The Global Outbreak Alert and Response Network (GOARN) was established by WHO in 2000.
- GOARN initially responded to national outbreaks such as cholera and yellow fever.
- Today GOARN is made up of more than 600 partners, including public health institutions, government agencies, NGOs, and labs specializing in epidemiology.

Through GOARN, the WHO's true impact was first realized with the coordination of the global response to the SARS epidemic in 2002 to 2003. From this response, the WHO established international networks and created standards for mutual assistance in anticipation of future threats (WHO, 2020d). The WHO Health Emergency Dashboard is an interactive web-based platform, refreshed every 15 minutes, that shares real-time information about global public health events and emergencies. Review current public health emergencies on the WHO public emergency dashboard at https://extranet.who.int/publicemergency.

International Health Regulations

In 2005, the International Health Regulations (IHR) of the WHO (2008) was accepted as a legally binding, international treaty between all member states. The IHR require that all countries will independently perform the following (Fig. 16-8):

- Detect: Make sure surveillance systems and laboratories can detect potential threats
- Assess: Work together with other countries to make decisions in public health emergencies
- Report: Report specific diseases, plus any potential international public health emergencies
- Respond: Respond to public health events (CDC, 2015)

Each nation has committed to meeting these four obligations within their own borders and to the development of an internal public health strategy and implementation plan for addressing domestic public health emergencies (WHO, 2020b).

Before public health events happen,

- The IHR direct the WHO (2020a) to provide tools, guidance, and training in support of any country.

During public health events,

- The WHO offers decision support to affected areas for rapid assessment, critical information, and communications, and
- GOARN coordinates sending teams with technical expertise upon request as needed.

According to the IHR reporting protocols, when there is a new reportable event, the affected nation first assesses the public health risk within 48 hours. If the event meets IHR reporting criteria, the country notifies the WHO within 24 hours. The WHO will then assess the event using the Emergency Response Framework (ERF). The ERF provides guidance for the level of response that is indicated. There are four response levels, from Ungraded (requiring no response or monitoring only) to Grade 3 requiring a major response across regions); see Table 16-2. The response needed is based on risk, as follows:

- Very low or low risk event: The WHO team may simply monitor the event. Mitigation, preparedness, and readiness may be part of the low-risk response.
- High or very high-risk event: The Incident Management System may be activated with an appropriately scaled response.

Public Health Emergencies of International Concern

Once Public Health Emergencies of International Concern (PHEIC) are declared, the WHO coordinates an active response with the reporting country and with other countries as indicated (WHO, 2020b). The response may include controlling borders as well as containing the source of the public health threat (WHO, 2020a). These were the steps followed in 2016 by Brazil with the Zika virus outbreak and in 2019 with the novel, SARS-CoV2 outbreak in Wuhan, China (CDC, 2020b, 2020d; CDC Division of Global Health Protection, 2019). Most epidemics or emergencies do not fulfill criteria to be considered a PHEIC. For example, WHO Emergency Committees (ECs) were not convened for the cholera outbreak in Haiti after the earthquake, for the use of chemical weapons in Syria, or following the Fukushima nuclear disaster in Japan (WHO, 2020b).

- Four critical diseases will always be considered extraordinary and require mandatory notification: smallpox, poliomyelitis due to wild-type poliovirus, human influenza due to a new subtype, and severe acute respiratory syndrome (SARS).
- Other conditions are potentially notifiable events according to IHR criteria, whether infectious disease, biological, radiological, or chemical events (CDC Division of Global Health Protection, 2019). See Figure 16-8.
- Review the IHR reporting requirements at https://wwwn.cdc.gov/nndss/ihr.html

Global Influenza Surveillance Network

Another important cooperative agency is the Global Influenza Surveillance and Response System (GISRS), a network of international laboratories established in 1952 by the WHO. GISRS has emerged as a critical player coordinating worldwide efforts for surveillance and control of influenza. Functions of GISRS include the following:

- Maintaining physical presence in 144 National Influenza Centres (NICs), 6 WHO Collaborating Centres, 4 Essential Regulatory Laboratories, and 13 WHO H5 reference laboratories (WHO, n.d., p. 1)
- Recommending the composition of twice yearly seasonal influenza vaccine, and aid in its development

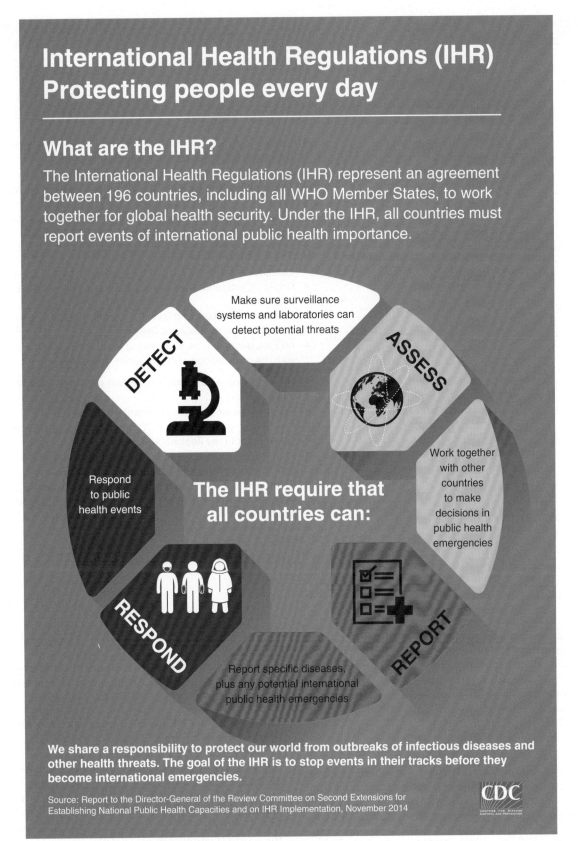

FIGURE 16-8 International health regulations. (Reprinted from CDC. (2015). *International Health Regulations (IHR). Protecting people every day*. Retrieved from https://www.cdc.gov/globalhealth/healthprotection/ghs/ihr/ihr-infographic.html)

TABLE 16-2 WHO Emergency Response Framework (ERF) Levels for Graded Emergencies

Level	Definition/WHO Response	Additional Information
Ungraded	A public health event or emergency ■ Monitoring only ■ **No** operational response	■ Does not require a WHO operational response
Grade 1	■ Single-country emergency ■ Requires **limited** response	■ Exceeds the usual country-level cooperation that the WHO Country Once (WCO) has with the Member State. ■ Most WHO response can be managed with in-country assets. ■ Organizational and/or external support required by the WCO is limited. ■ Provision of support to the WCO is coordinated by an Emergency Coordinator in the Regional Office.
Grade 2	■ Single-country or multiple-country emergency ■ Requires **moderate** response	■ The level of response required by WHO always exceeds the capacity of the WCO. ■ Organizational and/or external support required by the WCO is moderate. ■ Provision of support to the WCO is coordinated by an Emergency Coordinator in the Regional Office. ■ An Emergency Officer is appointed at WHO headquarters to assist with the coordination of Organization-wide support.
Grade 3	■ Single-country or multiple-country emergency ■ Requires **major or maximal** response	■ Organizational and/or external support required by the WCO is major. ■ Requires the mobilization of Organization-wide assets. ■ Provision of support to the WCO is coordinated by an Emergency Coordinator in the Regional Office(s). ■ An Emergency Officer is appointed at WHO headquarters to assist with the coordination of Organization-wide inputs. ■ On occasion, the WHE Executive Director and the Regional Director may agree to have the Emergency Coordinator based in headquarters. ■ For events or emergencies involving multiple regions, an Incident Management Support Team at headquarters will coordinate the response across the regions.

Source: WHO (2018a).

- Posting on an open access platform for the specific gene sequence of an influenza virus (reference viruses)
- Providing open access to confirmed lab protocols for testing and disease confirmation
- Developing test kits for shipping to requesting countries free of charge (Association of Public Health Labs, 2011)

Global Health Security Agenda

In 2014, the United States helped launch the Global Health Security Agenda (GHSA), an independent group of 67 countries, international organizations, nongovernmental organizations, and private sector companies who also have as their vision a world that is safe and secure from infectious diseases. The GHSA (n.d.) 2024 target is for 100 countries to complete assessment, planning, and mobilization to minimize gaps in health care services. Each country has agreed to demonstrate improvement in at least 5 of 11 technical areas according to measures within the WHO IHR Monitoring and Evaluation Framework. Because of GHSA partnerships, when SARS-CoV2 became a PHEIC, there was more information readily available to all nations than in any previous outbreak (CDC, 2020f). See Figures 16-9 and 16-10.

One Health

One Health is a coordinated approach, recognizing that PHEICs are increasingly related to the interconnectedness between humans, the health of animals, and our shared physical environment. The One Health initiative cuts across all sectors of society from local, regional, national, and global levels. It is especially crucial for low-resource emerging economies, but novel infectious diseases (e.g., Ebola, COVID-19) can impact many countries around the world (Gebreyes et al., 2014).

- The Food and Agricultural Organization of the U.N. (FAO, 2020) uses a One Health interconnected approach with an established early warning monitoring system to alert for changes in zoonotic diseases, food safety, and agricultural production.

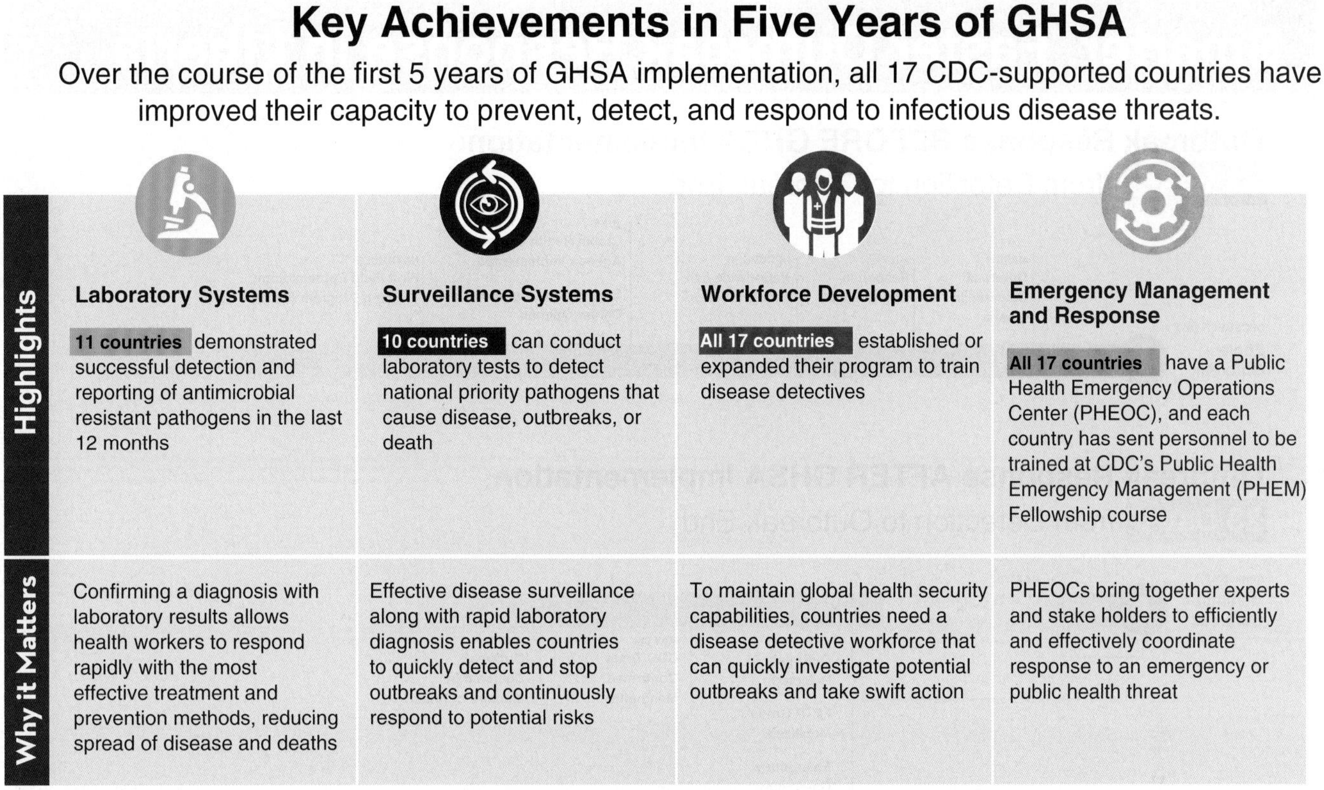

Key Achievements in Five Years of GHSA

Over the course of the first 5 years of GHSA implementation, all 17 CDC-supported countries have improved their capacity to prevent, detect, and respond to infectious disease threats.

	Laboratory Systems	Surveillance Systems	Workforce Development	Emergency Management and Response
Highlights	**11 countries** demonstrated successful detection and reporting of antimicrobial resistant pathogens in the last 12 months	**10 countries** can conduct laboratory tests to detect national priority pathogens that cause disease, outbreaks, or death	**All 17 countries** established or expanded their program to train disease detectives	**All 17 countries** have a Public Health Emergency Operations Center (PHEOC), and each country has sent personnel to be trained at CDC's Public Health Emergency Management (PHEM) Fellowship course
Why it Matters	Confirming a diagnosis with laboratory results allows health workers to respond rapidly with the most effective treatment and prevention methods, reducing spread of disease and deaths	Effective disease surveillance along with rapid laboratory diagnosis enables countries to quickly detect and stop outbreaks and continuously respond to potential risks	To maintain global health security capabilities, countries need a disease detective workforce that can quickly investigate potential outbreaks and take swift action	PHEOCs bring together experts and stake holders to efficiently and effectively coordinate response to an emergency or public health threat

FIGURE 16-9 Key achievements in 5 years of GHSA. (Reprinted from Centers for Disease Control and Prevention (CDC). (2020). *Key achievements in five years of GHSA*. Retrieved from https://www.cdc.gov/globalhealth/resources/factsheets/5-years-of-ghsa.html)

- In the United States, the CDC uses One Health to gain an understanding about how diseases spread among people, animals, and the environment.
- The foundation of One Health is three-fold: the multidisciplinary cooperation for communication, coordination of effort, and collaboration on activities at the animal–human–environment interface (CDC, 2018). See Figure 16-11.

Review the One Health in Action Web site: https://www.cdc.gov/onehealth/in-action/index.html

- Select one of the listed case studies. Identify the partnerships across disciplines, involved animals, and the environmental impact.
- What resolution for health was achieved? What was the role of cross-discipline cooperation?

The Centers for Disease Control and Prevention

In the United States, the Centers for Disease Control and Prevention (CDC, 2020b, 2020c) is the agency responsible for leading the federal response to an internal public health emergency. Each state is also required to have a strategic plan outlining the response of each local health agency (LHA). When a local public health event or emergency occurs somewhere within the United States, the LHA reports upstream to the state who then reports to the CDC. If the event has a potential international impact, the CDC evaluates the event according to the WHO IHR, as described above, and reports the concern to the WHO, as indicated for monitoring or mobilization of international support (CDC, 2017a, 2020e). See the infographic Anatomy of an Outbreak at http://thepoint.lww.com/Rector10e.

The CDC also has an outward facing global mission supporting global health security and disease outbreak investigation throughout the world. CDC scientists work collaboratively through 10 state-of-the-art global disease detection (GDD) Centers located in different regions of the world (CDC, 2017b). The expertise of the GDD centers evolved over the first four global epidemics of the 21st century (see Fig. 16-7).

The CDC plays a lead role in global health security when outbreaks occur anywhere. CDC disease experts join with stakeholders to address more than 400 diseases and health threats. Strengthening critical public health services globally protects Americans and saves lives worldwide. The CDC also maintains an emergency surge staff of responders ready to be deployed as needed. See Figure 16-12.

Partners in the CDC response effort include the following:

- Foreign governments and ministries of health
- Other U.S. government agencies
- The WHO and other international organizations
- Academic institutions
- Foundations
- Nongovernmental organizations (NGOs)
- Faith-based organizations
- Businesses and other private organizations

The C/PHN may participate with One Health principles anywhere and everywhere. The C/PHN's response

Smarter, Faster Outbreak Response in Liberia

Outbreak Response BEFORE GHSA Implementation:

+2 Years from Detection to Outbreak End

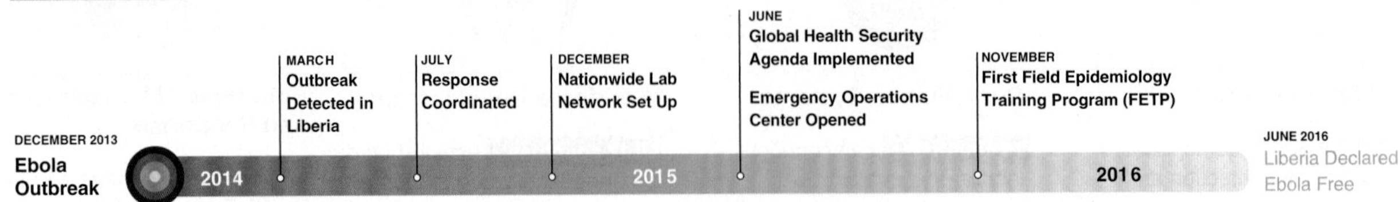

Outbreak Response AFTER GHSA Implementation:

23 Days from Detection to Outbreak End

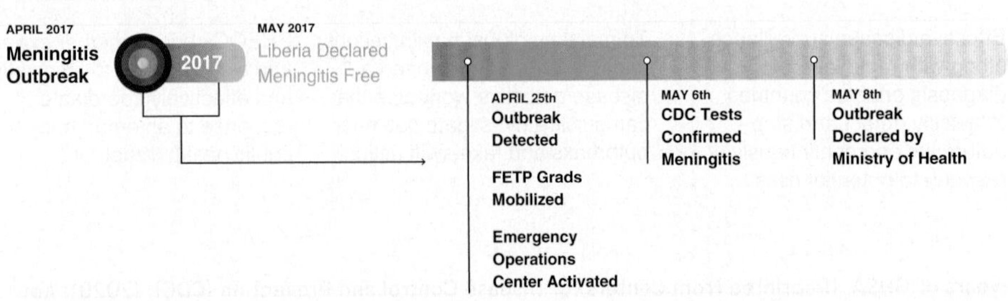

FIGURE 16-10 Outbreak response in Liberia before and after GHSA. (Reprinted from Centers for Disease Control and Prevention (CDC). (2020). Retrieved from https://www.cdc.gov/globalhealth/security/ghsa5year/outbreak-response.html)

during an infectious disease epidemic or pandemic may include one or more areas of focus as described by the WHO (2018a, 2018c):

Focus 1. Provide community education in support of an individual's response, such as wearing masks in public, handwashing, and physical distancing.

Focus 2. Explain evolving risk with communication to support life-saving actions using local data indicators.

Focus 3. Facilitate access to timely treatment for persons who display symptoms and ensure protection of the health care workforce.

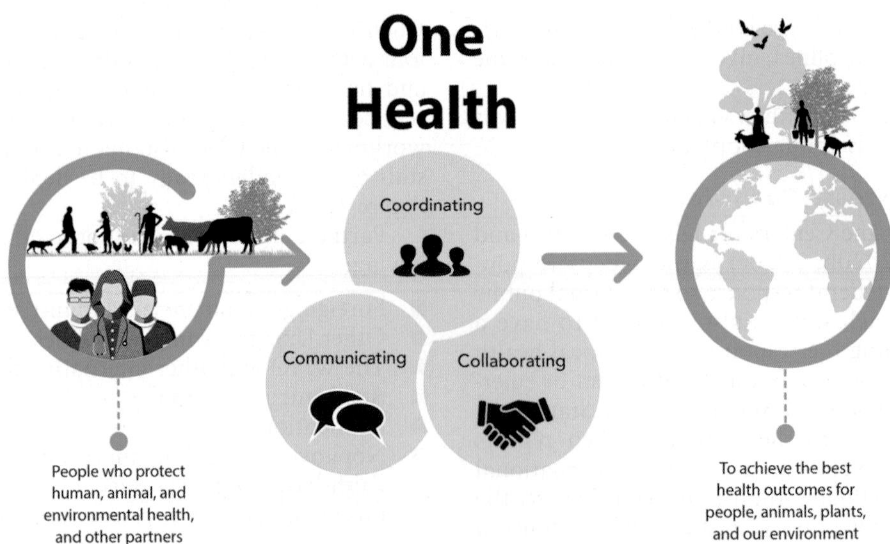

FIGURE 16-11 One health. (Reprinted from Centers for Disease Control and Prevention (CDC). (2018). Retrieved from https://www.cdc.gov/onehealth/images/multimedia/one-health-definition-graphic-with-bats.jpg)

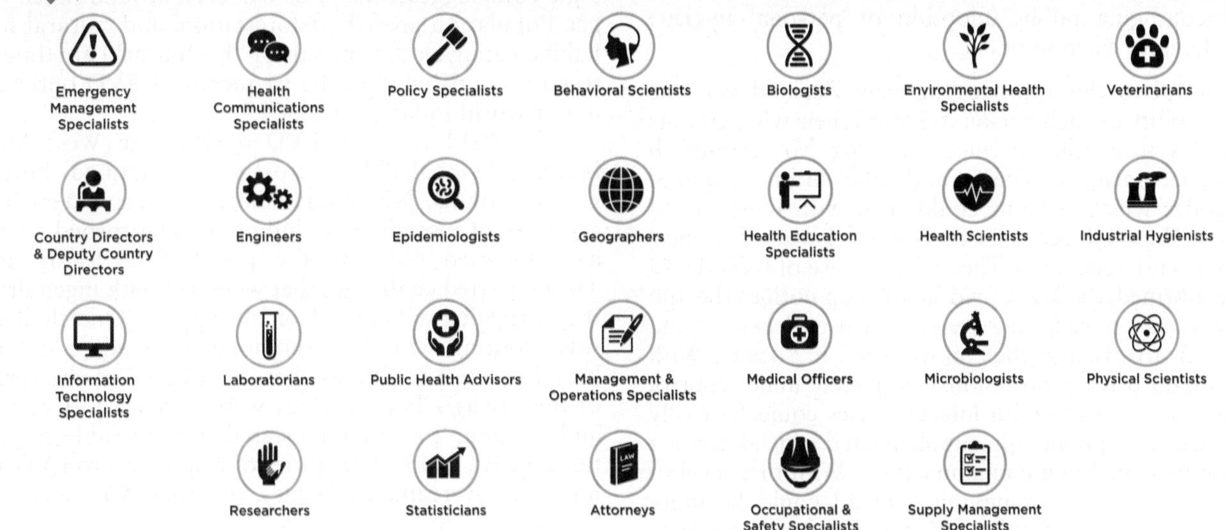

FIGURE 16-12 CDC's emergency response surge staff. (Reprinted from Centers for Disease Control and Prevention (CDC). (2017). Retrieved from https://www.cdc.gov/globalhealth/infographics/global-health-security/global-rapid-response-team.html)

Review the variety of disciplines represented in the CDC's Emergency Response Surge Staff (depicted in Fig. 16-12).

- Which disciplines are a surprise?
- Which surge staff role would you be interested in joining? Why?

View stories on creative global health partnerships with the CDC. https://www.cdc.gov/globalhealth/stories/

SARS-CoV2 (COVID-19)

In late December 2019, China gave an initial report to the WHO about an outbreak cluster of an unusual respiratory disease in the city of Wuhan. A week after the Chinese report, the WHO (2020h) announced to the world the preliminary identification of a previously unknown novel coronavirus named SARS-CoV2. At that time, nothing was known about where the virus came from or how it spread.

- Within 2 weeks of the report to the WHO in mid-January 2020, Chinese health officials posted the full genetic sequence of the virus online in the public genetic sequencing database, GenBank, at the National Institutes of Health (NIH). This made it possible for labs worldwide to develop lab tests and to make firm diagnoses on travelers from China who showed symptoms (National Center for Biotechnology Information [NCBI], 2020).
- By late January 2020, the CDC activated its Emergency Operations Center to assist in the global response to the epidemic. A few days later, the CDC had developed a real-time test to diagnose the disease using clinical specimens from affected patients. Several different lab assays from top labs worldwide were also posted online, providing lab protocols freely and globally (CDC, 2020c).
- The UK provided a large grant to the Coalition for Epidemic Preparedness Innovations (CEPI), a global pharmaceutical company whose goal was to release a vaccine within 6 to 8 months of the first announcement of the epidemic (CEPI, 2020). On the 11th of August, 2020, the Russian Federation reported approval of a vaccine (Sputnik V), bypassing the usual protocol of completing phase three trials before release. By the end of August, 2020 4 other vaccines were in phase three trials, 7 others were in phase two, and 15 others were in phase one. Additional vaccine candidates were in either early research or preclinical phases (Craven, 2020).

This initial response between the member states of the WHO in the first month after identification of the new disease demonstrated a coordinated worldwide action following the guidelines of the IHR. As the virus spread worldwide, different countries implemented their national plans in whole or in part, while some countries delayed their plans or ended efforts prematurely.

New Zealand was successful in eliminating COVID-19 within 6 months of the initial outbreak by embracing standard epidemiology measures (Ministry of Health–Manatū Hauora, 2020a). These actions included the following:

- Sequestering at home during the initial outbreak
- Maintaining robust border controls
- Implementing widespread testing of the population
- Providing rapid isolation of infected individuals

- Managing comprehensive contact tracing of patients with confirmed cases using public health informatics
- Launching a personal phone app for creating the digital diary of places visited (NZ Covid Tracer app)
- Enforcing quarantine of those who had contact with confirmed cases
- Encouraging public adoption of personal hygiene behaviors when in public

Central to the approach in New Zealand was the responsibility of each person to record their whereabouts every day to accelerate contact tracing. To accomplish their cyber-tracing, businesses and public locations posted QR codes which persons could scan with their smartphones. These QR scans created digital diaries of an individual's daily itineraries. Then when a case of COVID-19 was confirmed, the NZ Covid Tracer app notifies the app user that they have been exposed. The user decides if and to whom to disclose their movements in society. With strong data privacy provisions completely under control of the user, contacts with infected cases could be easily identified. The phone app supplemented official contact tracing by expediting communication. With that level of speedy notification, community spread could be more successfully managed as New Zealand society reopened.

New Zealand citizens were quick to participate, following the slogan of the app: "Protect yourself, your whānau [extended family], and your community" (Ministry of Health, 2020b, para. 1).

As stated by the New Zealand Ministry of Health (2020a, para. 1), their elimination strategy was a "sustained approach to keep it out, find it out, and stamp it out." The goals embraced standard public health epidemiology responses to prevent transmission of new cases from overseas travelers, develop effective treatments, and embrace an eventual vaccine.

- Watch a video explaining the use of the NZ Tracer App at https://youtu.be/j3GdnugLles.
- Explore this novel use of public health informatics at the NZ Tracer App Web site: https://tracing.covid19.govt.nz/.

As of early May 2020, no new, locally spread cases were reported in New Zealand, but a cluster of cases (about 30) erupted in early August 2020. The alert level was quickly raised to 3 in the affected Aukland area, and only essential movement was permitted, while the remainder of the country was raised to a level 2 that prohibited mass gatherings and promoted more social distancing. The search for the source of the outbreak was ongoing during early September (Lewis, 2020).

By August 31, 2020, the United States had 6,023,368 confirmed cases of COVID-19, and 183,431 confirmed deaths—the highest total numbers in the world. However, the U.S. case fatality ratio falls in the middle of the 20 most affected countries. Worldwide, a total of 25,344,339 confirmed cases were reported, and confirmed deaths were reported at 848,084 (Johns Hopkins Coronavirus Resource Center, 2020). For a world map indicating outbreaks, see: https://extranet.who.int/publicemergency.

Ebola

Ebola disease virus (EDV) is an infectious disease with repeated outbreaks, mostly in Africa. Although EDV was first identified in 1976 in an outbreak near the Ebola river in the Democratic Republic of Congo (DRC), epidemiologic data suggests the virus has been around much longer. Population growth, deforestation, and cultural food habits (eating exotic animals or "bushmeat") are thought to have contributed to the frequency of EVD outbreaks in our world today (CDC, 2019).

The 2014 to 2016 EVD outbreak in West Africa became a global PHEIC crossing international borders within months. Numerous emergency responders from a variety of disciplines including nursing rushed to help as teams tried to contain the spread of the deadly virus. They reported challenges that were met with ingenuity as they struggled without adequate supplies. One challenge was working with the communities to adapt cultural burial practice traditions that contributed to the spread of the disease. Two vaccines were ultimately developed and continue to be administered to vulnerable populations (CDC, 2019). For stories of responders to EVD and how they overcame challenges, visit these Web sites:

- Ebola outbreak responder stories: https://www.cdc.gov/about/24-7/cdcresponders/
- Ebola reports on overcoming challenges: http://www.cdc.gov/about/ebola/overcoming-challenges.html

Tuberculosis

Tuberculosis (TB) is an infectious disease caused by the tubercle bacillus (see Chapter 8). TB has been known for hundreds of years and was commonly referred to as *consumption*. Over time, the causative organism has become resistant to the medications used to treat it. TB continues as a world-wide chronic endemic disease. The WHO continues the Stop TB campaign that realized a milestone in 2018 when 7 million people were diagnosed and treated. There is an SDG to eradicate TB by 2030; however, large gaps in detection and treatment have led to an estimated 3 million people still not receiving the care they need (WHO, 2020k).

- One quarter of the world's population is thought to be infected, but only 5% to 15% of those become symptomatic within their lifetime.
- TB disproportionately affects poor people around the world.

Multidrug resistant TB (MDR-TB) is an increasing problem around the world.

- Globally, estimates of new cases of MDR-TB are 4.1%, with 240,000 deaths from MDR-TB in 2016.
- MDR-TB threatens to reverse progress made with the Stop TB campaign (WHO, 2020c).

Malaria

Malaria is a serious and sometimes fatal disease caused by the parasite *Plasmodium falciparum* or *Plasmodium vivax*. Malaria is a vector-borne disease spread by bites of the female Anopheles mosquito. Vaccines against

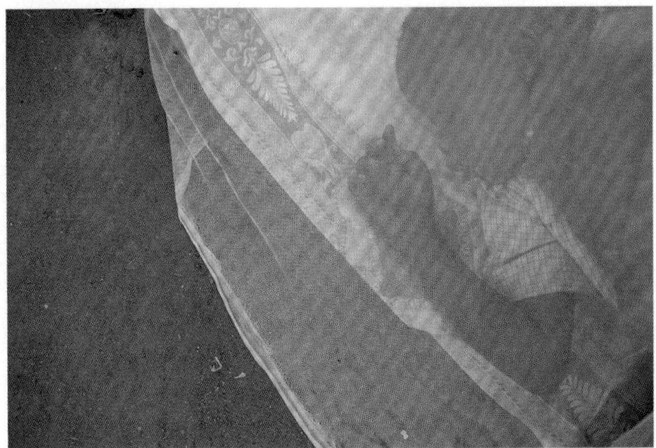

FIGURE 16-13 A child sleeping under a mosquito net in a refugee camp in South Sudan.

parasites are difficult to create. Even though it is a serious disease, illness and death from malaria can usually be prevented with appropriate interventions such as sleeping under bed nets (Fig. 16-13) and complying with medical treatment. Malaria disproportionately affects people living in poverty, especially impacting people of working age with damaging effects on emerging economies.

- In 1998, half the world was at risk for malaria. The Roll Back Malaria (RBM) Program, an ambitious international campaign, was launched with the goal to reduce the global burden of malaria (CDC, 2020g).
- Led by the WHO, UNICEF, UN Development Programme (UNDP), and the World Bank, 500 partners joined together in the RBM worldwide action plan.
- By 2003, RBM showed disappointing results.
- By 2010, a revised goal was accepted to reduce the incidence of malaria by 50% worldwide.
- In 2019, half the world remained at risk (End Malaria, n.d.).

Then, three interventions were developed in rapid order that gave the world hope that malaria could be entirely eliminated. A new campaign, End Malaria (EM), replaced RBM. The three ongoing interventions with EM are as follows:

1. Artemisinin-based oral drug therapy: An estimated 3 billion courses of therapy were completed between 2010 and 2018.
2. Insecticide-treated mosquito nets (ITNs): Between 2016 and 2018, 578 million ITNs were delivered globally.
3. Rapid diagnostic lab tests (RDTs): In 2018, 412 million RDTs were distributed globally (End Malaria, n.d.).

The End Malaria program was renewed to focus on endemic regions with the goal to control malaria by 2030.

- By 2018, 27 countries reported fewer than 100 indigenous cases.
- By 2019, the WHO awarded certification of elimination with zero indigenous cases to Paraguay, Uzbekistan, Algeria, Argentina, China, El Salvador, Iran, Malaysia, and Timor-Leste.
- Current focus is on sub-Saharan Africa to eliminate 228 million global cases and eliminate 405,000 deaths (End Malaria, n.d.).

The challenge remains in countries with emerging economies where there are large populations without sewer systems and clean water sources. Because people prefer to build their homes close to sources of water, mosquitoes that carry malaria are attracted to the standing water in those communities (Fig. 16-14).

The primary role of the C/PHN to end malaria is as a community educator. The topics of client education would cover simple measures:

- Proper placement and use of netting around a bed during the night
- Elimination of pools of standing water around the home
- Covering the body with light cotton clothes (Department of Health, Republic of South Africa, 2020).

Balami, Said, Zulkefli, Bachok, and Audu (2019) provided a malaria education program to pregnant women and found significant improvements in motivation, knowledge, and skills. Women were taught how to use insecticide-treated bed nets and received intermittent preventive medication during their clinic visits. See Box 16-4.

- Watch this video to see how the RBM campaign evolved. Partnership to End Malaria—20th Anniversary (2:23): https://youtu.be/iuq6-H1HuAM.
- Visit the Malaria Vaccine Initiative Web site to see the challenges for making a vaccine: https://www.malariavaccine.org/malaria-and-vaccines/vaccine-development/life-cycle-malaria-parasite.

Global HIV/AIDS Response

HIV has claimed the lives of more than 32 million people since HIV was identified in 1985. Between 2000 and 2018, as a result of global initiatives implementing evidenced-based practices, new HIV infections fell by 37% saving 13.6 million lives (WHO, 2020).

By the end of 2019, this was the global status of HIV/AIDS:

- New cases: approximately 800,000 new HIV cases confirmed with Sub-Saharan Africa accounting for nearly 66% of new infections globally

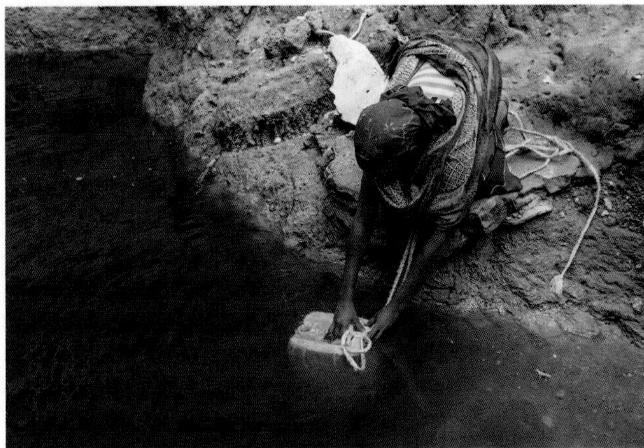

FIGURE 16-14 A woman gets water from a well to take back to her village.

- Living with HIV: an estimated 38 million people worldwide lived with HIV

Annual deaths: 690,000 million people died annually from HIV-related causes. (Avert, 2018; WHO, 2020g). Although there remains no cure for HIV infection, effective treatment controls the virus so people live productive lives. Treatment also helps prevent transmission. Current trends in HIV care focus on prevention, early testing, and treatment. With surveillance testing, people can know their status and take measures to either remain HIV negative or start treatment, thus preventing transmission to others. See Chapter 8.

- HIV is diagnosed through rapid diagnostic tests that provide same day results.
- Once HIV-positive status is known, treatment with antiretroviral therapy (ART) is initiated.
- Globally, in 2018, 62% of adults and 54% of children living with HIV were receiving ART.
- Concurrent assessment and treatment for possible TB infections and prevention of mother-to-child transmission have shown positive outcomes for improving maternal health and reducing HIV transmission to newborns (WHO, 2020a).

The success of HIV/AIDS management is noted by its change in status among the top 10 causes of death between 2000 and 2016, comparing the World to African and European Regions (Fig.16-15).

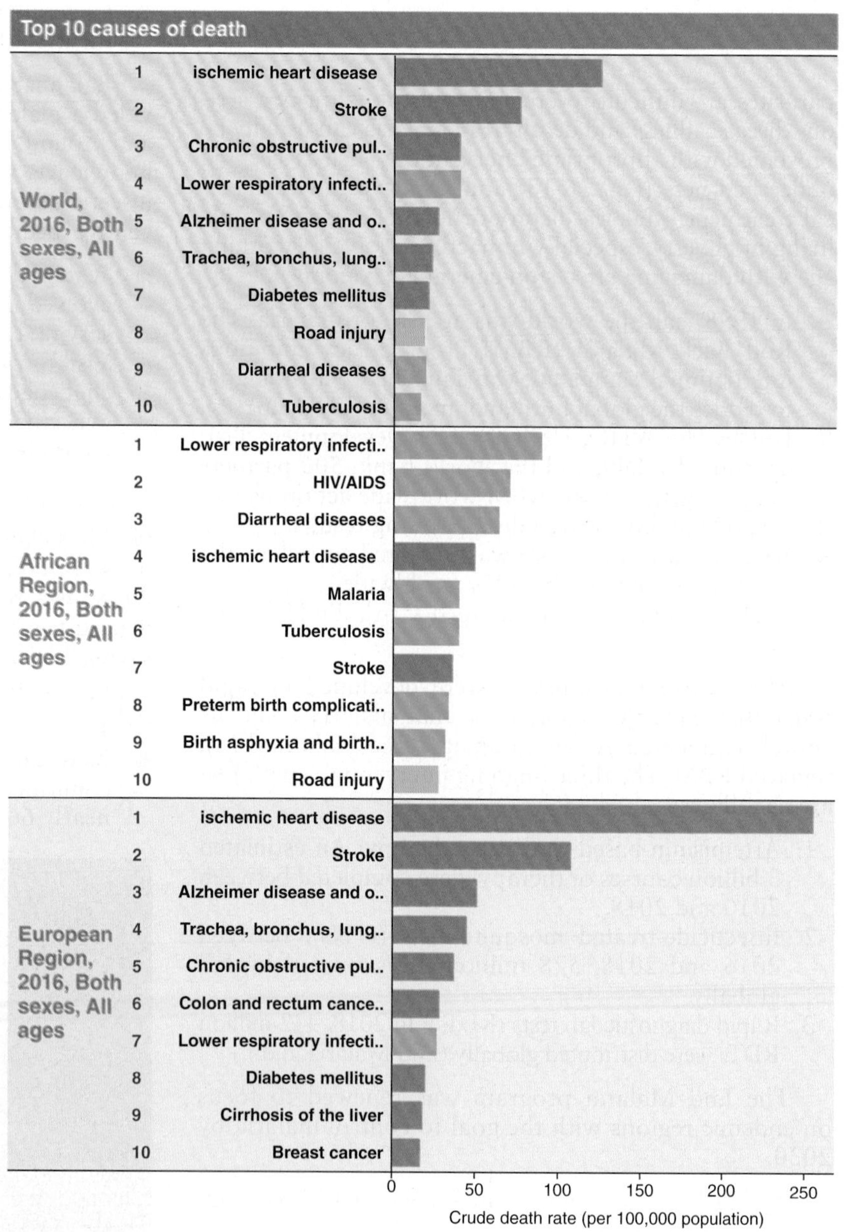

FIGURE 16-15 Ranking of 10 leading causes of death worldwide: European and African regions compared, all ages, both sexes, 2016. (Reprinted with permission from Global Health Observatory (GHO). (2018). *Top 10 causes of death* [Online interactive dashboard]. Available at https://www.who.int/gho/mortality_burden_disease/causes_death/top_10/en/)

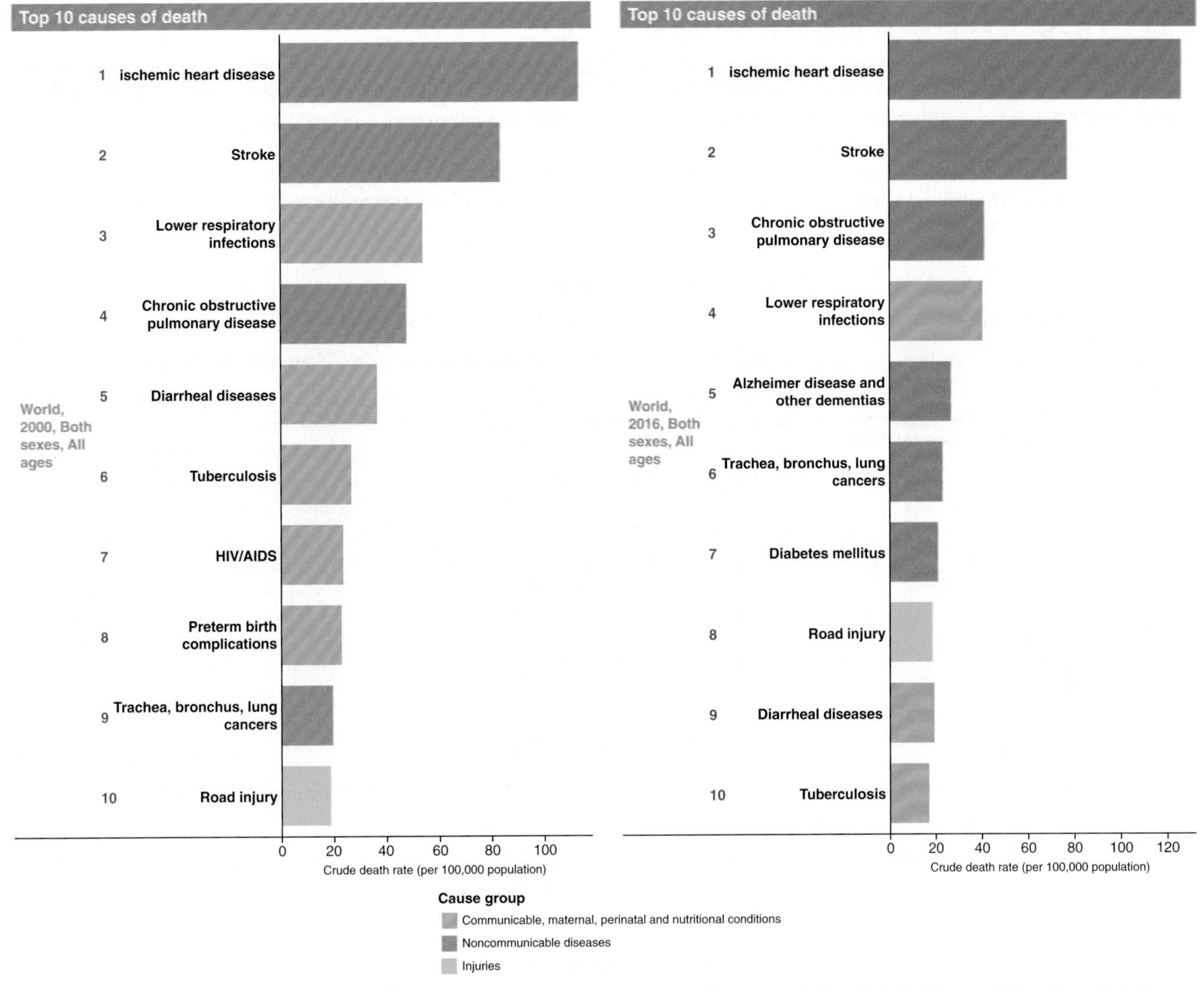

FIGURE 16-16 Global death rate per 100,000: Selected causes, 2000 and 2016 compared. (Reprinted with permission from Global Health Observatory (GHO). (2018). *Top 10 causes of death* [Online interactive dashboard]. Available at https://www.who.int/gho/mortality_burden_disease/causes_death/top_10/en/)

- Examine how other top 10 causes of death worldwide have changed between 2000 and 2016 (Fig. 16-16).
- Explore the WHO interactive webpage, Sexual and Reproductive Health and Rights and HIV (SRHHIV) linkages toolkit, to learn more about recent, relevant, and important resources: http://toolkit.srhhivlinkages.org/.

Acute Respiratory Tract Infections

The most common illness in the world and a leading cause of mortality is acute respiratory tract infection (ARI; Box 16-5). Pneumonia is the leading cause of death in children under 5 years of age, claiming nearly 1 million children annually. It is treatable, especially when caught early. Simple interventions such as vaccines, good nutrition, safe hygiene practices, and improved indoor air quality can help avoid ARI altogether (WHO, 2018b).

- Primary risk factors include low birth weight, poverty, crowding, lower educational levels, poor nutrition including early weaning, inadequate childcare practices, a lack of health education about ARI, and delays in seeking treatment.
- Additional risk factors include smoking and air pollution, both indoor and outdoor.
- Indoor air pollution is much higher among villages in areas experiencing poverty.
- Indoor air pollution is mostly from indoor cook stoves that use organic fuel and kerosene.
- Worldwide, over 2.4 billion people, mostly living in poverty, burn wood, coal, peat, and dung-cake inside their homes.
- Indoor cooking stoves kill 3.8 million people annually and are a contributing factor in 45% of all pneumonia deaths in children <5 years old.
- The risk of pneumonia in children is doubled with exposure to indoor air pollution (Ashwani & Kalosona, 2016; WHO, 2018b). See Fig. 16-17.

Measures for better control of ARI include immunizations, birth spacing, better nutrition including breast feeding, improved living conditions (including the use of smokeless cooking stoves), and immunizations.

BOX 16-5 LEVELS OF PREVENTION PYRAMID

Acute Respiratory Infection in Children

SITUATION: Acute respiratory tract infections (ARIs) that affect the lower respiratory tract and lungs, such as pneumonia and influenza, are among the leading causes of death in children worldwide.

GOAL: Prevent acute respiratory tract infections in children in developing countries. Using the three levels of prevention, partner with communities and families to avoid risk factors, to promptly diagnose and treat negative health conditions, and to restore health to the fullest possible potential.

Tertiary Prevention

Rehabilitation	*Treatment and Focused Prevention*	
	Health Promotion and Education	***Health Protection***
▪ Provide adequate nutrition. ▪ Provide adequate rest. ▪ Restore child to optimal level of functioning through the recovery period.	▪ Diagnose and treat ARIs early. ▪ Monitor for hypoxemia with pulse oximetry. ▪ Provide oxygen therapy with oxygen concentrators as indicated. ▪ Provide culturally appropriate symptomatic care. ▪ Reinforce compliance with treatment plan. ▪ Teach caregiver the signs and symptoms of complications.	▪ Educate for prevention of recurrence and spread of disease. ▪ Promote practices that prevent spread of disease among family members.

Secondary Prevention

Early Diagnosis	*Surveillance and Focused Prevention*
▪ Teach caregivers when to seek medical attention for an ARI. ▪ Refer early for prompt diagnosis of ARI to prevent further progression and ensure cost-effective management.	▪ Administer appropriate immunizations. ▪ Screen and monitor children for early signs and symptoms of ARI.

Primary Prevention

Health Promotion and Education	*Health Protection for Respiratory Conditions*
▪ Promote general health education among community members. ▪ Teach good hygiene and childcare practices. ▪ Promote child spacing and good prenatal care. ▪ Support exclusive infant breast-feeding with adequate nutrition after weaning. ▪ Eliminate poverty and household crowding.	▪ Promote early prenatal care to avoid low birth weight ▪ Promote healthy nutrition habits, including breastfeeding for infants. ▪ Treat all respiratory infections (HIV, TB, ARI). ▪ Reduce or avoid exposure to common respiratory risk factors such as indoor cook stoves without chimneys. ▪ Avoid direct or indirect exposure to smoke, including cigarette, cigar, or pipe smoking, and wood smoke.

One threat to reducing the incidence of pneumonia, however, is the increase in drug-resistant organisms. **Community health workers** (local people trained by health professionals) are being trained to diagnose and promptly treat early signs of pneumonia, when drugs will be the most effective, along with other environmentally related interventions. The C/PHN can also provide community education encouraging mothers to seek care and treatment early. See Figure 16-17.

These selected conditions show the impact when people are exposed to emerging health conditions with environmental impact. Global health issues become everyone's concerns when conditions spread within or beyond borders. When we commit resources to any country in need, we all benefit.

Interdependence of Nations During Migration

When hardships come, people would rather try to adapt and stay where they are, but if there is limited assistance from their government to remain, then people will leave. Populations may relocate within their own countries or move across borders or oceans to find safety after natural disasters. Climate change in today's world, which causes more frequent and severe wildfires (Fig. 16-18) and rising oceans

FIGURE 16-17 Protecting children from the environment. (Reprinted with permission from World Health Organization (WHO). (2020i). *Protecting children from the environment* [PHE Infographic]. Retrieved from https://www.who.int/phe/infographics/protecting-children-from-the-environment/en/)

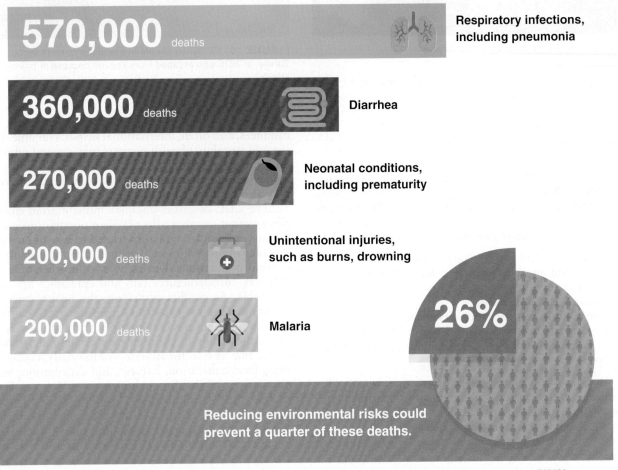

(from melting glacial ice), can result in population migration. Population movement may also be in response to

- Economic opportunities for workers and their families
- a nation's need to invite immigrants to offset low birthrates
- Large migrations of people fleeing violence or armed conflict (Fig. 16-19), or
- Food insecurity (UN Department of Economic and Social Affairs, 2017)

In each case, the challenge is to ensure that human rights are met first, followed by the maintenance of environmental law and refugee or migration law. In 2016, the UN adopted the Global Compact for Migration as a framework for international cooperation for orderly migration. Unfortunately, the actual migration process has become quite political. As of 2020, there were no global agreements or policies to support either present migration humanitarian crises or the impact on environmental rights breaches (Corendea, 2018; Gamlen & Gamlen, 2019).

- View the UN University video, *How-to Guide for Environmental Refugees*, describing the migration events of Carteret Islanders in Papua New Guinea at https://ourworld.unu.edu/en/how-to-guide-for-environmental-refugees

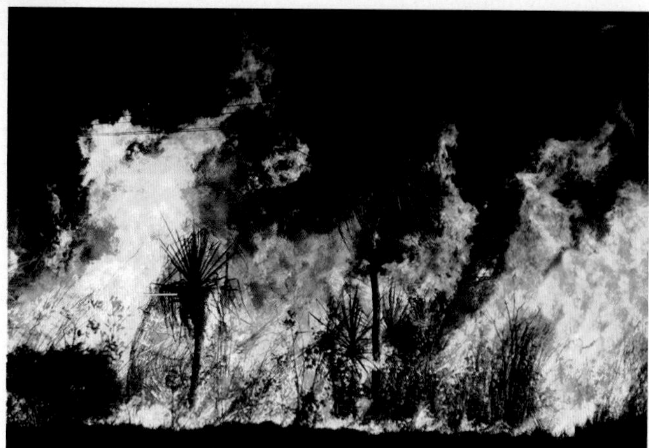

FIGURE 16-18 An Australian brushfire.

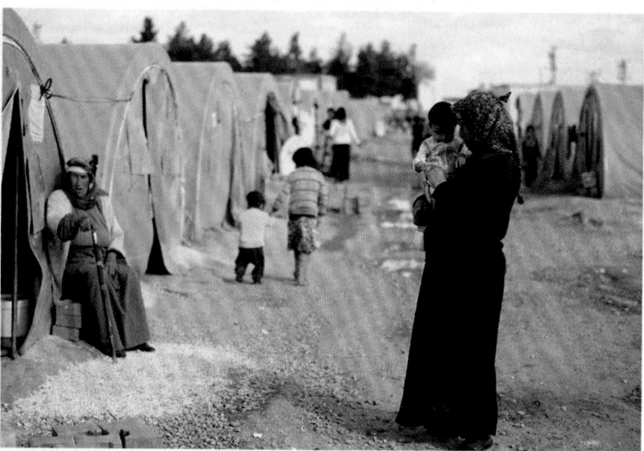

FIGURE 16-19 Syrian people in a refugee camp in Suruç, Turkey, in 2015 who escaped from Kobane because of Islamic state attack.

- Explore the Web site for the UN International Organization for Migration at: https://www.iom.int/wmr/

Armed Conflict, Uprisings, Wars, and Humanitarian Emergencies

An armed conflict is defined as major if the number of deaths has reached 1,000. Increasingly, conflicts are internal rather than between nations. Combatants seeking economic and political power often target the lives and livelihoods of civilians associated with opposing factions (Clark & Simeon, 2016; Themnér & Wallensteen, 2013).

- Armed conflicts and uprisings initially cause governments and agencies to place a high priority on injuries, but the ability to sustain routine health care is reduced as time goes on.
- The health infrastructure itself becomes vulnerable during conflicts and uprisings as a consequence of political instability. Often, opposing factions raid hospitals and clinics.

During national conflicts, health services become disorganized with decreased resources from disrupted supply chains. Such actions have been repeated over the years as conflicts have emerged. See Box 16-6.

C/PHNs need to become aware of who is involved in an immediate local conflict and who is influencing the situation from abroad. Outside help is needed in these instances, and often, international help is available. Funding and sustaining health projects may depend ultimately on a variety of factors, not the least of which is providing care when the safety and survival of patients and nurses may also be threatened.

The CDC describes complex humanitarian emergencies as situations that affect civilian populations and distinguishes them from factors related to war or civil strife, shortage of necessities such as food, and the displacement of local populations. During wars and other man-made disasters, infrastructures fail, and epidemics are almost inevitable. As conflict wears on, the health care needs of the combatants often take priority over health care needs of civilians. As communities and families are relocated, thousands of children may be injured, orphaned, or become at risk for disease. Additionally, conflict disrupts food cultivation, harvest, and distribution, leaving populations at risk for malnutrition, which can lead to disease (Clark & Simeon, 2016; WHO, 2017). These circumstances can result in complex humanitarian emergencies, with increased mortality rates beyond what is expected under normal circumstances (Abbas et al., 2018). See Box 16-7.

BOX 16-6 PERSPECTIVES

A World Health Organization Regional Advisor's Viewpoint on the Effect of War on International Cooperation

During the war in Yugoslavia, Bosnians and Serbs worked with the European Regional Office of the World Health Organization (WHO/EURO) in Copenhagen, Denmark, to develop interventions for women and children's health. WHO/EURO developed the training program to be held in Denmark but was not certain that the roads between Sarajevo and the coast would be open and safe for travel. Snipers had continued operating in the mountains surrounding Sarajevo and along the roads to the country's borders. Once the workshop started in Copenhagen, the nurses, physicians, and midwives, both Bosnians and Serbs, collaborated professionally during breakout sessions. However, the facilitator had to ensure separate dining spaces, because casual communication was difficult and awkward while the conflict was ongoing.

Marie, WHO regional advisor

BOX 16-7 WHAT DO *YOU* THINK?

Effects of Conflict on International Cooperation

In today's world, international cooperation could collapse due to changing national relationships, internal disruptions from natural disasters or violence, or political disagreements over policies such as withdrawal from the Paris Agreement on climate. What would be some of the social, political, and economic consequences in terms of health if international cooperation were diminished?

GLOBAL HEALTH ETHICS

Certain ethical considerations guide global health even as basic ethical principles guide the delivery of health care. Ethics of justice, equality, diversity, and inclusivity become even more important in an interconnected, multicultural world.

Clinical Service Learning for the C/PHN

Opportunities for participating in a global health activity may be offered for experiential learning. C/PHNs should familiarize themselves with global health ethical considerations whether engaging with global communities to conduct research or deliver clinical care in the community. Positive outcomes for the C/PHN from community and global health service learning include the following:

- Increased awareness caring for patients who are economically and socially disadvantaged
- Improved cultural awareness
- Increased interest in public health and primary care career-related opportunities.

Communities who host C/PHN students also enjoy documented benefits. These include the following:

- An influx of resources
- Extra hands
- Extra supplies and equipment

The presence of well-trained health volunteers can lead to skills transfer within the community, either intentionally through education or more indirectly through observation. Volunteers and host communities may develop a sense of solidarity. Sometimes the host community may gain social capital with nearby communities because foreign health care providers have spent time with them (Lasker et al., 2018).

Ethical Considerations for the Global Health Volunteer

C/PHNs and host communities. Enjoy mutual benefit when all parties are mindful of three main ethical considerations:

1. The weight of authority
2. The volunteer effect
3. The burden of hosting (Lasker et al., 2018, p. 22)

The weight of authority is a concept observed by Minkler in 2004 when, despite her positive intentions, she ended up creating distrust in a host community. This happened because she "was of a dominant culture (urban, white), received significant financial support…, and came from an outside institution" (Lasker et al., 2018, p. 22). Whether real or perceived, weight of authority can happen due to power differentials that often exist between volunteer students and the host community. As mentioned in the example, power differentials could be financial, racial, educational, or even institutional. Power dynamics are often deeply embedded in the political, social, and economic histories of the community, yet students might present themselves to the community without full awareness of these factors (Lough, Tiessen, & Lasker, 2018).

The volunteer effect happens when the C/PHN volunteer "travels to a community because the existing health care system there is weak or under resourced" (e.g., low-resources, disaster) (Lasker et al., 2018, p. 23). Volunteer nurses bring "donated equipment and supplies or provide education and training" to supplement the care that the existing system is unable to provide (Lasker et al., 2018, p. 23). Even though the volunteers are well-intentioned, their efforts might not be in tune with the area's health care system, or they may undermine local methods. Volunteer efforts may duplicate local services and thus waste important resources. It has been reported that some community members wait for volunteers to return rather than seek care from local health care sources, because the services of volunteers are free of charge. This devalues the local health care providers even further, creating dependency on the volunteers and their services The result is that the volunteer promotes "direct competition with local providers trying to make a living in their own communities" (Lasker et al., 2018, p. 23; Lough et al., 2018).

The burden of hosting is from the perspective of the host in the community who houses the C/PHN volunteer. Even though the C/PHN is providing services and activities at no cost, the host must provide housing, meals, transportation, and perhaps pay for a translator. In addition, hosts commit to accommodate learning experiences, often suspending their own work to do so. Typically, these learning opportunities are created for the student and are not spontaneous. Providing necessary support to "keep students safe, healthy, and productive during their time" with the community can place an extensive burden on the hosts (Lasker et al., 2018, p. 24). Volunteers should always be respectful to hosts and be helpful guests (Lough et al., 2018).

C/PHN volunteers should not presume that good intentions providing free health care activities or work exempt them from ethical concerns. Rather, regular self-reflection on how to embrace the ethical principle of "first do no harm" should come first before attempting to do good. Furthermore, it is important to consider that in any endeavor, we are all learners who first listen and observe, rather than begin with "doing" (Lasker et al., 2018, p. 24).

Individual Motivations

The C/PHN volunteer should honestly assess personal motivations when considering global health service. Motivations generally fall into one of two types: "volunteer-centric" focused on the volunteer's personal goals and interests and "community-centric" focused on the community's beneficial outcomes (Aluri et al., 2018; Lasker et al., 2018, p. 25; Philpott, 2010). See Table 16-3.

TABLE 16-3 Motivations for Global Health Service

Action	Motivational Focus	Seeking	Impact
Use Caution	▪ Volunteer centric ▪ Self-focused	Adventure and excitement more than offering help. Wants to share "superior" knowledge and skills with the population.	Looking for self-affirmation with an opportunity to prove themselves. Perhaps take a vacation doing medical or "poverty tourism" (p. 26).
Acceptable	▪ Volunteer centric ▪ Community-focused	A good global health learning experience. Can benefit both the volunteer and the host when the greater awareness is in favor of the community's goals. Seeks a sense of mutual reward and purpose, like-mindedness, and an opportunity to broaden clinical experience.	Linked with altruism that helps improve global understanding of health and disease. Bonus that the volunteer will better understand future patients, especially those who are immigrants (p. 27).
Optimal	▪ Community-centric ▪ Community-focused	Emphasis on global health learning experience focused on foundational global health principles	Community development, capacity building, partnership, and health system strengthening (p. 28).

Source: Lasker et al. (2018).

Consequences of Being a Global Health Volunteer

Global volunteering can be very expensive and may not offer long-term health or financial benefits to the communities served; it may actually be burdensome. Identifying opportunities that are both "ethical and sustainable" will preserve the dignity of the communities while supporting local empowerment and developing leadership opportunities (Lasker et al., 2018, p. 41). This approach will also provide a more meaningful experience for volunteers.

C/PHNs who develop and nurture community-centric positive motivations are in a position to make a positive impact on themselves and their host communities. The C/PHN volunteer is likely to acquire the state of mind of a global citizen (Lasker et al., 2018, p. 25; Philpott, 2010). The result for the C/PHN volunteer is as follows:

- Improved understanding of global health and disease
- Developing new partnerships and teamwork in challenging settings
- Implementing shared solutions
- Experiencing the scope of social determinants of health
- Acquiring specific skills, especially those of improved patience, listening, and observation.

Ultimately, optimal global health learning opportunities will provide C/PHNs with increased insights while developing experience with disease-specific interventions and activities. Overall, C/PHN contributions to community-led efforts can become part of the community's long-term sustainable goals. In the end, the outcomes will be better for communities. Global C/PHNs experience a more robust career where their unique skills and knowledge can be applied in a globalizing world (Lasker et al., 2018). Like transcultural nursing, described in Chapter 5, expanding one's horizons either in unfamiliar neighborhoods here or abroad (see Box 16-8) can promote a broader understanding and provide richer experiences for the C/PHN. Many of our clients are not far-removed from their countries of origin, and a global perspective provides C/PHNs with a more welcoming presence. The skills gained from global health experiences can help us better understand and work with all of our clients, wherever they may live.

BOX 16-8 PERSPECTIVES

A Student Nurse's Viewpoint on Studying Abroad in Ecuador

I never thought I would study abroad, but when the opportunity arose to take one of my nursing classes in Cuenca, Ecuador, I decided to embrace it, expecting a great learning experience. Little did I imagine that it was going to be anything short of life changing. Simply stated, it was humbling to be a guest in a host family's home, accepted like family. It was awesome to become immersed in a culture so different from our own. During our 1-month stay, our itinerary was packed with school as well as experiences in hospitals, clinics, school, and even an orphanage.

I recall a particular hospital where I assisted a compassionate nurse in giving bed baths with limited resources. I ripped three pairs of small-sized latex gloves before managing to keep a pair on my large hands. I learned that being a good nurse was not dependent on the availability of supplies but rather in maximizing the potential to deliver compassionate care in any circumstance.

I am happy I made the decision to study abroad. In addition to the learning experience, I gained insight, respect, humility, and gratitude for life and for others. It is as if I have become aware of what living fully is, something unattainable without the smells, sights, sounds, and interactions I encountered abroad.

Ella, student nurse

SUMMARY

- Community/public health nursing services are critical to the ultimate health of a community, providing important primary, secondary, and tertiary levels of health promotion and prevention throughout the world.
- Community assessment includes a comprehensive review of the patterns of care, demographic transitions, and epidemiologic transitions.
- Major principles of global health care include the global burden of disease (GBD), Health in All Policies (HiAP), Sustainable Development Goals (SDGs), and One Health.
- The GBD is calculated in a population or country by adding Years of Life Lost (YLL) to Years Lived With Disability (YLD) to determine the Disability-Adjusted Life Year (DALY). The higher the DALY, the greater the GBD.
- The United Nations and the World Health Organization are the integrating agencies for health around the world. Additional international agencies also support global health efforts.
- The International Health Regulations (IHR) guide the interdependence of nations at times of global epidemics or pandemics.
- Global ethical considerations include understanding of the weight of authority, the volunteer effect, and the burden of hosting.
- Global service-based learning requires careful self-reflection of one's own personal motivation behind volunteer efforts.

ACTIVE LEARNING EXERCISES

1. Describe three infectious diseases that are common around the world. What current efforts are being implemented to combat them? Over the last 25 years, what progress been made in reducing incidence, as well as morbidity and mortality for these diseases? List 4 (or more) of the 10 essential public health services that have been utilized to combat these infectious diseases.
2. Which of the worldwide leading risk factors for health are also present in the United States? Why? How can a local C/PHN address these risk factors? What partnerships could be developed locally that reflect international approaches? What interventional programs are available from your state or county health agencies that could be used to reduce these risk factors?
3. Conduct your own needs assessment in a familiar community. Use the community assessment framework described in this chapter to identify strengths of the community and gaps of care. After your assessment, select one C/PHN intervention as a priority for that community. Which of the 10 essential public health services support your proposed intervention? Provide a rationale for your choices.
4. Using the GBD, compare interactive tool at http://www.healthdata.org/data-visualization/gbd-compare, examine the most current results for a country with an emerging economy compared to the United States. Use all ages and both sexes in your comparison (e.g., all cause DALYs per 100,000 map; DALYs by causes treemap). How are the patterns different or similar? What factors could influence your findings? Compare the same two countries in 1990 and evaluate how the patterns of causes have changed for both.
5. Identify a country or community in which you would like to practice community/public health nursing. Before you begin a review of this country or community, write down your own knowledge, attitudes, and beliefs about the country or community, the people, and the culture. Examine your own motivations for wanting this experience. Identify how you might feel if you received services rather than provided services.

REFERENCES

Abbas, M., Aloudat, T., Bartolomei, J., Carballo, M., Durieux-Paillard, S., Gabus, L., ... Pittet, D. (2018). Migrant and refugee populations: A public health and policy perspective on a continuing global crisis. *Antimicrobial Resistance and Infection Control*, 7(113), 1. doi: 10.1186/s13756-018-0403-4.

Alkmim, M. B., Figueira, R. M., Marcolino, M. S., Cardoso, C. S., Abreu, M. P. D., Cunha, L. R., ... Ribeiro, A. L. P. (2012). Improving patient access to specialized health care: The Telehealth Network of Minas Gerais, Brazil. *Bulletin of the World Health Organization*, 90(5), 321–400. doi: 10.2471/BLT.11.099408.

Aluri, J., Moran, D., Kironji, A. G., Carroll, B., Cox, J., Chiung, C., ... DeCamp, M. (2018). The ethical experiences of trainees on short-term international trips: A systematic qualitative synthesis. *BMC Medical Education*, 18(1), 324.

Ashwani, K., & Kalosona, P. (2016). Effect of indoor air pollution on acute respiratory infection among children in India. *Social and Natural Sciences Journal*, 10(2), 1–8.

Association of Public Health Laboratories (APHL). (2011). *Lessons from a virus. Public health laboratories respond to the H1N1 pandemic.* Retrieved from https://www.aphl.org/aboutAPHL/publications/Documents/ID_2011Sept_Lessons-from-a-Virus-PHLs-Respond-to-H1N1-Pandemic.pdf#search=Lessons%20from%20a%20virus

Avert. (2018). *Global HIV and AIDS statistics.* Retrieved from https://www.avert.org/public-hub

Balami, A. D., Said, S. M., Zulkefli, N., Bachok, N., & Audu, B. (2019). Effects of a health educational intervention on malaria knowledge motivation, and behavioural skills: A randomized controlled trial. *Malaria Journal*, 18, 41.

Bill & Melinda Gates Foundation. (2019). *What we do*. Retrieved from http://www.gatesfoundation.org/What-We-Do

Breslow, L. (2006). Health measurement in the third era of health. *American Journal of Public Health*, *96*(1), 17–19.

Brundage, S. C., & Levine, C. (2019). *The ripple effect: The impact of the opioid epidemic on children and families*. Retrieved from https://uhfnyc.org/media/filer_public/59/b2/59b20ad0-6acf-4980-ba9a-07ad5f565386/uhf-opioids-20190307.pdf

Bureau of Justice Assistance, U.S. Department of Justice. (2019). *The resurgence of methamphetamines: Methamphetamine abuse associated with the opioid crisis*. Retrieved from https://it.ojp.gov/GIST/1212/The-Resurgence-of-Methamphetamines--Methamphetamine-Abuse-Associated-with-the-Opioid-Crisis

Centers for Disease Control and Prevention (CDC). (2015). *International Health Regulations (IHR): Protecting people every day [Infographic]*. Retrieved from https://www.cdc.gov/globalhealth/healthprotection/ghs/ihr/ihr-infographic.html

Centers for Disease Control and Prevention (CDC). (2017a). *Anatomy of an outbreak*. Retrieved from https://www.cdc.gov/globalhealth/infographics/global-health-security/anatomy-of-an-outbreak.html

Centers for Disease Control and Prevention (CDC). (2017b). *Global health security: Global disease detection centers*. Retrieved from https://www.cdc.gov/globalhealth/security/gdd.htm

Centers for Disease Control and Prevention (CDC). (2017c). *The public health system & the ten essential public health services*. Retrieved from https://www.cdc.gov/publichealthgateway/publichealthservices/essentialhealthservices.html

Centers for Disease Control and Prevention (CDC). (2018). *One Health basics*. Retrieved from https://www.cdc.gov/onehealth/basics/index.html

Centers for Disease Control and Prevention (CDC). (2019). *Ebola virus disease: Prevention*. Retrieved from https://www.cdc.gov/vhf/ebola/prevention/index.html

Centers for Disease Control and Prevention (CDC). (2020a). *2019 novel coronavirus (2019-nCoV) situation Summary*. Retrieved from https://www.cdc.gov/coronavirus/2019-nCoV/summary.html#cdc-response

Centers for Disease Control and Prevention (CDC). (2020b). *CDC COVID data tracker*. Retrieved from https://covid.cdc.gov/covid-data-tracker/#cases_totalcases

Centers for Disease Control and Prevention (CDC). (2020c). *CDC emergency operations center activations*. Retrieved from https://emergency.cdc.gov/recentincidents/

Centers for Disease Control and Prevention (CDC). (2020d). *Global disease detection from SARS to Zika*. Retrieved from https://www.cdc.gov/globalhealth/infographics/global-health-security/global-disease-detection-timeline.html

Centers for Disease Control and Prevention (CDC). (2020e). *Guidance for US CDC staff for the establishment and management of public health rapid response teams*. Retrieved from https://www.cdc.gov/coronavirus/2019-ncov/downloads/global-covid-19/RRTManagementGuidance-508.pdf

Centers for Disease Control and Prevention (CDC). (2020f). *Key achievements in five years of GHSA*. Retrieved from https://www.cdc.gov/globalhealth/resources/factsheets/5-years-of-ghsa.html

Centers for Disease Control and Prevention (CDC). (2020g). *Malaria*. Retrieved from https://www.cdc.gov/parasites/malaria/index.html

Centers for Disease Control and Prevention Division of Global Health Protection (CDC-DGHP). (2019). *International Health Regulations (IHR)*. Retrieved from https://www.cdc.gov/globalhealth/healthprotection/ghs/ihr/index.html

Centers for Disease Control and Prevention Global Health (CDC-GH). (2017). *Global disease detection by the numbers [Infographic]*. Retrieved from https://www.cdc.gov/globalhealth/infographics/uncategorized/global_disease_detection.htm

City-Data. (2020). *Montana languages*. Retrieved from http://www.city-data.com/states/Montana-Languages.html

Clark, T., & Simeon, J. C. (2016). War, armed conflict, and refugees: The United Nations' endless battle for peace. *Refugee Survey Quarterly*, *35*(3), 35–70.

Coalition for Epidemic Preparedness Innovations (CEPI). (2020). *CEPI to fund three programmes to develop vaccines against the novel coronavirus, nCoV-2019*. Retrieved from https://cepi.net/news_cepi/cepi-to-fund-three-programmes-to-develop-vaccines-against-the-novel-coronavirus-ncov-2019/

Colburn, C., & Seymour, B. (2018). Module 1: Global trends. In: B. Seymour, J. Cho, & J. Barrow (Eds.), *Toward Competency-Based Best Practices for Global Health and Dental Education: A Global Health Starter Kit*. A project of the Consortium of Universities for Global Health, Global Oral Health Interest Group. Retrieved from https://hsdm.harvard.edu/global-health-starter-kit

Corendea, C. (2018). *Regionalism, human rights, and migration in relation to climate change. Our World*. Retrieved from https://ourworld.unu.edu/en/regionalism-human-rights-and-migration-in-relation-to-climate-change

Craven, J. (August 27, 2020). *COVID-19 vaccine tracker. Regulatory Affairs Professionals Society*. Retrieved from https://www.raps.org/news-and-articles/news-articles/2020/3/covid-19-vaccine-tracker

Department of Health, Republic of South Africa. (2020). *Malaria prevention*. Retrieved from http://www.health.gov.za/index.php/malaria-prevention-treatment-advice

Doctors Without Borders USA. (n.d.). *Commitment to our supporters*. Retrieved from https://www.doctorswithoutborders.org/who-we-are/accountability-reporting/commitment-our-supporters

End Malaria. (n.d.). *RBM Partnership to end malaria: Overview*. Retrieved from https://endmalaria.org/about-us/overview

Food and Agriculture Organization of the United Nations (FAO). (2020). *Animal health*. Retrieved from http://www.fao.org/animal-health/en/

Gamlen, A., & Gamlen, M. (2019). International migration: Causes, challenges and policy responses. *Geodate*, *32*(1), 3–7.

Gebreyes, W., Dupouy-Camet, J., Newport, M., Oliveira, C., Schlesinger, L. S., Saif, Y., ... King, L. J. (2014). The global one health paradigm: Challenges and opportunities for tackling infectious diseases at the human, animal, and environment interface in low-resource settings. *PLoS Neglected Tropical Diseases*, *8*(11), e3257.

Global Health Observatory (GHO). (2016). *Top 10 causes of death [Online interactive dashboard]*. Retrieved from https://www.who.int/gho/mortality_burden_disease/causes_death/top_10/en/

Global Health Security Agenda. (n.d.). *Home*. Retrieved from https://ghsagenda.org

Haskins, J. (2017). *Healthy People 2030 to create objectives for health of nation: Process underway for next 10-year plan*. The Nation's Health. Retrieved from http://thenationshealth.aphapublications.org/content/47/6/1.1

Institute for Health Metrics and Evaluation (IHME). (2019a). *GBD 2017 resources*. Retrieved from http://www.healthdata.org/gbd/gbd-2017-resources

Institute for Health Metrics and Evaluation (IHME). (2019b). *GBD history*. Retrieved from http://www.healthdata.org/gbd/about/history

International Conference on Primary Health Care. (1978). *Declaration of Alma-Ata*. Paper presented at the International Conference on Primary Health Care, Alma-Ata, USSR. Retrieved from https://www.who.int/publications/almaata_declaration_en.pdf?ua=1

International Council of Nurses (ICN). (2020). *Who we are*. Retrieved from https://www.icn.ch/who-we-are/icn-mission-vision-and-strategic-plan

Johns Hopkins Coronavirus Resource Center. (August 31, 2020). *Tracking*. Retrieved from https://coronavirus.jhu.edu

Kaiser Family Foundation. (January 24, 2019). *The US government and the World Health Organization*. Retrieved from https://www.kff.org/global-health-policy/fact-sheet/the-u-s-government-and-the-world-health-organization/

Kenya Ministry of Health. (January 1, 2014). *Strategy for community health 2014–2019*. Retrieved from http://guidelines.health.go.ke/#/category/12/90/meta

Lasker, J., Evert, J., Adyatmaka, I., Bermúdez Mora, G., Woodmansey, K., Seymour, B. (2018). Module 5: Ethics and sustainability. In B. Seymour, J. Cho, & J. Barrow (Eds.), *Toward competency-based best practices for global health in dental education: A global health starter kit. A project of the Consortium of Universities for Global Health Global Oral Health Interest Group*. Retrieved from https://hsdm.harvard.edu/global-health-starter-kit

Lewis, D. (August 14, 2020). 'We felt we had beaten it': New Zealand's race to eliminate the coronavirus again. *Nature*. Retrieved from https://www.nature.com/articles/d41586-020-02402-5

Los Angeles Regional Adult Education Consortium. (2018). *Los Angeles Unified School District*. Retrieved from https://laraec.net/los-angeles-unified-school-district/

Lough, B. J., Tiessen, R., Lasker, J. N. (2018). Effective practices of international volunteering for health: Perspectives from partner organizations. *Globalization and Health*, *14*(1), 11. Retrieved from https://globalizationandhealth.biomedcentral.com/track/pdf/10.1186/s12992-018-0329-x

Marcolino, M. S., Figueira, R. M., Dos Santos, J. P., Cardoso, C. S., Ribeiro, A., & Alkmim, M. B. (2016). The experience of a sustainable large scale Brazilian telehealth network. *Telemedicine Journal and e-Health*, *22*(11), 788–908.

Ministry of Health–Manatū Hauora (New Zealand). (2020a). *COVID-19: Elimination strategy for Aotearoa New Zealand*. Retrieved from https://www.health.govt.nz/our-work/diseases-and-conditions/covid-19-novel-coronavirus/covid-19-current-situation/covid-19-elimination-strategy-aotearoa-new-zealand

Ministry of Health—Manatu (New Zealand). (2020b). *NZ COVID tracer app*. Retrieved from https://www.health.govt.nz/our-work/diseases-and-conditions/covid-19-novel-coronavirus/covid-19-resources-and-tools/nz-covid-tracer-app

Minkler, M. (2004). Ethical challenges for the "outside" researcher in community-based participatory research. *Health Education Behavior*, *31*(6), 684–697.

National Center for Biotechnology Information [NCBI]. (January 13, 2020). *Novel coronavirus complete genome from Wuhan outbreak now available from GenBank*. Retrieved from https://ncbiinsights.ncbi.nlm.nih.gov/2020/01/13/novel-coronavirus/

Omran, A. R. (2005). The epidemiologic transition: A theory of the epidemiology of population change. *Milbank Quarterly*, *83*(4), 731–757.

Pan American Health Organization (PAHO). (n.d.). *About the Pan American Health Organization (PAHO)*. Retrieved from https://www.paho.org/hq/index.php?option=com_content&view=article&id=91:about-paho&Itemid=220&lang=en

Partners in Health. (2020). *Our mission at PIH*. Retrieved from https://www.pih.org/pages/our-mission

Philpott, J. (2010). Training for a global state of mind. *AMA Journal of Ethics*, *12*(3), 231–236. Retrieved from https://journalofethics.ama-assn.org/article/training-global-state-mind/2010-03

Population Services International (PSI). (2014). *So, What's a DALY?* Retrieved from https://www.psi.org/publication/what-is-a-daly/

Shetty, R., Samant, J., Nayak, K., Maiya, M., & Reddy, S. (2017). Feasibility of telecardiology solution to connect rural health clinics to a teaching hospital. *Indian Journal of Community Medicine*, *42*(3), 170–173.

Simoes, J., Augusto, G. F., Frontiera, I., & Hernandez-Quevedo, C. (2017). Portugal: Health system review. *Health Systems in Transition*, *19*(2), 1–184. Retrieved from https://www.euro.who.int/__data/assets/pdf_file/0007/337471/HiT-Portugal.pdf?ua=1

Slogett, A. (2015). Demography on the world stage. In *Population Analysis for Policy and Programmes*. Paris: International Union for the Scientific Study of Population. Retrieved from http://papp.iussp.org/sessions/papp101_s01/PAPP101_s01_010_010.html

Themnér, L., & Wallensteen, P. (2013). Armed conflict, 1946–2012. *Journal of Peace Research*, *50*(4), 509–521. doi: 10.1177/0022343314542076.

U.S. Department of Health and Human Services (USDHHS). (2020). *Development of the national health promotion and disease prevention objectives for 2030*. Retrieved from https://www.healthypeople.gov/2020/About-Healthy-People/Development-Healthy-People-2030

UNICEF. (2016). *Transparency and accountability*. Retrieved from https://www.unicef.org/transparency/

United Nations (UN). (2020). *About the Sustainable Development Goals*. Retrieved from https://www.un.org/sustainabledevelopment/

United Nations Department of Economic and Social Affairs. (2017). *Population facts: Migration and population change—drivers and impacts*. Retrieved from https://www.un.org/en/development/desa/population/migration/publications/populationfacts/docs/MigrationPopFacts20178.pdf

United Nations Development Program. (2020). *Sustainable Development Goals*. Retrieved from https://www.undp.org/content/singapore-global-centre/en/home/sustainable-development-goals.html

United Nations Systems Chief Executives Board for Coordination (UNSCEB). (2016). *Directory of United Nations system of organizations*. Retrieved from https://www.unsceb.org/directory

Waddington, R. (2008). Portugal's rapid progress through primary health care. *Bulletin of the World Health Organization*, *86*(11), 817–908.

World Bank Group. (2020). *What we do*. Retrieved from http://www.worldbank.org/en/about/what-we-do

World Health Organization (WHO). (2006). *Constitution of the World Health Organization. Basic documents* (45th ed.). Retrieved from https://www.who.int/governance/eb/who_constitution_en.pdf

World Health Organization (WHO). (2008). *Annex 2 of the IHR, 2005. WHO guidance for the use of Annex 2 of the International Health Regulations (2005)* (p. 52). Retrieved from https://www.who.int/ihr/revised_annex2_guidance.pdf?ua=1

World Health Organization (WHO). (2014). *Metrics: Disability-adjusted life year (DALY)*. Retrieved from http://www.who.int/healthinfo/global_burden_disease/metrics_daly/en/

World Health Organization (WHO). (2017). *Diarrhoeal disease [Fact sheet]*. Retrieved from https://www.who.int/en/news-room/fact-sheets/detail/diarrhoeal-disease

World Health Organization (WHO). (2018a). Levels for graded emergencies [Table]. In *Managing epidemics: Key facts about major deadly diseases* (p. 222). License: CC BY-NC-SA 3.0 IGO. Retrieved from https://www.who.int/emergencies/diseases/managing-epidemics-interactive.pdf

World Health Organization (WHO). (2018b). *Newsroom: Household air pollution and health*. Retrieved from https://www.who.int/news-room/fact-sheets/detail/household-air-pollution-and-health

World Health Organization (WHO). (2018c). Response tips and checklists. In *Managing epidemics: Key facts about major deadly diseases* (pp. 31–50). License: CC BY-NC-SA 3.0 IGO. Retrieved from https://www.who.int/emergencies/diseases/managing-epidemics-interactive.pdf

World Health Organization (WHO). (2019a). *Maternal mortality: Levels and trends 2000-2017*. Retrieved from https://www.who.int/news-room/fact-sheets/detail/maternal-mortality

World Health Organization (WHO). (2019b). *Newsroom: Maternal mortality*. [Fact sheet]. Retrieved from https://www.who.int/news-room/fact-sheets/detail/maternal-mortality

World Health Organization (WHO). (2019c). *Review of 40 years of primary health care implementation at country level*. Retrieved from https://www.who.int/docs/default-source/documents/about-us/evaluation/phc-final-report.pdf?sfvrsn=109b2731_4

World Health Organization (WHO). (2020a). *About IHR: A global system for alert and response*. Retrieved from https://www.who.int/ihr/alert_and_response/en/

World Health Organization (WHO). (February 16, 2020b). *Coronavirus disease 2019 (COVID-19): Situation report—27*. Retrieved from https://www.who.int/docs/default-source/coronaviruse/situation-reports/20200216-sitrep-27-covid-19.pdf

World Health Organization (WHO). (2020c). *Drug-resistant TB: Global situation*. Retrieved from https://www.who.int/tb/areas-of-work/drug-resistant-tb/global-situation/en/

World Health Organization (WHO). (2020d). *Global Outbreak Alert and Response Network (GOARN)*. Retrieved from https://www.who.int/ihr/alert_and_response/outbreak-network/en/

World Health Organization (WHO). (2020e). *Health in All Policies: Framework for Country Action*. Retrieved from https://www.who.int/healthpromotion/frameworkforcountryaction/en/

World Health Organization (WHO). (2020f). *Health topics: Global burden of disease*. Retrieved from http://www.who.int/topics/global_burden_of_disease/en/

World Health Organization (WHO). (2020g). *HIV/AIDS [Fact sheet]*. Retrieved from https://www.who.int/en/news-room/fact-sheets/detail/hiv-aids

World Health Organization (WHO). (2020h). *Indoor air pollution and household energy*. Retrieved from https://www.who.int/heli/risks/indoorair/indoorair/en/

World Health Organization (WHO). (2020i). *Protecting children from the environment* [PHE Infographic]. Retrieved from https://www.who.int/phe/infographics/protecting-children-from-the-environment/en/

World Health Organization (WHO). (September 9, 2020j). *Timeline of WHO's reponse to COVID-19*. Retrieved from https://www.who.int/news-room/detail/29-06-2020-covidtimeline

World Health Organization (WHO). (2020k). *Tuberculosis (TB): Health topics*. Retrieved from https://www.who.int/tb/en/

World Health Organization (WHO). (2020l). *WHO called to return to the declaration of Alma-Ata. Social Determinants of Health*. Retrieved from https://www.who.int/social_determinants/tools/multimedia/alma_ata/en/

World Health Organization (WHO). (2020m). *WHO: Countries [Directory of Member States]*. Retrieved from https://www.who.int/countries/en/

World Health Organization (WHO). (n.d.). *GISRS Global Influenza Surveillance & Response System*. Retrieved from https://www.who.int/influenza/gisrs_laboratory/updates/GISRS_one_pager_2018_EN.pdf?ua=1

CHAPTER 17

Disasters and Their Impact

"If we do not succeed in understanding what it takes to make our societies more resilient to disasters, then we will pay an increasingly high price in terms of lost lives and livelihoods."

—Robert Glasser (2017), United Nations Disaster Risk Official

KEY TERMS

Biologic warfare
Casualty
Chemical warfare
Crisis intervention
Critical incident stress debriefing (CISD)
Directly impacted by disaster
Disaster
Disaster planning
Displaced persons
Incident command system (ICS)
Indirectly impacted by disaster
Intensity
Man-made disaster
Mass-casualty incident
Moulage
Multiple-casualty incident
Natural disaster
Phases of disasters
Posttraumatic stress disorder (PTSD)
Refugee
Resilience
Scope
Terrorism
Triage

LEARNING OBJECTIVES

Upon mastery of this chapter, you should be able to:

1. Describe a variety of disasters, including their causation, number of casualties, scope, and intensity.
2. Discuss three factors contributing to a community's potential for experiencing a disaster.
3. Identify the four phases of disaster management.
4. Describe the role of the community/public health nurse (C/PHN) in preventing, preparing for, responding to, and supporting recovery from disasters.
5. Use the levels of prevention to describe the role of the C/PHN in relation to acts of chemical, biologic, or nuclear terrorism.

INTRODUCTION

Have you, or someone you know, been affected by a recent disaster? In this millennium, we have witnessed multiple devastating natural disasters, such as Category 5 hurricanes, tsunamis, and earthquakes, and man-made destructive acts of terrorism (e.g., bombings) causing multiple fatalities. Natural and man-made disasters are ever-present possibilities regardless of where one lives or works, and health care professionals have an obligation to be skilled in disaster preparedness and response. This chapter will increase your understanding of the community/public health nurses (C/PHN's) role in preparing for, responding to, and recovering from natural disasters and terrorism.

DISASTERS

A **disaster** is any natural or man-made event that causes a level of destruction or emotional trauma exceeding the abilities of those affected to recover from without community assistance. Airplane crashes, mass shootings, and chemical explosions are all situations that are devastating to a community and, by definition, constitute disasters.

The geographic distribution and types of disasters vary around the world due to environmental, sociopolitical, and topographic factors. For example, California, Alaska, and Tennessee are associated with earthquakes and the Gulf Coast with hurricanes and oil spills. Similarly, it is not surprising to hear of drought in Ethiopia, floods in India during the monsoon season, or bombings in Afghanistan or Syria. When certain types of disasters are anticipated, communities are usually prepared for them. For instance, California has strict building codes to prevent destruction of structures in the event of earthquakes, but most California homes lack the basements and insulation that characterize homes east of the Rocky Mountains, which may be subject to severe storms or tornados. Similarly, residents of the northern United States, Germany, Austria, and Russia are better prepared for blizzards than are the southern regions of the United States and Europe.

Sadly, throughout history, disasters have affected every section of the globe. Table 17-1 lists only a few of them. However, technological advances, such as satellite data, have improved disaster management worldwide (International Charter, 2019).

Characteristics of Disasters

Disasters are often characterized by their cause.

- A **natural disaster** is caused by natural events, such as earthquakes and tsunamis.
- A **man-made disaster** is caused by human activity, such as mass shootings, the bombing of significant landmarks in major cities, or the riots in major cities after a sociopolitical event. Other man-made disasters include nuclear reactor meltdowns, industrial accidents, oil spills, construction accidents, and air, train, bus, and subway crashes. In fact, man-made disasters can and frequently do follow natural disasters, as occurred with the nuclear reactors in Japan following the earthquake and tsunami in 2011.
- A **casualty** is someone who has been injured or killed by or as a direct result of an accident or natural disaster.
- If casualties number more than two people but fewer than 100, the disaster is characterized as a **multiple-casualty incident**.
- Although multiple-casualty incidents may strain the health care systems of small or midsized communities, a **mass-casualty incident**—often involving many casualties—can completely overwhelm the health care resources of even large cities (DeNolf & Kahwaji, 2019).

Preparedness for mass-casualty incidents is essential for all communities. For instance, community leaders should closely track and report through various media the path and time of landfall of a hurricane to inform residents in the storm's path and support early evacuation of families and businesses. Communities can help minimize devastation from flooding by building reservoirs or refusing to grant building permits in flood-prone areas and by reinforcing areas around waterways with sandbags during rainy weather. In fire-prone areas, communities can heighten awareness of fire danger and enforce regulations supporting precautionary preventive measures

Unfortunately, some disasters occur without warning. For example:

- The terrorist attacks in New York City caught thousands of civilians by surprise. They were trapped in buildings with limited escape routes and very little time to retreat to safety.
- During the 2015 Paris terrorist attacks, survival depended on being in the right place at the right time.
- Coworkers were trapped in a building during the 2015 San Bernardino, CA terrorist attack when a married couple fired on them with automatic weapons. A total of 14 were killed and 27 were injured.
- Wildfires in California during 2017 and 2018, though not completely unanticipated, were uncharacteristically large, and control was hindered by drought conditions, along with heat and high winds.
- The mass shootings in Newtown, Connecticut; Aurora, Colorado; Las Vegas, Nevada; and Thousand Oaks, California occurred without warning and were the result of mentally unstable individuals acting alone.

Some disasters, such as the natural gas leak in a southern California community during 2015–2016, are at first unknown to the public. After residents began noticing headaches, nosebleeds, respiratory problems, and other symptoms, the Southern California Gas Company acknowledged that a deep well gas leak had occurred in a difficult-to-reach canyon miles away. The company assured the public that the leak did not pose an imminent health risk, although it had been occurring for months and would take several more months to stop. It was estimated that over 30,000 kg/hour of methane was released into the atmosphere, and the area became a no-fly zone per the Federal Aviation Administration (Reilly, 2016). The gas leak was finally stopped and "permanently sealed" in late February 2016 (Pamer, Wynter, & McDade, 2016, p. 4).

The **scope** of a disaster is the range of its effect, either geographically or in terms of the number of people impacted. The **intensity** of a disaster is the level of destruction and devastation it causes. For instance, an earthquake centered in a large metropolitan area and one centered in a desert may have the same numeric rating on the Richter scale yet have very different intensities in terms of the destruction they cause. As of seven months after its initial detection, the COVID-19 pandemic, stemming from a novel coronavirus that started in Wuhan, China in December 2019, had infected more than 12.5 million worldwide and caused over half a million deaths (CDC, 2020a).

The terrorist attacks on September 11, 2001 are the worst disaster in U.S. history, as a total of 2,996 people, including 19 terrorists, died in three attacks on U.S. soil. Terrorists took control of four airplanes and used them as missiles. Two planes hit the World Trade Center in New York City, killing 2,753 (Engel & Ioanes, 2020). The third plane hit the Pentagon, killing 125 in the Pentagon and the 64 aboard the plane. Passengers in the fourth plane, United Flight 93, were aware of the attacks and, once their plane was hijacked, attempted to take back the plane. The plane crashed in a field in Shanksville, Pennsylvania, killing 40 (Englel & Ioanes, 2019). Every year on September 11th, the country remembers those who perished in the attacks. Only 60% of the bodies have been identified thus far. The remains of firefighter Michael Haub were identified this year (Karimi, 2019). At least 200 firefighters have died to date from Ground Zero–related illnesses (Stanglin, 2019).

Persons Impacted by Disasters

Because disasters are so variable, there is no typical person impacted in a disaster, nor can anyone predict whether he or she will ever be impacted by a disaster. Those who are **directly impacted by disaster** experience the event firsthand, whether fire, flooding, mass shooting, vehicular accident, or bombing. They also constitute the

TABLE **17-1** Major Disasters: 2015 to 2020

Date and Location	Description
August to October 2015, Washington State, United States	Wildfires and mudslides in the state of Washington killed three firefighters and damaged or destroyed hundreds of homes.
October 2015, United States	Severe storms cause serious flooding in North and South Carolina, leading to 25 deaths and billions of dollars in property damage. Just prior to this, severe flooding in Kansas, Oklahoma, and Texas was responsible for 43 deaths and much destruction.
November 2015, Paris, France	A coordinated, multisite terrorist attack kills 130 people and injures over 350 people. Earlier, in January, terrorists attacked offices of a magazine and a Jewish market, killing 17.
January 2016, United States	Blizzard affected the northeast, mid-Atlantic, and southeast sections of the United States, killing 38 people.
March 2016, Belgium	Coordinated terrorist attacks at the airport and metro system killed 35 and injured over 250 people.
August 2017, Sierra Leone	Heavy rainfall and flooding sparked a huge mudslide, killing at least 600 and directly affecting more than 6,000
August 2017, Houston, TX	Hurricanes Harvey, Category 4 largest storm to hit the United States since the disastrous Hurricane Katrina in 2005
September 2017, Miami, FL	Hurricane Irma was the first Category 5 hurricane on record to strike the Leeward Islands. She made landfall on the Florida Keys as a Category 4 storm with a diameter covering Alabama, Georgia and South Carolina.
September 2017, Dominica, U.S. Virgin Islands, and Puerto Rico	Hurricane Maria hit the small Caribbean island of Dominica as a Category 5 storm, and then the U.S. Virgin Islands. The powerful storm made landfall in Puerto Rico as a Category 4 storm, the strongest hurricane to directly hit Puerto Rico since 1932. Millions of Puerto Ricans were without power for months after the hurricane made landfall.
September 2017, Mexico	7.1 magnitude earthquake in Mexico City, killing at least 225 people
October 2017, Las Vegas, NV	Mass shooting killing 58 and more than 500 injured (How the Las Vegas Strip shooting unfolded By Washington Post Staff https://www.washingtonpost.com/graphics/2017/national/las-vegas-shooting/?noredirect=on&utm_term=.2da5ecfb2ed1)
December 2017 to January 2018, Southern California	Thomas Fire: State's largest-ever wildfire, scorching more than 280,000 acres, or 440 square miles—nearly the size of New York City One month later the area experienced devastating mudslides closing major roadways, destroying hundreds of homes, and killing 17 people.
November 2018, Northern California	Camp Fire is one of the largest and deadliest fires in California history: 85 people died (Brekke, 2019), 19,000 buildings (mostly homes) were destroyed, and 153,336 acres were burnt (Miller, 2018).
November 2018, Southern California	Thousand Oaks, CA: Borderline Bar shooting; 12 people died and 128 injured (local college students) (Wilson, 2019). Two days later many of the families affected were told to evacuate due to the Woolsey Fire.
September 2019, Bahamas	Hurricane Dorian, a Category 5 hurricane, struck the Bahamas in which at least 53 people died, 1,300 are still missing, and 7,500 people are affected. The costs are expected to exceed $7 billion (Ailworth, 2019).
2019, California	6,190 incidents of fire, 198,392 estimated acres burned, with 732 structures damaged or destroyed, and 3 fatalities (https://www.fire.ca.gov/incidents/2019)
2019/2020, Australia	More than 240 days of wildfires left Australia with 25.5 million acres burned, thousands of homes destroyed, 33 people dead, and over a billion animals feared to have perished, including over 30,000 koalas. In the capital of Australia, the air quality index reached more than 23 times higher than air quality that is considered hazardous. (https://www.theverge.com/2020/1/3/21048891/australia-wildfires-koalas-climate-change-bushfires-deaths-animals-damage)
2020, global	The COVID-19 pandemic affected 210 countries and territories. As of July 14, 2020, there were 4,975,294 people currently infected worldwide. A total of 8,366,172 were closed cases, including 7% that were deceased. (https://www.worldometers.info/coronavirus/)

dead and the survivors of the event; these survivors are likely to have health effects from their experience, even if they are without physical injuries directly caused by the event. Some may be without shelter or food, and many experience serious psychological stress long after the event is over, such as victims of the Thomas Fire. This fire, California's largest wildfire to date, was started by sparks from powerlines during a powerful wind, destroyed 1,063 structures, and burned 281,893 acres (Box 17-1; Diskin, 2019).

Depending on the cause and characteristics of the disaster, some direct survivors may become displaced persons or refugees. **Displaced persons** are forced to leave their homes to escape the effects of a disaster. Usually, displacement is a temporary condition and involves movement within the person's own country. The term **refugee** is reserved for people who are forced to leave their homeland because of war or persecution (United Nations, n.d). Returning displaced persons or refugees can place economic and social strains on the county of origin. Along with needs for employment and shelter, these influx situations raise concerns, especially regarding early or forced marriages, child labor, and human trafficking (United Nations, n.d.). Whether the displacement of refugee status is permanent or not, the lasting impact to both the country of origin and the host country is significant.

Those who are **indirectly impacted by disaster** are the relatives and friends of persons directly impacted by the disaster. These supporters often undergo extreme anguish while trying to locate loved ones or accommodate their emergency needs. If bodies cannot be found or are unidentifiable, the supporting persons experience even greater anguish and may not be able to accept that a loved one did not survive. Family members of those killed on 9/11 in New York City worked with architects to develop a memorial that meets the expectations of most of those indirectly impacted by the attack and honors their loved ones. This effort, along with the Flight 93 National Memorial in Shanksville, PA, and the Pentagon Memorial, helps with the long healing process of the supporters and serves as a reminder of the impact that day had on each of our lives.

Factors Contributing to Disasters

It is useful to apply the host, agent, and environment model (epidemiological triad) to understand the factors contributing to disasters, because manipulation of these factors can be instrumental in planning strategies to prevent or prepare for disasters. See Chapters 7 and 8.

Host Factors

The *host* is the human being who experiences the disaster. Host factors that contribute to the likelihood of experiencing a disaster include age, general health, mobility, psychological factors, and socioeconomic factors. For instance, older residents of a mobile home community may be unable to evacuate independently in response to a tornado warning if they can no longer drive. Residents of a low-income apartment complex in a large city may be aware that their building is not compliant with city fire codes but avoid alerting authorities for fear of the complex being closed and being homeless due to their inability to afford new, safe housing.

Agent Factors

The *agent* is the natural or technologic element that causes the disaster. For example, the high winds of a hurricane and the lava of an erupting volcano are agents, as are radiation, industrial chemicals, biologic agents, and bombs.

Environmental Factors

Environmental factors are those that could potentially contribute to or mitigate a disaster. Common environmental factors include a community's level of preparedness; the presence of industries that produce harmful chemicals or radiation; the presence of flood-prone rivers, lakes, or

BOX **17-1** PERSPECTIVES

Viewpoint of a Victim of the Thomas Fire

Dry easterly winds and a spark of fire on the night of December 4, 2017 changed many lives, including my own. That spark of fire grew to be known as the Thomas Fire that destroyed over 500 structures, including our home of 20 years. The power had been out and the glow of flames appeared incredibly close—a setting for panic that told me to just get out. We left fast with only clothes for the next couple of days. My husband and I learned the next afternoon that our home had burned with nothing left but ashes and odd pieces of survival, like a whole wall of decorative master bathroom tile!

Over the next month, I felt a wave of emotions that included not only the obvious of sadness but a conflict between feeling both immense gratitude and highly overwhelmed from the countless people who reached out to us. It often seemed like I was just floating to get through the day yet appreciating the little things, like the smell of shower soap and taste of coffee at our daughter's home where we were staying. Interestingly, one word kept popping into my head over that immediate time period: resilience. I found strength in knowing I could be resilient through the kindness of others who truly cared.

Ever since the fire, I feel anxious during dry windy weather, the sound of fire department sirens and seeing the outbreak of fire. California has continued to be affected by devastating fires. The aftermath of fire destruction leads me to wonder where those people are at emotionally and physically in rebuilding their lives, knowing from personal experience how some plow through and others go through extreme grief. Each day I wake up taking a deep breath, reminding myself of having resilience, and knowing I have the ability to rebuild anew.

Colleen Nevins, DNP, RN

streams; above-average amount of rainfall or snowfall; above- or below-average high or low temperatures; proximity to fault lines, coastal waters, or volcanoes; and the presence or absence of political unrest.

Agencies and Organizations for Disaster Management

In 1803 the United States first recognized the need to prepare for emergencies through law and dedicated organizations. The first law was written as a direct response to a major disaster, the Portsmouth, New Hampshire fire of 1803, which swept through the seaport town. The majority of subsequent legislation was in response to specific crises and created many different agencies to respond to those disasters. The one constant was that the response of the federal government to disasters remained more reactive than proactive and was ad hoc in nature, only becoming coordinated with the establishment of the Federal Emergency Management Agency (FEMA) in 1979 and the passage of the Robert T. Stafford Disaster Relief and Emergency Assistance Act of 1988 (Haddow, Bullock, & Coppola, 2016). In response to World War II and the specter of all-out nuclear war with the Soviet Union, the United States created Civil Defense, a series of programs and agencies designed to protect the population from "counter-value" nuclear strikes and increase the survivability of a nuclear war. The U.S. Department of Health, Education, and Welfare (USDHEW), predecessor to the U.S. Department of Health and Human Services, created the *Handbook for Civil Defense Emergency Planning in Welfare Institutions*, which was a guide to protect individuals and help staff prepare for fallout from a nuclear event (USDHEW, 1961). Significant in this handbook was the attention given to family responsibilities and the likelihood that staff, including nurses, would choose family responsibilities over professional responsibilities. To help alleviate the problems associated with absenteeism as a result of the nurses' conflicting responsibilities, the handbook recommended:

- Reminding staff of their responsibility as public servants,
- Providing shelter for families within the institution,
- Planning for getting families to the shelter,
- Planning for families to assist the staff during a crisis (USDHEW, 1961).

Under the 1950 version for the United States Civil Defense Plan, health services were to remain under the control of existing health agencies to avoid unnecessary duplication of services and would be subject to the rules and regulations of civil defense. The U.S. Public Health Service (USPHS) was responsible for providing staffing for civil defense offices and would work for the state health officer who would have the lead. The roles have been in continual transition since that time, but the basic principles remain the same.

Public health has become recognized as a critical component of emergency planning, preparedness, and response. National public health response requires coordination with state and local authorities, to include nongovernmental agencies (Centers for Disease Control and Prevention [CDC], 2019a). The CDC website has an assortment of educational materials to explore disasters such as videos, online modules, and statistics.

Among disaster-relief organizations, perhaps none is as famous as the Red Cross, which is referred to as the American Red Cross in the United States and the Red Crescent Societies in Islamic countries. The American Red Cross was founded in 1881 by Clara Barton and was chartered by the U.S. Congress in 1905. It is authorized to provide disaster assistance free of charge across the country through its more than half a million volunteers and staff. The duties assumed by the Red Cross in the event of a disaster are to provide shelter, food, basic health and mental health services, and distribution of emergency supplies (American Red Cross, n.d.).

President George W. Bush sought to consolidate the roles and responsibilities of agencies and organizations involved in disaster response and to align them with emergency support functions (ESFs; Table 17-2).

- The Department of Homeland Security (DHS) was organized in 2002 and incorporates many of the nation's security, protection, and emergency response activities into a single federal department (DHS, 2015).
- In 2003, FEMA, along with parts of 23 agencies, became part of the DHS.
- FEMA, established in 1979, is the federal agency responsible for assessing and responding to disaster events in the United States and provides training and guidance in all phases of disaster management.
- The DHS includes other widely known agencies, including the Transportation Security Administration, U.S. Customs and Border Protection, U.S. Immigration and Customs Enforcement, U.S. Citizenship and Immigration Services, U.S. Coast Guard, and U.S. Secret Service (DHS, 2018).

FEMA provides oversight of the National Incident Management System (NIMS), developed to allow responders from different jurisdictions and disciplines to work more cohesively and proactively in response to natural disasters, emergencies, and terrorist acts.

NIMS is the National **Incident Command System (ICS)**, meaning that it takes a unified approach to incident management, incorporates standard command and management structures, and emphasizes preparedness, mutual aid, and resource management (Fig. 17-1; FEMA, 2017a). Nurses and other health care professionals must understand this system and are encouraged to take courses dealing with the ICS. These courses are available for free online from FEMA Emergency Management Institute at http://www.training.fema.gov/EMI/. The most important courses for a nurse are (1) IS-100 Introduction to the Incident Command System, (2) IS-200.C Basic Incident Command System for Initial Response, (3) IS-700 Introduction to the NIMS, and (4) IS-800.b Introduction to the National Response Framework. Students are encouraged to explore the FEMA distance learning platform at https://training.fema.gov/is/.

The Department of Health and Human Services (DHHS) is the lead federal agency for public health and medical services during a public health or medical disaster. Supplemental services are provided to state, local, and territorial governments and may include Disaster

TABLE 17-2 Emergency Support Functions Responsibilities

ESF	Scope	Coordinating Agency
1. Transportation	Coordinates the support of management of transportation systems and infrastructure, the regulation of transportation, management of the Nation's airspace, and ensuring the safety and security of the national transportation system	Department of Transportation
2. Communications	Coordinates government and industry efforts for the reestablishment and provision of critical communications infrastructure and services, facilitates the stabilization of systems and applications from malicious activity, and coordinates communications support to response efforts	DHS/Cybersecurity and Communications
3. Public works and engineering	Coordinates the capabilities and resources to facilitate the delivery of services, technical assistance, engineering expertise, construction management, and other support to prepare for, respond to, and recover from a disaster or an incident	Department of Defense—U.S. Army Corps of Engineers
4. Firefighting	Coordinates the support for the detection and suppression of fires. Functions include but are not limited to supporting wildland, rural, and urban firefighting operations	U.S. Department of Agriculture/U.S. Forest Service and DHS/ FEMA/ U.S. Fire Administration
5. Information and planning	Supports and facilitates multiagency planning and coordination for operations involving incidents requiring federal coordination	DHS/FEMA
6. Mass care, emergency assistance, temporary housing, and human services	Coordinates the delivery of mass care and emergency assistance	DHS/FEMA
7. Logistics	Coordinates comprehensive incident resource planning, management, and sustainment capability to meet the needs of disaster survivors and responders	General Services Administration and DHS/FEMA
8. Public health and medical services	Coordinates the mechanisms for assistance in response to an actual or potential public health and medical disaster or incident	Department of Health and Human Services
9. Search and rescue	Coordinates the rapid deployment of search and rescue resources to provide specialized lifesaving assistance	DHS/FEMA
10. Oil and hazardous materials response	Coordinates support in response to an actual or potential discharge and/or release of oil or hazardous materials	Environmental Protection Agency
11. Agriculture and natural services	Coordinates a variety of functions designed to protect the Nation's food supply, respond to plant and animal pest and disease outbreaks, and protect natural and cultural resources	Department of Agriculture
12. Energy	Facilitates the reestablishment of damaged energy systems and components, and provides technical expertise during an incident involving radiological/nuclear materials	Department of Energy
13. Public safety and security	Coordinates the integration of public safety and security capabilities and resources to support the full range of incident management activities	Department of Justice/Bureau of Alcohol, Tobacco, Firearms, and Explosives
14. Cross-sector business and infrastructure	Coordinates cross-sector operations with infrastructure owners and operators, businesses, and their government partners, with particular focus on actions taken by businesses and infrastructure owners and operators in one sector to assist other sectors to better prevent or mitigate cascading failures between them. Focuses particularly on those sectors not currently aligned to other ESFs (draft for 2019 4th ed.)	DHS/Cybersecurity and Infrastructure Security Agency
15. External affairs	Coordinates the release of accurate, coordinated, timely, and accessible public information to affected audiences, including the government, media, NGOs, and the private sector. Works closely with state and local officials to ensure outreach to the whole community	DHS

DHS, Department of Homeland Security; ESF, Emergency Support Functions; FEMA, Federal Emergency Management Agency; NGO, nongovernmental organization. Reprinted from The Department of Homeland Security. (2019 draft). *National response framework* (4th ed., pp. 39–42). Retrieved from https://www.fema.gov/media-library-data/1559136348938-063ec40e34931923814dd50df638b448/NationalResponseFrameworkFourthEdition.pdf

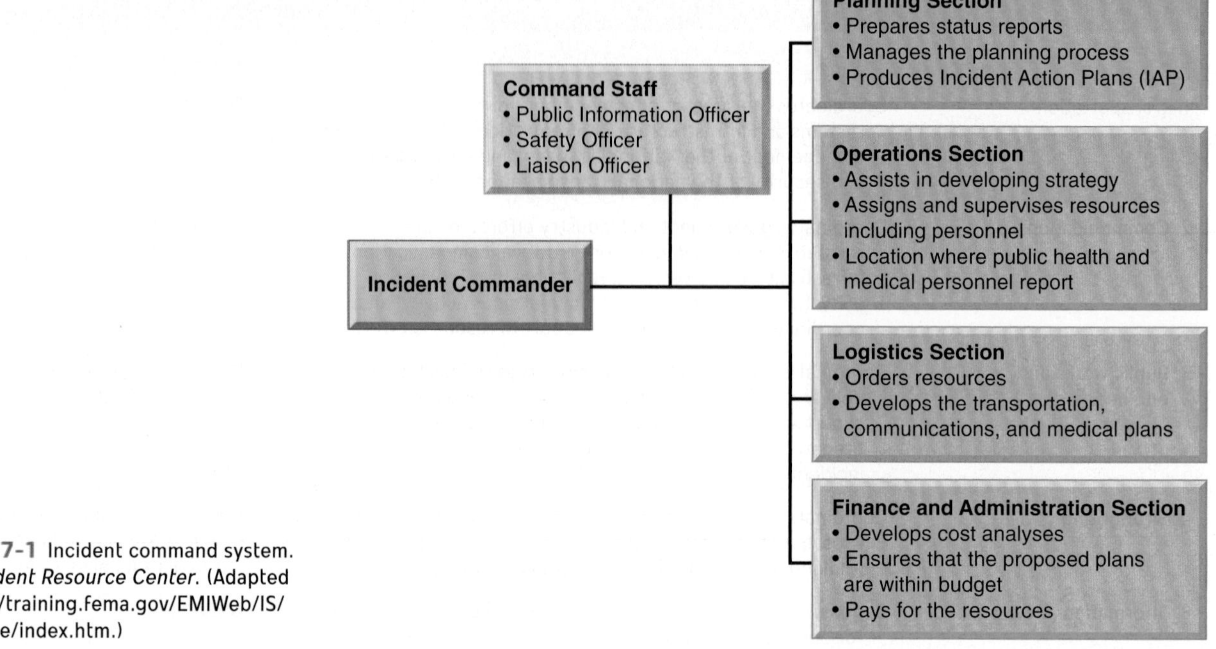
Planning Section
• Prepares status reports
• Manages the planning process
• Produces Incident Action Plans (IAP)
Command Staff
• Public Information Officer
• Safety Officer
• Liaison Officer
Operations Section
• Assists in developing strategy
• Assigns and supervises resources including personnel
• Location where public health and medical personnel report
Incident Commander
Logistics Section
• Orders resources
• Develops the transportation, communications, and medical plans
Finance and Administration Section
• Develops cost analyses
• Ensures that the proposed plans are within budget
• Pays for the resources

FIGURE 17-1 Incident command system. FEMA. *Incident Resource Center.* (Adapted from http://training.fema.gov/EMIWeb/IS/ICSResource/index.htm.)

Medical Assistance Teams (DMAT), USPHS officers, epidemiological personnel from the CDC, and veterinary support to name a few. Various international nongovernmental organizations (such as Doctors Without Borders, the International Medical Corps, and Operation Blessing), religious groups, and other volunteer agencies provide needed emergency care (Fig. 17-2; see Chapter 16).

Governments often send their military personnel and equipment in response to international disasters. However, political agendas may prevent aid typically accepted by countries experiencing catastrophe to reach the impacted communities. Fortunately, the USPHS Commissioned Corps was allowed to provide aid for the 2008 tsunami and earthquake survivors in Indonesia and Haiti. The USPHS has also worked collaboratively with the U.S. Navy to provide nursing and other medical care on combined humanitarian missions to South America and the South Pacific, and was sent to Africa to assist with the Ebola crisis (USPHS, 2019). See Chapter 28 for additional information about the role of the USPHS Commissioned Corps Nurses in emergency preparedness.

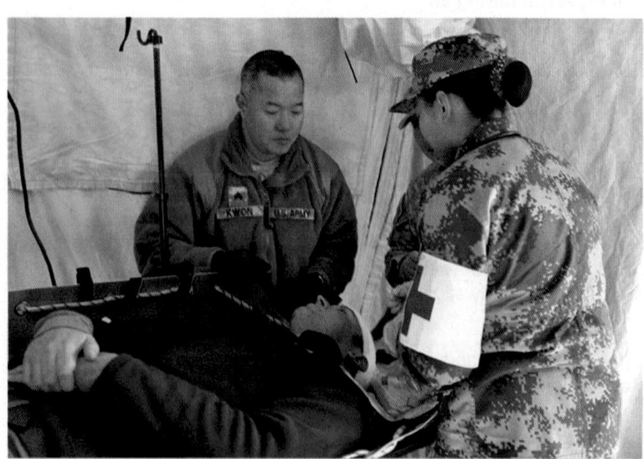
KWON
U.S. ARMY

FIGURE 17-2 Mobile hospitals are often deployed during disasters.

Phases of Disaster Management

In developing strategies to address the problem of disasters, it is helpful for the C/PHN to consider each of the four phases of disaster management: preventive/mitigation, preparedness, response, and recovery and become familiar with the language typically used in disaster preparedness (Emergency Management terms and definitions, FEMA, 2018).

Prevention or Mitigation Phase

Activities during this phase are focused on preventing future emergencies or minimizing their effects. The shaping of public policies and plans that either modify the causes of disasters or mitigate their effects on people, property, and infrastructure are critical activities during this phase. Mitigation activities take place *before* and *after* disaster emergencies.

To reduce our vulnerability to disasters, the United States has strengthened its disaster management activities over the past decade and continues to do so today (FEMA, n.d).

- The screening process at airports and shipping ports includes advanced imaging technology scanning and random hand-carried luggage or canine searches preboarding.
- Nonpassengers cannot go beyond the security entrance area, and photographic identification is required at two or more points before boarding.

Although globally we have experienced a pandemic and much will be learned from it, the Global Health Security has steps in place designed to help decrease the risk of pandemics. These steps include surveillance systems that detect possible threats, laboratories to identify the agent, a workforce for follow-up and containment, and emergency management systems to coordinate the activities (CDC, 2020b). To prevent possible contamination by Covid-19, individuals are advised to wash hands for 20 seconds, to wear a face mask when going out in public, and to maintain a 6 ft distance between each other (CDC, 2020c).

Preparedness Phase

Disaster *preparedness* involves improving community and individual reaction and responses, so that the effects of a disaster are minimized. Disaster preparedness includes plans for communication, evacuation, rescue, victim care, and recovery. Preparedness may be hazard-specific or a general all-hazard approach. For example, the Centers on Medicare and Medicaid Services (CMS) recommends that an "all-hazards approach" be taken by health care agencies when taking into consideration their location and disasters common to that area (CMS, 2017).

- For instance, although plans may differ in states at higher risk of earthquakes from those in tornado alley, the preparedness plans apply to numerous disasters.
- Communities must ensure that warning systems are tested routinely to ensure appropriate notifications to the residents of a tornado or hurricane, or any other potential threat.
- The Office of the Assistant Secretary for Preparedness and Response (2020) oversees the Strategic National Stockpile (SNS), which contains doses of vaccines, medical countermeasures, and needed medical supplies stored around the country in various strategic locations.
- The CDC reports that the SNS contains enough medications and medical supplies to manage a large public health emergency and protect the American public (CDC, 2016).
- Examples of preparedness include duck, cover, and hold during an earthquake and run, hide, or fight for an active shooter incident (FEMA, 2020a).

Nurses have a role in preparedness as well. Leaving one's home to assist in a disaster is difficult, especially if one, or one's family, is not prepared. Therefore, nurses need to be prepared with an individual and family plan and supplies that could possibly be needed. Enrolling in disaster classes or/and registering with a disaster agency such as the Red Cross, reinforces professional preparedness. On a community level, nurses can enhance preparedness by participating in community drills often held by public health agencies. Preparedness activities take place *before* an emergency occurs. We cannot provide adequate disaster relief until we are prepared on all three levels.

Response Phase

The *response phase* begins immediately after the onset of the disastrous event and *during* the emergency. Response is putting your preparedness plans into action immediately, with the goals of saving lives and preventing further injury or damage to property. Activities during the response phase include rescue, triage, on-site stabilization, transportation of injured, and treatment at local hospitals and clinics. Disaster triage differs from triage done in the emergency departments. START, the most commonly used technique in the United States, consists of triaging individuals in 30 to 60 seconds during a mass casualty. The four categories consist of the walking wounded/minor (green tag), delayed (yellow), immediate (red), and deceased (black). These categories are based on ambulation, respirations, perfusion, and mental status (Bazyar, Farrokhi, & Khankeh, 2019).

Response also requires recovery, identification, and refrigeration of deceased remains, until notification of family members is possible (USDHHS, 2020b). Persons trained in mortuary services are an essential part of any emergency planning and response effort. The mortuary teams includes pastoral personnel to ensure that remains are always treated with respect and in accordance with religious traditions. Supportive care, including food, water, and shelter for survivors and relief workers, is a critical element of the total disaster response. Veterinary response teams are essential to address the acute and long-term needs of the animals impacted by the disaster. Many shelters will not accept pets, causing confusion and delays in sheltering displaced persons (Fig. 17-3).

Individuals with chronic health conditions and/or mental illness may need specific interventions in recovery from a disaster. Those with serious mental illness such as bipolar disorder and schizophrenia are less likely to be prepared for disasters than the general population. Although these disorders are not caused by disasters, the effects of the disaster can cause higher hospitalizations and higher levels of avoidance behavior (SAMHSA, 2019). C/PHNs need to be aware of support agencies for this population because their needs may increase due to lack of support systems and poor coping skills. In recent years, it has become clear that all of us need to be have a plan in place so that we recover as quickly as possible if a disaster arises.

- Individuals on medications need at least a 3-day supply of medications. Special diet foods may be hard to locate during a disaster; therefore, advise patients to eat healthy as much as possible if their special diet foods are unavailable during a disaster.
- Be prepared for possible power outages (CDC, 2019a).

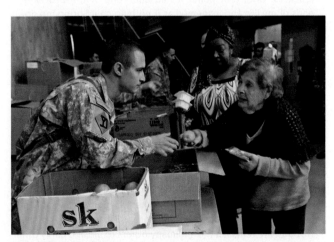

FIGURE 17-3 Victims of Superstorm Sandy receiving assistance at a temporary shelter.

- The Emergency Prescription Assistance Program helps to replace medications and equipment that is lost due to a disaster (Public Health Emergency, 2020).
- Knowledge of the community assists the C/PHN in ensuring all populations have services needed, with special attention paid to those who are most vulnerable.

Recovery Phase

During the *recovery phase*, the community joins together to repair, rebuild, or relocate damaged homes and businesses, and restore health, social, and economic vitality to the community. There will be many opportunities during this phase to enhance prevention and increase preparedness, thus reducing future vulnerabilities. Both survivors and relief workers may experience psychological trauma and should be offered mental health services to support their recovery (Box 17-2). The traumatic emotional scars may last a lifetime. The Substance Abuse Mental Health Services Administration (SAMHSA) offers guides and a disaster kit for managing stress in crisis for both professionals and victims (SAMHSA, 2011). Recovery activities take place *after* an emergency, and may extend over a period of months or even years.

During the recovery phase, special attention should be given to the needs of children who are approximately 25% of the population in the United States and even higher in other countries. The CDC has resources in English and Spanish to assist children that have experienced disasters. One example is the coloring book *Coping After a Disaster* (CDC, 2019b).

Role of the Community/Public Health Nurse

The C/PHN has a pivotal role in preventing, preparing for, responding to, and supporting recovery from a disaster (Association of Public Health Nurses [APHN] Public Health Preparedness Committee, 2014). After a thorough community assessment for risk factors, the C/PHN may initiate the formation of a multidisciplinary task force to address disaster prevention and preparedness in the community.

Preventing Disasters

Disaster prevention may be considered on three levels: primary, secondary, and tertiary (Box 17-3).

Primary Prevention. Primary prevention of a disaster means keeping the disaster from ever happening by taking actions that completely eliminate its occurrence—or, if that is not possible, to minimize damage through primary prevention. Primary prevention includes providing and participating in training sessions on prevention of disaster risk factors, knowing high-risk groups through community assessments, and working with community partners (CDC, 2019a). Primary prevention of disasters can be practiced in all settings in the workplace and home—with defined processes to reduce safety hazards and in the community, to monitor risk factors, reduce pollution, and encourage nonviolent conflict resolution (CDC, 2019b). Primary disaster prevention efforts should include awareness of a community's physical, psychosocial, cultural, economic, and spiritual stance. The C/PHN educates people at home, at work, at school, or

BOX **17-2** PERSPECTIVES

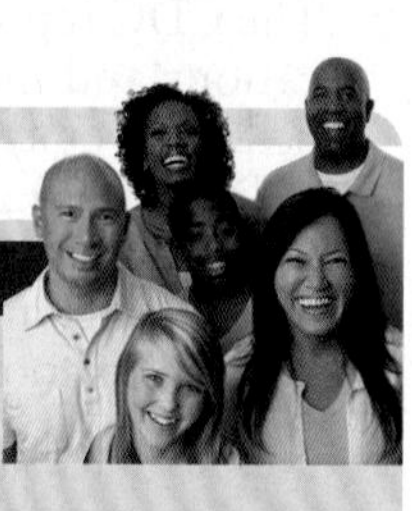

Viewpoint of a Survivor of the Route 91 Mass Shooting

As the first volleys of automatic gunfire rained down upon myself and the other 20,000 people watching Jason Aldean perform at the Route 91 Harvest Music Festival in Las Vegas, NV, my three friends and I looked around, trying to determine the source of the horrific sound that we had thought were firecrackers. Until that point, it had been one of the best weekends of my life and it seemed as if nothing could bring me down from the mountain of joy I felt. However, as Jason Aldean ran off stage and someone running past us yelled, "There's blood! That girl has been shot!" the mountain of joy came crumbling down and the devastation of what would eventually become an estimated 1,200 rounds of lethal ammunition, killing 58 beautiful souls, began to sink in.

Quickly, we moved towards the exit and stopped behind a barrier, trying to determine where the shooting was coming from and which way to go. As I looked back towards the emptying venue, I saw a young girl, shot through her eye, lying there. My work experience as an EMT kicked in, and a small group of strangers and I quickly carried her to the outer walls of the venue, passing her off to other strangers who said they had medical experience. From there, the adrenaline rushing through my veins led me and many others to aid and carry other gunshot victims out of what had become a war zone.

As the shooting eventually stopped and the only victims left inside the venue were those who were covered in a makeshift shroud to shield our eyes from the horror that lay underneath, the emotional roller coaster set in. I teetered between anger, extreme sadness, numbness, and confusion. I could not comprehend the magnitude of what had happened in front of my eyes. For weeks, it was all I could think about, replaying the steps I took, the sounds of gunfire, the cries, the feeling of a stranger's blood across my skin. Unless I was around my friends I had been at the concert with, I felt alone and uneasy in a crowded room. The posttraumatic stress was real, and it would take months of therapeutic counseling before I even felt remotely close to "normal."

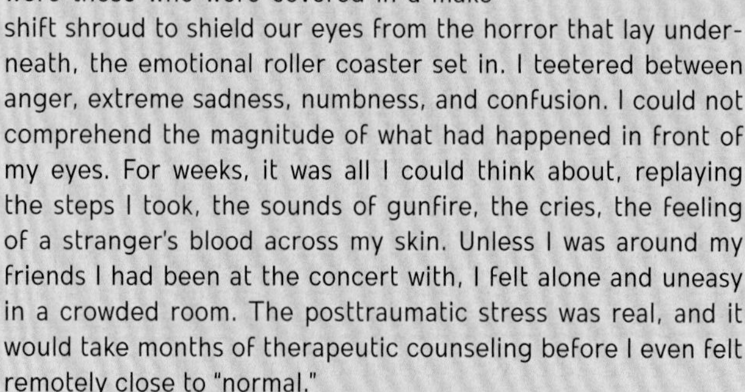

Over 2 years later, I still occasionally see a counselor to discuss the emotions and visions that are only a loud "pop" away. Though I do not bear any physical scars from the night of October 1, 2017, the emotional scars run deep and can be easily broken open. While I am able to function throughout my daily life and work life as an EMT in the emergency department seemingly fine, there is still not a day that goes by that I am not somehow reminded of that night.

Gabriel Mosse

BOX 17-3 LEVELS OF PREVENTION PYRAMID

Responding to a Tornado

SITUATION: A natural disaster—tornado

GOAL: Prepare, promptly diagnose, and treat and/or restore individuals, families, and communities to the fullest by using the three levels of prevention.

Tertiary Prevention

Rehabilitation	***Prevention***	
	Health Promotion and Education	***Health Protection***
▪ Remain safe during the immediate recovery period. ▪ Accept help from others—friends, family, and community services. ▪ Rebuild family lives through counseling and other services to reestablish stable life physically, emotionally, spiritually, and financially.	▪ Educate community members about the need to enhance planning against damage from future natural disasters, based on experiences with the current disaster.	▪ Keep recommended immunizations current. ▪ Community physical structures need rebuilding, with infrastructure planning and supports that improve ability to withstand natural disasters.

Secondary Prevention

Early Diagnosis	***Prompt Treatment***
▪ Remain in your position of safety until a community all-clear warning signal is sounded or until rescued. ▪ Leave a damaged building cautiously, if able and not seriously injured, and do not return until it is declared safe.	▪ Rescue individuals promptly and get appropriate care for those injured as soon as possible. ▪ The infrastructure of the community becomes/remains intact, keeping community members safe from hazards such as live wires, broken gas lines, and fallen debris.

Primary Prevention

Health Promotion and Education	***Health Protection***
▪ Increase community awareness. ▪ Increase community preparation through education. ▪ Each person is as prepared as possible both physically and emotionally.	▪ Community members know what to do and where to go, whether at home, work, school, or elsewhere in the community. ▪ Get to safety before the impact—southwest corner of a home's basement or an interior room away from windows and under heavy furniture.

in a faith community, and has a unique opportunity to be aware of the community perspective about safety and security focused on preventing a disaster. There are many prevention actions the C/PHN can initiate (APHN Public Health Preparedness Committee, 2014). These prevention actions can include the following:

- Completing a community assessment, including the residents with special needs and those in high-risk categories
- Collaborating with community leaders to provide general community prevention and preparation education activities. For instance, working with community partners C/PHNs promote policies that better prepare vulnerable populations. These relationships are built on trust and a common goal of serving the population. C/PHNs work closely with these community partners acting in a leadership role to ensure populations are assessed and have the services needed if a disaster occurs (APHN, 2014). The second aspect of primary disaster prevention is anticipatory guidance. Disaster drills and other anticipatory exercises help the community and relief workers experience some of the feelings of chaos and stress associated with a disaster before one occurs (APHN, 2014). It is much easier to do this when energy and intellectual processes are at a high level of functioning.
- The C/PHN has a role in community collaborative disaster drills through committee membership, organization of drills at the place of employment, or activism at the grassroots level to assist in holding community-wide disaster drills on a regular basis.

Secondary Prevention. Secondary disaster prevention focuses on the earliest possible detection and treatment. After a disaster, the local health department's C/PHNs work with the American Red Cross to coordinate and provide emergency assistance. Secondary prevention corresponds to immediate and effective response. Agencies who provided early evacuation, identified shelters for special-needs patients outside the high-risk area, implemented volunteer cascading communication systems, and conducted pre-event mock evacuation plans and included volunteers in their disaster plan were most successful with their response efforts. Recommendations to improve responses include identification of patients who may be reluctant to evacuate, the provision of adequate security at special-needs shelters, and, most importantly, practice drills (APHN, 2014; DHS, n.d.). Many local communities have developed preparedness programs to inform, prepare, and ensure residents are ready for any type of man-made or natural disaster, such as the City of New Orleans's NOLA READY (for more details, visit https://ready.nola.gov/home/).

Tertiary Prevention. Tertiary disaster prevention involves reducing the amount and degree of disability or damage resulting from a disaster. This level involves rehabilitative work and can help a community recover and reduce the risk of further disasters.

Since 9/11, the American Psychiatric Nurses Association has provided access to many resources for nurses dealing with traumatic events (American Psychiatric Nurses Association, 2016). Visit https://www.apna.org/m/pages.cfm?pageID=5196 for a detailed list of resources for dealing with traumatic events, and SAMHSA apps at https://store.samhsa.gov/product/samhsa-disaster for easy access when in the field. In addition to these references, the Office of the Assistant Secretary for Preparedness and Response (2019) offers a three-module series on compassion fatigue and secondary trauma for health care providers that can be found at https://files.asprtracie.hhs.gov/documents/aspr-tracie-dbh-self-care-for-health care-workers-modules-description-final-8-19-19.pdf

Preparing for Disasters

Disaster planning is essential for a community, business, and hospitals. Details of preparation and management by all involved, including community leaders, health and safety professionals, and lay people must be considered. Despite many disaster drills and numerous iterations of disaster plans before Hurricane Katrina, some hospitals in New Orleans were better prepared for terrorism events than for the hurricanes and flooding that were not uncommon to that geographic area. C/PHNs can be very instrumental in disaster preparedness (APHN, 2014). and must ensure they have their own family disaster preparation plan in place. For information on nurses' personal preparation for disaster and online courses on disaster preparedness, see Box 17-4.

Assessment for Risk Factors and Disaster History. The C/PHN is uniquely qualified to perform a community assessment for risk factors that may contribute to disasters (Quad Council Coalition, 2018). In addition, the nurse should review the *disaster history* and preparedness plans of the community. Have earthquakes, tornadoes, hurricanes, floods, blizzards, riots, or other disasters occurred in the past? If so, what (if any) were the warning signs? Were they heeded? Were people warned in time? Did evacuation efforts remove all people in danger? What were the community's on-site responses, and how effective were they? What programs were put in place to rehabilitate the community? Community health assessment tool may assist with identifying critical needs of the community (FEMA, 2020b).

Establishing Authority, Communication, and Transportation

- In addition to assessing for preparedness, the effective disaster plan follows the NIMS model and establishes a clear chain of authority, develops lines of communication, and delineates routes of transport. Establishing a clear and flexible chain of authority is critical for successful implementation of a disaster plan (CDC, 2018).
- Usually, the chain is hierarchical, with, for example, the community's governmental head (e.g., mayor) initiating the plan, alerting the media to broadcast warnings, authorizing the police to begin evacuations, and so on.
- Within each level of the organization, the hierarchy continues. For example, at the local hospital, the hospital administrator may be responsible for alerting nurse managers to call in additional personnel.
- Flexibility is essential, because key authority figures may themselves be survivors of the disaster. If the home of the chief of police is destroyed in an earthquake, his or her second-in-command must have equal knowledge of the community's disaster plan and be able to step in without delay.

Effective communication is often a point of breakdown for communities attempting to cope with major disasters. After the terrorist attacks in Oklahoma City and New York City, phone lines were damaged and cellular sites were overwhelmed, making communication difficult. Communication was possible only through handheld radios or by way of couriers on foot. At times of heightened chaos and stress, as well as after physical damage to communication facilities and equipment, misinformation and misinterpretation can flourish, leading to delayed treatment and increased loss of life.

Again, clarity and flexibility are the watchwords for establishing lines of communication.

- How will warnings be communicated?
- What backups are available if the normal communication systems are destroyed in the disaster?
- How will communication between relief workers at the disaster site, hospital personnel, police, and governmental authorities be maintained?
- What role will local media play, both in keeping information flowing to the outside world and in broadcasting needs for assistance and supplies?

BOX 17-4 Nurses' Personal Preparation for Disasters and Available Training

Nurses are ready, willing, and well positioned to respond to disasters; however, nurses receive minimal disaster-focused instruction as part of their formal education. Due to the reality that a disaster can occur at any time, it becomes all the more urgent for nurses to be well prepared through valid and low-cost education in disaster management (Brand, 2016).

American Nurses Association (ANA) has educational opportunities for nurses on disaster preparedness. When we are a prepared profession, we can cope and help our communities recover from disasters better, faster, and stronger. See https://www.nursingworld.org/practice-policy/work-environment/health-safety/disaster-preparedness/ for the following documents from the ANA:

- Position Statement Background Information: Registered Nurses' Rights and Responsibilities Related to Work Release During a Disaster
- Position Statement Background Information: Work Release During a Disaster—Guidelines for Employers

Other educational opportunities include:

- HHS Guidance for Mass Decontamination: Patient Decontamination in a Mass Chemical Exposure Incident: National Planning Guidance for Communities (available at http://www.phe.gov/Preparedness/responders/Documents/patient-decon-natl-plng-guide.pdf)
- A Nurse's Duty to Respond in a Disaster: Unresolved issues of legal, ethical, and professional considerations of disaster medical response remain a challenge, and could hamper the ability of nurses to respond. A concerted effort to solving these problems is needed, with nurses and stakeholders at the national, state, and local levels (available at https://www.nursingworld.org/~4ad845/globalassets/docs/ana/who-will-be-there_disaster-preparedness_2017.pdf).
- IOM Report on Establishing Crisis Standards of Care to use in Disaster Situations (PDF) (available at https://www.nursingworld.org/~4ad845/globalassets/docs/ana/stds-of-care-letter-report-2.pdf)

The American Nurses Association also offers the National Healthcare Disaster Certification (NHDP-BC); information on this program can be found at https://www.nursingworld.org/our-certifications/national-healthcare-disaster/. Nurses are able to take the certification exam once certain requirements are met.

Personal preparedness means that the nurse has read and understands workplace and community disaster plans and has developed a disaster plan for his or her own family (San Diego County Office of Emergency Services, n.d.). The prepared nurse should also have participated in disaster drills, have documented up-to-date vaccinations, be a certified basic life support (BLS) provider, and be able to provide basic first aid. Nurses preparing to work in disaster areas as "spontaneous volunteers" should have copies of their nursing license and driver's license, durable clothing, and basic equipment, such as stethoscopes, flashlights, and cellular phones to facilitate appropriate task assignments during the disaster response.

To increase understanding of and the ability to work within an emergency situation, every nurse should become familiar with the National Incident Management System (NIMS). The NIMS is "a systematic, proactive approach to guide all levels of government, NGOs, and the private sector to work together to prevent, protect against, mitigate, respond to, and recover from the effects of incidents." (FEMA, 2017a, p. 77). In essence, NIMS provides a framework for management of incidents in support of the national preparedness system. Free online courses are offered through FEMA at www.fema.gov. In addition to the FEMA courses, other options include the following

- CDC Emergency Preparedness and Response Training and Education: https://emergency.cdc.gov
- Federal Emergency Management Agency (FEMA): http://training.fema.gov/emi.aspx
- Public Health Foundation—Train.org: https://www.train.org
- National Institutes of Health—Radiation Emergency Medical Management: http://www.remm.nlm.gov/training.htm
- University of Minnesota, School of Public Health: http://www.sph.umn.edu/academics/ce/tools/

- Significant forms of communication have developed since the 9/11 terrorist attacks. Social media has become a critical method of communicating important health and safety information to the public since the 2001 terrorist attacks. Social media and disaster communication leaderships have collaborated and formed a partnership to disseminate information as quickly as possible (FEMA, 2020c).
- How will friends and family members be informed of the whereabouts or health status of loved ones?
- The CDC offers Crisis and Emergency Risk Communication (CERC) to ensure the correct messages by the correct authorities are communicated during emergencies. The training materials can be found on the CDC Web site at https://emergency.cdc.gov/cerc/index.asp.

The CDC Sample Single Overriding Communications Objective (SOCO) is an effective template to disseminate information concisely and quickly to the media during a disaster (see Box 17-5).

Closed or inefficient routes of transportation can also increase injury and loss of life. For example, if a single, narrow mountainous road is the only means of transporting firefighters to or evacuating residents from the scene of a forest fire, then disaster planners should propose widening the road or clearing a second road. Disaster planners must also consider what routes emergency vehicles will take when transporting disaster survivors to local and outlying hospitals or health care workers to the disaster site. What if the chosen routes are inaccessible because of floodwaters, advancing fires, mountain slides, avalanches, or building rubble? Are alternative routes designated? Also, how will people move about after the disaster? For example, after the Japanese earthquake and tsunami in 2011, Nakanishi, Matsuo, and Black (2013) examined planning methodologies and future

BOX 17-5 The CDC Sample Single Overriding Communications Objective (SOCO) Template

- In one BRIEF paragraph, state the key point or objective you want to accomplish by doing the interview. This statement should reflect what you, the author or speaker, would like to see as the lead paragraph in a newspaper story or broadcast report about your topic.
- What are the three or four facts or statistics you would like the public to remember as a result of reading or hearing about this story?
- Who is the main audience or population segment you would like this message to reach?

  Primary: General public   Secondary: Policy makers (awareness)
- What is the ONE message you want the audience to take away from this interview/report?

Reprinted from CDC. (n.d.). *Sample single overriding communications objective (SOCO).* Retrieved from https://www.cdc.gov/tb/publications/guidestoolkits/forge/docs/13_samplesingleoverridingcommunicationsobjective_soco_worksheet.doc

hypothetical disaster scenarios to help answer these types of questions.

Mobilizing, Warning, and Evacuating. In many natural disasters, local weather service personnel, public works officials, police officers, or firefighters have the earliest information indicating an increasing potential for a disaster. These officials typically have a plan in place for providing community authorities with specific data indicating increased risk (FEMA, 2018). They may also advise the mayor's office or other community leaders of their recommendations for warning or evacuating the public. Additionally, they may recommend actions the community can take to mitigate damage, such as spraying rooftops in the path of fires, sandbagging the banks of rising rivers, or imposing a curfew in times of civil unrest.

- Disaster plans must specify the means of communicating warnings to the public, as well as the precise information that should be included in warnings (DHS, 2016).
- Planners should never assume that all citizens can be reached by radio or television or that broadcast systems will be unaffected by the disaster. Broadcast media may indeed be a primary means of communicating warnings, but alternative strategies, such as social media or police and volunteers canvassing neighborhoods, should be considered.
- Social media options such as Facebook, Twitter, and blogs are reliable methods used by news stations and public health agencies that must not be ignored. Over 20 million tweets were sent by utilities after Hurricane Sandy, and Google's Web application, *Person Finder*, was especially helpful during the Boston Marathon bombings (SAMHSA, 2020a).
- In multilingual communities, messages should be broadcast in multiple languages.
- Not only homes but also businesses must be informed.
- Information that should be communicated includes the nature of the disaster; the exact geographic region affected, including street names if appropriate; and the actions citizens should take to protect themselves and their property.
- A study on the use of GPS devices in a simulated mass casualty found the devices useful in tracking patient locations throughout the drill (Gross et al., 2019). Technology improves tracking of injuries and fatalities.

An evacuation plan is an essential component of the total disaster plan (CDC, 2019a). The plan should include notification of the police, local military personnel, or voluntary citizens' groups of the need to evacuate people, as well as methods of notifying and transporting the evacuees. A plan should also be made for responding to citizens who refuse to evacuate. For example, will police authorities forcibly remove an elderly citizen from his home to a shelter? Will evacuation plans include household pets? If farms or ranches are in the path of fires or floods, will animals be evacuated? How? Who will do this and where will they be taken/sheltered?

Responding to Disasters

At the disaster site, police, firefighters, nurses, and other relief workers develop a coordinated response to rescue, triage, and treat disaster survivors. One of the first obligations of relief workers is to remove survivors from danger (Fig. 17-4).

Rescue. The job of rescue typically belongs to firefighters and urban search and rescue teams that have personnel with special training in search and rescue. Depending on the disaster agent, protective gear, heavy equipment, and special vehicles may be needed, and dogs trained to locate dead bodies may be brought in (Fig. 17-5). Sometimes, the immediate disaster site is not the best place for the disaster nurse, who can be far more effective in triage and treatment of survivors during this time. However, the C/PHN's population-based approaches, as well as knowledge of community resources and particularly vulnerable aggregates (Quad Council Coalition, 2018) are needed during this response phase.

Rescue workers face the logistically and psychologically difficult task of determining when to cease rescue

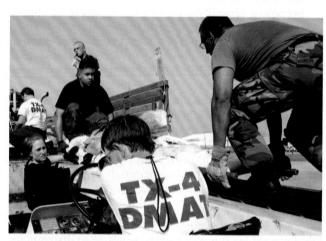

FIGURE 17-4 Rescue of a Hurricane Katrina victim.

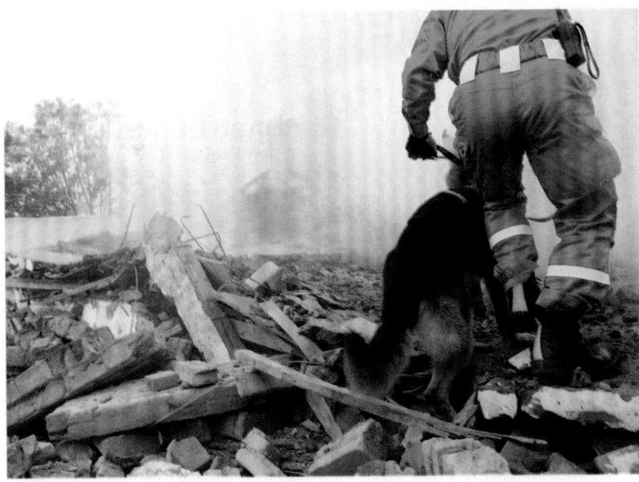

FIGURE 17-5 A firefighter-handler with a canine rescue dog.

efforts. Some factors to consider include increasing danger to rescue workers, diminishing numbers of survivors, and diminishing possibilities for survival. For example, after a plane crash on a snowy mountain, rescue efforts may cease if it is deemed that anyone who might have survived the crash would subsequently have died of exposure.

Triage. Knowing the prinicples and practices of triage allows the responding C/PHN to provide the most effectvie nursing skills (Wagner & Dahnke, 2015). Triage is the process of sorting multiple casualties in the event of a war or major disaster. It is required when the number of casualties exceeds immediate treatment resources. The goal of triage is to effect the greatest amount of good for the greatest number of people. For an image showing the four basic categories of the international triage system on a triage tag commonly used in disaster responses, visit thePoint.

- The most common method of triage used by first responders at a mass-casualty incident in the United States is the simple triage and rapid treatment (START) for adults and JumpSTART for pediatric patients. (For other triage methods, see thePoint.)
- START and JumpSTART are forms of triage used to sort victims into four categories (immediate, delayed, minor, or morgue/deceased) and are consistent with international triage system.

Prioritization of treatment may be very different in a mass-casualty event as opposed to an average day in a hospital emergency department. Under normal circumstances, a person presenting to a hospital emergency department with a myocardial infarction and showing no pulse or respirations would receive immediate treatment and have a chance of recovery. At a disaster site, a person without a pulse or respirations would most likely be placed in the nonsalvageable category.

- The term *mass casualty* refers to a number of persons impacted that is greater than that which can be managed safely with the available community resources, such as rescue vehicles and emergency facilities to serve disaster survivors while also meeting the needs of the rest of the community (Zarocostas, 2017).
- In mass-casualty occurrences, the broader community will need to become involved, including requests for rescue vehicles, firefighters, and police officers from neighboring towns, and/or the use of neighboring hospitals. Depending on the magnitude of the mass casualty, state and federal resources may also be needed.

This adds another layer of disaster management coordination that must be considered. The hurricane season of 2017 was one of the worst in US history (FEMA, 2017b) and, along with the California wildfires of 2017, stretched FEMA resources. FEMA provided support to millions of individuals. "By May 2018, nearly 4.8 million households...registered for assistance-more than the previous 10 years combined" (FEMA, 2018, p. 6). Based on the disasters of 2017, FEMA is revising the National Response Framework to improve relationships with the private sector and to improve their readiness outside the continental United States to name a few of the new revisions (FEMA, 2018).

C/PHNs should acquaint themselves with the phases of disaster a community experiences. According the Substance Abuse and Mental Health Services Administration (SAMHSA) there are six phases of disasters (Fig. 17-6; SAMHSA, 2018).

- Phase 1: Predisaster phase—fear and uncertainty
- Phase 2: Impact phase—range of intense emotional reactions
- Phase 3: Heroic phase—high level of activity with a low level of productivity
- Phase 4: Honeymoon phase—dramatic shift in emotion
- Phase 5: Disillusionment phase—realize the limits of disaster assistance
- Phase 6: Reconstruction phase—overall feeling of recovery

Immediate Treatment and Support. Disaster nurses provide treatment on-site at emergency treatment stations, at mobile field hospitals, in shelters, and at local hospitals and clinics (Box 17-6). In addition to direct nursing care, on-site interventions might include arranging for transport once survivors are stabilized, and managing the procurement, distribution, and replenishment of all supplies. The nurse may also manage provision or distribution of food and beverages, including infant formulas and rehydration fluids, and arrange for adequate, accessible, and safe sanitation facilities at the treatment location. Finally, the nurse often may also arrange for psychological and spiritual care of survivors of disasters (APHN Public Health Preparedness Committee, 2014).

Some survivors who seem physically uninjured may, in fact, be suffering from major injuries but be unable to relate their symptoms to a relief worker because of shock or anxiety. For instance, a father pulling debris away from his collapsed house after a tornado may be so worried about a missing child that he does not realize that he has a broken arm.

Other survivors may be so emotionally traumatized by the disaster that they act out, disrupting efforts to assist them and other survivors and possibly engaging in dangerous activities. These survivors must be assessed for head trauma and internal injuries, because their behavior may have a physiological cause (SAMHSA, 2020b).

Care of Bodies and Notification of Families. Identification and safe transport of the dead to a morgue or holding

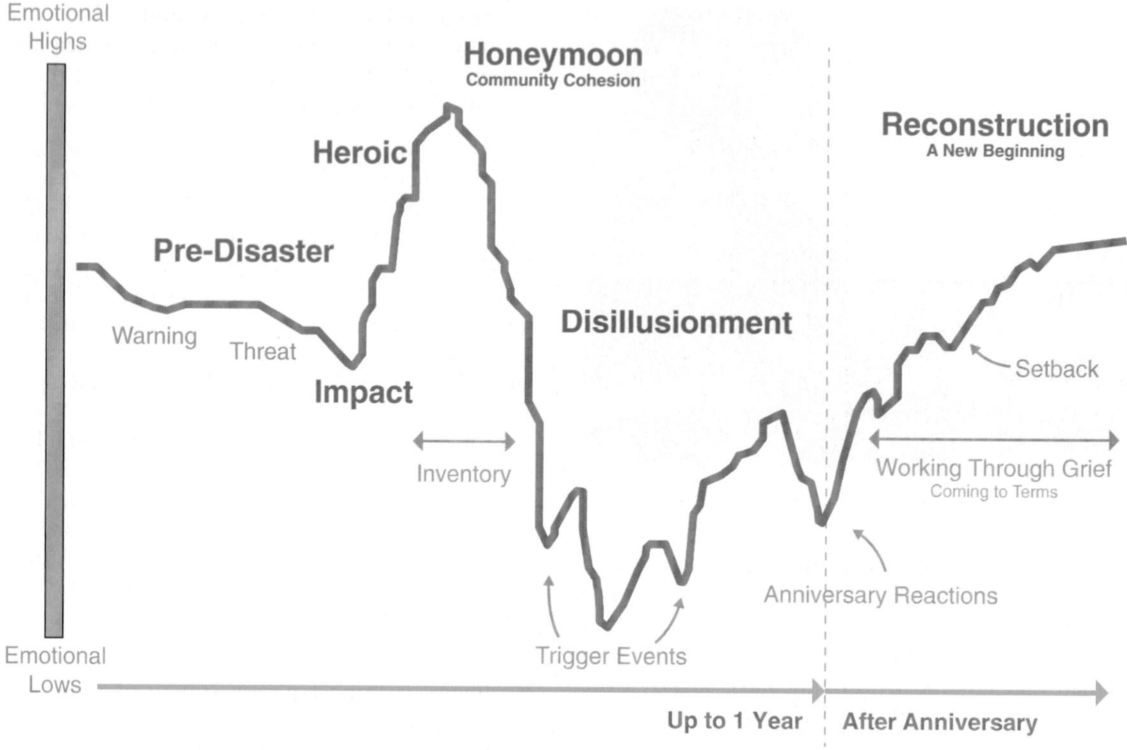

FIGURE 17-6 Six phases of disasters. (Reprinted from Substance Abuse and Mental Health Services Administration. (2020). *Phases of disasters.* Retrieved from https://www.samhsa.gov/dtac/recovering-disasters/phases-disaster. Adapted from Zunin & Myers as cited in DeWolfe, D. J. (2000). *Training manual for mental health and human service workers in major disasters* (2nd ed., HHS Publication No. ADM 90–538). Rockville, MD: U.S. Department of Health and Human Services, Substance Abuse and Mental Health Services Administration, Center for Mental Health Services.)

BOX 17-6 Mobile Field Hospital

On August 25, 2007, California featured the first state-owned mobile field hospital in a statewide disaster-training exercise. The tent hospital is one of three 200-bed hospitals purchased by California and prepositioned around the state in the event of a major emergency. The hospital can be deployed and on-site within 72 hours and comes equipped for 7 days of full patient care. Used together, the hospitals can be reconfigured into a 400- or 600-bed hospital, if needed. This is the same type of mobile field hospital used by the military, and it was modeled after the hospitals used by the Air Force and Navy. The various units within the hospital mirror services provided in any modern facility including emergency room, surgical suite, laboratory, x-ray, surgical intensive care, and even a pediatric unit.

More recently, mobile field hospitals were erected worldwide to treat patients with Covid-19, such as in New York's Central Park (below exterior view) and in Lombardia, Italy (below interior view).

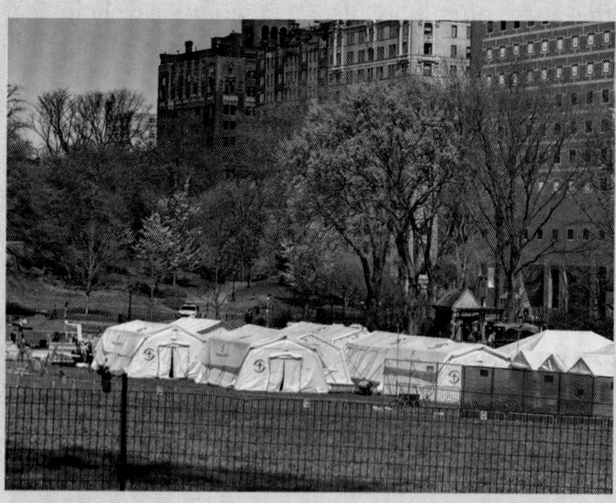

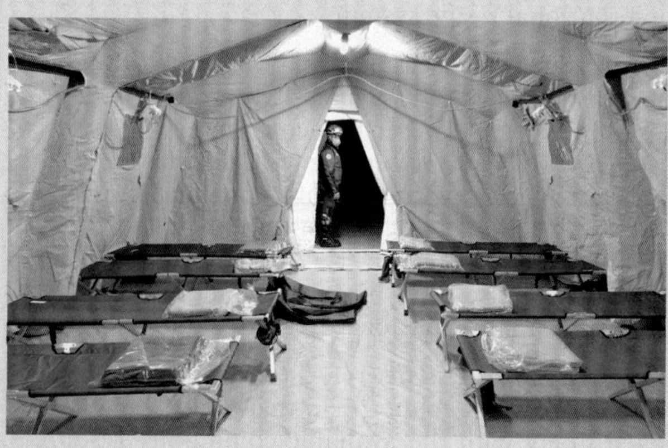

Source: Rodriguez (2016).

facility is crucial, especially if a contagion is feared, though this is rare in mass-casualty situations. Toe tags make documentation visible and accessible. Records of deaths must be accurately documented and maintained, and family members should be notified of their loved ones' deaths as quickly and compassionately as possible. If feasible, a representative from each of the area's faith communities should be available to assist families awaiting news of missing loved ones. A family's recovery from loss is often delayed when notification of their relative is not possible because the recovered bodies are badly damaged or not found (USDHHS, 2020b).

Supporting Recovery From Disasters

Disasters do not suddenly end when the rubble is cleared and the survivors' wounds are healed. Rather, recovery is a long, complex process often including long-term medical treatment, physical rehabilitation, financial restitution, case management, and psychological and spiritual support (FEMA, 2019).

Long-Term Treatment. Long-term treatment may be required for many survivors of disasters, straining the local rehabilitative care facilities and resources.

- Children who are survivors may have to deal with lifelong disabilities or scars from their ordeal, and families may be without adequate financial support for their child's medical care.
- Elderly citizens who had been in excellent health but who sustained serious injuries in the disaster might suddenly find that they can no longer live independently and must move to a long-term care facility.
- After floods, landslides, fires, or earthquakes, extensive property damage may cause some residents or businesses to relocate rather than rebuild on land they now deem to be disaster prone.
- A disaster that creates numerous persons impacted in a small community may alter the entire social fabric of that community permanently (SAMHSA, 2020b).

Long-Term Support. Immediately after a disaster, some survivors may be unable to concentrate on anything beyond fulfilling their immediate needs and those of their family. Disaster survivors may need funding to repair or rebuild their homes or to reopen businesses, such as stores, restaurants, childcare facilities, and other services needed by the community. Insurance settlements, FEMA funding, and private donations may assist in financing community rehabilitation. The FEMA Individual Assistance Program and Policy Guide can be found at: https://www.fema.gov/media-library-data/1551713430046-1abf12182d2d5e622d16accb37c4d163/IAPPG.pdf

Psychological support is often required after a disaster, both for survivors and for relief workers. Some individuals may experience posttraumatic stress disorder (PTSD). Many survivors, especially elderly persons displaced from their homes, may quietly lose their will to live and drift into apathy and malaise. Depression and anxiety are positively correlated in the elderly following earthquakes (Liang, 2017). While, some individuals may question their faith after a disaster, a systemic review found religion and spirituality may assist with coping and coming to terms with the disaster (Aten et al., 2019). These survivors in spiritual distress often require not only empathetic listening but also long-term skilled spiritual counseling. In assessing a community's citizens for counseling needs after a disaster, the PHN should not forget to include children. Often, children do not have words to express their feelings or fears and may act out in ways adults find difficult to understand, unless age-appropriate psychological intervention is provided. Medical responders to disasters are at risk of depression and PTSD with nurses being a greater risk than physicians. Risk factors included inadequate social support, inadequate coping skills, and insufficient training (Naushad et al., 2019).

Long-term support must be considered when assessing a community and planning for disasters. Each community may be unique in their needs, and each disaster requires a unique array of services and planning. Many communities may be efficient in providing services in quick response to a disaster; however, they often do not factor in the long-term needs and provide the structure and support (Reifels et al., 2015) needed by the community residents.

Need for Self-Care. Self-care, including stress education for all relief workers after a disaster, is a common practice and actively encouraged in many communities. Proponents report that stress education helps to reduce anxiety and put the situation into proper perspective. **Critical incident stress debriefing (CISD)** provides relief workers with professional debriefing that consists of phases followed by individual sessions and support services as needed (Harrison & Wu, 2017). CISD is generally provided between 24 and 72 hours after the disaster event. Proponents of CISD claim that it typically produces positive effects by:

- Accelerating the healing process
- Equipping participants with positive coping mechanisms
- Clearing up misconceptions and misunderstandings
- Restoring or reinforcing group cohesiveness
- Promoting a healthy, supportive work atmosphere
- Identifying individuals who require more extensive psychological assistance

A CISD addresses all components of the human response to trauma, including physiologic effects, emotions, and cognition (Occupational Safety and Health Administration, n.d.). The research on CISD has been mixed, but Mitchell (n.d.) reports that if the personnel providing the intervention are well trained and follow acceptable CISD practice standards, the outcomes are more positive. Self-care comes in many forms and is part of a prescription for emotional healing after a traumatic event. Self-care is for everyone touched by trauma including the rescue workers (CDC, 2018).

Trauma-informed care acknowledges the impact of various types of trauma on the individual's lifetime potential for health problems and "engaging in health-risk behaviors" (Menscher & Maul, 2016, para. 2). Both relief workers and recent trauma victims can benefit from this approach, which seeks to limit secondary traumatic stress by promoting empowerment and collaboration, as well as providing safety and choice. Earlier life experiences, such as abuse and neglect or systemic bias, may exacerbate experiences with traumatic events.

Psychological Consequences of Disasters

More research is needed in the monitoring of long term psychological effects and the evaluation of interventions following disasters (Généreux et al., 2019). It is estimated that 20% of Americans will experience a natural disaster (Wilson-Genderson, Heid, & Pruchno, 2018). Awareness of your perceptions and how your actions are viewed are essential in dealing with trauma victims. Fitzgerald & Hurst (2017) identify the prevalence of implicit bias even in health care providers. Their review of literature indicates that health care professionals exhibit the same amount of implicit bias as the general public and that diagnosis and treatment may be affected. In addition, trauma victims during a crisis may have previous trauma experiences related to power inequities, preventing a willingness to seek care or comply with medical instructions (Tello, 2018). Trauma-informed care requires the C/PHN to ask permission and be supportive (Tello, 2018). As health professionals, C/PHNs must be aware of their biases and prejudices (see https://implicit.harvard.edu/implicit/takeatest.html for a self-test for implicit bias).

Survivors of natural disasters experience a significant increase rate of psychological distress, PTSD, and depression (Beaglehole et al., 2018) The C/PHN and community mental health nurses, through education, screening, assessment, and referral, have an important role in the primary, secondary, and tertiary prevention of psychological disturbances due to a disaster.

Primary Prevention

Although a disaster, by its very nature, is often unforeseen, people's ability to cope with the disaster can be determined in part by their previous experiences and resources available.

Behavioral health is essential for overall health and wellness especially in the face of a disaster. Due to the uncertainty of when a disaster might occur, it is imperative to fortify personal and external resources before one happens. Interventions should include strengthening of cognitive, psychosocial, psychological, physical, and emotional domains of the individual and the community (Makwana, 2019). During these times, lessons learned from primary health education and interventions may help with the survival and recovery phases. Consideration must be given to the life stages of the survivors.

The American Psychological Association (2016) describes **resilience** as a process of behaviors, thoughts, and actions. The building of competency or resilience is an important primary prevention strategy, since a competent person or community can make informed decisions based on availability of resources and problem-solving skills. Community disaster training must include information on resiliency and resources to support individual and community resilience (APHN, 2014; CDC, 2019c; Makwana, 2019).

C/PHNs can contribute to primary prevention in the face of disaster by advocating for improving the social structure and economic conditions of the community, including housing, work, schools, child care, and recreational areas. it is also important for the C/PHN to advocate for the resources necessary for the community to meet both the physical and psychological challenges of a disaster.

Secondary Prevention

Survivors of disasters often feel anxious and overwhelmed and may be in *mental health crisis*, where the usual coping mechanisms are no longer effective in the face of the overwhelming disaster (Boyd, 2018). **Crisis intervention** is a secondary prevention intervention that the trained C/PHN can employ to minimize the stress and psychological consequences of the disaster (American Psychiatric Association [APA], 2016). Crisis intervention is a short-term intervention with the goal of alleviating negative effects of a disrupting, unexpected event such as disasters (APA, 2018) The phases of crisis interventions are closely related to the nursing process: assessment, planning of interventions, implementing the interventions, and evaluation and future planning (Townsend & Morgan, 2018).

Tertiary Prevention

People who have experienced or witnessed a disaster and have been unable to adequately cope with its consequences can develop *acute stress disorder* or the long-term effects of PTSD. According to the fifth edition of *Diagnostic and Statistical Manual of Mental Disorders* (DSM-5), text revision (American Psychiatric Association, 2019), both acute stress disorder and PTSD can occur after any traumatic event to which a person responds with intense fear, helplessness, or horror.

Posttraumatic stress disorder (PTSD), an anxiety disorder, occurs in some people after a traumatic event such as a disaster, crime, combat, or an accident (APA, 2019). It is important for the C/PHN to be aware of the symptoms of stress-related disorders and make referrals to the available mental health professionals.

TERRORISM AND WARS

At the start of the 21st century, the world is a global community. This is particularly evident with the increased international communication and travel practices. The incidence and sophistication of terrorist threats and acts around the world highlights our vulnerability, and dramatically emphasizes the need for increased preparedness within our communities for any type of biological, chemical, or nuclear terror attacks. One only needs to turn on the news to learn of terror attacks throughout the world.

History of Terrorism

The U.S. Federal Bureau of Investigation (FBI, n.d.b.) categorizes **terrorism** in one of two ways—as international terrorism or domestic terrorism. International terrorism is committed by persons or groups allied with foreign terrorist groups, whereas domestic terrorism is executed by individuals linked to U.S.-based extremist groups (FBI, n.d.b.). Generally, terrorism involves dangerous acts, violating laws, that are injurious to human life; it also involves a type of coercion or intimidation that affects government (U.S. Department of Justice, 2020). Terrorism and terrorist acts are not new. The term *terrorism* can be traced to 1798, and the use of terrorist tactics precedes this date. See Box 17-7 for a brief history of terrorist acts.

BOX 17-7 A Brief History of Terrorist Acts

- A highly organized religious sect called the *Sicarii* attacked crowds of people with knives during holiday celebrations in Palestine at about the time of Christ.
- During the French and Indian War of 1763, British forces gave smallpox-contaminated blankets to Native Americans.
- During World War I, the German bioweapons program developed anthrax, glanders, cholera, and wheat fungus as weapons targeting cavalry animals.
- In World War II, the Japanese tested biologic weapons on Chinese prisoners, and the Nazis conducted medical experiments with Jews forced into concentration camps (Spendlove & Simonsen, 2018).

Bioterrorism and Nuclear and Chemical Warfare

Three major countries operated offensive bioweapons programs in recent years: the United Kingdom until 1957, the United States until 1969, and the former Soviet Union until 1990. Iraq started its bioweapons program in 1985 and continued to develop weapons until 2003. Bioweapons include mustard gas, sarin, and VX gas, as well as anthrax (Spendlove & Simonsen, 2018). Terrorists typically use biologic or chemical agents, explosives, or incendiary devices to deliver the agents to their targets.

A terrorist attack using nuclear weapons or destruction of a nuclear plant would cause multiple and prolonged deaths with extensive damage and negative effects for decades.

Chemical warfare involves the use of chemicals such as explosives, nerve agents, blister agents, choking agents, and incapacitating or riot-control agents to cause confusion, debilitation, death, and destruction (Organisation for the Prohibition of Chemical Weapons [OPCW], 2020).

- Terrorists in the Middle East, willing to murder others and knowing they will be committing suicide, strap bombs to their bodies and detonate the explosives in or near targets.
- Others plant explosives at large outdoor events like the 2013 Boston Marathon (CNN, 2020) or crash vehicles loaded with explosives into crowds of people or into a building.
- The aircraft used on September 11, 2001, were incendiary devices because they were carrying thousands of tons of jet fuel.

The success of the mission depended on the surprise of the attack, severe damage to recognizable buildings, and the deaths of many people.

Biologic warfare involves using biologic agents to cause multiple illnesses and deaths. Biologic agents are graded as category A, B, or C by the CDC (see Table 17-3 for some examples). There are over 180 pathogens that have been used or studied as possible biologic warfare

TABLE 17-3 Categories of Biologic Agents

Category	Definition	Agents/Diseases
A	■ Pose highest risk to national security/public health: ■ Can be easily disseminated or transmitted from person to person ■ Result in high mortality rates and have the potential for major public health impact ■ Might cause public panic and social disruption ■ Require special action for public health preparedness	■ Anthrax (*Bacillus anthracis*) ■ Botulism (*Clostridium botulinum* toxin) ■ Plague (*Yersinia pestis*) ■ Smallpox (variola major) and other pox viruses ■ Tularemia (*Francisella tularensis*) ■ Viral hemorrhagic fevers
B	■ Second highest risk to national security: ■ Are moderately easy to disseminate ■ Result in moderate morbidity rates and low mortality rates ■ Require specific enhancements of CDC's diagnostic capacity and enhanced disease surveillance	■ Q fever (*Coxiella burnetii*) ■ Brucellosis (*Brucella* species) ■ Melioidosis (*Burkholderia pseudomallei*) ■ Psittacosis (*Chlamydia psittaci*) ■ Ricin toxin (*Ricinus communis*) ■ Epsilon toxin of *Clostridium perfringens* ■ *Staphylococcus* enterotoxin B (SEB) ■ Typhus fever (*Rickettsia prowazekii*) ■ Food- and waterborne pathogens
C	■ Third highest priority agents include emerging pathogens that could be engineered for mass dissemination in the future because of: ■ Availability ■ Ease of production and dissemination ■ Potential for high morbidity and mortality rates and major health impact	■ Nipah and Hantaviruses

CDC, Centers for Disease Control and Prevention.

Reprinted from the CDC Emerging Preparedness and Response. (2018). *Bioterrorism agents/disease.* Retrieved from https://emergency.cdc.gov/agent/agentlist-category.asp#b

(Smith, Hayoun, & Gossman, 2019). Typical biologic agents are anthrax, botulinum, bubonic plague, Ebola, and smallpox. These agents could be used to contaminate food, water, or air. Deliberate food and water contamination remains the easiest way to distribute biologic agents for the purpose of terrorism (American Academy of Pediatrics, 2020).

The United States is very concerned about the possibility of biologic warfare or bioterrorism. The anthrax infections and deaths that occurred after September 11, 2001, added to these concerns. It was years before the government investigation led to a scientist at Fort Detrick as the cause of this terroristic act. Although charges were never filed because of the individual's suicide, the FBI believes that he was solely responsible for this act of domestic terrorism (FBI, n.d.a.). Regardless of the source of terrorism, the outcomes are the same: fear, death, and destruction.

Trauma From the Warfront

Nurses, or men and women acting in that capacity, have provided comfort and care to soldiers long before Florence Nightingale arrived in the Crimea during the mid-19th century (see Chapter 3). Nurses continued to help during the Civil War and both World Wars, and their services continue today (Brooks & Hallett, 2015; Judd & Sitzman, 2014). Military nurses serving in the wars provide care to those with serious injuries and multiple casualties many times for extended periods of time. They may experience disturbing long-term psychological effects when returning home including feeling disconnected from civilian hospitals and feeling isolated upon their return (Finnegan, Lauder, & McKenna, 2016). It is important that appropriate psychological and physical interventions are provided for these servicemen and women (Krueger et al., 2015).

The trauma of warfare can be devastating and may continue to affect individuals for many years after completion of active service (Box 17-8; Magruder et al., 2016). Traumatic brain injury (TBI) is considered to be the "signature injury of the Iraq and Afghanistan wars" (Department of Defense, 2017, p. 3).

- Between 2000 and 2018, a staggering 383,947 Armed Service members were diagnosed with TBI peaking between 2011 and 2012 (Defense and Veterans Brain Injury Center, 2019).
- The most common causes of TBI include blast, object hitting head, and falls.
- TBI is associated with higher depression, PTSD, and suicidal ideation (Lindquist, Love, & Elbogen, 2017).
- Caregivers of veterans with traumatic brain injury are four times more likely to experience depression than the general population (Malec, Van Houtven, Tanielian, Atizado, & Dorn, 2017).
- Military personnel that have experienced a TBI are at a 4 times greater risk than personnel without a history of TBI (Loignon, Ouellet, & Belleville, 2020).
- One study found combat experiences and severity of PTSD were factors if the PTSD was chronic or not (Armenta et al., 2018).

BOX 17-8 STORIES FROM THE FIELD

Missed Opportunities for an Older Veteran

Tom Walton is a 70-year-old retired salesperson from an equipment manufacturer and a Vietnam veteran who served in the U.S. Navy. He has been a widower for the past year, and his adult children live out of state. Tom's health has declined dramatically since his wife's death, and he is struggling to control his hypertension and diabetes. Tom is noncompliant with medications and diet restrictions, and he seems to have more frequent outbursts of anger than usual.

Sadly, Tom's case is not one that is rare or unusual. I work at a Veteran's Administration (VA) clinic, and I often see cases like Tom's in our clinic. Many veterans do not deal with the traumas they experienced during warfare, and when support systems are weakened or they are no longer busy with work and family, these long-repressed feelings begin to reemerge. For Tom, his case could easily result in a deteriorating health care spiral that will ultimately lead to multiple hospitalizations or his demise. But, as a veteran, Tom may be a candidate for posttraumatic stress disorder (PTSD) treatment, mental health care treatment programs, or other proven treatment modalities offered by the VA. Unfortunately, many of our nation's veterans fail to take advantage of this resource, or even acknowledge that they may have this type of problem. In this case, having a working knowledge of the resources available to veterans in your community provides an opportunity for you, as a public health nurse, to assist Tom in accessing services that meet his health care needs and may prolong his life.

1. *What might you consider in providing care to veterans?*
2. *What resources are available in your area for veterans?*

—Bryan, VA Clinic Manager

C/PHNs should be aware of the needs of veterans, especially during disasters, terrorist attacks, and other traumatic events that may bring these past experiences to the forefront again. It is also important to ask patients if they have military experience during the initial assessment. This information may impact the planned interventions. C/PHNs should be aware of services available to veterans and treatments that are effective (Jain, McLean, Adler, & Rosen, 2016).

Factors Contributing to Terrorism

Political factors are the most common contributors to terrorism. Anti-American sentiment runs high in many foreign countries, especially those that perceive the United States as a threat to their military, economic, social, or religious self-determination. Terrorist acts are committed against American military installations abroad, in airports, in airplanes, at American embassies, and even on American soil targeting civilian populations. The war in Iraq in 2003 was based on information about suspected bioterrorism weapons and reports that Iraq was harboring anti-Western terrorists; these two pieces of information resulted in the toppling of the Saddam Hussein political regime. However, hundreds of military lives were lost and many thousands of civilians were killed, and no weapons of mass destruction were found (History, 2020).

Within the United States, domestic terrorism involves extremist views of a social, environmental, racial, political, or religious nature (FBI, n.d.b.). In 2019, a young man fatally shot 22 people at a Wal-Mart in El Paso, Texas. The FBI considers it an act of terrorism (Dilanian, 2019). As of November 2019 there have been 372 mass shootings, almost as many days in a year (Gun Violence Archive, 2020).

Role of the Community/Public Health Nurse

C/PHNs need to be prepared for the possibility of terrorist activity. They have a role in primary, secondary, and tertiary prevention.

Primary Prevention

C/PHNs are in ideal situations within communities to participate in surveillance. They must look and listen within their communities for antigroup sentiments, for example, antireligion, antigay, or antiethnic feelings, and appropriately report any untoward activities accordingly.

Nurses should be alert to signs of possible terrorist activity and develop the basic knowledge and skills to plan and respond to disasters including acts of terrorism (Veenema, 2018). The National Prevention Framework, produced by Homeland Security, provides guidelines to prevent or stop an act of terrorism. Pre- and postdisaster preparation to include critical, specific nursing competencies and evidence-based practices are strongly recommended by many hospitals and health care organizations for all health care personnel.. The American Nurses Association (ANA, 2016) has developed policies, resources, and educational opportunities for nurses on disaster preparedness acknowledging the importance of nurse preparation before a critical event (Fig. 17-7). The American Nurses Credentialing Center (ANCC) offers a certification in National Healthcare Disaster at https://www.nursingworld.org/our-certifications/national-healthcare-disaster/.

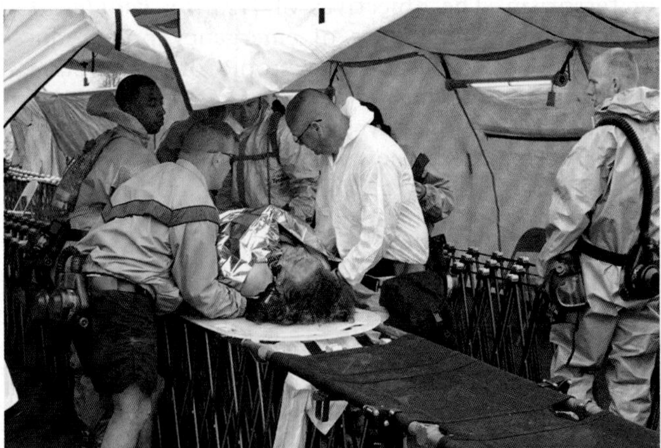

FIGURE 17-7 Disaster drills help prepare communities and health care workers.

Secondary and Tertiary Prevention

Although prevention of terrorist incidents is primarily the responsibility of the Department of Defense, the DHS, and public health and law enforcement agencies, C/PHNs must be ready to handle the secondary and tertiary effects of such attacks. Knowledge of the lethal and incapacitating chemical, biological, and radiological weapons potentially used by terrorists is important. Many of the communicable disease organisms that could be used by terrorists were discussed in Chapter 8.

Realizing that terrorist attacks may result in large numbers of casualties, the C/PHN must be prepared to act quickly, safely, and competently, and to access information and effectively use resources rapidly. Formulating, updating, and following a disaster plan is one of the most effective community-based strategies to minimize injury and mortality from terrorism. However, a recent systematic review discovered that nurses were unprepared to manage a disaster and did not feel confident (Labraque et al., 2018).

Most C/PHNs will not be on the front line of uncovering or immediately responding to terrorist activities; however, their skills will be needed with groups, families, or individuals who experience a terrorist-related event. C/PHNs provide direct care to survivors, help survivors with coping, or provide guidance to those who want to do something to help. After experiencing a traumatic event such as a terrorist attack, people do not know how to cope; they are warned to expect more attacks and to be vigilant. The terror we are fighting is often our own. This is a new experience for most people, and assistance from the C/PHN can help them cope effectively.

C/PHNs can make major differences in grassroots efforts to bring about change, on a day-to-day basis. For example, providing information on foods to avoid and nonmedical treatment options such as support groups, hypnosis, and biofeedback are a few examples of how nurses can assist with coping mechanisms. Community resilience is the goal of the interventions.

Current and Future Opportunities

There are many ways in which nurses, especially nursing students, can prepare both personally and professionally for emergency events in their own communities. Various governmental and educational programs are available as free online training covering a broad range of topics. Many schools of nursing have now begun to formalize their emergency preparedness plans in coordination with local hospitals, public health departments, or faith institutions. Nursing students should discuss their role, in the event of a local emergency with their faculty.

Knowing the nurse's role in an emergency will provide peace of mind regarding response capabilities and expectations. FEMA offers four particular courses within the incident command system (ICS 100, ICS 200, IS 700, & IS 800B), which are recommended for all health care personnel. Finally, make sure you have a family plan to reconnect with and care for children, spouses, and parents.

Increasingly, communities are conducting emergency preparedness exercises (e.g., mass-casualty exercises and tabletop exercises) in response to the need to prepare local resources to coordinate emergency response efforts for maximum effectiveness (CDC, 2016). Nursing students may be asked to participate in one of these exercises as a "victim." Take the opportunity anticipating the knowledge you gain from this experience will enhance your understanding of the process, and you may be able to help identify gaps in services or areas in need of improvement. You may be asked to have **moulage** applied to simulate injuries, and you will likely be given a brief description of your trauma (Box 17-9). Your assigned health problem may be emotional and not physical, allowing you to utilize your understanding of behavioral health issues and crisis intervention. Just as immunizations help fight against infections, participating in an emergency preparedness drill can build your tolerance and competency for responding appropriately in a real event.

Many organizations, both private and governmental, are seeking volunteers. If you wish to become more active in emergency preparedness volunteer efforts, the American Red Cross and your local Medical Reserve Corps are two options. You can continue your relationship with these organizations after you receive your nursing license, and your role with them will likely evolve.

BOX 17-9 What is Moulage?

Pronounced *mū-läzh*, the term *moulage* comes from the French word *mouler*, which means "to mold." In emergency preparedness training, moulage refers to the art of applying mock injuries for use in mass-casualty exercises. These injuries can be very simple or more complex, depending on available resources and the skills of the person applying the moulage. The use of moulage typically provides a more realistic experience for personnel participating in mass-casualty exercises.

Of the many online resources for information regarding equipment needed and how-to advice, one such Web site is Community Emergency Response Team (CERT) LAFD CERT, Moulage (https://www.cert-la.com/cert-training-education/moulage/).

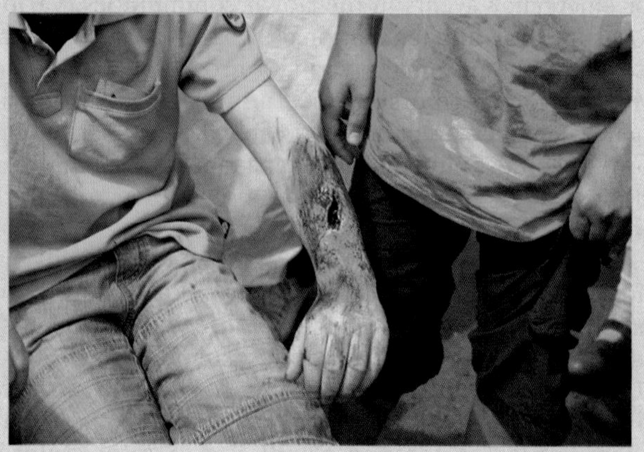

As a registered nurse, you may add your name to the registry along with your specialty training and contact information. Registration does not obligate you to any service; you agree only to be contacted if the need arises.

The APHN Public Health Preparedness Committee (2014) position paper, *The Role of the Public Health Nurse in Disaster, Preparedness, Response, and Recovery*, presented specific core competencies for public health nurses related to emergency preparedness, which can serve as a guide for students and practicing public health nurses. Please see thePoint for more information.

An adapted version of the 2014 position paper's table of disaster phases and corresponding nursing process actions is found in Box 17-10. Many options are available to you as both a student and a practicing nurse. What is important is that you are prepared. Assuring that you understand the role you may assume in the event of a local disaster or emergency situation is critical to your own welfare as well as to your community. You decide your level of participation, and be aware that resources are available for you to become as prepared as possible.

Objectives for *Healthy People 2030*

Healthy People 2030 includes four developmental objectives related to preparedness in disasters. These include (1) parents/guardians are aware of their children's school emergency and evacuation plans, (2) actions to take should a contagious disease occur, (3) adults who are aware of the transportation needs should a disaster occur and they need to evacuate, and (4) household emergency plan that includes vulnerable individuals (USDHHS, 2020a).

Healthy People 2010 focused upon increasing quality and years of healthy life and to eliminating health disparities. Formulated in the years before January 2000, many disasters, both natural and manmade, were unknown in recent times. The United States had not yet faced the national failures in the response to the hurricanes Katrina and Rita. We would also learn 18 months after the publication of *Healthy People 2010* that our nation was not immune from acts of terrorism. The objectives of *Healthy People 2020* directly addressed issues of emergency preparedness and response under the new topic of *Preparedness*. Additional topics also included preparedness activities, such as the objectives for public health infrastructure. The goal of the new topics and objectives were to improve our "ability to prevent, prepare for, respond to, and recover from a major health incident" (USDHHS, 2016, p. 1). Those specific objectives provide the support needed to enhance public health surveillance activities, laboratories, training, development of professional competencies, and performance standards for public health organizations. Healthy People 2030 builds on this with personal plans, awareness of the needs of vulnerable groups, and inclusion of contagions as part of a disaster response (USDHHS, 2020a). See Box 17-11.

BOX **17-10** C/PHN USE OF THE NURSING PROCESS

Disaster Preparedness, Response, and Recovery

Disaster Cycle	*Definition*	*Assessment*	*Planning*	*Implementation*	*Evaluation*
Preparedness	Includes Prevention, protection, mitigation What is needed to prevent a disaster or reduce the impact of one (lives lost, property damage)?	Do you have specific populations in your service area that are vulnerable and at risk because of problems with access and functional needs during disaster (e.g., physically/mentally disabled, those with Alzheimer's, frail elderly)? Determine any hazards or threats that pose risks.	Plan for additional assistance and accommodations for those at risk and vulnerable populations during disasters or other emergencies. Work with other stakeholders to meet their needs and the needs of your service area population (e.g., sheltering in place, evacuation, mass-casualty surge capabilities).	Conduct drills, trainings, and exercises regarding care of individuals, families, and communities during disasters. Focus on at-risk and vulnerable populations you have identified previously (e.g., physically/mentally disabled, those with Alzheimer's, frail elderly).	Evaluate the drills, trainings, and exercises in regard to care of at-risk and vulnerable populations. Identify gaps and any residual needs. Conduct evaluation of operational plans (e.g., preparedness, response, recovery for at-risk and vulnerable populations).
Response	Includes Lifesaving Protection of property Meeting basic human needs postdisaster What services and personnel are needed to save lives and protect property in a disaster? What services and personnel are needed immediately after the disaster to meet basic needs?	Using population-based triage, assess the impact of any communicable disease outbreak. Who is susceptible? Who has been exposed? Who is infected?	Work with stakeholders to develop or choose triage plans and methods of patient flow based on present symptoms and known history (e.g., COPD).	Work to organize PHNs and other trained personnel to provide care per triage plans. Perform ongoing rapid needs assessments during this phase, and ensure planning for community care support.	During the disaster, take part in continuing response planning and service planning. Ensure that necessary PHN care is provided.
Recovery	Includes assistance in recovery after a disaster What core skills and capacities are needed to ensure effective recovery?	Continue intermittent rapid needs assessment to ascertain health status and capacity for critical resources after the disaster (e.g., floods).	Together with stakeholders, make plans for any identified long-term health concerns, and pinpoint key resources needed for recovery.	Contribute to restoration of critical community services and sustaining the social and health infrastructures. Work to help the community achieve stabilization after the disaster.	Help with evaluation of disaster's long-term impact on the community. Through the work of PHNs, promote essential public health services.

Source: Association of Public Health Nurses, Public Health Preparedness Committee. (2014).

BOX **17-11** *HEALTHY PEOPLE 2030*

Objectives Related to Disaster Preparedness

Core Objectives

PREP-01	Increase the rate of bystander CPR for nontraumatic cardiac arrests
PREP-02	Increase the rate of bystander automated external defibrillator (AED) use for nontraumatic cardiac arrests in public places

Developmental Objectives

PREP-D01	Increase the proportion of parents and guardians who know the emergency or evacuation plan for their children's school
PREP-D02	Increase the proportion of adults who prepare for a disease outbreak after getting preparedness information
PREP-D03	Increase the proportion of adults who know how to evacuate in case of a hurricane, flood, or wildfire
PREP-D04	Increase the proportion of adults who have emergency plan for disasters

Reprinted from U.S. Department of Health & Human Services (USDHHS). (2020). *Healthy People 2030: Browse objectives.* Retrieved from https://health.gov/healthypeople/objectives-and-data/browse-objectives

SUMMARY

- A disaster is any event that causes a level of destruction that exceeds the abilities of the affected community to respond without assistance. Disasters may be caused by natural or man-made/technologic events and may be classified as multiple-casualty incidents or mass-casualty incidents.
- Persons impacted by disasters include those directly impacted (those injured or killed) and indirectly impacted (the loved ones of directly impacted). Displaced persons are those who are forced to flee their homes because of the disaster, and refugees are those who are forced to leave their homelands.
- Host factors that contribute to the likelihood of experiencing a disaster include age, general health, mobility, psychological factors, and socioeconomic factors. The disaster agent is the fire, flood, bomb, or other cause. Environmental factors are those that could potentially contribute to or mitigate a disaster.
- In developing strategies to address the problem of disasters, it is helpful for the C/PHN to consider each of the four phases of disaster management: mitigation, preparedness, response, and recovery.
- Communities experience six phases in a disaster: predisaster, impact, heroic, honeymoon, disillusionment, and reconstruction.
- An effective disaster plan establishes a clear chain of authority, develops lines of communication, and delineates routes and modes of transport. Plans for mobilizing, warning, and evacuating people are critical. At the disaster site, police, firefighters, nurses, and other relief workers develop a coordinated response to rescue survivors from further injury, triage survivors by seriousness of injury, and treat survivors on-site and in local hospitals. Care and transport of the dead bodies and support for the loved ones of the injured, dead, or missing need to be included in the disaster plan as well.
- Survivors of disasters suffer physical injuries and psychological trauma that can affect them for life. The importance of prevention, early crisis intervention, and ongoing treatment for those in need is evident. The C/PHN plays a key role in assessing individuals for symptoms of psychological trauma and intervening to prevent long-term consequences. Self-care, including stress education for all relief workers after a disaster, helps to lower anxiety and put the situation into perspective.
- Terrorism is the unlawful use of force or violence against persons or property to intimidate or coerce a government or civilian population in the furtherance of political or social objectives. Terrorism may be nuclear, biologic, or chemical and may involve the use of nerve agents and explosive devices. The C/PHN should be alert to signs of possible terrorist activity and prepared to address the secondary or tertiary effects of such attacks.
- Many opportunities are available for both student nurses and experienced C/PHNs to become involved in emergency preparedness and response efforts. Agencies such as the American Red Cross and the Medical Reserve Corps are options available to students and at a higher level of involvement, once licensed. With the development of *Healthy People 2030*, ongoing efforts to help communities prepare for disasters and emergencies will require more nurses willing and able to respond to a call for action.

ACTIVE LEARNING EXERCISES

1. Think about your own community and its residents. What environmental factors might be significant? What interventions could be included in a disaster plan to reduce these risk factors?
2. Think about your state and any sites that might be a target of terrorism. What is your state doing to address these issues? Examine Web sites (e.g., U.S. Homeland Security, Centers for Disease Control and Prevention, World Health Organization) for strategic planning or documents that could be helpful in assessing terror threats and preventing attacks. If an attack does occur, how would health professionals be most effective?
3. Using "Build a Diverse and Skilled Workforce" (1 of the 10 essential public health services; see Box 2-2), check with your local hospital about their disaster plan. Do they collaborate with your local health department and other agencies in designing and executing this plan? How often are "disaster drills" or simulations occurring? Who is involved in these? How many types of emergency situations do they cover?
4. As a C/PHN practicing in an area with a high concentration of veterans, what knowledge and skills do you think are necessary to provide culturally competent, evidence-based care to this segment of the population?
5. Interview a C/PHN who was involved in a disaster. Some topics to discuss might be—what kind of disaster preparedness did they have? Was their family affected by the disaster and what was it like to leave their family to help others?

REFERENCES

Ailworth, E. (2019). Opening the door to hell itself: Bahamas confronts life after Hurricane Dorian. *The Wall Street Journal*. Retrieved from https://www.wsj.com/articles/opening-the-door-to-hell-itself-bahamas-confronts-life-after-hurricane-dorian-11569176306

American Academy of Pediatrics. (2020). *Biological terrorism and agents*. Retrieved from https://www.aap.org/en-us/advocacy-and-policy/aap-health-initiatives/Children-and-Disasters/Pages/Biological-Terrorism-and-Agents.aspx

American Nurses Association. (2016). *Disaster preparedness & response*. Retrieved from http://www.nursingworld.org/disasterpreparedness

American Psychiatric Association (APA). (2016). *What are anxiety disorders?* Retrieved from http://www.psychiatry.org/patients-families/anxiety-disorders/what-are-anxiety-disorders

American Psychiatric Association (APA). (2018). *APA dictionary of psychology*. Retrieved from https://dictionary.apa.org/

American Psychiatric Association (APA). (2019). *Clinical practice guideline for the treatment of Post-Traumatic Stress Disorder (PTSD)*. Retrieved from http://www.apa.org/ptsd-guideline/patients-and-families/index.aspx

American Psychiatric Nurses Association. (2016). *Resources for dealing with traumatic events*. Retrieved from http://www.apna.org/i4a/pages/index.cfm?pageid=5196

American Psychological Association. (2016). *The road to resilience*. Retrieved from http://www.apa.org/helpcenter/road-resilience.aspx

American Red Cross. (n.d.). *American Red Cross guide to services*. Retrieved from http://www.redcross.org/images/MEDIA_CustomProductCatalog/m3140117_GuideToServices.pdf

Armenta, R. F., Rush, T., LeardMann, C. A., Millegan, J., Cooper, A., Hoge, C. W., & Millennium Cohort Study team. (2018). Factors associated with persistent posttraumatic stress disorder among U.S. military service members and veterans. *BMC psychiatry*, 18(1), 48. https://doi.org/10.1186/s12888-018-1590-5

Association of Public Health Nurses (APHN) Public Health Preparedness Committee. (2014). *The role of the public health nurse in disaster preparedness, response, and recovery* (2nd ed.). Retrieved from http://www.quadcouncilphn.org/wp-content/uploads/2016/03/2014_APHN-Role-of-PHN-in-Disaster-PRR-Ref-updated-2015.pdf

Aten, J. D., Smith, W. R., Davis, E. B., Van Tongeren, D. R., Hook, J. N., Davis, D. E., ... Hill, P. C. (2019). The psychological study of religion and spirituality in a disaster context: A systematic review. *Psychological Trauma Theory Research Practice & Policy*, *11*(6), 597–613. doi: 10.1037/tra0000431.

Bazyar, J., Farrokhi, M., & Khankeh, H. (2019). Triage systems in mass casualty incidents and disasters: A review study with a worldwide approach. *Open Access Macedonian Journal of Medical Sciences*, 7(3), 482–494. doi: 10.3889/oamjms.2019.119.

Beaglehole, B., Mulder, R. T., Frampton, C. M., Boden, J. M., Newton-Howes, G., & Bell, C. J. (2018). Psychological distress and psychiatric disorder after natural disasters: Systemic review and meta-analysis. *British Journal of Psychiatry*, *213*(6), 716–722. doi: 10.1192/bjp.2018.210.

Boyd, M. A. (2018). *Psychiatric nursing: Contemporary practice* (6th ed.). Philadelphia, PA: Wolters Kluwer.

Brand, R. (2016). *When disaster strikes*. Robert Wood Johnson Foundation. Retrieved from https://www.rwjf.org/en/library/research/2016/05/when-disaster-strikes.html

Brekke, D. (2019). *In remembrance: The names of those lost in the camp fire*. Retrieved from https://www.kqed.org/news/11710884/list-of-those-who-died-in-butte-county-paradise-camp-fire

Brooks, J., & Hallett, C. E. (Eds.). (2015). *One hundred years of wartime nursing practices, 1854–1953*. Manchester, UK: Manchester University Press.

Centers for Disease Control and Prevention (CDC). (2016). *Office of public health preparedness and response*. Retrieved from http://www.cdc.gov/phpr/

Centers for Disease Control and Prevention (CDC). (2018). *Emergency responders: Tips for taking care of yourself*. Retrieved from https://emergency.cdc.gov/coping/responders.asp#:~:text=Responder%20Self%2DCare%20Techniques&text=Write%20in%20a%20journal.,get%20adequate%20sleep%20and%20exercise

Centers for Disease Control and Prevention (CDC). (2019a). *Public health emergency preparedness and response capabilities: National standards for state, local, tribal, and territorial public health*. Retrieved from https://www.cdc.gov/cpr/readiness/00_docs/CDC_PreparednesResponseCapabilities_October2018_Final_508.pdf

Centers for Disease Control and Prevention (CDC). (2019b). *Coping after a disaster*. Retrieved from https://www.cdc.gov/cpr/readywrigley/documents/RW_Coping_After_a_Disaster_508.pdf

Centers for Disease Control and Prevention (CDC). (2019c). *Disaster planning: People with chronic disease*. Retrieved from https://www.cdc.gov/reproductivehealth/features/disaster-planning-chronic-disease/index.html

Centers for Disease Control and Prevention (CDC). (2020a). *WHO coronavirus disease (COVID-10) dashboard*. Retrieved from https://covid19.who.int/?gclid=Cj0KCQjw6ar4BRDnARIsAITGzlC07PXVBWo7aExbhEy1eIi0wXAKyhy8Ju0Z6amxvLOKwozDj_suCJcaAieyEALw_wcB

Centers for Disease Control and Prevention (CDC). (2020b). *Global health protection and security. Why it matters: The pandemic threat*. Retrieved from https://www.cdc.gov/globalhealth/healthprotection/fieldupdates/winter-2017/why-it-matters.html

Centers for Disease Control and Prevention (CDC). (2020c). *Coronavirus disease 2019: Covid-19. How to protect yourself and others*. Retrieved from https://www.cdc.gov/coronavirus/2019-ncov/prevent-getting-sick/prevention.html

Centers for Medicare and Medicaid Services (CMS). (2017). *Survey and certification group frequently asked questions (FAQs): Emergency preparedness regulation.* Retrieved from https://www.cms.gov/Medicare/Provider-Enrollment-and-Certification/SurveyCertEmergPrep/Downloads/FAQ-Round-Four-Definitions.pdf

CNN Editorial Research. (2020). *Boston marathon terror attack fast facts.* Retrieved from https://www.cnn.com/2013/06/03/us/boston-marathon-terror-attack-fast-facts/index.html

Defense and Veterans Brain Injury Center. (2019). *DoD worldwide numbers for TBI.* Retrieved from https://dvbic.dcoe.mil/dod-worldwide-numbers-tbi

DeNolf, R. L., & Kahwaji, C. I. (2019). *EMS, mass casualty management.* Retrieved from https://www.ncbi.nlm.nih.gov/books/NBK482373/

Department of Defense. (2017). Report to Congress in Response to Senate Report 114–263, Page 193, Accompanying S. 3000, The Department of Defense Appropriations Bill, 2017: Traumatic Brain Injury/Psychological Health. Retrieved from https://www.congress.gov/congressional-report/114th-congress/senate-report/263

Department of Homeland Security. (n.d.). *Hurricanes.* Retrieved from http://www.ready.gov/hurricanes

Department of Homeland Security (DHS). (2015). *Creation of the Department of Homeland Security.* Retrieved from https://www.dhs.gov/creation-department-homeland-security

Department of Homeland Security (DHS). (2018). *Operational and support components.* Retrieved from https://www.dhs.gov/operational-and-support-components

Department of Homeland Security (DHS). (2016). *Crisis communications plan.* Retrieved from https://www.ready.gov/business/implementation/crisis

Dilanian, K. (2019). *There is no law that covers 'domestic terrorism.' What would one look like?* Retrieved from https://www.nbcnews.com/politics/justice-department/there-no-law-covers-domestic-terrorism-what-would-one-look-n1040386

Diskin, M. (2019). What caused the Thomas Fire? Report reveals what sparked one of California's largest wildfires. *USA Today.* Retrieved from https://www.usatoday.com/story/news/nation/2019/03/13/thomas-fire-cause-report-released/3154686002/

Engel, P. & Ioanes,E. (2020, September). *What happened on 9/11, 19 years ago. Business Insider.* Retrieved from https://www.businessinsider.com/what-happened-on-911-why-2016-9

Federal Bureau of Investigation (FBI). (n.d.a.). *Amerithrax or Anthrax investigation.* Retrieved from https://www.fbi.gov/history/famous-cases/amerithrax-or-anthrax-investigation

Federal Bureau of Investigation (FBI). (n.d.b.). *Definitions of terrorism in the U.S. code.* Retrieved from https://www.fbi.gov/about-us/investigate/terrorism/terrorism-definition

Federal Emergency Management Agency (FEMA). (2017a). *National Incident Management System (NIMS).* Retrieved from https://www.fema.gov/media-library-data/1508151197225-ced8c60378c3936adb92c1a3ee6f6564/FINAL_NIMS_2017.pdf

Federal Emergency Management Agency. (2017b). *2017 Hurricane Season FEMA After-Action Report.* Retrieved from https://www.fema.gov/media-library-data/1531743865541-d16794d43d3082544435e1471da07880/2017FEMAHurricaneAAR.pdf

Federal Emergency Management Agency (FEMA). (2018). *2018–2022 Federal Emergency Management Agency strategic plan.* Retrieved from https://www.fema.gov/media-library-data/1533052524696-b5137201a4614ade5e0129ef01cbf661/strat_plan.pdf

Federal Emergency Management Agency (FEMA). (2019). *Fact sheet: Disaster case management program.* Retrieved from https://www.fema.gov/news-release/2019/02/12/fact-sheet-disaster-case-management-program

Federal Emergency Management Agency (FEMA). (2020a). *Individual and community preparedness division.* Retrieved from https://www.fema.gov/individual-and-community-preparedness-division

Federal Emergency Management Agency (FEMA). (2020b). *Hazard identification ad risk assessment.* Retrieved from https://www.fema.gov/hazard-identification-and-risk-assessment

Federal Emergency Management Agency (FEMA). (2020c). *Social media.* Retrieved from https://www.fema.gov/social-media

Finnegan, A., Lauder, W., & McKenna, H. (2016). The challenges and psychological impact of delivering nursing care within a war zone. *Nursing Outlook, 64*(5), 450–458. doi: 10.1016/j.outlook.2016.05.00.

Fitzgerald, C., & Hurst, S. (2017). Implicit bias in healthcare professional: A systematic review. *BMC Medical Ethics, 18*(19), 1–18. doi: 10.1186/s12910-017-0179-8.

Généreux, M., Schluter, P. J., Takahash, I. S., Usami, S., Mashino, S., Kayano, R., & Kim, Y. (2019). Psychosocial management before, during, and after emergencies and disasters-results from the Kobe Expert Meeting. *International Journal of Environmental Research and Public Health, 16*(8), 1309. doi: 10.3390/ijerph16081309.

Gross, I. T., Coughlin, R. F., Cone, D. C., Bogucki, S., Auerbach, M., & Cicero, M. X. (2019). GPS devices in a simulated mass casualty event, prehospital emergency care. *Prehospital Emergency Care, 23*(2), 290–295. doi: 10.1080/10903127.2018.1489018.

Gun Violence Archive. (2020). *Gun Violence Archive 2020.* Retrieved from https://www.gunviolencearchive.org/

Haddow, G. D., Bullock, J. A., & Coppola, D. P. (2016). *Introduction to emergency management* (6th ed.). New York, NY: Elsevier.

Harrison, R., & Wu, A. (2017). Critical Incident Stress Debriefing after adverse patient safety events. *The American Journal of Managed Care, 23*, 310–312. Retrieved from https://www.ajmc.com/journals/issue/2017/2017-vol23-n5/critical-incident-stress-debriefing-after-adverse-patient-safety-events

History.com. (2020). *War in Iraq begins.* Retrieved from https://www.history.com/this-day-in-history/war-in-iraq-begins

International Charter. (2019). *Charter activations.* Retrieved from http://www.disasterscharter.org/

Jain, S., McLean, C., Adler, E. P., & Rosen, C. S. (2016). Peer support and outcome for veterans with posttraumatic stress disorder (PTSD) in a residential rehabilitation program. *Community Mental Health Journal, 52*, 1089–1092. doi: 10.1007/s10597-015-9982-1.

Judd, D., & Sitzman, K. (2014). *A history of American nursing* (2nd ed.). Burlington, MA: Jones & Bartlett Learning.

Karimi, F. (2019). *A firefighter killed on September 11 is identified 18 years later.* Retrieved from https://www.cnn.com/2019/09/11/us/sept-11-firefighter-michael-haub-identified/index.html

Krueger, C. A., Rivera, J. C., Tennent, D. J., Sheean, A. J., Stinner, D. J., & Wenke, J. C. (2015). Late amputation may not reduce complications or improve mental health in combat-related, lower extremity limb salvage patients. *Injury, 46*(8), 1527–1532. doi: 10.1016/j.injury.2015.05.015.

Labraque, L. J., Hammad, K., Gloe, D. S., McEnroe-Petitte, D. M., Fronda, D. C., Obeidat, A. A., ... Mirafuentes, E. C. (2018). Disaster preparedness among nurses: A systematic review of literature. *International Nursing Review, 65*(1), 41–53. doi: 10.1111/inr.12369.

Liang, Y. (2017). Depression and anxiety among elderly earthquake survivors in China. *Journal of Health Psychology, 22*(14), 1869–1879. doi: 10.1177/135910531663943.

Lindquist, L. K., Love, H. C., & Elbogen, E. B. (2017). Traumatic brain injury in Iraq and Afghanistan veterans: New results from a National Random Sample Study. *The Journal of Neuropsychiatry and Clinical Neurosciences, 29*(3), 254–259. doi: 10.1176/appi.neuropsych.16050100.

Loignon, A., Ouellet, M. C., & Belleville, G. (2020). A systematic review and meta-analysis on PTSD following TBI among military/veteran and civilian populations. *The Journal of Head Trauma Rehabilitation, 35*, E21–E35. doi: 10.1097/HTR.000000000.

Magruder, K. M., Goldberg, J., Forsberg, C. W., Friedman, M. J., Litz, B. T., Vaccarino, V., ... Smith, N. L. (2016). Long-term trajectories of PTSD in Vietnam-era veterans: The course and consequences of PTSD in twins. *Journal of Traumatic Stress, 29*(1), 5–16.

Makwana, N. (2019). Disaster and its impact on mental health: A narrative review. *Journal of Family Medicine and Primary Care, 8*(10), 3090–3095. doi: 10.4103/jfmpc.jfmpc_893_19.

Malec, J. F., Van Houtven, C. H., Tanielian, T., Atizado, A., & Dorn, M. C. (2017). Impact of TBI on caregivers of veterans with TBI: Burden and interventions. *Brain Injury, 31*(9), 1235–1245. doi: 10.1080/02699052.2016.1274778.

Menscher, C., & Maul, A. (2016). Issue brief: Key ingredients for successful trauma-informed care implementation. *Center for Health Care Strategies.* Retrieved from https://www.samhsa.gov/sites/default/files/programs_campaigns/childrens_mental_health/atc-whitepaper-040616.pdf

Miller, S. (2018). Colossal California wildfire finally contained: grim search for bodies continues. *USA Today.* Retrieved from https://www.usatoday.com/story/news/nation/2018/11/25/california-wildfire-camp-fire-contained/2107829002/

Mitchell, J. T. (n.d.). *Critical incident stress debriefing.* Retrieved from http://www.info-trauma.org/flash/media-e/mitchellCriticalIncidentStressDebriefing.pdf

Nakanishi, H., Matsuo, K., & Black, J. (2013). Transportation planning methodologies for post-disaster recovery in regional communities: The East Japan earthquake and tsunami 2011. *Journal of Transport Geography, 31*, 181–191. doi: 10.1016/j.jtrangeo.2013.07.005.

Naushad, V. A., Bierens, J. J., Nishan, K. P., Firjeeth, C. P., Mohammad, O. H., Maliyakkal, A. M., ... Schreiber, M. D. (2019). A systematic review of the impact of disaster on the mental health of medical responders. *Prehospital and Disaster Medicine, 34*, 632–643. doi: 10.1017/S1049023X19004874.

Occupational Safety and Health Administration. (n.d.). *Critical incident stress guide.* Retrieved from https://www.osha.gov/SLTC/emergencypreparedness/guides/critical.html

Office of the Assistant Secretary for Preparedness and Response. (2019). *ASPR TRACIE disaster behavioral health self care for healthcare workers modules.* Retrieved from https://files.asprtracie.hhs.gov/documents/aspr-tracie-dbh-self-care-for-healthcare-workers-modules-description-final-8-19-19.pdf

Office of the Assistant Secretary for Preparedness and Response. (2020). *Public health emergency: Strategic national stockpile.* Retrieved from https://www.phe.gov/about/sns/Pages/default.aspx

Organisation for the Prohibition of Chemical Weapons (OPCW). (2020). *What is a chemical weapon?* Retrieved from https://www.opcw.org/our-work/what-chemical-weapon

Pamer, M., Wynter, K., & McDade, M. B. (2016). *SoCal Gas has permanently stopped leak in gas above Porter Ranch, state confirms*. Retrieved from http://ktla.com/2016/02/18/socal-gas-porter-ranch-leaking-well-announcement/

Public Health Emergency. (2020). *Emergency prescription assistance program*. Retrieved from https://www.phe.gov/Preparedness/planning/epap/Pages/default.aspx

Quad Council Coalition. (2018). *Community/Public Health Nursing [C/PHN] competencies*. Retrieved from http://www.quadcouncilphn.org/wp-content/uploads/2018/05/QCC-C-PHN-COMPETENCIES-Approved_2018.05.04_Final-002.pdf

Reifels, L., Bassilios, B., Spittal, M. J., King, K., Fletcher, J., & Pirkis, J. (2015). Patterns and predictors of primary mental health service use following bushfire and flood disasters. *Disaster Medicine and Public Health Preparedness, 9*(3), 275–282. doi: 10.1017/dmp.2015.23.

Reilly, K. (2016). *California residents fear long-term impact of gas leak*. Retrieved from http://time.com/4173516/california-gas-leak-resident-reaction/

Rodriguez, F. (2016, May 28). *Assembly votes to power up field hospitals*. Retrieved from https://a52.asmdc.org/press-release/assembly-votes-power-field-hospitals

San Diego County Office of Emergency Services. (n.d.). *Family disaster plan and personal survival guide*. Retrieved from https://www.readysandiego.org/content/dam/oesready/en/Resources/Family-Disaster-Plan-English.pdf

Smith, M. E., Hayoun, M. A., & Gossman, W. (2019). Biologic warfare agent toxicity. *StatPearles [Internet]*. Retrieved from https://www.ncbi.nlm.nih.gov/books/NBK441942/

Spendlove, J. R., & Simonsen, C. E. (2018). *Terrorism today: The past, the present, the future* (6th ed.). Boston, MA: Pearson Education, Inc.

Stanglin, D. (2019). *343 NYC firefighters died on 9/11. Since then, 200 have died from Ground Zero-related illnesses*. Retrieved from https://www.usatoday.com/story/news/nation/2019/07/19/nyfd-200th-firefighter-death-linked-9-11-related-illness-victims-compensation-fund/1776314001/

Substance Abuse and Medical Health Services Administration (SAMHSA). (2011). *SAMHSA's Disaster Kit*. Retrieved from https://store.samhsa.gov/product/samhsas-disaster-kit/sma11-disaster

Substance Abuse and Mental Health Services Administration (SAMHSA). (2018). *Phases of disasters*. Retrieved from https://www.samhsa.gov/dtac/recovering-disasters/phases-disaster

Substance Abuse and Mental Health Services Administration (SAMHSA). (2019). *Supplemental research bulletin: Disasters and people with serious mental illness*. Retrieved from https://www.samhsa.gov/sites/default/files/disasters-people-with-serious-mental-illness.pdf

Substance Abuse and Mental Health Services Administration (SAMHSA). (2020a). *Social media and disasters*. Retrieved from https://www.samhsa.gov/find-help/disaster-distress-helpline/social-media

Substance Abuse and Mental Health Services Administration (SAMHSA). (2020b). *Survivors of disaster resource portal*. Retrieved from https://www.samhsa.gov/dtac/disaster-survivors

Tello, M. (2018). Trauma-informed care: What is it, and why it's important. *Harvard Health Publishing*. Retrieved from https://www.health.harvard.edu/blog/trauma-informed-care-what-it-is-and-why-its-important-2018101613562

Townsend, M. C., & Morgan, K. L. (2018). *Psychiatric mental health nursing: Concepts of care in evidence based practice* (9th ed.). Philadelphia, PA: F.A. Davis.

United Nations. (n.d.). *Refugees*. Retrieved from https://www.un.org/en/sections/issues-depth/refugees/

U.S. Department of Health and Human Services (USDHHS). (2016). *Healthy People 2020 topics & objectives: Preparedness*. Retrieved from https://www.healthypeople.gov/2020/topics-objectives/topic/preparedness/objectives

U.S. Department of Health & Human Services (USDHHS). (2020a). *Healthy People 2030: Browse objectives*. Retrieved from https://health.gov/healthypeople/objectives-and-data/browse-objectives

U.S. Department of Health and Human Services (USDHHS). (2020b). *Management of the deceased*. Retrieved from https://chemm.nlm.nih.gov/deceased.htm

U.S. Department of Health, Education, and Welfare (USDHEW). (1961). *Handbook for civil defense emergency planning in welfare institutions (draft)*. Unpublished manuscript. National Archives.

U.S. Department of Justice. (2020). *Research on domestic radicalization and terrorism*. Retrieved from http://www.nij.gov/topics/crime/terrorism/pages/welcome.aspx

U.S. Public Health Service (USPHS). (2019). *U.S. Public Health Service Commissioned Corps*. Retrieved from https://www.hhs.gov/surgeongeneral/corps/index.html

Veenema, T. G. (2018). *Disaster nursing and emergency preparedness* (4th ed.). New York, NY: Springer Publishing Company.

Wagner, J. M., & Dahnke, M. D. (2015). Nursing ethics and disaster triage: Applying utilitarian ethical theory. *Journal of Emergency Nursing, 41*(4), 300–306.

Wilson-Genderson, M., Heid, A. R., & Pruchno, R. (2018). Long-term effects of disaster on depressive symptoms: Type of exposure on depressive symptoms: Type of exposure matters. *Social Science & Medicine, 217*, 84–91. doi: 10.1016/j.socscimed.2018.09.062.

Zarocostas, J. (2017). The cost of mass-casualty attacks. *The Lancet, 390*(10113), 2617–2618. doi: 10.1016/S0140-6736(17)33306-8.

CHAPTER 18

Violence and Abuse

"The right things to do are those that keep our violence in abeyance; the wrong things are those that bring it to the fore."

—Robert J. Sawyer (1960), Calculating God

KEY TERMS

Abusive head trauma (AHT)
Child abuse
Child maltreatment
Cycle of violence
Elder abuse
Emotional abuse
Implicit bias
Infanticide
Intimate partner violence (IPV)
Mandated reporters
Neglect
Neonaticide
Physical abuse
Protective factors
Risk factors
Sexual abuse
Spectrum of prevention

LEARNING OBJECTIVES

Upon mastery of this chapter, you should be able to:

1. Explain the dynamics of a crisis.
2. Discuss community risk factors and protective factors related to violence.
3. Describe the history of violence against women and children in the United States.
4. Identify the different types of violence against children and specific abusive situations.
5. Define intimate partner violence and explain the stages of the circle of violence.
6. Define elder abuse and discuss related vulnerability factors and prevention measures.
7. Identify other types of violence affecting individuals and communities.
8. Explain how each of the levels of prevention applies to addressing violence in individuals, families, and the community.
9. Use the nursing process to outline nursing actions in response to acts of violence.

INTRODUCTION

Violence is a global public health issue. It is not limited by sociodemographic or geographic factors—anyone may experience violence or abuse at any point in one's lifetime. For example, a toddler who is intentionally burned with a hot curling iron, a teenager who is being emotionally and physically bullied at school, an adult strangled by an intimate partner, an older adult restrained and left sitting for hours in urine and feces, a person stabbed during a physical assault, or a nurse violently attacked when triaging a patient. George Floyd, an African American man, died while being arrested by a white police officer. The deputy restrained Mr. Floyd by kneeling on his neck, causing neck compression and cardiopulmonary arrest; his death was ruled a homicide. The police officer has been charged with murder. This event set off largely peaceful demonstrations around the country highlighting Black Lives Matter, but in some cities, small groups looted, set fires, and committed other acts of violence (Eligon, Furber, & Roberston, 2020; Kazan, 2020). Acts of violence may occur once or multiple times and involve a single perpetrator or a group of perpetrators who may or may not be known to the person experiencing violence. Violence and abuse may occur in any setting—at home, in public, at work, or at school.

The World Health Organization (WHO, 2020a, para. 2) defines violence as "the intentional use of physical force or power, threatened or actual, against oneself, another person, or a group or community, that either results in or has a high likelihood of resulting in injury, death, psychological harm, maldevelopment, or deprivation." Violence is a complex phenomenon affecting individuals, groups, communities, and all of society. There is no single factor or group of factors to explain why a specific person is at risk of using violence or why one community experiences a higher incidence of violent acts than another community. Likewise, there is no single factor that specifically identifies an individual's or a community's vulnerability for experiencing violence.

In 1985, Surgeon General C. Everett Koop placed the concept of violence as a public health issue into the consciousness of the health care community and onto the national agenda. In 1992, the Centers for Disease Control and Prevention (CDC) formalized its role in addressing violence through the National Center for Injury Control and Prevention (https://www.cdc.gov/injury/index.html). Today, the CDC (2018c, para. 1) continues to address the public health issue of violence across the life cycle, stating: "Violence is a serious public health problem. From infants to the elderly, it affects people in all stages of life. Many more survive violence and suffer physical, mental, and or emotional health problems throughout the rest of their lives." These statements are supported by research findings, including the Adverse Childhood Experiences Study; the National Intimate Partner and Sexual Violence Survey; and other violence-related research. The effects of violence are seen across the biopsychosocial and spiritual continuums of health (CDC, 2020a). Community/public health nurses are uniquely positioned to respond to populations affected by violence through trauma-informed practices and violence prevention activities.

Acts of violence can result in a crisis, which is a stressful and disruptive event (or series of events) that comes with or without warning and disturbs the equilibrium of the individual, family, or community. A crisis can occur when usual problem-solving methods fail. Everyone experiences periods of crisis. If you reflect on your own history, you can probably identify one or more periods of crisis that you, your family, or your community experienced.

People respond to crises differently, including crises resulting from acts of violence. Some people approach a crisis as a challenge, an event to be reckoned with, whereas others may feel overwhelmed and defeated or give up. Some survivors of violence seek help and many experience minimal disruptions, perhaps perceiving themselves as even stronger than before the crisis occurred. Some people may have difficulty coping with the crisis, experience severe psychological distress, or express their feelings of rage, frustration, or powerlessness to others.

Regardless of their responses, people who are in crisis after experiencing violence need support, and C/PHNs have a unique opportunity and responsibility to provide support in a variety of situations and settings. For example, a nurse assisting a 15-year-old transgender patient at a free community-based sexually transmitted infection clinic refers to the patient using the patient's preferred name and pronoun and asks the patient when she last ate and whether she has a safe place to sleep that night. By being respectful and genuinely showing interest in the teen's well-being, the nurse gains the teen's trust and learns she is homeless and a victim of sex trafficking. Or, a pregnant woman reschedules her appointment at a community clinic twice and then arrives at the appointment with multiple faded bruises on her face and arms. The clinic nurse uses sensitivity and caring while screening for intimate partner violence (IPV) and identifying opportunities for appropriate referrals to community-based agencies.

Primary and secondary prevention measures used by C/PHNs that help prevent crises include teaching families communication skills and coping strategies and connecting them with community resources. In addition to assessment and education, C/PHNs provide tertiary responses with direct assistance during times of crisis or in the immediate aftermath of experiencing violence. This chapter discusses the knowledge and skills C/PHNs use in their practice of crisis prevention and intervention aimed at promoting improved health for individuals and communities who may be affected by acts of violence.

Throughout this chapter, difficult topics are discussed. Some topics may bring up unwanted memories, feelings of anger related to abuse, assault, implicit bias, compassion fatigue, or/and secondary trauma. Nurses are at risk for compassion fatigue when placed in stressful situations and the continuous offering of themselves (Peters, 2018). Compassion fatigue and secondary traumatic stress were closely related (Mottaghi, Poursheikhali, & Shameli, 2020). Health care providers that work with the abusers need to be aware of the higher level of **vicarious** trauma, the higher the risk for posttraumatic stress disorder (PTSD) (Newman, Eason, & Kinghorn, 2019). **Implicit bias**, or the "unconsciously held set of associations (or stereotypes) about a social group," can affect the quality of care C/PHNs provide their patients (Berghoef, 2019, para. 1). The Joint Commission's material on implicit bias can be found at https://www.jointcommission.org/-/media/deprecated-unorganized/imported-assets/tjc/system-folders/joint-commission-online/quick_safety_issue_23_apr_2016pdf.pdf?db=web&hash=A5852411BCA02D1A918284EBAA775988.

DYNAMICS AND CHARACTERISTICS OF A CRISIS

Each person is a dynamic system living within a given environment under the circumstances unique to that person alone. A person's conscious and subconscious behavior is gauged to maintain a balance within oneself and in one's relations with others. When an internal or external force disrupts one's balance and alters functioning, a loss of equilibrium occurs. The individual then attempts to restore equilibrium by using whatever resources are available to the individual, attempting to cope with the situation.

Coping refers to those actions and ways of thinking that assist people in dealing with and surviving difficult situations. If a person cannot readily cope with a stressful event, the person experiences a crisis (Boyd, 2018). Crises are usually resolved, either positively or negatively, within 4 to 8 weeks (Kanel, 2019). However, there may be long-term biopsychosocial health consequences related to experiences of violence and other adverse events. People's strong need to regain homeostasis and the intense nature of crises contribute to making the crisis itself a temporary condition.

Crises may be precipitated by a specific identifiable event that becomes too much for the problem-solving skills of those involved, may result from sudden unexpected or traumatic events, or may be related a person's perception of an event. Box 18-1 summarizes three common types of crisis.

BOX 18-1 Major Differences Between Types of Crisis

Developmental Crisis

- Part of normal growth and development that can upset normalcy
- Precipitated by a life transition point
- Gradual onset
- Response to development demands and society's expectations

Situational Crisis

- Unexpected period of upset in normalcy
- Event jeopardizes an individual's physical and psychological well-being
- Event may be internal (e.g., cancer) or external (being laid off)

Traumatic Crisis

- Unexpected, overwhelming and unusual event (e.g., disasters or acts of violence)
- Occurs to an individual or a group
- Events cause death, destruction, injury, or sacrifice

Source: Wheeler and Boyd (2018).

When a community crisis occurs on a large scale or is so unexpected that it also involves people who are hundreds of miles away, it can affect distant friends and relatives. Examples include an arson fire at an apartment building killing 12 people and injuring dozens of others; the terrorist attack in San Bernardino in 2015; the mass shooting at the Route 91 Harvest Music Festival in Las Vegas on October 1, 2017; and the terrorist attacks in New York City on September 11th, which indirectly affected people hundreds of miles away.

- A traumatic crisis is a stressful, unexpected, disruptive event arising from external circumstances that occur suddenly to a person, group, aggregate, or community. Typically, the external event requires behavioral changes and coping mechanisms beyond the abilities of the people involved (Wheeler & Boyd, 2018).
- The crisis occurs to people because of where they are in time and space. These events, which involve loss or the threat of loss, represent life hazards to those affected.
- C/PHNs may assist in a variety of traumatic crises, including those arising from acts of violence. In each situation, people feel overwhelmed and need help to cope. Skilled intervention can make the difference between a healthy and an unhealthy response to the crisis.

OVERVIEW OF VIOLENCE ACROSS THE LIFE CYCLE

Violence affects people across the life cycle, from birth through death. It may involve chronic or long-term acts of abuse, neglect, or maltreatment or situational acts of violence that may be unexpected and sudden. C/PHNs encounter many different types of violence, including child abuse and neglect, youth violence, gang violence, bullying, IPV, dating violence, sexual violence, and elder abuse and maltreatment. Multiple types of violence can occur within a single household, community, or neighborhood, affecting people at different stages in life.

As mentioned in the introduction, there is no single factor that can explain a specific act of violence. However, decades of research reveal that different types of violence are interconnected. For example:

- People who experience one form of violence are likely to experience other forms of violence.
- People who use violence in one context are likely to use violence in another context.
- Different types of violence share common short- and long-term biopsychosocial health effects that may contribute to chronic health conditions such as cancer, cardiovascular disease, lung disease, and diabetes.
- Different types of violence have shared risk factors and protective factors (CDC, 2016).

Violence is a complex phenomenon. Understanding the neurobiological effects, potential subsequent health effects, and overlapping causes of violence can help community health nurses to enhance protective factors and reduce risk factors and can help inform violence intervention and prevention activities.

Neurobiology of Trauma

Over the past few decades, neuroscience research has clarified the neurobiological response to trauma. This body of research has provided professionals responding to acts of violence a better understanding of human behavior and how people respond to trauma, contributed to trauma-informed practices, and enhanced the capacity of multidisciplinary responders to serve victims of violence. This knowledge is critical because many victims have been disregarded, not believed, dismissed, or revictimized through victim-blaming practices because well-intended professionals misunderstood what was normal human behavior after experiencing traumatic experiences.

An expanded definition of trauma includes all the events and experiences that are subjectively traumatic to an individual, which are different from person to person. Just as the brain is complex, so are a person's potential reactions and behaviors in response to an experience. This complexity is further compounded by many potential extraneous factors, such as substance use, past trauma, underlying pathologies, and established neural patterns. Although there are common responses, there are no absolute responses for all people; this is a fundamental concept behind trauma-informed care. Trauma-informed practices are improving how nurses interview victims, anticipate the support they need for coping with the physiological and psychological impact of traumatic experiences, and link them with community agencies (Wilson, Lonsway, & Archambault, 2016).

Protective Factors and Risk Factors

Many factors contribute to increasing or decreasing the occurrence of violence. **Risk factors** are factors known to increase the likelihood of experiencing violence. **Protective factors** are factors known to reduce the likelihood of experiencing violence or increase one's resilience when violence is experienced. Individual lived experiences and a person's own characteristics may also be risk factors or protective factors. For example, growing up in a high crime area and witnessing violence is a risk factor, whereas having communication and problem-solving skills that allow one to address conflict without using violence is a protective factor. The CDC (2020c) recognized the following protective factors and risk factors related to youth violence.

Protective factors:

- *Community protective factors* include coordinated resources and services among community agencies; access to mental health and substance abuse services; and community support and connectedness.
- *Relationship protective factors* include family support and connectedness; caring relationships between youth and adults; association with prosocial peers; and a commitment to or connection with one's school.
- *Individual protective factors* include skills that support solving problems nonviolently.

Risk factors:

- *Societal risk factors* include cultural norms supporting aggression toward others; depiction of violence in the media; societal income inequity; poor health, educational, economic, and social policies or laws; and harmful norms related to the concepts of masculinity and femininity.
- *Community risk factors* include neighborhood poverty; a high number of locations selling or providing alcohol; community violence; diminished economic opportunities and high unemployment rates; and poor neighborhood support and cohesion among residents.
- *Relationship risk factors* include social isolation and lack of social support; a poor parent–child relationship; family conflict; economic stress; associating with delinquent peers; and gang involvement.
- *Individual risk factors* include low educational achievement; lack of nonviolent problem-solving skills; poor behavioral control or impulsivity; history of violent victimization; witnessing violence; psychological and mental health problems; and substance use.

Community windshield surveys and other community-based learning opportunities often reveal community-level risk factors and protective factors. For example, the level of safety described by residents can greatly vary from one neighborhood to the next. There are neighborhoods in all cities where residents describe feeling unsafe and witnessing crimes. Such neighborhoods or communities are often referred to as high poverty or high crime areas. In these communities, residents experience an overwhelming number of community risk factors compared with protective factors. The CDC (2016) publication *Connecting the Dots* reveals the following:

- In neighborhoods where residents do not support or trust each other, residents are more likely to experience child maltreatment, IPV, and youth violence.
- People who are socially isolated and do not have supportive relationships with family, friends, or neighbors are at greater risk for using violence, including acts of child maltreatment, IPV, and elder abuse.
- A lack of economic and employment opportunities is associated with an increased risk for using violence, including acts of child maltreatment, IPV, self-directed violence, sexual violence, and youth violence.
- Communities in which societal norms support aggressive or coercive behaviors have an increased risk for violent acts such as physical assault of children, IPV, sexual violence, youth violence, and elder maltreatment.
- Witnessing community violence increases one's vulnerability for being bullied and the risk of using sexual violence against others.

To counteract community risk factors, residents need support to enhance their protective factors. For example, communities having coordinated resources and services among the different community agencies experience greater protective factors. Access to mental health and substance abuse services increases protective factors. Receiving community support and having connections within the community and with the family, prosocial peers, and school can also increase community protective factors and decrease individual vulnerability. What are some of the protective factors in your community?

HISTORY OF VIOLENCE AGAINST WOMEN AND CHILDREN

Violence against women and children is not new. For centuries, children were considered the property of their parents and most countries had animal welfare laws long before child welfare laws were adopted. The first documented case of child abuse occurred in 1874, involving Mary Ellen Wilson. However, due to the lack of child abuse laws of the period, her case was filed under the Animal Welfare Agency. This 9-year-old was so badly beaten and neglected by her foster mother that the public was shocked during the trial in the New York Supreme Court. This case changed public opinion on society's role in the protection of children and resulted in the forming of the Society for Prevention of Cruelty to Children in New York, the first organization of its kind (Smithfield, 2016). In the early 1900s, leaders concerned with child welfare issues promoted the development of international agencies focused on factors affecting the health of children. In 1924, the League of Nations adopted the Declaration of the Rights of the Child, which later informed the United Nation's Declaration of the Rights of the Child (1959) and the Convention on the Rights of the Child (1989). This committee meets three times yearly to address global concerns related to children's rights, including violence against children (Office of the United Nations High Commissioner for Human Rights, 2020).

Historically, women were also treated as property and often experienced gender-based violence resulting in biopsychosocial injuries. Recent global prevalence figures indicate that 35% of women worldwide have experienced IPV or nonpartner sexual violence in their lifetime (WHO, 2017). In 2010, the United Nation's Entity for Gender Equality and the Empowerment of Women was established and prioritized the prevention of and response to violence against women. The first global and regional estimates of violence against women were published in 2013, resulting in clinical and policy guidelines that have been widely disseminated, and 35 countries have participated in programs to build community capacity (WHO, 2016).

Public Laws and Protection in the United States

In the 1960s, the Children's Bureau began to focus on child abuse and supported the development of a mandatory child abuse reporting law that could be used as a model for state laws. The law required health professionals and childcare workers to report suspected child abuse to appropriate officials. In 1974, the Child Abuse Prevention and Treatment Act (CAPTA) was passed, becoming Public Law 93-247 (PL 93-247). This law served to reinforce the earlier mandatory reporting law model and was aimed at solving the growing problem of child abuse in the country. PL 93-247 has been amended several times since 1974. The CAPTA Reform Act of 1978 preceded the Family Violence Prevention and Services Act of 1984. Later, all three acts were consolidated into the Child Abuse Prevention, Adoption, and Family Services Act of 1988 (PL 100-294), and most recently, the Act (PL 108-36) was amended and reauthorized as the Keeping Children and Families Safe Act of 2003 (Child Welfare Information Gateway, 2019a). The Administration on Aging supports similar programs including the National Center on Elder Abuse (n.d.b) that works to educate and assist families, seniors, health care, and legal providers regarding elder abuse.

Myths and Truths About Violence and Abuse

Many myths about violence and abuse need to be dispelled. Strongly held myths by members of society, including C/PHNs and other health care providers, may interfere with their ability to help people in crisis get the help they need. Table 18-1 displays some common myths and truths about violence and abuse.

TABLE 18-1 Common Myths and Truths About Abuse in Families

Myth	Truth
Domestic abuse is only physical	Abuse can take all forms: physical, sexual, stalking, and psychological aggression
Men are the only abusers	Domestic violence has no gender boundaries on the batterer or battered
Domestic violence occurs most frequently among the low-income and uneducated families	Violence occurs across all incomes, educational levels, and across all racial, ethnic, and cultural groups
The situation must be bearable if the victim doesn't leave	Implies victim must be okay with the abuse. Victims stay because of fear of the abuser, fear of deportation, lack of money, or concern for children
Abusers cannot control their anger	Anger does not cause abuse. Abuse is a means to gain control

Source: Arizona Law (n.d.); Paisner (2018).

VIOLENCE AGAINST CHILDREN

- **Child abuse** is defined by the federal CAPTA (42 USCA, 5106g) as "any recent act or failure to act on the part of a parent or caretaker which results in death, serious physical or emotional harm, sexual abuse or exploitation; or an act or failure to act which presents an imminent risk of serious harm" (Child Welfare Information Gateway, 2019b, para. 1).
- **Child maltreatment** is defined as abuse and neglect toward a child under age 18 including "physical and/or emotional ill-treatment, sexual abuse, neglect, negligence and commercial or other exploitation, which results in actual or potential harm to the child's health, survival, development or dignity in the context of a relationship of responsibility, trust or power" (WHO, 2020c, para. 1).

Identifying and gathering worldwide data about child abuse is difficult because many cases are not investigated, death reports may not be classified as a result of abuse or homicide, and definitions of maltreatment may vary. Despite, this, the following global statistics reveal a concerning reality:

- A total of 25% of adults reported being physically abused during childhood, over 36% reported emotional abuse, and 16.3% reported neglect.
- Health effects of maltreatment include long-term physical and mental health impairments.
- Child maltreatment results in adverse social and occupational community outcomes (WHO, 2020c).

The National Child Abuse and Neglect Data System reported that 3.5 million referrals were investigated or had alternative responses by Child Protective Service departments in 2017 and 1,720 child fatalities due to abuse and neglect. Infants had the highest victimization rate at 25.3 per 1,000. Neglect (74.9%) continued as the category of highest occurrence followed by physical abuse (18.3%). Either one or both parents were responsible for almost 92% of all child maltreatment (Children's Bureau, 2019). Polyvictimization, experiencing two different types of maltreatment in a single report or different types of maltreatment across several reports, was reported in 14% of the cases of child maltreatment (Children's Bureau, 2019).

Nationally, measures have been taken to improve data gathering and information about violence toward children, as well as outcomes for these children. One of the largest investigations ever conducted to assess associations between childhood maltreatment and adult health and well-being is the Adverse Childhood Experiences (ACE) Study. The seminal 1998 study conducted by Felitti et al. (1998) has led to new research on the long-term consequences of maltreatment in children. Further information can be found on https://www.cdc.gov/violenceprevention/childabuseandneglect/acestudy/about.html.

Neglect

Neglect occurs when the physical, emotional, medical, or educational resources necessary for healthy growth and development are withheld or unavailable. Neglect is obvious to an observer if a very young child is playing unattended outside, is not dressed appropriately for the weather, or has an unkempt appearance (Box 18-2). However, neglect is not always so obvious (Psychology Today, 2019):

- Parents may refuse to buy eyeglasses for a child who needs them or to access dental care for severely decayed teeth (medical neglect).
- An 8-year-old may get to school only 3 days a week, possibly without breakfast and no lunch money or packed lunch (educational neglect).
- A family with three children may live in a sparsely furnished apartment with very little food available and only intermittent heat and multiple people coming and going in the residence, while the children may appear at school unwashed and without coats in winter weather (general neglect).
- Emotional neglect may be seen when demands placed on a child are excessive or inappropriate for his or her development, or the caretaker berates or verbally humiliates a child frequently and without reason.

C/PHNs need to assess if the neglect is due to lack of knowledge of child development, lack of finances, or lack of health care. Providing services such as WIC, education developed for health literacy level, and assisting parents to enroll children in a Child Health Insurance Program may provide the needed support for many families with children. Because of the invisibility of neglect, its prevalence is hard to estimate. Often, cases of neglect are brought to the attention of the proper authority only during the investigation of other forms of abuse or family issues.

BOX 18-2 Signs and Symptoms of Neglect and Emotional Abuse

Signs and Symptoms of Neglect

Neglect may be suspected if one or more of the following conditions exist:

- Lacks adequate medical (including immunizations), vision, or dental care.
- Often sleepy or hungry.
- Consistently dirty, demonstrates poor personal hygiene, or is inadequately dressed for weather conditions.
- There is evidence of poor or inadequate supervision for the child's age.
- The conditions in the home are unsafe or unsanitary.
- Malnourished, failure to thrive, poor weight gain.
- Substance abuse.

Signs and Symptoms of Emotional Abuse

Emotional abuse may be suspected if the child displays the following behavioral indicators:

- Shows extremes in behavior such as extremely demanding, passive, or compliant
- Inappropriately takes on parent role or infantile in behavior
- Physical or emotional development is delayed
- Depression or suicidal thoughts
- Unable to develop emotional bonds with others

Source: Child Welfare (2019); Stanford Medicine (2019).

Physical Abuse

Physical abuse is intentional harm to a child by another person that results in pain, physical injury, or death (Fig. 18-1). The abuse may include striking, biting, poking, burning, shaking, or throwing the child (Box 18-3). Some parents cannot control the degree of physical punishment they give their child (Child Welfare Information Gateway, 2019b). In one case, a mother repeatedly physically assaulted her young daughter while getting her into the car. The mother's behavior was recorded by the store's parking lot surveillance camera. Intervention and follow-up occurred, including incarceration and counseling for the mother and foster home placement for the child. If physical punishment is administered in anger, while the parent is under the influence of mind-altering substances or out of a sense of frustration, the punishment may cross over to become battering of the child. A parent or caregiver may claim the injuries are the fault of the child, such as a 2-week-old rolling off the bed and hitting their head. C/PHNs need to be knowledgeable about the stages of developmental growth to understand if a child is capable of performing such a skill.

Sexual Abuse

- **Sexual abuse** of children includes acts of sexual assault or sexual exploitation of a minor and may consist of a single incident or many acts over a long period. Sexual abuse is considered "The employment, use, persuasion, inducement, enticement, or coercion of any child to engage in, or assist any other person to engage in, any sexually explicit conduct or simulation of such conduct for the purpose of producing a visual depiction of such conduct" (Legal Information Institute, n.d., para. 1).
- Rape, molestation, prostitution, and human trafficking of minors are included in the definition.

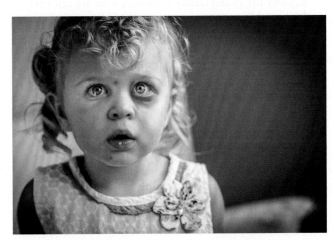

FIGURE 18-1 Young girl with signs of physical abuse.

BOX 18-3 Signs and Symptoms of Physical Abuse

Does the Child or Caregiver...Important Questions to Ask Yourself

- Frequent emergency department visits
- Caregiver blames child for injuries
- Delay in seeking health/medical care or changes provider frequently
- Explanation changes, doesn't match the child's developmental ability, or contradicts injuries

Signs of Physical Abuse

The most common systems affected are the integumentary, skeletal, and central nervous system.

Health care providers including C/PHNs must consider language and cultural differences when interviewing a child and parent. Interviewing with a translator is important with these cases.

- Has unexplained injuries, explanation does not match the injury, or injuries are inconsistent with medical diagnosis. such as
- Injuries may include bruises, bite marks, abrasions, lacerations, head injuries, internal injuries, and fractures
- Bruising from defensive injuries to forearms
- Burns from cigarettes, ropes, or immersion into hot water or hot grid
- Traumatic alopecia with possible hematoma area and is tender to touch
- Trauma to ear
- Appears depressed, withdrawn, anxious, or aggressive
- Appears scared of parent and does not want to go home

Behavioral Indicators of Physical Abuse

These behaviors are often exhibited by physically abused children:

- Attempts to hide injuries; child wears excessive layers of clothing, especially in hot weather.
- Frequently absent from school or misses physical education classes.
- Fearful, clingy, anxious, withdrawn, hypervigilant, or aggressive.
- The child is apprehensive when other children cry.
- Wary of physical contact with adults.
- Exhibits drastic behavioral changes in and out of parental/caretaker presence.
- The child suffers from seizures or vomiting.
- Exhibits depression, self-mutilation, suicide attempts, substance abuse, or sleeping and eating disorders.
- Fearful of going home.

Other indicators of physical abuse may include the following:

- A statement by the child that the injury was caused by abuse (chronically abused children may deny abuse).
- Knowledge that the child's injury is unusual for the child's specific age group (e.g., any fracture in an infant).
- Knowledge of the child's history of previous or recurrent injuries.
- Parent or caregiver shows little concern for the child or seeking or fails to seek medical care for the child's injury.

Source: Child Welfare (2019); Stanford Medicine (2019).

In a behavioral analysis of perpetrators, grooming is often used to gain access to child. Depending on the age of the child either the child or the parents are groomed. If these tactics do not work, the perpetrator may become more aggressive (Bryce, Robinson, & Petherick, 2019).

- Incest is sexual abuse among family members who are related by blood (e.g., parents, grandparents, older sibling). Intrafamilial sexual abuse refers to sexual activity involving family members who are not related by blood (e.g., stepparents, partner of a parent).

Child sexual abuse accounts for 6.7% of all maltreatments against children (Children's Bureau, 2019). The child may blame himself or herself for tempting or provoking the abuser. Indicators of sexual abuse are expressed in various ways, and attention should be given to a history of sexual abuse, sexual behavior indicators, behavioral indicators in younger children and behavioral indicators of sexual abuse in older children and adolescents, and physical symptoms of sexual abuse (Box 18-4). As **mandated reporters**, C/PHNs should be aware that sexual abuse of a child may surface through a broad range of physical, behavioral, and social symptoms. Some of these indicators, taken separately, may not be symptomatic of sexual abuse and should be examined in the context of other behaviors or situational factors (Box 18-5).

Care for children who have been sexually abused varies, as the duration of the molestation, the age, and symptoms of the child will influence their care measures. Long-term consequences of CSA have been well documented. A recent study found adolescent males who had been sexually abused were at a greater risk of substance use; while, girls were more likely to be suicidal and depressed (Gray & Rarick, 2018). Parents may also need counseling and support following the investigation and proceedings involving their child's victimization.

Commercial Sexual Exploitation

- Commercial sexual exploitation of children (CSEC) is "a range of crimes and activities involving the sexual abuse or exploitation of a child for the financial benefit of any person or in exchange for anything of value (including monetary and nonmonetary benefits) given or received by any persons" (Office of Juvenile Justice and Delinquency Prevention [OJJDP], n.d. para.1).
- Nonmonetary items may include food, shelter, clothing, drugs, transportation, or protection from another person. Forms of CSEC include child sex trafficking (prostitution of children), child sex tourism, production of child pornography, and transmission of live video of a child engaged in sexual acts in exchange for something of value. Internet-based marriage brokering, early age marriages, and performing in sex-related venues are also forms of CSEC (OJJDP, n.d.).

BOX 18-4 Indicators of Sexual Abuse

Physical Signs

- Sexually transmitted infections.
- Trauma to the perineal area including bleeding, bruising, or pain. Blood may be seen on sheets or undergarments.
- Discharge from genitals or anus.
- Pain during bowel movements or urination.

Behavioral Signs

- Enuresis and/or fecal soiling in bed when behavior has been outgrown
- Inappropriate sexual behavior for age
- Not wanting to be left alone with certain people or fearful to leave parent or caregiver
- Refuses to remove clothing
- Has money, gifts, or toys unexpectedly
- Self-injury/suicide attempts
- Sexually promiscuity in teens
- Substance use

Emotional Signs

- Nightmares or fear of being left alone at night
- Extreme worry or fear
- Sexually explicit language or explicit knowledge about sexual topics beyond age of child
- Mood changes

Nursing students are encouraged to research the topic to learn more.

Source: RAINN (2019); Stop It Now! (2019).

Emotional or Psychological Abuse

- **Emotional abuse** of children involves psychological mistreatment or neglect, which impairs a child's self-worth and sense of security and being loved. Types of psychological abuse includes rejection, scorn, terrorism, isolation, exploitation, lack of emotional response, exposure to domestic violence, and verbal threats or void of loving comments (Gluck, 2019).
- Emotional abuse alone is rarely reported because it is another hidden form of abuse. However, mandated reporters are required by law to report *suspected* cases of severe emotional neglect or abuse or deprivation in addition to *suspected* neglect and physical or sexual abuse (Child Welfare Information Gateway, 2019b).

Specific Abusive Situations

The previous information addressed the major types of child abuse in families, yet other patterns of abuse against children need to be discussed. Abusive head trauma, Munchausen syndrome by proxy, and parental filicide are uncommon, but by the time the symptoms are recognized, it is often too late. Diagnoses may be made at autopsy or after resulting comorbidities have developed. Technology-facilitated crimes against children are an increasingly common fear of parents. Technology-related crimes against children are occurring more often as children and adolescents have increased time, and access to computers such as when both parents (or a single parent) are at work and children are alone or with sitters. Another area of growing concern for parents and communities is school violence (Bryce et al., 2019).

BOX 18-5 PERSPECTIVES

A School Nurse's Viewpoint on Child Sexual Abuse—Emily's Secret

I am a school nurse at the only K-3 school in a small, rural town. Every child in those grades attends this school (1,000 children). I have a busy school nurse office, but I try to be observant to subtle cues. Sadly, sometimes it's so busy that I worry I miss things. Emily, a third grader, came to my office with stomachaches and vague complaints off and on for several months. Thinking back, this usually happened within the last hour of school. After school, she walked to her aunt's house and stayed there for a few hours until her mother picked her up after work. Emily was a petite child, well behaved, very quiet, and usually only responded with a few words when I asked about her ailments.

One day Emily came in with another stomachache and wanted to lie down. When I asked what was going on, she shrugged her shoulders and didn't really respond. When the final bell rang, I told her if she didn't feel well enough to walk home, I could call her aunt. The aunt was the emergency contact, so the procedure was to start there. She just seemed to really be avoiding going to her aunt's house and wanted me to call her mom at work.

I had a feeling something was wrong. I remembered from a recent workshop on child sexual abuse that sometimes the hardest thing was to break through the guilt and shame for the child to open up. I told Emily she "could tell me anything, and I wouldn't think she was bad." She began talking. Well, it was more like "verbal vomiting"—the words just came spilling out. She told me her uncle had been "touching her" and she "didn't want to go back there." She began crying, and I told her we would call her mom and someone from CPS to help her. I also sent someone to get her teacher, a person she felt comfortable and safe with, who stayed with Emily through the lengthy process.

Later, as I thought about the constant stream of children coming into my office every day, I wondered how many of those kids with subtle, vague complaints might have something going on that is as serious as Emily's secret. Now I try to be even more vigilant and open to their concerns—whatever they may be.

Zoey, school nurse

Abusive Head Trauma

- **Abusive head trauma (AHT)**, sometimes called shaken baby syndrome, is the intentional action of violently shaking a child, usually 2 years of age or younger; children 1 year of age and younger are at the greatest risk. AHT is the leading cause of death related to physical child abuse (CDC, 2020b).
- Injuries related to shaking, blunt impact, or a combination of both may result in neurological injury to the child (Vinchon, 2017). These types of injury very seldom occur through play, as in minor falls or as a result of being tossed into the air.
- Symptoms of AHT may include bilateral retinal hemorrhage, subdural or subarachnoid hematomas, the absence of other external signs of abuse, breathing difficulties, seizures, dilated pupils, lethargy, and unconsciousness (American Association of Neurological Surgeons [AANS], 2020).

The National Center on Shaken Baby Syndrome at https://www.dontshake.org offers resources for parents and health care providers. Explanations for injuries are often vague such as stating the baby was "fine" and then suddenly went into respiratory arrest or began having seizures—both common symptoms of AHT—or they may attribute the injuries to falling out the crib or off of the sofa. In the United States, approximately 1,300 children annually are injured or die due to AHT (National Center on Shaken Baby Syndrome [NCSBS], 2020). Children who survive AHT may require lifelong care, with approximately 80% having learning, physical, visual, and speech disabilities; hearing impairment; cerebral palsy; cognitive impairment; and seizures (NCSBS, 2020). Considering perpetrators of AHT are most often a parent or caregiver, C/PHNs can play a critical role in caregiver education and preventative mental health referrals.

Munchausen Syndrome by Proxy

Munchausen syndrome by proxy is a mental illness in which the parent or caregiver attempts to bring attention to self by injuring or inducing illness in their child. About 85% to 98% of perpetrators are the child's biological mother, who often forms close bonds with health care providers. Many of these abusers have a mental health illness or a history of abuse as a child (Boyd, 2018). The following scenarios can be typical of these cases:

- Serious medical problems or conditions that have no medical basis.
- The child experiences "seizures" or "respiratory arrest" only when the parent or caretaker is present.
- While the child is hospitalized, the parent or caretaker shuts off intravenous tubes or life-support equipment, causing the child distress, and then turns everything back on and summons help.
- The parent or caretaker induces illness by introducing a mild irritant or poison into the child's body.
- The child may have many school absences and a complicated medical history according to the child's mother or father who may seem overinvolved or demanding.

Child Murder by Mother or Father

- *Filicide* is a rare yet concerning type of child death, defined as child murder by a parent. **Infanticide** is defined as the murder of a child during the first year of life, whereas **neonaticide** is the murder of an infant within the first 24 hours of life. Maternal filicide is known to occur in all areas of the world. The United States has the highest rate of child murders than any developed country with the parent being the main perpetrator (Resnick, 2016).
- Risks factors include the maternal age of 19 or younger, lack of prenatal care, less than a high school diploma poverty, social isolation, depression, or suicidality (Debowska, Boduszek, & Dhingra, 2015; Resnick, 2016).
- In 2017, homicide was among the top 15 leading causes of death for children from birth to 18 years. In the United States, the child homicide rate is 7.2 deaths per 100,000 infants under the age of 5. Infants are most likely to be killed by their mother during the first week of life, but thereafter are more likely to be killed by a male perpetrator (Kochanek, Murphy, Xu, & Arias, 2019).

Measures for prevention and support to mothers include parenting classes, emotional support, providing emergency numbers for support, as well as treating maternal substance abuse and postpartum depression. Safe haven laws are in place to prevent infant abandonment, leading to potential injury or death, by denoting safe places to relinquish a newborn infant, such as a fire or police station (Child Welfare Information Gateway, 2017). See Box 18-6 for two examples of neonaticide.

Internet Crimes Against Children

Internet and technology-facilitated crimes are insidious because they come right into the home (Fig. 18-2). Children may unintentionally or intentionally access a chat room or Web site developed or used by perpetrators. The perpetrator establishes contact, usually pretending to be a teenager or young man who has similar interests and is affectionate and understanding about the youth's "problems." After gaining the child's trust, the perpetrator may engage in sexually explicit dialogue with the minor. Many minors find the attention from this stranger inviting or exciting and make plans to meet the person. When this happens, the minor falls victim to this individual, putting the child/adolescent at great risk for harm. Technology-enabled child abuse has led to the U.S. Attorney General authorizing a national awareness and justice program focusing solely on technology-facilitated sexual exploitation and abuse against children, named *Project Safe Childhood* (USDOJ, 2020) and the creation of Internet Crimes Against Children (ICAC) task forces. ICAC task forces assist federal, state, and local law enforcement agencies by enhancing their ability to investigate technology-facilitated crimes against children.

C/PHNs can assist families to prevent technology-facilitated crimes by the following:

- Encouraging parents to openly discuss with their children the dangers of online friendships that seek face-to-face meetings; downloading photos or uploading/posting photos to people they do not know; giving identifiable information about themselves (name, phone number, school they attend, home address); responding to e-mails, instant messages, or tweets

BOX 18-6 STORIES FROM THE FIELD

Neonaticide

Case 1

After realizing she was pregnant, a 17-year-old honor student chose not to tell her parents, friends, or boyfriend. She kept her pregnancy a secret by wearing loose clothing and complaining about "gaining weight" over the holidays. While home alone after school, she went into labor sitting on the toilet. She lay down on the bathroom floor and labored for several hours, experiencing significant blood loss. After delivering the newborn, she used scissors to cut the umbilical cord. She was afraid because she had not stopped bleeding. Blood was everywhere. She got the keys to the car and drove herself to a local hospital. On the way, she became dizzy and felt like she passed out. Coming to, she continued to drive to the hospital. Upon admission, she was treated to control the hemorrhaging. Later, an emergency department nurse asked about the newborn and the girl said, "I left it, It's on the bathroom floor." Police located the dead newborn as described and no formal charges were filed.

Case 2

A 16-year-old girl became pregnant after having sex with her boyfriend. She thought she was having stomach or GI problems and her mother took her to the pediatrician's office. The doctor prescribed medication for her symptoms, but she still felt ill. Concerned about being pregnant, she took an over-the-counter pregnancy test. The result was negative. A friend encouraged her to go to a walk-in clinic for a pregnancy test, the test result was inconclusive, and she began spotting. She continued to take her birth control pills, thinking she was not pregnant. A few months later during a family barbeque, she felt like she is getting the "stomach flu" and told her mother she was going to bed. Before going to bed, she tried to have a bowel movement, but nothing happened. She thought she might be in labor and lay down on the floor of the bathroom. To her shock and horror, she gave birth, quickly stabbed the newborn, and hid it in a trash bin where the body was later discovered. A court psychiatrist examined the girl, and she described "watching the birth and the stabbing from a vantage point above her body." Her defense was limited to testimony about whether she noticed the newborn's fingers moving and trying to counter the pathologist's findings that the lungs had inflated. Her attorney was not allowed to bring up issues surrounding her pregnancy and *neonaticidal syndrome.* The jury found her guilty of murder, and she was sentenced to prison for a life term.

1. *What are your thoughts about the two cases?*
2. *Have you seen examples like these in your local or regional newspapers or online news sources?*
3. *What preventive programs and policies might be helpful in addressing this issue? Are there EBP population-focused interventions available to address this problem?*

Source: Malmquist (2013).

that are suggestive or harassing; and, being aware of phishing and other forms of attempted identity theft.

- Establishing parent–child contracts for devices that can connect to web-based applications (e.g., computer, tablet, smartphone, gaming systems).
- Blocking or only permitting specific phone numbers for smartphone and web-based application calls and regularly checking for deleted phone calls and texts.
- Monitoring the amount of time that a child uses Internet accessible devices and reviewing user history for applications used and Web sites visited.

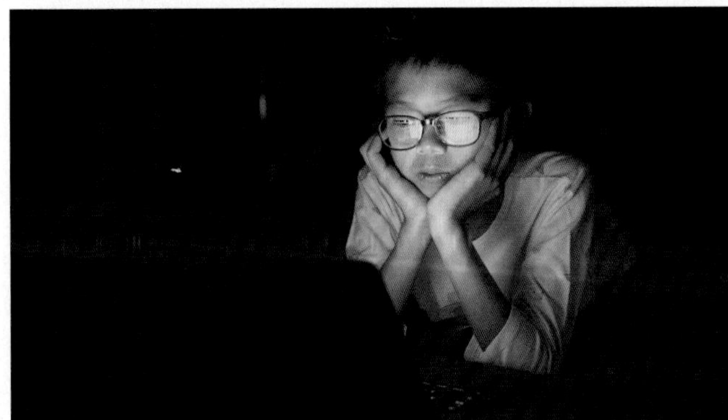

FIGURE 18-2 Children and youth can be victims of Internet crimes.

- Placing computer and gaming consoles in a high-traffic area in the home, affording easy observation of usage by the child.
- Using available parental controls or blocking software on all devices with Internet connectivity.
- Installing a firewall, antivirus, and malware/spyware programs that increase privacy and restrict usage.
- Discouraging downloading of apps, games, and other media that might contain hidden applications or programs that enable remote access by unauthorized users.
- Having access to their child's e-mail and other web-based accounts; randomly checking e-mails and text messages. Being aware of safeguards in place at their child's school, public areas the child frequents, and homes of their friends (Federal Bureau of Investigation [FBI], n.d.a).

There is a constant stream of news around cyberbullying and cyberstalking incidents. Cyberstalking is "the use of electronic communication to harass or threaten someone with physical harm" (Merriam-Webster, 2020, para. 1). Nationwide nearly 15% of all students have been cyberbullied including with slightly <20% of high school girls and 10% of boys being victims (CDC, 2018d). Effects of cyberbullying can be more far-reaching than those of traditional schoolyard bullying. Nurses can ensure families are prepared to identify and appropriately respond to cyberbullying, sexting, and threats from online predators.

- The destructive effects of cyberbullying were highlighted in the news when a 12-year girl committed suicide after receiving texts saying she was fat, had no friends, and that she should kill herself (Gillis, 2019).
- In 2019, a 21-year-old young man jumped from a parking structure at the university he was to graduate from in 20 hours. His girlfriend is being charged with manslaughter for sending him tens of thousands text messages telling him to kill himself (Boston25News, 2019).
- These stories put a face on a recent study that found that being a victim of cyberbullying increases the risk of suicidality (Chang, Xing, Ho, & Yip, 2019).

Parents can contact the Cyber Tip Line at (800) 843-5678 or access their Web site (www.cybertipline.com) if they suspect an online predator has contacted their child (National Center for Missing and Exploited Children, 2020).

Child Abduction

Although child abduction by a stranger happens infrequently, it remains one of the greatest fears for parents. Intense media coverage gives the impression that such crimes occur frequently, and this causes great stress among parents and community members. Child abduction by family members or intimate partners is more common. Nationally, the Amber Alert program and the Child Abduction Response Teams (CART) were established to provide an informed, prompt, and professional response to child abduction. Amber Alerts are sent through the radio, television, road signs, and the Wireless Emergency Alerts (WEA) system to millions of cell phone users. The goal of the Amber Alert is to provide instant collaboration and partnership in the community to assist in the search and safe recovery of the child and, as of May 2020, a total of 988 children have been rescued (USDOJ, n.d.a).

Prevention of child abduction is difficult, and at times, parents who think they have taught their children well may have a false sense of security.

C/PHNs can help parents improve their child's safety by promoting close supervision of young children and practicing behaviors to promote anonymity, such as:

- Placing the child in the seat of a shopping cart and holding their hand when in malls or stores
- Keeping a young child in sight always when playing outside
- Sharing parental supervision with another parent when children play
- Do not put the child's name or initials on clothing or backpacks
- Teaching the child a "password," which only the parents and child know, to use when a different person is picking them up from an activity
- Teaching children to recognize when they feel unsafe and to go get help
- Involving children in making safety plans and having them practice getting help
- Helping children understand when it is okay to give personal information (e.g., at school, medical office, lost in a store) and when it is not (e.g., a stranger they don't know)
- Practicing "think first" and "keep walking" activities with their children (Kidpower, 2020)

Older children and teens who go outside the home unattended by parents should be encouraged to use the following behaviors that promote safety: staying with groups of other children or teens, having a cell phone, leaving an itinerary with the parents, and not changing their plans without contacting parents.

Crimes Against Children by Babysitters

Abuse by caretakers is a fear of parents who work and leave their children with others. The C/PHN can help parents assess childcare settings by providing them descriptors for finding good childcare providers. Parents who use neighbors as babysitters should get references and drop by the home or childcare setting at various times during the day. They should assess their infants and follow up on any bruises, rashes, burns, conditions, or behaviors they observe that are not normal for their child. Parents need to listen to their children and ask about their day and activities. Parents must not ignore signs, such as a child's fear of going to the babysitter or reports of spankings, being shouted at, or other inappropriate treatment.

Childcare centers and many home childcare programs are licensed by the state. When parent complaints have been filed with licensing agencies, those programs are monitored more closely and the state is mandated to make changes or close the facility if necessary. Parents need to know that their child is safe and cared for when they leave them to pursue their employment or educational activities. A daycare owner was recently arrested for hiding 26 toddlers behind a fake wall in the basement of her home; there were only 2 care providers, and the business was only licensed for 6 children. When notified by law enforcement to pick up their children, parents were shocked to find their children in filthy conditions in the basement. One mother told reporters when she dropped off her child the home was clean; she had no idea the owner cared for children in the basement. The owner had previously lost her license to operate daycare centers in California for similar violations (Jensen, 2019).

School Violence

Violence in the school setting is an area of growing concern for parents and communities. Violence in schools may range from bullying, slapping, or punching to weapon use (CDC, 2019h). Random shootings and hostage situations in schools over the past decades have fueled fears about the safety of students and promoted research on how to prevent this type of community violence affecting children.

- Since the 1999 shootings at Columbine High School in Colorado where 13 students died, a total of 11 mass shootings in which 4 or more persons were killed has resulted in 127 student deaths through 2014 (Keneally, 2019).
- Seventeen more died during a mass shooting at the high school in Parkland, Florida in 2018 (Andone, 2020).
- The largest mass shooting event occurred in 2017 at an outdoor concert in Las Vegas where 58 people were killed and almost 1,000 injured (Romo, 2019).

Shootings have occurred at large universities, small community colleges, high schools, and elementary schools.

They have taken place throughout the country and no segment of the population is immune. The mass shootings have occurred in public and private schools, including the killing of 5 young girls at an Amish one room schoolhouse in Pennsylvania (Walters, 2016).

- Bullying is defined as "any unwanted aggressive behavior(s) by another youth or group of youths, who are not siblings or current dating partners, involving an observed or perceived power imbalance and is repeated multiple times or is highly likely to be repeated" (CDC, 2019b, p. 1).
- Bullying can be verbal, social, or physical or happen through electronic communication (cyberbullying).
- Children at high risk of being bullied may have delayed puberty, be gender nonconforming, have a unique physical appearance, or be socially rejected and isolated (Simms, Bushman, & Pederson, 2020).
- Gay, lesbian, bisexual, and transgender youth were more likely than were heterosexual youth to report high levels of bullying (CDC, 2017a).
- Bullying is interconnected with other types of youth violence including gang violence (Simms, Bushman, & Pederson, 2020).

The Youth Risk Behavior Survey collects information about health and prevention issues among adolescents. Included in the survey are questions about violence risks such as fighting, use of illegal drugs, carrying a weapon, and being threatened or injured with a weapon on school property. In 2017, of a national representative sample of youth in grades 9 to 12 found the following:

- 8.5% of 9th through 12th graders reported being in a physical fight on school property in the 12 months before the survey.
- 19% reported being bullied on school property and 14.9% reported being bullied electronically.
- 6.7% missed 1 or more days of school because they felt unsafe at school or on their way to and from school.
- 3.8% reported carrying a weapon on school property in the 30 days before the survey.
- 6.0% reported being threatened or injured with a weapon on school property (Kann et al., 2018).

School violence has immediate and long-term effects on students demonstrated by an increase in depression, anxiety, psychological problems, and fear (CDC, 2016). See Chapter 20 for more on school-age children and adolescents.

The U.S. Department of Education, the Department of Health and Human Services, and the Department of Justice have collaborated to provide funding, programs, and training that improve school safety through the *Safe Schools Healthy Students Framework*. Five elements identified for attention in building safe school climates are as follows:

- Create a safe and *violence* free school environment.
- Prevent behavioral health problems.
- Promote emotional, mental, and behavioral health.
- Provide early childhood psychosocial and emotional development programs.
- Connect communities, schools, and families (National Center for Healthy Safe Children, 2019).

Similar to community risk factors, those factors surrounding youth violence can be categorized as individual risks, relationship risks, and community or societal risks. Individual risks for perpetrating youth violence may include a history of violent victimization; a history of early aggressive behaviors, attention deficit, hyperactivity, or learning disorders; an association with delinquent peers; gang involvement; high emotional distress; social rejection; family violence and conflict; or poor behavioral control (CDC, 2020c). Low parental involvement, parental substance abuse or criminality, poor supervision, low emotional attachment to the parent, and harsh, lax, or inconsistent forms of discipline increase a child/adolescent's risk for violence. Community and societal risk factors for youth violence are associated with diminished economic opportunities, a high concentration of poverty, transiency, and family disruption, with low levels of community participation (CDC, 2020c).

Youth development programs address these risk factors in schools and communities, as well as promoting activities to help students in meeting individual needs. Mentoring programs are beneficial for at-risk teens when the mentors are appropriately trained and supported. Social skills, conflict resolution, and programs supporting student sports, arts, and extracurricular interests decrease an individual's risk of being involved in violence. School and societal strategies include surveillance, maintenance of facilities, and consistent classroom management techniques, along with adequate student supervision (USDHHS, n.d.). Parent involvement and education are expanding through programs such as *Healthy Start* and parent-participation preschools, *Loving Solutions* for elementary age students, and the *Parent Project* for parents of difficult adolescents (The Parent Project, 2019).

INTIMATE PARTNER VIOLENCE

Intimate partner violence (IPV) is the abuse or aggression that occurs within close relationships that are either current or previous. There are four types of IPV: physical violence, sexual violence, stalking, and psychological aggression (CDC, 2019d).

- 1 in 4 women and 1 in 10 men have experienced physical and/or sexual violence and/or stalking.
- 1 in 5 women and 1 in 7 men have been victims of severe physical violence.
- 1 in 5 women and 1 in 12 men have experienced sexual violence.
- 16% of all homicides have been committed by an intimate partner.
- 10% of women and 2% or men have been stalked.
- 43 million women and 38 million men have experienced psychological aggression (CDC, 2019f).

According to the WHO (2017), global prevalence figures for women indicate the following:

- IPV is a leading cause of morbidity and mortality in women worldwide, as well as a public health and human rights issue 35% of women have experienced either IPV or nonpartner sexual violence in their lifetime.

- 30% of women report being physically abused by an intimate partner at some point in their lives.
- 38% of all women who were murdered were murdered by their intimate partner.

While research related to IPV against members of the LGBTQ community is limited (Rollè, Giardina, Caldarera, Gerino, & Brustia, 2018), the most recent in-depth study conducted by the CDC (2010) found the following:

- A total of 26% of gay men and 37% of bisexual men experienced rape, physical violence, and/or stalking by an intimate partner at some point in their lifetime.
- Individuals who self-identify as lesbian, gay, and bisexual have an equal or higher prevalence of experiencing IPV, SV, and stalking as compared to self-identified heterosexuals.
- A total of 44% of lesbian women and 61% of bisexual women experienced rape, physical violence, and/or stalking by an intimate partner in their lifetime.
- Approximately 1 in 8 lesbian women (13%) and nearly half of bisexual women (46%) have been raped in their lifetime.
- A total of 40% of gay men and nearly half of bisexual men (47%) have experienced SV other than rape in their lifetime. The Human Rights Campaign (2020, para. 1) found that approximately 47% of transgender people are sexually assaulted "at some point in their lifetime."

Researchers often describe domestic violence, a form of IPV, as punching, grabbing, shoving, slapping, choking, kicking, biting, hitting with a fist or some other object, being beaten, or being threatened with a knife or gun by a spouse or cohabiting partner. The USDOJ (n.d.b, para. 2) defines domestic violence as "a pattern of abusive behavior in any relationship that is used by one partner to gain or maintain power and control over another intimate partner"; it may be emotional, economic, physical, psychological, or sexual in nature (Box 18-7).

Because of the nature of IPV, the problems are difficult to study and believed to be underreported. Much remains unknown about factors that increase or decrease the likelihood that one person will use violence against another person within an intimate relationship or in the course of seeking that relationship. However, models have been developed to aid in the understanding of the repetitive cycles often seen in intimate partner and domestic violence.

Cycle of Violence

The **cycle of violence** is a repetitive, cyclic pattern of abuse seen in domestic violence situations (Box 18-8). Developed by Walker in 1979, the cycle is still in use today. The cycle includes the tension-building phase, the explosion (acute battering incident), and the honeymoon phase (SexInfo Online, 2017; White Ribbon, 2019). For more information, refer to https://sexinfo.soc.ucsb.edu/article/cycle-domestic-violence. The psychological dynamics of these three phases help explain why the person experiencing abuse feels guilty and ashamed of their partner's violence toward them, and why they find it so difficult to leave, even when their lives are in danger.

Often, as the cycle of violence continues, the frequency of the cycle increases, with the tension-building phase and the acute battering incident occurring more often and diminishment or elimination of the loving reconciliation phase. Without intervention, this shorter, more violent cycle becomes increasingly risk-filled for outcomes that may lead to injury or maiming of a partner, incarceration, or death. Although early research focused on women who experience violence by men, the same descriptive cycle holds true regardless of the victim's or the aggressor's gender (Hinsliff-Smith & McGarry, 2017).

The Domestic Abuse Intervention Project in Duluth, Minnesota, developed a wheel of violence, identifying power and control at the center and citing eight categories of perpetrator behaviors (Fig. 18-3). This model is a useful tool for visualizing the multidimensional nature of abuse in which threats, coercion, isolation, blaming, intimidation, and use of children, male privilege, and economics convene to control the victim.

Reducing violence and its effects happens strategically at all three levels of prevention.

BOX 18-7 PERSPECTIVES

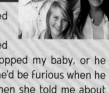

Viewpoint of a Victim of Intimate Partner Violence

My family was always shouting at each other. The hitting wasn't nearly as bad as all the yelling. Now here I am in the same boat all over again—the yelling, the hitting, but now I've got this new baby to take care of. I'm just so tired.

When the nurse showed up today to check on me and the baby, I swore to myself that I wouldn't tell her about last night. Then she looked at me and asked if I felt safe and that triggered me...I said "NO!" before I realized my mouth was even open. I told her how he punched me here in my side when I was changing the baby's diaper. That nurse was so nice. She helped me look at my options. Because I was holding the baby when he hit me, she said she was required to make a report of child abuse.

That was just awful news and I started crying; but like she said, I could have dropped my baby, or he could have missed me and hit her. I knew he'd be furious when he found out and I really started to panic. Then she told me about this place, a place downtown where I can stay with my baby. Then she helped me make arrangements. I'm so tired and scared, but I know now that I have to keep my baby safe. I still don't know what made me tell that nurse—I guess it was because she asked.

Angie

BOX 18-8 The Cycle of Violence

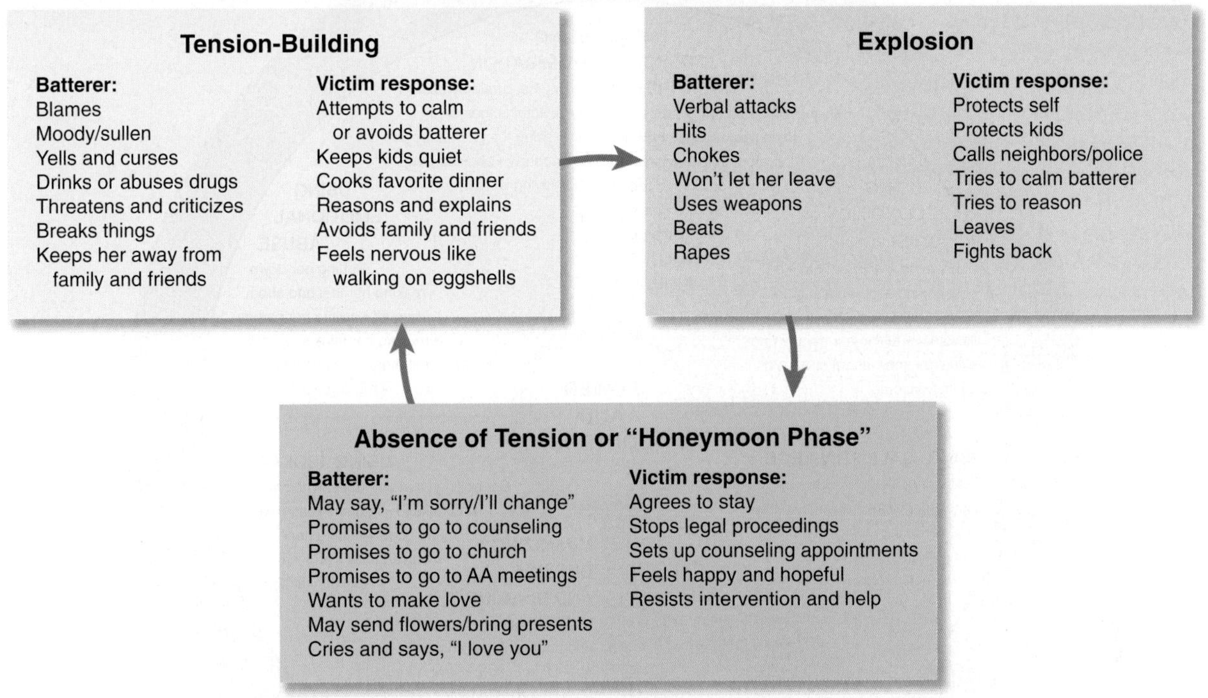

Tension-Building

Batterer:
Blames
Moody/sullen
Yells and curses
Drinks or abuses drugs
Threatens and criticizes
Breaks things
Keeps her away from family and friends

Victim response:
Attempts to calm or avoids batterer
Keeps kids quiet
Cooks favorite dinner
Reasons and explains
Avoids family and friends
Feels nervous like walking on eggshells

Explosion

Batterer:
Verbal attacks
Hits
Chokes
Won't let her leave
Uses weapons
Beats
Rapes

Victim response:
Protects self
Protects kids
Calls neighbors/police
Tries to calm batterer
Tries to reason
Leaves
Fights back

Absence of Tension or "Honeymoon Phase"

Batterer:
May say, "I'm sorry/I'll change"
Promises to go to counseling
Promises to go to church
Promises to go to AA meetings
Wants to make love
May send flowers/bring presents
Cries and says, "I love you"

Victim response:
Agrees to stay
Stops legal proceedings
Sets up counseling appointments
Feels happy and hopeful
Resists intervention and help

Tension-Building Phase

- Considered the longest of the phases—up to several weeks.
- Victim may feel they are "walking on eggshells."
- Abuser is edgy, negative mood, verbally abusive, and controlling.
- Minor augments occur.
- Victim attempts to appease partner in hopes calming situation and to avoid the acute explosion phase.

Acute Explosion Phase

- Shortest phase usually lasting 1 to 2 days.
- Most violent phase as tension is released.
- Violence may take many forms such as sexual, physical, verbal, psychological, and emotional abuse.
- Phase is triggered by an external event or the abuser's state of mind.
- Abuser may blame victim for the abuse.
- Victim may fight back, leave the person, or try and placate the abuser.

Honeymoon Phase

- Abuser may feel embarrassed and become withdrawn or attempt to justify actions.
- Abuser expresses remorse and pledges it will not happen again.
- Abuser promises to make behavioral changes such as work less, stop drinking, and be more attentive to victim.
- Abuser is excessively romantic to victim such as giving expensive gifts, flowers, candy.
- Victim forgives abuser.
- Intimacy may increase.
- Tension-building phase begins again.

Denial

- Common in each phase.
- Used to minimize seriousness of behavior.
- Creates a false sense of reality in victim.
- Family and friends use denial to lessen their responsibility.
- Abuser uses denial to diminish the abuse is their fault, that it wasn't abusive behavior, or the behavior was deserved.

Source: White Ribbon Australia (2019); SexInfo Online (2017). Figure reprinted with permission from Hatfield, N. T., & Kincheloe, C. (2018). *Introductory maternity and pediatric nursing* (4th ed., Fig. 16-3). Philadelphia, PA: Wolters Kluwer.

- Primary prevention efforts attempt to identify risk factors, reduce risks, and increase social support to prevent violence from occurring.
- Secondary prevention effort involves developing an immediate response to violence that addresses the short-term consequences through emergency response and medical care.
- Tertiary prevention interventions work to address the long-term effect of trauma through counseling and rehabilitation (CDC, 2019a).

Health care providers have a responsibility and opportunity to assess and initiate a safety plan when these patients report experiencing violence. A compendium of assessment tools for IPV can be found on the CDC Web site.

Teen Dating Violence

Teen dating violence includes physical violence, sexual violence, psychological aggression, and stalking between teenagers who are or have been in a casual or serious

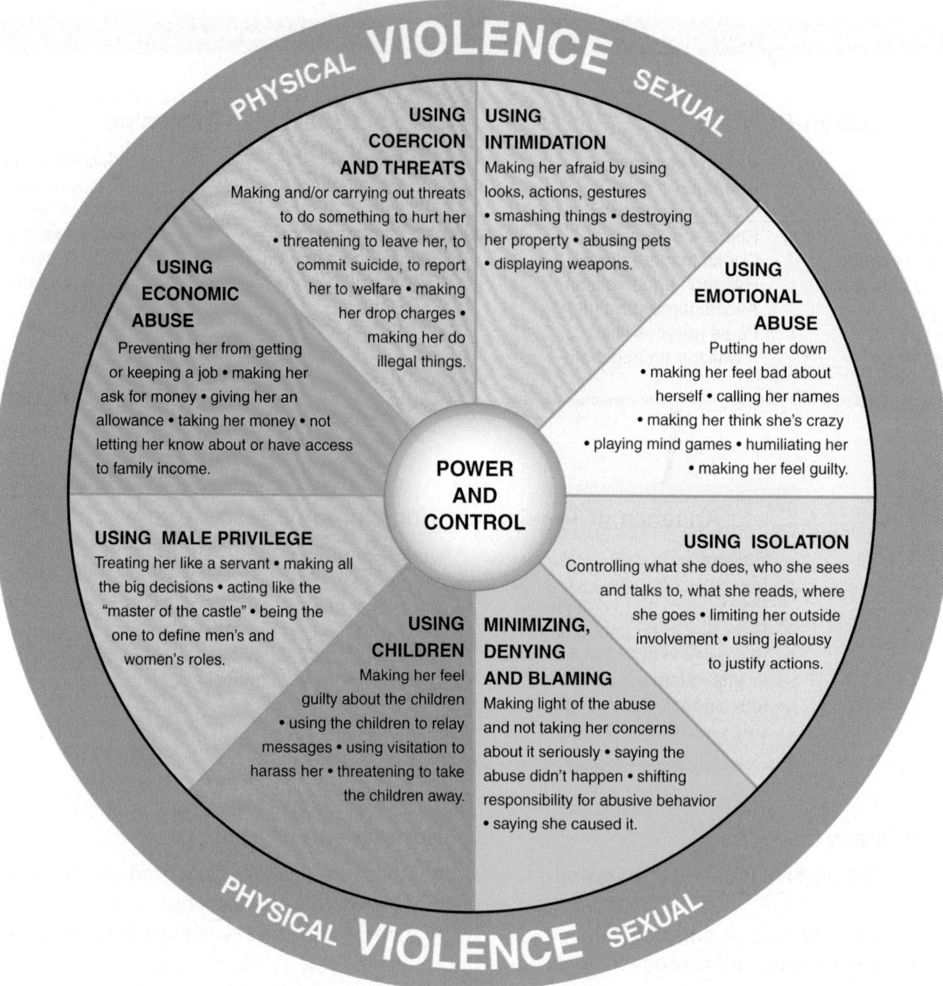

FIGURE 18-3 Wheel of violence.

dating relationship. It can be electronic or in person and might occur between a current or former partner (CDC, 2019f).

- The 2017 National Youth Risk Behavior Study revealed that 8% of high school students reported physical dating violence and 7% reported sexual dating violence in the past 12 months; furthermore, people who experience dating violence in adolescence are at higher risk for dating violence in college (CDC, 2018d).
- Documented risk factors include poverty, limited education, substance abuse, poor family functioning, child maltreatment, and childhood exposure to IPV (Stewart, Vigod, & Riazantseva, 2016).
- Research on male aggressors found that those who exhibited physical and psychological dating aggression often had a history of suicide attempts, reports of past physical aggression, and low relationship satisfaction/instability and jealousy (Collibee & Furman, 2016).

Teens, regardless of gender, who experience dating violence in adolescence, are more at risk for binge drinking, suicide attempts, doing poorly in school, physical fighting, and sexual activity (CDC, 2018a). Programs through schools and communities, such as *Dating Matters*, are part of a national effort to address harmful beliefs about dating violence and promote healthy and respectful dating relationships (CDC, 2018a). Dating violence in adolescent relationships is a serious problem and because of its prevalence, community health nurses should include screening for dating violence in all encounters with teens.

Stalking

Stalking may occur by either partner in a relationship, demonstrated as a "pattern of repeated and unwanted attention, harassment, contact, or any other course of conduct directed at a specific person that would cause a reasonable person to feel fear" (USDOJ, n.d.d, para. 2). Approximately, 17% of women report a lifetime prevalence of being a victim of stalking behavior, and 5.9% of men (CDC, 2018b). Cyberstalking, a technology-based attack, can also take many forms that can involve harassment, embarrassment, and humiliation of the victim. Twenty-five percent of those stalked were cyberstalked as well (Bureau of Justice Statistics [BJS], n.d.)

Violence During Pregnancy

IPV during pregnancy increases the vulnerability of the woman and the fetus. For example, when abusive partners target a woman's abdomen, not only are they hurting the women but also potentially jeopardizing the pregnancy (WHO, 2017).

- Worldwide the exact number of women abused during pregnancy may never be known. While a U.S. study of more than 36,500 pregnant women found <2% experienced IPV, the consequences of IPV during pregnancy are grave (CDC, 2017b).
- Victims of physical abuse and sexual abuse during childhood increases the risk of IPV during pregnancy. Violence during pregnancy increases risk of depression, anxiety, and negative self-image (Hrelic, 2019). Additionally, abuse during pregnancy results in higher rates of intrauterine growth retardation and preterm labor that can lead to low birth weight and neonatal risks (WHO, 2017). See Chapter 19 for more on maternal–child health issues.
- Pregnant teens are at a greater risk of IPV. One study found that among teenage couples 64% had no IPV, while the remaining couples experienced either the males, mutual, or females as the perpetrators of the violence (Lewis et al., 2017).

The prenatal care visit is one of the few times when providers have an important opportunity to identify women who are abused and therefore at risk for homicide. It is imperative that nurses conduct an assessment for danger and lethality so that the women can be aware of their level of risk and take safety precautions as needed. A series of questions requiring a "yes" or "no" response and inquiries about occurrences of abuse, escalation of abuse, frequency, severity, weapons, drugs or alcohol use by the perpetrator, and safety of other children should be incorporated into prenatal home visit assessments. All health care providers, including C/PHNs, should have regular training on IPV. According to The American College of Obstetricians and Gynecologist (ACOG) (2019), when choosing a tool to assess for IPV, avoid ones that include words such as "abuse," "rape," or "violence" as they may cause the person to feel stigmatized. The ACOG offers sample of a tool on their Web site. Numerous tools can also be located in *Intimate Partner Violence and Sexual Violence Victimization Assessment Instruments for Use in Healthcare Settings* (https://www.cdc.gov/violenceprevention/pdf/ipv/ipvandsvscreening.pdf). Annual screenings for IPV and providing interventions and referrals are part of the Women's Preventive Services Guidelines (HRSA, 2019). These are especially important for women who have not followed through with prenatal care, thereby allowing health care professionals to monitor the progress of their pregnancies. C/PHNs are uniquely situated to screen for IPV during pregnancy, particularly through *Healthy Start* and *Nurse Family Partnership Programs.*

Batterer Characteristics

Although a person of any gender may become a batterer, many studies and statistics are specific to male aggressors. The following attributes represent personal characteristics often seen in male aggressors of IPV:

- Poor sense of self-worth
- Low earnings or unemployed
- Not doing well in academics or dropping out of school
- Conduct disorders as a child
- Heavy substance use
- Mood disorders such as depression
- Exhibiting angry and hostile behavior
- Personality disorders (PD) such as borderline and antisocial PDs
- Physically abusive to others
- A loner with few or no friends
- Emotional immaturity
- "Belief in strict gender roles (e.g., male dominance and aggression in relationships)
- A desire for power and control in relationships"
- Being a prior "victim of physical or psychological abuse—this is consistently one of the strongest predictors of perpetration" (CDC, 2019i, para. 4)

Relationship, community, and societal factors may also affect a perpetrator's risk for aggressive IPV behaviors.

- Relationship factors include marital fights and tension, divorce and separations, money problems, issues with jealousy/being possessive, and problematic and difficult family relationships, as well as the male's need for dominance and control in the relationship.
- Community factors involve a lack of resources in the community, failure or unwillingness of others to intervene or contact authorities when they are aware of the abuse, and factors associated with poverty, such as overcrowding and unemployment.
- Societal factors include strict role stereotyping about male and female roles in marriage (CDC, 2019i).

Victim Characteristics

Increasing the victim's abilities to manage and improve their behaviors and understanding of relationship patterns and abuse allows victims to change their risk of being further victimized. Individual risk factors for IPV victims include the following:

- A prior history of IPV
- Being female
- Young age, especially if pregnant
- From low-income household
- Witnessing or experiencing violence as a child
- Lower education level
- Unemployment
- Being a single parent with children or separated/divorced/previously widowed
- For men, having a different ethnicity from their partner
- For women, having a greater education level than their partner
- For women, being American Indian/Alaska Native or African American
- For women, being disabled
- Childhood sexual and/or physical violence
- For women, having a verbally abusive, jealous, or possessive partner
- Veterans and active-duty military
- Some research indicates higher levels of IPV (especially emotional victimization) in same-sex couples (Ludermir, Barreto de Araújo, Valongueiro, Muniz, & Silva, 2017; Yakubovich et al., 2018)

Marked differences between partner's incomes, levels of education, or job status place a victim more at risk for IPV. Community characteristics are similar to those of the perpetrator, revealing that those communities with fewer available resources, in areas of poverty, and having a lack of sanctions against violent behaviors increase one's risk; there is some indication that rates of IPV are higher in rural versus urban areas. Traditional gender roles, such as a belief that men work and women are submissive and should stay home, are societal risk factors associated with higher IPV risk (Zapata-Calvente, Megías, Moya, & Schoebi, 2019).

Effects of Violence on Children

A national study found that over 40% of children were physically assaulted within the last year (Finkelhor, Turner, & Shattuck, 2013). The consequences of exposure to violence and abuse hinder children's health and development and can have a lifelong impact, negatively affecting health and increasing the risks of further victimization and becoming a perpetrator of violence (Box 18-9; WHO, 2020c).

Literature reviews consistently suggest that a positive correlation exists between children's witnessing IPV and some aspects of impaired child development. Young children are particularly vulnerable to the effects of violence, as they lack the ability to understand the trauma and are likely to exhibit somatic complaints (e.g., headaches, eating or sleep problems) and/or behavior regression, such as clinging, whining, or becoming nonverbal (National Child Traumatic Stress Network, n.d.). Meanwhile, school-age children and adolescents are more likely to either act out with delinquent behaviors or withdraw. Children in families with domestic violence are at risk for depression, negative mental health effects, and consequences that last far into their adult lives. These maladjustments may be behavioral (aggression and conduct problems), emotional (withdrawal, anxiousness, fearfulness), social, cognitive (learning disabilities), and/or physical.

- Researchers have linked physical alterations in the child's brain (e.g., cerebral cortex, limbic system, corpus callosum, hypothalamus) with PTSD following child exposure to domestic violence (Tsavoussis, Stawicki, Stoicea, & Papadimos, 2014).
- For some children, high cortisol and other hormonal responses may lead to chronic levels of arousal, aggression, anxiety, depression, eating disorders, and other problems (e.g., self-harm, general irritability). In others, during adulthood, attempts to adjust to new stressors may lead to down-regulation of receptors and the ability to only respond minimally to stress hormones (Tsavoussis et al., 2014).

Providers who work with children need to listen in a sincere, nonjudgmental manner and provide ongoing support when assisting the child and family with resources, such as counseling, education, or community violence prevention programs.

BOX **18-9** EVIDENCE-BASED PRACTICE

Generational Transmission of Intimate Partner Violence

About one quarter of women will experience intimate partner violence (IPV) or domestic violence during their lifetime (CDC, 2019d), and research has linked child exposure to IPV and later adult domestic violence behavior (CDC, 2019i). Some posit that children adopt behaviors that have been role modeled by parents; however, most children who have witnessed IPV do not abuse their partners in adulthood.

Others found that abused children, compared to IPV-exposed children, have a similar or even higher risk of becoming perpetrators of IPV as adults. Research has also indicated that there may be an even greater effect for those children who are both abused and who witness interparental violence.

Eriksson and Mazerolle (2015) wanted to know if examining gender role–specific behavior would give a clearer indication of generational transmission. Their research revealed a possible gender-specific connection to male IPV perpetration (e.g., male children who observe their fathers beating their mothers are more likely to do the same as adults).

- Given this evidence and after examining other research on this topic, what interventions might you consider when working with families dealing with domestic violence?

Source: Center for Disease Control and Prevention (CDC) (2019d); Eriksson and Mazerolle (2015).

ELDER ABUSE AND MALTREATMENT OF OLDER ADULTS

Elder abuse is the "intentional act, or failure to act, by a caregiver or another person in a relationship involving an expectation of trust that causes or creates a risk of harm to an older adult" (CDC, 2019c, para. 1). Examples include physical, sexual or abusive sexual contact, emotional or psychological abuse, neglect, financial or material exploitation, confinement, passive neglect, and willful deprivation (CDC, 2019c; National Council on Aging, n.d). As with other types of abuses against vulnerable populations, the true incidence and prevalence of elder abuse is not known.

- A total of 90% of adults over the age of 65 live in the community on their own or with family (USDOJ, 2018b).
- It is estimated that 1 in 10 older adults experience some type of abuse (USDOJ, 2018a). Worldwide estimates are as high as 1 in 6 adults over age 60 experience abuse (WHO, 2020b).
- Approximately two thirds of elder abuse victims are women, often about half of individuals have dementia (USDOJ, 2018a).
- Risk factors include low social support, dementia, poor physical health, and functional impairment (NCEA, n.d.b).
- Perpetrators are often adult children or spouses, male, history of substance disorders, or mental health issues (NCEA, n.d.b).
- The most reported abuse includes neglect, followed by financial exploitation and emotional abuse (USDOJ, 2018a).

- Two thirds of staff employed in skilled or assisted nursing facilities admitted to abusing residents within the past year (WHO, 2020b).

Forms of physical abuse include rough handling during caregiving, pinching, hitting, and slapping. Emotional abuse, which can take many forms, included being shouted at or threatened and having needed care withheld. Older adults may also be sexually assaulted or sexually abused. Some elders are neglected by those they depend on to meet their caregiving needs. Elders with dementia and those requiring assistance for all activities of daily living are more vulnerable to experiencing maltreatment due to caregiver stress or burnout, factors known to increase risk for maltreating older adults. A neglected older adult may appear unwashed and unkempt, be malnourished or dehydrated, or have pressure sores. Financial exploitation includes theft of Social Security or retirement money, savings or investments, and the use of these funds by the abuser. Criminals often approach elders with get-rich-quick schemes, sham investment opportunities, overpriced home repairs, or pose as collectors for illegitimate charities, thereby preying on the trusting nature of older adults (USDOJ, 2018a; NCEA, n.d.b). See Chapter 22 for more on older adults.

Vulnerability Factors

Individual characteristics associated with vulnerability of abuse include poor health, increased age, and disability. Lesbian, gay, bisexual, and transgender older adults and those who are residents of an assisted living facility are also more vulnerable to experiencing maltreatment (NCEA, n.d.a). The older LGBT community experiences discrimination due to age and sexual orientation leading to social isolation. This population may experience abuse and discrimination from medical providers and law enforcement (Bloemen et al., 2019). Dementia and newly diagnosed cognitive impairment correlate with occurrences of abuse. If violence or threats of violence by the elder toward the caregiver accompany dementia, this contributes to the elder's risk for abuse. Harmful effects of abuse for this vulnerable population include longer convalescence period, permanent damage, premature death, depression, and anxiety (WHO, 2020b).

The *invisibility* of elders in general, and abused elders specifically, increases an older adult's vulnerability of being abused. Reasons for invisibility among the elderly are multifaceted. Older adults may have less contact with the community, they are no longer in the workforce or in public on a regular basis, which keeps their problems hidden longer. Older adults are reticent to admit to being abused or neglected. Because the abuser is often a family member, the elder attempts to protect the abuser to avoid being entirely alone. On the other hand, the elder may fear reprisal from the abuser for coming forward with a self-report of abuse or telling someone about the home situation. Cultural and societal values also contribute to keeping "family matters" private, while shame and embarrassment make it difficult for many elders to tell others of the abuse (New York City Elder Abuse Center, 2013).

- Older adults may be considered a vulnerable population for several reasons. Individuals may experience a diminished capacity in self-determination, impaired cognitive ability, decreased physical strength, lack of or inadequate education including low health literacy, and lack of resources (Barbosa et al., 2017).
- Many elders who are frail are dependent on others for some aspect of their day-to-day survival. The degree to which an older adult needs assistance is often kept hidden from others because the elder fears being removed from his present living situation and being placed in a more restrictive environment.
- Additionally, vulnerability in elders is increased when any of the following characteristics are present: (1) being female, (2) 85 years and older, (3) widowers, (4) a decrease in health, (5) low income, and (6) lack of education and low health literacy (Barbosa et al., 2017).

Prevention of Elder Abuse

Elders who are dependent on others for their care often do not report abuse for fear of being abandoned. They feel powerless and at a loss about how to attain help. They often fear reprisal from the perpetrator if they tell others about the abuse. Awareness of elder abuse and education about the types of abuse via public and professional media campaigns has improved community recognition of the problem. C/PHNs need knowledge in screening procedures and risk factors for abuse and perpetrators. Respite care can provide valuable relief to family members. Training for caregivers as well as health care and social service providers that focus on recognizing stress and initiating intervention measures has developed a new understanding of effective interventions. Statutory requirements for reporting abuse and providing crisis hotlines for reporting elder abuse are also integral aspects of a community's response to the problem of elder abuse (WHO, 2020b). World Elder Abuse Awareness Day has been designated as an annual observance on June 15th to promote public awareness and prevention education regarding elder abuse (United Nations, n.d.).

OTHER FORMS OF VIOLENCE

Additional forms of violence include self-directed violence (including suicide), homicide, sexual assault, and human trafficking.

Self-Directed Violence

Self-directed violence (SDV), an intentional act to cause injury to one's self, is a public health issue worldwide. SDV is considered a range of behaviors involving fatal and nonfatal self-harm. Examples of self-harm include cutting, head banging or hitting, self-scratching, self-biting, burning self, attempted suicide, and suicide. Suicidal ideation, although not a behavior, is often included due to an association with SDV (CDC, 2019e).

Suicide is taking action that causes one's own death. According to the CDC, suicide rates are rising in every state in the United States. In 2017 alone, more than 47,000 people committed suicide in the United States. It touches all age groups; it is

- Second leading cause of death among 10- to 34-year-olds
- Fourth leading cause of death among 35- to 54-year-olds
- Eighth leading cause of death among 55- to 64-year-olds (CDC, 2019e)

In 2017, 10.6 million individuals in the United States considered suicide, of those 3.2 million had a plan and 1.4 million attempted suicide (CDC, 2019e).

It is important to be aware of warning signs of potential suicide when working with people in crisis. The strongest risk for suicide is a previous suicide attempt (WHO, 2019a). Warning signs fall into three categories: what the person talks about, types of behaviors, and mood. The more warning signs, the greater the risk (American Foundation for Suicide Prevention [AFSP], 2020). An individual may talk about not having a reason to live, feeling trapped, or suicide. Threats or comments that indicate a plan or giving personal items away are potential indicators of a person contemplating suicide. Isolation, sleeping too much, acting recklessly, and increased use of alcohol or drugs are high-risk behaviors for suicide. Moods that may reflect increased risk are depression, irritability, rage, humiliation, and anxiety.

Community awareness campaigns and education programs are needed to help a person recognize the risks and the importance of initiating prevention for someone who is suicidal (Box 18-10). Crisis hotlines with 24-hour access are a vital resource for a distraught individual, friend, or loved one to contact and find help during a crisis and to learn about local resources to contact.

BOX **18-10** STORIES FROM THE FIELD

Helping Youth Build the Strength to Prevent Suicide

Mark LoMurray is the founder and Executive Director of *Sources of Strength*, a youth suicide prevention program that address bullying, violence, and substance abuse. The program uses peer leaders with adult advisors in the school setting. The peer leaders help their classmates address emotions they're grappling with and cultivate strengths to use to change. The goal is to remove suicide intervention from the crisis mode and focus on development of appropriate coping skills. The main focus is positivity; instead of dwelling on negative emotions, strengths are emphasized. There are 8 strengths students can use to help develop coping skills. Arranged in a wheel the 8 sources of strength include mentors, positive friends, family support, mental health, medical access, spirituality, generosity, and healthy activities. Students are taught to reframe stressful situations to what will help the situation using the 8 strengths as a guide. A variety of modalities are used, for instance, playing games, talking, use of social media, and art. More information can be found at https://sourcesofstrength.org/.

1. *As you read this chapter, how might this program decrease violence in our communities?*
2. *Examine the 8 strengths and identity 3 to 4 that may have helped you in a stressful situation.*
3. *The Sources of Strength address several Healthy People 2030 objectives. After examining the topic areas of Health Behavior, Populations, and Social Determinants of Health, reflect on how Sources of Strength addresses these objectives.*

Source: ODPHP (2020a).

Homicide

Homicide is any non–war-related action taken to cause the death of another person. In 2017, globally, intentional homicide took the lives of 464,000 people (United Nations Office on Drugs and Crime, 2019). In 2017, there were 19,510 homicides reported in the United States alone. It was the 16th leading cause of death among all age groups and the 3rd leading cause of death of young people between the ages of 15 and 24 years (Kochanek, Murphy, Xu, & Arias, 2019).

Evidence suggests that violence can be prevented by measures aimed at individuals, families, relationships, community, and society. The Guide to Community Preventive Services (Community Guide) provides evidence-based recommendations and interventions for 22 health topics including or violence prevention for each level of prevention (USDHHS, n.d.). Although biologic and personal factors may influence one's predisposition to violence, an interaction between one's family, community, cultural, and other factors combine to create violence (WHO, 2019b). The WHO cites four key steps in developing a public health approach to violence. These steps include the following:

- Define the problem
- Discover the causes and risk factors
- Develop and test interventions
- Implement and scale effective interventions (WHO, 2019b)

Prevention methods include education programs for preschool, school-aged children, and adolescents to decrease bullying and improve social skills; parent education courses and parent resources such as advice lines, support groups, or a crisis nursery; and community measures that improve firearm safety and reduce firearm injuries.

Sexual Assault

Sexual assault is defined as "any nonconsensual sexual act proscribed by Federal, tribal, or State law, including when the victim lacks capacity to consent" (USDOJ, n.d.c, para. 2). According to the U.S. Department of Justice (USDOJ) (2016), this definition includes threats of sexual violence, attempted rape, and rape. The percent of sexual assaults are staggering:

- 30% of sexual assault victims were raped.
- 23% experienced attempted rape.
- 24% were sexually assaulted.
- 18% of victims received threats of sexual assault.
- 6% experienced "unwanted sexual contact without force."
- 19% of women and 1.5% of men… "have been victims of rape or attempted rape."
- For close to 78% of females who were raped, the assault was recorded before they turned 25.
- Over 67% of males who were sexually assaulted, victimization occurred before age 25 (USDOJ, 2016, p. 17).

The majority of perpetrators were either current or former intimate partners or acquaintances.

Community measures useful in preventing sexual assault involve education and prevention provided through state sexual assault coalitions, sexual assault programs for adolescents and college students, dating violence education, hotlines staffed to provide help for victims of sexual assault and interpersonal violence, and having trained professionals, such as Sexual Assault Response Team (SART) members, on hand (CDC, 2019g). Rape crisis centers and state sexual assault coalitions work together with law enforcement, health care providers, and community-based organizations (CBOs) to provide community education and care and support to victims. SART (Sexual Assault Response Team) consists of multidisciplinary members that are trained to understand the psychological and physical assessment needs of the victim, as well as the legal requirements for an investigation and court proceeding (National Sexual Violence Resource Center [NSVRC], 2018). The CDC's Rape Prevention and Education program provides current tools, training, and support works (CDC, 2019g). Unfortunately, only 33% of sexual assaults are reported to law enforcement (USDOJ, 2016).

A common role in the SART is a sexual assault nurse examiner (SANE). A SANE's role is more explicit than that of the C/PHN in assisting people who are affected by sexual violence, including victims, suspects, and the accused. For people who have experienced sexual assault, SANEs provide forensic medical exams and appropriate follow-up referrals based on the patient's individual needs. SANEs may specialize in pediatrics, adolescents, adults, or a combination of all three. A SANE represents one subspecialty of forensic nursing practice; forensic nurses work in a variety of community settings and specialize in many different types of patient populations affected by violence including elder abuse, IPV, homicide, human trafficking, and more (Adams & Hulton, 2016; DailyNurse®, 2019).

Human Trafficking

Human trafficking of adults and children on a national and international scale is recognized by the United States in the Trafficking Victims Protection Act (TVPA) of 2000.

- This federal law defined human trafficking as the "recruitment, harboring, transportation, provision, or obtaining of a person" for compelled labor or commercial sex or for labor or services through the "use of force, fraud, or coercion" (National Human Trafficking Hotline, n.d., para. 5). The law specifically identified any child <18 years who engaged in commercial sex as a victim of trafficking when coerced or forced.
- Since 2000, a total of 11 laws, revisions, and reauthorizations of the TVPA have been implemented; the most recent in 2018 (USDOS, 2019). Victims of human trafficking are not associated with any one specific demographical factor. Victims can be anyone of any age, ethnicity, economic status, or gender and are trafficked into various forms of human abuse such as commercial sex, medically assisted reproduction, many types of physical labor, and more.

In February 2020, during a weeklong investigation, federal, state, and county officials in California made over 500 arrests in a human trafficking sting operation. Twenty-seven suspects and 270 customers were arrested for sex trafficking. A total of 11 children and 76 adults were rescued (City News Service, 2020). Despite the significant number of known cases, the actual prevalence of human trafficking is not known. This, combined with the well-established negative health consequences, have made this into a public health problem, and one that is difficult to mitigate. Research shows that the majority of victims have encounters with health care providers. However, victims of human trafficking most often do not self-identify as victims during the health care encounter and health care providers do not readily recognize them as potential victims of human trafficking (Chisolm-Straker et al., 2016). This places nurses at the forefront of screening for human trafficking victims and also facilitating effective response protocols. A major response measure implemented by the USDHHS was the establishment of the National Human Trafficking Hotline (n.d.) at https://humantraffickinghotline.org/. The center is responsible for the 24-hour crisis line available in over 200 languages, plus additional texting (233733), live chat, and online resources to assist in the recognition and response to victims.

Gang Violence

According to the FBI (n.d.b), there are 33,000 violent gangs in the United States, consisting of street, motorcycle, and prison gangs. Violent activities involve prostitution, human trafficking, drug sales, robberies, and gun trafficking. Los Angeles City and County combined are considered the gang capital of the world with a total of 450 violent gangs comprising 45,000 individuals (Los Angeles Police Department [LAPD], 2019). Since 2016, there have been 491 homicides, 5,510 robberies, 98 rapes, and 7,050 felony assaults (LAPD, 2019). Teens join gangs for several reasons:

- Identity or recognition
- Fellowship
- Intimidation
- Protection
- Criminal activity (Office of Justice Programs [OJP], n.d.)

Teens involved in gangs are at higher risk of not graduating from high school, teen parenthood, and unemployment (OJP, n.d.).

Gun Violence

- A Pew Research Center Survey discovered 30% of Americans own a firearm, 11% live with someone that owns a firearm, nearly 60% have friends that own guns, and 72% of those that responded to the survey have fired a gun (Gramlich & Schaeffer, 2019).
- Most gun owners cite the Second Amendment to the Constitution as their right to own a firearm. Reasons for owning a firearm include protection (67%), followed by hunting, sport shooting, collector, and requirement of job (Gramlich & Schaeffer, 2019).
- In 2016, death from firearms was estimated to be 251,000 worldwide (Naghavi, 2018). The countries that account for 50% of these deaths include Brazil, the United States, Mexico, Colombia, Venezuela, and Guatemala. Homicide was the leading cause of firearm deaths at 64%, with suicides at 27%, and unintentional deaths by guns at 9% (Naghavi, 2018).

- In 2017, the United States had 39,800 deaths due to firearms; the highest number since 1993 (Gramlich & Schaeffer, 2019).

Of the 7,639 bills introduced in Congress from January to August 2019, 110 related to guns (Desjardins, 2019). The two bills with the most support were the Bipartisan Background Checks Act and the Concealed Carry Reciprocity Act. Grassroots movements include Moms Demand Action (https://momsdemandaction.org/), a movement to protect against gun violence by public safety measures; Everytown For Gun Safety (https://everytown.org/), a group that advocates for changes in gun laws; and March For Our Lives (https://marchforourlives.com/), whose Web site opens to voter registration and was started by the students of Marjory Stoneman Douglas high school in Parkland, Florida, after a mass shooting there that killed 17 and injured 17 in 2018 (Marjory Stoneman Douglas High School Public Safety Commission, 2019).

Workplace Violence

Workplace violence is defined as "any act or threat of physical violence, harassment, intimidation, or other threatening disruptive behavior that occurs at the work site" (OSHA, n.d., para. 2). The violence can take the form of threats, verbal abuse, physical assaults, or homicide. According to the U.S. Department of Labor, those at greatest risk include health care providers, customer service workers, employees working in small groups or alone, public service employees, and law enforcement officers (OSHA, n.d.).

Workplace injuries due to violence account for 12% of injuries among registered nurses. While this figure may appear low, it is three times greater than injuries due to violence when compared to any other occupation. Nurses employed in nursing and residential care are at greater risk, followed by hospitals and ambulatory care clinics (U.S. Bureau of Labor Statistics, 2018). In hospitals, those nurses working in emergency departments and in-patient psychiatric units have the highest risk of injuries due to violence. Health care workers underreport workplace violence by patients because of unclear definitions of workplace violence, feeling that the patient was not responsible for actions due to mental status, or believing violence is part of the job (JCAHO, 2018). The Joint Commission on Accreditation of Healthcare Organizations (JCAHO) standards and recommendations related to workplace violence are located at https://www.jointcommission.org/resources/patient-safety-topics/sentinel-event/sentinel-event-alert-newsletters/sentinel-event-alert-59-physical-and-verbal-violence-against-health-care-workers/.

The phrase "nurses eat their young" has long been a lament of novice nurses (Colduvell, 2017). Bullying or incivility among nurses is a common occurrence. It is estimated 44% of nurses have been bullied within the health care setting (JCAHO, 2016). In a CINAHL search of "bullying" and "nurses" between 2017 and 2019, a total of 375 results were found. Several countries were represented including the United States, Russia, Iran, Korea, and Australia demonstrating this is an epidemic in health care. While, incivility is considered part of the job by some, it has a negative impact on health care. Horizontal and vertical bullying increases burnout, turnover rate, patient care errors (e.g., medication errors and higher infection rates), and costs (JCAHO, 2016). However, the bullying can have fatal consequences. In 2018, a registered nurse in Wales committed suicide related to workplace bullying (Stephenson, 2018).

C/PHN Self-Care

The American Nurses Association (ANA) announced 2017 as the Year of the Healthy Nurse. Each month focused on a different topic of health such as sleep, happiness, mental health wellness, physical activity, and healthy eating (ANA, n.d.). Practicing these health promotion themes throughout our careers place us a better position to handle individual, family, community, and global violence. These topics should be a part of every C/PHN daily routine. Unfortunately, due to work requirements and family commitments nurses may not practice self-care techniques even though we teach these practices to our communities (Ross, Bevans, Brooks, Gibbons, & Wallen, 2017). Nurse leaders need to highlight and encourage self-care practices in the workplace (Ross et al. 2017); for instance mediation lunches, walking groups, or infographics on self-care.

HEALTHY PEOPLE 2030 AND VIOLENCE PREVENTION

The problem of violence is pervasive, affecting the people who experience violence directly and family members and society indirectly. Progress on selected violence and abuse objectives for *Healthy People 2030* include the following (Office of Disease Prevention and Health Promotion [ODPHP], 2020b):

- Reduce homicides: In 2018, the baseline for homicides was 5.9/100,000. The target for 2030 is to decrease this to 5.5/100,000.
- Reduce emergency department visits for nonfatal self-harm injuries: Reduce these emergency department visits from 182.7/100,000 in 2017 to 144.7/1,000 for person 10 years and older.
- Reduce gun carrying among adolescents: In 2017, 4.8% of students in grades 9 through 12 carried an firearm at least 1 day within the past year. The target for 2030 is 3.7%.

See Box 18-11 for selected Healthy People 2030 violence-related objectives.

LEVELS OF PREVENTION: CRISIS INTERVENTION AND FAMILY AND INTIMATE PARTNER (IP) VIOLENCE

C/PHNs are in a unique position to prevent, identify, and intervene during crisis situations involving family violence. Because C/PHNs encounter people in their own settings, a more accurate assessment with direct observation, discussion, and intervention can occur. The nurse's assessment skills, familiarity with the community, and access to resources enhance his ability to help families in crisis. By using the three levels of prevention, the nurse can assist families in a variety of ways to counter problems arising from family and IP violence (Box 18-12).

BOX **18-11** *HEALTHY PEOPLE 2030*

Selected Violence-Related Objectives

Core Objectives

IVP-09	Reduce homicides
IVP-10	Reduce nonfatal physical assault injuries
IVP-11, 12	Reduce physical fighting and gun carrying among adolescents
IVP-13	Reduce firearm-related deaths
IVP-14	Reduce nonfatal firearm-related injuries
IVP-15	Reduce child abuse and neglect deaths
IVP-16	Reduce nonfatal child abuse and neglect
IVP-17	Reduce adolescent sexual violence by anyone
IVP-18	Reduce sexual or physical adolescent dating violence
OSH-05	Reduce work-related assaults

Developmental Objectives

IVP-D04	Reduce intimate partner violence
AH-D03	Reduce the proportion of public schools with a serious violent incident

Reprinted from Office of Disease Prevention and Health Promotion (ODPHP). (2020a). *Healthy People 2030: Browse objectives.* Retrieved from https://health.gov/healthypeople/objectives-and-data/browse-objectives.

Primary Prevention

The cycle of violence can be interrupted. Primary prevention is the most effective level of intervention in terms of promoting clients' health and containing costs. Primary prevention reflects a fundamental human concern for well-being and includes planned activities undertaken by the nurse to prevent an unwanted event from occurring, to protect current health and healthy functioning, and to promote improved states of health for all members of a community. For the C/PHN, any activity that fosters healthful practices will counteract unhealthful influences, thereby empowering an individual or family to avoid or better respond to a crisis. Health promotion considerations include the biopsychosocial and spiritual needs of the individual and family.

Opportunities for interventions include promoting positive relationships and parenting practices, improving communication skills, and developing positive self-esteem. Healthy self-esteem also improves education and occupational success. If poverty is a contributing factor to the violence being experienced, adequate educational preparation and having a successful employee role may help to eliminate this stressor. Parenting influences children's coping strategies, decision-making, and sense of self-confidence. Parenting classes are an important resource, particularly for parents who are at high risk, such as teens, people with no exposure to children in their upbringing, and people raised in violent and abusive families. Parenting classes offer an opportunity for parents to discuss challenges, while learning new strategies for managing their children's behaviors and appropriate physical, emotional, and developmental expectations for their children's ages (Dutton, James, & Kelley, 2015).

Home visiting has been formalized into community/public health nursing model programs around the country, based on two decades of work by David Olds (Nurse-Family Partnership, 2020) and others. This evidenced-based program has shown that nurse follow-up and interventions during the pregnancy and for the first 2 years of the child's life was effective in preventing child abuse, decreasing the mother's reliance on government assistance, having mothers with longer spacing between their children and fewer subsequent pregnancies, and improving health habits, such as less smoking by mothers (USDHHS, 2019). To date, the NFP has served over 309,000 families in the United States (Nurse-Family Partnership, 2019). See Chapter 4. For more information on this unique partnership, refer to https://www.nursefamilypartnership.org. The effectiveness of home visit programs to pregnant women and families with a child from birth to 5 years are evaluated yearly by the Office of Planning, Research, and Evaluation (Sama-Miller, Akers, Mraz-Esposito, Coughlin, & Zukiewicz, 2019). This report provides an in-depth evaluation of home visit programs across the United States and is a valuable tool when starting a home visit program.

The interrelatedness between families and communities cannot be overlooked or underestimated. Neighborhoods need to be enfranchised, developed, and attentive to the needs for health and safety for all community members. Empowered families and communities can take back their neighborhoods from criminals, and their empowerment acts as a source of growth for other families.

Secondary Prevention

Early diagnosis and prompt treatment of the effects of family crisis or violence is the focus of secondary level prevention strategies. Secondary prevention seeks to reduce the intensity and duration of a crisis and to promote adaptive behavior. By creating a positive relationship with family members in their homes, the C/PHN can often uncover and intervene in a crisis or stop abusive situations.

Those affected by a violence-related crisis is rendered temporarily helpless and unable to cope on their own and are especially receptive to outside influence. C/PHNs can implement crisis resolution models to assist clients at the secondary level. The following process outlines a proven crisis intervention process (James & Gilliland, 2017):

1. Establish rapport.
2. Assess the individual and the problem for lethality.
3. Identify major problems and intervene.
4. Deal with feelings.
5. Explore alternatives and coping mechanisms.
6. Develop an action plan.
7. Follow up, including anticipatory planning for coping with future crises.

People in crisis will seek and generally receive some kind of help, but the nature of that help may act in favor of or against a healthy outcome from which the participants can grow and evolve. A client's desire for assistance gives the helping professional a prime opportunity to intervene; this opportunity also presents a challenge to make the

BOX 18-12 LEVELS OF PREVENTION PYRAMID

Promoting Crisis Resolution

SITUATION: Traumatic crisis due to act of violence regarding a mass shooting
GOAL: To use the three levels of prevention, to avoid promptly diagnose and treat the community's negative health conditions, and to restore the fullest possible potential.

Tertiary Prevention (Postcrisis)

Rehabilitation	*Primary Prevention* — *Health Promotion and Education*	*Primary Prevention* — *Health Protection*
■ Promote adaptation to a changed level of community wellness ■ Identification and use of additional resources	■ Yearly review of safety measures ■ Reinforce newly learned coping strategies ■ Continue to promote educational programs that promote safety	■ Reevaluate affected community members' mental health ■ Educate on the prevention of violence

Secondary Prevention (Crisis)

Early Diagnosis	*Prompt Treatment*
■ Get a prompt diagnosis on situation	■ Assist with reaction to the event ■ Allow for feelings of anger and grief ■ Set goals with clients and community ■ Refer to resources ■ Ensure safety—follow orders of police ■ Partner with community and agencies to provide needed services

Primary Prevention (Precrisis)

Health Promotion	*Health Protection*
■ Promote education on gun violence ■ Lobby for gun restrictions and bans on certain models ■ Teach and reinforce new coping strategies ■ Reinforce protective factors in the community	■ Educate public on steps to increase safety ■ Provide anticipatory guidance by conducting active shooter drills at job and school sites ■ Reinforce newly learned behaviors and lifestyle changes

intervention as effective as possible. Behaviors found to be helpful in these interventions include the following:

- Respect the client's confidentiality.
- Listen to the client and validate the client's experiences.
- Acknowledge any violation and oppression.
- Allow clients to make their own decisions.
- Assist the client and the client's family to plan for future safety.
- Promote access to community services (James & Gilliland, 2017).

The Quality and Safety Education for Nurses Project [QSEN] provides a guide for preparing future nurses to improve the quality and safety of the health care system in which they work (QSEN Institute, 2020). Knowledge, skills, and attitudes are delineated for the domain of safety. Although framed specifically for acute care settings, the domain of safety identifies factors that create a culture of safety such as communication and reporting systems (i.e., mandatory reporting). Effective use of strategies to assess and reduce harm is important when working with families in crisis. Valuing safety, vigilance, monitoring, and reporting are skills necessary for community/public health nursing practice.

- One goal of crisis intervention should be to help clients reestablish a sense of safety and security while allowing them to share their feelings and have those feelings validated. This process helps reestablish equilibrium at as healthy a level as possible and can result in client change and growth.
- Minimally, the goal is to resolve the immediate crisis and restore clients to their precrisis level of functioning. Overall, intervention seeks to improve their functioning to a healthier, more mature level that will enable them to cope with and prevent future crises.
- As discussed earlier, crises tend to be self-limited; intervention time generally lasts from 4 to 8 weeks, with resolution within 2 or 3 months (James & Gilliland, 2017).
- The urgency of the situation represents a window of opportunity that invites prompt, focused attention by the client and nurse in working together to achieve intervention goals.

At times, the nurse may be responding to a referral regarding suspected abuse; at other times, an abusive or neglectful situation may be uncovered on a home visit made for another reason. In any case, the C/PHN has an important role in reporting suspected abuse and encouraging the child, partner/spouse, or elder to go to the appropriate facility to seek care and to file required documentation about the abuse (Box 18-13).

Reporting Abuse

All states have reporting laws for suspected abuse, although states differ on aspects of the timeline for reporting, who to notify, and the sequence of events. The following steps represent one state's guidelines for reporting suspected child abuse (California Department of Education, 2020):

1. All mandated reporters must report known or suspected abuse or neglect.
2. Immediately, or as soon as practically possible, the designated agency such as the local child protective agency (police department after normal working hours) must be contacted by telephoned and given a verbal report. During this verbal report, mandated reporters must give their name—which is kept confidential and may be revealed only in court or if the reporter waives confidentiality (others can give information anonymously)—the name and age of the child, the present location of the child, the nature and characteristics of the injury, and any other facts that led the reporter to suspect abuse or that would be helpful to the investigator.
3. The mandated reporter must notify the appropriate agency immediately or as soon as possible, followed by a written report within 36 hours. It is imperative that nurses know their state laws for reporting. If a mandated reporter fails to report known or suspected instances of child abuse, they may be subject to criminal liability, punishable by up to 6 months in jail or/and a fine of $1,000.

Similar steps are required for nurses when reporting elder abuse and other vulnerable adults. Such cases of suspected maltreatment are reported to a local area agency on aging, Adult Protective Services, or to the police, and a screening/documentation form is used to

BOX 18-13 STORIES FROM THE FIELD

Community/Public Health Nursing and a Potential Family in Crisis

You are a PHN employed be the Smithville Health Department. You are following up on a referral from a community clinic's family planning clinic involving a 19-year-old woman, Sarah, who exhibited inappropriate behaviors with her 6-month-old daughter during a clinic visit. Per the referral, staff observed the mother shouting at the child, accusing her of "being spoiled rotten," the mother appeared quite anxious, and seemed to have difficulty waiting the 15 minutes for her examination. Although the behaviors described were insufficient to warrant a report to social services, the staff felt that this young mother would benefit from intervention on the part of the nurse.

In preparation for the home visit, you review the medical records of Sarah and her child to determine whether the family has had previous involvement with social service agencies such as Child Protective Services (CPS). You find that the maternal grandparents made a referral to child welfare staff on behalf of Sarah when she was 15. The grandparents were concerned about a sexual relationship between Sarah and her stepfather. The findings of the investigation were inconclusive, and the charges were never pursued.

You discuss the case with family planning and immunization clinic staff, because the family receives services at both clinics. The staff are familiar with Sarah and her husband Jacob. Their only interaction with Jacob was during a family planning clinic visit 2 months ago. They report Sarah appeared anxious and rushed, stating, "I really need to hurry, Jacob is waiting in the car, and he gets impatient." Shortly after that, the staff tell you, Jacob came running into the clinic shouting, "What the hell is taking you people so long?" He reportedly glared at Sarah, and the two quickly exited the clinic.

You phone the client and introduce yourself as a nurse with the local health department, explaining that nurses often visit new mothers to assist them in finding resources. You add that as a PHN, you will be available to talk with her about her child's growth and development. The client expresses interest in the visit and states, "I want you to show me some things about feeding her and stuff. I need help figuring out what to do at night, she still isn't sleeping much and it's driving me crazy." You advise the client that you will be happy to discuss those issues with her and that you will bring information to review together. Noting that the father of the baby is living in the home, you assure her that she may involve other family members, including the father of the baby, in the home visit. You jointly decide that the visit will occur the following day at 10:30 AM and that the father of the baby will be present if his work schedule allows.

On the day of the visit, as you walk up the stairs toward the apartment, you notice someone looking at you through the curtains. As you near the apartment door, the curtains close. Your repeated knocking on the door is met with no response. You call the client's name but there is no answer.

1. *Does this scenario provoke anxiety for you? How would you deal with your reaction?*
2. *How is this different from being in a hospital setting where a supervisor is readily available?*
3. *Given this scenario, what actions will you take?*
4. *If you had been working in the family planning clinic on the day that Jacob came in, what, if anything, would you have done differently?*
5. *As young parents, Jacob and Sarah are part of an aggregate that has unique risk factors for parenting. List as many of these risk factors as you can think of and brainstorm about possible community/public health nursing interventions for each.*
6. *What methods would you suggest the clinic staff utilize to detect signs and symptoms of physical, sexual, or emotional abuse among this aggregate?*

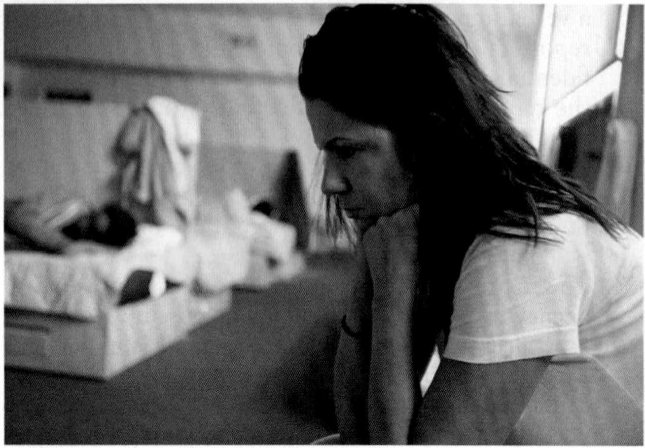

FIGURE 18-4 Public health nursing client in a homeless shelter.

gather and record pertinent information. Guidelines for filing the report and agency notification are specific within each state. In cases of partner/spousal abuse, adults who are mentally competent cannot be removed involuntarily from the abusive situation. The C/PHN can communicate concern for the client's safety, emphasize the importance being in a safe environment, and provide information regarding community resources, such as a shelter (Fig. 18-4). If the adult has a life-threatening injury or illness, medical follow-up must be encouraged; however, the victim may still be reluctant to seek help.

Tools

Assessment of suspected abuse cannot be overemphasized. The C/PHN may be the only person entering the home of a family in crisis where abuse is occurring. Asking the right questions, being a careful observer, and following the correct reporting process and recording procedures may mean the difference between life and death for a person or family experiencing violence. (See http://thepoint.lww.com/Rector10e for the following sample tools: a Suspected Child Abuse Report, a two-page Medical Report of Suspected Child Abuse, and a Domestic Violence Screening/Documentation Form.)

C/PHNs must be observant for hazards and personal safety. Follow agency policy if ever feel in harm's way. Some agencies assign nurses to go in pairs or with law enforcement to ensure safety. If the batterer is in the home, meet the victim in a public place and not in the home.

Tertiary Prevention

Tertiary prevention focuses on the rehabilitation of the person or family from the violence and crisis they have experienced. They may be alone, such as a trafficked teenager estranged from his family. Or, they may never again have the same relationships because partners may separate—by choice, motivated by fear or hatred; by court order, if the perpetrator is incarcerated; or due to a death. Regardless of an individual, or a couple or a family, long-term intervention may be needed to establish a climate more conducive to normalcy. Many of the services discussed as part of the secondary level of prevention are continued into the tertiary prevention phase to promote healing and to restore and promote family growth.

If incarceration is a part of tertiary prevention, the effects of having one person living in this environment must be factored into the services and support provided by the C/PHN to the other people involved (see Chapter 28 for information on working in correctional facilities). If children are involved, even if the partner/spouse has separated from the perpetrator, the perpetrator usually has legal rights to see the children. This may mean that other family members, usually from the abuser's side of the family, can bring the children to the prison to visit their parent. Making arrangements for these visits can create stress for adult survivors, children, and the visitors. The C/PHN needs to be aware of the complicated dynamics and emotional stress such difficult situations can produce for all family members. The victim–perpetrator relationship is as complex as the forces that created the violence and abuse (NCADV, n.d.b).

VIOLENCE FROM OUTSIDE THE HOME

There has always been some degree of violence that affects people in their homes, such as burglaries, murder, or abduction (Fig. 18-5). *Home invasion,* the purposeful and sudden entry into a home by force while people are home and awake, is a form of terror that relies on surprise. Confrontation is often sought, and offenders are often younger (under age 30) and male, working in small groups. They often look for victims who may be more vulnerable and are believed to have money or desired goods that they can pawn or sell (Heinonen & Eck, 2012). Motivation may be material or thrill; household belongings are frequently stolen while members of the home are incapacitated by being bound, blindfolded, and/or gagged. In some cases, people are murdered. Often, the perpetrators are under the influence of drugs or alcohol, and at times, the violence may be gang related.

Other forms of violence include the potential for terrorist activities through planned community violence (e.g., 9/11 attacks, Sandy Hook school shooting, Route 91 Harvest Music Festival) and biologic, chemical, or radioactive actions (see Chapter 17). Communities have developed resources such as the National Organization for Victim Assistance (NOVA) and crisis response teams (CRT), to

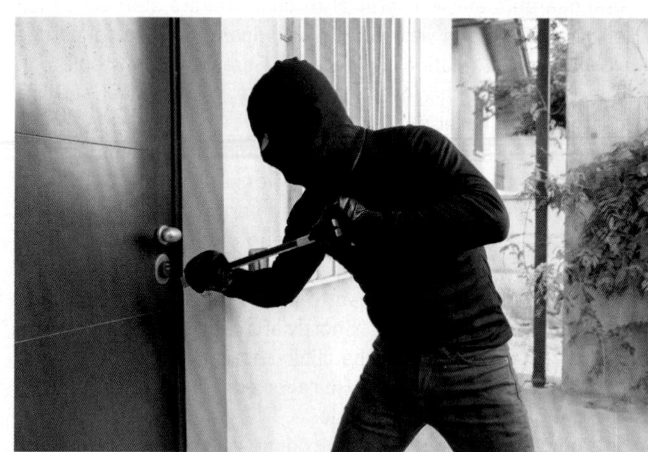

FIGURE 18-5 Crime is a type of community violence that can affect families.

assist individuals and groups experiencing a disaster or violent event (e.g., child murder or school shootings).

The *Global Study on Homicide 2019* provides an in-depth investigation into crime. Lethal violence can create a climate of fear and uncertainty. Intentional homicide victimizes individuals, families, and the community of the victim (United Nations Office on Drugs and Crime, 2019). Fear of violence can create psychological and physiologic stress reactions. These fears should not be ignored.

Historically, society has depended on the criminal justice system to respond to community violence with emphasis on deterrence and incarceration, which has limited prevention capacity. Today, violence is considered a public health issue requiring more than a criminal justice action. To put primary prevention into practice, an integrated multifaceted approach is required.

- The **spectrum of prevention** offers a systematic framework for developing effective and sustainable primary prevention programs.
- Developed by Larry Cohen, the spectrum of prevention identifies multiple levels for community intervention: strengthening individual knowledge and skills; promoting community education; educating providers; fostering coalitions and networks; changing organizational practices; and influencing policy and legislation.
- When used together, these levels are complementary and create synergy that results in greater effectiveness (Prevention Institute, n.d.).

Nurses may work at each level of the spectrum, by educating individuals and high-risk target populations, working on coalitions to foster increased awareness and use of screening tools by health care providers, and working with multisector partnerships to foster change in workplace, organizational, and community policy. Nurses may work with extended family members of the victims or families who have reported such an incident in their neighborhood and are now fearful of a reoccurrence. See Chapters 11 and 12.

THE NURSING PROCESS

Assessment and Nursing Diagnosis

Initially, the nurse must assess the nature of the crisis and the client's or community's response to it in a focused community assessment. How severe is the problem, and what are the risks? Who is at risk? Assessment must be rapid but thorough and focused on specific areas.

- First, the nurse concentrates on the immediate problem during the assessment. Why have clients asked for help right now? What are the injuries? How do they define the problem? What precipitated the crisis? When did it occur?
- Next, the nurse focuses on the clients' perceptions of the event. What does the crisis mean to them, and how do they think it will affect their future? Are they viewing the situation realistically? When a crisis occurs to a family or group, some members see the situation differently from others.
- Determine who is available to offer support to the individual or family. Consider family, friends, clergy, other professionals, community members, and agencies. Who are the clients close to, and whom do they trust?
- Finally, the nurse assesses the clients' or community's coping abilities and resources. Have they had similar kinds of experiences in the past? What techniques have they tried in this situation, and if they did not work, why not? Clients should be encouraged to think of other stress-relieving techniques, perhaps ones they have used in the past, and to try them.

After the assessment, a nursing diagnosis is developed. Nursing diagnosis priorities should focus on Maslow's (1971) Hierarchy of Needs at the Physiological and Safety levels related to the act of violence. Ineffective coping related to the client's or community's traumatic event provides a means to increase coping skills. When the violence problem is more community centered, the Omaha System of documentation and information management may be useful as a nomenclature as it comprehensively includes the family and community as clients or modifiers. The system consists of three relational, reliable, and valid components used together: The Problem Classification Scheme, Intervention Scheme, and the Problem Rating Scale for Outcomes (Omaha System, 2019). The Problem Classification Scheme includes neighborhood/workplace safety in the environmental domain. See Chapters 12 and 15.

Planning Interventions

Several factors influence clients' reaction to crises. Nurses should try to determine what factors are affecting clients before making intervention plans. The major balancing factors—clients' perceptions of the event, social supports, human resources, and clients' coping skills—have been assessed in the first step (James & Gilliland, 2017). While continuing to explore these, the nurse now also considers the clients' age, past experiences with similar types of situations, sociocultural and religious influences, general health status, and the actual assets and liabilities of the situation. This assessment helps clarify the situation and gives the nurse an opportunity to further encourage the clients' participation in the resolution process. If clients are defensive, resistant, and rigid, they are not processing clearly and can complete only simple tasks. It will take time before these clients can begin to solve problems related to the effects of the crisis on themselves and the loss they are experiencing, but the nurse will want to encourage them to reach this level.

A plan is based on multiple factors:

- The crisis
- The effect the crisis is having on clients' lives
- Where they are in coming to resolution of the crisis
- The ways in which significant others are affected and respond
- Their level of preparation for such a crisis
- The clients' strengths and available resources

Implementation of Interventions

During implementation, the partnership between the nurse and clients is important. Discussions about what is happening, reviewing the family's plan and rationale for this approach, and making appropriate changes are necessary. Know the resources in the community so as to make referrals as needed. Referrals may include social workers, mental health practitioners, clergy, law enforcement, or support groups. The C/PHN needs to:

- *Demonstrate acceptance of clients.* Clients need to feel the support of a positive, caring person who does not judge their feelings or behavior.
- *Use therapeutic communication.* Verbal and nonverbal therapeutic communication allows clients to feel safe in expressing their feelings of fear, anger, guilt, or other negative emotions.
- *Assist client in making and reaching achievable goals by using strengths.*
- *Communicate changes with client prior to making them.*
- *Do not offer false reassurance.* Clients need to face reality, not avoid it. A statement such as "Don't worry, it will all work out" is demeaning and meaningless.
- *Discourage clients from blaming others.* Clients often blame others as a way to avoid reality and the responsibility for problem solving.
- *Help clients learn new coping skills by providing alternatives.* Explore and test old and new techniques to reduce stress and anxiety. Ask questions.
- *Encourage clients to accept help from their social support system and spiritual resources as needed.* Denial in the early phases of crisis cuts off help. Encouraging clients to acknowledge the problem is a first step toward acceptance of help.
- *Promote development of new positive relationships.* Clients who have lost significant others through unintentional or intentional death, divorce, incarceration, or an act of perpetrated violence should be encouraged to find new connections, purpose, and people to fill the void and provide needed supports and satisfactions (Ackley, Ladwig, & Makic, 2017).

Evaluation

In the final step, clients and the nurse evaluate, stabilize, and plan for the future. Evaluating the outcome of the intervention might address the following:

- Are the clients using effective coping skills and exhibiting appropriate behavior?
- Are adequate resources and support persons available?
- Is the diagnosed problem solved?
- Have the desired outcomes been met?
- Are modifications needed in the assessment, outcomes, or interventions?

Analysis of these outcomes will provide a greater understanding for coping with future crises.

Clients' plans for the future should include setting realistic goals and means to implement them. Review with clients how their handling of the present crisis can help them cope with, minimize, or preferably prevent future crises.

SUMMARY

- Violence affects individuals, families, groups, communities, and all of society. Experiencing violence may result in a crisis, a temporary state of severe disequilibrium for persons who face a threatening situation.
- A crisis is a state that individuals can neither avoid nor solve with their usual coping abilities and occurs when some force disrupts normal functioning, thereby causing a loss of balance or normalcy in life. Crises create tension; subsequently, efforts are made to solve the problem and reduce the tension. If such efforts meet with failure, people feel upset, redefine the situation, and try other solutions, and if failure continues, the person eventually reaches the breaking point.
- Violence is a global public health issue. It is not limited by sociodemographic or geographic factors—anyone may experience violence or abuse at any point in their lifetime.
- Acts of violence can result in a crisis—a *crisis* is a stressful and disruptive event (or series of events) that comes with or without warning and disturbs the equilibrium of the individual, family, or community.
- Understanding the neurobiological effects, potential subsequent health effects, and the overlapping causes of violence can help community nurses to enhance protective factors, reduce risk factors, and inform violence intervention and prevention activities.
- Child abuse occurs among children of all ages, from infancy through the teen years, and may be physical, emotional, and/or sexual. Neglect and sexual exploitation are additional forms of child abuse.
- Community violence creates fear and uncertainty and impacts individuals and families that may live, work, play, and pray in close proximity.
- Maltreatment of older adults, often called elder abuse, may involve physical, sexual, emotional or psychological abuse; neglect; abandonment; financial or material exploitation; or self-neglect or any combination of these mistreatments.
- Community health nurses use three levels of prevention when working with families.
  - Primary prevention focuses on providing people with the skills and resources to prevent violent situations.
  - Secondary prevention involves immediate intervention at the time of the violent episode. Secondary level prevention may include medical attention, emotional support, police, and social services involvement.
  - Tertiary prevention offers rebuilding services and helps establish equilibrium with a structure that may be different, but healthier. The spectrum of prevention offers a multidimensional approach to building community capacity to address issues of violence.
- People in crisis need and often seek help.
  - Crisis intervention builds on these two phenomena to achieve its primary goal—reestablishment

of equilibrium. Crisis intervention begins with assessment of the situation, followed by planning a therapeutic intervention. The nurse then implements and carries out the intervention, building on the strengths and self-care ability of clients. Crisis intervention concludes with resolution and anticipatory planning to avert possible future crises.

- Regardless of the method of intervention used by the C/PHN, the steps of the nursing process provide an intervention framework. Assessing the assets and liabilities, a person's willingness to change, and the nature of the violence help the nurse form a nursing diagnosis. With this diagnosis, the nurse can begin to plan appropriate interventions and implement plans. Evaluation of the intervention techniques provides the nurse with new data to assist with ongoing assessment of the progress and additional anticipatory guidance needs.

ACTIVE LEARNING EXERCISES

Some activities may be uncomfortable to participate in, please give yourself the freedom to decline on any that cause undue stress.

1. Acts of violence affect the individual, the family, and the community. C/PHNs may practice or live in the area affected by the violence. As registered nurses, it is imperative that we engage in self-care so as to care for our clients. What are some successful self-care methods you have practiced? Is there research that confirms your self-care practice? How might you use that research to help your clients?
2. Gun violence in schools and social events have become part of society. Research legislative bills dealing with gun violence in your community or state. Write a letter in favor of or against the bill based in current statistics and facts.
3. Research "Assess and Monitor Population Health" and "Investigate, Diagnose, and Address Health Hazards and Root Causes" (2 of the 10 essential public health services; see Box 2-2) in relationship to racism and inequity in your community. As a C/PHN, what other essential public health services might you use to make changes?
4. A classmate comes to class with a black eye and upper arm bruising. Describe what you would, or would not, do and why. Role play with a classmate if possible. Although, gender was not mentioned did you assume the classmate was female? Do your actions differ if your classmate is a male? Research what your local community offers on the three levels of prevention of IPV. Where do you see the gaps and how might you correct them?
5. After reviewing your state's child abuse reporting form what do you think would be the most difficult about the process?
   - Research what your state and county laws are regarding filing.
   - What is the policy at your clinical agency?
   - Does your agency follow state law?
   - Self-care is important when working with children abuse cases. Does your agency use debriefing methods?

REFERENCES

Ackley, B. J., Ladwig, G. B., & Makic, M. B. F. (2017). *Nursing diagnosis handbook* (11th ed.). St. Louis, MO: Elsevier.

Adams, P., & Hulton, L. (2016). The sexual assault nurse examiner's interactions within the sexual assault response team: A systematic review. *Advanced Emergency Nursing Journal, 28*(3), 213–217. doi: 10.1097/TME.0000000000000112.

American Association of Neurological Surgeons (AANS). (2020). *Shaken baby syndrome*. Retrieved from https://www.aans.org/en/Patients/Neurosurgical-Conditions-and-Treatments/Shaken-Baby-Syndrome

American College of Obstetricians and Gynecologist (ACOG). (2019). *Intimate partner violence*. Retrieved from https://www.acog.org/clinical/clinical-guidance/committee-opinion/articles/2012/02/intimate-partner-violence

American Foundation for Suicide Prevention (AFSP). (2020). *Risk factors and warning signs*. Retrieved from http://afsp.org/about-suicide/risk-factors-and-warning-signs/

American Nurses Association (ANA). (2017). *Year of the Healthy Nurse: Resources to support nurses to take care of their health*. Retrieved from https://www.nursingworld.org/practice-policy/hnhn/2017-year-of-the-healthy-nurse/#:~:text=Practice%20%26%20Advocacy,-Nursing%20Excellence&text=ANA%20is%20declaring%202017%20to,all%20of%20us%20can%20improve

Andone, D. (February 14, 2020). It's been two years since the deadly shooting at a high school in Parkland, Florida. *CNN*. Retrieved from https://www.cnn.com/2020/02/14/us/parkland-shooting-marjory-stoneman-douglas-2-years/index.html

Arizona Law. (n.d.). *Myths and realities of domestic abuse*. Retrieved from https://law.arizona.edu/sites/default/files/myths_and_realities_of_domestic_abuse.pdf

Barbosa, K. T., Costa, K. N., Pontes, L., Batista, P. S., Oliveira, F. M., & Fernandes, M. G. (2017). Aging and individual vulnerability: A panorama of older adults attended by the family health strategy. *Texto & Contexto - Enfermagem, 26*(2). Retrieved from https://www.scielo.br/scielo.php?script=sci_arttext&pid=S0104-07072017000200306#fn1

Berghoef, K. (2019). *Implicit bias: What it means and how it affects behavior*. Retrieved from https://www.thoughtco.com/understanding-implicit-bias-4165634

Bloemen, E. M., Rosen, T., LoFaso, V. M., Lasky, A., Church, S., Hall, P., … Clark, S. (2019). Lesbian, gay, bisexual, and transgender older adults' experiences with elder abuse and neglect. *Journal of the American Geriatrics Society, 67*(11), 2338–2345. doi: 10.1111/jgs.16101.

Boston25News.com. (2019). *Former Boston College student charged for her alleged role in boyfriend's suicide*. Retrieved from https://www.wsbtv.com/news/former-boston-college-student-charged-in-suicide-death-of-boyfriend/1002758183

Boyd, M. A. (2018). *Psychiatric nursing: Contemporary practice enhanced update* (6th ed.). Philadelphia: Wolters Kluwer.

Bryce, I., Robinson, Y., & Petherick, W. (Eds.). (2019). *Child abuse and neglect: Forensic issues in evidence, impact, and management*. San Diego, CA: Academic Press, Elsevier.

Bureau of Justice Statistics (BJS). (n.d.). *Stalking*. Retrieved from https://www.bjs.gov/index.cfm?ty=tp&tid=973

California Department of Education. (2020). *Child abuse and identification reporting guidelines*. Retrieved from https://www.cde.ca.gov/ls/ss/ap/childabusereportingguide.asp

Centers for Disease Control and Prevention (CDC). (2010). *NISVS: An overview of 2010 findings on victimization by sexual orientation*. Retrieved from: https://www.cdc.gov/violenceprevention/pdf/cdc_nisvs_victimization_final-a.pdf

Centers for Disease Control and Prevention (CDC). (2016). *Preventing multiple forms of violence: A strategic vision for connecting the dots*. Retrieved from https://www.cdc.gov/violenceprevention/pdf/strategic_vision.pdf

Centers for Disease Control and Prevention (CDC). (2017a). *LGBTQ youth programs at a glance*. Retrieved from https://www.cdc.gov/lgbthealth/youth-programs.htm

Centers for Disease Control and Prevention (CDC). (2017b). *Prevalence of selected maternal and child health indicators for all PRAMS sites, Pregnancy Risk Assessment Monitoring System (PRAMS), 2016-2017*. Retrieved from https://www.cdc.gov/prams/prams-data/mch-indicators/states/pdf/Selected-2016-2017-MCH-Indicators-Aggregate-by-Site_508.pdf

Centers for Disease Control and Prevention (CDC). (2018a). *Dating Matters®*. Retrieved from https://www.cdc.gov/violenceprevention/intimatepartnerviolence/datingmatters/index.html

Centers for Disease Control and Prevention (CDC). (2018b). *Preventing stalking*. Retrieved from https://www.cdc.gov/violenceprevention/datasources/nisvs/preventingstalking.html

Centers for Disease Control and Prevention (CDC). (2018c). *Violence prevention*. Retrieved from https://www.cdc.gov/violenceprevention/index.html

Centers for Disease Control and Prevention (CDC). (2018d). Youth Risk Behavior Surveillance-United States, 2017. *Morbidity and Mortality Weekly Report, 67*(8), 1–113. Retrieved from https://www.cdc.gov/healthyyouth/data/yrbs/pdf/2017/ss6708.pdf

Centers for Disease Control and Prevention (CDC). (2019a). *Help stop violence before it happens*. Retrieved from http://vetoviolence.cdc.gov

Centers for Disease Control and Prevention (CDC). (2019b). *Preventing bullying*. Retrieved from https://www.cdc.gov/violenceprevention/youthviolence/bullyingresearch/fastfact.html

Centers for Disease Control and Prevention (CDC). (2019c). *Preventing elder abuse*. Retrieved from https://www.cdc.gov/violenceprevention/elderabuse/definitions.html

Centers for Disease Control and Prevention (CDC). (2019d). *Preventing intimate partner violence*. Retrieved from https://www.cdc.gov/violenceprevention/intimatepartnerviolence/fastfact.html

Centers for Disease Control and Prevention (CDC). (2019e). *Preventing suicide*. Retrieved from https://www.cdc.gov/violenceprevention/suicide/fastfact.html

Centers for Disease Control and Prevention (CDC). (2019f). *Preventing teen violence*. Retrieved from https://www.cdc.gov/violenceprevention/intimatepartnerviolence/teendatingviolence/fastfact.html

Centers for Disease Control and Prevention (CDC). (2019g). *Rape Prevention and Education (RPE) program*. Retrieved from https://www.cdc.gov/violenceprevention/sexualviolence/rpe/

Centers for Disease Control and Prevention (CDC). (2019h). *Understanding school violence: Fact sheet*. Retrieved from http://www.cdc.gov/violenceprevention/youthviolence/schoolviolence

Centers for Disease Control and Prevention (CDC). (2019i). *Violence prevention: Risk and protective factors for perpetration*. Retrieved from https://www.cdc.gov/violenceprevention/intimatepartnerviolence/riskprotectivefactors.html

Centers for Disease Control and Prevention (CDC). (2020a). *CDC advances violence prevention research*. Retrieved from https://www.cdc.gov/violenceprevention/publichealthissue/fundedprograms/researchawards.html

Centers for Disease Control and Prevention (CDC). (2020b). *Preventing abusive head trauma in children*. Retrieved from https://www.cdc.gov/violenceprevention/childabuseandneglect/Abusive-Head-Trauma.html

Centers for Disease Control and Prevention (CDC). (2020c). *Youth violence: Risk and protective factors*. Retrieved from http://www.cdc.gov/violenceprevention/youthviolence/riskprotectivefactors.html

Chang, Q., Xing, J., Ho, R. T. H., & Yip, P. S. F. (2019). Cyberbullying and suicide ideation among Hong Kong adolescents: The mitigating effects of life satisfaction with family, classmates and academic results. *Psychiatry Research, 274*, 269–273. doi: 10.1016/j.psychres.2019.02.054.

Child Welfare. (2019). *What is child abuse and neglect? Recognizing the signs and symptoms*. Retrieved from https://www.childwelfare.gov/pubpdfs/whatiscan.pd

Child Welfare Information Gateway. (2017). *Infant safe haven laws. State statutes current through December 2016*. Retrieved from https://www.childwelfare.gov/pubPDFs/safehaven.pdf#page=2&view=Safe%20haven%20providers

Child Welfare Information Gateway. (2019a). *About CAPTA: A legislative history*. Retrieved from https://www.childwelfare.gov/pubPDFs/about.pdf

Child Welfare Information Gateway. (2019b). *Definitions of child abuse and neglect*. Retrieved from https://www.childwelfare.gov/pubPDFs/define.pdf#page=1&view=Introduction

Children's Bureau. (2019). *Child Maltreatment 2017*. Retrieved from https://www.acf.hhs.gov/cb/resource/child-maltreatment-2017

Chisolm-Straker, M., Baldwin, S., Gaïgbé-Togbé, B., Ndukwe, N., Johnson, P. N., & Richardson, L. D. (2016). Health care and human trafficking: Seeing the unseen. *Journal of Health Care for the Poor and Underserved, 27*(3), 1220–1233. Retrieved from https://muse.jhu.edu/article/628131

City News Service. (2020). *Statewide human trafficking task force nets more than 500 arrests*. Retrieved from https://www.nbclosangeles.com/news/statewide-human-trafficking-task-force-nets-more-than-500-arrests/2303874

Colduvell, K. (April 14, 2017). *Nurse bullying: Stand up and speak out*. Retrieved from https://nurse.org/articles/how-to-deal-with-nurse-bullying/

Collibee, C., & Furman, W. (2016). Chronic and acute relational risk factors for dating aggression in adolescence and young adulthood. *Journal of Youth and Adolescence, 45*(4), 763–776. Retrieved from https://www.ncbi.nlm.nih.gov/pmc/articles/PMC4788968/

DailyNurse®. (2019). *From forensics to advocacy: What's it like to be a SANE (Sexual Assault Nurse Examiner)*. Retrieved from https://dailynurse.com/from-forensics-to-advocacy-what-its-like-to-be-a-sexual-assault-nurse-examiner-sane/

Debowska, A., Boduszek, D., & Dhingra, K. (2015). Victim, perpetrator, and offense characteristics in filicide and filicide-suicide. *Aggression and Violent Behavior, 21*, 113–124. doi: org/10.1016/j.avb.2015.01.011.

Desjardins, L. (2019). *Congress has 110 gun bills on the table. Here's where they stand*. Retrieved from https://www.pbs.org/newshour/politics/congress-has-110-gun-bills-on-the-table-heres-where-they-stand

Dutton, M. A., James, L., & Kelley, M. (2015). Coordinated public health initiatives to address violence against women and adolescents. *Journal of Women's Health, 24*(1), 80–85. Retrieved from https://www.ncbi.nlm.nih.gov/pmc/articles/PMC4302966/

Eligon, J., Furber, M., & Robertson, C. (2020). *Appeals for calm as sprawling protests threaten to spiral out of control*. Retrieved from https://www.nytimes.com/2020/05/30/us/george-floyd-protest-minneapolis.html

Eriksson, L., & Mazerolle, P. (2015). A cycle of violence? Examining family-of-origin violence, attitudes, and intimate partner violence perpetration. *Journal of Interpersonal Violence, 30*(6), 945–964.

Federal Bureau of Investigation (FBI). (n.d.a). *Parent guide to Internet safety*. Retrieved from https://www.cfalls.org/docs/FBI%20%20Parent%20Guide%20to%20Internet%20Safety.pdf

Federal Bureau of Investigation (FBI). (n.d.b). *What we investigate: Gangs*. Retrieved from https://www.fbi.gov/investigate/violent-crime/gangs

Felitti, V. J., Anda, R. F., Nordenberg, D., Williamson, D. F., Spitz, A. M., Edwards, V.,... Marks J. S. (1998). Relationship of childhood abuse and household dysfunction to many of the leading causes of death in adults: The adverse childhood experiences (ACE) study. *American Journal of Preventive Medicine, 14*(4), 245–258. doi: 10.1016/s0749-3797(98)00017-8.

Finkelhor, D., Turner, H. A., & Shattuck, A. (2013). Violence, crime, and abuse exposure in a national sample of children and youth: An update. *JAMA Pediatrics, 167*(7), 614–621. Retrieved from https://jamanetwork.com/journals/jamapediatrics/fullarticle/1686983

Gillis, M. E. (2019). Cyberbullying on rise in US: 12-year-old was 'all-American little girl' before suicide. *Fox News*. Retrieved from https://www.foxnews.com/health/cyberbullying-all-american-little-girl-suicide

Gluck, S. (May 2, 2019). *What is psychological abuse of a child?* Retrieved from https://www.healthyplace.com/abuse/child-psychological-abuse/what-is-psychological-abuse-of-a-child

Gramlich, J., & Schaeffer, K. (2019). FactTank: 7 facts about gun violence. *Pew Research Center*. Retrieved from https://www.pewresearch.org/fact-tank/2019/10/22/facts-about-guns-in-united-states/

Gray, S., & Rarick, S. (2018). Exploring gender and racial/ethnic differences in the effects of child sexual abuse. *Journal of Child Sexual Abuse, 27*(5), 570–587. doi: 10.1080/10538712.2018.1484403.

Health Resources & Services Administration (HRSA). (2019). *Women's preventive services guidelines*. Retrieved from https://www.hrsa.gov/womens-guidelines-2016/index.html

Heinonen, J. A., & Eck, J. E. (2012). *Home invasion robbery: Guide no. 70. Arizona State University, Center for Problem Oriented Policing*. Retrieved from https://popcenter.asu.edu/content/home-invasion-robbery-0

Hinsliff-Smith, K., & McGarry, J. (2017). Understanding management and support for domestic violence and abuse within emergency departments: A systematic review from 2000-2015. *Journal of Clinical Nursing, 26*(23–24), 4013–4027. doi: 10.1111/jocn.13849.

Hrelic, D. A. (August 13, 2019). *Intimate partner violence in pregnancy*. Retrieved from https://www.americannursetoday.com/intimate-partner-violence-in-pregnancy/

Human Rights Campaign. (2020). Sexual assault and the LGBTQ community. Retrieved from https://www.hrc.org/resources/sexual-assault-and-the-lgbt-community

James, R. K., & Gilliland, B. E. (2017). *Crisis intervention strategies* (8th ed.). Boston, MA: Cengage Learning.

Jensen, K. T. (December 26, 2019). Colorado day care owner allegedly used 'false wall' to hide 26 toddlers in a basement. *Newsweek*. Retrieved from https://www.newsweek.com/colorado-day-care-owner-allegedly-used-false-wall-hide-26-toddlers-basement-1479220

Joint Commission on Accreditation of Healthcare Organizations (JCAHO). (June 20, 2016). *Sentinel event alert 24: Bullying has no place in health care*. Retrieved from https://www.jointcommission.org/resources/news-and-multimedia/newsletters/newsletters/quick-safety/quick-safety-issue-24-bullying-has-no-place-in-health-care/

Joint Commission on Accreditation of Healthcare Organizations (JCAHO). (2018). *Sentinel event alert 59: Physical and verbal violence against health care workers*. Retrieved from https://www.jointcommission.org/resources/patient-safety-topics/sentinel-event/sentinel-event-alert-news-letters/sentinel-event-alert-59-physical-and-verbal-violence-against-health-care-workers/

Kanel, K. (2019). *A guide to crisis intervention* (6th ed.). Stamford, CT: Cengage Learning.

Kann, L., McManus, T., Harris, W., Shanklin, S., Flint, K., Queen, B., ...Ethier, K. (2018). Youth risk behavior surveillance—United States, 2017. *Morbidity and Mortality Weekly, 67*(8), 1–114.

Kazan, O. (June 2, 2020). Why people loot: On who looters are, what they want, and why some protests are more likely to include them. *The Atlantic*. Retrieved from https://www.theatlantic.com/health/archive/2020/06/why-people-loot/612577/

Keneally, M. (April 19, 2019). The 11 mass deadly school shootings that happened since Columbine. *ABC News*. Retrieved from https://abcnews.go.com/US/11-mass-deadly-school-shootings-happened-columbine/story?id=62494128

Kidpower. (2020). *Protecting children from stranger abduction/kidnapping*. Retrieved from https://www.kidpower.org/library/article/safety-tips-kidnapping/

Kochanek, K. D., Murphy, S. L., Xu, J., & Arias, E. (2019). Deaths: Final data for 2017. *National Vital Statistics Reports, 68*, 9. Retrieved from https://www.cdc.gov/nchs/data/nvsr/nvsr68/nvsr68_09-508.pdf

Legal Information Institute. (n.d). U.S. Code 5106g. Definitions. *Cornell Law School*. Retrieved from https://www.law.cornell.edu/uscode/text/42/5106g

Lewis, J. B., Sullivan, T. P., Angley, M., Callands, T., Divney, A. A., Magriples, U., ... Kershaw, T. S. (2017). Psychological and relational correlates of intimate partner violence profiles among pregnant adolescent couples. *Aggressive Behavior, 43*(1), 26–36. Retrieved from https://www.ncbi.nlm.nih.gov/pmc/articles/PMC5493138/

Los Angeles Police Department (LAPD). (2019). *Gangs*. Retrieved from http://www.lapdonline.org/search_results/content_basic_view/1396

Ludermir, A. B., Barreto de Araújo, T. V., Valongueiro, S. A., Muniz, M. L. C., & Silva, E. P. (2017). Previous experience of family violence and intimate partner violence in pregnancy. *Revista de Saúde Pública, 51*(85). Retrieved from https://www.scielo.br/scielo.php?script=sci_arttext&pid=S0034-89102017000100276

Malmquist, C. (2013). Infanticide/neonaticide: The outlier situation in the United States. *Aggression and Violent Behavior, 18*, 399–408.

Marjory Stoneman Douglas High School Public Safety Commission. (2019). *Initial report submitted to the governor, speaker of the house of representatives and senate president*. Retrieved from http://www.trbas.com/media/media/acrobat/2018-12/70135058816260-12074125.pdf

Merriam-Webster. (2020). *Cyberstalking*. Retrieved from https://www.merriam-webster.com/legal/cyberstalking

Mottaghi, S., Poursheikhali, H., & Shameli, L. (2020). Empathy, compassion fatigue, guilt, and secondary traumatic stress in nurses. *Nursing Ethics, 27*(2), 494–504. doi: 10.1177/0969733019851548.

Naghavi, M. (2018). Global mortality from firearms, 1990-2016. *JAMA, 320*(8),792–814. Retrieved from https://jamanetwork.com/journals/jama/fullarticle/2698492

National Center for Missing and Exploited Children. (2020). *CyberTipline*. Retrieved from http://www.cybertipline.com

National Center on Elder Abuse (NCEA). (n.d.a). *Mistreatment of lesbian, gay, bisexual and transgender (LGBT) elders: Research brief*. Retrieved from http://www.centeronelderabuse.org/docs/ResearchBrief_LGBT_Elders_508web.pdf

National Center on Elder Abuse (NCEA). (n.d.b). *Statistics and data*. Retrieved from https://ncea.acl.gov/What-We-Do/Research/Statistics-and-Data.aspx

National Center for Healthy Safe Children. (2020). *Safe Schools/Healthy Students (SS/HS) framework*. Retrieved from https://healthysafechildren.org/sshs-framework

National Center on Shaken Baby Syndrome (NCSBS). (2020). *Learn more*. Retrieved from https://www.dontshake.org/learn-more

National Child Traumatic Stress Network. (n.d.). *What is child trauma?* Retrieved from https://www.nctsn.org/what-is-child-trauma

National Council on Aging. (n.d.). *Elder abuse facts*. Retrieved from https://www.ncoa.org/public-policy-action/elder-justice/elder-abuse-facts/

National Human Trafficking Hotline. (n.d.). *Human trafficking*. Retrieved from https://humantraffickinghotline.org/type-trafficking/human-trafficking

National Sexual Violence Resource Center (NSVRC). (2018). *Sexual assault response team*. Retrieved from https://www.nsvrc.org/sarts

New York City Elder Abuse Center. (June 4, 2013). *Podcast: A conversation with Ashton Applewhite on ageism and elder justice*. Retrieved from http://nyceac.com/elder-justice-dispatch-nyceac-podcast-a-conversation-with-ashton-applewhite-on-ageism-elder-justice/

Newman, C., Eason, M., & Kinghorn, G. (2019). Incidence of vicarious trauma in correctional health and forensic mental health staff in New South Wales, Australia. *Journal of Forensic Nursing, 15*(3), 183–192. doi: 10.1097/JFN.0000000000000245.

Nurse-Family Partnership. (2019). *National snapshot: Families served*. Retrieved from https://www.nursefamilypartnership.org/wp-content/uploads/2019/07/NFP_Snapshot_April2019.pdf

Nurse-Family Partnership. (2020). *The David Olds story*. Retrieved from https://www.nursefamilypartnership.org/about/program-history/

Occupational Safety and Health Administration (OSHA). (n.d.). *Workplace violence*. Retrieved from https://www.osha.gov/SLTC/workplaceviolence/

Office of Disease Prevention and Health Promotion (ODPHP). (2020a). *Healthy People 2030: Browse Objectives*. Retrieved from https://health.gov/healthypeople/objectives-and-data/browse-objectives

Office of Disease Prevention and Health Promotion (ODPHP). (2020b). *Healthy People 2030: Violence prevention*. Retrieved from https://health.gov/healthypeople/objectives-and-data/browse-objectives/violence-prevention

Office of Justice Programs (OJP). (n.d.). *National criminal justice reference service: Special feature—Gangs*. Retrieved from https://www.ncjrs.gov/gangs

Office of Juvenile Justice and Delinquency Prevention (OJJDP). (n.d.). *Commercial sexual exploitation of children*. Retrieved from https://www.ojjdp.gov/programs/csec_program.html

Office of the United Nations High Commissioner for Human Rights. (2020). *Committee on the rights of the child*. Retrieved from https://www.ohchr.org/EN/HRBodies/CRC/Pages/CRCIntro.aspx

Omaha System. (2019). *The Omaha System. Solving the clinical date-information puzzle*. Retrieved from http://www.omahasystem.org/overview.html

Paisner, S. R. (2018). Five myths about domestic violence. *The Washington Post*. Retrieved from https://www.washingtonpost.com/outlook/five-myths/five-myths-about-domestic-violence/2018/02/23/78969748-1819-11e8-b681-2d4d462a1921_story.html

Peters, E. (2018). Compassion fatigue in nursing: A concept analysis. *Nursing Forum, 53*(4) 466–480. doi: 10.1111/nuf.12274.

Prevention Institute. (n.d.). *The spectrum of prevention*. Retrieved from https://www.preventioninstitute.org/tools/spectrum-prevention-0

Psychology Today. (February 22, 2019). *Child neglect*. Retrieved from https://www.psychologytoday.com/us/conditions/child-neglect

QSEN Institute. (2020). *Quality and safety education for nurses*. Retrieved from https://qsen.org/

RAINN. (2019). *Warning signs for young children*. Retrieved from https://www.rainn.org/articles/warning-signs-young-children

Resnick, P. J. (2016). Filicide in the United States. *Indian Journal of Psychiatry, 58*(Suppl 2), S203–S209. Retrieved from https://www.ncbi.nlm.nih.gov/pmc/articles/PMC5282617/?report=reader

Rollè, L., Giardina, G., Caldarera, A. M., Gerino, E., & Brustia, P. (2018). When intimate partner violence meets same sex couples: A review of same sex intimate partner violence. *Frontiers in Psychology, 9*, 1506. doi: 10.3389/fpsyg.2018.01506.

Romo, V. (January 29, 2019). FBI finds no motive in Las Vegas shooting, closes investigation. *NPR*. Retrieved from https://www.npr.org/2019/01/29/689821599/fbi-finds-no-motive-in-las-vegas-shooting-closes-investigation

Ross, A., Bevans, M., Brooks, A. T., Gibbons, S., & Wallen, G. R. (2017). Nurses and Health-Promoting Behaviors: Knowledge May Not Translate Into Self-Care. *AORN journal, 105*(3), 267–275. https://doi.org/10.1016/j.aorn.2016.12.018

Sama-Miller, E., Akers, L., Mraz-Esposito, A., Coughlin, R., & Zukiewicz, M. (September 30, 2019). Home visiting evidence of effectiveness review: Executive summary. *Mathematica*. Retrieved from https://www.mathematica.org/our-publications-and-findings/publications/september-2019-home-visiting-evidence-of-effectiveness-review-executive-summary

SexInfo Online. (2017). *The cycle of domestic violence*. Retrieved from https://sexinfo.soc.ucsb.edu/article/cycle-domestic-violence

Simms, L., Bushman, S., & Pedersen, S. (2020). Bullying: How to prevent it and help children who are victims. *National Center for Health Research*. Retrieved from http://www.center4research.org/bullying-prevent-help-children-victims/

Smithfield, B. (2016). The case of Mary Ellen—The first documented case of child abuse in the US was reported to the Animal Welfare Agency in 1874. *The Vintage News*. Retrieved from https://www.thevintagenews.com/2016/11/09/the-case-of-mary-ellen-the-first-documented-case-of-child-abuse-in-the-us-was-reported-to-the-animal-welfare-agency-in-1874/

Stanford Medicine. (2019). *Child abuse: Signs and symptoms of abuse/neglect*. Retrieved from http://childabuse.stanford.edu/screening/signs.html

Stephenson, J. (August 22, 2018). Nursing director to meet with family of 'bullied' suicide nurse. *Nursing Times*. Retrieved from https://www.nursingtimes.net/news/workforce/nursing-director-to-meet-with-family-of-bullied-suicide-nurse-22-08-2018/

Stewart, D. E., Vigod, S., & Riazantseva, E. (2016). New developments in intimate partner violence and management of its mental health sequelae. *Current Psychiatry Reports, 18*(1), 4. doi: 10.1007/s11920-015-0644-3.

Stop It Now! (2019). *Tip sheet: Warning signs of possible sexual abuse in a child's behavior*. Retrieved from https://www.stopitnow.org/ohc-content/tip-sheet-7

The Parent Project. (2019). *Who we are*. Retrieved from https://www.google.com/search?client=safari&rls=en&q=Healthy+Start+and+Loving+Solutions&ie=UTF-8&oe=UTF-8

Tsavoussis, A., Stawicki, S. P. A., Stoicea, N., & Papadimos, T. J. (2014). Child-witnessed domestic violence and its adverse effects on brain development: A call for societal self-examination and awareness. *Frontiers in Public Health, 2,* 178. Retrieved from https://www.ncbi.nlm.nih.gov/pmc/articles/PMC4193214/

U.S. Bureau of Labor Statistics. (November, 2018). *Occupational injuries and illnesses among registered nurses*. Retrieved from https://www.bls.gov/opub/mlr/2018/article/occupational-injuries-and-illnesses-among-registered-nurses.htm

U.S. Department of Health and Human Services (USDHHS). (2019). *Home visiting evidence of effectiveness review: Executive summary, September 2019*. Retrieved from https://homvee.acf.hhs.gov/sites/default/files/2019-09/HomeVEE_Executive_Summary_2019_B508.pdf

U.S. Department of Justice (USDOJ). (2016). *Sexual Assault Services Formula Grant Program, 2016 Report*. Office of Violence Against Women. Retrieved from https://www.justice.gov/ovw/page/file/1086476/download

U.S. Department of Justice (USDOJ). (2018a). *Elder Justice Initiative: Research and data*. Retrieved from https://www.justice.gov/elderjustice/eappa

U.S. Department of Justice (USDOJ). (2018b). *Rural and tribal elder justice. Summit event briefing*. Retrieved from https://www.justice.gov/elderjustice/book/file/1110846/download

U.S. Department of Health and Human Services (USDHHS). (n.d.). *The community guide*. Retrieved from https://www.thecommunityguide.org/

U.S. Department of Justice (USDOJ). (n.d.a). *Amber Alert. America's missing: Broadcast emergency response*. Retrieved from http://www.amberalert.gov/

U.S. Department of Justice (USDOJ). (n.d.b). Domestic violence. Retrieved from http://www.justice.gov/ovw/domestic-violence

U.S. Department of Justice (USDOJ). (n.d.c). *Sexual assault*. Retrieved from https://www.justice.gov/ovw/sexual-assault

U.S. Department of Justice (USDOJ). (n.d.d). *Stalking*. Retrieved from http://www.justice.gov/ovw/stalking

U.S. Department of Justice (USDOJ). (2020). *Project safe childhood*. Retrieved from https://www.justice.gov/psc

United Nations. (n.d.). *World Elder Abuse Awareness Day: 15 June*. Retrieved from https://www.un.org/en/observances/elder-abuse-awareness-day/

U.S. Department of State (USDOS). (2019). *International and Domestic Law. Office to monitor and combat trafficking in persons. U.S. Laws on trafficking in persons*. Retrieved from https://www.state.gov/international-anddomestic-law/

United Nations Office on Drugs and Crime. (2019). *Global study on homicide 2019*. Retrieved from https://www.unodc.org/unodc/en/data-and-analysis/global-study-on-homicide.html

Vinchon, M. (2017). Shaken baby syndrome: What certainty do we have? *Child's Nervous System, 33*(10): 1727–1733. doi: 10.1007/s00381-017-3517-8.

Walters, J. (October 2, 2016). 'The happening': 10 years after the Amish shooting. *The Guardian*. Retrieved from https://www.theguardian.com/us-news/2016/oct/02/amish-shooting-10-year-anniversary-pennsylvania-the-happening

Wheeler, S. R., & Boyd, M.A. (2018). Crisis, loss, grief, response, bereavement, and disaster management. In M. A. Boyd (Ed.), *Psychiatric nursing* (pp. 302–317). Philadelphia, PA: Wolters Kluwer.

White Ribbon Australia. (2019). *Cycle of violence: What is the cycle of violence?* Retrieved from https://www.youtube.com/watch?v=cFa0l1Zlio8

Wilson, C., Lonsway, K. A., & Archambault, J. (2016). Understanding the neurobiology of trauma and implications for interviewing victims. *Center for Victim Research*. Retrieved from https://www.evawintl.org/Library/DocumentLibraryHandler.ashx?id=842

World Health Organization (WHO). (2016). *Global plan of action: Health systems address violence against women and girls*. Retrieved from https://www.who.int/reproductivehealth/publications/violence/gpa-booklet/en/

World Health Organization (WHO). (2017). *Violence against women*. Retrieved from https://www.who.int/news-room/fact-sheets/detail/violence-against-women

World Health Organization (WHO). (2019a). *Suicide*. Retrieved from https://www.who.int/news-room/fact-sheets/detail/suicide

World Health Organization (WHO). (2019b). *Violence and injury prevention*. Retrieved from https://www.who.int/violence_injury_prevention/violence/en/

World Health Organization (WHO). (2020a). *Definition and typology of violence*. Retrieved from https://www.who.int/violenceprevention/approach/definition/en/

World Health Organization (WHO). (2020b). *Elder abuse*. Retrieved from https://www.who.int/news-room/fact-sheets/detail/elder-abuse

World Health Organization (WHO). (2020c). *Violence against children: Child maltreatment*. Retrieved from http://www.who.int/violence_injury_prevention/violence/child

Yakubovich, A. R., Stöckl, H., Murray, J., Melendez-Torres, G. J., Steinert, J. I., Glavin, C. E. Y., & Humphreys, D. K. (2018). Risk and protective factors for intimate partner violence against women: Systematic review and meta-analyses of prospective-longitudinal studies. *American Journal of Public Health, 108*(7), e1–e11. doi: 10.2105/AJPH.2018.304428.

Zapata-Calvente, A. L., Megías, J. L., Moya, M., & Schoebi, D. (2019). Gender-related ideological and structural macrosocial factors associated with intimate partner violence against European women. *Psychology of Women Quarterly, 43*(3), 317–334. doi.org/10.1177/0361684319839367.

UNIT 5

Aggregate Populations

CHAPTER 19

Maternal—Child Health

"Be gentle with the young."

—Juvenal (55–127 AD)

KEY TERMS

Abusive head trauma
Alcohol-related birth defects
Alcohol-related neurodevelopmental disorder
Child abuse
Environmental tobacco smoke (ETS)
Fetal alcohol effects
Fetal alcohol spectrum disorders (FASDs)
Fetal alcohol syndrome (FAS)
Gestational diabetes mellitus (GDM)
Head Start
High-risk families
Infant
Low birth weight (LBW)
Preschooler
Shaken baby syndrome
Sudden infant death syndrome (SIDS)
Toddler
Very low birth weight (VLBW)

LEARNING OBJECTIVES

Upon mastery of this chapter, you should be able to:

1. Identify major health problems and concerns for childbearing women, infants, toddlers, and preschoolers globally and in the United States.
2. Discuss major risk factors and special complications for childbearing families.
3. Describe the important considerations in developing effective health promotion programs to fit the needs of diverse maternal—child populations.
4. Describe various roles of a public and community/public health nurse (C/PHN) in serving the maternal—child population.
5. Recognize resources available regarding recommended immunization schedules for infants and children.
6. Discuss methods and interventions the C/PHN might use in working with infants, toddlers, and preschoolers to help promote their health.
7. Give examples of methods and interventions the C/PHN might use in working with infants, toddlers, and preschoolers to help promote their health.

INTRODUCTION

Maternal and child populations have always been priorities for public health and community and public health nurses (C/PHNs). These populations consist of childbearing women (including pregnant adolescents), infants, children, and adolescents. In this chapter, the focus is specifically on childbearing women (including adolescents) and children from birth through age 4 years. Often, more than half of the practice of C/PHNs in official public health agencies involves primary prevention work with mothers, such as family planning, preconception care, provision of prenatal care, and monitoring infant health. Why should maternal–infant populations require this amount of attention from C/PHNs? Despite advanced technology and availability of excellent perinatal services in the United States, we often have less than optimal birth outcomes—for instance, 318,847 low birth weight and 381,321 preterm infants were born in 2014 (Centers for Disease Control and Prevention [CDC], 2016d). Also, certain segments of the maternal and infant populations, such as adolescent mothers, those who are economically disadvantaged, and women and children of color, remain at high risk for disparities in regard to maternal deaths and complications and child risk and illness. Although some women receive excellent prenatal care and benefit from diagnostic and technological resources, many others lack access to prenatal care.

This chapter addresses major areas of concern regarding population health for maternal–infant clients. It also explores the global needs of and related services available to the youngest and thus most vulnerable of society's members. Health services that are commonly available in the United States for pregnant and postpartum women, infants, toddlers, and preschoolers are examined, and the role of the C/PHN in providing those services is explored.

HEALTH STATUS AND NEEDS OF PREGNANT WOMEN AND INFANTS

C/PHNs constitute a key group of health professionals involved in both program planning and the actual delivery of services to mothers and babies in the community. In the public health sector, these nurses are the largest group of professionals practicing public health. A solid understanding of vital statistics and other data regarding mothers and infants is important to determine the appropriateness and the effectiveness of programs and services. A review of some global and national vital statistics provides insight into the major problems facing maternal and child populations.

Global Overview

Maternal and newborn health has been thrust into the global community spotlight since the publication of the Sustainable Development Goals in 2015 (Global Burden of Disease 2015 Maternal Mortality Collaborators, 2016). The goal was to improve women's and children's health on a global scale through 17 sustainable development goals. The main key to decreasing maternal mortality is to increase prenatal care benefits and coverage.

Maternal Mortality Rate

One of the major indicators of population health is maternal health, which is often measured by the maternal mortality rate (MMR). The MMR is a measure of obstetric risk and is determined by dividing the number of maternal deaths by the number of live births per 100,000. Most maternal deaths are the result of direct causes (complications of pregnancy, labor, and delivery), hypertensive disorders, intervention omissions or incorrect treatment, the chain of events resulting from any one of these, and unsafe abortions. In developing countries, the MMR is 239 per 100,000 live births, compared with developed countries, where the MMR is around 12 per 100,000 live births—a very wide disparity (World Health Organization [WHO], 2018a). The U.S.'s MMR has risen from 7.2 per 100,000 live births in 1987 to 16.9 per 100,000 live births in 2016, although it has fluctuated between a low of 14.1 and a high of 17.8 per 100,000 live births since 2002 (CDC, 2018j). Although worldwide the MMR has decreased since 1990 by 44%, the worldwide goal is to eliminate preventable maternal death by 2030 (WHO, 2018a). This goal is achievable because most countries have implemented successful policies to eliminate maternal–child inequities (Box 19-1).

Infant Mortality Rate

Another critical population health indicator is the infant mortality rate (IMR). Globally, 4.2 million children under 5 years of age died in 2016, which is a significant decrease from the 8.8 million who died in 1990 (WHO, 2018b). Of these 4.2 million deaths, 44% took place during the neonatal period and were primarily caused by preterm

BOX **19-1** EVIDENCE-BASED PRACTICE

Reducing Child Mortality in Bangladesh

Child mortality rates have declined significantly in Bangladesh over the last 25 years. Bangladesh has experienced a 76% reduction in the under-five mortality rate from 144 per 1,000 in 1990 to 34 per 1,000 in 2016. Additionally, the neonatal mortality rate was decreased by 68% from 64 per 1,000 in 1990 to 20 per 1,000 in 2016 (World Bank Group, 2018). Routine childhood immunizations, oral rehydration therapy, and supplementation of vitamin A are inventions that have significantly influenced this reduction in child mortality rates. Full vaccination of children 12 to 23 months increased from 60% in 2000 to 84% in 2014. Children receiving oral rehydration therapy for diarrhea increased from 74% in 2000 to 84% in 2014 (Ministry of Health & Family Welfare, 2015). Vitamin A supplementation increased from 49% in 1994 to 62% in 2014. Furthermore, the government of Bangladesh implemented a nutrition plan in its National Health Strategy. Children who were underweight decreased from 43% in 2004 to 33% in 2014. Although these improvements are dramatic, additional developments in sustainable trends and equity are essential (Baruah et al., 2013).

Source: Baruah et al. (2013); Ministry of Health and Family Welfare, Bangladesh, Partnership for Maternal, Newborn, & Child, WHO, World Bank and Alliance for Health Policy and Systems Research (2015); World Bank Group (2018).

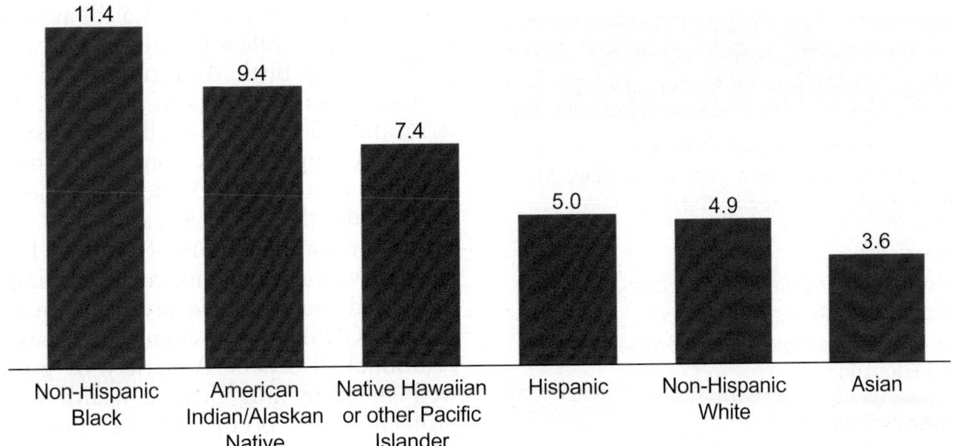

FIGURE 19-1 Infant mortality rates by race and ethnicity, 2016. (Reprinted from Centers for Disease Control and Prevention. (n.d.). *User guide to the 2016 Period Linked Birth/Infant Death Public Use File* (p. 80). Retrieved from https://www.cdc.gov/reproductivehealth/maternalinfanthealth/infantmortality.htm)

birth, birth asphyxia, and infection. More than half of the deaths for children under 5 years of age are preventable and the interventions are affordable (WHO, 2018b). In the United States, the IMR was 5.9 per 1,000 live births in 2016 (CDC, 2018j). Although this is a decrease from years past, 23,000 infants still died in 2016 in the United States. See Figure 19-1 for U.S. IMR ethnic comparison data.

National Overview

In the United States, the birth rate has decreased each year since 2007; in 2018, nearly 3.8 million women gave birth, a decline in the birth rate of 2% from the previous year (Martin, Hamilton, Osterman, & Driscoll, 2019). The general fertility rate declined to a total of 59.1 births per 1,000 women aged 15 to 44 years. Birth rates declined for non-Hispanic White, Hispanic, and African American women. Just over 40% of births were to unmarried women (Martin et al., 2019). When unmarried women rely on a single income, financial resources are more limited, and many of these women raise their children at poverty or near-poverty income levels, which impacts their health and their children's health over the life course of both (Fig. 19-2).

Child Health USA (U.S. Department of Health and Human Services [USDHHS], Health Resources and Services Administration [HRSA], Maternal and Child Health Bureau [MCHB], 2014) reports that adequate prenatal care is associated with adequate health insurance. In 2012, 88% of privately insured women and 83% of Medicaid-insured women received adequate prenatal care (defined as four or more provider visits during pregnancy). Seventy-two percent of those who were uninsured were least likely to receive adequate prenatal care. This correlates with health inequity characteristics such as race and ethnicity, poverty, and low maternal education levels (less than high school education).

Historically, the health of U.S. women and children has largely fallen under the umbrella of Title V of the Social Security Act, enacted in 1935. (For more on the Social Security Act, see Chapter 6.) Funding for state Maternal and Child Health and Crippled Children programs was part of this original legislation, as was some provision for child welfare services. Title V is "the longest-standing public health legislation in American history" and came to fruition after other legislation established a National Birth Registry; provided *Infant Care*, the first educational pamphlet; established the Children's Bureau; and provided protection against child labor practices (i.e., the first Child Labor Law of 1916; MCHB, n.d.b, para. 4). For an illustration of MCHB functions and programs, see Box 19-2.

In 1909, formal prenatal care was first provided in Boston by the Instructive District Nursing Association and spread across the country to outpatient clinics (MCHB, n.d.a). Since the inception of Title V, many programs have been developed with the goal of improving the health of women of childbearing age, as well as infants and children. Research areas have included prenatal and pregnancy health, child development and parenting, and improving health care systems and delivery of care, as well as obesity,

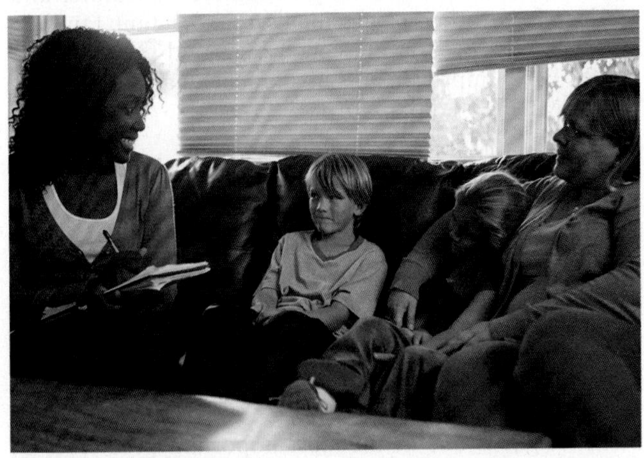

FIGURE 19-2 Support for mothers and children helps ensure healthier families.

BOX 19-2 Types of Services Offered Through Federal Maternal–Child Health Funding

Direct Health Care Services (Gap Filling)
Examples: Basic Health Services and Health Services for Children with Special Health Care Needs (CSHCN)

Enabling Services
Examples: Transportation, Translation, Outreach, Respite Care, Health Education, Family Support Services, Purchase of Health Insurance, Case Management, Coordination with Medicaid, WIC, and Education

Population-Based Services
Examples: Newborn Screening, Lead Screening, Immunization, Sudden Infant Death Syndrome Counseling, Oral Health, and Injury Prevention

Infrastructure Building Services
Examples: Needs Assessment, Evaluation, Planning, Policy Development, Coordination, Quality Assurance, Standards Development, Monitoring, Training, Applied Research, Systems of Care, and Information Systems

Source: U.S. Department of Health and Human Services (2008).

nutrition, medical homes, school services and outcomes, and behavioral health (MCHB, n.d.b). Healthy Start grants were first awarded in 1991 to 15 agencies, with the goal of reducing rates of infant mortality, low birth weight, premature births, and maternal deaths (MCHB, n.d.c). Evaluation of Healthy Start programs reveals that almost all programs provide home visitation to prenatal clients, and most continued these visits to infants and toddlers. Health education, smoking cessation counseling, services for perinatal depression, and involvement of male partners are hallmarks of most programs.

In 2017, \$374.4 million in grants were awarded to expand the Maternal, Infant, and Early Childhood Home Visiting Program (Home Visiting Program). This program provides C/PHN visits, assistance from social workers, teaching from early childhood educators, and services from other professionals to expectant families, much like the program designed by David Olds (HRSA, 2018). Early improvements in six benchmark areas were noted (MCHB, n.d.d, p. 3):

- Maternal and newborn health
- Child injuries, child maltreatment, and emergency department visits
- School readiness and achievement
- Crime or domestic violence
- Family economic self-sufficiency
- Service coordination/referrals for other community resources/support

Birth Weight and Preterm Birth

Birth weight is one of the most important predictors of infant mortality. **Low birth weight (LBW)** refers to babies who weigh <2,500 g (or <5.5 lb) at birth; **very low birth weight (VLBW)** refers to babies who weigh <1,500 g (or <3 lb 4 oz) at birth. An estimated 15 million infants are born prior to 37 weeks of gestation, making them preterm, and this number is still on the rise (Fig. 19-3; WHO, 2018b). Complications from infants born preterm led to 1 million deaths in 2015 and are the number-one cause of death under the age of 5 years.

Infant complications of preterm birth include hearing and vision problems; acute respiratory, gastrointestinal, and immunologic problems; and central nervous system (CNS), motor, cognitive, behavioral, and socioemotional disorders. A variety of growth concerns as well as acute and chronic health and developmental problems often occur, and the families of these infants are burdened with additional economic and emotional costs. In a study of children from birth to age 2 years who were preterm as infants, those with feeding difficulties or at risk for feeding difficulties had significant neurodevelopmental problems, such as impaired cognition and impaired language, motor, and socioemotional skills, that led to increased parental stress, poorer maternal mental health, or increased family stressors compared with those preterm infants who did not have feeding difficulties. Maternal mortality, LBW, and VLBW are three areas requiring attention by health care providers and the public health system. Nurses can contribute to reducing these rates and societal costs through outreach, surveillance, health teaching, counseling, and referral (Save the Children, n.d.).

In addition to infant deaths and LBW, the effects of pregnancy and childbirth on women are other important indicators of health and reflect discrepancies in access to reproductive health care. The United States is not ranked among the top 10 countries in maternal–child health in the *2015 Mother's Index*. It is ranked 33rd out of the more developed countries. The U.S. ranking is largely due to poorer scores on the indices of maternal and child health. The Eastern European countries of Slovakia, the Czech Republic, Belarus, and Croatia and the developing countries of Peru and Ethiopia rank higher than the United States (Save the Children, n.d.).

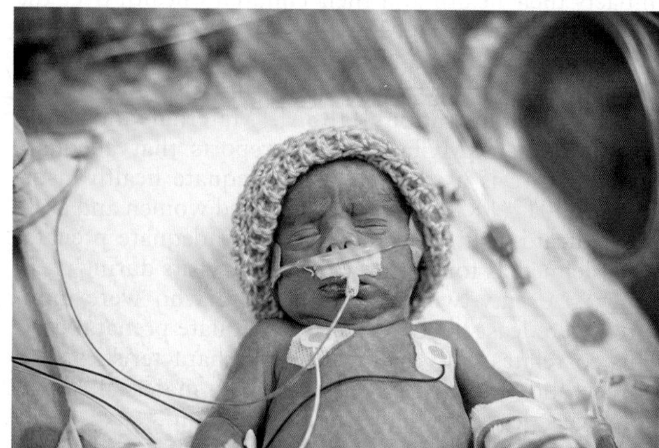

FIGURE 19-3 Infant in the neonatal intensive care unit.

In the United States, the MMR is higher than in other developed countries, mostly because of the disparities found among women of color. The MMR for Blacks (42.4 per 100,000 live births) is between three and four times greater than that for Whites (13.0), and the gap has continued to widen since 1986, when the MMR surveillance was initiated (CDC, 2020e). Pregnancy-related death risk increases with age and with lack of prenatal care for women of every race, but the risk of pregnancy-related death for U.S. Black women is three to four times greater than for White women. Even though the rate of maternal deaths is low, most maternal deaths are preventable.

One of the maternal–child objectives for *Healthy People 2030* is to improve the proportion of infants who are breast-fed. Breast-feeding is beneficial to both mother and infant, and recently, 79.2% of mothers reported ever breast-feeding. Only 49.4% of U.S. infants were breast-fed for the recommended 6-month period, and 18.8% were breast-fed exclusively for this 6-month period. It is estimated that if 90% of U.S. families would comply with the recommended American Academy of Pediatrics guidelines regarding exclusive breast-feeding, $3.7 billion in direct and indirect pediatric health costs and $10.1 billion in costs related to premature death resulting from pediatric disease would be saved (AmericanPregnancy.org, 2018). See Box 19-3 for *Healthy People 2030* maternal, infant, and child health objectives.

BOX **19-3** *HEALTHY PEOPLE 2030*

Objectives for Maternal, Infant, and Child Health

Improve the health and safety of infants; prevent pregnancy complications and maternal deaths; improve women's health before, during, and after pregnancy; and improve the health and well-being of children.

Core Objectives

MICH-01	Reduce the rate of fetal deaths at 20 or more weeks of gestation
MICH-02	Reduce the rate of all infant deaths
MICH-03	Reduce the rate of deaths in children and adolescents aged 1–19 years
MICH-04	Reduce maternal deaths
MICH-05	Reduce severe maternal complications identified during delivery hospitalizations
MICH-06	Reduce cesarean births among low-risk women with no prior births
MICH-07	Reduce preterm births
MICH-08	Increase the proportion of pregnant women who receive early and adequate prenatal care
MICH-09	Increase abstinence from alcohol amongst pregnant women
MICH-10	Increase abstinence from cigarette smoking among pregnant women
MICH-11	Increase abstinence from illicit drugs among pregnant women
MICH-12	Increase the proportion of women of childbearing age who get enough folic acid
MICH-13	Increase the proportion of women who had a healthy weight before pregnancy
MICH-14	Increase the proportion of infants who are put to sleep on their backs
MICH-15	Increase the proportion of infants who are breastfed exclusively through age 6 months
MICH-16	Increase the proportion of infants who are breastfeed at 1 year
MICH-17	Increase the proportion of children who receive a developmental screening
MICH-18	Increase the proportion of children with autism spectrum disorder who receive specail services by age 4 years
MICH-19	Increase the proportion of children and adolescents who receive care in a medical home

Developmental Objectives

MICH-D01	Increase the proportion of women who get screened for postpartum depression
MICH-D02	Reduce the proportion of women who use illicit opioids during pregnancy
MICH-D03	Increase the proportion of infants who are put to sleep in a safe sleep environment

Reprinted from U.S. Department of Health & Human Services (USDHHS). (2020). *Healthy People 2030: Browse objectives.* Retrieved from https://health.gov/healthypeople/objectives-and-data/browse-objectives

Adolescent Mothers

In 1991, after a steady 5-year upward trend, the United States reached a 20-year high in the number of children born to teen mothers (aged 15 to 19 years) of 61.8 per 1,000. That trend then reversed, with 2007 marking a decline in teen birth rates to 41.5 per 1,000. In 2018, the trend continued, with 17.4 births per 1,000 females aged 15 to 19 years (Martin et al., 2019). Furthermore, 38 states saw a decrease in birth rates among this age group (Martin et al., 2019). The decrease in teen birth rate can be attributed to several behavioral changes, such as decreased sexual activity, increased use of contraception at first sex and at most recent sex, and the increased use of contraception methods. Although the United States has seen a decrease in teen births, the country continues to have much higher teen birth rates compared with other developed countries, including Canada with a birth rate of 6.6 per 1,000 (Elflien, 2019). See Chapter 20 for more on adolescent pregnancy.

The *Healthy People 2030* (USDHHS, 2020) document encompasses specific goals and objectives for the maternal–child population, based on the previous achievements in the same or similar areas. After years of working toward improving maternal–child health, the United States has made limited progress. One objective, however, has been met; 70% of infants are now sleeping on their backs, up from a 35% baseline. The rate for sudden infant death syndrome had dropped by over 50% since 1994. This can be attributed to the national public health education campaign known as "Back to Sleep" (Eunice Kennedy Shriver National Institute of Child Development and Health, 2016).

Risk Factors for Pregnant Women and Infants

Most pregnant women in the United States are healthy; they have normal pregnancies and produce healthy babies. Many factors contribute to the health problems of those mothers and babies who figure in the statistics on infant mortality and LBW. The factors associated with LBW and infant mortality can be grouped into three categories (CDC, 2017b):

1. Lifestyle: Smoking, secondhand smoke exposure, inadequate nutrition, alcohol consumption, substance abuse, late prenatal care, environmental toxins, stress, violence, and lack of social support
2. Sociodemographic: Maternal age below 15 or above 35 years, low educational level, poverty, domestic violence, and unmarried status
3. Medical and gestational history: Primiparity, multiple gestation, short interpregnancy intervals, premature rupture of the membranes, uterine abnormality, febrile illness during pregnancy, spontaneous abortion, genetic factors, gestation-induced hypertension, less-than-ideal weight gain during pregnancy, and diabetes

It is in the area of lifestyle choices that nurses can have the most significant impact on pregnancy outcomes such as LBW, preterm birth, and infant mortality. Programs that provide access to and funding for C/PHNs are available through federal, state, and local funding (Box 19-4).

BOX **19-4** EVIDENCE-BASED PRACTICE

Home Visiting

There are many ways C/PHNs can help moms and babies. One of the programs in which a nurse can do this, in a very fundamental way, is through the Nurse-Family Partnership (NFP) program. The program was created by Dr. David Olds and came out of his experience working in a daycare. He quickly realized that to make an impact, he needed to reach families earlier in life. Thus, the NFP was born. Dr. Olds has done research to test and improve the program in Elmira, NY; Memphis, TN; and Denver, CO. The results have been consistent; NFP improves the lives of both moms and babies through the tenacious work of a registered nurse (RN). The program is guided by a robust theoretical framework that includes; self-efficacy, human ecology, and attachment theories. Nurses follow a curriculum based on these theories from the time the client finds out she is pregnant until the baby turns 2 years old. NFP nurses go through a rigorous and well-planned training curriculum. This training includes courses in Denver, Colorado at the National Service Office, in a way that ensures fidelity to the NFP model.

Previous research has been completed in 2002, 2004, and 2014 examining both paraprofessionals and nurses visiting clients. The studies showed that RNs had a more significant impact on varying outcomes of the program. The relationship that is formed between the RN and the client is one based on trust and support. The client begins to see the nurse as part of the family, and someone that she can go to with any concern. The NFP nurse home visitor becomes a life coach, lifting the client up in one of the toughest parts of a women's life pregnancy and the first 2 years of motherhood. NFP nurses offer praise and screen the baby to make sure milestones are being met. Parenting skills are taught, references are made, if needed, and encouragement is given. Clients can contact their NFP nurse with questions about their bodies, their babies, future plans, relationships, and so much more. The program provides the kind of consistency and advocacy that many of the clients have never experienced. The NFP nurse is a true ally and fierce advocate for both mom and baby in the critical early years of motherhood.

Source: Nurse-Family Partnership (2018a, 2018b); Olds et al. (2002, 2004, 2013).

Substance Use and Abuse

Another area of concern is substance use and abuse among the childbearing population. The range of adverse consequences associated with the use of tobacco, alcohol, and illicit drugs during pregnancy is wide and includes preterm birth, LBW, and fetal alcohol spectrum disorders (described later in this chapter). This puts these women and their unborn children in double jeopardy; not only are they at risk from the consequences of alcohol or drug use, but also they do not receive the preventive prenatal care that can eliminate or reduce other obstetric complications. This is most often related to the pregnant woman's concerns about legal ramifications of substance use while pregnant if they do seek care.

Substance abuse during pregnancy is a problem with staggering social and medical implications, such as preterm births, LBW, miscarriage, placental abruption, developmental delays, and child behavior and learning problems later in life (American Pregnancy Association, 2016). The precise rate of substance abuse among pregnant women is difficult to determine. In a large study (*n* = 27,874) of substance abuse and pregnancy, 26.3% of the women reported previous use and 2.6% current use. Adverse outcomes of these pregnancies included LBW, preterm birth, babies born small for gestational age, and admissions to neonatal intensive care units (NICUs).

The United States has seen an increased incidence of neonatal abstinence syndrome (NAS) as a result of heroin or other opioid use in pregnancy, with a NAS diagnosis every 25 minutes (Anbalagan & Mendez, 2020). The U.S. Agency for Healthcare Research and Quality (2019) reports 7 per 1,000 newborns are hospitalized for NAS. Between 1999 and 2014, there was a 333% increase in NAS (Anbalagan & Mendez, 2020). The states with the highest numbers of newborns hospitalized include West Virginia (48.1), Maine (33.1), Delaware (26.4), and Kentucky (22.9), with South Dakota at the lowest with 1.5 (U.S. Agency for Healthcare Research and Quality, 2019). Yet, not all states mandate the reporting of NAS, and/or states may differ in the NAS definition, which causes problems in determining rates (Anbalagan & Mendez, 2020). NAS occurs as a result of the sudden discontinuation of fetal exposure to substances such as heroin or other opioids during pregnancy. Withdrawal symptoms experienced by these infants include irritability, excessive or high-pitched crying, tremors, and gastrointestinal problems such as diarrhea. In the event that nonpharmacologic care does not alleviate these symptoms, morphine is the most commonly used pharmacologic treatment for withdrawal symptoms related to NAS. The long-term effects of NAS are not fully understood known due to socioeconomic and environmental factors of the mother, but these children may have poor school performance, vision problems, cognitive disabilities, neurodevelopmental delays, and higher mortality rates (Anbalagan & Mendez, 2020). It is clear more research needs to be done on this vulnerable population.

A lifestyle choice that includes the use of drugs during pregnancy and results in maternal addiction has placed millions of children at risk. These children are seen in NICUs, foster care, special education programs in the public schools, and later in the juvenile court system. Family structure patterns are altered because grandparents may find themselves primary caregivers for their grandchildren. A woman who uses alcohol or drugs may lose her inhibitions and engage in high-risk sexual behaviors, which can introduce other public health problems, such as acquisition of sexually transmitted infections (STIs), including HIV, and possible spread of the infection to the fetus or others (CDC, 2019g). The primary, secondary, and tertiary prevention interventions of the C/PHN cannot be underestimated when drug use takes such a high toll on every aspect of society.

Alcohol Use

Another societal problem is the use of and addiction to alcohol. It is difficult to establish accurate statistics on the number of women who drink during pregnancy, but results from the 2011 to 2013 Behavioral Risk Factor Surveillance System indicate that roughly 1 in 10 pregnant women drank alcohol within the past 30 days, compared with 53.6% of nonpregnant women. Prevalence of binge drinking was 18.2% for nonpregnant women and 3.1% for pregnant women, with a 4.6-times greater rate for unmarried pregnant women (CDC, 2015b).

The conditions that can occur in a child due to maternal drinking of alcohol during pregnancy are collectively known as **fetal alcohol spectrum disorders (FASDs)**. The most severe type of FASD is **fetal alcohol syndrome (FAS)**, which can result in facial abnormalities, delayed growth and development, neurologic defects, learning and sensory problems, and even death. What was once termed **fetal alcohol effects**, characterized as causing some but not all of the symptoms of FAS, is now separated into the more descriptive categories of **alcohol-related birth defects**, indicating problems with hearing, bones, heart, and kidneys, and **alcohol-related neurodevelopmental disorder**, represented by mental or functional problems, including cognitive and/or behavioral abnormalities (CDC, 2020b). Physical signs of FASDs are often much more subtle than in cases of FAS. However, those with FASD may have one or more of the following behaviors or characteristics (CDC, 2020c):

- Small size for gestational age or small stature in relation to peers
- Facial abnormalities (e.g., smooth philtrum)
- Poor coordination
- Hyperactivity, attention problems, and learning disabilities
- Difficulties in school, especially with math
- Developmental disabilities (e.g., speech and language delays)
- Intellectual disability or low intelligence quotient (IQ)
- Vision and hearing problems; problems with heart, kidneys, and bones
- Poor reasoning and judgment skills
- Sleep and sucking disturbances in infancy

It is important to provide evidence-based primary prevention before pregnancy and to reach women before drinking becomes such a part of their lives that they are unable or unwilling to abstain during pregnancy. For example, the Pregnancy Risk Assessment Monitoring System (PRAMS) is a surveillance system developed by the CDC and state health departments to collect population-based information on maternal preconception, prenatal, pregnancy, and postpartum behaviors and experiences. Data collected from 2016 revealed that <10% of women used tobacco 3 months prior to conception, and 7.1% continued to smoke while in the first trimester. This percent dropped in each trimester, with a decrease to 5.7% in the third trimester (Kondracki, 2019). Children are also at risk based on maternal alcohol use during childrearing, especially for adolescent mothers aged 15 to 19 years.

Working with women of childbearing age to improve their general health behaviors and promote better preparation for pregnancy is essential. For those pregnant women and mothers already using substances, maternal drug and alcohol treatment programs that focus on supportive parent–child attachment, enhancement of parenting and child-rearing capabilities, and encouragement of the use of support systems that can improve child health and cognitive development are needed. In-home family skills training and parenting education programs that are evidence based and promote C/PHN and client rapport can be effective methods of working with substance-abusing mothers and their at-risk children; however, more studies are recommended. In a systematic review of home visitation with alcohol- and drug-using mothers, there was no significant reduction of substance abuse among mothers entering drug and alcohol rehabilitation programs compared with those receiving home visitation. However, individual studies showed significance of home visitation in reducing these mothers' involvement with Child Protective Services, indicating a positive effect on parenting and childcare practices even if it did not effectively diminish the addictive behavior (Dauber et al., 2017).

Tobacco Use

Tobacco use has increased dramatically among women, especially since the women's movement of the 1970s, inevitably affecting maternal and newborn health. The nicotine in tobacco is a major addictive substance, and smoking is an addiction that many people find difficult to stop. Although the risk factors of smoking are well documented, many pregnant women continue to smoke. Smoking during pregnancy is one of the most studied risk factors in obstetric assessment. Women, who may have started smoking as adolescents, often continue to smoke in response to life stressors. From a population and C/PHN perspective, one study found that the higher the density of tobacco stores in a neighborhood, the higher the prevalence of smoking among pregnant women (Galiatsatos et al., 2020). The use of e-cigarettes, or vaping, is considered to be a health danger for pregnant women and developing fetuses. This nicotine delivery system poses threats to the baby. Also, the exhaled aerosol that is advertised to be "water vapor" actually contains nicotine and other chemicals such as metals, nitrosamines, and volatile organic compounds (CDC, 2016b).

Passive smoking or **environmental tobacco smoke (ETS)**—exposure to tobacco smoke from other people smoking in one's environment—also puts a person at risk for smoking-related disease. The Surgeon General has outlined major conclusions related to ETS based on years of research findings. One conclusion is that there is no risk-free level of secondhand smoke. Related to children and ETS, there is an increased risk of SIDS, more acute respiratory infection, ear disease, worse asthma, and risk for poor lung growth (Dede & Cinar, 2016). If a pregnant woman lives with a smoker, she and her fetus can be negatively affected by the other person's addiction. An initial health history of a pregnant woman should always include the assessment of tobacco use, smoking status, and exposure to smoke in the personal environment.

C/PHNs and other health care professionals must be involved in the control of tobacco products on many levels, especially in health policy development, community outreach, education, and advocacy. It is very common to see smoking incentives and advertisements in poorer neighborhoods and communities of color. It is also important to have skills in smoking risk assessment, cessation options, and symptom management interventions for smoking withdrawal. Nurses should serve as positive nonsmoking role models and to be active in research implementation using clinical guidelines and evidence-based practices. In the case of tobacco control, health policy development has made important strides at the grassroots level (see Chapter 13).

The C/PHN must not only advise clients to quit smoking but also offer supportive and empathetic approaches to stress reduction during smoking cessation, including methods or interventions that can help other symptom management that is associated with smoking cessation. For example, the C/PHN may counsel clients individually, refer for behavioral therapy, provide self-help manuals, or recommend nicotine replacement therapy or medication. Other approaches, such as support groups, can be helpful. Any permanent reduction in the number of cigarettes smoked, amount of secondhand smoke inhaled, or amount of smokeless tobacco products used is helpful in improving the health of the mother and her fetus. Particular attention should be paid to adolescent mothers (15 to 19 years), as their rates of smoking are much higher than for adolescents of similar age who are not mothers (Substance Abuse & Mental Health Services Administration, 2014).

Intimate Partner Violence

Intimate partner violence (IPV) is any sexual, physical, economic, and/or psychological abuse taken by someone against an intimate partner or ex-partner (New York City Department of Health and Mental Hygiene, 2020). Pregnancy is a vulnerable period for women and can increase their risk for IPV. It is estimated that 1 in 6 pregnant women from all walks of life experience IPV per year (March of Dimes, n.d.). Reasons for increased IPV during pregnancy can be an unintended pregnancy, increased stress related to supporting a child, and jealousy. These women may also avoid prenatal care services for a variety of reasons such as injuries, control by their partners, and a lack of resources such as transportation or money for mass transit. Pregnant women who experience psychological IPV have a 1-fold increase in the risk of suicidal ideation (Tabb et al., 2018). IPV can also have effects on the newborn and infant. In a longitudinal study of women who had experienced IPV, posttraumatic effects were found to have negative effects on the infants' and toddlers' language and neurologic development (Udo, Sharps, Bronner, & Hossain, 2016; see Chapter 18).

Sexually Transmitted Infections and Sexually Transmitted Diseases

Although STI and STD have been used interchangeably for some time, there are differences between the two terms. STIs refer to a person being infected but asymptotic, and sexually transmitted disease (STD) is used when symptoms are present (Rudderown, 2019). The CDC estimates the prevalence of all STI cases in the general population to be 110 million, with an annual incidence of 20 million, and health care costs of $16 billion. The CDC (2016e) has recommended STD screening of all pregnant women at the initial prenatal visit for *Chlamydia*, hepatitis B (and hepatitis C for high-risk mothers), HIV, and syphilis. Further, they recommend screening high-risk pregnant women for gonorrhea.

STIs can pass from mother to baby. Syphilis can cross the placenta and infect the fetus, as can HIV—which can also be passed to the infant through breast-feeding (CDC, 2016e). Congenital syphilis (CS) is on the rise at alarming rates. Between 2012 and 2017, the rate of CS increased 750% in California (California Department of Public Health, 2019). This increase is seen across the United States, where there has been a 153% increase from 2013 to 2017 to 918 cases (Schmidt, Carson, & Jansen, 2019). Other STIs (e.g., gonorrhea, hepatitis B, *Chlamydia*, genital herpes) can infect the baby as it passes through the birth canal during delivery. LBW, stillbirth, conjunctivitis, blindness, deafness, neurologic damage, chronic liver disease, and cirrhosis, along with neonatal sepsis and pneumonia, are possible infant complications of maternal STIs. Mothers may have premature rupture of membranes and resultant infection or may have a premature onset of labor. Some STIs can lead to cervical and other cancers, pelvic inflammatory disease, infertility, chronic hepatitis, and many other health problems (CDC, 2019f).

A pregnant woman who discovers she has an STI often feels ashamed, betrayed, embarrassed, and angry. Those who are asymptomatic may not realize they are infected or deny the existence of the disease and fail to carry out the treatment plan after diagnosis. Although educating the pregnant client about the effects of STIs is critical, providing information alone is not enough. The C/PHN has a pivotal role in enhancing the empowerment of women so they can act on the information they receive. The C/PHN engages with pregnant clients and helps them understand that they have control over their bodies. Usually, STIs are first discovered in pregnancy during routine prenatal screening, which places the clinic nurse and the nurse who may make home visits in the position to take an affirmative approach to treatment and follow-up.

HIV and AIDS

There are 36.9 million individuals living with human immunodeficiency virus (HIV). Almost 70% of all cases are found in sub-Saharan Africa (WHO, 2016). Most children with acquired immunodeficiency syndrome (AIDS) are children of HIV-positive mothers (WHO, 2020). Mother-to-child transmission (MTCT) of HIV can be almost fully prevented with antiretroviral treatment for mother and infant (WHO, 2020). To reduce MTCT, women must seek prenatal care early enough in their pregnancies for the antiretroviral drug to be effective. Antiretroviral therapy was provided to an estimated 20.9 million persons in 2017 (HIV.gov, 2018).

Early detection of HIV/AIDs and antiviral therapy has shown decline in the number of infants born with HIV since the height of the epidemic. A large-scale study conducted from 2005 to 2012 examining the association between mother and child HIV transmission in 15 jurisdictions of the United States found that 2% were diagnosed with HIV. It was concluded that there was an increased risk of having an HIV-infected infant among those mothers who received late testing/prenatal care or no prenatal antiretroviral therapy (Camacho-Gonzalez et al., 2015). An HIV-positive woman who is pregnant or who has delivered a baby requires special nursing management of the pregnancy and of the family after the birth of the newborn. There are many teaching opportunities for the C/PHN during a high-risk pregnancy, such as helping the client identify, change, or curtail high-risk behaviors and promoting adherence to prenatal and HIV care. Success in changing behaviors often requires an interdisciplinary approach of health care, social, emotional, and financial resources (Bungay, Massaro, & Gilbert, 2014; CDC, 2015a).

In the United States and other developed nations, HIV-infected women are advised not to breast-feed their infants because there is a chance that the infants will become infected with HIV from breast milk (CDC, 2020d). The C/PHN focuses teaching on providing a safe, available, and low-cost form of infant formula. In developing countries, the lack of clean water still makes formula feeding dangerous, and breast-feeding is usually recommended. The infection rate for HIV from breast-feeding and the mortality rate from formula made with impure water are about the same, resulting in a dilemma for women and health care providers in developing countries.

Poor Nutrition, Weight Gain, and Oral Health

Research has demonstrated a positive correlation between weight gain during pregnancy and normal birth weight in the babies. In 2009, the Institute of Medicine (IOM) released new guidelines for weight gain during pregnancy based on body mass indices (BMIs). Weight gain between 25 and 35 lb during pregnancy is recommended for women with BMIs ranging from 18.5 to 24.9, and the recommendation is 28 to 40 lb for underweight women with a BMI under 18.5, whereas overweight women with a BMI between 25 and 29 should gain 15 to 25 lb, and obese women with a BMI over 30.0 should hold their weight gain to between 11 and 20 lb (IOM, 2009). The American College of Obstetricians and Gynecologists (ACOG) reaffirmed in 2016 that the 2009 IOM gestational weight gain guidelines are important for clinicians to use. It is recommended that clinicians determine a woman's BMI at the initial prenatal visit and discuss weight gain, diet, and exercise goals initially and throughout the pregnancy (Fig. 19-4; ACOG, 2013 and reaffirmed in 2016).

Obesity currently affects about 39.8% of all adults (CDC, 2018a). Studies have shown that about 48% of pregnant women in the United States gain more than the recommended amount of weight (CDC, 2016f). Gestational diabetes poses the greatest risk to obese pregnant women and increases the risk for preterm birth (CDC, 2017c). C/PHNs who work with morbidly obese pregnant women can help them most by emphasizing good nutrition and by encouraging them to maintain their pre-pregnant weight without drastically reducing caloric intake. This can be accomplished primarily by a marked decrease in consumption of "empty calories" from junk food and replacing with increased intake of fruits,

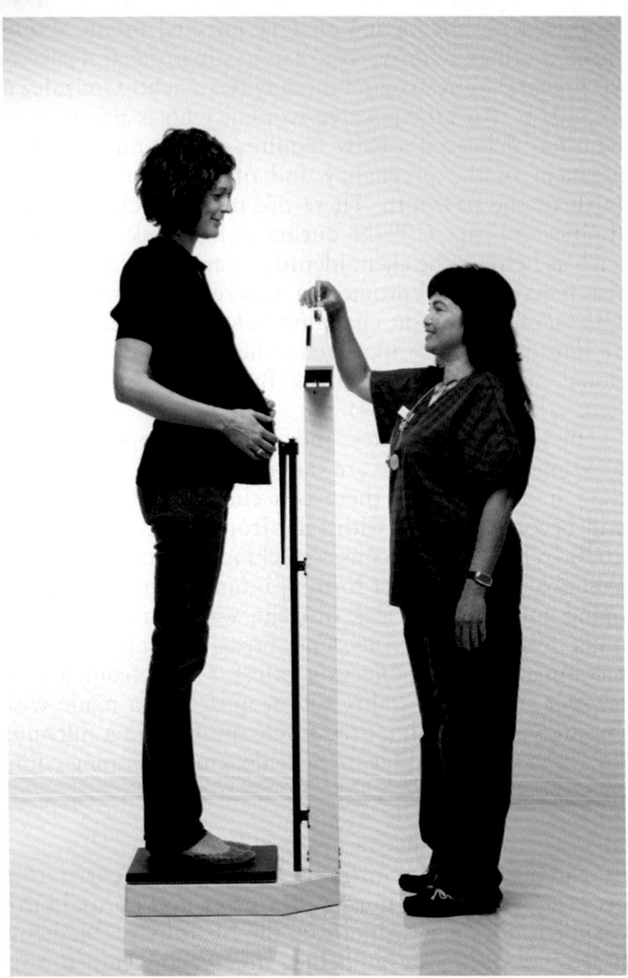

FIGURE 19-4 Weight gain during pregnancy should be monitored regularly.

vegetables, and low-fat sources of calcium. Pregnancy is never a time for dieting. Nutritional counseling can have an additional benefit in that it may ultimately decrease the risk of obesity or eating disorders in the client's children. For women who are prone to gaining too much weight, nutrition-rich, low-calorie foods are recommended.

Exercise during pregnancy is essential and can moderate maternal weight gain and improve overall fitness that is desirable for the labor and delivery process. After assessment, the C/PHN can determine whether the unwanted weight gain is related to the consumption of additional calories, to limited activity, or to fluid retention. Each cause must be managed differently. Underweight women have twice as many LBW babies as women whose weight is within normal range. Nutritional teaching is part of the C/PHN's role when working with a pregnant woman who has difficulty gaining the recommended weight during pregnancy. Finding ways to add calories to foods and increasing the woman's desire to eat are effective methods to improve maternal weight gain. Insufficient caloric intake in pregnant adolescents (who themselves are still growing) is an additional concern for their future health and health of the infant over the life course.

Periodontal infection may affect around 40% of women of childbearing age and is especially common among disadvantaged and ethnic or racial minorities who may not have adequate access to dental health care. Maternal periodontal disease has been linked to preterm birth, LBW, preeclampsia, and early fetal loss; however, recent studies have not shown the reduction of preterm birth or LBW among those infants whose mothers received periodontal therapy in pregnancy. Although the research is conflicting, it is evident that dental health procedures have generally been found to be effective and safe for pregnant women, especially during the second trimester (because of possible nausea during the first trimester and being uncomfortable in the third trimester) (Mark, 2018). Not only is dental health important during pregnancy, but poor dental hygiene and disease have been linked to health conditions, such as cardiovascular disease and diabetes. High maternal levels of the bacteria that cause cavities have been associated with a greater chance of subsequent dental caries in the infant (CDC, 2019d).

C/PHNs should teach women of childbearing age the importance of regular dental health checkups and proper dental hygiene, along with making referrals for dental treatment when needed. Because there is frequently a shortage of dental providers to see vulnerable or low-income women, the nurse sometimes has to advocate for pregnant women who have major oral health treatment problems, such as gingivitis or dental caries or infections. Dental health should be a part of general primary preventive education for all childbearing-age women and a major teaching and screening element of prenatal care.

Socioeconomic Status and Social Inequality

As noted earlier, poverty plays a role in pregnancy and birth outcomes. Social and economic disparities are factors in preterm birth in both developed and developing nations and reflect some of the social determinants of health (SDOH). These relationships may be more indirect, as poorer women often lack health insurance, have less access to quality prenatal care services, have poorer nutrition, and are exposed to more situational and psychological stressors. In the United Kingdom, a retrospective study with a very large sample ($n = 59{,}487$) was done that focused on the poorly understood factors that delay seeking antenatal care and engagement in that care. Findings indicated that higher parity, pregnancy during the teenage years, non-White ethnic background, unemployment, unmarried, poor social support, and smoking were significantly associated with late access to antenatal services and poor fetal outcomes (Kapaya et al., 2015). Prenatal stress is difficult to research because of the multiple variables that can affect prenatal stress. All areas of perceived stressors should be assessed (e.g., unintended pregnancy; nutrition; chronic stress and daily hassles; levels of social support; mental health issues, such as depression or anxiety, work stressors, racism, or discrimination; and any significant life events, such as death or other significant losses).

A systematic review of literature looked at SDOH and pregnancy of young people. Within the review, 17 of the studies found a link between at least one SDOH and pregnancy among young people with the area of poverty and family structure most represented (Maness

& Buhi, 2016). Other critical areas identified within the SDOH include neighborhood-built environment (crime and violence and environmental conditions), social and community context (family structure and incarceration/institutionalization), economic stability (poverty and housing stability), and education (high school graduation rates) (Maness & Buhi, 2016). The American College of Obstetricians and Gynecologist identify the role of SDOH and the impact it has on outcomes of health (ACOG, 2019). Social, economic, political, and cultural structures contribute to reproductive health issues. Practices that address inequalities are necessary for improving health outcomes while addressing national morbidity and mortality inequalities. Consider the following example. A C/PHN discovers during the interview that a pregnant patient with gestational diabetes has not been checking her blood sugar routinely. Rather than labeling the patient noncompliant, the nurse asks the patient what challenges she has encountered that prevent her from completing this task and discovers that the woman lacks a stable living environment in which to keep her supplies. The C/PHN makes arrangements with social services to address the housing concerns (ACOG, 2019).

The C/PHN can play a role in reproductive health care and equity. Nurses can inquire regarding structural determinants such as access to food and safe water. Does the client have utility needs, and is the home and community environment safe? Nurses can ensure access to social services and other services to support needs (ACOG, 2019).

Prenatal care is crucial to ensure good outcomes of pregnancy. Studies continue to reiterate the need for regular care visits, showing an association between regular and early care and fewer preterm deliveries and higher infant birth weights. Significant disparities in prenatal care are present among Black, Hispanic, and American Indian/Native American women (HRSA, n.d.). Access to obstetrical and gynecologic health care is difficult in many areas of the country. It is at crisis levels in some rural areas. Lack of adequate access to prenatal care leaves many pregnant women in danger (Box 19-5). Other factors, outlined in more detail in Chapter 25, may also affect the health of both mothers and babies.

Adolescent Pregnancy

Pregnancy during the adolescent years (13 to 19 years old) is considered a health risk because of the ongoing physical growth and the demands of psychosocial development during these years. The United States leads most developed nations in the rates of teenage pregnancy, abortion, and childbearing. Young maternal age at time of pregnancy and birth creates several medical risks for the mother and baby. Teen pregnancy is discussed further in Chapter 20.

Maternal Developmental Disability

For couples that are developmentally disabled, having a child puts increased stress on a system that is already burdened. Parenting requires attending to not just the child's physical care but socialization and developmental stimulation, well-child and illness health care, emotional nurturing, and age-appropriate supervision. Depending on the social support, and coping skills of the developmentally delayed parent, the stress and need for emotional

BOX **19-5** PERSPECTIVES

A Nursing Student's Viewpoint on the Dangers of Childbirth

I began working as a nurse's aide at our local hospital when I started nursing school. I learned firsthand the dangers of childbirth and the consequences that can result. One night, a female reported to the emergency room in labor and was admitted to the labor and delivery department. The young mother-to-be was very excited. Her contractions continued, though she did not progress with the labor process, so she was to be started on oxytocin (Pitocin) to increase the effectiveness of her labor. The nurse midwife checked on her patient frequently, but problems began after the first 8 hours of labor. As the dosage was increased, the fetus reacted with bradycardia, and the nurse midwife did not notify the physician. The Pitocin dosage was decreased and then the heart rate stabilized; this process continued for three cycles. The nurse midwife signed off her 12-hour shift and handed care of the patient over to the nurse midwife coming on shift. Again, whenever the Pitocin dosage was increased to the point of becoming effective, the fetus would respond with bradycardia. The physician in charge was still not notified. After 24 hours of a failed labor process and at this point severe bradycardia, and the fetus was in irreversible distress. The physician was finally notified of an emergency and reported to the bedside within 5 minutes. An emergency cesarean section was performed. The Apgar scores at delivery were 0, 0, 0, and 3 after 15 minutes of resuscitative effort. The infant was severely neurologically damaged. I found out later that the infant was diagnosed with severe cerebral palsy and will never walk, talk, or feed normally. She cannot swallow and will require suctioning, gastrostomy tube feeding, and total care throughout her lifetime. She is also cortically blind. A multimillion-dollar award was given, and the nurses and nurse midwives employed by the hospital were fired due to negligence. It is sad to think that this tragedy could have been avoided with prudent nurse–patient advocacy, reporting, and appropriate documentation—the things our nursing instructors are always drumming into our heads. I know that as a new graduate, I am now in a position of responsibility to make decisions to notify the physician or not. I have decided that the choice should always be to notify the physician. Even though it may seem inconvenient, it really should be done. I will never forget this case and its long-reaching consequences for the child and family, as well as for the nursing staff and nurse midwives.

Lyndsay, student nurse

control and positive decision-making can be monumental. Evidence from a seminal cohort study in Britain found that, for 4- to 6-year-olds, there was "no association of parental IQ with conduct or emotional problems" in the children; however, for children age 7 into adolescence, "strong evidence was observed" between lower parental IQ and child "conduct, emotional, and attention problems" (Whitley, Gale, Deary, Kivimaki, & Batty, 2011, p. 1032). Confounding variables included the environment of the home, parental affect, and child IQ. Even though there may not be strong evidence for these problems, children are still at risk for under-stimulation and environmental insecurity. Parent training/childcare skills programs, peer-to-peer support groups, community agencies, and careful home monitoring can reduce the risk of child abuse and neglect and promote more effective parenting (Promising Practices Network, n.d.).

How does the C/PHN work with developmentally disabled parents effectively? Most importantly, nursing support must enhance the natural resilience of the family.

The establishment of a trusting relationship between the nurse and the family is of foremost importance. Teaching by demonstration with many visual aids and prompts, along with games and creative approaches to engage and sustain attention, can challenge the nurse's creativity. Modeling of appropriate parenting behavior needs to occur on each visit. Supervision and monitoring of family functioning must continue until the child reaches adulthood. As part of the transition to other systems of care, C/PHNs often advocates for families with maternal developmental disability regarding the plan of care, interpreting it for other professionals and multiple disciplines. Many agencies employing nurses cannot provide the intensive follow-up that such a family requires. It is then necessary to make referrals to organizations that can provide support, such as the American Association of Retarded Citizens or Exceptional Parents Unlimited. The nurse may stay involved as a consultant to the paraprofessionals or make periodic home visits at times of developmental or situational crisis.

Complications of Childbearing

Some maternal deaths are not preventable (e.g., amniotic fluid embolism). Morbidity is also a factor, and although some major risk factors among pregnant women and infants have been discussed, several common medical complications of childbearing bear mentioning. The effects of hypertensive disease in pregnancy, gestational diabetes, postpartum depression, and grief in families who have lost a child are important areas in which the C/PHN can intervene effectively.

Hypertensive Disease in Pregnancy

Hypertension in pregnancy may be chronic or related specifically to pregnancy. Chronic is diagnosed prior to 20 weeks of gestation, and gestational (pregnancy related) is diagnosed after 20 weeks but goes away by 6 weeks postpartum. Chronic hypertension affects 1% to 5% of pregnancies and gestational about 5% to 10% (Friel, 2017).

Preeclampsia results in new-onset high blood pressure and protein in the urine, along with nondependent edema, and can result in eclampsia (characterized by convulsions and/or coma), pulmonary edema, liver rupture, renal failure, disseminated intravascular coagulopathy, and cortical blindness, as well as maternal death. The effects from pregnancy-induced hypertension on infants are often serious because placental health is associated with fetal growth (Dulay, 2017). Preeclampsia occurs in about 3% to 7% of pregnancies, with 25% of cases developing in the postpartum period (Dulay, 2017). Various methods are employed to attempt to prevent and control hypertension during pregnancy, namely, careful and constant monitoring of blood pressure, use of blood pressure medications if needed, frequent prenatal visits with monitoring of lab tests, a diet rich in fresh fruits and vegetables, lower sodium food choices, adequate fluid intake, weight gain limitations, rest, and regular exercise. Intermittent fetal monitoring may be required. These remain the most common preventive suggestions that C/PHNs, in collaboration with the clients' primary health care providers, can give to their pregnant clients. A calm environment, periods of rest, and the pregnant woman either elevating her feet or reclining in a left side lying position are also recommended. Additional assessment data may guide the nurse to focus teaching on stress reduction techniques and modification or elimination of smoking. As care providers C/PHNs can provide frequent monitoring of blood pressure and other symptoms and encourage the client to be vigilant in keeping prenatal appointments. However, medication or even hospitalization may be necessary. The C/PHN can offer support and understanding while continuing to be a resource for the client as the pregnancy progresses and the infant is born.

Gestational Diabetes

Gestational diabetes mellitus (GDM) occurs in pregnant women who have never had a problem with high blood glucose but do during pregnancy. The average onset for GDM is around the 24th week of pregnancy (American Diabetes Association, n.d.). GDM is estimated to occur in about 2% to 10% of pregnancies in the United States (CDC, 2017b). For the mother with GDM, there is a higher risk of hypertension, preeclampsia, urinary tract infections, cesarean section, and future risk of type 2 diabetes. As far as pathophysiology, GDM is similar to type 2 diabetes, and 50% of women with GDM eventually develop type 2 diabetes during their lifetimes. Because growth and maturation of the fetus are closely associated with the delivery of maternal nutrients, particularly glucose, maintenance of appropriate glucose levels is essential to the health of the fetus. Daily self-monitoring of blood glucose levels is recommended. Women should be encouraged to monitor blood glucose levels regularly 6 weeks postpartum and periodically throughout their life (CDC, 2017c).

The infant is at increased risk for fetal death because GDM has been associated with macrosomia, or large-for-gestational-age babies, birth injuries such as broken shoulders, breathing problems, and abnormally low blood sugars at birth (CDC, 2017c). The C/PHN can help in the control of GDM by encouraging early prenatal care, adequate nutrition, rest and exercise, and adherence to the particular dietary, activity, and blood glucose monitoring regimen suggested by the woman's health care provider. Those C/PHNs working with pregnant women should provide education on early warning signs for GDM and the importance of regular prenatal care, reminder about getting the glucose tolerance test around the 24th week of pregnancy, and follow-up.

Postpartum Depression

Although most people recognize the common fleeting mood swings immediately after childbirth known as "baby blues," high-profile cases like Andrea Yates, who suffered from postpartum psychosis and drowned her five small children, are rare (1 or 2 per 1,000 births) but nonetheless tragic (Criminal Justice, n.d.). Actresses Chrissy Tiegen and Reese Whitherspoon, among others, have discussed their postpartum depression and treatment with antidepressant medications, making this condition more visible and less stigmatizing (Davis, 2016).

According to need studies, one in seven women will experience postpartum depression (Lieber, 2018). Also, depression and posttraumatic stress disorder have been found in both mothers and fathers subsequent to a healthy birth following a prior perinatal loss (Gundersen Health, n.d.). Risks for postpartum depression include a family history of psychiatric illness, poor social support, stressful life events, anxiety during pregnancy, the personality traits of neuroticism, and more recently perfectionism (National Institute of Mental Health [NIMH], n.d.). Depression can affect anyone, even women without a history of prior depression. Perinatal depressive symptoms may not indicate major clinical depression. Nevertheless, symptoms may cause considerable psychological distress, such as irritability and restlessness; feeling hopeless, sad, and overwhelmed; having little energy or motivation and crying unexpectedly; sleeping and eating too little or too much; problems with cognition (memory, decision-making, focus); loss of pleasure or interest in usually pleasant activities; and withdrawal from family and friends (Fig. 19-5).

There are several nonpharmacologic interventions the nurse can initiate in addition to the ones mentioned above. First, caffeine can lead to sleep disturbance, and alcohol is a depressant that has been implicated in depression. A simple yet helpful suggestion is the elimination of both. Getting adequate sleep is important because sleep deprivation exacerbates psychiatric symptoms. Napping when the baby naps, resting when possible throughout the day, and going to bed early (albeit with the knowledge that sleep may be interrupted two or more times to feed the infant) will provide more hours of rest and sleep. Exercise is helpful and raises levels of endorphins. Anxiety symptoms often coexist with depression. Relaxation techniques that reduce anxiety can be helpful, including listening to relaxing music, doing yoga, or performing a simple exercise routine. Having a daily routine and setting realistic goals are also helpful (NIMH, n.d.). Participation in a support group allows women to identify with others who may be experiencing similar difficulties. Through discussion, women provide each other with both emotional and practical support.

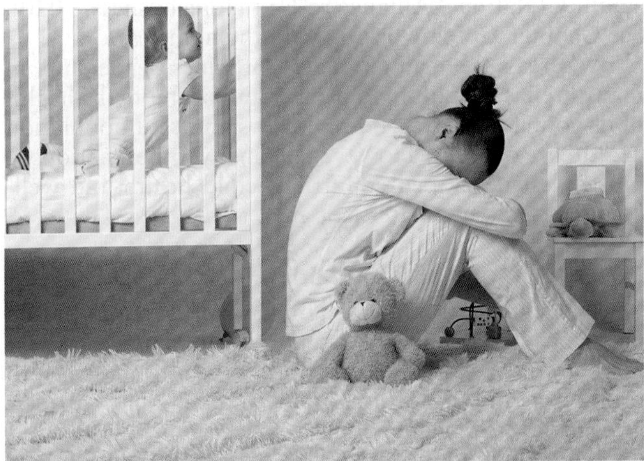

FIGURE 19-5 C/PHNs need to watch for signs of postpartum depression among their clients and offer assistance.

C/PHNs can intervene by initiating primary preventive mental health and coping measures that promote mental health throughout pregnancy and the postpartum period. Helping pregnant women to appreciate themselves and their strengths, embrace their new body changes, and positively anticipate their new role is primary preventive intervention for good mental health and promotion of attachment to their infant. If women are assessed to be at risk, mental health resources can be identified, and then, positive mental health outcomes may be fostered by supporting their self-esteem, optimizing the quality of their primary intimate relationships, anticipatory guidance on issues that may arise during pregnancy and the postpartum period, and reducing day-to-day stressors. At times, the nurse's efforts alone are not sufficient, and a referral to community mental health services for early detection and treatment is essential for the women and their children.

Fetal or Infant Death

An infrequent role for nurses in maternal–child health is that of grief counselor, but this may be a role for the advanced practice nurse in certain settings or communities. A couple may experience a miscarriage or ectopic pregnancy, stillbirth, or the death of an infant from **sudden infant death syndrome (SIDS)**. The exact cause of SIDS is not certain, but it may be associated with brainstem control of heart and lung functions (Illinois Department of Public Health, n.d.). It is more common in boys and most often occurs in infants between 1 and 4 months of age (Safe to Sleep, n.d.). Increased rates of SIDS are associated with side/stomach sleeping position, exposure to cigarette smoke, premature birth, cosleeping, having a sibling that died of SIDS, and soft bedding in the crib. SIDS is the leading cause of death for infants from 1 to 12 months of age; about 2,000 infants die annually from SIDS. Since 1990, the SIDS rate has dropped, but the rates for Black and American Indian/Alaska Native infants are disproportionately higher (Illinois Department of Public Health, n.d.).

In each situation of loss, the C/PHN has an important supportive role. People respond to grief in a variety of ways: some express deep sadness, shock, or disbelief; some weep and are unable to talk; and others talk incessantly about regrets or guilt. Even if a miscarriage occurs early in a pregnancy, the bonding between the mother and fetus has begun, and expressions of grief may be as intense as with the loss of an infant or child. Women often have feelings of abandonment, bereavement, and guilt, thinking that they did something wrong. When parents are unable to identify the exact cause of their fetal loss, they have a more difficult time letting go of grief and anxiety. Increased anxiety levels are also found, sometimes more frequently than depression. Psychological counseling has been associated with greater decreases over time in levels of worry, grief, and self-blame (Gundersen Health, n.d.). For couples that have delivered a stillborn baby, the shock is compounded by the experience of carrying the pregnancy to full term, along with the anticipation of an imminent delivery and the expectation of an addition to the family. This is especially true if all signs before the birthing event itself were positive.

Mothers who experience stillbirths recognize the need for spiritual and psychosocial support from professional caregivers. Families must acknowledge the death of the child and integrate the loss into their family lives. Home visitation and simply being there for the family and listening well are invaluable nursing interventions. Referral to mental health counseling or support groups specific to parents of stillborn children where they can share their feelings may be very helpful (March of Dimes, 2019). Providing continuity and support to the family for months after the death of an infant gives the C/PHN an opportunity to assess the family for signs of unresolved grief. Grieving families may find comfort, support, and helpful information from support groups and resources such as Compassionate Friends or First Candle. When a family experiences loss of an infant after the baby has been brought home from the hospital, grief and guilt are compounded by the loss of an anticipated future and the disrupted continuity in family life. An infant may die of SIDS, a congenital anomaly, an infection, or an accident. There are constant reminders of the infant's presence in the home from memories, photos, videos, and accumulated possessions. This death disrupts family homeostasis and the psychological and physiologic equilibrium of the family. In many cases, the police are involved, and an autopsy is required, contributing to the anguish of the grieving family. This promotes both guilt and loss of self-esteem and can even threaten the marriage.

INFANTS, TODDLERS, AND PRESCHOOLERS

Healthy children are a vital resource to ensure the future well-being of nations. They are the parents, workers, citizens, leaders, and decision makers of tomorrow, and their health and safety depend on today's decisions and actions. Their futures lie in the hands of those people responsible for their well-being, including the C/PHN, whose dominant responsibility is to the community and populations, such as dependent children.

The well-being of children has been a subject of great public health concern globally and in the United States. Its importance has been emphasized through development of numerous laws and services, yet the needs of many children continue to go unmet. Young children (up to age 4 years) are totally dependent on their caregivers. This contributes to their vulnerability during these years. Many young children often go to bed hungry; some infants and toddlers do not receive even the most basic immunizations before they reach school age. Accidents and injuries are a leading cause of death; preventable communicable diseases increase mortality among the very young.

Adverse childhood events (ACE) are potentially traumatic events that occur in childhood (aged 0 to 17 years) such as experiencing violence or abuse, witnessing violence in the home or community, and having a family member attempt or die by suicide (CDC, 2019e). Any aspect of a child's environment that can undermine their sense of safety, stability, and bonding are linked to chronic health issues, mental illness, and substance abuse as an adult. According to the CDC (2019e), 61% of adults surveyed in 25 states reported experiencing at least one type of ACE; one in six reported experiencing four or more types of ACEs. Women and minority groups are at greater risk for experiencing four or more types of ACEs. The CDC-Kaiser Permanente Adverse Childhood Experiences (ACE) study is the largest investigation of childhood neglect and abuse showing the effects of violence exposure and later-life health and well-being (Felitti et al., 1989). This seminal study identified seven categories of adverse childhood experiences that were corelated with multiple health risk factors later in life. ACE can have lasting and negative effects on children, increasing the risk of injury, maternal and child health problems, teen pregnancy, sex trafficking, STIs, and a wide range of chronic diseases. It is estimated that the effects of ACEs can cost families, communities, and society billions of dollars each year (CDC, 2019e).

Home environment and safety are current areas of concern for many children and families. Children in families make up approximately 33% of the homeless populations (National Alliance to End Homelessness, 2020). Point in time data show 56,342 family households identified as homeless, with approximately 16,000 families living on the street, in a car, or in other places not designated for human habitation. Typically, homeless families are headed by single women as head of household with limited education (National Alliance to End Homelessness, 2020). Children who are homeless have higher levels of emotional and behavioral problems and may have lower academic performance due to transience. Access to services and transition into permanent housing provides stability (National Alliance to End Homelessness, 2020). See Chapter 26 for Working with the homeless.

Whereas the United States provides leadership in many arenas, its failure to protect and promote the health of its youngest citizens represents a significant population health breakdown. However, in many other nations—mostly less-developed countries—child health and well-being are in even greater jeopardy.

Global History of Children's Health Care

Only recently in the history of the world have children been considered valuable assets, even in countries where there are now well-developed programs of infant health promotion and protection, infant and child day care services, and strict educational expectations for all children. In some countries today, however, female infants and children or those born with congenital anomalies are not valued. Countries, such as India and China, provide inequitable care for male and female children. Gender-selective abortions or infanticide also occur. Some birth, growth, and developmental rituals are harsh and would be considered illegal if judged by Western standards. Cultural practices that are fostered by political forces prevent many countries from improving the health of infants and young children (Save the Children, n.d.). For these reasons, there are great differences globally in child health care systems. The health of children in one country can affect that of children in other countries, including the United States. Major natural disasters place whole populations at risk, especially the very young and the very old.

National Perspective on Infants, Toddlers, and Preschoolers

The **infant** (birth to 1 year), **toddler** (aged 1 to 2 years), and **preschooler** populations (aged 3 to 4 years) are generally healthy years. Most U.S. children have a usual source of health care (96.9%), and their parents report them to be in excellent or very good health (CDC, 2017b; Larson, Cull, Racine, & Olson, 2016). Growth and development of infants and young children should be monitored regularly. Pediatricians and C/PHNs often provide anticipatory guidance for parents so that they better understand what to expect as their child grows and can plan for safety issues that may arise. See thePoint for a link to online growth charts.

The mortality rate for children ages 5 to 14 years is 13.0 per 100,000. Major causes are unintentional injuries (motor vehicle crashes, falls, drowning, fires, and burns), cancer, and suicide (CDC, 2016c). Some variation in mortality rates continues among racial/ethnic groups.

Accidents and Injuries

Toddlers and preschoolers are at risk for many types of accidents and unintentional injuries, such as those caused by unsafe toys, falls, burns or scalding, drowning, motor vehicle crashes, and poisonings. These unintentional injuries are the leading cause of mortality and morbidity for children from age birth to 19 years (CDC, 2016c). Male children have higher rates of death from injuries than females; it is almost twice the rate. Causes of injury deaths vary across age groups. For those children under age one, about 66% are caused by suffocation. Between ages 1 and 4, drowning is the leading cause. In 15- to 19-year-olds, being a passenger in a motor vehicle crash was the most frequent cause of injury death. American Indian/Alaska Native children had the highest death rates from injury, and Asian/Pacific Islander children had the lowest. The loss of children's lives resulting from all injuries combined represents a staggering number of productive life years lost to society. Childhood unintentional injuries lead to almost 12,175 deaths annually (CDC, 2017b).

The *National Action Plan for Child Injury Prevention* addresses child safety and provides an agenda for injury prevention (CDC, 2012). It brings together 60 partners in implementing injury prevention activities and providing a blueprint for collecting/interpreting data and surveillance and plans to promote research and enhance communication/education/training on injury prevention. Improving the outcomes of childhood injuries by working with health care and health systems and supporting strong policies to prevent injuries are further goals. Risks for childhood injuries that increase child vulnerability include "poverty, crowding, young maternal age, single parent households, and low maternal educational status" (CDC, 2012, p. 9). Using a public health model, the three levels of prevention are utilized to prevent injuries from occurring (e.g., safety latches on cabinets containing cleaning supplies or medications), minimize injuries (e.g., child safety seats), and improve emergency response and care after injury occurs (e.g., paramedic, trauma care). For instance, to prevent infant suffocation and SIDS, infants should go to sleep on their backs, in a crib or child-friendly bed without soft bedding or pillows, and parents should be cautioned about risk factors for SIDS and the potential dangers of sleeping with their babies. Information about the SIDS prevention campaign *Back to Sleep* should be provided to all parents of infants, and education should begin with hospital nurses and continue with C/PHNs in the community.

Burn injuries can affect children of all ages. Bath water that is too hot can also cause serious scalding injuries. Cigarette lighters and matches are fascinating to young children. Toddlers or preschoolers may be able to start a flame, injuring or killing themselves or others. The sound of a smoke alarm may frighten young children, and it is important for C/PHNs to instruct parents not only to teach their young children about fire prevention but also to be aware of the sound of the alarm and know what actions to take when they hear it, such as the *Stop Drop and Roll* program taught in Head Start and other preschool programs (National Fire Protection Association, n.d.). The C/PHN should also take every opportunity on home visits and in other health education settings to ask or observe if parents have a functional smoke detector in their home. Most community fire departments will install and test smoke detectors for free. Preventing the sources of injury or death from burns may be accomplished by eliminating opportunity and source. Through child supervision, safe storage of matches and lighters, and keeping children away from stoves and electrical outlets, burns and fires can be prevented.

Drowning is another category of unintentional injury in children. Brief lapses in supervision can have disastrous consequences. Young children are at risk for drowning wherever water occurs in depths exceeding a few inches—such as in toilet bowls, bathtubs, mop buckets or cans filled with rainwater, puddles, ponds, spas, and swimming pools. Lakes, rivers, streams, and irrigation ditches or canals are other water hazards. Infants, toddlers, and preschool-aged children are especially vulnerable because they are not aware of water dangers and they explore without fear. Poor children, especially children of color, are at higher risk for drowning because of lack of access to swimming lessons. The C/PHN can work with community groups and recreation centers to promote swimming for children. Parents need to provide a drown-free environment. Guidelines include the following (American Academy of Pediatrics, 2016; CDC, 2020a; Government of Alberta, 2018):

- Bathe young children in shallow water.
- Never leave young children unattended during a bath.

- Keep toilet lids down and bathroom doors closed—preferably secured with childproof safety handles.
- Never leave full mop buckets unattended.
- Eliminate water collection sites around the home by turning over or removing empty buckets, containers, flowerpots, and other items that can collect rainwater.
- Fence swimming pool areas and install childproof locks or alarm devices that sound when the water is disturbed.
- Promote water safety measures, including teaching young children to swim.
- Be aware of the dangers of open pool drains and suction outlets that can lead to drain entrapment and hair entanglement and ensure that drain covers and safety vacuum-release systems are installed.
- Vigilant supervision of young children at play to prevent involvements with neighborhood water sources

Supervising children in or around bathtubs, spas, pools, or other water receptacles is critical and requires close (arm's length) distances. Parents of young children should be encouraged to get cardiopulmonary resuscitation training. The real dangers of accidental drowning are related in Box 19-6.

BOX **19-6** STORIES FROM THE FIELD

Mop Bucket Drowning

I am a Head Start nurse, and one of my assigned centers is located within a farm-labor camp. There are many large, hardworking families in the camp. Older siblings often watch over young children and help with household chores. Most families keep their cinder block homes tidy and clean, and floors are constantly being mopped (no one has carpeting—it is a bare-minimum type of accommodation). One day, several children were absent from school, and when I made home visits to determine the cause of the absences, I discovered that one of the Garcia family's children, a toddler named Miguel, had unexpectedly died. Because many of the absent children were cousins, parents had kept them home while attending to the family. I knew the Garcia family well, and when I stopped by to check on them, they told me that Miguel had fallen into a large mop bucket the older sister had been using to clean the kitchen floor. She had gone outside for just a minute to separate the 5-year-old twins who were fighting, and when she returned, she found Miguel headfirst in the bucket. She tried to revive him but could not. The parents were working, trying to earn extra money for an elderly grandmother who needed surgery, and only learned of the tragedy when they returned home at the end of a long day. It was a very sad situation, and it reminded me of how even an everyday item can become deadly. Safety and prevention of unintentional injuries, especially with curious toddlers and preschoolers, is extremely important to teach all families.

1. *Address levels of prevention as this concept relates to childhood accidents. What could you do now to assist this family?*
2. *What strategies can C/PHNs use in their community to prevent drowning situations like this from happening again?*

Myra, Head Start nurse

Injuries and deaths from motor vehicle crashes continue to be a major safety problem in the United States. Of the 23,714 vehicle fatalities in 2016 only about 53% to 62% of drivers and passengers were wearing safety restraints (CDC, 2017d). A recent study found that more than 685,000 children ages 0 to 12 were not correctly placed in child safety seats or boosters as least at some point (CDC, 2017a). Many families have them and use them regularly but do not install them properly, placing the child at as much risk as if there were no restraint. The most current recommendations for safety seat use are categorized by age. For children birth up to age 2 years, a rear-facing seat should be used (placed in car's back seat); the child should continue in rear-facing seat until reaching the height or weight limit of the seat placed in the back seat; age 2 to at least 5 years, child should use forward-facing car seat until reaching upper weight and height limit for the seat; age 5 years and up, keep child in back seat with a seat belt–buckled booster seat until they reach height limit of 57 in. and can use a car seat belt alone; seat belts are considered to be properly fitting when the lap belt portion lays across the upper thighs (not stomach area) and the seat belt lays across the chest and not the neck (CDC, 2016a). There is much opportunity in this area for the C/PHN to educate the public and ensure that parents have the information and skills to secure their children properly when traveling by car. Safety seat clinics, where installations are checked and corrected, can help to promote the proper use of age-appropriate child restraints (Box 19-7).

Poisoning is a constant safety concern for young children, and toddlers are most often at risk. Sources of poisoning include household plants, prescription medications, over-the-counter drugs, unintentional medication overdoses, household cleaning products, other chemicals stored within a child's reach, and lead. Parents should be provided with the number for the Poison Help Hotline (1-800-222-1222) and encourage them to post it next to each telephone and call immediately in the event of a suspected poisoning or overdose (American Association of Poison Control Centers [AAPCC], n.d.b). They can also educate and demonstrate for parents how to childproof the home by eliminating major sources of poisoning. This includes keeping plants out of a child's reach or eliminating them from the home until the child is older, locking up household chemicals (e.g., toilet bowl cleaner, bleach, mouthwash, oven and drain cleaners, pesticides, gasoline, paint thinner, hair products) and storing them out of a child's sight and reach, using childproof medication containers, and storing all medicines in a locked box with a key that is kept out of reach (AAPCC, n.d.a). Alcoholic beverages should also be kept out of reach, as should tobacco products. Outside hazards, such as wild mushrooms and poisonous plants, flowers, and berries, must also be considered (AAPCC, n.d.b). It is also important to eliminate sources of lead in and around the home.

Lead Poisoning

Lead poisoning historically resulted in encephalopathy and death. Today, morbidity from lead poisoning is subtle and most often affects the child's CNS with long-term changes in behavior and IQ. The CDC estimates that half

BOX 19-7 EVIDENCE-BASED PRACTICE

Getting Families to Use Child Booster Seats

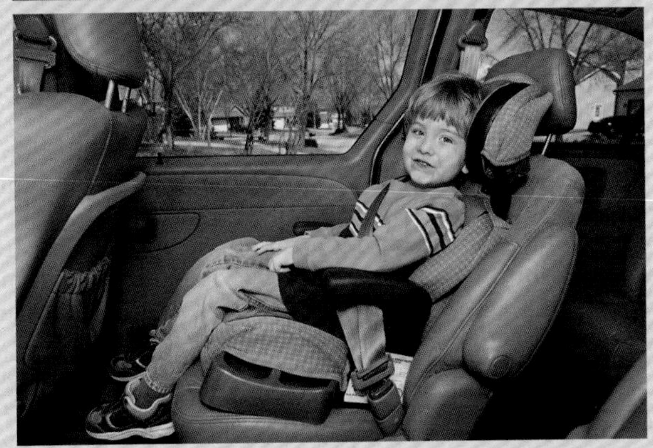

Many health departments, law enforcement, and social service agencies educate parents about the laws and benefits related to the use of child safety seats. Still, not every family consistently uses them. Education and awareness are essential to increase the use of child safety seats.

The Strike Out Child Passenger Injury (Strike Out) intervention program provided booster seat education for children ages 4 to 7 years at instructional baseball programs in four states. Twenty communities participated in the nonrandomized, controlled trial. The study tested the effectiveness of the education program before and after baseball season in increasing proper restraint use among participating children.

Findings revealed that the intervention program did increase the use of child restraint use in three of the four participating states (Alabama +15.5%, Arkansas +16.1%, and Illinois +11.0%). The study reinforces the importance that unique interventions can positively influence child safety use. It is essential for C/PHNs to use evidence and a variety of approaches to combat public health problems. For more information on selecting the proper car seat for children according to age and size, visit: https://www.cdc.gov/features/passengersafety/index.html.

Source: Aitken et al. (2013).

a million children between the ages of 1 and 5 years have elevated blood lead levels, or 5 μg of lead per deciliter of blood (CDC, 2018i). Lead in paint, dust, and soil can be inadvertently consumed, and lead also crosses the placental barrier. It can be transferred in breast milk and is also found in some infant formulas (American Academy of Pediatrics, 2018b). Lead is one cause of childhood poisoning. There is no safe level of lead, and the elimination of elevated blood lead levels in children is a U.S. Health Goal. The primary sources of lead exposure in preschool-aged children continue to be lead-based paint and lead-contaminated soil and house dust. The critical age of exposure (or peak level) is thought to be between ages 18 and 36 months. Levels generally begin to decline after age 3 years. Children who live in poverty and play in substandard housing areas remain at risk for direct exposure to significant sources of lead. Lead safety and housing code enforcement, along with periodic monitoring to detect new lead hazards, can help prevent future lead exposures. C/PHNs working together with environmental health sanitarians, should promote opportunities for blood lead screening, especially if it is suspected that children in certain homes, apartments, or neighborhoods are at risk for lead poisoning. Children have also been exposed to lead in some toys, candies, cosmetics, traditional medicines, and eating or drinking utensils imported from other countries. Many of these have been tested and revealed to have high levels of lead. Education and public awareness campaigns can help prevent this type of lead poisoning. The C/PHN can alert clients to the dangers of lead and its sources and work as an advocate for policies to reduce this danger for infants and children. See Chapter 9 for more on lead poisoning and water contaminated with lead.

Child Maltreatment

An estimated 678,000 children were victims of **child abuse** or maltreatment in 2018 (National Children's Alliance, 2019). Child maltreatment includes physical, emotional, and sexual abuse and neglect (e.g., withholding feeding or medical care) that occurs in anyone under 18 years old. Neglect is more an act or acts of omission in which a child's basic needs are not met. Children under age 4 years are at the greatest risk for severe abuse and neglect (CDC, 2018k). **Shaken baby syndrome** is often an overlooked form of abuse. **Abusive head trauma**, which includes shaken baby syndrome, is the leading cause of all child maltreatment deaths (National Center of Shaken Baby Syndrome, 2020). Shaken baby syndrome can be suspected in infants or toddlers who exhibit traumatic brain injuries caused by violent shaking or impact, is characterized by a triad of symptoms: retinal hemorrhage, subdural hemorrhage, and/or subdural hemorrhage with few signs of external trauma (American Academy of Pediatrics, 2018a). The soft brain tissues are injured as they move violently against the rough cranial bones as the infant is shaken or thrown against a hard object. The C/PHN has an important role in the prevention of shaken baby syndrome by providing parents with education regarding the triggers and intervention strategies. Educating parents that baby crying patterns are more severe in the first few months and progressively improve along with baby soothing techniques are essential before and after delivery (CDC, 2018k).

Failure to thrive (FTT) is characterized by slowing growth rate in height and weight, as well as head circumference among infants and toddlers. If an infant's growth rate is consistently below 3rd to 5th percentiles, drops more than two percentiles, or is lower than the 80th percentile of median weight for height, a diagnosis of FTT may be made. Problems with growth may be due to food insecurities and many behavioral or physiologic etiologies for infants but can also be related to child neglect or abnormal maternal–infant bonding. Child neglect differs from child abuse in that the action of the parent or guardian is more one of omission with neglect rather than commission as in the case of an injury related to abuse. Risk factors that point to child neglect as the basis for

FTT include those most often cited for abuse and neglect, along with specific concerns about parents intentionally withholding food, being resistant to recommended interventions, and having rigid beliefs about nutrition and health regimens that may jeopardize the infant. The exact incidence of FTT is difficult to determine, and no accurate estimates are available. The C/PHN can take a careful nutritional history and determine the mother's knowledge of basic infant needs, as well as checking for developmental milestones. A psychosocial history is also helpful (e.g., income/poverty level, cultural beliefs, social support networks, domestic abuse, substance abuse, mental health disorders), with careful attention to maternal bonding and feeding practices. Growth problems in the first 2 months of life may result in cognitive, language/speech, and fine motor deficits in childhood, and early intervention programs that involve home visitation have been effective in attenuating the long-term effects of FTT (Homan, 2016).

C/PHNs play a role in the prevention and management of child abuse and maltreatment. Preventive strategies such as parent education should begin prenatally and continue throughout the life span. Parent training programs can help teach parents to cope and child sexual abuse prevention programs may also be helpful. Home visiting programs that provide anticipatory guideline education will also help to prevent abuse and neglect. Early recognition and reporting of suspected abuse or/and neglect is a responsibility of C/PHNs.

See Box 19-8 and Chapter 18 for more on child abuse and neglect.

Communicable Diseases

Infants, toddlers, and preschool-aged children experience a high frequency of acute illnesses, more so than any other age group. Acute conditions commonly seen from birth to age 5 include sore throat, ear pain, urinary tract infection, skin infection, and respiratory infections (including ear infections, colds, influenza). Communicable diseases are prevalent in these age groups, as very young children are building an immune system and are just beginning to come in contact with a greater number of people outside their families (Fig. 19-6; American Academy of Pediatrics, 2017).

Acute respiratory illnesses are common in children under the age of 5 years. C/PHNs need to emphasize that over-the-counter cough and cold medications should not be used for children under age 2. The U.S. Food and Drug Administration (FDA) questioned their safety and effectiveness at a hearing in October 2007, and manufacturers removed medication targeted to infants and toddlers; they also changed labels all cold and cough medications to read that they should not be used in children under age 4 (FDA, 2018). Parents need to be informed of the dangers and suggest safer interventions.

Bronchiolitis is the most common type of lower respiratory infection among infants and starts with a

BOX 19-8 Reports of an Emergency Foster Home

The following are examples of the various situations from which abused and neglected children come, as reported by a couple who had an emergency foster home for the county department of social services. The examples represent children placed with them over a 2-year period in which they cared for 256 children.

- 2-Week-old Jose was taken to their home because the parents (under the influence of drugs) were found swinging Jose upside down in circles in an infant carrier as they walked along a downtown street at 3 AM. After being returned to his parents, he returned to foster care 1 month later after being found abandoned in an infant carrier at the county fair.
- Andre, Otis, and Selma, ages 8, 5, and 4, went to the foster home when the social services agency discovered they had been living with their father in an abandoned car for 2 years. They stayed for 3 weeks while the social worker found suitable housing for this family and counseling for the father.
- Victoria, 5 years old, a loving and passive child, arrived wearing a diaper and appeared developmentally delayed. She had a history of being physically and sexually abused. Her family was very dysfunctional, and it took the social worker several weeks to sort out relatives and their intentions before placing Victoria in a long-term foster home.
- Ronald and Randall, 6-year-old twin boys who were forced to "sexually please their mother" for several years, came to the emergency foster home before being placed with relatives while their mother underwent psychiatric treatment. The boys began counseling during their stay in the emergency foster home.
- Antoinette, age 7, had severe asthma and was very withdrawn. She came to the emergency foster home because her mother (and the mother's boyfriend) refused to care for her. The child came with every photograph of herself and personal mementos because the mother wanted no reminders of the child. The social worker located a grandmother who would be the child's guardian.
- 13-Year-old Robert came home from school one day and found his mother and all their furniture gone. After a few weeks of Robert living in the basement of the apartment building, someone alerted the social services agency, and he was placed in the emergency foster home for 2 months. His mother finally called social services after 6 weeks, saying Robert was too difficult for her to handle, but she may want to see him again someday. Robert was eventually placed in a group home for boys.
- Quyn, a 17-year-old Laotian girl, came into foster care after being referred by the school nurse because of wounds observed on her wrists and ankles. Quyn reported being strapped to a chair for 12 or more hours at a time by her father because she was not following the old ways and was shaming the family by being seen in public with a boy, and without a chaperone. Several meetings were held between the parents, a Southeast Asian community leader, and the social worker to resolve this situation so that Quyn could go home safely.

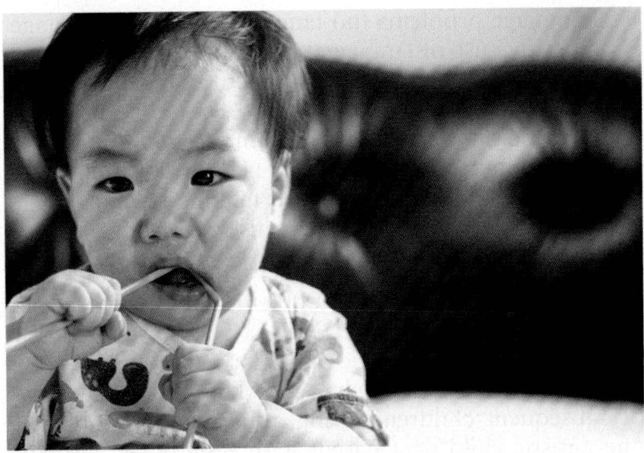

FIGURE 19-6 Infants, toddlers, and preschoolers are constantly putting things in their mouths and sharing items with others, contributing, in part, to the increased incidence of accidents and infections among them.

runny nose, fever, and cough. It is a common cause of hospitalization in this age group; about 2% of children with respiratory syncytial virus (RSV), the most common cause of bronchiolitis, are hospitalized every year. The majority of hospitalizations for bronchiolitis are for infants 6 months and younger. RSV is the cause in 70% of cases and can rise to 100% during winter epidemics. Although wheezing, tachypnea, and chest retractions can be frightening to parents, most healthy infants survive (95%). However, C/PHNs working with at-risk infants need to work with parents and pediatricians to ensure that palivizumab (monoclonal antibody) or RSV immunoglobulin is given to preterm infants or those born closer to term but exposed to environmental pollution or to other children. An effective RSV vaccine has not yet been found, but palivizumab (Synagis) can be used to help prevent the most severe cases of RSV in high-risk infants (e.g., premature, congenital heart problems) and is given monthly by injection during RSV season (CDC, 2018l).

Vaccine-Preventable Diseases

Vaccines are one of the greatest achievements of public health. Since 1980, there has been a 99% or greater decrease in deaths because of the vaccine-preventable diseases of mumps, pertussis, tetanus, and diphtheria and 80% or greater decline in deaths associated with vaccines instituted since 1980: hepatitis A and B, *Haemophilus influenzae* type B (HiB), and varicella. Worldwide, vaccine coverage has increased because of effects of manufacturers and philanthropists (e.g., Bill & Melinda Gates Foundation). The WHO has specific disease eradication and vaccine promotion programs around the world (see Chapter 16). Smallpox has been eradicated worldwide, and the viruses for polio, rubella, and measles are no longer endemic in the United States. Newborns immature immune systems and lack of exposure to antigens, along with somewhat porous physical barriers to microbes, put them at high risk of infection. By the age of 4 to 6 months, however, a brisker antibody response to vaccines becomes possible. Successful infant and childhood immunization programs have been responsible for high vaccine coverage and the subsequent decline in morbidity and mortality from these preventable diseases.

State-level immunization registries help track vaccine coverage at all age levels. Because day care centers and schools require proof of immunization, vaccination rates have improved over the last two decades. The financing of immunizations for infants and children has significantly improved as a result of two major initiatives. The Vaccines for Children Program and the Child Health Insurance Program (CHIP) cover children on Medicaid, uninsured children, and American Indian/Alaska Native children. In addition, underinsured children who receive immunizations at federally qualified health centers and rural health clinics are covered. Additional state programs and funds help provide free or low-cost vaccines for children who are not covered by the other programs. There are several ways for C/PHNs to help all families obtain free or low-cost immunizations and contribute to maintaining adequate levels of community immunity to communicable disease (see Chapters 8, 10, and 12).

Even if financial barriers are removed, there are other barriers. Transportation is a significant problem for some parents, especially in rural areas and for families in urban areas who have several children and need to take public transportation. All 50 states provide for medical exceptions to mandatory vaccination, and 47 allow religious exemptions; 18 permit philosophical or personal exemptions (National Conference of State Legislatures, 2017). Despite public health announcements in the media, some mothers remain unaware of the disabling consequences of diseases such as polio and do not realize the importance of fully vaccinating their children. Also, as more vaccines become available and the deadly diseases they prevent become a distant memory in the public's mind, more concerns about the safety of vaccines emerge. There has not been any link established between thimerosal, a vaccine preservative, and autism (CDC, 2018e). The use of thimerosal has been reduced or completely curtailed; single-dose packaging does not require the ethyl mercury preservative (CDC, 2018e) (see Chapter 8 for information about vaccine hesitancy). Numerous Web sites have emerged that advise against childhood immunization and provide graphic horror stories about the handful of severe reactions to vaccination. Media coverage and online Web sites about vaccine adverse events also contribute to decreased compliance on the part of parents in getting their children immunized. C/PHNs and other health professionals are encouraged to provide parents of very young children with meaningful stories of preventable deaths because of vaccines and to educate parents about scientifically based Web sites and resources rather than relying solely on dispassionate facts and figures.

Chronic Diseases

Infants and young children can be afflicted with chronic diseases that affect their quality of life.

Dental caries is the most common chronic disease among the 6 to 19 year age group (CDC, 2019c). Young children's diets, often unreasonably high in sugar, increase the incidence of dental caries in this population group. The practice of allowing infants to feed from the bottle beyond 15 to 16 months, or to fall asleep with a bottle, can lead to *baby bottle tooth decay* or *nursing caries*. Baby bottle tooth decay occurs when others persist in giving toddlers and preschool-aged children milk, juice, sodas, or sugared drinks continually throughout the day (American Academy of Pediatrics, 2018d). Frequent snacking and sippy cups filled with juice or sugary drinks can lead to cavities. It is recommended that sugary foods be eaten at mealtimes and not as snacks and that regular snack times be established. Also, between ages 6 and 12 months, sippy cups are often used to wean infants from the breast or bottle, but between-meal drinks should consist of water or milk. Nighttime breast-feeding beyond what is needed for nutrition can also lead to increased risk of dental caries (American Dental Association, 2016). Parents of infants older than 6 months who have several erupted teeth should be instructed to rub the infant's gums with a damp, clean cloth and to begin tooth brushing, using a soft pediatric toothbrush with a very small amount of fluoride toothpaste—about the size of a grain of rice. The first dental examination should be made within 6 months of the first tooth eruption. Addressing parental misconceptions about dental health and understanding cultural beliefs and practices related to dental health and hygiene are important (American Academy of Pediatrics, 2018d).

Dental caries is a preventable condition that can be addressed with proper nutrition and hygiene. The younger the age when dental caries first appear, the greater the risk for future tooth decay that increases the risks of chronic health conditions due the inflammatory response. Untreated dental caries can also lead to serious infections. Pain can interfere with learning at school. Many health departments are using fluoride varnishes as a means of preventing dental caries in young children. Dental hygienists and C/PHNs may be trained to apply the sealants and varnishes while making home visits, or children and families may visit clinics for treatment (American Academy of Pediatrics, 2018d).

Asthma symptoms may begin in infants and toddlers. Approximately 6 million children ages 0 to 17 years have asthma (CDC, 2018c). Inner-city, low-income, and minority children are disproportionately affected, and asthma hospitalizations are common. C/PHNs can assist families in finding appropriate health care providers and encourage proper administration of asthma medications and treatments. They can also teach families to reduce the presence of asthma triggers in their homes (see Chapters 9 and 20 for more information on environmental triggers, asthma, and other chronic diseases of childhood and adolescence).

Autism is a developmental spectrum disorder that is often first noticed in toddlers. Parents become aware that the child's communication and interaction with others are different and that the child may also display obsessive and narrow interests. Autism spectrum disorder (ASD) is a complex developmental disorder, and spectrum of ASD indicates that symptoms for each child varies and may range from mild to severe (CDC, 2018b). A child's communication skills and interaction with others are most often affected, along with obsessive behavior and narrowed interests. Behaviors associated with autism include:

- Language problems (no language, delay in language, repetitive use of language)
- Motor mannerisms (often repetitive rocking, hand flapping, object twirling)
- Fixation on objects (restricted interests)
- No spontaneous play or make-believe play (Fig. 19-7); no interest in peers (problems making friends)
- Little or no eye contact (may also resist hugging)

Boys are four times more likely than girls to develop autism. An estimated 16.4/1,000 children were identified to have ASD in 2014 (CDC, 2018c). The causes of autism are unclear—some genetic links have been found, but environment may also be a factor. There is a higher risk of subsequent children having autism in a family with one autistic child or a parent with ASD (CDC, 2018b). It is often associated with other disorders (e.g., congenital rubella syndrome, Down syndrome, fragile X syndrome, tuberous sclerosis), but the exact causes are not fully understood (CDC, 2018b). Families may need to be referred to early educational intervention programs and social service agencies for assistance. Parents need to be vigilant with daycares and preschools about their child's environmental sensitivities. It is important for C/PHNs to educate parents that parenting practices are *not* a cause of autism and that multiple, large-scale research studies on childhood immunizations have shown that there is no relationship between immunizations and autism (CDC, 2018d).

Sickle cell disease, an inherited blood disorder, affects thousands of children in the United States, most often those of African or Hispanic Caribbean ancestry. The characteristic chronic and severe anemia are common in young children with this condition, and it can affect memory, learning, and behavior. Children can also exhibit jaundice, gallstones, and joint pain. When both parents have the genetic mutation, the newborn will be afflicted with the disease. Those with the sickle cell trait have no symptoms of the disease but can pass it on to their offspring. In many states, routine newborn screening for sickle cell anemia is offered. Because sickle cell anemia can lead to splenic sequestration (or pooling of blood in the spleen), many children either have nonfunctioning spleens or have had them surgically removed.

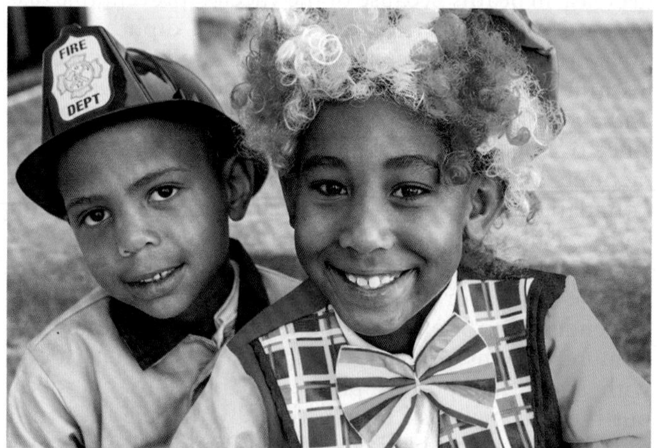

FIGURE 19-7 Dress-up and playtime are important for toddler and preschooler development.

Risk of infection is always a concern when this occurs before age 5 (CDC, 2019a). C/PHNs working with populations at risk for this disease can educate and refer families for diagnosis and treatment.

Food allergies is a growing problem in children. Infants with close family members who have atopic diseases are at risk for development of allergies. Prolonged breast-feeding for 1 year is recommended for these infants or the use of hypoallergenic infant formula. The CDC (2018m) does not recommend a delay in the introduction of the most allergic foods (milk, eggs, and peanuts) for infants past the usual 4 to 6 month of age as this will not prevent a child from developing an allergy. Fortunately, once allergies are diagnosed, they can be managed through dietary changes and by avoidance of allergy-producing foods. Parents need to be educated, so that they can consistently read food labels and alert family members to the young child's allergy so that inappropriate foods are avoided.

Muscular dystrophy (MD) and *cystic fibrosis* (CF) are two diseases that not only affect quality of life but also severely shorten the child's life. MD is a constellation of genetic disorders characterized by progressive atrophy and weakening of skeletal muscles. The onset of some forms of MD begins in infancy or early childhood, and MD is more common in boys (1 in than 3,500 male births). Girls are usually carriers, but a few may be "manifesting carriers" that have milder symptoms of muscle weakness (National Organization of Rare Disorders, 2016). *Duchenne MD* usually begins before age 6 and progresses rapidly until most boys are wheelchair bound and require a ventilator (NINDS, 2017). Recently in 2016 and 2017, the FDA released a disease-modifying drug, eteplirsen for DMD followed by deflazacort for the treatment of DMD (Muscular Dystrophy Association, 2018). Genetic testing can determine who is a carrier of the gene and can aid in confirming the clinical diagnosis.

CF is a genetic disease that usually begins in infancy—about 1,000 new CF cases are diagnosed annually and 75% are diagnosed before a child reaches age two (Cystic Fibrosis News Today, 2018). CF is characterized by a persistent cough or wheeze, shortness of breath, poor weight gain despite a good appetite, and a salty taste to the skin. Sticky, thick mucus builds up in the lungs and digestive tract. Respiratory infections become increasingly more frequent as the child ages. It is the major cause of severe chronic lung disease in children. Chest physiotherapy to help mobilize secretions is performed daily, usually by the parents. Sometimes, a vibrating inflatable vest is used that loosens mucus. Aerosolized antibiotic treatments and mucus-thinning medications help to improve lung function and reduce respiratory infections. Mucus also affects the pancreas and prevents release of digestive enzymes needed to digest food and absorb nutrients. Pancreatic enzyme supplements help with nutrient absorption (University of Pittsburgh Medical Center, 2018). C/PHNs reinforce these techniques and teach the family to avoid exposure to respiratory infections and to initiate prescribed antibiotic prophylaxis promptly. As much as feasible, the young child should be involved in his own care, offered valid choices, and encouraged to participate in decision-making. The family needs genetic counseling and emotional support as members work through feelings of anticipatory grief.

Nutrition

Proper nutrition is foundational to well-being later in life. The American Association of Pediatrics recommends exclusive breastfeeding for the first 6 months of life then gradually adding solid foods along with breastfeeding until 1 year of age (2018d). Bonding between mother and infant and overall maternal health are predictors of infant weight gain. Both nutrition and bonding can be accomplished by breastfeeding (Fig. 19-8). Along with convenience and no to low cost, there are other benefits of breastfeeding which include the following (American Academy of Pediatrics, 2016):

- *Nutrition*: Breast milk provides sugar, fat, and protein; the proteins are easily digested, and fats are well absorbed; it is the most complete form of nutrition for human infants.
- *Anti-infective and anti-allergic properties*: Breast milk contains immunoglobulins, enzymes, and leukocytes that protect against pathogens, and it decreases the incidence of allergy by eliminating exposure to potential antigens. Babies exclusively breast-fed for 6 or more months have fewer respiratory illnesses, ear infections, and cases of diarrhea. The chance of hospitalization for infants that are breast-fed for more than 4 months is reduced.
- *Infant growth*: Breast-fed babies usually gain weight at a more moderate rate and are leaner than bottle-fed babies; rapid weight gain in infancy has been associated with later chronic diseases.
- *Long-term health effects*: Breast-feeding exclusively for at least 6 months is associated with reduced risk of overweight in later life, and less change of developing atopic dermatitis, asthma, and leukemia and lymphoma. There has also been a 36% reduction in the risk of SIDS among breastfed babies and a decreased incidence of type 1 diabetes.
- *Benefits for mothers*: Breast-feeding burns extra calories, helps to reduce postpartum bleeding, and delays ovulation and menstruation; it also lowers the risk of later ovarian and breast cancers. Studies show that

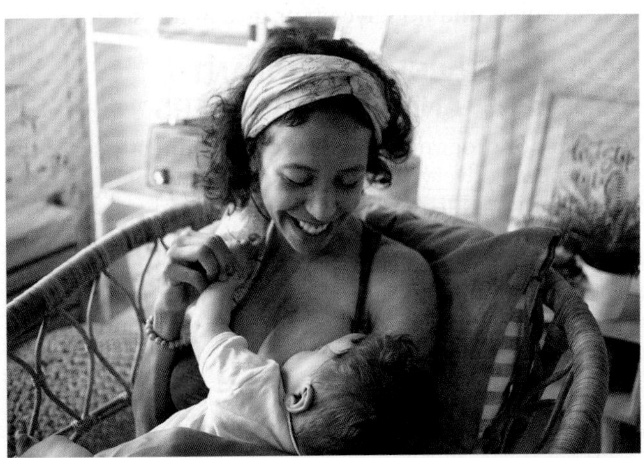

FIGURE 19-8 Breastfeeding has many benefits for both infant and mother.

the longer the period of lactation, the lower chance she has of developing hyperlipidemia, hypertension, cardiovascular disease, and diabetes.

The C/PHN can encourage pregnant women to consider the benefits of breast-feeding their infants and provide education and interventions to assist them with the most common barriers: concern about insufficient supply of breast milk, problems with the baby latching onto the breast, painful nipples, and scheduling problems. Women often choose to breastfeed their babies when they fully understand the health effects for their infants and themselves and when they receive positive influence from family and friends. The C/PHN can join with labor and delivery nurses and lactation consultants in promoting breast-feeding among mothers in the community. Nurses can lobby local hospitals to educate new mothers about the benefits of breastfeeding and stop the routine distribution of free samples of infant formula.

Child and adolescent obesity prevalence in 2015 to 2016 was 18.5% (Hales, Carroll, Fryar, & Ogden, 2017). In 2015 to 2016, there was a higher prevalence of obesity among Hispanic children and adolescents (25.8%) and non-Hispanic Blacks (22%) than among non-Hispanic Whites (14.1%) and non-Hispanic Asians (11%) (Hales et al., 2017). The Orr et al. (2019) study identified food insecurities associated with childhood obesity as mediated through feeding practices and beliefs. Families from insecure households were more likely to provide food to stop a baby from crying or to console a child. Another study identified that weight compared to length decreased from 14.5% in 2010 to 12.3% in 2014 among infants aged 3 to 23 months enrolled in Women, Infants, and Children (WIC) programs (Freedman et al., 2017).

Overfeeding can lead to nutrition problems and poor infant growth. The pattern of growth may also be important, such as growth problems in infancy along with overweight in later childhood. The most common sources of energy and nutrients for infants and toddlers are breast milk, formula, and milk. Fortified foods (e.g., grain-based foods with added vitamin A, folate, and iron) become increasingly more significant in toddler diets. In general, most nutrition recommendations include providing for a wide variety of foods for children. C/PHNs can encourage parents to continue to introduce new healthy foods to their toddlers and not give up or give in too soon.

HEALTH SERVICES FOR INFANTS, TODDLERS, AND PRESCHOOLERS

A variety of programs that directly or indirectly serve the health needs of very young children may be found in most communities. Nurses play a major and vital role in delivering these services especially for the working poor and vulnerable populations. In public and community health, programs fall into three categories, which approximate the three priorities of C/PHN practice: prevention, protection, and promotion.

Preventive Health Programs

Neighborhood community centers found in urban and rural settings provide families with parenting education, health and safety education, immunizations, various screening programs, and family planning services. In some areas, nurse-run clinics are established at local schools or community centers to assist in outreach services to the community. In collaboration with an interdisciplinary team, C/PHNs are often the primary care providers in these programs. The major goals are to keep communities healthy by focusing on primary and secondary prevention services. Three examples of preventive health programs for infants and young children are immunization programs, parent training programs, and quality day care health services.

Immunization Programs

Health departments, community clinics, and private health care providers continue to offer immunizations against the major childhood infectious diseases—measles, mumps, rubella, varicella, polio, diphtheria, tetanus, pertussis, hepatitis A and B, and Hib—some of which can cause permanent disability and even death. Pneumococcal, meningococcal, and influenza vaccines are also recommended, as is the vaccine for rotavirus (CDC, 2018h). Many of these diseases no longer plague infants and children, and newer vaccines offer an even greater promise of health. The current immunization schedule is available at https://www.cdc.gov/vaccines/schedules/easy-to-read/child-easyread.html (CDC, 2018k).

Although the threat of these diseases has been substantially reduced, vigilance is still essential. Low immunization levels in many areas of the United States, particularly among the poor and medically underserved, and increased disease rates signal the need for constant surveillance, outreach programs, and innovative educational efforts. The C/PHN can help young families find low-cost vaccinations by using the Vaccines.gov Web site (https://www.vaccines.gov/getting/where). Whenever infants and young children come in contact with public health and other community clinics, it is always important to check immunizations and provide the necessary vaccines. C/PHNs are deeply involved in preventive activities that promote immunizations. One important intervention is to provide each parent with immunization record that they can keep so that they have a record of their children's immunizations. Immunization information systems are in place but vary from state to state; therefore, it is essential that parents maintain a record (CDC, 2018g).

Parent Training Programs

Parent education and training programs have been useful in providing parents with the tools needed to deal with the stresses and challenges of parenting effectively. These programs provide education regarding appropriate growth and developmental milestones, anticipatory guidance, positive discipline techniques, parenting skills, appropriate play, and parent–child interaction promotion (Child Welfare Information Gateway, n.d.c). There are a variety of programs available for parents at local, state, and national levels with resources available at https://www.childwelfare.gov/topics/preventing/prevention-programs/parented/

Quality Day Care and Preschool Programs

It is estimated that 24% of children under the age of 5 spend time in center-based child care (Center for

American Progress, 2018). Quality child care centers improve school readiness, reduce family stress, and result in overall improvements in health and well-being for children and their families (The Children's Cabinet, 2018a).

Although safe, affordable child care is important, the long-term benefits of early childhood education are numerous. These benefits include higher rates of high school completion, college attendance, and full-time employment and lower rates of felony arrests, convictions, and incarcerations (The Children's Cabinet, 2018b). **Head Start**, a federally funded program that offers early childhood education to low-income children between ages 3 and 5, has consistently demonstrated significant improvements in preschoolers' social, emotional, and cognitive development, and those attending Head Start do better on several developmental and educational measures. Head Start children are also more likely to receive dental and health screenings, to have up-to-date immunization coverage, to have better school attendance, and to be less likely to be held back in school. The benefits of Head Start extend to families because more Head Start parents read more frequently to their children than do parents of children not enrolled in the program (National Head Start Association, 2018). However, the quality of day care and preschool programs varies considerably; licensing laws can regulate only minimum safety and health standards. In addition, numerous childcare operations are too small to require licensing, leaving quality and compliance unevaluated. As educators, C/PHNs play a role in providing education and referrals. Also, nurses can influence and advocate for quality of day care and preschool programs through active childcare consultation efforts that focus on health educational efforts for staff, monitoring of health and safety standards, and working to improve the state's or community's role in passing stronger licensing laws.

Health Protection Programs

Health protection programs for infants and young children are designed to protect them from illness and injury. Ultimately, these programs may even protect their lives.

Safety and Injury Protection

Accident and injury control programs serve a critical role in protecting the lives of children. Efforts to prevent motor vehicle crashes, a major cause of death, may include driver education programs, better highway construction, improved motor vehicle design and safety features, and continuing research into the causes of various types of crashes. Injury prevention and reduction have been addressed through strategies such as state laws requiring the use of safety restraints (e.g., seat belts, child safety seats), availability of front and side driver and passenger airbags, substitution of other modes of travel (air, rail, or bus), lower speed limits, stricter enforcement of drunk-driving laws, safer automobile design, and helmets for motorcyclists, bicycle riders, and skaters.

For infants, toddlers, and preschool-aged children to be safe when traveling in vehicles, they must be restrained in an approved infant carrier, child restraint seat, or booster seat. General guidelines recommend that all children under the age of 2 years ride in rear facing car seats. Forward facing seats with a harness are to be used when children have outgrown the rear-facing height and weight limit requirements. It is recommended that children use these as long as possible as allowed by the car safety seat manufacturer. Car seats must be positioned and secured as described by the manufacturer; used at all times, even for the shortest distances; and installed in the appropriate position (facing rear or front) based on the weight or age of the infant or young child. Belt positioning booster seats are recommended when weight or height requirements have exceeded forward facing car seat limits. All children younger than 13 should ride in the back seat (American Academy of Pediatrics, 2018c). C/PHNs collaborate with other community agencies, hospitals, law enforcement, and other community agencies to provide training, education, and child safety seat checks.

Lead poisoning prevention programs can be found in most state and local health departments. The Lead Contamination Control Act of 1988 provided for CDC funding and programs to eliminate childhood lead poisoning (CDC, 2018e). The CDC provides technical assistance, training, and surveillance at a national level. Another role of the C/PHN is to help with targeted screening and case management and provide education to clients and communities about lead poisoning at the local level. They also work with environmental health personnel and epidemiologists to reach out to neighborhoods and communities at risk for testing. See more on this in Chapter 9.

Protection From Child Abuse and Neglect

Services to protect children from abuse and neglect begin with a collaborative approach that includes social services, law enforcement, education, community health providers, and child advocacy. Protection begins with prevention efforts. Child abuse and maltreatment can be prevented by strengthening family economic and social support systems. Furthermore, C/PHNs must advocate for policies that support improved family economic and social systems (CDC, 2018g). "Policies that strengthen household financial security can reduce child abuse and neglect by improving parents' ability to satisfy children's basic needs (e.g., food, shelter, medical care), provide developmentally appropriate child care, and improve parental mental health, support positive parenting, ensure quality education and healthcare for children" (Fortson, Klevens, Merrick, Gilbert, & Alexander, 2016, p. 15). Additionally, social support systems and quality childcare and early education programs for children in communities are essential for prevention of child abuse and maltreatment. Working alongside community leaders, C/PHNs strive to ensure that communities have adequate resources to support healthy development of children (CDC, 2018g). Protecting children from abuse and maltreatment also includes the importance of early recognition of the signs of abuse and reporting this to authorities (see Chapter 18). Nurses along with day care providers, teachers, social workers, doctors, clergy, coaches, and all others working with children that suspect child abuse or maltreatment are required by law to report it. In addition, animal humane workers and commercial photograph developers are mandated reporters. Child abuse or maltreatment should be reported to local child protective services or law enforcement agency when it is suspected. Most states have hotline or toll-free numbers available for reporting (Child Welfare Information Gateway, n.d.b).

To promote safe and nurturing relationships and environments where children live and play free from abuse and violence, ACE must be addressed in our communities. C/PHNs must recognize those at risk for ACE and history of ACE in adults referring clients and families to resources; ACE is preventable. To combat ACE in the community, Washington state has directed efforts to addressing ACE in the community through legislation that aims to reduce prevalence through primary prevention of child maltreatment and community engagement to improve the public's health. Secondary measures include policy enacted through TANF to strengthen ACE families through Head Start parenting programs. Tertiary efforts include additional support for juvenile high-ACE offenders through functional family programs (CDC, 2019b).

Primary Prevention. Primary prevention measures include the use of social norming that promote positive parenting, family support groups, and public awareness campaigns about child maltreatment and how to report it, along with establishing community education to enhance the general well-being of children and their families. Educational-type services are designed to enrich the lives of families, to improve the skills of family functioning, and to prevent the stress and problems that might lead to dysfunction and abuse or neglect (CDC, 2018g).

Primary prevention also focuses on parent preparation during the prenatal period; practices that encourage parent–child bonding during labor, delivery, the postpartum period, and early infancy; and provision of information regarding support services for families with newborns. This is often the ultimate outcome sought by home visitation programs carried out or managed by C/PHNs. It is also helpful to provide parents of children of all ages with information regarding child-rearing strategies, anticipatory guidance for developmental milestones and tasks, and community resources.

Secondary Prevention. Services are designed to identify and assist families who may have risk factors for impaired parenting to prevent abuse or neglect. **High-risk families** are those families that exhibit the symptoms (risk factors) of potentially abusive or neglectful behavior or that are under the types of stress associated with abuse or neglect. These can include families living in poverty, substance abuse or mental health problems, parents who were abused when they were children, and parents or children with developmental disabilities. Early intervention with high-risk families can improve emotional and functional coping and help prevent further problems. High school parent education programs for pregnant adolescents, home visitation programs targeted to at-risk families, and respite care for families of children with disabilities are all examples of secondary prevention actions. Family resource centers in schools or community centers located in low-income neighborhoods can offer resource and referral services to families who may be dealing with multiple sources of stress. Evidence-based home visitation programs, such as the Nurse–Family Partnership, Early Head Start, and Healthy Families America, provide parental support and education and promote healthier family functioning and have resulted in decreased rates of child abuse and neglect (Child Welfare Information Gateway, n.d.a).

Tertiary Prevention. Intervention and treatment services are designed to assist a family in which abuse or neglect has already occurred, so that further abuse or neglect may be prevented, and the consequences of abuse or neglect may be minimized. There are several evidence-based programs that have been found effective in reducing the reoccurrence of child abuse. *Safe Environment for Every Kid (SEEK)* is an example of an enhanced primary care program; *Parent–Child Interaction Therapy*, *SafeCare*, and *The Incredible Years* are examples of behavioral training programs; and Trauma-Focused Cognitive Behavioral Therapy (TF-CBT) helps to reduce the consequences of post-traumatic stress disorder and depression after abuse has occurred (Fortson et al., 2016). Often, families are referred to mental health counselors to improve family communication and functioning. Some families may require crisis respite when they feel they cannot manage the stresses of child care. Parent mentoring programs can provide support and coaching to these parents (Child & Family Services, 2018).

The C/PHN and school nurse have major roles in all levels of prevention of child maltreatment. In addition, the nurse is in a unique position to detect early signs of neglect and abuse. The nurse must establish rapport with families and assist with appropriate interventions and referrals at the secondary and tertiary levels of prevention. The advanced practice nurse may also work with families of abused and neglected children as part of an interdisciplinary approach with teachers, the department of social services, the judicial system, foster families, and other health care providers if needed. The effectiveness of local programs depends, in large measure, on the willingness of health professionals to increase their awareness and work as a team to detect, report, develop, and evaluate interventions for the perpetrators and victims of abuse and neglect. Ongoing education of health care providers is recommended to increase awareness of changing child abuse patterns, new reporting laws, and resources available to families.

Health Promotion Programs

Early childhood development and intervention programs are designed to have positive effects on the outcomes of children's cognitive and social development. Some health promotion programs have considered children's physical health, and fewer have focused on parent–child interaction and child social development. All are considered important health promotion programs from birth through preschool years.

Infant Brain Development Research and Parent–Child Interactions

Research into the normal brain development of infants and toddlers has revealed that brain maturation in the first few years of life is very rapid: the brain grows to 80% of adult size by age 3, and the myelination pattern of an 18- to 24-month-old child is similar to that of an adult (Gilmore, Santelli, & Gao, 2018). The prefrontal cortex of 4-year-olds is already functional and becomes more organized throughout later adolescence. Early environment exerts a lasting influence on brain development, even in the womb. Appropriate early nutrition and stimulation promotes healthy development.

Early in life, rapid myelination is taking place, children need higher fat levels in their diet (50% of total calories should come from fat). Breast milk or formula will provide this fat during the first year of life, then breast milk or whole milk can be used after the first birthday. After age 2, children should reduce fat content to no more than 30% of calories coming from fat and 1% or 2% milk should be used (Zero to Three, 2018). Meaningful parent–child interactions should be established early; they include holding, rocking, comforting, touching, talking, and singing. When parents talk to infants and read to young children, children later demonstrate more advanced language and literacy skills. Providing a caring and supportive environment, with opportunities to learn and explore, is supportive of healthy brain development and promotes secure infant attachment (CDC, 2018g). Important parental behaviors that promote social development include gazing into an infant's eyes, paying attention to and interacting with toddlers, and listening to and answering preschoolers' questions. Providing infants and young children with secure, learning-rich environments where they can use their senses to discover new things helps them to maximize their potential. Emotional comfort and a secure environment ensure that young children will better deal with their feelings. It is important for the C/PHN to provide information to parents on the most current research results about brain development as well as tangible suggestions such as low-cost brain-stimulating toys and community resources to encourage quality parent–child interactions that promote appropriate physical growth and cognitive and social development.

Developmental Screening

With the emphasis on infant and early childhood development, C/PHNs often routinely carry out developmental screenings (Fig. 19-9). The American Academy of Pediatrics recommends developmental screening surveillance for children at each health visit along with an evidence-based developmental screening tool used at 9, 18, and 30 months, or anytime there is a concern. Autism-specific screenings are recommended at 18 and 24 months and social-emotional screenings should be conducted at regular intervals (2018e). There are a variety of screening tools available with resources available at https://screeningtime.org/star-center/#/screening-tools.

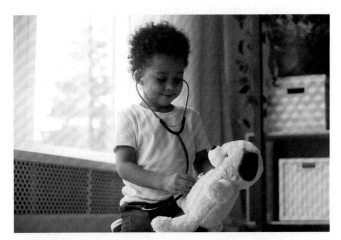

FIGURE 19-9 Allowing children to play with health care equipment can help alleviate fear and anxiety.

Developmental screening tools are also helpful in educating parents about normal child development and can provide a means of anticipatory guidance on developmental milestones and future safety issues. *Bright Futures*, an important resource for nurses and parents, provides tools to help families determine appropriate developmental milestones and expected behaviors, along with suggestions about when to seek help from professionals. A variety of screening tools available to nurses and other health professionals, ranging from parent report instruments to those that involve direct assessment of behaviors and skills, can examine overall physical and cognitive development or screen for such things as temperament, behavior, autism, and speech and language problems. It is important for the C/PHN to use tools that have reported validity and reliability. Early identification of problems can lead to interventions such as enrollment in early intervention programs and help children with school readiness. These early intervention programs are available in most communities or through the public school system (Bright Futures, 2018).

Programs for Children With Disabilities

Many children have special needs. They may have a congenital or acquired developmental disability, birth defect, or a chronic emotional, mental, or physical disease. About 1 in every 33 U.S. infants are born with a birth defect each year (CDC, 2018f). Some children suffer injuries after birth (Box 19-9). Autism and other mental or behavioral disorders develop after infancy and may require special services. Educational, health, and social or recreational services should be available for all children.

Federal law mandates early identification and intervention services for those with a variety of developmental disabilities. Developmental delays are characterized by slower development in one or more areas. The Individuals with Disabilities Education Act (IDEA) provides early intervention services, usually at home, for those from birth to age 2 who have developmental delays in physical, cognitive, communication, social/emotional, and adaptive development. Intervention services are also available to children with a mental or physical problem that is likely to result in a developmental delay. Newborns can receive infant stimulation services at home or in some schools specially designed to meet the needs of the very young. These programs are offered on a part-time basis for 1 to 2 hours, two to three times a week. Special education preschools are available for young children from ages 3 to 5. By preschool age, children may advance to half-day programs. Additional services can be provided to assist the families in getting children to the programs. Door-to-door bus service in specially equipped small buses or vans safely transports young children who

BOX 19-9 STORIES FROM THE FIELD

A Case of Kernicterus

A young mother was hospitalized for the birth of her second daughter, a beautiful little girl born without incident. The infant had difficulty latching on for breast-feeding and was not an active feeder. The mother told her obstetrical nurse that the infant seemed very different from her first child. The infant was irritable, but the nurse reassured the mother that the baby was fine and "not all babies are alike." Still, the new mother was concerned.

By the second day, the mother noticed that the baby was not very alert and did not want to feed. She also noticed that the baby's color was "yellowish," and the mother notified the nurse. Again, the nurse reassured the mother that this was "normal" for infants of Asian descent. The baby still was not feeding well, and there was yellowish-orange color stool in the baby's diaper. The mother notified the nurse and asked the nurse to call the doctor. The nurse refused and told the mother that she was "overreacting." The nurse again reassured the mother that the baby was "fine" and no action was taken. The young mother was not satisfied with the nursing care and requested additional assistance. A referral was made to the breast-feeding specialist at the hospital to help the new mother feed her infant. There were no phone calls documented to the physician nor was there documentation of the "yellowish-orange" stool. (The young mother kept the diaper for further proof of her concerns, though.) There was no documentation of irritability, inability to breast-feed, lethargy, or jaundiced appearance of the skin. The physician discharging the infant did not receive any information regarding irritability, yellowish stool, and yellowish tone of lower extremities and abdomen. No blood work was done. No referrals were made to home health or public health for follow-up.

Within 48 hours of discharge, the young mother brought her lethargic baby to the hospital's emergency room. On day 4 of life, the infant's bilirubin was 46. The infant was severely neurologically damaged, and the brain damage that resulted was irreversible. She was diagnosed with severe cerebral palsy, secondary to kernicterus (excessive bilirubin). The child has normal intelligence but will never be able to walk or talk. She will be fed through a gastrostomy tube for the rest of her life. The family was devastated.

The physician and hospital (nurses) were sued. The nurses on duty could not defend their actions with their charting or lack thereof. The attorneys for the hospital, representing the physician and nurses, could not defend the actions of their clients. A multimillion-dollar settlement was granted, and the nurses were fired. Unfortunately, this is not an isolated case. The irreversible brain damage that occurs as a result of untreated hyperbilirubinemia should not occur in the 21st century. This was a no-win situation that could have been avoided with proper nursing intervention. Hyperbilirubinemia should always be in the forefront of newborn assessment during the first few days of life.

The nurses involved in this case were not acting as the patient's advocate. The physician should have been notified immediately when signs and symptoms were first noted. Incorrect assumptions were made because of the nationality of the patient, an indication of lack of cultural competence. Home health nursing or public and community health nursing care should have been arranged for infant follow-up after discharge.

Linda O., certified life care planner, nurse consultant

1. *As a new C/PHN, what services do you think this family needs? Do you believe these services will change over time? If so, what type of anticipatory guidance should you provide the family and child?*
2. *This family may not have any trust of health care providers. How can you earn this family's trust?*
3. *How can you become culturally competent when working with a culture you are not familiar with?*

arrive at school in wheelchairs or with other assistive devices (Parlakian, 2018).

Availability of health services for children with disabilities varies with the size of the community. In small rural communities, children and their parents may have to travel long distances to receive specialized services, and in inner-city neighborhoods, lack of money for transportation can make even nearby services equally inaccessible. Accessibility is also influenced by lack of knowledge, attitudes, and prejudices. The nurse must recognize the power of these immobilizing factors and be able to deal with them effectively to make positive changes. See Chapter 23 for more on barriers to health care.

Most communities offer additional social and recreational programs for children that are disabled. For example, American Lung Association affiliate offices sponsor camping programs for children with asthma or other lung diseases. Often, these are camps for school-aged children that may last up to 1 week and be located in mountain or beach areas, but they may also be day camps, with parents in attendance for preschoolers. Many of these camps have C/PHNs either working or volunteering. Nationwide programs, such as the Special Olympics, offer recreational competition for the children in a variety of sports, such as bowling, track and field, skiing, and swimming. The C/PHN best serves families as a resource for such programs. Some parents are not aware of the rights or services available for their children with disabilities. Nurses can advocate for parents and help establish services in communities where needed services are lacking.

Nutritional Programs

Adequate nutrition must begin before birth. One of the most productive health promotion programs is the Special Supplemental Food Program for Women, Infants, and Children (WIC). In addition to supporting women and young children with nutritious foods and achieving the initial goals of decreasing the rates of preterm and LBW babies, increasing the length of pregnancy, and reducing the incidence of infant and child iron deficiency anemia, WIC also improves pregnant women's nutritional status.

BOX 19-10 LEVELS OF PREVENTION PYRAMID

Prenatal and Newborn Care

SITUATION: Desire for a healthy, full-term infant

GOAL: Using the three levels of prevention, avoid negative health conditions, and promptly diagnose, treat, and/or restore the fullest possible potential.

Tertiary Prevention

Rehabilitation	*Health Promotion and Education*	*Health Protection*
▪ The parents and significant others begin to bond with the newborn. ▪ Parents get to know the newborn and establish a successful breast- or bottle-feeding routine. ▪ The infant returns home in an age-appropriate infant car seat, which is used properly when traveling. ▪ The infant's birth is celebrated according to cultural and religious preferences. ▪ Parents resume sexual intercourse using a family planning method of their choice. ▪ The parents enjoy the new life they have created.	▪ Educate about benefits of early postpartum care. ▪ Set goals with client to make and keep appointments for postpartum and newborn visits to health care providers.	▪ Educate to avoid exposure to people with infectious diseases. ▪ Educate and follow up to assure that infant immunization schedule begins on time and continues through childhood.

Secondary Prevention

Early Diagnosis	*Prompt Treatment*
▪ The mother starts prenatal care early in the first trimester and continues care at regular intervals throughout the pregnancy.	▪ The mother does not use alcohol, tobacco, or other mood-altering substances during the pregnancy. ▪ The mother takes a daily prenatal vitamin with folic acid. ▪ Parents avoid exposure to people with infectious disease. ▪ The mother has adequate nutrition, rest, sleep, and exercise. ▪ The mother begins supportive services if eligible (WIC, Temporary Assistance for Needy Families). ▪ Family and significant others continue to be supportive. ▪ The parents attend labor preparation, infant care, and parenting classes. ▪ Name(s) is selected for the infant. ▪ Delivery method and location are selected. ▪ The home is prepared for the infant, e.g., adequate infant furnishings and supplies are acquired within the parents' budget. ▪ Preparations and plans are made regarding breast- or bottle-feeding. ▪ A pediatrician or pediatric nurse practitioner is selected. ▪ An infant car seat is acquired and properly installed. ▪ Plans are made to get to the chosen health care facility when in labor.

Primary Prevention

Health Promotion and Education	*Health Protection*
▪ The pregnancy is planned. ▪ Pregnancies are spaced 2 years (or more) apart. ▪ Mother has a positive attitude going into the pregnancy. ▪ A health care provider is chosen. ▪ There are financial resources to meet the expanding family's needs. ▪ Family and significant others are supportive. ▪ Mother's weight is as close to ideal as possible before conception.	▪ Parents do not use alcohol, tobacco, or other mood-altering substances when planning to conceive. ▪ The mother begins a vitamin regimen containing folic acid before the pregnancy.

WIC is not an entitlement program, but rather, Congress sets funding and eligibility requirements yearly (U.S. Department of Agriculture, 2018).

WIC provides information to parents about eating healthfully and promoting healthy rates of growth. Parents become more aware of the need to reduce consumption of saturated fat, salt, sugar, and over-processed foods. The C/PHN, through nutrition education, reinforcement of positive practices, and referral, plays a significant role in promoting the health of infants and young children (Box 19-10). For more information about WIC, see Chapter 20.

ROLE OF THE C/PHN

C/PHNs face the challenge of continually assessing each population's current health problems as well as determining available and needed services. Interventions are implemented for the maternal, infant, toddler, and preschool populations that focus on health promotion, health protection, and early intervention. Interventions may include work in family planning or high-risk clinics, telephone information services and hotlines, outreach interventions, child care consultation, or home visitation programs. The nurse uses educational and health coaching interventions when teaching family planning, nutrition, safety precautions, and appropriate health seeking or childcare skills. Such interventions involve providing information and encouraging client groups (parents and young children) to participate in their own health care. Other interventions include strategies in which the nurse uses a greater degree of persuasion or positive manipulation, such as conducting voluntary immunization programs, working in a lead screening program, encouraging smoking cessation during pregnancy, preventing communicable diseases, and encouraging appropriate use of child safety devices such as car seats. Finally, the nurse may use interventions that motivate people into adherence with laws that require certain immunizations or mandate reporting of suspected child abuse and environmental health standards violations, such as sanitation issues. Home visiting programs are effective in addressing needs of high-risk and hard to reach families (USDHHS, 2018). See Chapter 6 for new programs available through health care reform.

The C/PHN acts as an advocate and a resource for childbearing women and couples and families of young children. The nurse may be called upon to provide information to young mothers about infant temperament, sleep schedules, colic, parenting, discipline, toilet training, television or video choices, and nutrition and feeding. The nurse should be aware of federal, state, and local laws that preserve and protect the rights of children and families. Knowledge about educational, medical, social, and recreational services needed by young families is helpful. The nurse works to secure these services in the community. Ensuring that families have the resources to provide a safe and healthy environment for their children can take many forms. The nurse may lobby to change existing laws, initiate the effort needed to establish programs and services in the community, and teach families about infant safety or the importance of immunizations. The C/PHN also has skills of community and neighborhood assessment. These skills are vital to health departments and community-based organizations and primary care centers for development of programs needed for women and children (Aston et al., 2016).

SUMMARY

- Maternal–child health clients are an important population group to C/PHNs because their physical and emotional health is vital to the future of society.
- The United States does not fare well in comparison to other developed nations on maternal–child health indicators.
- Problems of substance abuse, STIs, and teen pregnancy can lead to less than optimal outcomes for newborns.
- Complications of pregnancy and childbirth, such as hypertension, gestational diabetes, postpartum depression, and fetal or infant death, offer opportunities for C/PHNs to provide education, outreach, monitoring, and support.
- IMRs in the United States are higher than those in many other countries around the world. Toddler and young child mortality and morbidity are often related to unintentional injuries
- Preventive services include immunization programs, along with quality day care and preschool.
- Health protection services include accident and injury prevention and control, as well as services to protect children from child abuse.
- Health promotion services include infant development through effective parent–child interaction, developmental screening, and services to children with special needs.

ACTIVE LEARNING EXERCISES

1. Using "Assess and Monitor Population Health" (1 of the 10 essential public health services; see Box 2-2), how do your county's statistics compare with those of others in your state on (1) infant mortality rates (collectively and by specific ethnic groups), (2) incidence of low birth weight and very low birth weight in infants, and (3) incidence of birth defects? What is the major cause of death among infants, toddlers, and preschool-aged children in the United states, in your state or local area?
2. Locate some national Web sites that give you current information about progress toward meeting some of the ***Healthy People 2030*** goals with mothers, infants, toddlers, and preschool-aged children. Are we making progress? What can a C/PHN do locally to promote meeting these goals? What needs to be done on the regional, state, or national level?
3. What is the major cause of death among infants, toddlers, and preschool-aged children in the United states, in your state or local area? What community-wide

interventions could be initiated to prevent these deaths? Select one intervention for each age group and describe how you and a group of community health professionals might develop this preventive measure.

4. Look at the pertussis, maternal mortality rate, and maternal–child health vital statistics in your county or community. What do these statistics tell you about your community's health? What other related statistics are important to gather to determine if your community is a positive and healthy place for childbearing women and young children?

5. Go to the Centers for Disease Control and Prevention Web site (www.cdc.gov) and look up the current childhood immunization schedule for children ages 0 to 4 years. How would you determine how to modify the schedule for a 30-month-old who is missing his last set of immunizations?

REFERENCES

Aitken, M. E., Miller, B. K., Anderson, B. L., Swearingen, C. J., Monroe, K. W., Daniels, D., ..., Mullins, S. H. (2013). Promoting use of booster seats in rural areas through community sports programs. *Journal of Rural Health, 29*(s1), s70–s78.

American Academy of Pediatrics. (2016). *Where we stand: Breastfeeding.* Retrieved from https://www.healthychildren.org/English/ages-stages/baby/breastfeeding/Pages/Where-We-Stand-Breastfeeding.aspx

American Academy of Pediatrics. (2017). *10 common childhood illnesses and their treatments.* Retrieved from https://www.healthychildren.org/English/health-issues/conditions/treatments/Pages/10-Common-Childhood-Illnesses-and-Their-Treatments.aspx

American Academy of Pediatrics. (2018a). *Abusive head trauma (shaken baby syndrome).* Retrieved from https://www.aap.org/en-us/about-the-aap/aap-press-room/aap-press-room-media-center/Pages/Abusive-Head-Trauma-Fact-Sheet.aspx

American Academy of Pediatrics. (2018b). *Blood lead levels in pregnant and breastfeeding moms.* Retrieved from https://www.healthychildren.org/English/ages-stages/prenatal/Pages/Blood-Lead-Levels-in-Pregnant-Breastfeeding-Moms.aspx

American Academy of Pediatrics. (2018c). *Car seat information for families.* Retrieved from https://www.healthychildren.org/English/safety-prevention/on-the-go/Pages/Car-Safety-Seats-Information-for-Families.aspx

American Academy of Pediatrics. (2018d). *How to prevent tooth decay in your baby.* Retrieved from https://www.healthychildren.org/English/ages-stages/baby/teething-tooth-care/Pages/How-to-Prevent-Tooth-Decay-in-Your-Baby.aspx

American Academy of Pediatrics. (2018e). *Screening recommendations.* Retrieved from https://www.aap.org/en-us/advocacy-and-policy/aap-health-initiatives/Screening/Pages/Screening-Recommendations.aspx

American Association of Poison Control Centers (AAPCC). (n.d.a). *Prevention.* Retrieved from http://www.aapcc.org/prevention/

American Association of Poison Control Centers (AAPCC). (n.d.b). *Working with AAPCC.* Retrieved from http://www.aapcc.org/working-aapcc/

American College of Obstetricians and Gynecologists (ACOG). (2013). *Committee opinion: Weight gain during pregnancy. Reaffirmed in 2016.* Retrieved from https://www.acog.org/clinical/clinical-guidance/committee-opinion/articles/2013/01/weight-gain-during-pregnancy

American College of Obstetricians and Gynecologists (ACOG). (2019). *Social determinants of health play a key role in outcomes.* Retrieved from https://www.acog.org/About-ACOG/News-Room/News-Releases/2017/Social-Determinants-of-Health-Play-a-Key-Role-in-Outcomes?IsMobileSet=false

American Dental Association. (2016). *Statement on early childhood caries.* Retrieved from http://www.ada.org/en/about-the-ada/ada-positions-policies-and-statements/statement-on-early-childhood-caries

American Diabetes Association. (n.d.). *Gestational diabetes.* Retrieved from http://www.diabetes.org/diabetes-basics/gestational

American Pregnancy Association. (2016). *Using illegal drugs during pregnancy.* Retrieved from http://americanpregnancy.org/pregnancy-health/illegal-drugs-during-pregnancy/

Anbalagan, S., & Mendez, M. (2020). *Neonatal abstinance syndrome.* Statpearls publishing. Retrieved from https://www.ncbi.nlm.nih.gov/books/NBK551498/

Aston, M., Etowa, J., Price, S., Vukic, A., Hart, C., MacLead, E., & Rande, P. (2016). Public health nurses and mothers challenge and shift the meaning of health outcomes. *Global Qualitative Nursing Research, 3*(2), 1–10.

Baruah, S., Haines, S., Hewitt, S., Holly, L., Jensen, P., Johnson, R., ... Olayemi, D. (2013). *Lives on the line: An agenda for ending preventable child deaths,* London, UK: Save the Children.

Bright Futures. (2018). *Developmental, behavioral, psychosocial, screening, and assessment forms.* Retrieved from https://brightfutures.aap.org/materials-and-tools/tool-and-resource-kit/Pages/Developmental-Behavioral-Psychosocial-Screening-and-Assessment-Forms.aspx

Bungay, V., Massaro, C. L., & Gilbert, M. (2014). Examining the scope of public health nursing practice in sexually transmitted infection prevention and management: What do nurses do? *Journal of Clinical Nursing, 23*(21/22), 3274–3285.

California Department of Public Health. (2019). *The congenital syphilis morbidity & mortality review toolkit.* Retrieved from https://www.cdph.ca.gov/Programs/CID/DCDC/CDPH%20Document%20Library/Congenital_Syphilis_Morbidity_and_Mortality_Review_Toolkit.pdf

Camacho-Gonzalez, A., Kingbo, M., Boylan, A., Eckard, A., Chahroudi, A., & Chakraborty, R. (2015). Missed opportunity for prevention of mother-to-child transmission in the United states. *AIDS, 29*(12), 1511–1515.

Center for American Progress. (2018). *Fact sheet: Child care.* Retrieved from https://www.americanprogress.org/issues/economy/news/2012/08/16/11978/fact-sheet-child-care/

Centers for Disease Control and Prevention (CDC). (2012). *National action plan for child injury prevention.* Retrieved from https://www.cdc.gov/safechild/pdf/National_Action_Plan_for_Child_Injury_Prevention-a.pdf

Centers for Disease Control and Prevention (CDC). (2015a). *HIV and substance use in the United States.* Retrieved from http://www.cdc.gov/hiv/risk/substanceuese.html

Centers for Disease Control and Prevention (CDC). (2015b). *One in 10 pregnancy women in the United States reports drinking alcohol.* Retrieved from https://www.cdc.gov/media/releases/2015/p0924-pregnant-alcohol.html

Centers for Disease Control and Prevention (CDC). (2016a). *Child passenger safety: Get the facts.* Retrieved from http://www.cdc.gov/motorvehiclesafety/child_passenger_safety/cps-factsheet.html

Centers for Disease Control and Prevention (CDC). (2016b). *Dual use of tobacco products.* Retrieved from http://www.cdc.gov/tobacco/campaign/tips/diseases/dual-tobacco-use.html

Centers for Disease Control and Prevention (CDC). (2016c). *National action plan for child injury prevention.* Retrieved from https://www.cdc.gov/safechild/nap/index.html

Centers for Disease Control and Prevention (CDC). (2016d). *National Center for Health Statistics: Birth weight and gestation.* Retrieved from http://www.cdc.gov/nchs/fastats/birthweight.htm

Centers for Disease Control and Prevention (CDC). (2016e). *STDs & pregnancy: CDC fact sheet detailed.* Retrieved from https://www.cdc.gov/std/pregnancy/stdfact-pregnancy-detailed.htm

Centers for Disease Control and Prevention (CDC). (2016f). *Weight gain during pregnancy.* Retrieved from http://www.cdc.gov/reproductivehealth/maternalinfanthealth/pregnancy-weight-gain.htm

Centers for Disease Control and Prevention (CDC). (2017a). *Child passenger safety: Get the facts.* Retrieved from https://www.cdc.gov/motorvehiclesafety/child_passenger_safety/cps-factsheet.html

Centers for Disease Control and Prevention (CDC). (2017b). *Early release of selected estimates based on data from the 2018 national health interview survey.* Retrieved from https://www.cdc.gov/nchs/data/nhis/earlyrelease/earlyrelease201705.pdf

Centers for Disease Control and Prevention (CDC). (2017c). *Gestational diabetes*. Retrieved from https://www.cdc.gov/diabetes/basics/gestational.html

Centers for Disease Control and Prevention (CDC). (2017d). *Seat belts: Get the facts*. Retrieved from https://www.cdc.gov/motorvehiclesafety/seatbelts/facts.html

Centers for Disease Control and Prevention (CDC). (2018). *Facts about birth defects*. Retrieved from https://www.cdc.gov/ncbddd/birthdefects/facts.html

Centers for Disease Control and Prevention (CDC). (2018a). *Adult obesity facts*. Retrieved from https://www.cdc.gov/obesity/data/adult.html

Centers for Disease Control and Prevention (CDC). (2018b). *Asthma in children*. Retrieved from https://www.cdc.gov/vitalsigns/childhood-asthma/index.html

Centers for Disease Control and Prevention (CDC). (2018c). *Autism spectrum disorder (ASD)*. Retrieved from https://www.cdc.gov/ncbddd/autism/facts.html

Centers for Disease Control and Prevention (CDC). (2018f). *Facts about birth defects*. Retrieved from https://www.cdc.gov/ncbddd/birthdefects/facts.html

Centers for Disease Control and Prevention (CDC). (2018g). *Immunization information systems*. Retrieved from https://www.cdc.gov/vaccines/programs/iis/about.html

Centers for Disease Control and Prevention (CDC). (2018h). *Immunization schedules*. Retrieved from https://www.cdc.gov/vaccines/schedules/easy-to-read/child-easyread.html

Centers for Disease Control and Prevention (CDC). (2018i). *Lead*. Retrieved from https://www.cdc.gov/nceh/lead/default.htm

Centers for Disease Control and Prevention (CDC). (2018j). *Pregnancy mortality surveillance system*. Retrieved from https://www.cdc.gov/reproductivehealth/maternalinfanthealth/pregnancy-mortality-surveillance-system.htm

Centers for Disease Control and Prevention (CDC). (2018k). RSV for *healthcare professionals*. Retrieved from https://www.cdc.gov/rsv/clinical/index.html

Centers for Disease Control and Prevention (CDC). (2018l). *Vaccines do not cause autism*. Retrieved from https://www.cdc.gov/vaccinesafety/concerns/autism.html

Centers for Disease Control and Prevention (CDC). (2018m). *When, what, and how to introduce solid foods*. Retrieved from https://www.cdc.gov/nutrition/infantandtoddlernutrition/foods-and-drinks/when-to-introduce-solidfoods.html

Centers for Disease Control and Prevention (CDC). (2019a). *Complications and treatments of sickle cell disease*. Retrieved from https://www.cdc.gov/ncbddd/sicklecell/treatments.html

Centers for Disease Control and Prevention (CDC). (2019b). *Learning from Washington's adverse childhood experiences (ACE) story*. Retrieved from https://www.cdc.gov/violenceprevention/acestudy/pdf/ACE_Case_Study_Washington.pdf

CDC (2019c). Oral health. Retrieved from https://www.cdc.gov/oralhealth/basics/childrens-oral-health/index.html#:~:text=1%20of%207%20(13%25),least%20one%20untreated%20decayed%20tooth.&text=Children%20aged%205%20to%2019,%2Dincome%20households%20(11%25).

Centers for Disease Control and Prevention (CDC). (2019d). *Pregnancy and oral health*. Retrieved from https://www.cdc.gov/oralhealth/publications/features/pregnancy-and-oral-health.html

Centers for Disease Control and Prevention (CDC). (2019e). *Preventing adverse childhood experiences*. Retrieved from https://www.cdc.gov/violenceprevention/childabuseandneglect/aces/fastfact.html?CDC_AA_refVal=https%3A%2F%2Fwww.cdc.gov%2Fviolenceprevention%2Fchildabuseandneglect%2Facestudy%2Faboutace.html

Centers for Disease Control and Prevention (CDC). (2019f). *STDs in women and infants*. Retrieved from https://www.cdc.gov/std/stats18/womenandinf.htm

Centers for Disease Control and Prevention (CDC). (2019g). *Substance use during pregnancy*. Retrieved from https://www.cdc.gov/reproductivehealth/maternalinfanthealth/substance-abuse/substance-abuse-during-pregnancy.htm

Centers for Disease Control and Prevention (CDC). (2020a). *Drowning prevention*. Retrieved from https://www.cdc.gov/safechild/drowning/index.html

Centers for Disease Control and Prevention (CDC). (2020b). *Fetal Alcohol Spectrum Disorders (FASDs)*. Retrieved from https://www.cdc.gov/ncbddd/fasd/

Centers for Disease Control and Prevention (CDC). (2020c). *Fetal Alcohol Spectrum Disorders Alcohol Use in Pregnancy*. Retrieved from https://www.cdc.gov/ncbddd/fasd/alcohol-use.html

Centers for Disease Control and Prevention (CDC). (2020d). *Human Immunodeficiency Virus (HIV)*. Retrieved from https://www.cdc.gov/breastfeeding/breastfeeding-special-circumstances/maternal-or-infant-illnesses/hiv.html

Centers for Disease Control and Prevention (CDC). (2020e). *Pregnancy mortality surveillance system*. Retrieved from https://www.cdc.gov/reproductivehealth/maternal-mortality/pregnancy-mortality-surveillance-system.htm

Child & Family Services. (2018). *Parent mentor*. Retrieved from https://childfamilyservices.org/parent-mentor-program/

Child Welfare Information Gateway. (n.d.a). *Home visiting programs*. Retrieved from https://www.childwelfare.gov/topics/preventing/prevention-programs/homevisit/homevisitprog/

Child Welfare Information Gateway. (n.d.b). *How to report suspected child maltreatment*. Retrieved from https://www.childwelfare.gov/topics/responding/reporting/how/

Child Welfare Information Gateway. (n.d.c). *Parent education programs*. Retrieved from https://www.childwelfare.gov/topics/preventing/prevention-programs/parented

Criminal Justice. (n.d.). *Postpartum depression, psychosis, and infanticide*. Retrieved from http://criminal-justice.iresearchnet.com/crime/domestic-violence/postpartum-depression-psychosis-and-infanticide/

Cystic Fibrosis News Today. (2018). *Cystic fibrosis stats*. Retrieved from https://cysticfibrosisnewstoday.com/cystic-fibrosis-statistics/

Dauber, S., Ferayorni, F., Henderson, C., Hogue, A., Nugent, J., & Alcantara, J. (2017). Substance use and depression in home visiting clients: Home visitor perspectives on addressing clients' needs. *Journal of Community Psychology, 45*(3), 396–412. doi: 10.1002/jcop.21855.

Davis, A. (2016). *Pregnancy 101: 11 celebrities who battled postpartum depression*. Retrieved from http://www.health.com/health/gallery/0,20448173,00.html/view-all

Dede, C., & Cinar, N. (2016). Environmental tobacco smoke and children's health. *Iranian Journal of Pediatrics, 26*(5), e5935. Retrieved from https://doi.org/10.5812/ijp.5935

Dulay, A. T. (2017). Preeclampsia and eclampsia. *Merck Manual*. Retrieved from https://www.merckmanuals.com/professional/gynecology-and-obstetrics/abnormalities-of-pregnancy/preeclampsia-and-eclampsia

Elflien, J. (2019). Fertility rate of teenagers in Canada from 2014 to 2018. *Statista*. Retrieved from https://www.statista.com/statistics/937516/teen-age-fertility-rate-canada/

Eunice Kennedy Shriver National Institute of Child Development and Health. (2016). *Back to sleep public education campaign*. Retrieved from http://www.nichd.nih.gov/sids/

Felitti, V., Anda, R., Nordenberg, D., Williamson, D., Spits, A., Edwards, V., ..., Marks, J. (1989). Relationship of childhood abuse and household dysfunction to many leading causes of death in adults. *American Journal of Preventive Medicine, 14*(4), 245–258.

Fortson, B. L., Klevens, J., Merrick, M. T., Gilbert, L. K., & Alexander, S. P. (2016). *Preventing child abuse and neglect: A technical package for policy, norm, and programmatic activities*. Atlanta, GA: National Center for Injury Prevention and Control, Centers for Disease Control and Prevention.

Freedman, D. S., Sharma, A. J., Hamner, P. L., Panzera, A., Smith, R. B., & Blanck, H. M. (2017). Trends in weight-for-length among infants in WIC from 2000-2014. *Pediatrics, 139*(1), 1–23.

Friel, L. A. (2017). Hypertension in pregnancy. *Merck Manual*. Retrieved from https://www.merckmanuals.com/professional/gynecology-and-obstetrics/pregnancy-complicated-by-disease/hypertension-in-pregnancy

Galiatsatos, P., Brigham, E., Krasnoff, R., Rice, J., Van Wyck, L., Sherry, M., ..., McCormack, M. (2020). Association between neighborhood socioeconomic status, tobacco store density and smoking status in pregnant women in an urban area. *Preventive Medicine, 136*, 106107. Retrieved from https://doi.org/10.1016/j.ypmed.2020.106107

Gilmore, J. H., Santelli, R. K., & Gao, W. (2018). Imaging structural and functional brain development in early childhood. *Nature Reviews Neuroscience, 19*(3), 123–137.

Global Burden of Disease 2015 Maternal Mortality Collaborators. (2016). Global, regional and national levels of maternal mortality, 1990-2015: A systematic analysis for the Global Burden of Disease Study 2015. *Lancet, 388*(10053), 1775–1812. Retrieved from https://doi.org/10.1016/S0140-6736(16)31470-2

Government of Alberta. (2018). *Child safety: Preventing drowning*. Retrieved from https://myhealth.alberta.ca/Health/Pages/conditions.aspx?hwid=ue5148spec

Gundersen Health. (n.d.). *Bereavement support*. Retrieved from http://www.gundersenhealth.org/resolve-through-sharing/about-us/

Hales, C. M., Carroll, M. D., Fryar, C. D., & Ogden, C. L. (2017). *Prevalence of obesity among adults and youth: United States 2015-2016. NCHS data brief, no 288*. Hyattsville, MD: National Center for Health Statistics.

Health Resources and Services Administration (HRSA). (April 2018). *Home visiting*. Retrieved from https://mchb.hrsa.gov/maternal-child-health-initiatives/home-visiting-overview

Health Resources and Services Administration (HRSA). (n.d.). *Prenatal—First trimester care access*. Retrieved from http://www.hrsa.gov/quality/toolbox/measures/prenatalfirsttrimester/

HIV.gov. (July 17, 2018). The global HIV/AIDS epidemic. *Global Statistics*. Retrieved from https://www.hiv.gov/hiv-basics/overview/data-and-trends/global-statistics

Homan, G. J. (2016). Failure to thrive: A practical guide. *American Family Physician, 94*(4), 295–299.

Illinois Department of Public Health. (n.d.). *Sudden infant death syndrome and infant mortality*. Retrieved from http://www.idph.state.il.us/sids/sids_factsheet.htm

Institute of Medicine (IOM). (2009). *Weight gain during pregnancy: Reexamining the guidelines*. Retrieved from http://www.iom.edu/Reports/2009/Weight-Gain-During-Pregnancy-Reexamining-the-Guidelines.aspx

Kapaya, H., Mercer, E., Boffey, F., Jones, G., Mitchell, C., & Anumba, D. (2015). Deprivation and poor psychosocial support are key determinants of late antenatal presentation and poor fetal outcomes: A combined retrospective and prospective study. *BMC Pregnancy and Childbirth, 15*(1), 309. doi: 10.1186/s12884-015-0753-3.

Kondracki, A. J. (2019). Prevalence and patterns of cigarette smoking before and during early and late pregnancy according to maternal characteristics: The first national data based on the 2003 birth certificate revision, United States, 2016. *Reproductive Health, 16*, 142. Retrieved from https://doi.org/10.1186/s12978-019-0807-5

Larson, K., Cull, W. L., Racine, A. D., & Olson, L. M. (2016). Trends in access to health care services for US children: 2000-2014, *Pediatrics*. Retrieved from http://pediatrics.aappublications.org/content/early/2016/11/11/peds.2016-2176

Lieber, A. (2018). *Postpartum depression: A guide to common depression after childbirth*. Retrieved from https://www.psycom.net/depression.central.post-partum.html

Maness, S., & Buhi, E. (2016). Associations between social determinants of health and pregnancy among young people: A systematic review of research published during the past 25 years. *Public Health Reports, 131*, 86–99.

March of Dimes. (2019). *Loss and grief: Stillbirth*. Retrieved from https://www.marchofdimes.org/complications/stillbirth.aspx

March of Dimes. (n.d.). *Abuse during pregnancy*. Retrieved from https://www.marchofdimes.org/pregnancy/abuse-during-pregnancy.aspx

Mark, A. M. (2018). Dental care during pregnancy. *Journal of the American Dental Association*. Retrieved from https://doi.org/10.1016/j.adaj.2018.09.006

Martin J. A., Hamilton B. E., Osterman M. J. K., & Driscoll, A. K. (2019). Births: Final data for 2018. *National Vital Statistics Reports, 68*(3). Hyattsville, MD: National Center for Health Statistics. Retrieved from https://www.cdc.gov/nchs/data/nvsr/nvsr68/nvsr68_13-508.pdf

Maternal and Child Health Bureau (MCHB). (n.d.a). *Historical timeline*. Retrieved from http://www.mchb.hrsa.gov/timeline/

Maternal and Child Health Bureau (MCHB). (n.d.b). *Healthy start*. Retrieved from http://mchb.hrsa.gov/programs/healthystart/

Maternal and Child Health Bureau (MCHB). (n.d.c). *Overview of funded projects*. Retrieved from http://mchb.hrsa.gov/research/about-projects.asp

Maternal and Child Health Bureau (MCHB). (n.d.d). *The Maternal, Infant, and Early Childhood Home Visiting Program: Partnering with parents to help children succeed*. Retrieved from https://mchb.hrsa.gov/sites/default/files/mchb/MaternalChildHealthInitiatives/HomeVisiting/pdf/programbrief.pdf

Ministry of Health and Family Welfare, Bangladesh, Partnership for Maternal, Newborn, & Child, WHO, World Bank and Alliance for Health Policy and Systems Research. (2015). *Success Factors for Women's and Children's Health: Bangladesh*. Retrieved from https://www.who.int/pmnch/knowledge/publications/bangladesh.pdf

Muscular Dystrophy Association. (2018). *Duchenne muscular dystrophy (DMD)*. Retrieved from https://www.mda.org/disease/duchenne-muscular-dystrophy

National Alliance to End Homelessness. (2020). *Children and families*. Retrieved from https://endhomelessness.org/homelessness-in-america/who-experiences-homelessness/children-and-families/

National Center of Shaken Baby Syndrome. (2020). *Learn more*. Retrieved from https://www.dontshake.org/learn-more#2019

National Children's Alliance. (2019). *National statistics on child abuse*. Retrieved from https://www.nationalchildrensalliance.org/media-room/national-statistics-on-child-abuse/

National Conference of State Legislatures. (2017). *Vaccination policies: Requirements and exemptions for entering school*. Retrieved from http://www.ncsl.org/documents/legisbriefs/2017/lb_2548.pdf

National Fire Protection Association. (n.d.). *Know when to stop, drop, and roll*. Retrieved from http://www.nfpa.org/public-education/resources/education-programs/learn-not-to-burn/learn-not-to-burn-grade-1/know-when-to-stop-drop-and-roll

National Head Start Association. (2018). *Head Start facts and impacts*. Retrieved from https://www.nhsa.org/facts-and-impacts

National Institute of Mental Health (NIMH). (n.d.). *Postpartum depression facts*. Retrieved from https://www.nimh.nih.gov/health/publications/postpartum-depression-facts/index.shtml

National Institute of Neurological Disorders and Stroke (NINDS). (2017). *Muscular dystrophy information page*. Retrieved from https://www.ninds.nih.gov/Disorders/All-Disorders/Muscular-Dystrophy-Information-Page

National Organization of Rare Disorders (NORD). (2016). *Duchenne muscular dystrophy*. Retrieved from https://rarediseases.org/rare-diseases/duchenne-muscular-dystrophy/

New York City Department of Health and Mental Hygiene. (2020). *Intimate partner violence*. Retrieved from https://www1.nyc.gov/site/doh/providers/resources/public-health-action-kits-ipv.page

Nurse-Family Partnership. (2018a). *The David Olds story: From a desire to help people, to a plan that truly does*. Retrieved from https://www.nursefamilypartnership.org/about/program-history/

Nurse-Family Partnership. (2018b). *Guiding theories: Three theories that guide the Nurse-Family Partnership*. Retrieved from https://www.nursefamilypartnership.org/nurses/guiding-theories/

Olds, D. L., Robinson, J., O'Brien, R., Luckey, D. W., Pettitt, L. M., Henderson, C. R., Jr., ..., Talmi, A. (2002). Home visiting by paraprofessionals and by nurses: A randomized controlled trial. *Pediatrics, 110*(3), 486–496.

Olds, D. L., Robinson, J., Pettitt, L. M., Luckey, D. W., Holmberg, J., Ng, R. K., ..., Henderson, C. R., Jr. (2004). Effects of Home Visits by Paraprofessionals and by Nurses: Age Four Follow-up Results of a Randomized Trial. *Pediatrics, 114*(6), 1560–1568.

Orr, C., Ben-Davies, M., Ravanbakht, S., Yin, H., Sanders, L., Rothman, R., Delamater, A., Wood, C., & Perrin, E. (2019). Parental feeding beliefs and practices and household food insecurity in infancy. *Academic Pediatrics, 19*(1), 80–89.

Parlakian, R. (2018). *What you need to know: Early intervention*. Retrieved from https://www.zerotothree.org/resources/2335-what-you-need-to-know-early-intervention

Promising Practices Network. (n.d.). *Infant health and development programs*. Retrieved from http://www.promisingpractices.net/program.asp?programid=136

Rudderown, L. C. (2019). STD and STI—What's the difference? *Nursing Center Blog*. Lippincott Nursing Center. Retrieved from https://www.nursingcenter.com/ncblog/january-2019/std-and-sti

Safe to Sleep. (n.d.). *Fast facts about SIDS*. Retrieved from https://www.nichd.nih.gov/sts/about/SIDS/Pages/fastfacts.aspx

Save the Children. (n.d.). *Global child protection*. Retrieved from https://savethechildren.org/us/what-we-do/global-programs/protection

Schmidt, R., Carson, P. J., & Jansen, R. J. (2019). Resurgence of Syphilis in the United States: An assessment of contributing factors. *Infectious Diseases, 12*. Retrieved from https://doi.org/10.1177/1178633719883282

Substance Abuse & Mental Health Services Administration. (2014). *Results from the 2013 national survey on drug use and health: Summary of national findings* (NSDUH Series H-48, HHS Pub No. [SMA] 14-4863). Rockville, MD: U.S. Department of Health and Human Services. Retrieved from http://www.samhsa.gov/data/sites/default/files/NSDUHresultsPDFWHTML2013/Web/NSDUHresults2013.pdf

Tabb, K., Huang, H., Valdovinos, M., Toor, R., Ostler, T., Vanderwater, E., ..., Faisal-Cury, A. (2018). Intimate partner violence is associated with suicidality among low-income postpartum women. *Journal of Women's Health, 27*(2), 171–178.

The Children's Cabinet. (2018a). *Why is quality childcare important?* Retrieved from http://www.childrenscabinet.org/child-care-resources/for-parents/why-is-quality-child-care-important/

The Children's Cabinet. (2018b). *Why is quality childcare important for school readiness?* Retrieved from http://www.childrenscabinet.org/wp-content/uploads/2013/04/School-Readiness.pdf

U.S. Agency for Healthcare Research and Quality. (2019). *HCUP Fast Stats—Map of Neonatal Abstinence Syndrome (NAS) among newborn hospitalizations*. Retrieved from https://www.hcup-us.ahrq.gov/faststats/NASMap

U.S. Department of Agriculture. (2018). *Women, Infants, and Children (WIC)*. Retrieved from https://www.fns.usda.gov/wic/women-infants-and-children-wic

U.S. Department of Health and Human Services. (2008). *State MCH-Medicaid Coordination: A Review of Title V and Title XIX Interagency Agreements* (2nd ed.). Retrieved from http://mchb.hrsa.gov/pdfs/statemchmedicaid.pdf

U.S. Department of Health and Human Services (USDHHS). (2018). *Home visiting*. Retrieved from https://mchb.hrsa.gov/maternal-child-health-initiatives/home-visiting-overview

U.S. Department of Health & Human Services (USDHHS). (2020). *Healthy People 2030: Browse objectives*. Retrieved from https://health.gov/healthypeople/objectives-and-data/browse-objectives

U.S. Department of Health and Human Services, Health Resources and Services Administration, Maternal and Child Health Bureau. (2014). *Child Health USA 2014*. Rockville, MD: U.S. Department of Health and Human Services.

U.S. Food & Drug Administration (FDA). (2018). *Use caution when giving cold and cough products to kids*. Retrieved from https://www.fda.gov/drugs/resourcesforyou/specialfeatures/ucm263948.htm

Udo, I. E., Sharps, P., Bronner, Y., & Hossain, M. B. (2016). Maternal intimate partner violence: Relationships with language and neurological development of infants and toddlers. *Maternal and Child Health Journal, 20*(7), 1424–1431. Retrieved from https://doi.org/10.1007/s10995-016-1940-1

University of Pittsburgh Medical Center. (2018). *Cystic fibrosis symptoms and treatment*. Retrieved from http://www.chp.edu/our-services/transplant/liver/education/liver-disease-states/cystic-fibrosis

Whitley, E., Gale, C., Deary, I., Kivimaki, M., & Batty, D. (2011). Association of maternal and paternal IQ with offspring conduct, emotional, and attention problem scores: Transgenerational evidence from the 1958 British Birth Cohort Study. *Archives of General Psychiatry, 68*(10), 1032–1038.

World Bank Group. (2018). *Mortality rate, under-5 (per 1000 live births)*. Retrieved from https://data.worldbank.org/indicator/SH.DYN.MORT?locations=BD

World Health Organization (WHO). (2016). *Global health observatory (GHO) data: HIV/AIDS*. Retrieved from http://www.who.int/gho/hiv/en/

World Health Organization (WHO). (2018a). *Fact sheet: Maternal mortality*. Retrieved from http://www.who.int/news-room/fact-sheets/detail/maternal-mortality

World Health Organization (WHO). (2018b). *Infant mortality: Situation and trends*. Retrieved from http://www.who.int/gho/child_health/mortality/neonatal_infant_text/en/

World Health Organization (WHO). (2020). *HIV/AIDS*. Retrieved from https://www.who.int/en/news-room/fact-sheets/detail/hiv-aids

Zero to Three. (2018). *How does nutrition affect the developing brain?* Retrieved from https://www.zerotothree.org/resources/1372-how-does-nutrition-affect-the-developing-brain

CHAPTER 20

School-Age Children and Adolescents

"Youth is the spirit of adventure and awakening. It is a time of physical emerging when the body attains the vigor and good health that may ignore the caution of temperance. Youth is a period of timelessness when the horizons of age seem too distant to be noticed."

—Ezra Taft Benson

KEY TERMS

Adverse childhood experiences (ACE)
Anorexia nervosa
Asthma action plan
Attention deficit hyperactivity disorder (ADHD)
Autism spectrum disorder (ASD)
Binge eating
Bulimia nervosa
Learning disorders
Obese
Overweight
Pediculosis

LEARNING OBJECTIVES

Upon mastery of this chapter, you should be able to:

1. Explain how poverty is a significant social determinant of health in children and adolescents.
2. Identify major health problems and concerns for U.S. school-age children and adolescents.
3. Discuss the relationship of academic achievement to health status.
4. Describe and analyze mortality and injury trends among school-age children and adolescents.
5. Evaluate *Healthy People 2030* objectives affecting children and adolescents and the barriers that may be involved in attaining these objectives.
6. Evaluate health promotion programs and services for school-age children and adolescent populations at the primary, secondary, and tertiary levels.

INTRODUCTION

According to Erick Erickson's developmental framework, the school-age and adolescent years are a time of task mastery and development of competence and self-identity. During these years, children grow physically, as well as emotionally and socially. They move from being under the total control of parents and families during the infant and toddler years to being more and more influenced by those outside the home—classmates, teachers, peers, and other groups (Hockenberry, Wilson, & Rodgers, 2019).

Poverty, a significant social determinant of health, poses a challenge to the health of many school-age children and adolescents. Other challenges for this population include chronic diseases, behavioral and learning problems, emotional and mental health issues, disabilities, injuries, communicable diseases, developmental issues, school concerns, and the risk behaviors characteristic of teenage years. This chapter explores the health needs of school-age children and adolescents and describes various services that address those needs, along with the community health nurse's role in assisting families with children.

SCHOOL: CHILD'S WORK

Children and adolescents spend most of their waking hours in school. The quality of their educational experiences (e.g., teacher–child interactions) can influence learning, and their academic success can predict future education, employment, and income. Therefore, their future success as tomorrow's parents, workers, leaders, and decision-makers depends in good measure on the achievement of their educational goals today.

Child health has been linked to school success—healthy children are found to be more motivated and prepared to learn (Centers for Disease Control and Prevention [CDC], 2017a)—and coordinated school health programs are linked to academic achievement (CDC, 2019a). This is well known to school nurses and community and public health nurses (C/PHNs) that work in schools.

In 2018, approximately 56.6 million school-age children and adolescents (5 to 18 years old) attended elementary and secondary schools in the United States. Of these students, approximately 50.7 million are educated in public schools and 5.9 million in private schools (National Center for Education Statistics [NCES], 2018a).

In 2016, the U.S. population aged 0 to 17 years was 51.1% White/non-Hispanic, 13.8% Black/non-Hispanic, 4.9% Asian/non-Hispanic, 24.7% Hispanic, and 4.2% all other groups (Federal Interagency Forum on Child and Family Statistics [FCFS], 2019c).

POVERTY: A MAJOR SOCIAL DETERMINANT OF HEALTH IN SCHOOL-AGE CHILDREN AND ADOLESCENTS

Although the United States is making strides against poverty, around 21% of children still live in poverty. In 2016, 44% of children under the age of 3 years lived in low-income families and 21% lived in poor households. Moreover, this burden of poverty is not equally shared among racial and ethnic groups. In comparison with White children, children of color are almost three times as likely to live in a poor household. One of every ten White children live below the poverty line and approximately one of every three Black, Hispanic, and Native American children live below the poverty line (National Center for Children in Poverty [NCCP], 2018).

Poverty has profound and lasting effects on children, as research has consistently shown over many years. In the most recent NCCP report, Dr. Heather Koball stated, "We're seeing promising movements in the year-to-year measurements of child poverty and economic stability.... But while the number of children experiencing poverty is on the decline, the rate of poverty for kids still remains stubbornly high, compared to the size of the population. Children are also more likely to suffer the material hardships associated with living in poverty; the anxiety, depression, and constant stress of being financially vulnerable leaves a lasting mark on children as they grow to adulthood, affecting earnings potential and health outcomes as adults" (NCCP, 2018).

Children living in poverty have poorer health overall and are more likely to experience:

- Chronic health condition (e.g., asthma, anemia)
- Injuries and accidents
- Behavioral problems, including academic failure, alcoholism, antisocial behavior, depression, substance abuse, and adolescent pregnancy
- Poor brain growth, neurodevelopment, and learning
- Developmental delay
- Exposure to environmental toxins, parental substance abuse and neglect, maternal depression, trauma and abuse, divorce, violent crime, low-quality child care, inadequate nutrition, and decreased cognitive stimulation and exposure to vocabulary in early childhood and infancy, all of which can contribute to social, emotional, and behavioral problems (Center for the Study of Social Policy, 2017; Van Ryzin, Fishbein, & Biglan, 2018)
- Lead poisoning
- Iron deficiency anemia
- Increased susceptibility to illness
- Family and community violence, leading to a view of the world as a hostile and dangerous place and mental health issues (Child Trends Databank, 2018a, 2018b)

Social determinants of health (SDOH)—which are the social, economic, and physical conditions in which children live—can affect their health and well-being; "Growing up in poverty is a powerful SDOH because it can affect children's access to many [of these] health-promoting conditions" (Francis et al., 2018, para 1). Children growing up in impoverished and unhealthy conditions can stress a child's response system, increasing the risk for poor physical, behavioral, social–emotional, and cognitive health (Francis et al., 2018). The relationship between lower socioeconomic status (SES) and poor health persists throughout childhood and adolescence into adulthood. Children who spend half of their life in poverty are 40% more likely to be living in poverty by the age of 35 years. As adults, these children are less likely to have completed high school and more likely to have lower occupational status and lower wages.

A classic longitudinal study, along with a series of preliminary studies, on the many stresses of childhood poverty (e.g., crowded homes/classrooms, inadequate child care, low socioeconomic status, family/peer problems) found that levels of the stress hormone cortisol influenced results on school readiness testing and affected cognitive functioning (e.g., impulse/emotional control, planning, attention), which, in turn, affects school success (Blair, 2012). For more affluent children, other stressors (e.g., divorce, learning disabilities, harsh parenting) can affect stress levels and outcomes. Continuing periods of high stress can lead to either high levels of cortisol or levels that are immediately high but then drop very low and that blunt children's responses to new challenges. Both those with blunted responses and those with very high cortisol responses were found to have lower executive function and more problems with writing, math, and reading, as well as poor self-control in class. The reverse was found for those with more characteristic patterns of cortisol response (elevated with a stressful event and then normalized afterward).

The children in this study were tested in Head Start and again in kindergarten. Parenting style was also examined, and parents of lower socioeconomic status were more prone to harsher forms of discipline that demanded obedience. Their children had lower executive functioning and either high or blunted cortisol levels. Parents using a more sensitive approach, who interacted with children during play and allowed more exploration, had children with better executive function and normal cortisol response. Researchers saw this as evidence that parenting style was an important part of child stress response. They noted that psychological stress in childhood "can substantially shape the course of their cognitive, social, and emotional development ... and impair specific learning abilities in children, potentially setting them back in many domains of life" (p. 67).

The negative impact of childhood poverty on learning and later income along with health continues to be well documented. Van Ryzin et al. (2018) indicate, "Researchers found that attaining economic security later in life did not completely attenuate this link between early poverty and health problems, suggesting that poverty and adverse social experiences early in life made the strongest contribution to negative long-term health effects" (p. 130).

Because the lifelong effects of poverty can be deeply rooted in children and adolescents, countering its effects requires a multilayered public health approach. Prevention programs that increase childhood nurturing have been shown to decrease behavioral, emotional, cognitive, and neurophysiological problem development and may be either family or school based.

Family-based prevention programs focus on teaching family management skills and improving family relationships. Change outcomes associated with these programs involve cultivating skills for monitoring and managing child behavior, negotiating conflicts, and improving overall family environment quality. Studies indicate that parenting programs can alter cortisol rhythms, improve stress regulation, and improve standard of living over time. One of these programs, the Nurse Family Partnership program has directly led to decreased use of welfare and other governmental assistance, improved employment for mothers, and improved birth spacing (see Chapter 4).

School-based programs focus on child development and the need to remediate the effects of low-income and deficient home environments. Change outcomes involve social–emotional and character development, such as improving decision-making skills, improving management of difficult situations, and establishing positive relationships. An example of a school-based program is Cooperative Learning, which focuses on instructional strategies and can be used in elementary, secondary, and postsecondary education settings. It involves group learning methods such as peer tutoring, reciprocal teaching, and collaborative reading. Teachers design their own small-group activities that focus on "positive interdependence." Members of the group are each responsible to achieve their goals and the success of the group. Such activities improve friendships, increase personal acceptance, and foster academic achievement (Van Ryzin et al., 2018).

Reaching families in need and disseminating programs to larger populations require policy initiatives and funding at the local, state, and national levels. Prevention programs can be implemented through improved access to health care systems. Using new technology strategies such as telehealth enables health service access and reduces provider-level barriers to health care. All of the strategies and programs discussed require ongoing evidence-based practice and community partnerships to educate public and policy makers, with the goal of disrupting the intergenerational effect of poverty (Van Ryzin et al., 2018). For more on poverty, see Chapter 23.

Several government programs and legislative reforms have provided assistance to the poor and attempted to help them move out of poverty. Welfare reforms enacted in 1996 (i.e., the Personal Responsibility and Work Opportunity Reconciliation Act) have been successful in moving many families from welfare to work. With a combination of welfare time limits, increasing work requirements/sanctions, and reducing financial disincentives for work, welfare reform and work success programs were projected to lead to greater employment. After 22 years, however, many are questioning whether the resulting safety net of Temporary Assistance for Needy Families (TANF) is adequate. The number of families receiving cash assistance through TANF decreased since its implementation from 68 of every 100 families in poverty receiving cash assistance in 1996 to 23 of every 100 families in poverty receiving cash assistance in 2016 (Center on Budget and Policy Priorities [CBPP], 2018). The majority of TANF adult recipients are single mothers with young children, and Hispanic children represented the greatest number of recipient children in 2015 (CBPP, 2018; Child Trends Databank, 2018a).

The Supplemental Nutrition Assistance Program (SNAP), formerly the Food Stamp Program, is one of the largest programs offered by federal Food and Nutrition Services. In 2016, the number of children receiving SNAP benefits was approximately 19 million. Positive health benefits for children are linked with SNAP. These positive outcomes include improved birth outcomes and improved adult health and self-sufficiency. However, the effectiveness of this program is also being questioned, as many families exhaust the resource by the end of the month and fall short of groceries (Child Trends Databank, 2018b).

Safety-net programs such as TANF and SNAP have demonstrated a reduced risk of nutrition-related problems (e.g., anemia, nutritional deficiency, failure to thrive), improved overall health, and decreased health care costs. They have also been associated with a reduction in the risk of child abuse and neglect. Research regarding SNAP and TANF programs suggests that increased evaluation is needed regarding the effectiveness at reducing poverty, the overall effect for children's health, and the use of health care services (Carlson & Keith-Jennings, 2018). Public insurance now covers the majority of poor and low-income children. In 2016, the rates of uninsured children reached an historic low, with only 5.3% of U.S. children lacking health insurance. Although Medicaid and Children's Health Insurance Program offer insurance coverage for low-income children, insurance premiums are associated with increased numbers of uninsured children (Dubay & Kenney, 2018; Kaiser Family Foundation, 2019). See Chapters 6 and 23 for more on insurance and vulnerable populations.

HEALTH PROBLEMS OF SCHOOL-AGE CHILDREN

The well-being of children is a concern both nationally and internationally. Many organizations have focused their resources on improving the health and well-being of children, including the World Health Organization (WHO), United Nations International Children's Education Fund, and U.S. governmental agencies, nonprofit groups, and charitable foundations. Unfortunately, the

BOX 20-1 *HEALTHY PEOPLE 2030*

Objectives to Improve the Health and Well-Being of Children

Core Objectives

EMC-01	Increase the proportion of children and adolescents who communicate positively with their parents
EMC-02	Increase the proportion of children whose parents read to them at least 4 days per week
EMC-03	Increase the proportion of children who get sufficient sleep
EMC-04	Increase the proportion of children with developmental delays who get intervention services by age 4 years

Research Objectives

EMC-R01	Increase the proportion of children with developmental delays who get intervention services by age 4 years

Developmental Objectives

EMC-D01	Increase the proportion of children who are developmentally ready for school
EMC-D02	Reduce the proportion of children and adolescents who are suspended or expelled

Reprinted from U.S. Department of Health & Human Services (USDHHS). (2020). *Healthy People 2030: Browse objectives.* Retrieved from https://health.gov/healthypeople/objectives-and-data/browse-objectives

needs of millions of children in the United States and worldwide remain unmet.

The *Healthy People 2030* framework for children is shown in Box 20-1.

Even in the wealthiest nations, many children face complex and often chronic health problems that cause them to miss school days or marginally participate in the classroom. Childhood is a critical period during which certain health behaviors or conditions can develop that can lead to more serious adult illnesses. The chronic health problems of children younger than age 18 years are characterized by the duration and persistence of symptoms and their impact on social functioning. Examples of chronic conditions in school-age children include:

- Asthma
- Autism spectrum disorder (ASD)
- Diabetes
- Neuromuscular disorders
- Poor oral health
- Seizure disorders
- ADHD
- Nutritional problems—anemia or obesity/overweight
- Food allergies
- Mental illness (CDC, 2017b)

Chronic Diseases

Stomachaches, headaches, colds, and flu are frequent complaints of school-age children. Common problems such as hay fever, sinusitis, dermatitis, tonsillitis, and hearing difficulties are also seen. Chronic health problems can affect a child's ability to learn and/or his or her physical and social development. Other more serious conditions, such as asthma, diabetes, hypertension, seizure disorders, food allergies, and poor oral health, have effects on academic achievement and educational attainment, affect the entire family, and can lead to developmental and social issues for children, as well as missed school days and eventual school failure. Understanding the influence of chronic diseases in children and families is key for public health and school nurses as they assist children and families in managing health (CDC, 2019a; Leroy, Wallin, & Lee, 2017; Miller, Coffield, Leroy, & Wallin, 2016).

With the prevalence of childhood chronic conditions increasing over the past two decades, approximately 25% of school-age children in the United States now have chronic health conditions and 5% have multiple chronic conditions. An increasing prevalence of asthma, food allergies, epilepsy, diabetes, and hypertension are common in the school setting (Table 20-1; Miller et al., 2016). Three common chronic disorders in children directly influenced by socioeconomic status and environment are (Food, Allergy, Research, and Education, n.d.):

- Asthma
- ADHD
- ASD

These chronic disorders have been evaluated according to social determinant influences such as poverty. Recent studies indicate that impoverished children have higher-than-average reported prevalence of asthma, ADHD, and comorbid health conditions. Prevalence of and comorbidities associated with ASD were comparable across income levels (Pulcini, Zima, Kelleher, & Houtrow, 2017).

In a study examining the prevalence and health care–related costs for children ages birth to 18 years with asthma, epilepsy, hypertension, food allergies, and diabetes; gender and ethnic variances were noted.

- Females had a higher prevalence of all chronic conditions except diabetes.
- African American children had nearly 50% higher rates of asthma than did White children, and the odds of having diabetes were 85% higher for White children than for Asian children and 60% lower for Hispanic children than for non-Hispanic children.
- Prevalence of epilepsy was higher in Hispanic children than in non-Hispanic children, and adolescents and children ages birth to 5 years had 29% greater odds of having epilepsy than adolescents aged 12 to 18 years.

TABLE 20-1 Prevalence of Common Chronic Conditions in School-Age Children

	Asthma	Food Allergies	Epilepsy	Diabetes	Hypertension
Percentage of school-age children with condition	7.3%–9.5%	4%–8%	0.7%	0.3%	0.17%

Source: Miller et al. (2016).

- Food allergy prevalence was comparable across races, with American Indian children and adolescents having the greatest percentage at 0.50% (Miller et al., 2016).

With the numbers of children with chronic conditions increasing, more children with significant health problems are present in schools (Leroy et al., 2017). Some children require specialized physical health care procedures, such as catheterization, suctioning, or ventilator care while in the school setting, even though school nurses are not always present in each school building every day (Toothaker & Cook, 2018).

The Individuals with Disabilities Education Act (IDEA) and Section 504 of the Rehabilitation Act of 1973 mandate that services must be provided for children identified as *disabled*. Many conditions may be characterized as disabling under these two laws, including autism, deafness or hearing impairment, blindness or vision impairment, emotional disturbances, mental retardation, specific learning disabilities, speech or language impairments, or other health impairments (e.g., ADHD, asthma). Once identified as disabled, children may qualify for special educational services. Children with chronic health conditions that can affect learning (e.g., diabetes, seizure disorders) may receive medications or other related services while in school to maintain health and promote ability to learn (U.S. Department of Education, 2018).

Many children with chronic health conditions take multiple medications at home and at school. This is a critical time for teens to develop schedules and optimal health behaviors. Medication adherence challenges can be particularly daunting for adolescents as they prepare to manage health as an adult. Common medication adherence barriers may include medication adverse effects, scheduling challenges, desire to appear "normal," and lack of family, social, or medical support. One recommendation to engage adolescents and improve medication adherence is the use of mobile technology-based interventions (Badawy, Thompson, & Kuhns, 2017). Home visits and consultations by C/PHNs and school nurses could also be helpful to parents and children or youth with chronic health conditions. See Chapter 28 for more on school nursing.

Asthma

Asthma is one of the most common chronic diseases of childhood. It is estimated that 8.4% of children younger than age 18 have been diagnosed with asthma. Childhood asthma rates steadily increased over the past two decades. Although reasons for increased asthma rates are somewhat unclear, experts speculate that better recognition and diagnosis of the disease, overcrowded conditions, and exposure to air pollution (indoor or outdoor), allergens, and irritants in the environment are probable culprits and may trigger asthma attacks.

Recent research indicates that prenatal and early postnatal exposure to environmental triggers and even prenatal stress and gender may increase asthma susceptibility. Children and adolescents with asthma may have attacks triggered by infections, exposure to cigarette smoke, stress, strenuous exercise, or weather changes (e.g., cold, wind, rain). Asthma disproportionately affects minority groups and families living below the poverty level (Bose et al., 2017; Miller & Lawrence, 2018; National Heart, Lung, and Blood Institute, 2018).

Children with asthma incur greater health care costs associated with increased emergency department visits and hospitalizations. Treatment for chronic asthma usually includes cromolyn sodium, leukotriene modifiers, inhaled and oral corticosteroids or long-acting beta agonists, and anti-immunoglobulin E therapy, but acute symptoms may involve inhaled beta$_2$ agonists and sometimes anticholinergics (National Heart, Lung, and Blood Institute, 2018). Asthma education programs are central to effective disease control and management. In 2018, the National Center for Environmental Health of the CDC published "EXHALE: A Technical Package to Control Asthma." The EXHALE program focuses on the following evidence-based strategies:

- E—Education on asthma self-management (AS-ME)
- X—X-tinguish smoking and secondhand smoke
- H—Home visits for trigger reduction and asthma self-management education
- A—Achievement of guidelines-based medical management
- L—Linkages and coordination of care across settings
- E—Environmental policies or best practices to reduce asthma triggers from indoor, outdoor, and occupational sources

School nurses and C/PHNs often work with students, families, and physicians to develop an **asthma action plan** to control, prevent, or minimize the untoward effects of acute asthma episodes. It is hoped that professionals in public health, health care, education, social services, and nongovernmental organizations will use the EXHALE program tools to improve asthma control/management and monitor and evaluate program success (Hsu, Sircar, Herman, & Garbe, 2018).

C/PHNs are in a unique position to implement many of the EXHALE strategies, especially education for children and their families. Education should include foundational asthma self-management (AS-ME) concepts including medication use, asthma self-management techniques, symptom recognition and appropriate treatment, and asthma trigger reduction.

Monitoring asthma medications and teaching proper methods of inhaler use are vital school nursing or C/PHN functions. Evidence indicates that AS-ME results in better asthma control, improved medication adherence, decreased health care costs, and fewer missed school days (Healthy Schools Campaign, 2018; Hsu et al., 2018).

Autism Spectrum Disorder

Autism spectrum disorder (ASD) is a complex developmental disorder frequently noticed within the first few years of life and typically lasts throughout a person's lifetime. The spectrum of ASD indicates that symptoms for each child varies and may range from mild to severe and from gifted to severely challenged (CDC, 2020a). A child's communication skills and interaction with others are most frequently affected, along with obsessive behavior and narrowed interests. Behaviors associated with autism include the following:

- Social issues such as
  - Does not respond to name by 12 months of age
  - Avoids eye contact
  - Prefers to play alone
  - Has flat or inappropriate facial expressions
  - Does not understand personal space boundaries
- Communication issues such as
  - Language problems—delay in language, repetitive use of words
  - Talks in flat, robot-like or sing-song voice
  - Does not pretend in play
- Unusual interests and behaviors
  - Is very organized
  - Has to follow certain routines
  - Fixation on objects and/or interests
  - Repetitive motions such as rocking or spinning (CDC, 2020a)

Autism has become an urgent public health concern with prevalence estimated at 1 of every 59 children by the age of 8 years. The disorder varies among racial/ethnic groups and communities with greater prevalence among males than females, and whites than minority group, although gender and ethnic prevalence differences are decreasing (Baio et al., 2018).

The yearly expense for autistic children is approximately $11.5 billion to $60.9 billion (2011 US dollars). This estimate includes a variety of costs including health care, special education, and lost parental productivity. Health care costs for children and adolescents with ASD are 4.1 to 6.2 times greater than for those without ASD, and when intensive behavioral therapy is required, the cost differential is even greater (CDC, 2020b).

The cause of autism is not clear—some genetic links have been found, but environment may also be a factor. There is a higher risk of subsequent children having autism in a family with one autistic child or a parent with ASD and for children born to older parents (CDC, 2020b).

ASD is frequently associated with genetic and chromosomal disorders, but the exact causes are not fully understood (CDC, 2020b). Through the CDC sponsored multi-year Study to Explore Early Development (SEED), additional autism risk factors are being identified. These include a family history of immune conditions and birth spacing (Croen et al., 2019; Schieve et al., 2018).

C/PHNs may come in contact with families dealing with autism through work in well-child or immunization clinics. It is important to assist families in accessing services for their children (early intervention is advantageous). It is also important to educate that parenting practices are *not* a cause of autism and that multiple, large-scale research studies on childhood immunizations do not indicate a relationship between immunization and autism (CDC, 2019b).

Diabetes

Although diabetes ranks lower as a prevalent childhood chronic illness, it is associated with significant complications and self-management challenges.

- Type 1 diabetes mellitus (T1DM) is usually diagnosed in early childhood and is the leading cause of diabetes in children and adolescents with non-Hispanic Whites having the greatest number of new cases.
- Type 2 diabetes mellitus (T2DM) is generally diagnosed later in life and associated with metabolic syndrome and being overweight. It is more prevalent in U.S. minority groups than non-Hispanic Whites (CDC, 2018a; Miller et al., 2016).
- Both type 1 (T1DM) and type 2 diabetes (T2DM) are found in school-age children, with T2DM rising almost exponentially in this age group, leading some scientists to call this a major public health crisis. This epidemic is thought to stem from increasing rates of childhood obesity, sedentary lifestyle, and the predisposition of certain ethnic groups (e.g., African American, Native American/Alaska Native, Hispanic/Latino, Pacific Islander) to the disease. A family history of T2DM and having one or more conditions related to insulin resistance also plays a role (CDC, 2017d).

A recent review by Mayer-Davis et al. indicates that the health burden of T1DM and T2DM among children and adolescents has increased substantially, especially among minority racial and ethnic groups. These findings are parallel to an increased prevalence of obesity and reflect an increased need for public health interventions to reduce the disease burden disparity. It is possible that variations in the prevalence of obesity will contribute to variations in insulin resistance and an increasing incidence of T2DM. Over time, there will be a substantial increase in U.S. youth with diabetes, especially in minority groups (Mayer-Davis et al., 2017).

Yoshida and Simoes (2018) discuss the increasing evidence about the relationship between sugar-sweetened beverages (SSB), obesity, and T2DM in children and adolescents. Their report indicates that the intake of SSB by children and adolescents corresponds with the rising obesity prevalence. Public health solutions that are all-inclusive and wide-ranging are needed to combat the obesity and T2DM epidemic. Programs that limit the availability and access to SSBs, improve the quality of all foods available in schools, and increase physical activity are being evaluated. Initiatives involving SSB taxation and healthy beverages subsidization are being considered.

It is hoped that such a program will increase revenue available for health promotion and develop awareness of SSB consumption health risks. Multiple challenges for these programs exist, including inconsistency among school wellness and nutrition policies, SSB substitution by other high-calorie drinks, increased student calorie intake at home, and opposition from the beverage industry (Yoshida & Simoes, 2018).

Research continues on the pathophysiology of diabetes and prevention strategies (e.g., lifestyle changes, causes of autoimmunity), as well as refining methods of diagnosis and treatment (e.g., insulin pumps, continuous glucose monitoring, closed loop systems).

- School-based interventions focusing on lifestyle modifications, weight loss, healthy eating, and exercise have effectively decreased T2DM risk factors short term. Additional research to determine long-term effects is recommended (Geria & Beitz, 2018).
- Studies regarding oral medication adherence in children and adolescents with T2DM demonstrate that self-management and medication adherence is similar to youth with other chronic diseases. Social and family support, pairing medication dosing with daily routines, and developing personal problem-solving skills improved self-management (Venditti et al., 2018).

Younger children with T1DM, especially those who use insulin pumps, may need careful monitoring, something that is not always possible for the school nurse assigned to several school sites. It is important for C/PHNs and others working with children and youth who have diabetes to consider their psychosocial needs, as well as their physical needs (Box 20-2). A multidisciplinary team approach coordinating family, school staff, and physician collaboration is optimal. See Chapter 28 for more on the school nurse's role with school-age children with diabetes.

Children and adolescents with diabetes may be reluctant to comply with their medical regimen, but strict adherence has proved to reduce later microvascular complications. Intensive insulin regimens are recommended for T1DM and for some cases of T2DM. Automated insulin delivery systems should be considered and glucose levels monitored multiple times each day.

Research is ongoing regarding the long-term effects of diabetes and best management strategies. It is important for school nurses and C/PHNs to understand each child's unique needs and circumstances and keep in mind a child's developmental stages. In addition to meeting the obvious emergency health–related concerns for diabetic children, it is imperative to teach children and families that proper diet, oral antidiabetic medications or insulin administration, physical activity, and blood glucose testing are vital strategies to keep blood glucose levels as close to normal as possible. This includes alerting teachers and school personnel to the signs and symptoms (as well as treatment) of hypoglycemia. Alerting teachers to these concerns may help them better understand the academic complications of this disease and ensure their support (Chiang et al., 2018).

The prevention of T2DM through education and improvement in exercise, nutrition, and lifestyle can be one of the most important areas of focus for health professionals who work with the school-age population—including C/PHNs who may come into contact with them during immunization or child health clinics (Box 20-3). Health education and health promotion to decrease

BOX 20-2 EVIDENCE-BASED PRACTICE

Emotional Impact on Children and Youth of Having Diabetes

Children and adolescents with diabetes (both T1DM and T2DM) cope with unique disease self-management and health challenges. They are required to pay stricter attention to their health and management of their chronic condition. In addition, there are emotional challenges such as anxiety.

In a descriptive pilot study, nurses Elertson, Liesch, and Babler (2016) explored expressing emotion through drawings by youth with T1DM. Participating youth were given a blank piece of white paper and asked, "If diabetes had a face, what would it look like?" A variety of emotions and self-expression were portrayed through pictures depicting sadness, tears, helplessness, frustration, and even monster-like images. Some of the drawings portrayed happiness, guilt, anger, judgment, and resentment. Some included written messages describing their experience with diabetes, for example, "Diabetes is my blood sucking monster"; "mad, angry, scared, it hurts"; and "diabetes has an effect on everyone, even people you don't think about" (Elertson et al., 2016, p. 36).

In another study, youth with T1DM are at increased risk of mental health symptoms. Nurses Rechenberg, Whittemore, and Grey (2017) wanted to better understand the emotional impact of children with diabetes. They conducted an integrative review of the literature about anxiety in youth with T1DM. Their research indicates that approximately 20% of youth with T1DM are positive for significant anxiety and depressive symptoms. The review evaluated health outcomes and anxiety-related symptoms including hypoglycemia fears, family conflict, glycemic control, depressive symptoms, blood glucose monitoring, general anxiety, quality of life, and interventions.

Rechenberg et al. (2017) found that it is important to distinguish the anxiety type when designing interventions. For example, state anxiety ("transient experience of the physiological arousal associated with feelings of dread and tension") has been more highly associated with depressive symptoms, and trait anxiety ("likelihood to respond anxiously to a stimulus") is associated with fear of hypoglycemia (Rechenberg et al., 2017, pp. 66, 69). Hypoglycemia fears are more prominent in girls and linked to poorer HbA1c levels and worse self-management. Social anxiety was associated with a poorer quality of life and decreased adherence. Promising interventions included behavioral–cognitive therapy and feasible implementations that strengthen connectedness among youth with T1DM. Adults (e.g., parents, caretakers, nurses) need to be aware of children's physical needs and offer assistance. They also must consider their emotional and psychosocial needs.

Source: Elertson et al. (2016); Rechenberg et al. (2017).

BOX 20-3 LEVELS OF PREVENTION PYRAMID

Prevention of Type 2 Diabetes Mellitus in School-Age Children

SITUATION: The public health nurse and children with type 2 diabetes (T2DM)
GOAL: By using the three levels of prevention, avoid or promptly diagnose and treat negative health conditions and/or restore the fullest possible potential.

Tertiary Prevention

Rehabilitation

- Monitor the child's health
- Work closely with the child, family, physician, and teacher to ensure proper follow-up
- Be alert to monitor for any possible complications (e.g., medication side effects)

Primary Prevention

Health Promotion and Education

- Continue to promote a healthy lifestyle that includes appropriate food choices, daily physical activity within the limitations of T2DM, and medication adherence

Health Protection

- Educate teachers on safety precautions for children diagnosed with T2DM in their classroom
- Monitor children taking medications for T2DM (e.g., over- or underdosage and adverse reactions)

Secondary Prevention

Early Diagnosis

- Teach older children to calculate their body mass index (BMI)
- Monitor BMI scores
- Yearly screenings for height and weight (calipers are useful)
- Complete health histories on at-risk children

Prompt Treatment

- Initiate referrals for health care provider follow-up in collaboration with parents of students at risk for T2DM
- Initiate referrals to health care providers in collaboration with parents of students with signs and symptoms of T2DM

Primary Prevention

Health Promotion and Education

- Educate to promote good nutrition and a physically active lifestyle
- Provide classroom contact in the early primary grades to encourage children to make good food choices
- Limit passive activities and increase sports and physical activity
- Teach older children how to make better food choices at fast-food restaurants

Health Protection

- Advocate for policies that limit access to sugary beverages and snacks at school and programs that raise awareness and family involvement in better nutrition and promote physical activity for families
- Organize T2DM prevention programs, focusing on healthy nutrition and physical activity

childhood obesity and sedentary lifestyles may help stem the tide of T2DM in children and adolescents (Geria & Beitz, 2018).

Seizure Disorders

Seizure disorders are fairly common in the school-age population. Epilepsy is a disorder of the brain in which neurons sometimes transmit abnormal signals. Epilepsy is considered to be one of the most common disabling neurologic conditions, and it is most common in the very young and in elderly populations.

Approximately 3.4 million people in the United States live with seizures, and of those, 470,000 are children (Epilepsy Foundation, n.d.). Lifetime prevalence of seizure disorders/epilepsy is estimated at 48 per 100,000, and new cases are most common in younger children and families of low-socioeconomic status.

Those with seizure disorders have an increased risk for developmental (ASD, delays), mental health (e.g., anxiety, depression, ADHD, conduct disorders), and physical comorbidities (e.g., headaches) (Epilepsy Foundation, n.d.).

Although there are some instances of intractable or drug-resistant epilepsy, many children diagnosed with seizure disorders/epilepsy can have their seizures controlled with antiepileptic medications. Treatment is based upon many factors including the type of seizures, history, and physical status. Vagus nerve stimulators, deep brain stimulation, and ketogenic diets are used in some cases after other treatments have failed (Mayo Clinic, 2018b).

Rectal diazepam is commonly prescribed for younger children and those with developmental disabilities, yet nurses are not always available to make an appropriate nursing assessment of the child before the drug is given to stop a seizure. Often, school staff is trained to give the emergency medication—highlighting the conflict between education laws and nurse practice acts (CDC, 2017b; see more on this in Chapter 28).

Parents may be reluctant to disclose a seizure diagnosis due to associated stigma. Children and adolescents with seizure disorders may feel embarrassed or be the victims of teasing or bullying. They may exhibit signs of school avoidance, or they may have problems learning. Seizure activity, along with the side effects of antiepileptic medications, may lead to problems with memory and learning, as well as changes in behavior. Moreover, seizures can affect short-term memory or language functions. Health care providers are in a position to educate and support families as they cope with the unique challenges of epilepsy (Benson, Lambert, Gallagher, Shahwan, & Austin, 2017; Kerr & Fayed, 2017). It is important to monitor medication adherence and teach school staff about first-aid measures for seizure victims. When teachers are anxious about having a child with epilepsy in the classroom, educational programs for them and other school staff members can be provided. Community health nurses or school nurses can help allay fears and promote appropriate and timely care.

Childhood Cancers

In 2017, cancer was the second leading cause of death from disease among U.S. children between infancy and age 14 years. Leukemias and brain, central nervous system, and neuroblastoma cancers are the most common types of childhood cancers. Childhood cancers, especially leukemias, now have better outcomes than ever before. Five-year survival rates for childhood cancers have increased by 0.6% each year since 1975 (Simon, 2018).

More children are surviving childhood cancers, and concern has shifted to later complications of treatment rather than about cancer recurrence. Survivors are at greater risk of cognitive and vision impairments, pituitary problems, delayed growth, and heart disease. Also, children who have been treated with chemotherapy and/or radiation may develop a second primary cancer, and the risk of leukemia may be increased (American Cancer Society, 2017a).

The cause of most childhood cancers remains unknown; however, high levels of ionizing radiation, Down syndrome, and other genetic syndromes (e.g., Beckwith-Wiedemann syndrome) have been linked to a higher risk for some childhood cancers. Pesticide exposure may be a factor, but research findings have not been decisive. Parental smoking may be linked to an increased cancer risk, but evidence for this is also inconclusive (National Cancer Institute [NCI], 2017).

Because many children return to school after initial hospitalization and treatment for cancer, school nurses or C/PHNs can help make this transition easier by educating classmates about cancer (e.g., it is not contagious), helping the children make necessary adjustments, and vigilantly protecting any immunocompromised students from communicable diseases (American Cancer Society, 2017b).

Behavioral and Learning Problems

Other childhood health problems, less easy to detect and measure but often just as debilitating, are those of emotional, behavioral, and intellectual development. Although these problems are not new, awareness and concern have increased as the rates of occurrence for other life-threatening childhood diseases have diminished. Emotional or behavior problems and learning disabilities are prevalent in childhood. It is estimated that one of every five children in the United States has learning and attention issues and yet only a few are actually identified (National Center for Learning Disabilities [NCLD], 2017).

Learning Disorders

Children with attention and learning issues come from all income levels and all nationalities (NCLD, 2017). **Learning disorders (LDs)**, also known as learning disabilities, are often recognized as the child progresses in school, and special education services may be needed. The cause of LDs is not known; however, differences in brain structure have been noted. Maternal alcohol or substance abuse during pregnancy, poor nutrition, childhood exposure to toxins, and traumatic brain injury may also contribute to LDs (Eunice Kennedy Shriver National Institute of Child Health and Human Development, 2018a).

Some LDs are apparent in early school years, whereas others do not present problems until early adolescence. Battles over homework, poor grades, acting out in school, or frequent child complaints about school, teachers, or schoolwork are often harbingers of LDs. Children with LDs are more likely to repeat a school grade, miss multiple school days, be suspended from school, and drop out (NCLD, 2017). Early identification and intervention are key to the success of a child with LDs. Students must first be carefully identified through specialized testing; then, special education or resource teachers can build on the child or adolescent's strengths while working to compensate for weaknesses.

The recently legislated Research Excellence and Advancements for Dyslexia Act and the Every Student Succeeds Act provide initiatives and strategies for early identification and response for struggling students (NCLD, 2017).

Common signs of LDs are (Eunice Kennedy Shriver National Institute of Child Health and Human Development, 2018b; NCLD, 2017):

- Reading problems (Fig. 20-1)
- Writing problems (fine motor control and handwriting; problems with spelling, grammar, punctuation, capitalization; difficulty controlling flow of thoughts)
- Math problems (problems learning and understanding concepts, missing steps or sequencing of problems, and placement of numbers in columns)
- Language problems (cannot quickly process what is heard, problems with multiple instructions, difficulty organizing thoughts and speaking in classroom situations)

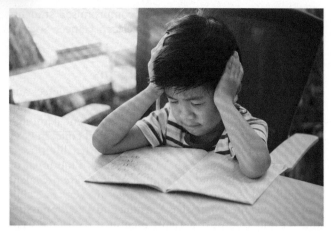

FIGURE 20-1 Reading is important to education and may be problematic for children with learning disabilities.

- Motor problems (problems with fine motor planning activities, such as tying, cutting, coloring; gross motor planning, such as jumping and running; trouble with visual–motor activities, such as hitting or catching a ball)
- Sequencing (getting letters or numbers out of order); organization (messy binders)
- Memory (difficulty retaining what was learned); abstraction (confused or not understanding what was said)

If LDs are not dealt with in childhood and adolescence, they can lead to later, more serious, problems related to employment, relationships, and quality of life in adulthood (NCLD, 2017). The C/PHN and school nurse can assist individuals and families in recognizing LDs and locating necessary resources. Some students with significant LDs may qualify for special education services, and school nurses can be helpful in facilitating this process along with teachers and learning specialists.

Attention Deficit Hyperactivity Disorder

Attention deficit hyperactivity disorder (ADHD), a common childhood disorder, is a cluster of problems related to hyperactivity, impulsivity, and inattention (National Institute of Mental Health [NIMH], n.d.a). The number of children with ADHD has increased over time; however, due to variations in testing and survey criteria, it is difficult to ascertain if percentages reflect the numbers of children with ADHD or the numbers of children diagnosed.

It is estimated that in 2016, 9.4% children ages 2 to 17 years had ever been diagnosed with ADHD, representing 1.6 million U.S. children. Of children with ADHD, approximately 62% were taking medications, 60% were being treated with behavioral therapy, and nearly 64% had a co-occurring condition such as anxiety, autism, depression, or behavioral issues (CDC, 2018b).

Diagnosis of ADHD involves a several-step process and should include reports from parents/guardians, teachers, and mental health providers if applicable. The primary care clinician generally makes the final diagnosis after considering all symptoms and reports, and ruling out other possible symptom causes. Boys are often recognized as having ADHD in early elementary grades, because they most often exhibit hyperactivity symptoms. Girls, on the other hand, are at increased risk for not receiving appropriate services because they exhibit lack of attention more frequently than hyperactivity (CDC, 2019c).

The exact cause of ADHD remains unknown. Research indicates, however, that a number of factors may be linked, including:

- Genetics and heredity
- Fetal exposure to cigarette smoking, alcohol use, drug use, or environmental toxins during pregnancy
- Childhood exposure to environmental toxins, such as high levels of lead
- Premature birth and/or low birth weight
- Brain injuries and/or central nervous system development problems (Mayo Clinic, 2018a; NIMH, 2018)

At each stage of development, those with ADHD are presented with distinct challenges. For example, children in elementary school may be involved in conflicts with peers and have problems organizing tasks. They may be more prone to accidents and may have more school-related problems, such as grade retention and suspension or expulsion. As adolescents, they may show less hyperactivity but continue to have restlessness, difficulty focusing, and impulsivity. These symptoms often continue into adulthood. Compared with non-ADHD teens, they may have more conflict with their parents, poorer social skills, and ongoing problems at school. They are also more likely to use tobacco and alcohol and have delinquent behaviors. As young adults, they are less likely to be enrolled in college and more likely to experience lower job performance ratings than their peers. In adulthood, they tend to have more marital and occupational problems (Mayo Clinic, 2018a; NIMH, 2018).

In a recent longitudinal cohort study, the frequency of digital media-use among adolescents was associated with subsequent ADHD symptoms. Researchers recommend that this area of research be expanded for further insights to ADHD causes (Ra et al., 2018).

Collaboration among the child's family, school, and physician is needed to diagnose ADHD and to plan appropriate interventions and educational accommodations. Although parents have a wealth of knowledge about the child, teacher confirmation of ADHD-related behaviors is very important. School nurses and C/PHNs can assist parents in recognizing the symptoms of ADHD and in obtaining appropriate treatment and follow-up.

A multimodal treatment approach is recognized as most effective. The main goals of medical treatment are to strengthen positive behaviors and decrease unwanted behaviors. Treatment strategies include medication, usually methylphenidate (Ritalin, Metadate, or Concerta), dextroamphetamine (Dexedrine), or combined dextroamphetamine and amphetamine (Adderall); school accommodations for learning problems; and social skills training for the child with ADHD.

Nonstimulant medications, such as clonidine, atomoxetine (Strattera), and guanfacine hydrochloride (Intuniv), are also used in children and adolescents (Mayo Clinic, 2018a; NIMH, 2018).

Family and individual counseling, parent support groups, and training in behavior management techniques, as well as family education about the condition, are also essential features of this treatment method. Recent research indicates that highly effective treatment includes group parent behavior therapy and/or individual parent behavior therapy with child participation (CDC, 2019c).

Parental resistance to treatment may result from side effects (e.g., problems with sleep, appetite, greater anxiety) or stem from fears about later abuse of substances. Alternative treatments that have been tried but not proven effective through research include yoga or meditation; special diets with decreased sugar and allergens such as wheat or milk, vitamin or herbal supplements, or increased omega-3 oils; and increased exercise (Mayo Clinic, 2018a). School nurses and C/PHNs can work closely with school staff, parents, and physicians in determining the efficacy of treatment regimens.

Behavioral and Emotional Problems

Good mental health is important to our overall health and well-being. Monitoring and understanding children's mental health is an important public health issue. Approximately 13% to 20% of U.S. children experience a mental health disorder each year. The lifetime prevalence of any mental disorder among 13- to 18-year-olds is 49.5%, and of those diagnosed, 22.2% have severe impairment. It is estimated that one out of every seven U.S. children between the ages of 2 and 8 years has had a diagnosed mental, behavioral, or developmental disorder (CDC, 2019d; NIMH, 2017).

Living in an environment where children are not safe or that undermines their stability or ability to bond—such as households with mental health issues, substance misuse, or separation due to prisons—can have lasting and negative effects on their health and well-being (CDC, 2020c). **Adverse childhood experiences (ACE)** are traumatic events that occur in childhood (ages 0 to 17), such as violence, abuse, or having a family member attempt or die by suicide. ACE is linked to mental illness, substance misuse, and chronic health problems; it can also negatively impact employment opportunities and education (CDC, 2020c). Associated conditions related to ACE (such as food insecurities or living in under-resourced or racially segregated neighborhoods) compound an already stressful environment, leading to toxic stress. As children grow up, they may have difficulty forming healthy or stable relationships, with these effects being passed on to their children; this chain reaction can result in such individuals or their children being more likely to perpetrate or be the victims of acts of violence (CDC, 2020c). ACE is preventable through education, strong economic support for families, legislation that protects against violence, and community support for safe and nurturing environments for children.

Of the millions of children living with mental health issues, ADHD (see previous section) is the most prevalent among children and youth ages 3 to 17 years. Children between the ages of 3 and 17 years of age experience additional types of mental health disorders including behavioral or conduct disorders (3.5%), anxiety (3.0%), depression (2.1%), ASD (1.1%), Tourette's syndrome (0.2% ages 6 to 17 years), and posttraumatic stress disorder (PTSD). Disruptive behavior disorders include oppositional defiant disorder (ODD) and conduct disorder (CD). Coexistence of ODD or CD with ADHD occurs in 1/3 to ½ of all children with ADHD. Males are more frequently diagnosed with both disorders as well as children of divorced parents and lower socioeconomic status. These children are more likely to be aggressive and hostile and have an increased risk of serious school or social delinquency. Early recognition, treatment, family support, school management, and child and family therapy increase the child's success (National Resource Center on ADHD, 2018). It is important to find referral sources for these children and their families, and this may be difficult in more rural or outlying areas.

Children are barometers of their environment. About 40% to 50% of couples in the United States divorce, and the second marriage rate of divorce are even higher. In 2016, 65% of children age 0 to 17 years lived with two married parents, 23% of children lived only with their mothers, 4% lived only with their fathers, 4% lived with unmarried parents, and 4% did not live with either parent. Children of divorce are more likely to exhibit behavior problems, with children who are products of highly contentious divorces most at risk (FCFS, 2019b).

Being aware of a child's family situation and living arrangements is helpful for understanding social, economic, and developmental well-being. C/PHNs can be alert to early symptoms and refer parents to marital counseling or suggest family therapists. Some schools also offer support groups for children of divorce.

School refusal, where a child develops a pattern of refusing to go to school or remain in school for the entire school day, is common in school-age children and differs from truancy. Unlike truancy, school refusal is commonly associated with symptoms of emotional distress—usually anxiety or depression—but may also be associated with oppositional defiant disorder, ADHD, or other disruptive behavior disorders. Often, the children complain of headaches, stomachaches, or other physical ailments, but some are motivated to miss school to gain parental attention. School refusal is most commonly found in children between ages 5 and 7 or ages 11 and 14. Transitional periods, such as school entry or moving to middle school or high school, are often the most difficult.

Children usually present to the school nurse or C/PHN with headaches and/or abdominal pains. They may throw tantrums, cry, or exhibit panic and fear to their parents in an attempt to stay home from school. Sometimes, children are afraid of something in the school environment (e.g., bullies, teachers, test taking), or they may have separation anxiety (American Academy of Child & Adolescent Psychiatry [AACAP], 2018). Family enmeshment or detachment, or high levels of family conflict, may contribute to school refusal problems, as well as parental anxiety disorders like agoraphobia and panic disorder (Maynard et al., 2015).

The best interventions include early return to school, with parental involvement in school, systematic desensitization (graded exposure to the classroom), relaxation training, emphasize positive aspects of going to school, and counseling being the most effective (ADAA, n.d.). If symptoms persist, evaluation by a mental health provider is recommended. C/PHNs and school nurses can serve as a liaison with the child, family, school, and health care/mental health care providers to promote a positive outcome.

Disabilities

In 2014 to 2015, the number of children ages 3 to 21 years served under IDEA was approximately 6.7 million—accounting for 13% of the total school-age population. Specific learning disabilities and speech or language difficulties were the two most common disabilities reported, followed by other health impairments (asthma, chronic illnesses), autism, intellectual disability, developmental delay, and emotional disorders. American Indian/Alaska Native children (17%) had the highest prevalence, followed by Black (16%), White (14%), Hispanic and Pacific Islander (both at 12%), and Asian (7%) (NCES, 2018b).

Many children with perceived disabilities or problems are referred for assessment and considered for placement in special education programs each year. School nurses often serve as a liaison between parents, physicians, and educators and are part of the team developing an individualized education plan (IEP) for children who qualify for special education services. Most children receive special services in a regular classroom because *full inclusion* or *mainstreaming* legislation mandates that fewer children be segregated into special classes or separate schools.

See Chapter 24 for more on clients with disabilities and Chapter 28 for more on school nursing.

Injuries

The loss of children's lives that results from all injuries combined suggests a staggering loss to society in the number of years of productive life lost. An injury is damage to the body, either unintentional or intentional, but use of the word accident is considered incorrect, as injuries may be prevented through environmental, individual behavioral, legislative, and institutional policy changes.

In the United States, unintentional injuries are the leading cause of death and disability for children between the ages of 1 and 19 years. Approximately 31.3% of deaths between age 1 and 9 years and 39.6% of deaths between age 10 and 24 years result from unintended injuries (Heron, 2017). Falls are the leading cause of injury between the ages of 1 and 14 years, followed by being struck by or against an object or person (FCFS, 2019c). Injuries not resulting in death often cause permanent disabilities or emotional and physical consequences for children and their families. (See thePoint for an infographic and a link to more information on falls in children and youth.)

Although injury death rates have dropped over the past two decades, injuries are responsible for approximately 75% of deaths during adolescence.

- Being struck by or against an object is the leading cause of injury between the ages of 15 and 19 years, followed by falls, motor vehicle crashes (MVC), overexertion, and being cut or pierced (FCFS, 2019d).
- During 2015, the leading causes of adolescent deaths were motor vehicle accident or firearms related (FCFS, 2019a).
- Suicide was the second leading cause of death of 15- to 19-year-olds during 2016 and homicide ranked third. Firearms were involved in 44.5% of teen suicides and 88.7% of teen homicides (CDC, 2020d).

Disparities exist among racial and ethnic groups. In 2014, homicide was the second leading cause of death among ages 1 to 24 years. In 2014, it was the leading cause of early death for non-Hispanic Black males, the second leading cause of Hispanic male death, and the third leading cause of death among non-Hispanic White males (CDC, 2017c). (See thePoint for an infographic and a link to more information on the homicide rate in this age group.)

Two public health concerns contributing to child and adolescent MVC are alcohol use and cell phone use while driving. A large-scale study examining the relationship between alcohol policies and fatal motor vehicle crashes (MVCs) found that alcohol was a factor in more than 25% of cases of motor vehicle fatalities involving children, adolescents, and young adults <21 years of age. Research indicated that restrictive alcohol policies are associated with reduced alcohol-related MVC among youth (Hadland et al., 2017).

Another concern for adolescents (and the general population) is use of cell phones while driving (Fig. 20-2). Adolescent cell phone use while driving has been legislatively banned in several states and yet reports indicate

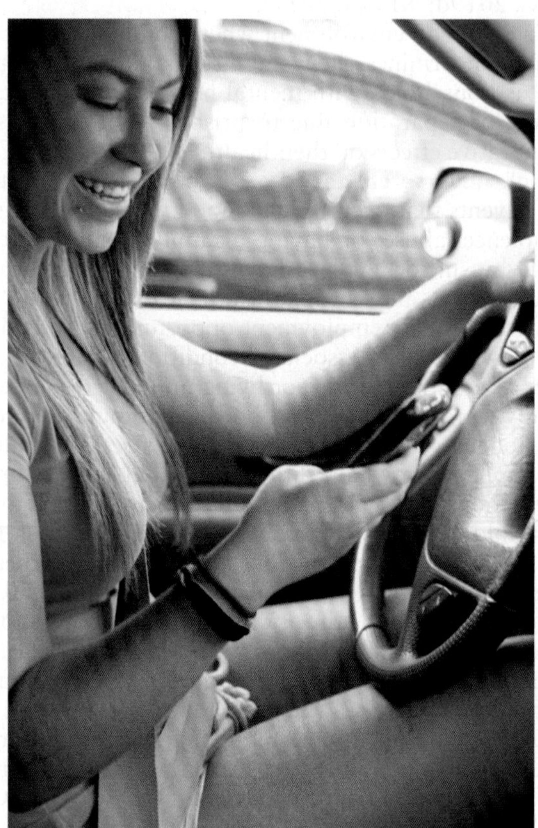

FIGURE 20-2 Cell phone use while driving—whether talking, texting, or using an app—is dangerous.

continued cell phone use while driving. Research investigating self-reported cell phone use indicates decreased handheld cell phone use but continued adolescent texting while driving—perhaps because of decreased visibility to officers and difficulty in enforcing bans. Increased education and intervention are recommended public health interventions for the adolescent population (Rudisill, Smith, Chu, & Zhu, 2018).

Cell phone use while driving is dangerous, especially for inexperienced adolescent drivers (Fig. 20-2).

In 2015 to 2016, approximately 69% of public schools reported one or more violent incidences. Fifty-seven percent of primary schools, 88% of secondary schools, and 90% of high schools reported violent incidents as defined by criminal incidents, violent victimization, and physical violence (NCES, 2017).

C/PHNs can promote injury prevention and control through education, promotion of safety engineering and environmental protection strategies, and legislative advocacy.

- C/PHNs can advance the prevention of unintentional injuries and deaths by working with families to initiate consistent use of seat belts and child safety seats in vehicles and the use of helmets and other protective gear for children riding bikes and skateboarding (Box 20-4).
- Where water is a natural hazard, wearing life jackets while boating and swimming can help decrease accidental drowning.
- Promotion of smoke and carbon monoxide detectors, poison prevention, and sudden infant death syndrome (SIDS) education can help to further decrease injury death rates.
- Teaching parents about presetting hot water heaters to lower than 130°F, recognizing the hazards of infant walkers, storing matches and lighters safely, and using pool fencing can help to prevent common unintentional injuries (Safe Kids Worldwide, 2018).
- Advocacy for stricter seat belt and child safety seat enforcement, as well as programs to provide child safety seats and bicycle helmets, has been shown to positively affect mortality and injury rates. Enforcement of seatbelt laws, graduated driver licensing programs, and adolescent education about MVC causes are also effective (CDC, 2020e).

Community health nurses can work with their local health departments and community action groups to provide seats and helmets to families who cannot afford them, organize clinics to educate about proper installation and use, and encourage local law enforcement to enforce seat belt and safety seat laws.

Communicable Diseases

The mortality rates of school-age children 5 to 14 years old are comparatively low and have decreased substantially over the last century, a reduction that can be attributed to the effective prevention and control of the acute infectious diseases of childhood, a significant achievement in the last century. Although mortality rates are low in this country, worldwide mortality because of communicable diseases continues with lower respiratory infections the most deadly. Globally, among children ages 5 to 14 years, the risk of dying from communicable disease has significantly decreased, whereas the prevalence of mortality related to injuries has increased to 25% (WHO, 2018b).

It is estimated that immunizations save 33,000 lives, prevent 14 million causes of disease, and save approximately $40 billion. The U.S. public health efforts (Healthy People 2030) focus on reducing vaccine-related illnesses and disease. School-age children must show proof of required vaccinations before they are allowed to enroll in school, although most states still allow exemptions for personal or religious beliefs (for information on which states allow religious and philosophical exemptions, visit: http://www.ncsl.org/research/health/school-immunization-exemption-state-laws.aspx). Vaccine hesitancy by parents has been linked to outbreaks such as measles; however, individual cases in 2017 to 2018 were similar to recent years (CDC, 2019e, 2020f).

BOX 20-4 STORIES FROM THE FIELD

Why Parents and Caregivers Are Inconsistent in Their Use of Car Restraints for Children

A leading cause of childhood injury and death continues to be motor vehicle crashes (MVC). The use of restraints (seatbelts, infant car seats, child booster seats) has been shown to be an effective population-level intervention that reduces fatalities and serious injuries (CDC, 2019k). I was part of a team of nurses, epidemiologists, and physicians from an eastern center for injury research and prevention who studied factors about parent and caregiver use of booster seats. Our goal was to understand why parents and caregivers inconsistently use car restraint systems. Our group designed a cross-sectional online survey with a convenience sample of parents in the United States. Survey participants were >18 years of age, spoke and read English, were the parent or caregiver of a child between 4 and 10 years of age, and had driven their child at least six times in the past 3 months. Participants answered questions about the situational use of car seats and booster seats with their child age 4 to 10 years and carpooling children. Our research found that parents and caregivers using booster seats did not fully restrain a child due to practical reasons more often than parents/caregivers using car seats did. Practical situations for not using a CRS included driving short distances, too many people in the car, and not having a CRS in the car. Decreased use of CRS puts children at a high risk of injury. It is imperative that health care providers continue to educate parents/caregivers and implement programs to promote CRS use.

—*Catherine, RN*

1. *As a C/PHN, what resources would you provide to a family with young children using a car seat?*
2. *What does the data in your community indicate regarding childhood morbidity and mortality for MVA? What strategies would work best for prevention in your community?*

Source: CDC (2019k); McDonald et al. (2018).

- Results from a 2016 national immunization survey revealed that around 90% of children between ages 19 and 35 months received vaccinations for polio, MMR, varicella, and hepatitis B.
- Non-Hispanic Black children were less likely to receive the full immunization series than non-Hispanic White children. Children in poverty, those covered by Medicaid, and children without insurance were also less likely to receive the full immunization series (see CDC for childhood immunization schedule, available at https://www.cdc.gov/vaccines/schedules/easy-to-read/child.html).

The National Immunization Survey–Teen (NIS-Teen) indicates that adolescent vaccination coverage in the United States has gradually increased. However, disparities continue with teens living in nonmetropolitan statistical areas undervaccinated (see CDC adolescent immunization schedule available at https://www.cdc.gov/vaccines/schedules/easy-to-read/preteen-teen.html).

Over the past several decades, the incidence of vaccine-preventable deaths has decreased; however, infectious diseases continue as a major cause of childhood illnesses, disability, and death. Vaccines are one of the most cost-effective health promotion services (ODPHP, 2018). Strong campaigns have been taken by health departments to get children immunized.

- Strategies shown to improve vaccination rates include the Vaccine for Children (VFC) Program, cost reduction, home visits, and linking vaccination opportunities with WIC visits.
- Public health professionals should continue to focus on eliminating socioeconomic barriers, strengthening school-entry requirements, and addressing vaccine misinformation.
- A Cochrane review by Jacobson Vann, Jacobson, Coyne-Beasley, Asafu-Adjei, and Szilagyi (2018) indicates that vaccination increases are seen in all age groups when reminders by telephone or text message, letter, or postcard are used. Combinations of reminders were also effective; however, reminding people over the phone are the most effective.
- Cancer prevention for preteens and adolescents through HPV vaccinations is effective. While HPV immunization rates have increased 5% from 2016 to 2017 with 66% of adolescents receiving the first dose to start the vaccine series, and 49% of adolescents completing all vaccinations in the series, there is still room for improvement. Parental resistance and a focus on vaccinating only girls can inhibit successful immunizations efforts in communities (CDC, 2018c).

Community-acquired methicillin-resistant *Staphylococcus aureus* (CA-MRSA) is another communicable illness seen in the school-age children population. C/PHNs and school nurses must be alert when skin infections or other conditions do not resolve quickly in children and adolescents. Sports teams, for instance, may spread this infection as team members come into close contact or use common-use facilities such as swimming pools. Referral to an infectious disease specialist may need to be considered (CDC, 2019f).

Pediculosis (head lice), another highly communicable disease, is a frustrating and common problem for many preschool and school-age children, and the incidence has been increasing with approximately 6 to 12 million 3- to 11-year-olds infected annually.

- Preschoolers and elementary-age children and their caretakers and family members are at highest risk for head lice.
- Close crowded conditions can also be a risk factor. Although lice are wingless, because children frequently play close to each other, they easily move from child to child.

Head lice may be white, gray, or brown in color—about the size of a sesame seed. They attach to the scalp and lay eggs (nits) in the hair. Nits typically hatch within 8 to 9 days. They reach adulthood during the next 9 to 12 days and live about 30 days. Without treatment, the cycle repeats every 3 weeks. Complete eradication generally requires that all viable nits be removed along with lice; family and close contacts should be checked for head lice and, if found, treated at the same time. Treatment typically involves over-the-counter insecticide shampoos (or pediculicides), such as pyrethrin-based *RID and Nix* or prescribed medications such as *Ulesfia, Natroba, or Sklice* (U.S. Food & Drug Administration [FDA], 2017).

School nurses and C/PHNs also need to educate families about reducing re-infestations by careful application of pediculicides, retreating in 2 weeks if necessary, and cleaning of any fomites (e.g., combs, hats, towels, sheets, clothing, and upholstered furniture) and removal of any viable nits. Drying sheets, blankets, and towels on high heat and washing all hats and clothing are effective measures. It is not necessary to use fumigant sprays, as they can be toxic (U.S. Food & Drug Administration [FDA], 2017).

Other Health Problems

Other health problems found in this age group include nutritional problems (primarily overeating and inappropriate food choices) and poor dental health. Obesity often begins in childhood and is a risk factor for CVD, diabetes, cancer, stroke, and osteoarthritis later in life. The percentage of children and adolescents has more than tripled in the last 40 years. Risk factors contributing to childhood obesity include genetics, metabolism, short sleep duration, eating and physical activity behaviors, and community environment (CDC, 2018d).

Food allergies can also play a role in poor nutritional status, especially with school-age children and adolescents. Researchers estimate that about 6 million children have food allergies, with teens and young adults being at greatest risk of anaphylactic reactions (Food, Allergy, Research, and Education [FARE], n.d.). Food allergies can be especially problematic in the school setting as strict avoidance of the food is the only way to prevent a reaction (see Chapter 28). It is recommended that parents and adolescents carefully read labels at the time of each use and that education systems have a plan to prevent allergic reactions and an response plan if an emergency should arise (CDC, 2018d; FARE, n.d.).

Dental caries is another common problem among school-age children. Approximately 18.6% of U.S. schoolchildren (5 to 19 years) have untreated cavities. In 2015, 84.7% of children age 2 to 17 visited a dentist during the year (CDC, 2017e).

Childhood Obesity

- About one in five U.S. children are obese, making childhood obesity a national concern. The CDC uses the term **overweight** for children and youth at or above the 85th percentile and less than the 95th percentile for youth the same age and gender. Children with a BMI greater than the 95th percentile are defined as **obese** (see Box 20-5 for an explanation and examples).
- Obese children are more likely to become obese adults and are at increased risk of chronic health diseases such as asthma, sleep apnea, bone and joint problems, metabolic syndrome, type 2 diabetes, cancer, and heart disease. They are also more likely to be teased, bullied, and suffer from social isolation, depression, and poor self-esteem (CDC, 2018d).

Preventive measures and early management of cardiovascular risk factors are now considered more effective forms of treatment than just clinical treatment of the disease complications after the fact.

- Multiple factors influence childhood obesity including genetics, decreased physical activity, increased television time, familial weight, poor nutrition knowledge, food insecurity, parental smoking, not having family mealtime, perceived neighborhood safety, and low economic status.
- Early childhood may be the best time to modify preventable factors influencing obesity. Studies recommend that health care providers begin discussing behaviors such as family mealtime and parental smoking with families of young children to reduce the risk of childhood obesity (Williams et al., 2018, p. 515).

Schools have been identified as a setting to promote healthy behaviors and provide nutrition for children. The Healthy, Hunger-Free Kids Act of 2010, authorized funding for foundational child nutrition programs at schools. A legislative goal was to provide balanced nutrition for children and reduce childhood obesity. Ninety percent of schools now report that they meet updated national meal provision standards, school lunch revenues have increased, and children are being educated to choose healthier food options (USDA Food & Nutrition Service, 2017). Centeio et al. (2018) examined the influence of the "Building Healthy Communities: Elementary School Program" on 5th grade children. This comprehensive program focused on physical activity, health education, and creating a healthy school culture. Study outcomes demonstrated decreased body mass index (BMI) and waist-to-height ratio (WHtR). School culture change and sustainability are predicted as school personnel were mentored to maintain the program (Centeio et al., 2018). Practice applying the nursing process to the problem of childhood obesity is shown in Box 20-6.

The causes of childhood obesity are multifactorial, and as a result, health care providers should take a multiple health behavior approach. Parental support and influence are key. Parents can help their younger children develop healthy eating habits by following recommendations of the American Heart Association (2018) and the CDC (2020g), for example:

- "Eat the Rainbow." Provide a variety of fruits and vegetables. Let children pick fruits/vegetables and have them help cook or prepare it.
- Choose lean meats, poultry, beans for protein.
- Watch out for added sugars. Avoid/limit sugar-sweetened drinks.
- Help kids be physically active at least 60 minutes each day (Fig. 20-3).
- Serve whole-grain/high-fiber cereals and breads.
- Serve low-fat and fat-free dairy products (two to three cups of milk daily).
- Read food nutrition labels—pick healthy nutritional foods.
- Be a role model—help your child develop healthy habits early (American Heart Association, 2018; CDC, 2020g).

The benefits of following a healthy diet, increasing physical activity, and maintaining a healthy diet are well-documented. Research has also shown that there is a link between obesity, cognition, and school achievement among children. A recent systematic review by Martin et al., (2018) explored the connection between cognition, school achievement, and school-based interventions to reduce weight and improve nutrition with child and adolescent obesity/weight. Their research indicated the following:

- School and community-based physical activity benefited cognitive function of obese or overweight children.

BOX 20-5 Explanation and Examples of Overweight Classification for Children and Teens

BMI is used as a screening tool to identify weight problems in children and teens. The criteria are different from those used for adults, as body fat differs between boys and girls and the amount of body fat changes with age. BMI-for-age growth charts for boys and girls are available at https://www.cdc.gov/growthcharts/clinical_charts.htm.

Weight Status Category	Percentile Range
Underweight	Less than the 5th percentile
Healthy weight	5th percentile to less than the 85th percentile
At risk of overweight	85th to less than the 95th percentile
Overweight	Equal to or greater than the 95th percentile

Source: Centers for Disease Control and Prevention (2018m).

BOX **20-6** C/PHN USE OF THE NURSING PROCESS

Addressing Childhood Obesity

James Lopez is entering 3rd grade. His teacher comes to you, the school nurse, because she is concerned about his poor performance in school. He frequently comes to school late and often puts his head on his desk and appears to be falling asleep. You notice that James has gained a significant amount of weight over the summer. His face is much fuller now than in his 2nd grade picture.

Assessment (Initial Visits)

You do the following:

- Call James' mother and make an appointment for a home visit.
- Complete a health history, noting family history of diabetes, current eating, activity, and sleeping patterns for James and the family, and determine whether he has a regular physician and insurance or Medicaid.
- Assess his vital signs, height and weight, hearing, and vision.
- Talk with James' teacher about his playground activity level and any signs of excessive thirst, hunger, or general fatigue.

Nursing Diagnoses

After a home visit, a meeting with James' teacher, and two observations and interviews with James, you decide a nursing diagnosis would look at:

- James' body requirements are more than what is required. James has a sedentary lifestyle, and he may be eating as a way to cope.
- Changes in the family's home life. Mother is single and attending truck-driving school necessitating several days' absence at a time. James cared for by a married teenage sister and her husband.

Findings, Plan, and Implementation

For the past 3 months, since his mother started her training, James has been eating large quantities of snack food and fast-food meals. He stopped participating in soccer and baseball because of lack of transportation. James' bicycle was recently stolen, and he now spends a lot of time playing video and computer games. James says that he misses his mother when she is away and that he "stays up late watching television" and has "trouble getting up for school" when he is at his sister's house.

You plan to work with the family to refer James to his physician to rule out diabetes. A family meeting is scheduled to provide health education on childhood obesity and inactivity. You discuss some possible interventions that the family can put into place:

- Decrease reliance on fast-food meals.
- Have a regular evening mealtime and encourage less snacking.
- Provide fresh fruit and vegetable snacks and decrease purchases of high-calorie, high-fat snack foods.
- Decrease sedentary activity (e.g., video and computer games, television viewing) and increase physical activity (e.g., team sports, walking, bicycling, active outdoor games).
- Establish a reasonable bedtime and consistently enforce it.
- Offer referral for family counseling so James can discuss his feelings in a safe environment.
- With the family's input, seek ways to improve contact between James and his mother and opportunities for his sister to improve understanding of good parenting practices.
- Meet with the teacher, family, and James to discuss ways to help with school performance.
- Continue to monitor James' progress with monthly height and weight checks, personal interviews, home visits, and teacher conferences.

Evaluation

The physician reported that James does not have diabetes; however, if he continues to gain weight and remains inactive, he is at a higher risk for type 2 diabetes. Evaluation of nursing diagnoses 1 and 2 includes the following goals:

- The family will report less reliance on fast-food and more meals cooked at home.
- The family will report more purchases of fresh fruits and vegetables and fewer purchases of high-calorie, high-fat snacks.
- James will report more physical exercise (by the use of a calendar) and fewer hours spent in sedentary activity (corroborated by family).
- James will exhibit less tardiness and fewer signs of sleep deprivation at school, and his school performance will improve.
- James and his family will complete sessions with a family counselor.
- James' weight will remain stable or will decrease as his height increases over time.

- School-based dietary interventions may benefit general school achievement.
- Nutritional diets at school can lead to improved general school achievement.
- Future studies should assess academic and cognitive outcomes along with physical outcomes.

Inadequate Nutrition

Poor nutritional status of schoolchildren is a global issue but also a problem in this country. Undernutrition can also have serious consequences, including effects on the cognitive development and academic performance of children and chronic health. Irritability, lack of energy, and difficulty concentrating are only some of the problems that arise from skipped meals or consistently inadequate nutrition. Infection and illness that lead to loss of school days can affect academic progress and interfere with the acquisition of basic skills, such as reading and mathematics. Food insecurity has been associated with child development problems, psychological and

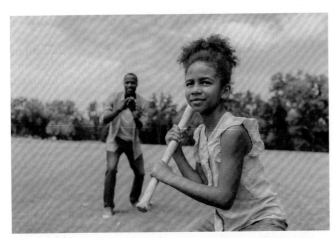

FIGURE 20-3 Physical activity is important for health and in childhood obesity prevention.

social issues, and poor general health (Shankar, Chung, & Frank, 2017).

- About 21.0% of U.S. households reported some degree of food insecurity in 2017, representing approximately 40 million people.
- Approximately 15.7% of households with children were food insecure, and of those headed by single women with children, 30.3% reported food insecurity (USDA, 2018).

A national study by Lee, Scharf, and DeBoer (2018) suggests that there is an association between food insecurity and obesity in school-age children (kindergarten through 3rd grade). A study by Rongstad, Neuman, Pillai, Birstler, and Hanrahan (2018) provide additional validation that there is a significant relationship between food insecurity and chronic diseases such as obesity and metabolic syndrome, ADHD, and anemia.

Undernutrition is frequently associated with poverty and hunger, but social pressure to be thin can also spark purposeful undernutrition. Because prepubertal children often exhibit a period of adiposity before a growth spurt, they are at risk for developing eating disorders. Along with childhood obesity, prevention of eating disorders is also a high priority in this age group.

- Some sources find pediatric eating disorders to be more prevalent than T2DM, and minority groups, boys, and younger children have higher rates. An estimated 5.4% of children between 13 and 18 years will suffer from an eating disorder. Of children with a lifetime prevalence of an eating disorder, 3.8% will be female and 1.5% will be male (James, 2017).
- The 2017 Youth Risk Behavior Survey indicates that 47.1% of students are trying to lose weight. The prevalence of trying to lose weight was higher in females than males, and higher among Hispanic students than White or Black students (CDC, 2017d).
- Yilmaz et al. (2017) indicated that there is increased prevalence of disordered among adolescents with ADHD. Authors recommend health care providers monitor youth with ADHD for disordered eating symptoms and early identification of eating disorders.

Research also indicates that youth with a history of obesity are at a higher risk of disordered eating. Signs of disordered eating include food rituals, refusal to eat foods once enjoyed, avoiding meals, overexercising, secret eating, preoccupation with food, calorie counting, fear of becoming fat, binge eating, and food phobias. Other concerning behaviors include depression, irritability, sudden mood changes, and anxiety around food and eating. Parents and health care providers alike should be aware of symptoms and seek evaluation of the child or adolescent (Dawson, 2017).

- School nurses and C/PHNs should be aware of signs and symptoms of this disorder, noting that T1DM children may be at higher risk, and watch for unexplained weight loss, stunting of normal growth patterns, concerns about body image, delayed puberty, and abnormal or restrictive eating.
- They can provide families with necessary information to promote healthful eating and exercise, as well as provide guidance for parental and child support (Dawson, 2017). Some school districts include BMI screening programs as part of healthy lifestyle promotion.
- The CDC recommends that schools have a series of safeguards in place before launching a BMI measurement program. This includes fostering a safe and supportive environment for all students and a comprehensive program to prevent and reduce obesity (CDC, 2017f).

Inactivity

An association between poor eating habits and physical inactivity has been found in numerous research studies. More television watching, fewer family meals eaten together at home, and living in an unsafe neighborhood were shown to be associated with overweight (Williams et al., 2018).

- The YRBS revealed that approximately 70% of children surveyed who were enrolled in physical education classes did not attend class on a daily basis.
- In addition, fewer than 15.4% of respondents stated that they were physically active for 60 minutes daily.
- About 22% watched 3 or more hours of television daily and 43% used a computer (other than for schoolwork) or played a video game on a daily basis (CDC, 2017d).

School nurses and C/PHNs can work with families to increase their levels of physical activity and to encourage limited television viewing for school-age children. They can also advocate for increased physical education in the school setting and for increased safe recreational opportunities in all neighborhoods.

Dental Caries

Dental caries is thought to be the most prevalent chronic childhood infectious disease.

- Caries affect 45.8% of children between the ages of 2 and 19 years with 84.7% of children age 2 to 17 years with a dental visit in the past year.

- Hispanic children have the highest rates of decay and non-Hispanic Black youth have the highest prevalence of untreated caries (Fleming & Afful, 2018).

The prevalence of dental caries in school-age children has decreased significantly since the early 1970s because of community fluoridation projects and the use of fluoride toothpaste. Fluoridated drinking water, the availability of school-provided fluoride rinse or gel, and dental sealant programs are cost-effective, proven methods of reducing dental caries in school-age children (National Institute of Dental & Craniofacial Research, 2018).

The peak incidence of dental caries is found among school-age children and adolescents, although the effects of decay are observed in adulthood as caries activity recurs or various restorations fracture or wear out and must be replaced.

- In 2016, 84.7% of children aged 2 to 17 years visited a dentist in the past year; but for children living in poverty, the percentage remains lower (FCFS, 2019e).
- Over time, these rates have improved with coverage through the State Children's Health Insurance Program and preventive programs such as community water fluoridation and the expansion of sealant programs.
- In a nationally, representative study of children and adolescents, Slade, Grider, Maas, and Sanders (2018) reaffirm the importance of fluoridated drinking water. Their study results support the continuation of community water fluoridation (CWF) policies and provide evidence for CWF as a key public health intervention.

Yet, access to dental care is still problematic. Barriers to dental care are more prevalent among the poor. Financial barriers, lack of education, and limited numbers of dentists accepting Medicaid lead to poor dental health values and adversely affect the appropriate use of early dental services and conscientious personal oral health care (Simmer-Beck, Wellever, & Kelly, 2017).

- A recent strategy for improving oral health of low-income children provided preventive services by registered dental hygienists in school-based clinics. Both adults and children are seen at the clinic; however, during school hours, at least 80% of the appointments were for children.
- Success of the program suggests that changes in licensing policies provide increased RDH autonomy in the public health setting (Simmer-Beck et al., 2017).

C/PHNs and other community health nurses working with school-age children and families can promote good dental health through education and advocacy, as well as through collaboration to provide adequate dental services to uninsured children and promotion of fluoridation and sealant programs.

ADOLESCENT HEALTH

Adolescence is a time of self-discovery, movement toward self-reliance, increasing opportunities, and pivotal choices that can affect the remainder of an individual's life.

- Adolescence generally begins with puberty and encompasses the ages between 10 and 24; it consists of early adolescence (aged 10 to 14), middle adolescence (15 to 17), and late adolescence (18 to mid-20s).
- Adult society largely segregates adolescents and often has ambiguous expectations for them. Adolescents are part of a subculture, one with its own language, dress, social mores, and values.
- The tasks of adolescence remain fairly constant: adolescents must become autonomous, come to grips with their emerging sexuality and the skills necessary to attract a mate, and acquire skills and education that can prepare them for adult roles, all while resolving identity issues and developing values and beliefs (ODPHP, 2018; Office of Adolescent Health, 2017a).
- The search for and expression of developing identity, along with the strong drive for social acceptance, are evident in the personal home pages and blogs of adolescents on social networking Internet sites such as Twitter and Facebook (Nesi, Choukas-Bradley, & Prinstein, 2018).

Adolescents and young adults make up 22% of the nation's population. Adolescents are generally healthy, but multiple health-related behaviors and social problems begin during this stage of development. Examples include mental health disorders, substance abuse, tobacco use, nutrition-related disorders, sexually transmitted diseases, unintended pregnancy, homelessness, homicide, suicide, and motor vehicle crashes (ODPHP, 2018).

- The leading causes of morbidity and mortality for U.S. youth are related to health risk-taking behaviors. Six health-related adolescent and young adult behaviors are monitored by the Youth Risk Behavior Surveillance System (YRBSS). These include behaviors contributing to unintentional injuries and violence; tobacco use, alcohol use, and substance abuse; sexual behaviors including unintended pregnancy and sexually transmitted diseases; dietary behaviors; and physical activity.

During the period that generally encompasses the teen years, adolescents encounter many complex changes physically, emotionally, cognitively, and socially. Rapid and major developmental adjustments create a variety of stresses with concomitant problems that have an impact on health and risk-taking.

- Because the amygdala influences adolescent brains more than the frontal cortex, teens base their decisions more on emotion—solving problems differently than adults. As a result, it is important to guide adolescents through the decision-making process before they engage in risky behaviors.
- The U.S. Office of Adolescent Health (2018a) explains that in stressful situations, adolescents are more likely to:
  - Think one way but act or feel differently
  - Misinterpret social cues
  - Participate in risky behaviors

Unintentional injuries were the leading cause of death in the 10- to 24-year age group. Most deaths in this adolescent/young adult age group are due to preventable causes.

- In 2016, 74% of adolescent deaths related to injury, with motor vehicle collision (MCV) accounting for approximately 22% of deaths, unintentional injuries (20%), suicide (17%), and homicide (15%).
- Although MVC deaths have decreased, they remain a significant cause of injury with adolescents and young adult drivers disproportionately represented in the data (Figs. 20-4 and 20-5). Teen males are two times more likely to be involved in an MVC than female adolescents are.
- In 2017, 5.5% of U.S. students reported using alcohol while driving, 13% of students reported using marijuana while driving, and 39.2% of students reported texting or e-mailing while driving a car (Kann et al., 2018).

Public health interventions are key to reducing teen injuries. A recent study investigated the effectiveness of the Save A Life Tour (SALT) program implemented in high schools. SALT is a safe-driving awareness program designed to educate about the harmful effects of distracted driving and drunk driving. Researchers concluded that that annual education regarding teen driving while intoxicated or distracted might reduce the morbidity and mortality associated with MVC. Key components of the program were to deliver a clear message of dangers and provide ongoing education (Layba, Griffin, Jupiter, Mathers, & Mileski, 2017).

Unintentional injuries also cause the greatest level of adolescent morbidity; the largest cause being transportation (drivers and passengers, bicyclists, pedestrians). Other causes include being struck by/against something, falling, poisoning, overexertion, and cutting/piercing.

- Emergency rooms treat approximately 22,000 children daily for nonfatal injuries. These injuries are highest among adolescents aged 15 to 19 years and can have a lasting effect for the children, their families, and society.
- The most common cause of unintentional injury for 10- to 19-year-olds (250,000 youth) is assault—being struck by/against, sexual assault, cut/pierce, and firearms. It is important to note that disparities exist between race/ethnicity.
- Black youth are significantly more at risk of homicide. This may be related to social determinants of health such as poverty, neighborhood crime, limited educational and occupational opportunities, and racism (Ballesteros, Williams, Mack, Simon, & Sleet, 2018).

Social stressors and strained relations with peers and parents are also linked to adolescent health complaints.

- Common complaints of adolescents include sleep deprivation, fatigue, chronic insomnia, acne, and concerns about weight and body image (Hockenberry et al., 2019). As children become adolescents, their sleep patterns change—they move from early risers/sleepers to staying up later and sleeping in later or catching up on sleep over weekends. This transition becomes more apparent through high school.
- Scientists believe that these changes in circadian and homeostatic sleep regulation support this delayed sleep phase, and there are concerns about consistent lack of sleep (Hale & Troxel, 2018).

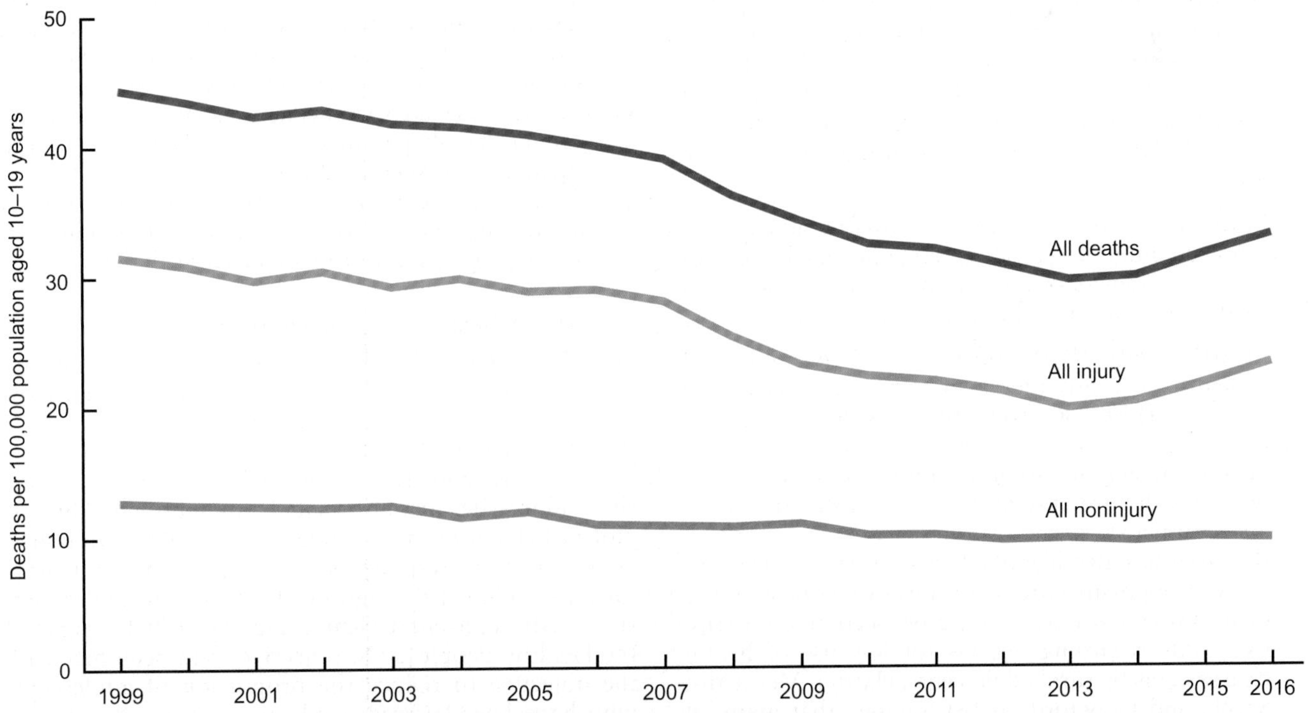

FIGURE 20-4 Total injury and noninjury death rates for children and adolescents aged 10 to 19 years: United States, 1999 to 2016. (Reprinted from CDC. [2018]. *Recent increases in injury mortality among children and adolescents aged 10 to 19 years in the United States, 1999–2016*. Retrieved from https://www.cdc.gov/nchs/data/nvsr/nvsr67/nvsr67_04.pdf)

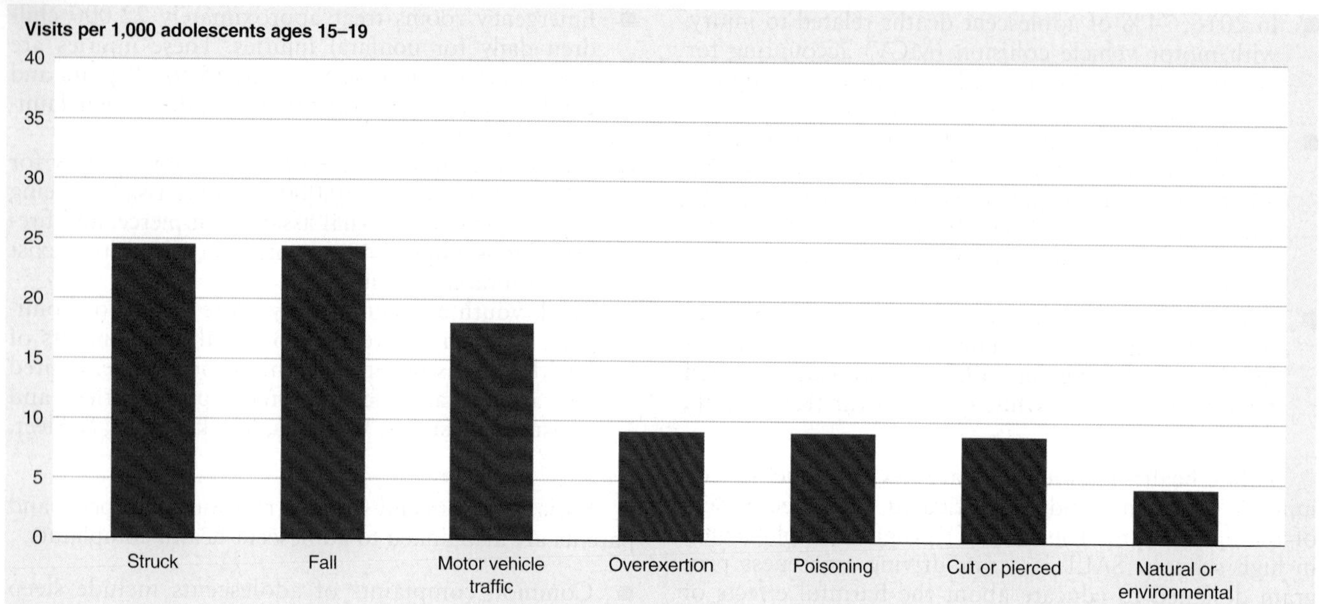

FIGURE 20-5 Emergency department visit rates for adolescents ages 15 to 19 by leading cause of injury, 2014 to 2015. (Reprinted from https://www.childstats.gov/americaschildren/phys_fig.asp#phy8b)

- Recent studies confirm the support for delaying adolescent school start times and indicate several health risks associated with sleep deprivation including being overweight, drinking alcohol, using drugs and tobacco, and poor academic performance (CDC, 2018e).
- A review of literature showed support for delayed start time for adolescents with improvement seen in attendance and tardiness, less falling asleep in class, improvement in grades, and reduction in MVA (Wheaton, Chapman, & Croft, 2016). Even modest delay times can be beneficial for student outcomes and supports development of evidenced-based policies for school districts and communities. Hale and Troxel (2018) suggested that, based on confirming research, later school times are also a social justice issue.

In the past, routine health care visits by adolescents were not commonplace. Newer recommended vaccines and better awareness of the health needs of adolescents have led to improvement, but concerns remain.

- In 2016, only 19.4% of 12- to 17-year-olds had a health care provider visit within the past year (CDC, 2017g). Reasons for underutilization of health care services may be related to lack of transportation, lack of parental support, past experience with health care system, lack of health care insurance, and cost.
- Research has also identified trust of health care providers as a possible reason for low or inconsistent use of health care services. In a cross-sectional, descriptive study regarding reasons for low use of health care systems by rural adolescents, Hardin, McCarthy, Speck, and Crawford (2018) founded that many of the barriers regarding adolescent access to care were resolved by a school-based health clinic.

Health literacy during adolescence is another important consideration. Teens are frequent users of mass media (Internet, television, radio, text messaging), and specific health-related educational interventions can be targeted to them by using these media. Although social media offers benefits such as health education, it can also put youth at risk for exposure to violence and risky behavior examples, opportunistic bullying, sexually explicit material, sexual solicitation, and Internet addiction.

- Research estimates that 92% of teens are online daily, with 88% belonging to at least one social networking site, and 88% having access to a cell phone.
- Increased use of social media designates it as a unique context that shapes an adolescent's behavior and life experience (Nesi et al., 2018).
- C/PHNs can help young people find reliable sources of information, as well as work with families to ensure proper monitoring of social media use.

Health Objectives for Adolescents

Healthy People 2030 objectives are focused on improving the health of all Americans. Goals and objectives for adolescent health have been developed (Box 20-7). Because much of the mortality and morbidity in this age group stems from risk-taking behaviors, many objectives addressing alcohol-related unintentional injuries, violent behaviors, and suicide and mental health issues, as well as more responsible reproductive health behaviors, are included throughout the document under Substance Abuse, Mental Health, etc. As of 2017, eight of the Healthy People 2020 objectives had been met with the objective to reduce the proportion of adolescents who have been offered, sold, or given an illegal drug on school property being met for the first time (Kann et al., 2018).

BOX **20-7** *HEALTHY PEOPLE 2030*

Objectives to Improve the Health and Well-Being of Adolescents

Core Objectives

AH-01	Increase the proportion of adolescents who had a preventative health care visit in the past year
AH-02	Increase the proportion of adolescents who speak privately with a provider at a preventative medical visit
AH-03	Increase the proportion of adolescents who have an adult they can talk to about serious problems
AH-05	Increase the proportion of 4th-graders with reading skills at or above the proficient level
AH-06	Increase the proportion of 4th-graders with math skills at or above the proficient level
AH-07	Reduce chronic school absence among early adolescents
AH-08	Increase the proportion of high school students who graduate in 4 years

Developmental Objectives

AH-D01	Increase the proportion of trauma informed early childcare settings and elementary and secondary schools
EMS-D04	Increase the proportion of children and adolescents who get appopriate treatment for anxiety or depression
EMC-D05	Increase the proportion of children and adolescents who get appropriate treatment for behavioral problems

Research Objectives

AH-R02	Increase the proportion of adolescents in foster care who show signs of being ready for adulthood
AH-R04	Increase the proportion of 8th-graders with reading skills at or above the proficient level
AH-R05	Increase the proportion of 8th-graders with math skills at or above the proficient level
AH-R06	Increase the proportion of youth with special health care needs, ages 12–17, who receive services to support their transition to adult health care
AH-R07	Increase the proportion of secondary schools with a start tie of 8:30 AM or later
AH-R08	Increase the proportion of secondary school with a full-time registered nurse
AH-R09	Increase the proportion of public schools with a counselor, social worker, and psychologist

Reprinted from U.S. Department of Health & Human Services (USDHHS). (2020). *Healthy People 2030: Browse objectives.* Retrieved from https://health.gov/healthypeople/objectives-and-data/browse-objectives

Emotional Problems and Suicide

The adolescent years are a time of rapid growth and change. Complex developmental changes physically, emotionally, cognitively, and socially may cause a teen to be emotional and unpredictable at times (Office of Adolescent Health, 2018a). The influence of peers increases, and peer pressure may influence behavior. Teens test family rules and generally search for their own identity and individuality apart from the family. Most parents and teens ride out this period with love and understanding and no long-term negative effects. For some children, however, a real or perceived lack of emotional support can lead to temporary or permanent emotional problems. Additionally, increased risk behaviors such as suicide, risky sexual behavior, and mental health disorders are associated with child and adolescent maltreatment. Because adolescents have less contact with the health care system than children, many conditions may go undetected. The transition from high school into early adulthood is often difficult and individuals with mental health issues often have worse outcomes than those with physical conditions (Jordan et al., 2018; Office of Adolescent Health, 2018a).

- Depression, anxiety disorders, and eating disorders may first appear during adolescence. It is estimated that one in five adolescents have mental health disorders with depression being the most commonly reported diagnosis.

- Prevalence rates of depression vary (Fig. 20-6). About 35% of high school students report feelings of sadness or hopelessness every day for longer than 2 weeks. Of those reporting symptoms, 41.1% are female and 21.4% are male.
- Anxiety disorders such as OCD, posttraumatic stress disorder, social anxiety disorders, and phobias are reported by approximately 32% of students between ages 13 and 18 years. Of concern is research indicating that the percentage of youth using alcohol after a major depressive episode is double that of youth not experiencing a major depressive episode (Office of Adolescent Health, 2018a).

Many adolescents are reluctant to seek help for emotional problems, or help may not be readily available to them. Most mental health disorders are treatable; however, in 2016, only 41% of adolescents experiencing depression received treatment. Barriers to treatment may include social stigma, cultural norms, and lack of qualified providers.

- Survey results indicate that 12.7% of youth aged 12 to 17 have been given some type of mental health services, but the usual disparities apply (e.g., ethnicity, income level, rural vs. urban locale).
- Treatment for serious mental health problems may include hospitalization or placement in a group home. Use of a team-based Collaborative Care program has improved mental and physical health outcomes.
- Mental health disorders experienced during adolescence may persist into adulthood, becoming more difficult to treat. It is critical to identify negative adolescent mental health behaviors, provide access to services, and educate teens about healthy physical and mental health skills (Office of Adolescent Health, 2018a).

The presence of major depressive disorder (MDD) is common in children and teens; it is associated with suicide and self-injury. It is more common in adolescents with chronic disease and can result in obesity, suicidal thoughts and attempts, and academic performance.

- Major depressive disorder is most commonly associated with lifetime prevalence of adolescent suicidal ideation, plans, and attempts. Health care providers can play an integral part in identifying adolescent depression and those at risk for suicide.
- Recent stressful events and preoccupation with suicide, as well as substance use, are also important to note. Being bullied, a history of sexual or physical abuse, aggressive conduct disorders, and personality disorders are risk factors for adolescent suicide attempts. When evaluating adolescent mental health, the broader context of school, social, and family influences needs to be considered (Diamond et al., 2017).

Suicide is the second leading cause of death in 10- to 19-year-olds.

- Between 2007 and 2015, suicide deaths increased by 130% in the 10- to 14-year-old group and 46% in the 15- to 19-year-old age group.
- Overall, male suicide rates are higher than female rates, and American Indian and Alaskan Native adolescent suicide rates are the highest. Ethnic disparity may result from social and environmental factors such as discrimination, exposure to others' suicides, and inadequate health care system access (Ballesteros et al., 2018).
- In 2017, 17.2% of high school students reported that they seriously considered suicide in the previous 12 months, and 7.4% made at least one suicide attempt. Approximately 2.4% made an attempt that required medical attention. Suicide attempt rates for adolescent female versus male students were higher (9.3% vs. 5.1%) (CDC, 2018f).

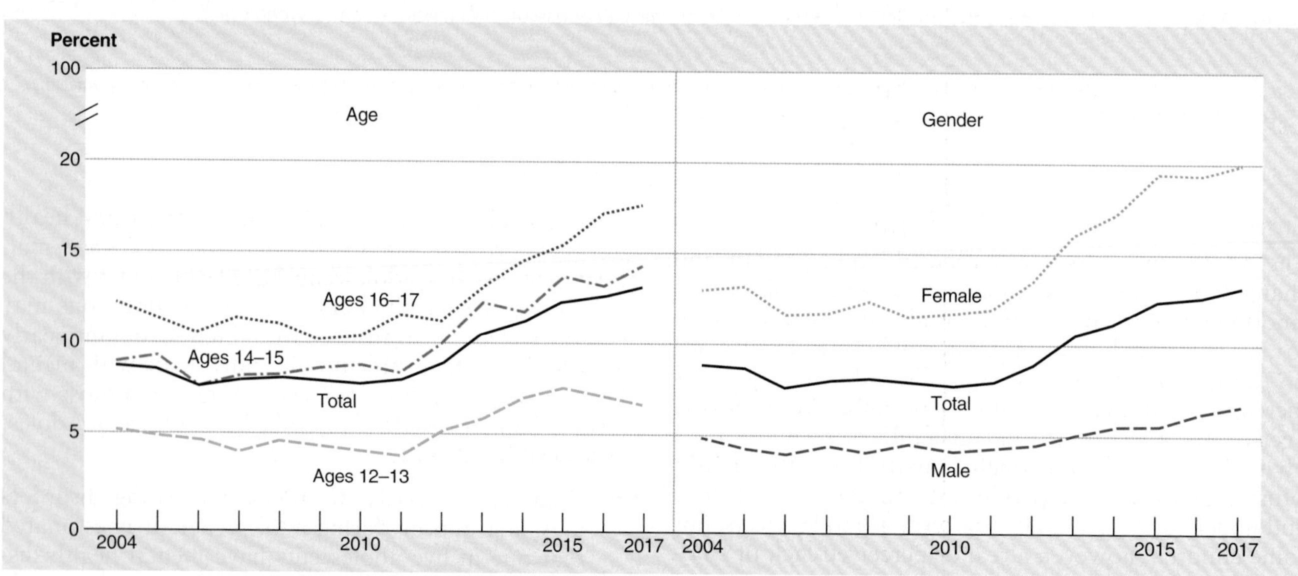

FIGURE 20-6 Percentage of youth ages 12 to 17 who had at least one major depressive episode in the past year by age and gender, 2004 to 2017. (Reprinted from https://www.childstats.gov/americaschildren/health_fig.asp#health4a)

School-based programs to educate adolescents about depression and suicide prevention have been useful. C/PHNs and school nurses often participate in the development or administration of these types of programs.

- Suicide prevention programs and direct intervention by counselors or school nurses to determine an adolescent's suicide intentions may be effective school-based interventions. It is important for counselors to identify markers for attempted suicide, such as a precipitating event, intense affective state, suicide ideation or actions, deterioration in social or academic functioning, or increased substance abuse.

C/PHNs and community mental health counselors may serve as consultants to schools in the development of sound prevention programs.

- Hallmarks of good prevention programs include student education on suicide awareness and intervention; coping and problem-solving skills training; skill building by reinforcement of strengths and protective factors while dealing with risk-taking behaviors; and teaching about the association between suicide and mental health (especially depression). Suicide screening is often thought to be effective in reducing suicidal ideation (Bhatta, Champion, Young, & Loika, 2018).

Youth suicide has been of great concern over the past several decades. Communities across the nation have been urged to implement effective school-based suicide prevention programs. There is some evidence that universal school-based programs decrease the number of adolescent suicide attempts.

- The SOS Signs of Suicide program is an evidence-based school-based intervention that educates adolescents about poor mental health, suicide, and coping mechanisms. It has been shown to decrease self-reported suicide attempts.
- Skills training programs that target a broader range of problems (e.g., depression, anxiety, negative self-perceptions) have been effective in teaching adolescents how to monitor feelings, identify triggers, and avoid and reframe negative thoughts. Relaxation skills training, learning how to seek out help from others, and promoting healthier responses to stress have also been successful in impacting internalizing behaviors.
- The Substance Abuse and Mental Health Services Administration (SAMHSA) awards grants in support of youth suicide prevention programs. SAMHSA has also developed a suicide prevention toolkit to help school around the nation implement programs (available online at https://store.samhsa.gov/product/Preventing-Suicide-A-Toolkit-for-High-Schools/SMA12-4669) (County Health Rankings & Roadmaps, 2018).

A behavior that can sometimes accidentally result in suicide is *self-injury* or *cutting* (Fig. 20-7). Adolescents with this abnormal behavior who overdose, head bang, cut, burn, brand, mark, or otherwise dangerously harm themselves are attempting to find relief from profound psychological pain. The physical injury distracts them from these painful emotions, often giving them a feeling of control or providing a means of feeling emotions when they are cut off from them.

- Emergency room visits for adolescents with nonfatal injuries have significantly increased in the United States since 2009. CDC research indicates that self-inflicted injuries among male adolescents remained stable, while female adolescents have increased about 8.4% each year between 2009 and 2015.
- For female youth aged 10 to 14, the percentage increased by 18.8% each year. This behavior most often begins in early adolescence or late childhood and can continue into adulthood.
- It is more common in those with a family history of suicide, self-injury, or maternal depression. Isolation, neglect, or abuse may predispose an adolescent to this behavior. Depression, poor quality of relationships, excessive seeking of reassurance, and eating disorders are often associated with self-injury (Stockwell, 2018).

C/PHNs and school nurses can provide education to adolescents and families about this condition and can work with schools to promote prevention strategies, such as early detection and referral to mental health providers.

Violence

Youth violence is defined as "the intentional use of physical force or power to threaten or harm others by young

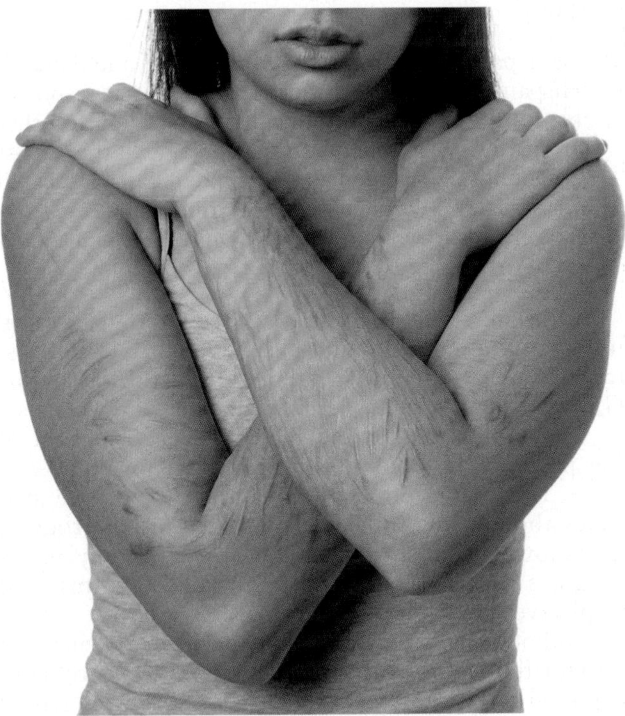

FIGURE 20-7 An adolescent girl with evidence of "cutting" self-injury.

people ages 10–24" (CDC, 2020h). The physical, emotional, and social effects of youth violence can be severe and long lasting. Youth violence affects entire communities and has become a leading cause of death for U.S. youth. The Youth Risk Behavior Surveillance Survey—United States, 2017, indicated that:

- 15.7% of high school students carried a weapon at least 1 day within 30 days of the survey.
- Male students (24.2%) carried a weapon more than female students (7.4%), with prevalence higher among White male students (29.0%), followed by Hispanic male students (18.4%), and Black male students (15.3%).
- In 2017, 3.8% of students did not go to school on at least 1 day prior to the survey because of safety concerns (Kann et al., 2018).
- It is not uncommon for children (0 to 17 years) to be exposed to more than one type of violence. Within the past year, approximately 37% of children were physically assaulted and 5% were sexually victimized (FCFS, 2019a).
- Homicide is a leading cause of death for adolescents and youth (aged 15 to 24). It is the leading cause of death for African American youth, the second leading cause of death for Hispanic youth, and the third leading cause of death for American Indian/Alaska Native (CDC, 2020h).
- Unfortunately, in the United States, more than 33% of homicide victims are young adults, meaning that approximately 13 adolescents are murdered each day.

Gangs are often associated with teen violence. In the United States, with a rise in gang membership to approximately 750,000 members, gangs are found in all 50 states.

- Gang participants are often young, male, and Black or Hispanic. Authorities believe that gangs are responsible for up to 13% of homicides, in addition to other crimes and drug sales. A survey of some of the largest city police departments in the United States indicated "significant criminal activity by youth gangs or gang-like groups of young people" (United States Department of Justice, 2018).

Multiple successful antigang programs have been implemented in communities including Gang Resistance Education and Training (G.R.E.A.T.). The G.R.E.A.T. program is taught by local law officials to students in middle and high schools. The goal of the program is to teach students how to avoid violence, resist gang pressure, and improve positive attitudes about law enforcement. This promising program has shown promising results as it successfully meets its goals (Bureau of Alcohol, Tobacco, Firearms, and Explosives [ATF], 2018).

Although gang members may engage in violence and intimidation, other instances of school violence have captured greater media attention. Incidents of high school shootings are of great concern to parents, teachers, communities, and the nation. These high-profile events are becoming more common and bring attention to the need for change (University of Virginia, 2018).

School violence has been linked to bullying and the overall school environment and should be addressed quickly.

- Bullying can result in depression, social anxiety, internalizing and psychosomatic symptoms, loneliness, and poor school performance (Jordan et al., 2018).
- In 2017, bullying incidents were reported by 19% of students in public schools, cyberbullying was reported by 14.9% of students, and 6.7% of students did not feel safe going to school.
- In 2017, 6.0% of adolescents reported being threatened or injured with a weapon; this statistic has decreased significantly since 2007.
- Males were more likely to be involved in carrying weapons and fighting. Another form of violence found among adolescents and young adults is dating violence.
- In 2017, 8.0% of high school students reported physical violence while dating. This is significantly higher than the percentage reported in 2013 (CDC, 2018f).

Of recent concern is the growing prevalence of school shootings and the effects this can have on students' well-being. Many students and their parents fear a shooting could occur in their school; nonwhite teens expressed a higher level of concern than white counterparts, and girls a greater concern than boys (Pew Research Center, 2018). School-aged children have become involved in the debate surrounding gun violence, where proposals focus on addressing mental illness, assault-style weapon ban, and the use of metal detectors in schools. To address this issue, researchers examined the relationship between 36 high schools' shootings and student achievement in 14 states and found that academic achievement was associated with standardized test scores in math and English, which were lower in affected schools 3 years following a deadly shooting (Beland & Kim, 2016). In addition, students' parents were likely to change their school selection due to a shooting; enrollment dropped for 9th grade students following a deadly shooting. Graduation and suspension rates showed no significant impact, despite a reduction in students' standardized test scores.

Cultural and environmental influences on youth include the violence to which children and adolescents are exposed. Increased aggressive behavior among children and teens has been attributed to violence in the environment, the home (spousal and child abuse), and the community, as well as to what children see on television and in movies. The effects of family violence (domestic violence, child maltreatment) can lead to internalizing and externalizing behaviors among youth.

- Personally experiencing or witnessing violence as a child is a risk factor for adolescent behaviors such as school dropout, running away from home, attempting suicide, and delinquency (Fix, Alexander, & Burkhart, 2018).

- School climate is important in reducing the levels of violence in this age group, as is adequate parental support. Family cohesion can also be a mediating factor for delinquency as a consequence of childhood effects of violence.
- The Functional Family Therapy (FTT) 3-month program used with adolescents with behavioral issues such as delinquency, and drug and alcohol abuse, has been adapted for adolescents with gang involvement and those at risk for gang involvement. A study found that prevention of gang involvement, subsequent delinquency, and decreased substance abuse were all positive outcomes of the program (Gottfredson, Thornberry, Slothower, & Devlin, 2018).

Substance Abuse

Why do adolescents turn to alcohol or illicit drugs? Substance abuse is one of the greatest threats to adolescent health (Fig. 20-8).

- In 2017, 14.0% of high school students reported using illicit drugs including cocaine, inhalants, heroin, methamphetamines, hallucinogens, or ecstasy. This is a significant decrease over the past 10 years in the United States (CDC, 2018f).
- There are many influences associated with adolescent substance use including influence and monitoring by parents and guardians, family structure, history of physical abuse and maltreatment, adult example and parental substance use, and teen peer influence.
- Some research indicates that friend and peer influences become an even stronger predictor of substance abuse as teens age (Henry, Fulco, Agbeke, & Ratcliff, 2018).
- Depression has also been linked to alcohol and substance use. Increased emphasis on family values was noted to be a protective factor for alcohol use. This includes not only the parenting style of the adolescent's parents but also the parenting influences of the teen's friend's parents (Office of Adolescent Health, 2018b).

Alcohol is the most frequently used substance for U.S. adolescents—it is often their first drug of choice. As adolescents get older, they are more likely to drink. Although rates of adolescent drinking have decreased since 2002, in 2017, 33% of 12th grade students report drinking, as compared to 20% of 10th grade students, and 7% of 8th grade students (Office of Adolescent Health, 2018b).

- The teen brain is very susceptible to the damaging effects of alcohol and a number of social, physical, and academic are associated with its use. Early drinkers more often report damaged family relationships, academic problems, problems with concentration and memory, use of other substances, and delinquent behavior in middle and high school.

2019 Monitoring the Future Survey
Key Findings: Percent Reporting Use of Selected Substances

	8th Grade	10th Grade	12th Grade
Vaping, Any			
Past Year	20.1	35.7	40.6
Past Month	12.2	25.0	30.9
Vaping, Nicotine			
Past Year	16.5	30.7	35.3
Past Month	9.6	19.9	25.5
Vaping, Marijuana			
Past Year	7.0	19.4	20.8
Past Month	3.9	12.6	14.0
Vaping, Just Flavoring			
Past Year	14.7	20.8	20.3
Past Month	7.7	10.5	10.7
Cigarettes			
Past Month	2.3	3.4	5.7
Daily	0.8	1.3	2.4
1/2 Pack +/Day	0.2	0.5	0.9

	8th Grade	10th Grade	12th Grade
Tobacco w/Hookah			
Past Year			5.6
Past Month	1.3	2.4	4.0
Flavored Little Cigars			
Past Month	2.2	3.7	7.7
Narcotis Other than Heroin			
Past Year			2.7
Past Month			1.0
Marijuana			
Past Year	11.8	28.8	35.7
Past Month	6.6	18.4	22.3
Daily	1.3	4.8	6.4
Alcohol			
Past Month	7.9	18.4	29.3
Daily	0.2	0.6	1.7
Binge	3.8	8.5	14.4

Change from 2018 to 2019

Significant Increase Significant Decrease

Source: University of Michigan, 2019 Monitoring the Future Study

FIGURE 20-8 2019 Monitoring the Future Survey key findings: percent reporting use of selected substances. (Reprinted from https://www.drugabuse.gov/publications/drugfacts/monitoring-future-survey-high-school-youth-trends)

- Early use of alcohol, even sipping/tasting with parental permission, was found to be a marker for increased alcohol use later in and the associated alcohol-related behaviors/problems (Colder, Shyhalla, & Frndak, 2018). It is important to stress education and prevention in late childhood to delay the initiation of alcohol use (Box 20-8).
- Family drinking, perceived family norms, and neighborhood societal contexts related to drinking have been found to affect adolescents' perceptions of the benefits of drinking. This perception, in turn, predicts their drinking behavior. Parenting practices (e.g., monitoring, discipline, enforcing rules related to alcohol use) have also been found to have an influence on adolescent drinking behavior (Cambron, Kosterman, Catalano, Guttmannova, & Hawkins, 2018; Colder et al., 2018).

Adolescents who are engaged emotionally and connected to school usually have better outcomes. Positive parenting practices such as open communication, monitoring adolescent activities, and teaching methods of self-control have also been associated with a reduction in adolescent alcohol use.

- Family mealtimes have been shown to promote family cohesion and problem- and emotion-focused coping by encouraging parents to help their children feel part of the family and allowing them valuable time to coach them in effective methods for dealing with daily stresses and problems. The benefits of family mealtime include improved self-esteem, improved mental health, decreased alcohol and substance abuse, and decreased depression (Youth.Gov, n.d.). To promote the health and welfare of adolescent children, it is vital to stress to families with young children the continued importance of family meals throughout adolescence.

Marijuana is the most commonly used illicit drug among 14- to 17-year-olds—35.6% of high school students reported ever using marijuana (Fig. 20-9).

- Marijuana use during adolescence has been associated with a much greater likelihood of drug abuse and dependency, poorer mental health, poorer academic performance, increased delinquency, and neurocognitive deficits (D'Amica, Rodriquez, Tucker, Pedersen, & Shih, 2018).
- Marijuana use has negative health effects, including anxiety, panic attacks, increased heart rate, frequent respiratory infections, impaired memory and learning, and tolerance. Regular marijuana smokers often have respiratory complications similar to those of tobacco smokers—cough, phlegm, respiratory infections, and airway obstruction (National Institute of Drug Abuse for Teens, 2017a).

BOX **20-8** POPULATION FOCUS

Using Evidence-Based Practice to Design Substance Abuse Prevention Strategies for Adolescents

School nursing runs in my family. In the 1980s, when my mother was a school nurse in a small, rural school district located in an agriculturally dependent county, there was only one high school in the small town of about 10,000 people. School personnel were aware of some "keg parties" after football games and the occasional alcohol-related fight on school property between some of the rougher students, but they were not fully aware of the substance abuse problems. The school psychologist conducted an anonymous survey and found, much to the surprise of teachers and administrators, that most of the teens involved in alcohol and drug abuse were the athletes and cheerleaders. They had assumed that the lower-income, trouble-making kids were much more involved, but this was not necessarily the case. My mother worked with the psychologist to implement health education classes in the high school and eventually the middle school and elementary schools to address this issue and health promotion in general.

I am a school nurse at a suburban, larger school district serving over 30,000 students with four high schools, a charter high school and a continuation high school. Each high school has a full-time school nurse, and the middle schools have one most of the week. We utilize evidence-based practice as school nurses, and there are many resources available to us. We are aware of national surveys on substance use among adolescents (e.g., YRBSS) and have conducted some ourselves to better understand our students' needs. Although alcohol is still a concern, drug use has increased since my mom's school nursing experience. A national survey found that 14.0% of high school students use some type of illicit drugs (CDC, 2018f).

The district school nurses met with our advisory board, parent groups, school administration, and eventually the school board to discuss the problem and address potential interventions. We discussed our population demographics, our various cultural and ethnic influences, and our community statistics. After examining the best research-based methods, we found screening, brief interventions (SBI), and referral to treatment is key to delaying and decreasing substance abuse in teens. Additionally, family-focused prevention programs often provide skills to parents (e.g., parenting, helping children develop social resistance skills, monitoring/rule setting). Parental education and family-centered interventions have been found to be most effective in preventing risk behaviors and promoting self-regulation among teens and early adults (Stormshak, DeGarmo, Chronister, & Caruthers, 2018).

Based on the evidence, our school district decided to implement SBIRT and a family-based prevention program for upper elementary students and their parents. I hope we can eventually encourage a more community-based approach to population health for our children and adolescents. I feel that with the resources we have today, we can really make a difference in the lives of our students and their families. I know my mother is proud of the work I am doing, and I hope my daughter considers carrying on the family tradition!

Holly, age 30, school nurse

Source: Centers for Disease Control and Prevention (CDC) (2020l); Lunstead et al. (2017); Stormshak et al. (2018).

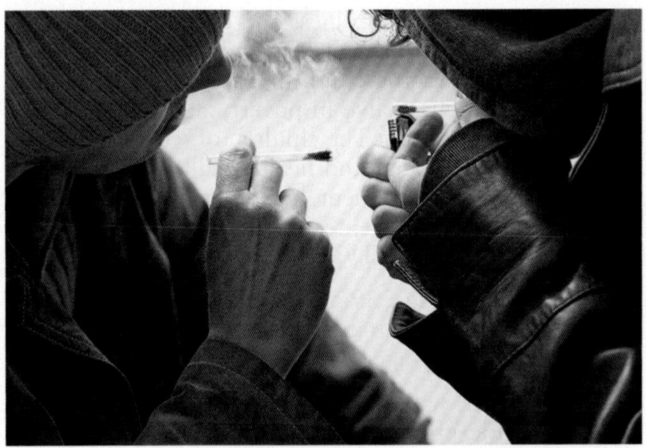

FIGURE 20-9 Marijuana use is common among adolescents.

Inhalant abuse is very common and frequently used by young teens. Inhalant use begins in early adolescence—more 12- and 13-year-olds reported using inhalants than any other illicit drug.

- The most commonly reported inhalants used were shoe polish, glue or toluene, spray paints, and lighter fluid or gasoline.
- Other inhalants commonly used include amyl nitrite "poppers"; locker room deodorizers or "rush"; cleaning fluid, degreasers, or correction fluid; halothane, ether, or other anesthetics; lacquer thinner or other paint solvents; butane or propane gases; nitrous oxide or "whippets"; and other aerosol sprays.
- Inhalant abuse can result in severe nervous system damage or death. Control of legal products, such as spray paint, lighter fluid, household solvents, gasoline, and glue, is difficult, making this problem almost impossible to monitor adequately (National Institute of Drug Abuse for Teens, 2017b).

Other drugs that are used by adolescents and young adults include "club drugs" such as MDMA (Ecstasy), a synthetic drug with amphetamine and hallucinogenic properties, and its purer form "Molly" often glamorized by singers and musicians. Visits to the ED and deaths have occurred from the use of many of these drugs. Cocaine and heroin use has significantly decreased since 1999 with 1.2% of teens using cocaine and <0.03% of teens using heroin in the last month. Methamphetamine use is also down with <0.03% of teens using in the last month and 0.06% use in a year (National Institute of Health, 2017). Methamphetamine labs are a public health hazard. Prolonged exposure to methamphetamine can result in cognitive deficits and psychosis (National Institute of Drug Abuse for Teens, 2017c, 2017d). C/PHNs should be aware of this when making home visits.

Another drug used by adolescents is anabolic steroids. The illicit use of anabolic steroids is difficult to monitor; however, 0.6% of 8th graders, 0.7% of 10th graders, and l.1% of 12th graders reported using steroids in a national survey (National Institute of Drug Abuse for Teens, 2017e). The Youth Risk Behavior Surveillance—United States, 2017 noted that use was higher in males, and more prevalent among Hispanic (3.5%) than White (2.2%) students.

- The prevalence of nonprescription steroid use increased between 1991 and 2001 and then decreased during 2001 to 2017 (Kann et al., 2018).
- Adverse effects of illicit steroid use include irritability, increased risk-taking behavior, extreme mood swings, paranoia, jealousy, and euphoria, as well as psychiatric conditions that may be intensified or induced (National Institute of Drug Abuse for Teens, 2017e).
- Because steroids are often readily available through Internet pharmacies, policymakers, health educators, and parents must make adolescents aware of the dangers, such as altered serotonin levels and increased aggression.

Adolescents are becoming more involved with prescription drugs, often found in their parents' medicine cabinets, purchased on the Internet or bought from friends at school. Secondary too marijuana and alcohol, they are the most commonly abused substances by teens. Medications are often mixed with alcohol, and adolescents often mistakenly believe prescription medications are safer than street drugs when used to produce a high. The Youth Risk Behavior Surveillance—United States, 2017 indicated that adolescent misuse of prescription drugs ranges from 7.8% to 19.3% across 36 states (Kann et al., 2018). Prevalence of prescription drug misuse by 12th grade students decreased significantly between 2014 and 2017; however, this remains one of the most commonly abused substances by all Americans aged 14 years and older (National Institute of Drug Abuse for Teens, 2017f).

Tobacco products are also easily acquired, often from parents. Approximately 28.9% high school seniors report ever trying a cigarette.

- Between 1991 and 2017, the overall rates of adolescents currently using cigarettes significantly decreased from 27.5% to 8.8%.
- In 2017, 1.6% of teens reported using smokeless tobacco such as chewing tobacco, snuff, dip, snus, or dissolvable products, and 8% of students reported smoking cigars.
- Electronic cigarettes (e-cigarettes) are becoming increasingly used in the adolescent population. In 2017, 42.2% of adolescents reporting that they had ever used an electronic vapor product, and 13.2% reported using e-cigarettes in the past 30 days (Kann et al., 2018).
- Research regarding adolescent e-cigarette use indicates an association between e-cigarette use and the subsequent use of tobacco (Soneji et al., 2017; Wills et al., 2017).

Social disapproval and heightened perception of health risks are thought to help contribute to the downward trend of smoking and smokeless tobacco use, along with price increases and advertising bans. But tobacco marketing continues to be problematic, as the tobacco industry has joined with convenience stores to more prominently display tobacco products, and even though state and federal taxes comprise about half the cost of a pack of cigarettes, states have not always sufficiently invested these funds in adolescent tobacco prevention (Cruz et al., 2018). Flavored nicotine products are marketed to youth luring children with such flavors as bubble gum and cotton candy (Tobacco Free Kids, 2017).

- Risk factors associated with cigarette smoking include being an older adolescent, male, and white. Also, having parents without college education and adolescent lack of college education plans (Office of Adolescent Health, 2017b).

Primary health care providers do not always question adolescents about smoking, drinking, and use of other substances. Some evidence highlights the effectiveness of brief interventions by health care providers in encouraging smoking cessation and improvement in other risk behaviors. Research recommends that health care professional counseling be provided as a preventive measure to adolescent tobacco users.

- Important to note is research indicating that education regarding the harmful effects of tobacco use are more effective than messages about the benefits of not smoking. This research may prove influential regarding the risk warning on tobacco products and in social media (Mays, Hawkins, Bredfeldt, Wolf, & Tercyak, 2017).
- C/PHNs and community health nurses can provide information to teens about smoking cessation programs and promote primary prevention by educating children and adolescents to choose not to smoke or engage in other health risk behaviors. They can also encourage physicians and parents to question and monitor adolescents about smoking and the use of tobacco products.

Teen Sexuality and Pregnancy

Teenage pregnancies, sexually transmitted diseases (STDs), and HIV/AIDS are public health concerns associated with the sexual activity of adolescents.

- In the 2017 YRBSS, 39.5% of high school students reported ever having sexual intercourse, and 53.8% used a condom during their last sexual intercourse.
- About 10% reported having had sexual intercourse with four or more persons, and 20.7% used birth control pills to prevent pregnancy (Kann et al., 2018).

Adolescent birth rates differ by age, racial and ethnic group, and country region. The downward trend in teen birth rates has continued over the past 25 years; however, the rate in the United States remains higher than many other developed countries.

- In 2016, teens (aged 15 to 19) experienced 209,809 pregnancies, with 74% of all teen births occurring to 18- to 19-year-olds.
- Teen births are more prevalent among Hispanic and Black females, although this rate has decreased in recent years.
- Preventive teenage pregnancy factors include being engaged in learning and after school activities, having a positive attitude toward learning and school, academic excellence, and living in a wealthier neighbor with higher income levels (Office of Adolescent Health, 2017c).

Teenage pregnancy is associated with increased health risks to both the mother and the child. These risks include increased risk of illness and death, increased risk of mother's death from violence, and increased developmental concerns of the child. In addition, young mothers are more likely to live in poverty and to be delayed in their own education. The children of teen mothers are at risk of several social and health challenges, including lower academic achievement, health problems, incarcerations during adolescence, teenage pregnancy, and young adult unemployment (CDC, 2019g).

- By 19 years of age, 39.5% of males and females have had sexual intercourse. Approximately 3.4% of teens have had sex by age 13.

As such, it would be appropriate for U.S. society to provide effective sexuality education. There is often debate about the virtues of comprehensive versus abstinence-only educational programs. Despite the controversy about the subject, in 2014, 72% of private and public schools in the United States taught pregnancy prevention as part of required health education. Most adolescents (aged 15 to 19) received education about STDs and abstinence (76%), 61% were taught about contraceptives, and 35% were taught how to use a condom. Many sexually active teens have no instruction on contraception before their first sexual experience (40% girls, 45% boys) (Guttmacher Institute, 2017). Teaching about contraception has not been shown to increase the risk of adolescent sexual activity or STIs, but it may decrease the risk of pregnancy. A systematic review and meta-analysis assessing the effectiveness of school-based programs found that sex education, of any type, when compared to no education was associated with delayed adolescent sexual intercourse. Research, however, was divided regarding effectiveness in preventing teen pregnancy (Marseille et al., 2018). Besides formal education through schools, adolescents note that peers, the media, and parents are also sources of information on sexual health. Between 70% and 78% of teens report talking with a parent about sex, although girls more often talk with parents about how to say no to sex or use birth control (Guttmacher Institute, 2017).

Pregnancy prevention programs can be effective in reducing teen pregnancy and birth rates (Fig. 20-10), as well as in reducing the number of second births to teenage mothers. Research regarding the effectiveness of a multicomponent, community-wide teen pregnancy prevention (TPP) program focusing on 15- to 19-year African American and Latino/Hispanic youth found that key elements influenced the success of a community mobilization program. Learnings included:

1. Communities are generally willing to "'face' the issue of teen pregnancy."
2. Support of the program by key stakeholders was critical to success.
3. Collaboration of health and human service agencies strengthened the program.
4. Education of and establishing trust within the community was essential.
5. Engagement of youth teams and extensive training for youth leaders was imperative.

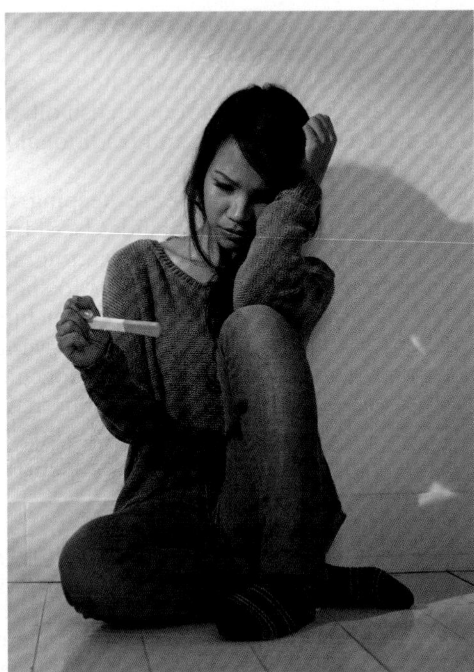

FIGURE 20-10 Pregnancy prevention programs can be helpful in decreasing rates of adolescent pregnancy.

Review of the TPP intervention research by project coordinators was positive, "*The model was important in creating a network of community partners and concerned citizens—including the youth of the community—who would contribute to normalizing TPP within their communities*" (Saunders, 2018). Health promotion professionals were important allies throughout the TPP community mobilization program through direct service, community advocacy and networking, and being actively involved in health promotion (Saunders, 2018).

Primary care providers often miss opportunities to provide counseling on prevention of pregnancy, HIV, and STDs, as well as other risk factors for unintentional injury. Nurses can provide information and counseling on birth control and emergency contraception to adolescent clients and collaborate with schools to promote effective pregnancy prevention programs. It is important for C/PHNs to provide education and health counseling on these subjects. A recent study by Rabbitte & Enriquez (2018) demonstrated the importance of nursing collaboration in high school sexual education and counseling, stating "*If implemented correctly, sex education teaches students about anatomy and physiology, healthy relationships, hygiene, positive self-image, how to handle uncomfortable situations, and about health resources available to them. School nurses are in a unique position to play a critical role in policy change with regard to sex education*" (p. 10).

Sexually Transmitted Infections

STI and HIV infections are epidemic among adolescents worldwide (WHO, 2018a). More than 20 diseases can be transmitted sexually; only the most common are reportable.

- Each year, about half of the STD cases occur among the 15- to 24-year-old age group, even though they represent only 27% of the population of sexually active individuals. These diseases include syphilis, gonorrhea, *Chlamydia*, HPV, and herpes simplex virus.
- Almost all sexually active people will get an HPV infection in their lifetime. HPV infections can lead to several types of cancer in both men and women and other health-related problems (CDC, 2018g).

Chlamydia, gonorrhea, and syphilis are other STDs/STIs found in the adolescent population.

- Of the 19 million new cases of STDs annually, about half are among adolescents (15 to 24 years old), and 21% of 13- to 24-year-olds in reporting states had a new HIV infection in 2016.
- In the adolescent population, STIs are more common among those engaging in sexual risk behaviors. In 2017, 40% of high school students reported ever having sexual intercourse and 30% were active within the previous 3 months.
- About 10% had sex with four or more partners, and 54% used a condom with their last sexual contact (CDC, 2020i).
- Gonorrhea is the most commonly reported STD (70%), followed by *Chlamydia* (63%), HPV (49%), genital herpes (45%), HIV (26%), and syphilis (20%) (CDC, 2018g).

About one in four sexually active adolescent females have an STD. Compared with adults, adolescents (10 to 19 years) and young adults (20 to 24 years) are at increased risk for acquiring STDs. Reasons for this may include a greater likelihood of multiple sex partners, unprotected intercourse, and selection of higher-risk partners. Immature biology makes adolescents more vulnerable to infection and earlier sexual initiation.

- Barriers to prevention and care include social and cultural conditions such as lack of health insurance and transportation, concerns about confidentiality, and lack of quality STD prevention services.
- Adolescent girls also have a physiologically amplified susceptibility to *Chlamydia* infection because of increased cervical ectopy.
- Serious complications from STDs include pelvic inflammatory disease (PID), sterility, increased risk of cancers of the reproductive system, and, with syphilis, blindness, mental illness, and death. There are also complications for the unborn children of those infected with STDs (CDC, 2018g).

Even though death rates from HIV/AIDS have dramatically fallen, new HIV infections reported annually do not reflect the same steep decline.

- It is estimated that as many as 51% of youth with HIV are not aware of their infection. Adolescents and young adults (aged 13 to 24) comprised 21% of all new cases of HIV infection in 2016 and young gay and bisexual men accounted for 81% of the new cases.
- As a result, in 2017, the CDC granted approximately $11 million per year/5-year community-based organizations for HIV testing of young gay and bisexual

men. The goal of these grants is to identify undiagnosed HIV infections and connect those diagnosed with HIV to appropriate health care resources (CDC, 2020j).

As noted earlier, sex education is effective at both delaying the onset of sexual activity and possibly increasing the use of contraception in adolescents who are already sexually active. It is also effective in increasing safer sex practices, knowledge of birth control method efficacy, and overall sexual knowledge when that content is taught (Rabbitte & Enriquez, 2018; Saunders, 2018). Prevention strategies identified by the CDC to reduce sexual risk behaviors included:

- Targeting behaviors that are most easily amenable to change (e.g., condom use, decreased number of sexual partners, abstinence)
- Tailoring programs to the target population, using theory as a guide in development of programs (e.g., modeling discussions with partners about condom use, skill building by role-playing situations, increasing self-efficacy)
- Addressing a broader content than just STI/HIV prevention education (e.g., problem-solving, social skills, gender pride, capacity building)

Evidence-based prevention interventions are the most effective (CDC, 2018h). See Chapter 28 for the school nurse's role with STD/HIV.

Acne

Acne is a skin disease that primarily affects adolescents going through puberty.

- The prevalence of acne in the adolescent population is nearly 95%. The precise cause of acne is not fully understood. It is often related to several factors. Genetics play a part (there is often a family history of acne), hormonal influences are also a factor (especially an increase in male hormones), and greasy cosmetics may plug cells of follicles, producing a plug.
- Acne usually begins during puberty (10 to 12 years of age) with the increase in circulating male hormones that stimulate sebaceous glands in the skin. It often affects adolescent men more than females (Skroza et al., 2018).

Common acne treatment includes skin cleansers, peelers, and medications to decrease sebaceous gland activity. Topical retinoids are the first-line drugs of choice because of their anti-inflammatory properties. Benzoyl peroxide is used to kill bacteria on the skin and in the pores. It may be sold over the counter (OTC) or by prescription. Other OTC medications include salicylic acid and resorcinol. Retin-A (a topical vitamin A ointment), glycolic acid, and alpha-hydroxy acids help to peel the impacted cells from the pores. Antibiotics (oral or topical), such as tetracycline or doxycycline, may be prescribed to help control bacteria on the skin. Isotretinoin reduces the size and activity of sebaceous glands but can cause liver or kidney dysfunction. Because of an extremely high risk of birth defects, female adolescents taking Isotretinoin are prescribed oral contraceptives and must participate in a Food and Drug Administration–approved risk management program. Corticosteroids may be injected directly into the comedones. Some adolescents choose to try complementary therapies such as tea tree oil, fish oil, or brewer's yeast, as well as biofeedback and traditional Chinese medicine (Cao et al., 2017).

The best preventive measures are keeping the skin clean, eating a balanced diet that includes fresh fruits and vegetables, drinking lots of water, and getting adequate sleep. It is important for male adolescents to shave carefully and for all teens with acne to avoid touching their faces or picking at their blemishes. They may want to use skin and hair products that are noncomedogenic. Adolescents with severe acne may need to be referred to dermatologists who specialize in this skin disorder (Mayo Clinic, 2017).

Poor Nutrition and Eating Disorders

Poor nutrition and obesity are common among adolescents, whose diets often consist of snacks with limited nutritional value interspersed among unhealthful meals. The nutritional needs of adolescents increase as their growth rate and body composition changes with puberty. Many things, from psychosocial factors, family and peers, availability of fast-food, and mass media marketing, influence the eating behaviors of adolescents. Research indicates that two thirds of adolescents are not aware of dietary needs, sources of nutrients, and diet–disease relationship (Demory-Luce & Motil, 2018).

- Girls are more at risk for problems with nutrition for several reasons: they tend to diet inappropriately, to have more finicky eating habits, and to be less physically active than teenage boys.
- Approximately 5.4% of adolescents (13 to 18 years) suffer from an eating disorder, with the majority being female. Issues with body image and control are at the heart of anorexia nervosa and bulimia nervosa, common problems for adolescent girls.
- **Anorexia nervosa** is an eating disorder with an emotional etiology that is characterized by body image disturbance (i.e., girls see themselves as fat, although they may be extremely thin), an intense fear of becoming fat or gaining weight, and refusal to maintain adequate body weight.
- **Bulimia nervosa** is an eating disorder characterized by recurrent episodes of binge eating with repeated compensatory mechanisms to prevent weight gain, such as vomiting (purging type) and fasting or exercise (nonpurging type) (National Institute of Mental Health, n.d.b).
- **Binge eating**, also a recognized eating disorder, involves recurrent episodes of binge eating without fasting, self-induced vomiting, or other compensatory measures. Self-esteem, depressive symptoms, and emotional eating are very sensitive predictors of binge eating. Low levels of support from peers can also be linked to binge eating, and binge eating is associated with an increased risk of becoming overweight or obese (National Institute of Mental Health, n.d.b).

These diseases affect both male and female adolescents. Research indicates that they are caused by multiple factors including genetics, biological, behavioral, psychological, and social elements. Nutrition education, psychological counseling, and cognitive–behavioral techniques that teach clients how to control stimuli, substitute alternative behaviors, and use positive visualization are all part of treatment; development of a support network is also important. Family and individually based treatments are most often used for severe cases of adolescent eating disorders and have been studied most often. Medications (e.g., antidepressants) have been used to treat some adolescents with eating disorders, when co-occurring illnesses exist (National Institute of Mental Health, n.d.b).

HEALTH SERVICES FOR SCHOOL-AGE CHILDREN AND ADOLESCENTS

A number of programs serve the health needs of school-age children and adolescents. Community health nurses play a major and vital role in delivering these services. Such programs fall into three categories that approximate the three practice priorities of community health nursing practice: illness prevention, health protection, and health promotion.

Preventive Health Programs

Among programs to prevent physical illness and other health problems among adolescents are immunizations and TB testing, as well as school- and community-based education, and support programs. Private and public counseling programs and other social services are also geared to promote health and prevent illness.

Immunizations and Tuberculosis Testing

C/PHNs are deeply involved in each of the preventive activities of immunizations and tuberculosis testing. Health departments and schools often work collaboratively to provide immunization services. Compulsory immunization laws are helpful in carrying out these preventive services, but recent survey results reveal that not all adolescents are fully covered.

- A national immunization survey revealed mixed results for adolescent vaccination. There were significant increases in vaccination rates for varicella, tetanus/diphtheria/acellular pertussis (Tdap), and meningococcal conjugate vaccine. HPV coverage also increased with 65.1% of females and 56% of males being vaccinated (Walker et al., 2017).

It is important for adolescents, as well as adults, to get a single dose of Tdap to protect themselves and infants who may be around them from whooping cough. Although pertussis in adolescents or adults often manifests as an upper respiratory infection with a chronic cough, for infants who have not yet been fully immunized, it can lead to serious complications.

In the recent past, adolescents were only given "catch-up" vaccinations (those missed in childhood), except for a tetanus/diphtheria booster. Recommended immunizations now include Tdap, meningococcal vaccine, pneumococcal polysaccharide vaccine, both hepatitis A and B, influenza vaccine, and HPV vaccine for both boys and girls. Additionally, any missed vaccines such as polio and varicella are recommended (for immunization tables, see thePoint).

Often, school nurses and community health nurses work with nurse volunteers to provide immunization clinics at elementary and middle schools; these are convenient for adolescents and their parents. School-based clinics are also great places to catch adolescents who need updated immunizations. There is some evidence that adolescent vaccinations are becoming more available at retail pharmacies. Researchers note, however, that higher levels of medical and health needs are met when children and adolescents have an annual visit with a health care provider (Office of Adolescent Health, 2018c). Routine visits give the health care provider an opportunity to discuss risk behaviors and health concerns with adolescents and to intervene early as problems arise. Annual tuberculosis (TB) testing is often recommended for children and adolescents from high-risk populations. Targeted TB skin testing identifies adolescents and children at risk for latent TB who could benefit from treatment to prevent progression of the disease (CDC, 2018h). See Chapter 8 for more on TB skin testing.

Education and Social Services

The health education of school-age children and adolescents includes a wide variety of approaches and can range from the basics of handwashing for elementary school students to health risk behavior for adolescents. Parental support services are commonly available through many public and private agencies, including churches. These services can have long-range effects on the health of school-age children, because emotionally healthy parents and stable families offer a healthful environment and support system for children and can facilitate their progress in school. In most states, community health nurses provide teaching and counseling services to parents in their homes and in groups. School nurses, school mental health counselors, and school psychologists also organize parent support groups in local schools. This is particularly important during periods of transition (e.g., from elementary to middle school, from middle to high school). Discussing parenting concerns and increasing parents' understanding of normal child growth and development help to allay fears and prevent problems. Through such efforts, family violence and abuse can be averted. Reduction in rates of divorce and the attendant consequences may also be a benefit of strengthening family resilience.

Family planning programs, often stationed strategically in inner cities, near schools, or in school-based clinics, provide birth control information and counseling to young people.

- In some communities, the school-based clinic dispenses condoms. In many states, adolescents have the right to consent for sexual and reproductive health care without parental permission. It is important that health care providers be aware of local and regional options for counseling.
- C/PHNs, in collaboration with an interdisciplinary team, are usually the primary care providers in these programs. Their major goals are to prevent teenage pregnancy, educate teens about reproduction and contraception, and encourage responsible sexual behavior.

- Schools can foster evidence-based health education and create healthy, safe, and nurturing school environments, especially when implementing policies and programs regarding reproductive health and health risk behaviors.
- Collaborative efforts by the student, family, school, community, and society are essential to promoting adolescent health. Developing healthy and safe health education environments will influence adolescent health and academic achievement (CDC, 2019h).

Children and adolescents can be influenced by adults' smoking in the home.

C/PHNs should educate parents about the effects of smoking in the home and its relationship to adolescent smoking. Youth tobacco use is also associated with peer approval, mental health (strongly associated with depression, anxiety, and stress), lower socioeconomic status, lower academic achievement, accessibility, and tobacco advertising.

- Multiple programs to reduce and prevent teen smoking have been implemented in recent years. Successful activities include higher tobacco costs, indoor smoking prohibition, raising minimum age of tobacco sales, social media, and community antitobacco programs (CDC, 2019i).

It is essential that C/PHNs work with law enforcement officials, school district administrators, and other community agencies to ensure compliance with local regulations and prevent or delay the use of tobacco products. Information on smoking cessation and resources to help prevent tobacco use by children and adolescents is available through the CDC and the Foundation for a Smokefree America.

Health Protection Programs

Safety and Injury Prevention

Accident and injury control programs serve a critical role in protecting the lives of school-age children and adolescents. They are cost-effective: seat belt laws, child safety seats, and helmet laws have saved millions of dollars in medical care. Efforts to prevent motor vehicle accidents, a major cause of adolescent death, include driver education programs, better highway construction, improved motor vehicle design and safety features, and continuing research into what causes various types of crashes.

- Injury prevention and reduction have been addressed through multiple strategies. These include state laws requiring the use of safety restraints; installation of driver and front passenger airbags; substitution of other modes of travel (air, rail, or bus); lower speed limits; stricter enforcement of drunk driving laws; graduated drivers licenses (GDLs) for teenagers; safer automobile design; and helmets for motorcyclists, bicycle riders, and skaters (Ballesteros et al., 2018).
- In developing interventions, community health nurses need to recognize that adolescents are prone to risk-taking/novelty-seeking behaviors as a result of their cognitive, physical, and psychosocial developmental stage (Nesi et al., 2018).
- A campaign from the CDC, "Parents are the Key," focuses on the influence of parents, pediatricians, and communities as safety features for teens (CDC, 2017h). Communities can also work with law enforcement officials to ensure compliance with mandatory seat belt laws and to promote safe speeds and appropriate driving behaviors near schools.

Safety programs also seek to protect school-age children and adolescents from the hazards of poisonings, ingestion of prescription or OTC drugs, product-related accidents (unsafe toys, bicycles, skateboards, skates, playground equipment, and furniture), and recreational accidents, including drowning and sports-related injuries. Safety services assume various forms. Poison control centers in many localities offer information and emergency assistance. Whereas the federal Consumer Product Safety Commission monitors the safety of products, education programs in schools or through local fire or police departments teach school-age children about bicycle and water safety, fire dangers, and hazards related to poisoning. Generally, the community health nurse can educate families to recognize potentially hazardous situations and encourage efforts to eliminate them. Working with school nurses and school district officials to reduce playground hazards can contribute to the reduction of school-related injuries.

Environmental hazards and other dangers await school-age children and adolescents in the workforce.

- There were approximately 19.3 million workers under age 24 in 2016, and 403 workers under age 24 died from a work-related injury in 2015. Hospitals treated nearly double the number of workers aged 15 to 19 years, as compared to workers over age 25; it is necessary to reduce the number of occupational-related injuries among 15- to 19-year-olds (The National Institute for Occupational Safety and Health (NIOSH), 2018).
- C/PHNs can join with occupational health nurses and school nurses to teach parents and children about the dangers and risks inherent in the workplace, and they can work with local employers to ensure safe working conditions and reasonable hours of employment that do not interfere with school.

Infectious Disease Prevention

Programs that protect school-age children and adolescents against infectious diseases encompass such efforts as closing swimming pools that have unsafe bacteria counts, conducting immunization campaigns in conjunction with influenza or measles outbreaks, and working with hospital pediatric units to reduce the incidence and threat of iatrogenic disease. Prevention of community-acquired MRSA is a new challenge for public schools, and C/PHNs may work with school nurses or others to provide educational programs covering a variety of infectious diseases. Epidemiologic investigations, especially with school sports teams, may be necessary to determine the cause of outbreaks (CDC, 2019f).

Child Protective Services

The Children's Bureau collects and analyzes information on child abuse and neglect, serves as an information clearinghouse, publishes educational materials on the subject, offers technical assistance, and conducts research into the problem (Administration on Children and Families [ACF], 2018a).

- In 2016, an estimated 4.1 million referrals were made alleging child abuse and/or neglect of approximately 7.4 million children.
- Approximately 58% of these referrals were screened, and almost 3.5 million cases had an investigation or alternative response. This reflects a Child Protective Services (CPS) response increase of 9.5% since 2012.
- Most victims suffered from neglect (74.6%), approximately 18.2% were physically abused, and 8.5% were sexually abused.
- There were 2.36 deaths per 100,000 children, and 70% of children were under age 3. More than 70% of deaths were attributed to neglect or a combination of neglect and another form of maltreatment.
- Nearly 45% of deaths were attributed to physical abuse or a combination of physical abuse and another form of maltreatment. Most perpetrators of child abuse and maltreatment (78%) were biological parents (ACF, 2018b).

Consequences for affected children include lower self-esteem, depression, suicide, self-abuse, substance abuse, eating disorders, less empathy for others, antisocial behavior, delinquency, aggression, violence, low academic achievement, and sexual maladjustment. Long-term emotional, social, cognitive, and physical consequences are well documented, and often follow abused children into adolescence and adulthood. Posttraumatic stress disorder, poor attachment and problems with trust, difficulties with language development and abstract reasoning, high-risk health behaviors, and abusive or violent behavior may be seen later in life (CDC, 2020k). These findings were first noted in a large-scale, landmark research study, the Adverse Childhood Experiences study (Felitti et al., 1998).

In some areas, C/PHNs are working together with social workers, mental health workers, and substance abuse counselors as part of a team that provides services to families. Improved training of mandated reporters, such as teachers and physicians, has led to better reporting of abuse; as professionals and the public become more aware of the problem, an increase in reporting has occurred. Child abuse prevention programs can be found in many public health departments and through some school districts as a primary preventive intervention. Primary prevention of child maltreatment can also occur through home visiting programs utilizing C/PHNs. These visits can also help to connect high-risk families to the community and promote better child outcomes when an appropriate curriculum is followed (Matone et al., 2018). Programs that target at-risk families, especially adolescent mothers and young couples prone to partner violence or harsh parenting practices, may help to prevent later child abuse. C/PHNs and school nurses must be vigilant for signs of family stress, harsh parenting practices, family violence, and other risk factors for child abuse and neglect, and must provide resources and respite as needed (for additional information, see Chapters 18 and 19).

Oral Hygiene and Dental Care

Fluoridation of drinking water, school-provided fluoride rinse or gel, and dental sealant programs are cost-effective and can reduce dental caries.

- Fluoride makes teeth less susceptible to decay by increasing the resistance of tooth enamel to the bacterially produced acid in the mouth. School-based programs that provide fluoride rinses and dental sealants and promote tooth brushing and nutrition education for dental health can be found in most areas of the country.
- Fluoridation of community water supplies is considered the most effective, safe, and low-cost means of protecting the dental health of children and adolescents.
- Although most dental care is focused on children, adolescents remain in need of dental health services. In addition to regular dental care, good nutrition, and proper oral hygiene, C/PHNs can promote public water fluoridation as an important program for protecting children's dental health. Nurses can also recommend that parents talk with their primary health care provider and dentist about fluoride varnish or supplements (CDC, 2019j).

Health Promotion Programs: Nutrition and Exercise

Nutrition and weight control programs form another important set of health promotion services. Children need to learn sound dietary habits early in life to establish healthy lifelong patterns. Being overweight during childhood or adolescence may persist into adulthood and may increase the risk for some chronic diseases later in life.

- A number of weight control programs for overweight children and adolescents are available through schools, health departments, community health centers, health maintenance organizations, and private groups (Geria & Beitz, 2018; Williams et al., 2018).
- Children and adolescents are particularly vulnerable to media and peer pressures with regard to their food choices. Because of increased rates of childhood obesity and a greater awareness of the need for better nutrition in adolescence, district-level policies to increase the availability of healthy foods at public schools is growing (Micha et al., 2018).

The C/PHN, through nutrition education and reinforcement of positive practices and policy advocacy, plays a significant role in promoting the health of children.

SUMMARY

- The physical and emotional health of children and adolescents can affect not only their academic achievement but also the future of society. Children and adolescents need the guidance and direction provided by community health nurses.
- Poverty is a significant social determinant of health that has been shown to contribute to many physical, psychological, and behavioral problems in children and adolescents. There is concern that government assistance programs are not sufficiently meeting the needs of poor children and adolescents.
- Health problems that affect learning and achievement in school-age children include chronic diseases, behavioral and learning problems, disabilities, injuries, communicable diseases, dietary and physical activity concerns, and poor dental health.
- The federally and state-mandated immunization program for school-age children and adolescents is one measure to prevent communicable diseases. Among vaccines given on schedule throughout childhood are those that prevent polio, smallpox, diphtheria, tetanus, typhoid, and many other diseases.
- Mortality rates for children and adolescents have decreased dramatically since the early 1900s, but morbidity rates remain high. Children and adolescents are vulnerable to many illnesses, injuries, and emotional problems, often as a result of a complex and stressful environment.
- Violence against children and deaths because of homicide occur in the United States at alarming rates. Unintentional injuries, suicide, and homicide are the leading threats to life and health for adolescents.
- Other health problems include alcohol and drug abuse, unplanned pregnancies, STIs and HIV/AIDS, and poor nutrition. All of these problems create major challenges for the community health nurse who seeks to prevent illness and injury among children and adolescents and to promote their health.
- *Healthy People* objectives for children and adolescents provide key goals for reduction of alcohol-related unintentional injuries; declines in violent behaviors, suicide, mental health issues; and more responsible reproductive health behaviors. Barriers to achieving these goals vary and include economic inequities; lack of sufficient immunization, educational, and community-supported health programs; and the presence of risk behaviors typical among developing youth.
- Community health nurses play a large role in promoting the health of adolescents, their families, and communities, through education programs and by developing strategies to support healthy growth and development and prevent risky behaviors that lead to injury, teen pregnancy, and sometimes death.
- Health services for children and adolescents span three categories: prevention, health protection, and health promotion. The community health nurse plays a vital role in each.
  - Preventive services may include immunization programs, parental support services, family planning programs, services for those with STIs, and alcohol and drug abuse prevention programs.
  - Health protection services often include accident and injury control, programs to reduce environmental hazards and control infectious diseases, and services to protect children and adolescents from child abuse and neglect.
  - Health promotion services may include programs in nutrition and weight control, along with HIV/AIDS prevention and smoking, alcohol, and drug abuse education.
- C/PHNs are integral to the health and well-being of children and adolescents, through their work with families, schools, and other community agencies.

ACTIVE LEARNING EXERCISES

1. You are a community health nurse assigned to work at a school. You learn that more than 20% of the students in this school district are receiving medications for treating attention deficit hyperactivity disorder (ADHD). Why is this significant? Explain your reasoning. What evidence-based information will you use to prepare an individualized health care plan for each child?
2. You are working in a rural health department and are researching the leading causes of death among children and adolescents. Where can you find national and state data for your search? What evidence-based public health interventions have been successful in preventing childhood deaths? Select one intervention for children or adolescents and describe how you and a group of community health professionals might develop effective preventive measures.
3. A 14-year-old girl from a middle-class family and a 14-year-old girl from a poor family both come to the health department clinic where you work. The girls have similar symptoms that suggest gonorrhea. Would your assessment and intervention be the same for the two girls? What personal assumptions or biases might influence your plan of care? Compose a sexually transmitted infections prevention instruction document for this population group.
4. Your school district is searching for ways to improve adolescent nutrition and diet. What influencing factors should you consider (e.g., student behaviors, environment/cultural influences, school policies)? What key stakeholders should you include as you research and develop a health improvement plan? Describe an evidence-based program that you could implement to increase physical activity and improve nutrition for school-age children and adolescents.
5. You are assigned to work with a rural elementary school with repeated outbreaks of head lice and limited access to health care. Search credible online

resources for causes of recurrent head lice infestations and effective over-the-counter treatment products. Describe two head lice treatments and the supporting evidence. What are the advantages and disadvantages of each treatment?

6. Apply "Utilize Legal and Regulatory Actions" (1 of the 10 essential public health services; see Box 2-2), to the following: Your school district allows personal exemptions for vaccination (i.e., parents can refuse to get mandatory vaccinations for their children based on personal, not solely religious, beliefs). The public health department has informed you that there is a measles epidemic in your county. What information do you need to promote a safe and healthy school environment? Outline your concerns and formulate a health intervention for your school.

REFERENCES

Administration on Children and Families. (2018a). *Child abuse & neglect*. Retrieved from http://www.acf.hhs.gov/programs/cb/focus-areas/child-abuse-neglect

Administration on Children and Families. (2018b). *Child maltreatment 2013*. Retrieved from https://www.acf.hhs.gov/cb/resource/child-maltreatment-2016

American Academy of Child & Adolescent Psychiatry (AACAP). (2018). *School refusal*. Retrieved from https://www.aacap.org/AACAP/Families_and_Youth/Facts_for_Families/FFF-Guide/School-Refusal-007.aspx

American Cancer Society. (2017a). *Late effects of childhood cancer treatment*. Retrieved from https://www.cancer.org/treatment/children-and-cancer/when-your-child-has-cancer/late-effects-of-cancer-treatment.html

American Cancer Society. (2017b). *Returning to school after cancer treatment*. Retrieved from https://www.cancer.org/treatment/children-and-cancer/when-your-child-has-cancer/after-treatment/returning-to-school.html

American Heart Association. (2018). *Daily tips to help your family eat better*. Retrieved from http://www.heart.org/en/healthy-living/healthy-eating/eat-smart/nutrition-basics/daily-tips-to-help-your-family-eat-better

American Psychological Association. (n.d.). *Effects of poverty, hunger, and homelessness on children and youth*. Retrieved from http://www.apa.org/pi/families/poverty.aspx

Anxiety and Depression Association of America (ADAA). (n.d.). *School refusal*. Retrieved from https://adaa.org/living-with-anxiety/children/school-refusal

Badawy, S. M., Thompson, A. A., & Kuhns, L. M. (2017). Medication adherence and technology-based interventions for adolescents with chronic health conditions: A few key considerations. *Journal of Medical Internet Research (JMIR), 5*(12), e202.

Baio, J., Wiggins, L., Christensen, D. L., et al. (2018). Prevalence of autism spectrum disorder among children aged 8 years—Autism and developmental disabilities monitoring network, 11 Sites, United States, 2014. *Morbidity and Mortality Weekly Report Surveillance Summaries, 67*(SS-6), 1–23. doi: 10.15585/mmwr.ss6706a1.

Ballesteros, M. E., Williams, D. D., Mack, K. A., Simon, T. R., & Sleet, D. A. (2018). The epidemiology of unintentional and violence-related injury morbidity and mortality among children and adolescents in the United States. *International Journal of Environmental Research and Public Health, 15*, 616. doi: 10.3390/ijerph15040616.

Benson, A., Lambert, V., Gallagher, P., Shahwan, A., & Austin, J. K. (2017). Parent perspectives of the challenging aspects of disclosing a child's epilepsy diagnosis to others: Why don't they tell? *Chronic Illness, 13*(1), 28–48. doi: 10.1177/1742395316648749.

Blair, C. (2012). Treating a toxin to learning. *Scientific American Mind, 23*, 64–67.

Bureau of Alcohol, Tobacco, Firearms, and Explosives. (2018). *Fact sheet—Gang Resistance Education and Training (G.R.E.A.T.) Program*. Retrieved from https://www.atf.gov/resource-center/fact-sheet/fact-sheet-gang-resistance-education-and-training-great-program

Bhatta, S., Champion, J., Young, C., & Loika, E. (2018). Outcomes of depression screening among adolescents accessing school-based pediatric primary care clinic services. *Journal of Pediatric Nursing, 38*, 8–14.

Beland, L., & Kim, D. (2016). The effect of high school shootings on schools and student performance. *Education and Policy Analysis, 38*(1), 113–126. doi: 10.3102/0162373715590683.

Bose, S., Chiu, Y. M., Hsu, H. L., Di, Q., Rosa, M. J., Lee, A., …, Wright, R. J. (2017). Prenatal nitrate exposure and childhood asthma. Influence of maternal prenatal stress and fetal sex. *American Journal of Respiratory Critical Care Medicine, 196*(11), 1396–1403. doi: 10.1164/rccm.201702-0421OC.

Cambron, C., Kosterman, R., Catalano, R. F., Guttmannova, K., & Hawkins, D. J. (2018). Neighborhood, family, and peer factors associated with early adolescent smoking and alcohol use. *Journal of Youth and Adolescence, 47*, 369–382. doi: 10.1007/s10964-017-0728-y.

Cao, H. Yang, G., Wang, J., Liu, J., Smith, C., Luo, H., & Liu, Y. (2017). Complementary therapies for acne vulgaris. *Cochrane Database of Systematic Reviews*, (1). Art. No.: CD009436. doi: 10.1002/14651858.CD009436.pub2.

Carlson, S., & Keith-Jennings, B. (2018). SNAP is linked with improved nutritional outcomes and lower health care costs. Center on Budget & Policy Priorities. Retrieved from https://www.cbpp.org/research/food-assistance/snap-is-linked-with-improved-nutritional-outcomes-and-lower-health-care

Centeio, E. E., McCaughtry, N., Moore, W. G., Kulik, N., Garn, A., Martin, J., …, Fahlman, M. (2018). Building healthy communities: A comprehensive school health program to prevent obesity in elementary schools. *Preventive Medicine, 111*, 210–215. doi: 10.1016/j.ypmed.2018.03.005.

Center for the Study of Social Policy. (2017). *Poverty and early childhood fact sheet*. Retrieved from http://nccp.org/topics/childhood.html

Centers for Disease Control and Prevention (CDC). (2017a). *Health and academics*. Retrieved from https://www.cdc.gov/healthyschools/health_and_academics/

Centers for Disease Control and Prevention (CDC). (2017b). *Research brief: Addressing the needs of students with chronic health conditions: Strategies for schools*, 2017. Retrieved from https://www.cdc.gov/healthyschools/chronic_conditions/pdfs/2017_02_15-How-Schools-Can-Students-with-CHC_Final_508.pdf

Centers for Disease Control and Prevention (CDC). (2017c). *Leading causes of death in males, 2014*. Retrieved from https://www.cdc.gov/nchs/fastats/adolescent-health.htm

Centers for Disease Control and Prevention (CDC). (2017d). National, Regional, State, and selected local area vaccination coverage among adolescents aged 13–17 years, United States, 2016. *Morbidity and Mortality Weekly Report (MMWR), 66*(33), 874–882. Retrieved from https://www.cdc.gov/mmwr/volumes/66/wr/mm6633a2.htm?s_cid=mm6633a2_w

Centers for Disease Control and Prevention (CDC). (2017e). *Dental caries and sealant prevalence in children and adolescents in the United States, 2011–2012*. Retrieved from http://www.cdc.gov/nchs/products/databriefs/db191.htm

Centers for Disease Control and Prevention (CDC). (2017f). *Healthy schools: Body mass index (BMI) measurement in schools*. Retrieved from https://www.cdc.gov/healthyschools/obesity/bmi/bmi_measurement_schools.htm

Centers for Disease Control and Prevention (CDC). (2017g). *Ambulatory Care Use and Physician office visits. Summary Health Statistics Tables for U.S. Children: National Health Interview Survey, 2016, Table C-8c*. Retrieved from https://www.cdc.gov/nchs/fastats/physician-visits.htm

Centers for Disease Control and Prevention (CDC). (2017h). *Parents are the key to safe teen drivers*. Retrieved from https://www.cdc.gov/parentsarethekey/index.html

Centers for Disease Control and Prevention (CDC). (2018a). *National Diabetes Statistics Report*, 2017. Retrieved from http://www.cdc.gov/diabetes/data/statistics/statistics-report.html

Centers for Disease Control and Prevention (CDC). (2018b). *Prevent type 2 diabetes in kids*. Retrieved from https://www.cdc.gov/features/prevent-diabetes-kids/index.html

Centers for Disease Control and Prevention (CDC). (2018c). *Understanding HPV coverage*. Retrieved from https://www.cdc.gov/hpv/hcp/vacc-coverage/index.html

Centers for Disease Control and Prevention (CDC). (2018d). *Obesity*. Retrieved from https://www.cdc.gov/healthyschools/obesity/facts.htm

Centers for Disease Control and Prevention (CDC). (2018e). *Schools start too early*. Retrieved from https://www.cdc.gov/features/school-start-times/index.html

Centers for Disease Control and Prevention (CDC). (2018f). *Youth Risk Behavior Survey Data Summary & Trends Report 2007-2017*. Division of Adolescent and School Health. Retrieved from https://www.cdc.gov/healthyyouth/data/yrbs/pdf/trendsreport.pdf

Centers for Disease Control and Prevention (CDC). (2018g). *Sexually transmitted diseases: Adolescents and young adults*. Retrieved from https://www.cdc.gov/std/life-stages-populations/adolescents-youngadults.htm

Centers for Disease Control and Prevention (CDC). (2018h). *Tuberculosis (TB): TB in children*. Retrieved from https://www.cdc.gov/tb/topic/populations/tbinchildren/default.htm

Centers for Disease Control and Prevention (CDC). (2019a). *Health and academics: Healthy students are better learners*. Retrieved from https://www.cdc.gov/healthyyouth/health_and_academics/index.htm

Centers for Disease Control and Prevention (CDC). (2019b). *Autism spectrum disorder: Frequently asked questions*. Retrieved from https://www.cdc.gov/ncbddd/autism/topics.html

Centers for Disease Control and Prevention (CDC). (2019c). *Data and statistics about ADHD*. Retrieved from https://www.cdc.gov/ncbddd/adhd/data.html

Centers for Disease Control and Prevention (CDC). (2019d). *Key findings: Children's mental health report*. Retrieved from https://www.cdc.gov/childrensmentalhealth/features/kf-childrens-mental-health-report.html

Centers for Disease Control and Prevention (CDC). (2019e). *NoroSTAT data*. Retrieved from https://www.cdc.gov/norovirus/reporting/norostat/data.html

Centers for Disease Control and Prevention (CDC). (2019f). *Methicillin-resistant Staphylococcus aureus (MRSA)*. Retrieved from https://www.cdc.gov/mrsa/community/schools/index.html

Centers for Disease Control and Prevention (CDC). (2019g). *Adolescent and school health—Why schools? The right place for a healthy start*. Retrieved from https://www.cdc.gov/healthyyouth/about/why_schools.htm

Centers for Disease Control and Prevention (CDC). (2019h). *About teen pregnancy*. Retrieved from https://www.cdc.gov/teenpregnancy/about/index.htm

Centers for Disease Control and Prevention (CDC). (2019i). *Youth and tobacco use*. Retrieved from https://www.cdc.gov/tobacco/data_statistics/fact_sheets/youth_data/tobacco_use/index.htm

Centers for Disease Control and Prevention (CDC). (2019j). *Children's oral health*. Retrieved from https://www.cdc.gov/oralhealth/basics/childrens-oral-health/index.html

Centers for Disease Control and Prevention (CDC). (2019k). *Child passenger safety: Get the facts*. Retrieved from https://www.cdc.gov/motorvehiclesafety/child_passenger_safety/cps-factsheet.html

Centers for Disease Control and Prevention (CDC). (2020). *Tips to help children maintain a healthy weight*. Retrieved from https://www.cdc.gov/healthyweight/children/index.html

Centers for Disease Control and Prevention (CDC). (2020). *CDC's alcohol screening and brief intervetnio efforts*. Retrieved from https://www.cdc.gov/ncbddd/fasd/alcohol-screening.html

Centers for Disease Control and Prevention (CDC). (2020a). *What is spectrum disorder*. Retrieved from https://www.cdc.gov/ncbddd/autism/facts.html

Centers for Disease Control and Prevention (CDC). (2020b). *Data & statistics on ASD*. Retrieved from https://www.cdc.gov/ncbddd/autism/data.html

Centers for Disease Control and Prevention (CDC). (2020c). *Violence prevention*. Retrieved from https://www.cdc.gov/violenceprevention/childabuseandneglect/aces/fastfact.html

Centers for Disease Control and Prevention (CDC). (2020d). *Fatal injury data*. Retrieved from https://www.cdc.gov/injury/wisqars/fatal.html

Centers for Disease Control and Prevention (CDC). (2020e). *Motor vehicle safety*. Retrieved from https://www.cdc.gov/motorvehiclesafety/

Centers for Disease Control and Prevention (CDC). (2020f). *Measles cases and outbreaks*. Retrieved from https://www.cdc.gov/measles/cases-outbreaks.html

Centers for Disease Control and Prevention (CDC). (2020g). Tips to help children maintain a healthy weight. Retrieved from https://www.cdc.gov/healthyweight/children/index.html

Centers for Disease Control and Prevention (CDC). (2020h). *Preventing youth violence*. Retrieved from https://www.cdc.gov/violenceprevention/youthviolence/fastfact.html

Centers for Disease Control and Prevention (CDC). (2020i). *Sexual risk behaviors: HIV, STD, & teen pregnancy prevention*. Retrieved from https://www.cdc.gov/healthyyouth/sexualbehaviors/

Centers for Disease Control and Prevention (CDC). (2020j). *HIV among youth*. Retrieved from https://www.cdc.gov/hiv/group/age/youth/index.html

Centers for Disease Control and Prevention (CDC). (2020k). *Child abuse and neglect: Consequences*. Retrieved from https://www.cdc.gov/violenceprevention/childabuseandneglect/consequences.html

CDC (2020l). *CDC's alcohol screening and brief intervention efforts*. Retrieved from https://www.cdc.gov/ncbddd/fasd/alcohol-screening.html

Center on Budget and Policy Priorities (CBPP). (2018). *Chart book: Temporary assistance for needy families*. Retrieved from https://www.cbpp.org/research/family-income-support/chart-book-temporary-assistance-for-needy-families

Center for the Study of Social Policy. (2017). Poverty and Early Childhood Fact Sheet. Retrieved from http://nccp.org/topics/childhood.html

Chiang, J. L., Maahs, D. M., Garvey, K. C., Hood, K. H., Laffel, L. M., Weinzimer, S. A., ..., Schatz, D. (2018). Type 1 diabetes in children and adolescents: A position statement by the American Diabetes Association. *Diabetes Care, 41*(9), 2026–2044.

Child Trends Databank. (2018a). *Child recipients of welfare (AFDC/TANF)*. Retrieved from https://www.childtrends.org/indicators/child-recipients-of-welfareafdctanf

Child Trends Databank. (2018b). *5 important things to know about children and the Supplemental Nutrition Assistance Program (SNAP)*. Retrieved from https://www.childtrends.org/child-trends-5/5-important-things-know-children-supplemental-nutrition-assistance-program-snap

Colder, C. R., Shyhalla, K., & Frndak, S. E. (2018). Early alcohol use with parental permission: Psychosocial characteristics and drinking in late adolescence. *Addictive Behaviors, 76*, 82–87. Retrieved from http://dx.doi.org/10.1016/j.addbeh.2017.07.030

County Health Rankings and Roadmaps. (2018). *Universal school-based suicide awareness & education programs*. Retrieved from http://www.countyhealthrankings.org/take-action-to-improve-health/what-works-for-health/policies/universal-school-based-suicide-awareness-education-programs

Croen, L. A., Qian, Y., Ashwood, P., Daniels, J. L., Fallin, D., Schendel, D., ..., Zerbo, O. (2019). Family history of immune conditions and autism spectrum and developmental disorders: Findings from the study to explore early development. *Autism Research, 12*(1), 123–135. doi: 10.1002/aur.1979.

Cruz, T. B., McConell, R., Wagman, B., Unger, J. B., Pentz, M. A., Urman, R., ..., Barrington-Trimis, J. L. (2019). Tobacco marketing and subsequent use of cigarettes, e-cigarettes, and hookah in adolescents. *Nicotine and Tobacco Research, 21*(7), 926–932. doi: 10.1093/ntr/nty107.

Dawson, R. (2017). Addressing eating disorders and weight control in children and adolescents. *Pediatric Annals, 46*(5), e176–e179. doi: 10.3928/19382359-20170424-01.

D'Amica, E. J., Rodriquez, A., Tucker, J. S., Pedersen, E. R., & Shih, R. A. (2018). Planting the seed for marijuana use: Changes in exposure to medical marijuana advertising and subsequent adolescent marijuana use, cognitions, and consequences over seven years. *Drug and Alcohol Dependence, 188*, 385–391.

Demory-Luce, D., & Motil, K. J. (2018). Adolescent eating habits. *UpToDate*, February 2018. Retrieved from https://www.uptodate.com/contents/adolescent-eating-habits#H14

Diamond, G. S., Herres, J. L., Ewing, E. S., Atte, T. O., Scott, S. W., Wintersteen, M. B., & Gallop, R. J. (2017). Comprehensive screening for suicide risk in primary care. *American Journal of Preventive Medicine, 53*(1), 48–54.

Dubay, L. C., & Kenney, G. M. (2018). When the CHIPs are down—Health coverage and care at risk for U.S. children. *New England Journal of Medicine, 378*(7), 597–599. doi: 10.1056/NEJMp1716920.

Elertson, K. M., Liesch, S. K., & Babler, E. K. (2016). The "face" of diabetes: Insight into youths' experiences as expressed through drawing. *Journal of Patient Experience, 3*(2), 34–38. doi: 10.1177/2374373516654771.

Epilepsy Foundation. (n.d.). *About epilepsy: Who gets epilepsy*. Retrieved from https://www.epilepsy.com/learn/about-epilepsy-basics/who-gets-epilepsy

Eunice Kennedy Shriver National Institute of Child Health and Human Development. (2018a). *What causes learning disabilities?* Retrieved from https://www.nichd.nih.gov/health/topics/learning/conditioninfo/causes

Eunice Kennedy Shriver National Institute of Child Health and Human Development. (2018b). *What are the signs of learning disabilities?* Retrieved from https://www.nichd.nih.gov/health/topics/learning/conditioninfo/symptoms

Federal Interagency Forum on Child and Family Statistics (FCFS). (2019a). *America's children: Key national indicators of wellbeing, 2017: America's children at a glance*. Retrieved from https://www.childstats.gov/americaschildren/glance.asp

Federal Interagency Forum on Child and Family Statistics (FCFS). (2019b). *Family structure and children's living arrangements*. Retrieved from https://www.childstats.gov/americaschildren/family1.asp

Federal Interagency Forum on Child and Family Statistics (FCFS). (2019c). *America's children: Key national indicators of wellbeing, 2017: Child injury and mortality*. Retrieved from https://www.childstats.gov/americaschildren/phys7.asp

Federal Interagency Forum on Child and Family Statistics (FCFS). (2019d). *America's children: Key national indicators of wellbeing, 2017: Adolescent injury and mortality*. Retrieved from https://www.childstats.gov/americas-children/phys8.asp

Federal interagency Forum on Child and Family Statistics (FCFS). (2019e). *America's children: Key national indicators of wellbeing, 2017: Oral health*. Retrieved from https://www.childstats.gov/americaschildren/care4.asp

Felitti, V. J., Anda, R. F., Nordenberg, D., Williamson, D. F., Spitz, A. M., Edwards, V., …, Marks, J. S. (1998). Relationship of childhood abuse and household dysfunction to many of the leading causes of death in adults: The adverse childhood experiences (ACE) study. *American Journal of Preventive Medicine, 14*(4), 245–258.

Fix, R. L., Alexander, A. A., & Burkhart, B. R. (2018). From family violence exposure to violent offending: Examining effects of race and mental health in a moderated mediation model among confined male juveniles. *International Journal of Offender Therapy and Comparative Criminology, 62*(9), 2567–2585. doi: 10.1177/0306624X1773110.

Fleming, E., & Afful, J. (2018). Prevalence of Total and Untreated Dental Caries Among Youth: United States, 2015–2016. NCHS Data Brief, 307. Retrieved from https://www.cdc.gov/nchs/data/databriefs/db307.pdf

Food, Allergy, Research, and Education (FARE). (n.d.). *Food allergy facts and statistics*. Retrieved from https://www.foodallergy.org/life-with-food-allergies/food-allergy-101/facts-and-statistics

Francis, L., De Priest, K., Wilson, M., & Gross, D. (2018). Child poverty, toxic stress, and social determinants of health: Screening and care coordination. *Online Journal Issues Nursing, 23*(3). doi: 10.3912/OJIN.Vol23No03Man02.

Geria, K., & Beitz, J. M. (2018). Application of a modified diabetes prevention program with adolescents. *Public Health Nursing, 35*, 337–343.

Gottfredson, D. C., Thornberry, T. P., Slowthower, M., & Devlin, D. (2018). *Reducing gang violence: A randomized trial of functional family therapy*. Made publically available through the Office of Justice Programs' National Criminal Justice Reference Service. Retrieved from https://www.ncjrs.gov/pdffiles1/nij/grants/251754.pdf

Guttmacher Institute. (February 2017). *Facts on American teens' sources of information about sex*. Retrieved from https://www.guttmacher.org/sites/default/files/factsheet/facts-american-teens-sources-information-about-sex.pdf

Hadland, S. E., Xuan, Z., Sarda, V., Blanchette, J., Swahn, M. H., Heeren, T. C., …, Naimi, T. S. (2017). *Pediatrics, 139*(3). pii: e20163037. doi: 10.1542/peds.2016-3037.

Hale, L., & Troxel, W. (2018). Embracing the school start later movement: Adolescent sleep deprivation as a public health and social justice problem. *American Journal of Public Health, 108*(5), 599–600.

Hardin, H. J., McCarthy, V. L., Speck, B. J., & Crawford, T. N. (2018). Diminished trust of healthcare providers, risky lifestyle behaviors, and low use of health services: A descriptive study rural adolescents. *Journal of School Nursing, 34*(6), 458–467. doi: 10.1177/1059840517725787.

Healthy Schools Campaign. (2018). *School health services matter more than ever*. Retrieved from https://healthyschoolscampaign.org/health/

Henry, K. L., Fulco, C. J., Agbeke, D. V., & Ratcliff, A. M. (2018). Intergenerational continuity in substance abuse: Does offspring's friendship network make a difference? *Journal of Adolescent Health, 63*, 205–212.

Heron, M. (2017). Deaths: Leading causes for 2015. *National Vital Statistics Report, 66*(5). Retrieved from https://www.cdc.gov/nchs/data/nvsr/nvsr66/nvsr66_05.pdf

Hockenberry, M. J., Wilson, D., & Rodgers, C. C. (2019). *Wong's nursing care of infants and children* (11th ed.). St. Louis, MO: Elsevier.

Hsu, J., Sircar, K., Herman, E., & Garbe, P. (2018). *EXHALE: A technical package to control asthma*. Centers for Disease Control and Prevention, National Center for Environmental Health. Retrieved from https://www.cdc.gov/asthma/pdfs/EXHALE_technical_package-508.pdf

Jacobson Vann, J. C., Jacobson, R. M., Coyne-Beasley, T., Asafu-Adjei, J. K., & Szilagyi, P. G. (2018). Patient reminder and recall interventions to improve immunization rates. *Cochrane Database of Systematic Reviews, 1*, Art. No.: CD003941. DOI: 10.1002/14651858.CD003941.pub3.

James, J. (2017). *Adolescent growth: Eating disorder statistics 2017*. Retrieved from https://adolescentgrowth.com/eating-disorder-statistics/

Jordan, J. W., Stalgaitis, C. A., Charles, J., Madden, P. A., Radhakrishnan, A. G., & Saggese, D. (2018). Peer crowd identification and adolescent health behaviors: Results from a statewide representative study. *Health Education & Behavior*, 1–13. doi: 10.1177/1090198118759148.

Kaiser Family Foundation. (2019). *Key facts about the uninsured population*. Retrieved from https://www.kff.org/uninsured/fact-sheet/key-facts-about-the-uninsured-population/

Kann, L., McManus, T., Harris, W. A., Shanklin, S. L., Flint, K. H., Queen, B., …, Ethier, K. K. A. (2018). Youth risk behavior surveillance—United States, 2017. *Morbidity and Mortality Weekly Report (MMWR), 67*(8), 1–114. Retrieved from https://www.cdc.gov/mmwr/volumes/67/ss/ss6708a1.htm

Kerr, E. N., & Fayed, N. (2017). Cognitive predictors of adaptive functioning in children with symptomatic epilepsy. *Epilepsy Research, 136*, 67–76.

Layba, C., Griffin, L. W., Jupiter, D., Mathers, C., & Mileski, W. (2017). Adolescent motor vehicle crash prevention through a trauma center-based intervention program. *Journal of Trauma and Acute Care Surgery, 83*(3), 850–853.

Lee, A. M., Scharf, R. J., & DeBoer, M. D. (2018). Association between kindergarten and first-grade insecurity and weight status in U.S. children. *Nutrition, 51–52*, 1–5. Retrieved from https://doi.org/10.1016/j.nut.2017.12.008

Leroy, Z. C., Wallin, R., & Lee, S. (2017). The role of school health services in addressing the needs of students with chronic health conditions. *Journal of School Nursing, 33*(1), 64–72. doi: 10.1177/1059840516678909. Retrieved from https://www.ncbi.nlm.nih.gov/pubmed/27872391

Lunstead, J., Weitzman, E. R., Kaye, D., & Levy, S. (2017). Screening and brief intervention in high schools: School nurses' practices and attitudes in Massachusetts. *Substance Abuse, 38*(3), 257–260.

Marseille, E., Mirzazadeh, A., Biggs, M. A., Miller, A. P., Horvath, H., Lightfoot, M., Malekinejad, M., & Kahn, J. G. (2018). Effectiveness of school-based teen pregnancy prevention programs in the USA: A systematic review and meta-analysis. *Prevention Science, 19*, 468–489. Retrieved from https://doi.org/10.1007/s11121-017-0861-6

Martin, A., Booth, J. N., Laird, Y., Sproule, J., Reilly, J. J., & Saunders, D. H. (2018). Physical activity, diet and other behavioural interventions for improving cognition and school achievement in children and adolescents with obesity or overweight (Review). *Cochrane Database of Systematic Reviews, 3*. Art No.: CD009728. doi: 10.1002/14651858.CD009728.pub4.

Matone, M., Kellom, K., Griffis, H., Quarshie, W., Faerber, J., Gierlach, P., …, Cronholm, P. F. (2018). A mixed methods evaluation of early childhood abuse prevention within evidence-based home visiting programs. *Maternal and Child Health Journal*, 22(S1), S79–S91. Retrieved from https://doi.org/10.1007/s10995-018-2530-1

Mayer-Davis, E., Lawrence, J., Dabelea, D., Divers, J., Dolan, L., Imperatore, G., …, Wagenknecht, L. (2017). Incidence trends of type 1 and type 2 diabetes among youths, 2002–2012. *New England Journal of Medicine, 376*(15), 1419–1429. doi: 10.1056/NEJMoa1610187.

Maynard, B. R., Brendel, K. E., Bulanda, J. J., Heyne, D., Thompson, A., & Pigott, T. D. (2015). Psychosocial interventions for school refusal behavior with elementary and secondary school students: A systematic review. *Campbell Systematic Reviews, 12*. doi: 10.4073/csr.2015.12.

Mayo Clinic. (2017). *Acne treatment*. Retrieved from https://www.mayoclinic.org/diseases-conditions/acne/diagnosis-treatment/drc-20368048

Mayo Clinic. (2018a). *Attention-deficit/hyperactivity (ADHD) disorder in children*. Retrieved from https://www.mayoclinic.org/diseases-conditions/adhd/symptoms-causes/syc-20350889

Mayo Clinic. (2018b). *Epilepsy: Diagnosis & treatment*. Retrieved from https://www.mayoclinic.org/diseases-conditions/epilepsy/diagnosis-treatment/drc-20350098

Mays, D., Hawkins, K. B., Bredfeldt, C., Wolf, H., & Tercyak, K. P. (2017). The effects of framed messages for engaging adolescents with online smoking prevention interventions. *Translational Behavioral Medicine, 7*(2), 196–203.

McDonald, C. C., Kennedy, E., Fleisher, L., & Zonfrillo, M. R. (2018). Situational use of child restraint systems and carpooling behaviors in parents and caregivers. *International Journal of Environmental Research and Public Health, 15*, 1788. Retrieved from doi.org/10.3390/ijerph15081788

Micha, R., Karageorgou, D., Bakogianni, I., Trichia, E., Whitsel, L. P., Sroty, M., …, Mozaffarian, D. (2018). Effectiveness of school food environment policies on children's dietary behaviors: A systematic review and meta-analysis. *PLoS One, 13*(3), e0194555. Retrieved from https://doi.org/10.1371/journal.pone.0194555

Miller, G. F., Coffield, E., Leroy, Z., & Wallin, R. (2016). Prevalence and costs of five chronic conditions in children. *Journal of School Nursing, 32*(5), 357–364. doi: 10.1177/1059840516641190.

Miller, R. L., & Lawrence, J. (2018). Understanding root causes of asthma: Perinatal environmental exposures and epigenetics. *Annals of American Thoracic Society, 15*(S2), S103–S108.

National Cancer Institute. (2017). *Cancer in children and adolescents*. Retrieved from https://www.cancer.gov/types/childhood-cancers/child-adolescent-cancers-fact-sheet

National Center for Children in Poverty (NCCP). (2018). *Basic facts about low-income children: Children under 18 years, 2016*. Retrieved from http://www.nccp.org/publications/pub_1194.html

National Center for Education Statistics (NCES). 2017. *Indicators of school crime and safety*. Retrieved from https://nces.ed.gov/programs/crimeindicators/

National Center for Education Statistics (NCES). (2018a). *Fast facts: Back to school statistics*. Retrieved from https://nces.ed.gov/fastfacts/display.asp?id=372

National Center for Education Statistics (NCES). (2018b). *Students with disabilities*. Retrieved from https://nces.ed.gov/programs/coe/indicator_cgg.asp

National Center for Learning Disabilities (NCLD). (2017). *The state of learning disabilities: Understanding the 1 in 5*. Retrieved from https://www.ncld.org/the-state-of-learning-disabilities-understanding-the-1-in-5

National Heart, Lung, and Blood Institute. (2018). *Asthma*. Retrieved from https://www.nhlbi.nih.gov/health-topics/asthma

National Institute of Dental & Craniofacial Research. (2018). *The tooth decay process: How to reverse it and avoid a cavity*. Retrieved from https://www.nidcr.nih.gov/health-info/childrens-oral-health/tooth-decay-process

National Institute of Drug Abuse for Teens. (2017a). *Marijuana*. Retrieved from https://teens.drugabuse.gov/drug-facts/marijuana

National Institute of Drug Abuse for Teens. (2017b). *Inhalants*. Retrieved from https://teens.drugabuse.gov/drug-facts/inhalants

National Institute of Drug Abuse for Teens. (2017c). *MDMA (ecstasy or molly)*. Retrieved from https://teens.drugabuse.gov/drug-facts/mdma-ecstasy-or-molly

National Institute of Drug Abuse for Teens. (2017d). *Methamphetamine*. Retrieved from https://teens.drugabuse.gov/drug-facts/methamphetamine-meth

National Institute of Drug Abuse for Teens. (2017e). *Anabolic steroids*. Retrieved from https://teens.drugabuse.gov/drug-facts/anabolic-steroids

National Institute of Drug Abuse for Teens. (2017f). *Prescription drugs*. Retrieved from https://teens.drugabuse.gov/drug-facts/prescription-drugs

National Institute of Health (NIH). (2017). *Monitoring the future study: Trends in prevalence of various drugs*. Retrieved from https://www.drugabuse.gov/trends-statistics/monitoring-future/monitoring-future-study-trends-in-prevalence-various-drugs

National Institute of Mental Health (NIMH). (n.d.a). *NIMH pages about attention deficit hyperactivity disorder (ADHD)*. Retrieved from http://www.nimh.nih.gov/topics/topic-page-adhd.shtml

National Institute of Mental Health (NIMH). (n.d.b). *Eating disorders*. Retrieved from https://www.nimh.nih.gov/health/topics/eating-disorders/index.shtml#part_145414

National Institute of Mental Health (NIMH). (2017). *Mental illness*. Retrieved from https://www.nimh.nih.gov/health/statistics/mental-illness.shtml

National Institute of Mental Health (NIMH). (2018). *Suicide*. Retrieved from https://www.nimh.nih.gov/health/statistics/suicide.shtml

National Institute of Occupational Safety and Health. (2018). Home page. Retrieved from https://www.cdc.gov/niosh/index.htm

National Resource Center on ADHD (CHADD). (2018). *Disruptive behavior disorders*. Retrieved from http://www.chadd.org/about-adhd/disruptive-beghavior-disorders/

Nesi, J., Choukas-Bradley, S., & Prinstein, M. (2018). Transformation of adolescent peer relations in the social media context: Part 1—A theoretical framework and application to dyadic peer relationships. *Clinical Child and Family Psychology Review, 21*, 267–294. Retrieved from https://doi.org/10.1007/s10567-018-0261-x

Office of Adolescent Health. (2017a). *Adolescent development e-learning module*. Retrieved from https://www.hhs.gov/ash/oah/resources-and-training/online-learning-modules/adolescent-development/index.html

Office of Adolescent Health. (2017b). *Tobacco use in adolescence*. Retrieved from https://www.hhs.gov/ash/oah/adolescent-development/substance-use/drugs/tobacco/index.html

Office of Adolescent Health. (2017c). *Trends in teen pregnancy and childbearing*. Retrieved from https://www.hhs.gov/ash/oah/adolescent-development/reproductive-health-and-teen-pregnancy/teen-pregnancy-and-childbearing/trends/index.html

Office of Adolescent Health. (2018a). *Mental health in adolescents*. Retrieved from https://www.hhs.gov/ash/oah/adolescent-development/mental-health

Office of Adolescent Health. (2018b). *How common is adolescent alcohol use?* Retrieved from https://www.hhs.gov/ash/oah/adolescent-development/substance-use/alcohol/how-common/index.html

Office of Adolescent Health. (2018c). *Where teens receive preventive health care*. Retrieved from https://www.hhs.gov/ash/oah/adolescent-development/physical-health-and-nutrition/clinical-preventive-services/where-teens-receive-care/index.html

Office of Disease Prevention and Health Promotion (ODPHP). (2018). *Healthy people 2020: Adolescent health*. Retrieved from https://www.healthypeople.gov/2020/topics-objectives/topic/Adolescent-Health

Pew Research Center. (2018). *A majority of U.S. teens fear a shooting could happen at their school, and most parents share their concern*. Retrieved from https://www.pewresearch.org/fact-tank/2018/04/18/a-majority-of-u-s-teens-fear-a-shooting-could-happen-at-their-school-and-most-parents-share-their-concern/

Pulcini, C. D., Zima, B. T., Kelleher, K. J., & Houtrow, A. J. (2017). Poverty and trends in three common chronic disorders. *Pediatrics, 139*(3), e20162539.

Ra, C. K., Cho, J., Stone, M., De La Cerda, J., Goldenson, N., Moroney, E., …, Leventhal, A. (2018). Association of digital media use with subsequent symptoms of Attention-Deficit/Hyperactivity Disorder among adolescents. *Journal of the American Medical Association, 320*(3), 255–263. doi: 10.1001/jama.2018.8931.

Rabbitte, M., & Enriquez, M. (2018). The role of policy on sexual health education in schools: Review. *The Journal of School Nursing, 1*, 12. Retrieved from https://doi-org.erl.lib.byu.edu/10.1177/1059840518789240

Rechenberg, K., Whittemore, R., & Grey, M. (2017). Anxiety in youth with type 1 diabetes. *Journal of Pediatric Nursing, 32*, 64–71.

Rongstad, R., Neuman, M., Pillai, P., Birstler, J., & Hanrahan, L. (2018). Screening pediatric patients for food insecurity: A retrospective cross-sectional study of comorbidities and demographic characteristics. *Wisconsin Medical Journal, 117*(3), 122–125.

Rudisill, T. M., Smith, G., Chu, H., & Zhu, M. (2018). Cellphone legislation and self-reported behaviors among subgroups of adolescent U.S. drivers. *Journal of Adolescent Health, 62*, 618–625.

Safe Kids Worldwide. (2018). *Safe kids worldwide safety tips*. Retrieved from http://www.safekids.org/safetytips

Saunders, E. J. (2018). Mobilizing communities in support of teen pregnancy prevention: "Communitywide Initiatives" findings. *Health Promotion Practice, 19*(1), 16–22. doi: 10.1177/1524839916662602.

Schieve, L. A., Tian, L., Drews-Botsch, C., Windham, G. C., Newschaffer, C., Daniels, J. L., …, Fallin, M. D. (2018). Autism Spectrum Disorder and birth spacing: Findings from the study to explore early development (SEED). *Autism Research, 11*(1), 81–94. doi: 10.1002/aur.1887.

Shankar, P., Chung, R., & Frank, D. A. (2017). Association of food insecurity with children's behavioral, emotional, and academic outcomes: A systematic Review. *Journal of Developmental and Behavioral Pediatrics, 38*(2), 135–150. doi: 10.1097/DBP.0000000000000383.

Simmer-Beck, M., Wellever, A., & Kelly, P. (2017). Using registered dental hygienists to promote a school-based approach to dental public health. *American Journal of Public Health, 107*(S1), 5556–560.

Simon. (2018). *Facts & figures 2018: Rate of deaths from cancer continues decline*. Retrieved from https://www.cancer.org/latest-news/facts-and-figures-2018-rate-of-deaths-from-cancer-continues-decline.html

Skroza, N., Tolino, E., Mambrin, A., Zuber, S., Balduzzi, V., Marchesiello, A., …, Potenza, C. (2018). Adult acne versus adolescent acne. *Journal of Clinical and Aesthetic Dermatology, 11*(1), 21–25. Retrieved from https://www.ncbi.nlm.nih.gov/pmc/articles/PMC5788264/

Slade, G. D., Grider, W. B., Maas, W. R., & Sanders, A. E. (2018). Water fluoridation and dental caries in U.S. children and adolescents. *Journal of Dental Research, 97*(10), 1122–1128. doi: 10.1177/0022034518774331.

Soneji, S., Barrington-Trimis, J. L., Wills, T. A., Leventhal, A. M., Unger, J. B., Gibson, L. A., …, Sargent, J. D. (2017). Association between initial use of e-cigarettes and subsequent cigarette smoking among adolescents and young adults: A systematic review and meta-analysis. *Journal of American Medical Association Pediatrics, 171*(8), 788–797. doi: 10.1001/jamapediatrics.2017.1488.

Stockwell, S. (2018). ED visits for self-harm by girls are on the rise. *American Journal of Nursing, 118*(3), 13. doi: 10.1097/01.NAJ.0000530923.41338.ce.

Stormshak, E., DeGarmo, D., Chronister, K., & Caruthers, A. (2018). The impact of family-centered prevention on self-regulation and subsequent long-term risk in emerging adults. *Prevention Science, 19*, 549–558. Retrieved from https://doi.org/10.1007/s11121-017-0852-7

The National Institute for Occupational Safety and Health (NIOSH). (2018). *Young worker safety and health*. Retrieved from https://www.cdc.gov/niosh/topics/youth/default.html

Tobacco Free Kids. (2017). *The flavor trap*. Retrieved from https://www.tobaccofreekids.org/microsites/flavortrap/full_report.pdf

Toothaker, R., & Cook, P. (2018). A review of four health procedures that school nurses may encounter. *National Association School Nurse (NASN) School Nurse, 33*(1), 19–22. doi: 10.1177/1942602X17725885.

United States Department of Justice. (2018). *Gang statistics*. Retrieved from https://www.justice.gov/jm/criminal-resource-manual-103-gang-statistics

U.S. Department of Agriculture (USDA) Food & Nutrition Service. (2017). *FACT SHEET: Healthy, Hunger-Free Kids Act School Meals Implementation*. Retrieved from https://www.fns.usda.gov/pressrelease/2014/009814

U.S. Department of Agriculture (USDA). (2018). *Food security in the United States: Key statistics & graphics*. Retrieved from https://www.ers.usda.gov/topics/food-nutrition-assistance/food-security-in-the-us/key-statistics-graphics.aspx

U.S. Department of Education. (2018). *IDEA: Individuals with disabilities education act*. Retrieved from https://sites.ed.gov/idea/

U.S. Department of Health and Human Services (USDHHS). (2020). *Healthy People 2030: Browse objectives*. Retrieved from https://health.gov/healthypeople/objectives-and-data/browse-objectives

U.S. Food & Drug Administration (FDA). (2017). *Treating and preventing head lice*. Retrieved from https://www.fda.gov/ForConsumers/ConsumerUpdates/ucm171730.htm

University of Virginia. (2018). *Virginia Youth Violence Project: Reports and Research Summaries*. Retrieved from https://curry.virginia.edu/faculty-research/centers-labs-projects/research-labs/youth-violence-project/youth-violence-project-0

Van Ryzin, M. J., Fishbein, D., & Biglan, A. (2018). The promise of prevention science for addressing intergenerational poverty. *Psychology, Public Policy, and Low, 24*(1), 128–143.

Venditti, E. M., Tan, K., Chang, N., Laffel, L., McGinley, G., Miranda, N., …, Delahanty, L. (2018). Barriers and strategies for oral medication adherence among children and adolescents with Type 2 diabetes. *Diabetes Research and Clinical Practice, 139*, 24–31.

Walker, T. Y., Elam-Evans, L. D., Singleton, J. A., Yankey, D., Markowitz, L. E., Fredua, B., …, Stokley, S. (2017). National, regional, state, and selected local area vaccination coverage among adolescents aged 13–17 years—United States, 2016. *Morbidity and Mortality Weekly Report (MMWR), 66*(33), 874–882. Retrieved from https://www.cdc.gov/mmwr/volumes/66/wr/mm6633a2.htm

Wheaton, A. G., Chapman, D. P., & Croft, J. B. (2016). School start times, sleep, behavioral, health, and academic outcomes: A review of the literature. *Journal of School Health, 86*(5), 363–381. Retrieved from https://www.ncbi.nlm.nih.gov/pubmed/27040474

Williams, A. S., Bin, G., Petroski, G., Kruse, R. L., McElroy, J. A., & Koopman, R. J. (2018). Socioeconomic status and other factors associated with childhood obesity. *Journal of the American Board of Family Medicine, 31*(4), 514–521.

Wills, T. A., Knight, R., Sargent, J. D., Gibbons, F. X., Pagano, I., & Williams, R. J. (2017). Longitudinal study of e-cigarette use and onset of cigarette smoking among high school students in Hawaii. *Tobacco Control, 26*(1), 34–39. doi: 10.1136/tobaccocontrol-2015-052705.

World Health Organization. (2018a). *Sexually transmitted infections among adolescents: The need for adequate health services*. Retrieved from http://www.who.int/maternal_child_adolescent/documents/9241562889/en/

World Health Organization. (2018b). *The top 10 causes of death*. Retrieved from http://www.who.int/news-room/fact-sheets/detail/the-top-10-causes-of-death

Yilmaz, Z., Javaras, K. N., Baker, J. H., Thornton, L. M., Lichtenstein, P., Bulik, C. M., & Larsson, H. (2017). Association between childhood to adolescent attention deficit/hyperactivity disorder symptom trajectories and late adolescent disordered eating. *Journal of Adolescent Health, 61*(2), 140–146.

Yoshida, Y., & Simoes, E. (2018). Sugar-sweetened beverage, obesity, and type 2 diabetes in children and adolescents: Policies, taxation, and programs. *Current Diabetes Reports, 18*(6), 31. doi: 10.1007/s11892-018-1004-6.

Youth.Gov. (n.d.). *Substance abuse prevention: Risk and protective factors*. Retrieved from https://youth.gov/youth-topics/youth-mental-health/risk-and-protective-factors-youth

CHAPTER 21

Adult Health

"Male and female represent the two sides of the great radical dualism. But in fact, they are perpetually passing into one another. Fluid hardens to solid, and solid rushes to fluid. There is no wholly masculine man, no purely feminine woman."

—Margaret Fuller (1810–1850), Woman in the Nineteenth Century, 1845

KEY TERMS

Adult
Anorexia nervosa
Binge eating
Bisexual
Bulimia nervosa
Cancer
Cardiovascular disease (CVD)
Chronic lower respiratory disease (CLRD)
Diabetes mellitus
Erectile dysfunction (ED)
Life expectancy
Menopausal hormone therapy (MHT)
Menopause
Myalgic encephalomyelitis/chronic fatigue syndrome (ME/CFS)
Osteoporosis
Perimenopause
Prostate
Substance use disorder (SUD)
Transgender
Unintentional injuries

LEARNING OBJECTIVES

Upon mastery of this chapter, you should be able to:

1. Identify key demographic characteristics of women and men throughout the adult life span.
2. Discuss the concepts of life expectancy, health disparities, and health literacy and how they apply to adult women and men living in the United States.
3. Discuss the major chronic illnesses found in adult women and men in the United States.
4. Compare and contrast the manifestations of chronic illnesses in adult women and men.
5. Discuss factors affecting the health of adult women and men in the United States.
6. Identify primary, secondary, and tertiary health promotion activities designed to improve the health of women and men across the life span.
7. Identify the *Healthy People 2030* objectives for adult women and men.
8. Describe the role of the community health nurse in promoting the health of adult women and men across the life span.

INTRODUCTION

Mrs. Anderson is a relatively healthy middle-aged woman, with no chronic health conditions. Her family history is positive for type 2 diabetes mellitus, cardiovascular disease, and colon cancer. She tries to eat healthy, but her moderately stressful career and busy family make it difficult to find time to cook and exercise. Over the past few years, she has noticed weight gain and is concerned that this, along with her family history, may lead to the development of chronic disease. What are considerations for Mrs. Anderson based on her age, risk factors, and current health status? What preventative services and screenings might she need?

Community and public health nurses (C/PHN) are in a key position to educate clients like Mrs. Anderson on health promotion and disease prevention and inform them of U.S. Preventative Services recommendations. This teaching impacts community health by improving the health of individuals.

The term *adult* has many different meanings in society. To children, an **adult** is anyone in authority, including a 14-year-old babysitter. As people age, they tend to redefine the term upward. It is not unusual, for example, to hear an older person describe a couple in their mid-30s as "kids." The U.S. criminal justice system distinguishes between adults and juveniles for purposes of delimiting types of crimes and possibilities for punishment, and labor legislation provides different protections for children than for adult workers. Even hospitals and health care systems vary somewhat as to the ages at which they distinguish pediatric and geriatric clients from middle-aged adults.

How would you characterize an adult? Does your definition rest solely on age or is it influenced by other factors, such as marital status, employment status, financial independence, amount of responsibility for self and others, and so on?

- For the purposes of this chapter, an adult is defined as anyone 18 years of age or older. Obviously, there are tremendous differences in health profiles and health care needs as people age.
- As adults enter their middle years (35 to 65), they experience many normal physiologic changes. However, some changes are the result of disease, environment, or lifestyle and can be modified through behavior change.

Throughout history, the health care needs of women and men have differed more often than shown similarities (Fig. 21-1). Many health promotion and health protection programs are designed specifically for women or for men, as the examples below illustrate.

- Mammography screening programs and prenatal clinics are designed with women's health in mind.
- Teaching about testicular self-examination (TSE) and prostate cancer screening is typically included in health promotion programs for men.
- Programs in many areas, such as cardiac rehabilitation, stress management, and dating violence prevention, may have initially targeted one gender but are now established as programs for both genders.

Despite areas of overlap in women's and men's health, morbidity and mortality statistics, historical development of research foci, and workforce changes require that the health care needs of women and men be examined separately. This chapter focuses on the health of women and men across the adult life span. A physical profile of middle-aged adults is organized by body systems and can be found on thePoint®.

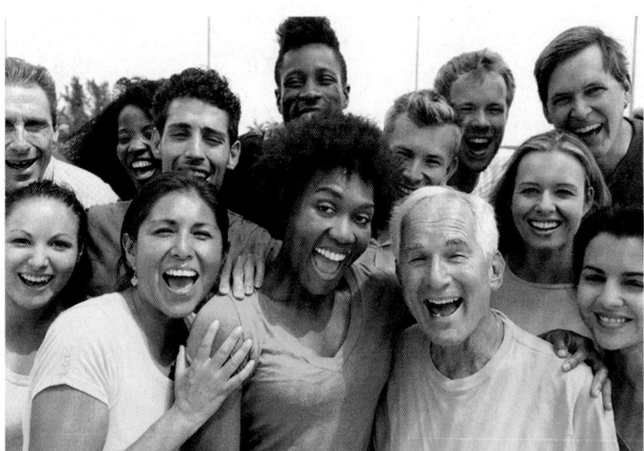

FIGURE 21-1 Health care needs of men and women of varying ages are often different.

DEMOGRAPHICS OF ADULT WOMEN AND MEN

Examining mortality statistics provides key information to understanding changes in the health and well-being of a population. In 2016, a total of 2,744,248 people died in the United States. The age-adjusted death rate was 728.8 per 100,000 for all ages (Kochanek, Murphy, Xu, & Arias, 2017). Causes of death varied by age, gender, and ethnicity, but the 10 leading causes of death for all people in rank order are shown in Table 21-1.

Since the beginning of the 21st century, the major causes of death have remained fairly consistent. This was a major shift from the turn of the 20th century, when communicable diseases, such as tuberculosis and pneumonia, were leading causes of death. The shift from communicable to chronic illness can be attributed to the significant advances in public health, prevention, technology, pharmacotherapy, and biomedical research (see Chapters 1 and 7).

- In 2016, 74% of all deaths in the United States were attributed to the 10 leading causes (Heron, 2018).
- Diseases of the heart and malignant neoplasms are the top two causes of death for both men and women and accounted for 44.9% of deaths in 2016.

Differences included the following:

- Cerebrovascular diseases (stroke) were the third leading cause of death for women.
- Unintentional injuries (accidents) were the leading cause of death for all adults aged 25 to 44 years and the third leading cause of death for men.
- Cancer was the leading cause of death in adults aged 45 to 65 years (Heron, 2018; National Center for Health Statistics [NCHS], 2019).

TABLE 21-1 The 10 Leading Causes of Death for All Ages in 2017

Cause of Death (in rank order)	Number of Deaths
1. Diseases of the heart (heart disease)	647,457
2. Malignant neoplasms (cancer)	599,108
3. Unintentional injuries (accidents)	169,936
4. Chronic lower respiratory diseases	160,201
5. Cerebrovascular diseases (stroke)	146,383
6. Alzheimer's disease	121,404
7. Diabetes mellitus (diabetes)	83,564
8. Influenza and pneumonia	55,672
9. Nephritis, nephritic syndrome, and nephrosis (kidney disease)	50,633
10. Intentional self-harm (suicide)	47,173

Source: National Center for Health Statistics (2017).

LIFE EXPECTANCY

Life expectancy is the average number of years that an individual member of a specific cohort (usually a single birth year) is projected to live. It is another standard measurement used to compare the health status of various populations and is typically calculated based on age-specific death rates. Health statistics often report life expectancy figures at birth and at 65 and 75 years of age (Table 21-2).

- In the United States, life expectancy increased consistently over time until 2015, when for the first time in 25 years it decreased for both males and females (Xu, Murphy, Kochanek, & Arias, 2018).
- Women have a higher life expectancy than men, but the gap has narrowed from 7.0 years in 1990 to 5.0 years in 2016.
- There also continue to be differences in life expectancy based on race and ethnicity in the United States. In 2016, individuals of Hispanic origin had a life expectancy of 81.8 years, whereas the life expectancy for Whites was 78.5 years and for Blacks was 74.8 years, indicating a disproportionate burden of morbidity and mortality (NCHS, 2019).

Globally, life expectancy in the United States trails that of many countries (Table 21-3). Japan reports the highest life expectancy for males and females. In all countries, disparities exist between male and female life expectancy. The smallest disparity can be found between women and men living in Iceland, at 2.6 years (NCHS, 2019).

TABLE 21-3 Life Expectancy at Birth for Selected Countries by Sex, 2015

	Female	Male	Disparity
Japan	87.1	80.8	6.3
France	85.5	79.2	6.3
Switzerland	85.1	80.8	4.3
Spain	85.8	80.1	5.7
Australia	84.5	80.4	4.1
Iceland	83.8	81.2	2.6
Germany	83.1	78.3	4.8
Greece	83.7	78.5	5.2
Korea	85.2	79.0	6.2
United States	81.1	76.3	4.8

Reprinted from National Center for Health Statistics. (2017). *Heath, United States, 2017.* Retrieved from https://www.cdc.gov/nchs/data/hus/2017/014.pdf

HEALTH DISPARITIES

The overarching goal of the *Healthy People* initiative is to eliminate health disparities and improve the health of all Americans. A health disparity is defined as a difference in health status that occurs by gender, race/ethnicity, education or income, disability, geographic location, or sexual orientation (Orgera & Artiga, 2018). Health disparities occur when one segment of the population has a higher rate of disease or mortality than another or when survival rates are less for one group when compared with another (National Institutes of Health [NIH], 2019a). Often, persons with the greatest health burden have the least access to health care services, adequate health care providers,

TABLE 21-2 Life Expectancy at Birth and 65 Years of Age According to Sex: United States, Selected Years, 1900–2017

	At Birth			At 65 Years		
Year	Both Sexes	Male	Female	Both Sexes	Male	Female
1900	47.3	46.3	48.3	—	—	—
1950	68.2	65.6	71.1	13.9	12.8	15.0
1960	69.7	66.6	73.1	14.3	12.8	15.8
1970	70.8	67.1	74.7	15.2	13.1	17.0
1980	73.7	70.0	77.4	16.4	14.1	18.3
1990	75.4	71.8	78.8	17.2	15.1	18.9
2000	76.8	74.1	79.3	17.6	16.0	19.0
2010	78.7	76.2	81.0	19.1	17.7	20.3
2016	78.7	76.2	81.1	19.4	18.0	20.6
2017	78.6	76.1	81.1	19.4	18.0	20.6

—, data not available.

Reprinted from National Center for Health Statistics (NCHS). (2019). *Health, United States 2017.* Retrieved from https://www.cdc.gov/nchs/data/nvsr/nvsr68/nvsr68_07-508.pdf

information, communication technologies, and supporting social services. Interdisciplinary, collaborative, public, and private approaches as well as public–private partnerships are needed to develop strategies to address the health disparity goal of *Healthy People 2030*. Chapter 23 discusses health disparities in more detail.

HEALTH LITERACY

Health literacy is defined as the degree to which individuals have the capacity to obtain, process, and understand basic health information and services needed to make appropriate health-related decisions. The ability to read and understand health information is key to managing health problems. Low health literacy contributes to health disparities and has been documented as an increasing problem among certain racial and ethnic groups, non–English-speaking populations, and persons over 65 years of age in the United States. Low health literacy is directly associated with (Health Resources & Services Administration, 2019; NIH, National Library of Medicine, n.d.):

- Poorer health outcomes
- Higher use of emergency service
- More frequent hospitalizations
- Increased risk of death

See Chapter 10 for additional information on health literacy.

MAJOR HEALTH PROBLEMS OF ADULTS

Morbidity and mortality among adults vary substantially by age, gender, and race/ethnicity. Several leading causes of death are presented in this section. Heart disease is the first-leading cause of death in adults and is presented along with stroke. Malignant neoplasms, chronic lower respiratory diseases (CLRDs), unintentional injuries, and diabetes mellitus are among the top 10 leading causes of death and are discussed separately. Other selected major causes of death are covered in detail in other chapters: suicide (Chapter 25), Alzheimer's disease (Chapter 22), and homicide (Chapter 18).

Coronary Heart Disease and Stroke

Cardiovascular disease (CVD) describes a group of heart and blood vessel disorders including hypertension, coronary heart disease (CHD), stroke, arrhythmias, valvular heart disease, peripheral vascular disease, and cardiomyopathies (World Health Organization [WHO], 2019). Over the last three decades, cardiovascular mortality in the United States has declined by about 50%. These gains are attributed to increased use of evidence-based medical therapies for secondary prevention and reduction in risk factors associated with lifestyle and environment (Box 21-1). Despite these gains, approximately one third of all deaths in the United States are still due to CVD. Currently, an estimated 92.1 million adults are living with one or more types of CVD and over half of these individuals are 60 years of age or older. It is estimated that every 36 seconds, an American will die from CVD, accounting for 2,300 deaths each day (Fig. 21-2; Benjamin et al., 2018; Centers for Disease Control and Prevention [CDC], 2017a).

In the United States, racial/ethnic minority populations continue to encounter more barriers to CVD diagnosis and care, receive lower-quality treatment, and experience worse health outcomes. Such disparities are linked to complex factors such as income and education, genetic and physiological factors, access to care, and communication barriers. Although it appears as though the disparity gap may be declining, this is likely not due to gains made by racial/ethnic minority populations, but worsening cardiovascular health in Whites (Brown et al., 2018). To tackle inequalities in CVD morbidity and mortality, actions that focus on the social determinants of health are needed. This includes development and implementation of health and social policy interventions that improve access to and quality of health care services and a reduction in poverty and unemployment (Dong, Fakeye, Graham, & Gaskin, 2018).

According to the American Heart Association (AHA), risk factors for CVD can be separated into three categories:

BOX 21-1 EVIDENCE-BASED PRACTICE

Landmark Research on Cardiovascular Disease

The hallmark Framingham Heart Study identified major risk characteristics associated with the development of CVD and the effects of related factors such as blood triglycerides, gender, and psychosocial issues. The study began in 1948 under the direction of National Heart Institute, now known as the National Heart, Lung, and Blood Institute (NHLBI). At that time, the death rates from CVD were rising, but little was known about the general causes of heart disease and stroke. The Framingham Heart Study researchers recruited 2,336 men and 2,873 women between the ages of 30 and 62 in an effort to identify common factors or characteristics that contribute to CVD. All participants lived in the town of Framingham, Massachusetts. Every 2 years, these individuals were scheduled for an extensive medical history, physical examination, and laboratory tests. In 1971, the study enrolled 5,124 of the original participants' adult children and their spouses (offspring cohort) (Framingham Heart Study, 2018).

In an effort to reflect the changing demographics that occurred in the town of Framingham since the original cohort was enrolled, researchers implemented a new study in 1994. This study included individuals of Black, Hispanic/Latino, Asian, Indian, Pacific Islander, and Native American origin (Omni cohort). In 2002, a third generation (the children of the offspring cohort) was recruited and a second group of Omni participants was enrolled in 2003. Over the last several years, investigators expanded their research into the role of genetics and CVD. The Framingham Heart Study celebrated its 70th anniversary in 2018, with 15,447 participants covering three generations and 3,698 peer-reviewed research articles since it began in 1948. Fortunately, findings from the Framingham Heart Study will continue to make important scientific contributions about the causes and treatment of CVD and related health issues (Framingham Heart Study, 2018).

Source: Framingham Heart Study (2018).

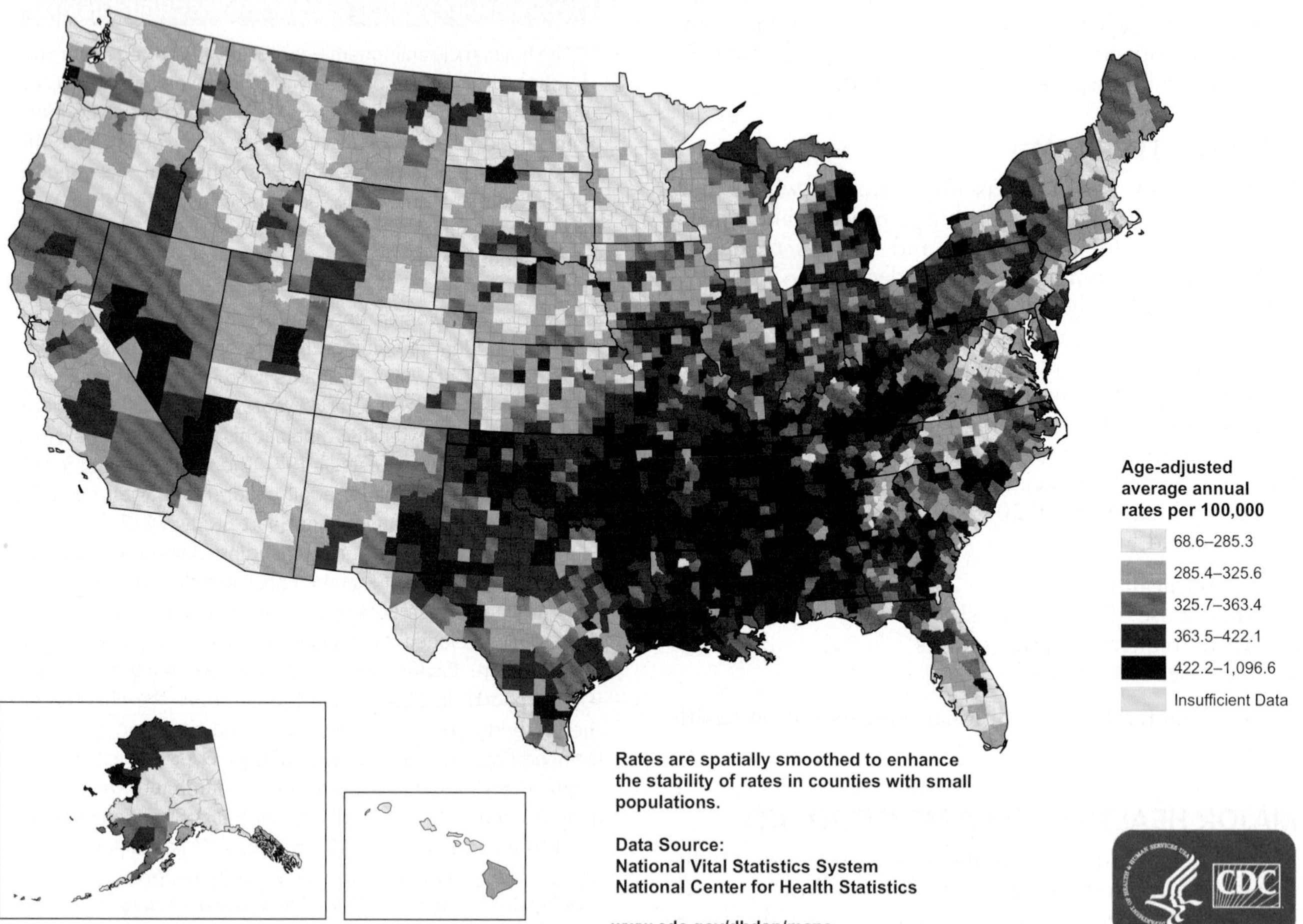

FIGURE 21-2 Heart disease death rates, 2015–2017 adults, ages 35+ by county. (Source: Centers for Disease Control and Prevention, Division for Heart Disease and Stroke Prevention. (2019). *Quick maps of heart disease, stroke, and socio-economic conditions*. Retrieved from http://www.cdc.gov/dhdsp/maps/national_maps/hd_all.htm)

major risk factors that cannot be changed, modifiable risk factors, and contributing risk factors (2016).

- Major risk factors that cannot be modified or treated include heredity (family history, race), increasing age, and gender (male).
- Risk factors that can be modified, treated, or controlled include high blood cholesterol, high blood pressure, smoking tobacco, physical inactivity, diabetes, and obesity/overweight.
- Risk factors that are known to contribute to heart disease are stress, alcohol consumption, and diet and nutrition.

About half of all Americans (49%) have at least one of the three key risk factors for heart disease: high blood pressure, high cholesterol, and cigarette smoking. The likelihood of heart disease or stroke multiplies with the increasing number of risk factors present (CDC, 2019a).

Stroke ranks fifth among all causes of death in the United States and is a leading cause of serious physical and cognitive long-term disability in adults (Box 21-1).

- Approximately 795,000 Americans experience a new or recurrent stroke each year—610,000 of these are first attacks and 185,000 are recurrent attacks. On average, someone in the United States has a stroke every 40 seconds.
- Disparities exist among people who are at risk for having a stroke. For example, women have a higher lifetime risk of having a stroke compared with men, with approximately 55,000 more women than men experiencing a stroke each year.
- The risk of having a first stroke is nearly twice as high for Blacks than Whites, and Blacks are more likely to die following a stroke than are their White counterparts. The risk for stroke among Hispanics/Latinos falls between that of Whites and Blacks, with stroke mortality increasing in this population since 2013.
- In the Southeastern United States (the "Stroke Belt"), stroke death rates are higher than in any other part of the country. Strokes cost the United States about $34 billion each year. This total includes the cost of health care services, medications, and missed days of work (Benjamin et al., 2018; CDC, 2020a).

Cancer

Cancer is a major chronic illness and remains the second leading cause of death in the United States (Xu et al., 2018).

- The National Cancer Institute's (NCI) Surveillance, Epidemiology, and End Stage Program (SEER) (2020) estimated that, in 2015, there were approximately 15.1 million Americans living with cancer.
- It was estimated that in 2018, 1,735,350 new cancer cases would be diagnosed, and of these cases, 609,640 persons were expected to die.
- Approximately 87% of all cancers are diagnosed in persons 50 years of age and older, and as individuals age, they are more likely to develop cancer.
- Among ethnic groups, Blacks are more likely to develop and die from cancer.
- Over their lifetime, men living in the United States are more likely to develop cancer than women.
- The Agency for Healthcare Research and Quality estimated the total expenditures for cancer in 2015 at $80.2 billion (American Cancer Society [ACS], 2019; NCI, 2020).

Cancer is caused by internal and external factors.

- Internal factors are inherited gene mutations, hormones, immune conditions, and gene mutations that occur from metabolism.
- External factors include tobacco and alcohol use, chemicals, radiation, infectious organisms, and poor lifestyle choices.
- These factors can occur in isolation or together to initiate illness.
- Screenings can reduce the cancer mortality rate, especially malignancies associated with the breast, colon, rectum, cervix, and lung (ACS, 2019).

While the lung cancer death rate continues to decline, it remains the number one cause of cancer deaths among adults in the United States. In 2018, there were an estimated 234,030 new lung cancer cases and 154,050 deaths, attributing to more than 25% of all cancer deaths in the United States (ACS, 2019).

Cigarette smoking is the predominant risk factor for lung cancer. The quantity of cigarettes smoked and the number of years a person smoked both increase an individual's risk of developing lung cancer. Other risk factors include occupational or environmental exposure to secondhand smoke, radon, or asbestos; genetic susceptibility (disease at an early age); and a history of tuberculosis. Annual screening for lung cancer using low-dose computed tomography scan is recommended for individuals 55 to 74 years of age who currently smoke or have smoked in the past 15 years and have at least a 30-pack history. Shared decision-making in screening and smoking cessation counseling for current smokers are key factors in the success of screening and prevention (Smith et al., 2018; Wood et al., 2018).

Colon and rectal cancers are the third most common cancers in adults. In 2018, an estimated 97,220 cases of colon and 43,030 cases of rectal cancers were expected to occur, resulting in 50,630 deaths (ACS, 2019).

- The risk of developing colorectal cancer increases with age, and 90% of all cases are diagnosed in individuals 50 years of age or older.
- There are several modifiable factors associated with the increased risk of colorectal cancer. These factors include obesity, physical inactivity, a diet high in red or processed meat, alcohol consumption, long-term smoking, and low intake of whole grains, fruits, and vegetables.
- Other risk factors include certain inherited genetic mutations, personal or family history of polyps or colorectal cancer, and personal history of chronic inflammatory bowel disease.
- The U.S. Preventative Services Task Force (USPSTF, 2016a) recommends that screening for colon and rectal cancer should begin at age 50 years for men and women who are at average risk (see Screenings and Checkup Schedule for Women and Men on thePoint®).

Chronic Lower Respiratory Diseases

Chronic lower respiratory disease (CLRD) comprises three major conditions: chronic bronchitis, emphysema, and asthma. CLRD is the third leading cause of death in the United States. The term chronic obstructive pulmonary disease (COPD) includes emphysema and chronic bronchitis. COPD is a leading cause of death, affecting over 16 million adults in the United States. The COPD National Action Plan identified educational interventions to inform the public on ways to prevent, diagnose, and treat this disease (NIH, National Heart, Lung, and Blood Institute [NHLBI], 2019). By 2020, the annual cost of medical care for adults living with COPD will be more than $49 billion (CDC, 2018a).

- Cigarette smoking is the major risk factor for developing COPD, accounting for 85% to 90% of cases. Pipe, cigar, and other types of tobacco smoke also can cause COPD, especially if the smoke is inhaled.
- The remaining COPD cases are attributable to environmental exposures and genetic factors (American Lung Association [ALA], 2020a).
- Since 2000, the number of women dying from COPD has surpassed the number of men. Women are more vulnerable to lung damage from cigarette smoke and other pollutants because their lungs are smaller, and research has found that estrogen plays a role in worsening the disease (ALA, 2020a).
- The exact cause of asthma is unknown, but research indicates that both genetic and environmental factors contribute to its cause. In the United States, approximately 20.4 million adults have been diagnosed with asthma and 6.1 million children under 18 years of age have asthma. The prevalence of asthma is higher in women (10.7%) than in men (6.5%), respectively (ALA, 2020b; CDC, 2016).

Unintentional Injuries

Unintentional injuries refer to any injury that results from unintended exposure to physical agents, including heat, mechanical energy, chemicals, or electricity. They are the fifth leading cause of death overall and the leading cause of death for persons 44 years of age and younger. The top three causes of unintentional injuries include motor vehicle crashes, poisoning, and falls. Approximately 214,000 Americans die from injury each year—one person every 3 minutes (Fig. 21-3; CDC, 2017a, 2017b).

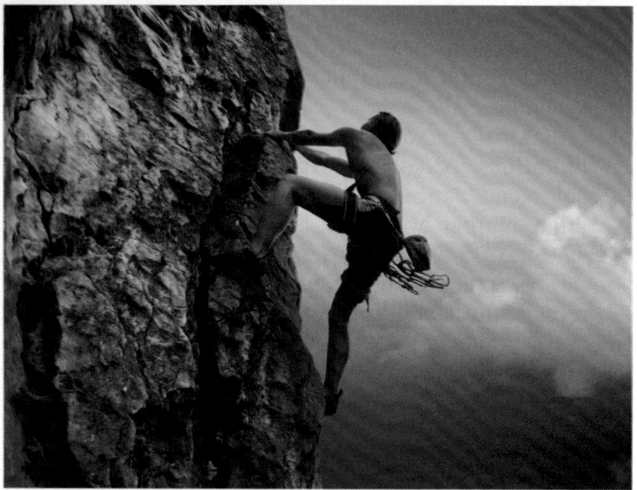

FIGURE 21-3 Unintentional injuries such as falls are the leading cause of death for those aged 44 years and younger.

TABLE 21-4 Estimated Diagnosed and Undiagnosed Diabetes Among People Ages 18 Years or Older, United States, 2020

Group	Number Who Have Diabetes and Rate per 1,000
Ages 18–44 years old	4.2%
Ages 45–64 years old	17.5%
Ages 65 years or older	26.8%
Men	14%
Women	12%

Source: Center for Disease Control (2020e).

- In 2015, 2.8 million people were hospitalized due to injuries and 27.6 million were treated in emergency departments. The costs associated with fatal injuries were $214 billion, whereas nonfatal injury costs were over $457 billion.
- Males account for the majority of fatal injury costs (78% or $166.7 billion), as well as nonfatal injury costs (63% or $287.5 billion; CDC, 2017a, 2017b, 2020b).
- Drugs, both pharmaceutical and illicit, cause the vast majority of poisoning deaths in the United States, and the number of drug-related deaths continues to increase. Two out of three deaths from drugs involve opioids.
- Overdose deaths from opioids have increased more than six times since 1999. In 2017, 47,000 people died from an opioid death in the United States (CDC, 2020c).

The CDC advocates for preventing opioid overdose by improving opioid prescribing, reducing exposure to opioids, preventing misuse of opioids, and improving treatment modalities for opioid use disorder (CDC, 2017c). See Chapter 25 for more on substance use.

In the United States, motor vehicle accidents are a leading cause of death. In 2015, more than 2.5 million individuals were treated in emergency rooms due to injuries from motor vehicle accidents.

- The costs of medical care and productivity losses due to motor vehicle accidents in a 1-year period exceeded 63 billion dollars (CDC, 2020d).
- Efforts to decrease motor vehicle injuries are directed toward prevention of motor vehicle crashes through education and policies related to seat belts, impaired driving, distracted driving, older adult drivers, teen drivers, and motorcycle and bicycle safety (2017f).

Diabetes Mellitus

Diabetes mellitus is the seventh leading cause of death in the United States. This chronic health condition puts individuals at risk for other serious health conditions, including heart disease, stroke, hypertension, blindness, kidney disease, and nervous system disease (i.e., neuropathy, which is a loss of sensation or pain in the feet or hands).

- According to the CDC (2017g), over 30 million Americans have type 1 or type 2 diabetes. Of these, 9.2 million have not been diagnosed yet.
- Additionally, more than 84 million adults have prediabetes and are at risk to develop type 2 diabetes.
- Risk factors for type 2 diabetes include family history, being overweight, age >45 years, not getting enough physical activity, and history of gestational diabetes.
- Races/ethnicities at increased risk for developing type 2 diabetes are African American, Hispanic/Latino, American Indian, and Alaska Native (Table 21-4; CDC, 2020e, 2020f).
- The American Diabetes Association (2018) recommends screening for diabetes for all people beginning at age 45 years and repeated every 3 years if test results are normal and for asymptomatic adults who are overweight and/or obese. Individuals with more than one risk factor may need to be screened more frequently.

Arthritis

Arthritis is a common term used to describe joint pain or joint disease; there are, in fact, more than 100 types of arthritis conditions, with the most common being osteoarthritis, rheumatoid arthritis, and psoriatic arthritis (Arthritis Foundation, n.d.). Over 54 million or 23% of all adults have some type of arthritis, with the condition occurring more often in women and more frequently as we age. Symptoms include swelling, pain, stiffness, and decreased range of motion; however, symptoms come and go and may be mild, moderate, or severe (CDC, 2019b). Arthritis may cause visible permanent joint changes such as knobby finger joints or may be less visible and detected only through x-ray (Arthritis Foundation, n.d.). The disease may occur with other conditions such as diabetes, heart disease, and obesity (CDC, 2019b). Arthritis can affect daily life including a person's ability to work, walk, or climb stairs. Over 140 billion is spent on medical costs related to this disease each year. Approaches to reducing arthritis pain and managing independence may include (CDC, 2019b):

- Being active
- Maintaining a healthy weight
- Protecting your joints
- Staying educated
- Pharmacological and nonpharmacological treatment options

Staying active is an important part of mitigating health issues such as arthritis. The CDC works with national organizations such as the YMCA to provide fitness classes that reach over 200,000 adults; efforts to address health disparities includes bringing classes to low income and underserved communities (CDC, 2019b).

Obesity

Obesity is defined as having a body mass index (BMI) of 30 or greater and is recognized as a national health threat and a major public health challenge in the United States. This condition is a major risk factor for CVD, along with certain types of cancer, type 2 diabetes, obstructive sleep apnea, and premature death (CDC, 2020g).

- According to the *National Health and Nutrition Examination Survey*, in 2015–2016, the prevalence of obesity among adults was 39.8%. Middle-aged adults (40 to 59 years old) had a higher prevalence of obesity at 42.8% than young adults (20 to 39 years old) at 35.7%. The prevalence of obesity in adults over age 60 years was 41.09% (Hales, Carroll, Fryar, & Ogden, 2017).
- Some groups have higher rates of obesity than others. Adults from lower socioeconomic and education levels have a higher prevalence of obesity, as do non-Hispanic Black and Hispanic adults (CDC, 2017c; Hales et al., 2017).
- Additionally, certain geographic regions have higher obesity rates than others in the United States. The South (32.4%) and Midwest (32.3%) have the highest prevalence of obesity, and at least 35% of adults in Alabama, Arkansas, Iowa, Louisiana, Mississippi, Oklahoma, and West Virginia are obese (CDC, 2019c).

Being obese can have serious health consequences; it is the leading cause of death in the United States and worldwide (CDC, 2019d), and it is associated with reduced quality of life and poorer mental health outcomes. In addition, those that are obese are at increased risk for mortality, hypertension, elevated LDL, dyslipidemia, stroke, type 2 diabetes, gallbladder disease, osteoarthritis, CHD, sleep apnea, some cancers, and difficulty with physical functioning (CDC, 2019d). There are also economic and societal consequences from obesity, including medical costs associated with related health issues and productivity concerns related to absenteeism, as well as premature mortality and morbidity (CDC, 2019d). Healthy behaviors that include healthy diet patterns and regular physical exercise should be incorporated into lifestyle habits. Community environment that are safe and offer healthy food and places for physical activity are also necessary (CDC, 2019d).

Healthy People 2030 has several objectives targeting obesity, some of which are shown in Box 21-2.

BOX 21-2 *HEALTHY PEOPLE 2030*

Select Objectives Related to Obesity

OA-01	Increase the proportion of older adults with physical or cognitive health problems who get physical activity
NWS-03	Reduce the proportion of adults with obesity
NWS-05	Increase the proportion of health care visits by adults with obesity that include counseling on weight loss, nutrition, or physical activity
PA-02	Increase the proportion of adults who do not have enough aerobic physical activity for substantial health benefits
PA-04	Increase the proportion of adults who do enough muscle-strengthening activity

Reprinted from U.S. Department of Health & Human Services (USDHHS). (2020). *Healthy People 2030: Browse objectives.* Retrieved from https://health.gov/healthypeople/objectives-and-data/browse-objectives

According to current guidelines, adults should receive a minimum of 150 minutes (2.5 hours) of moderate intensity or 75 minutes of vigorous aerobic exercise every week, in addition to 2 days muscle-strengthening exercises (USDHHS, 2018). Community health nurses play an important role in combatting obesity through educating adults on the importance of maintaining a healthy weight, or weight reduction if indicated, through physical activity and proper nutrition.

Substance Use

- In 2017, 30.5 million people aged 12 years or older used an illicit drug, or about 1 in 9 Americans. In 2017, illegal drug use was marked primarily by marijuana use and the misuse of prescription pain relievers. Smaller numbers of individuals were current users of cocaine, hallucinogens, methamphetamine, inhalants, or heroin or were misusers of prescription stimulants or sedatives (Substance Abuse and Mental Health Services Administration [SAMSHA], 2017a).
- Men are more likely than women to use illegal drugs and have higher rates of use or dependence on illicit drugs and alcohol than do women (National Institute of Drug Abuse [NIDA], 2018). Not all people who abuse illegal drugs, however, develop a substance abuse disorder (see Chapter 25).

According to SAMHSA (2019), a **substance use disorder (SUD)** occurs when the recurrent use of alcohol and/or drugs causes clinically and functionally significant impairment such as health problems, disability, and failure to meet major responsibilities at work, school, or home. SUD is a serious and continuing problem among adult women and men living in the United

States. Women are just as likely as men to develop a SUD (NIDA, 2018).

- In 2017, an estimated 19.7 million people aged 12 or older had a SUD related to their use of alcohol or illicit drugs in the past year in the United States.
- The abuse of opioids, leading to opioid use disorder, has become a national epidemic and public health concern. Approximately 2.1 million people had an opioid use disorder, including 1.7 million people with a prescription pain reliever use disorder and 0.7 million people with a heroin use disorder (SAMSHA, 2017a).
- The medical diagnosis of alcohol use disorder (AUD) refers to a chronic relapsing brain disease characterized by compulsive alcohol use, loss of control over alcohol intake, and a negative emotional state when not using. To be diagnosed with AUD, a person must meet certain criteria as delineated in the Diagnostic and Statistical Manual of Mental Disorders (DSM).

Under the current version of the DSM (DSM-V), anyone meeting 2 of the 11 criteria during the same 12-month period can be diagnosed with AUD. The severity of AUD is outlined as mild, moderate, or severe based on the number of criteria met (National Institute on Alcohol Abuse and Alcoholism [NIAAA], 2017). In the United States, it is estimated that 16 million people have AUD. Approximately 15.1 million adults in the United States ages 18 and older had AUD in 2015. This includes 9.8 million men and 5.3 million women. Adolescents can also be diagnosed with AUD. In 2015, an estimated 623,000 adolescents ages 12 to 17 years had AUD (NIAAA, 2018).

Tobacco use is another major public health problem and the leading cause of preventable diseases and deaths in the United States.

- More than 16 million Americans are living with a disease related to smoking.
- Smoking causes cancer, heart disease, stroke, lung diseases, diabetes, and COPD. Cigarette smoking is responsible for more than 480,000 deaths per year in the United States, including more than 41,000 deaths resulting from secondhand smoke exposure. This is about 1,300 deaths every day (CDC, 2020h).
- In 2017, an estimated 48.7 million people aged 12 years or older were current cigarette smokers, including 27.8 million people who smoked cigarettes daily (NIAAA, 2018). When examining cigarette smoking based on gender, men (17.5% of males) are more likely to smoke cigarettes than women (13.5% of females).
- The total economic cost of smoking is more than $300 billion a year, including approximately $170 billion in direct medical care for adults and $156 billion in lost productivity due to premature death and exposure to secondhand smoke (CDC, 2020h).
- E-cigarettes (also known as e-cigs, e-hookahs, mods, vape pens, vapes, tank system, and electronic nicotine delivery systems) are used by 2.8% of adults in the United Sates; the product is largely used by young adults. The product produces an aerosol by heating liquid, which usually contains nicotine; users then inhale this aerosol. E-cigarettes are not considered safe because they contain "harmful and potentially harmful substances, including nicotine, heavy metals like lead, volatile organic compounds, and cancer-causing agents" (CDC, 2020h, para. 2). Adults may use e-cigarettes to reduce craving for regular cigarettes, but the FDA has not approved e-cigarettes as an aid to quit smoking (CDC, 2020i).

Because of the significance of the problem, 28 of the *Healthy People 2030* objectives are related to tobacco use.

The illegal use of prescription opioids, synthetic opioids (fentanyl), and heroin is a major public health concern in the United States. A serious national crisis exists due to the abuse and addiction of opioids.

- Every day, 130 people die due to opioid overdose in the United States. In 2017, 47,600 individuals died from an overdose of opioids and an estimated 1.7 million people experience the disease (NIDA, 2019).
- This rise in opioid overdose deaths is due to increased prescribing of opioids in the 1990s, the rise in heroin use beginning in 2010, and synthetic opioid (such as fentanyl) abuse stemming from 2013 (CDC, 2017c, 2019e; NIDA, 2019).
- The economic aftermath of prescription opioid misuse in the United States is estimated at $78.5 billion a year, including the costs of health care, lost productivity, addiction treatment, and criminal justice involvement (NIDA, 2019).

The full extent of the damage of the opioid crisis goes beyond economics, influencing family and community life and placing an extreme strain on community resources, including first responders, emergency rooms, hospitals, and treatment centers.

In response to the opioid crisis, the USDHHS is focusing efforts on:

1. Improving access to treatment and recovery services
2. Promoting use of overdose-reversing drugs
3. Strengthening understanding of the epidemic through improved public health surveillance
4. Providing support for innovative research on pain and addiction
5. Initiating better practices for pain management

In 2018, the NIH launched HEAL (Helping to End Addiction Long-term) Initiative, an aggressive, trans-agency effort to increase scientific solutions to positively impact the national opioid public health crisis (NIH, 2018).

WOMEN'S HEALTH

Women have not been the focus of medical attention throughout history. Health benefits achieved by women were incidental compared with those of men. Advances in women's health are very recent and primarily an advantage for women living in Western countries, where the women's or feminist movement has made major inroads (Fig. 21-4).

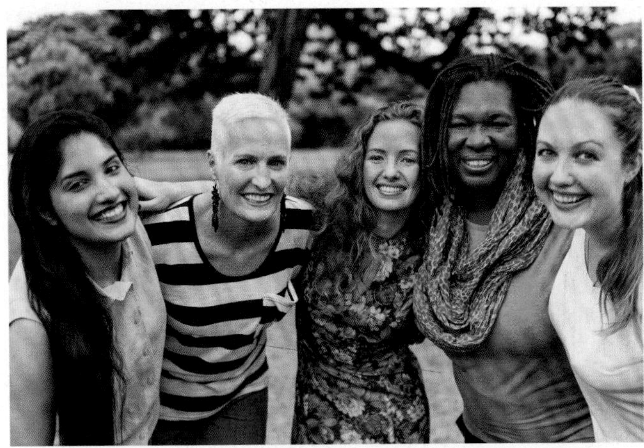

FIGURE 21-4 Women's health has not historically been the focus of health care research.

Overview of Factors Influencing Women's Health

Women's rights in the United States started in the second half of the 19th century and over time addressed issues directly or indirectly impacting the health of women: voting rights, labor laws, reproductive rights, and violence against women (International Women's Day, n.d.). This section of the chapter examines women's health concerns over the adult life span, the major causes of acute and chronic illness and death, and the issues, trends, and policies that have affected and currently affect women. For a discussion of how research in genomics and pharmacogenomics is being applied to women's health, see Box 21-3.

Women's health is still overlooked in much of the world. Only in the past few decades has the health of women been a formidable issue in the United States, coming not so coincidently with the modern women's feminist movement that began in the 1960s.

- The landmark 1963 publication *The Feminine Mystique* helped launch the modern women's movement by critically examining the role of women in American society (Foster, 2015; Friedan, 2013). The Boston Women's Health Book Collective's *Our Bodies, Ourselves* (initially released in 1973) represented the first book to explore women's health issues, exclusively written by and for women. In addition, this publication served as a model for women who wanted to learn about themselves, communicate their findings with doctors, and challenge the medical establishment to change and improve the care that women received (Our Bodies Ourselves, n.d.).
- To further expand the dialogue regarding women's health, consumer activists created the National Women's Health Network in 1975, primarily to shape health policy and support consumer health decisions (National Women's Health Network, 2018). These historical occurrences likely contributed to more female researchers and women as participants in research.
- Feminists paved the way for women to have their voices heard on many health, social, and political issues. Women sought out higher-education opportunities in greater numbers and entered workplaces once solely occupied by men, especially during and after World War II.
- These positive changes escalated women toward greater equality, and with equality came the freedom—and pressure—for women to compete with men in their social and work settings. Issues related to women's health were discovered as a result of research that now more regularly includes women.
- The importance of women's health research was reaffirmed in the NIH's Revitalization Act of 1993, Subtitle B—clinical research equity regarding women and minorities to "identify projects for research on women's health that should be conducted or supported by the national research institutes; identify multidisciplinary research relating to research on women that should be so conducted or supported ..." (NIH, 1993, section 486).

Women's Health Research

In response to changing priorities, researchers have designed and implemented major studies that focus exclusively on women. Five significant studies have provided and continue to provide important health information about women:

- The *Women's Health Initiative* (WHI) was a major research program addressing the most common causes of death, disability, and poor quality of life in postmenopausal women—CVD, cancer, and osteoporosis (WHI, n.d.).
- The *Women's Health Study* (WHS) evaluated the effects of vitamin E and low-dose aspirin therapy in primary prevention of CVD and cancer in apparently healthy women (WHS, n.d.).
- The *Nurses' Health Study (NHS) I* involved investigating risk factors for cancer and CVD, and the *NHS II* researched diet and lifestyle risk factors in a population younger than the original NHS cohort (NHS, 2016).
- The *NHS III* is currently investigating women's health issues related to lifestyle fertility/pregnancy, environment, and nursing exposures (NHS, 2016).

The WHI addressed CVD, cancer, and osteoporosis and was one of the largest prevention studies of its kind in the United States, starting in 1991 and spanning 15 years. This study was sponsored by the NIH and the NHLBI, involved 161,808 women ages 50 to 79 years, and was considered to be one of the most far-reaching clinical trials for women's health ever undertaken. To date, more than 616 publications have been associated with findings from this study, which address coronary artery calcium, breast cancer risk, colorectal cancer, venous thrombosis, peripheral arterial disease risk, risk of CHD, dementia and cognitive function, and the effects of estrogen alone in reducing the risk of CHD (National Center for Biotechnology Information, 2017; WHI, n.d.).

The WHS was a randomized, double-blind, placebo-controlled clinical trial sponsored by the NHBLI and the NCI. It was the first large clinical trial to study the use of low-dose aspirin to prevent heart attack and stroke in women 45 years of age and older. This study began in

BOX 21-3 EVIDENCE-BASED PRACTICE

Genomics and Pharmacogenomics

An individual's genome consists of their entire set of DNA, including all genes. Genomics considers how a person's genes interact with each other, the individual's environment and their behaviors, such as diet and exercise, to influence growth, development, and health (WHO, n.d.). This is different than genetics, which considers the function and composition of a single gene. Discoveries made in the field of genomics allow health care providers to translate research to clinical practice. For example, genomics has increased understanding of why individuals with the same disease may not respond similarly or have the same treatment outcomes, guiding individualized treatment. It also assists in the identification of individuals with increased risk for the development of certain diseases based on gene mutation, gene interaction, and environment, to develop individualized prevention and treatment strategies. These advances in science and technology have allowed health care to increase its focus on the delivery of individualized care and prevention, known as precision medicine (CDC, 2020n; NIH, 2019b; NIH, NCI, 2017).

Nurses and other health care providers use genomics routinely in practice. In the community setting, the nurse may educate women about breast cancer and risk factors, providing information about genetic testing for women with a family history. Health care providers partner with women who have BRCA1 or BRCA2 gene mutations to individualize breast and ovarian cancer prevention and screening. The same is true for those with a strong family history of heart disease. Careful family and personal health histories may guide health care providers to recommend testing for Familial Hypercholesterolemia (FH). Individuals with gene mutations causing FH need targeted treatment to prevent adverse cardiac events. Nurses play a key role in patient education to assist the individual with FH in reducing or eliminating modifiable risk factors that could also contribute to cardiovascular disease.

Another important aspect of genomics is pharmacogenomics, which considers information about an individual's genome to guide decision-making in medication and dose selection. The utilization of pharmacogenomics to guide treatment has become routine for some disease states and/or medications. Examples of utilizing pharmacogenomics to guide treatment include:

- Avoiding primaquine and other medications known to cause acute hemolytic anemia in individuals with G6PD deficiency, caused by an alteration of the G6PD gene.
- Choosing an HIV medication other than abacavir for individuals with an HLA-B*57:01 allele due to increased risk for developing a severe hypersensitivity reaction.
- Adjusting warfarin dose in individuals with CYP2C9 or VKORC1 gene variations to avoid increased bleeding risk (Dean, 2018; FDA, 2018b; NORD, 2017).

Individualizing patient care based on genomics and pharmacogenetics will continue to increase as the availability of genomic data expands. It is essential for nurses to have an understanding of genomics and pharmacogenomics in order to answer questions appropriately and provide appropriate and individualized health promotion and disease prevention education.

Source: Centers for Disease Control and Prevention (2020n); Dean (2018); Food and Drug Administration (FDA) (2018b); National Institutes of Health (NIH) (2019b); National Institutes of Health, National Cancer Institute (NIH, NCI) (2017); National Organization for Rare Diseases (NORD) (2017); World Health Organization (WHO) (n.d.).

1991 and continued through March 2009 for additional observation and follow-up of the original 28,345 participants. Findings indicated that low-dose aspirin does not prevent first heart attacks or death from cardiovascular causes in women; however, stroke was found to be 17% lower in the aspirin group. More than 110 professional articles are associated with this investigation. Recent publications address the association of dietary fat intake with risk of atrial fibrillation in women and the novel protein glycan biomarker and future CVD events (WHS, n.d.).

The NHS (three separate phases) represents the longest running study related to women's health in the world, investigating factors that influence the health of women.

- The *NHS I*, a prospective study that began in 1976, enrolled registered nurses aged 30 to 55 years. Every 2 years, participants received a follow-up questionnaire with questions about diseases and health-related topics including smoking, hormone use, and menopausal status. Later in the study, questions regarding diet and nutrition and quality of life were added.
- The *NHS II* represented women who started using oral contraceptives in adolescence, a population with long-term exposure during early reproductive years. Women, aged 25 to 42 years, were enrolled and followed forward in time. Every 2 years, participants received a follow-up questionnaire and were surveyed about diseases and health-related topics including smoking, hormone use, pregnancy history, and menopausal status.
- The *NHS III* began recruitment in 2010 and will continue until 100,000 nurses (registered and licensed practical, 22 to 45 years of age) are enrolled. Also, nurses from Canada are participants and the study aims to be more representative of the diverse backgrounds of nurses. These studies are supported by major nursing organizations, with more than 280,000 participants to date (NHS, 2016).

Women's Health Promotion Across the Life Span

What health care needs do women have that are different from those of men? Is there a need to look at health promotion throughout the life cycle of adult women? How is the health of an 18-year-old different from that of a 50-year-old woman? Most of us would have no trouble agreeing that women have different health care needs that must be considered and that these concerns vary with age. Knowing what the needs are is essential to knowing how to help women promote their health.

Healthy People 2030 Goals for Women

As a nation, we have been focusing on improving the health of all citizens through the *Healthy People* initiatives, commencing with the 1979 Surgeon General's report, *Healthy People: The Surgeon General's Report on Health Promotion and Disease Prevention*, providing measurable population objectives. *Healthy People 2000* set a standard for change and improvement in objectives that were met or exceeded in some areas and were far from being reached in others. In that initiative, objectives in 14 areas focused specifically on women's health. *Healthy People 2010* focused on two overarching goals: increasing the quality of life and eliminating health disparities, containing 25 objectives relating to women. *Healthy People 2020* reaffirmed the goals of *2010* and added two additional goals: quality of life, healthy development, along with healthy behaviors across the life span and creating social and physical environments that promote good health (USDHHS, 2015). In the nation's fourth generation of health planning, 35 objectives pertain to the health of women (Box 21-4). As the community health nurse works with women at various stages in the life cycle, the objectives in *Healthy People 2030* can give structure to program planning and services offered to women in the community at the primary, secondary, and tertiary levels of prevention.

BOX **21-4** *HEALTHY PEOPLE 2030*

The Objectives for Women

Core Objectives

C-04	Reduce the female breast cancer death rate
C-05	Increase the proportion of females who get screened for breast cancer
C-09	Increase the proportion of females who get screened for cervical cancer
MICH-04	Reduce maternal deaths
MICH-05	Reduce severe maternal complications during delivery hospitalizations
MICH-06	Reduce cesarean births among low-risk women with no prior births
MICH-07	Reduce preterm births
MICH-08	Increase the proportion of pregnant women who receive early and adequate prenatal care
MICH-10	Increase abstinence from cigarette smoking among pregnant women
MICH-11	Increase abstinence from illicit drugs among pregnant women
MICH-12	Increase the proportion of women of childbearing age who get enough folic acid
MICH-13	Increase the proportion of women who had a healthy weight before pregnancy
FP-01	Reduce the proportion of unintended pregnancies
FP-02	Reduce the proportion of pregnancies conceived within 18 months of a previous birth
FP-09	Increase the proportion of women who get needed publicly funded birth control services and support
FP-11	Increase the proportion of women at risk for unintended pregnancy who use effective birth control
STI-01	Increase the proportion of sexually active female adolescents and young women who get screened for chlamydia
STI-03	Reduce the syphilis rate in females
STI-04	Reduce congenital syphilis
STI-06	Reduce the proportion of adolescents and young adults with genital herpes
STI-07	Reduce pelvic inflammatory disease in female adolescents and young women
HIV-03	Reduce the number of new HIV diagnoses

Developmental Objectives

FP-D01	Increase the proportion of publicly funded clinics that offer the full range of reversible birth control
MICH-D01	Increase the proportion of women who get screened for postpartum depression
MICH-D02	Reduce the proportion of women who use illicit opioids during pregnancy

Reprinted from U.S. Department of Health & Human Services (USDHHS). (2020). *Healthy People 2030: Browse objectives*. Retrieved from https://health.gov/healthypeople/objectives-and-data/browse-objectives

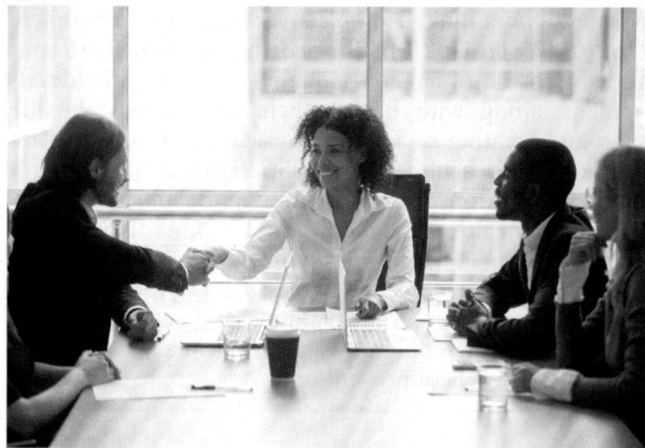

FIGURE 21-5 Choosing a career path is one developmental task for young adults.

Young Adult Women (18 to 35 Years)

Women in the earlier years of adulthood have different tasks to accomplish and issues to address than women in later adulthood, and the transition from adolescence to adulthood can be stressful. There are major developmental tasks that young women need to accomplish such as forming an identity and the development of intimacy. Behaviors associated with young adulthood include completing postsecondary education, choosing and establishing a career (Fig. 21-5), choosing a significant other for the long term, establishing a household, and planning for children by using a variety of parenting models (childbirth, adoption, foster parenting). During this time, women also develop a personal philosophy that encompasses meaningful and comforting spiritual beliefs that are consistent with day-to-day living (Berk, 2018).

Women in this age group tend to be healthy. Unfortunately, during this period, many women engage in health risk behaviors such as physical inactivity, eating poorly, participating in unprotected sexual intercourse, and smoking (Box 21-5). Some, if not all, of these behaviors may have been established in adolescence and represent modifiable behaviors. If not addressed, poor lifestyle choices can contribute significantly to the leading causes of morbidity and mortality: diseases of the heart and vascular systems, cancers, chronic respiratory diseases, and diabetes (CDC, 2019f). The majority of health concerns for many women in this age group are related to eating disorders, reproductive health and sexually transmitted infections (STIs), physical activity, mental health and mood disorders, and substance use.

BOX **21-5** WHAT DO *YOU* THINK?

Fad Diets

Each year, approximately 45 million Americans begin a diet. Fad diets have been around for centuries and don't seem to be going anywhere. Every year new diets promise results, but do they work and are they safe?

In 2018, the ketogenic diet (keto) made its way back into mainstream. This is a high-fat, low-carbohydrate diet that eliminates sugar, grains/starches, fruits, beans/legumes and encourages high-fat foods such as eggs, nuts, meats/fish, full-fat dairy and cheeses, and healthy oils. Low-carb vegetables are also encouraged. The goal is to reach ketosis by replacing dietary carbs with fats. Benefits may include weight loss and decreased glucose and insulin levels. There are conflicting studies reporting benefits and risks of the ketogenic diet. While individuals adhering to this diet lose weight, once carbohydrates are re-introduced, the resulting side effect is often weight gain. Research has shown both increase and decrease in LDL cholesterol, as well as the development of insulin resistance, and nonalcoholic fatty liver disease.

The paleolithic diet is known by a few different names and continues to be a popular option among individuals trying to lose weight. This is a low-carbohydrate, high protein diet that encourages high consumption of lean meats and vegetables, moderate consumption of fruits, nuts, and seeds, and abstinence from dairy, legumes, and grains. While it has many of the same attributes of keto, it is higher in protein and lower in fat. Evidence suggests that maintaining a low carbohydrate diet, such as the paleo or ketogenic diet, long term may increase mortality from cardiovascular disease, stroke, and cancer, when compared to higher carbohydrate diets. However, the source of carbohydrate intake, whole-food versus highly processed, must be considered and whole-food sources recommended as an individual's main carbohydrate intake.

The plant-based, or vegan, diet has gained momentum in recent years and eliminates all animal products including meat, eggs, and dairy. It is rich in fruits, vegetables, nuts, seeds, legumes, and plant proteins. While there are variations of veganism, such as whole-food plant-based or raw, there are many vegan "junk foods" or processed vegan replacement foods that can cause more harm than good. Adherence to a plant-based diet that is not heavily based on processed vegan foods may reduce weight and help manage or eliminate chronic disease.

Other recent dieting trends include intermittent fasting, juicing, detoxing, and gluten-free diet. Whether individuals ask about the health benefits or adverse effects of diets they are following or considering, it's important to encourage them to research potential nutritional deficiencies certain diets may cause. This allows for intentional monitoring for dietary deficiencies and supplementation if needed. For example, individuals following a ketogenic diet may not be consuming sufficient amounts of fiber or vitamins and minerals found in fruits and vegetables. Vegans may need to supplement or be intentional about consuming vitamins B12 and D3, omega-3 fatty acids, iron, and calcium.

Do you know someone who seems to always be trying the latest diet? Is that person successfully losing weight or in a constant weight loss/weight gain cycle? As a C/PHN, how would you approach this subject?

Source: Gunnars (2018); Kosinski and Jarnayvaz (2017); Mauer (2018); Mazidi, Katsik, Mikhailidis, and Banach (2018); T. Collin Campbell Center for Nutrition Studies (2018).

Eating Disorders. Eating disorders are complex, chronic illnesses primarily affecting young women. There is no single cause of these disorders; however, several things may contribute: culture, personal characteristics, emotional disorders, stressful events, biology, and families. The three most common are anorexia nervosa, bulimia nervosa, and binge eating.

- **Anorexia nervosa** is characterized by marked by weight loss, emaciation, a disturbance in body image, and a fear of weight gain. Persons affected lose weight either by excessive dieting or by purging themselves of ingested calories. This illness is typically found in industrialized nations and usually begins in the teen years. Young women are 10 to 20 times more likely than young men to experience anorexia. Refusal to maintain body weight can be life threatening due to electrolyte disturbances, anemia, and secondary cardiac arrhythmias. Low body weight can impair insulin production, leading to amenorrhea (absent menstrual periods) and decreased bone density (National Institute of Mental Health, 2016, 2018; Office on Women's Health, 2018a).
- **Bulimia nervosa** is characterized by recurrent episodes of binge eating, self-induced vomiting and diarrhea, misuse of laxatives or diuretics, excessive exercise, strict dieting or fasting, and an excessive concern about body shape or weight. Females in cultures where emphasis is placed on a certain ideal of beauty, individuals who have been sexually abused or come from families with a history of eating disorders, and individuals with low self-esteem and a history of not being "in control" or with communication and emotional difficulties are at greater risk (Office on Women's Health, 2018b; SAMHSA, 2017b).
- **Binge eating** is the most common eating disorder in the United States, with typical onset in late adolescence and early 20s. It is characterized by repeated episodes of uncontrolled eating including eating large amounts quickly, when not hungry, and until comfortably full. Many individuals with this disorder have difficulty expressing their feelings, have difficulty controlling impulses and stress, and feel depressed about overeating. Obesity is common because purging is not a characteristic of this disorder. This disorder results in increased risk for type 2 diabetes, high cholesterol, osteoarthritis, kidney disease or renal failure, heart disease, and hypertension (Office on Women's Health, 2018c; SAMHSA, 2017b).

In general, females have a higher rate of eating disorders than males. However, millions of men and boys battle all forms of this illness. The community health nurse can play a vital role in identifying affected persons and refer these individuals to appropriate health care providers, mental health counselors, and self-help groups. Screening tools that may help identify individuals requiring referral for further assessment are available (National Eating Disorder Association, 2018).

Reproductive Health. During the reproductive years, it is important for both women and men to be as healthy as possible (Fig. 21-6). During this time, healthy habits

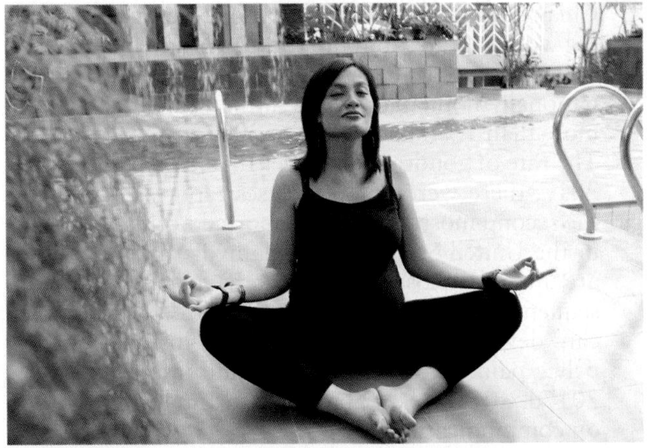

FIGURE 21-6 Good health is important during pregnancy.

can be initiated, and unhealthy habits resolved to ensure the best health during the years individuals focus on having children. Preconception health is important for all women of reproductive age, not just those planning to become pregnant, because it focuses on getting healthy and staying healthy (CDC, 2020j).

Although preconception care is addressed in *Healthy People 2030*, many of the preconception objectives are related to family planning and maternal health. The CDC has developed a checklist for women of reproductive age to commit to healthy preconception activities including (CDC, 2020j):

- Make a plan and take action
- See a health care provider
- Take 400 µg of folic acid every day
- Stop smoking, using drugs, and drinking excessive amounts of alcohol
- Avoid toxic substances
- Reach and maintain a healthy weight
- Get help for violence
- Learn family history
- Get mentally healthy
- When ready, plan pregnancy

Community health nurses have been at the forefront of maternal and child health care for decades, and they must continue to strive to incorporate components of preconception care into their practices. Nurses must also advocate for clients to influence public policy, which has the potential to improve access to care for many women and improve pregnancy outcomes.

Sexual health and STIs are important health concerns for young women. Sexual activity typically commences in adolescence and continues throughout the life span. STIs are epidemic in the United States, especially among young adults (see Chapter 8).

- Human papillomavirus (HPV) is the most common STI in the United States. Approximately 79 million Americans are infected with HPV, resulting in 10,800 cases of cervical cancer and 300,000 high grade cervical lesions annually. Gardasil 9 is a two or three dose vaccine that can prevent 90% of cervical cancers, as well as anogenital warts. Gardasil 9 is now approved for individuals 9 to 45 years old (CDC, 2019g; FDA, 2018a).

- Chlamydia and gonorrhea are also common STIs affecting women. Rates for both these STIs have increased in women in recent years. Chlamydia is the most reported nationally notifiable disease in the United States, with more than 1.7 million cases in 2017.
- The rate of gonorrhea is lower than chlamydia, but in 2017, there were 555,608 cases reported, making it the second most nationally reported notifiable disease in the United States. Both chlamydia and gonorrhea are underdiagnosed, which can have deleterious consequences for women. If treatment is delayed, women can develop pelvic inflammatory disease, chronic pelvic pain, ectopic pregnancy, and infertility (CDC, 2017d, 2018b). See Chapter 8 for more information on communicable diseases.

Routine screening recommendations for STIs in women include the following:

- HPV: screen women 30 to 65 years old every 5 years with high-risk HPV testing (alone or with cytology screening; USPSTF, 2018a)
- Chlamydia and gonorrhea: annual screening for women under age 25 years or older women with risk factors (CDC, 2017d; USPSTF, 2016b)
- HIV: screen individuals aged 15 to 65 years; annual screening if high risk; younger or older depending on risk factors (USPSTF, 2018b)

Community health nurses working with adult women should provide factual information to increase women's knowledge of STI risk. This information should be a part of frank discussions regarding condom use, sexual partners (male and female), type of sexual activity (oral, anal, vaginal), life-threatening consequences of an undiagnosed STI, and undesirable pregnancy outcomes. Outside of abstinence, condom use is the first line of prevention against STIs. See Chapter 8 for more on communicable diseases.

Adult Women (35 to 65 Years)

Women in the adult age group of 35 to 65 years have established themselves into patterns of living that have served them well or ill. During this period, the results of years of choices may present themselves in the form of chronic illnesses. Nevertheless, many women in this age group have time to change health habits to possibly reverse encroaching chronic illnesses (Fig. 21-7). For other women, lifestyle choices and undetected diseases have shortened their life spans, and large numbers of women in this age group are dying prematurely.

Adult women demographics are shifting. An increasing number of educated women are having children, and they are having them later in life; they are also spending more time in the work force before they have children. Births within the United States are decreasing; however, foreign-born births are increasing. In the United States, one in four mothers is solo mother, raising children on their own. Typical stereotypes are also shifting as working women face pressure to be more involved as mothers, while men are more involved in childcare and housework than in the past (Pew Research Center, 2020a). Women in the developmental stage between 35 and 65 years of age may face many challenges including:

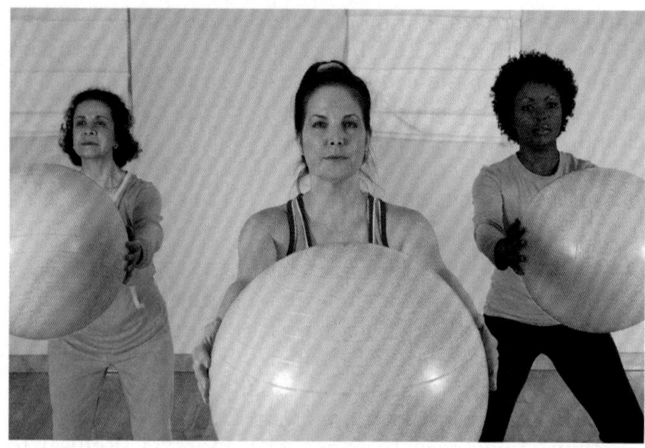

FIGURE 21-7 Menopause is transitional period in a woman's life, and healthy diet and exercise are important.

- Caring for aging parents
- Supporting young adult children
- Family–work role conflict
- Economic burden for single mothers
- Gender gap
- Parenting pressure (Pew Research Center, 2020b)

Menopause and Hormone Replacement Therapy

- **Perimenopause**, or menopausal transition, is the period of time leading up to the last menstrual cycle and is characterized by cycle changes and irregularity. Women typically begin to notice symptoms of perimenopause in their 40s. Menstrual flow may be light or heavy, and spotting may occur, depending on varying estrogen and progesterone levels. Women may also have vasomotor symptoms such as hot flashes (flushes) or night sweats and climacteric symptoms such as experience sleep disturbances and vaginal and urinary tract changes (American College of Obstetricians and Gynecologists [ACOG], 2018a; Martin & Barbieri, 2019). The average length of perimenopause is 4 years but may last up to 10 years.
- **Menopause** is a time that marks the permanent cessation of menstrual activity (last menstrual period). The average age is 51 years (range = 45 to 58); however, it can occur earlier (Office on Women's Health, 2018d). Natural menopause is defined as cessation of menstrual periods for 12 consecutive months, with no other apparent cause.
  - Menopause symptoms differ among women and may last months to years. They range from hardly noticeable in some women to very severe in others. Symptoms include nervousness or anxiety, hot flashes (flushes), chills, excessive sweating (often at night), excitability, fatigue, mood disorders (apathy, mental depression, crying episodes), insomnia, palpitations, vertigo, headache, numbness, tingling, myalgia, urinary disturbances, and vaginal dryness (ACOG, 2018a; Office on Women's Health, 2018d).
  - According to the *Study of Women's Health Across the Nation* (SWAN), hot flashes and some of the other menopausal symptoms last an average of 7.4 years, persisting 4.5 years once menopause is

reached. However, these symptoms may persist for longer, particularly in African American women and those who are overweight or obese (Santoro, 2016).

The Endocrine Society recommends diagnosis of menopause based on the cessation of menstruation for 12 consecutive months. Recommendations for women in the menopausal transition include discussions about menopausal symptoms, osteoporosis, cancer screening, and assessment for CVD; along with a determination of the need for appropriate **menopausal hormone therapy (MHT)** (Stuenkel et al., 2015). For women under age 60, or who are <10 years past onset of menopause, with bothersome menopausal symptoms, MHT may be an appropriate treatment option. Health care providers must take patient risk for CVD, venous thromboembolic events, and breast cancer into account when considering initiation or continuation of MHT and should use a shared decision-making approach (Martin & Barbieri, 2019). At this time, ACOG recommends against the use of MHT as primary or secondary prevention of heart disease or osteoporosis (ACOG, 2018b). Women who are not candidates for oral MHT may be able to use transdermal routes or nonhormonal therapies to relieve symptoms, depending on risk factors and contraindications.

- Some women choose to use bioidentical hormone therapy—chemically similar hormones derived from plants—that may (e.g., micronized estradiol and progesterone) or may not be approved (e.g., Triest, Biest, pregnenolone) by the Food and Drug Administration (FDA).
- Current evidence does not support the use of bioidentical hormone therapy over conventional MHT (ACOG, 2018c; Martin & Barbieri, 2019).
- Women may also choose natural products (e.g., phytoestrogens, black cohosh, DHEA, dong quai, vitamin E) for symptomatic relief. Women choosing natural or herbal supplements should be counseled on lack of evidence supporting efficacy and long-term safety, as well as potential side effects and drug interactions (National Center for Complementary and Integrative Health, 2018).
- Other complementary health approaches women may choose for menopausal symptom relief includes hypnotherapy, meditation, yoga, and acupuncture.

Osteoporosis

- A gradual loss in bone density is known as **osteoporosis**. Typically, bone mass stops increasing around age 30 years. As women age, bones may weaken and easily fracture as estrogen levels decrease.
- In the United States, 1 in 4 women over the age of 65 years has *osteoporosis* (CDC, 2020k). Therefore, it is important for women to build strong bone early. Bone density is influenced by many factors such as heredity, race/ethnicity, physical activity, and nutrition. It is important for women of all ages to maintain a healthy diet that is rich in calcium and vitamin D, engage in physical activity, and avoid smoking.
- There are several classes of medications that can be used to treat osteoporosis: bisphosphonates (helps build bone mass), selective estrogen receptor modulators (slows rate of bone loss), calcitonin (slows rate of bone loss), and teriparatide (helps build up new bone).
- The USPSTF recommends screening for osteoporosis in women over the age of 65 years, or in postmenopausal women under age 65 years with increased risk for osteoporosis-related fractures (USPSTF, 2018b). See Chapter 22 for more on osteoporosis in older women.

Heart Disease

- Heart disease is the number one killer of women, causing the death of 295,995 females in 2016 (Xu et al., 2018). The most common heart problem, CHD, is underdiagnosed, undertreated, and under-researched in women.
- In addition, women have a higher mortality rate after heart attack and poorer outcomes than do men, and this may be related to delayed diagnosis and treatment.
- Risk factors for heart disease in women are age, family history, race/ethnicity, physical inactivity, sleep apnea, obesity, diabetes mellitus, high blood pressure, high cholesterol, and cigarette smoking (Office on Women's Health, 2018e).

Family history, race/ethnicity, and advancing age cannot be changed, but women can make lifestyle changes to alter other risk factors. The remaining risk factors are issues that the community health nurse can discuss with female clients in this age group. Community health nurses can help raise awareness regarding heart disease when working with women at the individual, family, or aggregate levels. Some important facts that can be shared are as follows:

- Heart disease accounts for 1 in 5 female deaths in the United States (CDC, 2019c).
- In the United States, approximately 1 in 16 Black, White, and Hispanic women over the age of 20 years have CHD (CDC, 2019c).
- The average age for first heart attack in females is 72.0 years (Benjamin et al., 2018).
- In all age groups, mortality rate for women following a heart attack is higher than in men (Office on Women's Health, 2018d).
- Almost two thirds of women who suddenly die from heart disease have had no previous symptoms (CDC, 2019c).
- Heart disease is sometimes thought of as a "man's disease," but about the same number of women and men die each year of heart disease (CDC, 2019c).
- Women may have atypical heart symptoms or less acute chest pain, which may delay them from seeking care (Office of Women's Health, 2019).
- MHT may increase risk of heart attack, stroke, and blood clots (Office of Women's Health, 2018f).
- Nine out of 10 women have at least one risk factor for heart disease (NIH, NHLBI, 2019).

An excellent lay resource is "*Go Red for Women*," a public awareness program of the AHA to help improve knowledge (AHA, 2018). Also, *Well-Integrated Screening and Evaluation for Women across the Nation*

(WISEWOMAN), a CDC program that helps women with little or no health insurance reduce their risk for heart disease, stroke, and other chronic diseases (located in 21 sites across 19 states), can be helpful. The program assists women ages 40 to 64 in improving their diet, physical activity, and other behaviors (Fig. 21-8). This program also provides cholesterol tests and other screening (CDC, 2020K, 2020L).

Cancer

- Cancer is the second leading cause of death for women, estimated to kill 286,010 females in the United States in 2018. The majority of cancers (87%) occur in persons 50 years of age and older.
- An estimated 38% of women in the United States will develop cancer in their lifetime. To help address this disparity, community health nurses can provide more opportunities for education and screening for this population. Screening has reduced the deaths for cancers of the breast, colon, rectum, and cervix (ACS, 2019).
- Breast cancer is the most common cancer among women; however, more women die of lung cancer. In 2018, it is estimated that 40,920 deaths related to breast cancer will occur (SEER, n.d.a).

Overall, the death rates from breast cancer have declined since 1990, and the biggest decline was among women under 50 years of age (Table 21-5). This can be attributed to early detection and improvements in treatment. The sooner breast cancer is discovered, the more successfully it is treated. By obtaining regular clinical breast exams and mammograms, eating a diet low in fat and high in fruits and vegetables, breast-feeding (if possible), and avoiding prolonged use of MHT, a woman is doing what she can to promote breast health.

- Although breast self-examination (BSE) is no longer a routine screening recommendation, it is important that women are familiar with their breasts. This allows them to recognize any overt changes in their breasts, especially changes related to size, shape, symmetry, and nipple discharge. The community health nurse has many resources available to provide information and to teach women breast awareness in their homes, small groups in clinics, or in various other community settings to enhance knowledge of breast health (ACS, 2020a). See Chapters 11 and 12 for more on breast cancer screening.

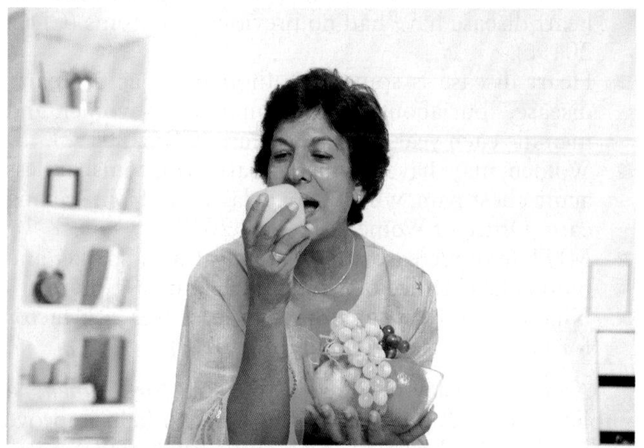

FIGURE 21-8 A healthy diet is an important part of health promotion.

TABLE 21-5 Breast Cancer Death Rates Among All Women: 2013–2017

Women	Rate
Age-Adjusted Rates per 100,000	
All races	20.3
Black	27.6
White	19.8
American Indian/Alaska Native	14.6
Hispanic	14.0
Asian/Pacific Islander	11.4

Source: Cancer Statistic Center (2018); Surveillance, Epidemiology, and End Stage Program (SEER) (n.d.a).

Breast cancer screening is important for early detection when tumors are likely to be smaller and confined to the breast. Early detection is associated with better prognosis for survival. The USPSTF (2016c) published the following breast cancer screening recommendations for women of average risk:

- Women, age younger than 50 years: should be an individual decision and the patient's context (risk for disease) should be taken into account (Grade C).
- Women, aged 50 to 74 years: biennial screening with mammography (Grade B).
- Women, aged 75 years and older: evidence is insufficient to assess the benefits and harms of screening mammography (Grade I; USPSTF, 2016c).
- Women who have a first-degree relative with breast cancer (mother, sister), have a breast cancer gene (*BRCA1* or *BRCA2*), or have had previous breast cancer are at a higher risk for developing the disease than other women in the general population. Therefore, these individuals need to consult their physicians regarding timelines for screenings (ACS, 2020a).

Cervical cancer screening has improved early detection and prevention of cervical cancer dramatically. Both the incidence and the death rates for cervical cancer have declined in recent decades because of treatment of preinvasive cervical lesions. The major risk factors for this disease are infection with certain types of HPV, unprotected intercourse at an early age, and multiple sex partners. In 2018, it is estimated that 13,240 new cases of invasive cervical cancer will be diagnosed in the United States, contributing to 4,170 deaths among women from this disease. The 5-year survival rate for this cancer, if prompt treatment is initiated, is 66.2% for all stages and 91.7% for local infiltration, making it one of the most successfully treated cancers (SEER, n.d.b). The USPSTF published the following cervical cancer screening recommendations:

- Women younger than 21 years: recommend against screening (Grade D)
- Women age 21 to 29 years: every 3 years with cervical cytology (Grade A)
- Women age 30 to 65 years: every 3 years with cervical cytology alone, or every 5 years with high-risk human papillomavirus testing (hrHPV), or every 5 years with hrHPV and cytology combination (Grade A)
- Women older than 65 years: recommend against screening with adequate screening previously and not at high risk (Grade D) (USPSTF, 2018c)

C/PHN can continue to improve screening and early diagnosis through education and advocating for low-cost screening, which will allow at-risk low-income and rural women access to regular cervical cancer screenings. In addition to screening, educating women about the HPV vaccine is an important strategy to reduce the incidence of cervical cancer. The Gardasil 9 vaccine protects against 9 HPV virus types that may cause cervical cancer and anogenital warts. It is started as early as age 9 and given as two (age 9 to 13) or three doses (age 14 and older) over 6 months. Previously, the HPV vaccine was only available for individuals age 9 to 26; however, in 2018, the FDA approved the expanded use of Gardasil 9 to also cover males and females age 27 to 45 years (FDA, 2018a; Merck Sharp & Dohme Corporation, 2018).

- Ovarian cancer contributes to more deaths than any other cancer of the female reproductive system and accounts for 5% of cancer deaths among women. In 2018, a total of 22,240 cases were anticipated and 14,070 deaths were expected.
- The primary risk factor for this disease is heredity, or a strong family history of breast or ovarian cancer. The 5-year survival rate is 47.4% compared to cervical (66.2%) and breast (89.9%) cancers.
- The USPSTF recommends against routine screening for ovarian cancer in women who do not have symptoms. However, women considered at high risk should receive a pelvic exam, a transvaginal ultrasound, and a blood test for the tumor marker CA 125. Therefore, C/PHNs need to continue to stress the importance of early detection (SEER, n.d.c; Torre et al., 2018; USPSTF, 2018d).

Myalgic Encephalomyelitis/Chronic Fatigue Syndrome

- **Myalgic encephalomyelitis/chronic fatigue syndrome (ME/CFS)** is a chronic and debilitating disease characterized by fatigue lasting for 6 or more months, worsening of symptoms after exertion and unrefreshing sleep. Other symptoms may include cognitive impairment, orthostatic intolerance, frequent sore throat, headache, painful muscles, and joint pain. It is estimated that between 836,000 and 2.8 million persons in the United States have ME/CFS, with women affected up to four times more than men.
- Symptoms may last for months or years, waxing and waning and are difficult to validate objectively, but they are subjectively debilitating. Because the cause is unknown, there is no specific treatment and no prevention suggestions.
- Treatment is focused on supportive care for the associated pain, depression, and insomnia. The Solve ME/CFS Initiative provides support and information for women and is one of seven organizations that contributed to *Impact of Chronic Overlapping Pain Conditions on Public Health and the Urgent Need for Safe and Effective Treatment*, a report that raises awareness of chronic pain conditions that disproportionately impact women.

The community health nurse can assess activity level and degree of fatigue, emotional response to the illness, and coping ability. Emotionally supportive family members and health care providers are helpful. Referring women to mental health counseling or a local support group is useful for many women and within the role of the community health nurse (CDC, 2019h; Chronic Pain Research Alliance, 2015; Institute of Medicine, 2015; Solve ME/CFS Initiative, 2018).

MEN'S HEALTH

Gender is among the numerous factors that influence health. More male neonates die at birth, and men are more likely to die earlier from a chronic illness than women (Fig. 21-9). This is evidenced by the difference in life expectancy between men and women in the United States; women survive an average of 5 years longer than men (CDC, 2017e; Xu et al., 2018).

Overview of Factors Influencing Men's Health

Masculinity is an influencing factor in men's health. Men are socialized to be independent and conceal their vulnerability. Therefore, even when they are aware of personal physical or mental health problems, they are less likely to access the health care system. How the male identity is maintained can include activities that are hazardous to their health, and the result is a high death rate from unintentional injuries among young men. Examples of these activities include substance use, use of firearms, excessive alcohol consumptions, and smoking (CDC, 2017e; Xu et al., 2018).

Men's Health Promotion Across the Adult Life Span

In the early years of young adulthood (between 18 and 35 years), men continue to grow and mature. Adult men aged 35 to 65 years have reached maturity, the peak of

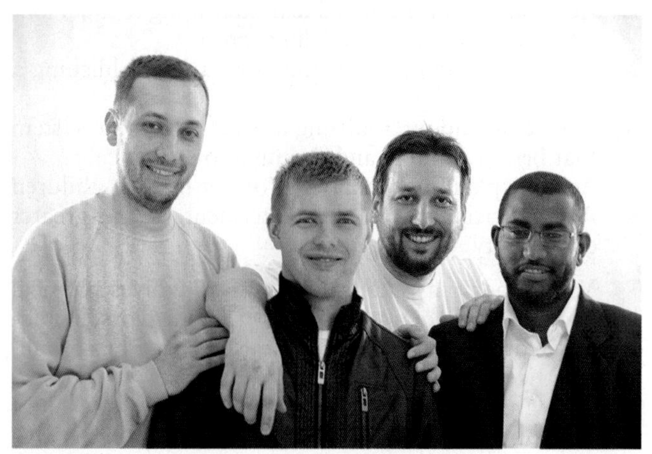

FIGURE 21-9 Men have different health care needs at various stages of life.

BOX **21-6** *HEALTHY PEOPLE 2030*

The Objectives for Men

Core Objectives

C-07	Increase the proportion of adults who get screened for colorectal cancer
C-08	Reduce the prostate cancer death rate
STI-05	Reduce the syphilis rate in men who have sex with men
HIV-03	Reduce the number of new HIV diagnoses
LGBT-01	Increase the number of national surveys that collect data on lesbian, gay, and bisexual populations
LGBT-02	Increase the number of national surveys that collect data on transgender populations
PA-02	Increase the proportion of adults who do enough aerobic physical activity for substantial health benefits
TU-01	Reduce current tobacco use in adults
SU-03	Reduce drug overdose deaths
SU-13	Reduce the proportion of people who had alcohol use disorder in the past year
SU-15	Reduce the proportion of people who had drug use disorder in the past year
NWS-03	Reduce the proportion of adults with obesity
MHMD-08	Increase the proportion of primary care visits where adolescents and adults are screened for depression

Reprinted from U.S. Department of Health & Human Services (USDHHS). (2020). *Healthy People 2030: Browse objectives.* Retrieved from https://health.gov/healthypeople/objectives-and-data/browse-objective

their physical and intellectual development, and their greatest earning power. What specific needs do men in these age groups have? Are their needs being met through provided services?

Healthy People 2030 Goals for Men

Healthy People 2030 addresses men's health through family planning, STD, LGBT, and adult health issues such as mental health, substance abuse and opioids, tobacco, nutrition, physical activity, chronic diseases, and cancer (Box 21-6).

Young Adult Men (18 to 35 Years)

The young adult male has many tasks to accomplish including:

- Acquisition of training/education leading to a personally and financially rewarding career
- Selecting a compatible companion and establishing a life together (Fig. 21-10)
- Practicing and internalizing a belief and value system that brings comfort and meaning to existence
- Actively planning for having (or not having) children
- And participating in the betterment of the greater community

Young men may choose work that involves physical labor, office work, or a variety of other endeavors, including active duty military. They may also be veterans of military service.

Young men engage in risk taking behaviors without thinking about the consequences. Depending on his attitudes and practices before a man enters young adulthood, he may or may not be enticed to experiment or continue with the use of tobacco, alcohol, or illicit drugs. Experimentation or usage of these substances can occur while in college, the military, or working at a full-time job. In addition, young men respond to challenges such as drag racing and exceeding speed limits. This is an important age group for the C/PHN to reach with health information because decisions made in these formative years affect how young men live the rest of their lives. The nurse can meet with young adult men in work settings, college campuses, military bases, health clubs and bars, and at single-adult groups sponsored by religious communities and other organizations.

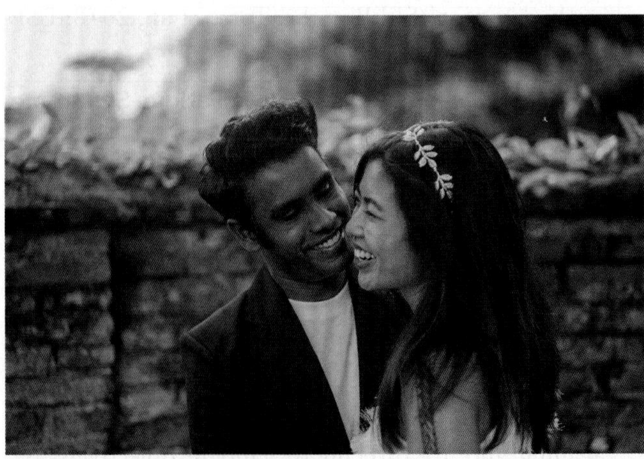

FIGURE 21-10 Choosing a significant other is a developmental task of young adulthood.

Another issue to address during the early years is the young man's attitudes and beliefs toward sex and sexual experimentation. Young men may question their sexuality as they mature. During this stage, some men come to the realization that they are homosexual—a person who has sexual interest in or sexual intercourse exclusively with members of his or her own gender. Some men who have sex with men (MSM), women, or both often do not consider themselves to be bisexual. When taking a sexual history, community health nurses must ask men if they have sex with women, men, or both, and they should be aware of issues affecting the lesbian, gay, bisexual, and transgender (LGBT) population.

Transgender, another term associated with sexuality, describes individuals who experience and/or express their gender differently and often does not correspond with the person's apparent or birth gender. An example is when a presumed male chooses to put on makeup and clothes that a female would traditionally wear. Some transgender individuals define themselves as *female to male* or *male to female* and may take hormones and/or undergo medical procedures to enhance or make permanent their gender selection, including gender reassignment surgery. Others prefer to simply be called *male* or *female*—the gender they present to others, whether or not they have undergone permanent gender reassignment.

Sexual experimentation, whether heterosexual or homosexual, can place young men at risk for diseases that affect long-term health or is life threatening. Men who are sexually active can reduce the possibility of being infected with an STI by limiting the number of sexual partners and using condoms consistently and correctly. Condoms also serve as a form of birth control for men. *Monogamy*, having sex with only one partner and abstinence can further reduce or eliminate the chance of contracting an STI. Public health nurses can serve as a resource for young men and can help them obtain free or low-cost condoms and treatment for STIs.

Human Immunodeficiency Virus. From 2012 through 2016, the rates of diagnoses of HIV infection in the Northeast and the Midwest decreased. The rates in the South and the West remained stable. In 2017, rates were 16.1 in the South, 10.6 in the Northeast, 9.4 in the West, and 7.4 in the Midwest (CDC, 2017f). Because the percentage of persons diagnosed with HIV varies by geographic region, it is important that prevention, testing, and treatment interventions be tailored for each area's distinctive needs. https://www.cdc.gov/hiv/statistics/overview/geographicdistribution.html

- Despite advances in the prevention and treatment of human immunodeficiency virus (HIV), the disease continues to disproportionately impact men in the United States.
- In 2016, the rate of HIV infected men was 570.1 per 100,000 compared to 169.9 in females. Of the 754,218 infected males in 2016, 72% of infections were attributed to male-to-male sexual contact (CDC, 2017f).
- The highest rate of new infection was seen in blacks/African Americans, followed by Hispanics/Latinos.
- HIV new infection was most prevalent in persons aged 25 to 29 years followed by those persons aged 20 to 24 years (CDC, 2019i).
- When examining trends in the disease based on race/ethnicity and age, the burden of the disease is highest among men of color and young adults.

Alcohol and illicit drug use are known to decrease social inhibitions and increase the risk for HIV transmission through risky sexual behaviors (e.g., lack of condom use) and the sharing of needles or other injection equipment (CDC, 2019i). Community health nurses must be able to talk openly and nonjudgmentally with men about their use of substances and their sexual relationships. These conversations can be challenging, but they have to occur if the number of HIV infections is to be reduced.

Testicular Cancer

- The risk for testicular cancer is a health problem that young men should be aware of even before early adulthood. The disease occurs most often in men between 20 and 34 years of age.
- A few risk factors have been identified that increase a young man's chance of developing testicular cancer including a personal history of an undescended testicle, abnormal testicular development, family history of testicular cancer, race/ethnicity (White), and age, (ACS, 2018).
- It is a rare form of cancer and is not on the list of objectives for men in *Healthy People 2030*. However, if detected early, this cancer is highly curable.
- According to the Testicular Cancer Society (2020), it may be beneficial to the overall health of a young man to know how to perform a testicular self-exam. For more information on TSE, visit the following Web site of the Testicular Cancer Society: https://testicularcancersociety.org/pages/self-exam-how-to

The choices a young adult man makes during these years establish healthy eating, work, rest, and exercise habits that will benefit him for a lifetime. A man should follow the dietary food guidelines that are recommended by U.S. Department of Agriculture (2016). Establishing a pattern of rest that allows his body to recover and refresh from a day full of meaningful activities will help him look forward to each day. He should establish an exercise routine that meets his personal needs, fits his skills and talents, and includes some physical activities that involve his family (Fig. 21-11). These choices provide him with the knowledge that he is doing everything he can to keep himself healthy and to prevent the two major killers of men—heart disease and cancer. Typically, young adult clients have few interactions with health care providers in any given year. It is important for people in this age group to have regular health checkups, be assessed for early signs of disease, and engage in health promotion activities.

Adult Men (35 to 65 Years)

Men in the developmental stage between 35 and 65 years of age face many challenges including:

- Caring for their own families and children
- Caring for aging parents and in-laws

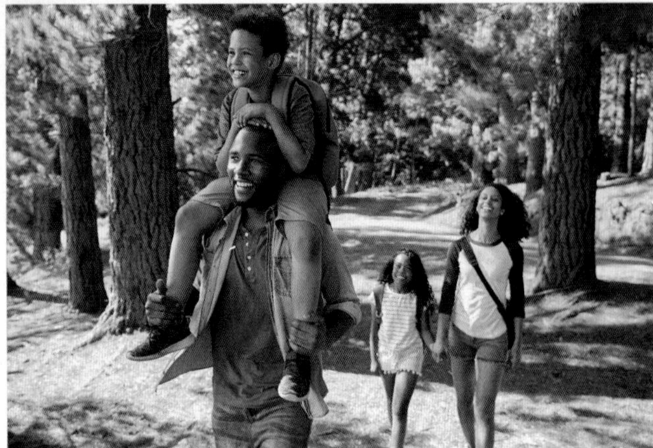

FIGURE 21-11 Adult men are encouraged to maintain good health through eating a healthy diet and getting regular exercise.

- Economic burdens of putting children through college
- Adjusting to the reality that their career path is probably set, and many life choices have been made

The term "midlife" is applied to the first half of this age period, 35 to 49 years during which many men experience a "midlife crisis." This period of time can be a difficult stage of life due to:

- Reappraisal of values, priorities, and personal relationships
- Doubt and anxiety realizing that his life is half over
- Beliefs he has not accomplished enough
- Struggles to find new meaning or purpose in his life
- Boredom with his personal life, job, or partners
- Desires to make life changes in personal life, job, or partners

In fact, men in midlife are at higher rates for suicide behavior than the general population (SAMHSA, 2018).

The later years in this stage, ages 50 to 64, involve preparation for retirement. In anticipation of retirement, these years are marked by:

- Expanded social relationships
- Pursuit of new hobbies to fill increased leisure time
- Finishing a career and accumulation of the best retirement benefits
- Making life altering decisions
- Potential health problems
- Loss of loved ones, particularly a spouse or long-term companion

Successful navigation of this stage can be fulfilling but may require a man to enhance his self-care skills. This includes having a positive attitude toward aging, one that examines the benefits of maturity, finds a balance between work and home, and maintains a healthy lifestyle by eating balanced meals and obtaining regular exercise. The community health nurse can provide anticipatory guidance to men approaching this stage and provide them with information on ways to manage life more effectively.

Reproductive Health. As mentioned earlier in this chapter, during the reproductive years, both women and men should strive to be as healthy as possible. During this stage, especially when a man has decided that his family is complete (Fig. 21-12), he may choose a permanent form of birth control through a surgical procedure called *vasectomy*. A vasectomy entails:

- Removal of all or a segment of the vas deferens
- Sperm cannot be released
- Routinely conducted on an outpatient basis
- Minimally invasive
- Takes about 30 minutes (CDC, 2017g)

Compared to tubal ligation (a surgical form of contraception for women), vasectomy is equally effective in preventing pregnancy, but vasectomy is simpler, faster, safer, and less expensive. A vasectomy is not protective against STIs and almost all can be reversed (NIH, 2016). Because these methods, however, are intended to be irreversible, all women and men should be counseled about the permanency of these procedures (CDC, 2017g).

Erection problems are common among men of all ages but especially in men as they age. **Erectile dysfunction (ED)**, sometimes called *impotence*, is the repeated inability to get or keep an erection firm enough for sexual intercourse. The word impotence may also be used to describe other problems that interfere with sexual intercourse, such as lack of sexual desire and problems with ejaculation or orgasm. Using the term *erectile dysfunction* makes it clear that these other issues are not involved (AUA, 2018; Urology Care Foundation, 2018). Because an erection requires a specific sequence of events, ED can occur when any of the associate events are disrupted. The sequence includes nerve impulses in the brain, spinal column, and areas around the penis, as well as response in muscles, fibrous tissues, veins, and arteries in and near the corpora cavernosa. Damages to nerves, arteries, smooth muscles, and fibrous tissues, often as a result of disease, are the most common causes of ED. Comorbidities such as diabetes, kidney disease, chronic alcoholism, multiple sclerosis, atherosclerosis, vascular disease, and neurologic disorders are primary health risk factors for ED (AUA, 2018; Urology Care Foundation, 2018).

Lifestyle choices that contribute to heart disease and vascular problems also increase the risk of ED. Smoking,

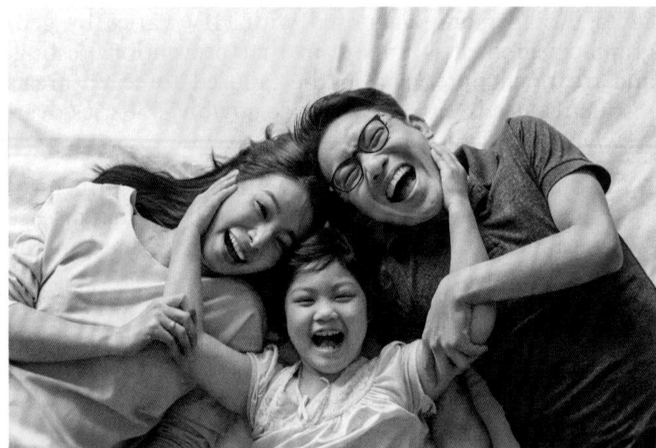

FIGURE 21-12 Reproductive health is an important consideration for men.

being overweight, and lack of exercise are possible causes of ED. Surgery (especially radical prostate and bladder surgery for cancer) can injure nerves and arteries near the penis, causing ED. Injury to the penis, spinal cord, prostate, bladder, and pelvis can lead to ED by harming nerves, smooth muscles, arteries, and fibrous tissues of the corpora cavernosa. In addition, many common medicines—antihypertensive, antihistamines, antidepressants, tranquilizers, appetite suppressants, and cimetidine—can produce ED as a side effect. In diagnosing ED, the medical provider will do a thorough health history including a lifestyle assessment. Specific questions related to the cardiovascular system and the nature of ED will be addressed (AUA, 2018; Urology Care Foundation, 2018).

Drugs for treating ED can be taken orally, injected directly into the penis, or inserted into the urethra at the tip of the penis. Current medical treatment consists of approved sildenafil citrate (Viagra), the first pill to treat ED. Since then, vardenafil hydrochloride (Levitra [oral], Staxyn [sublingual]), tadalafil (Cialis), and avanafil (Stendra) have been created and belong to a class of drugs called phosphodiesterase (PDE) type 5 inhibitors. These medications are currently the first line of therapy for treating ED. The drugs work by relaxing smooth muscles in the penis during sexual stimulation and allow increased blood flow. They can be taken as needed before sexual activity, up to once a day. Low-dose daily dosing rather than "on-demand" dosing has been found to be beneficial for some couples (Urology Care Foundation, 2018).

Cardiovascular Disease. Heart disease is the leading cause of death in men across most racial/ethnic groups. Despite a decline in the overall death rate from CVD, the burden of disease among men remains high.

- In 2013, CVD caused 310,000 deaths in men (CDC, 2020m).
- Approximately 70% to 89% of sudden cardiac events occur in men, and 50% of these men have no previous symptoms of disease.
- The average age for a first heart attack among men is 66 years.
- About 8.5% of White men, 7.9% of Black men, and 6.3% of Mexican American men have some coronary disease.
- The rate of a first cardiovascular event rises from 3 per 1,000 men at 35 to 44 years of age to 74 per 1,000 men at 85 to 94 years of age.
- It is interesting to note, if all forms of major CVD were eliminated, life expectancy among all persons would increase by almost 7 years (CDC, 2020m).

Major risk factors for heart disease in men include hypertension, hyperlipidemia (high LDL), tobacco use, diabetes, obesity/overweight, lack of physical activity, excessive alcohol consumption, stress, and low daily fruit and vegetable consumption (Box 21-7). When working with adult men, the community health nurse should educate men about the importance of modifying factors that increase their risk of developing CVD (CDC, 2020m). C/PHNs should discuss the signs and symptoms of a heart attack and how to access emergency medical treatment with adult males.

BOX 21-7 EVIDENCE-BASED PRACTICE

Church-Based Blood Pressure Interventions for Young Black Males

Hypertension is a significant disorder among Black males in the United States who experience early-onset and multiple comorbidities. Black males are less likely to engage in healthy lifestyles and seek medical advice and treatment. Interventions directed at young black males to decrease the incidence and severity of hypertension are limited.

A community-based participatory research study was conducted (Carter-Edwards et al., 2018) in the southeastern United States to explore using the church as a venue to offer blood pressure interventions for young black men. Focus group participants consisted of 19 men, 9 were aged 18 to 35 years and 10 were aged 36 to 50. Focus group questions explored lifestyle and self-management behaviors related to hypertension. The analysis of the focus group data revealed that most lifestyle behaviors were perceived to be manageable although participants admitted to added stress in managing busy work and family-related activities. Interestingly, another major theme generated was understanding hidden sodium.

Although the findings confirm persistent challenges of engaging young black men for blood pressure interventions, the results imply that programs should utilize the church infrastructure as a means to disseminate information and implement health care interventions. Prayer, supportive family systems, church leaders, mentors, and peers may help young black men increase their knowledge and achieve optimal lifestyles related to their blood pressure (Carter-Edwards et al., 2018).

Nurses were not included in the study, yet community health nurses would be an invaluable resource, as they can form partnerships to educate young black males on healthy lifestyles. Nurses are in a key position to recognize concerns touching the health and well-being of patients, determine health configurations across patient populations, connect patients with community resources and social services, and develop comprehensive interventions (Bachrach & Thomas, 2016).

Source: Bachrach and Thomas (2016); Carter-Edwards et al. (2018).

Prostate Health. Prostate health is another concern that may occur later in this life stage. The **prostate** is a doughnut-shaped gland located at the bottom of the bladder, about halfway between the rectum and the base of the penis. The prostate encircles the urethra. The walnut-sized gland produces most of the fluid in semen. Men can experience infection (prostatitis), prostate enlargement (benign prostatic hyperplasia [BPH]), and prostate cancer (ACS, 2020b).

- BPH is very common among men.
- The primary risk factor for developing BPH is age. Nearly 50% of men over 50 years of age report symptoms that are related to prostate gland enlargement.
- Symptoms of BPH are caused by an obstruction of the urethra and gradual loss of bladder function, which results in incomplete emptying of the bladder. The most commonly reported symptoms of BPH involve lower urinary tract symptoms (LUTS), such

as hesitant, interrupted, or weak urinary stream, urgency or leaking of urine, and more frequent urination, especially at night.

- Men often report the symptoms of BPH before the physician diagnoses it through a digital rectal examination (DRE).
- Treatment for BPH can include medication or surgery to reduce the size of the prostate (Urology Care Foundation, 2019).

Prostate cancer is the most frequently diagnosed cancer in men and the second leading cause of cancer death.

- According to the ACS, 1 man in 7 will get prostate cancer during his lifetime and 1 man in 38 will die from the disease.
- However, most prostate cancers grow slowly and do not cause any health problems in men who have them.
- More than 2.9 million men in the United States who have been diagnosed with prostate cancer at some time in their lives are still alive today.
- Prior to age 40, prostate cancer is very rare, but the chance of having prostate cancer rises rapidly after age 50.
- About 6 cases in 10 are diagnosed in men 65 years of age and older.
- Age is the strongest risk factor for prostate cancer, but family history and ethnicity also need to be considered.
- Prostate cancer occurs more often in Black men than in men of other races and occurs less often in Asian and Hispanic/Latino men.

The reasons for these racial and ethnic differences are not clear. Starting at age 50, all men should talk to their health care provider about the pros and cons of screening for prostate cancer. This discussion should start at age 45 if a man is Black or has a father or brother who had prostate cancer before age 65. Men with two or more close relatives who had prostate cancer before age 65 should talk with their health care provider about screening for prostate cancer at age 40 (ACS, 2020b; CDC, 2019j). The effectiveness of the screening test, prostate-specific antigen (PSA), has been brought into question, and the USPSTF (2015) has outlined a framework for further study and review.

Treatment for prostate cancer depends on the man's age, overall health status, and stage of disease (Tabayoyong & Abouassaly, 2015).

- Treatment options include surgery to remove all or part of the prostate (prostatectomy), radiation, and hormone therapy.
- Surgery, radiation, and hormone therapy all have the potential to disrupt sexual desire and performance, temporarily or permanently.
- Urinary dysfunction and incontinence are common side effects that occur after surgery or radiation.
- Rather than immediate treatment, watchful waiting or active surveillance is an option that may be appropriate for older men with limited life expectancy and/or less aggressive tumors (Filson, Marks, & Litwin, 2015).

A community health nurse can reinforce or clarify information shared with the man by his health care provider, discuss his treatment options with him and his family, and provide the support they may need if prostate cancer is diagnosed.

ROLE OF THE COMMUNITY HEALTH NURSE

The community health nurse works with adults in all age groups using the three levels of prevention—primary, secondary, and tertiary—as a guide. Interventions are conducted at the individual, family, group, and aggregate levels to make progress toward the *Healthy People 2030* objectives (Box 21-8).

Client teaching by the community health nurse is a major factor in preventing and managing chronic diseases. The challenge to the nurse is to be prepared to discuss issues, backed up with knowledge of and access to the appropriate community resources, to meet client needs. What the nurse can accomplish can be quite dramatic in terms of reducing days in the hospital because of chronic disease, improving quality of life for the chronically ill person, and preventing a combination of unhealthy habits from becoming causative factors in new cases of chronic disease. A nursing care plan matrix can guide the community health nurse in discussing areas of health promotion and protection with the client. An example of a nursing care plan matrix for young adults can be found in Box 21-9.

Primary Prevention

- Primary prevention activities focus on education to promote a healthy lifestyle. Much of the community health nurse's time is spent in the educator role.
- When working with individuals, the C/PHN should encourage routine health examinations, healthy eating habits, adequate sleep, moderate drinking, and no smoking. Among aggregates, the community health nurse focuses on community needs for services and programs that will keep that population healthy, such as providing flu vaccine clinics, teaching sexual responsibility, and preventing STIs.

The community health nurse may collaborate with community leaders and other stakeholders in designing programs, work with committees to secure funding, or approach the state legislature to lobby for needed changes to state laws and policies governing the health of adults. At other times, the nurse works with small groups of adults who could benefit from making healthy choices in diet, relaxation, and physical activity. Likewise, it is not unusual for the C/PHN to work with an individual to promote healthy living. An example of available resources on smoking cessation to those working with the veteran population is shared in Box 21-10.

Secondary Prevention

- Secondary prevention focuses on screening for early detection and prompt treatment of diseases. Throughout the life span, screening tests can help adults identify disease early (see Screenings and Checkup Schedule for Women and Men on thePoint®).
- A significant amount of the community health nurse's time is spent in assessing the need for planning,

BOX 21-8 LEVELS OF PREVENTION PYRAMID

Breast Cancer

SITUATION: Breast cancer.

GOAL: Using the three levels of prevention, avoid or promptly diagnose and treat negative health conditions and restore the fullest potential.

Tertiary Prevention

Rehabilitation	*Health Promotion and Education*	*Health Protection*
▪ Recovery at home with return to activities of daily living within 2 wk	▪ Maintains periodic follow-up with health care provider, follow-up mammogram at 6 and 12 mo, and as recommended by health care provider ▪ Education regarding risk for other cancers (cervical, ovarian, uterine, etc.)	▪ Practice breast awareness and receive mammograms as recommended; receives screening for ovarian cancer—transvaginal ultrasonography and blood test for tumor marker CA 125

Secondary Prevention

Early Diagnosis	*Prompt Treatment*
▪ Identification of lump in left breast, appointment made with health care provider for evaluation ▪ Receives mammogram and sonogram	▪ Needle aspiration of lump followed by cytologic studies ▪ Lumpectomy with removal of two suspicious lymph nodes ▪ Low-dose radiation

Primary Prevention

Health Promotion and Education	*Health Protection*
▪ Education regarding breast awareness and mammograms, as needed ▪ Education regarding environmental exposure and breast cancer (smoking, alcohol, chemicals) ▪ Education regarding low-fat diet and maintaining a body mass index <29	▪ Avoidance of environmental exposures that may contribute to cancer ▪ Maintains breast awareness and obtains mammogram when appropriate

implementing, or evaluating programs that focus on the early detection of diseases.

- This is followed with teaching to prevent further damage from the disease in progress or to prevent the spread of the disease, if it is communicable. Examples of secondary prevention programs include establishing mammography clinics, teaching breast and TSE, and screenings—blood pressure, blood glucose, BMI, and cholesterol. Wherever adults gather in groups, this is a good place to provide both primary and secondary health care and prevention services.

Tertiary Prevention

- The tertiary level of prevention focuses on rehabilitation and preventing further damage to an already compromised system. Many adults with whom a community health nurse works have chronic diseases, conditions resulting from another disease, or long-standing injuries with resulting disability.
- Ideally, negative health conditions can be prevented. If not, the next best thing is for them to be diagnosed early, without damage to an individual's health. But if negative health conditions have not been treated or brought under control, then the individual is at a tertiary level of prevention. At this level of prevention, the nurse focuses on maintaining quality of life.

Depending on the client's age, tertiary prevention can be simple or very complex. A 19-year-old man who breaks his leg while skiing needs information about using crutches safely, a reminder to eat protein foods for bone healing, and an appointment to return to his health care provider if he experiences various symptoms and to get the cast removed. He generally needs no additional help from others. Tertiary prevention in this case is uncomplicated. On the other hand, a 62-year-old woman who is 70 lb overweight with out-of-control blood glucose levels, symptoms of congestive heart failure, and difficulty walking more than 20 ft has much to accomplish in order to feel healthy. Can the nurse help the woman lose weight? Will weight loss bring her diabetes under control and alleviate congestive heart failure symptoms? With some weight reduction, will she be able to walk

BOX 21-9 Nursing Care Plan Matrix for Health Promotion, Young Adults: 18 to 35

Community health nurses can use this matrix to individualize teaching, services, and/or care to young adult clients. Use the questions to stimulate the development of an individualized approach that is client focused and client driven with the community health nurse acting as the catalyst. In any or all of these areas, the community health nurse may (1) discuss issues and commend the client for positive attitudes and behaviors (e.g., when the client is making healthful decisions, such as condom use for his/her health and the health of significant others); (2) discuss the issues and guide the client to resources that will enhance more positive behaviors and decisions (e.g., flu shot clinic or healthy lifestyle program for adults); or (3) discuss the issues and inform the client that immediate changes must be made to protect the health of self or others and inform/utilize the appropriate resources as soon as possible (e.g., follow-up for symptoms related to suspected STI).

1. *Life partner.* Ascertain whether the client is looking for a life partner or is choosing to live a single life. Discuss how the single life is satisfying for the client and ways to make it richer.
   Discuss settings in which client can meet others (male or female, based on sexual preference) with similar interests, philosophy, and outlook, such as work settings, school settings, faith communities, recreational communities, and the like.
   Discuss what the client is looking for in a potential life partner, expectations for the relationship, what the client contributes, how the client compromises and resolves conflict, and other issues. If in a relationship, what is good, what needs improving, and how to initiate change.
2. *Life's work.* How is the client preparing for his/her life's work (education, formal training, on the job training)? Will the life's work provide resources for client's life plans? Will the work choice provide long-term satisfaction? Is the work choice a "stepping stone" to another work role? How will/does he/she handle work and rearing children? What needs changing or can be improved in the work/children arrangement?
3. *Planning for children.* What knowledge does he/she have about family planning? What methods fit best with his/her philosophy, religious beliefs, and lifestyle? What are the long-term effects of the choices? How many children is the client planning to rear? Has he/she thought through the ramifications of this number? If choosing not to have (or unable to have) children, how will he/she deal with this? Does he/she want alternative suggestions for raising a child (adoption, foster parenting) or information about interacting with children (volunteering)?
4. *Maintaining physical and mental health.* In this area, the community health nurse needs to explore all areas of health promotion and protection. This will include discussions regarding primary and secondary prevention. Primary prevention discussions could include:
   - Diet and nutrition
   - Physical and leisure activities
   - Safe sex practices
   - Periodic health examinations
   - Personal safety—seat belts, protective helmets, dating violence, etc.
   - Immunizations
   - Regular use of sunscreen
   - Stress reduction activities

   Secondary prevention discussions could include:
   - Screening for sexually transmitted infections
   - Testicular self-examination
   - Smoking cessation
   - Pelvic exams and Pap smears
   - Counseling and support at times of stress
5. *Developing a life's philosophy.* Discuss client's personal life satisfaction, which may include religiosity and spirituality, living in congruence with cultural/ethnic/family beliefs and expectations, and coming to a comfortable level of satisfaction with life choices, having few regrets.

BOX 21-10 POPULATION FOCUS

Public Health and the Veteran Population

The Office of Patient Care Services within the Veterans Health Administration provides a public health focus on health promotion and disease prevention for the veteran population. The mission is accomplished through education and outreach, public health policy development, population-based surveillance, performance measurement and improvement, clinical guidelines, and research. Current focus areas for the veteran population include reducing complications from military exposures, hepatitis C, HIV/AIDS, influenza, women's health issues, and tobacco cessation. The veteran population is disproportionately affected by smoking-related illnesses. Many veterans began using tobacco during military service or deployment. The U.S. Department of Veterans Affairs Mental Health Web site "Tobacco and Health" was developed specifically for the veteran population to provide evidence-based information and helpful resources for veterans interested in improving their health by quitting the use of tobacco. The Web site is resource rich and can be accessed by any veteran or health care professional at http://www.mentalhealth.va.gov/quit-tobacco/index.asp. Two particularly meaningful resources for the veteran population are the SmokefreeVET (a text messaging program utilizing daily advice and support) and Stay Quit Coach (a mobile app to help Veterans deal with issues arising in tobacco cessation).

—*Cory, VA Staff Nurse*

Source: Veterans Health Administration, U.S. Department of Veterans Affairs (2019).

more easily? Or, will the woman feel better with physical therapy and a different medication regimen? Is there a quicker, safer, and better approach? On assessment, the nurse discovers that the woman has been as much as 80 lb overweight for 40 years. Will this information alter the nurse's approach to helping this woman? What additional information does the nurse need?

Caring for people at the tertiary level of prevention can become quite complicated because many body systems may be involved. In addition, all people function within many social systems, which may include family expectations, roles people have within the family, expected behaviors, community system knowledge and involvement, personal expectations, motivation, and support. Working at the tertiary level involves all of the nurse's skills in addition to community resources and a client who can be or wants to be motivated.

SUMMARY

- The 20th century saw a shift in the leading causes of death, from communicable to noncommunicable diseases. Currently, the five leading causes of death in adults are diseases of the heart, malignant neoplasms, unintentional injuries, CLRDs, and cerebrovascular diseases—none of which are communicable.
- The health care needs of adults are of great concern. Many needs are the same for both women and men, but the important differences were addressed in this chapter.
- Adults have health care needs that change as they age. Diet and exercise, obesity, substance use, safety, and healthy lifestyle choices are issues that adults must consider throughout their lives.
- Genomics refers to how a person's genetic makeup and environment predispose an individual to the development of disease. Understanding a person's genetic risk and environmental factors that may further influence and increase risk allows community health nurses to provide targeted education on disease prevention. Heart disease and cancers remain important concerns for both men and women, and health decisions made as a young adult can have a major impact on persons as they age.
- Chronic illness is an issue of increasing concern for both men and women as life expectancies increase. C/PHN should use the three levels of prevention to promote health across the life span. Primary prevention activities focus on education to promote a healthy lifestyle. Secondary prevention focuses on screening for early detection and prompt treatment of diseases.
- The C/PHN role at this stage is to assess needs; to plan, implement, or evaluate programs that focus on the early detection of diseases; and to educate clients to prevent further damage from or spread of disease. The tertiary level of prevention focuses on rehabilitation and prevention of further damage to an already compromised system. At this level of prevention, the nurse focuses on maintaining quality of life.

ACTIVE LEARNING EXERCISES

1. Using journals or online sources, select three articles that relate to a preventable chronic disease. For each article, summarize the content, identify the likely cause, and describe how the disease may have been prevented.
2. You are asked to offer a weight control program for 12 young adults who are residents in an apartment complex that has monthly programs related to health and wellness. The ages of the intended participants range from 20 to 30. What steps would you take to develop a successful program? What would be important to emphasize with this age group? What resources (e.g., smartphone apps, online information) might be useful to them in adhering to a healthy diet and exercise program?
3. Apply "Assess and Monitor Population Health" (1 of the 10 essential public health services; see Box 2-2) as follows: Using nursing and other health care databases, research a chronic disease associated with men or women aged 35 to 65. In a small group discussion with your classmates, identify selected concerns and discuss both personal responsibility and societal responsibility regarding management of this health problem.
4. In a small group, determine screening recommendations for a male and female at 50 years of age. Which recommendations are similar? Which are different?
5. Complete a health history on an adult, including medical, family, social history, and environmental history. Based on the information collected, determine the individual's personal risk factors. Which risk factors are modifiable? Which are not modifiable? Which chronic diseases is he or she at risk for developing? What education would you provide to help the individual reduce his or her risk?

thePoint: Everything You Need to Make the Grade!

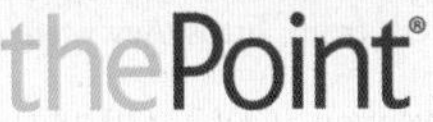

Visit http://thePoint.lww.com/Rector10e for NCLEX-style review questions, journal articles, supplemental materials, study aids for all learning styles, and more!

REFERENCES

American Cancer Society (ACS). (2018). *Testicular cancer*. Retrieved from http://www.cancer.org/cancer/testicularcancer/detailedguide/testicular-cancer-detailed-guide-toc

American Cancer Society (ACS). (2019). *Cancer facts and figures 2019*. Retrieved from https://www.cancer.org/content/dam/cancer-org/research/cancer-facts-and-statistics/annual-cancer-facts-and-figures/2019/cancer-facts-and-figures-2019.pdf

American Cancer Society (ACS). (2020a). *American cancer society recommendations for early detection of breast cancer*. Retrieved from https://www.cancer.org/cancer/breast-cancer/screening-tests-and-early-detection/american-cancer-society-recommendations-for-the-early-detection-of-breast-cancer.html

American Cancer Society (ACS). (2020b). *Prostate cancer*. Retrieved from https://www.cancer.org/cancer/prostate-cancer.html

American College of Obstetricians and Gynecologists (ACOG). (2018a). *The menopause years*. Retrieved from https://www.acog.org/store/products/patient-education/pamphlets/womens-health/the-menopause-years

American College of Obstetricians and Gynecologists (ACOG). (2018b). *Committee opinion: Hormone therapy and heart disease*. Retrieved from https://www.acog.org/Clinical-Guidance-and-Publications/Committee_Opinions/Committee_on_Gynecologic_Practice/Hormone_Therapy-and-Heart-Disease

American College of Obstetricians and Gynecologists (ACOG). (2018c). *Committee opinion: Compounded bioidentical menopausal hormone therapy*. Retrieved from http://www.acog.org/Resources-And-Publications/Committee-Opinions/Committee-on-Gynecologic-Practice/Compounded-Bioidentical-Menopausal-Hormone-Therapy

American Diabetes Association (ADA). (2018). Classification and diagnosis of diabetes: Standards of medical care—2018. *Diabetes Care, 41*(Suppl 1), S13–S27. doi: 10.2337/dc18-S002.

American Heart Association (AHA). (2016). *Understand your risks to prevent a heart attack*. Retrieved from https://www.heart.org/en/health-topics/heart-attack/understand-your-risks-to-prevent-a-heart-attack

American Heart Association (AHA). (2018). *Go red for women*. Retrieved from https://www.goredforwomen.org

American Lung Association (ALA). (2020a). *Lung health and diseases: What causes COPD*. Retrieved from http://www.lung.org/lung-health-and-diseases/lung-disease-lookup/copd/symptoms-causes-risk-factors/what-causes-copd.html

American Lung Association (ALA). (2020b). *Lung health and diseases: Asthma*. Retrieved from http://www.lung.org/lung-health-and-diseases/lung-disease-lookup/asthma/

American Urological Association (AUA). (2018). *Erectile dysfunction: AUA guideline (2018)*. Retrieved from https://www.auanet.org/guidelines/male-sexual-dysfunction-erectile-dysfunction-(2018)

Arthritis Foundation. (n.d.). *What is arthritis?* Retrieved from https://www.arthritis.org/health-wellness/about-arthritis/understanding-arthritis/what-is-arthritis

Bachrach, C., & Thomas, T. (2016). Training nurses in population health science: What, why, how? Presentation at the 133rd meeting of the National Advisory Council for Nurse Education and Practice, Rockville, MD.

Benjamin E. J., Virani S. S., Callaway C. W., Chang A. R., Cheng S., Chiuve S. E., ... Muntner, P. (2018). Heart disease and stroke statistics—2018 update: A report from the American Heart Association. *Circulation, 137*(12), e67–e492. doi: 10.1161/CIR.0000000000000558.

Berk, L. E. (2018). Emotional and social development in early adulthood. In *Development through the lifespan* (7th ed., pp. 468–506). Hoboken, NJ: Pearson Education.

Brown, A. F., Liang, L., Vassar, S. D., Escarce, J. J., Merkin, S. S., Cheng, E., ... Longstreth, W. T. (2018). Trends in racial/ethnic and nativity disparities in cardiovascular health among adults without prevalent cardiovascular disease in the United States, 1988–2014. *Annals of Internal Medicine, 168*, 541–549. doi: 10.7326/M17-0996.

Cancer Statistic Center. (2018). *Estimated deaths, 2013–2017*. Retrieved from https://cancerstatisticscenter.cancer.org/#!/cancer-site/Breast

Carter-Edwards, L., Lindquist, R., Redmond, N., Turner, C. M., Harding, C., Oliver, J., ... Shikany, J. M. (2018). Designing faith-based blood pressure interventions to reach young black men. *American Journal of Preventive Medicine, 55*, 5. doi: 10.1016/j.amepre.2018.05.009.

Centers for Disease Control and Prevention (CDC). (2016). *National Center for Health Statistics*. Retrieved from https://www.cdc.gov/nchs/fastats/asthma.htm

Centers for Disease Control and Prevention (CDC). (2017a). *Injury prevention and control: Data and statistics. Key injury and violence data*. Retrieved from https://www.cdc.gov/injury/wisqars/overview/key_data.html

Centers for Disease Control and Prevention (CDC). (2017b). *National Center for Health Statistics: Accidents or unintentional injuries*. Retrieved from http://www.cdc.gov/nchs/fastats/accidental-injury.htm

Centers for Disease Control and Prevention (CDC). (2017c). *Opioid overdose: Overdose prevention*. Retrieved from https://www.cdc.gov/drugoverdose/prevention/index.html

Centers for Disease Control and Prevention (CDC). (2017d). *Chlamydia—CDC fact sheet*. Retrieved from https://www.cdc.gov/std/chlamydia/std-fact-chlamydia.htm

Centers for Disease Control and Prevention (CDC). (2017e). *Mortality in the United States, 2017*. Retrieved from https://www.cdc.gov/nchs/products/databriefs/db328.htm

Centers for Disease Control and Prevention (CDC). (2017f). *HIV Surveillance Report, 2017* (Vol. 29). Retrieved from https://www.cdc.gov/hiv/pdf/library/reports/surveillance/cdc-hiv-surveillance-report-2017-vol-29.pdf

Centers for Disease Control and Prevention (CDC). (2017g). *US selected practice recommendations for contraceptive use, 2016*. Retrieved from https://www.cdc.gov/reproductivehealth/contraception/mmwr/spr/summary.html

Centers for Disease Control and Prevention (CDC). (2018a). *Chronic obstructive pulmonary disease (COPD)*. Retrieved from https://www.cdc.gov/copd/infographics/copd-costs.html

Centers for Disease Control and Prevention (CDC). (2018b). *Sexually Transmitted Disease Surveillance 2017*. Atlanta, GA: U.S. Department of Health and Human Services.

Centers for Disease Control and Prevention (CDC). (2019a). *Heart disease fact sheet*. Retrieved from http://www.cdc.gov/dhdsp/data_statistics/fact_sheets/fs_heart_disease.htm

Centers for Disease Control and Prevention (CDC). (2019b). *Arthritis*. Retrieved from https://www.cdc.gov/chronicdisease/resources/publications/factsheets/arthritis.htm

Centers for Disease Control and Prevention (CDC). (2019c). *Adult obesity prevalence maps*. Retrieved from https://www.cdc.gov/obesity/data/prevalence-maps.html

Centers for Disease Control and Prevention (CDC). (2019d). *Overweight and obesity*. Retrieved form https://www.cdc.gov/obesity/adult/causes.html

Centers for Disease Control and Prevention (CDC). (2019e). *Morbidity and mortality weekly report: Drug and opioid-involved overdose deaths—United States, 2013–2017*. Retrieved from https://www.cdc.gov/mmwr/volumes/67/wr/mm675152e1.htm?s_cid=mm675152e1_w

Centers for Disease Control and Prevention (CDC). (2019f). *About chronic disease*. Retrieved from https://www.cdc.gov/chronicdisease/about/index.htm

Centers for Disease Control and Prevention (CDC). (2019g). *Genital HPV infection—fact sheet*. Retrieved from https://www.cdc.gov/std/hpv/stdfact-hpv.htm

Centers for Disease Control and Prevention (CDC). (2019h). *Myalgic encephalomyelitis/chronic fatigue syndrome: Symptoms*. Retrieved from https://www.cdc.gov/me-cfs/symptoms-diagnosis/symptoms.html

Centers for Disease Control and Prevention (CDC). (2019i). *HIV risk and prevention*. Retrieved from http://www.cdc.gov/hiv/risk/

Centers for Disease Control and Prevention (CDC). (2019j). *Who is at risk for prostate cancer?* Retrieved from https://www.cdc.gov/cancer/prostate/basic_info/risk_factors.htm

Centers for Disease Control and Prevention (CDC). (2020a). *Stroke in the United States*. Retrieved from http://www.cdc.gov/stroke/facts.htm

Centers for Disease Control and Prevention (CDC). (2020b). *Injury prevention and control: Data & statistics. Costs of injuries and violence in the United States*. Retrieved from http://www.cdc.gov/injury/wisqars/overview/cost_of_injury.html

Centers for Disease Control and Prevention (CDC). (2020c). *Opioid overdose: Data overview*. Retrieved from https://www.cdc.gov/drugoverdose/data/index.html

Centers for Disease Control and Prevention (CDC). (2020d). *Motor vehicle safety: Cost data and prevention policies*. Retrieved from https://www.cdc.gov/motorvehiclesafety/costs/index.html

Centers for Disease Control and Prevention (CDC). (2020e). *National Diabetes Statistics Report, 2020: Estimates of Diabetes and Its Burden in the United States*. Atlanta, GA: U.S. Department of Health and Human Services. Retrieved from https://www.cdc.gov/diabetes/pdfs/data/statistics/national-diabetes-statistics-report.pdf

Centers for Disease Control and Prevention (CDC). (2020f). *Diabetes: Who's at risk?* Retrieved from https://www.cdc.gov/diabetes/basics/risk-factors.html

Centers for Disease Control and Prevention (CDC). (2020g). *Adult obesity causes and consequences*. Retrieved from https://www.cdc.gov/obesity/adult/causes.html

Centers for Disease Control and Prevention (CDC). (2020h). *Smoking & tobacco use: Fast facts*. Retrieved from https://www.cdc.gov/tobacco/data_statistics/fact_sheets/fastfacts/index.htm

Centers for Disease Control and Prevention (CDC). (2020i). *Smoking and tobacco use*. Retrieved from https://www.cdc.gov/tobacco/basic_information/e-cigarettes/about-e-cigarettes.html

Centers for Disease Control and Prevention (CDC). (2020j). *Before pregnancy: Women*. Retrieved from https://www.cdc.gov/preconception/women.html

Centers for Disease Control and Prevention (CDC). (2020k). *Does osteoporosis run in your family?* Retrieved from https://www.cdc.gov/features/osteoporosis/index.html

Centers for Disease Control and Prevention (CDC). (2020l). *WISEWOMAN*. Retrieved from https://www.cdc.gov/wisewoman/index.htm

Centers for Disease Control and Prevention (CDC). (2020m). *Men and heart disease fact sheet*. Retrieved from https://www.cdc.gov/dhdsp/data_statistics/fact_sheets/fs_men_heart.htm

Centers for Disease Control and Prevention (CDC). (2020n). *Genomics and health*. Retrieved from https://www.cdc.gov/genomics/disease/genomic_diseases.htm

Chronic Pain Research Alliance. (2015). *Impact of chronic overlapping pain conditions on public health and the urgent need for safe and effective treatment*. Retrieved from http://www.chronicpainresearch.org/public/CPRA_WhitePaper_2015-FINAL-Digital.pdf

Dean, L. (2018). *Warfarin therapy and VKORC1 and CYP genotype. Medical Genetics Summaries*. Retrieved from https://www.ncbi.nlm.nih.gov/books/NBK84174/

Dong, L., Fakeye, O. A., Graham, G., & Gaskin, D. J. (2018). Racial/ethnic disparities in quality of care for cardiovascular disease in ambulatory settings: A review. *Medical Care Research and Review*, *75*(3), 263–291. doi: 10.1177/1077558717725884.

Filson, C. P., Marks, L. S., & Litwin, M. S. (2015). Expectant management for men with early stage prostate cancer. *CA: A Cancer Journal for Clinicians*, *65*(4), 264–282. doi: 10.3322/caac.21278.

Food and Drug Administration (FDA). (2018a). *FDA approves expanded use of Gardasil 9 to include individuals 27 through 45 years old*. Retrieved from https://www.fda.gov/NewsEvents/Newsroom/PressAnnouncements/ucm622715.htm

Food and Drug Administration (FDA). (2018b). *Table of pharmacogenomic biomarkers in drug labeling*. Retrieved from https://www.fda.gov/downloads/Drugs/ScienceResearch/UCM578588.pdf

Foster, J. E. (2015). Women of a certain age: "Second wave" feminists reflect back on 50 years of struggle in the United States. *Women's Studies International Forum*, *50*, 68–79. doi: 10.1016/j.wsif.2015.03.005.

Framingham Heart Study. (2018). *Framingham heart study*. Retrieved from https://www.framinghamheartstudy.org

Friedan, B. (2013). *The feminine mystique* (50th anniversary ed.). New York, NY: W. W. Norton and Company.

Gunnars, K. (2018). *The paleo diet: A beginner's guide plus meal plan*. Retrieved from https://thepaleodiet.com/the-paleo-diet-premise/

Hales, C. M., Carroll, M. D., Fryar, C. D., & Ogden, C. L. (2017). Prevalence of obesity among adults and youth: United States, 2015–2016. In *NCHS Data Brief, 288*. Retrieved from https://www.cdc.gov/nchs/data/databriefs/db288.pdf

Health Resources & Services Administration. (2019). *Health literacy*. Retrieved from https://www.hrsa.gov/about/organization/bureaus/ohe/health-literacy/index.html

Heron, M. (July 26, 2018). Deaths: Leading causes for 2016. *National Vital Statistic Report*, *67*(6). Retrieved from https://www.cdc.gov/nchs/data/nvsr/nvsr67/nvsr67_06.pdf

Institute of Medicine. (2015). *Beyond Myalgic Encephalomyelitis/Chronic Fatigue Syndrome, redefining an illness, report guide for clinicians*. Retrieved from https://pubmed.ncbi.nlm.nih.gov/25695122/

International Women's Day. (n.d.). *About International Women's Day (March 8)*. Retrieved from https://www.internationalwomensday.com/About

Kochanek, K. D., Murphy, S. L., Xu, J., & Arias, E. (2017). Mortality in the United States. In *NCHS Data Brief, 293*. Retrieved from https://www.cdc.gov/nchs/products/databriefs/db293.htm

Kosinski, C., & Jarnayvaz, F. R. (2017). Effects of ketogenic diets on cardiovascular risk factors: Evidence from animal and human studies. *Nutrients*, *9*(5), 517. doi: 10.3390/nu9050517.

Martin, K. A., & Barbieri, R. L. (2019). *Preparations for menopausal hormone therapy*. Retrieved from https://www.uptodate.com/contents/preparations-for-menopausal-hormone-therapy

Mauer, R. (2018). *The ketogenic diet: A beginner's guide to keto*. Retrieved from https://www.healthline.com/nutrition/ketogenic-diet-101#foods-to-eat

Mazidi, M., Katsik, N., Mikhailidis, D. P., & Banach, M. (2018). Low-carbohydrate diets and all-cause and cause-specific mortality: A population-based cohort study and pooling prospective studies. Abstract presented at the European Society of Cardiology Congress 2018, Munich, Germany.

Merck Sharp & Dohme Corporation. (2018). *Patient information about Gardasil 9*. Retrieved from https://www.merck.com/product/usa/pi_circulars/g/gardasil_9/gardasil_9_ppi.pd

National Cancer Institute (NCI). (2020). *Surveillance, Epidemiology, and End Stage Program (SEER)*. Retrieved from https://seer.cancer.gov/

National Center for Biotechnology Information (NCBI). (2017). *Women's health initiative clinical trial and observational study SHARe*. Retrieved from https://www.ncbi.nlm.nih.gov/projects/gap/cgi-bin/study.cgi?study_id=phs000200.v11.p3

National Center for Complementary and Integrative Health (NCCIH). (2017). *Menopausal symptoms: In depth*. Retrieved from https://www.nccih.nih.gov/health/menopausal-symptoms-in-depth

National Center for Health Statistics (NCHS). (2017). *Leading causes of death*. Retrieved from https://www.cdc.gov/nchs/fastats/leading-causes-of-death.htm

National Center for Health Statistics (NCHS). (2019). *Health, United States, 2017*. Retrieved from https://www.cdc.gov/nchs/data/nvsr/nvsr68/nvsr68_07-508.pdf

National Eating Disorder Association (NEDA). (2018). *Eating disorders screening tool*. Retrieved from https://www.nationaleatingdisorders.org/screening-tool

National Institute on Alcohol Abuse and Alcoholism (NIAAA). (2017). *Alcohol use disorder*. Retrieved from https://www.niaaa.nih.gov/alcohol-health/overview-alcohol-consumption/alcohol-use-disorders

National Institute on Alcohol Abuse and Alcoholism (NIAAA). (2018). *Alcohol facts and statistics*. Retrieved from https://www.niaaa.nih.gov/alcohol-health/overview-alcohol-consumption/alcohol-facts-and-statistics

National Institute of Drug Abuse (NIDA). (2018). *Substance use in women*. Retrieved from https://www.drugabuse.gov/publications/research-reports/substance-use-in-women/sex-gender-differences-in-substance-use

National Institute of Health (NIDA). (2019). *Opioid overdose crisis*. Retrieved from https://www.drugabuse.gov/drugs-abuse/opioids/opioid-overdose-crisis

National Institutes of Health (NIH). (1993). *National Institutes of Health Revitalization Act of 1993, Subtitle B—Clinical research equity involving women and minorities*. Retrieved from https://www.ncbi.nlm.nih.gov/books/NBK236531/

National Institutes of Health (NIH). (2016). Vasectomy: Other FAQs. Retrieved from https://www.nichd.nih.gov/health/topics/vasectomy/conditioninfo/faqs

National Institutes of Health (NIH). (2018). NIH launches new initiative, doubles funding to accelerate scientific solution to stem national opioid epidemic. Retrieved from https://www.nih.gov/news-events/news-releases/nih-launches-heal-initiative-doubles-funding-accelerate-scientific-solutions-stem-national-opioid-epidemic

National Institutes of Health (NIH). (2019a). *Health disparities*. Retrieved from https://medlineplus.gov/healthdisparities.html

National Institutes of Health (NIH). (2019b). *What is a genome?* Retrieved from https://ghr.nlm.nih.gov/primer/hgp/genome

National Institutes of Health, National Cancer Institute (NIH, NCI). (2017). *Precision medicine in cancer treatment*. Retrieved from https://www.cancer.gov/about-cancer/treatment/types/precision-medicine

National Institutes of Health, National Heart, Lung, and Blood Institute (NIH, NHLBI). (2019). *Listen to your heart*. Retrieved from https://www.nhlbi.nih.gov/health-topics/education-and-awareness/heart-truth/listen-to-your-heart

National Institutes of Health, National Library of Medicine. (NIH, NLM). (n.d.). *Health literacy*. Retrieved from https://nnlm.gov/initiatives/topics/health-literacy

National Institute of Mental Health. (2016). *Eating disorders*. Retrieved from https://www.nimh.nih.gov/health/topics/eating-disorders/index.shtml

National Institute of Mental Health. (2018). *Eating disorders: About more than food*. Retrieved form https://www.nimh.nih.gov/health/publications/eating-disorders/index.shtml

National Organization for Rare Diseases (NORD). (2017). *Glucose-6-phosphate dehydrogenase deficiency*. Retrieved from https://rarediseases.org/rare-diseases/glucose-6-phosphate-dehydrogenase-deficiency/

National Women's Health Network. (2018). *About the National Women's Health Network*. Retrieved from https://www.nwhn.org/about-us/

Nurses' Health Study (NHS). (2016). *History*. Retrieved from https://www.nurseshealthstudy.org/about-nhs/history

Office on Women's Health. (2018a). *Anorexia nervosa fact sheet*. Retrieved from https://www.womenshealth.gov/files/documents/fact-sheet-anorexia.pdf

Office on Women's Health. (2018b). *Bulimia nervosa fact sheet*. Retrieved from https://www.womenshealth.gov/files/documents/fact-sheet-bulimia.pdf

Office on Women's Health. (2018c). *Binge eating disorder fact sheet*. Retrieved from https://www.womenshealth.gov/files/documents/fact-sheet-binge-eating.pdf

Office on Women's Health. (2018d). *Menopause*. Retrieved from https://www.womenshealth.gov/menopause

Office on Women's Health. (2018e). *Heart disease risk factors*. Retrieved from https://www.womenshealth.gov/heart-disease-and-stroke/heart-disease/heart-disease-risk-factors

Office on Women's Health. (2018f). *Heart attack and women*. Retrieved from https://www.womenshealth.gov/heart-disease-and-stroke/heart-disease/heart-attack-and-women

Office on Women's Health. (2019). *Heart attack symptoms*. Retrieved from https://www.womenshealth.gov/heart-disease-and-stroke/heart-disease/heart-attack-and-women/heart-attack-symptoms

Orgera, K., & Artiga, S. (2018). *Disparities in health and health care: Five key questions and answers*. Retrieved from https://www.kff.org/disparities-policy/issue-brief/disparities-in-health-and-health-care-five-key-questions-and-answers/

Our Bodies Ourselves. (n.d.). *History*. Retrieved from http://www.ourbodiesourselves.org/history/

Pew Research Center. (2020a). *6 Facts about moms*. Retrieved from https://www.pewresearch.org/fact-tank/2019/05/08/facts-about-u-s-mothers/

Pew Research Center. (2020b). *Chapter 5: Balancing work and family*. Retrieved from https://www.pewsocialtrends.org/2013/12/11/chapter-5-balancing-work-and-family/

Santoro, N. (2016). Perimenopause: From research to practice. *Journal of Women's Health*, *25*(4), 332–339. doi: 10.1089/jwh.2015.5556.

Smith, R. A., Andres, K. S., Brooks, D., Fedewa, S. A., Manassaram-Baptiste, D., Saslow, D., ... Wender, R. C. (2018). Cancer screening in the United States, 2018: A review of current American Cancer Society guidelines and current issues in cancer screening. *CA: A Cancer Journal for Clinicians*, *68*(4), 297–316. doi: 10.3322/caac.21446.

Solve ME/CFS Initiative. (2018). *About the disease*. Retrieved from https://solvecfs.org/about-the-disease/

Stuenkel, C. A., Davis, S. R., Gompel, A., Lumsden, M. A., Murad, M. H., Pinkerton, J. V., & Santen, R. J. (2015). Treatment of symptoms of the menopause: An Endocrine Society Clinical Practice Guide. *Journal of Clinical Endocrinology & Metabolism*, *100*(11), 3975–4011. doi: 10.1210/jc.2015-2236.

Substance Abuse and Mental Health Services Administration (SAMHSA). (2017a). *Key substance use and mental health indicators in the United States: Results from the 2017 National Survey on Drug Use and Health*. Retrieved from https://www.samhsa.gov/data/report/2017-nsduh-annual-national-report

Substance Abuse and Mental Health Services Administration (SAMHSA). (2017b). *Eating disorders*. Retrieved from https://www.samhsa.gov/treatment/mental-disorders/eating-disorders

Substance Abuse and mental Health Service Administration (SAMHSA). (2018). *Suicide prevention*. Retrieved from https://www.integration.samhsa.gov/clinical-practice/suicide-prevention-update

Substance Abuse and Mental Health Services Administration (SAMHSA). (2019). *Mental health and substance use disorders*. Retrieved from https://www.samhsa.gov/find-help/disorders

Surveillance, Epidemiology, and End Stage Program (SEER). (n.d.a). *Cancer stat facts: Female breast cancer*. Retrieved from https://seer.cancer.gov/statfacts/html/breast.html

Surveillance, Epidemiology, and End Stage Program (SEER). (n.d.b). *Cancer stat facts: Cervical cancer*. Retrieved from https://seer.cancer.gov/statfacts/html/cervix.html

Surveillance, Epidemiology, and End Stage Program (SEER). (n.d.c). *Cancer stat facts: Ovarian cancer*. Retrieved from https://seer.cancer.gov/statfacts/html/ovary.html

T. Collin Campbell Center for Nutrition Studies. (2018). *Living a whole-food, plant-based life*. Retrieved from https://nutritionstudies.org/whole-food-plant-based-diet-guide/

Tabayoyong, W., & Abouassaly, R. (2015). Prostate cancer screening and the associated controversy. *Surgical Clinics of North America*, *95*(5), 1023–1039. doi: 10.1016/j.suc.2015.05.001.

Testicular Cancer Society. (2020). *Testicular self-exam*. Retrieved from https://testicularcancersociety.org/pages/self-exam-how-to

Torre, L. A., Trabert, B., DeSantis, D. E., Miller, K. D., Samimi, G., Runowicz, C. D., Guaden, M. M., ... Siegel, R. L. (2018). Ovarian cancer statistics, 2018. *CA: A Cancer Journal for Clinicians*, *68*(4), 284–296.

Urology Care Foundation. (2018). *What is erectile dysfunction?* Retrieved from https://www.urologyhealth.org/urologic-conditions/erectile-dysfunction

Urology Care Foundation. (2019). *What is Benign Prostatic Hyperplasia (BPH)?* Retrieved from https://www.urologyhealth.org/urologic-conditions/benign-prostatic-hyperplasia-(bph)

U.S. Department of Agriculture. (2016). *MyPlate*. Retrieved from https://www.choosemyplate.gov/MyPlate

U.S. Department of Health and Human Services (USDHHS). (2015). *Healthy People 2020: Disparities*. Retrieved from https://www.healthypeople.gov/2020/about/foundation-health-measures/Disparities

U.S. Department of Health and Human Services (USDHHS). (2018). Active adults. In *Physical Activity Guidelines for Americans* (2nd ed., pp. 55–65). Washington, DC: U.S. Department of Health and Human Services. Retrieved from https://health.gov/paguidelines/second-edition/pdf/Physical_Activity_Guidelines_2nd_edition.pdf#page=55

U.S. Department of Health & Human Services (USDHHS). (2020). *Healthy People 2030: Browse objectives*. Retrieved from https://health.gov/healthypeople/objectives-and-data/browse-objectives

U.S. Preventative Services Task Force. (2016a). *Final update summary: Colorectal cancer screening*. Retrieved from https://www.uspreventiveservicestaskforce.org/uspstf/recommendation/colorectal-cancer-screening

U.S. Preventative Services Task Force. (2016b). *Final update summary: Chlamydia and gonorrhea: Screening*. Retrieved from https://www.uspreventiveservicestaskforce.org/Page/Document/UpdateSummaryFinal/chlamydia-and-gonorrhea-screening?ds=1&s=chlamydia

U.S. Preventative Services Task Force. (2016c). *Final recommendation statement: Breast cancer: Screening*. Retrieved from https://www.uspreventiveservicestaskforce.org/Page/Document/RecommendationStatementFinal/breast-cancer-screening1

U.S. Preventative Services Task Force. (2018a). *Final update summary: Human immunodeficiency virus (HIV) infection: Screening*. Retrieved from https://www.uspreventiveservicestaskforce.org/Page/Document/UpdateSummaryFinal/human-immunodeficiency-virus-hiv-infection-screening

U.S. Preventative Services Task Force. (2018b). *Final recommendation statement: Osteoporosis to prevent fractures: Screening*. Retrieved from https://www.uspreventiveservicestaskforce.org/Page/Document/RecommendationStatementFinal/osteoporosis-screening1#consider

U.S. Preventative Services Task Force. (2018c). *Final update summary: Cervical cancer screening*. Retrieved from file:///Users/joey-stanleyhotmail.com/Downloads/cervical-cancer-final-rec-statement.pdf

U.S. Preventative Services Task Force. (2018d). *Final update summary: Ovarian cancer*. Retrieved from https://www.uspreventiveservicestaskforce.org/uspstf/recommendation/ovarian-cancer-screening

Veterans Health Administration, U.S. Department of Veterans Affairs. (2019). *Tobacco and health*. Retrieved from https://www.mentalhealth.va.gov/quit-tobacco/

Women's Health Initiative (WHI). (n.d.). *About WHI*. Retrieved from https://www.whi.org/about/SitePages/About%20WHI.aspx

Women's Health Study (WHS). (n.d.). *Overview of women's health study (WHS) study design*. Retrieved from http://whs.bwh.harvard.edu/images/WHS%20website-Overview%20of%20study.pdf

Wood, D. E., Kazerooni, E. A., Baum, S. L., Eapen, G. A., Ettinger, D. S., Hous, L., ... Hughes, M. (2018). Lung cancer screening, version 3.2018: Clinical practice guidelines in oncology. *Journal of the National Comprehensive Cancer Network*, *16*(4), 412–441. doi: 10.6004/jnccn.2018.0020.

World Health Organization (WHO). (2019). *Cardiovascular disease*. Retrieved from https://www.who.int/cardiovascular_diseases/about_cvd/en/

World Health Organization (WHO). (n.d.). *Human genomics in global health*. Retrieved from https://www.who.int/genomics/geneticsVSgenomics/en/

Xu, J. Q., Murphy, S. L., Kochanek, K. D., Bastian, B., & Arias, E. (2018). Deaths: Final data for 2016. *National Vital Statistics Reports*, *67*(5). Hyattsville, MD: National Center for Health Statistics.

CHAPTER 22

Older Adults

"In the end, it's not the years in your life that count. It's the life in your years."

—President Abraham Lincoln (1809–1865)

KEY TERMS

Age dependency ratio
Ageism
Aging in place
Alzheimer's disease (AD)
Arthritis
Assisted living
Beta-amyloid
Case management
Chronic conditions
Continuing care retirement communities (CCRCs)
Custodial care
Elder abuse
Geriatrics
Gerontological
Hospice
Long-term care
Nursing home
Osteoporosis
Palliative care
Polypharmacy
Respite care
Senility
Tau protein
Universal design

LEARNING OBJECTIVES

Upon mastery of this chapter, you should be able to:

1. Describe the global and national health status of older adults.
2. Identify and refute at least three common misconceptions about older adults.
3. Describe characteristics of healthy older adults.
4. Provide an example of primary, secondary, and tertiary prevention practices in the older adult population.
5. Identify four chronic conditions most commonly found in the older adult population.
6. Describe initial steps for reporting elder abuse.
7. Describe various types of living arrangements and care options as older adult's age in place.
8. Describe the importance of integrating palliative care into aspects of care for older adults.

INTRODUCTION

Ms. Barbara is still in the apartment she and her husband shared for many years after they retired. At 94, Ms. Barbara tends her parakeet, Bert, and visits her neighbors regularly. Because she does not drive anymore, she orders her groceries online for delivery. Her apartment has a universal design with safety bars and a pull string for quick assistance. She loves card games and plays bridge and Scrabble regularly with others in the retirement community. Her health has had its ups and downs, but with the support of an automated pill box and frequent visits from her daughter, Ms. Barbara is able to remain independent in her apartment.

Older adults constitute a large and rapidly growing population group in the United States, one that you will join eventually. Perhaps your parents or grandparents are part of that group now. Improved medical care, advances in public health standards, and a focus on prevention have contributed to dramatic increases in life expectancy in the United States. A child born in 2016 could expect to live 78.6 years, about 30 years longer than a child born in 1900 (Administration for Community Living, 2019b). A second reason for the huge growth in the number of older adults began in 2011 as the baby boomers (people born after World War II between the years of 1946 and 1964) reached age 65. One out of four of these baby boomers will live past age 90 (Administration for Community Living, 2019b). Older adults represent 15.2% of the U.S. population or about one in every seven Americans (over 50 million); this number is expected to double by 2060, when older adults will outnumber young children.

Racial and ethnic minority populations will increase to approximately 28% of older adults by 2030 (U.S. Department of Health and Human Services, 2020b). The health status of racial and ethnic minorities of all ages lags far behind that of nonminority populations. For a variety of reasons, older adults may experience the effects of health disparities more dramatically than any other population group.

Looking forward to these changing health needs of the nation, *Healthy People 2030*, the road map for health in the United States, lists five overarching goals, all of which focus on healthy aging:

1. Attain health and well-being, free from preventable disease, disability, injury, and premature death.
2. Eliminate disparities, and achieve health equity for all.
3. Create environments that promote full potential for health for all.
4. Promote healthy development and healthy behaviors across all life stages
5. Engage leadership, constituents, and the public to take action to improve health for all (ODPHP, 2020).

The future older population is expected to be better educated than the current one. The increased levels of education may accompany better health, higher incomes, more wealth, and consequently a higher standard of living in retirement.

Baby boomers bring much to the conversation about retirement, including an interest in the solvency of Medicare and Social Security programs and an interest in **aging in place** in their communities. At the end of the 2008 recession, which impacted many retirement plans, about one half of working adults aged 50 to 64 years reported that they were not prepared to retire and were delaying retirement, according to a national survey by the Pew Research Center's (2016).

In addition to financial preparation for retirement and older age, many older adults view marriage through a different lens than older generations before them. Given that many baby boomers are divorced or have never been married, they have a different opinion about the definition of family, including how obligated they feel about taking care of an older family member (Reuters, 2017). Single adults may not have the same preparation for retirement that married adults do.

Another factor affecting the health of the current generation of older adults is ever-rising health care costs in the United States (Fig. 22-1). These costs have a disproportionately greater impact on older adults because the cost of providing health care for an American 65 years or older is three to five times greater than the cost for someone younger (Peterson-Kaiser Health System Tracker, 2016).

The growth of the aging population presents opportunities for public health nurses to work with communities to strengthen and expand programs and services targeted to seniors, to advocate for the needs of the aging population with government agencies and other organizations, and to assure access to quality health care services that address their unique and complex problems (United Nations, 2017).

This chapter first examines the characteristics of the aging population in the United States and the global challenge of an aging society. Ageism is discussed in the context of misconceptions about older adults. Next, the primary, secondary, and tertiary health needs of older adults are explored. Diseases common among older adults are reviewed, with a focus on Alzheimer's and other dementias. Elder abuse is reviewed with a focus on financial abuse and abuse reporting. Finally, population-based health services and nursing interventions applied to the health of the aging population are discussed in light of cost containment and comprehensive care.

GERIATRICS AND GERONTOLOGY

Nurses trained in the specialty of gerontological nursing are needed to care for our aging population. **Gerontological** nursing encompasses all aspects of the aging process, including economic, social, clinical, psychological, and spiritual factors. Gerontological nursing focuses on

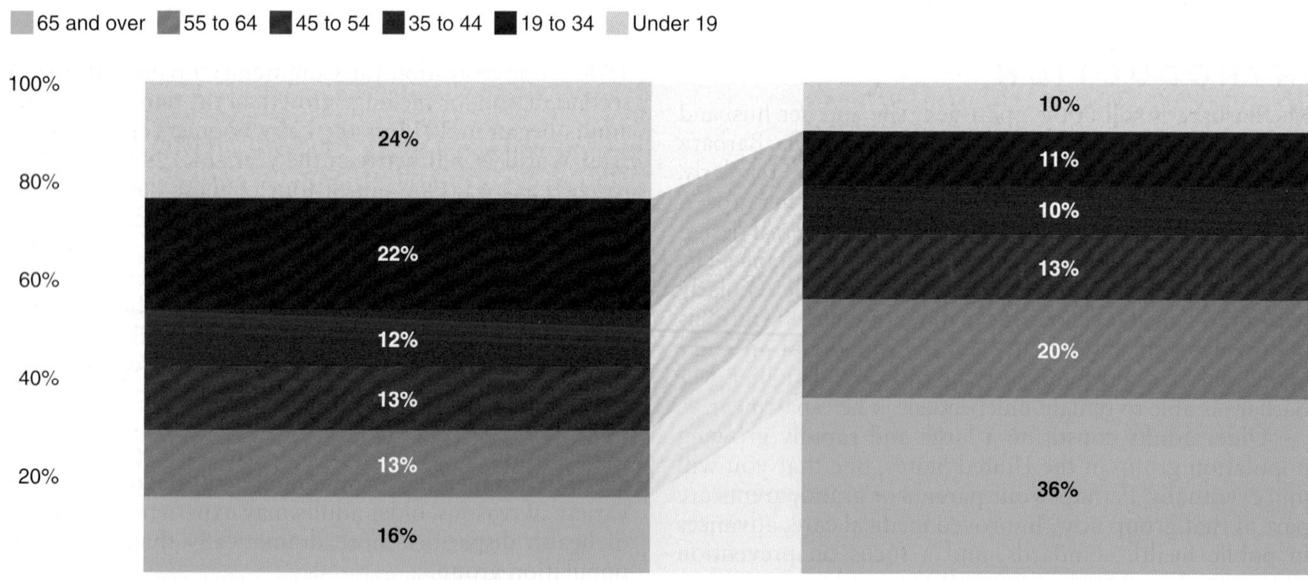

FIGURE 22-1 Share of total health spending by age group and share of the population. (Peterson-Kaiser Health System Tracker. (2016). *How do health expenditures vary across the population?* Reprinted with permission from the Kaiser Family Foundation. Retrieved from https://www.healthsystemtracker.org/chart-collection/health-expenditures-vary-across-population/?sf_data=results&_sft_category=spending&sf_paged=2#item-whites-have-higher-health-spending-in-most-age-categories-than-people-in-other-groups_2016)

promoting and improving the health of older adults. This holistic approach includes evaluating the impact of these factors on the older adult and society. Health is defined by the person and may include the ability to age in place or sustain maximum functioning.

In contrast, **geriatrics** is a medical specialty. Like other medical specialties, geriatrics focuses on abnormal conditions and the treatment and cure of those conditions. A geriatrician is a medical doctor with specialized training in geriatrics.

A C/PHN works with older adults at the individual, family, and group levels. In one instance, the nurse may work to promote and maintain the health of a vigorous 80-year-old man who lives alone in his home. However, a community/public health perspective must also concern itself with the aggregate of older adults. There are many groups of seniors with whom the nurse may choose to work, such as those who attend a memory day care center, those who belong to a retirement community, those who live in a nursing home, or members of a caregiver support group. Other groups include residents of a senior citizens' apartment building; those with cognitive, vision, or hearing impairments; homeless men and women; and veterans. Work with clients can also involve political advocacy. The possibilities for C/PHNs to work with older adults are vast and ever expanding.

HEALTH STATUS OF OLDER ADULTS

People are living longer as a result of improved health care, eradication and control of many communicable diseases, use of antibiotics and other medicines, healthier dietary practices, safer global water supplies, regular exercise, and accessibility to a better quality of life via education and social services. Increased life expectancy reflects, in part, the success of public health interventions. However, community/public health programs must now respond to new challenges, such as the following: the growing burden of chronic illness, physical and cognitive impairments, increasing concerns about future caregiving, coordinating care across providers and settings, and rapidly rising health care costs.

Chronic diseases, often referred to as **chronic conditions**, affect older adults at a disproportionately higher rate. They contribute to disability, diminish quality of life, and increase health care costs. Two out of three older Americans have multiple chronic conditions, with treatment for this group resulting in 66% of the U.S. health care budget (Centers for Disease Control and Prevention [CDC], 2017a).

C/PHNs have the opportunity to address key challenges faced by the older population. They can work to meet the long-term needs of individuals with cognitive and physical impairments, coordinate care across providers, oversee the adequacy of services, and support family caregivers in the plan of care. In this way, C/PHNs can help older adults live in the communities, a more cost-effective and desirable outcome.

Global Demographics

The unprecedented growth in the number of older adults is not limited to the United States but is happening worldwide. In 2010, an estimated 524 million people were aged 65 years or older—8% of the world's population. By 2050, this number is expected to nearly triple, to about 1.5 billion, representing 16% of the world's population (United Nations, 2017).

Life expectancy at birth around the world now is 67. A child born in Myanmar or in Brazil can expect to live 20 years longer than one born 50 years ago. And in Iran, only 1 person in 10 is currently older than 60 years, but in 35 years' time, this will change to 1 in 3 (Beard et al., 2016).

Although more developed countries have the oldest population profiles, the vast majority of older people—and the most rapidly aging populations—are in less developed countries. Between 2010 and 2050, the number of older people in less developed countries is projected to increase more than 250%, compared with a 71% increase in developed countries (United Nations, 2017).

Because of this demographic shift, along with altered societal expectations, changes in attitudes and social policies worldwide are needed. Many countries have few or no social programs, pensions, or health care services available for their older adult populations.

National Demographics

As a result of demographic transitions, including declining infant and childhood mortality, lower fertility rates, and improvements in adult health, the shape of the global age distribution is changing. The age distribution in developed countries, such as the United States, includes a larger proportion of older adults than does the age distribution in less developed countries.

By 2025, the United States is expected to have 80% more older adults than in 2000, but the number of working-age adults will grow by only 15% (Ortman, Velkoff, & Hogan, 2014). This is often represented by an **age dependency ratio**. By looking at Figure 22-2, you can see that over the years, an increasing number of younger, working-age adults are needed to provide support for older adults (15 working-age persons for 1 older adult in 1960 vs. 23 in 2015). However, the age dependency ratio does not take into consideration that many older adults may still be working or have other sources of income.

Despite the overall trend toward increased life expectancy, disparities exist among various subgroups in the population. Life expectancy is highest for White Americans and lowest for Black Americans, who have the highest death rates of any of the racial and ethnic groups in the United States. The Hispanic, Black, and Asian populations have been expanding and are projected to grow substantially through 2025 (U.S. Census Bureau, 2015). Although the older population is not expected to become majority–minority in the next four decades, it is projected to be 42% minority in 2050, up from 20% in 2010 (U.S. Census Bureau, 2015).

The health status of racial and ethnic minorities of all ages lags behind that of nonminority populations. For a variety of reasons, older adults may experience the effects of health disparities more dramatically than any other population group (Box 22-1). To help address these health disparities, the Racial and Ethnic Approaches to Community Health (REACH) (CDC, 2020b) program supports community-based coalitions in the design, implementation, and evaluation of innovative strategies to reduce or eliminate health disparities among racial and ethnic minorities. The goal of REACH is to achieve health

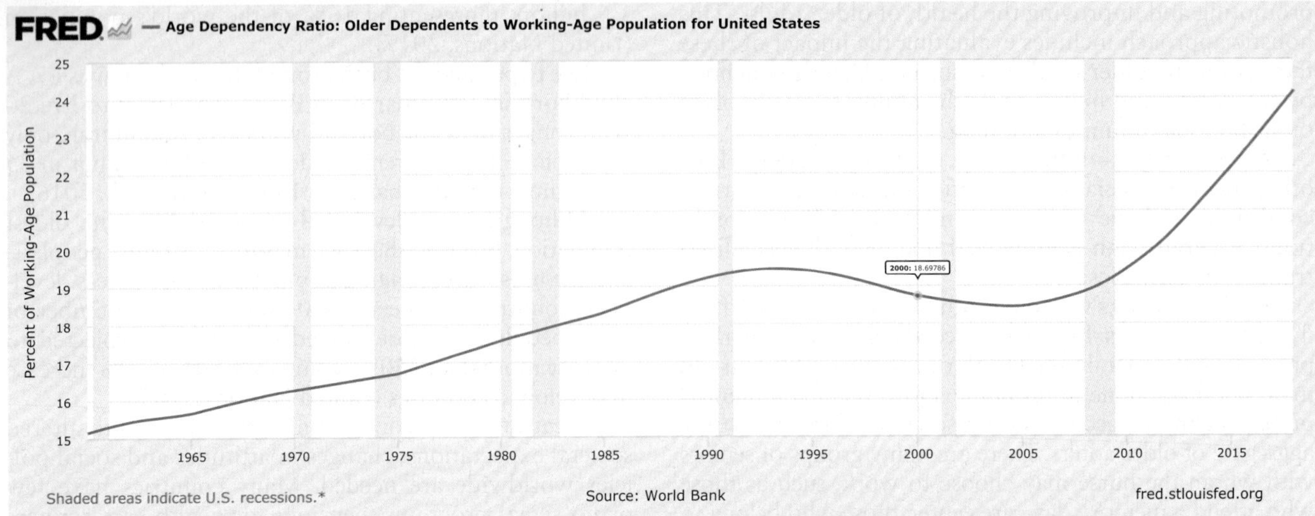

FIGURE 22-2 World Bank, Age Dependency Ratio: Older Dependents to Working-Age Population for the United States [SPPOPDPNDOLUSA]. (Retrieved from FRED, Federal Reserve Bank of St. Louis; https://fred.stlouisfed.org/series/SPPOPDPNDOLUSA, January 24, 2019. FRED® and the FRED® logo are registered trademarks of the Federal Reserve Bank of St. Louis. Used with permission. FRED® chart provided courtesy of the Federal Reserve Bank of St. Louis.)

equity, eliminate disparities, and improve the health of all groups (CDC, 2020b).

Growth in the number of older adults will significantly affect health care resources, housing options for older adults, and national longevity statistics. As the number of older people increases, so, too, will their need for assistance with activities of daily living (ADLs) and other services, especially those persons with Alzheimer's and other dementias. Many will serve as caregivers to family members who need assistance in attending to ADLs such as dressing, eating, toileting, and bathing, and researchers are seeking effective methods for providing respite to caregivers and reducing costs. Laws pertaining to health care and social services

BOX 22-1 EVIDENCE-BASED PRACTICE

Health Risks Faced by Older Adults

Below are three examples of research findings related to health risks faced by older adults that are relevant to community/public health nurses (C/PHNs).

Suicide

Assessment of older adults for suicide risk is an important consideration for community health nurses and C/PHNs. Although suicide attempts are less frequent in older adult populations, the completion rate is high, with 25% of older adults, both male and female, succeeding. Nurses need to understand the known risk factors for suicide, such as depression, anxiety, and bipolar disorder. However, many older adults may not have diagnosable symptoms and may not be assessed for mental illness. C/PHNs need to understand the losses that may contribute to suicidal ideation, such as the loss of a spouse or friend or physical problems with vision, hearing, or untreated pain. They should also know of key supports for older adult: supportive family and friends, spiritual practices, and connection to the community. This article discusses assessment, screening, and reducing risk by connecting clients to resources.

Health Complications Related to Homelessness

The proportion of homeless who are older adults is increasing by virtue of the aging of the general population. According to the research study indicated below, conducted in Oakland, California, one half of single homeless adults are aged 50 years or older and have the kinds of chronic conditions that typically occur in housed adults aged 75 years or older. This study considers participants who stayed in four primary environments: unsheltered, shelters, and homeless hotels, with family or friends, and in rentals following a period of homelessness. Nearly 40% had problems with at least one activity of daily living, and 25% had cognitive impairment. Many had vision and hearing problems and urinary incontinence. This study highlights the needs of older homeless adults who do not have supportive living environments to meet their needs.

Chronic Illness and Functional Disabilities

Consider the influence of Programs that offer All-Inclusive Care for the Elderly (PACE) sites in communities and what occurs after a PACE site closed. PACE activities are organized around a day center that provides medical and social services to avoid institutionalization of older people with chronic illnesses and functional needs. Outcomes of PACE site closures lead to higher numbers of emergency department visits, hospitalizations, and nursing home placements. C/PHNs need to learn about comprehensive programs such as PACE, which can be effective in reducing health care costs.

Source: Diggle-Fox (2016); Brown et al. (2017); Meunier et al. (2016).

are being passed to better address the needs of older adults, most of whom will remain in the community. The Administration on Community Living, along with the National Family Caregivers Support Project Program (NFCSP), provides grants to states and territories to provide five types of services (Administration for Community Living [ACL], 2019a):

- Information to caregivers about available services
- Assistance to caregivers in gaining access to the services
- Individual counseling, organization of support groups, and caregiver training
- Respite care
- Supplemental services, on a limited basis

These services are designed to work with other state- and community-based services to provide a coordinated set of supports. Studies have shown that these services can reduce caregiver burnout and stress and keep them healthy, delaying the need for costly **assisted living** or **nursing home** care (Administration for Community Living, 2019b).

Many older adults live in poverty; over 4.5 million older adults (9%) were below the federal poverty level in 2016. This poverty rate represents a statistically significant increase from the poverty rate of 8.5% in 2013 (Kaiser Family Foundation, 2018). However, in 2017, the Supplemental Poverty Measure (SPM) from the U.S. Census Bureau, which was adjusted for regional costs of living and nondiscretionary expenses, revealed a poverty level for older adults of 14.1% (over 5% higher than the official 9% rate). This increase is mainly due to adding medical out-of-pocket expenses, which were not included in the original poverty level calculations (U.S. Census Bureau, 2018).

The education level of the older population is rising. Between 1970 and 2016, the percentage of older persons who had completed high school increased from 28% to 85%. In 2014, about 28% had a bachelor's degree or higher. Considerable racial and ethnic differences were found in the proportion completing high school (i.e., 90% of non-Hispanic Whites, 80% of Asians, 77% of African Americans, 71% of American Indian/Alaska Natives, 54% of Hispanics). In comparison, only 30% of older Whites and 9% of older African Americans had high school diplomas in 1970 (Administration for Community Living, 2019b). With higher levels of education come broader health consumerism and improved quality of life.

DISPELLING AGEISM

Ageism is negative stereotyping of older adults and discrimination because of older age. These stereotypes often arise from negative personal experiences, myths shared over time, and a general lack of current information. A majority of older adults report having experienced ageism in the form of being patronized, ignored, or treated as if they were incompetent (Applewhite, 2016).

By becoming more aware of the myths and realities of older age, C/PHNs can improve the health and quality of life of the growing population of older adults. C/PHNs must guard against ageism in their practice by dispelling common myths and misconceptions (Table 22-1).

TABLE **22-1** Myths About Older Adults

Myth	Reality
Senility: *It's normal for older adults to become confused, childlike, and forgetful. They become "senile."*	Certain parts of the brain do shrink, and some blood flow is reduced. Regardless, many older adults continue to think well. **Senility** and dementia are often equated. However, not all older adults develop dementia. Alzheimer's dementia is the most common of all dementias (Alzheimer's Association, 2020).
Rocking chair: *As age increases, older adults withdraw, become inactive, and cease being productive.*	People live longer, work later, and live well with chronic conditions. People over 50 are firing up the longevity economy with "encore careers" (AARP, 2017a).
Homogeneity: *As older adults age, they lose their individual differences and become progressively more alike.*	"Young" and "Old" are helpful when one considers living a long or a short period of time. However, despite looking different, older people feel about the same inside as they did when young. The move to slow or stop aging may not be helpful.
The old benefitting at the expense of the young: *Older people are pulling down the economy. We cannot afford longevity.*	The economy profits more from the wisdom of older workers than ever before (AARP, 2017a). Many grandparents care for their children and grandchildren, and Medicare and Medicaid keep older adults independent during the time that younger people are raising their own families. The federal government established an advisory council to help older adults raising grandchildren in the Supporting Grandparents Raising Grandchildren Act (2018). Organizations on aging concur that we can provide for health care and retirement if we use our resources wisely (Lindland, Fond, Haydon, & Taylor-Kendall, 2015).
Inability: *Older adults are unable to learn new things and are set in their old ways of doing things.*	Learning is a lifetime ability that continues into old age. Although older adults may experience some difficulty with short-term (or working) memory as they get older, their long-term memory generally remains sound. People at any age can learn new information and skills. Although some are slower to adopt technology, once older adults join the online world, they use their technology most every day (Narushima, Liu, & Diestelkamp, 2018).

The aging process among older adults is individual, subtle, gradual, and lifelong. One can see remarkable differences among individuals in the rate of aging. Even in a single individual, various systems of the body age at different rates. Therefore, chronologic age cannot readily be a reliable indicator of health needs. Methods for calculating your "real" or biological age can give you a better picture of your body's true state of health (see http://www.biological-age.com/about.html for a calculator you can use for yourself and your clients). For information on how to make a healthy transition into older age, see Box 22-2.

MEETING THE HEALTH NEEDS OF OLDER ADULTS

Many factors contribute to healthy aging, including a lifetime of healthy habits and circumstances, a strong social support system, and a positive emotional outlook. Most people recognize a healthy older person when they meet one.

What is healthy old age? Would you consider Minerva Blackstone in Box 22-3 to have a healthy old age? The vast majority (94%) of older adults in the United States, even those with chronic diseases or other disabilities, are

BOX 22-2 LEVELS OF PREVENTION PYRAMID

Transitioning to Older Age

SITUATION: Making a healthy transition into a satisfying old age

GOAL: Using the three levels of prevention, prevent or delay chronic diseases, promptly diagnose and treat conditions, and restore the fullest possible potential.

Tertiary Prevention

Rehabilitation

- Adapt to changed roles with spouse and significant others.
- Maintain health while assessing increasing dependency needs, including alternative housing, modifications in transportation, and changing health care needs.

Health Promotion and Education

- Periodically review and update will, insurances, and other important documents as needed.
- Keep beneficiaries or executors aware of changes in and location of documents and personal wishes regarding end-of-life care and funeral/burial arrangements.

Health Protection

- Review medications, prescription and over-the-counter, on a regular basis.
- Explore and provide community resources as needs change.

Secondary Prevention

Early Diagnosis

- See Chapter 21 recommendations for screenings for adults.
- Follow the U.S. Task Force Recommendations for regular screening of potential health problems (USPSTF, 2018a).
- Focus on results of the Medicare Annual Wellness Visit (Cordell et al., 2013) results or screen for cognitive impairment and depression symptoms.
- Assess for social engagement: volunteerism, faith-based activities, family, and support of others.
- Assess for caregiver health and burden levels.

Prompt Treatment

- Provide resources for social engagement: healthy, satisfying, and enriching activities.
- Follow up on any abnormal findings, keeping any family or caregivers informed.
- Manage vision, hearing problems.
- Provide strategies for behaviors resulting from cognitive problems.
- Provide community resources to prevent caregiver burnout.

Primary Prevention

Health Promotion and Education

- Begin preparations early—emotional, spiritual, and financial.
- Plan ahead for changes in health status and potential need for long-term care.
- Complete documents, such as a will and a living will.

Health Protection

- Regularly assess health status.
- Follow the recommended schedule for immunizations of the Centers for Disease Control and Prevention (2020c; https://www.cdc.gov/vaccines/schedules/hcp/adult.html).
- Medicare Wellness visit.
- Include oral examination in routine medical and nursing visits.
- Implement a health-promoting regimen that includes diet and exercise.
- Assess living environment for comfort and safety hazards.

BOX 22-3 STORIES FROM THE FIELD

Minnie Blackstone

I am a public health nurse (PHN) and live next door to Minerva Blackstone, affectionately called Minnie by her friends. Minnie is a lively 87-year-old woman who enjoys life. Every day, except in bad weather, she walks a half mile to visit her granddaughter Karen. There, she works on the quilt she is making for Karen. Twice a week, Minnie takes the city bus to the senior citizens' center to join her friends in an exercise class. Minnie has noticed that her vision and her hearing are not what they used to be. She can no longer crochet in the evening with low lighting but has found a bright magnifying lamp to help her continue her hobby. As for her hearing, Karen has set up an appointment with the audiologist. Do you know how much hearing aids will cost Minnie? Will Medicare pay for them?

Minnie is a happy person but is not content unless she is up on the latest political developments. She never misses the news and talks about current events at every chance. She has a good appetite and generally sleeps well. Minor arthritis does not hamper her activities nor does the hypertension that she controls by independently taking her medication daily. Right now Minnie is enjoying a healthy old age. What planning needs to be made for Minnie when and if her arthritis or other chronic conditions disable her?

Carole, District PHN

living outside institutions and are relatively independent. Good health in the older adult means maintaining the maximum possible degree of physical, mental, and social vigor. It means being able to adapt, to continue to handle stress, and to be active and involved in life and living. In short, healthy aging is being able to function, even when disabled, with the assistance of others as needed.

Wellness among the older population varies considerably. It is influenced by many factors, including personality traits, life experiences, current physical and cognitive health, current societal supports, and personal health behaviors

Areas of focus for Healthy People 2030 for older adults (USDHHS, 2020a) include the following:

- Increase physical activity for those who have reduced physical and cognitive function
- Reduce pressure ulcer–related hospital admissions
- Reduce emergency department visits due to falls
- Reduce inappropriate medication use
- Reduce hospital admissions due to diabetes
- Reduce hospital admissions for pneumonia
- Reduce hospital admissions for urinary tract infections

In 2016, the category dementias, including Alzheimer's disease (AD), was added to Healthy People 2020 topics and objectives and is in the objectives for Healthy People 2030 (USDHHS, 2020a). This chapter discusses AD in depth (see Diseases and Conditions Common in Old Age). Important steps for the care of those with dementia and their caregivers include earlier diagnosis, reduction of severity of both cognitive and behavioral symptoms, and supporting caregivers (Healthy People 2020, 2020b; USDHHS, 2020a).

Other actions that can increase healthy aging include addressing health disparities among older adults, encouraging people to plan for end-of-life care and communicate their wishes through advance directives, improving oral health and increasing physical activity among seniors by promoting environmental changes, increasing adult immunization levels, and preventing falls. Some older adults demonstrate maximum adaptability, resourcefulness, optimism, and activity. Others, often those from whom we tend to draw our stereotypes, have disengaged and present a picture of dependence and resignation. Most older adults are somewhere in between these two extremes. Although the level of wellness varies among older adults, that level can be raised.

The goals in community health nursing are to maximize the wellness potential of older adult clients and to support their highest level of functional ability. Nurses must analyze and build on an older person's strengths rather than focus on the difficulties or deficits.

LEVELS OF PREVENTION

Older adults, like any age group, have certain basic needs: physiologic and safety needs, as well as the needs for love and belonging, self-esteem, and self-actualization. Their physical, emotional, and social needs are complex and interrelated. The following sections discuss these needs according to primary, secondary, and tertiary prevention activities.

Primary Prevention

Primary prevention activities involve those actions that keep one healthy. Such primary prevention activities as health education, follow-through of sound personal health practices (e.g., flossing, seat belt use, exercise), recommended routine screenings, and maintenance of an appropriate immunization schedule ensure that older adults are doing all that they can to maintain their health.

Nutrition and Oral Health Needs

People who have maintained sound dietary habits throughout their life have little need to change in old age. Adults aged 80 years and over had the lowest rate of obesity, 26.7%, from 2013 to 2016 (Healthy People, 2020b). The U.S. Department of Agriculture (USDA, n.d.) replaced the food pyramid with MyPlate as a visual to guide the food intake of Americans. Tufts University has modified MyPlate for older adults (Fig. 22-3). The modifications include an emphasis on drinking plenty of fluids, including water, tea, and coffee, and consuming a diet high in fiber. Although multivitamins are not meant to replace food as a source of nutrients, taking them as a supplement to food to achieve recommended intakes may be a good idea (Tufts University, 2015).

It is generally believed that older people need to maintain their optimal weight by eating a diet that is low in fats, moderate in carbohydrates, and high in proteins with a daily calorie count of 1,200 to 1,600 (Fig. 22-4). Older adults need less vitamin A but more calcium and vitamin D (for healthy bones), more folic acid, and more vitamins B_6 and B_{12} (for cognitive health) than younger adults. Many communities offer meals to seniors, either at senior centers or by way of

Meals on Wheels, through grants provided by the Older Adult Nutrition Program (Administration for Community Living, 2020).

Oral health is integral to general health and well-being throughout one's life. Major advances in the field of oral health—including community water fluoridation, advanced dental technology, better oral hygiene, and more frequent use of dental services—have had a substantial impact on the number of older adults who retain their natural teeth. The percentage of older adults who have lost all their natural teeth has declined to 18%, surpassing the *Healthy People 2020* target of no more than 20% (CDC, 2017b). The percentage of adults aged 65 or over with a dental visit in the past year was 60.6% (CDC, 2017b). Healthy People 2030 guidelines addresses oral health and maintenance, with a focus for older adults on receiving treatment for root decay (USDHHS, 2020a).

Poor oral health has been associated with peripheral vascular disease, diabetes, and risk for death caused by pneumonia in nursing homes (Almirall, Serra-Prat, Bolibar, & Balasso, 2017). Even those with dentures must be vigilant in maintaining oral health, as they are still at risk from inflammatory processes leading to diseases such as pneumonia. Many older adults, especially those who are disadvantaged or have limited incomes, have decreased nutritional and fluid intake, changes in gums, and increased periodontal disease, as well as a higher incidence of dry mouth.

Fluid intake and oral hygiene are appropriate topics for anticipatory guidance from C/PHNs working with older adults. Take the time to assess the older adult's oral cavity, including mucosa, denture fit, and any complaints about chewing or swallowing.

In addition to maintaining a healthy diet, older adults are cautioned to limit the use of alcohol. Any person can have a problem with alcohol, and it is not unusual for older adults to have an alcoholic drink. Use of alcohol can lead to falls or car crashes (National Institute for Aging [NIA], 2020a). As with all adults, older persons should avoid tobacco, drink fluoridated water or use flu-

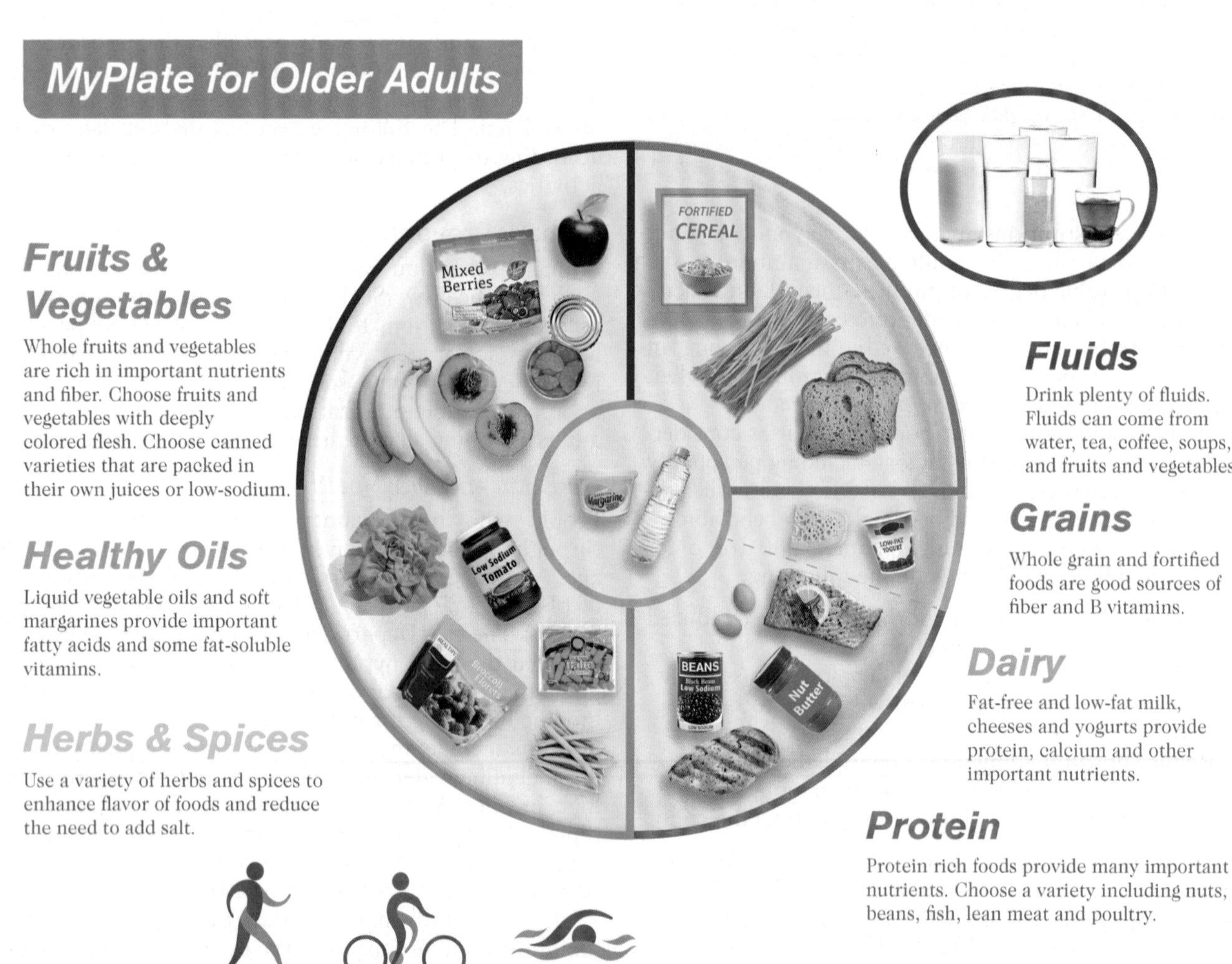

FIGURE 22-3 MyPlate for older adults. (Reprinted with permission. Available at https://hnrca.tufts.edu/myplate/("My Plate for Older Adults" Copyright 2016 Tufts University, all rights reserved. "My Plate for Older Adults" graphic and accompanying website were developed with support from the AARP Foundation. "Tufts University" and "AARP Foundation" are registered trademarks and may not be reproduced apart from their inclusion in the "My Plate for Older Adults" graphic without express permission from their respective owners.)

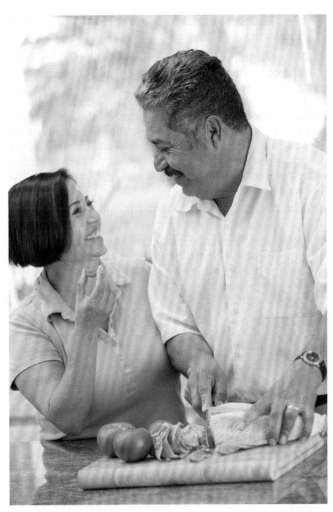

FIGURE 22-4 Healthy nutrition for older adults. Preparing and eating meals should be an uncomplicated, natural process, best shared with others.

oride toothpaste, practice good oral hygiene, and have regular dental checkups (CDC, 2017b). They should also avoid the habitual use of laxatives, instead adding more fluids, fiber, and bulk to their diet with fresh fruits and vegetables. Also, inadequate fluid intake can contribute to bowel and bladder problems. Increased physical activity and exercise help maintain regularity of bowel function in older adults.

Exercise Needs

Older adults need to exercise; in fact, they thrive when exercise is incorporated into their daily routine (National Institute on Aging, 2020b). Research demonstrates that exercise and increased physical activity have multiple benefits for the older adult, including:

- Arthritis relief, restoration of balance and reduction of falls, strengthening of bone, proper weight maintenance, and improvements in glucose control, cognitive and brain function, and overall mortality (Macera, Cavanaugh, & Belletiere, 2017)
- A healthy state of mind, improved sleep, and reduced risk of heart disease (Roitto et al., 2018)
- Decreased incidence of osteoporotic fractures due to a reduced risk of falling, with an exercise routine that includes activities to improve strength, flexibility, and coordination, even among the very old

The C/PHN should explore the kinds of activity that appeal to older adults, including walks. A wide variety of activities are appropriate for and benefit older adults:

- In one study, older adults who were informed about the benefits of walking walked more than those who were reminded of the negative consequences of not walking (Notthoff & Carstensen, 2017).
- Exercise may occur with others in connection with such activities as homemaking chores, gardening, hobbies, or recreation and sports.
- Resistance training (with small dumbbells or resistance bands), along with either Tai Chi or regular walking, has been shown to increase muscle strength, stability, and functional ability among seniors (Healthfinder.gov, 2020).
- Physical disabilities need not be a barrier to exercise, as there are specialized exercise programs (e.g., chair aerobics, wheelchair fitness).

Sleep

Sleep is another area of focus in *Healthy People* and is important to older adults for the following reasons:

- In older adults, adequate sleep is necessary to fight off infection and support the metabolism of sugar to prevent diabetes or to work effectively and safely.
- Sleep timing and duration affect a number of endocrine, metabolic, and neurological functions that are critical to the maintenance of individual health.
- Untreated, sleep disorders and chronic short sleep are associated with an increased risk of depression, heart disease, high blood pressure, obesity, diabetes, and all-cause mortality (Gulia & Kumar, 2018).

Some changes in sleep are natural with aging, such as:

- Decreased slow-wave or deep sleep due to the body producing lower levels of growth hormone
- Altered circadian rhythms (the internal clock that tells one when to sleep and when to wake up), causing the older adult to want to go to sleep earlier in the evening
- Nighttime wakefulness and interrupted sleep due to pain, the need to void, medications, and snoring, which may worsen with age (Gulia & Kumar, 2018)

The C/PHN can assess and help older adults having sleep challenges by:

- Asking them to keep a sleep journal
- Investigating their nighttime voiding patterns
- For men, assessing for the possibility of an enlarged prostate, which can cause problems with complete bladder emptying and may need treatment

Objectives for Healthy People 2030 focus on reduction of accidents due to driving while drowsy, providing treatment for those with obstructive sleep apnea, and sufficient sleep (USDHHS, 2020a).

Economic Security Needs and Poverty

Economic security is a major need for older adults. Many older adults work beyond retirement age for reasons of enjoyment and purpose, but they may also be concerned about having financial stability through the rest of their lives. Factors affecting economic security in older adults include the following:

- Having to spend retirement resources caring for elderly parents or grandchildren
- Limited income and reliance on Social Security and Supplemental Security Income, with half of all people on Medicare in 2016 having incomes of <$26,200 (Kaiser Family Foundation, 2018)

Fearing the potential cost of major illness and wanting to avoid being a burden on family or friends, many older people conserve their limited finances by practices that may threaten their health:

- Adopting frugal eating patterns
- Skipping or taking only partial doses of medications
- Limiting the use of home heating and cooling
- Spending little on themselves, in general

For older adults today who have lived many years past retirement without sufficient financial security to maintain them throughout these additional years, fears are not unfounded. More than a quarter of Hispanic older adults and nearly a quarter of Black older adults lived in poverty in 2016, compared with around 1 in 10 White adults aged 65 or older (Kaiser Family Foundation, 2018).

Many older adults are not aware that there are important preventive health measures and community-based programs that can maximize function and help older adults maintain health at a higher level (U.S. Preventive Services Task Force [USPSTF], 2018b). C/PHNs should be familiar with and share with their clients local support services that may provide housing, food, and utilities for older people in need, which can do much to help relieve the source of that stress and anxiety.

Psychosocial and Spiritual Needs

All human beings have psychosocial needs that must be met for their lives to be rich and fulfilling. Typically, aging is seen as a time of loss and decline, and much research focuses on the physiological and psychological impact of multiple losses and decline. However, some research indicates that older adults actually pay attention to and remember positive information and memories more than younger people do (American Psychological Association, 2020). There may be biological and psychological reasons for this:

- The amygdala in the brain reacts to emotions, and biological research indicates that older adults may not react at a brain level to negative information in the way the younger adults do (Mather, 2016), meaning that they may be more likely to gather and hold onto only their good memories.
- For many, old age may be a time of life reflection, review, and reevaluation of what gives meaning and satisfaction in life. Knowing that they have limited time, older adults may choose to focus on positive emotions.

However, with a lack of healthy relationships with other people, life can be very lonely and diminished in quality for older people.

Holistic nursing is a hallmark of community and public health nursing. This means a focus on the body, mind, and spirit. The word spirit comes from the Latin meaning "breath" and refers to the core of an individual, the part that gives meaning to life (New World Encyclopedia, n.d.). Although related, religion and spirituality are distinct concepts:

- A spiritual component exists in all people but not everyone is religious.
- Religion is generally recognized to be the practical expression of spirituality or the organization, rituals, and practice of one's beliefs.
- Religion includes specific beliefs and practices, whereas spirituality is far broader.

According to the Pew Forum, belief in God continues to be very important to older adults, including the younger baby boomers, even though religious practices vary (Pew Research Center, 2018). Whereas other sources of well-being decline, religion may become more important over time. Individuals within different cultures have varying philosophies and practices of spirituality but derive similar positive outcomes.

Faith-based nursing is one of the community nursing roles that epitomizes this holistic approach of caring for one's clients, many of whom are older adults. See Chapter 29 for an in-depth discussion of faith community nursing.

Coping With Multiple Losses and Suicide. Older adults may experience multiple losses, including loss of income and purpose from a career once practiced, loss of the economic stability of employment, and loss of space due to replacement of a larger residence, where the older adult may have raised a family. The loss of a spouse after 50 years of marriage may have a huge impact on the remaining partner. Short- or long-term declines in health may result in pain or limited mobility and may necessitate multiple moves, such as a move to a child's home, a move to an assisted living facility, and a move to a skilled living facility. Repetitive losses occur as significant others, relatives, friends, and acquaintances die. There is no right or wrong way to grieve, but there are healthy and unhealthy ways to cope with the pain. Assisting older adults with handling these losses is an important role of the public health nurse. To do this, C/PHNs need to be aware of some of the facts about grief.

As Kübler-Ross (1969) stated in her classic work, there are five stages of grief: denial, anger, bargaining, depression, and, finally, acceptance. Inadequate coping with the compounding losses can make an older person believe that life holds no meaning. Depression may be a difficult problem for older adults. Social and emotional withdrawal can often occur, as can suicide.

- Among the risk factors for suicidal behavior in older adults are the loss of a spouse; having other mental

disorders, such as dementia and depression; physical illnesses or decline; and social isolation.
- Although older populations have a much lower rate of suicide attempts than younger age groups do, the rate of completed suicide is high (Conejero, Olie, Courtet, & Calati, 2018). The rates of suicide may be underreported, given the negative stigma around suicide, especially in older adults.

Community health nurses should be observant of risk factors and be prepared to ask questions, including whether the client is suicidal, as older adults are not likely to talk about the subject (Diggle-Fox, 2016). Asking someone whether he or she is suicidal does not put the idea in the person's head. This is a myth. Most people are grateful that they have been asked. If you think someone is suicidal, do not let them be left alone; seek further services for the older adult.

Older adults who have maintained good health and developed a supportive system of family and friends have more fulfilled lives (Fig. 22-5). Churches, universities, and senior service programs often have volunteers who regularly meet with isolated seniors either in their homes or **long-term care** facilities, increasing social support for those who have no family members nearby.

Explore the senior services available in your community on the Internet. Good examples are the local Area Agency on Aging (AAA), the local health department, senior community centers, and the YMCA. Some counties have a senior resources guide. The Eldercare Locator, available at https://eldercare.acl.gov/Public/Index.aspx, can provide current information on local caregiver services and resources.

Maintaining Independence. The need for autonomy—to be able to assert oneself as a separate individual—is important for all people. Independence helps to meet the need for self-respect and dignity. Older adults need to have their ideas and suggestions heard and acted upon, and they ought to be addressed by their preferred names in a respectful tone of voice. Respect for the older adult is not a strong value in American society, but it is highly valued in Asian, Italian, Hispanic, and Native American cultures. Older people represent a rich resource of wisdom, experience, and patience that is often unacknowledged in the United States.

Older adults who are in poverty, minorities, or veterans and who experience poorer health need support at home to remain independent. Communities work with local, state, and federal agencies to create programs to provide support to older adults who need assistance but want to remain in their home communities. A good example of a program supporting older veterans at home is the Veteran in Charge program in Colorado Springs, Colorado. This program allows veterans to receive community-based services to continue living in their homes as long as possible and gives them control of the who, what, when, and how much related to the care (https://www.theindependencecenter.org/veterans/).

Interaction, Companionship, and Purpose. Baby boomers, who started to reach the retirement age of 65 in 2011, have changed the face of aging. Nearly 75% of boomers feel that full-time retirement is not for them. This may be, in part, because they are not financially prepared to live another 20 years past retirement (AARP, 2016). As the largest and healthiest aging cohort, they may also be the most engaged.

However, not everyone will be employed after the age of 65. Some may be challenged with physical or mental impairments or caring for spouses or parents. A new phrase in our language is "Grand families." It is possible that grandparents and even great grandparents may be cutting into their own finances to care for grandchildren whose parents may have been deployed or are struggling with substance abuse.

Programs exist to support older adult caregivers. Examples include the federally supported Foster Grandparents and Senior Companions programs, which engage millions of Americans in service (Fig. 22-6). These older adults work part-time offering companionship and guidance to handicapped children, the terminally ill, and

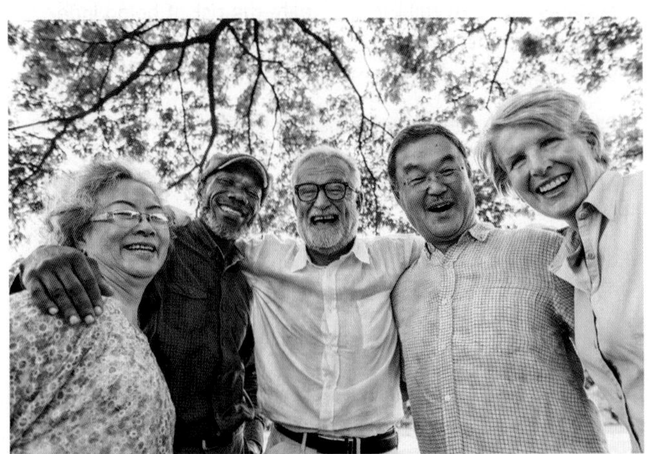

FIGURE 22-5 A supportive system of family and friends helps older adults meet their psychosocial needs.

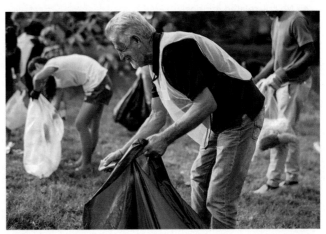

FIGURE 22-6 Volunteering can be a rewarding experience for older adults.

other people in need (Corporation for National & Community Service, n.d.).

In cases where family and social networks have weakened, C/PHNs and others can help to improve their psychosocial health by working at individual, family, and community levels. The problem is of greatest significance for women, who outnumber men considerably in the later years and who more frequently live alone. Take time to explore skills that older adults can do from home: letter writing, volunteer phone calling, or crafting for others who are ill.

Safety and Health Needs

Safety issues are a major concern for older adults and the C/PHNs who work with them. Several areas of focus are discussed here: personal health and safety, home safety, and community safety.

Personal health and safety includes three major areas: immunizations, home safety and prevention of falls, and drug safety (Box 22-4).

Immunizations. Older adults are at increased risk for many vaccine-preventable diseases. Preventable illnesses cause substantial morbidity and mortality in older patients, who tend to have more medical comorbidities and are at higher risk for complications. Acute respiratory infections, including pneumonia and influenza, are the eighth leading cause of death in the United States, accounting for 56,000 deaths annually (CDC, 2019a).

Nonetheless, vaccination rates in the United States do not meet targets for vaccination against flu and pneumonia, such as the *Healthy People 2020* target of 90%. Healthy People 2030 objectives target a reduction in hospital admissions due to pneumonia by older adults (USDHHS, 2020a). Although influenza does kill an estimated 36,000 people per year, in older adults, it is the exacerbating effect it has on other conditions (e.g., pneumonia, congestive heart failure, or chronic obstructive pulmonary disease [COPD]) that is of greatest concern (National Foundation for Infectious Diseases, 2018).

Racial and ethnic disparities exist among older adults receiving influenza and pneumonia vaccines; therefore, it is important to engage in outreach efforts to these populations, such as culturally targeting communication, reaching out to those providers serving this population, and offering vaccination clinics in underserved sections of the community. The CDC regularly updates immunization guidelines for older adults (CDC, 2020c).

Attempts to improve immunization coverage involve changing provider knowledge, attitudes, and behavior through reminders and standing orders, so that "missed opportunities" when seeing clients are prevented.

BOX 22-4 C/PHN USE OF THE NURSING PROCESS

Nursing Care Plan For Community Older Adults: Example of Risk For Falls: Ms. Belmont

Ms. Belmont lives with the companionship of an elderly Dalmatian dog. She goes out with her daughter occasionally for lunch and for appointments. Generally she and her dog are at home. At 94 years old, she states that she isn't as strong as she used to be and has mentioned concern that she may trip over her dog.

Problem Statement

- Fall prevention

Desired Outcomes

- No falls
- No fall-related injuries
- Can demonstrate preventive measures (take up any loose rugs, remove electric cords, etc.)
- Implements strategies to prevent falls at home (e.g., coaches the dog verbally to stay in front of her walker, locks the cellar door to remind herself to avoid the stairs)

Contributing Factors

- Altered mobility and physical impairments: osteoporosis, neuropathy, impaired balance
- Sensory and cognitive impairments: profound hearing loss, macular degeneration, mild cognitive impairment
- Sleep problems
- Home safety: dog in the way
- Environmental concerns: bathroom and bedroom setup, distance to kitchen

Nursing Interventions	Rationale
Assess for conditions that increase risk: changes in mental status; medication changes; worsening vision, hearing, or cognition; poor hydration or nutrition status.	Proper assessment is key to prevention.
Consider a safety bracelet/necklace/device to call for assistance should a fall occur.	A safety device would mitigate the risk of being independent with her companion at home.
Review the dog safety issue: is the training adequate to keep the dog out of Ms. Belmont's way?	The dog is family, supporting psychosocial needs.
Educate about medications and other fall risk issues.	Identification of drug interactions and side effects can improve safety.
Integrate Ms. Belmont's daughter into the safety planning.	The presence of family can provide an early alert system as well as protect Ms. Belmont from activities that increase her risk of falls.

Additional opportunities for vaccinating people exist beyond the primary care setting, as C/PHNs are well aware. Regardless of the site, a method for tracking and communicating vaccinations is needed so that vaccination information may be documented and shared with the elder's primary care provider.

Shingles is caused by the varicella–zoster virus (VZV); this is the same virus that causes chickenpox. Anyone who has had chickenpox can develop shingles because VZV remains in the nerve cells of the body after the chickenpox infection clears, and VZV can reappear many years later causing shingles. Shingles is a very painful localized skin rash, often with blisters. The disease most commonly occurs in people 50 years or older, people who have medical conditions that keep the immune system from working properly, or people who receive immunosuppressive drugs. A new shingles vaccine called Shingrix (recombinant zoster vaccine) was licensed by the U.S. Food and Drug Administration (FDA) in 2017. The CDC recommends that healthy adults aged 50 years or older get two doses of Shingrix, 2 to 6 months apart (CDC, 2018a). Shingrix provides strong protection against shingles, and C/PHNs should advise clients about this vaccine.

Fall Prevention. According to the CDC STEADI fact sheet, every 20 minutes an older adult dies from a fall, and one in five falls causes a serious injury, such as a head trauma or a fracture. Furthermore, fewer than half of fallers talked to the primary provider about the fall. Medicare costs for fall injuries total over $31 billion dollars annually (CDC, 2019b). In fact, falling once can double your chances of falling again. In 2017, medical costs for falls exceeded 50 billion dollars, with Medicare and Medicaid responsible for 75% of these costs (CDC, 2017c). Although not all falls cause serious injuries, effects from falls, such as decreased mobility and excessive bleeding due to taking medications such as blood thinners, lead to additional concerns (CDC, 2017c).

Environmental hazards (e.g., lack of nonslip surfaces and handrails) and host conditions (e.g., poor vision, problems with balance) are often the causative factors in falls. Falls are a preventable problem. The CDC STEADI initiative has a toolkit that includes screening tools and other clinician and patient resources to guide you in preventing falls in older adults (2019b).

We have all heard stories about older adults who have fallen and fractured a hip and who were not wearing technology that could have helped them call for assistance, such as a pendant alert. Today, more than in any other time, older adults can be safer and more comfortable at home or in a facility as the result of smart home technology and wearable monitoring. Smart homes may include environmental, activity, and physiological sensors, with more affordable systems being developed in a rapidly expanding market (Boxes 22-5 and 22-6; Majumder et al., 2017). Smart homes have been purported as a method to safeguard senior safety through alerts and notification related to falls, first aid, and detection of unattended cooking (Wong, Skitmore, & Buys, 2017). One study looked at the use of smart home technologies in older individuals in Hong Kong. Seniors reported concerns related to confidence in the use of machines specifically, technical problems, and the inability to fix a problem. However, seniors did like automation processes such as reminders, because this reduced the need for outside assistance (Wong et al., 2017).

Risk factors for falls include (CDC, 2017c, para, 4) the following:

- Difficulty with walking and balance
- Vitamin D deficiency
- Medications that effect balance such as tranquilizers, sedative, or antidepressants
- Vision problems
- Poor footwear
- Hazards such as throw rugs, clutter, and uneven steps

Medications. Medications are often prescribed to control the effects of chronic conditions. A significant safety issue for the older adult arises from the use of prescription and over-the-counter (OTC) drugs. Problems can arise from a single difficulty or a combination of issues such as:

- Number of medications taken daily
- Absorption rate of medications
- Drug interactions
- Side effects

In addition, the more medications taken daily, the higher the rate of nonadherence to the schedule (Chou, Tong, & Brandt, 2019). This problem is compounded when older adults have visual or cognitive impairments. Older adults often have multiple chronic diseases for which they take prescription medications. It is not unusual for older people to be taking four to six medications daily. The use of multiple drugs, called **polypharmacy**, is defined as using from 5 to 10 prescription drugs (Golchin, Frank, Vince, Isham, & Meropol, 2015). For example, an older adult with two chronic diseases, such as heart failure and COPD, is likely to take more than five medications.

Older adults often receive multiple prescriptions from multiple providers and sometimes from multiple pharmacies, including mail-order pharmacies. They are less likely to see the pharmacist in person, and these circumstances put older adults at risk of receiving the same or similar medications in error. For example, an older adult living in the community has arthritis and heads to the pharmacy for pain management. Many of the pain medications the older adult considers contain acetaminophen (Tylenol). However, this older adult is already taking prescribed pain medication that contains acetaminophen and thus is at risk of overdosing.

Medication side effects or drug interactions can lead to falls and further disability. Older adults need education about the drugs they take and their possible effects. They also need proper supervision of their overall medication intake, including complementary and alternative therapies (e.g., herbal treatments) and OTC drugs. It is also important for all seniors to keep a list of their current medications and doses and to have this available in the event of an emergency. This is an area in which the community health nurse can intervene very effectively (Box 22-7).

BOX 22-5 Guidelines for Assessing the Safety of the Environment

Illumination and Color Contrast

- Is the lighting adequate but not glare producing?
- Are the light switches easy to reach and manipulate?
- Can lights be turned on before entering rooms?
- Are night-lights used in appropriate places?
- Are there working flashlights close by (bedroom, kitchen, bath, living room)?
- Is color contrast adequate between objects such as a chair and floor?

Hazards

- Are there throw rugs, highly polished floors, or other hazardous floor coverings?
- If area rugs are used, do they have a nonslip backing and are the edges tacked to the floor?
- Are there cords, clutter, or other obstacles in pathways?
- Is there a pet that is likely to be running underfoot?

Furniture

- Are chairs the right height and depth for the person?
- Do the chairs have armrests?
- Are tables stable and of the appropriate height?
- Is small furniture placed well away from pathways?

Stairways

- Is lighting adequate?
- Are there light switches at the top and bottom of the stairs?
- Are there securely fastened handrails on both sides of the stairway?
- Are all the steps even?
- Are the treads nonskid?
- Should colored tape be used to mark the edges of the steps, particularly the top and bottom steps?

Bathroom

- Are grab bars placed appropriately for the tub and toilet?
- Does the tub have skid-proof strips or a rubber mat in the bottom?
- Has the person considered using a tub seat?
- Is the height of the toilet seat appropriate?
- Has the person considered using an elevated toilet seat?
- Does the color of the toilet seat contrast with surrounding colors?
- Is toilet paper within easy reach?

Temperature

- Is the temperature of the room(s) comfortable?
- Can the person read the markings on the thermostat and adjust it appropriately?
- During cold months, is the room temperature high enough to prevent hypothermia?
- During hot weather, is the room temperature cool enough to prevent hyperthermia?

Overall Safety

- How does the person obtain objects from hard-to-reach places?
- How does the person change overhead light bulbs?
- Are doorways wide enough to accommodate assistive devices?
- Do door thresholds create hazardous conditions?
- Are telephones easily accessible, especially for emergency calls?
- Would it be helpful to use a cordless portable phone or a cellular phone?
- Would it be helpful to have some emergency call system available?
- Does the person wear sturdy shoes with nonskid soles?
- Are smoke alarms present and operational?
- Is there a carbon monoxide detector (if the house has gas appliances)?
- Does the person keep a list of emergency numbers by the phone?
- Does the person have an emergency exit plan in the event of fire?

Bedroom

- Is the height of the bed appropriate?
- Is the mattress firm at the edges to provide enough support for sitting?
- If the bed has wheels, are they locked securely?
- Would side rails be a help or a hazard?
- When side rails are in the down position, are they completely out of the way?
- Is the pathway between the bedroom and bathroom clear of objects and adequately illuminated, particularly at night?
- Would a bedside commode be useful, especially at night?
- Does the person have sufficient physical and cognitive ability to turn on a light before getting out of bed?
- Is furniture positioned to allow safe use of assistive devices for ambulation?
- Is a telephone situated near the bed?

Kitchen

- Are storage areas used to the best advantage (e.g., are objects that are most frequently used in the most accessible places)?
- Are appliance cords kept out of the way?
- Are nonslip mats used in front of the sink?
- Are the markings on stoves and other appliances clearly visible?
- Does the person know how to use the microwave oven and other appliances safely?

Assistive Devices

- What assistive devices are used?
- Is a call light available, and does the person know how to use it?
- Would the person benefit from any assistive devices that are not being used?
- Are assistive devices being used safely and properly, or do they present additional hazards?

Source: Miller (2019).

BOX 22-6 QSEN: FOCUS ON QUALITY

Safety for Older Adults

Safety: Minimizes risk of harm to patients and providers through both system effectiveness and individual performance (Cronenwett et al., 2007, p. 126).

(See https://qsen.org/competencies/pre-licensure-ksas/#quality_improvement for the knowledge, skills, and attitudes associated with this QSEN competency.)

Nurses must deliver safe and effective care. Not only must they be vigilant in the safety of the care they provide, they are also tasked with proving a safe environment for the patient. In the community setting this can be difficult, because patients and families may need assistance or education regarding home safety. C/PHNs may be able to identify issues or concerns based on home visits and discussions with patients and their families and are positioned to provide support and education.

For example, a C/PHN working in a metropolitan city makes a home visit to Margaret, a 90-year-old woman living alone, following her hospitalization for a fall. The nurse discovers that despite using a walker, "Maggie" is spry, alert, and attentive. In the 900-square-foot home, the nurse notes many small rugs scattered around and furniture cluttered within every room, limiting walking space. Maggie states that she has lived in this house for 70 years and is not moving. The daughter is present for the home visit, and the son lives two blocks away; both check in on their mother daily.

1. *What risks are presented in this situation?*
2. *How would you address safety for the patient and her family?*

Source: Cronenwett et al. (2007); Dolansky and Moore (2013).

Research evidence indicates that polypharmacy in older adults is being addressed by the use of appropriate screening tools such as the Beer's criteria and STOPP Screening tool (https://consultgeri.org/try-this/general-assessment/issue-16). C/PHNs can help by doing a thorough medication review with older adults (Box 22-7).

Safety in the Community. Safety can involve many things, such as pedestrian and driving issues, crime and fear of crime against older adults, and environmental factors such as sun exposure, pollution, heat, and cold.

Because of age-related changes in vision, hearing, and mobility and the effects of polypharmacy, older adults are at risk in the community as pedestrians and as drivers. Automobile crashes and pedestrian injuries can be life-threatening events when elders are involved. As pedestrians, older adults must be increasingly vigilant to traffic patterns, sidewalk irregularities, and the possibility of being a victim of street crime.

Often out of necessity and pride, older people may drive longer than their abilities permit. The C/PHN may recommend resources for families who need to talk about driving safety https://www.aarp.org/auto/driver-safety/we-need-to-talk/ (AARP, n.d.).

Although many older adults are fearful of being victims of crime, rates of nonfatal violent crime and property crime against the elderly are lower than in all younger age groups. See Box 22-8 for actions the C/PHN can take to assist elders with a fear of crime.

Secondary Prevention

Secondary prevention focuses on early detection of disease and prompt intervention (see Chapter 1). Much of the C/PHN's time is spent in educating the community on preventive measures and positive health behaviors. This includes encouraging individuals to obtain routine screening for diseases such as hypertension, diabetes, or cancer, which, if identified early, can be treated successfully. Many nurses, working in collaboration with community agencies, are in positions to establish screening programs based on the desires and demographics of the community and agency focus, making them accessible to the population being served.

BOX 22-7 **Preventing Polypharmacy in Older Adults**

Below are some strategies you can use to help patients reduce the risk of polypharmacy.

Recommendations

- Use the correct medication, at the correct dose, and for the shortest duration.
- AMOR
  - **A**ssess medications and review for interaction.
  - **M**inimize nonessential medications.
  - **O**ptimize by noting duplication.
  - **R**eassess patient for function, cognition, clinical status, and medical adherence.
- *Start low and go slow* is recommended for medication prescriptions of older adults.

Nurse's Role

- Look for duplications in drugs—same category or drug classification.
- Are the medication dosages therapeutic?
- Are there any interactions such as drug–drug, drug–food, or drug–disease?
- Are any nondrug therapies being used?

Source: Smith and Kautz (2018).

BOX 22-8 Simple Steps to Prevent Crime and Identity Theft

- Never open the door automatically; always keep doors and windows locked.
- Use neighborhood watch to keep an eye on your neighborhood.
- Don't leave notes on the door when going out.
- Let someone know when you are away and cancel deliveries.
- Keep the lights on at night and use a timer.
- Keep an inventory of serial numbers and photographs of valuable items; keep copies in a safe place.
- Ask for proper identification of delivery persons or strangers. Do not let a stranger in your home.
- Never give out information on the phone letting someone know you are alone.
- Use direct deposit as much as possible, and keep valuables in a safe deposit bank box.
- Be wary of unsolicited offers to fix your home. It could be a scam. If it happens, report it to the police right away.

Older adults need to be encouraged to follow the routine health screening schedule prescribed by their clinic or health care provider. See Chapter 21 for information on adult screenings (see http://www.cdc.gov/vaccines/schedules/hcp/imz/adult.html for a recommended immunization schedule for older adults).

Diseases and Conditions Common in Old Age

Four of five older adults experience at least one chronic condition, and many suffer multiple chronic conditions as they progress into older age. Cardiovascular disease, cancer, diabetes, and obesity are common to all adults and are discussed in depth in Chapter 21. AD is covered in this chapter as a disease of older adults, as well as arthritis, sensory loss, depression, and osteoporosis. Common chronic conditions seen in older adults are as follows:

- Alzheimer's disease
- Arthritis
- Cardiovascular disease
- Depression
- Diabetes
- Hearing loss
- Obesity
- Osteoporosis

The prevalence of chronic disease and resulting disability in older adults require health promotion behaviors and guidance. Chapter 21 covers appropriate preventive services recommended for older adults (see Screenings and Checkup Schedule for Women and Men in on thePoint of Chapter 21).

Alzheimer's Disease. Alzheimer's disease (AD) is the most common form of dementia in older adults, first described in 1907 by Dr. Alois Alzheimer, who depicted many of the symptoms that are now known as Alzheimer's dementia. AD is the sixth leading cause of death and the only disease among America's top 10 that cannot be prevented or cured.

- Ethnically diverse older adults face a higher risk: African Americans are twice as likely and Hispanics one and one-half times more likely to develop AD than Whites (Mayeda et al., 2016).

Although much is still unknown about this devastating age-related disease, the Alzheimer's Association (AA, 2020a) annually releases a report of the current scientific findings. To identify AD, a comprehensive examination is needed (see Box 22-9). AD causes more deaths than breast and prostate cancer combined. Yet less than half of those diagnosed with AD or their caregivers report being told of their diagnosis, in contrast to 90% of persons with any of the four most common types of cancer being told.

Between 2017 and 2025, every state is expected to see at least a 14% rise in the AD prevalence (AA, 2020b). Because of this growth, *Healthy People 2020* designated

BOX 22-9 Annual Cognitive Assessment

Although there is no single test to identify Alzheimer's disease (AD) (AA, 2020b), annual cognitive assessment recently became a mandatory component of the Annual Wellness Visit (AWV) required for all Medicare and Medicaid enrollees (Borson et al., 2013; Scott & Mayo, 2018). It is recommended that health care providers offer a comprehensive examination during this AWV (Wiese & Williams, 2015). A complete health and family history—including cognitive, behavioral, and psychiatric, physical exam, lab tests, neurologic, functional, and mental status assessments—are essential. A comprehensive assessment is needed because many conditions, including some that are treatable or reversible (e.g., thyroid disease, depression, brain tumors, drug reactions), may cause dementia-like symptoms.

C/PHNs are well positioned to initiate a discussion about memory with their clients and family members as the first step of assessment for cognitive decline, followed by a brief 5-minute screening using one of several methods recommended by an AA workgroup (Cordell et al., 2013; Scott & Mayo, 2018), such as Borson's (2013) Mini-Cog, which involves a clock-drawing test and recall of three words. Another tool is the Quick Dementia Rating Scale (Galvin, 2015), which asks family members 10 questions regarding the client's functional ability; the patient's responses give a clear indication of dementia risk. If an AD diagnosis is given, the nurse can provide anticipatory guidance on managing potential behavior changes and help the family to plan for future care needs. Early and accurate diagnosis could save up to 7.9 trillion in care costs by 2050 (AA, 2020b).

Dr. Lisa Wiese, Assistant Professor, Florida Atlantic University

dementias, including AD, as a focus area (*Healthy People 2020, 2020c*). Healthy People 2030 guidelines highlight the need for early identification, reduction in preventable hospitalizations, and communication with a provider regarding care and treatment (USDHHS, 2020a).

The occurrence of AD is not a normal development in the aging process. Damage to the brain from AD can begin 20 years prior to the onset of symptoms (AA, 2020b). One of the major contributors to AD is the slow accumulation of "plaques and tangles" that interfere with brain function. A concentration of **tau proteins** result in tangles and block the transport of essential nutrients inside the neurons. Plaques result from an excess amount of **beta-amyloid**, which are thought to interrupt the neuronal communication at brain synapse. The increased presence of tau proteins and beta-amyloid activates the production of microglia, which are charged with clearing these toxins. Unfortunately, the microglia are overwhelmed by the amount of proteins and debris left by dying cells, and a harmful chronic inflammatory response ensues. The result is even more cell death and brain atrophy. Another contributor to decreased brain function is the consequent decreased ability of the brain to metabolize its main fuel, glucose. Persons with diabetes and cardiovascular disease were recently found to have a higher risk for AD and related dementias (ADRD). This led to the additional findings that a combination of a person's health, environmental factors, and lifestyle choices in addition to age-related and genetic factors influence the onset and progression of AD (AA, 2020b).

- There is a simple means of describing the difference between the normal forgetfulness of aging and AD. We may forget where we have placed our keys, but upon finding them, we remember why we needed the keys, whereas a person with AD loses immediate recall.
- People in the preclinical Alzheimer's stage eventually notice that they are forgetting recent activities or events, or names of familiar things or people (AA, 2020b).
- In the mild stage, persons may be able to work, drive, and participate in well-known activities but may become lost or forget commonly used words. A typical sign of Alzheimer's is the difficulty in creating new memories, as the limbic system where memories are stored is often the area affected first by beta-amyloid plaques and neurofibrillary tangles.
- As the disease advances, the symptoms become serious enough to cause people with AD or their family members to recognize that things are "not right" and that help is needed. The moderate stage is characterized by struggles to complete routine tasks, wandering, and behavior and personality changes. Persons may become agitated, experience paranoia, and begin to lose the ability to complete ADLs.
- Persons in the severe stage of Alzheimer's dementia become bedbound and cannot communicate in words that can be understood by others (AA, 2020b).
- On average, a person with AD lives 4 to 8 years after diagnosis but can live as long as 20 years, depending on other factors (AA, 2020b). Contrary to the myth, persons with AD are still the same person they once were, but their current reality is different.

Several medications have been approved for use with persons diagnosed with Alzheimer's dementia. Medications called cholinesterase inhibitors are prescribed for mild to moderate AD. Memantine is prescribed for moderate to severe stages, often in combination with donepezil. However, these drugs only delay the progression of symptoms for a limited time. At best, available medications "turn back the clock somewhat" with the disease worsening at a slower rate, or the drugs control some of the client's behaviors that jeopardize safety, thereby promoting caregiver management.

How does this disease impact the role of the C/PHN? First, the C/PHN can conduct family teaching regarding health behaviors that may reduce the risk of ADRD, such as staying active, exercising, healthy eating habits, adequate sleep, and managing cardiovascular risk factors (diabetes, smoking, obesity, and hypertension (AA, 2020b)). The C/PHN can stress the importance of completing the Medicare Annual Wellness Visit, including routine cognitive screening to detect early signs and symptoms of MCI, which provide the opportunity to investigate other possible causes of decline. Early detection benefits also include the following:

- Effective management of coexisting conditions
- Appropriate use of available treatment regimens and holistic modalities
- Pursing health-promoting activities; brain games, exercise, improved nutrition, and sleep patterns
- Coordination of care between all members of the health care team, including providers and caregivers
- Encouraging the client and family to participate in activities that bring joy/are meaningful
- Accessing support services, day centers, and caregiver support groups

Learning about the illness and ADRD management that will decrease care costs is essential, where nearly one in every five Medicare dollars is spent. Average per person Medicare spending for those with ADRD is three times higher than average per person spending across all other seniors. Medicaid payments are 19 times higher (AA, 2020b). These 2018 figures did not include caregivers, who provide 83% and over 18 billion hours of unpaid care to those with ADRD, valued at $232 billion (Black et al., 2018).

- The person with dementia often exhibits depression, agitation, sleeplessness, and anxiety, which disrupt the caregiver's normal routine, greatly adding to caregiver stress. Caregiver burden is multiplied by new or worsening illness, creating a further demand on health care resources. Caregivers experience twice the rate of anxiety and depression as other caregivers (Zhu et al., 2015).
- In many situations, the main caregiver is an aged spouse. The C/PHN can make a difference in health outcomes for both the person with ADRD and their caregiver by helping to connect families to community resources (Box 22-10).

BOX 22-10 C/PHN USE OF THE NURSING PROCESS

Resources for Managing Alzheimer's Disease

Assessment

Mr. and Mrs. Boxwell are in their early 80s and have lived modestly on a fixed income since Mr. Boxwell's retirement. However, their budget has been strained this year as they have had $300 to $400 a month in out-of-pocket expenses for prescription medications. Mrs. Boxwell confessed to you (the C/PHN visiting them after receiving a referral from the senior center) that during some months, they will skip medication doses to "make ends meet." Mrs. Boxwell is diabetic, Mr. Boxwell has heart failure, and they both take medications for hypertension. They live in a small, older home, and their older model car is seldom driven as they report "the traffic is getting worse" and they have "come close to having a car crash two times" lately. They are receptive to your suggestions and are trying to stay healthy and independent.

Problem Statements

1. Health status altered as a result of insufficient finances to purchase needed medications for chronic diseases
2. Altered safety and diminished driving skills

Plan and Implementation

Problem Statement 1

The C/PHN will explore the clients' eligibility for Medicare Part D and Medicaid. It is possible that these clients are eligible, yet unaware of these programs. The nurse will look at Benefits CheckUp, a service of the National Council of Aging that has information on benefits programs for older adults (benefitscheckup.org).

The C/PHN will consult with the clients' primary health care provider and ask for a change in prescriptions from brand names to generic. Also, ordering some medications in larger doses that come in scored tablets may be less expensive, and the client can safely break the larger pills in half. Mrs. Boxwell will check with her present distributor of diabetic supplies about getting larger quantities, generic brands of syringes, alcohol pads, etc.

Problem Statement 2

Mr. Boxwell will look into selling the car and exploring the bus schedule and other senior shuttle services that can be used to travel to the doctor and grocery store. Mr. and Mrs. Boxwell's daughter spends a day with them monthly and takes them wherever they want to go, as long as it is "a fun outing," and they will look into coordinating errands with her.

Evaluation

The couple is eligible for Medicare Part D, and this will help defray the out-of-pocket costs for medications. They have reduced medication costs as much as possible and report not missing any prescribed medications.

They sold their car and are negotiating the bus in good weather and using a taxi in the winter or when it is raining (they figured they save $1,000 a year in auto insurance, auto maintenance, and gasoline, whereas the bus and taxi cost them about $22 a month).

Because the couple is receptive to the help you have provided, you initiate a discussion regarding their long-term plans for housing needs as they get older. They are not opposed to a senior housing option and have been talking about it with their daughter. They are going to talk with a realtor about selling their house, explore some senior apartments with their daughter on her monthly visits, and review their budget.

Arthritis. Arthritis encompasses more than 100 diseases and conditions that affect joints, surrounding tissues, and other connective tissues and is the leading cause of disability for adults in the United States (CDC, 2018b).

- Types of arthritis include osteoarthritis (OA), rheumatoid arthritis (RA), gout, and fibromyalgia. With OA, the number of cartilage cells diminishes, cartilage becomes ulcerated and thinned, and subchondral bone is exposed. The bony surfaces rub together resulting in joint destruction with subsequent pain and stiffness (National Institute of Arthritis and Musculoskeletal and Skin Diseases [NIAMS], 2019).

Gentle exercise is helpful for clients with OA, following treatment for pain. Acetaminophen is the first drug of choice; however, clients often find a combination of medications and daily routines that helps them the most. The nurse can best assist these clients by assessing the safety of a particular regimen and suggesting treatment changes as new research becomes available: new medications, surgical options for joint replacement, and dietary changes, such as vitamins and foods high in essential fatty acids (NIAMS, 2017).

RA is a progressive chronic condition that begins during young adulthood and becomes disabling as the disease continues, attacking tissues of the joints and causing systemic damage in the later years (NIAMS, 2017). This form of arthritis is an autoimmune disease that causes inflammation, deformity, and crippling. RA is treated with anti-inflammatory agents, corticosteroids, antimalarial agents, gold salts, and immunosuppressive drugs. Joint discomfort is often relieved by gentle massage, heat, and range-of-motion exercises.

The C/PHN needs to be aware of the major differences between these two prevalent forms of arthritis. Recommended treatments, including physical therapy, diet, and medication, change as more evidence-based research is conducted on arthritis (NIAMS, 2017).

Depression. Depression is not a normal part of growing older, yet it is common among older adults (CDC, 2017d). Health care providers can miss depression and mistake it for a natural response to grief/loss or illness.

The nurse needs to keep in mind the many potential causes of depression. Medical conditions, such as stroke, cancer, vitamin B_{12} deficiency, diabetes, chronic pain with dependence on prescription painkillers, or insomnia, may lead to depressive symptoms. Many prescription drugs can trigger or exacerbate depression. These include blood pressure medications, sleeping pills, calcium channel blockers, ulcer, and pain medications. Screening for depression is within the scope of responsibility of the C/PHN. The Geriatric Depression Scale (GDS) is available and revised for 2019 (https://consultgeri.org/try-this/general-assessment/issue-4.pdf).

C/PHNs can help elders prevent the overwhelming signs and symptoms of depression related to losses by working with community groups. Through senior centers, adult housing units, senior day care centers, or men's and women's groups at religious centers, the C/PHN can meet with seniors to offer support, teach strategies to improve the quality and quantity of support systems, invite mental health speakers to discuss the topic of depression prevention, and generally assess the holistic health status of the elders in that setting.

Osteoporosis. Osteoporosis is a disease of aging bone in which the amount of bone is decreased and the strength is reduced. Osteoporosis means "porous bone," meaning that the condition enlarges the holes, and the bones become brittle.

- Researchers estimate that one in five women in the United States has osteoporosis and that half of the women over 50 will have a fracture of the hip, wrist, or vertebrae; it is considered a major public health threat for approximately 44 million U.S. adults over age 50 (International Osteoporosis Foundation, n.d.).

Proper diet and weight-bearing exercise throughout life are now recognized as the most effective measure to maintain bone health. There is growing evidence that calcium and vitamin D supplementation can help lower rates of fractures and reduce bone loss in the elderly. Higher protein intake may also help prevent bone loss (International Osteoporosis Foundation, n.d.). There are many FDA-approved drugs to treat osteoporosis that can be prescribed by a primary care provider. Therefore, identification of risk factors and regular screenings is essential to prevent the progression of this debilitating disease (International Osteoporosis Foundation, n.d.).

Sensory Loss. Older adults complain about losing their "taste buds" and have deficits in smell. This is why it is not unusual for older adults to over-salt their food or reach for sweet foods they can taste.

- The prevalence of hearing loss (as high as 75%) and vision impairments (18%) is high in adults >70 years old (Correia et al., 2016). Most hearing loss happens slowly over time, and the older adult may not recognize their hearing problem. These losses of hearing and vision are correlated with depression, social isolation, physical function, cognitive impairment, and quality of life (Contrera, Wallhagen, Mamo, Oh, & Lin, 2016).

C/PHNs can assess for hearing and vision loss using simple tests. For vision, a simple reading of text from a book or newspaper with glasses can suffice. Problems like macular degeneration or glaucoma can cause blindness and need medical care, while presbyopia can be solved with drugstore readers. For hearing, check to see if the older adult uses well-fitted hearing aid, and that they have a good supply of batteries. A family member may be able to supply information about how well the older adult is hearing, but a referral to a clinic may be helpful. Cost for hearing aids is significant in the decision for improvement of hearing. Some amplification help can be found with smartphone application or necklace type amplifiers. But these and hearing aids are not yet paid for by Medicare (Contrera et al., 2016) and can be quite expensive. Medicaid will pay for some hearing solutions, should the older adults have dual eligibility.

Tertiary Prevention

Tertiary prevention involves follow-up and rehabilitation after a disease or condition has occurred or been diagnosed and initial treatment has begun. Chronic diseases that are common among older adults, such as heart failure, stroke, diabetes, cognitive impairment, or arthritis, cannot always be prevented but can frequently be postponed into the later years of life through a lifetime of positive health behaviors. However, when they occur, the debilitating symptoms and damaging effects can be controlled through healthy choices encouraged by the C/PHN and recommended by the primary care practitioner.

- Although many older adults are considered generally healthy, 80% have at least one chronic condition and 50% have at least two (National Council on Aging [NCOA], 2018).
- A small proportion suffer more disabling forms of disease, such as COPD, cerebral vascular accidents (CVAs), cancer, or DM, with some requiring extensive care and ongoing medical management.

Heart disease and cancer pose their greatest risks as people age, as do other chronic diseases and conditions, such as stroke, chronic lower respiratory diseases, AD, and diabetes. Influenza and pneumonia also continue to contribute to older adult deaths among older adults, despite the availability of effective vaccines. While the risk for disability from disease clearly increases with advancing age, poor health is not the inevitable outcome of aging. Many older adults manage chronic conditions well throughout the remainder of their lives.

HEALTH COSTS FOR OLDER ADULTS: MEDICARE AND MEDICAID

As the number of older adults grows, so do costs for health care (see Chapter 6 Medicare and Medicaid). Older adults generally pay about 13% of health care from out of pocket, and the rest comes from insurances, especially Medicare. There is a concern that older adults, especially those with low incomes, will have much higher out-of-pocket costs (Hatfield, Favreault, McGuire, & Chernew, 2018). See Figure 22-7 for total federal outlays for Medicare spending in 2017. With the addition of Social Security, Medicaid, ACA, and CHIP, half of the pie is spent annually (Kaiser Family Foundation, 2017).

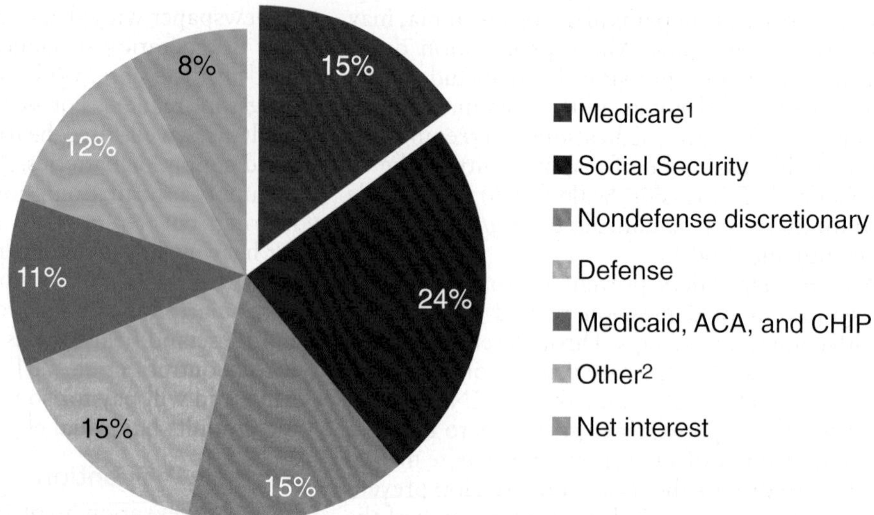

8%
15%
12%
11%
24%
15%
15%
Medicare1
Social Security
Nondefense discretionary
Defense
Medicaid, ACA, and CHIP
Other2
Net interest
Total Federal Outlays, 2018: $4.1 trillion
Net Federal Medicare Outlays, 2018: $605 billion
NOTE: All amounts are for federal fiscal year 2018.1 Consists of mandatory Medicare spending minus income from premiums and other offsetting receipts.2 Includes spending on other mandatory outlays minus income from offsetting receipts. ACA is Affordable Care Act. CHIP is Children's Health Insurance Program.
SOURCE: KFF analysis of federal spending from Congressional Budget Office, The Budget and Economic Outlook, 2019 to 2029 (May 2019).

FIGURE 22-7 Total Federal outlays for Medicare Spending in 2018. (Reprinted with permission from the Kaiser Family Foundation. Retrieved from https://www.kff.org/medicare/issue-brief/the-facts-on-medicare-spending-and-financing/#:~:text=Medicare%20spending%20was%2015%20percent,same%20as%20the%202018%20projection)

Medicare or Medicaid does not cover all health care costs for older adults. It is predicted that by 2050, the numbers of older adults, especially those over 85 years of age and those with cognitive impairment, will need support with ADLs. Most of care is done by informal unpaid caregivers. This is often done at a heavy physical and financial cost, including lost opportunities for employment, health insurance, and retirement savings. Services for older adults are very expensive.

Medicare

Although Medicare does cover many services for older adults, there can be significant out-of-pocket costs. Some are surprised that Medicare does not cover long-term or custodial care, most dental care and dentures, eye examinations for prescribing glasses, and hearing aids and examinations (Medicare.gov, n.d.).

Medicare Part A covers inpatient care and rehabilitation expenses, hospice care services, and some home health care services. Hospitalizations and rehospitalizations are a significant expense for the Medicare program. A major theme of health care reform was the prevention of hospitalizations by providing more supportive care at home.

Medicare Part B covers outpatient and primary care visits. When enrolling for Medicare Part B, older adults will pay 20% of the monthly expenses. Medicare premiums for medical insurance (Part B) are $11,608 per person per year for most beneficiaries and are higher for those with incomes above $85,000 (Medicare.gov, 2018). See Chapter 6 for more details on Medicare.

Medicaid

Although the majority of people enrolled in Medicaid are children and families, most Medicaid spending goes for services provided to people aged 65 years and over and people with disabilities (Kaiser Family Foundation, 2018) (see Fig. 22-7).

Most people believe that Medicaid is a program for the poor, whereas Medicare is for those who are financially secure. In FY 2010, 14% of all Medicaid beneficiaries—9.6 million—were "dual eligible" seniors and younger persons with disabilities who are covered by Medicare as well. One of every five Medicare beneficiaries is a dual eligible client. Dual eligible beneficiaries are very poor, and many have high health and long-term care needs. Medicaid assists them with their Medicare premiums and cost sharing and covers full Medicaid benefits for a large majority of them—most importantly, long-term services and supports at home or in a care facility, which Medicare does not cover (Kaiser Family Foundation, 2018). See Chapter 6 for more details on Medicaid.

ELDER ABUSE

Elder abuse or mistreatment (i.e., abuse and neglect) is defined as intentional actions that cause harm or create a serious risk of harm to a vulnerable elder by a caregiver or another person who stands in a trust relationship with the older adult.

Signs of elder abuse may be missed by professionals working with older adults because of lack of training

BOX **22-11** WHAT DO *YOU* THINK?

Mrs. Stetson's Story

The C/PHN has been visiting Mrs. Stetson for a wound dressing for the past few weeks. After Mr. Stetson passed away, her son, John, offered to help her with the finances. She was no longer able to see well enough to do the bank deposits. John took her to the bank to be added as a signer on the account. When Mrs. Stetson's daughter from out of town arrived several months later for a visit, she wanted to do some Christmas shopping with her mother for the grandchildren. Upon arrival to the bank with her daughter, Mrs. Stetson found that her checking account and substantial amount of her savings were drained. She shared this information with the C/PHN. What should the C/PHN do? Review the steps for reporting elder abuse in your state: What is your professional responsibility?

on elder mistreatment or lack of reporting. In addition, older adults themselves may be unwilling to speak up for fear of retaliation, physical inability to report, cognitive impairment, or they do not want to get the abuser (90% of whom are a family member) in trouble. See Chapter 18 for comprehensive discussion of all types of elder abuse and mistreatment.

It is notable that financial abuse often accompanies one of the other forms of abuse (see Box 22-11). The financial abuse of seniors is a growing problem, often called the "crime of the 21st century." A senior can be financially stable and living independently and may suddenly become destitute and forced out of the home as a result of financial abuse. The most common perpetrators of elder abuse are spouses or partners of elders, often in a relationship with long-term domestic violence. Family members account for 76% of reported mistreatment. Abusers, particularly adult children, are often dependent on the victim for financial assistance, housing, or because of personal problems such as mental illness, alcohol, or drug abuse (NIA, 2020c).

Various state, local, and county agencies investigate and enforce elder abuse laws. The first agency to respond to a report of elder abuse in most states is APS. In some states, certain professionals are required or encouraged to report elder abuse; there are generally doctors and nurses, psychologists, police officers, social workers, and employees of banks and other financial institutions. In 2017, APS in Texas received funding to improve elder abuse reporting by using telehealth to connect virtually with clients who were reported to the state as suspected victims of elder abuse. In the first 8 months, 300 clients were referred for assessments by a team of physicians that provided mental health assessments, guardianship filings, employee misconduct reviews, and other medical assessments. This approach reaches older adults in rural and hard-to-reach areas (Burnett, Dyer, Clark, & Halphen, 2018).

APPROACHES TO OLDER ADULT CARE

As we noted in the introduction to this chapter, the United States and the world is experiencing unprecedented growth in the number of aging older adults. Current costs of care in facilities, price of long-term care insurance, and the limits on amounts of support in community services will demand new or improved models of care. Case management can focus on primary, secondary, and tertiary services to enhance the quality of care by decreasing fragmentations, maximizing resources, and providing the highest quality of care possible.

Case Management and Needs Assessment

Case management involves assessing needs, planning and organizing services, and monitoring responses to care throughout the length of the caregiving process, condition, or illness. Nurses have stepped into the case management role to coordinate and manage patient care across the continuum of health services. Following the nursing process, nurses as case managers assure quality outcomes and cost containment as well as coordination of care. They work with the health care team including social work as each discipline has "...different training, different skills, and see patients from a different perspective" (Christie 2018, para, 4).

Social workers use case management to address their clients' social needs, including their financial problems. Provisions of the Affordable Care act support home- and community-based services by providing Medicaid coverage for home services coordinated by a case manager. This funding is available through states who opt in to the ACA Community First Choice (Medicaid.gov, 2015). When covered by a community program like the First Choice option, case managers and C/PHNs can support the family members of an older adult who will be paid for caregiving for their family member, a great cost saving when compared with a nursing home.

The C/PHN is part of the case management team and should be prepared to assess the needs of older adults with valid instruments:

- The Older Americans Resources and Services Information System (OARS), developed by Duke University Center for the Study of Aging and Human Development (Duke University, 2014), utilizes two sections of one tool—OARS Multidimensional Functional Assessment Questionnaire (OMFAQ)—to determine levels of functioning in five areas (mental health, physical health, economic resources, social resources, and ability to perform ADLs).
- The Katz Index of ADLs is based on an evaluation of the functional independence or dependence of clients with respect to bathing, dressing, toileting, and related tasks (Katz, 1963).
- The Lawton Instrumental ADLs Scale looks at an older adult's ability to perform such activities as using the telephone, shopping, doing laundry, and handling finances (Graf, 2008).
- Times Up and Go Test (TUG) is a measurement of the time in seconds for a person to rise from sitting from a standard armchair, walk 10 ft, turn, walk back to the chair, and sit down. The person wears regular footwear and walking supports (cane, walker). The test is predictive of falls in older adults (Kang et al., 2017).

- Cognitive Screens: to screen for the need for further testing, should the client or family be worried. Open this link and try the MiniCog (https://consultgeri.org/try-this/general-assessment/issue-3.1).
- Vision and hearing screens: The test is familiar to older adults. A simple test of reading with corrective lenses if used will suffice to know if the older adult can read directions, pill bottles. This would not screen for eye problems like macular degeneration. For hearing, the Whisper Test may be used, with hearing aids if the older adult uses them (https://geriatrics.ucsf.edu/sites/geriatrics.ucsf.edu/files/2018-06/whispertest.pdf).
- Spiritual assessment: Spiritual needs can be assessed using many different instruments or questionnaires. Try FICA (Faith, Importance, Community, Address) for example (Dameron, 2005).

HEALTH SERVICES FOR OLDER ADULT POPULATIONS

How well are the needs of older adults being met? To answer this question, other questions must be raised. Do health programs for older adults encompass the full range of needed services? Are programs both physically and financially accessible? Do they encourage clients to function independently? Do they treat older people with respect and preserve their dignity? Do they recognize older adults' needs for companionship, economic security, and social status? If appropriate, do they promote meaningful activities instead of overworked games or activities such as bingo, shuffleboard, and ceramics? Are health care services and other social services provided based on evidence and research? Effective services for older adults should be comprehensive, coordinated, and accessible and demonstrate evidence-based quality.

Criteria for Effective Service

Several criteria help to define the characteristics of an effective community health service delivery system. Four, in particular, deserve attention. In order to be effective, it should be *comprehensive*. Many communities provide some programs, such as limited health screening or selected activities, but do not offer a full range of services to more adequately meet the needs of their senior citizens (see Box 22-12). A comprehensive set of services should provide the following:

1. Affordable housing options
2. Adult day and memory care programs
3. Access to high-quality health care services (prevention, early diagnosis and treatment, rehabilitation)
4. Health education (including preparation for retirement) and centralized resources for information
5. In-home services that promote aging in place
6. Recreation and activity programs that promote healthy nutrition and socialization
7. Specialized transportation services
8. Safe and outdoor spaces that promote activity and enjoyment

A second criterion for a community service delivery system is *coordination*. A good example of efforts toward effective and coordinated services is the Age Friendly Cities and Communities programs (AARP, 2019a). Communities that apply for Age-Friendly demonstrate that the community addresses the above listed services. In 2018, 301 communities are designated age-friendly (AARP, 2020a).

A coordinated information and referral system provides another link. Most communities need this type of information network, which contains a directory of all resources and services for the older adult and includes the name and telephone number of a contact person with each listing. An example of this network is 2-1-1. This number connects the caller to services, and many communities have their own. San Diego 2-1-1 is a good illustration (https://211sandiego.org/).

A third criterion is *accessibility*. Too often, services for seniors are inconveniently located or are prohibitively expensive. Some communities are considering multiservice community centers to bring programs and services for low-income elderly closer to home. The Program of All-Inclusive Care of the Elderly (PACE) is one example of this (National PACE Association, 2020). Comprehensive services are offered to eligible nursing home patients, including personal, health care, and housing. Other services such as transportation, in-home services (home health aides, homemakers, grocery and meal delivery) may further solve accessibility problems for many older adults.

Finally, an effective community service system for older people should promote *quality* programs. This means that services should truly address the needs and concerns of a community's senior citizens and be based on evidence of good outcomes. A range of housing types, from luxurious retirement communities with all ameni-

BOX 22-12 WHAT DO *YOU* THINK?

Services in your Community

Have you wondered whether or not you should intervene if you see an older adult in a situation where they might need help? Or perhaps a neighbor will tell you about someone who might be in trouble. As a nurse, these kinds of situations come to our attention regularly. Silver Key SOS of Colorado Springs, Colorado offers an SOS (Senior Outreach Service). Anyone can contact Silver Key if there is a concern about an older person who may need help (https://www.silverkey.org/services/senior-assistance/silver-key-sos/). The reporting person need not be identified to the referred older adult. Once notified, a case manager will contact the older person and connect them with appropriate services, if the older adult is willing. Services include counseling for many problems, community resources, treatment for depression or misuse of drugs or prescriptions, teach your peers and family to recognize some warning signs: confusion, physical problems, signs of home/person neglect, social isolation, and economic problems.

Look for these kinds of services in your community. Do they exist under city services? Perhaps the County Health Department? How would you go about connecting families or older adults to services?

ties for the active and wealthier senior to secure and more modestly priced or low-income apartments for independent senior living, are being built in most communities. However, affordable rental apartments and homes for older adults and low-income families are in short supply in many communities, putting some older adults in homeless situations. Age-friendly communities are focusing on this problem with an array of solutions, including "tiny houses," "granny flats," and redesigning current homes to **universal design**, that is, usable by anyone of any age, whether a disability or not (e.g., wider door frames, less steps up).

Services for Older Adults by Level of Care Required

There is increased emphasis on providing needed services for older people at home, the essence of aging in place. Today's emphasis on cost control gives added support for providing services at home. Given the increase in longevity, the potential for cost savings appears significant if care for dependent older people can be supported where they live (see Table 22-2).

Maintaining functional independence should be the primary goal of services for the older population. Assessment of needs, ability to function, and the use of assessment tools to form the basis for determining appropriate services is necessary. Although many well older people can assess their own health status, some are reluctant to seek help. Therefore, outreach programs serve an important function in many communities, as they locate people in need of health or social assistance and refer them to appropriate resources.

- Independent living is a general term for any housing arrangement designed exclusively for seniors. Types of independent living facilities include subsidized senior housing, retirement communities, Continuing Care Retirement Communities, and age-restricted apartments (55+). The senior housing industry is rethinking these older models to come up with inter-

TABLE 22-2 Senior Residential and Home Health Care Service Comparison

Senior Living facilities types	Assisted Living Can be a few residents or a large building, great variety in types and services	Skilled Nursing Facility (SNF) Skilled rehabilitation	Custodial Care (Nursing Home/Facility) about 4.2% of >65 years old live in nursing homes CDC (2020a)	Home Health Care
Model	Social housing model	Medical model	Both	Both
Services provided (AARP, 2019c, 2019d)	▪ Care and supervision ▪ Room and board ▪ Activities ▪ Assist ADLs ▪ Stores/may provide medication assistance ▪ Dementia care ▪ May have a dementia unit	▪ 24-hour nursing ▪ Room and board ▪ Assistance with ADLs ▪ Activities ▪ Dispenses/administers medications ▪ Provides rehab care: PT, OT, and Speech post hospitalization ▪ No dementia care	▪ 24-hour nursing ▪ Room and board ▪ Assistance with ADLs ▪ Activities ▪ Dispenses/administers medications ▪ May have a dementia unit	▪ Homemaker ▪ Home health aide ▪ Nursing services ▪ Provides rehab care: PT, OT, and Speech post hospitalization ▪ Limited dementia care
Skilled professionals (CMS, 2020)	Varies by state, with some states. LVNs, RNs may not be required	Nursing staff are required by law	RNs per 8-hour shift LVNs 24 hours daily CNAs Dieticians States may have additional requirements	Varies by state: licensure for providers. Can be for profit or nonprofit, or a subdivision of an agency or a hospital
Licensure authority (CMS, 2020)	State driven: Department of Public Health or Human Services	Federal oversight-U.S. Department of Health and CMS	State Department of Health and Federal CMS	State and federal
Average cost/month (Genworth, 2018)	$4,000	$5,500-$6,5000	$7,441-$8,365	$4,004-$4,195 $21.00-$22.00 hourly
Who pays? (CMS, 2020)	▪ Private pay ▪ Long-term insurance ▪ Medicaid in indigent cases is limited by space	▪ Medicare limited days ▪ Private pay ▪ Medicaid in indigent cases, limited by space	▪ Medicare limited days ▪ Private pay ▪ Medicaid in indigent cases, limited by space	▪ Private pay ▪ Long-term insurance ▪ Medicaid in indigent cases

generational community models, as baby boomers tend to be less interested in senior-only communities.

- The concept of **continuing care retirement communities (CCRCs)**, sometimes referred to as total life care centers, allows older people to "age in place," with flexible accommodations designed to meet their health and housing needs (AARP, 2019b). CCRCs are the most expensive long-term care solution available to seniors; however, they provide all levels of living, from total independence to the most dependent.
- Assisted living communities provide care to residents who need support with ADLs (these could include eating, dressing, bathing, mobility, toileting, grooming, and assistance with medications). These communities typically provide cooked meals in a shared dining hall, housekeeping, laundry, and transportation. Some communities include additional services such as salon/barbershops, art/activities, or a theater (Dementia Care Central, 2019).
- Memory care units are for individuals with dementia who require skilled care and supervision. These units or living spaces provide 24/7 supervision by staff who are specifically trained to care for patients with memory loss (Dementia Care Central, 2019).

Residents entering CCRCs sign a long-term contract that provides for housing, services, and nursing and dementia care. Many seniors enter into CCRC contracts while they are healthy and active, knowing they will be able to stay in the same community and receive nursing care should this become necessary. Currently, CCRCs are redesigning their homes and apartments to fit the needs of the baby boomers, who want more of a village feel. Dedicated memory care units in long-term and assisted living are part of the redesign. Older adults who invest in a CCRC need to have financial means to support the entrance and monthly fees. Entrance fees can be as high as $1,000,000 (AARP, 2019b).

- The growing *Village Concept* is a relatively new, self-supporting solution for independent living in which older adults live in their own homes, in a neighborhood, or in some cases high rise city apartment buildings. Neighbors share services such as transportation, grocery shopping, or helping with household chores provided by village providers, either professional or volunteer. The village encourages socialization with a wide offering of activities among the members, and some hold wellness activities. This option requires a membership fee, on average, about $450 a year to provide services (AARP, 2017b).

Older adults who remain in their homes or apartments may rely on smart home technology to improve their autonomy (Majumder et al., 2017). Other older people may live with family members or participate in home sharing (https://www.seniorhomeshares.com/about). They may attend an adult or memory day care center during the day. Sometimes being able to stay home or return home includes short-term living arrangements. This could be a rehabilitation hospital for recovery and physical therapy related to a hip fracture, or respite care, which gives the usual caregiver a much-needed rest from 24-hour-a-day caregiving and helps prevent "burnout" (see Box 22-13).

Many nurses do not know the difference between an SNF and a **custodial care** nursing home. They often exist within the same building.

- SNFs are reimbursed for 30 days by Medicare for rehabilitation for conditions such as post stroke, spinal cord injury, IV therapy, and PT, OT, and Speech (CMS, 2020).
- When an older adult has a long-term chronic condition that cannot be managed in the community, a nursing home is an option. There is 24-hour nursing and nursing assistant care in both SNF and nursing homes, but the payment model is quite different (see Table 22-2).

Nursing home reform was legislated in the late 1980s, putting increased demands on facilities to provide competent resident assessment, timely care plans, quality improvement, and protection of resident rights (Omnibus Budget Reconciliation Act, 1987). This increased

BOX 22-13 Family Caregiving Concerns

Finances

Taking time off from work to care and loss of income; most caregivers are working women who will not be contributing to their own retirement accounts for possibly long periods of time. The Credit for Caring Act is proposed legislation that would create a $3,000 tax credit for caregivers who work and care for their parents (AARP, 2019d).

Payment for Caregiving

Caregivers are often not paid. Medicaid eligible and veterans may get assistance, which varies by state. Long-term care insurance is often out of the financial reach of many families.

Hospice and End-of-Life Guidance

This concern centers on how to have the conversations with family members.

Caregiver Life Balance

This concern involves the daily work of caregiving, especially when it falls on one family member, can result in depression, anxiety, fatigue, guilt, and anger.

Resources

These include adult day programs, support groups, dementia care, and respite care.

Safety as We Age

These concerns include aging parents driving as well as home safety (AARP, 2020d).

complexity of services has resulted in increased costs in these facilities. Staffing needs increase as care becomes more complex and the resident population grows. Licensed personnel must be knowledgeable decision-makers, managers of unskilled staff, staff educators, and role models, as well as efficient and effective administrators in an essentially autonomous practice setting. And, as the population grows, the need for greater numbers of both licensed and attendant staff becomes more evident.

END OF LIFE: ADVANCE DIRECTIVES, HOSPICE, AND PALLIATIVE CARE

A final need of older adults is preparing for a dignified death. In her classic work, *On Death and Dying*, Elisabeth Kübler-Ross (1969) described death as the final stage of growth and one that deserves the same measure of quality as other stages of life.

- Although death is a natural part of life, many older people fear death as an experience of pain, humiliation, discomfort, or financial concern for loved ones. Sometimes, very aggressive and heroic medical treatments are offered to those near the end of their lives, often at the urging of family members.
- Planning for a dignified death is an important issue for many older people, and C/PHNs can facilitate conversations among family members and provide necessary information and resources. Look up www.theconversationproject.org, a very helpful toolkit to help individuals and families have the conversation about wishes for end of life.

The C/PHN will need to be aware of the laws around physician-assisted suicide and patient self-determination around death. The Death with Dignity Web site is very helpful: https://www.deathwithdignity.org/learn/access/. In addition, there are personal and professional decisions around this topic and nursing practice that a C/PHN might want to think about (Stokes, 2016).

Advance Directives

Living wills and advance health care directives (AHCDs), sometimes referred to as *advance directives*, are legal documents that instruct others about end-of-life choices should an individual be unable to make decisions independently. The forms for advance directives are available for every state online through AARP (2020b).

An AHCD only becomes effective under the circumstances specified in the document. This document allows for appointment of a health care agent who will have the legal authority to make health care decisions on behalf of the patient and for specific written instructions for future health care in the event of any situation in which the patient can no longer speak for himself or herself. Examples include the following:

- The use of dialysis and breathing machines
- Use of resuscitation if breathing or heartbeat stops
- Tube feeding
- Organ or tissue donation

Having such documents prepared and making them known to significant others can ensure that wishes will be honored. These documents can provide clear directions for families and health care professionals and are gaining more recognition and importance as a result of increasing ethical dilemmas and challenges brought on by advances in technology (American Medical Association, 2020). Advance directives can be revoked or replaced at any time, as long as the individual in question is capable of making his or her own decisions. It is recommended that these documents be reviewed every 2 years or so, or in the event of a change in health status and revised to ensure that they continue to accurately reflect an individual's wishes.

Projections indicate that by 2030, close to one half of older adults greater than the 85 years of age will have dementia and may not have a spouse or family living with them (Meunier et al., 2016). C/PHNs and other health care professionals will be faced with choices around end-of-life decisions. The education and decisions need to come far in advance for older adults.

Hospice

Hospice is an option that takes a multidisciplinary approach to end-of-life care and needs. Hospice is more a concept of care than a specific place, although some hospice organizations provide individuals with a place to die with dignity if they have no home or choose not to die at home. Hospice is an option for people with a "projected" life expectancy of 6 months or less and often involves palliative care (pain and symptom relief) as opposed to ongoing curative measures.

Chapter 30 details hospice care. The C/PHN can be a helpful resource in connecting clients with hospice services before end of life in imminent, and hospice is most beneficial for all.

Palliative Care

Palliative care consists of comfort and symptom management and does not provide a cure. For most chronic ongoing health conditions—such as diabetes, high blood pressure, congestive heart failure, arthritis, and COPD—there are no cures, only symptom relief. Palliative care should not be viewed as synonymous with hospice or end-of-life care. Rather, palliative care should be viewed as any care primarily intended to relieve the burden of physical and emotional suffering that may accompany illness associated with aging. Palliative care should be a major focus of illness care throughout the life span and in any community setting, regardless of whether a client is a hospice patient or not (National Consensus Project, 2020). There is an excellent summary of palliative care in Chapter 30.

CARE FOR THE CAREGIVER

The burden of caregiving is receiving more attention in recent years because it is such a demanding and costly role. An increasing number of older people are cared for in their home by a spouse or other family member, often referred to as an informal caregiver, on an unpaid basis.

Almost 75% of persons receiving care at home rely exclusively on informal caregivers, usually women between the ages of 45 and 64 (Schultz & Eden, 2016). The demands of caregiving exact a toll on the caregiver, who not only may miss important screening and health care

BOX 22-14 STORIES FROM THE FIELD

Case Management: Role of the C/PHN

Mr. Jessup is 94 years old and lives with his wife, age 86, in a small mobile home on some acreage in a rural area of our county. He is hard of hearing, but he only needs glasses for reading. Mr. Jessup was diagnosed with prostate cancer 20 years ago and has some bowel incontinence as a result of radiation treatments; he manages this well with pull-up protective underwear. They have one son who lives in the same town; they speak by phone every other day, and he comes by to visit when he can. Their three grandsons are all away at college and they rarely see them.

Mrs. Jessup has recently been having memory lapses, and some difficulty remembering to turn off the stove and close the refrigerator door. She has trouble with a number of daily tasks. She likes to have someone bring them fast-food as a treat every week, and they are beginning to require assistance with errands and housekeeping tasks.

Recently, Mr. Jessup noticed that he was having more difficulty doing his outside chores. He seems more "weak" and "tired" and he has recently had quite a bit of "nausea and vomiting." The Jessup's son took them for an appointment with his urologist, and it was determined that his prostate-specific antigen (PSA) was elevated.

You are a district C/PHN and have recently been assigned to the Jessup family to assess their functional limitations and provide them with information on resources they might need over the next few months.

1. *How would you begin your visit?*
2. *What assessments could be helpful (social, spiritual, mental/cognitive, etc.)?*
3. *What resources and services might be helpful to them?*

visits for self but also often give up a social life. Because of the toll of caregiving on their own health, caregivers for those with AD and dementia had $7.9 billion in additional health care costs (AARP, 2020c). Their own decline in health compromises their ability to be a caregiver unless they get some relief (see Chapter 32; Box 22-13).

Respite care is a service that is receiving increasing attention. Although there are different approaches to respite care, all have the same basic objective: to provide caregivers with planned temporary, intermittent, substitute care, allowing for relief from the daily responsibilities of caring for the care recipient (AARP, 2020c). Long-term care insurance may cover some costs of respite care. The 2000 Older Americans Act Amendments provided funding for states to work through NFCSP to address respite care specifically on the local level (ACL, 2019a).

THE COMMUNITY HEALTH NURSE IN AN AGING AMERICA

C/PHNs can make a significant contribution to the health of older adults. The nurse may function as a collaborator, case manager, advocate, and educator to assist older adults and their families to maintain or improve health. Because these nurses are in the community and already have contact with many seniors, they are in a prime position to carry out a comprehensive needs assessment, culminating in a nursing diagnosis and holistic plan for the health care needs of this group. Case management is often a critical aspect of the nurse's role because the C/PHN must know what resources are available and when and how to make referrals for these older clients (see Box 22-14).

SUMMARY

- C/PHNs work with older adults and families in many settings, wherever they find them, and with whatever health needs are present. While the priority of community/public health nursing is health promotion and disease prevention, community nurses work with older adults with chronic health conditions who are aging in place to help them achieve their maximal health potential. Because the trend for older adults is to remain in community, C/PHNs need to assess their living situations and find out as much as possible about the community's support systems, available resources, and gaps in services.
- As the number of older adults in America grows, the need for health care services and health professionals that serve older people in communities will escalate.
- Healthy longevity is the goal for the aging population and is a focus of *Healthy People*. This means being able to function as independently as possible; maintaining as much physical, mental wellness, and social engagement as possible while adapting to chronic conditions and functional impairments.
- Through advocacy, education counseling, case management, and collaboration with clients, families, and health services and providers, the community health nurse can be effective in improving quality of care and social conditions for older adults.
- Older adults prefer to age in place and live independently in the community. Public health nurses deliver health care services to a large and rapidly growing segment of the population.
- Alzheimer's dementia is the sixth leading cause of death and the only disease among America's top 10 that cannot be prevented or cured. Between 2017 and 2025, every state is expected to see at least a 14% rise in the AD prevalence (AA, 2020b). The C/PHN will support families and caregivers who need support caring for older adults with this devastating disease.
- A variety of living arrangements and care options are available from which to choose and can be tailored to the older person's desires and needs. These include continuing care communities, villages, day and memory care centers, PACE programs, assisted living, skilled and SNF long-term care centers, and hospice.

- The community health perspective includes a case management approach that offers a centralized system for assessing the needs of older people and then matching those needs with the appropriate services. The C/PHN should also seek to serve the entire older population by assessing the needs of the population, examining the available services, and analyzing their effectiveness. The effectiveness of programs can be measured according to four important criteria (targeted to the specific needs of the population): comprehensiveness, effective coordination, accessibility, and quality.

ACTIVE LEARNING EXERCISES

1. On the Internet, search for and download instructions for filling out your own advance directive. Complete the form for your state and discuss your wishes with someone who is likely to be involved in your health care.
2. Picture an older adult you know well or know a great deal about. Make a list of characteristics that describe this person. How many of these characteristics fit your picture of most senior citizens? What are your biases (ageisms) about them?
3. As part of your regular community health nursing workload, you visit a senior day care center one afternoon each week. You take the blood pressures of several people who are taking antihypertensive medications and do some nutrition counseling. The center accommodates 60 senior clients, and you would like to serve the health needs of the aggregate population. List five potential health needs of this group. What actions might you consider taking at an aggregate level? With whom would you consult as you plan programs at the center?
4. Using "Strengthen, Support, and Mobilize Communities and Partnerships" (1 of the 10 essential public health services; see Box 2-2), discover examples of innovative community programs for elders at the primary, secondary, and tertiary levels of care. Determine whether such programs could work in your own community. Discuss with C/PHNs and local stakeholders or key informants.

REFERENCES

Administration for Community Living (ACL). (2019a). *National Family Caregiver Support Program*. Retrieved from https://acl.gov/programs/support-caregivers/national-family-caregiver-support-program

Administration for Community Living. (2019b). *2018 Profile of older Americans*. Retrieved from https://acl.gov/news-and-events/announcements/now-available-2018-profile-older-americans

Administration for Community Living. (2020). *Nutrition program*. Retrieved from https://acl.gov/programs/health-wellness/nutrition-services

Almirall, J., Serra-Prat, M., Bolibar, I., & Balasso, V. (2017). Risk factors for community-acquired pneumonia in adults: A systematic review of observational studies. *Respiration, 94*(3), 299–311. doi: 10.1159/000479089.

Alzheimer's Association. (2020a). *Alzheimer's disease facts and figures*. Retrieved from https://www.alz.org/alzheimers-dementia/facts-figures#:~:text=More%20than%205%20million%20Americans%20of%20all%20ages%20have%20Alzheimer's,10%25)%20has%20Alzheimer's%20dementia

Alzheimer's Association. (2020b). *How is alzheimer's disease diagnosed?* Retrieved from https://www.alz.org/alzheimers-dementia/diagnosis

American Association of Retired People (AARP). (2016). *You call this retirement? Boomers still have work to do*. Retrieved from https://www.aarp.org/work/retirement-planning/info-2014/boomer-retirement-little-savings-means-working.html

American Association of Retired People (AARP). (2017a). *Smash the stereotypes of aging*. Retrieved from https://www.aarp.org/health/healthy-living/info-2017/aging-stereotypes-longevity-book.html

AARP. (2017b). *The age-in-place vilalge movement*. Retrieved from https://www.aarp.org/home-family/friends-family/info-2017/age-in-place-village-movement-fd.html

American Association of Retired People (AARP). (2019a). *Introducing the age-friendly network*. Retrieved from https://www.aarp.org/livable-communities/network-age-friendly-communities/info-2014/an-introduction.html

American Association of Retired People (AARP). (2019b). *How continuing care retirement communities work*. Retrieved from https://www.aarp.org/caregiving/basics/info-2017/continuing-care-retirement-communities.html

American Association of Retired People (AARP). (2019c). *Financial and legal: Bill would give some family caregivers financial relief*. Retrieved from https://www.aarp.org/caregiving/financial-legal/info-2017/credit-for-caring-act.html

American Association of Retired People (AARP). (2019d). *Financial and legal: Long-term care calculator: Compare costs, types of service in your area*. Retrieved from https://www.aarp.org/caregiving/financial-legal/info-2017/long-term-care-calculator.html

American Association of Retired People (AARP). (2020a). *The AARP network of age-friendly communities: Member list*. Retrieved from https://www.aarp.org/livable-communities/network-age-friendly-communities/info-2014/member-list.html

American Association of Retired People (AARP). (2020b). *Advanced Directive Forms*. Retrieved from https://www.aarp.org/caregiving/financial-legal/free-printable-advance-directives/

American Association of Retired People (AARP). (2020c). *Caregiver life balance*. Retrieved from https://www.aarp.org/caregiving/life-balance/info-2017/finding-respite-care.html

American Association of Retired People (AARP). (2020d). *Family caregiving*. Retrieved from https://www.aarp.org/caregiving/

American Association of Retired People (AARP). (n.d.). *Auto/driver safety: We need to talk*. Retrieved from https://www.aarp.org/auto/driver-safety/we-need-to-talk/

American Medical Association. (2020). *Advance care directives*. Retrieved from http://www.ama-https://www.ama-assn.org/delivering-care/ethics/advance-directives

American Psychological Association (2020). *Memory chagnes in older adults*. Retrieved from https://www.apa.org/research/action/memory-changes

Applewhite, A. (2016). *This chair rocks: A manifesto against ageism*. Networked Books.

Beard, J. R., Officer, A., Carvalho, I., Sadana, R., Pot, A., Michel, J., et al. (2016). The world report on ageing and health: A policy framework for healthy ageing. *Lancet, 387*(10033), 2145–2154. doi: 10.1016/S0140-6736(15)00516-4.

Black, C. M., Fillit, H., Xie, L., Hu, X., Kariburyo, M. F., Ambegaonkar, B. M., ... Khandker, R. K. (2018). Economic burden, mortality, and institutionalization in patients newly diagnosed with Alzheimer's disease. *Journal of Alzheimer's Disease, 61*(1), 185–193.

Borson, S., Frank, L., Bayley, P. J., Boustani, M., Dean, M., Lin, P. J., ... Ashford, J. W. (2013). Improving dementia care: The role of screening and detection of cognitive impairments. *Alzheimer's and Dementia, 9*, 151–159. https://doi.org/10.1016/j.jalz.2012.08.008

Brown, R., Hemati, K., Rile, E., Lee, C., Ponath, C., Tieu, L., ... Kushel, M. (2017), Geriatric conditions in a population-based sample of older homeless adults. *The Gerontologist, 57*(4), 757–766. doi: 10.1093/geront/gnw011.

Burnett, J., Dyer, C. B., Clark, L. E., & Halphen, J. M. (2018). A statewide elder mistreatment virtual assessment program: Preliminary data. *Journal of the American Geriatrics Society, 67*(1), 151–155. doi: 10.1111/jgs.15565.

Centers for Disease Control and Prevention (CDC). (2017a). *Older persons' health*. Retrieved from http://www.cdc.gov/nchs/fastats/older-american-health.htm

Centers for Disease Control and Prevention (CDC). (2017b). *Oral and dental health*. Retrieved from http://www.cdc.gov/nchs/fastats/dental.htm

Centers for Disease Control and Prevention (CDC). (2017c). *Import facts about falls*. Retrieved from https://www.cdc.gov/homeandrecreationalsafety/falls/adultfalls.html

Centers for Disease Control and Prevention (CDC). (2017d). *Depression is not a normal part of growing older*. Retrieved from https://www.cdc.gov/aging/mentalhealth/depression.htm

Centers for Disease Control and Prevention (CDC). (2018a). *Vaccines and preventable diseases: Shingrix recommendations*. Retrieved from https://www.cdc.gov/vaccines/vpd/shingles/hcp/shingrix/recommendations.html

Centers for Disease Control and Prevention (CDC). (2018b). *Arthritis basics*. Retrieved from http://www.cdc.gov/arthritis/basics/index.html

Centers for Disease Control and Prevention (CDC). (2019a). *People 65 years and older & influenza*. Retrieved from https://www.cdc.gov/flu/about/disease/65over.htm

Centers for Disease Control and Prevention (CDC). (2019b). *STEADI: Stopping elderly accidents, deaths & injuries*. Retrieved from https://www.cdc.gov/steadi/

Centers for Disease Control and Prevention (CDC). (2020a). *People that live in a nursing home or long-term care facility*. Retrieved from https://www.cdc.gov/coronavirus/2019-ncov/need-extra-precautions/people-in-nursing-homes.html

Centers for Disease Control and Prevention (CDC). (2020b). *Racial and ethnic approaches to community health (REACH)*. Retrieved from www.cdc.gov/nccdphp/dch/programs/reach

Centers for Disease Control and Prevention (CDC). (2020c). *Recommended adult immunization schedule, by vaccine and age group*. Retrieved from http://www.cdc.gov/vaccines/schedules/hcp/imz/adult.html

Centers for Medicare and Medicaid Services (CMS). (2020). *Nursing homes*. Retrieved from https://www.cms.gov/Medicare/Provider-Enrollment-and-Certification/CertificationandComplianc/NHs.html

Christie, E. (2018). *RN case managers, social workers should work as a team with clearly defined roles*. Retrieved from https://www.reliasmedia.com/articles/141672-rn-case-managers-social-workers-should-work-as-a-team-with-clearly-defined-roles

Chou, J., Tong, M., & Brandtm N. J. (2019). Combating polypharmacy through deprescribing potentially inappropriate medications. *Journal of Gerontological Nursing, 45*(1), 9–15. doi: 10.3928/00989134-20190102-01.

Conejero, I., Olie, E., Courtet, P., & Calati, R. (2018). Suicide in older adults: Current perspectives. *Clinical Interventions in Aging 13,* 691–699. doi: 10.2147/CIA.S130670.

Contrera K. J., Wallhagen M. I., Mamo, S. K., Oh, E. S., & Lin, F. R. (2016). Hearing loss health care for older adults. *Journal of American Board of Family Medicine, 29*(3), 394–403. doi: 10.3122/jabfm.2016.03.150235.

Cordell, C. B., Borson, S., Boustani, M., Chodosh, J., Reuben, D., Verghese, J., ... Medicare Detection of Cognitive Impairment Workgroup. (2013). Alzheimer's Association recommendations for operationalizing the detection of cognitive impairment during the Medicare Annual Wellness Visit in a primary care setting. *Alzheimer's & Dementia, 9*(2), 141–150.

Corporation for National & Community Service. (n.d.). *Foster grandparents*. Retrieved from http://www.nationalservice.gov/programs/senior-corps/foster-grandparents

Correia, C., Lopez, K. J., Wroblewski, K. E., Huisingh-Scheetz, M., Kern, D., Chen, R., ... Pinto, J. M. (2016). Global sensory impairment among older adults in the United States. *Journal of the American Geriatrics Society, 64*(2), 306–313. doi: 10.1111/jgs.13955.

Cronenwett, L., Sherwood, G., Marnsteiner, J., Disch, J., Johnson, J., Mitchell, P., ... Warren, J. (2007). Quality and safety in education for nurses. *Nursing Outlook, 55*, 122–131. Retrieved from https://digitalcommons.sacredheart.edu/cgi/viewcontent.cgi?article=1123&context=nurs_fac

Dameron, C. M. (2005). Spiritual assessment made easy..with ACRONYMS! *Journal of Christian Nursing, 22*(11), 14–16. doi: 10.1097/01.CNJ.0000262323.59843.2e.

Dementia Care Central. (2019). *Residential care for dementia: Assisted living, memory care, nursing homes & other options*. Retrieved from https://www.dementiacarecentral.com/memory-care-vs-assisted-living/#memory-care

Diggle-Fox, B. S. (2016). Assessing suicide risk in older adults. *The Nurse Practitioner, 41*(10), 35–36. doi: 10.1097/01.NPR.0000502853.23307.25.

Dolansky, M. A., & Moore, S. M. (2013). Quality and safety education for nurses (QSEN): The key is systems thinking. *The Online Journal of Issues in Nursing. 18*(3). Manuscript 1. doi: 10.3912/OJIN.Vol18No3Man01.

Duke University. (2014). *Older Americans resources and services (OARS): The methods and its uses*. Center for the Study of Aging and Human Development. Retrieved from http://centerforaging.duke.edu/services/141

Galvin, J. E. (2015). The Quick Dementia Rating System (QDRS): A rapid dementia staging tool. *Alzheimer's & Dementia: Diagnosis, Assessment & Disease Monitoring, 1*(2), 249–259.

Golchin, N., Frank, S. H., Vince, A., Isham, L., & Meropol, S. B. (2015). Polypharmacy in the elderly, *Journal of Research in Pharmacy Practice, 4*(2), 85–88.

Graf, C. (2008). The Lawton Instrumental Activities of Daily Living Scale. *American Journal of Nursing, 108*(4), 53–62.

Gulia, K. K., & Kumar, V. M., (2018). Sleep disorders in the elderly: A growing challenge. *Psychogeriatrics, 18*(3), 155–165. https://doi.org/10.1111/psyg.12319

Hatfield, L. A., Favreault, M. M., McGuire, T. G., & Chernew, M. E. (2018). Modeling heath care spending growth on older adults. *Health Services Research, 53*(1), 138–155. doi: 10.1111/1475-6773.12640.

Healthfinder.gov. (2020). *Lower your risk of falling*. Retrieved from https://health.gov/myhealthfinder/topics/everyday-healthy-living/safety/lower-your-risk-falling

Healthy People 2020. (2020a). *Older adults data details*. Retrieved from https://www.healthypeople.gov/node/3493/data-details

Healthy People 2020. (2020b). *Healthy People 2020 leading health indicators: Progress update*. Retrieved from http://www.healthypeople.gov/2020/leading-health-indicators/Healthy-People-2020-Leading-Health-Indicators%3A-Progress-Update

Healthy People 2020. (2020c). *Dementias, including Alzheimer's disease*. Retrieved from https://www.healthypeople.gov/2020/topics-objectives/topic/dementias-including-alzheimers-disease

International Osteoporosis Foundation. (n.d.). *Facts and statistics*. Retrieved from http://www.iofbonehealth.org/facts-statistics

Kaiser Family Foundation. (2017). *Income and Assets of Medicare Beneficiaries, 2016–2035*. Retrieved from https://www.kff.org/medicare/issue-brief/income-and-assets-of-medicare-beneficiaries-2016-2035/

Kaiser Family Foundation. (2018). *How many seniors live in poverty*? Retrieved from http://kff.org/medicare/issue-brief/poverty-among-seniors-an-updated-analysis-of-national-and-state-level-poverty-rates-under-the-official-and-supplemental-poverty-measures/

Kang, L., Han, P., Wang, J., Ma, Y., Jia, L., Fu, L., ... Guo, Q. (2017). Timed Up and Go Test can predict recurrent falls: A longitudinal study of the community-dwelling in China. *Clinical Interventional Aging, 12*, 2009–2016. doi: 10.2147/CIA.S138287.

Katz, S. (1963). Studies of illness in the aged. The index of ADL: A standardized measure of biological and psychosocial function. *Journal of the American Medical Association, 185*, 914–919.

Kübler-Ross, E. (1969). *On death and dying*. Touchstone, NY: Scribner.

Lindland, E., Fond, M., Haydon, A., & Kendall-Taylor, N. (2015). *Gauging aging: Mapping the gaps between expert and public understandings of aging in America*. Washington, DC: FrameWorks Institute.

Macera, C. A., Cavanaugh, A. C., & Bellettiere, J. (2017). State of the art review: Physical activity and older adults. *American Journal of Lifestyle Medicine*. Retrieved from https://journals.sagepub.com/doi/pdf/10.1177/1559827615571897

Majumder, S., Aghayi, E., Noferesti, M., Memarzadeh-Tehran, H., Mondal, T., Pang, Z., & Deen, J. (2017). Smart homes for elderly healthcare-recent advances and research challenges. *Sensors (Basel), 17*(11), 2496. doi: 10.3390/s17112496.

Mather, M. (2016). The affective neuroscience of aging. *Annual Review of Psychology 67*, 213–238. doi: 10.1146/annurev-psych-122414-033540

Mayeda, E. R., Glymour, M. M., Quesenberry, C. P., & Whitmer, R. A. (2016). Inequalities in dementia incidence between six racial and ethnic groups over 14 years. *Alzheimer's & Dementia, 12*(3), 216–224.

Medicaid.gov. (2015). *Community First Choice (CFC) 1915 (k)*. Retrieved from https://www.medicaid.gov/medicaid/hcbs/authorities/1915-k/index.html

Medicare.gov. (n.d.). *What's not covered by part A & part B*? Retrieved from https://www.medicare.gov/what-medicare-covers/not-covered/item-and-services-not-covered-by-part-a-and-b.html

Medicare.gov. (2018). *Part B costs*. Retrieved from https://www.medicare.gov/your-medicare-costs/part-b-costs

Meunier, M., Brant, J., Audet, S., Dickerson, D., Gransbery, K., & Ciemins, E. (2016). Life after PACE (Program of All-Inclusive Care for the Elderly): A retrospective/prospective, qualitative analysis of the impact of closing a nurse practitioner centered PACE site. *Journal of the American Association of Nurse Practitioners, 28*, 596–603. doi: 10.1002/2327-6924.12379.

Miller, C. A. (2019). *Nursing for wellness in older adults* (8th ed.). Philadelphia, PA: Wolters Kluwer.

Narushima, M., Liu, J., & Diestelkamp, N. (2018). Lifelong learning in active ageing discourse: Its conserving effect on wellbeing, health and vulnerability. *Ageing Society, 38*(4), 651–675. doi: 10.1017/S0144686X16001136.

National Consensus Project. (2020). *Clinical practice guidelines for quality palliative care: 4th edition.* Retrieved from http://nchpc.conferencespot.org/

National Council on Aging (NCOA). (2018). *Healthy aging.* Retrieved from https://www.ncoa.org/wp-content/uploads/2018-Healthy-Aging-Fact-Sheet-7.10.18-1.pdf

National Foundation for Infectious Diseases. (2018). *Influenza.* Retrieved from http://www.nfid.org/influenza/

National Institute of Arthritis and Musculoskeletal and Skin Diseases (NIAMS). (2017). *Arthritis.* Retrieved from http://www.niams.nih.gov/Health_Info/Arthritis/default.asp

National Institute of Arthritis and Musculoskeletal and Skin Diseases (NIAMS). (2019). *Rheumatoid arthritis.* Retrieved from http://www.niams.nih.gov/Health_Info/Rheumatic_Disease/default.asp

National Institute on Aging. (2020a). *Facts about aging and alcohol.* Retrieved from https://www.nia.nih.gov/health/facts-about-aging-and-alcohol#:~:text=Alcohol%20is%20a%20factor%20in,or%20coordination%20should%20not%20drink

National Institute on Aging. (2020b). *Exercise and physical activity.* Retrieved from http://www.nia.nih.gov/healthy/publications/excercise-phsycal-activity/introduction

National Institute on Aging. (2020c). Elder abuse. Retrieved from https://www.nia.nih.gov/health/elder-abuse

National PACE Association. (2020). *Is PACE for you?* Retrieved from http://www.npaonline.org/pace-you

New World Encyclopedia. (n.d.). *Spirit.* Retrieved from http://www.newworldencyclopedia.org/entry/Spirit

Notthoff, N., & Carstensen, L. (2017). Promoting walking in older adults: Perceived neighborhood walkability influences the effectiveness of motivational message. *Journal of Healthy Psychological, 22*(7), 834–843. doi: 10.1177/1359105315616470.

Office of disease Prevention and Health Promotion. (2020). *Healthy People 2030 framework.* Retrieved from https://www.healthypeople.gov/2020/About-Healthy-People/Development-Healthy-People-2030/Framework

Omnibus Budget Reconciliation Act. (1987). *Federal nursing home reform act from the Omnibus Budget Reconciliation Act of 1987.* Retrieved from www.ncmust.com/doclib/OBRA87summary.pdf

Ortman, J., Velkoff, V., & Hogan, H. (2014). *The older population in the United States, current population reports,* 25–1140. U.S. Census Bureau. Retrieved from https://www.census.gov/prod/2014pubs/p25-1140.pdf

Peterson-Kaiser Health System Tracker. (2016). *How do health expenditures vary across the population?* Retrieved from https://www.healthsystemtracker.org/chart-collection/health-expenditures-vary-across-population/?sf_data=results&_sft_category=spending&sf_paged=2#item-start

Pew Research Center. (2016). *More older Americans are working, and working more, than they used to.* Retrieved from https://www.pewresearch.org/fact-tank/2016/06/20/more-older-americans-are-working-and-working-more-than-they-used-to/

Pew Research Center: Religion and Public Life. (2018). *Religious landscape study: Generational cohort.* Retrieved from http://www.pewforum.org/religious-landscape-study/generational-cohort/

Reuters. (2017). Baby Boomers are over marriage. *New York Post.* Retrieved from https://nypost.com/2017/04/07/baby-boomers-are-over-marriage/

Roitto, H. M., Kautiainen, H., Ohman, H., Savikko, N., Strandberg, T. E., Raivio, M., ... Pitkala, K. H. (2018). Relationship of neuropsychiatric symptoms with falls in Alzheimer's Disease...Does exercise modify the risk? *Journal of the American Geriatric Society, 66*(12), 2377–2381. doi: 10.1111/jgs.15614.

Schultz, R., & Eden, J. (Eds). (2016). *Committee on family caregiving for older adults: Board on Health Care Services, Health and Medicine Division, National Academies of Sciences, Engineering, and Medicine.* Washington, DC: National Academies Press.

Scott, J., & Mayo, A. M. (2018). Instruments for detection and screening of cognitive impairment for older adults in primary care settings: A review. *Geriatric Nursing, 39*(3), 323–329. doi: 10.1016/j.gerinurse.2017.11.001.

Smith, D., & Kautz, D. (2018). Protect older adults from polypharmacy hazards. *Nursing 2018, 48*(2).

Stokes, F. (2016). The emerging role of nurse practitioners in physician-assisted death. *Journal of Nurse Practitioners, 13*(2), 150–155. https://doi.org/10.1016/j.nurpra.2016.08.029

Supporting Grandparents Raising Grandchildren Act of 2018, S. 1091, 115th Cong., Second Sess. (2018). Retrieved from https://acl.gov/sites/default/files/about-acl/2018-10/BILLS-115s1091enr%20-%20SGRG.pdf

Tufts University. (2015). *MyPlate for older adults.* Retrieved from http://now.tufts.edu/news-releases/tufts-university-nutrition-scientists-unveil-

211San Diego. (n.d.). *What is 211?* Retrieved from https://211sandiego.org/

U.S. Census Bureau. (2015). *The next four decades: The older population in the United States: 2010 to 2050.* Retrieved from https://www.census.gov/prod/2010pubs/p25-1138.pdf

U.S. Census Bureau. (2018). *The Supplemental Poverty Measure: 2017.* Retrieved from https://www.census.gov/content/dam/Census/library/publications/2018/demo/p60-265.pdf

USDA (n.d.). *Choose My Plate.* Retrieved from https://www.choosemyplate.gov/

U.S. Department of Health & Human Services (USDHHS). (2020a). *Healthy People 2030: Browse objectives.* Retrieved from https://health.gov/healthypeople/objectives-and-data/browse-objectives

U.S. Department of Health & Human Services (USDHHS). (2020b). *Older Adults.* Retrieved from https://www.healthypeople.gov/2020/topics-objectives/topic/older-adults

U.S. Preventive Services Task Force. (2018a). *USPSTF A and B recommendations.* Retrieved from https://www.uspreventiveservicestaskforce.org/Page/Name/uspstf-a-and-b-recommendations/

U.S. Preventive Services Task Force. (2018b). *Information for health professionals.* Retrieved from http://www.uspreventiveservicestaskforce.org/Page/Name/tools-and-resources-for-better-preventive-care

United Nations. (2017). *The 2017 revision of world population prospects.* Retrieved from https://www.un.org/development/desa/publications/world-population-prospects-the-2017-revision.html

Wiese, L., & Williams, C. (2015). Annual cognitive assessment for older adults: Update for nurses. *Journal of Community Health Nursing, 32,* 1–13. doi: 10.1080/07370016.2015.1087244.

Wong, J., Leung, J., Skitmore, M., & Buys, L. (2017). Technical requirements of age-friendly smart home technologies in high-rise residential buildings: A systematic intelligence analytical approach. *Automation in Construction, 73,* 12–19.

Zhu, C. W., Scarmeas, N., Ornstein, K., Albert, M., Brandt, J., Blacker, D., ... Stern, Y. (2015). Health-care use and cost in dementia caregivers: Longitudinal results from the Predictors Caregiver Study. *Alzheimer's & Dementia, 11*(4), 444–454.

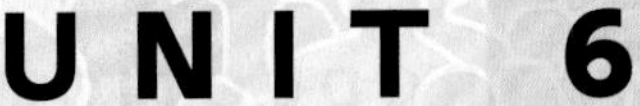

UNIT 6

Vulnerable Populations

CHAPTER 23

Working With Vulnerable People

"How far you go in life depends on your being tender with the young, compassionate with the aged, sympathetic with the striving, and tolerant of the weak and the strong—because someday you will have been all of these."

—George Washington Carver (1860–1943), Botanist and Scientist

KEY TERMS

Differential vulnerability hypothesis
Empowerment strategies
Environmental resources
Health disparities
Human capital
Marginalized populations
Racial/ethnic disparities
Racism
Relative risk
Social capital
Social determinants of health
Socioeconomic gradient
Socioeconomic resources
Vulnerability
Vulnerable populations

LEARNING OBJECTIVES

Upon mastery of this chapter, you should be able to:

1. Describe the term "vulnerable populations."
2. Discuss the effects of vulnerability and relative risk.
3. Differentiate between the concepts of social capital and human capital.
4. List three of the most common factors related to vulnerability.
5. Identify two strategies to solicit and evaluate input from vulnerable populations when planning health care programs and services.
6. Explain the socioeconomic gradient in health.
7. Describe three types of health disparities.
8. Describe four C/PHN roles or behaviors that help promote client empowerment.

INTRODUCTION

The concept of **vulnerability** is an important one for nurses because of its implications for health, no matter where they practice. Often, vulnerable populations are subpopulations, such as ethnic or racial minorities, the uninsured, those with HIV/AIDS, children, older adults, the poor, and those who are homeless (American Public Health Association, 2017; Stafford & Wood, 2017). These subpopulations often have higher morbidity and mortality rates, less access to health care (and disparities in outcomes of health care), shorter life expectancy, and an overall diminished quality of life compared with the population in general (Agency for Healthcare Research and Quality [AHRQ], 2015; American Public Health Association, 2017).

In this chapter, we examine popular models and theories of vulnerability, important concepts, and contributing factors. We also briefly discuss health disparities that are more common among vulnerable members of society and the role of C/PHNs working with these groups. This chapter provides an overview of this subject and lays the foundation for other chapters.

THE CONCEPT OF VULNERABLE POPULATIONS

In this section, we consider several key models and theories related to vulnerability, the criteria used to determine who is considered vulnerable, and causative factors linked to vulnerability.

Models and Theories of Vulnerability

Key models and theories of vulnerability that have been proposed include the vulnerable populations conceptual model developed by Flaskerud and Winslow in 1998 (Box 23-1; Fig. 23-1), the Behavioral Model for Vulnerable Populations (Box 23-2; Fig. 23-2), the differential vulnerability hypothesis (Kessler, 1979; Box 23-3), the concept of social capital (Fig. 23-3), a general model of vulnerability, and Maslow's Hierarchy of Needs.

The importance of **social capital** is sometimes missed, as it can be subtle and less obvious than the lack of money or jobs (Fig. 23-3). But the presence of friends and family or someone to rely on in case of an emergency can be invaluable in assisting individuals through many of life's difficulties. Social support, or a close confidante, can promote social and psychological health and help counteract the effects of stressful events. In our mobile society, many people live great distances from family members and have difficulty establishing new friendships. Those who live alone or who are socially isolated are at greatest risk of vulnerability, increased morbidity and mortality, and decreased overall health (Lubben, Gironda, Sabbath, Kong, & Johnson, 2015); thus, C/PHNs should be aware of this and strive to provide additional support and resources.

A general model of vulnerability helps to explain individual and community risk factors that lead to vulnerability, as well as problems with access to care and quality of care received that impact health outcomes on both an individual and community level, as described in a seminal article by Shi, Stevens, Lebrun, Faed, and Tsai (2008). According to this model, vulnerable populations often experience clusters of risk factors, and these are viewed as cumulative. The specific combinations of risks

BOX 23-1 Vulnerable Populations Conceptual Model (Flaskerud & Winslow, 1998)

Flaskerud and Winslow (1998) developed a popular conceptual framework of vulnerability (see Fig. 23-1) that contains three related concepts: resource availability, relative risk, and health status. The model provides evidence of the link between poor health status and socioeconomic resource availability through the loss of income, jobs, and health insurance. The following concepts are supported by this model:

- Lack of resources (e.g., socioeconomic and environmental) increases a population's exposure to risk factors and reduces individuals' ability to avoid illness.
- **Socioeconomic resources** include **human capital** (e.g., jobs, income, housing, education), social connectedness or integration (e.g., social networks or ties; social support or the lack of it, characterized by marginalization), and social status (e.g., position, power, role).
- **Environmental resources** deal mostly with access to health care and the quality of that care.
- Limited access or lack of access to care can arise from many sources, including crime-ridden neighborhoods, insufficient transportation systems, lack of adequate numbers and types of providers, limited choices of health care plans, or no health insurance.
- **Relative risk** refers to exposure to risk factors identified by a substantial body of research as lifestyle, behaviors and choices (e.g., diet, exercise, use of tobacco, alcohol and other drugs, sexual behaviors), use of health screening services (e.g., mammogram, colonoscopy), and stressful events (e.g., crime, violence, abuse, firearm use).

Source: Flaskerud and Winslow (1998).

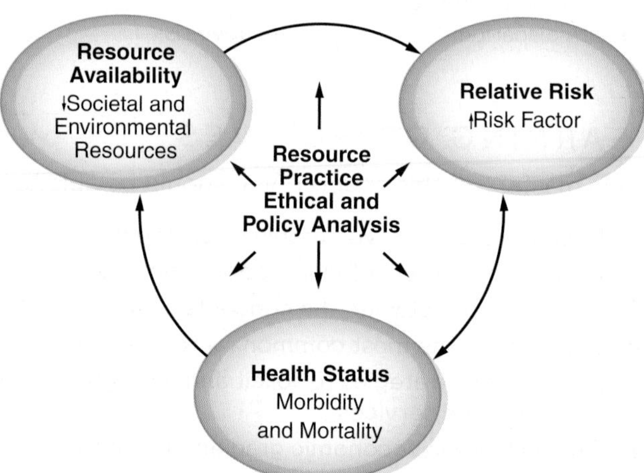

FIGURE 23-1 Vulnerable populations conceptual model. (Adapted from Flaskerud, J. H., & Winslow, B. J. (1998). Conceptualizing vulnerable populations health-related research. *Nursing Research, 47*(2), 69–78.)

BOX 23-2 The Behavioral Model for Vulnerable Populations (Gelberg, Andersen, & Leake, 2000)

Gelberg et al. (2000) advanced another classic model, the Behavioral Model for Vulnerable Populations; this model looks at population characteristics (predisposing and enabling factors and needs) as an explanation for health behaviors and eventual health outcomes (Burg & Oyama, 2016). The following concepts are supported by this model:

- Predisposing factors included demographic variables (e.g., gender, age, marital status), social variables (e.g., education, employment, ethnicity, social networks), and health beliefs (e.g., values and attitudes toward health and health care services, knowledge of disease).
- Social structures (e.g., acculturation and immigration), sexual orientation, and childhood characteristics (e.g., mobility, living conditions, history of substance abuse, criminal behavior, victimization, or mental illness) were also considered predisposing factors.
- Enabling factors included personal and family resources, as well as community resources (e.g., income, insurance, social support, region, health services resources, public benefits, transportation, telephone, crime rates, social services resources).
- Perceived health needs and population health conditions also were considered, as were health behaviors including diet, exercise, tobacco use, self-care, and adherence to care.
- The use of health services (e.g., ambulatory and inpatient care, long-term care, alternative health care) and personal health practices (e.g., hygiene, unsafe sexual behaviors, food sources) combined with the other factors to produce outcomes such as perceived and evaluated health and general satisfaction with health care services.

The model has been used in research with homeless adults (Doran et al., 2014) and in examining barriers to interconceptual care (Rhoades et al., 2014), with mixed results. See Figure 23-2, interrelated pathways linking education to health.

Source: Burg and Oyama (2016); Doran et al. (2014); Gelberg et al. (2000); Rhoades et al. (2014).

(e.g., low income, low education) are more detrimental to health outcomes, as is the greater number of risk factors that accumulate over time.

Most nursing students are familiar with Maslow's Hierarchy of Needs (Maslow, 1987), with physiological needs (e.g., water, food, air) as the base of a pyramid, and the needs for safety, belonging, esteem, and self-actualization building from the basic needs. Chronic poverty, environments of crime and violence, or disenfranchisement, racism, and discrimination (vulnerability) can keep people from meeting the higher needs (Bates, 2016). **Racism** is largely defined as believing that race is the primary

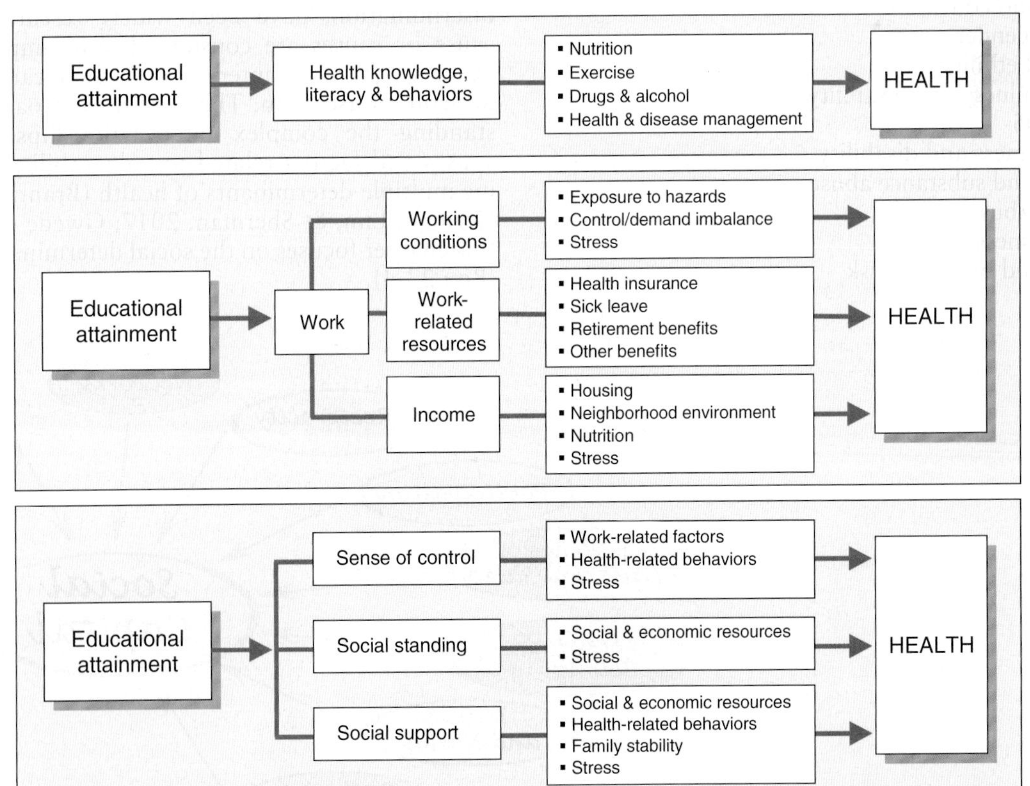

FIGURE 23-2 Interrelated pathways linking education to health. (From Braveman, P., Ergerter, S., & Williams, D. R. (2011). The social determinants of health: Coming of age. *Annual Review of Public Health, 32*, 381–398, used with permission.)

BOX 23-3 The Differential Vulnerability Hypothesis (Kessler, 1979)

Kessler's (1979) **differential vulnerability hypothesis** states that there is a relationship between social status and psychological distress; a person's psychological distress is determined by the impact of the stressor event as influenced by social status (this includes class, sex, marital status, and rural vs. urban). The formula $P_i = V_i (S)_i + a_i$ is defined as (Kessler, 1979, p. 101): "(P) Psychological distress is the result of varying exposure to environmental stress events or situations (S) acting on individuals who possess varying vulnerabilities to stress (V); (a) represents the residual influence of constitutional makeup of the mental health of person (i) independent of any environmental stresses he/she might experience" (Kessler, 1979, p. 101).

The hypothesis has been used in research with racial inequity (Roxburgh & MacArthur, 2014; Wickrama, Bae & Walker, 2016).

Source: Kessler (1979); Roxburgh and MacArthur (2014); Wickrama et al. (2016).

factor of our capacities and traits as humans and that any racial differences result in feelings of either superiority or inferiority.

Who Is Considered Vulnerable?

In her classic book, Aday (2001) included the following factors and populations in the description of who is considered vulnerable:

- Income and education
- Age and gender
- Race and ethnicity
- Chronic illness and disability
- HIV/AIDS
- Mental illness and disability
- Alcohol and substance abuse
- Familial abuse
- Homelessness
- Suicide and homicide risk
- High-risk mothers and infants
- Immigrants and refugees
- Military personnel

Other authors considered the uninsured and underinsured as **vulnerable populations** because of their difficulties with health care access and the potential for poor health outcomes, as well as victims of bullying and crime, children in foster care, those in the gay and lesbian community, veterans and returning military personnel, and victims/survivors of torture and terrorism (Hong, Pequero, & Espelage, 2018; Koven, 2018; Mohatt et al., 2018; Scherrer et al., 2018).

- Although many segments of the population may be considered vulnerable at some point in their lives, some population segments are more often identified as vulnerable because of their long-term situations (de Chesnay & Anderson, 2016). The very young and the very old have particular risk factors that increase their chances of poor health, as well as unique issues with access to health care.
- An extensive body of research substantiates the reality of higher morbidity and mortality rates for racial and ethnic minorities than for the White population, thus demonstrating **racial/ethnic disparities** in health (Gwede, Quinn, Green, 2016; Institute of Medicine [IOM], 2003; Neumayer & Plümper, 2015).

Prevalence of Vulnerable Populations and Causative Factors

Root causes of vulnerability, such as low socioeconomic status (SES), lack of insurance coverage, racism, and discrimination, have been widely researched. Which cause or causes are considered most important? The exact weight of the interaction of these causes has been difficult to ascertain. The current approach to understanding the complex interrelationships among the causes and factors related to vulnerability is to examine multiple determinants of health (Brantley, Kerrigan, German, Lim, & Sherman, 2017; Gwede et al., 2016); this chapter focuses on the social determinants of health (Box 23-4).

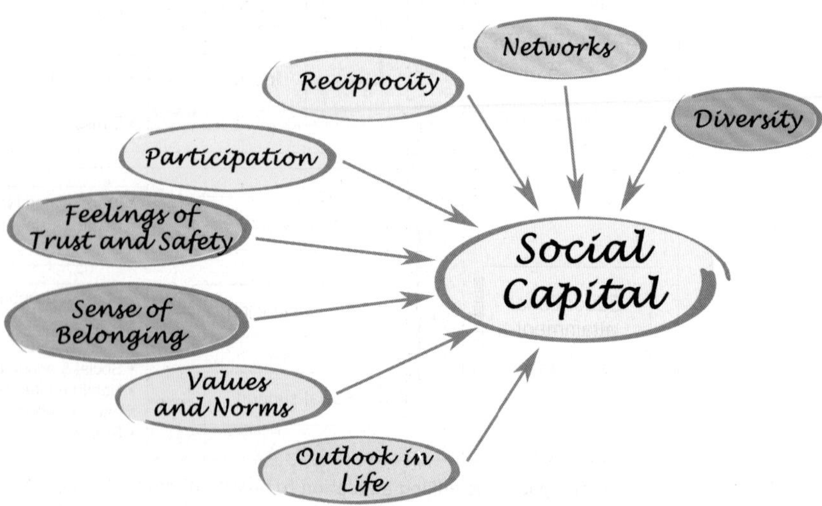

FIGURE 23-3 Social capital is a network of relationships where one lives and works.

BOX 23-4 STORIES FROM THE FIELD

Teen Pregnancy

Teen pregnancy is viewed as a social issue that impacts families for generations. Although the teen pregnancy rate has been declining over the past few decades, the United States still has the highest teen pregnancy rate among developed nations (Watson & Vogel, 2017). Teen mothers are less likely to receive prenatal care and more likely to live in poverty and have more than one child before age 20, and their children are more prone to behavioral issues (Watson & Vogel, 2017).

One teenage mother describes being a teenage mother at school as follows:

"I feel like an ant ... traveling the whole world. I have to get around the world by trying to get a boat to get across the water, trying to get some food so I don't fall over and die. .... [I]t's the hardest battle you're ever going to face." (Watson & Vogel, 2017)

1. *Discuss vulnerable populations. What risk factors apply to this situation?*
2. *What primary, secondary, and tertiary interventions can be applied to this scenario?*

Source: Watson and Vogel (2017).

Poverty

If only one indicator is measured—poverty—it is evident that vulnerability touches a large segment of the global population and the population in the United States (see Fig. 23-4):

- According to the latest figures from the World Bank (2015), an estimated 767 million people are living in extreme poverty (living on $1.90 or less a day), and 2.1 billion are living in moderate poverty (living on between $1.90 and $3.10 a day).
- The official poverty rate in the United States is 12.7%, which represents an estimated 43.1 million people (Center for Poverty Research, University of California Davis [UCD], 2017).
- Poverty thresholds in the United States are $12,486 for a single individual under age 65, $14,507 for a household of two people with a householder 65 years or older with no children, and $24,339 for a family of four with two children under 18 (Center for Poverty Research, UCD, 2017).
- According to the National Center for Children in Poverty (2017), 36% of the children in poverty are Black, or African American, 33% American Indian, 30% Hispanic or Latino, 12% White, and 12% Asian or Pacific Islander.

How does poverty make one vulnerable to poor health outcomes? The answer to this question is complex:

- One supposition is that having less money means being less able to afford most aspects of a quality life, including adequate housing in a safe neighborhood. This living situation may lead to fewer opportunities for exercise, especially if walking outside puts one at risk of becoming a victim of violence.
- Fewer community resources are usually available, such as grocery stores, quality schools, recreation facilities, and health care providers. Lower income level is associated with lower levels of education and often results in a person having to work at jobs where he or she is exposed to higher risks (e.g., mining), or the need to work at more than one job to make ends meet, and often without health insurance coverage (Centers for Disease Control & Prevention [CDC], 2015a).

Data from the National Health Interview Survey showed that from 2013 to 2015, the percentage of adults aged 18 to 64 years (Martinez & Ward, 2016):

- Who were uninsured decreased for poor (40.0% to 26.2%), near-poor (37.8% to 23.9%), and not-poor (11.7% to 7.7%) adults
- Who had a usual place to go for medical care increased for poor (66.9% to 73.6%) and near-poor (71.1% to 75.9%) adults
- Who had seen or talked to a health professional in the past 12 months increased for poor (73.2% to 75.8%) and near-poor (71.9% to 75.9%) adults
- Who did not obtain needed medical care due to cost at some time during the past 12 months decreased for poor (16.8% to 12.4%), near-poor (14.6% to 11.0%), and not-poor (4.9% to 3.8%) adults

Research has shown that those groups with the lowest income and least education were consistently less healthy than were those with the most income and education (World Health Organization, 2020a). Poverty and race/ethnicity are often intertwined, but SES is considered a consistent and robust variable related to health and death (Brantley et al., 2017; Montez, Zajacova, & Hayward, 2017; Montez, Zhang, Zajacova, & Hamilton, 2018; Neumayer & Plümper, 2015; Williams, Priest, & Anderson, 2016):

- Low-income minority neighborhoods with poor access and poor walkability to fresh fruits, vegetables, and lean proteins are associated with a significant increase in cardiovascular disease mortality and type 2 diabetes (Gaglioti et al., 2018; Haynes-Maslow, Ammerman & Leone, 2017). Many of these neighborhoods are termed food deserts due to the lack of available supermarkets (Fig. 23-5).
- Research has shown that fast food restaurants are more prevalent in low-income neighborhoods, and this prevalence has been shown to have a positive correlation with obesity and type 2 diabetes (Michimi & Wimberly, 2015; Rummo et al., 2017).

Another risk factor for vulnerability that is associated with poverty is exposure to pollution and smoking:

- One finding indicates that the highest amount of pollution is most often found in neighborhoods where there is more poverty, lower education levels, and higher rates of unemployment (CDC, 2015a).
- Others note an association between SES and poorer respiratory health, often due to living conditions, such as ambient air pollution and smoking (Berry, Nickerson, & Odum, 2017), and because of a higher smoking prevalence among those with lower SES (Lowe et al., 2018).

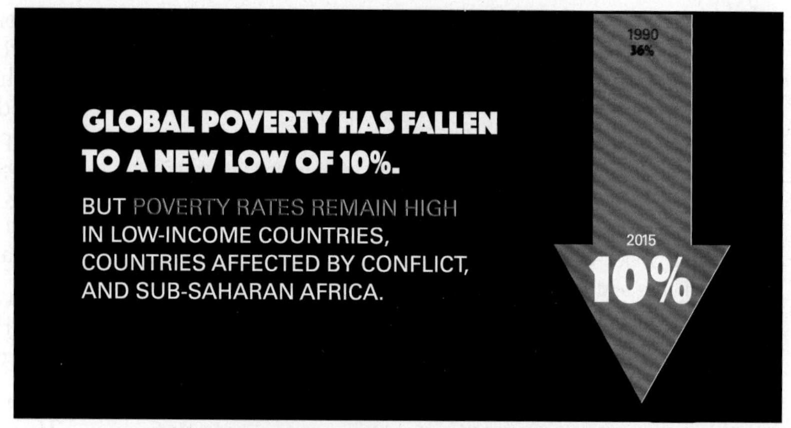

GLOBAL POVERTY HAS FALLEN TO A NEW LOW OF 10%.
BUT POVERTY RATES REMAIN HIGH IN LOW-INCOME COUNTRIES, COUNTRIES AFFECTED BY CONFLICT, AND SUB-SAHARAN AFRICA.

NEW STANDARDS FOR A GROWING WORLD

Half of the countries for which the World Bank monitors poverty have now reduced extreme poverty to below 3%, but that doesn't mean poverty is nonexistent in these countries.

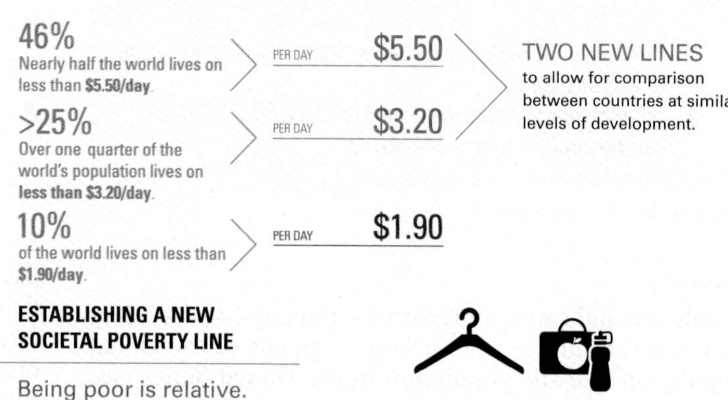
46%
Nearly half the world lives on less than **$5.50/day**.
PER DAY $5.50
>25%
Over one quarter of the world's population lives on **less than $3.20/day**.
PER DAY $3.20
10%
of the world lives on less than **$1.90/day**.
PER DAY $1.90
TWO NEW LINES
to allow for comparison between countries at similar levels of development.
ESTABLISHING A NEW SOCIETAL POVERTY LINE

Being poor is relative.

n a poor country, one may only need clothing and food to perform work, whereas in a richer society, one may also need access to Internet, a phone, and a vehicle.

In 2015, about 2.1 billion people were poor relative to their societies.

-VS-

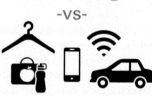

BEYOND MONETARY POVERTY

Poverty isn't just about money. It's about measuring people's well-being—not just their income or consumption.

MULTIDIMENSIONAL POVERTY

electricity

income/consumption

sanitation

water

education

FIGURE 23-4 Infographic: Poverty and Shared Prosperity 2018: Piecing together the poverty puzzle. (Adapted with permission from World Bank. (2018). Retrieved from https://www.worldbank.org/en/news/infographic/2018/10/17/infographic-poverty-and-shared-prosperity-2018-piecing-together-the-poverty-puzzle). See thePoint for the complete infographic.

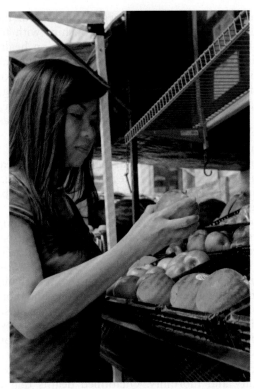

FIGURE 23-5 Income and race/ethnicity influence access to healthy food.

- Also, research has shown that lower SES groups are as likely as higher ones to attempt smoking cessation but are less likely to be successful (Perelman et al., 2017). The lower success in the ability to quit smoking is being examined to find more effective evidence-based treatment for low-income populations (Evans et al., 2015).

At the population level, increases in total income and reductions in poverty levels are "strongly associated with subsequent improvements in population health" (Aday, 2005, p. 190). This is proven out in a systematic review of maternal mortality outcomes. Financial barriers and lack of maternal health education for the mother and partner were shown to negatively impact maternal-child outcomes (Banke-Thomas, Banke-Thomas, & Ameh, 2017). Income affects health, and poor health can affect the income of an individual as well as that of a nation (see Chapter 6).

Uninsured and Underinsured

If the uninsured are also classified as a vulnerable population, even more Americans join the ranks, because the majority of those without health insurance are working adults who are not eligible for Medicaid or Medicare.

- The percentage of uninsured in 2013 was estimated at 16.7%. In 2016, 10.3% of people in the United States were without health insurance (Kaiser Family Foundation, 2019).
- The decline in the percentage of uninsured is attributable in great part to the Patient Protection and Affordable Care Act (ACA), signed into law by President Barack Obama on March 23, 2010. This law requires most U.S. citizens and legal residents to have health insurance coverage, along with many other provisions (Knickman & Kovner, 2015). See Chapter 6 & 13 for more on the ACA.
- Although the improvement in health insurance coverage is encouraging, disparities in access to health care continue.
  - In 2014, 31 million people were underinsured in the United States, which was unchanged from 2010.
  - In 2003, only 1% of privately insured adults had a deductible of $3,000 or more, but that increased to 11% in 2014 (Collins, Rasmussen, Beutel, & Doty, 2015) and 13% in 2016 (Commonwealth Fund Report, 2017).
- Also, most health care experts feel that there will still be disparities in quality, access, and outcomes for those who are more vulnerable (Gwede et al., 2016).

How does having inadequate or no health insurance lead to poor health outcomes? As explained in Chapter 6, those with few or no resources in this area do not use early screenings and preventive measures, and they delay getting treatment in an effort to save money. Those without health insurance receive care only for the problem at hand and not always for underlying causes. They do not get regular physical examinations and may be inadequately immunized against common diseases. Thus, they are at risk for poorer general health. Also, when examination and subsequent treatment are delayed, diseases, such as cancer or cardiovascular illness, may result in earlier death.

Race and Ethnicity

The United States is a multiracial, multiethnic country. About one third of the population belongs to a racial or ethnic minority group, and this proportion will continue to increase, as minorities are projected to constitute more than half of all children by 2023 (Frey, 2018; Laun, 2019).

- Hispanics represent the largest minority group (16% of the total population, up from 13% in 2000 census), and they are also the fastest-growing group, with a lifetime average number of children per woman of 2.53, compared with 1.71 for White women (Pew Research Center, 2015).
- Blacks in the United States account for a higher proportion of new HIV diagnoses, those living with HIV, and those who have ever received an AIDS diagnosis, compared with other races and ethnicities (CDC, 2015b). In 2016, Blacks accounted for 44% of HIV diagnoses, though they comprise only 12% of the U.S. population (CDC, 2015b).
- There is a disparity in the prevalence of preterm births in the United States, with 12.7% of infants born to Black mothers being premature compared with only 8.0% among White mothers (McKinnon et al., 2016).
- Infant mortality is much higher among African Americans at 10.9% when compared with 4.9% among White Americans (U.S. Department of Health and Human Services, 2019).
- Hypertension increases the prevalence of cardiovascular disease outcomes, such as stroke, congestive heart failure, kidney failure, and cognitive impair-

ment/dementia, and Blacks are disproportionately more affected by hypertension and its comorbid conditions. In the United States, the prevalence of hypertension is 40% to 50% in African Americans compared with 25% to 30% in Whites (Osei & Galliard, 2017).

- Blacks have higher prevalence of heart failure, by twofold, stroke, by twofold to fourfold, and kidney failure, by twofold to fourfold, in the United States (Osei & Gaillard, 2017).

Why does simply being a member of a racial or ethnic minority group make someone vulnerable? The reasons are complex and just beginning to be understood. Williams et al. (2016) found in a review of the scientific research that racism affects the health of minority racial populations in multiple ways.

- Institutional racism in policies and procedures reduced access to housing, neighborhood and educational quality, employment opportunities, and other societal resources.
- Cultural racism affects economic status and health by creating a policy environment adverse to equal policies.
- Experiences of racial discrimination are a type of psychosocial stressor that can increase health risks.

Recent immigrants have healthier exercise and dietary patterns than do those born inside the United States.

- A systematic review of acculturation, obesity, and health behaviors among recent migrants showed that there was evidence across multiple studies for a positive association between acculturation (measured with standard measures or as duration of stay) and obesity (Alidu & Grunfeld, 2017).
- Others note the generational link between minority group membership and low educational attainment (e.g., father's education level) and the tie between education and health (Hahn & Truman, 2015).
- A majority of Hispanics and Blacks have spent a lifetime at a lower level of educational attainment and continue to lag behind in most areas.
- One bright spot is that the percentages of Hispanics and African Americans enrolled in college have increased significantly over the past two decades. From 1997 to 2016, for instance, the percentage of Black young adults enrolled in college has increased by 6% and the percentage of Hispanic young adults has increased by 17% (Digest of Education Statistics, 2016).

VULNERABILITY AND INEQUALITY IN HEALTH CARE

Various social factors, known as the social determinants of health, including SES, affect a person's vulnerability to poor health. Specific areas in which inequities in health outcomes result from these social factors are known as health disparities.

Social Determinants of Health

The World Health Organization has defined the **social determinants of health** as "...factors such as where we live, the state of our environment, genetics, our income and education level, and our relationships with friends and family all have considerable impacts on health...," including the available health system (World Health Organization, 2020b, para. 1). Commonly acknowledged factors, such as social norms or attitudes (e.g., discrimination, racism); exposure to crime, violence, and social disorder; and concentrated poverty, are associated with health outcomes and are recognized as social determinants of health (CDC, 2015a; USDHHS, n.d.). The connection between social inequalities and health is illustrated in the Bay Area Regional Health Inequalities Initiative (BARHII) conceptual framework: http://barhii.org/framework (BARHII, 2015).

The unequal distribution of these factors among certain groups is thought to contribute to health disparities that are persistent and pervasive. The IOM report *For the Public's Health: The Role of Measurement in Action and Accountability* called for addressing the underlying factors, not only the data, related to morbidity and mortality (2010). When we address health disparities, we must consider these social determinants and work on all levels—individual, aggregate, community, and population—to reduce them.

Social determinants of health are related to both morbidity and mortality. Quantified deaths that could be attributed to social factors in the United States were reported:

- The authors found that life expectancy in the United States for the top and bottom 1% of the income distribution varies by 15 years for men and 10 years for women (Price, Khubchandani, & Webb, 2018).
- Moreover, it is estimated that only 10% to 15% of the increase in length of life in Western nations can be attributed to improved medical care, according to Raphael's classic treatise (2003).
- Between 2001 and 2014, life expectancy increased by 2.34 years for men and 2.91 years for women in the top 5% of the income distribution, but by only 0.32 years for men and 0.04 years for women in the bottom 5% (Chetty et al., 2017).
- Life expectancy for low-income individuals varied substantially across local areas. In the bottom income quartile, life expectancy differed by approximately 4.5 years between areas with the highest and lowest longevity (Chetty et al., 2017).
- Geographic differences in life expectancy for individuals in the lowest income quartile were significantly correlated with health behaviors such as smoking. Life expectancy for low-income individuals was correlated with the local area fraction of immigrants, fraction of college graduates, and government expenditures (Chetty et al., 2017).
- Life expectancy can also be linked to where you live as predicted through zip code (Robert Wood Johnson Foundation, 2018a, 2018b).

To improve the health of disadvantaged groups, early public health efforts addressed determinants of health such as sanitation and poverty, along with living conditions and other environmental issues, as noted in Chapters 3 and 9. The present need to address underlying

BOX **23-5** *HEALTHY PEOPLE 2030*

Social Determinants of Public Health

- Economic stability
- Education access and quality
- Health care access and quality
- Neighborhood and built environment
- Social and community context

Reprinted from USDHHS (2020). *Social determinants of health.* Retrieved from https://health.gov/healthypeople/objectives-and-data/social-determinants-health

social conditions to improve health status is borne out by current research on race and socioeconomic class (Hahn & Truman, 2015). It is now widely acknowledged that to truly have an impact on the health of the population, there is a need to improve social conditions (Bharmal, Derose, Felician, & Weden, 2015; CDC, 2018). Political action and participatory action research are vital tools in reducing the effects of these conditions, as are methods of community empowerment (World Health Organization, 2020b; see Chapters 4 and 13). Healthy People 2030 addresses the context to which people's lives influence their health (see the social determinants of health in Box 23-5).

Socioeconomic Gradient of Health

In a series of large-scale, longitudinal studies in England, the now classic Whitehall studies, British civil servants were divided into socioeconomic groups based on their occupational status, from executives to unskilled workers. What the investigators discovered was an improvement in mortality and morbidity rates as the level of one's occupation and pay increased. Those at the lowest levels had the poorest health, but as they moved up the salary scale and occupational level, their health improved. What makes this so interesting is that all of the workers had basic health insurance coverage and free medical care—no real problems with access to health care existed. Although less pronounced, even when the researchers adjusted for diet, exercise, and smoking, the gradient persisted (Marmot, Ryff, Bumpass, Shipley, & Marks, 1997; Marmot & Wilkinson, 2006). The investigators of one study found higher prevalence of heart disease for all participants at the lower end of the social stratus. The researchers also found death rates for diabetic participants to be about 200% higher in the lowest social group when compared with the highest (Chaturvedi, 1998).

A U.S. study, following up on children of Framingham study subjects, found an association between lower socioeconomic position and coronary heart disease. A later study found higher odds of smoking, excess consumption of alcohol, and obesity, which "may contribute to adult cardio metabolic disease" by the predisposition of these unhealthy behaviors (Loucks et al., 2009; Non et al., 2016, para. 5).

This direct relationship between social class or income and health has been termed the **socioeconomic gradient** (Hajizadeh, Mitnitski, & Rockwood, 2016). It has been found in populations around the world, although not always unfailingly, and has been related to

- Poor health outcomes regarding cardiovascular disease in European countries (Lenhart, Wiemken, Hanlon, Perkett, & Patterson, 2017)
- Cancer incidence, mortality, and survival in Western countries (Olver & Roder, 2017)
- Injury rates, such as blunt and penetrating injuries (Chikani et al., 2015)
- Increased burden of chronic illness among Kenyan, South African, and Indian citizens (Mendenhall, Kohrt, Norris, Ndetei, & Prabhakaran, 2017)
- Outcomes of adult asthma, chronic obstructive pulmonary disease, and rhinitis (Torres-Duque, 2017)
- Behaviors, such as smoking, that are highest among those who are from the working class and who have low-income and low educational levels (Psaltopoulou et al., 2017)
- Chronic conditions in older adults, with individuals in the poorest neighborhoods in Canada being more likely to have more chronic conditions and die as a result of those conditions (Lane, Maxwell, Grunier, Bronskill, & Wodchis, 2015)
- Higher rates of in-hospital mortality in U.S. pediatric patients and Iranian acute coronary syndrome patients (Abbasi et al., 2015)
- Lower levels of education and income being associated with higher rates of low birth weight, whereas higher levels of occupation and income being associated with lower rates of infant mortality (Elder, Goddeeris, & Haider, 2016)

Health Disparities

Health disparities are differences in the quantity of disease, burden of disease, and other adverse health conditions present in different groups (Zhang et al., 2017).

- Health disparities may be unavoidable, such as health-damaging behaviors that are chosen by an individual despite health education and counseling efforts, but most are thought to be due to inequities that can be corrected (Mueller, Purnell, Mensah, & Cooper, 2015).
- A long-held belief about health inequities, adopted by the World Health Organization (2017), is that they are unnecessary and avoidable as well as unjust and unfair, so that the resulting health inequalities also lead to inequity in health.
- Health disparities can be objectively viewed as a disproportionate burden of morbidity, disability, and mortality found in a specific portion of the population in contrast to another.
- The topic of social determinants of health was added to *Healthy People 2020* (Office of Disease Prevention and Health Promotion, 2020a). The *National Healthcare Quality and Disparities Report* revealed that disparities persist, but several racial disparities in rates of childhood immunizations and adverse events associated with procedures have been eliminated (AHRQ, 2015).
- Reported disparities exist in the areas of quality of health care, access to care, levels and types of care,

and care settings; they exist within subpopulations (e.g., elderly, women, children, rural residents, disabled) and across clinical conditions.

- Promoting healthy choices does not eliminate health disparities; action must be taken to improve the conditions within people's environments. That is why Health People 2030 has increased its focus on SDOH (USDHHS, n.d.). In fact, one of Healthy People's 2030 goals focuses on SDOH: "Create social, physical, and economic environments that promote attaining the full potential for health and well-being for all" (USDHHS, n.d., para 4).

Poor access to quality care and overt discrimination are examples of disparities. Discrimination can occur during service delivery if health care providers are biased against a specific group or hold stereotypical beliefs about that group. Providers may also not be confident about providing care for a racial or ethnic group with whom they are unfamiliar. Language may be a problem, as can cultural values and norms that are unfamiliar to providers. Patients can also react to providers in a way that promotes disparities; patients may not trust the information given to them and may not follow it as explained, leading to inadequate care (Mueller et al., 2015).

Access to Care

The landmark IOM (2003) report *Unequal Treatment: Confronting Racial and Ethnic Disparities in Health Care* noted a large body of research highlighting the higher morbidity and mortality rates among all racial and ethnic minority groups when compared with Whites. This report drew attention to an issue that continues today and remains relevant. Differences in health care access were also explained, whether due to inadequate or no health insurance, problems getting health care, poorer quality of care, fewer choices in where to go for care, or the lack of a regular health care provider. For instance, because there are fewer numbers of health care providers in minority neighborhoods, finding a primary care provider is more difficult for those living in these areas. Providing low-cost or free clinics within low-income neighborhoods has been shown to improve the management of chronic conditions and decrease rates of hospitalization (Hutchinson et al., 2018).

Progress in this area has remained slow. The Institutes of Medicine's Progress Report highlights the following mechanisms to address 21st century health care needs: better coordination of care, nurses to practice to the full extent of their license, increased educational levels of nurses (including more doctorate and bachelor's prepared nurses), increased workforce diversity, and nurse engagement in leadership roles (National Academy of Sciences, 2019).

Residential segregation, although illegal, still exists and can play a role in health disparities. Many vulnerable populations, especially racial and ethnic minority groups and low-income populations, find health care at safety-net hospitals and community clinics where they are at the mercy of balanced budgets and vast bureaucratic systems (AHRQ, 2015). However, more recent data showed that the ACA is improving access for uninsured individuals to safety-net clinics in states with expanded Medicaid coverage (Angier et al., 2015).

Other geographic factors can affect access to health care services. For example, a classic study by O'Mahony et al. (2008) found that only 25% of pharmacies in non-White neighborhoods, compared with 72% in predominately White neighborhoods, stocked sufficient opioid drugs to meet the needs of palliative care patients in different New York neighborhoods.

Health care access is also problematic for other vulnerable groups. For example, services and resources for the mentally ill and substance abusers are often fragmented and inadequate, as are those for abusing families and homeless persons. Refugees and immigrants may have difficulty finding affordable and easily accessible health care, largely because of their lack of health insurance and the need to find care at free clinics or emergency rooms (Richard et al., 2016). When vulnerable individuals cannot get appropriate health care or treatment for illness or disease, for whatever reason, they are more likely to have health deficits.

Quality of Care

Quality of care is another area in which health disparities persist. One aspect of quality care is the comfort level patients have with their providers. Research indicates that racial and ethnic minority clients feel more comfortable and satisfied with care from a health care provider who comes from the same racial and/or ethnic group (Fig. 23-6; AHRQ, 2015). However, a shortage of ethnically diverse health care providers exists. Despite racial and ethnic minorities constituting 37% of the U.S. population, only 19% of registered nurses are from minority racial and ethnic groups (American Association of Colleges of Nursing, 2015).

Lack of quality health care services is common among racial and ethnic minority groups. A recent study on Black and White older adult Medicare general surgical patients showed that Blacks had higher 30-day mortality, in-hospital mortality, in-hospital complications, and failure-to-rescue rates, longer length of stay, and more 30-day readmissions (Silber et al., 2015). The researchers suggested that poorer health of Blacks on surgical presentation was a major contributing cause for the disparities (Silber et al., 2015).

Communication can also be a factor in poor quality of care. Marginalized vulnerable populations, such as substance abusers, at-risk mothers and infants, abusing families, suicide- and homicide-prone individuals, and the mentally ill or disabled, may feel they are treated as "second-class

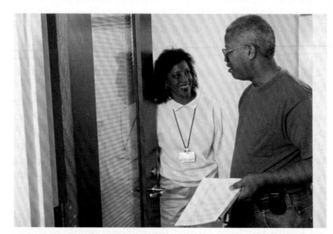

FIGURE 23-6 Racial and ethnic minority clients often prefer health care providers from the same racial and ethnic background.

citizens," and cultural barriers and misunderstandings can lead to a discontinuation of recommended regimens. Poor health outcomes may result as effectiveness of health care for vulnerable populations is not often considered or even well defined (Hutchinson et al., 2018).

WORKING WITH VULNERABLE POPULATIONS

Through the day-to-day provision of care and participation in larger efforts in the community, the nurse can help improve health outcomes for vulnerable populations (see Box 23-6).

The Role of Public Health Nurses

C/PHNs can work to improve the health of vulnerable populations by empowerment, facilitating external support from patient's family and friends, and engaging in evidence-based practice.

Empowerment

Because vulnerability often equates with feelings of powerlessness, the actions of C/PHNs can either promote engagement or destroy chances for rapport. C/PHNs can use **empowerment strategies** in their work with clients once trust and rapport have been established (Box 23-7). The personal values, experiences, characteristics, and actions of both nurses and clients influence the speed at which this process takes place and the eventual level of connection. Helping clients identify their fears and clearly defining the C/PHN role with the client and family are also important.

Building and preserving relationships with clients is a central focus of C/PHN home visits. It requires building trust and rapport and helping them to feel accepted, engaged, and ready. The building phase involves working with individual clients to improve their social connections, build their strengths, and work toward their goals. Building self-efficacy, motivation, and health literacy are essential in this stage, as are helping them with coping skills and giving encouragement as they build resilience.

Extending strategies include helping clients to use new strategies and apply them in other situations. Phone calls and other methods of checking in with clients are used to help them change behaviors and access services. Negotiation and teamwork approaches are helpful in this stage. Keeping a focus on solutions rather than problems helps build client strengths. Six principles of solution-focused nursing, built on mental health nursing concepts, are helpful (McAllister, 2010):

- Focus on the person, not the problem.
- Do not focus solely on problems. Begin with an emphasis on strengths, as this can build client hope and self-confidence.
- Resilience is just as important as vulnerability.
- Work to change unjust societal and cultural forces.
- Nurses should assist clients as they adapt and grow and not focus solely on care and illness.
- Encourage a proactive approach that uses the three stages of client involvement: joining, building, and extending.

These solution-focused nursing principles of client empowerment are exemplified in a study directed by

BOX **23-6** QSEN: FOCUS ON QUALITY

Patient-Centered Care for Working With Vulnerable Populations

Patient-Centered Care: Recognize the patient or designee as the source of control and full partner in providing compassionate and coordinated care based on respect for patient's preferences, values, and needs (Cronenwett et al., 2007, p. 123).

(See https://qsen.org/competencies/pre-licensure-ksas/#quality_improvement for the knowledge, skills, and attitudes associated with this QSEN competency.)

C/PHNs work with many vulnerable groups, including the homeless population. Vulnerable groups within the community may be marginalized and lack access to quality health care services. To build rapport and trust, nurses must provide respectful understanding and care while focusing on the needs of the client. How do the QSEN competencies assist nurses in demonstrating patient-centered care to the homeless?

Students in a community health clinic spent time working with homeless clients and their families in a homeless center. Some students had limited previous exposure to diverse populations and were aware only of stereotypes and misconceptions regarding this population. Homeless women heads-of-household and their children made up 60% of the population using this facility. Students were unaware of the variance of demographics and backgrounds regarding this vulnerable group.

In conjunction with the homeless center, student identified clients' needs and provided an educational health fair. Local agencies supplied free needed items; education stations were then created to support heath issues surrounding the donated items (e.g., an oral health education station provided free travel-size toothbrushes).

While offering health education, students engaged with clients and their families, which gave them the opportunity to learn about vulnerability. One student had a conversation with a mother about how she became homeless. The woman shared that after her husband died, she had no family or support systems for herself or her child with severe asthma. The woman lost her home and insurance, so she was unable to pay for her child's medical bills. Another student talked with a man about how long he had been homeless. This man was a veteran and suffered from PTSD and drug misuse; alienated from his family and friends, he had been homeless for several years.

In speaking with clients, students identified issues that prevented use of shelters by some clients, such as lack of privacy or rules prohibiting pet dogs. Students learned valuable skills related to working with a vulnerable group and breaking through fears related to stereotypes and biases.

Source: Cronenwett et al. (2007).

BOX 23-7 Community/Public Health Nurse Actions to Promote Client Empowerment

Which community/public health nursing activities/actions are most effective in promoting empowerment among nurses' vulnerable clients? In Falk-Raphael's (2001) well-known qualitative study of public health nurses (C/PHNs) and their clients, several themes were noted as components of the C/PHN role:

- *Empowerment* is "an active, internal process of growth" that is reached by actualizing the full potential inherent within each client, and this occurs "within the context of a nurturing nurse–client relationship" (p. 4). C/PHNs describe the process of empowerment as a two-way street with clients not only gaining knowledge and skills and "acting on informed choices" but also further empowering the nurse to continue the work of the empowerment (p. 6).
- *Having a client-centered approach*, denoted by flexibility in dealing with clients, for example, "meeting them where they are," "communicating at their level," and "backing off and following client's agenda" (p. 6)
- *Developing a trusting relationship* based on mutual respect and dignity, for example, clients as active partners with the C/PHN assuming more or less responsibility as needed; being empathetic, nonjudgmental, and "creating a safe environment" (p. 7)
- *Employing advocacy*, both at an individual level as well as political advocacy, for example, using their role and power as a professional to cut through bureaucratic red tape, connecting clients with available community resources, supporting clients in reaching their health goals, making their expertise available, and being a client resource as someone who is open and "available" (p. 8)
- *Being a teacher and role model*, using a variety of strategies and providing opportunities for clients to safely practice new skills. For example, using strategies such as teaching classes, providing individual coaching, providing positive reinforcement and support, demonstrating skills such as assertiveness, and encouraging community action/participation are helpful
- *Capacity building* through encouraging and supporting of clients' work toward attaining health goals, for example, "reflective listening and an empathetic approach" focusing on strengths, not limitations; facilitating client "self-exploration" and providing encouragement for them to "act on their choices" while being "realistic about barriers to success"; or having expectations for client accountability regarding their decisions and actions (p. 9)

Source: Falk-Raphael (2001).

the American Academy of Nursing. In examining the commonalities of nurse-designed models of health care, the authors of this study found four common elements (Mason, Jones, Roy, Sullivan, & Wood, 2015, p. 548):

- Health holistically defined
- Individual-, family-, and community-centric approaches to care
- Relationship-based care
- Group and public health interventions (Box 23-8)

While empowering clients, nurses should also remember to empower themselves through collaboration with others and self-care. Working with disadvantaged populations can be challenging and exhausting. Often, novice community health nurses feel overwhelmed and suffer "compassion fatigue" when confronted with the crushing realities that their vulnerable, disenfranchised clients face on a daily basis. Feelings of guilt sometimes surface when nurses contrast their own life experiences with those of their clients. To be effective in working with vulnerable populations, it is often more helpful to donate money and items on a group level rather than an individual level and to work for substantial changes in community attitudes and policies. Also, it is vital to remain grounded to continue to have the necessary energy and compassion (Box 23-9).

BOX 23-8 PERSPECTIVES

A C/PHN's Viewpoint on Community/Public Health Nursing

I have been a C/PHN for many years and been fortunate enough to work with various populations. I remember a case when I learned that although experience is a valuable asset, sometimes this contributes to assessment miscues. I had an established relationship with a socioeconomically disadvantaged postpartum client, who was experiencing anxiety, feelings of being overwhelmed, and insomnia. The interventions that I had successfully used for so many other moms in similar situations with postpartum depression had failed with this client. It was not until I inquired about a picture of my client, Nancy, in her military uniform that she shared with me that she had served for a few years in the Middle East. She further stated that she did not like to discuss her past, she regretted not being physically able to continue her military career, and she just wanted to "get some sleep." Long story short, we were able to get Nancy into a Veteran's Administration (VA) residential treatment program for substance abuse and medical treatment for traumatic brain injury (TBI). I learned through this encounter that experience coupled with a patient-centered assessment, minus my internal preconceptions, results in the best outcomes for patients. Nancy had more than the usual stressors affecting her, and I was glad that I was finally able to pick up on those clues and address her needs more completely.

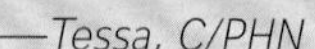
—*Tessa, C/PHN*

BOX **23-9** EVIDENCE-BASED PRACTICE

Caring and Compassion

Dmytryshyn, Jack, Ballantyne, Wahoush, and MacMillan (2015), studying public health nurses (C/PHNs) working with a Nurse–Family Partnership program, found that compassion fatigue could be problematic for nurses working with vulnerable young mothers in this long-term home visiting program (described in more detail in Chapter 4). C/PHNs generally found the nurse–client relationship rewarding but needed to adapt their philosophy and definition of client success to see clients as the experts of their own individual lives. In this qualitative study, C/PHNs expressed personal costs of worrying about clients and doubting their own effectiveness in their ability to address concerns of clients. When they were able to shift the focus to the client, they reported greater satisfaction in the nurse–client relationship and in watching the successes of their clients over time.

Source: Dmytryshyn et al. (2015).

In one study, outcomes of empowerment for clients included increased self-esteem and confidence, improved self-efficacy, and the ability to "reframe situations in a positive way" (Falk-Raphael, 2001, p. 10). Clients also subsequently made better choices regarding their health and used resources more appropriately. They were better able to seek information and services and became more politically active. Clients' focus became more proactive than reactive, and they felt that they could communicate more effectively to define boundaries or express feelings. Consequently, clients were also better able to collaborate with their health care providers, becoming more trusting partners in care by demonstrating ownership for their actions and their health. Some clients noted a newfound ability to see their communities in a more holistic way and looked for ways to change things for the better. A large part of C/PHN practice is to work with the vulnerable and encourage them to become more self-reliant and responsible for their health.

Facilitating External Support

The degree of external support clients have, along with their temperament and other individual factors, affects their ability to cope with stress and adverse situations. The support can be from family members, neighbors, friends, teachers, or others. C/PHNs can help clients establish external support at both the individual and population levels (Boxes 23-10 and 23-11). (For an interactive map that provides information on the degree to which specific U.S. communities are affected by external stresses on human health, see the CDC's Social Vulnerability Index at https://svi.cdc.gov/.)

Using Evidence to Reduce Vulnerability

Community health nurses can help vulnerable populations, communities, individuals, and families reduce their vulnerability by using evidence from research, expert

BOX **23-10** STORIES FROM THE FIELD

A View of Disasters

When disaster strikes the communities of those who are struggling to survive, the effects are devastating, and the recovery is long and challenging. Communities with poorly built homes, without strong foundations or storm windows, are less safe during tornadoes and hurricanes. Floods impact low-lying, low-income neighborhoods the hardest (Lowrey, 2019). The high cost of living in California has encouraged low-income individuals to migrate to less expensive and remote fire-prone areas (Lowrey, 2019).

In 2018, the most destructive fire in California history incinerated the town of Paradise within a matter of hours. The poor were the hardest hit, and 2 months after the disaster, because of inadequate housing for the poor, there were still hundreds living in shelters. Many of those impacted were elderly and disabled, living in trailer homes. Local hospitals and other health care facilities were also incinerated, impacting access to health care. A nurse who was interviewed after the disaster, referring to the struggling poor impacted by the devastating fire, likened the incident to a house of cards; when removing a card, the whole house collapses (Lowrey, 2019).

In 2017, Hurricane Harvey caused catastrophic flooding and many deaths in Houston, Texas. The New York Times interviewed a survivor of this disaster 1 year later. She spoke about the experience of losing her home and living in a trailer. The survivor had no savings to use for recovery, and the support she received from the government, nonprofit groups, and volunteers was not enough for her and her family to return to a sense of normalcy. The survivor and her family were left feeling sad, broken, and confused (Fernandez, 2018).

In 2005, Hurricane Katrina broke through the levee system in New Orleans, Louisiana, causing massive flooding. Many of the poor residents did could not flee because they did not have a car, and they didn't have money to pay for a hotel and other necessities. Health issues related to the aftermath of the hurricane included concerns about contamination of local waters with solid waste, pesticide use for vector control from an abundance of mosquitoes, and reduction in air quality from mold and dust. The poor bore the brunt of the disaster, and the few facilities that existed to quickly help the victims became miserable and dangerous places (Schake, Sommers, Subramanian, Waters, & Arcava, 2019). Moving from large shelters to trailer homes negatively affected the mental health of some survivors and caused a great strain on family relationships. A Hurricane Katrina survivor who was born and raised in a housing project in New Orleans was relocated, as many were, to Houston, where she had no family, social support, nor means of transportation (Voice of a Witness, 2019).

Source: Fernandez (2018); Lowrey (2019); Schake et al. (2019); Voice of a Witness (2019).

BOX 23-11 Foundational Public Health Services (FPHS) Model

The FPHS model is a conceptual framework describing the capacities and programs that state and local health departments should be able to provide to all communities and for which costs can be estimated.

Foundational Public Health Service

Foundational Areas

- Environmental Health[a]
- Chronic Disease
- Injury Prevention
- Maternal, Child Health
- Access Linkage
- Communicable Disease

Foundational Capabilities

- All Hazards
- Communications
- Policy Development
- Assessment
- Community Partnership
- Organizational Competencies

Other Health/Services

- Critical Care
- Environmental Protection[a]
- Behavioral Health
- Disability Related
- Other Services

[a]"Environmental Health" refers to prevention (permitting, education, regulation) activities. "Environmental Protection" refers to remediation and environmental quality.

Adapted with permission from Resnick, B. A., Fisher, J. S., Colrick, I. P., and Leider, J. P. (2017). The foundational public health services as a framework for estimating spending. *American Journal of Preventive Medicine, 53*(5), 646–651.

opinion, and best practices (see Chapter 4 on evidence-based practice). Often, evidence is embedded in policies, procedures, and clinical guidelines. Thus, the first place to locate evidence for practice is in the specific agency documentation for nursing practice. Sometimes, a community need is discovered that requires creative thinking and evidence-based interventions (Box 23-12).

Many areas for improvement of the lives of vulnerable populations lie in areas related to prevention and health promotion, as described above. Primary prevention is readily available in the form of immunizations for children, adolescents, and adults. Nursing activities to promote increasing immunization levels among vulnerable people will result in greater economic and social returns for the whole community. Similar is the involvement of nurses in smoking prevention and smoking cessation activities. Also, some vulnerable subpopulations require additional insight and experience, such as veterans (Box 23-13) and victims of human trafficking (Box 23-14).

Veterans who have experienced trauma may not recognize dysfunctional coping styles such as social isolation and mistrust of others as symptoms of mental health disorders but as functional coping strategies. Increase in alcohol and substance use has been shown to parallel and increase in PTSD symptoms (Koven, 2018). Military sexual trauma (MST) increases PTSD symptoms

BOX 23-12 POPULATION FOCUS

Improving Health Care Professionals' Caring for LGBTQ Persons

Karen and Lisa had been together for 17 years. They lived in a state where same sex marriage is not legal but they were registered domestic partners. Together they had three children ages 9, 11, and 15. Their children were conceived through artificial insemination. Two of the children were conceived by Lisa and one by Karen.

For their summer vacation, they decided to visit a well-known amusement complex for a week. Three days into their vacation, Karen suddenly complained of a severe headache and within minutes, was unresponsive. She was taken by ambulance to a local hospital.

When Lisa arrived at the hospital with their children, she was stopped by the emergency room admissions clerk, who said she needed her insurance information. After providing the information, she asked to see her partner. The admissions clerk found the charge nurse who asked Lisa what her relationship was to Karen. When Lisa told her they were partners, the charge nurse told her that only immediate family would be allowed in to see her and she was not considered family. Lisa tried to explain that she was Karen's only immediate family, that both her parents were dead and that they had been together for 17 years. Again, the charge nurse refused to allow her in. Lisa spent the next couple hours on the phone with friends back home, sending one of them to their home to find their official domestic partnership paperwork.

After the paperwork had been faxed to the admissions clerk, Lisa approached the charge nurse again asking to see Karen. In a condescending tone, the charge nurse told Lisa that her paperwork is not recognized in this state and she again refused to allow her to see Karen. She did, however, agree to allow the 9-year-old daughter (the only one of the children Karen gave birth to) to come into the emergency room, but Lisa was concerned that this would be too traumatic for her since she could not go with her nor could her older siblings.

Karen had been intubated immediately upon arrival to the emergency room and underwent CT imaging, which revealed a massive intracranial hemorrhage, likely from an AV malformation. Four hours after her arrival at the hospital, Karen died. Alone.

1. *How do you define family?*
2. *How would you react to this policy?*
3. *What would you do to meet the needs of the patient and the patient's family?*

—*Marla Seacrist, PhD, RN*

Source: National LGBT Health Education Center (2015, 2016, n.d.); The Fenway Institute (2015).

BOX 23-13 POPULATION FOCUS

Veterans Health

Veterans are a unique and diverse population in the community. There are approximately 20 million veterans living in the United States, with almost 2 million of those being women (VetPop, 2016). Veterans are older in comparison to non-Veterans (NCVAS, 2018), have shorter life expectancy, lower amounts of education, and household income when compared to the general U.S. population (NCVAS, 2017). The military culture (deployments, service commitments, training, and battlefield exposure) and the subsequent impact on the health of veterans and their families can only be experienced by this population. The current veteran population is diverse, with representation from varying gender and sexual orientations, ethnicities and races, ages, and geographies (Veterans Health Administration, 2018). These characteristics have historically resulted in greater health disparities and therefore constitute veterans as a vulnerable population. Veterans can experience long-lasting negative effects because of their time in the military. These negative effects are often the result of traumatic stress and can create vulnerabilities that result in mental health disorders, alcoholism, substance abuse, dysfunctional relationships, homelessness, depression, and unemployment (Koven, 2018).

Traumatic exposures can lead to posttraumatic stress disorder (PTSD). PTSD has been associated with an increased risk for depression, anxiety, attachment avoidance, obesity, type 2 diabetes, and substance abuse (Scherrer et al., 2018). PTSD has been associated with a nearly 200% increase in hospitalizations among active duty service members between 2006 and 2012, and it is a leading diagnosis in the U.S. Department of Veterans Affairs medical settings (Armenta et al., 2018). These statistics may underestimate the impact of PTSD because many service members in need of treatment might not seek care.

- Symptoms of PTSD and depression overlap significantly (Sher, Braqualais, & Casas, 2012).
- Common features of depression include diminished interest or participation in significant activities, irritability, sleep disturbance, difficulty concentrating, restricted range of affect, and social detachment (Sher et al., 2012).
- Veterans who live in rural communities are more socially isolated and are 20% more likely to commit suicide than veterans who live in urban areas (Mohatt et al., 2018).
- Obesity is twice as common in patients with PTSD compared to those without PTSD and those with PTSD were 30% more likely to report being diagnosed with type 2 diabetes than those without traumatic exposure (Scherrer et al., 2018).
- Traumatic brain injuries have resulted in frontal lobe deficits that are linked to impulsive behaviors such as aggression and violence (Kois, et al., 2018; Mohatt et al., 2018).

Cory Church, PhD, RN-BC

Source: Armenta et al. (2018); Kois et al. (2018); Koven (2018); Mohatt et al. (2018); NCVAS (2017, 2018); Scherrer et al. (2018); Sher et al. (2012); Veterans Health Administration (2018); VetPop (2016).

BOX 23-14 Human Trafficking

Each year, approximately 14,500 to 17,500 women, men, and children are trafficked into the United States for the purposes of forced labor or sexual exploitation (American Civil Liberties Union, 2018). The Global Slavery index (2018) estimates that on any given day in 2016, there were 403,000 people living in conditions of modern slavery in the United States, a prevalence of 1.3 victims of modern slavery for every thousand.

Human trafficking has significant effects on both physical and mental health. Victims of human trafficking rarely come forward to seek help because of language barriers, fear of the traffickers, and/or fear of law enforcement. Traffickers use force, fraud, or coercion to lure their victims and force them into labor or commercial sexual exploitation. Traffickers look for people who are susceptible for a variety of reasons, including psychological or emotional vulnerability, economic hardship, lack of social safety net, natural disasters, or political instability.

Victims of human trafficking often have untreated medical problems, including physical injuries associated with abuse and torture (e.g., burns, lacerations, missing or broken teeth), malnutrition, dehydration, substance use disorders, depression, anxiety, and PTSD (Nursing for Women's Health, 2016; Richards, 2014). It is estimated that 80% human trafficking victims are women and girls (Nursing for Women's Health, 2016). Female victims are at increased risk for gynecologic and obstetric problems, including persistent or untreated sexually transmitted infections, unintended pregnancies, repetitive abortions or miscarriages, trauma to the rectum or vagina, and infertility (Nursing for Women's Health, 2016; Richards, 2014).

Nurses are ideally positioned to screen, identify, care for, provide referral services for, and support victims of human trafficking. It is imperative for nurses who provide care to human trafficking victims to have knowledge of local organizations specializing in working with trafficked women; free health services (general practice, reproductive health, hospital, and mental health); sources of advice on housing and other social services; legal aid/immigration advice services; local churches/community support organizations; language training centers; and nongovernmental organizations in the victim's home country (U.S. Department of the State, 2018). Screening patients for human trafficking in private, safe, health care settings and, if needed, utilizing professional interpreter services are imperative in providing care to this vulnerable group of people. During interviews and care encounters with these victims, it is key for nurses to be respectful and nonjudgmental.

Source: American Civil Liberties Union (2018); Nursing for Women's Health (2016); Richards (2014); U.S. Department of the State (2018).

and attachment anxiety, causing issues with intimacy and trust (Holiday, et al., 2018). MST is defined by the Veterans Health Administration as sexual assault and repeated, threatening sexual harassment occurring during military service (Veterans Health Administration, 2018). The prevalence of MST among veterans is estimated to be 21.5% among women and 1.1% among men (Kimmerling et al., 2007).

Along with physical and psychological injuries, war has the capacity to affect veterans spiritually and morally. Veterans exposed to combat can experience moral injury. Moral injury has been defined as "perpetrating, failing to prevent, bearing witness to, or learning about acts that transgress deeply held moral beliefs and expectations" (Drescher et al., 2011, p. 10). Some of the symptoms reported among combat veterans with PTSD in the literature that arguably might be related to moral injury include (Drescher et al., 2011)

- Negative changes in ethical attitudes and behavior
- Change in or loss of spirituality, including negative attributions about God
- Guilt, shame, and forgiveness problems
- Anhedonia and dysphoria
- Reduced trust in others and in social/cultural contracts
- Aggressive behaviors
- Poor self-care or self-harm

A greater understanding of the emotional scars experienced by veterans and their greater risk for comorbidities will help improve and direct care, resulting in better outcomes.

Women veterans are also increasing in the community and are the fastest-growing population within the veteran community (U.S. Department of Veterans Affairs [USDVA], 2015). In the last 10 years, women enrolled in health care service through the Veterans Health Administration have doubled. Women veterans are younger and more racially and ethnically diverse in comparison with male veterans (Northern Center for Veteran's Analysis and Statistics [NCVAS], 2016). Higher numbers of female veterans have experienced MST (USDVA, 2010). The Veterans Health Administration is working to address strategic priorities in the areas of primary care, health education, and reproductive health. Each Veterans Health Administration health care system contains an MST coordinator and a Women Veterans Program manager to advise and advocate for female veterans' health care services. Nurses in both acute and primary care areas can seek out these services for their patients.

It is evident that Veterans have multiple determinants that affect health and access to care. The Veterans Health Administration health care system is working to improve disparities among vulnerable populations and increase access to care (USDVA, 2016). Nurses in all care settings can call the Veterans Health Administration to determine access and benefits for veterans. It is equally important for nurses to assess military service in patients and the impact of service on one's health.

The *Military Health History Pocket Card for Clinicians* (USDVA, 2017) provides an easy guide for clinicians to understand veterans' unique medical problems and concerns associated with military service. Nurses can ask, "Would it be ok if I talked with you about your military experience? Did you have any illnesses or injuries while in the service?" The pocket card can help nurses understand if veterans are seeking compensation and benefits for their care, or the current living situation of a veteran. These questions help a nurse determine the level of care needed for veterans in the community. Finally, the pocket card can help establish rapport and collaborative relationships with veterans (Box 23-15).

Improving Health Literacy

In addition to immunizations, smoking cessation, and other preventive interventions, the following topics are highlighted as evidence-based concepts shown to improve the health status of vulnerable populations: health literacy, access to nursing services, and policy.

People living in low-income communities often have low educational levels that are related to low literacy and low health literacy levels. An estimated 80 million

BOX **23-15** PERSPECTIVES

An Emergency Room Nurse's Viewpoint on Community/Public Health Nursing

I have been an emergency room nurse for several years and been fortunate enough to work with various populations. As a beginning emergency nurse, I did not understand that I would advocate for services and resources of patients that sought care in the emergency department. I remember a patient who was experiencing depression, anxiety, and having suicidal ideation came to the local county hospital. Fortunately, I read through the patient's social and medical history only to find that the patient had prior military experience and posttraumatic stress disorder. I brought up the patients' military experience, and this was a way for us to establish a nurse–patient relationship. After speaking with the veteran, I was able to determine that he wanted to seek mental health care through the Veterans Health Administration (VHA), but the nearest hospital was several hours away. Through collaboration with the nursing case manager, we were able to establish transportation to the VHA hospital for inpatient mental health treatment. I learned through this encounter that assessing military history in patients is key, especially in individuals in the community with mental health concerns. I was finally able to understand my role in advocating for resources and help for individuals in the community.

—*Cory Church, PhD, RN-BC*

Americans have limited health literacy. Because clients have difficulty obtaining, processing, and understanding health information, it is not surprising that low health literacy is associated with poorer health outcomes and poorer use of health care services. A systematic review found that low health literacy was associated with more emergency care use, higher hospitalization rates, fewer instances of influenza vaccine and mammography, poorer ability to read labels and interpret health messages, and greater inability to demonstrate appropriate medication administration, as well as higher mortality and poorer overall health status among senior citizens (AHRQ, 2015).

Assisting vulnerable groups and communities to improve health literacy is one approach for reducing vulnerability and improving health outcomes. Many cities have literacy programs that use volunteers to provide tutoring. This is an excellent way for nurses to give back to the community. Literacy training contributes to health literacy by improving reading, writing, and comprehension skills. A crucial aspect of improving health literacy is improvements in public schools so that more students graduate with adequate skills for higher education and employment. See Chapters 10 and 11 for more on health literacy.

Improving Access to Nursing Services

The benefits of home health are well known (Olds et al., 1997). Home visiting can be provided from almost any setting that provides services to communities. The usual settings are local health departments, home health care agencies, community-based hospice agencies, and visiting nurse associations. In addition, school nurses, ambulatory nurses, parish or faith-based nurses, and other nurses have recently provided limited home visiting services to clients or families seen in a variety of settings, including outpatient clinics, Head Start programs, places of worship, and health centers. Expanding home visiting to all vulnerable groups holds promise for improving the health of many individuals and communities (Fig. 23-7).

School-based health centers (SBHCs) are considered one of the most effective strategies for delivering preventive care, especially for difficult-to-reach populations such as adolescents. Numerous evaluations have shown that SBHCs achieve marked improvements in adolescent health care access when compared with that in other settings (Shackleton et al., 2016). These clinics are included in health care reform funding, largely because of their proven track record for accessibility and quality.

Nurse-led clinics (NLCs) have also increased access to care for communities and provided care that is more affordable, convenient, and with reduced patient waiting times. The nursing role in such clinics involves patient assessment, admission, health-related education, treatment and monitoring, discharge, and referral to other health care professionals. Findings indicate that NLCs were well received by patients, with positive experiences reported by patients (Randall, Crawford, Currie, River, & Betihavas, 2017). See Chapters 28 and 29. Improving access to nursing care in the community has been shown to have benefits for population and individual health.

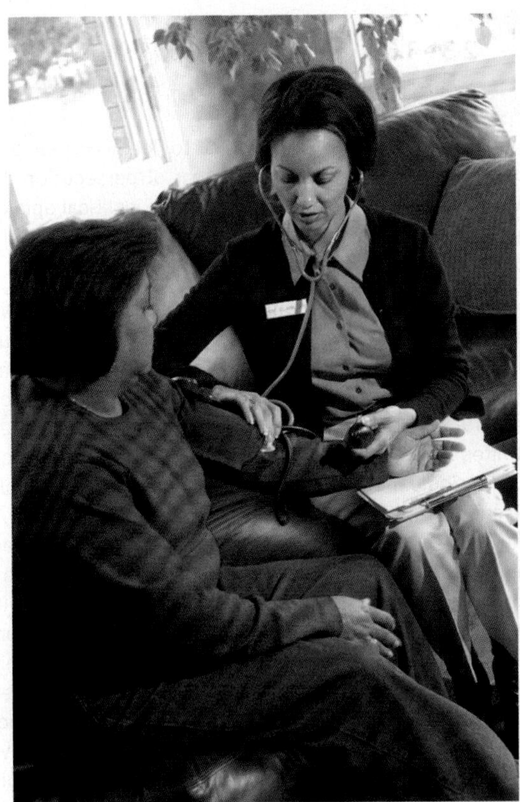

FIGURE 23-7 Home visiting has been shown to have positive outcomes for a variety of vulnerable populations. Results from over three decades of research have demonstrated that home visiting by registered nurses is effective in improving outcomes for low-income women and children.

Improving Health and Public Policy

Policies to reduce vulnerability for individuals, families, and communities have been shown to be effective at all levels: local, state, and national. Policy based on evidence is an important component of reducing vulnerability for communities and individuals. This section addresses health and public policy, including policy in schools, cities, counties, and health care settings. Policy includes social, economic, environmental, and health aspects. See Chapter 13 for an expansive discussion of policy.

Small changes in policy can make a big difference in outcomes for vulnerable communities. For example, policies to provide healthy foods in school vending machines provide healthier choices for all students, not just those considered vulnerable. Mandatory physical activity time for school children contributes to preventing obesity and enhancing learning in all children and it is essential that future research and policy makers continue to recognize the school environment as a way to improve health for all (Cisse-Egbuonye et al., 2016; Owen, Kerner, Newson, & Fairclough, 2017).

Communities that lack safe places for physical activities need to have attention directed to the appropriate governing bodies, such as the city council or the department of recreation. Community residents can be effective in bringing about change that improves a total community (Hood, Gennuso, Swain, & Catlin, 2016).

BOX **23-16** POPULATION FOCUS

Challenges for Community/Public Health Nursing Related to Refugee Resettlement

"A refugee is a person who has had to flee his or her country of origin due to a well-founded fear of persecution due to war, race, religion, ethnicity, nationality, political opinion, or association with a particular group." (UNHCR, 1951 Refugee Convention)

Currently, there are large numbers of displaced people worldwide. The United Nations High Commission for Refugees (UNHCR) registered 70.8 million displaced persons, 25.9 million refugees, and 3.5 million asylum seekers in its database for the year 2019 (UNHCR, 2020). Refugees granted resettlement in the United States are among the most vulnerable refugee cases, including single mothers, children, the elderly, survivors of violence and torture, and people with acute medical needs.

Refugee women, in particular, have been exposed to extreme levels of poverty, deprivation, violence, and trauma, which often remain unaddressed after resettlement (COE, 2020). Displacement from one's home and country of origin, loss of family through civil unrest or other traumatic events, as well as loss of familiar cultural norms are enormous challenges for this population (UNHCR, 2020). Further stressors include concerns about poor job opportunities and a fear of poverty. Low literacy skills, language barriers, differences in cultural practices, and lack of knowledge about health care limit access to physical and mental health care services (Riggs, Yelland, Duell-Piening, & Brown, 2016). A lack of culturally appropriate mental health services, providers, and psychosocial programs to address these issues further complicate provision of care for this population.

When assessing the needs of a local population, nurses need to take into consideration both the traumatic events that individuals have experienced as well as the resiliency that they demonstrate in adapting to their new homes. Innovation and creativity are key in developing appropriate interventions for delivery of care to the resettled refugee population. To be effective, community interventions and quality improvement programs must be designed in collaboration with local refugee resettlement organizations that have expertise in working with this population. Appropriate nurse-led interventions might include psychosocial support groups (Felsman, 2016), health literacy programming for English as a Second Language (ESL) classes, individual health coaching for persons with chronic illness, and doula services for pregnant refugee women.

THE STORY OF ESTER (NAME CHANGED FOR PRIVACY)

Rebels kidnapped Ester's husband in the Democratic Republic of Congo during the civil war one evening. Soon after, rebel forces came back, took her and her children to the forest, and attempted to rape her and her daughter. When she resisted, the rebels shot her in the hip, crippling her. The rebel leader kidnapped her daughter and took her as his wife. Her son, niece, and nephew ran into the forest. She was rescued and taken to a hospital by a kind person on a bicycle. She eventually made her way to a UNHCR refugee encampment, where she registered as an official refugee and lived for many years.

Ester now lives in the United States in a small city, learning how to negotiate a new language, culture, foods, and health care system. She did eventually find her son and speaks to him by phone when she can. Wheelchair bound, she struggles to make a living; her goal is to reunite her family in America, but it will take a lot of money.

What is the best plan of care for Ester as a new refugee?

Irene Felsman, DNP, MPH, RN

Source: COE (2020); Felsman (2016); Riggs et al. (2016); UNHCR (2020).

One model that addresses both individual and social determinants of health is the County Health Rankings Model (Fig. 1-3; Robert Wood Johnson Foundation, 2018a).

SOCIAL JUSTICE AND PUBLIC HEALTH NURSING

Social justice occurs when a society provides for the overall health and well-being of all people by treating people fairly. It involves an equal societal bearing of burdens and reaping of benefits, and it is a widely held view that social justice is the foundation of public health nursing (Box 23-16; Matwick and Woodgate, 2017).

- Community health nurses who practice social justice have broad and holistic views of health; they have strong convictions that health care is a basic human right and that improving the health of communities is an example of social justice.
- Social justice ensures the distribution of resources that benefits **marginalized populations** and holds in check the self-interest of more privileged populations. Impartiality is the goal.
- For instance, C/PHNs concerned with social justice include socially marginalized and vulnerable populations (e.g., criminal justice involved, undocumented residents) in their influenza pandemic planning processes. Not to do so would constitute discrimination and would be morally indefensible.

SUMMARY

- Vulnerable populations are at risk for poor health outcomes, including increased risk for morbidity and mortality.
- Various models or theoretical frameworks examine personal and environmental resources and risks relative to vulnerability.

- Leading factors that make aggregates vulnerable are poverty, age, gender, race or ethnicity, being uninsured or underinsured, being a single parent, and having little or no education.
- Social determinants of health are factors strongly associated with health outcomes and include social norms or attitudes, such as discrimination and racism; exposure to crime, violence, and social disorder; and concentrated poverty.
- The socioeconomic gradient, a direct relationship between social class/income and health, has been repeatedly demonstrated in research conducted around the world.
- Health disparities are defined as differences in access to quality health care and in health outcomes, particularly along income/class and racial/ethnic lines, and are usually characterized as avoidable and unfair.
- To be effective, C/HNs must establish a sense of trust and rapport with their clients by finding common ground.
- Empowerment strategies with individual clients can help them to meet their full potential while also providing empowerment to the nurses working with them.
- Community health nurses can provide individual support as well as support and leadership for vulnerable communities.
- Nurses can use evidence-based practice when addressing health disparities among vulnerable populations.
- C/PHNs should be concerned with improving the health literacy, access to health care, and health outcomes through political action.
- C/PHNs must be aware of the value of cultural, racial, and socioeconomic differences and that these differences are often turned into discrimination in health care services and policies. With a focus on social justice, they must be determined to ensure equitable access to care for all.

ACTIVE LEARNING EXERCISES

1. Identify at least four vulnerable groups within your community. Using one of the models of vulnerability depicted in this chapter, determine the health status for each of these groups. Describe the relative risk for each group.
2. Using "Communicate Effectively to Inform and Educate" (1 of the 10 essential public health services; see Box 2-2), find available community resources for each of the groups you identified in exercise 1. Where are the resources located? How easily accessible are they? What outreach services do they provide for the vulnerable population they serve? Describe some socioeconomic resources. What areas are most deficient?
3. Talk to two expert C/PHNs and discuss the concept of empowerment with them. What strategies have they used with clients? Ask them to share examples of when they felt that they made a real difference in the lives of their clients. Note any similarities between these nurses' responses and the roles and behaviors of C/PHNs and client empowerment strategies described in this chapter.
4. Check with the health department about any interagency groups or committees that may be addressing the needs of vulnerable populations in your community. What issues are most important to this group? Who are the members? Note the agencies represented. Are there any community members present? If possible, attend a meeting or access minutes of a recent meeting and determine the types of issues being discussed. Is there a sense of community involvement and participation?
5. Search for a current evidence-based article on vulnerable populations based on ideas from this chapter. Discuss the main points of each article and how they may relate to vulnerable populations (e.g., health disparities, socioeconomic gradient), as well as individual clients you may be seeing in your clinical rotations (e.g., empowerment, health literacy). Based on the research findings, what interventions might be most helpful? Are they feasible in your area? With your specific populations?

REFERENCES

Abbasi, S. H., De Leon, A. P., Kassaian, S. E., Karimi, A., Sundin, O, Jalali, A., ... Macassa, G. (2015). Introducing the Tehran Heart Center's premature coronary atherosclerosis cohort: THC-PAC study. *International Journal of Preventive Medicine*, 6, 36.

Aday, L. A. (2001). *At risk in America: The health and health care needs of vulnerable populations in the United States* (2nd ed.). San Francisco, CA: Jossey-Bass.

Aday, L. A. (Ed.). (2005). *Reinventing public health: Policies and practices for a healthy nation*. San Francisco, CA: Jossey-Bass.

Agency for Healthcare Research and Quality (AHRQ). (2015). *2014 National healthcare quality and disparities report (AHRQ Pub. No. 15–0007)*. Rockville, MD: Author.

Alidu, L., & Grunfeld, E. (2017). Gender differences in beliefs about health: a comparative qualitative study with Ghanaian and Indian migrants living in the United Kingdom. *BMC Psychology*, *5*(1). doi: 10.1186/s40359-017-0178-z.

American Association of Colleges of Nursing. (2015). *Fact sheet: Enhancing diversity in the nursing workforce*. Retrieved from https://www.aacnnursing.org/News-Information/Fact-Sheets/Enhancing-Diversity

American Civil Liberties Union. (2018). *Human trafficking: Modern enslavement of immigrant women in the united states*. Retrieved from https://www.aclu.org/other/human-trafficking-modern-enslavement-immigrant-women-united-states

American Public Health Association. (2017). Retrieved from https://www.apha.org

Angier, H., Hoopes, M., Gold, R., Bailey, S. R., Cottrell, E. K., Heintzman, J., ... DeVoe, J. E. (2015). An early look at rates of uninsured safety net clinic visits after the Affordable Care Act. *Annals of Family Medicine*, *13*(1), 10–16. doi: 10.1370/afm.1741.

Armenta, R., Rush, T., Leard-Mann, C., Millegan, J., Cooper, A., & Hoge, C. (2018). Factors associated with persistent posttraumatic stress disorder among U.S. military service members and veterans. *BMC Psychiatry*, *18*, 48.

Banke-Thomas, O., Banke-Thomas, A., & Ameh, C. (2017). Factors influencing utilization of maternal health services by adolescent mothers in low-and middle-income countries; a systematic review. *BMC Pregnancy and Childbirth*, *17*(1). doi: 10.1186/s12884-017-1246-3.

Bates, B. (2016). *Learning theories simplified and how to apply them to teaching*. Thousand Oaks, CA: Sage.

Bay Area Regional Health Inequalities Initiative (BARHII). (2015). *Framework*. Bay Area Regional Health Inequalities Initiative.

Berry, M., Nickerson, N., & Odum, A. (2017). Delay discounting as an index of sustainable behavior; devaluation of future air quality and implication for public health. *International Journal of Environmental Research and Public Health*, *14*(9). doi: 10.3390/ijerph14090997.

Bharmal, N., Derose, K. P., Felician, M., & Weden, M. M. (2015). *Working paper: Understanding the upstream social determinants of health*. Santa Monica, CA: RAND Health.

Brantley, M., Kerrigan, D., German, D., Lim, S., & Sherman, S. (2017). Identifying patterns of social and economic hardship among structurally vulnerable women: a latent class analysis of HIV/STI risk. *AIDS and Behavior*, *21*(10), 3046–3056. doi: 10.1007/s10461-017-1673-1.

Burg, M. A., & Oyama, O. (2016). *The behavioral health specialist in primary care: Skills for integrated practice*. New York, NY: Springer Publishing Co.

Center for Poverty Research, University of California, Davis. (2017). *What is the current poverty rate in the United States?* Retrieved from poverty.ucdavis.edu/faq/how-many-people-are-poor

Centers for Disease Control and Prevention (CDC). (2015a). *CDC health disparities and inequalities report, United States, 2013*. Retrieved from http://www.cdc.gov/mmwr/pdf/other/su6203.pdf

Centers for Disease Control and Prevention (CDC). (2015b). *HIV among African Americans*. Retrieved from http://www.cdc.gov/hiv/group/racialethnic/africanamericans/

Centers for Disease Control and Prevention (CDC). (2018). *Social determinants of health*. Retrieved from https://www.cdc.gov/socialdeterminants/index.htm

Chaturvedi, N. (1998). Socioeconomic gradient in morbidity and mortality in people with diabetes: Cohort study findings from the Whitehall study and the WHO multinational study of vascular disease in diabetes. *British Medical Journal*, *316*(7125), 100–105.

Chetty, R., Stepner, M., Abraham, S., Lin, S., Suderi, B., & Turner, N. (2017). The association between income and life expectancy in the United States 2001-2014. *JAMA*, *15*(16), 1750–1766. doi: 10.1001/jama.2016.4226.

Chikani, V., Brophy, M., Vossbrink, A., Hussani, K., Salvino, C., Skubic, J., et al. (2015). Association of insurance status with health outcomes following traumatic injury: statewide multicenter analysis. *Western Journal of Emergency Medicine*, *16*(3), 408–413. doi: 10.5811/westjem.2015.1.23560.

Cisse-Egbuonye, N., Liles, S., Schmitz, K., Kassem, N., Irvin, V., & Hovell, M. (2016). Availability of vending machines and school stores in California schools. *Journal of School Health*, *86*(1), 48–53. doi: 10.1111/josh.12349.

Collins, S. R., Rasmussen, P. W., Beutel, S., & Doty, M. M. (2015). *The problem of underinsured and how rising deductibles will make it worse—findings from the Commonwealth Fund biennial health insurance survey, 2014*. Retrieved from www.commonwealthfund.org/publications/issue-briefs/2015/may/problem-of-underinsurance

Commonwealth Fund Report. (2017). *Underinsured rate increased sharply in 2016; more than two of five marketplace enrollees and a quarter of people with employees health insurance plans are now underinsured*. Retrieved from https://www.commonwealthfund.org/press-release/2017/underinsured-rate-increased-sharply-2016-more-two-five-marketplace-enrollees-and

Council on Europe (COE). (2020). *Migrant and refugee women and girls*. Retrieved from https://www.coe.int/en/web/genderequality/migrant-and-refugee-women-and-girls

Cronenwett, L., Sherwood, G., Marnsteiner, J., Disch, J., Johnson, J., Mitchell, P., ... Warren, J. (2007). Quality and safety in education for nurses. *Nursing Outlook*, *55*, 122–131. doi: 10.1016/j.outlook.2007.02.006.

De Chesnay, M., & Anderson, B. A. (Eds.). (2016). *Caring for the vulnerable: Perspectives in nursing theory, practice, and research* (4th ed.). Burlington, MA: Jones & Bartlett Learning.

Digest of Education Statistics. (2016). *Digest of education statistics*. Retrieved from https://nces.ed.gov/programs/digest/

Dmytryshyn, A., Jack, S. M., Ballantyne, M., Wahoush, O., & MacMillan, H. L. (2015). Long-term home visiting with vulnerable young mothers: An interpretive description of the impact on public health nurses. *BMC Nursing*, *14*, 12.

Doran, K., Schumway, M., Hoff, R., Blackstock, O., Dilworth, S., & Riley, E. (2014). Correlates of hospital use in homeless and unstably housed women: the role of physical health and pain. *Women's Health*, *24*(5), 535–541. doi: 10.1016/j.whi.2014. 06.003.

Drescher, P., Foy, D., Kelly, C., Leshner, A., Schutz, M., & Litz, B. (2011). An exploration of the viability and usefulness of the construct of moral injury in war veterans. *Traumatology*, *17*(1), 8–13.

Elder, T., Goddeeris, J., & Haider, S. (2016). Racial and ethnic infant mortality gaps and the role of socio-economic status. *Labour Economics*, *43*, 42–54.

Evans, S. D., Sheffer, C. E., Bickel, W. K., Cottoms, N., Olson, M., Piti, L. P., ... Stayna, H. (2015). The process of adapting the evidence-based treatment for tobacco dependence for smokers of lower socioeconomic status. *Journal of Addiction Research & Therapy*, *6*(1). doi: 10.4172/2155-6105.1000219.

Falk-Rafael, A. R. (2001). Empowerment as a process of evolving consciousness: A model of empowered caring. *Advances in Nursing Science*, *24*(1), 1–16.

Felsman, I. C. (2016). Supporting health and well-being for resettled refugee women: The global women's group. *Creative Nursing*, *22*(4), 226–232. doi: 10.1891/1078-4535.22.4.226.

Fernandez, M. (2018). *A Year After Hurricane Harvey, Houston's Poorest Neighborhoods Are Slowest to Recover*. New York Times. Retrieved from https://www.nytimes.com/2018/09/03/us/hurricane-harvey-houston.html

Flaskerud, J. H., & Winslow, B. J. (1998). Conceptualizing vulnerable populations health-related research. *Nursing Research*, *47*(2), 69–78.

Frey, H. (2018). *The U.S. will become "minority white" in 2045, census projects*. Retrieved from https://www.brookings.edu/blog/the-avenue/2018/03/14/the-us-will-become-minority-white-in-2045-census-projects/

Gaglioti, A., Xu, J., Rollins, L., Baltrus, P., O'Conel, L., Cooper, D., ... Akentob, T. (2018). Neighborhood environmental health and premature death from cardiovascular disease. *Preventing Chronic Disease*, *15*, E17. doi: 10.5888/pcd15.170220.

Gelberg, L., Andersen, R., & Leake, B. (2000). The behavioral model for vulnerable populations: Application to medical care use and outcomes for homeless people. *Health Services Research*, *34*(6), 1273–1302.

Global Slavery Index. (2018). *Prevalence*. Retrieved from https://www.globalslaveryindex.org/2018/findings/country-studies/united-states/

Gwede, C., Quinn, G., & Green, B. (2016). Highlighting health disparities in racial and ethnic minorities and other underserved populations. *Cancer Control: Journal of the Moffitt Cancer Center*, *23*(4), 323–325. doi: 10.1177/107327481602300402.

Hahn, R., & Truman, B. (2015). Education improves public health and promotes health equity. *International Journal of Health Services*, *45*(4), 657–678. doi: 10.1177/002073145585986.

Hajizadeh, M., Mitnitski, A., & Rockwood, K. (2016). Socioeconomic gradient in health in Canada: Is the gap widening or narrowing? *Health Policy*, *120*(9), 1040–1050. doi: 10.1016/j.healthpol.2016.07.019.

Holiday, R., Smith, N., & Monteith, L. (2018). An initial investigation of nonsuicidal self-injury among male and female survivors of military sexual trauma. *Psychiatry Research*, *268*, 335–339.

Hong, J., Pequero, A., & Espelage, D. (2018). Experiences in bullying and/or peer victimization of vulnerable, marginalized, and oppressed children and adolescents: an introduction to the special issue. *American Journal of Orthopsychiatry*, *88*(4), 399–401. doi: 10.1037/ort0000330.

Hood, C. M., Gennuso, K. P., Swain, G. R., Catlin, B. B. (2016). County health rankings: Relationships between determinant factors and health outcomes: relationships between determinant factors and health outcomes. *American Journal of Preventive Medicine*, *50*(2), 129–135.

Hutchinson, J., Thompson, M., Troyer, J., Elnitsky, C., Coffman, M., & Thomas, L. (2018). The effect of North Carolina free clinics on hospitalizations for ambulatory care sensitive conditions among the uninsured. *BMC Health Services Research*, *18*(1). doi: 10.1186/s12913-018-3082-1.

Institute of Medicine (IOM). (2003). *Unequal treatment: Confronting racial and ethnic disparities in healthcare*. Washington, DC: The National Academies Press.

Kaiser Family Foundation. (2019). *Key facts about the uninsured population*. Retrieved from https://www.kff.org/uninsured/issue-brief/key-facts-about-the-uninsured-population/

Kessler, R. (1979). Psychological consequences of stress. *Journal of Health and Social Behavior*, *20*, 100–108.

Kimmerling, R., Gima, K., Smith, M., Maguen, S., Litz, Street, A., et al. (2007). The Veterans Health Administration and military sexual trauma. *American Journal of Public Health*, *97*(12), 2160–2166.

Knickman, J. R., & Kovner, A. R. (Eds.). (2015). *Jonas & Kovner's health care delivery in the United States* (11th ed.). New York, NY: Springer.

Kois, L., Blakey, S., Brett, O., Gardner, M., Johnson, J., Hamer, R., et al. (2018) Neuropsychological correlates of self-reported impulsivity and informant-reported maladaptive behaviour among veterans with posttraumatic stress disorder and traumatic brain injury history. *Brain Injury*, *23*, 1–8.

Koven, S. (2018). Veteran treatments; PTSD interventions. *Healthcare (Basel)*, 6(3), 94.

Lane, N., Maxwell, C., Grunier, A., Bronskill, S., & Wodchis, W. (2015). Absence of socioeconomic gradient in older adults survival with multiple chronic conditions. *eBioMedicine*, 2(12), 2094–2100. doi: 10.1016/j.ebiom.2015.11.018.

Laun, L. (2019). *Population reference bureau's exclusive preview of the upcoming decennial census reveals population shifts with major implications for the nation's political, social, and economic future*. Retrieved from https://www.prb.org/what-the-2020-u-s-census-will-tell-us-about-a-changing-america/

Lenhart, C., Wiemken, A., Hanlon, A., Perkett, M., & Patterson, F. (2017). Perceived neighborhood safety related to physical activity but not recreational screen-based sedentary behavior in adolescents. (Report). *BMC Public Health*, 17(1), 1–9. doi: 10.1186/s12889-017-4756-z.

Leone, L., Haynes-Maslow, L., & Ammerman, A. (2017). Veggie van pilot study: impact of a mobile produce market for underserved communities on fruit and vegetables access and intake. *Journal of Hunger & Environmental Nutrition*, 12(1), 89–100.

Loucks, E. B., Lynch, J. W., Pilote, L., Fuhrer, R., Almeida, N. D., Richard, H., ... Benjamin, E. J. (2009). Life-course socioeconomic position and incidence of coronary heart disease: The Framingham Offspring Study. *American Journal of Epidemiology*, 169(7), 829–836.

Lowe, K., Make, B., Crapo, J., Kinney, G., Hokanson, J., Kim, V., ... Regan, E. (2018). Association of low income with pulmonary disease progression in smokers with and without chronic obstructive pulmonary disease. *ERJ Open Research*, 4(4). doi: 10.1183/23120541.00069-2018.

Lowrey, A. (2019). *What the camp fire revealed*. The Atlantic. Retrieved from httpps://www.theatlantic.com/ideas/archive/2019/01/why-natural-disasters-are-worse-poor/580846/

Lubben, J., Gironda, M., Sabbath, E., Kong, J., & Johnson, C. (2015). *Social isolation presents a grand challenge for social work. Working paper no. 7*. Cleveland, OH: American Academy of Social Work and Social Welfare.

Marmot, M., & Wilkinson, R. (Eds.). (2006). *Social determinants of health*. Oxford, UK: Oxford University Press.

Marmot, M., Ryff, C. D., Bumpass, L. L., Shipley, M., & Marks, N. F. (1997). Social inequalities in health: Next questions and converging evidence. *Social Science and Medicine*, 44(6), 901–910.

Martinez, M., & Ward, B. (2016). *Health care access and utilization among adults aged 18-64, by poverty level: United States, 2013-2015*. Hyattsville, MD: U.S. Department of Health and Human Services, Centers for Disease Control and Prevention, National Center for Health Statistics.

Maslow, A. (1987). *Motivation and personality* (3rd ed.). New York, NY: Addison-Wesley.

Mason, D. J., Jones, D. A., Roy, C., Sullivan, C. G., & Wood, L. J. (2015). Commonalities of nurse-designed models of health care. *Nursing Outlook*, 63(5), 540–553.

Matwick, A., & Woodgate, R. (2017). Social justice: A concept analysis. *Public Health Nursing*, 34(2), 176–184.

McAllister, M. (2010). Solution focused nursing: A fitting model for mental health nurses working in a public health paradigm. *Contemporary Nurse*, 34(2), 149–157.

McKinnon, B., Seungmi, Y., Kramer, M., Bushnik, T., Sheppard, A., & Kaufman, J. (2016). Comparison of black-white disparities in preterm birth between Canada and the United States. *Canadian Medical Association Journal*, 188(1), E19–E26. doi: 10.1503/cmaj.150464.

Mendenhall, E., Kohrt, B., Norris, S., Ndetei, D., & Prabhakaran, D. (2017). Non-communicable disease syndemics: poverty, depression, and diabetes among low-income populations. *Lancet*, 389(10072), 951–963. doi: 10.1016/S0140-6736(17)30402-6.

Michimi, A., & Wimberly, M. C. (2015). The food environment and adult obesity in US metropolitan areas. *Geospatial Health*, 10(2), 368. doi: 10.4081/gh.2015.368.

Mohatt, N., Billera, M., Demers, N., Monteith, L., & Bahraini, N. H. (2018). A menu of options: Resources for preventing veteran suicide in rural communities. *Psychological Services*, 15(3), 262–269.

Montez, J., Zajacova, A., & Hayward, M. (2017). Disparities in disability by educational attainment across US states. *American Journal of Public Health*, 107(7), 1101–1108. doi: 10.2105/AJPH.2017.303768.

Montez, J., Zhang, W., Zajacova, A., & Hamilton, T. (2018). Does college major matter for women's and men's health in midlife? Examining the horizontal dimensions of educational attainment. *Social Science & Medicine*, 198, 130–138. doi: 10.1016/j.socscimed.2018.01.005.

Mueller, M., Purnell, T., Mensah, G., & Cooper, L. (2015). Reducing racial and ethnic disparities in hypertension prevention and control: what will it take to translate research into practice and policy? *American Journal of Hypertension*, 28(6), 699–716. doi: 10.1093/ajh/hpu233.

National Academy of Sciences. (2019). *Accessing progress on the institute of medicine report the future of nursing*. Retrieved form https://www.nap.edu/read/21838/chapter/1

National Center for Children in Poverty. (2017). *Basic facts about low income children*. Retrieved from http://www.nccp.org/publications/pub_1170.html

National Center for Veterans Analysis and Statistics (NCVAS). (2016). *Profile of Women Veterans: 2015*. Retrieved from https://www.va.gov/vetdata/docs/SpecialReports/Women_Veterans_Profile_12_22_2016.pdf

National Center for Veterans Analysis and Statistics (NCVAS). (2017). *Mortality rates and life expectancy of Veterans*. Retrieved from https://www.va.gov/vetdata/docs/SpecialReports/Mortality_study_USVETS_2015_1980_2014.pdf

National Center for Veterans Analysis and Statistics (NCVAS). (2018). *Profile of Veterans: 2016*. Retrieved from https://www.va.gov/vetdata/docs/SpecialReports/Profile_of_Veterans_2016.pdf

National LGBT Health Education Center. (2015). *Top 10 things: Creating inclusive health care environments for LGBT people*. Retrieved from https://www.lgbthealtheducation.org/wp-content/uploads/Ten-Things-Brief-Final-WEB.pdf

National LGBT Health Education Center. (2016). *Affirmative care for transgender and gender non-conforming people: Best practices for front line health care staff*. Retrieved from https://www.lgbthealtheducation.org/wp-content/uploads/2016/12/Affirmative-Care-for-Transgender-and-Gender-Non-conforming-People-Best-Practices-for-Front-line-Health-Care-Staff.pdf

National LGBT Health Education Center. (n.d.). *Providing inclusive services and care for LGBT people: A guide for health care staff*. Retrieved from https://www.lgbthealtheducation.org/wp-content/uploads/Providing-Inclusive-Services-and-Care-for-LGBT-People.pdf

Neumayer, E., & Plümper, T. (2015). Inequalities of income and inequalities of longevity: A cross-country study. *American Journal of Public Health*, 106(1), 160–165.

Non, A. L., Roman, J. C., Gross, C. L., Gilman, S. E., Loucks, E. B., Buka, S. L., et al. (2016). Early childhood social disadvantage is associated with poor health behaviors in adulthood. *Annals of Human Biology*, 43(2), 144–153.

Nursing for Women's Health. (2016). Human trafficking. *Nursing for Women's Health*, 20(3), 324–326.

O'Mahony, S., McHenry, J., Snow, D., Cassin, C., Schumacher, D., & Selwyn, P. A. (2008). A review of the barriers to utilization of the Medicare hospice benefits in urban populations and strategies for enhanced access. *Journal of Urban Health*, 85(2), 281–290.

Office of Disease Prevention and Health Promotion. (2020a). *Social determinants of health*. Retrieved from https://www.healthypeople.gov/2020/topics-objectives/topic/social-determinants-of-health

Olds, D. L., Eckenrode, J., Henderson, C. R., Jr., Kitzman, H., Powers, L, Cole, R., ... Luckey, D. (1997). Long-term effects of home visitation on maternal life course and child abuse and neglect. Fifteen-year follow-up on a randomized trial. *Journal of the American Medical Association*, 278(8), 637–643.

Olver, I. (2017). Cancer control-a global perspective. *European Journal of Cancer Care*, 26(1). doi: 10.1111/ecc.12654.

Olver, I., & Roder, D. (2017). History, development and future cancer screening in Australia. *Pubic Health Research and Practice*, 27(3), e2731725. doi: 10.17061/phrp2731725.

Osei, K., & Galliard, T. (2017). Disparities in cardiovascular disease and type 2 diabetes risk factors in black and whites; dissecting racial paradox of metabolic syndrome. *Frontiers in Endocrinology*, 8, 20. doi: 10.3389/fendo.2017.00204.

Owen, M., Curry, W., Kerner, C., Newson, L., & Fairclough, S. (2017). The effectiveness of school-based physical activity interventions for adolescent girls: A systematic review and meta-analysis. *Preventive Medicine*, 105, 237–249. doi: 10.1016/j.ypmed.2017.09.018.

Perelman, J., Timo-Koija, D., Moor, I., Frederico, B., Kulpers, M., Richter, M., ... Lorant, V. (2017). The association between personal income and smoking among adolescents: a study in six European cities. *Addiction*, 112(12), 2248–2256. doi: 10.1111/add.13930.

Pew Research Center. (September 26, 2015). *Total fertility rate for population estimates and projections, by race-Hispanic origin and generation: 1965–1970; 2015–2020; 2060–2065*. Retrieved from http://www.pewhispanic.org/2015/09/28/modern-immigration-wave-brings-59-million-to-u-s-driving-population-growth-and-change-through-2065/9-26-2015-1-30-23-pm-2/

Price, J., Khubchandani, J., & Webb, F. (2018). Poverty and Health Disparities: What can public health professionals do? *Health Promotion Practice*, 19(2), 170–174.

Psaltopoulou, T., Hatzia, G., Papgeorgiou, N., Androulakis, E., Briasoulis, A., & Tousoulis, D. (2017). Socioeconomic status and risk factors for cardiovascular disease: impact of dietary mediators. *Hellenic Journal of Cardiology*, 58(1), 32–42. doi: 10.1016/j.hjc.2017.01.022.

Randall, S., Crawford, T., Currie, J., River, J., & Betihavas, V. (2017). Impact of community based nurse-led clinics on patient outcomes, patient satisfaction, patient access and cost effectiveness: A systematic review. *International Journal of Nursing Studies*, 73, 24–33. doi: 10.1016/j.ijnurstu.2017.05.008.

Raphael, D. (2003). A society in decline. In R. Hofrichter (Ed.), *Health and social justice: Politics, ideology, and inequity in the distribution of disease* (pp. 59–88). San Francisco, CA: Jossey-Bass.

Rawlett, K. (2011). Analytical evaluation of the health belief model and the vulnerable populations conceptual model applied to a medically underserved, rural population. *International Journal of Applied Science and Technology*, *1*(2), 15–21.

Rhoades, H., Wenzel, S., Golinelli, D., Tucker, J., Kennedy, D., & Ewing, B. (2014). Predisposing, enabling and need correlates of mental health treatment utilization among homeless men. *Community Mental Health Journal*, *50*(8), 943–952. doi: 10.1007/s10597-014-9718-7.

Richard, L., Furler, J., Densley, K., Haggerty, J., Russell, G., Levesque, J., et al. (2016). Equity of access to primary healthcare for vulnerable populations: The IMPACT international online survey of innovations. *International Journal for Equity in Health*, *15*(1). doi: 10.1186/s12939-016-0351-7.

Richards, T. (2014). Health implications of human trafficking. *Nursing for Women's Health*, *18*, 155–163. doi: 10.1111/1751-486x12112.

Riggs, E. Yelland, J., Duell-Piening, P., & Brown, S. (2016). Improving health literacy in refugee populations. *The Medical Journal of Australia*, *204*(1), 9–10. doi: 10.5694/mja15.01112.

Robert Wood Johnson Foundation. (2018a). *Could where you are born influence how long you live?* Retrieved from https://www.rwjf.org/en/library/interactives/whereyouliveaffectshowlongyoulive.html

Robert Wood Johnson Foundation. (2018b). *County health ranking's model*. Retrieved from http://www.countyhealthrankings.org/county-health-rankings-model

Roxburgh, S., & MacArthur, K. (2014). Childhood adversity and adult depression among the incarcerated: Differential exposure and vulnerability by race/ethnicity and gender. *Child Abuse and Neglect*, *38*, 1409–1420.

Rummo, P., Guilkey, D., Ng, S., Meyer, K., Popkin, B., Reis, J., ... Gordon-Larsen, P. (2017). Does unmeasured confounding influence associations between the retail food environment and body mass index over time? The coronary artery risk development in young adults (CARDIA) study. *International Journal of Epidemiology*, *46*(5), 1456–1464. doi: 10.1093/ije/dyx070.

Schake, M., Sommers, B., Subramanian, S., Waters, M., & Arcava, M. (2019). Effects of gentrification on health status after Hurricane Katrina. *Health & Place*, *15*, 102237.

Scherrer, J., Sales, J., Lustman, P., Berk-Clark, C., Schnurr, P., Tuerk, P., ... Chard, K. (2018). The role of obesity in the association between posttraumatic stress disorder and incident diabetes. *JAMA Psychiatry*, *75*(11), 1189–1198.

Shackleton, N., Jamal, F., Viner, R., Dickson, K., Patton, G., & Bonell, C. (2016). School-Based Interventions Going Beyond Health Education to Promote Adolescent Health: Systematic Review of Reviews (Report). *Journal of Adolescent Health*, *58*(4), 382–396. doi: 10.1016/j.jadohealth.2015.12.017.

Sher, L., Braqualais, D., & Casas, M. (2012). Posttraumatic stress disorder, depression, and suicide in veterans. *Cleveland Clinic Journal of Medicine*, *72*(2), 92–97.

Shi, L., Stevens, G., Lebrun, L., Faed, P., & Tsai, J. (2008). Enhancing the measurement of health disparities for vulnerable populations. *Journal of Public Health Management and Practice*, *14*(Suppl), s45–s52.

Silber, J., Rosenbaum, P., Kelz, R., Gaskin, D., Ludwig, J., Ross, R., ... Fleisher, L. (2015). Examining causes of racial disparities in general surgical mortality: Hospital quality versus patient risk. *Medical Care*, *53*(7), 619–629. doi: 10.1097/MLR.0000000000000377.

Stafford, A., & Wood, L. (2017). Tackling health disparities for people who are homeless? Start with social determinants. *International Journal of Environmental Research & Public Health*, *14*(2), 1535.

The Fenway Institute. (2015). *A toolkit for collecting data on sexual orientation and gender identity in clinical settings*. Retrieved from http://doaskdotell.org/

Torres-Duque, C. (2017). Poverty cannot be inhaled and it is not a genetic condition. How can it be associated with chronic airflow obstruction? *European Respiratory Journal*, *49*(6). doi: 10.1183/13993003.00823-2017.

U.S. Department of Health and Human Services. (2014). *Federal poverty guidelines for FFY 2015*. Retrieved from https://aspe.hhs.gov/2015-poverty-guidelines

U.S. Department of Health and Human Services (USDHHS) (n.d.). *Social determinants of health*. Retrieved from https://health.gov/healthypeople/objectives-and-data/social-determinants-health

U.S. Department of Veterans Affairs. (2010). *Top 10 things all healthcare & service professionals should know about VA services for survivors of military sexual trauma*. Retrieved from https://www.mentalhealth.va.gov/docs/top_10_public.pdf

U.S. Department of Veterans Affairs, Office of Health Equity. (2016). *National Veteran health equity report- FY 2013*. Retrieved from https://www.va.gov/HEALTHEQUITY/docs/National_Veterans_Health_Equity_Report_FY2013_FINAL_508_Comp.pdf

U.S. Department of Veterans Affairs, Veterans Health Administration, Office of Academic Affiliations. (2017). *Military health history pocket card for clinicians*. Retrieved from https://www.va.gov/OAA/archive/Military-Health-History-Card-for-print.pdf

U.S. Department of Veterans Affairs, Women's Health Services. (2015). *Study of barriers for women Veterans to VA healthcare*. Retrieved from https://www.womenshealth.va.gov/WOMENSHEALTH/docs/Womens%20Health%20Services_Barriers%20to%20Care%20Final%20Report_April2015.pdf

UNHCR. (1951). *Conference of plenipotentiaries on the status of refugees and stateless persons: Summary record of the thirty fourth meeting*. Retrieved from https://www.unhcr.org/en-us/protection/travaux/3ae68cdf0/conference-plenipotentiaries-status-refugees-stateless-persons-summary.html

UN Refugee Agency (UNHCR). (2020). *Figures at a Glance*. Retrieved from https://www.unhcr.org/en-us/figures-at-a-glance.html?query=25.9%20million%20refugees

United States Department of the State. (2018). *Trafficking persons report*. Retrieved from https://www.state.gov/reports/2018-trafficking-in-persons-report/

Veteran's Healthcare Administration. (2018). Retrieved for ptsd.va.gov, on August 16, 2018.

VetPop. (2016). *Data Catalog*. Retrieved from https://catalog.data.gov/dataset/vetpop2016

Voice of a Witness. (2019). *Voices of the storm: the people of New Orleans on Hurricane Katrina and its aftermath*. Retrieved from https://voiceofwitness.org/oral-history-book-series/voices-from-the-storm/

Watson, L., & Vogel, L. (2017). Educational resiliency in teen mothers. *Cogent Education*, *4*, 1–22. https://www.tandfonline.com/doi/pdf/10.1080/2331186X.2016.1276009?needAccess=true

Wickrama, K., Bae, D., & Walker, C. (2016). Black-white disparity in young adults' disease risk: An investigation of variation in the vulnerability of black young adults to early and later adversity. *Journal of Adolescent Health*, *59*, 209–214.

Williams, D., Priest, N., & Anderson, N. (2016). Understanding associations between race, socioeconomic status and health: Patterns and prospects. *Health Psychology*, *35*(4), 407–411. doi: 10.1037/hea0000242.

World Bank. (2015). *Overview*. Retrieved from www.worldbank.org/en/topic/poverty/overview

WHO. (2017). *Human rights and health*. Retrieved from https://www.who.int/news-room/fact-sheets/detail/human-rights-and-health

World Health Organization. (2020a). *Health Impact Assessment (HIA): The determinants of health*. Retrieved from http://www.who.int/hia/evidence/doh/en/

World Health Organization. (2020b). *Social determinants of health?* Retrieved from http://www.who.int/social_determinants/sdh_definition/en/

Zhang, X., Perez, E., Bourne, P., Peprah, E., Duru, O., Breen, N., ... Denny, J. (2017). Big data science: opportunities and challenges to address minority health and health disparities in the 21st century. *Ethnicity & Disease*, *27*(2), 95–106. doi: 10.18865/ed.27.2.95.

CHAPTER 24

Clients With Disabilities

"I choose not to place 'DIS,' in my ability."

—Robert M. Hensel (1969–, Disability Advocate)

KEY TERMS

- Activity limitations
- American Sign Language
- Americans with Disabilities Act (ADA)
- Assistive devices and technology
- Disability
- Environmental factors
- Family and Medical Leave Act
- Impairments
- Individuals with Disabilities Education Act (IDEA)
- International Classification of Functioning, Disability, and Health (ICF)
- National Council on Disability
- Participation restrictions
- Respite care
- Secondary conditions
- Social Security's Supplemental Security Income (SSI)
- Temporary Assistance for Needy Families (TANF)
- Universal design

LEARNING OBJECTIVES

Upon mastery of this chapter, you should be able to:

1. Discuss the national and global implications of disabilities.
2. Describe the economic, social, and political factors affecting the well-being of individuals with disabilities and their families.
3. Provide an example of primary, secondary, and tertiary prevention practices for individuals with disabilities.
4. Describe the laws that protect individuals with disabilities, such as the Americans with Disabilities Act.
5. Discuss the benefits of universal design for all persons.
6. Explain the role of the community health nurse when working with clients with disabilities.

INTRODUCTION

Currently, an estimated 61.4 million (25.7%; Fig. 24-1) of noninstitutionalized American adults live with **disabilities**, consisting of vision, hearing, mobility, self-care, cognitive, and independent living deficits (Centers for Disease Control and Prevention [CDC], 2018; Okoro, Hollis, Cyrus, & Griffin-Blake, 2018). Disability is an overarching term to describe limitations in activities, impairments, and restrictions in one's ability to participate; "Disability refers to the negative aspects of the interaction between individuals with a health condition (such as cerebral palsy and depression) and personal and environmental factors (such as negative attitudes, inaccessible transportation and public buildings, and limited social supports)" (WHO, 2011, p.7). Conditions such as an aging population and a higher risk for disabilities in older people, as well as a global increase in chronic health conditions, have led to a greater prevalence in disabilities.

> Across the world, people with disabilities have poorer health outcomes, lower education achievements, less economic participation and higher rates of poverty ... partly because people with disabilities experience barriers in accessing services..., including health, education, employment, and transport as well as information. These difficulties are exacerbated in less advantaged communities (WHO, 2011, p. 5).

According to the Census Bureau, disability status is determined by difficulties in these six areas: hearing, vision, cognitive, ambulatory, self-care, and independent living; children 5 to 14 can have difficulty in hearing, vision, ambulatory, and self-care; and children

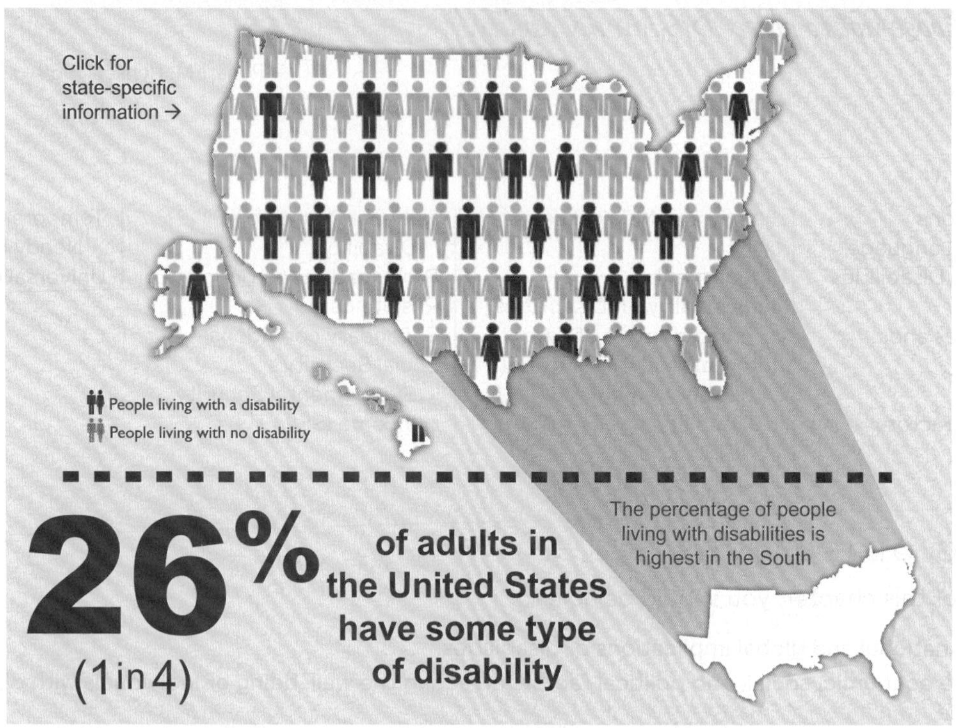

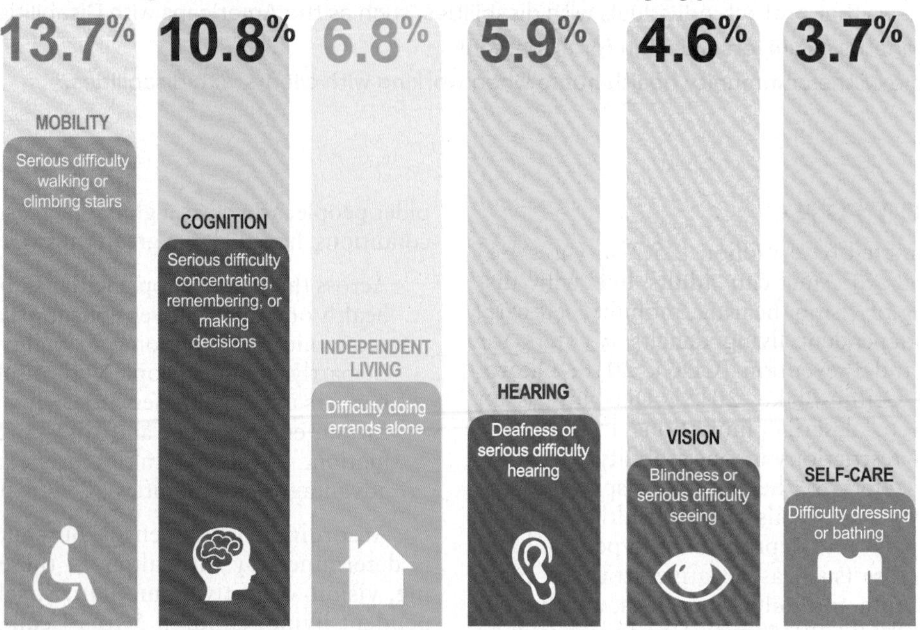

FIGURE 24-1 Disability impacts ALL of us. (Reprinted from Centers for Disease Control and Prevention. (n.d.). *Disability Impacts All of US*. Retrieved from https://www.cdc.gov/ncbddd/disabilityandhealth/documents/disabilities_impacts_all_of_us.pdf.)

<5 can have difficulties in hearing and vision (American Community Survey, 2015). Among young adults, cognitive disabilities were the most common, whereas mobility disabilities were more prevalent in those over the age of 45 (Okoro et al., 2018). Overall, disabilities related to mobility were the most prevailing (Kraus, Lauer, Coleman, & Houtenville, 2018; Okoro et al., 2018). The primary physical causes for limitations included back and neck pain and arthritis, whereas depression and anxiety were the leading psychiatric causes (Kennedy, Wood, & Frieden, 2017). In 2015, one of every five adults in the United States had been diagnosed by a health care provider with arthritis, most commonly osteoarthritis.

More than one third of those over the age of 65 have a disability (Kraus et al., 2018). As our populations age, these numbers will increase. There is little difference in gender in the likelihood of a disability, yet by race, American Indian/Alaskan Natives (17.7%) and Whites (14.1%) were more likely to report a disability (Pew Research Center, 2019). Some states are more likely to have people with disabilities than other states. Among the 50 states, Utah had the lowest percent of the population with disabilities at 9.9%, whereas West Virginia had the highest percent at 20.1% (Kraus et al., 2018). With population growth and an aging population, by 2030, the number of adults with arthritis is expected to increase to 67 million (CDC, 2019b).

Globally, 15% of the world's population has a disability (World Health Organization [WHO], 2019a). Worldwide, nonfatal injuries result in temporary or permanent disabilities in likely thousands of people yearly. In the adolescence age group, depression is the number one cause of disability and anemia is the number three cause of disability. Twenty percent of years lost to disability are due to mental illness (WHO, 2015). Disabilities in children and adults over 60 years were more common in low- to middle-income countries (Banks, Kuper, & Polack, 2018). Adult hearing loss and vision problems were the highest cause of disabilities worldwide. Mental illnesses, such as depression, bipolar disorder, schizophrenia, and alcohol use disorders, were in the top 20 causes of disabilities worldwide (GBD 2015 Disease and Injury Incidence and Prevalence Collaborators, 2016).

In addition to the human burden of disability, the related financial costs of direct medical care and associated indirect costs had significant impact on public and private payers of health and social insurance. Those living with disabilities are at a greater risk of poverty due to the high cost of medical care directly related to the disability, as well as the costs associated with secondary conditions, lower educational attainment, and a higher rate of unemployment or low-paying employment (American Psychological Association, 2019). Costs related to disabilities vary depending on the severity of the disability, the individual's age, and household composition (Mitra, Palmer, Kim, Mont, & Groce, 2017). Employment status varies depending on the type of disability. Individuals with hearing disabilities have the highest percent of employment, and those with self-care disabilities have the lowest rate of employment (Kraus et al., 2018). In 2016, 35.9% of those with disabilities were employed compared with 76.6% of persons without disabilities. Individuals with disabilities make a median income of $10,000 less than persons without disabilities (Kraus et al., 2018).

This chapter begins with an overview of disabilities, followed by a discussion of current national and global trends in addressing these issues. The various organizations that focus on improving the well-being of those affected by disabling conditions, the impact of these disabilities on families, and the role of the C/PHN in addressing the related needs of individuals, families, and aggregates are discussed. The benefits of universal design and issues of easy access for all ages and abilities are introduced.

PERSPECTIVES ON DISABILITY AND HEALTH

People with disabilities daily face negative societal views and stereotypes of disability, and many, along with their families, allies, and advocates, have challenged these views. New and more positive approaches continue to emerge that view individuals and their needs from a more person-centered, holistic standpoint. The diverse personal narratives of those living with disabilities emphasize the individual circumstances and unique responses to disability, and social support and potential inclusive care for the individual have a positive impact on engaging those with disabilities in settings such as work (Cook, Foley, & Semeah, 2016).

Individuals living with a disability must be included in clinical and population health strategies to prevent acquisition of additional chronic diseases or threats to their health (Mahmoudi & Meade, 2015; Reichard, Gulley, Rasch, & Chan, 2015). A literature review conducted on the benefits of park-based physical activities found improvement in the three domains of health: physical, social, and psycho-emotional and spiritual (Saitta, Devan, Boland, & Perry, 2019). In the landmark U.S. Surgeon General's *Call to Action to Improve the Health and Wellness of Persons with Disabilities* placed the health of persons living with disabilities equal in importance to the health of the nation, and today, disability remains a priority for the nation, as reflected in *Healthy People 2030* (Box 24-1; U.S. Department of Health and Human Services, 2020).

One area in which further development is needed to better meet the needs of people with disabilities is that of health and wellness apps, such as medical text messaging or mHealth. Although mHealth apps are helpful for those with chronic conditions such as hypertension or diabetes, they are limited in usefulness for persons with disabilities (Jones, Morros, & Deruter, 2018). Accessibility necessitates redesign of these apps for use by those with vision or hearing impairment, poor fine motor skills, or cognitive disabilities (Jones et al., 2018).

Another potential area of development is the use of technology to enhance the integration of persons with disabilities into society. Manzoor & Vimarlund (2018) completed a literature review on the use of digital technology to improve social inclusion. Results revealed that none of the articles discussed the level of user knowledge needed to use the technology or the cost associated with

BOX 24-1 *HEALTHY PEOPLE 2030*

Disability and Health—Objectives

Core Objectives

DH-01	Reduce the proportion of adults with disabilities who delay preventive care because of cost
DH-02	Reduce the proportion of adults with disabilities who experience serious psychological distress
DH-03	Reduce the proportion of people with intellectual and developmental disabilities who live in institutional settings with 7 or more people
DH-04	Increase the proportion of homes that have an entrance without steps
DH-05	Increase the proportion of students with disabilities who are usually in regular education programs

Research Objectives

DH-R01	Increase the proportion of national surveys with questions that identify people with disabilities
DH-R02	Increase the proportion of state and DC health departments with programs aimed at improving health in people with disabilities

Reprinted from U.S. Department of Health & Human Services (USDHHS). (2020). *Healthy People 2030: Browse objectives.* Retrieved from https://health.gov/healthypeople/objectives-and-data/browse-objectives

the technology. Only a few articles discussed technology that could assist in the job market, participation in social events, and accessing educational opportunities (Manzoor & Vimarlund, 2018). As technology advances, hopefully new and innovative solutions addressing these needs will emerge.

Healthy People 2030

In the United States, *Healthy People* is the most influential series of planning documents that seek to address health promotion and disease prevention as a basis for improving the health of all Americans (U.S. Department of Health and Human Services, 2020). *Healthy People* strives toward a vision of a society in which all people live long, healthy lives. Through its clearly delineated, science-based, and measurable objectives, the decennial *Healthy People* has had far-reaching influences on national and state health initiatives, health care policy, research priorities, and funding since its first efforts in 1979. The evolving American perspectives on disability and on chronic illness have been reflected in the changing focus of the Healthy People series. A comparison among Healthy People plans since its inception underscores the emergence of new approaches to both identifying priority areas and planning to improve the health of individuals with disabilities and chronic illness. In *Healthy People 2000*, only one priority area was devoted to disability and chronic illness: "Diabetes and Chronic Disabling Conditions" (USDHHS, 2016). One of the most influential aspects of the decade of Healthy People 2010 was to promote a change in thinking within the health care community about the health promotion and disease prevention needs of people with disabilities. This shift was essential to remedy the lack of existing health promotion and disease prevention activities for this population. Misconceptions of those with disabilities include the following: (1) all people with disabilities have poor health or may have chronic pain; (2) those with disabilities should be treated as different and special; (3) public health activities need to focus only on preventing disability; (4) people with disabilities are similar; (5) there is no need for a clear definition of "disability" or "people with disabilities" in public health practice; and (6) environment does not play a significant role in the disability process (Together We Rock, n.d.).

In *Healthy People 2020*, the section "Disability and Health" further strengthens *Healthy People*'s approach to disability to emphasize the principles of health promotion and disease prevention for those currently experiencing disabilities and/or chronic illnesses. Rather than narrowly defining individuals with disabilities and/or chronic illnesses through their limiting conditions, *Healthy People 2020* developers understand that individuals with disabilities and/or chronic illnesses have the potential to meet and exceed health promotion and disease prevention goals set for the nation's population as a whole. This approach is consistent with the multifaceted national goal of improving parity across all groups and among all individuals. For example, the goal of "Disability and Health" in *Healthy People 2020* is to engage those with disabilities of all ages to maintain the optimal state of health and prevent chronic conditions so that the highest quality of life can be maintained (ODPHP, 2016). For Healthy People 2030, 62 main objectives are identified across the following five broad categories:

- health conditions
- health behaviors
- populations
- settings and systems
- social determinants of health (U.S. Department of Health & Human Services, 2020)

These objectives reflect a growing emphasis on holistic approaches that recognize that life satisfaction is just as important to human health and well-being as are preventive services. In addition, Healthy People 2030 indicates a growing realization that healthy life-years for persons with disabilities equate to decreased health costs at local, state, and national levels, just as they do for persons without disabilities (ODPHP, 2016; Box 24-2).

Halfway between *Healthy People 2010* and *Healthy People 2020*, the 2005 *Midcourse Review* analyzed changes since implementation of *Healthy People 2010*. It recognized the issue with accommodations for those with disabilities in disaster management and disaster settings (USDHHS, 2016). The United States experienced a great deal of natural disasters in 2018 with the

BOX **24-2** PERSPECTIVES

Focus on Persons With Disabilities

Recent events from the COVID-19 pandemic and rolling electrical outages in California to prevent wildfires highlight the isolating effect events can have on the health and well-being of those with a disability, specifically those with limited mobility. Living independently can be difficult for those using wheelchairs and walkers and for those relying on care providers. The recent pandemic provided other aspects of care to consider such as good hygiene, cleaning and disinfecting, and preventing the spread of infection, as well as having plans for if the direct support provider gets sick, ways to ensure enough prescription medication is on hand, and how to obtain assistance with purchasing household items and groceries. Electrical outages required patients in the community to have backup medical equipment, generators, batteries, nonperishable food, and flashlights or lanterns.

It is imperative that clients with mobility limitations have a plan in place to support their care and well-being during these isolating events. A C/PHN's disaster preparedness plans must address such crises and provide resources for clients and their families so they are not forgotten.

Mark, a C/PHN case manager in the field

fires and mudslides in California, flooding in Maryland, and hurricane Florence in the Carolinas. Man-made disasters included mass shooting devastated the country in Thousand Oaks California in which 12 people were killed, mainly young adults, and in Pittsburgh Pennsylvania where a gunman killed 11 people in a synagogue. Smith and Notaro (2015) found individuals with disabilities are significantly less likely to be prepared for disasters than persons not disabled, and those with activity limitations or severe mental health illness are especially at risk of unpreparedness. The U.S. Department of Home Land Security (2018) met with individuals with disabilities and local agencies and advocacy groups for feedback on ways to improve disaster relief to the population with disabilities. Issues addressed included improved communication, involve persons with disabilities in the emergency planning, ensure shelters are accessible to all, and improve FEMA resources. Universities provide training to staff, faculty, and students on actions to take if an active shooter comes on campuses. This training meant to assist the population on what to do should an event occur may have unexpected outcomes for individuals with disabilities (Box 24-3).

The health of people with disabilities is influenced by many social and physical factors. Using the ICF and the WHO principles of action for addressing health determinants, *Healthy People 2020* identified three areas for public health action. These areas are listed below (ODPHP, 2020):

1. Promote full potential of health and well-being.
2. Eliminate health disparities among people with disabilities and those without disabilities.
3. Address determinants of health and address health equity for people with disabilities.

BOX **24-3** PERSPECTIVES

A Community Member Viewpoint on Active Shooter Response by Persons With Disabilities

I went to the "Active Shooter Response" workshop at work to stir things up. As a wheelchair user, I knew the currently popular "Run. Hide. Fight." model didn't take people like me into consideration. I was prepared to draw attention to every point that didn't apply to people with various disabilities and put the facilitator on the spot for alternative solutions. I wanted to make people think, but I quickly realized I had a lot of thinking to do myself.

The facilitator shared some interesting tactics that seemed useful, like creating obstacles between yourself and the shooter, finding a hiding place, and the difference between cover and concealment. Then it was time to test our new skills. I felt surprisingly good about adapting what I'd learned.

The first drill began with a police officer rushing in, screaming for everyone to "get down." I stood out like a spire when everyone else collapsed to the ground. My glaring vulnerability felt like a gut punch. I could drop out of my chair, but then I'd be stranded. My only hope to save myself is to stay in my chair, but where does that leave me with the officer? I'm at the mercy of his training and ability to quickly evaluate the situation.

We reset and drilled again. The "shooter" stormed in, and my colleagues ran from the room slinging furniture behind them, slowing down the faux assailant...and me! Their impromptu barricades effectively trapped me with an armed aggressor.

In that moment, my cautious optimism melted into terror. The well-intentioned light I meant to shed on the need for inclusive emergency preparedness seemed so petty when people were running for their lives. The A.D.A, accessibility, inclusion, even the kindness of strangers, all the social strategies I had come to rely on for helping me navigate life were suddenly off the table, and I can't even be upset.

My friends and neighbors have families they desperately want to go home to and lives they want to go on living just like I do. You can't really know how a person will react in a crisis, and I have no right to expect anyone to put themselves in danger for me. I don't even want that. In a world where active shooter drills have become necessary, and weather events are becoming more and more extreme, have I finally met my match?

My fellow disabled citizens and I will continue to keep an eye out for ways to disappear in a wheelchair and fight off attackers with crutches and canes, but we all must learn how to be aware of the people around us and create protocols that give everyone at least a chance to survive.

Amanda Timpson, who was diagnosed with bilateral spastic diplegia cerebral palsy as a toddler and became a wheelchair user at the age of 22 due to a car accident

International Classification of Functioning, Disability, and Health

The **International Classification of Functioning, Disability, and Health (ICF)** supports the more positive, emerging approaches to understanding disabling conditions (WHO, 2019b). The ICF (WHO, 2019b) is a universal classification system using standardized language that views the domains of health from a holistic viewpoint. It takes into account body functions and structures, activities and participation, environmental factors, and **personal factors**. This multidimensional approach supports a complex evaluation of an individual's circumstances in terms of functioning, disability, and health. By combining the "medical model" with the "social model," the ICF provides a biopsychosocial approach for assessing people with disabilities. Its approach emphasizes that no two people with the same disease or disability have the same level of **functioning**. The aims of the ICF are to provide a scientific basis for understanding and research, improve communication among providers and those with disabilities, allow for data comparisons, and provide a coding system for health information systems (WHO, 2019b).

The following concepts and related definitions further clarify the ICF view of health:

- **Body functions**: physiologic functions of body
- **Body structure**: anatomic parts of the body
- **Impairments**: problems in body function or structure
- **Activity**: task or action
- **Participation**: to be involved in a life situation
- **Activity limitations**: difficulty an individual may have with an activity
- **Participation restrictions**: limitations in involvement
- **Environmental factors**: the physical and social environments where people live and conduct their lives (WHO, 2019a)

For public health nursing practice, application of the ICF reinforces that disability and disease are additional factors to be considered in planning and implementing a care plan for individual clients and for population groups in the community. For individual clients, the ICF guides and facilitates assessment across a wide range of variables. Although two individuals may have the same apparent disability, such as a below-the-knee amputation, their health status and personal well-being can be quite different. One may have a more positive outlook, more social supports, or fewer additional health issues that complicate rehabilitation than another. The C/PHN must always consider the totality of the situation, including the biologic, psychological, sociocultural, and environmental realms of the whole person.

The World Health Report

World Report on Disability (WHO, 2011) addresses the barriers for those with disabilities and the role of the environment in facilitating or restricting participation for those with disabilities. The barriers include inadequate policies and standards, negative attitudes, lack of provision of services, problems with service delivery, inadequate funding, lack of accessibility, lack of consultation and involvement, and lack of data and evidence (WHO, 2011, pp. 9–10). According to the report, when those with disabilities encounter barriers, results may include poorer health outcomes, lower educational achievements, less economic participation, higher rates of poverty, and increased dependency and restricted participation. The WHO challenged the global community to address barriers and inequalities for those with disabilities in regard to health, rehabilitation, support and assistance, environments, education, and employment (WHO, 2011). In addressing the barriers to health care, the following provide for a more patient-centered care approach for the disabled: use of equipment with universal design, communication of information in appropriate formats, and using alternative models of service delivery provides. In addition, health service providers must have education and training to know how to provide care to those with disabilities. Services for care should focus on efficiency and effectiveness; increasing access to assistive technology increases independence and participation and may reduce costs. Those that are disabled must be empowered to manage their health and advocate on their own behalf. Additionally, policy responses must emphasize early intervention, the benefits of rehabilitation, and provision of services close to where people live (WHO, 2011).

In the seminal report by the, World Health Report (WHR) (WHO, 2002b) emphasized that health care providers worldwide should broaden their clinical and population health practices, rather than continue to focus narrowly on acute illness. Changes in lifestyles and behaviors that have key impacts on increasing healthy years of life should be emphasized. The 10 leading health risks identified by the WHO are as follows:

- air pollution and climate change;
- noncommunicable diseases;
- global influenza pandemic;
- fragile and vulnerable settings;
- antimicrobial resistance;
- ebola and other high-threat pathogens;
- weak primary health care;
- vaccine hesitancy;
- dengue; and
- HIV (WHO, 2019c).

Across the globe, these 10 health risks affect low- and middle-income countries; low levels of socioeconomic status are correlated to poor health and lower quality of life (WHO, 2019c). For those with disabilities, individuals and their families "...are at increased risk for poor health and quality-of-life outcomes when their disability status affects their socioeconomic standing" (American Psychological Association, 2019, para 6).

Environment now plays a role in the health of individuals, with drought, famine, conflict, and population displacement creating protracted crisis situations and contributing to lack of care, chronic illness, disability, and premature death (WHO, 2019c). Of the leading 10 health risks (above), six are directly related to pathogens:

- ebola
- global influenza pandemic

Vaccine hesitancy and increase in vaccine preventable diseases, dengue, HIV, and antimicrobial resistance (WHO, 2019a). Diabetes, cancer, and heart disease are responsible for over 41 million deaths each year and can be attributed to the use of tobacco, alcohol, unhealthy diets, and air pollution. Children are most at risk when unable to access basic health care. In addition, children in vulnerable settings may face famine, drought, and lack access to vaccinations. Malnutrition and deficits of important nutrients can lead to a wide array of preventable disabilities. For example, the leading cause of acquired blindness in children is vitamin A deficiency (Vijayaraghavan, 2018), and the leading cause of intellectual disability and brain damage is iodine deficiency (Georgieff, 2017).

The United Nations Convention on the Rights of Persons With Disabilities

An estimated 1 billion people across the globe live with disabilities, with 110 to 190 million (2.2% to 3.8%) people 15 years and older having significant difficulties in functioning (WHO, 2016). Factoring in the over 2 billion family members affected by disability, the WHO stressed that almost one third of the world population is directly impacted by disabilities. The sheer magnitude of this issue and the recognition that people with disabilities are significantly overlooked across the world led to the 2006 United Nations (UN) Convention on the Rights of Persons with Disabilities (CRPD). To date, 160 countries have signed the Convention or its Optional Protocol (UN, 2016). This document remains the standard for considering the rights of those with disabilities, regardless of age, race, gender, or other demographic considerations. Some of the key principles include respect for dignity and autonomy, nondiscrimination, inclusion into society, acceptance and

- respect for differences, equality of opportunity, accessibility, gender equality, and respect for children's capacities and preserving their identity (UN, 2016).

More information is located on their website: https://www.un.org/development/desa/disabilities/convention-on-the-rights-of-persons-with-disabilities.html.

Although the U.S. Congress passed legislation in support of the U.N. CRPD in 2009, this positive effort proved symbolic, because the effort fell short of the needed step to ratify the Convention. This happened because only Congress can ratify treaties. Despite a wide variety of successful legislation and program development at the national level (see Civil Rights Legislation, below), the United States has been unable to ratify the UN CRPD. As of January 2019, the CRPD is still pending in the U.S. Senate (U. S. Department of State, 2019).

The World Report on Disability

In 2011, the WHO and the World Bank reassessed global progress on disability since the 2006 CRPD (UN, 2016). The *Convention* provided guidance to governments globally and communicated that it was their responsibility to improve the lives of individuals and families living with disability. Citizens of every country must and need to participate in their country's development. People living with disabilities must advocate for the removal of barriers that prevent their full participation in their communities, including access to health, education, employment, transportation, and information services. To assure full participation of people with disabilities in their communities, stakeholders in each country—and globally—must establish an inclusive world characterized by enabling environments, rehabilitation and support services, adequate social protection, and relevant policies, programs, standards, and legislation (WHO, 2019a).

Specific recommendations include:

- Address unmet health care needs.
- Assess health risks for those with disabilities (such as comorbidities or engagement in health-risk behaviors).
- Advocate for those who have barriers to care (WHO, 2019a).

Citizens of every country, including Americans at every level, can become engaged in translating the World Health Organization into action. Even though government at every level must play a significant part, operationalizing the recommendations affords important roles for service providers, academic institutions, the private sector, communities, and especially people with disabilities and their families (WHO, 2019a).

HEALTH PROMOTION AND PREVENTION NEEDS OF PERSONS WITH DISABILITIES

Two ways that CHNs and other health care providers can better address the health care needs of people with disabilities are to take advantage of every opportunity to promote their quality of life and to work to eliminate disparities between their level of health care access and quality and that of people without disabilities.

Missed Opportunities by Health Care Providers to Affect Quality of Life

All of us, whether with or without disabilities, require basic elements to maintain health, including clean air and water, a safe place to live, sunshine, exercise, nutritious food, socialization, and the opportunity to be successful in life's pursuits. As self-evident as these health-promoting elements may seem, for the millions of persons who deal with disability, such basic needs too often take second place to other issues. It is equally problematic that health promotion and disease prevention measures, most notably at the primary and secondary levels, are often nonexistent or lacking (Fig. 24-2). Individuals with disabilities are more likely to experience difficulties accessing health care, dental services, mammograms, Pap tests, and fitness

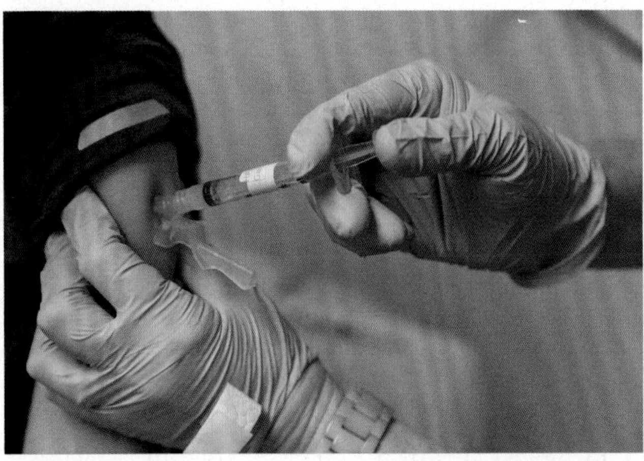

FIGURE 24-2 Preventive services, such as immunizations, are sometimes forgotten among the disabled population.

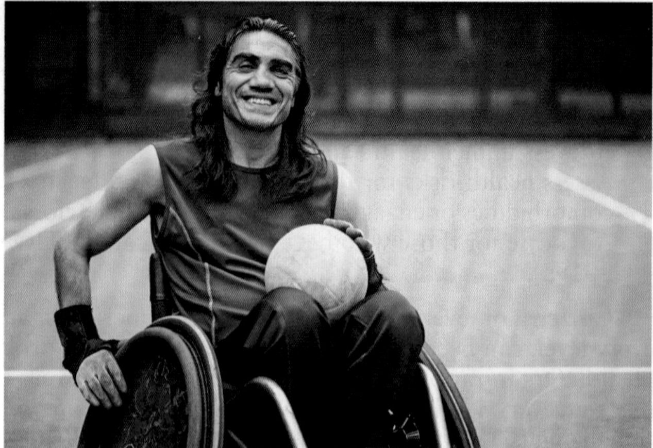

FIGURE 24-3 A disabled rugby player.

activities and are more likely to use tobacco, be overweight or obese, have hypertension, and have lower employment rates (ODPHP, 2016). Key to addressing these barriers is for people with disabilities to have an opportunity to participate in public health activities, receive appropriately timed health interventions, engage with the environment without restrictions, and be able to participate in life without limitations (Fig. 24-3; ODPHP, 2020).

The CDC is making an effort to reduce health disparities among persons with disabilities. Surveillance, or use of surveys, helps to determine the needs and problems that people with disabilities experience, and research programs help to prevent the development of secondary conditions. **Secondary conditions** include mental, emotional, social, medical, or family/community issues that may be experienced as a result of having a disabling condition. For instance, inadequate transportation was reported by 31% of adults with disabilities compared with only 13% of adults without disabilities; poverty is also a concern, as 26% of adults with disabilities report an annual income of under $15,000 compared with 9% of those without disabilities (CDC, 2020). The focus of the health care delivery system is increasingly skewed toward secondary and tertiary prevention efforts, and limited emphasis is placed on the primary prevention needs of this population. Health care providers often fail to address many issues related to health promotion and prevention with people with disabilities that they do cover with those without disabilities, which is a grave concern (CDC, 2020). For example, issues such as sexuality are often not explored with individuals with disabilities. Holland-Hall and Quint (2017) discovered that sexual health education was frequently ignored in the adolescent population with mild-to-moderate disabilities even though their sexual activity is equal to that of their peers.

Disability often serves as the presenting reason for an individual's encounter with the health care community, including the C/PHN. As a result, the disability often drives the selection of prevention efforts, to the possible exclusion of other, equally important health issues. Box 24-4 offers several examples of missed opportunities in the areas of primary and secondary prevention. It is of particular concern to the practice of community/public health nursing that the broad range of health promotion and prevention needs of all clients be addressed.

BOX 24-4 Missed Opportunities

Example 1

A 60-year-old woman, blind since birth, self-sufficient, and active all of her life, has developed severe arthritis. She encounters a health care system that far too often focuses on her "disabilities" and not her "abilities." The focus is placed squarely on her tertiary health promotion needs, often at the expense of health-promoting or lifestyle-enhancing needs. The result is a failure to recognize that the "disability" of arthritis is likely no less and no more an issue for her than for a sighted person. She receives the same medication therapy as does a sighted person but may not be offered a physical therapy program because of her disability. Her need for physical therapy is no less important, but locating an appropriate, safe, and easily accessible program requires some additional work on the part of her provider. At issue is that options potentially discussed with a sighted person are more apt to be omitted completely, which may negatively affect the client's overall health and well-being.

Example 2

A 20-year-old man with learning disabilities, who is employed at a local factory, receives a regularly scheduled physical examination with a new provider. He lives in a congregate care facility, which is an out-of-home facility that provides housing for people with disabilities in which rotating staff members provide care for 16 or more adults or any number of children/youth younger than 21 years of age. It excludes foster care, adoptive homes, residential schools, correctional facilities, and nursing facilities (U.S. Department of Health and Human Services [USDHHS], 2016). The major finding of the examination is that he is due for a tetanus booster and should also begin the series for hepatitis A, because he lives in a high-risk area of the western United States. He takes the referral slip and leaves the office. One year later, at his regularly scheduled visit, it becomes clear that he never received his immunizations. Apparently, he didn't know what he was supposed to do with the paper, because he has difficulty reading, and he had no idea where to go to get his "shots." The primary prevention elements were provided, but clearly not in a manner appropriate for this individual. With additional explanation and follow-up, perhaps the outcome would have been quite different.

Example 3

A 34-year-old woman, who has been severely obese since the birth of her last child (4 years ago), has not had a gynecologic examination since that birth. She is aware of the need to have regular examinations, yet she cannot bring herself to make an appointment. The reason is that she knows she will have to be weighed, and this terrifies her, especially because it is done in an open area where others can see. She finally gets the courage to call for an appointment and tells the clerk that she does not want to be weighed. The clerk's response is less than helpful, and she is essentially told that it is "policy." She makes the appointment but does not keep it. This situation could have been handled in a compassionate manner, recognizing the painful experience that weighing is for many individuals and suggesting alternatives, one of which could have been simply to bypass the scales until after the interview and examination. At that point, the woman may have been more amenable to the measurement and a more discrete area could have been offered. In this case, the opportunities to provide primary, secondary, and tertiary prevention were lost.

Gofine, Mielenz, Vasan, and Lebwohl (2018) documented the risk of missed opportunities for clinical preventive services among people with mobility disability. Americans 50 to 75 years old with a mobility disability were less likely to receive routine colorectal cancer screening. The researchers also discovered that age, comorbidities, and the severity of the disability played a role. Additionally, Na et al. (2017) determined that the care for chronic diseases and preventive care such as annual visits to the primary care provider, vision exams, and mammograms for women decreased as activity limitation increased for older adults receiving Medicare. Furthermore, women with intellectual and development disabilities were less likely to receive routine cervical cancer screenings, even if they had been sexually active, as evident by previous pregnancies (Brown, Plourde, Ouellette-Kuntz, Vigod, & Cobigo, 2016). In light of the *Healthy People 2030* guidelines, these studies indicate a need to focus concerted efforts on improving preventive health screenings and services for those with disabilities (U.S. Department of Health and Human Services, 2019).

Health Care Disparities

Individuals living with disabilities, along with their families and advocates, have embraced concerns about the type and quality of the health-related services to which they have access and the referral process they face. They also have concerns about the care they receive being appropriate to their individual circumstances. Lack of access to individualize, quality health care can result in increased illness and disability, as well as potentially decreased quality or length of life. It is important to consider the impact that access to care can have in the continuum of health and the **health care disparities** between those with disabilities and those without disabilities, such as the risk for unmet care needs. For example, the inability to access medical, dental, and prescription drug care is 57% to 85% higher in those with disabilities than in those without disabilities (Mahmoudi & Meade, 2015). The recent opioid epidemic also touches those with disabilities. When compared with adults without disabilities, adults with disabilities were prescribed opioids more frequently, misused opioids at a higher rate, misused the drug for pain, and received less treatment for opioid misuse (Lauer, Henly, & Brucker, 2019). This study highlights the need for health care providers to improve services and referrals for this population. Additional disparities may exist in services received by those with disabilities.

A **medical home** should provide care that is family centered and coordinated with a permanent health care provider, have any easy referral process, and be the usual source of care (Rosen-Reynoso et al., 2016). Ideally, services provided should be prompt and easy to navigate. However, only 43% of children with special health care needs and emotional, behavioral, or developmental disabilities had a medical home (Rosen-Reynoso et al., 2016). Several factors were found to negatively impact needed services: non-English speakers, male child with disability, severity of disability, at or below 200% of poverty level, uninsured, Black or Hispanic race, and single-parent households (Rosen-Reynoso et al., 2016). Reducing health disparities between those with disabilities and those without disabilities provides an opportunity for maximal health of those with disabilities, as well as for the general U.S. population.

Primary, secondary, and tertiary prevention activities are essential aspects of quality care for all persons. According to a recent literature review, researchers found that individuals with disabilities face four obstacles in accessing preventive care:

- the physical environment of the provider's office not being large enough for a wheelchair;
- transportation challenges, including expense, poor access, and late pick-ups;
- health care providers having a negative demeanor; and
- financial concerns (Marrocco & Krouse, 2017).

Those with disabilities require specialized attention to needs resulting from or related to their disabilities, yet they also require preventive care to attain healthier outcomes (Marrocco & Krouse, 2017). C/PHNs are in a prime position to advocate for needed changes for those with disabilities. Such changes include increased attention to health promotion and disease prevention needs, accessible and appropriate delivery of those services, and specialized treatment plans that incorporate the latest knowledge of a specific illness or disability (Box 24-5).

CIVIL RIGHTS LEGISLATION

Legislation is vital to ensure that every individual's rights are protected and that there is legal recourse to secure needs that have been denied. As is often true for other issues of equality, legislation is only one of many steps that must be taken. The movement to achieve civil rights for persons with disabilities in this country has gained momentum and continues to seek the influence and public attention that will improve the health and lives of those with disabilities and **handicaps**. The **Americans with Disabilities Act (ADA)** was signed into law in 1990 to protect the civil liberties of Americans living with disabilities and continues to updated, as recently as 2017, when movie theaters were required to provide captioning and audio description for movies that are produced with those features (United States Department of Justice [USDOJ], n.d.). This legislation and others, such as Section 504 of the Rehabilitation Act of 1973 and Individuals with Disabilities Education Act in 1990, resulted from a long and difficult struggle (Landmark, Zhang, Ju, McVey, & Ji, 2017). Individuals with disabilities and their advocates made their voices heard by repeatedly demanding an end to inferior treatment and lack of equal protection under the law, which have impeded their daily lives. The ADA has set the standard for a number of subsequent laws that, together with pre-ADA legislation, have become a broad spectrum of protections for people with disabilities. These laws, which are listed in Table 24-1, cover a variety of issues, including telecommunications, architectural barriers, and voter registration.

This federal law protects those with a disability, which is defined as "…a person who has a physical or mental impairment that substantially limits one or more major life activities, a person who has a history or record of such an impairment, or a person who is perceived by

BOX 24-5 PERSPECTIVES

A Nurse's Viewpoint on Community Health Nursing

I have worked supporting people with disabilities, different roles, such as home health, C/PHN home visitor, and public health nursing manager. As C/PHN, assessment and screening are essential interventions when interacting with disabling individuals and their families. Listening to parents and caregivers could make a difference to assess for early services. For example, I received a referral to check a toddler's development. Mom was concerned that something was wrong with her child. The initial bio-psycho-social assessment of the toddler and family did not show any red flags, but the mother needed health teaching, parenting, and connection with resources available for children zero to five.

Further developmental screenings identified caution in gross and fine motor skills that required a referral to the regional center, early intervention program. Through on-going case management, consulting with the medical providers, and advocating for specialty services due to lack of improvement, this toddler was finally connected with specialty services and diagnosed with a degenerative muscle disorder. The family applied to social security disability program to meet their child and family needs, find transportation, and modify the environment to accommodate a wheelchair, hospital bed, homeschooling, therapies, and medical services among others. The C/PHN interventions for this child and family, as a home visitor case manager, included collaboration with staff from multiple agencies, advocacy, and coordination with the children services' C/PHN care manager. Parents learned to voice their concerns, got involved with the community, and advocated for their child until the end of her life, several years later.

As C/PHN, we need to assess the needs of people with disabilities at the individual, family, community, and system level. C/PHN needs to keep in mind the developmental stages of people with disabilities and aspects of sexual health to prevent sexual, physical, and emotional abuse. Across the life span, people with disabilities have sexual health needs finding partners and forming their own family, which could be challenging and requires C/PHN interventions and referrals to agencies, including child and adult protective services. When working with people with disabilities, advocacy is one C/PHN intervention that is a common denominator. People with disabilities and their families need a voice, support, information, guidance, encouragement to get services from basic human needs of food and shelter to complex health care to maintain health and wellness, be active, surrounded, and supported by the community.

—*Claudia Pineda Benton, Supervising Public Health Nurse for Community Health Nursing Field and Maternal Child Adolescent Health Programs*

others as having such an impairment. The ADA does not specifically name all of the impairments that are covered" (USDOJ, 2009, page 2). The ADA does not list specific diagnoses but focuses on the impact the disability has on daily living, such as on the ability to care for self, perform manual tasks, see, hear, eat, sleep, walk, stand, lift, bend, speak, breathe, learn, read, concentrate, think, communicate, and work. Despite this specificity, there remains a broad range of interpretations and legal challenges with respect to who is actually covered by the ADA.

In addition to the uncertainty about who is actually protected by the ADA, there can also be confusion about who is required to comply with the provisions of the Act and what specific remedial actions are necessary. The ADA currently applies to all employers with 15 or more employees (including religious organizations), and all activities of state and local governments irrespective of their size. Public transportation, businesses that provide public accommodation, and telecommunication entities are also required to provide access for individuals with disabilities. It is important to note that the ADA does not override federal and state health and safety laws (U.S. Department of Labor [USDOL], n.d.a).

Individuals who believe that their legal rights under the ADA have been violated may seek remedy by filing a lawsuit or submitting a complaint to one of four federal offices, depending on the specific type of alleged violation: (1) the USDOJ, Civil Rights Division; (2) any U.S. Equal Employment Opportunity Commission field office; (3) the Office of Civil Rights, Federal Transit Administration; or (4) the Federal Communications Commission. The process for filing a complaint is not a simple task, and many seek the assistance of attorneys, legal aid societies, or various private organizations, some of which are discussed later in this chapter (Box 24-6).

The USDOJ published *A Guide to Disability Rights Laws* (2009). The guide provides information on federal civil rights laws for those with disabilities and is available in large print, CD, and Braille. The laws included are

- Americans with Disabilities Act (ADA)
- Telecommunications Act
- Fair Housing Act
- Air Carrier Access Act
- Voting Accessibility for the Elderly and Handicapped Act
- National Voter Registration Act
- Civil Rights of Institutional Persons Act
- Individuals with Disabilities Education Act (IDEA)
- Rehabilitation Act
- Architectural Barriers Act

The most challenging aspect of providing services for persons with disabilities is to alter the perceptions and misunderstandings of others about people with disabilities (Yee, 2016). The perspective of one community member offers one such example (Box 24-7).

The National Council on Disability (n.d) is an independent federal agency charged with advising the President, Congress, and other federal agencies regarding policies, programs, practices, and procedures that affect people with disabilities. Its policy areas include civil rights, cultural diversity, education, emergency management, employment, financial assistance and incentives, health care, housing, international issues, long-term services and

TABLE **24-1** Disability Rights Laws

Law	Summary	Contact
Americans with Disabilities Act (ADA) (1990)	Prohibits discrimination in 1. employment 2. state and local government 3. public accommodations, commercial facilities, transportation, and telecommunications	• U.S. Equal Opportunity Commission • Civil Rights Division • U.S. Department of Justice (USDOJ) • Office of Civil Rights, Federal Transit Administration
Telecommunications Act of 1996	Telecommunication equipment and services are accessible	Federal Communications Commission (FCC)
Fair Housing Act (amended 1988)	Prohibits housing discrimination	U.S. Department of Housing and Urban Development (HUD)
Air Carrier Access Act (1990)	Prohibits discrimination in air transportation by domestic and foreign carriers	U.S. Department of Transportation (DOT)
Voting Accessibility for the Elderly and Handicapped Act of 1984	Requires polling places to be physically accessible for federal elections	USDOJ, Civil Rights Division
National Voter Registration Act of 1993	"Motor Voter Act"—makes it easier to vote by increasing low registration rates by minorities and persons with disabilities	USDOJ, Civil Rights Division
Civil Rights of Institutionalized Persons Act (CRIPA) 1997	Right to receive care in the least restrictive setting	USDOJ
Individuals with Disabilities Education Act (1990)	Make available free public education in the least restrictive environment for all children with disabilities	U.S. Department of Education, Office of Special Education Programs
Rehabilitation Act (1973)	Prohibits discrimination in all federal programs or programs receiving federal financial assistance	• Employer's Equal Employment Opportunity Office • U.S. Department of Labor, Office of Federal Contract Compliance Programs • USDOJ
Architectural Barriers Act (1968)	Buildings constructed or altered with federal funds must meet federal accessibility standards	U.S. Architectural and Transportation Barriers Compliance Board
Accessible Design (2010 Standards)	Standards required for new construction and alterations under Title II and Title III	U.S. Architectural and Transportation Barriers Compliance Board
Revision of the ADA Title II and Title III regulations to implement the requirements of the ADA Amendments Act of 2008 (2016)	To clarify the meaning and interpretation of the ADA definition of "disability"	Civil Rights Division, U.S. Department of Justice (USDOJ)
Provide appropriate auxiliary aids and services for people with disabilities (2017)	Movie theaters provide closed captioning and audio description when showing a digital movie.	Civil Rights Division, U.S. Department of Justice (USDOJ)

Source: U.S. Department of Justice Civil Rights Division, Disability Rights Section (2020).

BOX 24-6 Office of Civil Rights: Compliance With the Americans With Disabilities Act

The responsibility of the U.S. Department of Justice, Office of Civil Rights (OCR), is to investigate complaints of alleged violations of the Americans with Disabilities Act (ADA). An example of one of those complaints involved a 22-year-old Connecticut woman with cerebral palsy. She had been placed in a nursing home because of changes in her living situation and health care status, but wanted to move back into the community. The OCR intervened to ensure that the woman secured appropriate housing and that counseling and intensive case management services were in place when she moved back into the community. Another example involved a man with traumatic brain injury (TBI) who was told he must remain in a hospital when he requested home health care services. OCR intervened and secured physical, occupational, and speech therapy for the client, as well as physical modifications needed for his home. A 32-year-old quadriplegic man had lived independently in his own apartment with a health aide's assistance, but suddenly lost his apartment and was transferred against his will to a facility. He was able to get a wheelchair accessible apartment but could not get health aide services. OCR intervened on his behalf and secured a personal care assistant so that he could live in his new apartment. Without the protection afforded under the ADA, the outcome could have been much different.

Source: USDHHS, Office for Civil Rights (September 2006).

support, technology, transportation, and youth issues. NCD's Web site has publications dating back to 1986 on civil rights. Information can be found at https://www.ncd.gov/policy/civil-rights.

FAMILIES OF PERSONS WITH DISABILITIES

Families that include a member with a disability face many challenges. Below we consider factors affecting families' ability to cope with the disability and the impact of caregiving on families.

Factors Affecting the Family's Ability to Cope

The parents of a child with disabilities must come to grips with many unknowns. Shenaar-Golan (2017) studied subjective well-being in parents of children with disabilities. Often times their financial stability is depleted and parents express concern for the future well-being of their child, especially as the parents age. The study found that the parents' level of hope and perception of the disability and the parental relationship affected their subjective well-being (Shenaar-Golan, 2017). The child's transition from a minor to an adult and the child's leaving the school setting, which provides a routine for the child, may cause anxiety for parents and the child. Parents may not have the necessary knowledge to ensure a smooth transition. Researchers found that a structured training period for parents of soon-to-be-adult children with autism increased their knowledge of services such as SSDI, housing, and Medicaid and made them feel more comfortable in advocating for their children and more empowered (Taylor, Hodapp, Burke, Waitz-Kudla, & Radideau, 2017). Families may also have little understanding of what services they are entitled to because of language barriers, difficult agency policies, or disjointed service delivery. These challenges may be magnified when a family member is newly diagnosed with a disability.

The C/PHN is usually not the first health care professional that the family encounters. They may already have been through a lengthy struggle to receive assistance. In these circumstances, the nurse may be confronted with

BOX 24-7 PERSPECTIVES

A Community Member Viewpoint on Hearing Loss

I lost my hearing as a young adult. By the time I was 28 years old, I had no natural hearing left. I received a cochlear implant when I was 32. Around the time I decided to have the implant, I was struggling so much to survive in the hearing world (phone usage, conversations with hearing people, etc.). The decision to receive a cochlear implant changed my life. I could now communicate with the hearing world again. While the cochlear implant has some amazing benefits, there are some negatives still. For one, I still do not have perfect hearing. I have enough hearing, though, for people to not realize I am deaf. This "hidden disability" can be problematic. Many people assume I am just stupid. It happens all the time. What they don't know is that I am actually well educated and very intelligent. Often, I hear my friends, family, and fellow students talk about how smart I am, but when I don't hear something I sound stupid. I might mishear the beginning of a conversation and respond with something totally off topic. This particular trait should be a red flag that the person may have a hearing loss. It is very demoralizing for people to treat you like you are stupid, when the reality is you just can't hear well. Another very difficult thing about having a cochlear implant is that when you can't wear it for some reason (dead battery, loss, medical procedure, etc.) you feel absolutely powerless, and often fearful, in the hearing world. I've most often experienced this in the health care environment. When I had to have surgical procedures that required removing my implant, I could not hear the instructions provided to me in preop. I could not hear the words that were intended to calm or comfort me. Instead, I was in a constant state of panic wondering if I was missing important information related to my health and safety. Hearing people should also realize that deaf people are extremely tuned to the visual world. We see your frustrated eye rolls, side glances, and facial expressions very acutely. It is very hurtful and frustrating to see this and not be able to do anything about it. Like many "hidden disabilities," imagining yourself in someone else's shoes would probably facilitate a more beneficial and pleasant interaction.

Veronica Russell

a frustrated family, reluctant to trust yet another health care provider. Nurses must earn the trust and confidence of the family by practicing consistency, following through with promised actions, and always being truthful. Not all problems that the family faces can be remedied, and even for problems that do have solutions, time and effort may be needed to obtain the desired result. Nageswaran and Golden (2018) uncovered four themes in the relationship between the caregivers (parents) and the home health nurse:

- the relationship developed over time;
- trust and communication were crucial;
- boundaries were difficult to maintain; and
- a good working relationship between the nurse and the caregiver decreased caregiver stress, lowered stress for the health care provider, and improved care of the child.

Additionally, when working with an older child and the family, the CHN needs to remain respectful to both parties. The child is a separate entity, and the child's wishes need to be considered as much as possible (Cureton & Silver, 2017).

The Impact of Caregiving on Families

Caring for a family member who is disabled, whether a child or an adult, is stressful. High levels of anxiety, stress, depression, and illness are often reported in these families (Dykens, 2015). Caregiver strain is common in families caring for a member with disabilities. These caregivers have multiple roles, associated with employment, caring for other children in the family, the parents' relationship, and providing care for the child with needs (Pilapil, Coletti, Rabey, & DeLaet, 2017). Caregiving affects the parents' physical and/or psychological health, financial status, and family function (Pilapil et al., 2017).

Hamilton, Mazzucchelli, and Sanders (2015) also examined parental support for children with disabilities. In the adolescent years, the needs of the child dramatically shift, as parenting styles that worked at a younger age are no longer effective. Parents report struggling to understand these needs and making accommodations for the transitions of their adolescent children, and this frustration leads to increased stress and feelings of grief. The study suggested that a targeted, evidence-based parenting program should be tailored for this special population. Nurses should be prepared to provide parenting support and referrals to parental support groups and educational programs that can assist the parents in providing the best care possible to their children with disabilities.

Nurses should also be aware of the physical needs of parents caring for children with disabilities. In a study by Garip et al. (2017), the researchers noted that mothers of children with cerebral palsy reported depression and lower quality of life associated with a high level of fatigue. Nurses should assess the mother's fatigue level and be watchful for signs and symptoms of depression to assure that the parent is able to provide the care needed for the child.

Caregivers of older adults tend to be spouses or adult children. One study found an average of 30 hours per week of care was provided (Wolff et al., 2018). Although caregivers reported less emotional, financial, and physical difficulties between 1999 and 2015 (Wolff, 2018), many suffer from poor physical health, depression, and anxiety (Riffin, Van Ness, Wolff, & Fried, 2019). Over half of caregivers reported caregiver burden related to the recipient's dementia (Riffin et al., 2019). Fewer than 10% of caregivers use supportive services or attend training on best practices in providing care (Riffin et al., 2019). C/PHNs working with this population should provide caregivers with community resource referrals such as in respite care, support services, and local classes for training.

Children and adults with disabilities are at risk of abuse due to many factors. The exact number of children with disabilities who are abused remains unknown. The abuse could be triggered by the parents being stressed with the obligations of caring for a disabled child or frustrated with the child's difficult behavior (CDC, 2018). Other risk factors for abuse include inadequate social support for the parents, financial burdens, and time constraints in caring for a child with disabilities (Prevent Child Abuse America, 2019).

Categories of elder abuse or dependent adult abuse include physical abuse, psychological abuse, neglect, and financial abuse. Platt et al. (2017) discovered that over 63% of men and 68% of women with developmental disabilities had been abused as adults. More women than men had been sexually abused, but for other types of abuse, there was no difference between genders (Platt et al., 2017). Health care providers may find it difficult to detect intimate partner violence (IPV) in women with disabilities. Health care staff need to be educated on communication skills with women who have experienced IPV to detect and treat these women (Ruiz-Pérez, Pastor-Moreno, Escribà-Agüir, & Maroto-Navarro, 2018). In a study conducted by Ballan, Freyer, and Powledge (2017), researchers discovered that men with disabilities experienced IPV at a higher rate than men or women without disabilities. More than 71% of the men described physical abuse as the most severe type of abuse and nearly half had seen a medical provider. Yet, fewer than 16% of these men had been referred to IPV assistance (Ballan et al., 2017). Clearly more needs to be done to protect this population from abuse.

Geographic differences were noted in a national survey of therapy services provided to infants and toddlers with developmental disabilities. Magnusson and McManus (2017) found that states differ in their ability to meet the needs of these children for physical, occupational, and speech therapy. IDEA requires states to provide early intervention services but allows the individual states to set their own criteria. Children living in states with narrow early intervention eligibility had a significant level of unmet therapy needs. Furthermore, children of racial/ethnic minorities had higher levels of unmet needs (Magnusson & McManus, 2017). Paying for needed resources places a financial burden on many families. Parents of children with special needs are more likely to be single, unemployed, or underemployed and to have incomes of <$50,000 per year (McRee, Maslow, & Reiter, 2017). The cost of care of a child with special needs is high and a financial burden to families even when considering only the obvious costs, such as health care provider and hospital bills, diagnostic testing, medical treatments, and prescription medicines (Price & Oliverio, 2016). However, the care often includes many less obvious costs, such as 24-hour supervision for activities of daily living, and these costs often do not end when these children reach the age of 18, but last for their lifetimes. Therapy, health care professionals, financial planners, support group facilitators, educational advocates, special education attorneys, and other professionals may be required for care.

Although *Healthy People 2030* directly addresses delays in receiving primary and preventative care, obstacles to obtaining **assistive devices and technologies** may still be encountered (U.S. Department of Health and Human Services, 2019). **Temporary Assistance for Needy Families (TANF)**, **Social Security's Supplemental Security Income (SSI)**, and Medicaid are three government assistance programs nurses should familiarize themselves with. TANF is a time-limited federal program that provides assistance to families that cannot meet basic needs. Each state determines how to use the funds (U.S. DHHS, n.d.). SSI is a federal program that provides income to persons with disabilities who have little or no income to meet their basic needs (Social Security Administration, 2018). Lastly, Medicaid provides affordable coverage as well as services not normally covered by provider insurance (Musumeci, 2018). Those with disabilities and their families often are unaware of eligible programs and confused about the rules and regulations of each program. CHNs working with this population need to educate themselves on government resources and nonprofit agencies that assist the family in attaining equipment and supplies. Advocating for our clients and providing case management provide a welcome relief to families.

Respite care is another resource of great importance for families. Due to the constant demands of providing care 24 hours per day, 7 days per week and the stress associated with numerous demands, respite offers relief and hope in regaining normalcy, not only for the primary caregiver, but for the siblings, as well (Whitmore & Snethen, 2017). When focus is placed on the needs of one family member, other children may feel that their own needs are not as important, which can lead to behavioral and health-related problems (Box 24-8). Although more spouses and adult children who care for older adults with disabilities are using respite care, only 15% of caregivers currently use it (Wolf et al., 2018). Respite care is vital to the family's health and should be considered a priority in the overall treatment plan. ARCH National Respite Network and Resource Center provides a list of respite services nationwide.

The issue of employment is generally of great significance to families, as employment options may be quite limited when a family member has special needs. The family may have to remain in a particular location to access needed health and social services, reducing the possibility of increased earning potential at a different location or in another field of employment. Although some legal protections are provided under the **Family and Medical Leave Act** of 1993, it does not apply in all situations. For instance, it is only available in companies with more than 50 employees and is most often used for birth and care of a newborn or newly adopted child or for temporary care of a family member with a serious health problem (spouse, parent, or child). More importantly, it allows only for time off; it does not mandate that employers continue a salary during those periods (USDOL, n.d.b). Family members may have to choose between taking unpaid time off and continuing to work while dealing with the needs of the family member as best they can. Some individuals choose to work part-time or not to work at all so that they can care for family members (Baillargeon, Bernier, & Normand, 2011). At a time when many families have two wage earners to help meet financial commitments, families engaged in caregiving may have to rely on only one income. Limitations in income are particularly challenging considering the myriad needs of those who are disabled, needs that may not be covered by any insurance.

Falk (2016) explored the relationship between welfare status and health. The researcher noted that families receiving TANF often were eligible for many programs and that the different policies and requirements are difficult for families to navigate.

Caregiver health needs and mental health status are another area of concern for families. The mental health of the mother as caregiver is documented to be an area of concern, and the expression of depression in this population is concerning (In Sook & Hyun Sook, 2015; Yamaoka et al., 2015). Although research often focuses on the mental health of the mother as caregiver, a line of research exploring paternal mental health when caring for a child with an intellectual disability is growing. This research suggests that the child's behavior problems, father's daily stress, low parenting satisfaction, and childcare needs are the biggest predictors for the father's mental health difficulties (Giallo et al., 2015). A study exploring family health of parents caring for a child with disabilities indicated that parent caregivers who experienced activity restriction and low social support and those families in the lowest quartile of monthly expenditure were more likely to experience psychological distress (Yamaoka et al., 2015). It is important for nurses to provide detailed information about the child's health needs, disease, disability, medical services available, and social support available to meet the needs of the child to decrease parental mental health stress and disorders. Recognizing that caregivers within a family are at increased risk for poor health outcomes, it is important that the C/PHN select appropriate interventions to address the health needs of all family members.

Families may experience financial difficulties, poor physical or mental health, and a variety of other challenges. For instance, a classic study on loss of family income related to having a child with autism spectrum disorder found an average decrease in annual income of 14% for these families (Montes & Halterman, 2008). Families are often ill prepared to deal with the complicated systems that must be accessed to obtain needed care. The C/PHN is in an optimal position to interpret those systems to the families and to advocate for the needed care, services, and equipment (Fig. 24-4). The nurse must view the family holistically, recognizing additional needs that may develop as a result of the situation currently faced, and include an assessment of caregiver and family work patterns when caring for families with a family member who is disabled.

Organizations Serving the Needs of Individuals With Disabilities and Their Families

Many governmental and privately funded organizations are dedicated to serving individuals with disabilities and

BOX 24-8 C/PHN USE OF THE NURSING PROCESS

Supporting a Family With a Child With Autism

ASSESSMENT

The local public health department received a referral from the school nurse requesting a home visit on the Smith family. The family recently moved to the area with three small children. The school nurse expressed concern because the children are late to school every morning, their clothes are dirty, and they arrive to school hungry. The C/PHN arrives to the home unannounced in order to assess the home life. Both parents are home but the father retreats into the bedroom when the nurse arrives. The mother of the children, Joanne, is 25 years old and has recently lost her job at a small boutique. The father, Richard, is 26 and has started working two jobs to pay the bills. The family recently moved to a new town 100 miles away from the wife's family who provided emotional support and help with childcare. The one-bedroom apartment is cluttered and dirty. The apartment is void toys and family photos. James the 5-year-old was diagnosed with autism at the age of two. He is seen hitting his head against wall and throwing clothes. Joanne is attempting to calm her son and is yelling to Richard to help without success. The other children are playing videos ignoring their mother's request for help. Joanne expresses being overwhelmed since the family moved away from her family and friends. The family has not connected with a medical home yet, finances are insufficient to pay bills, and they have no social support in the new neighborhood. The two older children ages 7 and 10 are sick with colds and have productive coughs. They have missed 4 days of school and are falling behind in their studies. The mother appears unconcerned about her children's health issues. The family does not have a medical home and the mother expresses being overwhelmed with the children's health issues, especially James. The C/PHN notices the lack of affection between members.

PROBLEM STATEMENTS

1. Ineffective parenting skills
2. Support for a healthy family management plan

PLAN/IMPLEMENTATION

Problem Statement 1

The C/PHN will:

- Assess the family support systems and refer the parents to support groups of children with disabilities.
- Provide resources for sliding scale family counseling and other governmental or private organizations.
- Provide information regarding respite care for parents to have time for themselves and the other children.
- Encourage parenting classes and role model communication techniques with children.
- Continue to assess parents stress level and assess for possible abuse.
- Schedule monthly follow-up visits to provide a resource and support to the parents.

Problem Statement 2

The C/PHN will:

- Assist the family in finding a medical home.
- Educate the parents in healthy behaviors such as exercise and proper nutrition.
- Assess health literacy of parents and provide information that best meets their needs and understanding.
- Acknowledge each family member's health concerns.

EVALUATION

The C/PHN conducted follow-up visits every 2 weeks to check on family progress. After 1 month, the C/PHN reported the family had a medical home that provided antibiotics for the older children's sinus infection. The two older children and the parents had gone to the park twice using a free respite service provided through a local church. The children are attending school and are doing well. The parents have joined support group for parents with children with disabilities and have made friends with group members. The mother is observed playing with children. The home while still cluttered is clean. The C/PHN informs the parents they are doing wonderful and will decrease her visits to monthly. She encourages the parents to contact her if they have any questions or concerns.

their families as well as educating the public on disabilities. These organizations provide nurses with a starting point for exploring specific topics pertinent to practice. As clients and families may also be accessing online content through personal or public internet access, it is important for nurses to prescreen and make recommendations to clients and families about reliable and accurate sites. Numerous organizations provide Web sites to assist individuals with disabilities and their families; a few key Web sites are listed in Table 24-2.

The C/PHN student is encouraged to explore these resources and to learn more about specific disabilities that can impact clients and their families. For example, parents may not realize their child has a hearing loss. It may take an outside family member, a neighbor, a teacher, or a nurse to notice a child who is not talking at an age-appropriate level or who does turn to the source of a sound. Children born prematurely and the elderly are at risk for hearing loss. Genetic syndromes and accidents can also cause unexpected loss of hearing. In fact, one out of every eight people in the United States has a hearing loss (CDC, 2019a). Luckily, there are screening tools, treatments, and interventions for those that are deaf or hard of hearing. In addition to technology such as hearing aids and cochlear implants, many people learn alternate ways to communicate such as sign language. Box 24-9 offers a brief summary of the purpose and use of **American Sign Language** and other signed languages, and Box 24-10 discusses Braille.

UNIVERSAL DESIGN

For those living with a disability or chronic disease and their family members, the issue of access is of utmost importance. **Universal design** is the concept of pur-

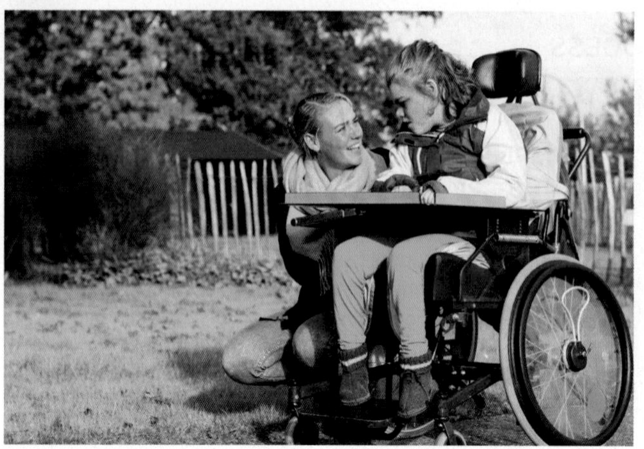

FIGURE 24-4 Public health nursing support for families with children with disabilities can be critical in helping them access resources and services.

posely creating environments in a way that they are accessible to all without the need for modifications. The term universal design has been attributed to Ron Mace, founder of the Center for Universal Design, based out of North Carolina State University. Mace, who had polio as a child, died suddenly in 1998, leaving behind a long legacy of advocacy on behalf of accessibility in design (Center for Universal Design, 2016). Universal design is at the core of the ADA, and it is important to note the relationship between inclusiveness and reduction of barriers to access (Hums, Schmidt, Bocak, & Wolff, 2016). Universal design is for everyone, not solely for those with disabilities.

The issue of accessibility is not new. The ADA, as discussed earlier, addresses issues of access in employment, governmental building, and public accommodations. The Fair Housing Accessibility Guidelines, effective beginning in 1991, provide for design and construction of multifamily dwellings (four or more units) in accordance with accessibility requirements (United States Department of Housing and Urban Development, n.d.). Provisions mandate that doorways be wide enough to accommodate wheelchairs, dwellings be readily accessible to and usable by persons with handicaps, and accessible routes be throughout buildings (Figs. 24-5 through 24-7; Fair Housing Accessibility First, n.d.). The specific provisions may be found at https://www.fairhousingfirst.org.

TABLE **24-2** Web sites to Assist Those With Disabilities and Their Families

Organization	Description	Website
Disabled World	Provides lists of disabled services within the United States	https://www.disabled-world.com/disability/foundations/us-organizations.php
American Deafness and Rehabilitation Association (ADARA)	National organization that assists and educates those who work with the deaf and hard of hearing	https://www.adara.org/
American Council of the Blind (ACB)	Mission is to increase independence and quality of life for the blind and visually impaired; has had a historical presence in state I local chapter since the 1880s	https://www.acb.org
The Arc	Works to support and protect the rights of those with intellectual and developmental disabilities	https://thearc.org/
National Organization on Disabilities	Works to increase employment opportunities for working-age disabled Americans	https://www.nod.org/
Easterseals	A resource for individuals with disabilities providing programs, services, early intervention, workforce development, and adult day care	https://www.easterseals.com
Special Olympics	Uses sports and activities to inspire and reach those with disabilities	https://www.specialolympics.org/
United Cerebral Palsy	Provides family assistance, education, financial assistance, and resources for those with a spectrum of disabilities	http://ucp.org/
Special Needs Alliance	National organization of attorneys who specialize in public benefits law and assist those with disabilities	https://www.specialneedsalliance.org/
National Center on Disability and Journalism	Provides links to many resources and services	https://ncdj.org/resources/organizations/#neurological-disorders-and-injury

BOX 24-9 Sign Language in Brief

- Sign language is the use of "handshapes" and gestures to communicate ideas or concepts.
- American Sign Language is a unique language with its own rules of grammar and syntax.
- American Sign Language is primarily used in America and Canada and is the natural language of the deaf community; in Britain, British Sign Language (BSL) is used.
- Sign languages are not universal.
- International Sign Language (Gestuno) is composed of vocabulary signs from various sign languages for use at international events or meetings to aid communication.
- Systems of Manually Coded English (i.e., Signed English, Signing Exact English) are not natural languages but systems designed to represent the translation of spoken language word for word.

Source: ASL University (n.d.); CDC (2014); National Institute on Deafness and Other Communication Disorders (2015).

For those with existing disabilities and as the population ages, ensuring easy accessibility to all in businesses, housing, and places of recreation is of paramount importance. Having the opportunities for healthy participation in physical activity may forestall or prevent the development of illness. For the community, having an environment that promotes rather than restricts a healthy lifestyle can be economically advantageous (Fig. 24-8).

BOX 24-10 What Is Braille?

Braille takes its name from Louis Braille, an 18-year-old blind Frenchman who created a system of raised dots on paper for reading and writing by modifying a system used on board sailing ships for night reading. The six raised dots of each Braille "cell" vary to form palpable letters and punctuation. Persons experienced in Braille can read at speeds of 200 to 400 words per minute, comparable to print readers. Braille text can be written (1) by hand with a slate and stylus; (2) with a Braille writing machine; or (3) with specialized computer software and a Braille-embossing device attached to the printer.

Source: National Federation of the Blind (n.d.)

Note: More information about Braille is available at: http://nfb.org/search/node/braille.

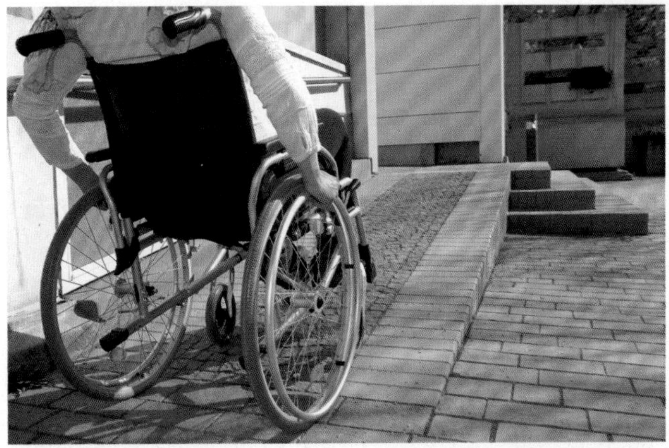

FIGURE 24-5 Ramps are needed for those using wheelchairs to gain access to buildings.

A healthier population may be achieved with attention to the environmental barriers that impede healthy lifestyles for all persons, including those with disabling conditions.

THE ROLE OF THE COMMUNITY/PUBLIC HEALTH NURSE

This section considers the various roles of the C/PHN working with this population. It is important to review these roles in the context of multilevel practice: the individual, the family, and the community. Chapter 2 first examined the broad spectrum of roles that the C/PHN assumes within the community (i.e., clinician, educator, advocate, manager, collaborator, leader, researcher), as well as the 10 essential services of public health. Consider an example of the variety of roles with respect to a 55-year-old female client who uses a wheelchair. The client has difficulty obtaining a gynecologic examination because of the lack of accessible examination tables at the

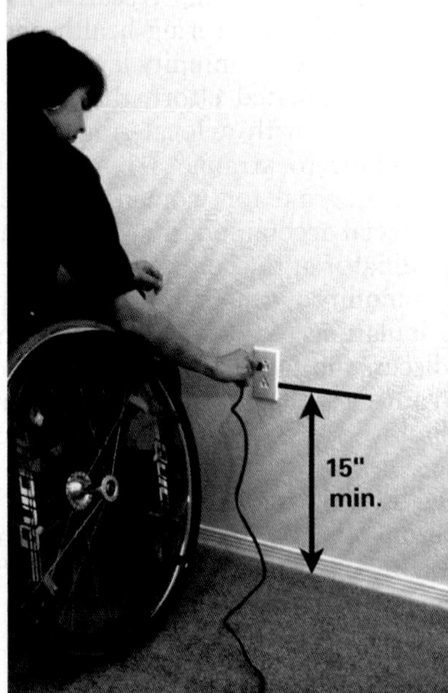

FIGURE 24-6 Recommended height of electrical outlet for ease of access for wheelchair-seated person. (From CDC Image Library. Retrieved from http://phil.cdc.gov/Phil/quicksearch.asp.)

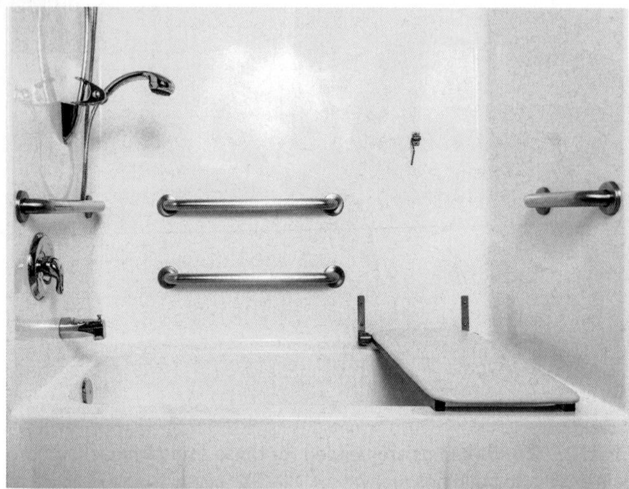

FIGURE 24-7 Handicap access shower. (CDC Image Library. Retrieved from http://phil.cdc.gov/Phil/quicksearch.asp.)

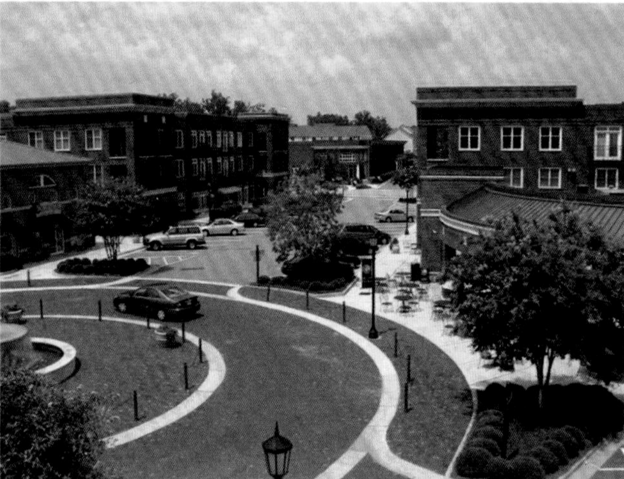

FIGURE 24-8 Planned, mixed-use development with curb cuts, well-marked crossings, sidewalks, and accessible commercial and public spaces. (Source: Center for Universal Design. CDC Image Library.)

local clinic; as a result, she has not had an examination for more than 20 years. Recognizing the need for a complete examination, the C/PHN arranges with the clinic to find appropriate alternatives that will aid the client in receiving the needed examination, possibly by ensuring that additional personnel are provided. The C/PHN is an advocate at the individual level providing the essential services of monitoring health. Because this solution is temporary and less than optimal, the nurse contacts a number of clinics in neighboring communities and finds one that has appropriate equipment for people who have difficulty transferring to a standard examination table. Unfortunately, this clinic is 1 hour away. The nurse then contacts a number of other C/PHNs and discovers that they also have a significant number of women clients with this problem who have not received a gynecologic examination in many years. The C/PHN discovers a need at the community level through research. Essential services provided include monitoring health and diagnosis and investigation at the community level.

Through a coordinated effort, the nurse is able to develop partnerships with a local transportation company and the clinic to arrange a twice-yearly gynecologic screening program for women in the community who require special accommodations. Acting as an advocate and coordinator at the community level, the C/PHN mobilizes community partnerships, develops policy, and links the population to needed services. Information sheets that discuss the need for annual gynecologic examinations and advertise the program are distributed to area C/PHNs, employers, and health clinics. Functioning in the educator role at the community level, the C/PHN is providing the essential services of informing, educating, and empowering others. Data collection on examinations provided over the next few years shows a 65% increase in the number of women with special needs who have received a gynecologic examination within the past year. Continuing in the role of researcher at the community level, the C/PHN practices the essential services of evaluating the services and reaching new solutions.

This is not an uncommon scenario in the practice of community/public health nursing. Often, the needs of an individual may open the door to areas of concern for many in a community and provide a basis for intervention that can benefit a larger population. The complexity of issues surrounding these conditions requires creativity, tenacity, honesty, and, most of all, knowledge. C/PHNs who are informed about the issues that affect those with disabilities at local, state, and national levels are prepared to offer assistance to their clients and to their communities.

Although successes at the individual level are laudable, the extent to which the health and well-being of those affected are improved must be the ultimate goal. Forming partnerships within the community places the C/PHN in a prime position to initiate and support efforts to improve the health status of those populations.

It is important for C/PHNs to consider population health among those with disabilities. As Grady (2011) reminds us, our U.S. population is living longer, is suffering multiple chronic illness and disabilities, and needs nurses trained to meet the requirements of this aging population. Population health promotion and prevention of secondary disabilities are also public health concerns across age groups and conditions (Ouellette-Kuntz, Cobigo, Balogh, Wilton, & Lunsky, 2015). Community-based interventions that help support all populations with self-management skills, improve health behaviors, and prevent secondary disabilities have been shown to be popular and can result in cost savings as well as improved health outcomes (Ravesloot et al., 2016).

SUMMARY

- The issues of disability are of growing importance in public health and to community/public health nursing, both nationally and internationally.
- Through the efforts of the WHO, the international community has been challenged to provide increased attention to health promotion and disease prevention.

- The aging of the U.S. population and the rise in lifestyle-related illnesses such as diabetes and obesity are often linked with increasing rates of disability. Health disparities and differing access to services are a focus of *Healthy People 2030*.
- *Healthy People* has placed increasing focus on individuals' well-being, helping those with disabilities to get support and services within the health care system, at work, home, and school. To improve quality of life, accessibility in our homes, schools and workplaces is essential.
- Legislation is but one step toward equality for those affected by disabilities and chronic illnesses. The IDEA and ADA secured many improvements in accessibility and specific legal protections for the disabled, but it is only the beginning.
- C/PHNs are in a prime position to advocate for the health needs of the disabled and chronically ill. With a long history of serving those who are most vulnerable, C/PHNs can help make needed changes at the individual, family, and community levels.

ACTIVE LEARNING EXERCISES

1. Interview an individual with a disability (e.g., hearing, vision, mobility) about the challenges that he or she has faced in interactions with nondisabled persons and in everyday activities.
2. Using "Utilize Legal and Regulatory Actions" (1 of the 10 essential health services), how does legislation effect the health and well-being of a disabled client and their family? Looking at disability rights, how would you address the essential services specific to Developing Policies and Enforcing Laws?
3. Take an inventory of your house or apartment and make a list of modifications you would need to make if you had a disability. Would you even be able to stay in your current residence (e.g., are you living in a second-floor apartment in a building that does not have an elevator)?
4. What resources are available in your community to assist disabled individuals and families?
5. Address health promotion activities for clients and their families in your community health clinical course who are either disabled or have a chronic illness. Examples of health promotion activities could include healthy eating, physical activity, and leisure-time activities. Does the public health department have any outreach services for disabled clients to encourage them to obtain routine preventable services? Ask some of your clients with disabilities and chronic illnesses about their experiences and feelings about preventive services.

REFERENCES

American Psychological Association. (2019). *Disability and socioeconomic status*. Retrieved from https://www.apa.org/pi/ses/resources/publications/disability

American Sign Language (ASL) University. (n.d.). *International sign language (Gestuno)*. Retrieved from http://www.lifeprint.com/asl101/pages-layout/gestuno.htm

An, R., Andrade, F., & Chiu, C. (2015). Overweight and obesity among U.S. adults with and without disability, 1999–2012. *Preventive Medicine Reports, 2*, 419–422. doi: 10.1016/j.pmedr.2015.05.001.

Andersen, S. L., Olsen, J., & Laurberg, P. (2015). Foetal programming by maternal thyroid disease. *Clinical Endocrinology Oxford, 83*(6), 751–758. doi: 10.1111/cen.12744.

Ballan, M. S., Freyer, M. B., & Powledge, L. (2017). Intimate partner violence among men with disabilities: The role of health care providers. *American Journal of Men's Health, 11*(5), 1436–1443. doi: 10.1177/1557988315606966.

Baillargeon, R. H., Bernier, J., & Normand, C. L. (2011). The challenges faced by caregivers of children with impairments of psychological functions: A population-based cross-sectional study. *Canadian Journal of Psychiatry, 56*(10), 614–620.

Banks, L., Kuper, H., & Polack, S. (2018). Poverty and disability in low- and middle-income countries: A systematic review. *PLoS One, 13*(9), e0204881.

Brolan, C. E., Boyle, F. M., Dean, J. H., Taylor-Gomez, M., Ware, R. S., & Lennox, N. G. (2012). Health advocacy: A vital step in attaining human rights for adults with intellectual disability. *Journal of Intellectual Disability Research, 56*(11), 1087–1097.

Brown, H. K., Plourde, N., Ouellette-Kuntz, H., Vigod, S., & Cobigo, V. (2016). Brief report: Cervical cancer screening in women with intellectual and development disabilities who have had a pregnancy. *Journal of Intellectual Disability Research, 60*(1), 22–27. doi: 10.1111/jir.12225.

Centers for Disease Control and Prevention (CDC). (2014). *Manually coded English (MCE)*. Retrieved from http://www.cdc.gov/ncbddd/hearingloss/parentsguide/building/manual-english.html

Centers for Disease Control and Prevention (CDC). (2015). *CDC's built environment and health initiative*. Retrieved from https://www.cdc.gov/nceh/information/built_environment.htm

Centers for Disease Control and Prevention (CDC). (2018a). *Disability and Health Data System (DHDS)*. Retrieved from http://dhds.cdc.gov

Centers for Disease Control and Prevention (CDC). (2018b). *Safety and Children with Disabilities: Childhood maltreatment among children with disabilities*. Retrieved from https://www.cdc.gov/ncbddd/disabilityandsafety/abuse.html

Centers for Disease Control and Prevention (CDC). (2019a). *Hearing loss in children*. Retrieved from https://www.cdc.gov/ncbddd/hearingloss/facts.html

Centers for Disease Control and Prevention (CDC). (2019b). *Arthritis*. Retrieved from http://www.cdc.gov/chronicdisease/resources/publications/aag/arthritis.htm

Centers for Disease Control and Prevention (CDC). (2020). *Disability and health promotion*. Retrieved from https://www.cdc.gov/ncbddd/disabilityandhealth/index.html

Center for Universal Design. (2016). *About the center: Ronald L. Mace*. Retrieved from https://www.ncsu.edu/ncsu/design/cud/about_us/usronmace.htm

Cobigo, V., Balogh, R., Wilton, A., & Lunsky, Y. (2015). The uptake of secondary prevention by adults with intellectual and developmental disabilities. *Journal of Applied Research on Intellectual Disabilities, 28*(1), 43–54.

Cody, P. J., & Lerand, S. J. (2013). Original study: HPV vaccination in female children with special health care needs. *Journal of Pediatric and Adolescent Gynecology, 26*, 219–223. doi: 10.1016/j.jpag.2013.03.003.

Cook, L. H., Foley, J. T., & Semeah, L. M. (2016). Research paper: An exploratory study of inclusive worksite wellness: Considering employees with disabilities. *Disability and Health Journal, 9*, 100–107. doi: 10.1016/j.dhjo.2015.08.011.

Cureton, A., & Silvers, A. (2017). Respecting the dignity of children with disabilities in clinical practice. *HEC Forum, 29*(3), 257–276. doi: 10.1007/s10730-017-9326-3.

Dykens, E. M. (2015). Family adjustment and interventions in neurodevelopmental disorders. *Current Opinion in Psychiatry, 28*(2), 121–126.

Fair Housing Accessibility First. (n.d.). *Requirements*. Retrieved from http://www.fairhousingfirst.org/fairhousing/requirements.html

Falk, G. (2016). *Temporary Assistance for Needy Families (TANF): Size and characteristics of the cash assistance caseload*. Congressional Research Service: Report, 1. Retrieved from https://www.fas.org/sgp/crs/misc/R43187.pdf

Garip, Y., Ozel, S., Tuncer, O. B., Kilinc, G., Seckin, F., & Arasil, T. (2017). Fatigue in mothers of children with cerebral palsy. *Disability Rehabilitation, 39*(8), 757–762. doi: 10.3109/09638288.2016.1161837.

GBD 2015 Disease and Injury Incidence and Prevalence Collaborators. (2016). Global, regional, and national incidence, prevalence, and years lived with disability for 310 diseases and injuries, 1990–2015: A systematic analysis for the global burden of disease study 2015. *Lancet, 388*, 1545–1602. doi: 10.1016/S0140-6736(16)31678-6.

Georgieff, M. K. (2017). Iron assessment to protect the developing brain. *American Journal of Clinical Nutrition, 106*(Suppl 6), 1588S–1593S.

Giallo, R., Seymour, M., Matthews, J., Gavidia-Payne, S., Hudson, A., & Cameron, C. (2015). Risk factors associated with the mental health of fathers of children with an intellectual disability in Australia. *Journal of Intellectual Disability Research, 59*(3), 193–207. doi: 10.1111/jir.12127.

Gofine, M., Mielenz, T. J., Vasan, S., & Lebwohl, B. (2018). Use of colorectal cancer screening among people mobility disability. *Journal of Clinical Gastroenterology, 52*(9), 789–795. doi: 10.1097/MCG.0000000000000835.

Grady, P. A. (2011). Advancing the health of our aging population: A lead role for nursing science. *Nursing Outlook, 59*, 207–209.

Greenwood, V. J., Crawford, N. W., Walstab, J. E., & Reddihough, D. S. (2013). Immunisation coverage in children with cerebral palsy compared with the general population. *Journal of Paediatrics & Child Health, 49*(2), E137. doi: 10.1111/jpc.12097.

Hamilton, A., Mazzucchelli, T. G., & Sanders, M. R. (2015). Parental and practitioner perspectives on raising an adolescent with a disability: A focus group study. *Disability & Rehabilitation, 37*(18), 1664–1673. doi: 10.3109/09638288.2014.973969.

Hensel, R. M. (2016). The official Robert M. Hensel website. Retrieved from http://roberthensel.webs.com/myquotes.htm

Holland-Hall, C., & Quint, E. H. (2017). Sexuality and disability in adolescents. *Pediatric Clinics of North America, 64*(2), 435–449. doi: 10.1016/j.pci.2016.11.011.

Horner-Johnson, W., Dobbertin, K., & Iezzoni, L. I. (2015). Disparities in receipt of breast and cervical cancer screening for rural women age 18 to 64 with disabilities. *Women's Health Issues, 25*(3), 246–253. doi: 10.1016/j.whi.2015.02.004.

Hums, M. A., Schmidt, S. H., Novak, A., & Wolff, E. A. (2016). Universal design: Moving the Americans with Disabilities Act from access to inclusion. *Journal of Legal Aspects of Sport, 26*(1), 36–51.

Iezzoni, L. I., Kurtz, S. G., & Rao, S. R. (2015). Trends in mammography over time for women with and without chronic disability. *Journal of Women's Health, 24*(7), 593–601. doi: 10.1089/jwh.2014.5181.

In Sook, C., & Hyun Sook, R. (2015). Factors affecting depression in mothers of children with disabilities. *Child Health Nursing Research, 21*(1), 46–54. doi: 10.4094/chnr.2015.21.1.46.

Jones, M., Morris, J., & Deruyter, F. (2018). Mobile healthcare and people with disabilities: Current state and future needs. *International Journal of Environmental Research and Public Health, 15*(3), E515. doi: 10.3390/ijerph15030515.

Kennedy, J., Wood, E. G., & Frieden, L. (2017). Disparities in insurance coverage, health services use, and access following implementation of the Affordable Care Act: A comparison of disabled and nondisabled working-age adults. *Inquiry: The Journal of Health Care Organization, Provision and Financing, 54*, 1–10. doi: 10.117/0046958017734031.

Kraus, L., Lauer, E., Coleman, R., & Houtenville, A. (2018). *2017 disability statistics annual report*. Durham, NH: University of New Hampshire.

Landmark, L. J., Zhang, D., Ju, S., McVey, T. C., & Ji, M. Y. (2017). Experiences of disability advocates and self-advocates in Texas. *Journal of Disability Policy Studies, 27*(4), 203–211. doi: 10.1177/1044207316657802.

Lauer, E. A., Henly, M., & Brucker, D. L. (2019). Prescription opioid behaviors among adults with and without disabilities- United States, 2015–2016. *Disability and Health Journal, 12*, 519–522. doi: 10.1016/j.dhjo. 2018.12.001.

Magnusson, D. M., & McManus, B. (2017). State-level disparities in caregivers-reported unmet therapy need among infants and toddlers with developmental delay in the United States. *HPA Resources, 17*(1), J3–J1.3. ISSN:1931-6313.

Mahmoudi, E., & Meade, M. A. (2015). Research paper: Disparities in access to health care among adults with physical disabilities: Analysis of a representative national sample for a ten-year period. *Disability and Health Journal, 8*, 182–190. doi: 10.1016/j.dhjo.2014.08.007.

Manzoor, M., & Vimarlund, V. (2018). Digital technologies for social inclusion of individuals with disabilities. *Health and Technology, 8*(5), 377–390. doi: 10.1007/s12553-018-0239-1.

Marrocco, A., & Krouse, H. J. (2017). Obstacles to preventive care for individuals with disability: Implications for nurse practitioners. *Journal of the American Association of Nurse Practitioners, 29*(5), 282–293. doi: 10.1002/2327-6924.12440.

McCann, D., Bull, R., & Winzenberg, T. (2015). Sleep deprivation in parents caring for children with complex needs at home: A mixed methods systematic review. *Journal of Family Nursing, 21*(1), 86–118. doi: 10.1177/1074840714562026.

McPherson, A. C., Keith, R., & Swift, J. A. (2014). Obesity prevention for children with physical disabilities: A scoping review of physical activity and nutrition interventions. *Disability & Rehabilitation, 36*(19), 1573–1587.

McRee, A. L., Maslow, G. R., & Reiter, P. L. (2017). Receipt of recommended adolescent vaccines among youth with special health care needs. *Clinical Pediatrics, 56*(5), 451–460. doi: 10.1177/0009922816661330.

Mitra, S., Palmer, M., Kim, H., Mont, D., & Groce, N. (2017). Extra costs of living with a disability: A review and agenda for research. *Disability and Health Journal, 10*(4), 475–484. doi: 10.1016/j.dhjo.2017.04.007.

Montes, G., & Halterman, J. S. (2008). Association of childhood autism spectrum disorders and loss of family income. *Pediatrics, 121*(4), e821–e826.

Musumeci, M. B. (2018). Medicaid's role for children with special health care needs. *The Journal of Law, Medicine, & Ethics, 46*, 897–905. doi: 10.1177/1073110518821987.

Nageswaran, S., & Golden, S. L. (2018). Establishing relationships and navigating boundaries when caring for children with medical complexity at home. *Home Health Care Now, 36*(2), 93–102. doi: 10.1097/NHH.0000000000000636.

Na, L., Hennessy, S., Bogner, H. R., Kurichi, J. E., Stineman, M., Streim, J. E., ... Pezzin, L. E. (2017). Disability stage and receipt of recommended care among elderly medicare beneficiaries. *Disability and Health Journal, 10*(1), 48–57. doi: 10.1016/j.dhjo.2016.09.007.

National Council on Disability (NCD). (n.d.). *About us*. Retrieved from https://www.ncd.gov/about

National Council on Disability (NCD). (2008a). *Finding the gaps: A comparative analysis of disability laws in the United States to the United Nations Convention on the Rights of Persons with Disabilities (CRPD)*. Retrieved from www.ncd.gov/publications/2008/May122008

National Council on Disability (NCD). (2008b). *National disability policy: A progress report*. Retrieved from https://www.ncd.gov/rawmedia_repository/ea8e79b7_17db_427b_a838_19030deb107e.pdf

National Council on Disability (NCD). (2014). *National disability policy: A progress report*. Retrieved from https://www.ncd.gov/progress_reports/10312014

National Federation of the Blind. (n.d.). *Braille–What is it? What does it mean to the blind?* Retrieved from http://www.nfb.org/images/nfb/Publications/fr/fr15/Issue1/f150113.html

National Institute on Deafness and Other Communication Disorders. (2015). *American sign language*. Retrieved from https://www.nidcd.nih.gov/health/american-sign-language

Office of Disease Prevention and Health Promotion (ODPHP). (2016). *Healthy People 2020: Disability and health*. Retrieved from https://www.healthypeople.gov/2020/topics-objectives/topic/disability-and-health

Office of Disease Prevention and health Promotion. (2020). *Health people 2030 framework*. Retrieved from https://www.healthypeople.gov/2020/About-Healthy-People/Development-Healthy-People-2030/Framework

Okoro, C. A., Hollis, N. D., Cyrus, A. C., & Griffin-Blake, S. (2018). Prevalence of disabilities and health care access by disability status and type among adults-United States, 2016. *Morbidity and Mortality Weekly Report (MMRW), 67*, 882–887. doi: 10.15585/mmwr.mm6732a3.

Ouellette-Kuntz, H., Cobigo, V., Balogh, R., Wilton, A., & Lunsky, Y. (2015). The uptake of secondary prevention by adults with intellectual and developmental disabilities. *Journal of Applied Research on Intellectual Disabilities, 28*(1), 43–54.

Pew Research Center. (2019). *Older American are More Likely to Have a Disability*. Retrieved from https://www.pewresearch.org/fact-tank/2017/07/27/7-facts-about-americans-with-disabilities/ft_17-07-27_disabledolderamericans/

Pilapil, M., Coletti, D. J., Rabey, C., & DeLaet, D. (2017). Caring for the caregiver: Supporting families of youth with special health care needs. *Current Problems in Pediatric and Adolescent Health Care, 47*(8), 190–199. doi: 10.1016/j.cppeds.2017.07.003.

Platt, L., Powers, L., Leotti, S., Hughes, R. B., Robinson-Whelen, S., Osburn, S., ... Nicolaidis, C. S. (2017). The role of gender in violence experienced by adults with developmental disabilities. *Journal of Interpersonal Violence, 32*(1), 101–129. doi: 10.1177/0886260515585534.

Prevent Child Abuse America. (2019). *Maltreatment of children with Disabilities-Fact sheet*. Retrieved from https://preventchildabuse.org/resource/maltreatment-of-children-with-disabilities-2/

Price, M. S., & Oliverio, P. (2016). The costs of raising a special needs child after divorce. *American Journal of Family Law, 30*(1), 25–31.

Ravesloot, C., Seekins, T., Traci, M., Boehm, T., White, G., Witten, M. H., ... Monson, J. (2016). Living well with a disability, a self-management program. *MMWR Supplement, 65*(1), 61–67.

Reichard, A., Gulley, S. P., Rasch, E. K., & Chan, L. (2015). Diagnosis isn't enough: Understanding the connections between high health care utilization, chronic conditions and disabilities among U.S. working age adults. *Disability and Health Journal, 8*(4), 535–546. doi: 10.1016/j.dhjo.2015.04.006.

Riffin, C., Van Ness, P. H., Wolff, J. L., & Fried, T. (2019). Multifactorial examination of caregiver burden in a national sample of family and unpaid caregivers. *Journal of the American Geriatrics Society, 67*(2), 277–283. doi: 10.1111/jgs.15664.

Robinson, L. R., Holbrook, J. R., Bitsko, R. H., Hartwig, S. A., Kaminski, J. W., Ghandour, R. M., ... Boyle, C. A. (2017). Differences in health care, family, and community factors associated with mental, behavioral, and developmental disorders among children aged 2–8 years in rural and urban areas—United States, 2011–2012. *Morbidity and Mortality Weekly Report. Surveillance Summaries, 66*(8), 1–11. doi: 10.15585/mmwr.ss6608a1.

Rosen-Reynoso, M., Porche, M. V., Kwan, N., Bethell, C., Thomas, V., Robertson, J., ... Palfrey, J. (2016). Disparities in access to easy-to-use services for children with special health care needs. *Maternal Child Health Journal, 20*(5), 1041–1053. doi: 10.1007/s10995-015-1890-z.

Ruiz-Pérez, I., Pastor-Moreno, G., Escribà-Agüir, V., & Maroto-Navarro, G. (2018). Intimate partner violence in women with disabilities: Perception of healthcare and attitudes of health professions. *Disability and Rehabilitation, 40*(9), 1059–1065. doi: 10.1080/09638288.2017.1288273.

Saitta, M., Devan, H., Boland, P., & Perry, M. A. (2019). Park-based physical activity interventions for persons with disabilities: A mixed-methods systemic review. *Disability and Health Journal, 12*(1), 11–23. doi: 10.1016/j.dhjo.2018.07.006.

Shenaar-Golan, V. (2017). Hope and subjective well-being among parents of children with special needs. *Child & Family Social Work, 22*(1), 306–316. doi: 10.1111/cfs. 12241.

Smith, D. L., & Notaro, S. J. (2015). Is emergency preparedness a 'disaster' for people with disabilities in the US? Results from the 2006–2012 behavioral risk factor surveillance system (BRFSS). *Journal of Disability and Society, 30*(3), 401–418. doi: 10.1080/09687599.2015.1021413.

Social Security Administration. (2018). *Supplemental Security Income Home Page-2018 Edition*. Retrieved from https://www.ssa.gov/ssi/

Stevens, G. A., Bennett, J. E., Hennocq, Q., Lu, Y., De-Regil, L. M., Rogers, L., ... Ezzati, M. (2015). Articles: Trends and mortality effects of vitamin A deficiency in children in 138 low-income and middle-income countries between 1991 and 2013: A pooled analysis of population-based surveys. *The Lancet Global Health, 3*, e528–e536. doi: 10.1016/S2214-109X(15)00039-X.

Taylor, J. L., Hodapp, R. M., Burke, M. M., Waitz-Kudla, S. N., & Radideau, C. (2017). Training parents of youth with Autism Spectrum Disorder to advocate for adult disability services: Results from a pilot randomized controlled trial. *Journal of Autism and Developmental Disorders, 47*(3), 846–857. doi: 10.1007/s10803-016-2994-z.

The Arc. (n.d.). *Public policy and legal advocacy: Policy issues affecting people with disabilities*. Retrieved from http://www.thearc.org/what-we-do/public-policy

Together We Rock. (n.d.). *Common myths and misconceptions about disability*. Retrieved from http://static1.squarespace.com/static/565dec2de4b0475ab00625b6/t/56cbc06a62cd94fc4bc447b3/1456193645073/Myths+and+Misconceptions+–+Accessible+Format+–+Jan+27%2C+2016.pdf

United Nations. (2016, May 30). *Treaty collection: Chapter IV: Human rights—Convention on the Rights of Persons with Disabilities*. Retrieved from https://treaties.un.org/Pages/ViewDetails.aspx?src=IND&mtdsg_no=IV-15&chapter=4&lang=en

U.S. Census Bureau. (2015). *American Community survey and Puerto Rico Community Survey 2015 Subject and Definitions*. Retrieved from https://www2.census.gov/programs-surveys/acs/tech_docs/subject_definitions/2015_ACSSubjectDefinitions.pdf

U.S. Department of Health and Human Services (USDHHS). (n.d.). *Category: Programs for Families and Children*. Retrieved from https://www.hhs.gov/answers/programs-for-families-and-children/index.html

U.S. Department of Health and Human Services (USDHHS). (2006). *Progress toward Healthy People 2010 targets: Disability and secondary conditions*. Retrieved from http://www.healthypeople.gov/2010/data/midcourse/html/focusareas/fa06progresshp.htm

U.S. Department of Health and Human Services (USDHHS). (2016). *Healthy People 2020: About Healthy People*. Retrieved from https://www.healthypeople.gov/2020/About-Healthy-People

U.S. Department of Health and Human Services (USDHHS), Office for Civil Rights. (2006, September). *Delivering on the promise: OCR's compliance activities promote community integration*. Retrieved from http://www.hhs.gov/civil-rights/for-individuals/special-topics/community-living-and-olmstead/compliance-activities-promote-integration/index.html

U.S. Department of Health & Human Services (USDHHS). (2020). *Healthy People 2030: Browse objectives*. Retrieved from https://health.gov/healthypeople/objectives-and-data/browse-objectives

U.S. Department of Home Land Security. (2018). *The Whole Community: Individuals with Disabilities in Disaster Response and Recovery*. Retrieved from https://www.dhs.gov/blog/2018/08/29/whole-community-individuals-disabilities-disaster-response-and-recovery

U.S. Department of Housing and Urban Development. (n.d.). *Fair housing accessibility guidelines*. Retrieved from http://portal.hud.gov/hudportal/HUD?src=/program_offices/fair_housing_equal_opp/disabilities/fhefhag

U.S. Department of Justice Civil Rights Division. (n.d.). *Information and Technical Assistance on the Americans with Disabilities Act*. Retrieved from https://www.ada.gov

U.S. Department of Justice Civil Rights Division. (2009). *A Guide to Disability Rights Laws*. Retrieved from https://www.ada.gov/cguide.htm

U.S. Department of Justice Civil Rights Division, Disability Rights Section. (2020). *A guide to disability rights law*. Retrieved from https://www.ada.gov/cguide.htm

U.S. Department of Labor (USDOL). (n.d.a). *Employers and the ADA: Myths and facts*. Retrieved from https://www.dol.gov/odep/pubs/fact/ada.htm

U.S. Department of Labor (USDOL). (n.d.b). *The Family and Medical Leave Act*. Retrieved from https://www.dol.gov/whd/regs/compliance/1421.htm

U.S. Department of State. (2019). *Treaties pending in the Senate (updated as of January 2, 2019)*. Retrieved from https://www.state.gov/s/l/treaty/pending

Vijayaraghavan, K. (2018). National control programme against nutritional blindness due to vitamin A deficiency: Current status & future strategy. *The Indian Journal of Medical Research, 148*(5), 496–502.

Whitmore, K. E., & Snethen, J. (2018). Respite care services for children with special healthcare needs: Parental perceptions. *Journal for Specialist in Pediatric Nursing, 23*(3), e12217. doi: 10.1111/jspn.12217.

Wolff, J. L., Mulcahy, J., Huang, J., Roth, D. L., Covinsky, K., & Kasper, J. D. (2018). Family caregivers of older adults, 1999–2015: Trends in characteristics, circumstances, and role-related appraisal. *Gerontologist, 58*(6), 1021–1032. doi: 10.1093/geront/gnx093.

World Health Organization (WHO). (2001). *International classification of functioning, disability and health*. Geneva, Switzerland: Author.

World Health Organization (WHO). (2002a). *Towards a common language for functioning, disability, and health*. Retrieved from http://www.who.int/classifications/icf/icfbeginnersguide.pdf?ua=1

World Health Organization (WHO). (2002b). *World health report: Reducing risks, promoting healthy life*. Geneva, Switzerland: Author.

World Health Organization. (2011). *World Report on Disability*. Retrieved from https://apps.who.int/iris/bitstream/handle/10665/70670/WHO_NMH_VIP_11.01_eng.pdf;jsessionid=E07AF4E7D44C47A86B7289C214FB404B?sequence=1

World Health Organization (WHO). (2015a). *WHO global disability action plan 2014-2021: Better health for all people with disability*. Retrieved from https://apps.who.int/iris/bitstream/handle/10665/199544/9789241509619_eng.pdf?sequence=1

World Health Organization (WHO). (2016). *What's disability to me? Personal narratives*. Retrieved from http://www.who.int/disabilities/en/

World Health Organization (WHO). (2019a). *Disability and Health*. Retrieved from https://www.who.int/news-room/fact-sheets/detail/disability-and-health

World Health Organization (WHO). (2019b). *International classification of functioning, disability and health*. Retrieved from https://www.who.int/classifications/icf/en/

World Health Organization. (2019c). *Ten threats to global health in 2019*. Retrieved from https://www.who.int/emergencies/ten-threats-to-global-health-in-2019

Yamaoka, Y., Tamiya, N., Moriyama, Y., Sandoval Garrido, F. A., Sumazaki, R., & Noguchi, H. (2015). Mental health of parents as caregivers of children with disabilities: Based on Japanese Nationwide Survey. *PLoS One, 10*(12), e0145200. doi: 10.1371/journal.pone.0145200.

Yee, S. (2016). *Where prejudice, disability, and "disabilism" meet*. Retrieved from http://dredf.org/news/publications/disability-rights-law-and-policy/where-prejudice-disability-and-disabilism-meet/

CHAPTER 25

Behavioral Health in the Community

"Mental health and mental disorders are not opposites, and mental health is not just the absence of mental disorder."

—World Health Organization

KEY TERMS

At-risk alcohol use
Behavioral health
Integrated behavioral health
Mental disorders
Mental health
Substance-related disorders

LEARNING OBJECTIVES

Upon mastery of this chapter, you should be able to:

1. Identify key mental disorders and describe their effect on individuals and the community.
2. Identify commonly used substances and their effect on health.
3. Follow the steps of the nursing process in detection of at-risk alcohol use and management of that risk.
4. Use prevalence data to inform the development of individual- and community-level interventions to address mental health and substance use disorders.
5. Use the Strategic Prevention Framework to guide the implementation of sustainable prevention activities to promote the behavioral health of the community.

INTRODUCTION

This chapter provides an overview of behavioral health, a term used to refer to both mental health and substance use. A comprehensive approach to behavioral health recognizes a continuum of care, from promotion to prevention, treatment, and recovery. Community/public health nursing practice is discussed, with a focus on individual-, community-, and policy-level interventions. The community/public health nurse has a key role in working with individuals, families, and communities to promote optimal behavioral health and thereby decrease the prevalence and incidence of mental and substance-related disorders (Box 25-1).

CONTEMPORARY ISSUES

From concerns over the opioid crisis and alcohol use and controversies over supervised injection sites and the legalization of marijuana to the integration of behavioral health services and the emergence of antistigma strategies, behavioral health issues have undeniably preoccupied the United States in recent years.

Opioid Crisis

A total of 63,632 Americans died of drug overdoses in 2016, and two thirds of these deaths involved a prescription or illicit opioid (Centers for Disease Control and Prevention [CDC], 2018a). As the supply of prescription opioids has been reduced, rates of deaths from heroin and fentanyl have rapidly increased (Hall & Farrell, 2018). Community and public health nurses (C/PHNs) have crucial roles to play in addressing this public health problem, including identifying persons at risk because of opioid use and providing education, support, and resources for this population (Fig. 25-1).

Supervised Injection Sites

Supervised injection sites, also known as safe consumption sites, have been found to mitigate overdose-related harms and unsafe drug use as well as facilitate the acceptance of treatment and other health services (Kennedy, Karamouzian, & Kerr, 2017). These services are available in Europe, Australia, and Canada and are beginning to emerge in the United States. The first supervised injection sites in North America were established in Vancouver, Canada, and the experience gained from them has informed the expansion of this harm reduction approach elsewhere. Proponents of these services view them as beneficial to public health and the community. Opponents believe these sites do nothing to deter drug use or help individuals stop opioid use. Contentious legislative battles are ensuing as federal law prohibits these services, and if such sites are opened, they will face action

BOX 25-1 Behavioral Health Terminology

- **At-risk alcohol use:** Thresholds for alcohol use are based on healthy individuals and those adults 21 years or older. Alcohol assumption that causes risk to a person's health or increases risk to others is unsafe. Health conditions and activities may indicate a lower level of alcohol consumption (Mahmoud, Finnell, Savage, Puskar, & Mitchell, 2017).
- **Behavioral health:** This term, which is used to refer to both mental health and substance use, looks at a comprehensive approach, recognizing a continuum of care, from promotion to prevention, treatment, and recovery.
- **Integrated behavioral health:** Integrated care blends medical and behavioral health factors in one setting. The advantage of an integrated system is coordination of care, and team communication of all health care providers as they work toward person-centered health goals (Agency for Healthcare Research and Quality, 2012a, 2012b).
- **Mental health:** *Healthy People 2030* addresses increased treatment for those with mental health. In addition, screening and early identification is essential for all including youth and the homeless (U.S. Department of Health and Human Services [USDHHS], 2020).
- **Mental disorders:** "Health conditions that are characterized by alterations in thinking, mood, and/or behavior that are associated with distress and/or impaired functioning. Mental disorders contribute to a host of problems that may include disability, pain, or death" (Office of Disease Prevention and Health Promotion, 2020)
- **Substance-related disorders:** Use of 10 separate classes of drugs that, when taken in excess, activate the brain reward system, resulting in neglect of normal everyday activities. This system influences the reinforcement of behaviors and the production of memories (American Psychiatric Association, 2013).

Source: Agency for Healthcare Research and Quality (2012a, 2012b); American Psychiatric Association (2013); Mahmoud et al. (2017); U.S. Department of Health and Human Services (USDHHS) (2018, 2020).

by the United States Department of Justice to close them. Box 25-2 identifies some of the tensions between harm reduction and public safety. Informed by the evidence related to health outcomes for persons who use these services and areas in which they are situated, C/PHNs will be able to advocate for best practices to promote the health of this population and society.

Legalization of Marijuana/Cannabis

Paralleling the opioid epidemic, there has been a rapid expansion of the legalization of cannabis in the United States, for both medical and recreational use. In 2012, Colorado and Washington became the first two states to legalize marijuana for recreational use. Since then, 33 states and Washington, DC have passed laws allowing use of marijuana for medical purposes and eleven states (Washington, Oregon, California, Nevada, Colorado, Alaska, Maine, Vermont, Massachusetts, Illinois, and Michigan) and Washington, DC have legalized recreational, or nonmedical, use by adults (Fig. 25-2; National Council of State Legislatures, 2020).

Marijuana helplines have been established to assist persons seeking information and help in several of these states. In their assessment of such helplines in four states, Carlini and Garrett (2018) reported that helpline staff had no knowledge about the effects and interactions of marijuana's two main components (tetrahydrocannabinol and cannabidiol), nor could they explain the differences

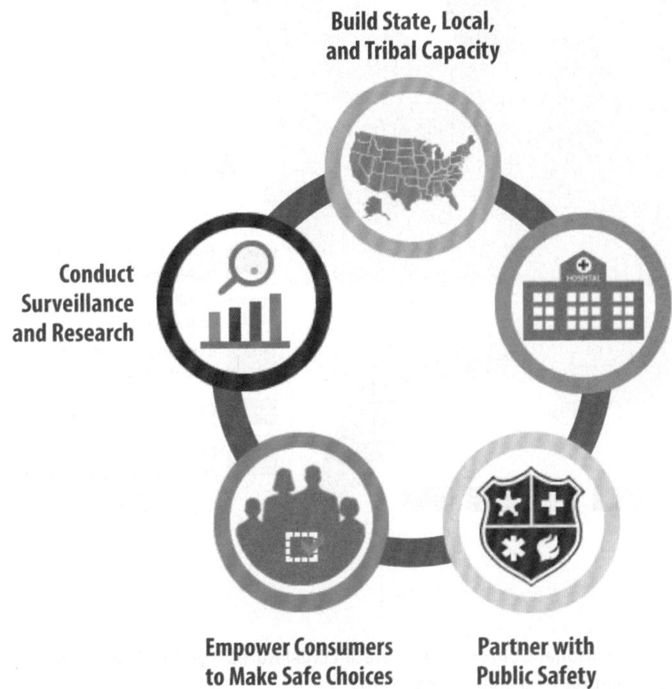

FIGURE 25-1 CDC's efforts to prevent opioid overdoses and other opioid-related harms. (Reprinted from Centers for Disease Control and Prevention. (2019). Retrieved from https://www.cdc.gov/opioids/pdf/Strategic-Framework-Factsheet_Jan2019_508.pdf)

BOX 25-2 Safe Consumption Sites: Tensions Between Harm Reduction and Public Safety

Harm Reduction

- Do safe consumption sites reduce drug overdose deaths?
- Do safe consumption sites encourage people who use opioids to seek help/treatment?

Safety Concerns

- Do safe consumption sites create social problems in neighborhoods?
- Do safe consumption sites encourage more people to use drugs?

Source: European Monitoring Centre for Drugs and Drug Addiction (2018).

in risk between smoking, eating, or vaporizing marijuana. It is essential for C/PHNs to have basic knowledge about marijuana components and methods of use. Educating individuals or the public with this information does not imply endorsement of marijuana use, but rather is an essential role that C/PHNs should assume.

Some also suggest that there may be a therapeutic role of cannabis in opioid use treatment.

- A study by Socías and colleagues (2018) concluded that at least daily cannabis use was associated with higher retention in opioid treatment when compared with less than daily consumption.
- Yet, this emerging area of research calls for further exploration because previous studies reported mixed results on this association (Timko & Cucciare, 2018).
- C/PHNs need to stay abreast with the trends in the care of persons with opioid use disorder and critically evaluate novel approaches to improve engagement in care for this population.

Alcohol Use

The emphasis on the opioid crisis has in some ways overshadowed concerns over alcohol use, which, according to the World Health Organization (WHO), contributes to 3 million deaths annually (WHO, 2018a). C/PHNs can provide evidence-based strategies to address this significant problem and help achieve the WHO goal of 10% reduction in the harmful use of alcohol globally by 2025 (WHO, 2018b) and the alcohol-related Healthy People goal of reducing alcohol use in the United States (Fig. 25-3).

Integration of Behavioral Health Services

For decades, primary care, mental health, and substance use services have been separated, requiring patients to seek services among multiple sites and providers to obtain comprehensive care. Recognizing that the needs of persons with mental health problems, substance use, and physical conditions were not being adequately met, provider organizations began to design and implement integrated services in their practice and communities.

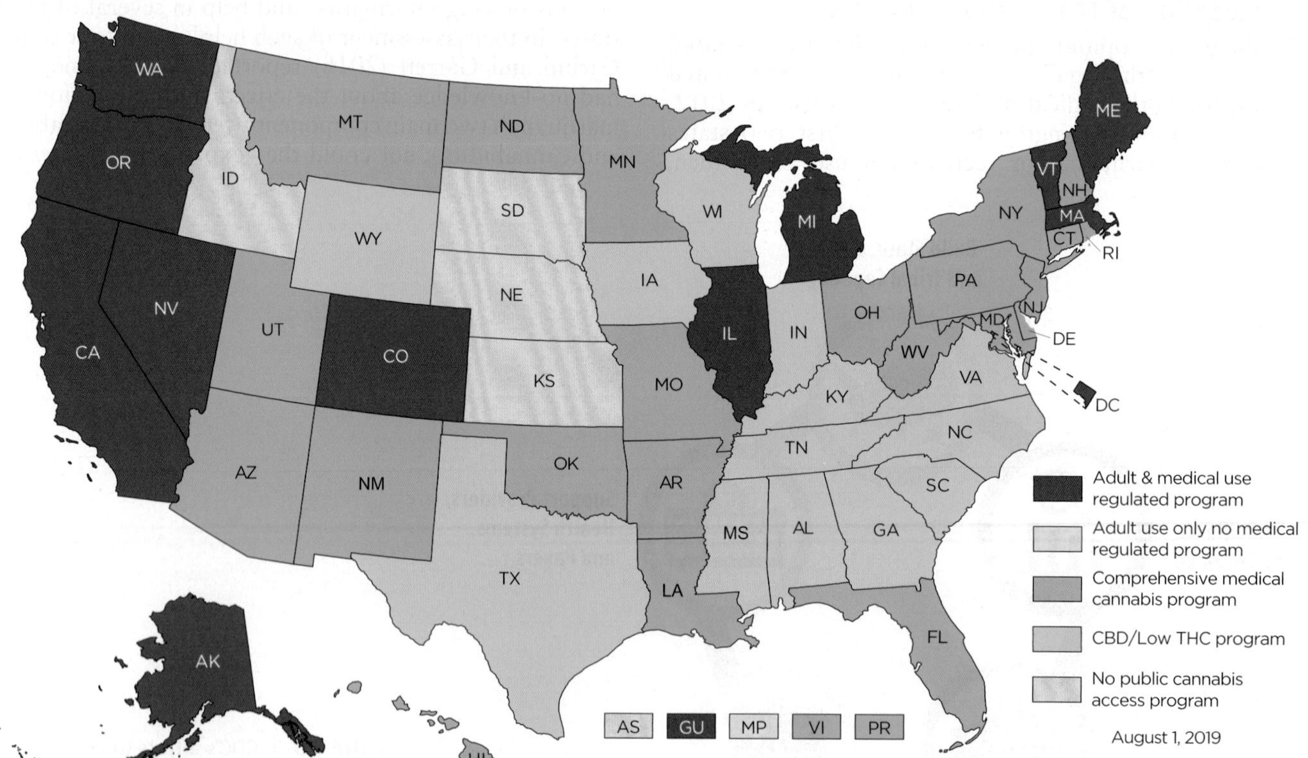

FIGURE 25-2 State cannabis programs. (Reprinted with permission from National Conference of State Legislatures. (2019). *State medical marijuana laws*. Retrieved from http://www.ncsl.org/research/health/state-medical-marijuana-laws.aspx)

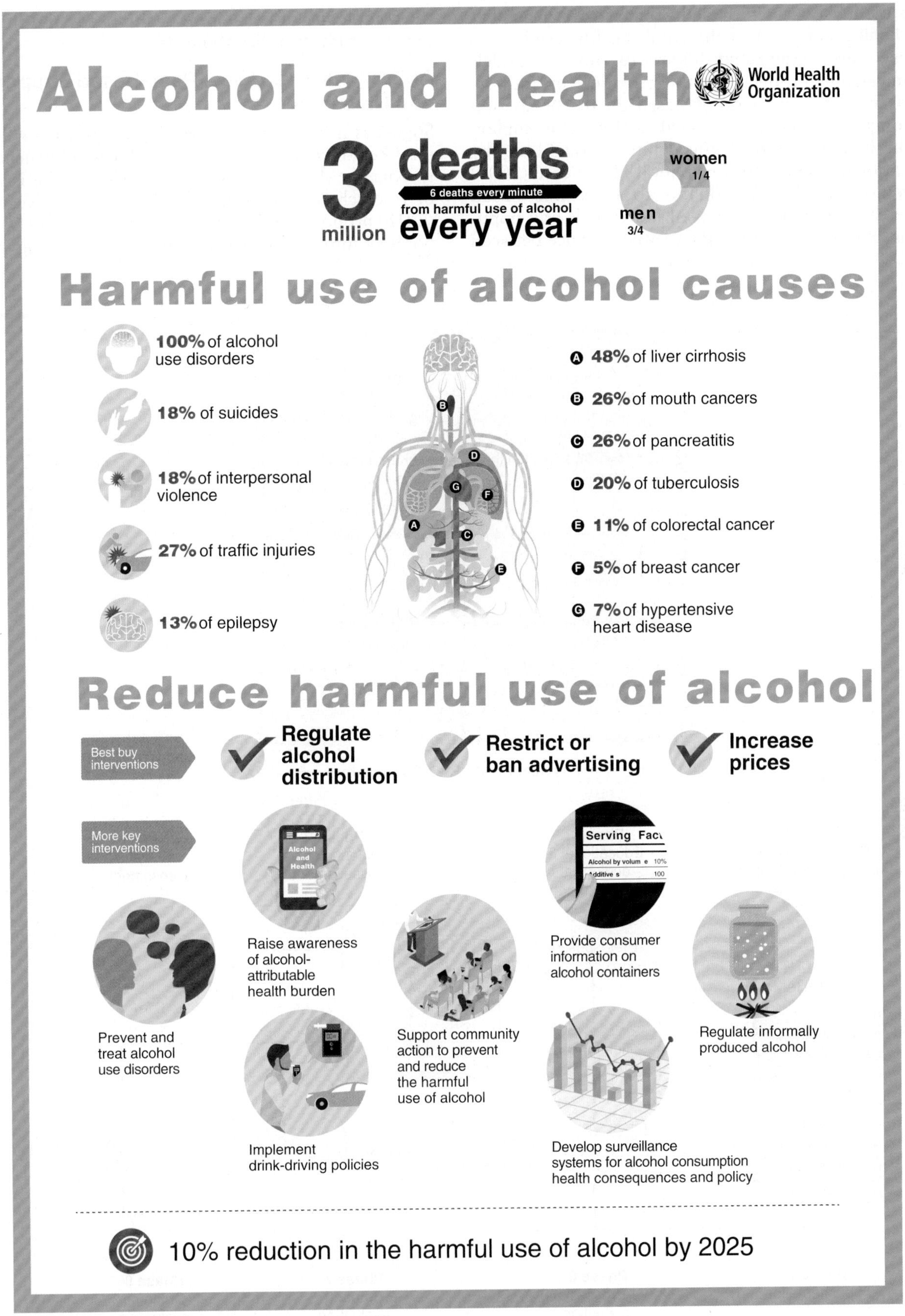

Alcohol and health

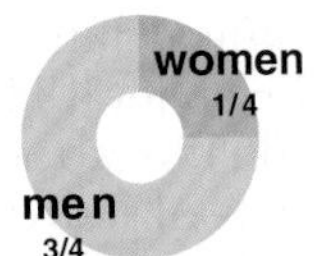

3 million deaths every year from harmful use of alcohol

6 deaths every minute

women 1/4

men 3/4

Harmful use of alcohol causes

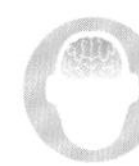
100% of alcohol use disorders

18% of suicides

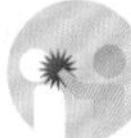
18% of interpersonal violence

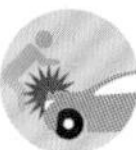
27% of traffic injuries

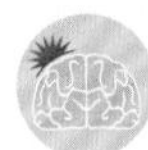
13% of epilepsy

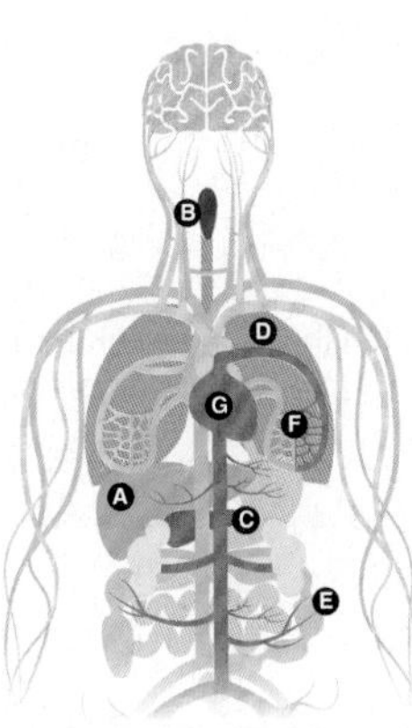

A **48%** of liver cirrhosis

B **26%** of mouth cancers

C **26%** of pancreatitis

D **20%** of tuberculosis

E **11%** of colorectal cancer

F **5%** of breast cancer

G **7%** of hypertensive heart disease

Reduce harmful use of alcohol

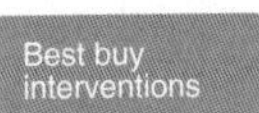

Regulate alcohol distribution

Restrict or ban advertising

Increase prices

More key interventions

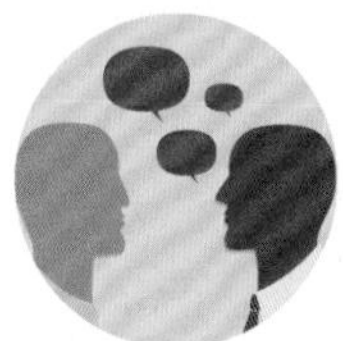
Prevent and treat alcohol use disorders

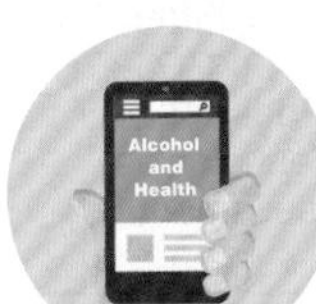

Raise awareness of alcohol-attributable health burden

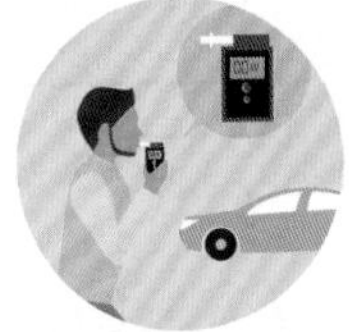
Implement drink-driving policies

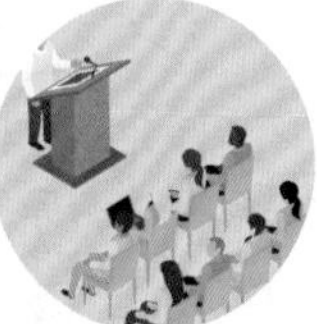
Support community action to prevent and reduce the harmful use of alcohol

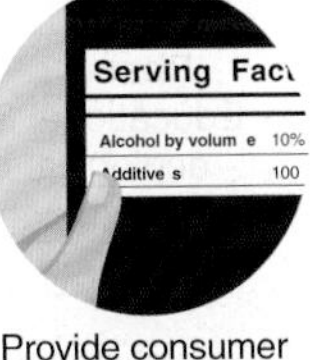

Provide consumer information on alcohol containers

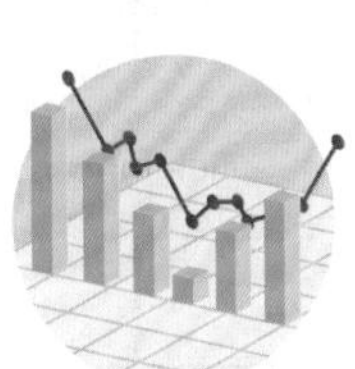
Develop surveillance systems for alcohol consumption health consequences and policy

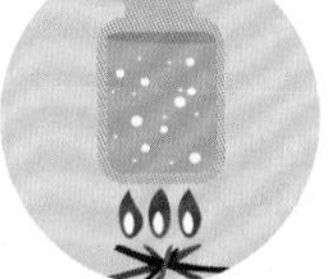
Regulate informally produced alcohol

10% reduction in the harmful use of alcohol by 2025

FIGURE 25-3 Alcohol and health. (Reprinted with permission from World Health Organization. (2018). *Global status report on alcohol and health*. Geneva, Switzerland: Author. Retrieved from http://www.who.int/substance_abuse/infographic_alcohol_2018.pdf?ua=1)

These model services provided primary care in **behavioral health** clinics or behavioral health services in primary care. **Integrated behavioral health** models of clinical integration guide the providers in addressing the need for populations based on the behavioral risk/complexity and the physical health risk/complexity. The Four Quadrant Clinical Integration Model by the National Council for Behavioral Healthcare (2009) serves as a guide for C/PHNs to determine broad approaches to meet the needs of individuals and populations. Figure 25-4 depicts the relative balance between the complexity of behavioral health needs and the complexity of physical health needs.

Antistigma Strategies, Peer-Based Support, and Naloxone

Stigma is a key barrier to seeking treatment for behavioral health conditions for many who could benefit from it (Knaak, Mantler, & Szeto, 2017), yet there is a lack of research on this topic. Corrigan and Nieweglowski (2018) proposed antistigma strategies that could be incorporated into public health programs targeting opioid

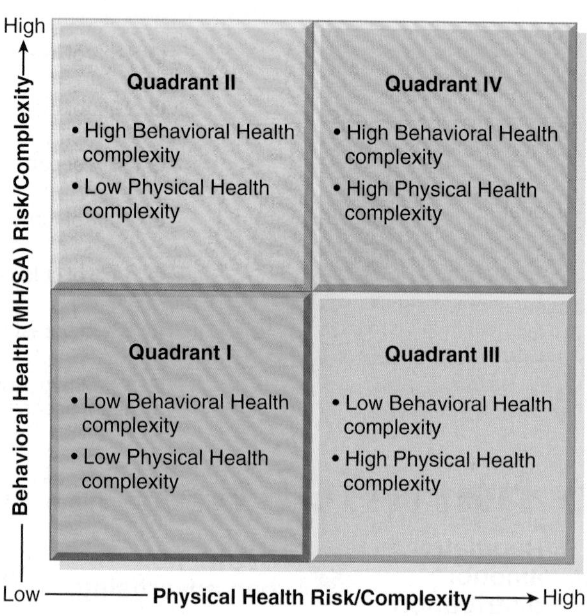

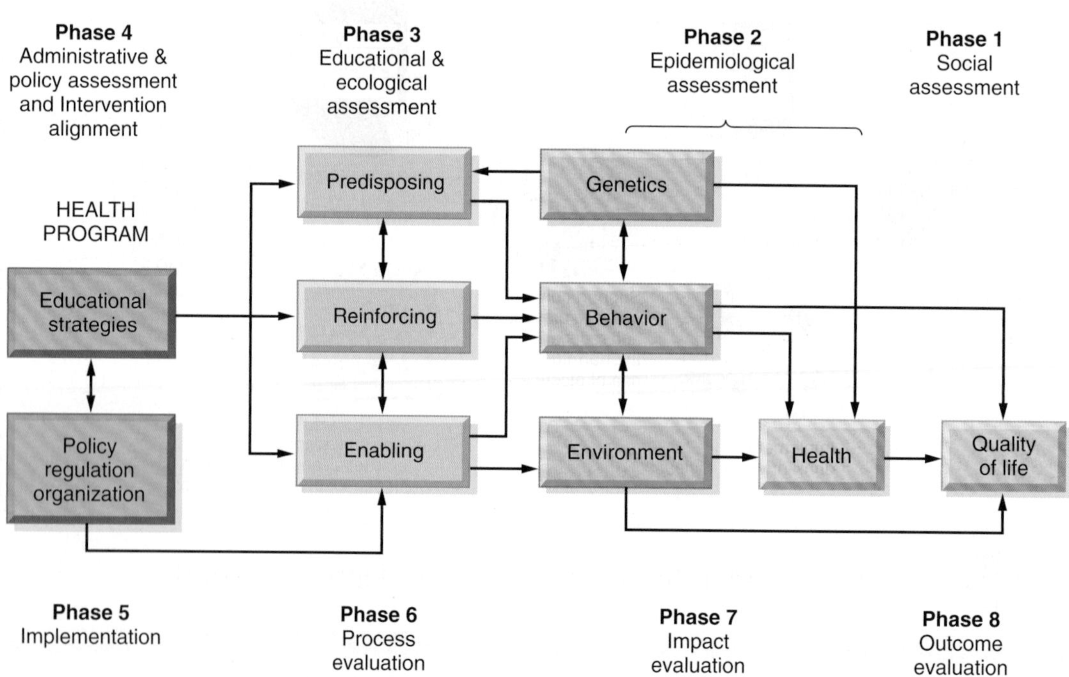

FIGURE 25-4 Four Quadrant clinical integration model. (Adapted with permission from National Council for Behavioral Health. (2009). *Behavioral health/primary care integration and the person-centered healthcare home.* Washington, DC: Author. Retrieved from https://www.samhsa.gov/sites/default/files/programs_campaigns/samhsa_hrsa/four-quadrant-model.pdf)

stigma. Such strategies may be relevant for C/PHNs to help resolve stigma that has persisted for decades. Stereotypes, prejudice, and discrimination underlie stigma, factors that, in part, can be confronted through education that dispels myths with facts.

- A study by Mahmoud and colleagues (2019) reported that after receiving education on how to detect and manage alcohol and opioid use, nursing students' stigma-related perceptions were favorably changed.
- Further, as these nursing students engaged with this patient population in the clinical setting, their attitudes toward working with these patients exhibited positive changes (Mahmoud et al., 2019).
- Contact with persons who are in treatment or in recovery may be a good addition to education programs that are meant to reduce stigma (Corrigan & Nieweglowski, 2018).
- C/PHNs are in key positions to apply these antistigma strategies when providing education to the public and engaging people in recovery.

Peer-based recovery support services provided by persons who have a lived experience and experiential knowledge of substance use disorders have proliferated over the past decade. These peer roles are garnering increased support in the face of the opioid epidemic.

Another trend is the increasing public availability of naloxone, an opioid-reversing drug (USDHHS, 2018). Given their presence in community settings, The C/PHN has a key role in the fight against the opioid epidemic (see Box 25-3). C/PHNs can and should carry and use naloxone as a key part of the public health response to the opioid crisis.

BOX 25-3 The C/PHN's Role in the Fight Against the Opioid Epidemic

Prescription of opioid pain medications has increased since the 1990s, with assurance from pharmaceutical companies that risk of addiction was low (Gale, 2016). Subsequently, overuse of both prescription and nonprescription opioids occurred with associated increase in overdose events of 30% to 70% from 2016 to 2017 (Vivolo-Kantor et al., 2018).

The Department of Health and Human Services (HHS) declared a public health emergency and proposed strategies to combat this opioid epidemic (Hargan, 2017). The accompanying community burdens associated with the loss of life, productivity, and health care treatment dollars as well as increased demands on criminal justice systems were deemed unsustainable. In response, the American Nurses Association (ANA) emphasized the nurse's role in assessment and formulation of plans to decrease the impact of this epidemic while still advocating for appropriate treatment for painful conditions (ANA, 2018).

As frontline caregivers to the opioid-using population, Cleveland Clinic nurses have taken lead roles in the opioid task force established in early 2017. The task force has multiple focus areas designed to change harmful behaviors (Consult QD, 2017).

First, nurses are studying the clinical settings, and describing patterns of those addicted to opioid medications. Integral to improvement of clinical care is incorporating alternative treatments to chronic pain as well as the provision of rescue medications in cases of overdose (Consult QD, 2017).

Next, health policy and laws that impact the availability of naloxone to first responders and pharmacists are addressed. In addition, policy is needed to facilitate treatment of addicted pregnant women and address associated child custody matters (Consult QD, 2017).

Finally, nurses provide prevention education in the community with nurse-led information sessions within public gathering facilities. In addition, nurses develop curricula and educate peers how to avoid "compassion fatigue," which frequently develops when providing care for those with substance abuse and addiction (Consult QD, 2017).

Source: American Nurses Association (ANA) (2018); Consult QD (October 16, 2017); Hargan (2017); Vivolo-Kantor et al. (2018).

PREVENTION OF SUBSTANCE USE AND MENTAL DISORDERS

Relevant to behavioral health, the Healthy People 2030 leading health indicators focus on mental health and mental disorders, substance abuse, and tobacco (U.S. Department of Health and Human Services, 2020). The overarching goals are to:

- Improve mental health through prevention and by ensuring access to appropriate quality mental health services
- Reduce substance abuse to protect the health, safety, and quality of life for all, especially children
- Reduce illness, disability, and death related to tobacco use and secondhand smoke exposure

Across these three major priority areas, C/PHNs can use evidence-based interventions to address the targeted outcomes. Interventions can be categorized according to the three levels of preventive behaviors, as shown in Box 25-4.

A comprehensive approach to behavioral health means seeing prevention as part of an overall continuum of care. The Behavioral Health Continuum of Care Model (Wisconsin Behavioral Health Association, n.d.), depicted in Figure 25-5, recognizes multiple opportunities for addressing behavioral health problems and disorders. The components of the model include promotion, prevention, treatment, and recovery.

- Promotion strategies reinforce the entire continuum of behavioral health services. These strategies are designed to create the environments and conditions that support behavioral health and help individuals overcome challenges.
- Prevention strategies, as characterized by Gordon (1983) in a classic article on prevention, may be grouped into three different categories, according to the level of risk that each addresses: universal, selective, and indicated.

BOX 25-4 LEVELS OF PREVENTION PYRAMID

The C/PHN Works With High-Risk Populations for Mental Disorders and Substance Abuse

SITUATION: Community and public health nurses play a key role in affecting the social determinants of health in vulnerable populations. The main goal of the C/PHN is to improve the population's health through highlighting prevention and addressing the determinants of health within that population.

GOAL: To provide examples of the three levels of prevention when working with high-risk populations for mental disorders and substance use. These examples are meant to provide a starting point for the C/PHN practice and will vary based on the population served. The first step in working with any aggregate is the development of trust.

Tertiary Prevention

- Provide classes on mental health and mental disorders to individuals and families.
- Provide resources and referrals to communities affected by substance use.
- Develop community partnerships to address these issues.
- Focus on the strengths of the community when developing interventions.

Secondary Prevention

Early Diagnosis	***Prompt Treatment***
■ Provide screening programs for the early detection of mental health concerns such as depression, suicidal thoughts, and substance use. ■ Ensure that all adolescents receive screenings in schools. ■ Increase referrals to inpatient and outpatient treatment programs. ■ Provide harm reduction by needle exchange programs.	■ Provide referrals and treatment that are culturally sensitive and in native language of the client. ■ Provide anticipatory guidance and ensure referrals are operational. ■ Provide educational material that is culturally sensitive and literacy-appropriate. ■ Offer clinic hours that meet the needs of the community such as after-work hours or weekends.

Primary Prevention

Health Promotion and Education	***Health Protection***
■ Ensure that educational material and health promotion take into account the health literacy level of the population and the individual. ■ Provide education and health promotion activities in partnership with the community members. Education topics should be relevant to the intended age group and community need. Topics may include coping skills, nutrition, exercise, wellness tips, mental health, and stress reduction.	■ Assess the community's social determinants of heath and how they affect mental health. ■ Hold town meetings to gain insight into the needs to the community. ■ Meet with community partners to decrease number of liquor stores in lower income neighborhoods. ■ Assist the population in navigating sign-ups for a medical home. ■ Achieving higher education has been shown to improve health and decrease poverty. Provide mentoring to middle-school and high-school students. ■ Nurse-run clinics in areas with low percentage of health care providers.

Charlene Niemi PhD, RN, PHN, CNE.

- *Universal prevention* includes those strategies delivered to broad populations wherein the benefits outweigh the costs and risks for everyone. Examples of this include public health campaigns related to suicide prevention, legislation related to impaired driving, and a minimum age for purchase of alcohol.
- *Selective strategies* are indicated when a person's risk of becoming ill is elevated. Through detection of risk, vulnerable subgroups of individuals can be identified. As a result, programs and practices can be provided to reduce the risk.
- *Indicated strategies* address specific risk conditions, focusing efforts on individual risk factors or behaviors that put individuals at high risk for developing a behavioral disorder.
- Treatment begins with case identification, which entails the ability to correctly identify those individuals

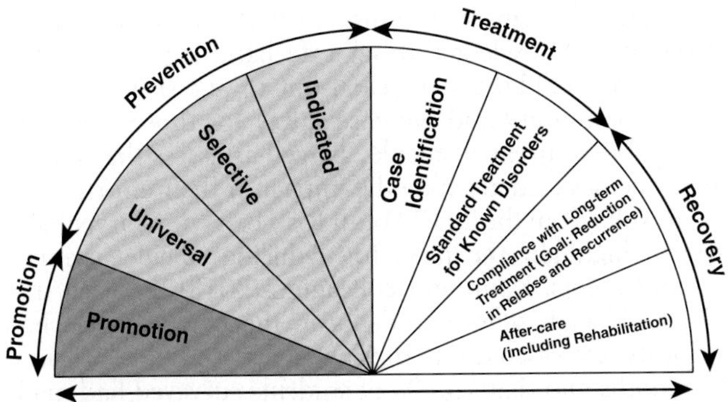

FIGURE 25-5 Behavioral health continuum of care model. (Reprinted with permission from Louis, L. *Oppor of parents lead.* Retrieved from http://www.parentslead.org/sites/default/files/ContinuumofCareModel.pdf)

who have a behavioral disorder with minimal false positives. Once identified, individuals who are at risk need to be referred for evidence-based treatments.

- Recovery focuses on promoting a high-quality and satisfying life in the community for all people. By engaging with individuals in recovery, C/PHNs can provide support and help them achieve their recovery goals, monitor progress toward and recognize when they are moving away from goals, and support their transitions throughout the recovery process. C/PHNs can foster activities that contribute to wellness and a meaningful life, enhancing ways that persons in recovery can connect with others in their communities.

MENTAL HEALTH

Improving **mental health** is a key goal of Healthy People 2030 (Box 25-5). Mental health is essential to personal well-being, family and interpersonal relationships, and the ability to contribute to community or society (U.S. Department of Health and Human Services, 2020). C/PHNs should understand the risk factors that challenge and undermine the health of individuals across the lifespan, such as adverse childhood experiences (Merrick et al., 2018) and social determinants of health (Walker & Druss, 2018). Early and regular mental health screenings are important for detecting emerging mental health problems. C/PHNs can engage the community in health-promoting activities and help establish community conditions to support health behaviors. These strategies are important for the prevention of **mental disorders**, which are associated with significant distress or disability in social, occupational, or other activities (American Psychiatric Association [APA], 2013).

Suicide

Two *Healthy People 2030* objectives related to mental health improvement are to (1) reduce the suicide rate and (2) reduce suicide attempts by adolescents (U.S. Department of Health and Human Services, 2020). Suicide is a leading cause of death in the United States. According to the CDC WISQARS data (CDC, 2020a), in 2018, suicide was the tenth leading cause of death overall, claiming the lives of 48,344 people, and by age groups, suicide was ranked as the

BOX 25-5 *HEALTHY PEOPLE 2030*

Selected Mental Health and Mental Disorders Objectives

Core Objectives

MHMD-01	Reduce the suicide rate
MHMD-02	Reduce suicide attempts by adolescents
MHMD-03	Increase the proportion of children with mental health problems who get treatment
MHMD-04	Increase the proportion of adults with serious illness who get treatment
MHMD-05	Increase the proportion of adults with depression who get treatment
MHMD-06	Increase the proportion of adolescents with depression who get treatment
MHMD-07	Increase the proportion of people with substance use and mental health disorders who get treatment for both
MHMD-08	Increase the proportion of primary care visits where adolescents and adults are screened for depression

Developmental Objectives

MHMD-D01	Increase the number of children and adolescents with serious emotional disturbance who get treatment

Research Objectives

MHMD-R01	Increase the proportion of homeless adults with mental health problems who get mental health services

Reprinted from U.S. Department of Health & Human Services (USDHHS). (2020). *Healthy People 2030: Browse objectives.* Retrieved from https://health.gov/healthypeople/objectives-and-data/browse-objectives

- Second leading cause of death for persons aged 10 to 34 years
- Fourth leading cause of death for persons aged 35 to 54 years
- Eighth leading cause of death for persons aged 55 to 64 years

The National Violent Death Reporting System collects data regarding violent deaths, including those resulting from suicide. Recognizing at-risk groups is an important first step in reducing suicide rates. C/PHNs can use report summaries to develop, implement, and evaluate programs and policies to prevent suicides and other violent deaths. For example, the report by Ertl and colleagues (2019) provides information related to the circumstances preceding suicides reported in 32 states in 2016. The most common precipitating circumstances included substance use and current depressed mood in the individual. More than one fourth of these individuals were receiving mental health treatment at the time of their death (Ertl et al., 2019). Demographic characteristics are also important considerations for suicide prevention. Based on deaths occurring in 2016, the overall suicide rate for males was nearly 3.5 times the rate for females, and non-Hispanic American Indian/Alaska Natives had the highest rates of suicide (Ertl et al., 2019).

The method of suicide and location of the injury can also be important data for C/PHNs developing prevention strategies. Firearms have been reported to be used in nearly half (49.4%) of suicides, followed by hanging/strangulation/suffocation (27.8%) and poisoning (14.4%) (Ertl et al., 2019). Houtsma, Butterworth, and Anestis (2018) discussed strategies to mitigate the risks related to firearms, including decreasing their availability through removal and safe storage and educating professionals and individuals within the firearm community so that they can, in turn, disseminate knowledge about safe handling and storage of firearms. C/PHNs can reach out to at-risk individuals in the community and increase safety for those who may be capable of firearm suicide, as well as assess the rates of such suicides to determine the impact of their efforts.

Results from the 2017 Youth Risk Behavior Surveillance System highlight the need for reducing suicide attempts by adolescents. Kann and colleagues (2018) reported that 17.2% of high school students in the United States had seriously considered attempting suicide in the previous 12 months and that 13.6% of students surveyed had made a plan about how they would attempt suicide. The CDC has developed a technical package that provides evidence-based strategies for preventing suicide (Stone et al., 2017). C/PHNs can lead programs to provide children, youth, and adults with skills to resolve problems and negative influences that are associated with suicide. Evidence-based strategies discussed by Stone et al. (2017) include the following:

- Strengthen economic supports.
- Strengthen access and delivery of suicide care.
- Create protective environments.
- Promote connectedness.
- Teach coping and problem-solving skills.
- Identify and support people at risk.
- Lessen harms and prevent future risk.

Major Depressive Episode

In 2018, about 17.7 million U.S. adults (those aged 18 years or older) reported experiencing at least one major depressive episode; of those, 37% reported that they received no treatment (SAMHSA, 2019a). As seen in Figure 25-6, the prevalence was higher among adult

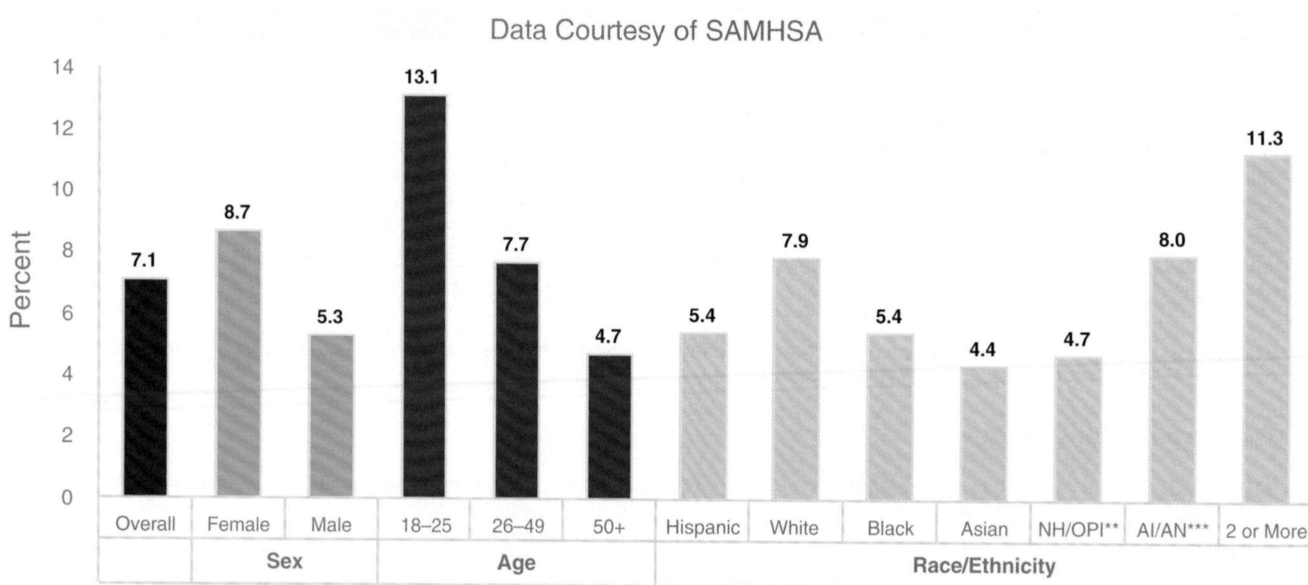

FIGURE 25-6 Past year prevalence of major depressive episode among US adults (2017). (Reprinted from NIMH. (2017). *Major depression. Past year prevalence of major depression episode among US adults (2017)*. Retrieved from https://www.nimh.nih.gov/health/statistics/major-depression.shtml)

females than males, in individuals aged 18 to 25 years, and among adults reporting two or more races.

Among adolescents, 14.4% of the U.S. population aged 12 to 17 years reported at least one major depressive episode (SAMHSA, 2019a). As seen in Figure 25-7, the prevalence was higher among adolescent females than males, with increasing prevalence from age 12 to 16 years and highest among White adolescents and those reporting two or more races. Of adolescents with major depressive episode, nearly 60% reported that they received no treatment (SAMHSA, 2019a).

What can C/PHNs do to help reduce the proportion of persons who experience major depressive episodes and increase the proportion who receive treatment?

- A systematic review and meta-analysis by Deady and colleagues (2017) reported that a range of eHealth cognitive behavioral programs have small, but positive effects on symptoms reduction for depression at both indicated/selective and universal prevention levels. The authors suggest that eHealth has potential for more reach with fewer resources than more traditional approaches because it is better able to overcome a range of financial, geographic, and time barriers (Deady et al., 2017).
- Technology-supported interventions for depression, such as Step-by-Step, developed by the WHO, are feasible to deliver to communities, adaptable, evidence based, and scalable in multiple settings (Carswell et al., 2018). This online psychological intervention is directed toward people with depression, includes informational and interactive exercises, and is designed to be a minimally guided self-help intervention (Carswell et al., 2018).
- C/PHNs could have a valuable role in providing support to end users to help them overcome any barriers to using or navigating through the content of such applications and encouraging their engagement by sending personalized messages and feedback (Fuller-Tyszkiewicz et al., 2018).

National Depression Screening Day is held annually during Mental Illness Awareness Week in October (http://screening.mhanational.org/screening-tools). C/PHNs can be actively involved by hosting an event in the community, conducting screenings, and providing information to help youth and adults identify the signs and symptoms of depression in themselves, their family members, and their peers. The Patient Health Questionnaire is the most commonly used depression screening instrument in the United States (O'Connor et al., 2016). Because the U.S. Preventive Services Task Force recommends there be adequate systems in place to ensure accurate diagnosis, effective treatment, and appropriate follow-up (Siu et al., 2016), C/PHNs should document a list of resources in the community where adults and adolescents can be evaluated and treated for major depression.

SUBSTANCE USE

The *Diagnostic and Statistical Manual of Mental Disorders* 5th Edition (*DSM*; APA, 2013) provides diagnostic criteria for **substance-related disorders** encompassing 10 classes of drugs: alcohol; caffeine; cannabis; hallucinogens; inhalants; opioids; sedatives, hypnotics, and anxiolytics; stimulants; tobacco; and other or unknown substances. A departure from the previous edition of the *DSM,* the fifth edition shifted from categorizing the severity as "abuse" or "dependence" to recognizing substance use along a continuum from "mild" to "moderate" to "severe" based on the corresponding symptoms that are reported (APA, 2013). For some, substance use may increase the risk of harm to their health or well-being and/or increase the risk of harm to others (Mahmoud et al., 2017), and as such, they may not meet the criteria for a

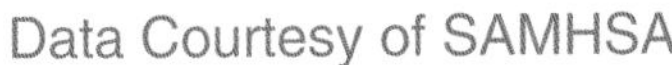

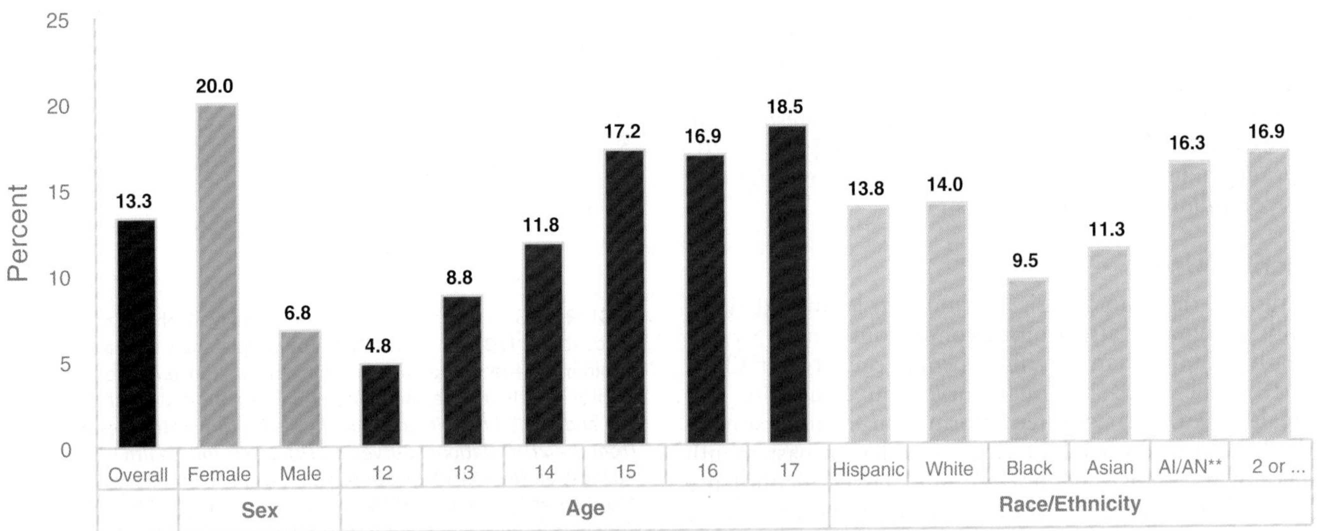

FIGURE 25-7 Past year prevalence of major depressive episode among US adolescents (2017). (Reprinted from NIMH. (2017). *Major depression. Past year prevalence of major depression episode among US adolescents (2017).* Retrieved from https://www.nimh.nih.gov/health/statistics/major-depression.shtml)

BOX 25-6 *HEALTHY PEOPLE 2030*

Selected Substance Use Objectives

Core Objectives

SU-01	Increase the proportion of people with a substance use disorder who got treatment in the past year
SU-02	Reduce cirrhosis deaths
SU-03	Reduce drug overdose deaths
SU-04	Reduce the proportion of adolescents who drank alcohol in the past month
SU-05	Reduce the proportion of adolescents who used drugs in the past month
SU-06	Reduce the proportion of adolescents who used marijuana in the past month
SU-07	Reduce the proportion of adults who used drugs in the past month
SU-08	Reduce the proportion of adults who use marijuana daily or almost daily
SU-09	Reduce the proportion of people under 21 years who engaged in binge drinking in the past month
SU-10	Reduce the proportion of people aged 21 years and over who engaged in binge drinking in the past month
SU-11	Reduce the proportion of motor vehicle crash deaths that involve a drunk driver
SU-12	Reduce the proportion of people who misused prescription drugs in the past year
SU-13	Reduce the proportion of people who had alcohol use disorder in the past year
SU-14	Reduce the proportion of people who had marijuana use disorder in the past year
SU-15	Reduce the proportion of people who had drug use disorder in the past year

Developmental Objectives

SU-D01	Increase the number of admission to substance use treatment for injection drug use
SU-D02	Increase the proportion of people who get a referral for substance use treatment after an emergency department visit

Research Objectives

SU-R01	Increase the proportion of adolescents who think substance abuse is risky

U.S. Department of Health & Human Services (USDHHS). (2020). *Healthy People 2030*: Browse objectives. Retrieved from https://health.gov/healthypeople/objectives-and-data/browse-objectives

substance use disorder diagnosis. Healthy People 2030, as shown in Box 25-6, focuses on substance use. C/PHNs should know how to detect the level of risk associated with alcohol and other drug use and the skills to intervene accordingly. The sections below address the scope of the problem associated with each substance, how to screen for risk, and how to intervene accordingly. For commonly used substances, signs of use, and associated health risks, see https://www.drugabuse.gov/sites/default/files/Commonly-Used-Drugs-Charts_final_June_2020_optimized.pdf and https://www.drugabuse.gov/drug-topics/commonly-used-drugs-charts

Alcohol Use

Although the opioid crisis continues to loom and rightfully command attention, alcohol contributes to the death of more than 3 million people each year (WHO, 2018). The 2018 National Survey on Drug Use and Health (NSDUH) collected information from persons in the United States aged 12 years or older on past month alcohol use, binge alcohol use, and heavy alcohol use (SAMHSA, 2019a). Figure 25-8 displays the prevalence for each category and its definition.

The percent of alcohol varies by beverage. In screening for alcohol use, it is important to explain the definition of a standard drink. A graphic depiction of a

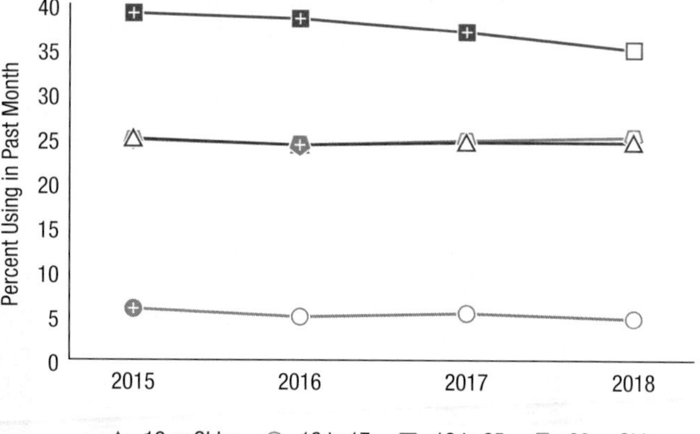

FIGURE 25-8 Past month binge and heavy alcohol use: percentages (2015 through 2018) for people aged 12 years or older, by age group. (Reprinted from Substance Abuse and Mental Health Services Administration. (2019). *Key substance use and mental health indicators in the United States: Results from the 2018 National Survey on Drug Use and Health* (HHS Publication No. PEP19-5068, NSDUH Series H-54). Rockville, MD: Center for Behavioral Health Statistics and Quality, Substance Abuse and Mental Health Services Administration. Retrieved from https://www.samhsa.gov/data/sites/default/files/cbhsq-reports/NSDUHNationalFindingsReport2018/NSDUHNationalFindingsReport2018.pdf)

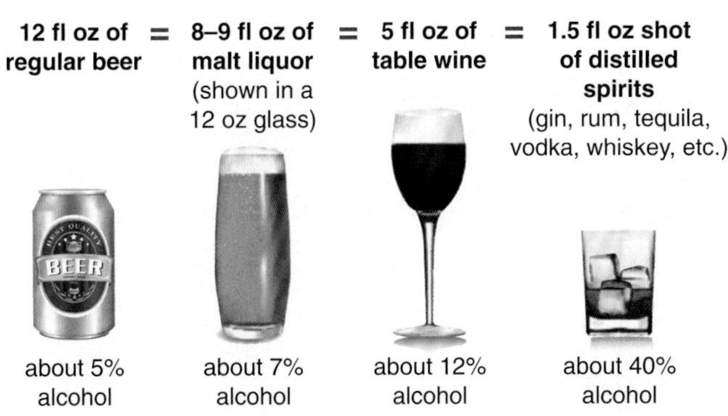

1.5 fl oz shot of distilled spirits (gin, rum, tequila, vodka, whiskey, etc.)

about 40% alcohol
Each beverage portrayed above represents one standard drink of "pure" alcohol, defined in the United States as 0.6 fl oz or 14 g. The percent of pure alcohol, expressed here as alcohol by volume (alc/vol), varies within and across beverage types. Although the standard drink amounts are helpful for following health guidelines, they may not reflect customary serving sizes.

FIGURE 25-9 What is a standard drink? (Reprinted from National Institute on Alcohol Abuse & Alcoholism (NIAAA). (n.d.a). *What is a standard drink?* Retrieved from https://www.niaaa.nih.gov/alcohol-health/overview-alcohol-consumption/what-standard-drink)

standard drink available from the National Institute on Alcohol Abuse and Alcoholism (n.d.a) is useful for providing this information (Fig. 25-9).

The National Institute on Alcohol Abuse and Alcoholism (n.d.b) has established low-risk alcohol consumption limits for healthy adults based on sex (Fig. 25-10). There are no safe limits for youth, and various health conditions and activities may warrant lower limits or no alcohol consumption at all. For example, alcohol consumption is contraindicated at any time during pregnancy (CDC, 2018b).

Grounded in an understanding of the nursing process, the definition of a standard drink, and recognition of the alcohol consumption limits for healthy adults, C/PHNs can promote the reduction of alcohol use by delivering evidence-based interventions. Box 25-7 illustrates the application of the nursing process to care of a patient with alcohol use disorder, including the standard steps of screening, brief intervention, and referral to treatment (SBIRT). This example illustrates how SBIRT can be used in public health nursing to help meet the Healthy People 2030 goal of reducing substance use. The National Institute on Alcohol Abuse and Alcoholism (NIAAA) publications, *Planning Alcohol Interventions Using NIAAA's CollegeAIM* (NIAAA, n.d.c) and *Alcohol Screening and Brief Intervention for Youth: A Practitioner's Guide* (NIAAA, 2020), provide step-by-step guidance and tools for the delivery of this set of clinical strategies.

At the community level, C/PHNs can organize and actively engage in the National Alcohol Screening Day. This annual event, an initiative of the National Institutes of Health, is conducted to provide information about alcohol and health as well as free anonymous screening (https://nationaldaycalendar.com/national-alcohol-screening-day-thursday-of-first-full-week-in-april/). C/PHNs can help identify and address gaps in the treatment system by surveilling the types of specialty treatment that are provided in the community and assessing the time to access treatment as well as other factors affecting one's ability to receive timely and affordable treatment.

Drug Use

The annual NSDUH for persons in the United States aged 12 years or older obtains information on drugs including marijuana, cocaine, heroin, hallucinogens, inhalants, and methamphetamine (SAMHSA, 2019a). C/PHNs should remain up to date on the prevalence of drug use in the community. The SBIRT clinical strategies can be used to identify and address drug use, including the use of a psychotherapeutic drug that is not as directed, including without a prescription of one's own. A single screening question begins the process (Smith, Schmidt, Allensworth-Davies, & Saitz, 2010); a positive response to that question triggers the administration of the Drug Abuse Screening Test (DAST; Skinner, 1982; Yudko, Lozhkina, & Fouts, 2007). To view the DAST, go to https://cde.drugabuse.gov/instrument/e9053390-ee9c-9140-e040-bb89ad433d69. The intervention is provided based on the level of risk per the DAST score.

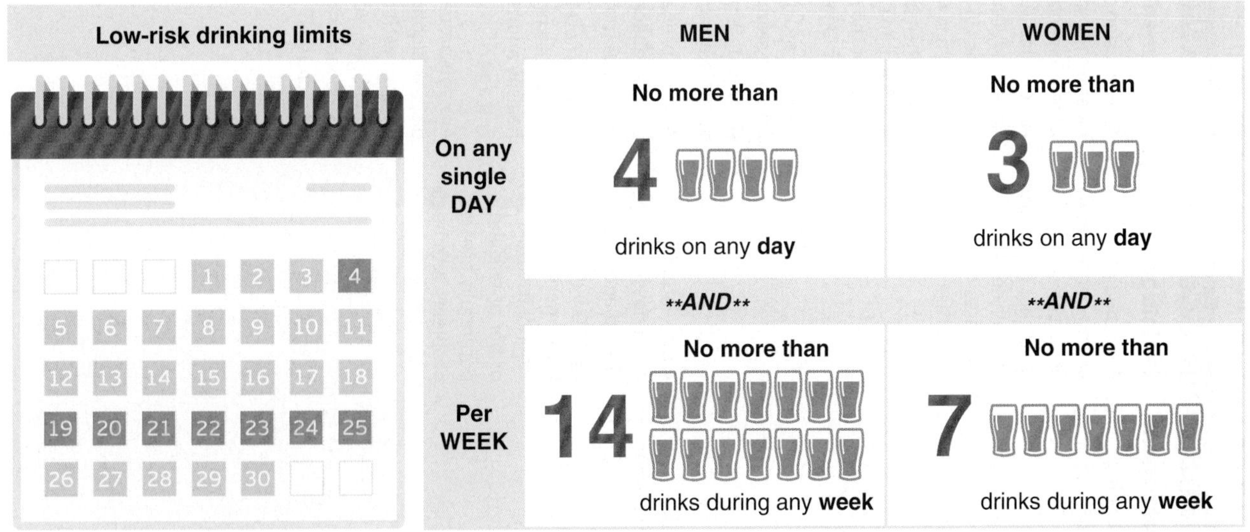

Low-risk drinking limits
MEN
WOMEN
On any single DAY
No more than
4
drinks on any day
No more than
3
drinks on any day
AND
AND
Per WEEK
No more than
14
drinks during any week
No more than
7
drinks during any week
No amount of alcohol or drug is safe if driving, pregnant, or a possible substance use disorder.

FIGURE 25-10 Low-risk alcohol consumption limits. (Reprinted from National Institutes of Health (NIH). (2016). *Rethinking drinking: Alcohol and your health.* Retrieved from https://pubs.niaaa.nih.gov/publications/RethinkingDrinking/Rethinking_Drinking.pdf)

BOX **25-7** C/PHN USE OF THE NURSING PROCESS

Detection and Management of At-Risk Alcohol Use

Component	Definition	Assessment	Planning	Implementation	Evaluation
Screening	A method of identifying people who use alcohol at a level that is harmful to their health or increases their risk for future harm	Are you using an established measure for screening, such as recommended by the National Institute on Alcohol Abuse and Alcoholism, "How many times in the past year have you had five (men) or four (women or patients over age 65) drinks or more in a day?" or the Alcohol Use Disorders Identification Test? Can you provide the definition of a standard drink or provide a graphic when administering the screen?	Have screening measure available for administration. Determine if you will screen all people or specific groups. Prepare to employ best practices during the screening process.	Perform screening based on best practices: • Explain that it is a part of the standard practice. • Ask their permission to screen. • Interact in a nonjudgmental manner. • Convey empathic verbal and nonverbal behaviors during screening. • Thank the patient for answering the questions.	Evaluate the person's response to screening. Ensure that you were neutral in your responses to the person's questions or statements that may have been challenging of the process.
Brief Intervention	A motivational, awareness-raising, shared agenda-setting conversation with a person whose alcohol use puts him or her at risk and potentially creates problems with health and wellness.	Are you prepared to provide feedback based on the results of the screening? Do you know the recommended alcohol limits for healthy adults based on sex and age? Are you prepared to discuss alcohol limits for persons with other health conditions including those on alcohol-interactive medications?	Develop your motivational interviewing skills. Practice those skills in a simulated environment and/or with experts.	Engage in the brief intervention based on best practices: • Ask permission to provide feedback about their alcohol use and screening results. • Use reflection and open-ended questions during the conversation. • Provide feedback about the risks associated with their alcohol use. • Negotiate a goal with the person based on the steps the person is willing to take. • Demonstrate the motivational interviewing spirit by: • Providing summary statements of the person's stated reasons for change • Negotiating a treatment plan in a collaborative manner • Affirming the person's strengths, ideas, and/or successes	Determine if a goal was established and accepted by the person. Evaluate your ability to convey the true spirit of motivational interviewing as opposed to using it as a technique.

Referral to Treatment	Establishing a clear method of follow-up with persons who may benefit from ongoing care because of risk or who need specialized treatment	Are you aware of your own limitations in terms of knowledge, skills and scope of practice to provide ongoing care for the person who is at high risk because of alcohol use? Do you know referral sources within and outside of your health care system?	Establish a list of potential resources for further assessment and/or treatment. Ensure that you are prepared to address questions about those resources, including access, cost, and what is provided. Engage in a discussion about potential barriers to acceptance of the referral and discuss ways to overcome them. Provide a warm handoff to the referral source or otherwise make a direct introduction of the person to the specialist provider.	Did you follow best practices below? • Recognize the person's need for alcohol treatment based on their screening score and/or medical/behavioral factors. • Suggest the use of specific community and specialty resources. • Arrange appropriate follow-up for ongoing evaluation.	Evaluate if the person is accepting of the recommendation for referral. At follow-up, ascertain if the person followed through with the referral, and if so, the outcome.

Source: Babor et al. (2001); Pringle et al. (2017).

Marijuana

The drug that survey respondents most commonly reported as having used in the past month is marijuana, used by 43.5 million people aged 12 years or older (SAMHSA, 2019a). Marijuana use was reported by 43.5 million, or 15.9%, of Americans aged 12 years or older reported in 2018; this percentage of use was higher than any of the percentages of use from 2002 to 2017 (SAMHSA, 2019a). With the emerging context of legalization of marijuana, it will be important for C/PHNs to continue to monitor the prevalence of marijuana use in their communities. Given the adverse health effects and harms associated with marijuana use (Memedovich, Dowsett, Spackman, Noseworthy, & Clement, 2018), C/PHNs need to educate the public on its impact on health. (See Boxes 25-8 and 25-9.)

Cocaine and Crack

In 2018, 2% (5.5 million) of 5.5 people aged 12 years or older reported current use of cocaine and 0.3% who reported current use of crack cocaine. Among those aged 12 to 17 years, 0.4% (11,200) used cocaine and fewer than 0.1% (4,000) used crack (SAMHSA, 2019a).

Heroin

Heroin use has increased in recent years. Roughly 800,000 people aged 12 years or older reported heroin use in 2018 (SAMHSA, 2019a). Until 2002, methadone was the primary medication used to treat individuals with heroin use disorder and was dispensed through licensed treatment facilities. The introduction of buprenorphine in 2002 allowed for an additional medication option and also increased access to treatment because this medication could be prescribed by physicians in their office or clinic setting. Access to buprenorphine was further increased with the passage of the Comprehensive Addiction and Recovery Act (P.L. 114-198), which allowed nurse practitioners to prescribe buprenorphine. The SUPPORT for Patients and Communities Act (Congress.gov, 2018) expanded access to this medication even further by allowing Certified Nurse Specialists, Certified Nurse Midwives, and Certified Nurse Anesthetists to prescribe buprenorphine for a 5-year period (American Academy of Physician Assistants [AAPA], 2018).

Hallucinogens

In 2018, about 5.6 million people aged 12 years or older reported the use of hallucinogens, or 2% of the population. Compared with all other age groups, the highest percentage of use was reported by people aged 18 to 25 years at 6.9% (SAMHSA, 2019a).

Inhalants

Respondents of the NSDUH survey are asked to report the use of inhalants to get high, but not to include accidental inhalation of a substance. In 2018, approximately 2 million people aged 12 years or older reported use of inhalants. Use was more common among adolescents aged 12 to 17 years than among people in other age groups (SAMHSA, 2019a).

BOX 25-8 QSEN: FOCUS ON QUALITY

Patient-Centered Care for Behavioral Health: Adolescent Access to and Use of Marijuana

Evidence-Based Practice: Integrate best current evidence with clinical expertise and patient/family preferences and values for delivery of optimal health care (Cronenwett et al., 2007, p. 123).

(See http://qsen.org/competencies/pre-licensure-ksas#quality_improvement for the knowledge, skills, and attitudes associated with this QSEN competency)

More states are permitting commercial production and sales of recreational, or retail, marijuana. A public health concern is a potential increase in adolescents' access to and use of marijuana given the evidence of negative health effects on this population. The National Survey on Drug Use and Health (NSDUH; https://nsduhweb.rti.org/respweb/homepage.cfm), conducted annually, asks questions about marijuana use for Americans ages 12 and older. Information from the NSDUH is used to support prevention and treatment programs, monitor substance use trends, estimate the need for treatment, and inform public health policy. In Colorado, the commercialization of medical marijuana allowed the proliferation of consumable marijuana products including candies, lozenges, baked goods, and beverages, with little attention paid to standardized dosing levels, guidance for novice users, food safety, and contamination issues. The legalization of marijuana cultivation for dispensaries has impacted growing conditions and horticultural practices with the goal of increasing the supply and the potency of the psychoactive ingredient tetrahydrocannabinol (THC).

1. *What are the harms associated with marijuana use among adolescents? How would you incorporate that evidence in educating the public?*
2. *Are strategies used to prevent unintentional poisoning transferrable to children and youth related to edible products and access to marijuana? If so, how would those be used in public health messages?*
3. *What data are needed to monitor impaired driving and risks of fatalities associated with marijuana use? Are limits for drivers' THC levels warranted?*
4. *What areas of the health care system should be under surveillance to monitor the impact of increased access to marijuana? How would data collected from those systems be used to inform public awareness campaigns or support policies and regulations to protect children, youth, and the community at large?*

Source: Cronenwett et al. (2007).

BOX 25-9 Marijuana Use in the United States

According to a 2018 Gallup poll, 66% of Americans favor legalizing the recreational use of marijuana (McCarthy, 2018). It is estimated that 43.5 million Americans between the ages of 12 and older used marijuana in 2018 (SAMHSA, 2019). *Delta-9-tetrahydrocannabinol* (THC) is the main psychoactive chemical found in the *Cannabis sativa* plant. Although usually smoked, it can be brewed in tea or mixed in foods called *edibles*. The THC content has steadily increased since 1976, when marijuana had an average of THC content of 0.72% (Marijuana Break, 2018). In 2014, this rose to 50% to 80% in some samples (NIDA, 2018).

Marijuana use disorders (MUD) account for about 30% of all users. Frequent users prior to age 18 are at a four to seven times greater risk of developing MUD. Roughly 4 million people in the United States have MUD (NIDA, 2018). Academic difficulties occur with use, including increased risk of skipping college classes, poorer grades, and poorer graduation rates (Arria, Caldeira, Bugbee, Vincent, & O'Grady, 2015), and cognitive difficulties were significantly related to the minutes of marijuana use (Conroy, Kurth, Brower, Strong, & Stein, 2015). Judgment and attention are impaired (NIDA, 2018).

Frequent use is associated with mental health problems including depression, increased anxiety with use (Keith, Hart, McNeil, Silver, & Goodwin, 2015), panic, fear, and paranoia (NIDA, 2018). When used in large doses, acute psychosis may occur.

THC affects several parts of the brain, including the hippocampus and the orbitofrontal cortex, causing impaired thinking and difficulty in absorbing new information. A 25-year study found that those with a lifetime exposure to marijuana had lower scores in verbal memory. The effects on the cerebellum and basal ganglia result in poor balance and coordination as well as slowed reaction time (NIDA, 2018).

THC stimulates the mesolimbic system to release a high level of the neurotransmitter dopamine producing the "high." When compared to nonusers, in marijuana users there was a higher incidence of other drug use such as alcohol (use including binge drinking), almost half used cocaine, and 30% used amphetamines (Keith et al., 2015).

Currently, 14 states and the District of Columbia have legalized recreational use of marijuana (National Conference of State Legislatures, 2020). Teens and young adults' perception of the risks of the drug have decreased partially due to the legalization of the drug for medical and recreational use in some states (NIDA, 2018). Research continues to shed light on the benefits and dangers of marijuana use. C/PHNs need to stay up-to-date on the community trends and research in order serve their communities.

Charlene Niemi, PhD, RN, PHN, CNE

Source: Arria et al. (2015); Conroy et al. (2015); Keith et al. (2015); Marijuana Break (2018); McCarthy (2018); National Institute on Drug Abuse (NIDA) (2018); Substance Abuse and Mental Health Services Administration (2017, 2019a); WHO (2020).

Methamphetamine

Most of the methamphetamine in the United States is produced and distributed illicitly, creating a serious public health and safety problem in the United States. Some suggest that the lull in the methamphetamine epidemic, at its peak in 2005, is swiftly ending, as this drug now accounts for 11% of the total number of opioid deaths (The Lancet, 2018). In 2018, about 1.9 million people aged 12 years or older reported current use of methamphetamine (SAMHSA, 2019a). About 43,000 adolescents aged 12 to 17 years reported methamphetamine use, or 0.7% of adolescents. The next-largest age group were 273,000 young adults aged 18 to 25 years who reported use in 2018; 1.6 million adults aged 26 years or older reported methamphetamine use also in 2018 (SAMHSA, 2019a).

Prescription Drugs

In the NSDUH, respondents are asked to report on any use of a prescription drug that is not used as directed, including use without a prescription of one's own. In 2018, this type of prescription drug use was reported by 16.9 million of the population aged 12 years or older. In 2018, among four different prescription drug categories, pain relievers were the most commonly reported, with 9.9 million persons aged 12 years or older reporting having used them in the past month, followed by prescription tranquilizers and sedatives (6.4 million), and prescription stimulants (5.1 million) (SAMHSA, 2019a).

Of greatest concern are prescription opioid analgesics (e.g., morphine, oxycodone), which along with heroin and fentanyl contribute to opioid-involved deaths. In 2018, close to 70% of the over 67,000 drug overdose deaths in the United States involved an opioid (CDC, 2020b). Various strategies have been undertaken to prevent overprescribing of opioids (Dowell, Haegerich, & Chou, 2016), improve drug monitoring programs (Bao et al., 2018), increase access to naloxone for opioid overdose reversal (Kerensky & Walley, 2017), increase linkages to harm reduction services and treatment (Hawk & D'Onofrio, 2018), and provide fentanyl test strips (Peiper et al., 2019). C/PHNs can assume important roles in promoting these strategies in the community and providing education to the public on the crisis and ways to mitigate it.

TOBACCO USE

Across the United States, tobacco consumption was the leading risk factor in terms of disability-adjusted life years (DALYs) for the years 1990–2016 (Mokdad et al., 2018). In 2016, about 63.4 million people aged 12 years or older reported tobacco use in the past month, the majority of whom smoked cigarettes (Fig. 25-11).

The use of electronic cigarettes is rapidly emerging among adolescents, along with concerns about its impact on the health of both the individual and the public. A literature review by Perikleous, Steiropoulos, Paraskakis, Constantinidis and Nena (2018) reported as risk factors for e-cigarette use among adolescents the following: being male, being an older adolescent, being able to afford e-cigarettes, being a regular or heavy smoker, and having peers who smoke. With e-cigarette use rising

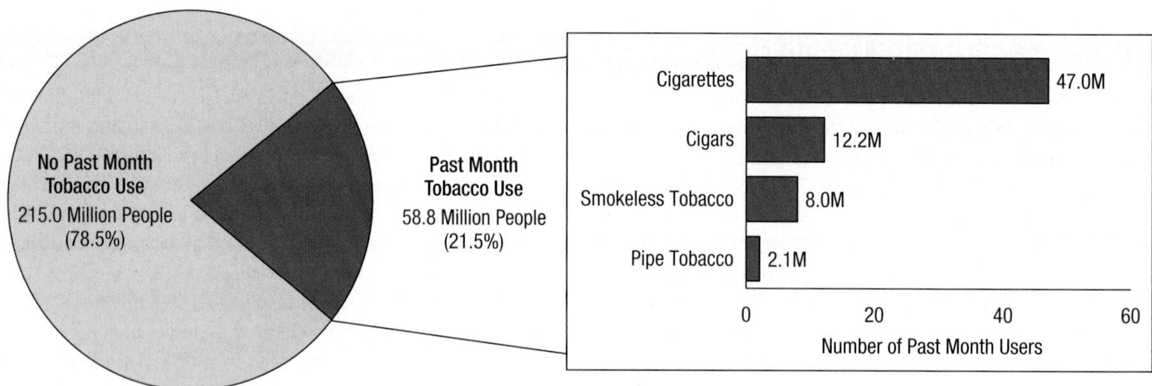

Note: The estimated numbers of current users of different tobacco products are not mutually exclusive because people could have used more than one type of tobacco product in the past month.

FIGURE 25-11 Past Month Tobacco Use among People Aged 12 or Older: 2018. (Reprinted from Substance Abuse and Mental Health Services Administration. (2019). *Key substance use and mental health indicators in the United States: Results from the 2018 National Survey on Drug Use and Health* (HHS Publication No. PEP19-5068, NSDUH Series H-54). Rockville, MD: Center for Behavioral Health Statistics and Quality, Substance Abuse and Mental Health Services Administration. Retrieved from https://www.samhsa.gov/data/sites/default/files/cbhsq-reports/NSDUHNationalFindingsReport2018/NSDUHNationalFindingsReport2018.pdf)

among high school students in 2018 to 3.05 million (U.S. Food and Drug Administration, 2020), C/PHNs need to be attentive to the attraction of this mode of tobacco use and provide educational initiatives targeting youth and young adults.

The U.S. Preventive Services Task Force (2017) recommends screening and providing brief intervention for tobacco use as part of standard routine health care for adults and women who are pregnant. The U.S. Department of Health and Human Services clinical practice guideline provides information about screening and interventions that can be provided based on the individual's willingness to quit. It is recommended that all patients be asked whether they use tobacco and, if so, whether they want to quit.

The Agency for Healthcare Research and Quality (2012a) recommends five major components for treating tobacco use and dependence:

- "Ask" about tobacco use
- "Advise" to quit
- "Assess" willingness to make a quit attempt
- "Aid" the person in quitting
- "Arrange" for follow-up

C/PHNs are encouraged to adopt these 5As as part of their standard care to address this major health problem in the United States and globally. Strategies for various populations are provided on the smokefree.gov Web site, including strategies for those who are willing to quit, those unwilling to quit, those who have recently quit, and specific populations (e.g., veterans, women, teens, those 60 years and older, and Spanish speakers).

COMMUNITY- AND POPULATION-BASED INTERVENTIONS

Interventions to promote behavioral health at the community level begin with a community assessment to establish a community diagnosis, followed by interventions that can address the specific public health issue identified in the diagnosis. The *Healthy People 2030* objectives serve as a starting point in the development of an intervention. Community interventions move beyond single interventions and outcomes at individual levels of health behavior change.

Depicted in Figure 25-12, the five steps of SAMHSA's A Guide to SAMHSA's Strategic Prevention Framework (SAMHSA, 2019b) can guide C/PHNs in a comprehensive process for addressing the behavioral health problems facing communities.

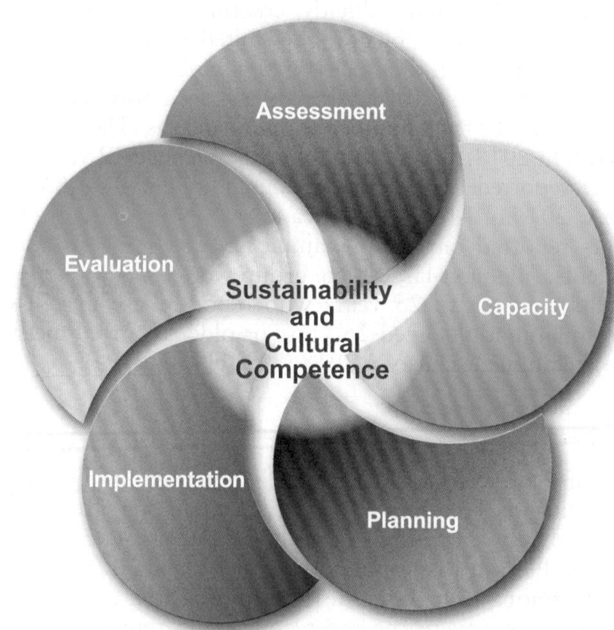

FIGURE 25-12 A guide to SAMHSA's Strategic Prevention Framework. (Reprinted from Substance Abuse and Mental Health Services Administration. (2019). *A guide to SAMHSA's strategic prevention framework.* Retrieved from https://www.samhsa.gov/sites/default/files/20190620-samhsa-strategic-prevention-framework-guide.pdf)

TABLE 25-1 Strategic Planning Framework: Step-by-Step Guidance for the C/PHN

Step	Description	Questions to Address	Information That Can Help Address the Questions
1. Assess	Assess the problem and related behaviors including risk and protective factors.	What substance misuse problems occur in the community? How often, where, and to which populations is this occurring?	State and local data collected within the community Identified risk and protective factors within the community Identify gaps given current community resources and their capacity.
2. Capacity	Build local capacity to address prevention.	Who are your stakeholders, and what information do they need? How can they be motivated to be involved? Who should be part of the prevention team? Can partnerships be created?	Identify all possible stakeholders within the community to raise awareness and support.
3. Plan	Formulate a plan and prioritize risk and protective factors.	How are risks and protective factors prioritized? Does the community have the resources to address the problem?	Create a plan that aligns to your logic model.
4. Implement	Delivery of evidence-based interventions and programs.	Can the community provide evidence-based solutions for required levels and needs within the community? What support is necessary for implementation?	Create evidence-based program and treatments that meet the needs of your community.
5. Evaluate	Conduct a process evaluation, looking at both process and outcomes.	How successful were the programs and practices? What was the effect of the program? Did changes occur, and if so, what were those changes? Were stakeholders included in the evaluation process with respect for all groups?	Create report based on process and outcomes of programs. Evaluation designs, instruments, and methods of evaluation used.

Source: Substance Abuse and Mental Health Services Administration (SAMHSA) (2019b).

Table 25-1 provides descriptions of each step of the process.

Community coalitions that have used the Strategic Prevention Framework include the following:

- Iowa Department of Public Health substance abuse program (https://idph.iowa.gov/substance-abuse/programs/spfrx/about): A program designed to raise awareness about the dangers of sharing medications and to work with the pharmaceutical and medical communities to communicate the risks of overprescribing to youth
- Kansas Prevention Coalition (http://kansaspreventioncollaborative.org/Coalitions/Strategic-Prevention-Framework): Using the Strategic Prevention Framework, offers community programs and resources on prevention (the Web site provides an overview of the framework, and the New and Highlights section of the Web site provides links to numerous community programs and resources)
- SAMHSA provides a *Collaborative Approach to the Treatment of Pregnant Women with Opioid Use Disorder,* offering communities guidance in developing interagency policies and practices to assist pregnant women and their infants in the health, safety, and recovery (SAMHSA, 2016).
- *Screening and Assessment of Co-occurring Disorders in the Justice System* provides direction and guidance to communities to assess and address symptoms of mental health and substance abuse disorder in offenders (SAMHSA, 2019c).
- *Medication-Assisted Treatment Programs in Criminal Justice Settings* are exemplified in New Jersey and Rhone Island. In an effort to stabilize individuals over the course of their sentences and after release, medications are prescribed to treat opioid use disorder (OUD) (SAMHSA, 2019d).
- Kentucky and Massachusetts use a relapse prevention focus, where criminal offenders with OUD are provided naltrexone before and after release to avoid the risk of relapse after reentry into the community (SAMHSA, 2019d).

SUMMARY

- Substance use disorders are linked to health problems. Healthy People 2030 focuses on strategies to prevent and access to treatment to mitigate health problems and deaths.
- At the individual level, C/PHNs can detect the person's level of risk via screening instruments, assess the individual, and intervene accordingly.
- The Strategic Prevention Framework serves to guide C/PHNs in community-level interventions to address behavioral health problems.

ACTIVE LEARNING EXERCISES

1. Develop your skills in assessing health education materials. Select a Healthy People 2030 objective related to mental health and mental disorders, substance use, or tobacco use. Search for accessible health education materials related to that behavioral health problem. Select one health education flyer, brochure, booklet, or Web site. Evaluate the material using the Suitability Assessment of Health Education Materials Scoring Sheet available at http://aspiruslibrary.org/literacy/SAM.pdf. Provide a summary narrative of your scoring and justification, based on the literature for your evaluation. Provide a list of the references used in your analysis of the health education materials.
2. Using "Enable Equitable Access" (1 of the 10 essential public health services; see Box 2-2), identify services for behavioral health in your community or state. What services are available, and how accessible are those services?
3. Examine the evidence related to safe consumption spaces. Assume a position on the pro or the con side and conduct a literature search to support that perspective.
4. Identify a health promotion topic based on one of the Healthy People 2030 objectives related to a behavioral health problem. Develop a 5-minute presentation on the topic preparing no more than 20 PowerPoint slides. The presentation can be in person or by creating an Ignite presentation that can be delivered online. Whichever format you select, the following resources will be useful in developing your talk.
   - https://www.youtube.com/watch?v=yGENcskRGRk&feature=youtu.be%2F
   - https://speakingaboutpresenting.com/content/fast-ignite-presentation/
   - http://www.lauramfoley.com/ignite/
5. Research behavioral health issues in your community. Gather data from local, state, and national agencies to determine incidence and prevalence of behavioral health concerns and morbidity and mortality rates. One source might be the CDC's Web-based Injury Statistics Query and Reporting System (WISQARS). Begin by going to the Web site: https://www.cdc.gov/injury/wisqars/index.html.
   - Select "Fatal Injury and Violence Data."
   - Select "Fatal Injury Reports 1981–2018."
   - Review the following areas and make selection(s) for each:
     - Year Range/Census Region
     - Intent or manner of the injury
     - Cause or mechanism of the injury
   - Complete the "Select-specific options" that are of interest for your report.
   - Submit the request to see the results.
   - Click "Download Results in a Spreadsheet CSV) File."

REFERENCES

Agency for Healthcare Research and Quality. (2012a). *Five major steps to intervention (The "5 A's")*. Retrieved from https://www.ahrq.gov/professionals/clinicians-providers/guidelines-recommendations/tobacco/5steps.html

Agency for Healthcare Research and Quality. (2012b). *Preventive services recommended by the USPSTF*. Retrieved from https://www.ahrq.gov/sites/default/files/publications/files/cpsguide.pdf

American Academy of Physician Assistants (AAPA). (2018). *President signs SUPPORT for patients and communities act*. Retrieved from https://www.aapa.org/news-central/2018/10/president-signs-support-patients-communities-act/

American Nurses Association (ANA). (2018). The opioid epidemic: The evolving role of nursing. *Issue Brief*. Retrieved from https://www.nursingworld.org/~4a4da5/globalassets/practiceandpolicy/work-environment/health--safety/opioid-epidemic/2018-ana-opioid-issue-brief-vfinal-pdf-2018-08-29.pdf

American Psychiatric Association. (2013). *Diagnostic and statistical manual of mental disorders* (5th ed.). Arlington, VA: Author.

Arria, A. M., Caldeira, K. M., Bugbee, B. A., Vincent, K. B., & O'Grady, K. E. (2015). The academic consequences of marijuana use during college. *Psychology of Addictive Behaviors, 29*(3), 564–575. doi: 10.1037/adh0000108.

Babor, T. F., Higgins-Biddle, J. C., Saunders, J. B., & Monteiro, M. G. (2001). *The alcohol use disorders identification test (AUDIT): Guidelines for use in primary care*. Geneva, Switzerland: World Health Organization, Department of Mental Health and Substance Abuse. Retrieved from http://www.who.int/substance_abuse/publications/audit/en/

Bao, Y., Wen, K., Johnson, P., Jeng, P. J., Meisel, Z. F., & Schackman, B. R. (2018). Assessing the impact of state policies for Prescription Drug Monitoring Programs on high-risk opioid prescriptions. *Health Affairs, 37*(10), 1596–1604. Retrieved from https://www.healthaffairs.org/doi/full/10.1377/hlthaff.2018.0512

Carlini, B. H., & Garrett, S. B. (2018). Drug helplines and adult marijuana users: An assessment in Washington, Colorado, Oregon, and Alaska. *Substance Abuse, 39*(1), 3–5. doi: 10.1080/08897077.2017.1355872.

Carswell, K., Harper-Shehadeh, M., Watts, S., van't Hof, E., Ramia, J. A., Heim, E., ... van Ommeren, M. (2018). Step-by-Step: A new WHO digital mental health intervention for depression. *Mhealth, 4*, 34. Retrieved from https://pubmed.ncbi.nlm.nih.gov/30225240/

Centers for Disease Control and Prevention (CDC). (2018a). *Drug overdose deaths continue to rise; increase fueled by synthetic opioids*. Atlanta, GA: CDC. Retrieved from https://www.cdc.gov/media/releases/2018/p0329-drug-overdose-deaths.html

Centers for Disease Control and Prevention (CDC). (2018b). *Alcohol use in pregnancy*. Retrieved from https://www.cdc.gov/ncbddd/fasd/alcohol-use.html

Centers for Disease Control and Prevention (CDC). (2020a). *10 leading causes of death, United States 2018, all races, both sexes*. Retrieved from https://webappa.cdc.gov/cgi-bin/broker.exe

Centers for Disease Control and Prevention (CDC). (2020b). *Opioid overdose*. Retrieved from https://www.cdc.gov/drugoverdose/index.html#:~:text=The%20number%20of%20drug%20overdose,a%20prescription%20or%20illicit%20opioid

Congress.gov. (2018). *H.R.6—SUPPORT for Patients and Communities Act 115th Congress (2017-2018)*. Retrieved from https://www.congress.gov/bill/115th-congress/house-bill/6

Conroy, D. A., Kurth, M. E., Brower, K. J., Strong, D. R., & Stein, M. D. (2015). Impact of marijuana use on self-rated cognition in young adult men and women. *The American Journal on Additions, 24*, 160–165. doi: 10.1111/ajad.12157.

Consult QD. (October 16, 2017). Nurses step up to fight opioid crisis. *Cleveland Clinic*. Retrieved from https://consultqd.clevelandclinic.org/nurses-step-up-to-fight-opioid-crisis/

Corrigan, P. W., & Nieweglowski, K. (2018). Stigma and the public health agenda for the opioid crisis in America. *International Journal of Drug Policy, 59*, 44–49. doi: 10.1016/j.drugpo.2018.06.015.

Cronenwett, L., Sherwood, G., Marnwsteiner, J., Disch, J., Mitchell, P., Sullivan, D., & Warrwn, J. (2007). Quality and safety in education for nurses. *Nursing Outlook, 55*, 122–131. doi: 10.1016/j.outlook.2207.02.006.

Deady, M., Choi, I., Calvo, R. A., Glozier, N., Christensen, H., & Harvey, S. B. (2017). eHealth interventions for the prevention of depression and anxiety in the general population: A systematic review and meta-analysis. *BMC Psychiatry, 17*(1), 310.

Dowell, D., Haegerich, T. M., & Chou, R. (2016). CDC guideline for prescribing opioids for chronic pain—United States, 2016. *JAMA, 315*(15), 1624–1645. doi: 10.1001/jama.2016.1464.

Ertl, A., Sheats, K. J., Petrosky, E., Betz, C. J., Yuan, K., & Fowler, K. A. (2019). Surveillance for violent deaths—National violent death reporting system, 32 States, 2016. *MMWR Surveillance Summaries, 68*(9), 1–36. doi: http://dx.doi.org/10.15585/mmwr.ss.6809a1.

European Monitoring Centre for Drugs and Drug Addiction. (2018). *Perspectives on drugs: Drug consumption rooms: An overview of provision and evidence*. Lisbon: Author. Retrieved from http://www.emcdda.europa.eu/system/files/publications/2734/POD_Drug%20consumption%20rooms.pdf

Fuller-Tyszkiewicz, M., Richardson, B., Klein, B., Skouteris, H., Christensen, H., Austin, D., ... Shatte, A. (2018). A mobile app–based intervention for depression: End-user and expert usability testing study. *JMIR Mental Health, 5*(3), e54. Retrieved from https://www.ncbi.nlm.nih.gov/pmc/articles/PMC6127496/

Gale, A. H. (2016). Drug company compensated physicians role in causing America's deadly opioid epidemic: When will we learn? *Missouri Medicine, 113*(4), 244–246.

Gordon, R. S., Jr. (1983). An operational classification of disease prevention. *Public Health Reports, 98*(2), 107. Retrieved from https://www.ncbi.nlm.nih.gov/pmc/articles/PMC1424415/

Hall, W. D., & Farrell, M. (2018). Reducing the opioid overdose death toll in North America. *PLoS Medicine, 15*(7), e1002626. Retrieved from https://www.ncbi.nlm.nih.gov/pmc/articles/PMC6067703/

Hargan, E. (2017). *Determination that a public health emergency exists*. Washington, DC: Department of Health & Human Services. Retrieved from https://www.hhs.gov/about/news/2017/10/26/hhs-acting-secretary-declares-public-health-emergency-address-national-opioid-crisis.html

Hawk, K., & D'Onofrio, G. (2018). Emergency department screening and interventions for substance use disorders. *Addiction Science & Clinical Practice, 13*(18). doi: 10.1186/s13722-018-0117-1.

Houtsma, C., Butterworth, S. E., & Anestis, M. D. (2018). Firearm suicide: pathways to risk and methods of prevention. *Current Opinion in Psychology, 22*, 7–11. Retrieved from https://doi.org/10.1016/j.copsyc.2017.07.002

Kann, L., McManus, T., Harris, W. A., Shanklin, S. L., Flint, K. H., Queen, B., ... Lim, C. (2018). Youth risk behavior surveillance—United States, 2017. *MMWR Surveillance Summaries, 67*(8), 1. Retrieved from https://www.cdc.gov/mmwr/volumes/67/ss/ss6708a1.htm

Keith, D. R., Hart, C. L., McNeil, M. P., Silver, R., & Goodwin, R. D. (2015). Frequent marijuana use, binge drinking and mental health problems among undergraduate. *The American Journal on Addictions, 24*, 499–506. doi: 10.1111/ajad.12201.

Kennedy, M. C., Karamouzian, M., & Kerr, T. (2017). Public health and public order outcomes associated with supervised drug consumption facilities: A systematic review. *Current HIV/AIDS Reports, 14*(5), 161–183. doi: 10.1007/s11904-017-0363-y.

Kerensky, T., & Walley, A. Y. (2017). Opioid overdose prevention and naloxone rescue kits: what we know and what we don't know. *Addiction Science & Clinical Practice, 12*(1), 4. Retrieved from https://ascpjournal.biomedcentral.com/articles/10.1186/s13722-016-0068-3

Knaak, S., Mantler, E., & Szeto, A. (2017). Mental illness-related stigma in healthcare: Barriers to access and care and evidence-based solutions. *Healthcare Management Forum, 30*(2), 111–116. doi: 10.1177/0840470416679413.

Mahmoud, K. F., Finnell, D., Lindsay, D., MacFarland, C., Marze, H., Scolieri, B. B., & Mitchell, A. M. (2019). Can Screening, Brief Intervention and Referral to Treatment (SBIRT) education and clinical exposure impact nursing students' stigma toward alcohol and opioid use? *Journal of American Psychiatric Nurses Association, 25*(6), 467–475. doi: 10.1177/1078390318811570.

Mahmoud, K. F., Finnell, D. S., Savage, C. L., Puskar, K. R., & Mitchell, A. M. (2017). A concept analysis of *Substance Misuse* to inform contemporary terminology. *Archives of Psychiatric Nursing, 31*(6), 532–540. Retrieved from https://www.sciencedirect.com/science/article/pii/S0883941717300109?via%3Dihub

Marijuana Break. (2018). *5 best and strongest marijuana strains of 2019*. Retrieved from https://www.marijuanabreak.com/best-and-strongest-marijuana-strains-of-2018

McCarthy, J. (2018). *Two in three Americans now support legalization marijuana*. Retrieved from https://news.gallup.com/poll/243908/two-three-americans-support-legalizing-marijuana.aspx

Memedovich, K. A., Dowsett, L. E., Spackman, E., Noseworthy, T., & Clement, F. (2018). The adverse health effects and harms related to marijuana use: An overview review. *CMAJ Open, 6*(3), E339–E346. doi: 10.9778/cmajo.20180023.

Merrick, M. T., Ford, D. C., Ports, K. A., & Guinn, A. S. (2018). Prevalence of adverse childhood experiences from the 2011-2014 Behavioral Risk Factor Surveillance System in 23 states. *JAMA Pediatrics, 172*(11), 1038–1044. doi: 10.1001/jamapediatrics.2018.2537.

Mokdad, A. H., Ballestros, K., Echko, M., Glenn, S., Olsen, H. E., Mullany, E., ... Kasaeian, A. (2018). The state of US health, 1990-2016: burden of diseases, injuries, and risk factors among US states. *JAMA, 319*(14), 1444–1472. doi: 10.1001/jama.2018.0158.

National Conference of State Legislatures. (2020). *State medical marijuana laws*. Retrieved from https://www.ncsl.org/research/health/state-medical-marijuana-laws.aspx

National Council of State Legislatures. (2020). *State medical marijuana laws*. Retrieved from https://www.ncsl.org/research/health/state-medical-marijuana-laws.aspx

National Institute for Alcohol Abuse and Alcoholism. (2020). *Professional educational materials*. Retrieved from https://www.niaaa.nih.gov/publications/clinical-guides-and-manuals

National Institute on Alcohol Abuse and Alcoholism. (n.d.a). *What is a standard drink*. Retrieved from https://pubs.niaaa.nih.gov/publications/practitioner/PocketGuide/pocket_guide2.htm

National Institute on Alcohol Abuse and Alcoholism. (n.d.b). *NIAAA strategic plan 2017-2021*. Retrieved from https://www.niaaa.nih.gov/strategic-plan/introduction

National Institute on Alcohol Abuse and Alcoholism. (n.d.c). *Alcohol alert*. Retrieved from https://pubs.niaaa.nih.gov/publications/aa65/aa65.htm

National Institutes of Health (NIH). (2016). *Rethinking drinking: Alcohol and your health*. Retrieved from https://pubs.niaaa.nih.gov/publications/RethinkingDrinking/Rethinking_Drinking.pdf

National Institute on Drug Abuse (NIDA). (2018). *Marijuana research report series*. Retrieved from https://www.drugabuse.gov/drugs-abuse/marijuana

O'Connor, E., Rossom, R. C., Henninger, M., Groom, H. C., Burda, B. U., Henderson, J. T., ... Whitlock, E. P. (2016). *Screening for depression in adults: An updated systematic evidence review for the U.S. Preventive Services Task Force*. AHRQ Publication No. 14-05208-EF-1. Rockville, MD: Agency for Healthcare Research and Quality. Retrieved from https://www.ncbi.nlm.nih.gov/books/NBK349027/

Office of Disease Prevention and Health Promotion. (2020). *Mental health and mental disorders*. Retrieved from https://www.healthypeople.gov/2020/topics-objectives/topic/mental-health-and-mental-disorders#:~:text=Mental%20disorders%20are%20health%20conditions,disability%2C%20pain%2C%20or%20death

Peiper, N. C., Clarke, S. D., Vincent, L. B., Ciccarone, D., Kral, A. H., & Zibbell, J. E. (2019). Fentanyl test strips as an opioid overdose prevention strategy: Findings from a syringe services program in the Southeastern United States.

International Journal of Drug Policy, 63, 122–128. Retrieved from https://doi.org/10.1016/j.drugpo.2018.08.007

Perikleous, E. P., Steiropoulos, P., Paraskakis, E., Constantinidis, T. C., & Nena, E. (2018). E-cigarette use among adolescents: An overview of the literature and future perspectives. *Frontiers in Public Health, 6*, 86. Retrieved from https://doi.org/10.3389/fpubh.2018.00086

Pringle, J. L., Seale, J. P., Shellenberger, S., Grasso, K. M., Kowalchuk, A., Laufman, L., & Bray, J. H. (2017). Development and evaluation of two instruments for assessing SBIRT competency. *Substance Abuse, 38*(1), 43–47.

Skinner, H. A. (1982). The drug abuse screening test. *Addictive Behaviors, 7*(4), 363–371.

Siu, A. L., Bibbins-Domingo, K., Grossman, D. C., Baumann, L. C., Davidson, K. W., Ebell, M., ... Krist, A. H. (2016). Screening for depression in adults: US Preventive Services Task Force recommendation statement. *JAMA, 315*(4), 380–387. doi: 10.1001/jama.2015.18392.

Smith, P. C., Schmidt, S. M., Allensworth-Davies, D., & Saitz, R. (2010). A single-question screening test for drug use in primary care. *Archives of Internal Medicine, 170*(13), 1155–1160. doi: 10.1001/archinternmed.2010.140.

Socías, M. E., Wood, E., Lake, S., Nolan, S., Fairbairn, N., Hayashi, K., ... Milloy, M. J. (2018). High-intensity cannabis use is associated with retention in opioid agonist treatment: A longitudinal analysis. *Addiction*, 113(12), 2250–2258. doi: 10.1111/add.14398.

Stone, D. M., Holland, K. M., Bartholow, B., Crosby, A. E., Davis, S., & Wilkins, N. (2017). *Preventing suicide: A technical package of policies, programs, and practices*. Atlanta, GA: National Center for Injury Prevention and Control, Centers for Disease Control and Prevention. Retrieved from https://www.cdc.gov/violenceprevention/pdf/suicideTechnicalPackage.pdf

Substance Abuse and Mental Health Services Administration (SAMHSA). (2016). *A collaborative approach to the treatment of pregnant women with opioid use disorders*. Retrieved from https://store.samhsa.gov/product/A-Collaborative-Approach-to-the-Treatment-of-Pregnant-Women-with-Opioid-Use-Disorders/SMA16-4978?referer=from_search_result

Substance Abuse and Mental Health Services Administration (SAMHSA). (2017). *SAMHSA's Center for the Application of Prevention Technologies (2017)*. Retrieved from www.samhsa.gov/capt/sites/default/files/resources/preventing-youth-marijuana-use-programs-strategies-2017.pdf

Substance Abuse and Mental Health Services Administration (SAMHSA). (2019a). *Key substance use and mental health indicators in the United States: Results from the 2018 National Survey on Drug Use and Health* (HHS Publication No. PEP19-5068, NSDUH Series H-54). Rockville, MD: Center for Behavioral Health Statistics and Quality, Substance Abuse and Mental Health Services Administration. Retrieved from https://www.samhsa.gov/data/sites/default/files/cbhsq-reports/NSDUHNationalFindingsReport2018/NSDUHNationalFindingsReport2018.pdf

Substance Abuse and Mental Health Services Administration (SAMHSA). (2019b). *A guide to SAMHSA's strategic prevention framework*. Retrieved from https://www.samhsa.gov/sites/default/files/20190620-samhsa-strategic-prevention-framework-guide.pdf

Substance Abuse and Mental Health Services Administration (SAMHSA). (2019c). *Screening and assessment of co-occurring disorders in the justice system*. Retrieved from https://store.samhsa.gov/product/Screening-and-Assessment-of-Co-Occurring-Disorders-in-the-Justice-System/PEP19-SCREEN-CODJS

Substance Abuse and Mental Health Services Administration (SAMHSA). (2019d). *Use of medication-assisted treatment for opioid use disorder in criminal justice settings*. Retrieved from https://store.samhsa.gov/product/Use-of-Medication-Assisted-Treatment-for-Opioid-Use-Disorder-in-Criminal-Justice-Settings/PEP19-MATUSECJS

The Lancet. (2018). Opioid and methamphetamine: A tale of two crises. *Lancet, 391*(10122), 713. doi: 10.1016/S0140-6736(18)30319-2.

Timko, C., & Cucciare, M. A. (2018). Commentary on Socias et al. (2018): Clinical research perspectives on cannabis use in opioid agonist treatment. *Addiction, 113*(12), 2259–2260. doi: 10.1111/add.14432.

U.S. Department of Health and Human Services (USDHHS). (2018). *Surgeon General's advisory on naloxone and opioid overdose*. Retrieved from https://www.surgeongeneral.gov/priorities/opioid-overdose-prevention/naloxone-advisory.html

U.S. Department of Health & Human Services (USDHHS). (2020). *Healthy People 2030*: Browse objectives. Retrieved from https://health.gov/healthypeople/objectives-and-data/browse-objectives

U.S. Food and Drug Administration (USFDA). (2020). *2018 NYTS data: A startling rise in youth e-cigarette use*. Retrieved from https://www.fda.gov/tobacco-products/youth-and-tobacco/2018-nyts-data-startling-rise-youth-e-cigarette-use#:~:text=E%2Dcigarette%20Use%20among%20High,using%20e%2Dcigarettes%20in%202018

U.S. Preventative Services Task Force (USPSTF). (2017). *Final recommendation statement: Tobacco smoking cessation in adults, including pregnant women: Behavioral and pharmacotherapy interventions*. Retrieved from https://www.uspreventiveservicestaskforce.org/Page/Document/RecommendationStatementFinal/tobacco-use-in-adults-and-pregnant-women-counseling-and-interventions1

Vivolo-Kantor, A. M., Seth, P., Gladden, R. M., Mattson, C. L., Baldwin, G. T., Kite-Powell, A., Coletta, M. A. (2018). Vital signs: Trends in emergency department visits for suspected opioid overdoses-United States, July 2016-September 2017. *Morbidity and Mortality Weekly Report (MMWR), 67*, 279–285. Retrieved from https://www.cdc.gov/mmwr/volumes/67/wr/mm6709e1.htm

Walker, E. R., & Druss, B. G. (2018). Mental and addictive disorders and medical comorbidities. *Current Psychiatry Reports, 20*(10), 86. doi: 10.1007/s11920-018-0956-1.

Wisconsin Behavioral Health Association. (n.d.). *Continuum of care*. Retrieved from https://www.wibha.org/our_aims/continuum_of_care.php#:~:text=A%20comprehensive%20approach%20to%20behavioral,behavioral%20health%20problems%20and%20disorders

World Health Organization (WHO). (2018a). *Global status report on alcohol and health*. Geneva, Switzerland: Author. Retrieved from https://apps.who.int/iris/bitstream/handle/10665/274603/9789241565639-eng.pdf?ua=1&ua=1

World Health Organization (WHO). (2018b). *WHO launches SAFER alcohol control initiative to prevent and reduce alcohol-related death and disability*. Retrieved from https://www.who.int/substance_abuse/safer/launch/en/

World Health Organization (WHO). (2020). *The health and social effects of nonmedical cannabis use*. Retrieved from https://www.who.int/substance_abuse/publications/cannabis_report/en/index4.html

Yudko, E., Lozhkina, O., & Fouts, A. (2007). A comprehensive review of the psychometric properties of the Drug Abuse Screening Test. *Journal of Substance Abuse Treatment, 32*(2), 189–198. doi: 10.1016/j.jsat.2006.08.002.

CHAPTER 26

Working with the Homeless

"We have come dangerously close to accepting the homeless situation as a problem that we just can't solve."

—Linda Lingle (1953), American Politician

KEY TERMS

Chronically homeless
Continuum of care
Deinstitutionalization
Doubling up
Homeless
Housing First
Literally homeless
Period prevalence counts
Point-in-time counts
Single-room occupancy (SRO) housing
Survival sex
Trauma-informed care
Unaccompanied youth
Unsheltered (hidden) homeless

LEARNING OBJECTIVES

Upon mastery of this chapter, you should be able to:

1. Define the concept of homelessness.
2. Describe the demographic characteristics of the homeless living in the United States.
3. Discuss factors predisposing persons to homelessness.
4. Compare and contrast the unique challenges confronting selected subpopulations within the homeless community.
5. Explain the effects of homelessness on health.
6. Analyze the extent and adequacy of public and private resources to combat the problem of homelessness.
7. Assess your beliefs and values toward homelessness.
8. Propose community-based nursing interventions to facilitate primary, secondary, and tertiary prevention in addressing the problem of homelessness.

INTRODUCTION

What was once considered unthinkable in a prosperous nation is now an expected occurrence in towns and cities across the United States. Drive through an inner city or suburban community on any given day, and you will see people on street corners holding signs stating "Hungry and homeless." Where is the public outcry in response to this scene? Has the American conscience been anesthetized to this form of human suffering? Or is the need simply too overwhelming and the problems too far reaching to mount an effective campaign to prevent such a tragedy?

The purpose of this chapter is to define the concept of homelessness, examine the factors contributing to homelessness, analyze the major issues confronting the homeless, and examine the role of the community health nurse (CHN) in addressing the needs of the homeless.

The McKinney-Vento Homeless Assistance Act (Title 42 of the U.S. Code) defines as **homeless** a person who lacks a fixed, regular, adequate nightly residence; this definition includes as homeless those who stay in supervised public or private shelters that provide temporary accommodations. Homeless individuals may also reside in institutional settings providing temporary shelter or in public or private places that are not designed for or used as a regular long-term sleeping accommodation for human beings (e.g., cars, parks, campgrounds; Fig. 26-1). Such individuals are often referred to as **literally homeless**. Incarcerated individuals are not considered homeless under this definition (McKinney-Vento Homeless Assistance Act, 1987).

The education subtitle of the McKinney-Vento Homeless Assistance Act expands on the definition of homelessness when addressing homeless children and youth. The Act includes as homeless those children who share housing with others because of economic hardship or loss of housing, are abandoned in hospitals, are awaiting placement in foster care, or are living in motels, trailer parks, or camping grounds. However, children awaiting foster care placement were removed from the definition of homeless in 2016 (National Center for Homeless Education, n.d.).

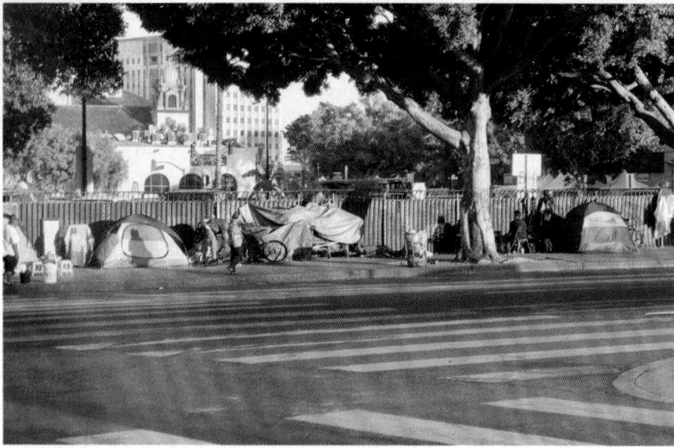

FIGURE 26-1 A row of tents and belongings of some of the over 30,000 homeless people who live in Los Angeles. Homeless individuals often struggle to find shelter.

The U.S. Department of Housing and Urban Development (USDHUD) defines homeless people as those living on the streets, in vehicles, in shelters or parks, or in transitional housing; unaccompanied youth or families with children who are defined as homeless under other federal statutes; or individuals facing imminent eviction (within 14 days; National Health Care for the Homeless Council [NHCHC], 2018). Although this definition may be appropriate for the urban homeless, who are more likely to live on the street or in shelters, persons living in rural areas tend to cohabit with relatives or friends in overcrowded, substandard housing (Housing Assistance Council [HAC], 2016). Box 26-1 outlines selected *Healthy People 2030* goals that relate to the homeless population.

SCOPE OF THE PROBLEM

It is difficult to estimate the number of people who are homeless, because homelessness is a temporary condition. Rather than trying to count the number of homeless people on a given night, or **point-in-time counts**, it may be more prudent to gauge the number of people who have been homeless over a longer time frame, such as over the course of a year, or **period prevalence counts** (Ontario Ministry of Housing, 2017; USDHUD, 2017b).

It is also difficult to locate and account for homeless people. Most estimates of homelessness are based on the number of people served in shelters or soup kitchens or the number of people who can easily be located on the streets. People who spend time at places that are difficult to reach (e.g., cars, campgrounds, caves, boxcars, wooded areas) are considered **unsheltered (hidden) homeless**. Many people are unable to access shelters because of overcrowding and limited capacity (Box 26-2). In rural areas, there are fewer housing options and resources for the homeless. As a result, people may be forced to live temporarily with friends or family (a practice known as **doubling up**). Although still experiencing homelessness, these individuals are not always counted in homeless statistics or considered eligible for homeless services (NHCHC, 2019).

BOX 26-1 *HEALTHY PEOPLE 2030*

Objectives Related to Homelessness

Objective	Description
MHMD-R01	Increase the proportion of homeless adults with mental health problems who get mental health services
HIV-01	Reduce the number of new HIV infections
Related Access to Care Objectives	
AHS-01	Increase the proportion of people with medical insurance
AHS-04	Reduce the proportion of people who can't get medical care when they need it
AHS-06	Reduce the proportion of people who can't get prescription medicines when they need them
AHS-07	Increase the proportion of people with a usual primary care provider
AHS-08	Increase the proportion of adults who get recommended evidence-based preventative health care
AHS-09	Reduce the proportion of emergency department visits with a longer wait time than recommended
AHS-R01	Increase the ability of primary care and behavioral health professional to provide more high-quality care to patients who need it

Reprinted from U.S. Department of Health and Human Services (USDHHS). (2020). *Healthy People 2030: Browse objectives.* Retrieved from https://health.gov/healthypeople/objectives-and-data/browse-objectives

The USDHUD, in its *Annual Homeless Assessment Report to Congress*, publishes the latest counts of homelessness nationwide. In 2017, on a single night in January, there were an estimated 553,742 sheltered and unsheltered homeless people across the nation (Fig. 26-2). Approximately 48% of people experiencing homelessness were in unsheltered locations. The number of homeless people in the nation decreased by 14% from 2007 to 2017, with the number of people in unsheltered locations declining by 25% and the number of people in sheltered locations declining by 8%. From 2016 to 2017, the number of homeless increased in major cities but declined elsewhere in the United States. From 2007 to 2017, the rate of homelessness has declined across all categories except for the sheltered homeless, which has increased by 4% in major cities (USDHUD, 2017b).

BOX **26-2** POPULATION FOCUS

Tent Cities and Solutions for the Homeless

After the Great Recession of 2007 to 2008, tent cities began springing up across many larger cities in the United States, some of them with mutually determined codes of conduct and social structures. These temporary communities were a similar phenomenon to the shantytowns of the Great Depression, and many cities have responded to these temporary encampments by criminalizing them, citing concerns for public health and safety (Herring, 2015; National Law Center on Homelessness and Poverty [NLCHP], 2017).

Imagine a world where it is illegal to sit down. Could you survive if there were no place you were allowed to fall asleep, store your belongings, or to stand still? Homeless people, like all people, must engage in activities such as sleeping or sitting down in order to survive. Yet in communities across the nation, these harmless, unavoidable behaviors are treated as criminal activity under laws that criminalize homelessness (NLCHP, 2017).

Between 2007 and 2016, the number of homeless encampments reported by the media has increased 1,342% (NLCHP, 2017). Encampments have been reported in every state across the nation and in the District of Columbia. Most of these temporary communities are illegal and under constant threat of eviction. The dramatic increase in encampments is a reflection of the growth in homelessness and the lack of accessible shelter.

Why do people live in tent cities? Most cities in the United States do not have sufficient shelter beds to accommodate the number of homeless in need of shelter. Many shelters limit admission based on gender. Others do not allow children. Some shelters do not allow personal belongings or have no provision for their safe storage. Other shelters lack accommodations for persons with disabilities. Many shelters have strict curfews that may make it difficult to hold down a job. Very few shelters allow pets (NLCHP, 2017).

Some states have adopted more tent city–friendly policies. Innovations in addressing the tent city crisis include hosting permanent encampments with colocated service centers, engaging religious organizations to temporarily host tent cities on their properties, and providing permits for temporary encampments on city property (NLCHP, 2017).

1. *Have you seen tent cities in your community? How do you feel when you see them?*
2. *What do you think could be done to address some of the issues raised by the proliferation of tent cities? Debate the issue with classmates.*
3. *How could C/PHNs be involved in helping to design feasible population-focused interventions?*

Source: Herring (December 2015); NLCHP, 2017.

Two thirds of the homeless are adults in households with no children. The remaining one third (33%) are homeless families (USDHUD, 2017b). Because of the transient nature of homelessness and the difficulty involved in locating and counting the homeless, it is unlikely that researchers will ever be able to estimate the exact magnitude of homelessness in America (NCH, 2018a).

There is a direct relationship between poverty and homelessness. In general, homelessness is decreasing due, in part, to the strides made over recent years to increase

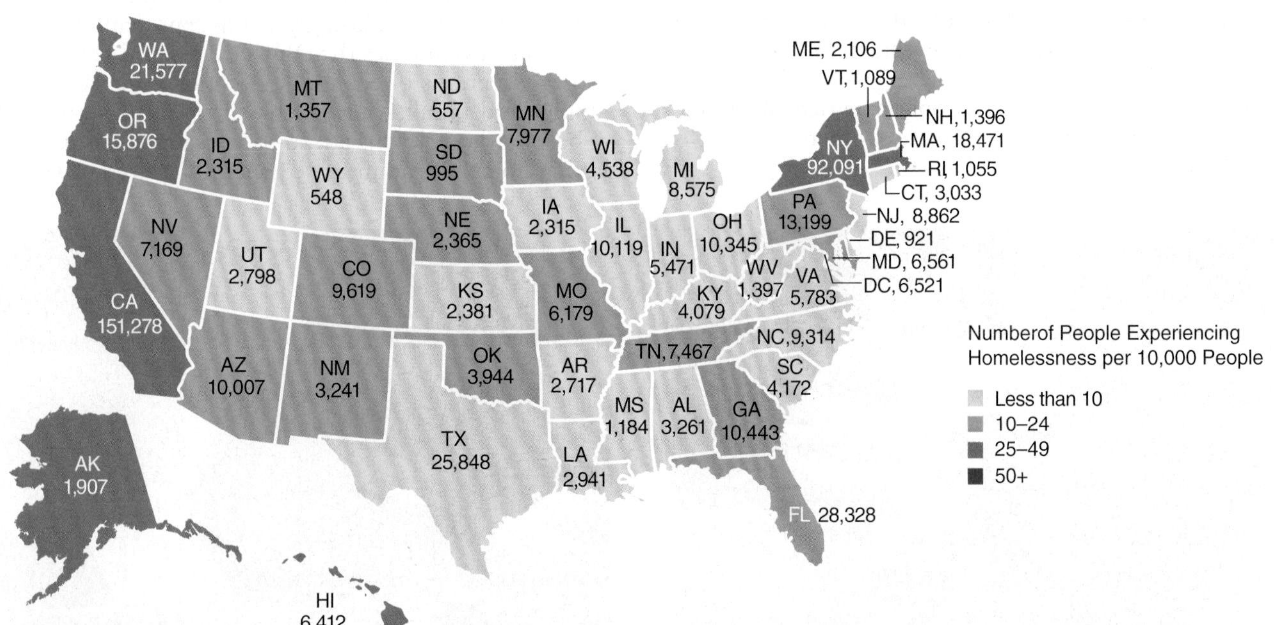

FIGURE 26-2 Estimates of homeless people by state, 2019. (Reprinted from U.S. Department of Housing and Urban Development (USDHUD). (2019). *The 2019 annual homeless assessment report to Congress.* Retrieved from https://files.hudexchange.info/resources/documents/2019-AHAR-Part-1.pdf)

federal funding for homeless prevention and assistance programs. Still, only one in five families eligible for federal housing assistance receive the help they need (National Low Income Housing Coalition [NLIHC], 2019). Despite improvements in employment and in the economy, those who are in poverty, living with friends and family, and paying over half their income for housing continue to be at risk for homelessness. Housing programs for the homeless have removed many homeless people from the streets, but the lack of affordable housing continues to present formidable challenges to eliminating homelessness (National Alliance to End Homelessness [NAEH], 2017, 2020e).

In 2016, The U.S. Conference of Mayors Task Force on Hunger and Homelessness reported its survey findings of 32 cities in 24 states across the nation. The survey revealed that the majority of cities followed the national trend of a declining rate of homelessness. The need for housing assistance and the lack of affordable housing were identified as the most pressing issues requiring improved resources to reduce the rate of homelessness (United States Conference of Mayors, 2016).

Demographics

Poverty is directly linked to homelessness (Fig. 26-3). Demographic groups more likely to be poor are also at greater risk of becoming homeless.

Age

- In 2017, 88% of individuals experiencing homelessness were adults over 24 years of age, 10% were 18 to 24 years old, and only 1% were under 18 years of age.
- Among the unsheltered homeless, 87% are over 24 years old and 1.6% are under 18 years of age (USDHUD, 2017b).

Gender

- The majority of homeless individuals are unaccompanied adult men. Men are more likely than women to be unsheltered.
- Approximately 61% of people experiencing homelessness are men and 39% are women (USDHUD, 2017b).
- From 2016 to 2017, homelessness declined by 1% among women but increased by 1% among men.
- Fewer than 1% of homeless individuals identify themselves as transgender or as not male, female, or transgender (USDHUD, 2017b).

Ethnicity

The racial and ethnic makeup of the homeless population varies based on geographic location.

- Nationally, 47% of people experiencing homelessness are non-Hispanic white, whereas approximately 41% are African American and 22% are Hispanic or Latino.
- Persons in sheltered situations are more likely to be African American, whereas those in unsheltered settings are more likely to be white (USDHUD, 2017b).
- Compared with the U.S. population, the sheltered homeless are more likely to be unaccompanied adult males, African Americans, and disabled (USDHUD, 2017c).

Families

- Families with children represented 33% of the homeless population in the United States in 2017.
- Over 20% of people experiencing homelessness are children.
- Approximately 59% of homeless people in families are children (under 18 years of age).
- More than 90% of homeless people in families reside in shelters.

The number of homeless people in families declined by 21% from 2007 to 2017. The number of homeless families declined by 26%, with the majority of the decline being in families with children in unsheltered locations (USDHUD, 2017b).

Although nearly 78% of adults experiencing sheltered homelessness as part of families with children are women, men are increasingly being represented in sheltered homeless families (USDHUD, 2017c). During recessions and periods of economic decline, more two-parent families and families headed by single fathers are likely to become homeless (Fig. 26-4). Because organizations serving homeless families are generally geared to serving

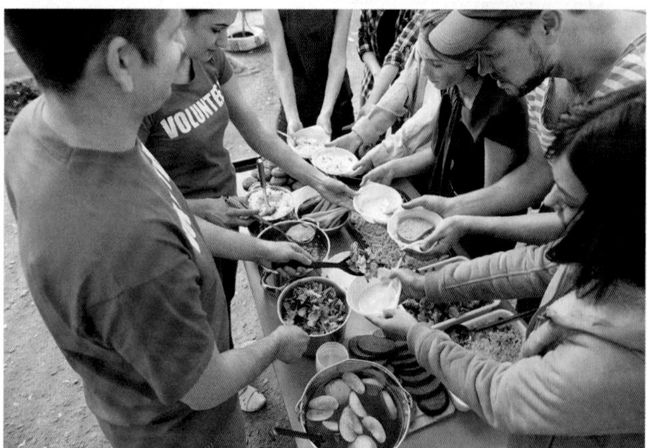

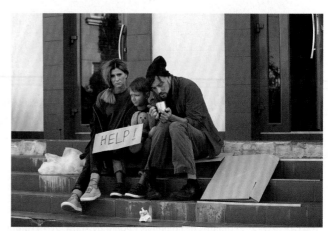

FIGURE 26-3 Volunteers sharing food with homeless people. Raising awareness about homelessness is an important step in seeking community solutions.

FIGURE 26-4 Homeless family sitting on the street. Families with children represent about one third of the homeless population in the United States.

single women with children, it may be difficult for intact families and families headed by men to access shelter (Zobel, 2016).

Contributing Factors

Persons are predisposed to homelessness because of a complex array of factors that result in individuals having to choose between necessities of daily living. Scarce resources limit choices. What would you do if you had to choose between eating and buying your child's medication? Housing consumes a huge portion of one's income and is often the first asset to be lost. Many families find they are only a paycheck away from homelessness (Boxes 26-3 and 26-4).

Poverty

In 2016 (Semega, Fontenot, & Kollar, 2017):

- Nearly 41 million people (or 12.7% of the U.S. population) were living in poverty.
- Eighteen percent of children (under 18 years old) lived in poverty.
- Poverty rates were highest among single female heads of household.

Factors impacting poverty include declining wages, loss of jobs that offer security and carry benefits, an increase in temporary and part-time employment, erosion of the true value of the minimum wage, a decline in manufacturing jobs in favor of lower-paying service jobs, globalization and outsourcing, and a decline in public assistance. As wages drop, the potential to secure adequate housing wanes (NCH, 2018c, 2019d).

Compounding the problem are a lack of affordable housing (particularly **single-room occupancy [SRO] housing** or housing units intended to be occupied by one person) and limited funding for housing assistance. A household seeking to afford a two-bedroom rental home in the United States must earn at least $21.21 per hour. This figure is nearly $14 higher than the federal minimum wage of $7.25 (NLIHC, 2018). The Raise the Wage Act of 2017 is expected to gradually raise the minimum wage to $15 per hour by 2024 (Economic Policy Institute, 2019).

When rental costs increase and the number of available low-rent units declines, the housing gap widens. Moreover, federal support for housing assistance is unable to keep pace with the high demand for housing (NCH, 2018a). As a result, many persons must pay

BOX **26-4** WHAT DO *YOU* THINK?

Street or Shelter? Which Would You Choose?

Many people wonder why so many homeless individuals choose not to use shelters. Walker (2018) discussed the following reasons why homeless persons may be reluctant to utilize shelter services: (1) lack of sufficient beds and overcrowding (many shelters require you to arrive at prescribed times and to wait in line to secure a space at night; if you have a job, you cannot always arrive in time, or you may work at night and need a place to sleep during the day); (2) fear of communicable diseases (e.g., bedbugs and other contagious diseases); (3) fear of having your belongings stolen; (4) having to leave your pets behind; (5) fear for one's safety and concerns regarding being attacked or abused; (6) fears of being proselytized or coerced to adopt particular faith perspectives; (7) having to be separated from one's spouse or loved ones, including older male children (who may not be allowed in a family shelter); and (8) difficulty adhering to sobriety requirements (for individuals who are active in their addiction).

1. *What do you think might be other reasons an individual would choose to sleep outside rather than in a homeless shelter?*
2. *How could some of these issues be effectively addressed?*
3. *How does your city address these issues and the overall problem of homelessness?*

Source: Walker (2018).

BOX **26-3** PERSPECTIVES

A Homeless Couple's Viewpoint on Living in Their Car

My name is Sally. Sam and I are in our fifties and have been homeless for 2 years. We became homeless when my husband's company downsized, and he lost his job. I had to go on medical disability because of my brittle diabetes. I could no longer work, and the medical bills just kept piling up. Eventually, we were unable to pay our rent and were evicted from our home. We have been living in our car. We park in the local SuperMart lot at night. This place is great. It is located in a safe area of town, and it is open 24 hours a day, so we always have access to restroom facilities. We stayed in a county shelter for a while. The social worker there tried to help us find housing, but we were afraid to go into the parts of town where the subsidized housing was located. The criminal activity there was so pervasive that we just figured we would be safer living in our car. We have been married for over 30 years, but we were separated at the shelter and told we could not demonstrate any physical affection. When we tried to apply for food stamps, we were told we needed to produce our rent and gas and electric bills, or we would be ineligible to receive this benefit. I kept telling them that we live in our car. We don't pay rent! We don't have a gas and electric bill! Many times, we were turned down from housing and other benefits, because we did not meet the eligibility criteria. We were not single parents. We had no children. We did not suffer from a severe mental health or addiction disorder. We were not veterans. It is so frustrating. There are resources, but there are so many barriers to accessing them.

Sally

high rents to obtain shelter. This situation leads to overcrowding and substandard housing. Because the demand for housing assistance exceeds federal housing assistance resources, there are often long waiting lists. Waiting lists may close when demand for housing exceeds the supply of subsidized units available for occupancy (NCH, 2019c; USDHUD, n.d.).

Lack of Affordable Health Care

In the absence of affordable health care coverage, a serious illness or disability can lead to job loss, savings depletion, and even eviction. In 2016, nearly 28 million Americans (9% of the population) were without health care coverage (Kaiser Family Foundation, 2020).

The Affordable Care Act has expanded Medicaid coverage to millions of previously uninsured people, reducing the number of uninsured in the United States from 44 million in 2013 to <28 million in 2016 (Kaiser Family Foundation, 2019).

The uninsured are less likely to receive preventive care or care for chronic health conditions. They are more at risk for preventable hospitalizations and missed diagnoses. Nearly half of all bankruptcies in the United States are due, in part, to medical debts (Kaiser Family Foundation, 2019). Those who are able to qualify for medical assistance may be reluctant to seek employment, fearing termination of benefits. Many others have limited coverage that requires higher co-pays or deductibles and does not cover major catastrophic illnesses. A catastrophic adverse health event can plunge one into a homeless condition.

Employment

Low-income wage earners may hold jobs with nonstandard work arrangements. Temporary employees, day laborers, independent contractors, and part-time employees are examples of those with work arrangements that tend to pay lower wages, offer few or no benefits, and have less job security.

For persons with few or no job skills, it is virtually impossible to compete for jobs that offer a living wage. Barriers to employment among the homeless include a lack of education or job skills; a lack of transportation, childcare, or other supportive services; a lack of access to technology; and disabilities that make it difficult to pursue or retain employment. To overcome homelessness and maintain employment, one must not only obtain a job that pays a living wage but also have access to supportive services such as childcare and transportation (NCH, 2018c).

Domestic Violence

Domestic violence is a major cause of homelessness among women. For victims of domestic violence, the choice is often between living in an abusive situation and leaving to face life on the streets. More than one third of domestic violence survivors report being homeless following separation from their intimate partners.

Victims of domestic violence are often isolated from social support networks and financial resources, rendering them especially vulnerable. They may lack a steady income or a stable employment record and often experience anxiety, depression, panic disorder, or substance abuse disorders. A major challenge facing service providers of homeless domestic violence victims is the need to ensure a safe and secure environment and to protect client confidentiality (NAEH, 2020b, 2020c).

Mental Illness

- Untreated mental illness may precipitate homelessness, and homelessness is a significant risk factor for poor mental health (Stafford & Wood, 2017).
- Approximately 112,000 homeless persons across the United States reported a severe mental illness in 2017 (USDHUD, 2017a).
- In January 2016, 20% of people experiencing homelessness had a serious mental illness (Substance Abuse and Mental Health Services Administration [SAMHSA], 2017a).

Deinstitutionalization (being released from institutions into the community) has contributed to the number of severely mentally ill persons represented in the homeless population (Howell, 2017). Some mentally ill persons self-medicate their disturbing symptoms using street drugs, placing them at increased risk of addictions and diseases transmitted through injection drug use. Mental illness and substance abuse are often comorbid conditions, which, coupled with poor physical health, makes it especially difficult to secure employment and safe, affordable housing (SAMHSA, 2017a).

Addiction Disorders

Rates of alcohol and drug abuse are disproportionately high among the homeless. In January 2016, 20% of people experiencing homelessness had a serious mental illness, and a similar percentage had a chronic substance use disorder (SAMHSA, 2017a).

For persons already at risk for homelessness, the behaviors associated with an addictive disorder can create instability and jeopardize family and employment support nets. Once homeless, persons may resort to drugs or alcohol to dull the pain of being homeless and ease the feelings of hopelessness that accompany such a desperate state. They may also turn to chemical substances to self-medicate the disturbing symptoms of an untreated mental illness. Fragmentation of services, limited access to care, lack of transportation, social isolation, and complex treatment needs make it difficult to receive the services needed to achieve a successful recovery (NAEH, 2020f).

Many shelters require sobriety to access services. There may be long waiting lists for addiction treatment, and homeless people who do not have a phone and are difficult to locate may be dropped from the waiting list. Lack of transportation and lack of documentation needed to access programs (i.e., birth certificates, social security cards) further exacerbate the problem. Denial of Supplemental Security Income or Social Security Disability Insurance to persons with substance abuse-related disabilities creates a huge barrier to achieving recovery support, proper medical care, and housing and income assistance. Moreover, the federal programs targeting homelessness, mental health, and addictions services (Box 26-5) lack the funding necessary to effectively address this problem on a national level.

BOX **26-5** PERSPECTIVES

A C/PHN's Viewpoint on Caring for the Homeless

I can't believe I am sitting around this table. What am I doing here? How did I end up on the Board of Directors of an organization that houses one of the largest residential addiction recovery programs for homeless men in the country? I have been a public health nurse for years. I know how to take care of homeless patients. But this is a whole different ball game. I'm looking at budgets and learning about capital campaigns. I even testified before a gubernatorial commission to advocate for funding for homeless services. And now I am chairing a Board level committee that is analyzing census tract data to determine the impact of its wellness center on public health. We are looking at emergency department utilization rates and rates of hospitalization for substance-related illnesses to see if our Wellness Center has an impact on our clients and the surrounding community. If we can demonstrate that our programs reduce hospitalizations and emergency room visits, we may be eligible to apply for population health funding and to partner with local hospitals in much bigger ways to make a positive impact in our community. This is exciting stuff!

Stan, C/PHN

Additional Variables

Additional variables impacting homelessness include personal and financial crises, natural disasters, immigration and refugee crises, and personal choice. For example, natural disasters or immigration crises may displace previously independent and self-sufficient individuals and families, rendering many homeless and in need of emergency shelter. See more on disasters and their aftermath in Chapter 17.

Homeless Subpopulations

Although many of the struggles the homeless face are universal, there are subpopulations within the homeless community that are uniquely vulnerable. Often, these groups face additional burdens because of their special needs and challenges.

Homeless Men

Approximately 61% of people experiencing homelessness are men (USDHUD, 2017b). The majority of homeless men are single adults.

Some men find themselves in a cycle of intermittent homelessness as they move back and forth between prisons, treatment centers, shelters, temporary housing, and the streets. Other men are at risk for becoming **chronically homeless**. Nearly one quarter of the homeless population in the United States is chronically homeless (USDHUD, 2017b). A chronically homeless adult is someone who has been homeless for long periods of time or has experienced repeated episodes of homelessness.

These individuals have a diagnosed disability such as mental illness, substance abuse, or a chronic medical condition and have been homeless for at least a year or have experienced at least four episodes of homelessness in the past 3 years. In 2017, the Annual Homeless Assessment Report to Congress recorded nearly 87,000 chronically homeless individuals in its point-in-time count (an 18% decline since 2010). Nearly 70% of these individuals were unsheltered (i.e., living on the street or in places not fit for human habitation; USDHUD, 2017b).

Homeless men are more likely to be treated with disdain than other homeless subgroups. Some people perceive the homeless male as largely to blame for his plight, believing that he is able bodied and should be able to work. Moreover, homeless men may have disabilities that are not severe enough to warrant eligibility for health and social services. Often health and social programs give priority to women and children (Myrick, 2016).

Homeless Women

Women, as single parents, lead most homeless families in the United States (Fig. 26-5). Nearly 80% of sheltered homeless families are led by women (USDHUD, 2017c). Domestic violence is a major cause of homelessness among women (USDHHS, 2016).

Lack of affordable housing forces many women to choose between living in an abusive home and facing life on the streets. Domestic violence victims often have poor credit and employment records due to the disruption caused by family violence. If violence is discovered in the home, landlords may evict tenants, forcing the family onto the streets (Family & Youth Services Bureau, 2016). Once on the street, a woman faces the risk of greater abuse. Moreover, the increased risk for exposure to violence and sexual assault on the streets increases the risk for sexually transmitted infections and traumatic injuries.

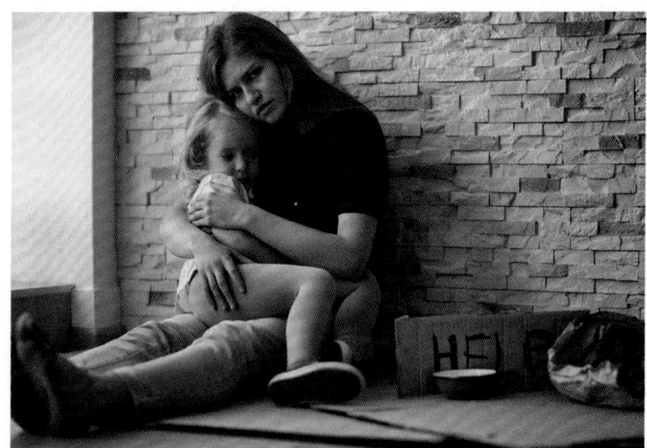

FIGURE 26-5 Homeless poor woman and her daughter asking for help. Most homeless families are headed by single female heads of household.

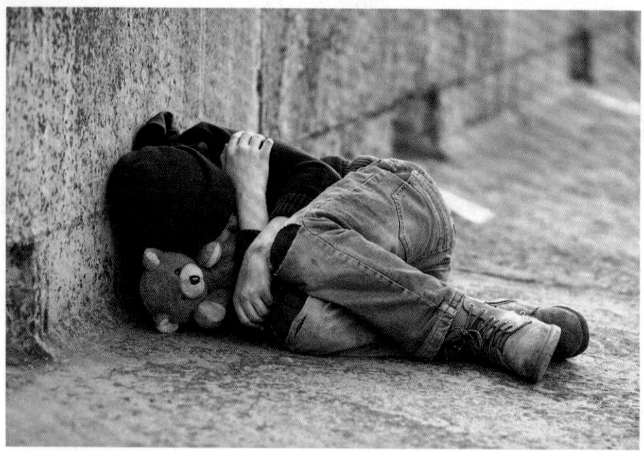

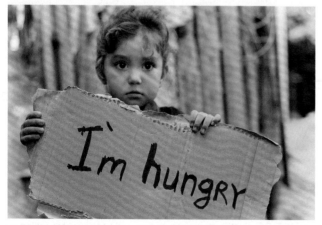

FIGURE 26-6 A young homeless boy sleeping on a bridge.

Homeless Children

- In 2017, there were nearly 41,000 unaccompanied homeless children and youth (those under the age of 25 years) in the United States, of whom 12% were under the age of 18 years (Fig. 26-6).
- One in 20 children under 6 years of age was homeless in 2014 and 2015 (USDHHS, 2017).
- From 2007 to 2016, the number of children in families living in poverty increased by 13% (USDHUD, 2017c).

The majority of homeless children and youth live in shelters, share housing with friends or relatives, or live in motels or campgrounds. Compared with their housed counterparts, homeless children are more likely to become ill, go hungry, and experience emotional and behavioral disorders (Fig. 26-7). They are also more likely to experience developmental delays and learning disabilities. Children in homeless families are more likely to experience parental separation, by being placed in either foster care or the care of friends or relatives. More than 25% of homeless children have witnessed violent acts (American Institute on Research, 2020; Child Trends Data Bank, 2015).

FIGURE 26-7 A 3-year-old homeless girl. Homeless children are more likely to go hungry than their housed counterparts.

Education is compromised when one is homeless. Homeless children are more than twice as likely to repeat grades in school as other children and more likely to drop out or be suspended or expelled (Child Trends Data Bank, 2015; NAEH, 2020a). They are also less likely to graduate from high school or college than their housed counterparts (Hayes, 2016). Barriers to education include transportation to and from the shelter, lack of academic and medical records required for registration, unstable living arrangements necessitating multiple moves, and urgent needs for food and shelter that take priority over education (Family & Youth Services Bureau, 2016).

Homeless children are more likely to get sick than other children. Not only are acute and chronic health problems more severe in homeless children, but these children are less able to access medical and dental care. Asthma, hyperactivity/inattention disorders, and behavioral problems are more prevalent in homeless children than in the general population (Child Trends Data Bank, 2015).

Homeless Youth

On a single night in January 2016, nearly 36,000 unaccompanied youth were experiencing homelessness in the United States (USDHUD, 2017c). **Unaccompanied youth** are defined as persons under 25 years of age who are not accompanied by either a parent or guardian and are not themselves a parent (USDHUD, 2017b).

These youths may have run away from home or been evicted by their parents. There may be conflicts in the home that make it dangerous for them to return home. Many have been victims of abuse and have spent time in foster care. They may be overlooked during homeless counts because they are often difficult to locate (Child Trends Data Bank, 2015). For more information on the road to youth homelessness, see Figure 26-8.

In a national survey, nearly one third of youth experiencing homelessness had experiences with the foster care system and nearly half had been incarcerated or in juvenile detention (Morton, Dworsky, & Samuels, 2017). Foster care placement is associated with homelessness among youth. Moreover, some youth who are discharged from residential or foster care with inadequate housing or income support may find themselves homeless (Ahmann, 2017).

Homeless adolescents may have difficulty accessing emergency shelter because of shelter policies that prohibit older youth from the facility or because of a lack of bed space. Due to lack of education or job training skills, many resort to prostitution or **survival sex** (exchanging sex for food, shelter, or other basic necessities). As a result, homeless youth are at higher risk for sexually transmitted infections. Homeless youth also suffer disproportionately from mental health disorders (Cima & Parker, 2017; NCH, 2019b; Oppong Asante, Meyer-Weitz, & Petersen, 2016).

It is not uncommon for homeless youths to be arrested for running away, breaking curfews, or being without supervision. As young people age out of the foster care system, they find themselves on the street with inadequate support systems and little opportunity for housing or employment (Box 26-6; Ahmann, 2017).

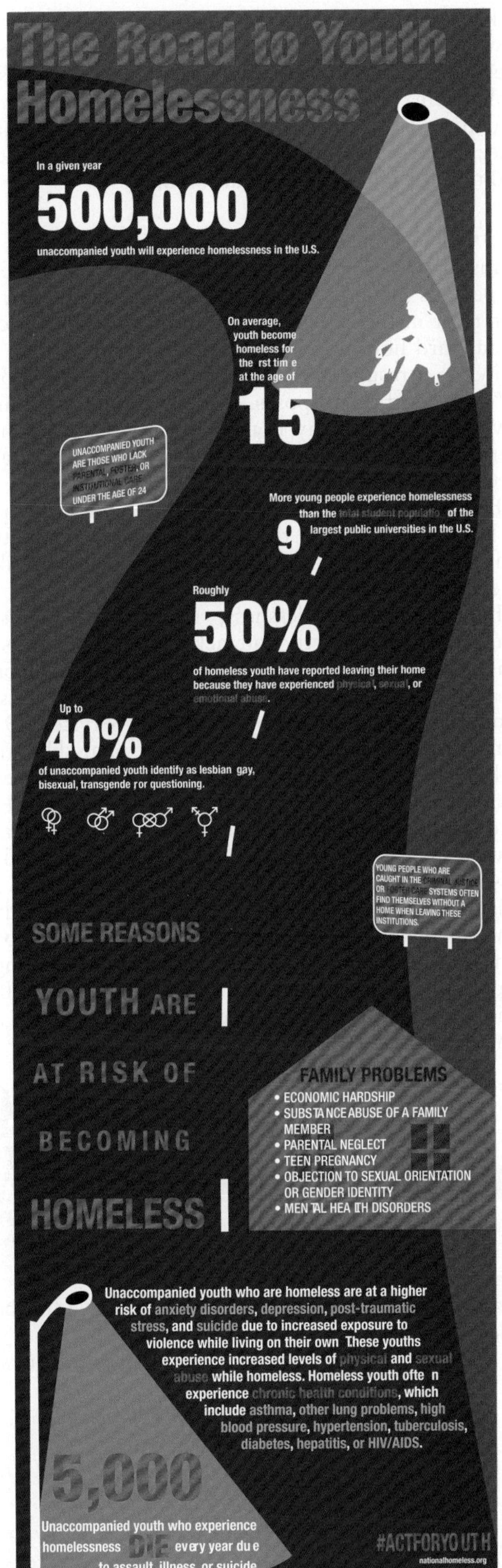

FIGURE 26-8 The road to youth homelessness. (Retrieved from https://nationalhomeless.org/wp-content/uploads/2014/12/Infographic1-FINAL.jpg. Used with permission.)

BOX 26-6 STORIES FROM THE FIELD

Crisis Shelter Intake of Roberto, a Homeless Youth

I sat across from Roberto in a darkened, gritty community room at the homeless teen drop-in center located in an edgy part of downtown. He had just gone through an hour-plus worth of intake questions from the shelter staff; he was tired of questions, though grateful to get one-to-one time with a caring adult and *very happy* to have food in his belly. The intake questionnaire painted a picture of how he landed in this shelter as a 16-year old: a history of being in foster care while in elementary school; a diagnosis of anxiety disorder; a housing history mostly living with a loving, single parent who struggled to pay for a place in this gentrified city; and an academic record moving from school to school with four siblings whom he cared about a lot. Still, he told the intake workers of wishes and hopes of going to college, continuing with his love of art, and finding his own housing "to take the burden of having another kid at home" off his mom.

I ran through his HEADDS assessment screening tool and a brief PHQ-9 to understand the background and status of his physical and mental health. Roberto told me about his extended family whom he loved very much but couldn't live with right now. He liked school and got decent grades, though he worried about paying for college. He played soccer as an extracurricular, but rarely stayed at a school long enough to become a starter on the varsity teams. He stayed away from drinking and drugs because his father had been a drunk and left the family while he was young. And despite having an on-again, off-again girlfriend, says he adheres to his Catholic faith and has never had sex. On his PHQ-9, he scored "moderate depressive" symptoms and noted his anxiety has been "pretty high" the past couple weeks, and especially today being in this new place, not knowing anyone in the shelter. He repeatedly says "thank you" as staff walk by to welcome him to the center and shows extreme gratitude to me as we wrap up our discussion.

1. *What are some other critical pieces of information would you like to know about Roberto before you take him back to the housing staff for case management planning?*
2. *What 1 to 2 health or social concerns do you want to address with him right now using motivational interview techniques? What are Roberto's top health concerns you would like to include in his case management plan for this shelter stay?*

Scott Harpin, PhD, MPH, RN, APHN-BC, FSAHM

Homeless Families

Poverty and the lack of affordable housing place families at risk of becoming homeless. Declining wages, changes in welfare programs, unstable employment, domestic violence, and a struggling economy have all contributed to the rise in family homelessness. Racial disparities and the challenge of single parenting also contribute to the growing trend in family homelessness (NAEH, 2020a).

Homelessness often breaks up the family unit. Families may be separated by shelter policies that prohibit admission to older boys or men. Sometimes, parents are forced to leave their children with family or friends or to place them in foster care to shelter them from becoming homeless (Child Trends Data Bank, 2015; United States Interagency Council on Homelessness, 2018).

A child is at greater risk for homelessness if the child's father becomes injured or ill, experiences a job loss, has a substance abuse issue, or becomes involved with the criminal justice system. Fifty percent of fathers of homeless children are unemployed, and 43% have problems with drugs or alcohol. Homeless children are at a high risk of being placed in foster care, and a personal history of foster care predicts family homelessness during adulthood. To assist homeless families, attention must be focused on promoting affordable housing; supporting education, job training, and childcare for parents; promoting access to school; expanding violence prevention and treatment services; and preventing unnecessary separation of families (American Institute on Research, 2020; Lenz-Rashid, 2017; NCFH, 2014; United States Interagency Council on Homelessness, 2018).

Homeless Veterans

- According to the 2017 Annual Assessment Report to Congress, 9% of homeless adults are veterans (USDHUD, 2017b).
- Female homeless veterans represent approximately 9% of the homeless veteran population (Box 26-7; USDHUD, 2017c).
- Homelessness among veterans declined 45% from 2009 to 2017 (USDHUD, 2017b).
- In 2009, the U.S. Department of Veterans Affairs established a goal to end homelessness among veterans by 2015.

The U.S. Department of Veterans Affairs administers programs that provide long-term care, emergency shelter, 2-year transitional housing, group homes, and work therapy for homeless veterans. These programs provide case management, residential treatment, and other services to homeless veterans and improve housing, employment, and access to care for the homeless veteran population. Unfortunately, the programs are often unable to keep pace with existing needs (NCH, 2019a; National Coalition for Homeless Veterans, n.d.).

The Rural Homeless

Because there are fewer shelters in rural areas, homeless persons living in rural areas are less likely to live in shelters or in the streets and more likely to live in cars, substandard housing, or "doubled up" with friends and family. As a result, they may not be considered "homeless" for reporting purposes. Moreover, the communities in which they live may not be able to access as much federal funding, because the statistics do not adequately reflect the magnitude of the problem.

Families with single mothers and children compose the largest segment of the rural homeless population. Native Americans and migrant workers are more likely to be among the rural homeless.

Like urban homelessness, rural homelessness is largely a result of poverty and lack of affordable housing. Although housing costs are lower in rural areas, incomes are also lower (HAC, 2016; 2017; National Advisory Committee on Rural Health and Human Services, 2014). Homelessness in rural areas may be precipitated by structural or physical housing problems that force families to relocate to safer but more expensive housing (Fig. 26-9). In addition, the lack of job opportunities, the distance between low-income housing and job sites, the lack of transportation, rising rents, geographic isolation, and the lack of resources compound the problem. To address the needs of the rural homeless, the definition of homelessness needs to be expanded to include people living in temporary or substandard housing (HAC, 2016, 2017; National Advisory Committee on Rural Health and Human Services, 2014).

BOX 26-7 PERSPECTIVES

A Homeless Female Veteran's Viewpoint

I am a female veteran, recently discharged from active duty service during which I was deployed to Iraq. I am now homeless. I am one of thousands of veterans who sleep on the streets of America every night. I did not know that I was at risk for homelessness when I joined the military; in fact, I thought a military career or enlistment would help me be successful in life. I did not know that women veterans are three to four times more likely to become homeless than nonveteran women. Or, that posttraumatic stress disorder (PTSD) is twice as likely to be diagnosed in women as in men. Considering that 14% of all deployed military personnel to Iraq and Afghanistan are women, I guess I should have known this was a possibility for me. But I was not prepared for what happened to me.

I am also a victim of sexual trauma, which is a trigger for PTSD, and this has profoundly impacted my ability to return to a normal life as a veteran.

Now, I never feel safe and I am not able to trust anyone or anything. I know you look at me and wonder why I am in this position. I am sure that you don't understand why I do not seem to be able to change my situation. Believe me, I have tried.

Sarah, a veteran

1. *What resources are available in the community for homeless female veterans?*
2. *Are there barriers to accessing these resources for certain veterans?*
3. *What are some of the common assumptions and stereotypes circulating in your community about homeless veterans?*
4. *What would you want to include in your assessment in order to identify risks and to implement treatment planning for homeless veterans like Sarah?*

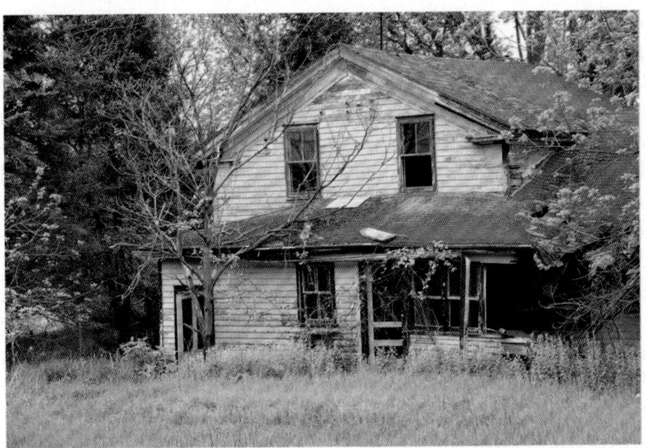

FIGURE 26-9 Rural housing may be structurally unsound or substandard.

The Older Homeless

- Only 4.7% of sheltered homeless individuals were 62 years or older in 2016 (USDHUD, 2017c).
- Even so, as the population ages, many more adults are aging into poverty (Goldberg, Lang, & Barrington, 2016).
- Although the percentage of older individuals in shelters is low, it has increased from 2.9% in 2007 to 4.7% in 2016 (USDHUD, 2017c).
- The percentage of individuals aged 51 to 61 years who are housed in shelters also increased from nearly 14% in 2007 to nearly 18% in 2016 (USDHUD, 2017c).
- Some researchers define the "older homeless" as homeless persons 50 years or older because of the declining physical health that accompanies street living (NCH, 2012b).

Many older people live on a fixed income. At the same time, housing has become increasingly more unaffordable. Moreover, the cost of health care continues to rise, leaving older adults at higher risk of poverty. Their restricted income renders them more vulnerable to unexpected financial crisis and even homelessness. The Social Security benefits to which many are entitled are inadequate to cover housing costs. Moreover, the waiting list for affordable housing for seniors is often 3 to 5 years (Goldberg et al., 2016; NCH, 2018b). Isolation also contributes to homelessness. Many older people live alone and lack a support network.

Homeless adults 50 years and older have health issues similar to those of housed adults who are 15 to 20 years older. Homeless older adults, compared with the general population, are more likely to experience difficulty in activities of daily living at a younger age. Shelter conditions, such as the use of bunk beds and shared bathing facilities, can also increase the risk of falls and injury.

Lesbian, Gay, Bisexual, and Transgender Homeless

Lesbian, gay, bisexual, transgender, and questioning (LGBTQ) persons often experience difficulty finding shelters that accept them. They are sometimes required to identify themselves as a particular gender. Transgender individuals may be turned away from shelters or subjected to physical, sexual, or verbal abuse. They are more likely to be victims of violence, abuse, and exploitation than their gender-conforming peers (NCH, 2018e).

Transgender youth account for 2% of the unaccompanied homeless youth population (USDHUD, 2017b). LGBTQ youth have a 120% increased risk of becoming homeless compared with youth who identify as heterosexual or cisgender (Morton et al., 2017).

HEALTH CARE AND THE HOMELESS

Acute and chronic health problems are prevalent among the homeless population, and they contribute to and result from homelessness. Conditions such as HIV/AIDS, diabetes, and heart disease are three to six times more prevalent in the homeless population than among the general population (NAEH, 2020d). Chronic health conditions require ongoing monitoring and are often difficult to treat in a population that is transient and lacks stable housing (NCH, 2018d; NHCHC, 2019).

Persons with HIV/AIDS are at higher risk of homelessness, because HIV-related illness can impact job stability. Moreover, health care costs associated with treating the illness can exact an enormous financial burden on a low-income family. Insufficient funds to adequately house the poor with HIV/AIDS may also contribute to homelessness among HIV-infected individuals. Substance abuse and sexual exploitation among the homeless increases the risk of HIV infection. Moreover, it is difficult to maintain adherence to complex HIV/AIDS medication regimens without access to good food, bathrooms, refrigeration, and clean water (Aidala, et al., 2016; NCH, 2012a).

Poverty, substance abuse, poor nutrition, and coexisting medical and psychiatric illnesses also predispose the homeless to severe oral health problems. Persons with poor access to dental treatment and preventive services have higher rates of oral disease. Poor oral health is also associated with lower levels of education and income (United States Department of Health and Human Services, 2019).

It is difficult for the homeless to adhere to complex treatment regimens. For example, where would a homeless person find a refrigerator to store insulin? Where would someone keep supplies for dressings? How could someone with no access to transportation keep regular appointments with health care providers? How does a homeless person keep track of multiple appointment dates? How is a shelter resident who receives the typical shelter diet high in carbohydrates, fats, and sodium to adhere to a low-salt or diabetic diet?

"Health Care for the Homeless" was a model for homeless health care developed through a 19-city demonstration project funded by the Robert Wood Johnson Foundation and the Pew Memorial Trust. In 1987, federal legislation (the McKinney-Vento Homeless Assistance Act) was passed that authorized federal funding for these programs. Grants are awarded to community-based organizations that deliver high-quality health care to homeless populations. Health Care for the Homeless projects exist across the nation to provide comprehensive primary care and supportive services, including substance abuse treatment, to medically underserved populations (Box 26-8; NHCHC, 2018).

BOX 26-8 EVIDENCE-BASED PRACTICE

Impact of Cell Phone Use on Coping and Social Connectedness Among Homeless Youth

Tyler and Schmitz (2017) examined the impact of cell phone data collection use on maintaining social connectedness and informational awareness among homeless youth in two mid-western cities in the United States. Participants completed a baseline interview and were then given a disposable cell phone that was activated for 28 to 30 days. Text questions were sent to them from an automated system. Participants were asked to respond to the text questions (11 texts per day) and received cash and/or gift cards for their participation.

A follow-up in person interview was used to assess benefits and cell phone usage patterns. Data revealed that the youth reported using the study phones to seek employment and housing and to schedule appointments. The phones also served as a source of comfort for them, as they had a lifeline for communicating with others in the event of an emergency. The cell phones also enhanced the participants' feelings of independence and autonomy and promoted a greater sense of emotional and social connectedness. The researchers concluded that cell phone ownership among homeless youth can promote positive mental health, improve coping skills, strengthen social support systems, and promote access to vital resources.

1. *What creative outreach approaches might the community health nurse (CHN) develop to improve coping skills, enhance communication and connectedness, and promote greater access to resources for the homeless?*
2. *What new technologies or communication devices might be used to enhance outreach efforts?*
3. *How can creative approaches be used to improve, not only health care delivery, but the delivery of other supportive services?*
4. *How might the CHN use research evidence to make a case for funding technologies that enhance communication and service delivery in the homeless population?*

Source: Tyler and Schmitz (2017).

RESOURCES TO COMBAT HOMELESSNESS

Both public and private sectors have promoted a variety of initiatives to address the problem of homelessness. These initiatives are intended to impact homelessness on the local, state, and national levels and to ensure a coordinated, comprehensive, and systematic approach to addressing the problem of homelessness.

Public Sector

The McKinney-Vento Homeless Assistance Act (PL100-77) was the first and only major piece of federal legislation intended to address the problem of homelessness on a national level. This landmark legislation Act, passed by Congress in 1987, originally consisted of 15 programs to address the major, pressing needs of the homeless. These needs included emergency shelter, transitional and permanent housing, job training, primary health care, education, and housing (NCH, 2006; NLIHC, 2019).

The current Act has been amended over the years to expand its scope and strengthen its impact. In particular, the amendments made to the Act in 1990 represented significant milestones in advocating for the needs of the homeless. These amendments included the creation of the Shelter Care Plus program, which provided for housing assistance for persons with disabilities, mental illness, AIDS, and drug and alcohol addiction. Another amendment created a demonstration program within the Health Care for the Homeless program to provide primary care and outreach to at-risk and homeless children. In addition, the Community Mental Health Services Program was amended and retitled: the Projects for Assistance in Transition from Homelessness.

Finally, the amendments made in 1990 strengthened access to public education for homeless children and youth. The McKinney-Vento Act authorized the U.S. Department of Education to administer the Education for Homeless Children and Youth program, which provides grants to schools to assist in identifying children who are homeless and to provide services to help them succeed in school (NLIHC, 2019). States are required to provide grant funding to local educational institutions to insure access to a free, appropriate education for homeless youth and children (NCH, 2006; NLIHC, 2019).

Over the years, Congress has appropriated funding to enable implementation of this federal legislation. The extent of federal funding has fluctuated over the years. Moreover, rising rental housing costs limit the impact of these limited resources. Although homeless advocates acknowledge that the Act was an important step in addressing homelessness, the lack of adequate funding over recent years threatens its impact on a national level (NLIHC, 2019).

The USDHUD oversees a number of programs established in the McKinney-Vento Act that provide rental, homeownership, and supportive housing for older, low-income, and disabled persons. The Department also manages grants for community development initiatives and helps to strengthen the housing market (NLIHC, 2019).

In many communities, this housing assistance is based on a **continuum of care** model, in which programs are developed to assist persons to transition from emergency to transitional to permanent housing. Emergency shelters provide temporary overnight shelter, whereas transitional housing provides up to 24 months of housing and supportive services. Rapid rehousing programs provide short-term rental assistance and supportive services, whereas permanent housing provides long-term housing and supportive services (NAEH, 2020h).

In recent years, a **Housing First** philosophy has guided much of the publicly funded housing initiatives. In a Housing First approach, housing is viewed as an immediate priority. The goal of Housing First is to end homelessness by providing stable, permanent housing as soon as possible and to provide supportive services to enable people to maintain their housing. Housing or supportive services are not contingent upon adherence to rigid rules or policies or to the maintenance of sobriety (NAEH, 2020h). See Box 26-2 on tent cities and successful approaches to Housing First.

The Homeless Emergency Assistance and Rapid Transition to Housing (HEARTH) Act of 2009 increased funding for McKinney-Vento programs that provide emergency, transitional, and permanent housing and supportive services to the homeless and resources to local school districts to coordinate services for homeless children (NCFH, 2014). The HEARTH Act also consolidated homeless programs at USDHUD and made the homeless assistance system more performance based (NLIHC, 2019).

On March 23, 2010, President Barak Obama signed into law the Affordable Care Act, federal legislation that extends health insurance coverage and gives states the option to expand Medicaid coverage to low-income individuals regardless of disability or family status. This landmark legislation enabled homeless individuals in many states to secure health care coverage (NAEH, 2020g). See Chapter 6.

Another significant milestone in federal initiatives to reduce homelessness occurred in 2001 when the federal government adopted the goal of ending chronic homelessness in 10 years. To meet this goal, annual funding was appropriated to create new permanent supportive housing. These resources helped to stimulate the production of housing. Many communities followed the lead of the federal government and developed their own 10-year plans (Burt, 2006; McEvers, 2016).

In 2010, the U.S. Interagency Council on Homelessness published the nation's first comprehensive federal strategic plan to prevent and end homelessness. The document, entitled "Opening Doors," outlined a comprehensive and ambitious plan aimed at eliminating homelessness on a national level. The goals of the plan included ending chronic homelessness in 10 years, preventing and ending homelessness for families, youth, and children in 10 years, preventing and ending homelessness among veterans in 5 years, and establishing a path to end all types of homelessness (USICH, 2015). This plan was updated and amended in 2012 and 2015. Progress reports on the plan attest to the effectiveness of this federal, coordinated initiative in reducing homelessness across the nation (USICH, 2017). Table 26-1 summarizes the nine titles of the McKinney-Vento Act. Table 26-2 presents selected federally sponsored programs for addressing the needs of the homeless.

Private Sector

The private sector has made a concerted effort to organize communities in the battle against homelessness by forming coalitions, alliances, and memberships that champion the causes of the homeless. These organized efforts are carried out at the national, state, and local levels to positively impact the problem of homelessness in communities across the nation. Table 26-3 presents a list and descriptions of selected resources in the private sector to combat homelessness.

ROLE OF THE C/PHN

C/PHNs maintain a long tradition of providing care to vulnerable populations and play a vital role in addressing the health needs of the homeless. Settings for care include shelters, clinics, soup kitchens, churches, community centers, social service agencies, and even the streets.

TABLE 26-1 McKinney-Vento Homeless Assistance Act Titles I to IX

Title I	Statement of findings by Congress and definition of homelessness
Title II	Establishes the Interagency Council on Homelessness, a council composed of 15 heads of federal agencies to address the needs of homeless populations
Title III	Authorizes the Emergency Food and Shelter Program, administered by the Federal Emergency Management Agency (FEMA)
Title IV	Authorizes the emergency shelter and transitional housing programs administered by the Department of Housing and Urban Development (HUD) including the Emergency Shelter Grant Program, the Supportive Housing Demonstration Program, Supplemental Assistance for Facilities to Assist the Homeless, and Section 8 Single Room Occupancy Moderate Rehabilitation
Title V	Requires federal agencies to make available federal land and buildings for states and local governments to use to assist the homeless
Title VI	Authorizes programs to provide health care services to the homeless, including Health Care for the Homeless program, Community Mental Health Services Block Grant Program, and two demonstration programs providing substance abuse and mental health treatment services to the homeless
Title VII	Authorizes the Adult Education for the Homeless Program, the Education of Homeless Children and Youth Program (administered by the Department of Education), the Job Training for the Homeless Demonstration Program (administered by the Department of Labor), and the Emergency Community Services Homeless Grant Program (administered by the Department of Health and Human Services)
Title VIII	Amends the Food Stamp Program to facilitate access by the homeless and expands the Temporary Emergency Food Assistance Program (administered by the Department of Agriculture)
Title IX	Extends the Veterans Job Training Act

Source: National Association for Education of Homeless and Youth (2018); National Coalition for the Homeless (2006).

TABLE 26-2 Federally Sponsored Programs for the Homeless

Program	Description
The U.S. Interagency Council on Homelessness	The United States Interagency Council on Homelessness coordinates the federal response to homelessness and creates a national partnership with public and private sectors to reduce and end homelessness in the United States. The Council is responsible for reviewing the effectiveness of federal initiatives and programs to assist the homeless, promoting better coordination of services between programs, and informing state and local governments and private sector organizations about sources of federal homeless assistance (www.usich.gov).
Substance Abuse and Mental Health Services Administration Center for Mental Health Services	The Center for Mental Health Services, a center of the federal Substance Abuse and Mental Health Services Administration (SAMHSA), supports states in facilitating access to mental health services and supports outreach and case management for the homeless mentally ill (SAMHSA, 2019). The Center for Mental Health Services also operates the Homelessness Resource Center, which provides resource information and information on the latest research and best practices for addressing the problem of homelessness (SAMHSA, n.d.a, n.d.b).
Projects for Assistance in Transition from Homelessness (PATH)	PATH is a SAMHSA grant program created under the McKinney Act to provide treatment and supportive services to persons with severe mental illnesses, including those who are homeless or at risk of becoming homeless. The grants support outreach, mental health and substance abuse treatment, and rehabilitation for the severely mentally ill (SAMHSA, 2017a, 2017b).
Health Care for the Homeless (HCH)	The HCH program (a provision of the McKinney Act) awards grants to community-based organizations that seek to provide quality, accessible health care to the homeless. The HCH program is administered by the United States Department of Health and Human Services Health Resource and Service Administration Bureau of Primary Care. HCH projects provide comprehensive primary care and supportive services to low-income populations in medically underserved communities (NHCHC, 2018).
The U.S. Department of Housing and Urban Development (HUD)	HUD provides funding for supportive housing for low-income individuals and families, including low-income elderly and disabled. Funds can be used for housing development or rental assistance. Grants are also provided to public housing agencies to renovate or replace dilapidated public housing. (www.hud.gov)

Source: NHCHC (2018); SAMHSA (n.d.a, n.d.b, 2016, 2017a, 2017b).

TABLE 26-3 Private Sector Initiatives to Combat Homelessness

Initiative	Description
National Coalition for the Homeless (NCH)	The National Coalition for the Homeless is the nation's oldest advocacy and direct service organization for the homeless. The mission of the Coalition is to prevent and end homelessness while ensuring the immediate needs of the homeless are met and their civil rights protected. (http://nationalhomeless.org)
The National Center on Family Homelessness (NCFH)	The National Center on Family Homelessness seeks to prevent and end family homelessness by advancing knowledge gained from research, programs, trainings, and collaborations with homeless shelter and service providers. The organization seeks to raise awareness of the causes and effects of homelessness and to inform local, state, and national solutions for the problem of homelessness. See http://www.familyhomelessness.org.
National Coalition for Homeless Veterans	The National Coalition for Homeless Veterans is a 501(c)(3) nonprofit organization that provides resource and technical assistance to service providers and local, state, and federal agencies that provide assistance to homeless veterans. The Coalition advocates for the needs of homeless veterans and for increased funding for federal homeless veteran assistance programs. See http://www.nchv.org.
National Alliance to End Homelessness (NAEH)	The National Alliance to End Homelessness seeks to end homelessness by advocating for policies that promote solutions to homelessness, providing technical assistance to local communities, and advancing data and research on best practices and solutions for combating homelessness. See http://www.endhomelessness.org.
Commission on Homelessness and Poverty, American Bar Association	This Commission is committed to educating the public and the legal community about the issue of poverty and homelessness and trains members of the legal community on how best to advocate for those in need. The Commission also advocates for public policies that protect and provide for the needs of the poor and homeless. See http://www.americanbar.org/groups/public_services/homelessness_poverty/about_us.html.
National Low-Income Housing Coalition	The National Low-Income Housing Coalition is dedicated to establishing housing stability and expanding the supply of low-income housing in America. A major priority of the coalition is to promote public policy that provides funding for housing for extremely low-income people. See http://www.nlihc.org.

BOX **26-9** QSEN: FOCUS ON QUALITY

Quality Improvement for Homeless Populations

Quality Improvement: Use data to monitor the outcomes of care processes and use improvement methods to design and test changes to continuously improve the quality and safety of health care systems (Cronenwett et al., 2007, p. 123).

(See https://qsen.org/competencies/pre-licensure-ksas/#quality_improvement for the definition and knowledge, skills, and attitudes associated with this QSEN competency.)

It is likely that you evaluate the quality of the care given to your patients in the acute care setting every day you are in a patient care environment. Biomarkers such as improvements in blood pressure and hemoglobin A1C levels, reduction in pain, or changes in function such as improvement in activities of daily living may serve as indicators of success when measuring the effectiveness of one's nursing interventions. But how is success measured when one is caring for large and diverse population groups such as the homeless?

To measure change in this context, one must first define what is meant by "success." For example, what are the markers for success when working with a population of homeless teen mothers? What about a population of homeless men with decade long histories of active addiction? Literature reviews, surveys, or focus groups may help point to measures of success. Interviews with key stakeholders also provide insight as to the most important measures for evaluating program effectiveness in a population.

Lashley (2018) examined the impact of length of stay among homeless men in recovery from chemical addiction in a faith-based recovery program on four quality of life indicators. A time series design was used to measure changes at program admission and at 3-, 6-, and 9-month intervals. Nicotine dependence, self-esteem, depression, and physical activity were evaluated at distinct times throughout the 1-year program to determine whether length of stay in the program impacted these measures. Each variable was measured using standardized instruments. The researcher found that self-esteem, depression, and physical activity all improved over time. Nicotine dependence scores also declined but not at a rate that was statistically significant. The author concluded that time spent in this recovery program had a significant impact on three of the four quality of life indicators.

1. *What outcomes do you believe are most important to track when caring for homeless populations?*
2. *How might you engage a target population to actively participate in the evaluation process?*

Source: Cronenwett et al. (2007); Lashley (2018).

Trust is an essential ingredient in the development of a therapeutic relationship with the homeless. However, it is sometimes difficult to establish trust with clients who have experienced negative encounters with the health care system. Often these negative perceptions are intensified by limited resources, inadequate access to care, or prejudicial views. As with other vulnerable populations, the homeless struggle with feelings of powerlessness, loss of control, and low self-esteem.

This lack of trust and self-esteem among the homeless often comes from experiencing disproportionately harsh consequences for violating the law. Behaviors that would ordinarily be considered lawful in the privacy of one's home become criminal activity when they are exhibited in public. For example, the homeless can be arrested for loitering, sleeping, urinating, or drinking alcohol in public. These behaviors can trigger a criminal record, thereby jeopardizing future employment or housing opportunities. Moreover, parents can be incarcerated for failing to pay child support (National Conference of State Legislators, 2018). Consider a man who is laid off from a low-wage job. He is unable to pay child support and is arrested. His violation generates a criminal record and compromises his ability to secure employment in the future. He becomes trapped in a cycle of poverty and homelessness that is difficult to escape.

To effectively address the multifaceted problems associated with homelessness, a comprehensive and holistic approach is needed (Boxes 26-9 to 26-11). As such, the CHN is responsible for implementing primary, secondary, and tertiary preventive measures to prevent homelessness or to assist those who are homeless to obtain needed services (Box 26-12).

BOX **26-10** WHAT DO *YOU* THINK?

Reflecting on Personal Beliefs and Values About Homelessness

Every nurse encounters new situations with prior assumptions, biases, and preunderstandings. When considering work with the homeless, it is important to clarify one's own beliefs and values about poverty, homelessness, addictions, and mental disorders.

1. *What has been your experience with the homeless?*
2. *Have you ever observed a homeless individual asking for money or holding up signs at a busy intersection?*
3. *What thoughts and feelings do encounters such as these provoke?*

It may be helpful to interview people who work with the homeless or to visit clinics, shelters, or other settings where the homeless congregate or access services.

1. *How are homeless people treated?*
2. *What is a typical day like for someone who is homeless?*
3. *How often do homeless persons hear their names?*
4. *How often are they touched in a way that is therapeutic, respectful, and affirming?*

By reflecting on your personal values and by allowing yourself to get closer to the people and places that are a part of the experience of homelessness, you will gain a deeper understanding of the homeless condition and be better equipped to serve those suffering from homelessness.

BOX **26-11** PERSPECTIVES

A Nurse's Viewpoint on Working With the Homeless

When I first decided to visit the homeless men's shelter, I was scared to death. Here I was, a veteran nurse with over 20 years of experience, but I was afraid. But, I thought to myself—afraid of what? I couldn't tell you. I suppose I harbored the stereotypes that most of us associate with homeless addicts. I remember passing this shelter years ago, looking out at the men hanging out on the street corner, and thinking to myself "Please God, don't let my car break down!" I remember thinking, "I would never step foot in a place like that."

Well, I believe God has a sense of humor. He was equipping me for work I could not have ever imagined. My views about homelessness were challenged to the core when I peered into the faces of those men, heard their stories, and began to feel their pain. Theirs were stories of broken lives and lost hope but also of courage in the face of suffering and the will to survive in the midst of great adversity. These men were as diverse as their stories. They were from all walks of life. They possessed incredible gifts and talents. They were musicians, artisans, businessmen, writers, and poets.

So here I am. Doing what I can to bring hope and healing. The irony is I came to bring hope and yet I am the one who is being healed. Healed in the broken areas of my life. I am so grateful to God for giving me this unique opportunity. It is a great privilege to serve these men.

Rita, C/PHN

BOX **26-12** C/PHN USE OF THE NURSING PROCESS

An On-Site Nursing Clinic for Homeless Women and Children

Sheila Hendricks, a public health nurse for the Manchester City Health Department, and her colleagues were brainstorming ideas for how to reach the growing population of homeless women and children in their jurisdiction. They arranged a meeting with the director of a local rescue mission in the area. The mission provided emergency shelter to 100 homeless women and children each night. The community health nurses negotiated with the rescue mission to establish an on-site nursing clinic twice a week that would provide health education, screenings, and referrals on a drop-in basis.

Assessment

After the clinic was in operation for 2 weeks, Sheila identified poor nutrition, lack of primary care services, depression, high rates of sexually transmitted infections, and addictions as priority health issues in the population.

Plan

Problem statement (in order of priority):

- Client does not have access to health and social services due to transportation, no insurance and comunity resources.
- Family difficulties with coping from addition, mental health, intimate partner violence, and hazards associated with street living.
- Client has not meet nutritional requirements due to addiction, chronic health issues, and limited resources for nutritional foods.

GOAL: To promote access to care by linking clients to essential health and social services

RATIONALE: If clients are able to access needed services, the other diagnoses can potentially be addressed (i.e., need for counseling, health care, housing, education).

Implementation

- Primary care services provided by nurse practitioner at the shelter
- HCH Clinic referrals made for more extensive follow-up
- Social worker engaged to assist clients in applying for housing and public assistance
- Referrals to local community mental health center for counseling
- Nurse-led health education and counseling sessions and on-site screenings with referrals to health department clinic as needed

Evaluation

90 days after the clinic had been in operation:

- 65 women and 28 children had frequented the clinic over the past 3 months. All 65 women received health promotion teaching and a resource packet for further reference.
- 80% of clients who required referrals to outside agencies were successful in accessing care.
- 25 women and 15 children were under the care of the nurse practitioner for acute or chronic health conditions.
- 10 cases of latent tuberculosis (TB) infection identified through TB testing with referrals to the City Health Department TB clinic for follow-up treatment.
- 7 abnormal PAP smears identified, and 8 clients diagnosed with sexually transmitted infections.
- 15 clients diagnosed HIV positive. 15 referrals to City Health Department or the local Health Care for the Homeless Clinic for treatment.
- 40 women applied for social service benefits. Awaiting receipt of benefits.

Primary Prevention

Primary prevention includes advocating for affordable housing, employment opportunities, and better access to health care to prevent the downward spiral into homelessness. Strategies for preventing homelessness may include financial counseling to assist clients to better manage their money, assistance in locating sources of legal or financial aid to prevent eviction (i.e., loans or grants for emergency funds to help pay for rent, utilities), or assistance in accessing social services, temporary housing, or health care to avoid a housing, health, or family crisis (Anderson & McFarlane, 2018).

Health education that addresses primary prevention may focus on positive parenting skills, violence prevention, anger management, coping skills, healthy eating, or principles of basic hygiene. Immunization programs can help to prevent communicable disease in this high-risk population. Counseling victims of intimate partner violence and helping them to locate safe shelter can also aid in the prevention of homelessness (Anderson & McFarlane, 2018). Addiction treatment is also important to prevent the likely consequences of untreated addiction: death, incarceration, institutionalization, or homelessness.

Secondary Prevention

The focus of secondary prevention measures is on the early detection and treatment of adverse health conditions. This requires a thorough assessment of client needs, including the need for housing, health care, education, social services, and employment (Box 26-13). Clients also benefit from secondary prevention measures such as screening for communicable and chronic diseases (i.e., hepatitis, tuberculosis, sexually transmitted infection, HIV, hypertension, diabetes, cancer).

Barriers to accessing services and the extent of community resources available to the homeless also need to be assessed (Anderson & McFarlane, 2018). Resources such as shelters, soup kitchens, medical clinics, social service agencies, and supportive housing should be readily accessible to the homeless population. Providers servicing homeless populations should be educated in **trauma-informed care**, a homeless service delivery model that recognizes the traumatic experiences associated with homelessness and the traumatic events that led to living on the streets. Strength-based interventions and skill building are used to assist homeless clients in regaining control of their lives (Davies & Allen, 2017).

Lack of transportation can be a major barrier to accessing care. Some programs have responded to this need by adopting mobile health vans that provide care on street corners and in neighborhoods (Yu, Hill, Ricks, Bennett & Oriol, 2017). Clinics have also been established in shelters to facilitate client access (Chatterjee et al., 2017). These clinics are often managed by nurses. Nurse-run community-based clinics are an effective means of promoting optimum care among disenfranchised populations (Randall, Crawford, Currie, River & Betihavas, 2017). Nursing students also play an important role in promoting access to care for the homeless.

The CHN should also consider the role of faith-based communities in providing physical and spiritual support to the homeless. Many places of worship have responded to the crisis of homelessness by offering food, shelter,

BOX 26-13 PERSPECTIVES

A C/PHN's Holistic Approach to Homelessness

I got a referral from our communicable disease coordinator regarding a homeless client with a lesion on his lower leg (wound botulism). I quickly learned that he had a long history of drug abuse, suicide attempts (13 known), and repeated hospitalizations for this wound. He was discharged from the hospital each time because he had no insurance, and he was also misdiagnosed.

I finally located him living on a friend's property in a disheveled travel trailer with a leaky roof and broken windows. It was a rainy week; during the winter months, and he and his small dog were trying to keep warm and dry. He used the oven for heat and a nearby field as his bathroom. His only relatives lived out of state, and he dumpster dived for food. He ate food from expired cans, when he could find them. He knew about the local food lunch program and health care at our county clinic, but he was seldom able to utilize these services, because of lack of transportation and difficulties with ambulation related to his leg wound.

As a C/PHN, your view of the patient is holistic and goes beyond the diagnosis. My C/PHN partner and I did the following:

- Reviewed his wound care.
- Assisted him in getting his medication, with money from the local Coordinating Council and Ministerial Association.
- Referred his case to two churches who provided him with assistance from their food pantries and a Pizza Hut gift card for his birthday (to cheer him up).
- Obtained tarps for his trailer, and a sleeping bag from a local service group.
- Assisted him with a disability application.
- Connected him to a mobile mental health unit and; updated his immunizations.
- We arranged for transport to another hospital for treatment, as the patient refused to go back to the original hospital that had misdiagnosed him and kept discharging him.

I remember that, after I graduated with my BSN, someone asked me why I was leaving the recovery room to go into public health nursing. At that time, I told the person "I didn't want my varicose veins popping out of my support hose before I retired." But, I love public health nursing and am so glad that I made this choice. And, as I am planning my retirement, I can truly say, "It's been quite a ride"!

Susan, a District C/PHN

BOX 26-14 STORIES FROM THE FIELD

Faith-Based Outreach

As a faith community nurse working in a large church congregation, you are invited to develop an outreach program to minister to the needs of an inner-city mission that is receiving financial support from the church. Approximately 500 homeless men in recovery from chemical addictions frequent the mission daily. Staff and residents have expressed concerns regarding a recent outbreak of boils among residents.

Assessment data reveal the following issues:

- Approximately 80% of clients have a history of injection drug use.
- Clients sleep in dormitory-style accommodations and share bathroom facilities.
- An on-site barbershop operated by the residents provides haircuts for a nominal fee.
- Clients have access to a small recreational area with donated exercise equipment.
- Laundry is typically washed in cold water, and at times the laundry runs out of detergent.

Consider the following questions:

1. *What additional data would you wish to gather to address the outbreak of boils at the shelter? How would you collect these data?*
2. *What host, agent, and environmental factors may have contributed to the outbreak of boils?*
3. *Discuss appropriate nursing interventions to address the outbreak. Consider the following levels of prevention: primary, secondary, and tertiary.*
4. *What advocacy role might the community health nurse play in addressing this issue?*

counseling, medical care, and social services within the context of the faith community. Clinics have been built within faith communities to promote access to care (Box 26-14).

Tertiary Prevention

Tertiary preventive measures attempt to limit disability and to restore maximum functioning. The goal is to provide rehabilitative care and support to clients who are already experiencing the consequences of homelessness. Often, homeless individuals have chronic health conditions that have gone untreated for long periods of time. This neglect in attending to health needs results in significant disease morbidity. Treating complications of advanced disease, providing rehabilitative and respite care, and offering counseling and support are important tertiary preventive strategies.

Case Management

At each level of prevention, the C/PHN functions as a case manager and coordinator of care to ensure seamless delivery of services as people transition from one level of care to another. It is often difficult for the homeless to keep track of multiple appointments, negotiate the bureaucracy of multiple agencies and services, and maintain communication with providers through follow-up phone calls, letters, or visits. With no permanent address or phone, homeless clients encounter obstacles to adhering to recommendations to follow up on test results or to notify their provider if symptoms persist or worsen. The C/PHN can help to bridge these gaps in service delivery and promote more effective adherence to therapeutic regimens.

Advocacy

Advocacy is a vital dimension of the C/PHN's role in working with the homeless. Advocacy entails working with different sectors of the community to develop innovative models for responding to the crisis of homelessness. Advocacy creates the broader system-wide changes needed to end homelessness (NCH, 2019e). The C/PHN acts as an advocate at each level of prevention to effect positive change (Box 26-15). For example, the nurse may advocate for mental health and substance abuse services to promote mental health and prevent homelessness (primary prevention). Alternatively, he or she may advocate for legislation to fund supportive housing, health care, or social services to benefit the homeless chronically mentally ill (tertiary prevention). The C/PHN can also assume an advocacy role by becoming involved in local, state, or national coalitions or organizations devoted to protecting the rights of the homeless or by speaking out on legislation that impacts the homeless (NCH, 2019e; NLIHC, 2019).

BOX **26-15** LEVELS OF PREVENTION PYRAMID

Preventing Illness Among Homeless Male Addicts

SITUATION: Promoting health and preventing illness among homeless male addicts

GOAL: To apply the three levels of prevention to avoid adverse health conditions, promptly diagnose and treat disorders, and assist the homeless male addict population to maintain or regain optimal health

Tertiary Prevention

- Provide case management of chronic health conditions.
- Advocate for expansion of counseling, rehabilitative services, and addictions treatment programs for the homeless.
- Advocate for supportive and transitional housing to enable homeless residents with addiction disorders to successfully transition back into the community.

Secondary Prevention

- Conduct mass screenings for diseases commonly found in homeless male population (tuberculosis, HIV, hepatitis, prostate cancer, colorectal cancer).
- Develop programs for health screening and early diagnosis and treatment in the community that are culturally sensitive and accessible to the homeless (i.e., mobile vans, faith community, or shelter-based clinics).

Primary Prevention

Health Promotion and Education

- Support employment and job training opportunities that assist clients to obtain jobs with livable wages and benefits.
- Advocate through housing coalitions and legislative efforts to promote affordable housing, employment opportunities, and better access to health care.
- Develop culturally sensitive health education programs that promote healthy coping, positive parenting, communication and relationship building, mental health, and injury and illness prevention.
- Promote programs that offer counseling and support to prevent continued high-risk behaviors as a result of untreated addiction.

Health Protection

- Advocate for legislation to protect citizens from environmental toxins and industrial wastes common to low-income areas.
- Provide immunization services to prevent communicable disease transmission.
- Counsel clients on proper nutrition, exercise, and basic hygiene to promote healthy lifestyles and prevent disease transmission
- Advocate for funding for nutrition programs for the homeless and for homeless shelters that would allow for the purchase of nutritious foods.

SUMMARY

- A homeless person is one who lacks a fixed, regular, adequate nightly residence; this definition includes as homeless those who stay in supervised public or private shelters that provide temporary accommodations.
- Although accurately estimating the number of homeless in the United States is challenging, a count performed on one night in 2017 indicated that there were 553,742 sheltered and unsheltered homeless people across the nation.
- Poverty, a lack of affordable health care, low-income and low-benefit employment, domestic violence, mental illness, addictions, personal and financial crisis, natural disasters, immigrant and refugee status, and personal choice are factors that may predispose persons to homelessness.
- Each subpopulation within the homeless community faces its own unique challenges with homelessness, including men, women, children, youth, families, veterans, rural homeless, older persons, and LGTB persons.
- Acute and chronic health problems plague the homeless and are difficult to treat because of the challenges associated with being homeless.
- Both the public and private sectors have launched concerted efforts to combat the problem of homelessness through the passage of federal legislation and through the formation of national, state, and local coalitions and alliances to champion the cause of the homeless.
- The C/PHN delivers primary, secondary, and tertiary preventive measures to prevent homelessness or to assist those who are homeless to obtain needed services.
- The C/PHN serves as a case manager to coordinate care and to assist clients to negotiate the bureaucracy of multiple agencies and services.
- The C/PHN acts as an advocate to promote the rights of the homeless and to speak out on legislation impacting homelessness.

ACTIVE LEARNING EXERCISES

1. Reflect in writing on the meaning of "home." Share your reflections with classmates either face to face or online. How similar are your responses?
2. Interview a homeless person regarding the most difficult choices he or she has had to make. What were the conditions surrounding these choices?
3. Volunteer to work at a soup kitchen or homeless shelter. Observe carefully the faces, sounds, attitudes, and activities. What is it like there? What would it be like to receive rather than give service?
4. Using "Assess and Monitor Population Health" (1 of the 10 essential public health services; see Box 2-2), analyze online census data to determine the rates of homelessness in your county, state, or region. How many people are homeless? What is the age and gender distribution? What policies exist to address the issue of homelessness in your community? Consider how you might address these issues in a letter or visit to your local city, county, or state legislator.
5. Perform a windshield survey in a low-income community. What resources are lacking? Where is the nearest bank, school, grocery store, or health clinic? What are the conditions of the roads, homes, and other buildings? How do you feel as you drive through the community? What do you think it would be like to live there?

REFERENCES

Ahmann, E. (2017). Supporting youth aging out of foster care. *Pediatric Nursing, 43*(1), 43–48.

Aidala, A. A., Wilson, M. G., Shubert, V., Gogolishvili, D., Globerman, J., Rueda, S., & ... Rourke, S. B. (2016). Housing status, medical Care, and health outcomes among people living with HIV/AIDS: A systematic review. *American Journal of Public Health, 106*(1), e1–e23.

American Institute on Research. (2020). *National Center on Family Homelessness (NCFH)*. Retrieved from https://www.air.org/center/national-center-family-homelessness

Anderson, E., & McFarlane, J. (2018). *Community as partner: Theory and practice in nursing* (7th ed.). Philadelphia, PA: Wolters Kluwer Health/Lippincott Williams & Wilkins.

Burt, M. (2006). *Testimony related to provisions of s. 1801, The Community Partnership to End Homelessness Act of 2005*. Retrieved from http://webarchive.urban.org/UploadedPDF/900937_burt_033006.pdf

Chatterjee, A., Obando, A., Strickland, E., Nestler, A., Harrington-Levey, R., Williams, T., & LaCoursiere-Zucchero, T. (2017). Shelter-based opioid treatment: Increasing access to addiction treatment in a family shelter. *American Journal of Public Health, 107*(7), 1092–1094.

Child Trends Data Bank. (2015). *Homeless children and youth: Indicators on children and youth*. Retrieved from http://www.childtrends.org/wp-content/uploads/2015/01/112_Homeless_Children_and_Youth.pdf

Cima, M. J., & Parker, R. D. (2017). Impact of homelessness and unstable housing on adolescent health. *Mental Health & Prevention, 7*, 8–11. doi:10.1016/j.mhp.2017.05.002

Cronenwett, L., Sherwood, G., Marnsteiner, J., Disch, J., Johnson, J., Mitchell, P., ... Warren, J. (2007). Quality and safety in education for nurses. *Nursing Outlook, 55*, 122–131. doi: 10.1016/j.outlook.2007.02.006

Davies, B. R., & Allen, N. B. (2017). Trauma & homelessness youth: Psychopathology & intervention. *Clinical Psychology Review, 54*, 17–28.

Economic Policy Institute. (2019). *Why American needs a $15 minimum wage*. Retrieved from https://www.epi.org/publication/why-america-needs-a-15-minimum-wage/

Family & Youth Services Bureau. (2016). *Domestic Violence and Homelessness: Statistics (2016)*. Retrieved from https://www.acf.hhs.gov/fysb/resource/dv-homelessness-stats-2016

Goldberg, J., Lang, K., & Barrington, V. (2016). How to prevent and end homelessness among older adults. *Justice in Aging*. Retrieved from www.justiceinaging.org

Hayes, J. (2016). Key amendments to McKinney-Vento Act take effect October 1. *United States Interagency Council on Homelessness*. Retrieved from https://www.usich.gov/news/key-amendments-to-mckinney-vento-act-take-effect-october-1

Herring, C. (December 2015). *Tent City, America*. Retrieved from https://placesjournal.org/article/tent-city-america/

Housing Assistance Council. (2017). *Rural voices: Action for a rapidly changing America*. Retrieved from www.ruralhome.org/storage/documents/rural-voices/rv-se-2017.pdf

Housing Assistance Council. (2016). *Rural voices: Rural homelessness*. Retrieved from http://www.ruralhome.org/component/content/category/145-rural-homelessness

Howell, D. (2017). The unintended consequences of deinstitutionalization. *American Criminal Law Review, 54*(17), 17–23. Retrieved from http://www.americancriminallawreview.com/files/7214/8856/2214/Howell_Deinstitutionalization.pdf

Kaiser Family Foundation. (2020). *Health insurance coverage of the total population*. Retrieved from https://www.kff.org/other/state-indicator/total-population/?currentTimeframe=0&sortModel=%7B%22colId%22:%22Location%22,%22sort%22:%22asc%22%7D

Kaiser Family Foundation. (2019). *Key facts about the uninsured population*. Retrieved from https://www.kff.org/uninsured/fact-sheet/key-facts-about-the-uninsured-population/

Lashley, M. (2018). Impact of length of stay on recovery measures in faith based addiction treatment. *Public Health Nursing, 35*(5), 396–403. Retrieved from https:/doi.org/10.1111/phn.12401

Lenz-Rashid, S. (2017). Supportive housing program for homeless families: Foster care outcomes and best practices. *Children and Youth Services Review*, 79, 558–563. doi:10.1016/j.childyouth.2017.07.012

McEvers, K. (February 1, 2016). *Utah reduced chronic homelessness by 91 percent: Here's how*. Retrieved from http://www.npr.org/2015/12/10/459100751/utah-reduced-chronic- homelessness-by-91-percent-heres-how

McKinney-Vento Homeless Assistance Act. (1987). *U. S. Congress, Public Law 100-77*. Retrieved from http://www.gpo.gov/fdsys/pkg/STATUTE-101/pdf/STATUTE-101-Pg482.pdf

Morton, M. H., Dworsky, A., & Samuels, G. M. (2017). *Missed opportunities: Youth homelessness in America. National estimates*. Chicago, IL: Chapin Hall at the University of Chicago. Retrieved from http://voicesofyouthcount.org/wp-content/uploads/2017/11/ChapinHall_VoYC_NationalReport_Final.pdf

Myrick, D. (2016). *Why are there more homeless men than women?* Retrieved from https://www.culturalweekly.com/homeless-men-women/

National Advisory Committee on Rural Health and Human Services. (2014). *Homelessness in rural America*. Retrieved from https://www.hrsa.gov/sites/default/files/hrsa/advisory-committees/rural/publications/2014-homelessness.pdf

National Alliance to End Homelessness. (2020a). *Children and families*. Retrieved from https://endhomelessness.org/homelessness-in-america/who-experiences-homelessness/children-and-families/

National Alliance to End Homelessness. (2020b). *Domestic violence*. Retrieved from https://endhomelessness.org/homelessness-in-america/what-causes-homelessness/domestic-violence

National Alliance to End Homelessness. (2020c). *Domestic violence*. Retrieved from http://www.endhomelessness.org/pages/domestic_violence

National Alliance to End Homelessness. (2020d). *Health*. Retrieved from https://endhomelessness.org/homelessness-in-america/what-causes-homelessness/health

National Alliance to End Homelessness. (2020e). *Housing*. Retrieved from https://endhomelessness.org/homelessness-in-america/what-causes-homelessness/housing/

National Alliance to End Homelessness. (2020f). *Mental illness and homelessness*. Retrieved from https://endhomelessness.org

National Alliance to End Homelessness. (2020g). *Policy priorities*. Retrieved from https:/endhomelessness.org/ending-homelessness/policy/priorities

National Alliance to End Homelessness. (2020h). *Resources*. Retrieved from https://endhomelessness.org/resources/

National Alliance to End Homelessness. (2017). *The state of homelessness in America 2015*. Retrieved from https://endhomelessness.org/homelessness-in-america/homelessness-statistics/state-of-homelessness-report-legacy/

National Association for Education of Homeless and Youth. (2018). *The McKinney-Vento Act and Title I, Part A, as amended by the Every Student Succeeds Act of 2015*. Retrieved from https://naehcy.org/essa/

National Center for Homeless Education. (n.d.) *The McKinney-Vento definition of homeless*. Retrieved from https://nche.ed.gov/mckinney-vento-definition/

National Center on Family Homelessness (NCFH). (2014). *America's youngest outcasts. A report card on child homelessness*. Retrieved from https://www.air.org/sites/default/files/downloads/report/Americas-Youngest-Outcasts-Child-Homelessness-Nov2014.pdf

National Coalition for the Homeless. (2018a). *Current state of homelessness*. Retrieved from http://nationalhomeless.org/wp-content/uploads/2018/04/State-of-things-2018-for-web.pdf

National Coalition for the Homeless. (2018b). *Elder homelessness*. Retrieved from http://nationalhomeless.org/issues/elderly/

National Coalition for the Homeless. (2018c). *Employment and income*. Retrieved from https://nationalhomeless.org/issues/economic-justice/

National Coalition for the Homeless. (2018d). *Health care*. Retrieved from http://nationalhomeless.org/issues/health-care/

National Coalition for the Homeless. (2012a). *HIV/AIDS and homelessness*. Retrieved from http://www.nationalhomeless.org/factsheets/hiv.html

National Coalition for the Homeless. (2012b). *Homelessness among elderly persons*. http://www.nationalhomeless.org/factsheets/elderly.html

National Coalition for the Homeless. (2019a). *No wrong doors for homeless veterans*. Retrieved from https://nationalhomeless.org/?s=veterans

National Coalition for the Homeless. (2019b). *Homeless youth*. Retrieved from https://nationalhomeless.org/issues/youth/

National Coalition for the Homeless. (2018e). *LGBT homelessness*. Retrieved from http://www.nationalhomeless.org/issues/lgbt

National Coalition for the Homeless. (2006). *McKinney-Vento Act*. Retrieved from http://www.nationalhomeless.org/publications/facts/McKinney.pdf

National Coalition for the Homeless. (2019c). *Take a number: The long wait for rental assistance*. Retrieved from https://nationalhomeless.org/take-a-number-the-long-wait-for-rental-assistance/

National Coalition for the Homeless. (2019d). *Why are people homeless?* Retrieved from https://nationalhomeless.org/about-homelessness/

National Coalition for the Homeless. (2019e). Take action. Retrieved from https://nationalhomeless.org/taking-action/

National Coalition for Homeless Veterans. (n.d.). *Grants*. Retrieved from http://nchv.org/index.php/service/service/grants/#HUDVASH

National Conference of State Legislators. (2018). *Child support and incarceration*. Retrieved from http://www.ncsl.org/research/human-services/child-support-and-incarceration.aspx

National Health Care for the Homeless Council (NHCHC). (2018). *FAQ*. Retrieved from https://nhchc.org/faq/

National Health Care for the Homeless Council (NHCHC). (2019). *Homelessness and health: What's the connection?* Retrieved from https://nhchc.org/wp-content/uploads/2019/08/homelessness-and-health.pdf

National Law Center on Homelessness and Poverty. (2017). *Tent City USA: The growth of America's homeless encampments and how communities are responding*. Retrieved from https://www.nlchp.org/Tent_City_USA_2017

National Low Income Housing Coalition. (2019). *Advocates guide 2018*. Retrieved from https://nlihc.org/sites/default/files/AG-2019/Advocates-Guide_2019.pdf

National Low Income Housing Coalition. (2018). *Out of reach 2017*. Retrieved from http://nlihc.org/oor/about

Ontario Ministry of Housing. (2017). *Guidelines for service manager homeless enumeration*. Ontario: Queen's Printer for Ontario. Retrieved from http://www.msdsb.net/images/ADMIN/correspondence/2017/SH_Guidelines_SM__Homeless_Enumeration_EN.pdf

Oppong Asante, K., Meyer-Weitz, A., & Petersen, I. (2016). Mental health and health risk behaviours of homeless adolescents and youth: A mixed methods study. *Child and Youth Care Forum, 45*(3), 433–449. doi:10.1007/s10566-015-9335-9

Randall, S., Crawford, T., Currie, J., River, J., & Betihavas, V. (2017). Impact of community based nurse-led clinics on patient outcomes, patient satisfaction, patient access and cost effectiveness: A systematic review. *International Journal of Nursing Studies, 73*, 24–33. doi:10.1016/j.ijnurstu.2017.05.008

Semega, J., Fontenot, K., & Kollar, M. (2017). *Income and poverty in the U.S.: 2016: U.S. Census Bureau current population reports. Washington, DC: U.S. Government Printing Office*. Retrieved from https://www.census.gov/content/dam/Census/library/publications/2017/demo/P60-259.pdf

Stafford, A., & Wood, L. (2017). Tackling health disparities for people who are homeless? Start with social determinants. *International Journal of Environmental Research and Public Health*, 14(12), 1535. Retrieved from https://doi.org/10.3390/

Substance Abuse and Mental Health Services Administration (SAMHSA). (n.d.a). *Homelessness Resource Center: About us*. Retrieved from https://www.samhsa.gov/homelessness-programs-resources

Substance Abuse and Mental Health Services Administration (SAMHSA). (n.d.b). *Homelessness Resource Center facts*. Retrieved from https://www.samhsa.gov/homelessness-programs-resources

Substance Abuse and Mental Health Services Administration. (2017a). *Homelessness and housing*. Retrieved from https://www.samhsa.gov/homeless-housing-resource-network

Substance Abuse and Mental Health Services Administration. (2017b). *PATH*. Retrieved from https://www.samhsa.gov/homelessness-programs-resources/grant-programs-services/path

Substance Abuse and Mental Health Services Administration (SAMHSA). (2019). *Resources for families coping with nebtal and substance use disorders*. Retrieved from https://www.samhsa.gov/families

Tyler, K., & Schmitz, R. (2017). Using cell phones for data collection: Benefits, outcomes, and intervention possibilities for homeless youth. *Children and Youth Services Review, 76*, 59–64.

United States Conference of Mayors. (2016). *The U.S. Conference of Mayors' Report on Hunger and Homelessness*. Retrieved from https://endhomelessness.atavist.com/mayorsreport2016

United States Department of Health and Human Services. (2016). *Domestic violence and homelessness*. Retrieved from https://www.acf.hhs.gov/domestic-violence-and-homelessness

United States Department of Health and Human Services. (2017). *Early childhood homelessness in the United States: 50-state profile*. Retrieved from https://www.acf.hhs.gov/sites/default/files/ecd/epfp_50_state_profiles_6_15_17_508.pdf

U.S. Department of Health and Human Services (USDHHS). (2020). *Healthy People 2030: Browse objectives*. Retrieved from https://health.gov/healthypeople/objectives-and-data/browse-objectives

United States Department of Housing and Urban Development. (n.d.). *Housing choice vouchers fact sheet*. Retrieved from http://portal.hud.gov/hudportal/HUD?src=/program_offices/public_indian_housing/programs/hcv/about/fact_sheet

United States Department of Housing and Urban Development. (2017a). *HUD 2017 Continuum of care homeless assistance programs homeless populations and subpopulations*. Retrieved from https://www.hudexchange.info/resource/reportmanagement/published/CoC_PopSub_NatlTerrDC_2017.pdf

United States Department of Housing and Urban Development. (2017b). *The 2017 annual homeless assessment report (AHAR) to Congress*. Retrieved from https://files.hudexchange.info/resources/documents/2017-AHAR-Part-1.pdf

United States Department of Housing and Urban Development. (2017c). *The 2016 Annual Homeless Assessment Report (AHAR) to Congress*. Retrieved from https://www.hudexchange.info/resources/documents/2016-AHAR-Part-2.pdf

United States Interagency Council on Homelessness. (2017). *Fiscal Year 2017 performance and accountability report*. Retrieved from https://www.usich.gov/resources/uploads/asset_library/FY2017_USICH_PAR_FINAL.pdf

United States Interagency Council on Homelessness. (2018). *Homeless in America: Focus on Families with Children*. Retrieved from https://www.usich.gov/resources/uploads/asset_library/Homeslessness_in_America_Families_with_Children.pdf

United States Interagency Council on Homelessness. (2015). *Opening doors: Federal strategic plan to prevent and end homelessness*. Retrieved from https://www.usich.gov/resources/uploads/asset_library/USICH_OpeningDoors_Amendment2015_FINAL.pdf

Yu, S., Hill, C., Ricks, M, Bennett, J., & Oriol, N. (2017). The scope and impact of mobile health clinics in the United States: A literature review. *International Journal of Equity and Health, 16*, 178. doi:10.1186/s12939-017-0671-2

Walker, C. (2018). *Why so many homeless refuse to stay in overnight shelters*. Retrieved from https://www.westword.com/news/reasons-why-denvers-homeless-sleep-outside-and-not-in-overnight-shelters-10987893

Zobel, S. (2016). LA family housing supports single fathers with children. *Substance Abuse and Mental Health Services Administration*. Retrieved from https://www.samhsa.gov/homelessness-programs-resources/hpr-resources/single-fathers-children-shelters

CHAPTER 27

Rural, Migrant, and Urban Communities

"No city should be too large for a man to walk out of in a morning."

—Cyril Connolly (1903–1974), British Critic

"Globalization is exposing new fault lines—between urban and rural communities, for example."

—Ban Ki-moon, United Nations Secretary General

KEY TERMS

Built environment
Critical access hospitals (CAHs)
Federally qualified health centers
Frontier area
Health professional shortage areas (HPSAs)
In-migration
Medically underserved areas
Medically underserved population
Migrant farmworkers
Migrant streams
Nomadic migrant workers
Out-migration
Population density
Rural
Rural health clinics
Seasonal farmworkers
Sustainable communities
Urban
Urban health
Urbanized area
Urban planning
Urban sprawl

LEARNING OBJECTIVES

Upon mastery of this chapter, you should be able to:

1. Define the terms *rural, frontier, migrant,* and *urban.*
2. Discuss the population characteristics of rural residents.
3. Describe five barriers to health care access for rural clients.
4. Describe the lifestyle of migrant farm workers and their families.
5. Identify at least three health problems common to migrant workers and their families.
6. Discuss barriers and challenges to migrant health care.
7. Identify common health disparities found among rural and urban populations.
8. Propose intervention strategies at the aggregate or community level to assure a healthier *built environment* in both rural and urban areas.
9. Explain the concept of *social justice* and how it relates to public health nursing in rural and urban areas.
10. Compare and contrast the challenges and opportunities related to rural and urban community health nursing practice.

INTRODUCTION

As a community/public health nurse (C/PHN), I enjoyed making home visits to see Alison. She was quiet at first, but slowly she would open up about herself when she knew I was there to help her and not judge. Alison lived in a small duplex in a big city in California surrounded by dense housing, a busy street that never slept, and constant noise—babies crying, sirens, and people's voices. She was used to the noises now, but it wasn't always that way, she said. Over 60 years ago, Alison moved here as a young bride of 20; the city provided opportunity for her and her husband to find work and raise a family. Many young families had moved there from the country. It was full of people even then, though not nearly the population it was when I spoke with her. Alison and her husband Jim moved from one of the rural communities further south. They left their families to start their own with hopes and dreams. Alison sighed as she shared stories of her childhood, staring off into the distance as she remembered the time her sister almost died because the family had to drive 90 minutes to a hospital as none existed in their small community. Although Alison said she missed the

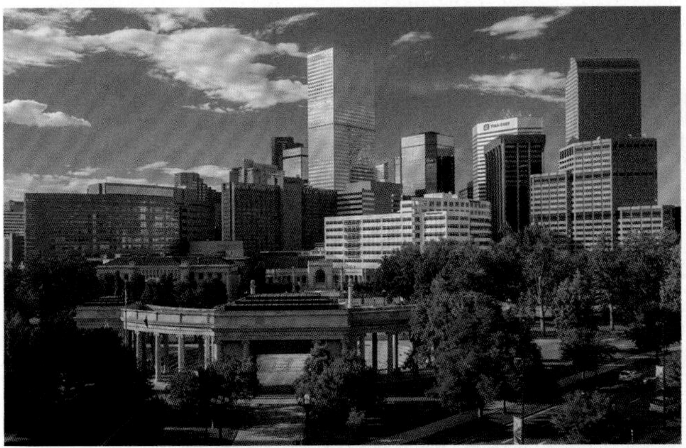

FIGURE 27-1 The Denver Tech Center skyline.

slow pace of a small community, she stated she might not have advanced her education had she not had access to a college in the big city.

Alison's story illustrates how different rural and urban life can be. About half of the population live in what is known as the suburbs, but the remainder live in one of two diametrically opposed areas: rural or urban (Fig. 27-1). There is a good chance that many of you reading this book live either in very densely populated, bustling urban areas or in sparsely populated, somewhat isolated rural areas. Public health nursing in urban and rural areas requires not only general public health nursing knowledge and skills but also a unique understanding of how these distinctive environments affect the health of the populations living there. Where you live can and does markedly affect your health outcomes, with rural and urban areas having distinctive problems and issues.

Rural nursing practice offers many opportunities. Nurses are respected community members—their judgment and opinions count. Rural nurses are key members of the health care team. They can make a difference in the lives of their neighbors, friends, and community. Rural C/PHNs often struggle with helping clients gain access to quality health care and the inherent transportation problems found in isolated areas. The challenges are many, but the rewards are great.

Urban C/PHNs often specialize in particular areas of interest. They deal with different types of problems, such as homelessness, overcrowding, bioterrorism threats, and violent crime. They are often called upon to advocate for their most vulnerable clients, and they develop collaborative relationships with other professionals. Urban community health nursing can also be very rewarding and satisfying.

An aggregate at risk, migrant workers suffer higher frequency of illness, greater complications, and more long-term debilitating effects. Exacerbated by a magnitude of environmental and work stressors, the health of migrant families is also compromised by limited access to health care, mobility, language and cultural barriers, low educational levels, and few economic and political resources. Because migrant health needs are largely manageable within community settings, C/PHNs are ideal health providers. C/PHNs must advocate for the health of migrant workers, who have very little economic or political power, and also guide them through the complexities of a changing health care system.

This chapter addresses the special health needs and concerns of rural, migrant, and urban clients and the ways in which a community health nurse can address those needs. After reading the chapter, you may come to appreciate the many advantages that rural nurses enjoy and consider rural nursing as a practice choice or you may find that being a C/PHN in an urban area offers you more opportunities for specialization and networking. Either way, your contributions can improve the health of populations living at both extremes.

DEFINITIONS AND DEMOGRAPHICS

Definitions

The U.S. government provides several definitions of rural. It is important to understand the terms and how they are used in federal programs and grant funding. The U.S. Department of Agriculture (USDA) (2020) rural–urban continuum examines metropolitan and nonmetropolitan areas on the basis of counties, and this provides different data apart from census reports (U.S. Census Bureau, 2016a). Nonmetropolitan areas have some type of combination that includes "open countryside," rural towns (<2,500 people), and **urban** areas (2,500 to 49,999 people; Fig. 27-2). State and federal agencies recognize county-level jurisdictions and governments and depend upon employment, income, and population data that are available on an annual basis. Many states have offices of rural health or other agencies dealing with issues specific to rural populations.

- For the purposes of this chapter, **rural** is defined as *communities with fewer than 10,000 residents and a county* **population density** *of <1,000 persons per square mile*. This definition of rural is arbitrary because rural clients do not merely consider population density or community size when defining their *ruralness*.
  They have a multitude of reasons for defining their community as rural, such as distance from a large city, major occupations in the area (e.g., agriculture), or number of students in the local schools. If you have access to a small community, ask some of the residents the reasons why they consider their community to be urban or rural (USDA, 2019a; Fig. 27-3).
- The term **frontier area** is used to designate sparsely populated rural places that are isolated from population centers and services, but specific definitions vary (Rural Health Information Hub [RHIH], 2018a). A common definition of a "frontier and remote area" (FAR) is one with six or fewer persons per square mile, but others include not only population density but also distance and travel time to market service areas.
  For instance, 60 miles or 60 minutes of driving on paved roads to the nearest 75-bed (or greater) hospitals could constitute a frontier area. The USDA (2019b) has developed FAR codes, based upon urban–rural census data and delineated by ZIP codes.
- There are four levels of FAR codes; level one includes a good number of people living far from city areas

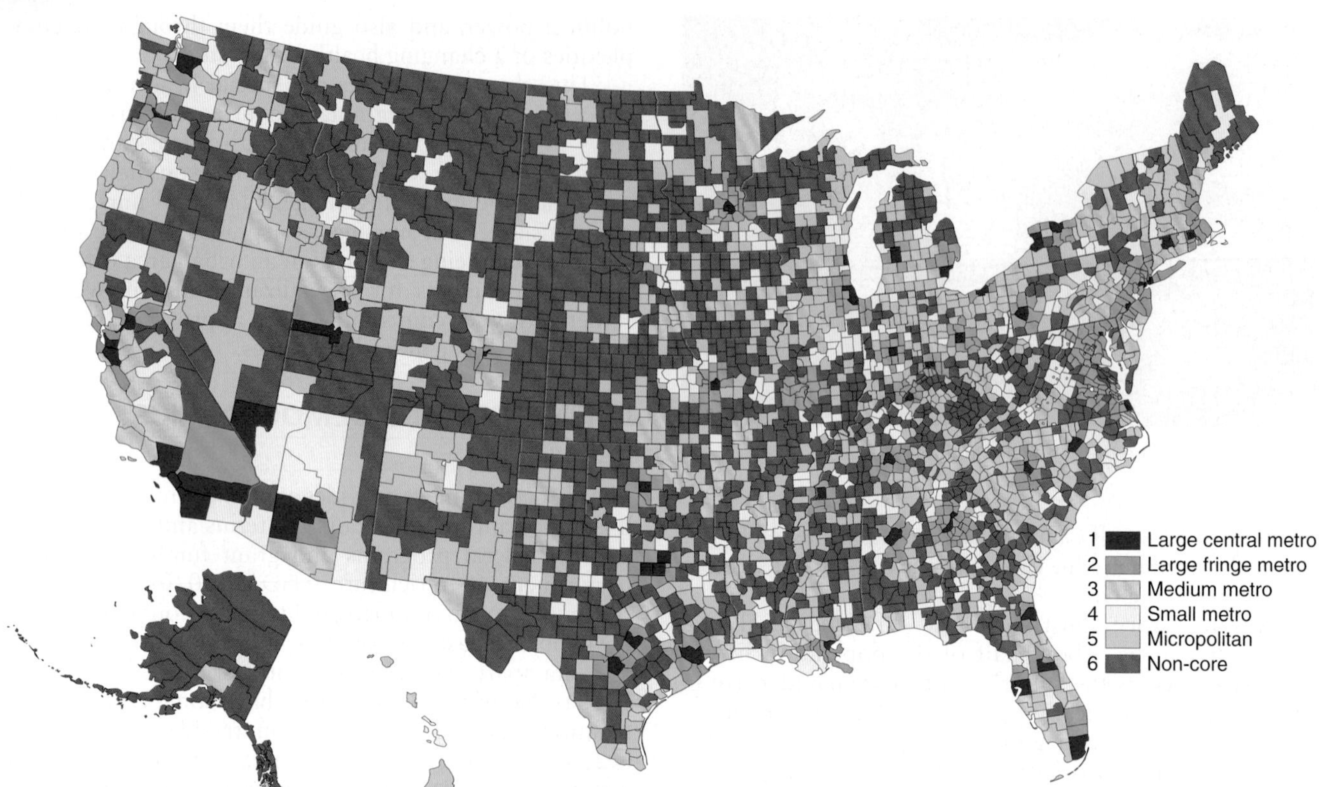

FIGURE 27-2 2013 urban–rural classification schemes for counties, 2017. (Reprinted from Centers for Disease Control and Prevention, National Center for Health Statistics. (2020). Retrieved from https://www.cdc.gov/nchs/images/popbridge/URv3.png)

where higher-level goods are available (e.g., regional airport hubs, stores with major household appliances, advanced medical care), whereas level four includes fewer people with a more significant level of remoteness (e.g., decreased access to stores selling gas or groceries, or basic medical care).

- The other two levels may also have access to movie theaters, car dealerships, and clothing stores. This is helpful to researchers and public health agencies in determining rural–urban status and designing programs to meet specific needs. Rural–urban commuting area (U.S. Census Bureau, 2019) is also used to designate remote areas (RHIH, 2020a).
- It is estimated that 3 million people (4% of population) live in frontier areas that comprise 56% of the U.S. land areas. States with more than 10% of their population in a frontier area include Idaho, Nebraska, Maine, Arkansas, Oklahoma, Alaska, Arizona, Montana, Wyoming, New Mexico, Colorado, North Dakota, and South Dakota (National Center for Frontier Communities, 2019).

Health issues of concern in rural areas may be of even greater concern for frontier areas. Sparsely populated areas may be less able to attract health care professionals.

- The term **health professional shortage areas (HPSAs)** is used to identify urban or rural geographic areas, population groups, or facilities with chronic shortages of medical, dental, or mental health professionals. The federal government determines which areas are HPSAs. As of 2015, there were 15,557 in the United States. Over 59 million people live in areas that have been designated as HPSAs for primary care, representing about 60% of need met. Over 90.3 million live in mental health HPSAs, and 47.4 million are in areas with shortages of dentists (Health Resources and Services Administration [HRSA], 2020; see also https://www.kff.org/other/state-indicator/primary-care-health-professional-shortage-areas-hpsas/?activeTab=map¤tTimeframe=0&selectedDistributions=total-primary-care-hpsa-designations&sortModel=%7B%22colId%22:%22Location%22,%22sort%22:%22asc%22%7D).
- In **medically underserved areas**, residents experience a shortage of health services; these areas are determined by the federal government using a score based on the shortage of primary care physicians, high infant mortality rates, high percentage of the population living below the poverty level, and a high proportion of residents over age 65.
- A **medically underserved population** includes those with economic and cultural/linguistic barriers to primary health care services (Fig. 27-3; HRSA, 2020).

Population Statistics

The number of persons living in urban areas of the United States tripled since the mid-1800s, to almost 60 million in 2000, and grew 10.8% from 2000 to 2010 (Table 27-1). About 81% of the total population can be found in urban areas (U.S. Census, 2016b).

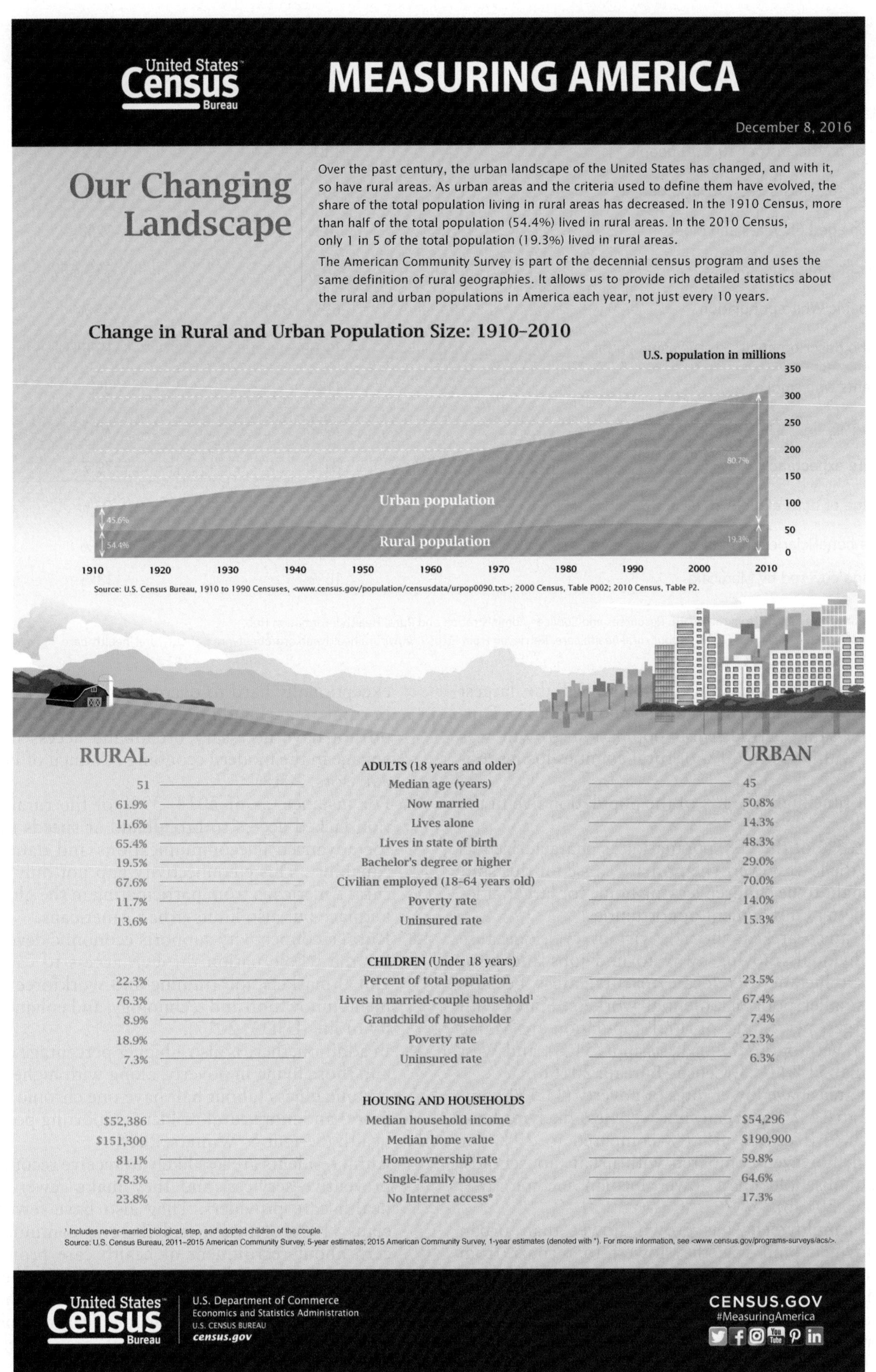

FIGURE 27-3 Change in rural and urban population size: 1910 to 2010. (Reprinted from U.S. Census Bureau. (2020). *Measuring America: Our changing landscape*. Retrieved from https://www.census.gov/library/visualizations/2016/comm/acs-rural-urban.html)

TABLE 27-1 A National Rural Health Snapshot: Rural Versus Urban

National Rural Health Snapshot	Rural	Urban
Percentage of population	19.3%	80.7%
Number of physicians per 10,000 people	13.1	31.2
Number of specialists per 100,000 people	30	263
Population aged 65 years and older	18%	12%
Average per capita income	$45,482	$53,657
Non-Hispanic White population	69%–82%	45%
Adults who describe health status as fair/poor	19.5%	15.6%
Adolescents who smoke	11%	5%
Male life expectancy in years	76.2	74.1
Female life expectancy	81.3	79.7
Percentage of dual-eligible Medicare beneficiaries	30%	70%
Medicare beneficiaries without drug coverage	43%	27%
Percentage covered by Medicaid	16%	13%

All information in this table is from the Health Resources and Services Administration and Rural Health Information Hub.
National Rural Health Association. (2018). *About rural health care.* Retrieved from https://www.ruralhealthweb.org/about-nrha/about-rural-health-care

- California, Arizona, and Texas showed the largest growth in suburbs of large metropolitan cities. During the same period, rural population growth was 4.5% with 46% to 60% of rural counties losing residents.
- An all-time high of 51% of the population live in the suburbs.
- Only 16% of the U.S. population is characterized as rural, the lowest ever. The primary cause for this shift is thought to be children leaving home for larger cities with better employment opportunities.
- Rural areas are caught in a vicious cycle, because of individuals moving away to find jobs and businesses reluctant to relocate to rural areas because of a smaller pool of potential workers. States with the largest percentage of rural population are Maine (61%), Vermont (61%), Mississippi (51%), and West Virginia (51%) (U.S. Census Bureau, 2016b).
- Rural areas have lower rates of poverty (11.7% compared to 14% for urban) but were less likely to have a bachelor's degree (19.5% compared to 29% for urban); however, compared with urban households, rural households had lower median income (U.S. Census, 2016b).

  Rural employment has grown slower than urban employment and was the slowest to recover from the recession in 2007. Many Americans living in rural communities continue to face barriers that prevent them from attaining the quality of life they deserve. Access to adequate transportation is difficult for many rural Americans. Insufficient access to medical care can lead to health problems; this can be exceptionally hard to overcome for Americans living in rural areas. In addition, too many rural Americans do not have necessary broadband access needed to engage in the modern economy (Council of Economic Advisors, 2018).
- For instance, as of 2014, 39% of the rural population lacked access to broadband at speeds necessary for advanced telecommunications and data transfer capability. This e-connectivity gap not only prevents rural Americans from participating in the global marketplace but also limits urban Americans.
- Rural e-connectivity supports economic development for the whole nation through access to capital and global markets, job training and workforce development, innovation and technology, and enhanced quality of life (USDA, 2017).
- In addition, there is also a higher percentage of elderly and those living in poverty, along with higher rates of chronic illness (about half have one chronic illness or more) and more rural residents reporting poor to fair health (Seright & Winters, 2015).

  Rural residents are less likely to receive recommended preventive services, and they make fewer visits to health care providers. They also have fewer physicians (10% of total), and there is continuous concern about recruitment of health care professionals in rural areas of the United States and other countries beyond what incentives (e.g., scholarships, forgivable loans) can offer (Rural Health Information Hub, 2018b). Specialized medical care is rarely found in rural areas. Of the 2,000 rural hospitals, 75% of them have 50 or fewer beds; most are designated

critical access hospitals (CAHs) as they have 25 or fewer beds (Rural Health Information Hub, 2018a). CAHs must provide 24-hour emergency care, with either MD on site or RN on site with MD on call and able to arrive within 30 minutes. They must also have 25 beds maximum and be over 35 miles from the next hospital or 15 miles if the terrain is difficult (Seright & Winters, 2015).

Recent solutions have been formulated to address these issues:

- The National Health Service Corp (NHSC) Program addresses long-standing primary care health professional shortages by providing physicians, APRNs, and other health professionals with scholarships and repayments of student loans in return for at least 2 years' service in communities facing shortages.
- Area Health Education Centers (AHECs) were developed by Congress in 1971 to recruit, train, and retain health care professionals committed to underserved populations, which includes rural areas. There are over 56 AHECs with more than 235 centers operating in almost every state. Many work collaboratively with medical schools, nursing programs, and allied health schools to improve health for underserved and underrepresented populations.
- **Federally qualified health centers** make up one of the largest health care systems for rural America and are frequently the only source of primary and preventive services in their communities. Fifty-three percent of these community health centers are located in rural and frontier areas. Nurses play a central role in all three of these initiatives, providing both direct primary and preventive care (Rural Health Information Hub, 2018a).

Changing Patterns of Migration

- Population changes in rural areas are usually related to natural increase through births or decrease through **out-migration**, the process of residents moving out of rural communities and into urban places. When America was a more rural country, there was more natural increase than out-migration, which caused continued growth in the rural population. Since the beginning of the 21st century, more rural counties have experienced out-migration, and rural towns in some areas have disappeared; this trend has slowed but continues overall (USDA, 2019a).
- The lack of **in-migration** is related to a decrease in retirees moving to rural areas, problems recruiting professionals and managers for local manufacturing companies, poverty, and low quality of life (USDA, 2017). Population trends have many implications for the health services needed by rural people. The patterns of rural migration change like shifting sand, adding to the challenge of planning resources for rural communities (U.S. Census Bureau, 2019).

  Although other sectors of the American economy have largely recovered from the Great Recession (Fig. 27-4), rural America has lagged in almost every indicator (Fig. 27-5). Today, rural areas are more economically diverse than in the past, reflecting the national trend to greater reliance on service jobs. While traditional rural occupations such as agriculture, mining, and manufacturing employ less of the rural population than before, they continue to anchor the economies of more than half the U.S. counties (USDA, 2017).

Demographics

Migrant farmworkers constitute a mobile population with shifting composition, and it is difficult to precisely determine their number or origins. These estimates also vary because of the influx of illegal and undocumented workers. A large number of seasonal and migrant farmworkers reside in the United States, 33% are U.S. citizens, and others have permanent resident status. Most of the estimated 3 million migrant (42%) and seasonal (58%) farmworkers tend to be either newly arrived immigrants, with few connections, or established legal residents, with limited opportunities and skills, who rely on farm labor for survival (NCFH, 2018a). In addition to male workers, who make up the majority, you may also see mothers bring infants and young children to work with them, and the children spend their days strapped to their mother's back or playing among the pesticide-laden fields.

- **Seasonal farmworkers** generally live in one geographic location and are temporarily employed in agriculture, whereas migrant farmworkers meet that classification while moving to find agricultural work throughout the year, usually from state to state, and establishing temporary residences (Migrant Clinicians Network, 2017a).
- Some live apart from their families, forming groups of single men; others travel with their entire families. The average migrant farmworker spends from June to September doing seasonal harvesting, with about 8 weeks on the road traveling from farm to farm for work, and is then unemployed unless other work, such as hauling or canning, is found.
- Work days begin before dawn and often last 12 hours or longer. Farmworkers cannot be paid for overtime, as federal laws exclude this category of work. Seventeen states do not require workers' compensation insurance for agricultural workers, 14 states require workers' compensation for all agricultural workers and the remainder requires it but provide exceptions for small employers (NCFH, 2018a).

Migrant farmworkers represent some of the most economically disadvantaged people in the United States. According to the 2013 to 2014 National Agricultural Workers Survey (NAWS) survey results, 30% of migrant worker families had total family income levels below the national poverty guidelines. The same survey found that 83% of these workers said that they were paid by the hour, 9% were paid by the piece, and 8% were salaried or had other payment methods. Using piece rate as a basis for payment is common in agricultural work when the crop being picked is easily weighed and measured, motivating workers work faster during such a short window of seasonal crop harvesting (NCFH, 2018a). Farmworkers paid at a per piece rate may earn as little as 40 cents for a bucket of tomatoes or sweet potatoes, therefore

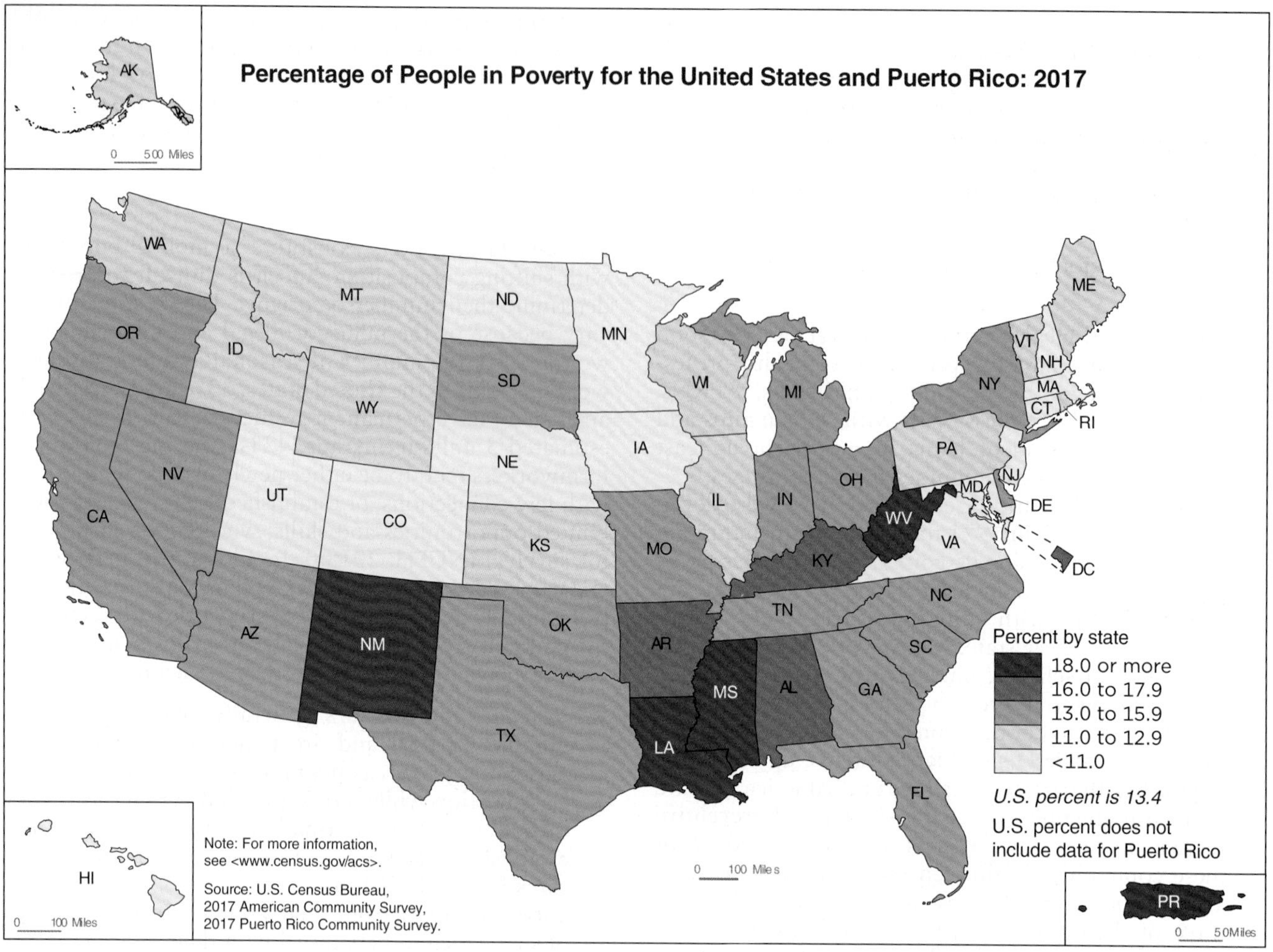

Percentage of People in Poverty for the United States and Puerto Rico: 2017

Percent by state
18.0 or more
16.0 to 17.9
13.0 to 15.9
11.0 to 12.9
<11.0

U.S. percent is 13.4

U.S. percent does not include data for Puerto Rico

Note: For more information, see <www.census.gov/acs>.

Source: U.S. Census Bureau, 2017 American Community Survey, 2017 Puerto Rico Community Survey.

FIGURE 27-4 Percentage of people in poverty for the United States and Puerto Rico: 2017. (From the U.S. Census Bureau. (2018). *Poverty: 2016 and 2017. Geography of poverty.* Retrieved from https://www.census.gov/content/dam/Census/library/publications/2018/acs/acsbr17-02.pdf)

needing to pick approximately 2 tons of produce (125 buckets) to earn 50 dollars (Student Action Farmworkers [SAF], 2011–2019). In addition to low wages, agricultural workers rarely have access to worker's compensation, occupational rehabilitation, or disability compensation benefits.

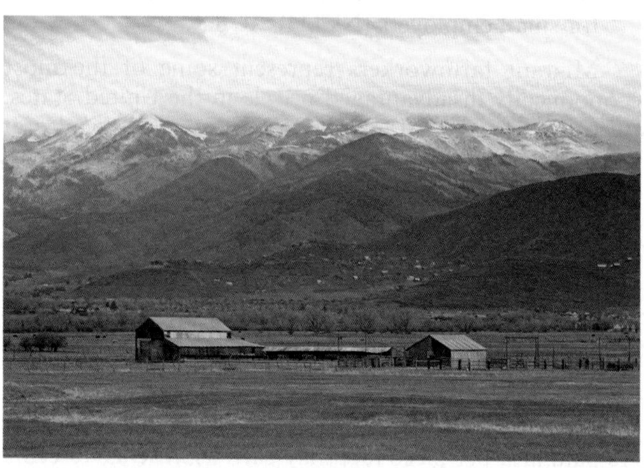

FIGURE 27-5 A farm in rural Utah.

Migrant Streams and Patterns

Migrant farmworkers usually have their permanent residence, or *home base*, in states with a traditionally high number of immigrants, like California, Texas, Florida, Washington, Oregon, and North Carolina (SAF, 2011–2019). From their home base, migrant farmworkers move to locations where new crops are ready for harvest, following the harvest seasons as they move from place to place along predetermined routes called **migrant streams** (Fig. 27-6). Some migrant farmworkers are multigenerational; their families have been farmworkers for several generations, traveling the same streams for many years. It is common for migrant farmworkers to send money back home to family members in other countries, like Mexico, China, India, and the Philippines. In fact, an estimated $625 billion dollars was sent by migrants to individuals in their home countries in 2017, a 7% increase from 2016. More specifically, more than 30 billion dollars was sent from the United States to Mexico by migrant workers (Pew Research Center, 2020). Of farmworkers in the United States, 75% were born in Mexico and 60% live apart from their immediate family members. Immigrant farmworkers often leave their home country to seek a better life for their families (SAF, 2011–2019).

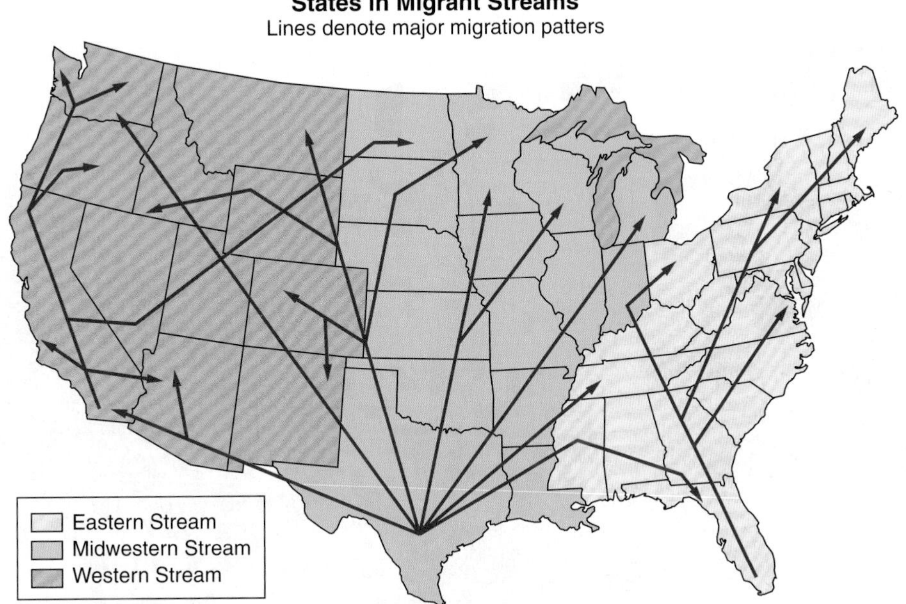

FIGURE 27-6 Migrant streams. (Source: Migrant Head Start Program, USHDHUD.)

Three principal streams formulate the agricultural routes that migrant laborers follow.

- The *eastern stream* originates in Florida, where most of their time is spent, and extends up the East Coast through North Carolina, Tennessee, Kentucky, Virginia, and other states east of the Mississippi, as far as north as Ohio, New Jersey, New York, Connecticut, Massachusetts, New Hampshire, Vermont, and Maine.
- The *midwestern stream* begins in southern Texas or northern Mexico and fans out across the United States, ending in the Northwestern and Midwestern states bordering Canada, both east and west of the Mississippi.
- The *western stream* originates in California and moves up the West Coast to all Western states and from central California into Oregon and Washington (NCFH, 2018a).
- California, Florida, and Texas are regarded as *sending states*, as they are often home states with long growing seasons where migrant streams begin and end (Fig. 27-7). Male workers may travel with the crops and leave their families in these home states (USDHUD, 2016). Workers move from areas with cotton, tree fruits and nuts, and vegetable crops to other areas where they harvest cherries, watermelons, cantaloupes, or potatoes.

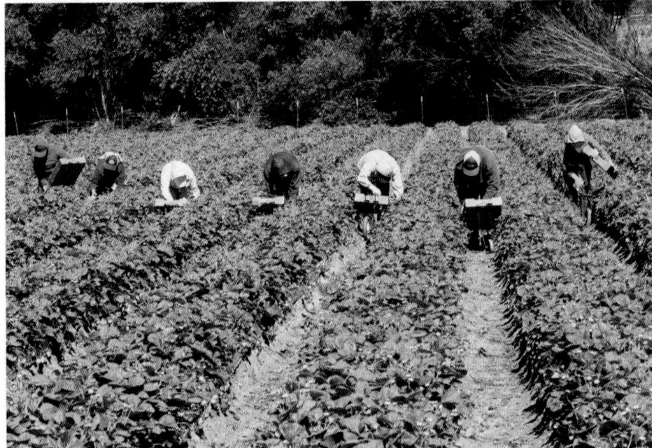

FIGURE 27-7 Migrant farm workers pick and package crops (strawberries) directly into boxes in the Salinas Valley of central California.

Nomadic migrant workers travel away from home for several years, working from farm to farm and crop to crop and relying on word of mouth about job opportunities. Some of these workers eventually settle in the areas to which they have migrated, whereas others return to their home base. A given ethnic group usually follows its own particular stream and pattern of migration. New growth states, like Utah, Minnesota, Wisconsin, Nebraska, Kansas, Tennessee, and Arkansas, have seen immigrant population's increase. Some migrant workers find work in service sector jobs and others labor in construction or landscaping, thus ending their need to constantly move with the crops. Married men, not living with their families, are more likely to migrate than those living with their families, often because of the need to send money back home.

RURAL HEALTH

Rural areas have historically had less racial diversity than urban areas. However, that is rapidly changing. More recently, rapid Hispanic growth areas are found in the South and Metropolitan areas (Fig. 27-8; Pew Research Center, 2018). California, Texas, and Florida are home to 55% of the U.S. Hispanic population, with 14.4 million living in California. In rural counties, the white

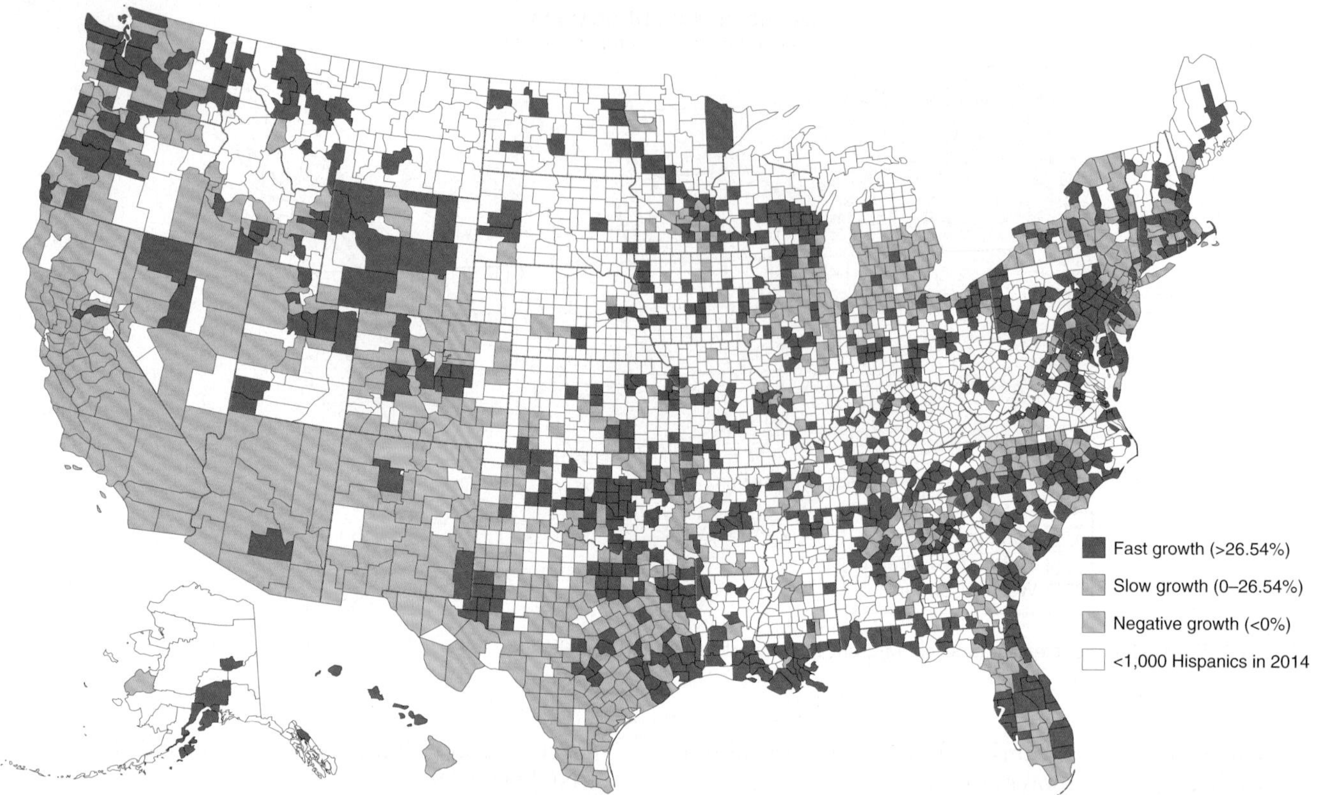

FIGURE 27-8 The fastest-growing Latino counties between 2007 and 2014 were largely located in the South and metropolitan areas. (Reprinted with permission from Stepler, R., and Lopez, M. H. (2016). *U.S. Latino population growth and dispersion has slowed since onset of the Great Recession.* Pew Research Center: Hispanic Trends. Retrieved from http://www.pewhispanic.org/2016/09/08/latino-population-growth-and-dispersion-has-slowed-since-the-onset-of-the-great-recession/ph_2016-09-08_geography-06/)

population has decreased, and other ethnic groups have increased in size, but still only 11% of rural counties are majority nonwhite (Pew Research Center, 2020).

Urban and rural disparities have changed over time. The National Rural Health Association (2019) identifies life expectancy to have shifted with those in rural areas living slightly longer than those in urban areas (Table 27-1). Health concerns of populations in rural areas are related to the environment, occupations, injuries, and distance from health care providers. Population trends have a direct relationship to the kinds of health services that are needed in rural communities. Growing families with young children need maternity, pediatric, and family health medical services, along with dental care and mental health services. They also can benefit from health promotion and disease prevention activities. The elderly, on the other hand, need health care to manage increased number of chronic health conditions. Rural communities need to provide access to nursing homes and rehabilitative services, as well as to hospitals, clinics, and health promotion programs that serve the elderly and the entire community.

The Built Environment in Rural Areas: Relationship to Health

Even with the advances of medicine and genomics, and the staggering percentage of our gross domestic product (GDP) spent on health care, scientists feel that we will not be able to significantly improve our overall health and quality of life without addressing how we plan our living spaces.

As discussed in Chapter 9, the **built environment** consists of the development of housing, highways, shopping areas, and other man-made features added to the natural environment.

As populated areas expand, stresses are placed on natural habitats, water supplies, and air quality. The built environment is inextricably related to health. Substantial scientific evidence gained in the past decade has shown that various aspects of the built environment can have profound, directly measurable effects on both physical and mental health outcomes, particularly adding to the burden of illness among ethnic minority populations and low-income communities (Hansen, Umstattd Meyer, Lenardson, & Hartley, 2015).

Urban sprawl is a concern in some rural areas, as people move from urban centers to more suburban environments. Urban encroachment into agricultural areas creates problems with air and water pollution, access to health care, and heat islands. *Heat islands* occur when green areas are exchanged for asphalt, resulting in temperature and ecosystem changes that can extend to more rural areas (Trivedi et al., 2015). Ozone levels are often highest just outside the city, because "ozone is formed relatively slowly by the action of sunlight on oxides of nitrogen and hydrocarbons" (p. 72). Urban sprawl also causes problems with water pollution and the availability of water. Encroachment of housing areas into natural habitats or farmlands can lead to wider human exposure to pesticides, herbicides, and other hazards such as mosquito-borne illnesses. Mass transit is not often available in suburban areas and almost never found in rural areas. Opportunities for health-promoting behaviors are often more limited in rural areas. Deteriorating (or no) sidewalks can be a barrier to walking in rural areas. Exercise or fitness facilities, bike paths, jogging trails, and other incentives for physical activity are also often lacking in rural communities.

- Trivedi and colleagues (2015) examined data from a large national survey and found that rural adults were 1.19 times more likely to be obese when compared to urban adults. The prevalence was 35.6% in rural residents versus 30.4% for urban residents, and that difference was also found for both males and females (37.7% vs. 32.5%; 33.4% vs. 28.2%).
- Exercise levels were lower among rural adults than for those in urban areas (Trivedi et al., 2015). Obesity is prevalent in rural areas, and the physical environment, along with diet, plays a role in this epidemic (Lenardson, Hansen, & Hartley, 2015).
- Eating out, especially at buffets, fast-food restaurants, and cafeterias, instead of cooking at home, as well as not participating in physical activity have been associated with higher rates of obesity (Lenardson et al., 2015). In fact, Bhutani, Schoeller, Walsh, and McWilliams (2018) found that for every 1-meal/week increase in fast-food and sit-down restaurant consumption was associated with an increase in BMI by 0.8 and 0.6 kg/m^2, respectively.

Rural roads are another concern because they are often narrow, without streetlights, and poorly maintained. More fatalities occur on rural roads and highways. While 19% of the country's population lived in rural areas in 2012, 54% of all road fatalities occurred there (National Highway & Traffic Safety Administration, 2018). Speeding, failure to use safety restraints, and alcohol are common causes of fatal crashes in rural areas. Over half of fatal crashes occurred during daylight hours in rural areas; the opposite is true in urban areas. Fifty-five percent of all fatal alcohol-related crashes occurred in rural areas, and 65% of rural occupant deaths in pickup trucks were not using restraints. Slow-moving farm equipment traveling on rural roads, along with speeding and failure to use safety restraints, are often fatal conditions for drivers in rural areas.

Self, Home, and Community Care in Rural Areas

Historically, self-management of health care problems has been the most common way for rural people to cope with illness (Fig. 27-9). This can be viewed as a type of strength, or it may be seen as a limitation.

- Rural residents are often viewed as hardworking, traditional, hardy, self-reliant, and resistant to accepting help or services from outside agencies regarded by them as welfare-type programs.
- Many rural clients are considered individualistic, independent, and resourceful. They often take care of illnesses or injuries on their own or have a supportive network to help them get their health needs met.
- Small communities commonly have strong social networks, but this type of familiarity may lead to problems with privacy and confidentiality, as well as stigma regarding mental health or substance abuse treatment.
- Because cost, travel, weather, and distance are barriers to obtaining health services from formal health care providers, rural clients may employ a variety of folk treatments and home remedies before consulting a nurse or a physician; such clients tend to visit providers at a much later stage than do people in urban areas.
- Rural residents may utilize physicians who are more likely to provide care that is outside their specialty areas.
- Compared with hospitals that are less rural, CAHs have been found to have significantly higher patient mortality rates.
- Patients living in rural areas are known to have higher risk for poor health outcomes, more likely to smoke and consume less healthy diets. These factors may contribute to higher mortality rates.
- Social determinants of health for rural dwellers, such as living environment, community health supports, distance to providers, and local economic prospects, can contribute to the mortality disparity (Heath, 2017).
- The low population density in rural areas makes service delivery more difficult, especially for those with special health needs. The greater treatment barriers when living in an isolated area are geography and lack of adequate transportation.
- Home health care (HHC) is particularly difficult in sparsely populated areas, for both patients and nurses. Locating addresses in very rural areas often takes additional skills. (See Box 27-1 for the story of a home health nurse trying to locate a client's home.) The benefits of HHC are worthwhile; it allows people to stay at home, supports their hardiness, and compensates for the long distance between home and formal health care.

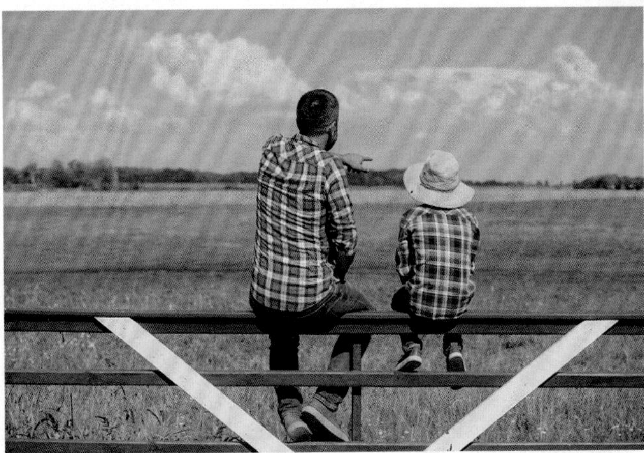

FIGURE 27-9 Life in a rural area may seem idyllic, but there are some significant risks of a rural lifestyle.

BOX 27-1 Locating a Rural Home Health Client

It can be difficult to locate a patient in the rural community. Directions may include structures such as barns, fences, and trees, or identification of stores that are familiar to the patient and their family but not the nurse. In addition, living quarters may be on long unmarked dirt roads or be an additional structure to an already existing address. Once I received directions from a patient who told me to "...take the second dirt road on the right after you get off the highway (after the Dairy Queen), you'll see a big oak tree with a swing. Continue down that road for about 5 maybe 6 minutes and turn right again at the red one-story house. Drive to you see the green barn, don't turn there, but turn left at the next barn. You'll see our house over the hill." Additional time may be needed to navigate rural residents because GPS systems may not be of assistance in these rural areas.

Major Health Problems in Rural Communities

Among major health problems affecting individuals in rural areas are cardiovascular disease (CVD), diabetes, and COPD. Geography, economics, and rural lifestyle factors may account for the higher rate of these major health problems.

Cardiovascular Disease

CVD is a leading cause of death in the United States (42%), and the total direct and indirect costs of CVD and stroke were estimated at over $351.3 billion in 2015 (American Heart Association, 2020). Research demonstrates that geography may play a role.

- Mortality because of heart disease is highest in the South, especially following the path of the Mississippi River (Bolin et al., 2015). Regional variations have been noted in prevalence of CVD and stroke. Studies have found increased stroke mortality in the South (stroke belt), and many researchers are focusing on the possible underlying risk factors related to geographical variations. One group of researchers wanted to better understand the effect of length of time living in the stroke belt and age at first exposure.
- Rural areas usually have less high-tech health care equipment available, which may affect outcomes for patients with cardiovascular emergencies. Being within 60 minutes of a Primary Stroke Center (PSC) can determine outcome for many patients. C/PHNs can advocate for better access to care and promote healthy lifestyle choices as well as population-targeted interventions to reduce stroke and CVD.
- Rural residents may ignore early cardiovascular symptoms and give little heed to preventive interventions such as exercise and low-fat diets.
- Several models of care are being implemented to address rural CVD. In Maine, community-based education is targeting the specific needs of low-income residents with CVD with attention given to socioeconomic status, and residents' local culture and education level. In Montana, pharmacists are working with rural clients to discuss medication management, nutrition, and other risk factors such as smoking with good success. In rural east Colorado, community health workers meet clients in local community facilities such as libraries and schools to provide screenings, referrals, services, and education (Rural Health Information Hub, 2019a).

Diabetes

Rural populations are disproportionately affected by diabetes and CVD (8.6% and 38.8%, respectively); the prevalence is generally greater in rural areas, and this is even more pronounced among Hispanics and Blacks. Mortality rates for diabetes were higher in the rural regions within the south and Midwest with 21% of deaths per 100,000 compared to 15.1% per 100,000 in the northwest and west (HRSA, 2018). Overall, the prevalence of diabetes is 15% to 17% higher in rural areas than in urban (HRSA, 2018).

- Rural areas have been cited as promoting obesity on a population level because of fewer opportunities for walking, as residents spend a great deal of time commuting to work or driving to essential services, and rural residence was positively correlated with BMI, distance to retail food, and commute times, among other things (Calancie et al., 2015).
- Lower physical activity rates and greater barriers to physical activity are commonly found in rural populations, as opposed to populations living in urban settings (Bolin et al., 2015).
- Rural populations also face greater barriers in diagnosis, treatment, and follow-up care. Some compliance issues with prescribed medication regimens may relate to the lack of health insurance and low-income levels in rural areas but could also be due to lower health literacy and education levels.
- Other problems with accessing care may involve transportation and weather. A lack of access to quality health care services has been a long-standing problem for rural Americans because of the significant difference in access to health care (HRSA, 2020).

Anderson, Saman, Lipsky, and Lutfiyya (2015), in a comparison study of people living in rural counties versus nonrural counties, found that rural residents had statistically lower scores in areas such as clinical care, morbidity factors, and general health behavior. For instance, a classic study by Krishna, Gillespie, and McBride (2010) highlighted the extreme complications encountered by rural residents who often have to travel great distances to access services for diabetes care, such as basic follow-up with podiatrists for diabetic foot care, ophthalmologists for retinal health, and nutritionists and health educators, as well as routine laboratory blood tests, to guide lifestyle choices. C/PHNs, especially in rural and frontier areas, often provide follow-up for diabetic clients who may be unable to regularly access their health care providers because of problems with distance or transportation. Home visits to check on their diet/exercise, blood glucose monitoring, and foot care are important safeguards for this population. Also, interventions targeted to behavior change can be helpful.

Chronic Obstructive Pulmonary Disease

Prevalence of COPD in rural counties is twice that of urban areas (8.2% vs. 4.7%) with high concentrations occurring in the Appalachia and the southern geographic regions (DHHS, 2018). Medicare beneficiaries aged 65 years and over in rural regions had higher COPD-related hospitalization than urban (13.8 to 11.4 per 100,000). Lack of access to care, limited transportation, decreased specialty services, and treatment options increase the disparity of COPD in rural versus urban areas. Environmental exposures can also affect COPD patients in rural communities (DHHS, 2018). Typical rural occupations expose people to very dusty or dirty air, chemicals, environmental pollutants, and occupational activities such as farming and coal mining. Even nonagricultural rural workers are much more likely to be exposed on the job to high levels of gases, dust, and fumes (27%) than urban workers (15%). In addition, a higher percentage of rural than urban people smoke, including exposure to secondhand smoke. Smoking among teen-agers is decreasing but remains considerably higher among rural young people. Other causative factors for high mortality rates from COPD include difficulties for rural people getting to basic and specialized medical care. Rural individuals may have to travel longer distances to received care and treatment (DHHS, 2018). Small rural hospitals may not have the equipment to measure and track changes in a person's breathing over time and may not have respiratory therapists to teach patients better ways to live with their damaged lungs (Myers, 2018). Environment issues particularly relate to agriculture and the health risks that accompany farming and other rural lifestyles.

Agriculture and Health

Although farming is not characteristic of all rural areas where agricultural production occurs, both direct and indirect effects on health can exist.

- In a classic summary sponsored by the Institute of Medicine (Merchant, Coussens, & Gilbert, 2006), it is noted that pesticides and fertilizers can affect water, air, and soil, and dust created from plowing for crops can affect the air quality. For instance, an "estimated 70% of antibiotics are used for nontherapeutic purposes in intensive livestock production," placing workers at risk for developing antibiotic-resistant infections (p. 4).
- Donham and Thelin (2016) focused their research on diseases commonly seen in agricultural workers, mainly arthritis (rheumatoid and osteoarthritis), injuries of the musculoskeletal system, skin cancer, burns, rural roadway crashes, and zoonotic diseases. Neurotoxicity can develop due to exposure to industrial chemicals and pharmaceuticals, leading to report of neuropsychiatric disorders, such as attention deficit hyperactivity disorder (ADHD) and autism.
- Exposure to these substances during early development may lead to adverse behavior effects manifested at a later time of life. Pesticides are a wide group of chemicals that are still actively used, and residues are found in the environment and in food products (Lee, Eriksson, Fredriksson, Buratovic, & Viberg, 2015).
- Pesticides are linked to disease and environmental risks through various routes (e.g., residues in food and drinking water). These hazards range from short term (e.g., skin and eye irritation, headaches, dizziness, and nausea) to chronic problems (e.g., cancer, asthma, and diabetes). Further, their risks are difficult to explain due to the involvement of various factors (e.g., period and level of exposure, type of pesticide) (Kim, Kabir, & Jahan, 2017).
- Lawsuits have been filed in California, Delaware, Florida, Hawaii, and Missouri against Monsanto over its popular herbicide, Roundup, with its active ingredient now thought to be a "probable human carcinogen" (Gillam, 2016, para. 8). The World Health Organization's International Agency for Research on Cancer has called glyphosate a "probable human carcinogen," and in 2017, the state of California added this weed killer to its list of cancer-causing chemicals (Cone, 2019).

Many rural residents depend on their own well water for drinking, and water quality is monitored only sporadically by well owners and then usually only for nitrates and coliform bacteria (Lee et al., 2015). About 30% of rural residents obtain drinking water from very small water systems, without the monitoring and regulations associated with large urban water suppliers. Testing of small water systems should be done at regular intervals in order to get a true picture of water quality (Wedgworth et al., 2015). In addition, agricultural-related morbidity and mortality are relatively high. Agriculture, forestry, and underground mining are ranked high in the rate of occupational injuries (U.S. Department of Labor, 2017).

It is estimated that 33,000 injuries to children are farm related, and approximately 100 of them are fatal. Of the fatal injuries to youth, 23% were machinery related (often tractors), 19% were vehicle related (including ATVs), and drowning was to blame in 16% of fatalities. Most fatalities (34%) were in the 16- to 19-year age group (Occupational Health & Safety Administration [OSHA], n.d.). Farming injuries can result from tractor rollovers, suffocations in grain bins, exposure to harmful substances, falls, fires or explosions, accidents with other farm equipment, and on- or off-road collisions. Some injuries result in permanent disability, and worker training programs to recognize hazards and prevent injuries are rare in rural areas. See Box 27-2 for farming accidents.

Access to Health Care in Rural Areas

Insurance, Managed Care, and Health Care Services

Health insurance in today's market is costly, especially for individual purchasers. Some people, therefore, forego health insurance for themselves and their families. Depending on their income, people may or may not be eligible for Medicaid or State Children's Health Insurance Programs (S-CHIPs). Even people who are eligible for government health assistance may not apply because of their belief that it is a sign of weakness to accept a handout. Historically, a traditional fee-for-service model delivered health care in rural and urban communities (see

BOX 27-2 Agricultural Accidents

Farm Tractor Accidents

In the old days before mechanical equipment, a farmer might be injured by one of his horses or mules, or accidently stabbed with a pitchfork. Today, tractors are involved in the majority of injuries and deaths. ROPS, or a roll cage over the tractor seat, can save lives; they were standard on every tractor manufactured in the country since 1985 (1959 in Sweden). If a farmer uses the seat belt and the tractor equipped with ROPS turns over, there is a good chance that he will survive the accident. Sadly, many farmers don't use seat belts, and many use older tractors without ROPS protection. There are many potential hazards on farms (e.g., falling bales of hay, heat stroke, dangerous equipment like hay balers, choppers, combines), but tractor rollovers and children falling from tractors are much too common and can often be prevented.

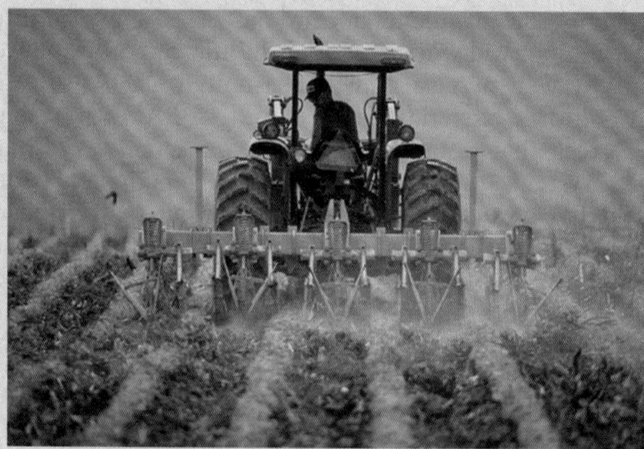

Death on the Farm

Agricultural deaths are not uncommon, elderly men, youths, and hired hands are the most affected. Agriculture industry has the highest fatal occupational injuries with 23.2 per 100,000 and nonfatal injuries 58,300 in 2016. Tractor rollovers are preventable; ROPS along with seatbelt use can eliminate these injures. Engineering controls along with policies, practices, and protective equipment can control agricultural workplace accidents. Currently, there are 4.2 million tractors in use with all new equipment manufactured with ROPS. As of 2006, 59% of tractors were equipped with ROPS. Due to longevity of equipment, retrofitting of equipment is an option, but cost, special clearance, tractor housings, and personal preferences are barriers for many farmers.

Source: Forst (2018).
(Photo source: USDA Agricultural Research Service.)

Chapter 6). However, that is changing, and it is challenging for rural providers to deliver the cost-effective, complex health care that rural persons need in small practices.

- Rural patients often utilize family practice clinics.
- The managed care model, which attempts to control costs and improve health care delivery, has slowly diffused into rural communities. In addition, rural practitioners are reluctant to become part of organizations that negotiate to reduce their payments, as many of them already see a disproportionate number of Medicaid and uninsured patients that impact their bottom line.
- Low population density makes this type of health care insurance less profitable.
- More states are moving to Medicaid managed care models, and Medicare offers this option to beneficiaries. This puts rural residents at a disadvantage, as they may have poor access to services because of distance and travel time.

Building provider networks in rural communities is both time- and effort-intensive because rural providers are often inexperienced with managed care organizations (MCOs). The federal government provides support for **rural health clinics** in areas designated as underserved and nonurban; differences in effectiveness and efficiency have been noted in larger clinics versus smaller clinics (RHIH, 2020a). These clinics have served rural clients for more than 30 years, and they are an important source of health care.

- Rural areas are characterized by a lack of core health care services (e.g., primary care, hospital care, emergency medical services, long-term care, mental health and substance abuse counseling services, dental care, and public health services).
- Shortages were noted for physicians, with urban areas having 263 specialists for every 100,000 residents and rural areas having 30 specialists for every 100,000 residents (Lahr, Neprash, Henning-Smith, Tuttle, Hernandez, 2019).
- In the United States, 56% of all rural counties do not have a pediatrician affecting the health status of children (Rural Health Information Hub, 2019a).
- Population health services in rural areas may be covered by a combination of public health departments, physicians in private practice, local hospitals, as well as various community agencies.
- In some rural or frontier areas, state health departments may offer services, as no local infrastructure may be present. Many rural residents depend heavily on public health department services. Seventeen percent of local health departments (LHDs) serve small towns (populations under 10,000), and 44% serve communities with populations between 10,000 and 49,999.
- These LHDs are less likely than larger health departments to provide environmental health services, but they often provide many of the other services (e.g., primary prevention, health services, epidemiology/surveillance) found in larger health departments (National Association of County and City Health Officials, 2016).
- Numerous states have sizable rural areas; this geographic isolation may restrict access to health care for vulnerable groups, especially minorities and those with disabilities. To adequately address health disparities, rural areas need to be better incorporated into discussions of geographic and racial inequality (Caldwell, Ford, Wallace, Wang, & Takahashi, 2016). See Box 27-3 for a hard lesson learned by one C/PHN student.

BOX **27-3** PERSPECTIVES

A NURSING STUDENT VIEWPOINT ON RURAL TRANSPORTATION

I live in a relatively large city of 450,000 people. When I started my community health nursing rotation, I was assigned to a rural county public health department in an adjoining county over 50 miles from my house. When I arrived for my first clinical day, my professor told me that I was assigned to see clients in an isolated community another hour away from the health department! There was nothing but farmland between the county seat and this small town.

After I got over my frustration about traveling such long distances, I began to visit some of my families and started to actually enjoy my time with them. They were so appreciative and open to my suggested interventions. I really seemed to be making a difference. One older gentleman, Armando, was a diabetic who spoke very little English. He lived with his wife of 50 years, who spoke almost no English. Their children had moved away in order to go to school and get better jobs. His diabetes was not well controlled, and the rural health clinic FNP suggested that he see a specialist (actually an internist) in the largest city in the county. I helped him make arrangements with the doctor for an early afternoon visit and made sure that he could catch the county bus that ran between the smaller communities and the county seat.

When I came back for a follow-up visit the next week, I was shocked to learn that Armando's appointment had been pushed back to 4:30 PM because of the doctor's involvement in hospital emergencies, and by the time Armando was finished with his appointment, the county bus service had ended. Armando, with no money and no one to call for a ride, began walking back to his home—over 52 miles away! About halfway home, a farm truck driver gave him a lift to the large cotton farm a few miles from his home. I never realized how difficult it was for rural people to get to their medical appointments. I thought that the bus would not be a problem, but I learned my lesson. Now, I make sure that the physician's office understands the patient's circumstances and the importance of getting them back to the bus stop in time to make the last bus.

Andrea, senior nursing student

Unpredictable weather adds to potential barriers for rural clients. Snow, ice, wind, flash floods, and rain can make travel dangerous, even over short distances.

- Parents may decide not to risk driving on poorly maintained roads to get their children immunized or to have their own hypertension evaluated (Fig. 27-10).
- Elderly people may choose to delay health care when long travel times, especially in isolated rural areas, are involved.
- Rural populations have disproportionately high injury mortality rates, much of which is due to motor vehicle accidents (APHA, 2018).
- In a more recent study by Chaiyachati et al. (2018), offering complimentary ridesharing services to Medicaid patients did not reduce rates of missed primary health care appointments. The acceptance of free rides was low, and rates of missed appointments remained unchanged at 36%. Study results indicated that efforts to reduce missed appointments due to transportation barriers may require more targeted approaches.
- Historically, rural communities have been somewhat overlooked in the transportation planning process. In fact, because of the way in which transportation dollars are allocated, rural states often receive less funding than more densely populated states (APHA, 2018).
- Inadequate phone service, dead zones in cell coverage, and the lack of adequate contact information for emergency physicians on staff are all problems frequently encountered in rural areas (Bolin et al., 2015).

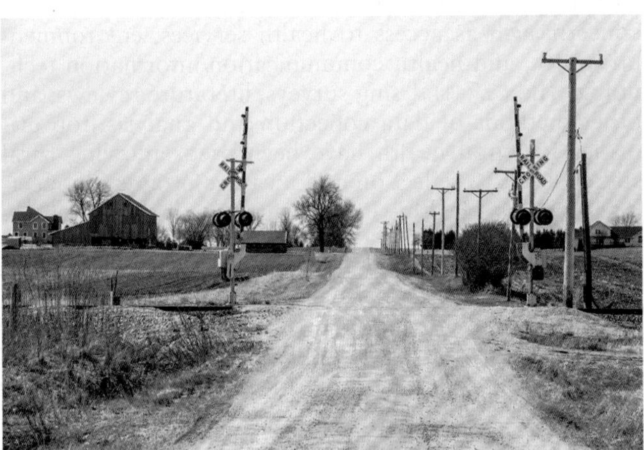

FIGURE 27-10 A railroad crossing along a dirt road across farmland on a winter day without snow in northern Illinois.

New Approaches to Improve Access

The *Healthy People 2030* document mandates improvements in access, health education, health screening, immunizations, environmental health, and disease morbidity for the United States. Creative ways of delivering these and other services to rural clients need to be explored. Access to care is a social justice issue: clients who live in rural areas should receive quality health care, regardless of where they choose to live. The *Healthy People 2030* plan of action includes investment in health and well-being for all individuals. The first three overarching goals of *Healthy People 2030* focuses on the elimination of health disparities, improving health access, and creating healthy environments.

- Attain healthy, thriving lives and well-being, free of preventable disease, disability, injury, and premature death
- Create social, physical, and economic environments that promote attaining full potential for health and well-being for all (USDHHS, 2020a).

Faith-based nursing has been a staple in rural areas, as well as with some urban communities, but is gaining momentum as more formal interventions are developed, for instance, mental health promotion for rural Latino immigrants (Stacciarini et al., 2016). Even informal support from other church members and friends may provide a compassionate environment for needed behavioral changes such as healthy diet and increased physical activity. See more on faith-based nursing in Chapter 29. Results indicate that perceived improvements in church nutrition environments were most strongly associated with decreases in unhealthy food consumption and stronger intentions to use physical activity resources at church. Perceived changes in the physical activity environment were unrelated to church or general behavior (Jacob et al., 2016).

One approach that has been successful in numerous rural areas is the use of *mobile clinics*. These clinics bring health care providers to remote places for health screenings, immunizations, dental care, mental health visits, and other services.

- Mobile health clinics are frequently staffed by NPs and can improve access to health care for low-income residents.
- They often are available to residents on evenings and weekends and offer culturally sensitive and bilingual outreach, as well as care for uninsured clients.
- Although the aim of the Affordable Care Act (ACA) includes increasing the number of insured individuals in the United States and overcoming health disparities, it has no provisions for mobile medical clinics, which appear to serve as an important component of health care delivery, especially to vulnerable populations.
- In addition, mobile dental clinics provide an innovative solution to providing dental to improve physical access to dental care for medically underserved population in poor urban and remote rural communities.
- Many mobile clinics provide existing dental clinics services at lower or no cost to the user.

School-based clinics can improve access for schoolchildren (and sometimes their families) but may be less prominent in rural areas (see more on school-based clinics in Chapter 28). These clinics provide available, community-based, affordable, and culturally acceptable care to well and sick children. Often, grant-supported, school-based clinics facilitate the receipt of health education and primary care by children who are otherwise without easy access to health services. More than 66% of school-based health centers offer primary care and behavioral health services. In addition, school-based health centers are associated with improved educational status, including higher grade point averages and higher rates of high school completion (National Conference of State Legislatures, 2020).

Telehealth, another approach to increasing access to care, provides electronically transmitted clinician consultation between the client and the health care provider. This option is especially useful for connecting home health nurses with their patients who need close monitoring at home. It is also useful for patient and professional health education, public health applications, and health administration. Specialty health care also may be accessed, with patients and providers connected via two-way audiovisual transmission over telephone lines or the Internet, thus obviating the need for patients to leave their residences. Streaming media, video conferencing, and store-and-forward imaging are just some of the applications commonly utilized (HRSA, 2020).

- Telehealth interventions for speech–language services to rural children were found by parents to be both feasible and acceptable. Parents found the teletherapy to be more frequent and consistent services, which in turn promoted their confidence and skill in assisting their children to achieve their speech and language goals (Fairweather, Lincoln, & Ramsdeb, 2016).
- Online counseling and remote counseling link rural clients with urban behavioral health services. Counseling services can also be provided online in Spanish (Rural Health Information Hub, 2020b).
- Telehealth is especially critical in rural and other remote areas that lack sufficient health care services, including specialty care. The range and use of telehealth services have expanded over the past decades, along with the role of technology in improving and coordinating care. Grants and other funding are available to promote the use of this technology (HRSA, 2020; RHIH, 2019b). See Chapter 10.

Healthy People 2030 Goals

The five overarching goals of *Healthy People 2030* are to:

- Attain healthy, thriving lives and well-being, free of preventable disease, disability, injury, and premature death
- Eliminate health disparities, achieve health equity, and attain health literacy to improve the health and well-being of all
- Create social, physical, and economic environments that promote attaining full potential for health and well-being for all
- Promote healthy development, healthy behaviors, and well-being across all life stages
- Engage leadership, key constituents, and the public across multiple sectors to take action and design policies that improve the health and well-being of all (USDHHS, 2020a, para. 11)

Because of the unique health issues facing rural America, *Healthy People 2030* identifies broad areas of concern such as access to health services, environmental health, and health communication/information technology (Box 27-4). Using surveys, literature reviews, and other methods of data collection and analysis, top priorities for rural health have been used, allowing rural stakeholders to reflect on and measure progress in meeting previous Healthy People rural goals (Bolin et al., 2015). In addition, there are data to substantiate continued problems with access to health care and insurance, as well as emergency services, in rural areas. And there is a higher rate of CVD and diabetes, along with obesity and tobacco use among rural populations (NRHA, 2019).

- A large longitudinal study of maternal and infant health in Maine revealed that access to prenatal care, along with pregnancy care and outcomes, was similar for rural and urban women over an 11-year period

BOX 27-4 *HEALTHY PEOPLE 2030*

Health Issues in Rural America

Access to Health Services

AHS-01	Increase the proportion of people with health insurance
AHS-02	Increase the proportion of people with dental insurance
AHS-05	Reduce the proportion of people who can't get the dental care they need when they need it
AHS-08	Increase the proportion of adults who get recommended evidence-based preventative health care
AHS-R02	Increase the use of telehealth to improve access to health services
ECBP-D06	Increase the number of community-based organizations providing population-based primary prevention services

Diabetes

D-09	Reduce the rate of death from any cause in adults with diabetes
D-D01	Increase the proportion of eligible people completing CDC-recognized type 2 diabetes preventative programs

Environmental Health

EH-06	Reduce the amount of toxic pollutants released into the environment

Health Communication and Health Information Technology

HC/HIT-06	Increase the proportion of adults offered online access to their medical record

Heart Disease and Stroke

HDS-01	Improve cardiovascular health in adults

Reprinted from U.S. Department of Health and Human Services (USDHHS). (2020a). *Healthy People 2030: Browse objectives.* Retrieved from https://health.gov/healthypeople/objectives-and-data/browse-objectives

(Harris, Aboueissa, Baugh, & Sarton, 2015). Rural mothers had higher BMIs prior to pregnancy and were generally younger, less well educated, unmarried, and living in low-income households. They were also more likely to smoke, but less likely to drink alcohol, and were not often sure of their pregnancies until later than urban mothers, but they still accessed prenatal care at similar times (Harris et al., 2015).

- Access to quality care is linked to availability of health insurance. Rural residents, when compared to urban counterparts, have higher rates of uninsured, higher out-of-pocket costs, and higher proportions of emergency room visit costs; they are also less likely to be covered through group health insurance or managed care plans and less likely to have prescription drug coverage (Bolin et al., 2015).
- Also, insurance instability (gaps in coverage) is correlated with increased use of emergency rooms, and this is particularly significant for rural residents who often have less access (Fields, Bell, Moyce, & Bigbee, 2015). Because of lower rates of insured rural residents, their preventive health care is often lacking (e.g., lower rates of mammograms, colonoscopies, vision examinations).
- Approximately 65% of primary care professional shortages occur in rural counties. Rural residents are also less likely than urban residents to have a usual source of primary care (Rural Health Information Hub, 2019a).
- Problems more commonly seen in rural areas include oral health and cigarette and smokeless tobacco use. Sixty percent of rural counties are considered professional shortage areas for dental health, and more dentists are over age 55 in rural areas (42% vs. 38% in urban) (Rural Health Information Hub, 2019a). Rural populations are less likely to have annual dental examinations. They are also more likely to have tooth or gum disease, often because of higher rates of cigarette and smokeless tobacco use, and they are more likely to use the emergency room because of dental caries than urban residents (Bolin et al., 2015).
- Rural teens have a higher rate of tobacco and alcohol use than their urban counterparts (Rural Health Information Hub, 2019a).
- Unintentional overdose deaths due to nonmedical use of prescription drugs disproportionately impact rural over urban settings in the United States. Specific geographic areas, such as Appalachia, parts of the West and the Midwest, and New England, have seen higher prevalence than other areas (United States Department of Health and Human Services, 2018).
- Drug overdose rates in the Central United States have grown dramatically over the last decade. Missouri, Oklahoma, and Wyoming have rates of overdose nearly double the rates of New York, California, Texas, or Virginia and nearly double the rates of Eastern rural states. Unfortunately, some central states still

do not make naloxone available to the public, nor have they passed "Good Samaritan" laws protecting bystanders who report overdose incidents to emergency services, or who administer naloxone to someone who has overdosed. Some Central U.S. states with high levels of overdose have taken action to make overdose deaths less likely by making naloxone more available and its use in an emergency more protected (Dombrowski, Crawford, Khan, & Tyler, 2016).

- Prescription opioid use and abuse is increasingly becoming a public health crisis across the United States. Over the last two decades, opioid-related deaths have increased dramatically to become a serious public health concern. Opioid-related mortality rates have reached epidemic levels in rural areas of the United States, such as Appalachia, New England, and the Mountain West with rural counties having an 87% higher chance of receiving an opioid prescription compared to persons living in large metropolitan areas (Mundell, 2019; Rigg, Monnat, & Chavez, 2018).
- Rates of opioid-related inpatient hospital stays, emergency room visits, and mortality are high in predominantly rural states like Maine, Kentucky, and West Virginia, but rates are lowest in other largely rural states such as Iowa and Nebraska (Weiss et al., 2017).
- Newer and less addictive types of pain control are needed (Dryden, 2016).

Cancer disparities are found in rural populations. Rural women are less likely to receive screening mammograms and Pap smears than urban women. In one study, cancer incidence was 447 cases per 100,000 in metropolitan counties and 460 per 100,000 in nonmetropolitan counties. Cancer mortality rates were 166 per 100,000 in metropolitan counties and 182 per 100,000 in nonmetropolitan counties. Higher incidence and mortality in rural areas were observed for cervical, colorectal, kidney, lung, melanoma, and oropharyngeal cancers (Blake, Moss, Gaysynsky, Srinivasan, & Groyle, 2017). Rural populations also have a lower proportion of colonoscopies to screen for colorectal cancer. Further, most rural physicians are trained as generalists, therefore not trained to perform colonoscopies (Evans et al., 2015).

Mental health is another concern in rural settings as 19.1% of rural residents 18 years and older had any mental health issue and 4.9% experienced serious thoughts of suicide (RHIH, 2020b). The prevalence of mental health is similar between rural and urban, yet there are limited services available to address this issue in rural communities. Accessibility of services, availability of services, and acceptability are all barriers for those residing in rural areas (RHIH, 2020b).

Rural C/PHNs need to consider the *Healthy People 2030* objectives priority areas as guides for improving the health status of clients in rural communities.

Community Health Nursing in Rural Settings

Most rural nurses working in the community are thought to have little education in public health, as the associate degree in nursing is often accepted by health departments in rural areas (Harris et al., 2015). However, rural areas promote a broad scope of C/PHN practice, as these nurses deal with a wide variety of issues—immunizations, home health, school nursing, maternal–child health, emergency preparedness, as well as communicable disease/epidemiology. Rural health departments are often lacking in technological and communication systems, but there is an even greater need for reliable communication capability and training opportunities for rural C/PHNs who provide the majority of care in rural and frontier communities (Knudsen & Meit, n.d.).

Rural community health nurses most often grew up in rural areas or lived for a time in small communities. They frequently have extended family, are active members of their community, and are highly respected professionals.

The rural community health nurse plays many roles:

1. *Advocate*: Assists rural clients, families, and populations in obtaining the best possible care
2. *Coordinator/case manager*: Connects rural clients with needed health and social services, often assisting with information on transportation
3. *Health teacher*: Provides education to individuals, families, or groups on health promotion or other health-related topics (e.g., prepared childbirth, parenting, diabetes maintenance, home safety)
4. *Referral agent*: Makes appropriate connections between rural clients and urban service providers
5. *Mentor*: Guides new community health nurses, nursing students, and other nurses new to the rural community
6. *Change agent/researcher*: Suggests new approaches to solving patient care or community health problems based on research, professional literature, and community assessment
7. *Collaborator*: Seeks ways to work with other health and social service professionals to maximize outcomes for individual clients and the community at large
8. *Activist*: With a deep understanding of the community and its population, takes appropriate risks to improve the community's health

Rural C/PHNs have the opportunity to use autonomy in daily practice. Nurses must rapidly assume independent and interdependent decision-making roles because of the small workforce and large workload. For nurses who live and work in rural areas, resources are limited and demands are many. Rural C/PHNs learn to prioritize tasks quickly and work efficiently with others to get the job done. Referrals to other rural providers are facilitated because providers frequently know one another. Rural C/PHNs may experience the challenge of physical isolation from personal and professional opportunities associated with urban areas. Rural nurses may also feel isolated in their clinical practices because of the scarcity of professional colleagues (Box 27-5).

The rural community health nurse often receives a salary that is lower than that of urban nurses in comparable positions (Harris et al., 2015). However, there are benefits to rural nursing. Housing costs are usually lower than in larger cities and long commutes to and from work on congested highways are often avoided, although rural driving can be hazardous. As a place to live and raise a family, rural communities offer a slower pace of life, open spaces, and friendly atmosphere. The smaller system of health care in a rural community can be advantageous

BOX **27-5** STORIES FROM THE FIELD

Frontier Nursing: Then and Now

As described in Chapter 2, Mary Breckinridge founded the Frontier Nursing Service in 1925, with nurse–midwives providing care to clients in their own homes. Nurses traveled by horseback and on foot into the sparsely populated hollows of Kentucky (American Association for the History of Nursing, 2018). Today, NPs working in nurse-managed clinics in rural Appalachian communities in Virginia were interviewed about their practices, in a classic study by Caldwell (2007), and spoke about their connections to the people and communities they serve. One said, "Here you get to know the whole family and that is rewarding...you know what is important to them...what their worries and concerns are....so you probably get closer to your patient in this area than you might outside here. It becomes an extended family, which is very rewarding" (p. 76).

Another NP described a man with severe COPD who visited her clinic. He was also a patient of another area provider, but when the NP examined the man, she noticed the gauze 4× 4 he had on the back of his neck and enquired about it. The man said he "cut himself shaving." The NP pressed the man to see the wound and found that he had "cancer with the bone exposed," describing it as "the most awful thing that I had ever seen in my life. I could put my fist in there. And you could see his carotids pulsating." She told the patient how serious this was and arranged for a plastic surgeon to see him right away. He had a total neck resection and recovered completely. She reflected, "What if I had accepted his story about the sore and it being all right? It was not what he was coming to see me for...I look at more than just the chief complaint" (p. 77).

1. *What factors are important to consider when caring for clients in a rural setting?*
2. *What situations have you seen in rural settings?*
3. *Knowing more about rural health, would you do anything differently in this scenario?*

to the C/PHN. It may be easier to understand the system and initiate planned change.

However, many rural areas find it difficult to recruit nurses and need to more effectively advertise their benefits. When RN to population ratios are high in both rural and urban areas, years of potential life lost and rates of poor health are significantly improved, as well as rates of teen births and mammography; however, this association was shown to improve even more as the level of rurality increased demonstrating the importance of adequate nurse staffing in all areas (Fields, Bigbee, & Bell, 2016).

MIGRANT HEALTH

Have you ever thought about the people who harvest the fruits and vegetables that you eat? Have you ever thought about who they are, where they come from, where they live, or what their health is like? What would happen to the complex system of agricultural production and distribution if workers were not available to pick crops at peak harvest times? Whatever your political, social, or ethical views on this subject, migrant workers and their families often cross paths with C/PHNs, and we need to understand them in order to effectively provide care (Box 27-6).

BOX **27-6** WHAT DO *YOU* THINK?

Undocumented Migrant Workers

There are many critics of undocumented migrant workers. Some feel that their willingness to work for low wages keeps overall wages lower for everyone working in agriculture, while others feel that migrants are taking jobs away from Americans. The United Farmworkers, an agricultural worker union, introduced the *Take Our Jobs* program in 2010 to address these issues. Unemployed Americans were invited to work in the fields along with migrant farmworkers, but very few accepted this invitation; those that did attempt it had a difficult time keeping up with the grueling pace of work. Stephen Colbert, a television show host and comedian, picked beans and packed corn as part of the challenge, and filmed some of his workday experiences for his late-night show. He also gave testimony to Congress on the need for better wages, living conditions, and visa programs for these workers. What do you think about the issue? You can view this testimony first-hand in the following video (https://www.youtube.com/watch?v=0TYyeNU8Wvc). You can also view Charlie LeDuff taking this migrant challenge in the San Joaquin, California fields (https://www.youtube.com/watch?v=J7TGWaHaUeU).

In addition, a government project was trialed in 1965, when the Bracero Agreement between the United States and Mexico, providing Mexican agricultural workers in the U.S. fields, expired. Farmers complained, stating that crops would rot in their fields. Therefore, project A-TEAM was created—Athletes in Temporary Employment as Agricultural Manpower. A nationwide call was placed to recruit high school boys, providing field labor as their summer job. Although initially 18,000 were registered, only 3,300 actually worked in the fields. Ironically, even though the initial intent was to recruit "jocks," many of the recruits were not athletes but just boys looking for summer jobs. The boys were paid minimum wage—$1.40 per hour at that time—plus a small stipend for filling crates with fruits or vegetables (i.e., 0.05 cents for every crate filled with 30 to 36 cantaloupe). Work was hard, days were long, temperatures were hot, and the boys were not allowed to return home until summer's end. Many of the boys did not last the entire stint. A university history professor, Lori Flores, was quoted as saying "The A-TEAM reveals a very important reality: It's not about work ethic for undocumented workers. It's about the fact that this labor is not meant to be done under such bad conditions and bad wages" (Arellano, 2018, p. 7). The A-TEAM was considered a giant failure and was never tried again!

Migrant farmworkers are an integral part of the farming community in the United States and across the world. In fact:

- The agricultural industry relies heavily on migrant workers to harvest the almost endless array of fresh produce that appears year-round in supermarkets across the United States as fresh, frozen, and canned fruits and vegetables.

- Opponents of immigration restrictions predict that imposing them would jeopardize the supply of labor available to farmers during critical plant and harvest seasons. They contend that more restrictive immigration policies could lead to reduced profits for some farms and threaten the sustainability of agricultural sectors that are heavily dependent on farm labor, especially fruit, tree nuts, vegetables, and horticulture (USDA, 2020).
- More than 3 million seasonal and migrant farmworkers provide labor for the $28 billion vegetable and fruit crops of the United States (National Center for Farmworker Health [NCFH], 2018a).
- Many of these workers are unauthorized or illegal immigrants to the United States, often from Mexico. The vast majority entered this country in an unauthorized manner.

Agricultural Labor and Immigration Policies Changing

Despite their importance to American agriculture, migrant workers often go unnoticed beyond the fringes of the camps and farms to which they travel in order to pursue their livelihood. The number of migrant agricultural workers there are in a particular region, state, or even in the nation is difficult to estimate due to high mobility, language and cultural differences, and varying levels of citizenship status (NCFH, 2018a). California, Texas, Washington, Florida, Oregon, and North Carolina currently have the highest number of migrant farmworkers (NCFH, 2018a). They come with the hope of bettering their impoverished lives. Some are legal residents, but most are undocumented aliens and live in fear of deportation. All endure backbreaking, menial labor for low wages and are often deprived of basic rights to safe working conditions, adequate sanitation/housing, health care, and a quality education for their children (see Boxes 27-7 and 27-8).

The United States has passed legislation affecting agricultural workers. States across the nation have implemented policies to address growing numbers of unauthorized workers, whether they work on farms or elsewhere. In over 20 states, legislatures have passed laws that penalize employers who knowingly hire unauthorized workers. At least 100 municipalities around the nation have proposed or enacted ordinances that penalize businesses for hiring and landlords for renting to unauthorized workers (USDA, 2018).

The H-2A Temporary Agricultural Program provides a legal means to bring foreign-born workers to the United States to perform seasonal farm labor on a temporary basis; these consist of crop farmers and producers of livestock. Employers must demonstrate, and the U.S. Department of Labor must certify, that efforts to recruit U.S. workers were unsuccessful. Employers must also pay a state-specific minimum wage, provide housing, and pay for transportation. One of the most significant indicators of the scarcity of farm labor is the fact that H-2A employment applications and certifications have quadrupled in the past 12 years, increasing from just over 48,000 positions certified in 2005 to 200,000 in 2017 (USDA, 2018). With the H-2A visa, there are restrictions against farmworkers changing employers, and this could affect their work safety climate (Arcury et al., 2015).

BOX 27-7 U.S. Migrant Worker Demographics

Origin and Nationality

- Most are foreign-born (73%), with about 69% from Mexico.
- Forty percent have been in the United States 20 or more years, while 35% for 10 to 19 years.
- Forty-seven percent of the crop workers are unauthorized, 31% are citizens, and 22% have work visas.

Age

- The age of agricultural workers in the United States has been increasing since 2000.
- Seventeen percent are between the ages of 14 and 24, compared to 35% in 1999 to 2000.
- Twenty-seven percent are between 25 and 34 years.
- Twenty-four percent are between 35 and 44 years.
- Eighteen percent are between 45 and 54 years.
- Fourteen percent are 55 years or more, compared to 5% in 1999 to 2000.

Sex/Marital Status/Offspring

- Seventy-two percent of agricultural workers are male, and 28% are female.
- Sixty-three percent are married, 29% are single, and 8% are divorced.
- Fifty-seven percent are parents, 29% have one to two children, and 14% have three or more children in the household.

Education

- Thirty-six percent have completed grades 1 to 6.
- Twenty-one percent have completed grades 7 to 9.
- Twenty-eight percent have completed grades 10 to 12.
- Eleven percent have completed education beyond grade 12.

English Language

- Twenty-seven percent cannot speak English "at all."
- Forty-three percent speak English "a little" or "somewhat."
- Thirty-one percent speak English "well."

Migrant Status and Seasonality

- Approximately 16% of farmworkers are considered migrant (traveling 75 miles to obtain farm jobs).
- Many travel to multiple farm sites within a year.
- About 84% are considered seasonal agricultural workers.
  - Most (41%) work in fruit and nut crops.
  - Others (22%) work in horticulture (22%) and vegetables (21%) (NCFH, 2018a).

Compensation

- Only 8% of U.S. migrant farmworkers are salaried.
- The majority are paid low hourly wages (83%) or by the piece (9%).

Source: National Center for Farmworker Health (NCFH) (2018a).

BOX 27-8 STORIES FROM THE FIELD

A Case of Active Tuberculosis in a Rural Community

As the C/PHN in a rural community, I received many types of referrals for families including maternal child, older adults, child abuse, or communicable disease cases. The small public health district office was located in a small agricultural town of approximately 20,000 people, with a large Spanish-speaking population. One day, I responded to a new, active tuberculosis (TB) case. A 20-year-old Hispanic male had been in the county hospital and was on respiratory isolation. I would need to examine his living conditions and his contacts.

Gregorio explained that he and his brothers had traveled from his home country of Chiapas, Mexico, to the United States. There were 20 names in total that were close contacts and needed follow-up. They lived in a two-bedroom home, without furniture, and each man took a spot on the floor to sleep at night. One by one, each was interviewed for TB risk assessment and a TB skin test was placed. On return to the home in 2 days, skin tests were read, and those who had positive tests were referred to the community health center for chest x-rays.

Gregorio was hospitalized until he was no longer communicable. The county health department instituted daily directly observed therapy (DOT) and assisted with transportation to medical appointments.

1. *What do you see as the role of the community health nurse in this situation?*
2. *Discuss how communicable disease control and surveillance looks different in a rural setting.*

—Judy H. Pedro, MSN, RN, APHN-BC

Migrant Farmworkers: Profile of a Nomadic Population

Maintaining a low public profile, migrant workers are often marginalized from mainstream society. They remain unseen, unheard, poorly understood, and excluded from many programs that provide health care assistance for low-income people.

- The migrant worker is a kind of disenfranchised person, for whom many do not want to take responsibility. Yet the needs of these workers are great. They are plagued with different, more complex, and more frequent health problems than the general population (Migrant Clinicians Network, 2017a).
- Common ailments include infectious diseases (e.g., TB, parasites), gastrointestinal disorders, dermatitis, pesticide exposure, emotional distress and depression, vision and eye problems, cancer, and chronic illnesses, such as asthma, bronchitis, diabetes, and hypertension.
- They are often afflicted by poverty, poor nutrition, substandard housing conditions, extended working hours, and grueling, often unsafe, working conditions.
- Their demographics, socioeconomic conditions, and lifestyle resemble those of a low-income country, despite the fact that they live and work in one of the most prosperous nations in the world.
- Although migrant families are in dire need of health resources, various economic, cultural, and language barriers prevent this aggregate from accessing available health services. Poverty, frequent mobility, low literacy, and language and cultural barriers impede farmworkers access to cost-effective health care and social services.
- Approximately 30% of all agricultural worker households had total family incomes below the U.S. government's poverty guidelines. The average wage earned by a migrant worker was $10.19 per hour. Further, only 51% of agricultural workers reported being covered by workers' compensation insurance (NCFH, 2018a).

Migrant workers often live and work in areas where health care practitioners are in short supply. Among Latino immigrants, common barriers to utilizing the health care system include access to insurance, limitations in the type of health care utilized, discrimination in health care services, immigration fears, stigmas, lack of social and financial capital, communication problems, and long waiting periods for access to health care (Migrant Clinicians Network, 2017a). Additional barriers include limited transportation, prejudice because of immigrant status, mistreatment because they are "undocumented," lack of time-efficient health care delivery methods, increasing cost of health care, and needing services not being offered (NCFH, 2018a). Migrant workers may use traditional cultural remedies and folk healers, if available, but often also use low-cost, over-the-counter medications, and professional health care systems, blending both traditional and U.S. health care practices (McCullagh, Sanon, & Foley, 2015).

Historical Background

Both historically and internationally, farmers have rarely been able to permanently employ the large workforces needed to harvest their crops.

- Throughout the 19th century, however, the small, family-owned farms typical in the United States got through the harvest by using schoolchildren, neighbors, and local day laborers. As time went by, this became more difficult to accomplish.
- During the 1920s, over half a million Mexicans migrated to the United States, many drawn to work in seasonal agriculture. With the Great Depression, many of the small, independently run farms went bankrupt, and citizens were concerned about limited employment opportunities.
- The United States has experienced farm labor shortages for the past century, becoming more severe during World War II. To meet the demand for farm laborers, the Bracero Program was created in 1942, which allowed over 4 million guest workers to come in from rural, poor areas in Mexico due to agricultural worker shortages in the United States.
- In 1964, the program was replaced by the H2 Temporary Guest Worker program, with H-2A being agricultural workers and H-2B being guest workers who perform nonagricultural work.

- In 2016, the U.S. Department of State certified 165,741 H-2A visas out of 172,654 that were requested (NCFH, 2018a).
- In 2016, the states with the highest numbers of H-2A workers were Florida, North Carolina, Georgia, and Washington (Figueroa, Moberg, & Hennen, 2017).
- Some studies have noted an increase in the agricultural worker population over the last decade, and the presence of agricultural workers has been shown to increase the overall economic output of the regions in which they work. In fact, research conducted about the agricultural economy of Michigan found that agricultural workers contributed over $23.3 million dollars to the state's economy annually by enabling farmers to produce higher-value crops, after wages and housing were deducted. Stringent immigration laws passed in Arizona and Georgia demonstrated the devastating impact of farm labor shortages (NCFH, 2018a).

Living apart from society, the plight of migrant farmworkers was largely ignored until exposure on a 1960 television documentary—Edward R. Murrow's *Harvest of Shame*—created a national outcry. This led to the passage of the Migrant Health Act of 1962, which addressed the specific health needs of migrant workers for the first time in U.S. history. This act authorized delivery of primary and supplementary health services to migrant farmworkers (NCFH, 2018a). Federally funded migrant health clinics serve areas in the United States where significant number of migrant farmworkers gather. In 2010, 165 migrant clinics served more than 863,000 seasonal and migrant farmworkers and members of their families, a number far below the estimated 3+ million farmworkers thought to be in this country. Eligibility for services at the clinics includes being principally employed in agricultural labor for the prior 24 months (Farmworker Justice, 2020). Services may be provided seasonally, on a temporary basis, or year-round. Staffing usually includes doctors, nurses, NPs, PAs, outreach workers, social workers, and dental and pharmacy workers, along with health educators.

Transportation may also be a component in some areas. Primary and preventive health care services are provided to migrant workers and their families throughout more than 500 clinic sites. However, funding is often inadequate, and many clinics are not sufficiently staffed or operated to meet the health needs of migrant farmworkers and their dependents. Most migrant health centers receive funding from a variety of sources, including Medicaid in some instances. Additionally, although these clinics exist throughout the United States, large geographic regions are not served well or at all. Other services, such as *promotora programs* that employ Hispanic lay health workers or nursing voucher programs providing health care services at participating clinics and nurse referrals to specialists, are available in some areas. Encouraging recruitment of these health workers targeting Latino communities, especially underserved ones, could potentially increase Latinas' interest in serving as promotoras, improve the quality of promotora work, and more fully engage Latinos in community health programs to address their health issues (Molokwu, Penaranda, Flores, & Shokar, 2016; Schwingel et al., 2017).

Migrant Lifestyle

To understand the health needs of migrant farmworkers and their families, it is important to realize their lifestyle. Migrant workers and their families endure a transient and uncertain life, with long hours, stressful working conditions, low wages, and poor health care. Substandard housing, unsafe working conditions, and language barriers make life even more difficult (USDHUD, 2016). In addition, about 25% of migrant farmworkers have been in the United States for under 1 year; therefore, American customs and behaviors may be foreign to them (Rao, Hancy, Velez, Freeman, & Davis, n.d.).

- Migrant workers are exposed to environmental hazards such as pesticides, extreme temperatures, and chemicals.
- Up to 20,000 pesticide injuries are reported yearly of the 2 million agricultural workers in the United States.
- Those in agriculture and farming are at risk for musculoskeletal injury. In addition, limited or no PPE may be provided.
- Workplace demands such as pressure to work without breaks coupled with fear of job insecurity and deportation affects workplace stress (Moyce & Schenker, 2018).

Depending on the economy and the crop, a migrant farmworker's income varies widely. Migrant farmworkers' average annual income is $11,000; for a family, it is approximately $16,000. This makes farm work the second lowest paid job in the nation (after domestic labor). Even so, despite their poverty, most farmworkers are not eligible for social services. Less than 1% of all farmworkers use general assistance welfare, 2% use social security, and fewer than 15% are Medicaid recipients (NCFH, 2018a).

Migrant Hero

César Chavez founded the National Farm Workers Association (NFWA; later changed to United Farm Workers [UFW]), the first union in agricultural labor history to successfully organize migrant farmworkers.

- As a child, he traveled with his family to harvest crops, but they rarely had enough food to eat and often lived in shacks.
- Work was frequently scarce, wages were low, and labor contractors cheated the family out of the money they earned.
- Moving to California during the Great Depression, the family became part of the migrant community.
- Chavez attended as many as 65 different schools and dropped out of school upon completing eighth grade, to help support his family by working full time in the fields (Biography, 2019).
- Chavez organized many successful strikes and boycotts, the most famous one being the boycott of California grapes as a protest against the indiscriminate use of spraying by growers in 1968. This boycott lasted for longer than 5 years, and on two occasions, he fasted as a protest against the use of agricultural pesticides. His efforts united people who, as individuals, had no significance in the power structure.

- His legacy is an example of how people can unite to build power together. He achieved great recognition, although he never had the financial trappings of success.
- Throughout his life, he ignored personal hardships to continue the struggle with union victories and losses. Chavez and his union won several victories for migrant farmworkers when many growers signed contracts with the union.
- As a labor leader, Chavez employed nonviolent means to bring attention to the plight of farmworkers. He led marches, organized boycotts, and went on several hunger strikes (Biography, 2019).

Health Risks of Migrant Workers and Their Families

Poverty, transient lifestyle, low literacy, language barriers, and cultural barriers impede migrant workers' access to social services and cost-effective health care (MCN, 2017a). In addition, migrant workers who use health services must overcome other issues: limited means of transportation, lack of time-efficient health care delivery methods, and the medical referral system. In some areas, federally funded health centers are available to provide serves to populations with limited access to health care. These include low-income populations, the uninsured, those with limited English proficiency, agricultural workers, individuals and families experiencing homelessness, and those living in public housing (NCFH, 2018a). In 2015, the Health and Resources Services Administration (HRSA) of the U.S. Department of Health and Human Services reported that the health center program provided health care to 910,172 agricultural workers and their families, with 92% covered by specific funds to provide services to this population. According to National Center for Farmworker Health (NCFH) (2018a) data, the most common diagnoses reported by these Health Centers for migrant workers included the following:

- Overweight/obesity
- Hypertension
- Diabetes mellitus
- Otitis media and eustachian tube disorders
- Depression and other mood disorders

Migrant workers who are lawfully in the United States (including H-2A workers) may receive coverage under the ACA. Legal farmworkers whose income is below 138% of the federal poverty line may receive health care through Medicaid. Workers unauthorized cannot receive health insurance (MCN, 2017a).

Undocumented migrant farmworkers are "10.7 and 3% less likely to use U.S. and foreign health care, respectively, compared to documented farmworkers" (Luo & Escalante, 2018, p. 923). Health insurance has been found to significantly increase hired migrant farmworkers' use of U.S. health care by 22.3%. Notably, compared to their documented working peers, undocumented migrant farmworkers are less likely to utilize private health clinics and are even less likely to rely on migrant health centers, even when these providers are their most viable sources of health services (Luo & Escalante, 2018). National statistics on migrant seasonal workers are sparse, with much of the data regional and only sporadically collected. Some of the statistics include the following:

- Migrant workers are a vulnerable and underserved population, with an average life expectancy of 49 years, compared to 77.2 years for most Americans. They have a greater disease burden than other populations and work in occupations with high hazard levels.
- TB rates tend to be 6 times higher for migrant workers and are at increased risk for contracting a viral, fungal, bacterial, and parasitic infections (La Cooperativa, 2020).
- Migrant children are often delayed for immunizations and have an increased incidence of TB; intestinal parasites and infections; nutritional deficiencies and malnutrition; skin, respiratory tract, and ear infections; dental problems; and pesticide and lead exposure (SAF, 2011–2019).
- Migrant workers have high rates of work-related conditions, such as musculoskeletal injuries, lacerations, falls, heat stress, eye injuries, hearing loss, and skin diseases, because of equipment use and exposure to pesticides and other chemicals, dust, exposure to hot and cold extremes, and sun exposure (MCN, 2017a).
- Migrant children are often exposed to heat and sun, musculoskeletal injuries, pesticides, and hazardous tools and machinery (NCFH, 2018b).
- The data indicate that HIV/AIDS is escalating among migrant farmworkers and that steps need to be taken to prevent the impact among the population and their families. Recommendations are provided for improving health outcomes among migrant workers, preventing HIV transmission, and providing continuous comprehensive care and support for HIV-infected migrant farmworkers (CDC, 2020).
- Poverty, migration patterns, lower educational level, and language barriers may make it harder for some Hispanics/Latinos to get HIV testing and care. Undocumented Hispanics/Latinos may be less likely to use HIV prevention services, get an HIV test, or get treatment for HIV because of concerns about being arrested and deported (CDC, 2020).
- Migrants disproportionately suffer from the effects of COVID-19 due to economic hardships brought on by shutdowns and social distancing; contagion risk due to overcrowding, predisposed health issues, lack of access to health care, and uninsured status; and as targets for hate and discrimination (Migrant Policy Institute, 2020).

Occupational Hazard

The hazards of agricultural employment, coupled with limited legal protection, jeopardize the health of the migrant farmworker. Migrant workers have higher rates of adverse job-related exposures and working conditions, which lead to poor health outcomes, injuries, and occupational fatalities. Health disparities of migrant workers are related to environmental and occupational exposures, as a result of language/cultural barriers, access to health care, documentation status, as well as the political climate of the host country (Moyce & Schenker, 2018). In a Canadian study with migrant workers, participants reported that they did not speak up when they saw unsafe workplace practices and even did not report their injuries for fear of losing employment and fear of retaliation (Yanar, Kosny, & Smith, 2018). Falls, cuts, muscle strains and sprains, and repetitive motion injuries (e.g., carpal tunnel syndrome) commonly afflict migrant laborers. Migrant and seasonal farm work typically requires stooping, long hours working in wet clothes, working with sometimes contaminated soil and water, climbing, carrying heavy loads, and exposure to the sun and the elements. Failure to perform these activities on a rigid timetable dictated by seasons and weather can result in crop loss. This urgency compels farmworkers to labor in all weather conditions, including extreme heat or cold, rain, bright sun, and high humidity.

- Migrant workers are among the most vulnerable members of society. They are often engaged in what are known as "3-D jobs—dirty, dangerous, and demanding (sometimes degrading or demeaning)"—and these workers are often hidden from the public eye and from public policy.
- They work for less pay, for longer hours, and in worse conditions than do nonmigrants and are often subject to human rights violations, abuse, human trafficking, as well as violence.
- Migrant workers are more likely to take greater risks on the job, do work without adequate training or protective equipment, and do not complain about unsafe working conditions (Moyce & Schenker, 2018).

Pesticide Exposure

Migrant farmworkers may be at higher risk of exposure to cancer-causing chemicals than the general population (Fig. 27-11). They are exposed to pesticides used routinely in the fields: picking produce that has been sprayed; walking behind farm equipment that is mobilizing dirt that has been treated; contact with pesticide spray from a neighboring field; bringing home pesticide residue on their clothes and shoes; or exposure to chemical residues in the soil, air, food, and well water (MCN, 2017a).

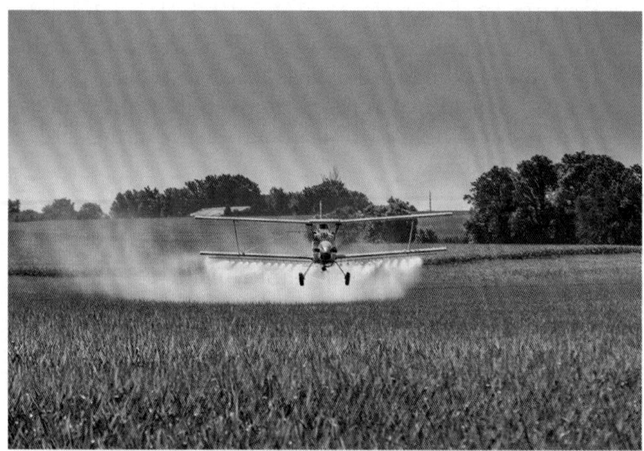

FIGURE 27-11 A crop duster applies chemicals to a field of vegetation.

- A large body of evidence exists on the role of pesticide exposures in the increased incidence of human diseases such as cancers, Alzheimer's disease, Parkinson's disease, amyotrophic lateral sclerosis, asthma, bronchitis, infertility, birth defects, ADHD, autism, diabetes, and obesity (Mostafalou & Abdollahi, 2017).
- A study by Butler-Dawson, Galvin, Thorne, & Rohlman (2016) indicated that children in farming communities are at increased risk from pesticides due to a parent working in agricultural. Further, organophosphate exposure may be associated with deficits in learning on neurobehavioral performance, especially in tests of motor function. Even though this pesticide is being phased out in the United States, we still see elevated levels in agricultural households.
- While research shows pesticide-associated cancers are higher in farmworkers, data strongly suggest that cancer is even higher in farmworker children. This is due to "a number of predisposing events occurring prior to conception, in utero, and/or after birth" likely resulting in a greater incidence of pesticide-related cancer in farmworker children (National Center for Farmworker Health, 2018b).

Pesticide exposure levels in reproductive-age farmworkers consistently exceed levels in the general population. It is estimated that thousands of farmworkers suffer pesticide poisoning each year, but exact counts are not possible because of inadequate surveillance systems and reluctance of farmworkers to report injuries (Farmworker Justice, 2020). Surveillance systems are only in place in 11 states; the Sentinel Event Notification System or Occupational Risk (SENSOR) is a means of reporting pesticide-related injuries as well as other occupational illnesses and injuries (CDC/National Institute for Occupational Safety & Health, 2017). Some farmworkers, primarily those without H-2A visas, were less likely to be provided pesticide safety equipment and often were not notified when pesticides were applied. Reporting of pesticide-induced morbidity and mortality is not required in every state. California has the oldest and most thorough pesticide surveillance system in the United States, beginning in 1971 that requires health care providers to contact their LHD whenever they suspect an illness or injury is related to pesticide exposure. The health department then alerts the county agricultural commissioner and also completes a Pesticide Illness Report (California Department of Pesticide Exposure, 2020).

But, even with reporting laws, many cases are never recognized because workers do not seek medical care. Pesticide burns and rashes often go untreated because of lack of education about the dangers of pesticides and lack of available services. Migrant workers are often unaware of the hazards of pesticides.

- Arcury et al. (2018) found that migrant farmworkers and nonfarmworkers had detections for pesticide and herbicide urinary metabolites.
- Griffith et al. (2018) compared children's pesticide exposures by expressing the child's pesticide metabolite concentration as a fraction of the adult's concentration living in the same household. Exposures in their community were consistently higher, often

above the 95th percentile of the exposures reported by the National Health and Nutrition Examination Survey (NHANES).

- Plascak et al. (2018) determined that dimethyl OP house dust concentrations were 400% higher within homes where at least two residents were agriculture workers.
- Pesticide drift has been shown to result in elevated levels of active compounds in both indoor air and house dust in homes near agricultural application areas. Houses closer to agricultural herbicide applications had significantly elevated levels of herbicides in house dust than in homes that were further away (Shelton & Hertz-Picciotto, 2015).
- Orchard air-blast applications of pesticides, along with wind direction, can influence pesticide drift from crops into agricultural residences; potential exposures can be analyzed through screening tests (U.S. Environmental Protection Agency, 2018).

Even though it may be required of health care providers to report pesticide poisoning, it is often misdiagnosed because the symptoms can mimic those of viral infections or heat-related illness. Symptoms of pesticide exposure include sore throat, runny nose, headache, fatigue, red/swollen/watery eyes, drowsiness, itchy skin, abdominal pain, and nausea or vomiting. More severe symptoms may include sweating, salivation, blurred vision or pinpoint pupils, fever, severe thirst, muscle twitching, or weakness and incontinence (especially with organophosphate or carbamate exposures). Finally, with the most severe exposures, seizures, respiratory depression, and unconsciousness or coma can occur. There are over 19,000 pesticide products registered with the EPA and more than one thousand active ingredients (U.S. Environmental Protection Agency, 2018). Only a few categories of pesticides account for more than half of the cases of acute illness; these include inorganic compounds, carbamates, pyrethroids, and organophosphates. Although the impact of acute pesticide poisoning is widely recognized, little is understood about the long-term effects of the repeated low-level exposures to which migrant farmworkers are constantly subjected. The Florida Department of Health lists the chronic effects of long-term pesticide exposure as birth defects, cancers, blood disorders, neurological problems, and reproductive issues. Extreme exposure can lead to loss of consciousness, coma, or death (NCFH, 2018a). Numerous studies have examined the link between exposure to pesticides and various neurologic problems and cancer—most often with organophosphate-based pesticides. Some evidence of an association between pesticide exposure and the incidence of diabetes has been found (Grice et al., 2017). Prenatal exposure to organophosphate pesticides has been significantly associated with slightly decreased intellectual development (Hertz-Picciotto & Sass, 2018). Today, it is more common for farmworkers to be exposed to "nonpersistent" pesticides that are metabolized in the body within days (NCFH, 2018a).

The Environmental Exposure History, I PREPARE in Chapter 9, is a helpful assessment tool for community health nurses working with migrant and seasonal workers to use to determine pesticide exposure. When a client presents with symptoms that may be suggestive of pesticide exposure, mnemonic prompts may help to clarify common symptoms (Box 27-9).

BOX 27-9 Mnemonic Prompts to Determine Cholinergic Symptoms of Organophosphate Exposure

Sludge

Salivation
Lacrimation
Urination
Defecation
Gastric secretions
Emesis

Dumbbels

Defecation
Urination
Miosis
Bronchorrhea
Bradycardia
Emesis
Lacrimation
Salivation/seizures/sweating (the four most acute symptoms: bradyarrhythmias, bronchospasm, muscle weakness, and bronchorrhea)

Source: Open Anesthesia (2020); Rajan (2016).

Pesticide exposure can be a single event, may occur multiple times, or can even be continuous. Health effects are thought to be a function of the frequency of exposure and the dose. Most migrant workers come into contact with pesticides through their work. However, exposure to pesticides does not affect only those working in the fields.

- Organophosphates decrease the levels of acetylcholinesterase, found in nerve endings, and can be absorbed through the skin, inhaled, or ingested. Most workers have metabolites present, and farm work and housing close to agricultural fields are common factors associated with exposure (Chem-Tox.com, 2019).
- Drifts from sprayed fields and residues on farmworker clothing, shoes, tools, and skin, as well as food brought from the fields, are all potential sources of exposure. Vehicles can also become contaminated, as can carpets and furniture. Contaminated clothing should be kept in separate hampers and laundered separately; workers need to be encouraged to leave boots and shoes outside their homes and to change clothing and shower before eating and playing with their children. Substandard housing is also a factor.

Agricultural fields are usually located in isolated areas on the outskirts of rural communities (Fig. 27-12). While in these isolated fields, migrant workers often are not provided with sanitation facilities or fresh drinking water. Farmworkers experience more heat fatalities than any other group of outdoor laborers. Migrant farmworkers are often paid by the piece instead of the hour, which incentivizes the workers to not stop for breaks. This is

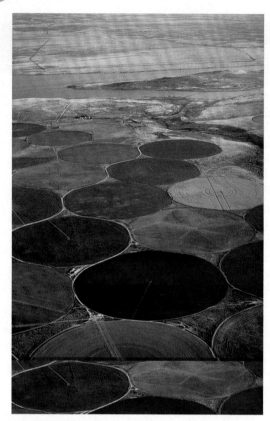

FIGURE 27-12 Fields in Eastern Oregon. (Source: USDA, Agricultural Research Service.)

a ploy that employers use to get the workers to work faster and harder (Moyce & Schenker, 2018). Migrant farmworkers also face many cultural barriers that leave them "marginalized and unempowered" (Kearney, Hu, Xu, Hall, & Balanay, 2016). These cultural barriers are often the reason that many employers do not offer sufficient safety education, shade, hydration, and cool-down rest to prevent heat-related illnesses. Employers must show the employees how important their safety and well-being is to them, while also take proactive measures to conduct risk assessments and health education to reduce unnecessary deaths and prevent heat-related injuries for agricultural workers (Kearney et al., 2016). In fact, it is the employer's responsibility to encourage workers to drink sufficiently to maintain hydration; to ensure water availability; to facilitate worker access to water, shade, and other resources; to provide regular rest breaks of appropriate duration for the work conditions; and to monitor workers for signs of illness (Kearney et al., 2016). California and Oregon have implemented such standards.

U.S. Laws Enacted to Protect the Migrant Farmworker

Below are some of the laws that have been enacted to protect migrant farmworkers and their families. Even so, despite difficult working conditions, farmworkers in the United States are excluded from many federal-level labor protections (Rodman et al., 2016).

- The Migrant and Seasonal Agricultural Worker Protection Act (MSPA) (1992/revised in 2015): protects migrant and seasonal agricultural workers through the establishment of standards relating to wages, housing, transportation, disclosures, and record-keeping. This act also mandates that farm labor contractors register with the U.S. Department of Labor (NCFH, 2018a).
- Occupational Safety and Health Act (1970): specifies that agricultural employers with 11 or more employees who conduct hand labor operations in a field must provide drinking water at a suitable drinking temperature, toilet and handwashing facilities within a reasonable, accessible distance, and the employee must be notified by the employer of the location of such facilities (NCFH, 2018a).
- Agricultural Worker Protection Standard (1992/revised in 2015): Enforced by the Environmental Protection Agency (EPA), this standard is primarily focused on the safe handling of pesticides. It now prohibits children under the age of 18 from handling pesticides, requires that workers do not enter areas recently sprayed with pesticides, and improves protection for workers from retaliation if they make complaints about standard violations (NCFH, 2018a).
- Immigration and Nationality Act: The H-2A portion of this act offers protections for H-2A workers concerning: pay rate; written notification of a work contract with beginning and end dates; the three-fourths guarantee (employee must guarantee employment for at least 75% of the contract period); housing will be provided at no cost to the employee; and the employer will be responsible for transportation to and from work as well as to and from their country of origin (NCFH, 2018a).
- Title VII of The Civil Rights Act of 1964: This act initially involved the prohibition of employment discrimination based on race, sex, color, national origin, and religion. Multiple amendments of this act are especially significant for female migrant farmworkers. Title VII protects employees of both sexes against sexual harassment such as: Quid pro quo (offering a professional benefit in exchange for sexual acts); hostile environments (sexual comments, suggestive physical contact, or showing sexual materials); and retaliation (punishment from the employer for reporting or formalizing a complaint on sexual harassment) (NCFH, 2018a).

Substandard Housing and Poor Sanitation

Quality of housing affects farmworker health (Wiltz, 2016). Formal demographic data on farmworker housing are often lacking. Migrant worker housing is often substandard or nonexistent.

- In 1989, the North Carolina Legislature passed the Migrant Housing Act of North Carolina, establishing minimum standards for agricultural worker housing. The Migrant Housing Act requires that any person owning or operating a housing unit for migrant workers and their dependents register with the North Carolina Department of Labor and have the housing inspected prior to the migrants moving in so that corrections needed can be made (Langley et al., 2017).

- Investigative reporting on migrant housing found that in seven states along the midwest and southern territories found mold, sewage, faulty electrical wiring, and pest infestation. To improve living conditions for workers some states have offered tax credit for investors who build farmworker housing (Wiltz, 2016). There is much room for sustained advocacy and action for migrant farmworker housing as access to adequate and safe employer-provided housing for migrant farmworkers is needed.
- Over the last decade, governmental agencies and nonprofit groups have become more interested in the improvement of agricultural worker housing conditions. The U.S. Department of Agriculture's Rural Housing Service, the U.S. Department of Labor, and the U.S. Department of Housing and Urban Development all provide housing services to agricultural workers and can be contacted with agricultural worker housing questions. Some of these programs include the Farm Labor Housing Loans and Grants Program, the National Farmworker Jobs Housing Assistance Program, and the Family Self-Sufficiency Program (NCFH, 2018a).
- In a classic article by Cole and Crawford (1991), a vivid example of one migrant camp in Alabama highlighted workers living in a converted chicken house. An upper portion of the wall had been removed for ventilation, creating easy access for insects and birds. A dirt floor, a single light bulb, and two portable toilets located a distance away were some of the other features. Two sinks in a common living area provided the only water for the almost 60 people who lived in the chicken house. Many did not have mattresses, and because the workers were harvesting potatoes, potato baskets often served as the only furniture.
- Such living situations still exist today. Living with 13 other workers in a three-bedroom home in Watsonville, California, a female farmworker remarked, "We have to put up with this because we can't afford anything else" (Holden, n.d., p. 40).

Migrant farmworkers move frequently, and often have great difficulty securing adequate housing. Farmers who hire workers on H-2A visas are required to provide free housing, but this accounts for only 2% to 5% of the workers. For farmworkers who don't live in state-licensed or inspected facilities, they may live in unregistered labor camps or rely on the private housing market (Wiltz, 2016).

Although data on migrant housing are scant, surveys have uncovered the following:

- Over 50% of all housing units surveyed were overcrowded (compared to only 3% of U.S. households), and 44% of mobile homes were substandard.
- Approximately 25% of the units surveyed had at least one broken appliance or fixture, and 11% had no working stove.
- Between 13% and 39% of housing is owned by employers, and for those lucky enough to find employer-owned housing, over half of those units were offered without charge.
- Agricultural employers most commonly own single-family homes (39%), apartments (14%), dorms/barracks (4%), motels (2%), and some even reported living conditions not meant for human habitation such as in cars, tents, and outdoors (2%).
- Over 25% of housing units were located adjacent to agricultural fields, and more than half of these had no working shower/tub.
- Families with children occupied 65% of moderately or severely substandard units (HAC, n.d.).

Substandard housing is not the only concern. Crowding is also a problem, as many farmworkers, unable to find sufficient numbers of rental units, share housing—sometimes paying per person costs. One of the few studies on migrant housing found that Minnesota seasonal vegetable workers' construction trailer barracks, housing 15 to 20 single migrant workers, rented for $90 per month per person (Migrant Housing, n.d.). When housing cannot be found, workers and families may have to resort to paying rent to live in garages, barns, sheds, chicken coops, or they may be forced to stay in their cars.

Poor Nutrition, Overweight, and Obesity

Migrant and seasonal farmworkers and their families have higher rates of obesity and are more likely to be obese and overweight (Lim, Song, & Song, 2017). Despite often working among fruit and vegetable crops, migrant families often have difficulty procuring food and maintaining a sufficient supply. Farmworkers constitute a vulnerable population with several characteristics that put them at risk for poor dietary quality: low income, food insecurity, rural isolation, poor housing, and lack of access to food subsidy programs. In addition, parental feeding styles may underlie poor dietary quality for children in farmworker families, where dietary quality is poor. Because of the connections of diet quality to obesity and the negative health outcomes of obesity, interventions to improve dietary quality for migrant farmworker families are necessary (Quandt et al., 2016). Quandt et al. (2018) also found that less than one in five migrant families supplement meals with garden produce and food from food pantries, farmers markets, and hunting, and fishing. Approximately one half of lunches and 25% of dinners are purchased from vendors or other commercial sources, while 20% report issues with food security. Food-related practices of migrant farmworkers require change to improve the inclusion of fresh produce and other nutrient-dense foods. Common health problems of migrant children are similar to their parents and include general poor nutrition, anemia, vitamin A deficiency.

Risks to Social, Emotional, and Behavioral Health

- Migrant children are often called upon by their families to stay home from school to care for younger children, attend to other household chores, or even to work alongside their parents in the fields. Many children of farmworkers report beginning as early as age 10 (MCN, 2017b).
- They may feel socially estranged, be constantly moving, have difficulty finding health-promoting

recreational activities, and have difficulty assimilating (MCN, 2017b). This causes stressors related to immigration status.

- Migratory patterns for farm worker's children make it difficult to complete credits and stay in school. The transient nature of farm working means children may leave the school year early or receive partial instruction for an academic year (Granados, 2018).

Migrant children are less likely to graduate from high school, because educational interruption and difficulty "catching up." Globally, children between the ages of 7 and 14 who live in a rural setting are less likely to attend school but more likely to work. The average level of education completed was the eighth grade (NCFH, 2018b).

Research on children whose parents have been arrested, detained, and/or deported has led to parental depression and poor cognitive and behavioral outcomes for children (Migration Policy Institute, 2015). According to the AAP policy Detention of Immigrant Children, children seeking refuge in the United States endure emotional and physical stress and should not be separated from families but instead should be treated with dignity and respect, according to the recently released. Separation from parents, siblings, and other relatives and caregivers could exacerbate the children's health problems and could also overwhelm the system and cause a crisis in care. The situation becomes even more complicated when one parent of legal children is born in the United States and is a legal citizen and the other is not. Mixed-status families are extremely vulnerable in terms of access to health care and increased chances of being impacted by family disruption through deportation removal (Vargas & Pirog, 2016).

Ramos, Carlo, Grant, Trinidad, & Correa (2016) study results indicated that stress and depression were positively associated with occupational injury. Further, occupational injury was a significant factor for depression. Participants who had been injured on the job were more than seven times more likely to be depressed. These results highlight the interconnection between the work environment and mental health.

Intimate Partner Violence

Intimate partner violence (IPV) is a serious public health problem with substantial consequences for women's physical, sexual, and mental health. Migrant farm-working women are particularly at risk in an intimate relationship because of cultural beliefs and environmental factors, which include challenges with the migratory lifestyle, limited finances, as well as poor working and living conditions. In addition, the migrant women are often less aware of resources to advocate for themselves within the health care system, making interventions difficult (MCN, 2017a). While health care provider screening for IPV increases the rates of identification, many providers do not effectively screen (Wilson et al., 2015). Research on domestic violence among this vulnerable population is scant, but more than 1,000 battered farmworker women in a multicenter study were interviewed and researchers identified the typical profile as:

- Childbearing age (15 to 40)
- Hispanic
- Afraid of their partner
- Married or living with partner
- Drug or alcohol use by partner

The overall incidence was 24.5%. Fifty percent of abused women were pregnant at the time of the abuse (MCN, 2017c). What makes farmworker domestic violence so significant is the fact that these women often experience language barriers, do not have adequate access to health care, live isolated lives with little social support, and fear deportation if they report the abuse—all factors that lead them to endure their violent situation in silence. One example is a migrant woman, who shared a one-room dwelling with her husband, infant, and five single men. Her husband became increasingly violent and unpredictable. He began to beat her and the baby, and she was unable to predict what would initiate a violent attack. She finally fled when one of the men living with them also began beating her. She attributed the aggressive behavior to the powerlessness felt by the men. The Violence Against Women Act of 1994 affords protection for undocumented battered women and children by allowing them to seek legal immigration status without the help of their abusers (MCN, 2017c). C/PHNs must be aware of these issues and what resources are available in the community (Box 27-10).

Infectious Diseases

- TB is a common infectious disease among farmworkers.
- The number of agricultural worker patients diagnosed with TB at Migrant Health Centers in 2016 was 261, equating to a prevalence rate of 30.3 cases per 100,000 patients.
- Research conducted with migratory workers near the U.S.–Mexico border found that 55% of the 109 workers tested positive for a latent TB infection (NCFH, 2018a). Because of their migrant patterns, it is difficult to be accurately diagnosed and to complete treatment regimens; they endure poor access to health care and social isolation.
- Many factors may prevent them from successfully completing a treatment regimen, and language barriers, along with cultural differences, may preclude them from fully understanding the impact of their disease on themselves and others. For instance, a Mexican migrant worker may be diagnosed with TB in California and begin treatment there but may move to Washington state to pick cherries and run out of medication before completing treatment. Moving back to California for summer work, he may again start treatment but may travel home to Mexico during the winter, only to be reinfected by an older, untreated member of his extended family.
- Migrant children are at increased risk for respiratory and ear infections, intestinal parasites, skin infections, TB, and delayed development (MCN, 2017b). Lack of awareness that minor symptoms, such as diarrhea, fever, or ear aches, may indicate a more serious underlying issue can be problematic. An earache is minor, but it can lead to a major problem, such as deafness, if left untreated. Delays in seeking medical attention, due to poverty and a lack of health insurance, can create long-standing health issues.

BOX **27-10** LEVELS OF PREVENTION PYRAMID

Domestic Violence in the Migrant Population

SITUATION: Although the migrant lifestyle can be difficult for the entire family, women and children suffer most from family violence that the migrant way of life promotes. Research is scant; however, informal discussions occur among women and health care providers. Outreach workers sometimes possess lists of men who are abusive and their victims. Isolation and subjugation to a patriarchal system usually prohibit migrant women from seeking help if they are abused. Fear of consequences and difficulty expressing negative views about their husbands prevent women from speaking out (MCN, 2017c).

GOAL: Prevent intimate partner violence.

Tertiary Prevention

Rehabilitation	*Health Promotion and Education*	*Health Protection*
▪ Promote family rehabilitation, with or without abuser in the home. ▪ Encourage ways to eliminate or reduce social and geographic isolation among vulnerable women.	▪ Alleviate stressors of the migrant lifestyle, such as overcrowding and substandard living conditions. ▪ Provide emotional support and educate on what constitutes abuse. ▪ Promote self-esteem and encourage women can take control of their situation.	▪ Encourage women to contact health care providers as they migrate. ▪ Encourage women to find appropriate lay community outreach workers for support. ▪ Encourage migrant women to unite and create an environment that allows them to speak out while supporting one another against abuse.

Secondary Prevention

Early Diagnosis	*Prompt Treatment*
▪ Promptly identify abused women—through self-identification or by other family members or professionals—remove from the dangerous situation.* ▪ Keep communication lines open, be culturally sensitive, and examine for injuries.	▪ Secure victim in a safe battered women's shelters. ▪ Assist victims to regain self-esteem.

*Secondary prevention is difficult because of limited financial resources, lack of transportation, no nearby friends or relatives for support, language barriers (e.g., non–English speaking), and limited safe shelters for battered women in rural areas.

Primary Prevention

Health Promotion and Education	*Health Protection*
▪ Create awareness of the harsh living conditions that migrant families endure. ▪ Advocate for improved and safe living conditions on state and national levels. ▪ Provide adequate housing that eliminates.	▪ Train bilingual and bicultural lay migrant women on the issues of spousal abuse and help them form support groups. ▪ Provide opportunities for women and men to improve self-esteem that will change attitudes toward each other.

Migrant workers are at greater risk of HIV infection due to inconsistent condom use; heterosexual contact with an infected male; use of commercial sex workers due to the shortage of women in the rural communities; and use of lay injections, where untrained peers will inject a migrant with vitamins and antibiotics and reuse needles (Rural Health Information Hub, 2018b). They also note that there is now a higher prevalence of HIV found in rural areas of Mexico, as workers bring the infection back to their homes. HIV-positive status may be misunderstood and, because of stigmatization and fears of deportation, may be purposely hidden from health officials. Estimated HIV rates are reported to be between 0.47% and 13%, depending on geographic area and personal risk factors like drug abuse; however, accurate national prevalence rates are almost impossible to attain (MCN, 2017a). Other infectious diseases (e.g., hepatitis, enteric diseases, and parasites) may commonly afflict migrant workers, often because of inadequate sanitation and hygiene facilities.

Whatever your viewpoint on this issue, it is important to the public's health that basic health care services be available to vulnerable populations. Continued efforts must be made to conduct research assessing risks and hazards, especially those of pesticide exposure. Many government publications document the despair and isolation of migrant workers, yet very little has been done to address the living and working environments that contribute to diminished health. Although migrant workers are a mobile population and difficult to study, they represent an important, integral part of our economy; infectious disease among this population increases health risks for all (NCFH, 2018a).

Unique Methods of Health Care Delivery and Primary Prevention

Because migrant health centers do not adequately meet the health needs of the entire migrant community, several innovative methods of health care delivery have been developed and implemented by community health nurses.

- Several programs are using promising models to intervene to address some of the social determinants of child health by utilizing existing programs and also linking community partners to better serve the community. An example is the partnership between Farmworker Justice and the Migrant Clinician's Network working together to monitor initiatives to improve children's health (MCN, 2017b). Migrant education programs, especially with Mexican American resource teachers as role models, have also been helpful.
- Mobile health vans staffed with bilingual community health nurses and lay workers can travel to migrant camps; this provides an effective strategy for outreach health screening and education. By going to migrant camps and delivering care during nonwork hours such as evenings and weekends, community health nurses increase health access and overcome barriers. Although migrant families receive only fragmented acute care, a nurses' outreach team can succeed in encouraging migrant farmworkers to prevent illness with immunizations, good nutrition, and healthy lifestyles. A viable alternative to traditional medical clinics, the mobile nursing clinic provides primary care to an underserved population through health promotion, disease prevention, and early treatment (Williams, 2017).
- Mobile dental vans can provide services to migrant worker's children, often with arrangements made through school nurses and dental care provided by dental schools or through partnerships. Barriers to good oral health include lack of insurance, high cost of services, language, immigration status, socioeconomic status, and fear/trust (Ponce-Gonzalez, Cheadle, Aisenberg, & Cantrell, 2019). Children of migrants are suffering from poor oral health; this disparity can be reduced by improving their parents' literacy in their primary language and educating parents regarding good oral health practices. An appropriate oral health policy remains crucial for marginalized populations (Reza et al., 2016). Migrant farmworkers were reported to have low levels of knowledge about oral cancer risk factors and signs/symptoms and to be less likely to seek preventive care (Dodd, Schenck, Chaney, & Padhya, 2016). Migrant preschoolers were found to have overall low-quality diets, with fewer than recommended levels of vegetables, fruits, and whole grains in one study (Quandt et al., 2016).
- Hispanic women have greater incidence and mortality rates of cervical cancer when compared with non-Hispanic Whites in the United States Fleming et al. (2018). Peer-led health instruction and coaching via Charles (talking circles) may improve cervical cancer screening and improve detection rates among farmworker communities.

Mobility impedes continuity of care, and the inadequate system of medical record keeping for the migrant population is frustrating and challenging. Data information systems are vital components for monitoring the health status of individual farmworkers as they migrate, as well as essential for generating research and follow-up care for long-range health planning. Data also help justify appropriation of monies to migrant health agencies. The Health Center Resource Clearinghouse (n.d.) is a 501c3 nonprofit organization that creates practical solutions intersecting poverty, migration, and health. They have instituted tracking systems and clinical tools for diabetes, CVD, cancer, and prenatal networks, to name a few. Another system, *TBNet* promotes the completion of TB treatment among migrant populations.

The medical histories of migrant children are often unknown to current providers. The U.S. Department of Education (n.d.) now offers the Migrant Student Information Exchange (MSIX) that permits states to transfer health and educational information on migrant students. The MSIX system was a part of the amended *No Child Left Behind Act* that was enacted by Congress to assist states in developing an effective method of tracking educational and health information as well as the number of migratory children in each state. However, the ability to track these children in the migratory lifestyle from one work location to another is often inconsistent. Early intervention for migrating children is not always feasible, but it can greatly improve outcomes.

MiVIA ("my way" in Spanish) is putting health records online and making them available to migrant workers and their health care providers. Workers get a photo identification card, and their records can be accessed only by the use of a personal password. They can access their medical files, medications, a medical reference guide (bilingual), and other resources, such as local clinics and doctors, public transportation, and housing online, no matter their location (MiVIA, 2016). The program began in California's wine country in 2002 but is spreading to more distant locations.

Community Health Nursing in Migrant Settings

Beyond barriers to health care, such as lack of health services, language, and cultural impediments, inadequate transportation, financial strains, underinsurance, and questionable residency status, which are by themselves formidable obstacles, the migrant lifestyle is troubled with challenges. Because of the insecurity and instability inherent in a mobile lifestyle, long-term health goals are difficult to establish and long-term follow-up of any chronic illness is problematic. Nonetheless, C/PHNs provide much-needed services using community resources, innovative thinking, tenacity, and sensitivity.

Strategies for improving the health status and resource use of migrant workers and their families include the following:

- Improving existing services
- Advocating and networking
- Practicing cultural sensitivity
- Using lay personnel for community outreach
- Utilizing unique methods of health care delivery
- Employing information tracking systems

Community health nurses are the major providers of migrant health services and have a crucial role in the development and management of interventions. In response to the growing need for available, accessible, and affordable health care for farmworker families, nurses are called on not only to understand the migrant lifestyle but also to help migrant families overcome the barriers to health care (Box 27-11).

In the past, male migrant workers traveled primarily in organized crews; now, they may travel in family units with women and children. Added attention must be given to family members exposed to the hazards of the migrant lifestyle. Even as many migrant workers settle into communities, the cycle of poverty continues as other workers arrive from impoverished countries. With a paucity of health resources, the C/PHN is sometimes the only health provider who provides care for this population.

Providing care for migrant workers presents a challenge, requiring nurses to be innovative and to go beyond the boundaries of traditional health services (Box 27-12). Although many resources and programs exist to help migrant families, the needs are still overwhelming. By aligning with the goals of *Healthy People 2030* to improve the health of one of the most underserved populations, the community health nurse will also be improving the health of the nation as a whole.

BOX 27-11 PERSPECTIVES

NURSE AND NURSING INSTRUCTOR VIEWPOINTS ON MIGRANT HEALTH

"I spoke with one of my students after clinical last week, and she told me about her work this semester with a 35-year-old single mother of two who had been discharged from the hospital following a lupus flare-up. The student felt that her client was a devoted mother, but she let her 8- and 12-year-old children stay home from school to help with family farm tasks in order to make ends meet. After weekly visits with her client for almost 2 months, she told me—'I was finally able to get her to trust me enough to help her trust others.' She has reached out to her neighbors and asked for help and they are more than willing to lend a hand. Now, her children can return to school and go back to being children instead of day laborers! I told her that sometimes, it takes a strong person to reach out for help and that she is a strong woman!"

Kevin, nursing faculty member, faith-based college, western Massachusetts

"I was having a conversation with students about how to "break the ice" when making home visits to families who have never had home health services. One student mentioned that at the beginning of the semester, she was afraid that her shyness would be her downfall. But in the week that followed, it occurred to her that the best way to establish trust with anyone is to express an interest in answering questions they have before you pose your own. The student now makes it a habit to ask every patient the three things they would like her to know about them that will help her to personalize their care. During week 8 of the clinical semester, the student stated—This was a real "icebreaker" and my patients have been much more open to listening and learning from me once I listen and learn about them!"

Betsy, community health nursing instructor in a northern California school of nursing

"First of all, a nurse should expect the unexpected. Because of the migratory way of life...clients do not always know where they will be next week or next month. Therefore, we must understand that they do not always have their medical records, immunization records, or income records. Hours are very irregular, depending on what time the workers get in from the fields and what time the shifts are. Because of the distances we travel, we work anywhere from 8 to 12 hours a day. The most rewarding part of the job is bringing health services to the underserved and uninsured. The people are so gracious and appreciative of whatever services we provide."

J. S., RN, Michigan

"Since farmworkers come to our area for only 4 months of the year, it is rare that I care for a migrant woman through her entire pregnancy. I may diagnose her pregnancy, I may see her for three or four prenatal visits, or I may meet her only once before she goes into labor and delivers her baby. I struggle with the desire to make a difference in a short period of time and with the disappointment of not being able to follow through."

C. K., CNM, RN, Pennsylvania

"I worked as a Head Start nurse for many years in an agricultural area of California. One of my assignments was a state/county migrant farm labor housing project. I was asked to make a home visit to check on a 4-year-old who hadn't come to preschool in a few days. When I arrived at the family's duplex, I found the sixth grader there, caring for all five of her younger siblings, including the 4-year-old and an 8-month-old baby. When I asked why she was home with all of the children, she guardedly informed me (after some coaxing) that her parents had been picked up in an immigration raid at the tree farm where they worked and had been taken back to Mexico. The children were now alone, with no family nearby. I worked with a nun at Catholic Social Services to provide care for the children until the parents returned to the United States so that the children, who were all U.S. citizens, would not be placed in foster care. The parents had not been allowed to contact their children before being placed on the bus to Mexico, but other workers, who were not undocumented, had seen them go and told the children about their plight. It was heartbreaking to see the fear in their eyes. I quickly went to work looking for resources for them."

Holly, Head Start nurse, California

BOX 27-12 C/PHN USE OF THE NURSING PROCESS

WORKING WITH MIGRANT FAMILIES

Background Data and Assessment

Tom Reynolds is a community health nurse in central Montana. He has three migrant camps in his service area that are homes for primarily Mexican residents. The men primarily work in strenuous construction jobs—masonry, landscaping, and in agriculture (cherry orchards, dairy farm, and ranches). The women work as housekeeping staff in private homes, motels, and hotels in the area. In the evenings, he would stop by the camps to catch up with residents and assess any current health concerns. At the end of a 3-week period, Tom had met with the residents in each of the three camps. The feedback from these informal conversations assisted Tom in the formulation and implementation of a nursing plan of care targeting the health promotion needs of this unique population of residents.

Problem Statements

1. Changes in the family health status secondary to language, transportation barriers, and health literacy barriers
2. Fear as it relates to deportation and separation from family members
3. Occupational and situational injury, illness, and stress because of extended work hours and poverty-level living conditions

Plan and Implementation

Tom researched funding options for a demonstration project that was sponsored by the local health department. The director of the health department agreed to support the project for 6 months if Tom could find matching funds for the project from a local foundation, recruit the needed personnel, and the results were positive.

Tom was able to recruit three other community health nurses, one of whom was bilingual and familiar with the cultural values and practices of the migrant workers. In addition, Tom reached out to the university's undergraduate nursing program and the community health instructor agreed to utilize the three camps as clinical sites for the upcoming semester. The nurses, students, and staff social worker from the health department coordinated weekly evening and weekend visits to each of the three camps. The teams completed a family assessment for each family: established health records, completed a community-based assessment for each of the three camps, administered immunizations, assisted with arranging transportation to and from medical appointments, and enrolled families in the Women, Infants, and Children Supplemental Food Program (WIC). In addition, the teams completed short teaching sessions on topics such as oral care, hand hygiene, family planning, and infant safety.

The students were inspired by Tom's energy and asked to utilize this experience to develop their Capstone Projects that centered on meeting an unmet need of the unique group of residents. The local farmworkers heard about all of the activities at the camp and they began to organize food and clothing drives to assist the residents in meeting the challenges of the warm Montana summers and snowy winters.

Evaluation

The evaluation of the interventions was so positive that the program became a permanent service of the health department. In the months that followed, a nurse practitioner and volunteer dentist were added to the team to provide on-site care and evaluations. With optimal health and a decrease in issues related to health disparities, several families were able to leave the camps and establish permanent homes in the local community.

URBAN HEALTH

Urban health is influenced by the interactions of citizens in three areas:

- Where they reside
- Where they work
- Where they gather for daily life events

According to the World Health Organization (WHO) (2020a) the following facts influence the social determinants of health in **urbanized area** settings:

- Poverty: Often, poor urban households may be hidden in urban areas of higher wealth. Many people are also likely to be pushed into poverty due to higher prices of essential commodities in urban areas.
- Slums: Approximately 33% of the developing world's urban population lives in slums, accounting for close to one quarter of the total global urban population. Slums are characterized by overcrowding, lack of access to safe water and sanitation, and safety concerns. Poor housing conditions, overcrowding, lack of access to safe water and sanitation, and a lack of secure tenure characterize slums. Lack of access to and use of safe, sustainable water and sanitation is globally one of the biggest contributors to ill-health and preventable mortality.
- Poor air quality: Data from >1,600 cities, 88% of the urban population are exposed to particulate matter levels in the air that exceed WHO Air Quality Guideline values.
- Child labor: Globally, 168 million children worldwide are child laborers. Child laborers comprise 11% of the child population as a whole. In urban settings, child domestic labor is a principal phenomenon.
- Health concerns: A range of acute and chronic health concerns and risk factors has emerged in urban settings, and these realities offset earlier gains. Noncommunicable diseases (NCDs) are pervasive to urban living.
- Transportation: Cities and towns within residential urban areas were designed for the convenience of private automobiles, which makes it extremely difficult today to provide efficient access to public services for older people, especially once they are no longer able to drive.
- Substance use and abuse (including alcohol, prescription, and illegal substances).

There is a direct relationship between the health of urban residents and the physical environment, the social influences within the environment, and access to services that support physical health and social well-being. Urban health considers those characteristics of the environment as they relate to the health of the population living within large cities. Characteristics that define urban areas such as size, density, and complexity come with advantages and disadvantages; large size in cities may mean that the public health system can efficiently reach large numbers of people for interventions but may also lead to incomplete coverage for services due to larger populations.

During recent decades, public health crises, such as the flooding from Texas to Arkansas due to excess rain (2019), the Flint, Michigan water crisis (2014) and wildfires in California (2018) powerfully demonstrate the convergence of race, place, and poverty in determining health outcomes. Tung, Cagney, Peek, and Chin (2017) described the Flint water crisis, as an urban nightmare marked by concentrated poverty, deteriorating housing conditions, infrastructure decay, and organizational failure in a city inhabited by predominately poor, black residents. See Chapter 9 for more on this.

Deaton (2018) documented the link between poverty, human rights, and the inequities of the U.S. health system. According to Deaton, 40 million people (12.7%) of the population live in poverty within the United States and that number is growing exponentially because of the inequities in our nation's health system. The following are some of the most astounding findings from his analysis:

- U.S. infant mortality rates are one of the highest in the developed world (ranking 33 out of 36) (America's Health Ranking, 2018).
- The United States has the highest prevalence of obesity in the developed world.
- In access to clean water and safe sanitation, the United States ranked 36th in the world.
- The United States has the highest income inequality rate of all Western nations.
- Eight million more Whites are poor in America than are African Americans living in poverty. Thirty-one percent of poor children are White, 24% are Black, and 36% are Hispanic.
- Seven million Americans making more than 150% of the poverty line ($31,000 for a family of three) dropped below the poverty line after paying medical costs between 2010 and 2014. Over half of them ended up below 50% of the poverty level.

How can the poorest of the poor Americans overcome the health disparities that surround their daily lives? The solution posed by Deaton and other health care advocates is to support the implementation of nationwide universal health coverage.

In 2000, the Johns Hopkins University founded the Urban Health Institute (JHI) as a means to bolster support among an inner-city population. The goals of the Institute (2018) include the following:

- *Facilitate collaborations* between JHI and the Baltimore community around research, community projects, program planning/implementation, and evaluation.
- *Improve the understandings* of JHI as they relate to the health needs and goals of the community and, concurrently, to improve the understandings of the community as to the work that JHI does that has the promise of improving the health and welfare of the community.
- *Strengthen the capacity* of the Baltimore community by bringing the knowledge and skills available through JHI to community-identified needs and issues.
- *Strengthen educational offerings* and opportunities within JHI as they relate to urban health and development.
- *Initiate long-term, cooperative interventions* that will improve the health and well-being of Baltimore and the East Baltimore community.

The New York Academy of Medicine (2020) has organized the Institute of Urban Health to the academy sponsors the *Journal of Urban Health*, a publication that focuses on population-based research with low-income and at-risk populations living in urban areas. But how did the health of these urban communities regress to such conditions that focused efforts are now required? The routes of these conditions trace their origins to the 1800s.

History of Urban Health Care Issues

An examination of urban health care issues requires an in-depth analysis of the vulnerabilities of urban dwellers that has existed for centuries. The following list provides a historical summary of these unique issues:

- Housing: During the mid-1800s and early 1900s, U.S. population increased dramatically due to the influx of millions of immigrants from large European and Eastern European countries. Groups of individuals and families began to congregate in urban tenements and ghetto housing buildings. The 1893 World's Columbian Exposition in Chicago introduced the "city beautiful" concept of replacing crumbling urban cities and tenements with more classical buildings and parks/lakes to address the crime and social problems of the day (Pain, 2016).
- Poverty: Today, Haitian and Middle Eastern families inhabit some of the same neighborhoods that were inhabited by the Eastern European immigrants during the early 1900s. However, many of the same buildings continue to provide less than optimal shelter for this new group of immigrants. Although ghetto living provides a sense of belonging, for many, it is temporary because it engenders more negatives than positives. Children and grandchildren of the original immigrants seek different lives for themselves, away from the urban areas that are often riddled with crime, unsafe housing, and disease. Others, because of poverty, drugs, or fear of being homeless, remain in urban slum areas.
- Access to health care: Access to care remains inequitable due to cultural, economic, and health literacy barriers that were not adequately addressed by many health care organizations.

Two connected disciplines, **urban planning** and public health, have addressed housing and health care issues from the 19th century to the present. Urban planning worked to improve the welfare of individuals and communities by supporting the growth of healthy, effective, appealing, and accessible places. Urban planners often address the community's needs related to diversification of the transportation system, housing, reducing air pollution and greenhouse gases, street network design, and built environment site design; in some large cities, these tasks are handled by separate departments that do not often interface with environmental or public health (Nieuwenhuijsen, 2016).

- *The American Public Health Association* (APHA, 2020) describes the mission of public health to "promote and protect the health of people and the communities where they live, learn, work, and play."
- Public health leaders promote wellness by encouraging healthy behaviors. Together, these disciplines addressed the needs of the identified vulnerable populations. Initially, during the late 19th and early 20th centuries, these two systems were linked in promoting health by facilitating physical activity through the creation of green space.
- They also designed cities to be less vulnerable to contagions. They joined together in preventing infectious diseases by ensuring healthful drinking water and sewage systems (Owens, 2016).
- The target of public health agencies shifted from investigating ways to improve the infrastructure to a focus on germ theories and immunizations, challenges that were easier for physicians to address than changing environments.

Objectives of specialists in urban planning and public health are to support sustainable urban development in developed nations are to mitigate climate change, minimize energy consumption, reduce pollution, protect natural areas, and provide a safe and healthy environment for the citizens, particularly those who comprise the most vulnerable populations. Leaders at the CDC are concerned with factors that affect people and their environments and support efforts that address the improvement of both physical and social environments as related to places to live, work, and play. The CDC's *Healthy Places* describes the components involved: interaction between environment and health, poorly planned growth leading to sprawl, and increased used of vehicles, and healthy community design that promotes health and well-being (2017).

The WHO provides education and information regarding strategies that will optimize the health of cities and their citizens (WHO, 2020b). WHO recognizes the opportunities that exist for urban residents regarding health, education, and safety while acknowledging the unique risks that face urban residents (WHO, 2020a). By 2050, 70% of the global population will live in cities (WHO, 2020a). Issues of overcrowding and lack of available sanitation facilities and clean water increase the risks of communicable diseases for urban residents who reside in urban slums and tenement housing projects. Additionally, there is an increased likelihood of substance use disorders, urban crime, violence, and mental illness due to global poverty issues and barriers posed by the limited health literacy of urban residents. WHO advocates for education and program initiatives that support the physical, emotional, and social health of all urban residents.

The *Healthy People 2030* document addresses societal determinants of health and the environments in which we live, work, and play. Notwithstanding the complexity of urban areas, particularly in large metropolitan cities, health promotion efforts and a focus on healthier environments are key components of this national health effort. Topical areas of concentration include global health, adolescent and older health, and the social determinants of health. These foci allow governmental policy leaders to assess, implement, and evaluate health programs regarding information and resources to optimize health in urban communities.

Emerging Issues in Access to Health Services

Access to health care in the United States is regarded as "unreliable" because many people do not receive the appropriate and timely care they need. The U.S. health care system, which was already overwhelmed, has faced an even greater influx of patients because health care reform was fully implemented in 2014; 20 million Americans have gained health insurance coverage yet millions still lack (U.S. Department of Health & Human Services [USDHHS], 2020b). Health care issues that should be monitored over the next decade include the following:

- Increasing and measuring insurance coverage and access to the entire care continuum (from clinical preventive services to oral health care to long-term and palliative care)
- Addressing disparities that affect access to health care (e.g., race, ethnicity, socioeconomic status, age, sex, disability status, sexual orientation, gender identity, and residential location)
- Assessing the capacity of the health care system to provide services for newly insured individuals
- Determining changes in health care workforce needs as new models for the delivery of primary care become more prevalent, such as the patient-centered medical home and team-based care
- Monitoring the increasing use of telehealth as an emerging method of delivering health care (USDHHS, 2020b, para. 10)

Urban Populations and Health Disparities

The majority of the world's populace now lives in cities, which is a change from long-held rural dominance (Fig. 27-13). An analysis of the mortality rate differences between high-poverty urban and high-poverty rural areas suggest that place characteristics influence health and health outcomes above and beyond the impact of the social determinants of health for those populations. However, it is important to note that these populations are not static in their residence and the dynamic nature of urban living directly influences the health of populations over time.

Along with urban living, other global challenges include health inequity, NCD, infectious disease, and the social determinants of health (Lee et al., 2018; Winchester et al., 2016). The greatest growth of large cities

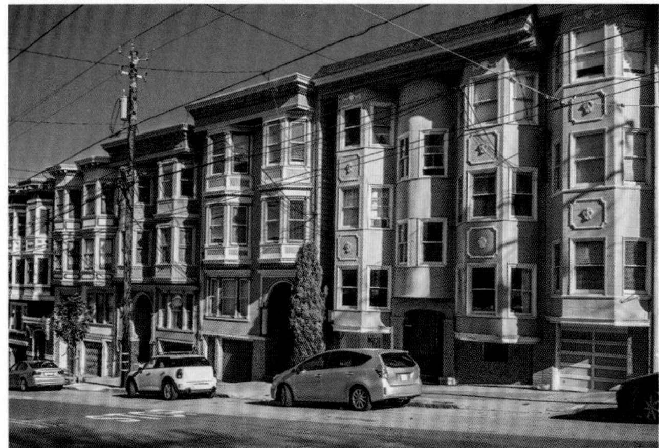

FIGURE 27-13 An example of urban housing: Colorful Victorian homes in San Francisco, California.

around the world is among less-wealthy nations, where urban slums are developing at a rapid rate, but leave many still impoverished and without piped water and sanitation (Ritchie & Roser, 2018). Depending upon the classification used, more than one third of the U.S. population lives in central cities.

In the United States, in 2018, 83.7% of the population is urban (273,368,693 people), which is expected to increase to 86.1% (305,356,412) by 2030 (Worldometers, 2017). According to the Pew Research Center (2020), in the United States, 14% of the population lives in rural areas (46 million), 31% are urban residents (98 million), and 55% live in the suburbs (175 million). Rural county populations have lagged in recent years, with one half having fewer residents now than in 2000 (Table 27-2).

One example of how changes in population can adversely affect large cities can be found in Baltimore. Between 2017 and 2018, the city lost 7,436 or 1.2% of its population and marks the 4th year for a population decline. Domestic migration, where the population moves out of the city to other cities and counties than those that move into the county, accounts for the decline (The Washington Post, 2019). Population loss leads to a smaller tax base and a greater proportion of poor residents, yet the city had the same maintenance expenses for sewers, water lines, and streets.

- Historically, movement to the suburbs began with the housing boom and highway expansion occurring after WWII.

TABLE **27-2** Urban Versus Rural Trends

Urban Dwellers	Rural Dwellers
▪ 17% live in poverty/14% for suburbs	▪ 18% live in poverty
▪ 35% have a college degree	▪ 19% have a college degree
▪ Smaller number of young adults	▪ Increased number of adults aged 65 years or older

- People moved from large cities to more suburban areas, and shopping malls and schools followed.
- Cars became even more essential, because public transportation did not always extend into suburban areas thereby leading to long commute times and traffic congestion.

Although not all suburban areas have remained attractive and vital, an income gap persists between city and suburban residents. Poverty is two times greater in large central cities than in corresponding suburban areas (19.6% vs. 11.2%); the suburban poor, or those living below the poverty line, grew by 57% between 2000 and 2015. By 2012, 59 of the top 95 metropolitan areas in the United States found the majority of their region's poor located in the suburbs. In 2015, 16 million poor people lived in suburban areas (Kneebone, 2017). This is indicative of a "suburbanization of poverty" (p. 12). Poverty rates were highest in metropolitan areas in the Midwest and South, and almost half of all large cities had significant increases in poverty rates. Only about one third of suburban areas recorded poverty rate increases.

Today, the declining urban situation is not confined to a few large cities. To achieve the vision of creating "social, physical, and economic environments that promote full potential for health and well-being for all" as an overarching goal of *Healthy People 2030*, more must be done to promote health and prevent disease in urban areas (USDHHS, 2020a, para. 11). The primary reason for health disparities, as mentioned in Chapter 23, is the disproportionate burden of certain health and social problems among different populations—in this instance, urban areas. Environmental exposure to air pollution contributes to illness and mortality including heart disease, cancer, and respiratory diseases. Consumer products (e.g., fast-food, alcohol, tobacco) are more readily available in urban and low-income areas and have been shown to be significant health risks that contribute to health disparities (Holleran, 2017).

Other environmental issues, such as extreme heat events where temperatures rise and lead to climate-related deaths, may amplify public health stressors and profoundly affect vulnerable populations. When examining urban form and its relationship to this weather phenomenon, exposures to dangerously high temperatures are a public health threat expected to increase with global climate change (CDC, n.d.).

- Heat waves can exacerbate the risks associated with heat exposure, and urban residents are more vulnerable to these threats due to the urban heat island effect. Urban planners are urged to consider construction limits in order to help with thermal regulation (Eagleview, 2016).
- Urban cities are often heat islands because of fewer green spaces and a larger proportion of asphalt. Extreme heat events not only lead to increased ED visits for heat-related illness, they can lead to increased hospitalizations for those with asthma and other chronic conditions, as well as death for elderly and other vulnerable populations (Matte et al., 2016; Soneja et al., 2016; Winquist, Grundstein, Chang, Hess, & Sarnat, 2016).

- Cities provide interventions such as extreme heat warnings and cooling centers but not all residents avail themselves of these services.
- Canadian researchers (Bélanger et al., 2016) interviewed almost 3,500 people in 1,647 buildings in disadvantaged areas across nine of the largest cities to determine their perception of adverse health effects of urban heat. Those with negative health impacts relied more on adaptation methods (e.g., eating iced foods, visiting air-conditioned places, taking showers to cooldown, turning off appliances). As with rural areas, the built environment greatly impacts urban neighborhoods.

Urban health equity depends on political empowerment of the people to strongly represent their interests and needs in order to challenge unfair distribution of resources. Further, with most of the world living within the built environment, this poses a major opportunity to improve urban health and equity (APHA, 2018). Poor social conditions and health inequalities have been recognized in urban areas around the world. Urban slums in low- and some middle-income countries provide social exclusion for many living in poverty and threaten development. For example:

- The Zika virus was, and continues to be, a disease of the urban poor. Slum-defining characteristics, such as poor water and sanitation, crowding, and poor structural quality of housing, offer ample opportunities for mosquitoes to breed and spread the Zika virus (Snyder et al., 2017).
- People in cities are also at risk for COVID-19 infections based on risk factors such as household overcrowding, race, ethnicity, low income, and underlying health conditions such as diabetes and obesity (NYU Langone Health, 2020).
- Inadequate urban housing and neighborhood disorder are related to poor-quality sleep among Latino adults (Chambers, Pichardo, & Rosenbaum, 2016).
- Prenatal exposure to particulate matter (diesel fuel, perchloroethylene) has been shown to affect math scores when the children reach third grade; researchers suggest "individual pollutants may additively impact health" (Stingone, McVeigh, & Claudio, 2016, p. 144).
- Indoor environmental exposures are contributors to childhood asthma morbidity. Indoor area pollutants have been associated with asthma symptoms in children, and reduction of indoor allergens and pollutants has shown improvements in asthma symptoms (Matsui, Abramson & Sandel, 2016).
- Urban indoor environments in multifamily housing units pose challenges as pollutants may be seen in many of the units and residents have limited ability to make changes (EPA, 2018).

In addition to concerns about housing, hazardous waste landfill sites are often located in or near urban areas. Noise exposure, often associated with large inner cities, has been linked to cardiovascular death, hypertension, and ischemic heart disease (Munzel et al., 2018). In Flint, Michigan, following pollution of their water system, soil lead data show higher lead values in the metropolitan city center, and seasonal blood lead variations indicate that resuspension of lead dust may be to blame (Laidlaw et al., 2016). See Chapter 9 for more on environmental health.

- Continued exposure to higher sound levels found in large cities can lead to noise-induced hearing loss as well as decreased levels of work performance, among other things (Recio, Linares, Banegas, & Diaz, 2016).
- Significantly lower psychomotor speed and reduced working memory were found in a sample of healthy adults when subjected to urban noise levels (Wright, Peters, Ettinger, Kuipers, & Kumari, 2016).
- Lead poisoning has been more often reported in older homes and apartments in large cities (Childers, 2017).
- A national study found that traffic-related air pollution (measured by nitrogen dioxide levels) was significantly associated with small for gestational age births and lower birth weights and may be a source of air pollution related to poor pregnancy outcomes in Canada (Fig. 27-14; Stieb et al., 2016).
- Another study examined the effects of long-term air pollution exposure on survival rates for acute myocardial infarctions (Chen et al., 2016). Researchers concluded 12.4% of deaths could have been prevented if the lowest measured concentration of ambient fine particulate matter in urban areas had been consistently achieved over the study period.
- The risk for major depressive disorder has also been shown to increase as exposure to particulate matter increased; this was true in the general population but was even more highly significant in people with chronic diseases (Kim et al., 2016).

While global data have often suggested that urban residents have better health on average than their rural counterparts, this benefit is truly only greater for those at the high end of the income scale. This only magnifies the disparities in urban areas between rich and poor or the social gradient. A more current view is that those living in urban slums, often in megacities outside the United States, have health outcomes that are either similar to or worse than those of their rural neighbors (Kneebone, 2017).

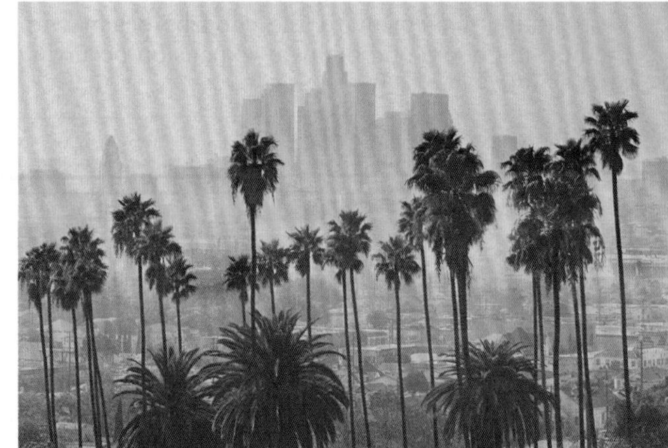

FIGURE 27-14 Air pollution is a common problem in metropolitan areas, as seen in this view of the Los Angeles skyline.

Violence is often associated with large metropolitan cities. After many years of a decline, the national rates for violent crimes increased from 2014 to 2016 or 361.6 per 100,000 in 2014 to 386.3 per 100,000 in 2016. Crimes increased by 4% in cities >1 million, decreased by 4% in cities from 500,000 to 999,000, and increased by 5% in smaller cities <50,000 (Congressional Research Service, 2018).

- In 2015, victimizations of people from urban areas accounted for 40% of all rapes and sexual assaults, 48% of robberies, and 40% of aggravated assaults.
- In contrast, victimizations of those living in rural areas accounted for 5% of rapes and sexual assaults, 5% of robberies, and 14% of aggravated assaults.
- Over a four-decade period, Parker and Stansfield (2015) found that increased population diversity in U.S. cities contributed to declining homicide rates; racial differences were noted with growing Hispanic presence in Black areas leading to lower Black homicide rates, but no differences were found in White homicide rates.

Among youth, Latinos/Hispanics are disproportionately represented among youth gangs, and substance use and sales are gang-related activities. Individuals who are exposed to urban violence may develop PTSD, and a study examining health-related quality of life among those with PTSD who were exposed to urban violence found that they had higher levels of anxiety and depression, more childhood traumas, and more new trauma experiences (Pupo, Serafim, & deMello, 2015). Supportive family members were shown to be associated with decreased levels of involvement with violence during adolescence. While those living in low-resource urban areas may be unable to avoid witnessing violence, having one supportive parent was a predictor for significantly less violence involvement (Culyba et al., 2016).

Inner cities are often thought to be places with low-income residents living in large, poorly maintained government housing projects. Dilapidated housing in central cities exposes residents to cracks in walls and ceilings, peeling paint, broken windows, leaking pipes, and pests such as cockroaches and rats. There is often limited access to adequate rental properties, and rent is often higher in large cities, making it difficult for low-income residents to find adequate housing.

- Nationwide, about one third of households live in rentals, but 43% of rental properties are in central cities. Median rents in 90 cities were over 30% of the gross median income; no more than 30% of one's household income is considered to be affordable rent (Pew Charitable Trusts, 2018).
- In Chicago, the average rental percentage increased from 21% to 31%, and New Orleans reported 35%. Miami rent is now 43% of the typical household income, despite efforts to increase the number of apartment buildings.
- Apartment rental growth has seen an increase nationally of 1.6% with some areas such as Phoenix and Las Vegas seeing additional growth. Rental rates have increased by 1.3% nationally with rent hikes of over 30% in Colorado and California (Salviati, 2020). Low-income housing, when available, is often plagued with construction and maintenance problems and is characterized by crowding, poor quality, high population density, and attendant health problems. Over 1.3 million U.S. households are located in public housing. Over one third of rental housing was built before 1960, and owners of multifamily rental properties that have lost tenants and income may scrimp on maintenance that decreases property values even more (Pew Charitable Trusts, 2018).
- Urban poor are often forced to live in neighborhoods that do not facilitate outdoor activity or have markets that provide healthy foods, such as fresh fruits and vegetables.
- A walk through most urban corner markets reveals that they do not always offer low-fat dairy products or fresh produce but generally do their best business selling lottery tickets, liquor, sodas, and cigarettes.
- In New York City, it is estimated that only half of residents consume two or more servings of fruits and vegetables daily, and typical interventions aimed at increasing consumption are not likely to be effective in neighborhoods with low education levels (Li, Zhang, & Pagán, 2016).

In a Philadelphia study of patients with high hospital utilization (≥3 inpatient admissions within 12 months; ≥6 chronic illnesses), 30% were found to be food insecure, and 25% were marginally food insecure (Phipps, Singletary, Cooblall, Hares, & Braitman, 2016). In the past 30 days, 40% were concerned that their food would run out, 17.5% said that they did not eat for a full day, and 10% reported being hungry and not eating some or all of the time. Food insecurity can have negative impacts on health, especially for those with chronic conditions. In a qualitative study of San Francisco area individuals with HIV/AIDS, participants discussed living on insufficient food supplies and being hungry, as well as having concerns about the potential poor health effects of eating a "cheap diet" (Whittle et al., 2015, p. 154). Some reported having to use socially and personally unacceptable means of getting food (e.g., trading sex for food, depending on friends/family/charities). High rents related to gentrification of their neighborhoods were cited as a cause of their food insecurity.

Sociologists Wilson and Kelling first proposed the *broken window theory* in 1982, noting that if a broken window goes unrepaired, soon more windows are broken, and this sends a powerful message to residents that no one cares. A classic research study by Keizer, Lindenberg, and Steg (2008) tested this theory in six-field experiments where neighborhoods, characterized by broken windows, litter, unreturned shopping carts, and graffiti, were studied. They found that when residents see others violating social norms or rules (e.g., disorderly or petty criminal behavior), they are then more likely to also violate norms and rules and that this is a cause for the spread of disorder.

Population density, complexity, and racial/ethnic diversity are associated with urban areas. Central cities are often home to a large proportion of poor people and those from different racial and ethnic groups. In the 21st century, America has evolved into a metropolitan nation with more than 8 out of 10 Americans living in metropolitan areas of varying sizes. Between 2010 and 2018, the fastest growing U.S. cities included The Villages, Florida; Myrtle Beach, South Carolina; Austin, Texas; Midland, Texas; Greeley, Colorado; St. George, Utah; Cape Coral/ Fort Myers, FL; and Redmond, Oregon. Conversely, the cities with the greatest rates of decline included Pine Bluffs, Arkansas; Johnstown, Pennsylvania; Charleston, West Virginia; Douglas, Arizona; and Beckley, West Virginia (Stebbins, 2018).

Urban poor have health problems characterized by accidental and violent injuries, as well as NCDs and chronic stress (Maxmen, 2016). As noted in Chapter 23, poverty makes a significant difference in health status. Neighborhood disadvantage and disorder (drug activity, violent crime) have been related to the rapid transition from no drug involvement to problem drug use (Reboussin et al., 2015). Neighborhood poverty has been associated with HIV diagnosis in a New York City study (Wiewel et al., 2016). Working class urban residents no longer can find industrial jobs, and a concerted effort to improve conditions in urban America is needed in the form of urban policy development. Over the past 25 years, cities and their suburbs have become more alike, and the demographic and health profiles that were previously uniquely urban are now shared by "edge cities" and suburbs populated by poor and minority families. Political power has shifted to more affluent suburban areas, where the tax base and spending practices are greater, at the expense of these cities.

Urban health disparities present a challenge that can be addressed only by the joint effort of public health and urban planning bodies. Coalitions of public health professionals, planners, builders, architects, along with transportation engineers and government officials, are needed to promote healthy, sustainable communities (Fig. 27-15).

- There is a move to make cities and their suburbs **sustainable communities**. These are seen as healthy places where both natural and historic resources are protected, employment is available, urban sprawl is contained, neighborhoods are safe, air pollution is minimized, lifelong learning is promoted, health care and transportation are easily accessible, and all citizens have the opportunity to improve their quality of life.

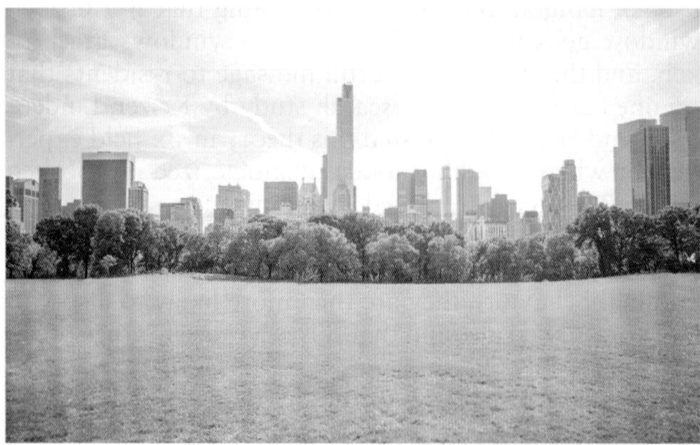

FIGURE 27-15 This view of New York City shows Central Park, a *green area* interspersed among densely populated areas—an example of good urban planning.

- A federal collaborative program, the Partnership for Sustainable Communities (2018), is a nonprofit organization that helps American cities become more socially, economically, and environmentally sustainable while focusing on land use planning, affordable housing, community development, energy use, and transportation.

As with all good plans, the sustainable development plan requires that the recipient of the planning be involved. Democratizing the practice of urban planning is vital to its success. Communities that have been victimized through ineffective planning must be included in the decision-making process. This process will require the inclusion of the practical experience that residents bring to the table, alongside expert input. The health of communities must be addressed from all levels of environmental impact (individual, community, and systems), and population health in the urban setting must be studied (Gottlieb et al., 2016). Data must be included from the various environments, such as homes, workplaces, schools, and community spaces. These approaches then bring such action in line with what is often referred to as *environmental justice* or the marriage of environmental health and civil rights (Agyeman, Schlosberg, Craven, & Matthews, 2016). A framework to ensure such justice requires that all individuals and communities have the right to work, play, and live in environments that are safe and healthy. It also requires that polluters are punished and required to provide compensation for damages and/ or renovation.

Community Health Nursing in Urban Settings

Urban public health nursing can be very rewarding, and many nurses are drawn to urban areas where salaries are higher and opportunities for advancement or additional education greater. In urban areas, there are a larger number of nurses, more schools of nursing, and more intensive recruitment efforts than in rural areas, although inner-city areas, much like rural settings, can have problems filling C/PHN vacancies.

- RN workforce studies reveal a higher rate of nurses (935 vs. 853 per 100,000 populations) and a greater proportion of nurses with a BSN (65% vs. 48%) in urban areas when compared with rural areas (HRSA, 2020).
- The current health care education system tends to be urban-centric, with the exception of online education programs.
- Urban areas sometimes draw people away from rural areas.

C/PHN practice is population-focused care that requires unique knowledge, competencies, and skills. C/ PHN roles have always extended beyond sick care, also encompassing advocacy, health education, community organization, collaboration with community agencies, as well as political and social reform. Primary prevention (health promotion) is a major focus. C/PHNs have a key role of working with populations to improve health and social conditions of vulnerable populations. These nurses practice in diverse settings such as community nursing centers, home health agencies, housing developments, local and state health departments, neighborhood centers, churches, schools, and worksites. C/PHNs can develop sustainable programs and build community capacity for health promotion in collaboration with community members. By utilizing a community-based participatory research (CBPR) model, C/PHNs can collaborate with community members, leaders, and stakeholders to identify resources and solutions to problems. Specific public health roles include advocates, collaborators, educators, partners, policy-makers, and researcher. An example is through the use of the "power of the pulpit." The Black Church is seen as an influential political and social force in the Black community. Church leadership often supports a history of promoting encouraging and facilitating community-based screening and health care programs (Bishop-McDaniel, 2017). Community health nurses collaborate with their clients to develop their facility for long-term health promotion and improvement of their quality of life. Their ultimate goal is to empower clients to be self-sufficient.

There are many points at which the community health nurse can make a difference in people's lives. Nurses provide services in deteriorating urban areas, with those living in poverty in all settings and among all vulnerable populations. Nurses first need to assess themselves for their attitudes and preconceptions. Although access to care can be improved for many low-income people in urban areas, many clients simply need an advocate. Our ability to envision solutions and join together with clients aids us in helping to create a healthier environment for all (Fullilove & Cantal-Dupart, 2016). The urban communities, and the poor or vulnerable people living in them, need strengthening and interventions that can be initiated by C/PHNs using the nursing process as a guide. See Chapter 23.

Self-assessment

Confronting poverty and caring for vulnerable people from diverse backgrounds, whether in rural or urban areas, necessitates reflective assessment of one's own assumptions and beliefs. Because poverty may be prevalent over a lifetime, nursing students may have personal or family experience of living in poverty. However, because the stigma is so great and faultfinding so pervasive in American society, acknowledging and reflecting on this experience may be painful. In contrast, because poverty is so hidden and frequently denied, some nursing students have lived apart from any knowledge of the human experience of poverty. They may have come to believe many of the negative stereotypes about poor people. Nursing students and practicing nurses need to ask such questions as "How have my judgments been shaped? How can I open myself to caring for those from whom most of society turns away?"

We learn from one another's stories (Box 27-13). First, learn from your classmates, friends, and neighbors

BOX **27-13** PERSPECTIVES

C/PHN Instructors' Viewpoints on Urban Health Nursing

- Ann, a nursing faculty member at a small Roman Catholic college, had a one-to-one postclinical conference with a student and relays this conversation. The student had made many visits to an African American teen mother of two thriving children. The young mother lived in a dangerous housing project, and, although she locked him out of her second-floor apartment, her abusive boyfriend had been known to climb up the drainage pipe and over the porch roof. Sometimes, he forced open a window and beat her. The mother worked every day at a fast-food establishment; her grandmother took care of the children. After a couple of months of weekly visits, the student exclaimed, "When I read her chart, I saw her as an immoral girl—a slut—and I expected her to be a loser. Now, I can't believe what I've learned about how strong she is. She just keeps fighting for herself and for her kids to survive! She's a great mom and I told her so!"
- Another faculty member, Sharon, who taught community health nursing in a Midwestern school of nursing, was having an informal discussion with a student who related her experience of trying to get comfortable making home visits with low-income young women. She was making brave attempts at home visits to a pregnant woman, about her age, living in the deteriorating outskirts of a major city. She thought she had established rapport and was making headway developing trust with the client. One day, the client asked the student, with concern in her voice, if she had "broken off her engagement." The flustered student then had difficulty explaining the absence of her engagement ring, which she had never mentioned, but the client had obviously noticed. During the previous week, she had suddenly realized she was wearing this special ring in marginal neighborhoods and thought it best to leave it at home. Of course, she thought that she had to fabricate another reason to tell the client but felt badly for being so judgmental when the client was identifying with the student and believed they had something in common.
- Lynn, a new public health nursing faculty member from a large state university in the West, was shocked and repulsed by the comment of one of her students during lecture one day. When discussing vulnerable populations in urban centers and rural areas, the point was made that poverty can be a generational phenomenon and that many of our clients may find it difficult to dig out of this circumstance. Social justice was discussed, along with the need for C/PHNs to become social activists in order to change political and socioeconomic factors that keep the status quo. One student, a Hispanic female from a middle-class family, spoke up stating "they should all get jobs at McDonalds." This spurred further discussion about population-focused versus individual-focused interventions and approaches and the need for all of us to be aware of our prejudices and stereotypical viewpoints.

who are courageous enough to tell you their own experiences of living in poverty. Ask them and listen intently. Then, let your clients teach you. One honor that nurses have is the opportunity to work with people from all walks of life. During your clinical experiences in community health, you are particularly likely to meet impoverished, vulnerable individuals and families living outside the mainstream. And you can join with them to empower them by helping to build skills and confidence and connecting them to resources.

Improving Access

Even with ACA and government-sponsored health insurance and services, extensive barriers prevent many people from accessing services. The community health nurse serves as an advocate and bridge for families who need to gain access. Barriers to access associated with the clients themselves include reluctance to seek coverage because of feelings of powerlessness; being unaware that such services exist or are worthwhile; lacking resources such as a telephone or transportation; being illiterate; and preoccupation with meeting survival needs and competing life priorities instead of health needs. Barriers associated with applying for health insurance include a system that is unfriendly and complicated. The process may require a car, a phone, and appointments at inconvenient times. Also, service interruptions are not uncommon, as wages vary over time. The nurse can intervene as a coach and guide, interpreting the system to the client and the client to the system. Likewise, nurses can serve as change agents to improve the system whenever possible.

Strengthening Communities

We are all connected. All of us as citizens have a stake in preventing the adverse hardships of poverty and ill health. All of society pays to support community members that do not contribute, to house those who are incarcerated, and to ignore the vulnerable. Many of us fear crime in our homes, schools, businesses, and communities. Society, as a whole, is impacted when adults are incapable of providing nurturing environments for their children. In addition, the alienation of many groups in society erodes our sense of community as a nation. Community health planning should seriously consider an organizing process that builds community and that focuses on developing neighborhood competence to solve problems and create solutions for itself (see the discussion of community development in Chapter 15).

SUMMARY

- Rural clients are a unique aggregate, and community health nurses are key to ensuring the delivery of appropriate health services to this population. There are numerous definitions of the term *rural*. In this chapter, some characteristics of rural communities include the following:
  - Communities with fewer than 10,000 residents.
  - A county population density of fewer than 1,000 people per square mile.
  - Rural areas often have less diversity than urban cities but that is changing in many areas.
  - Rural clients generally have lower educational levels than urban clients, due in part to less access to higher education and lower-paying jobs.
  - Income levels and housing costs are frequently lower in rural areas than in larger cities.
  - Many at-risk populations live in these communities, where there are often fewer employment opportunities, a lack of adequate housing, and limited access to health and social services.
  - Rural elders may have more limited alternatives for housing if they can no longer live alone.
  - Mental health services are inadequate, even though the need may be great. Numerous risks are associated with agriculture.
- Between the 2000 and 2010 censuses, urban population growth was about twice than in rural areas. The elderly are a rapidly growing population in rural communities.
- Urban health issues have existed for hundreds of years in the United States, and they continue today. Many disenfranchised and minority groups call inner cities home. Air pollution, poverty, discrimination, substandard housing, crime, substance use disorder, and social inequities often characterize life in urban settings.
- The built environment is an important consideration in urban as well as rural settings and can contribute to greater health risks. Some large cities have had marked decreases in population and significant problems with unemployment, although more people around the world live in urban areas now than in rural areas.
- Migrant farmworkers are an integral part of the agricultural community in the United States and the world but are often barely visible in society. As members of the community with varied and significant health needs, these are complicated by social isolation, occupational hazards such as pesticide exposure, poor working conditions, and working with dangerous farm equipment.
- Migrant workers and their families often endure substandard housing and poor sanitation, while living in high-risk environments. Migrant children are often educationally, socially, and physically disadvantaged. Migrant health care centers often do not adequately meet the health needs of the migrant community; therefore, innovative methods of health care delivery have been developed and implemented by community health nurses, including mobile health vans and information tracking systems.

ACTIVE LEARNING EXERCISES

1. Search for two recent journal articles relating to access to health care or quality of care for rural, urban, or migrant population. After summarizing the content, identify barriers to access that are common to both and those that are different. What are the main themes relating to health and access to care?
2. Discuss the common characteristics of rural, migrant, and urban clients. How can the C/PHN be better prepared to meet their unique needs? What are some specific challenges facing the C/PHN working in a rural area? In an urban area? Or with the migrant farmworker population?
3. Describe some of the benefits of rural public health nursing. Describe some of the benefits of urban public health nursing.
4. Discuss health, living, and working concerns of migrant workers. How does a nomadic lifestyle affect the needs of migrant workers?
5. Using "Create, Champion, and Implement Policies, Plans, and Laws" (1 of the 10 essential public health services; see Box 2-2), examine new or existing policies or laws and determine how they might affect today's migrant population.

REFERENCES

Agyeman, J., Schlosberg, D., Craven, L., & Matthews, C. (2016). Trends and directions in environmental justice: From inequity to everyday life, community, and just sustainabilities. *Annual Review of Environment and Resources, 41*, 321–340.

America's Health Ranking. (2018). *2018 annual report*. Retrieved from http://www.americashealthrankings.org/learn/reports/2018-annual-report/findings-international-comparison

American Association for the History of Nursing. (2018). *Mary Breckenridge*. Retrieved from https://www.aahn.org/breckinridge

American Heart Association. (2020). *2020 Heart disease and stroke statistics update fact sheet—at-a-glance*. Retrieved from https://professional.heart.org/idc/groups/ahamah-public/@wcm/@sop/@smd/documents/downloadable/ucm_505473.pdf

American Public Health Association (APHA). (2018). *At the intersection of public health and transportation: Promoting healthy transportation policy*. Retrieved from http://www.apha.org/NR/rdonlyres/43F10382-FB68-4112-8C75-49DCB10F8ECF/0/TransportationBrief.pdf

American Public Health Association (APHA). (2020). *What is public health?* Retrieved from https://www.apha.org/what-is-public-health

Anderson, T. J., Saman, D. M., Lipsky, M. S., & Lutfiyya, M. N. (2015). A cross-sectional study on health differences between rural and non-rural U.S. counties using the County Health Rankings. *BMC Health Services Research, 15*(1), 441. doi: 10.1186/s129113-015-1053-3.

Arcury, T., Chen, H., Laurienti, P., Howard, T., Barr, D., Mora, D., & Quandt, S. (2018). Farmworker and nonfarmworker Latino immigrant men in North Carolina have high levels of specific pesticide urinary metabolites. *Archives of Environmental Occupational Health, 73*(4), 219–227. doi: 10.1080/19338244.2017.1342588

Arcury, T. A., Summers, P., Talton, J. W., Nguyen, H. T., Chen, H., & Quandt, S. A. (2015). Job characteristics and work safety climate among North Carolina farmworkers with H-2A visas. *Journal of Agromedicine, 20*(1), 64–76.

Arellano, G. (August 23, 2018). *When the U.S. government tried to replace migrant farmworkers with high schoolers*. National Public Radio. 1-15. Retrieved from https://www.npr.org/sections/thesalt/2018/07/31/634442195/when-the-u-s-government-tried-to-replace-migrant-farmworkers-with-high-schoolers

Bélanger, D., Abdous, B., Valois, P., Gosselin, E., & Sidi, A. L. (2016). A multilevel analysis to explain self-reported adverse health effects and adaptation to urban heat: A cross-sectional survey in the deprived areas of 9 Canadian cities. *BMC Public Health, 16*, 144.

Bhutani, S., Schoeller, D. A., Walsh, M. C., & McWilliams, C. (2018). Frequency of eating out at both fast-food and sit-down restaurants was associated with high body mass index in non-large metropolitan communities in midwest. *American Journal of Health Promotion, 32*(1), 75–83.

Biography. (2019). *Cesar Chavez*. Retrieved from https://www.biography.com/people/cesar-chavez-9245781

Bishop-Mcdaniel, A. G. (2017). *Leadership consensus on successful obesity prevention programs in "The Black Church": A Delphi study*. (Dissertation Study). University of the Rockies.

Blake, K. D., Moss, J. L., Gaysynsky, A., Srinivasan, S., & Croyle, R. T. (2017). Making the case for investment in rural cancer control: An analysis of rural cancer incidence, mortality, and funding trends. *Cancer Epidemiology and Prevention Biomarkers, 26*(7), 992–997.

Bolin, J. N., Bellamy, G. R., Ferinand, A. O., Vuong, A. M., Kash, B. A., Schulze, A., & Helduser, J. W. (2015). Rural Healthy People 2020: New decade, same challenges. *Journal of Rural Health, 31*(3), 326–333.

Butler-Dawson, J., Galvin, K., Thorne, P. S., & Rohlman, D. S. (2016). Organophosphorus pesticide exposure and neurobehavioral performance in Latino children living in an orchard community. *Neurotoxicology, 53*, 165–172.

Calancie, L., Leeman, J., Jilcott Pitts, S. B., Kettel Khan, L., Fleishhacker, S., Evenson, K. R., ... Ammerman, A. (2015). Nutrition-related policy and environmental strategies to prevent obesity in rural communities: A systematic review of the literature, 2002-2013. *Preventing Chronic Disease, 12*, E57. Retrieved from https://www.cdc.gov/pcd/issues/2015/14_0540.htm

Caldwell, D. R. (2007). Bloodroot: Life stories of nurse practitioners in rural Appalachia. *Journal of Holistic Nursing, 25*, 73–79.

Caldwell, J., Ford, C., Wallace, S., Wang, M., & Takahashi, L. (2016). Intersection of Living in a rural versus urban area and race/ethnicity in explaining access to health care in the United States. *American Journal of Public Health, 106*(8), 1463–1469.

California Department of Pesticide Exposure. (2020). *Pesticide illness surveillance program*. Retrieved from http://www.cdpr.ca.gov/docs/whs/pisp.htm

CDC/National Institute for Occupational Safety & Health. (2017). *Pesticide illness and injury surveillance*. Retrieved from https://www.cdc.gov/niosh/topics/pesticides/default.html

Center for Disease Control. (n.d.). *Extreme heat can impact our health in many ways*. Retrieved from https://www.cdc.gov/climateandhealth/pubs/EXTREME-HEAT-Final_508.pdf

Center for Disease Control and Prevention. (2020). *Living with HIV*. Retrieved form https://www.cdc.gov/hiv/basics/livingwithhiv/index.html

Centers for Disease Control and Prevention (CDC). (2017). *Healthy places*. Retrieved from http://www.cdc.gov/healthyplaces/

Chaiyachati, K., Hubbard, R., Yeager, A., Mugo, B., Shea, J., Rosin, R., & Grande, D. (2018). Rideshare-based medical transportation for Medicaid patients and primary care show rates: A difference-in-difference analysis of a pilot program. *Journal of General Internal Medicine*, 2018;*33*(6), 863–868.

Chambers, E. C., Pichardo, M. S., & Rosenbaum, E. (2016). Sleep and the housing and neighborhood environment of urban Latino adults living in low-income housing: The AHOME study. *Behavioral Sleep Medicine, 14*(2), 169–184.

Chem-Tox.com. (2019). *Living near agriculture increases rates of serious health problems*. Retrieved from https://chem-tox.com/agriculture/

Chen, H., Burnett, R. T., Copes, R., Kwong, J. C., Villeneurve, P. J., Goldberg, M. S., ... Tu, J. V. (2016). Ambient fine particulate matter and mortality among survivors of myocardial infarction: Population-based cohort study. *Environmental Health Perspectives, 124*(9), 1421–1428.

Childers, L. (2017). *California health report*. Retrieved from http://www.calhealthreport.org/2017/02/18/new-report-finds-children-at-a-higher-risk-of-lead-exposure-in-several-california-cities/

Cole, A., & Crawford, L. (1991). Implementation and evaluation of the health resource program for migrant women in the Americus, Georgia area. In

A. Bushy (Ed.), *Rural nursing* (Vol. *1*, pp. 364–374). Newbury Park, CA: Sage Publications.

Cone, M. (April 4, 2019). *What you need to know about a popular weed killer's alleged link to cancer*. Kaiser Health Network. Retrieved from https://khn.org/news/popular-weed-killers-alleged-link-to-cancer-spreads-concern/

Congressional Research Service. (2018). *Recent violent crime trends in the United States*. Retrieved from https://fas.org/sgp/crs/misc/R45236.pdf

Council of Economic Advisors. (2018). *President Donald J. Trump is working to rebuild rural America*. Retrieved from https://www.whitehouse.gov/briefings-statements/president-donald-j-trump-working-rebuild-rural-america/

Culyba, A. J., Ginsburg, K. R., Fein, J. A., Branas, C. C., Richmond, T. S., Miller, E., & Wiebe, D. J. (2016). Examining the role of supportive family connection in violence exposure among male youth in urban environments. *Journal of Interpersonal Violence*, *34*(5), 1074–1088.

Deaton, A. (February 8, 2018). *Hiding in America's "Deep Poverty Problem" is health care*. Health Commentary: Exploring Human Potential. Retrieved from http://www.Healthcommentary.Org/2018/02/08/Hiding-Americas-Deep-Poverty-Problem-Health-Care/

Department of Health and Human Services. (2018). *Addressing the burden of chronic obstructive pulmonary disease in rural America*. Retrieved from http://hrsa.gov/sites/default/files/hrsa/advisory-committees/rural/publications/RuralCOPD.pdf

Dodd, V. J., Schenck, D. P., Chaney, E. H., & Padhya, T. (2016). Assessing oral cancer awareness among rural Latino migrant workers. *Journal of Immigrant and Minority Health*, *18*(3), 552–560.

Dombrowski, K., Crawford, D., Khan, B., & Tyler, K. (2016). Current rural drug use in the US Midwest. *Journal of Drug Abuse*, *2*(3), 22.

Donham, K. J., & Thelin, A. (2016). *Agricultural medicine: Rural occupational and environmental health, safety, and prevention*. Hoboken, NJ: John Wiley & Sons.

Dryden, J. (February 3, 2016). Scientists more effectively control pain by targeting nerve cell's interior. *Brain in the News*, *23*(3), 1–2.

Eagleview. (2016). *5 key factos in urban planning*. Retrieved from https://www.eagleview.com/newsroom/2016/08/5-key-factors-in-urban-planning/

Environmental Protection Agency (EPA). (2018). *Indoor air quality in multifamily housing*. Retrieved from https://www.epa.gov/indoor-air-quality-iaq/indoor-air-quality-multifamily-housing

Evans, D. V., Cole, A. M., & Norris, T. E. (2015). Colonoscopy in rural communities: A systematic review of the frequency and quality. *Rural and Remote Health*, *15*, 3057.

Fairweather, G. C., Lincoln, M. A., & Ramsdeb, R. (2016). Speech language pathology teletherapy in rural and remote education settings: Decreasing service in inequities. *International Journal of Speech-Language Pathology*, *18*(6), 1–11.

Farmworkers Justice. (2020). *Accessing healthcare*. Retrieved from https://www.farmworkerjustice.org/about-farmworker-justice/our-advisory-council/farmworker-justice-staff/

Fields, B. E., Bell, J. F., Moyce, S., & Bigbee, J. L. (2015). The impact of insurance instability on health service utilization: Does non-metropolitan residence make a difference? *Journal of Rural Health*, *31*(1), 27–34.

Fields, B. E., Bigbee, J. L., & Bell, J. F. (2016). Associations of provider-to-population ratios and population health by county-level rurality. *The Journal of Rural Health*, *32*(3), 235–244.

Figueroa, Moberg, & Hennen. (2017). *Health access for H-2A workers: Summary of current trends and strategies for community outreach*. Retrieved from http://www.ncfh.org/uploads/3/8/6/8/38685499/health_access_for_h-2a_workers.pdf

Fleming, K., Simmons, V. N., Christy, S. M., Sutton, S. K., Romo, M., Luque, J. S., ... & Meade, C. D. (2018). Educating Hispanic women about cervical cancer prevention: Feasibility of a promotora-led charla intervention in a farmworker community. *Ethnicity & Disease*, *28*(3), 169–176.

Forst, L. (2018). Tractor rollovers are preventable. *American Journal of Public Health*, *108*(11), 1436–1437.

Fullilove, M. T., & Cantal-Dupart, M. (2016). Medicine for the city: Perspective and solidarity as tools for making urban health. *Journal of Bioethical Inquiry*, *13*(2), 215–221.

Gillam, C. (May 6, 2016). *What killed Jack McCall? A California farmer dies and a case against Monsanto takes root*. Retrieved from http://www.huffingtonpost.com/carey-gillam/what-killed-jack-mccall-a_b_9852216.html

Gottlieb, A., Hoehndorf, R., Dumontier, M., & Altman, R. B. (2016). Ranking adverse drug reactions with crowdsourcing. *Journal of Medical Internet Research*, *17*(3), e80.

Granados, A. (2018). Education, unsettled. In *Education week*. Retrieved from https://www.edweek.org/ew/projects/education-unsettled-migrant-students.html

Grice, B. A., Nelson, R. G., Williams, D. E., Knowler, W. C., Mason, C., Hanson, R. L., ... & Pavkov, M. E. (2017). Associations between persistent organic pollutants, type 2 diabetes, diabetic nephropathy and mortality. *Occupational and Environmental Medicine*, *74*(7), 521–527.

Griffith, W., Vigoren, E., Smith, M., Workman, T., Thompson, B, Coronado, G., & Faustman, E. (2018). Application of improved approach to evaluate a community intervention to reduce exposure of your children living in farmworker households *to organophosphate pesticides. Journal of Exposure Science & Environmental Epidemiology*, *29*, 358–365.

Hansen, A. Y., Umstattd Meyer, M. R., Lenardson, J. D., & Hartley, D. (2015). Built environments and active living in rural and remote areas: A review of the literature. *Current Obesity Reports*, *4*(4), 484–493.

Harris, D. E., Aboueissa, A. M., Baugh, N., & Sarton, C. (2015). Impact of rurality on maternal and infant health indicators and outcomes in Maine. *Rural and Remote Health*, *15*(3), 1–17.

Health Center Resource Clearinghouse (n.d.). *Migrant clinicians network*. Retrieved from https://www.healthcenterinfo.org/our-partners/migrant-clinicians-network-mcn/

Health Resources and Services Administration (HRSA). (2018). *HRSA funded research shows diabetes mortality in rural American a significant cause for concern*. Retrieved from http://hrsa.gov/about/news/press-releases/hrsa-funded-research-shows-diabetes-mortality.html

Health Resources and Services Administration (HRSA). (2020). *Medically underserved areas and populations (MUA/Ps)*. Retrieved from https://bhw.hrsa.gov/shortage-designation/muap

Heath, S. (2017). *Which patient care barriers impact rural hospital mortality rates?* Patient Engagement HIT. Retrieved from https://patientengagementhit.com/news/which-patient-care-barriers-impact-rural-hospital-mortality-rates

Hertz-Picciotto, I., Sass, J., Engel, S., Bennett, D., Bradman, A., Eskenazi, B., ... & Whyatt, R. (2018). Organophosphate exposure during pregnancy and chld neurodevelopment: Recommendations for essential policy reforms. *PLoS Med*, *15*(10), e1002671. doi.org/10.1371/journal.pmed.1002671.

Holden, C. (n.d.). *Migrant health issues: Housing. Monograph No. 8*. Buda, TX: National Center for Farmworker Health.

Holleran, M. (2017). *How fast food chains supersized inequality*. In e New Republic. Retrieved from https://newrepublic.com/article/144168/fast-food-chains-supersized-inequality

Housing Assistance Council (HAC). (n.d.). *Farmworkers*. Washington, DC: Author. Retrieved from http://www.ruralhome.org/storage/documents/farmoverview.pdf

Jacob Arriola, K. R., Hermstad, A., St. Clair Flemming, S., Honeycutt, S., Carvalho, M. L., Cherry, S. T., ... & Kegler, M. C. (2016). Promoting policy and environmental change in faith-based organizations: Outcome evaluation of a mini-grants program. *Health Promotion Practice*, *17*(1), 146–155.

Johns Hopkins Urban Health Institute. (2018). *"About Us"*. Johns Hopkins Urban Health Institute. Retrieved from https://urbanhealth.jhu.edu/about/

Kearney, G. D., Hu, H., Xu, X., Hall, M. B., & Balanay, J. A. G. (2016). Estimating the prevalence of heat-related symptoms and sun safety-related behavior among Latino farmworkers in eastern North Carolina. *Journal of Agromedicine*, *21*(1), 15–23. doi: 10.1080/1059924X.2015.1106377.

Keizer, K., Lindenberg, S., & Steg, L. (2008). The spreading of disorder. *Science*, *322*(5908), 1681–1685.

Kim, K. H., Kabir, E., & Jahan, S. A. (2017). Exposure to pesticides and the associated human health effects. *Science of the Total Environment*, *575*, 525–535.

Kim, K. N., Lim, Y. H., Bae, H. J., Kim, M., Jung, K., & Hong, Y. C. (2016). Long-term fine particulate matter exposure and major depressive disorder in a community-based urban cohort. *Environmental Health Perspectives*, *124*(10), 1547–1553.

Kneebone, E. (2017). The changing geography of US poverty. *Testimony before the House Ways and Means Committee, Subcommittee on Human Resources February 15, 2017*. Retrieved from https://www.brookings.edu/testimonies/the-changing-geography-of-us-poverty/

Knudsen, A., & Meit, M. (n.d.). *Public health nursing: Strengthening the core of rural public health (Policy Brief)*. Kansas City, MO: National Rural Health Association.

Krishna, S., Gillespie, K. N., & McBride, T. M. (2010). Diabetes burden and access to preventive care in the rural United States. *The Journal of Rural Health*, *26*(1), 3–11.

La Cooperativa. (2020). *Health issues for migrant workers*. Retrieved from http://www.lacooperativa.org/health-issues-migrant-workers/

Lahr, M., Neprash, H. Henning-Smith, H., Tuttle, M. S., Hernandez, A. (2019). *Access to specialty care for Medicare beneficiaries in rural communities*. University of Minnesota Rural Health Research Center.

Laidlaw, M. A., Filippelli, G. M., Sadler, R. C., Gonzales, C. R., Ball, A. S., & Mielke, H. W. (2016). Children's blood lead seasonality in Flint, Michigan and soil-sourced lead hazard risks. *International Journal of Environmental Research & Public Health*, *13*(4), e358.

Langley, R., Hirsch, A., Cullen, R., Allran, J., Woody, R., & Bell, D. (2017). North Carolina state agencies working to prevent agricultural injuries and illnesses. *Journal of Agromedicine*, *22*(4), 358–363.

Lee, I., Eriksson, P., Fredriksson, A., Buratovic, S., & Viberg, H. (2015). Developmental neurotoxic effects of two pesticides: Behavior and neuroprotein studies on endosulfan and cypermethrin. *Toxicology*, *335*, 1–10.

Lee, J., Schram, A., Riley, E., Harris, P., Baum, F., Fisher, M., ... & Friel, S. (2018). Addressing health equity through action on the social determinants of health: A global review of policy outcome evaluation methods. *International Journal of Health Policy and Management, 7*(7), 581.

Lenardson, J. D., Hansen, A., & Hartley, D. (2015). Rural and remote food environments and obesity. *Current Obesity Reports, 4*(1), 46–53.

Li, Y., Zhang, D., & Pagán, J. A. (2016). Social norms and the consumption of fruits and vegetables across New York City neighborhoods. *Journal of Urban Health, 93*(2), 244–255.

Lim, Y., Song, S., & Song, W. (2017). Prevalence and determinants of overweight and obesity in children and adolescents from migrant and seasonal farmworkers families in the united states- a systematic review and qualitative assessment. *Nutrients, 9*(3), 1–17. doi: 10.3390/nu9030188.

Luo, T., & Escalante, C. L. (2018). Health care service utilization of documented and undocumented hired farm workers in the U.S. *The European Journal of Health Economics, 19*(7), 923–934.

Matsui, E., Abramson, S., & Sandel, M. (2016). Indoor environmental control practices and asthma management. *American Academy of Pediatrics, 138*(5), e20162589.

Matte, T. D., Lane, K., & Ito, K. (2016). Excess mortality attributable to extreme heat in New York City, 1997–2013. *Health Security, 14*(2), 64–70.

Maxmen, A. (2016). Stress: The privilege of health. *Nature, 531*(7594), s58–s59.

McCullagh, M. C., Sanon, M. A., & Foley, J. G. (2015). Cultural health practices of migrant seasonal farmworkers. *Journal of Cultural Diversity, 22*(2), 64.

Merchant, J., Coussens, C., & Gilbert, D. (2006). *Rebuilding the unity of health and the environment in rural America*. Washington, DC: National Academies Press. Retrieved from https://www.ncbi.nlm.nih.gov/books/NBK56972/

Migrant Clinicians Network. (2017a). *Migrant/seasonal farmworker*. Retrieved from https://www.migrantclinician.org/issues/migrant-info/migrant.html

Migrant Clinicians Network. (2017b). *Children's health*. Retrieved from https://www.migrantclinician.org/issues/childrenshealth

Migrant Clinicians Network. (2017c). *Women's health*. Retrieved from https://www.migrantclinician.org/issues/womenshealth

Migrant Housing. (n.d.). *Migrant center housing*. Retrieved from www.stancoha.org/Migrant.htm

Migrant Policy Institute. (2020). *Vulnerable to COVID-19 and in front-line jobs, immigrants are mostly shut out of U.S. relief*. Retrieved from https://www.migrationpolicy.org/article/covid19-immigrants-shut-out-federal-relief

Migration Policy Institute. (2015, September 21). *Deportation of a parent can have significant and long-lasting harmful effects on child well-being, as a pair of reports from MPI and the Urban Institute detail*. Retrieved from http://www.migrationpolicy.org/news/deportation-parent-can-have-significant-and-long-lasting-harmful-effects-child-well-being-pair

MiVIA. (2016). *Connecting patients and clinicians nationwide: Welcome to MiVIA*. Retrieved from https://www.ruralhealthinfo.org/rural-monitor/mivia-program-electronic-health-records/

Molokwu, J., Penaranda, E., Flores, S., & Shokar, N. K. (2016). Evaluation of the effect of a promotora-led educational intervention on cervical cancer and human papillomavirus knowledge among predominately Hispanic primary care patients on the US-Mexico border. *Journal of Cancer Education*, 31(4), 742–748. doi: 10.1007s13187-015-0938-5.

Mostafalou, S., & Abdollahi, M. (2017). Pesticides: An update of human exposure and toxicity. *Archives of Toxicology, 91*(2), 549–599.

Moyce, S. C., & Schenker, M. (2018). Migrant workers and their occupational health and safety. *Annual Review of Public Health, 39*, 351–365. doi: 10.1146/annurev-publhealth-040617-013714.

Mundell, E. J. (January 17, 2019). *Opioid prescriptions almost twice as likely for rural vs. urban Americans*. Retrieved from https://www.usnews.com/news/health-news/articles/2019-01-17/opioid-prescriptions-almost-twice-as-likely-for-rural-vs-urban-americans

Munzel, T., Sorensen, M., Schmidt, F., Schmidt, E., Steven, S., Kroller-Schon, S., & Daiber, A. (2018). The adverse effects of environmental noise exposure on oxidative stress and cardiovascular risk. *Antioxidants & Redox Signaling*, 28(9), 873–910.

Myers, W. (2018). *COPD: Speak your piece: Rural trend in lung disease heads in the wrong direction*. The Daily Yonder. Retrieved from http://www.dailyyonder.com/speak-piece-rural-trend-lung-disease-heads-wrong-direction/2018/12/28/29256/

National Association of County & City Health Officials. (2016). *2016 National profile of local health departments*. Retrieved from https://nacchovoice.naccho.org/2017/01/25/2016-national-profile-of-local-health-departments/

National Center for Farmworker Health (NCFH). (2018a). *Agricultural workers factsheet*. Retrieved http://www.ncfh.org/fact-sheets--research.html

National Center for Farmworker Health (NCFH). (2018b). *Maternal & child health fact sheet*. Retrieved from http://www.ncfh.org/uploads/3/8/6/8/38685499/fs-maternal_and_child_health_2018.pdf

National Center for Frontier Communities. (2019). Retrieved from https://www.ers.usda.gov/data-products/frontier-and-remote-area-codes/

National Conference of State Legislatures. (2020). *States implement health reform: School-based health centers*. Retrieved from https://www.ncsl.org/research/health/school-based-health-centers.aspx

National Highway & Traffic Safety Administration. (2018). *Traffic safety facts 2016 data: Rural/urban comparison*. Retrieved from https://crashstats.nhtsa.dot.gov/Api/Public/ViewPublication/812521#:~:text=Rural%20traffic%20fatalities%20decreased%20by,2007%20to%2017%2C656%20in%202016.&text=Speeding%2Drelated%20fatalities%20occurred%20in,in%20rural%20and%20urban%20areas.

National Rural Health Association (NRHA). (2019). *Rural health voices*. Retrieved from https://www.ruralhealthweb.org/blogs/ruralhealthvoices/july-2019/nrha-releases-2019-policy-papers

New York Academy of Medicine. (2020). *Institute for Urban Health*. Retrieved from https://www.nyam.org/journal-urban-health/

Nieuwenhuijsen, M. (2016). Urban and transport planning, environmental exposures and health-new concepts, methods and tools to improve health in cities. *Environmental Health, 15*(Supp 1), S38. doi: 10.1186/s12940-016-0108-1.

NYU Langone Health. (2020). *New COVID local risk index identifies neighborhoods at high risk of pandemic's impact*. Retrieved from https://nyulangone.org/news/new-covid-local-risk-index-identifies-neighborhoods-highest-risk-pandemics-impact

Occupational Safety & Health Administration (OSHA). (n.d.). *Agricultural operations standards: Field sanitation*. Retrieved from https://www.dol.gov/sites/dolgov/files/WHD/legacy/files/whdfs51.pdf

Open Anesthesia. (2020). *Organophosphate poisoning: Diagnosis and treatment*. Retrieved from https://www.openanesthesia.org/organophosphate_poisoning_diagnosis_and_treatment/

Owens, C. (January 29, 2016). *Reconnecting urban planning and public health*. Retrieved from https://nextcity.org/daily/entry/urban-planning-public-health-collaborating

Pain, S. (2016). The rise of the urbanite. *Nature, 531*(7594), 550–551.

Parker, K. F., & Stansfield, R. (2015). The changing urban landscape: Interconnections between racial/ethnic segregation and exposure in the study of race-specific violence over time. *American Journal of Public Health, 105*(9), 1796–1805.

Partnership for Sustainable Communities. (2018). *Partnership for sustainable communities: Five years of learning from communities and coordinating federal investments*. Retrieved from https://www.epa.gov/smartgrowth/partnership-sustainable-communities-five-years-learning-communities-and-coordinating

Pew Charitable Trusts. (2018). *American families face a growing rent burden*. Retrieved from https://www.pewtrusts.org/-/media/assets/2018/04/rent-burden_report_v2.pdf

Pew Research Center. (2018). *Social and demographic trends*. Retrieved from https://www.pewsocialtrends.org/2018/05/22/demographic-and-economic-trends-in-urban-suburban-and-rural-communities/

Pew Research Center. (2020). *Global attitudes and trends*. Retrieved from https://www.pewresearch.org/global/

Phipps, E. J., Singletary, S. B., Cooblall, C. A., Hares, H. D., & Braitman, L. E. (2016). Food insecurity in patients with high hospital utilization. *Population Health Management, 19*(6), 414–420. doi: 10.1089/pop.2015.0127.

Plascak, J. J., Griffith, W. C., Workman, T., Smith, M. N., Vigoren, E., Faustman, E. M., & Thompson, B. (2018). Evaluation of the relationship between residential orchard density and dimethyl organophosphate pesticide residues in house dust. *Journal of Exposure Science & Environmental Epidemiology*, 29(3), 379–388.

Ponce-Gonzalez, I., Cheadle, A., Aisenberg, G., & Cantrell, L. F. (2019). Improving oral health in migrant and underserved populations: Evaluation of an interactive, community-based oral health education program in Washington state. *BMC Oral Health, 19*(1), 30.

Pupo, M. C., Serafim, P. M., & deMello, M. F. (2015). Health-related quality of life in posttraumatic stress disorder: 4 years follow-up study of individuals exposed to urban violence. *Psychiatry Research, 228*(3), 741–745.

Quandt, S. A., Groeschel-Johnson, A., Kinzer, H. T., Jensen, A., Miles, K., O'Hara, H. M., ... & Arcury, T. A. (2018). Migrant farmworker nutritional strategies: Implications for diabetes management. *Journal of Agromedicine, 23*(4), 347–354.

Quandt, S. A., Trejo, G., Suerken, C. K., Pulgar, C. A., Ip, E. H., & Arcury, T. A. (2016). Diet quality among preschool-age children of Latino migrant and seasonal farmworkers in the United States. *Journal of Immigrant and Minority Health, 18*(3), 505–512.

Ramos, A., Carlo, G., Grant, K., Trinidad, N., & Correa, A. (2016). Stress, depression, and occupational injury among migrant farmworkers in Nebraska. *Safety*, 2(4), 23.

Rao, Hancy, Velez, Freeman, & Davis (n.d.). *HIV/AIDS and Farmworkers in the U.S. White Paper*. Retrieved from https://www.migrantclinician.org/files/HIVWhitePaper08.pdf

Reboussin, B. A., Green, K. M., Milam, A. J., Furr-Holden, D. M., Johnson, R. M., & Ialongo, N. S. (2015). The role of neighborhood in urban Black adolescent marijuana use. *Drug & Alcohol Dependence*, *154*, 69–75.

Recio, A., Linares, C., Banegas, J. R., & Diaz, J. (2016). Road traffic noise effects on cardiovascular, respiratory, and metabolic health: An integrative model of biological mechanisms. *Environmental Research*, *146*, 359–370.

Reza, M., Amin, M. S., Sgro, A., Abdelaziz, A., Ito, D., Main, P., & Azarpazhooh, A. (2016). Oral health status of immigrant and refugee children in North America: A scoping review. *Journal of the Canadian Dental Association*, *82*(g3), 1488–2159.

Rigg, K. K., Monnat, S. M., & Chavez, M. N. (2018). Opioid-related mortality in rural America: Geographic heterogeneity and intervention strategies. *International Journal of Drug Policy*, *57*, 119–129.

Ritchie, H., & Roser, M. (2018). Urbanization. In *Our World in Data*. Retrieved from https://ourworldindata.org/urbanization

Rodman, S. O., Barry, C., Clayton, M. L., Frattaroli, M. L., Neff, R. A., & Rutkow, L. (2016). Agricultural exceptionalism at the state level: Characterization of wage and hour laws for U.S. farmworkers. *Journal of Agriculture, Food Systems, and Community Development*, 6(2), 89–110.

Rural Health Information Hub. (2018a). *Recruitment and retention for rural health facilities*. Retrieved from https://www.ruralhealthinfo.org/topics/rural-health-recruitment-retention

Rural Health Information Hub. (2018b). *Rural migrant health*. Retrieved from https://www.ruralhealthinfo.org/topics/migrant-health

Rural Health Information Hub. (2019a). *Critical access hospitals*. Retrieved from https://www.ruralhealthinfo.org/topics/critical-access-hospitals

Rural Health Information Hub. (2019b). *Telehealth use in rural healthcare*. Retrieved from https://www.ruralhealthinfo.org/topics/telehealth

Rural Health Information Hub (RHIH). (2020a). *Your first stop for rural health information*. Retrieved from https://www.ruralhealthinfo.org/

Rural Health Information Hub (RHIH). (2020b). *Rural mental health*. Retrieved from http://ruralhealthinfo.org/topics/mental-health

Salviati, C. (2020). *Apartment list national rent report*. Retrieved from https://www.apartmentlist.com/rentonomics/national-rent-data/

Schwingel, A., Wiley, A. R., Teran-Garcia, M., McCaffrey, J., Gálvez, P., & Vizcarra, M. (2017). Promotoras and the semantic gap between Latino community health researchers and Latino communities. *Health Promotion Practice*, *18*(3), 444–453.

Seright, T. J., & Winters, C. A. (2015). Critical care in critical access hospitals. *Critical Care Nurse*, *35*(5), 62–67.

Shelton, J. F., & Hertz-Picciotto, I. (2015). Neurodevelopmental disorders and agricultural pesticide exposures: Shelton and Hertz-Picciotto respond. *Environmental Health Perspectives*, *123*(4), A79–A80.

Snyder, R. Boone, C., Cardoso, C., Aguiar-Alves, F., Neves, F., & Riley, L. (2017). Zika: A scourge in urban slums. *PLos Negl Trop Dis*, *11*(3), e0005287. doi: 10.1371/journal.pntd.0005287.

Soneja, S., Jiang, C., Fisher, J., Upperman, C. R., Mitchell, C., & Sapkota, A. (2016). Exposure to extreme heat and precipitation events associated with increased risk of hospitalization for asthma in Maryland. *Environmental Health*, *15*, 57.

Stacciarini, J. M., Vacca, R., Wiens, B., Loe, E., LaFlam, M., Pérez, A., & Locke, B. (2016). FBO leaders' perceptions of the psychosocial contexts for rural Latinos. *Issues in Mental Health Nursing*, *37*(1), 19–25.

Stebbins, S. (May 26, 2018). *USA Today. Migrations and growth: The fastest growing (and shrinking) cities in the U.S.* Retrieved from https://www.usatoday.com/story/money/economy/2018/05/26/fastest-growing-and-shrinking-us-cities/34813515/

Stieb, D. M., Chen, L., Hystad, P., Beckerman, B. S., Jerrett, M., Tjepkema, M., ... Dugandzic, R. M. (2016). A national study of the association between traffic-related air pollution and adverse pregnancy outcomes in Canada, 1999-2008. *Environmental Research*, *148*, 513–526.

Stingone, J. A., McVeigh, K. H., & Claudio, L. (2016). Association between prenatal exposure to ambient diesel particulate matter and perchloroethylene with children's 3rd grade standardized test scores. *Environmental Research*, *148*, 144–153.

Student Action Farmers (SAF). (2011-2019). *U.S. farmworker factsheet*. Retrieved from http://safeunite.org/content/united-states-farmworker-factsheet

The Washington Post. (2019). Baltimore sees biggest population lost in single year since 2001, census estimates show. Retrieved from https://www.washingtonpost.com/local/baltimore-sees-biggest-population-loss-in-single-year-since-2001-census-estimates-show/2019/04/21/f601f560-62b9-11e9-9ff2-abc984dc9eec_story.html?noredirect=on&utm_term=.0a98c28167b3

Trivedi, T., Liu, J., Probst, J., Merchant, A., Jhones, S., & Martin, A. B. (2015). Obesity and obesity-related behaviors among rural and urban adults in the USA. *Rural and Remote Health*, *15*(4), 3267.

Tung, E., Cagney, K., Peek, M., & Chin, M. (2017). Spatial context and health inequity: Reconfiguring race, place, and poverty. *Journal of Urban Health*, *94*(6), 757–763. doi: 10.1007/s11524-017-0210-x.

U.S. Department of Agriculture (USDA). (2017). *Report to the President of the U.S. from the task force on agriculture and rural prosperity*. Retrieved from https://www.usda.gov/sites/default/files/documents/rural-prosperity-report.pdf

U.S. Department of Education. (n.d.). *Migrant student records exchange initiative (MSIX)*. Retrieved from https://www2.ed.gov/admins/lead/account/msixbrochure.pdf

U.S. Department of Health & Human Services (USDHHS). (2020a). *Healthy people 2030 framework*. Retrieved from https://www.healthypeople.gov/2020/About-Healthy-People/Development-Healthy-People-2030/Framework

U.S. Department of Health & Human Services (USDHHS). (2020b). *Access to health services*. Retrieved from https://www.healthypeople.gov/2020/topics-objectives/topic/Access-to-Health-Services

U.S. Department of Health and Human Services. (2018). *The opioid crisis and economic opportunity: Geographic and economic trends*. Retrieved from https://aspe.hhs.gov/system/files/pdf/259261/ASPEEconomicOpportunity-OpioidCrisis.pdf

U.S. Department of Housing & Urban Development (USDHUD). (2016). *Common questions about migrant/farmworkers*. Retrieved from https://www.hud.gov/states/florida/working/farmworker/commonquestions

U.S. Department of Labor. (2017). *Bureau of labor statistics*. Retrieved from https://www.bls.gov/iif/oshwc/osh/os/summ1_00_2017.htm

United States Census Bureau. (2016a). *New census data show differences between urban and rural population*. Retrieved from https://www.census.gov/newsroom/press-releases/2016/cb16-210.html

United States Census Bureau. (2016b). *Measuring American: Our changing landscape*. Retrieved from https://www.census.gov/library/visualizations/2016/comm/acs-rural-urban.html?CID=acs-rural-urban

United States Census Bureau. (2019). *Census Flows Mapper*. Retrieved from https://flowsmapper.geo.census.gov/

United States Department of Agriculture (USDA). (May, 2018). *Farm labor*. Retrieved from https://www.ers.usda.gov/topics/farm-economy/farm-labor/#size

United States Department of Agriculture (USDA). (2019a). *What is rural?* Retrieved from https://www.nal.usda.gov/ric/what-is-rural

United States Department of Agriculture (USDA). (2019b). *Frontier and remote area codes*. Retrieved from http://www.ers.usda.gov/data-products/frontier-and-remote-area-codes.aspx

United States Department of Agriculture (USDA). (2020). *Rural education*. Retrieved from https://www.ers.usda.gov/topics/rural-economy-population/employment-education/rural-education/

Vargas, E. D., & Pirog, M. A. (2016). Mixed-status families and WIC uptake: The effects of risk of deportation on program use. *Social Science Quarterly*, *97*(3), 555–572.

Wedgworth, J. C., Brown, J., Olson, J. R., Johnson, P., Elliott, M., Grammar, P., & Stauber, C. E. (2015). Temporal heterogeneity of water quality in rural Alabama water supplies. *Journal-American Water Works Association*, *107*(8), e401–e415.

Weiss A. J., Elixhauser, A., Barrett, M. L., Steiner, C. A., Bailey, M. K., & O'Malley, L. (2017). *Opioid-related inpatient stays and emergency department visits by state, 2009–2014*. HCUP Statistical Brief #219, Rockville, MD: Agency for Healthcare Research and Quality. Retrieved from https://www.hcup-us.ahrq.gov/reports/statbriefs/sb219-Opioid-Hospital-Stays-ED-Visits-by-State.jsp

Whittle, H. J., Palar, K., Hufstedler, L. L., Seligman, H. K., Frongillo, E. A., & Weiser, S. D. (2015). Food insecurity, chronic illness, and gentrification in the San Francisco Bay area: An example of structural violence in United States public policy. *Social Science & Medicine*, *143*, 154–161.

Wiewel, E. W., Bocour, A., Kersanske, L. S., Bodach, S. D., Xia, Q., & Braunstein, S. L. (2016). The association between neighborhood poverty and HIV diagnoses among males and females in New York City, 2010-2011. *Public Health Reports*, *131*(2), 290–302.

Williams, J. (2017). *Mobile clinical offers care for migrant workers*. In UNC Health Care. Retrieved from http://news.unchealthcare.org/news/2017/may/mobile-clinic-offers-care-to-farm-workers

Wilson, J. B., Rappleyea, D. L., Hodgson, J. L., Brimhall, A. S., Hall, T. L., & Thompson, A. P. (2015). Healthcare providers' experiences screening for intimate partner violence among migrant and seasonal farmworking women: A phenomenological study. *Health Expectations*, *19*(6), 1277–1289. doi: 10.1111/hex.12421.

Wiltz, T. (2016). *States struggle to provide housing for migrant farmworkers*. In PEW. Retrieved from https://www.pewtrusts.org/en/research-and-analysis/blogs/stateline/2016/05/02/struggle-to-provide-housing-for-migrant-farmworkers

Winchester, M. S., BeLue, R., Oni, T., Wittwer-Backofen, U., Deobagkar, D., Onya, H., ... & Airhihenbuwa, C. (2016). The Pan-University Network for Global Health: Framework for collaboration and review of global health needs. *Globalization and Health*, *12*(1), 13.

Winquist, A., Grundstein, A., Chang, H. H., Hess, J., & Sarnat, S. E. (2016). Warm season temperatures and emergency department visits in Atlanta, Georgia. *Environmental Research*, *147*, 314–323.

World Health Organization. (2020a). *About social determinants of health*. Retrieved from https://www.who.int/social_determinants/sdh_definition/en/

World Health Organization (2020b). *Healthy cities*. Retrieved from http://www.who.int/healthpromotion/conferences/9gchp/healthy-cities/en/

Worldometers. (2017). Retrieved from http://www.worldometers.info/world-population/us-population/

Wright, B. A., Peters, E. R., Ettinger, U., Kuipers, E., & Kumari, V. (2016). Moderators of noise-induced cognitive change in healthy adults. *Noise & Health*, *18*(82), 117–132.

Yanar, B., Kosny, A., & Smith, P. (2018). Occupational health and safety vulnerability of recent immigrants and refugees. *International Journal of Environmental Research and Public Health*, *15*(9).

UNIT 7

Settings for Community/Public Health Nursing

CHAPTER 28

Public Settings

"Public health nursing is the practice of promoting and protecting the health of populations using knowledge from nursing, social, and public health sciences."

—The Definition and Practice of Public Health Nursing: A Statement of the APHA Public Health Nursing Section, 2013

KEY TERMS

Correctional nurses
Indian Health Service (IHS)
Individualized education plans (IEPs)
Individualized health plans (IHPs)
Local health departments (LHDs)
School-based health centers (SBHCs)
School nurse
Section 504 plans
Student study teams (SSTs)
U.S. Public Health Service (USPHS) Commissioned Corps

LEARNING OBJECTIVES

Upon mastery of this chapter, you should be able to:

1. Explain the focus of the nursing process and how community/public health nurses (C/PHNs) and other nurses working in the publicly funded sector use the tool to provide care in their communities.
2. Describe how federal, state, and local public health infrastructures influence the population's health.
3. Evaluate the potential benefits of school-based health centers and possible parental or community objections.
4. Compare and contrast common roles and functions of C/PHNs, school nurses, and correctional nurses.

INTRODUCTION

Many nursing students are not aware of the vast employment opportunities available outside the hospital in publicly funded settings. This chapter discusses several of these publicly funded health settings and the opportunities nurses can garner, particularly in services such as public health nursing, school nursing, and correctional nursing. Although these nursing opportunities differ greatly from one another, they have several characteristics in common. Community nurses who work in a setting supported through public funds (e.g., taxpayer-funded):

1. Still use the nursing process, just with a population or group of people rather than an individual.
2. Emphasize *prevention* of disease or disability.
3. Work with a variety of people, usually vulnerable populations.
4. Focus on population-based care and must be able to network and collaborate with other agencies and disciplines (e.g., a nurse working in a correctional facility collaborating with mental health workers and correctional officers).
5. May advocate for individuals and the community and serve on regional task forces or advisory boards.
6. Must be autonomous, flexible, creative thinkers who are self-directed and able to prioritize and use the nursing process and evidence-based practices to make decisions and plan efficient care for their respective populations.

PUBLIC HEALTH NURSING

A C/PHN is a nurse who works to promote and protect the health of an entire population (American Nurses Association [ANA], 2013). An estimated 231,000 to 341,000 workers compose the U.S. public health workforce (University of Michigan Center of Excellence in Public Health Workforce Studies, 2018). This workforce consists of epidemiologists, nurses, environmentalists, laboratory professionals, nutritionists, dental workers, social workers, and other health care providers.

Approximately 18% of all registered nurses (RNs) are employed in public or community health settings (Beck & Boulton, 2016). The trends of inadequate access to health care and rising costs of health care have contributed to more nurses working in these settings. Unfortunately, many are unaware of the employment opportunities available in the public sector. This section describes the roles and opportunities for RNs at the local, state, and federal levels of government, with particular focus on governmental agencies, as these facilities employ the majority of C/PHNs.

Education

The ANA (2013) recommends that an entry-level C/PHN should have a bachelor's degree in nursing. This is important because baccalaureate programs provide additional training in public health and leadership. Some states, such as California, require nurses to take additional classes and obtain certification beyond a bachelor's degree if the Bachelor of Science in Nursing program does not offer specific content (e.g., child abuse, public health didactic, and practicum). C/PHNs working with specific populations or in administration should hold a master's degree.

Key Functions of the C/PHN in the Public Setting

Public health nursing practice consists of many areas of expertise, including:

- Focusing on the health of populations
- Reflecting the needs and priorities of the community
- Establishing caring relationships with individuals, families, communities, and systems
- Being grounded in cultural sensitivity, compassion, social justice, and a belief in the worth of all people (e.g., vulnerable populations)
- Having a basic understanding of all aspects of health (e.g., physical, emotional, mental, social, spiritual, and environmental)
- Using strategies to promote health that are motivated by epidemiologic evidence
- Using individual, as well as collaborative, strategies to achieve results

In brief, the role of the C/PHN is to focus on the health of the public. C/PHNs combine their nursing and clinical knowledge of disease and the human response to it, along with public health skills, to accomplish their goals (ANA, 2015). They apply the nursing process, not only with individuals but also with populations. C/PHNs are a critical link between data tracking (e.g., epidemiology) and developing a clinical understanding of a disease or condition and use the data to prioritize their interventions to stop the spread of diseases, such as measles, and also to intercede with other concerns (e.g., childhood obesity). For example, C/PHNs may develop a campaign for children to wear bike helmets after an increase of fatal head injuries is noted in their area. A key emphasis of the C/PHN is prevention, and a key focus is educating and empowering the community.

The Council of Public Health Nursing Organizations (CPHNO) (https://www.cphno.org), formerly the Quad Council, developed the first Competencies for Public Health in 2010. The organization is composed of these organizations: Association of Community Health Nursing Educators (ACHNE), Association of Public Health Nurses (APHN), Rural Nurse Organization, American Nurses Association (ANA), Alliance of Nurses for Healthy Environment, American Public health Association—Public Health Nursing Section (APHA). These competencies have been updated and are used as a tool in education and for agencies in orienting new C/PHNs (Quad Council Coalition, 2018). See Box 28-1 for community settings for C/PHNs.

C/PHNs may focus on a population that is a geographic community (e.g., a state or municipality) or a focus group (e.g., adolescents or older persons) spanning all socioeconomic levels. To accomplish this, C/PHNs often work with individuals or families at highest risk, and their motive is to improve, protect, and promote the health of the entire population. A distinctive goal of C/PHNs relative to the goals of other nursing disciplines is achieving the greatest good for the majority of people (ANA, 2015) (See Chapter 23 for an in-depth discussion of social justice). This requires priority planning and a basic knowledge of the community. It can also create ethical dilemmas for C/PHNs when they have personal and passionate issues that they would like to pursue but which are not the top priority for the majority of community members.

For example, a child in a community may have been hit by a car while riding his bike without a helmet, while at the same time, in the same community, there may be

BOX 28-1 Community Settings for Public Health Nurses

Community/Public health nurses (C/PHNs) can be found working in communities advocating for environmental, transportation, and safety policies in collaboration with community organizations.

- C/PHNs may work in schools, public health clinics/departments, or local government agencies advocating for elimination of health disparities.
- C/PHNs are increasingly seen working on global health issues as the international borders are rapidly disappearing due to increased, rapid international travel and enhanced electronic communication technology (American Public Health Association, 2013).
- Visiting nursing is an opportunity for family health education and one-to-one educating for managing specific illness.
- Geriatric nursing is a growing specialty as the care for older adults in assisted living skilled care facilities or through home care is increasing with the aging baby boomer population.
- Correctional nursing provides an opportunity to impact community health by promoting healthy lifestyle practices and effective management of communicable diseases are implemented during incarceration prior to release.

10 births to teen moms, 20 instances of drug overdose, and an outbreak of pertussis. The C/PHNs in that community must prioritize which issue to address first by deciding which issue impacts the most people and what interventions will help the population thrive (ANA, 2015). Because each community is different, once all factors are taken into account, the priorities will vary among communities. Hence, *assessment* is a critical component of public health and a key tool for the nurses who work in the public sector (ANA, 2015; Turnock, 2016).

Another way Community/public health nursing differs from other areas in nursing is that C/PHNs must actively seek out and identify potential problems and situations (ANA, 2015). Nurses who work in a hospital setting address the issues that come to them. A nurse in the intensive care unit of a hospital works with an assigned patient load. C/PHNs, on the other hand, are out in the community identifying the problems, not waiting for problems to come to them. For example, C/PHNs may participate in visits to childcare centers to note any safety hazards and ensure that rules and regulations are being followed and that children are properly immunized. These visits are part of the priority of *assurance* (Turnock, 2016).

C/PHNs cannot perform all these activities alone. They need to collaborate with other partners and optimally use often limited resources. C/PHNs are in a unique situation because they work with their populations (i.e., clients) and with others to find the best solutions for a situation or problem. For instance, C/PHNs may notice an increase in the number of measles cases in their community. They may then work with families to identify where and how the children were exposed to the disease and with local health care providers to provide treatment and vaccinations for those at highest risk of exposure to and damage from measles. C/PHNs also work with school nurses and other school personnel to exclude from school attendance those children who are not adequately immunized against measles. This helps decrease the spread and potential harm because of measles. C/PHNs educate a variety of groups, such as parent–teacher associations and city or school officials, as to how measles spreads, what can be done to treat the disease, and the importance of herd immunity in protecting the public. Education thus empowers each group to be part of the solution. Finally, C/PHNs can work with public health officials to develop a policy for all new school entrants to receive a second booster of measles vaccine. *Policy development* is the third critical component of public health (Turnock, 2016).

PUBLIC HEALTH FUNDING AND GOVERNMENTAL STRUCTURES

Well-functioning public health departments are critical entities in the effort to build a healthy nation. Accurate estimations of essential funding to support public health adequately are difficult to determine. Because C/PHNs can work at any and all levels of government, it is important to understand the organizational structure, communication, and funding streams between the federal, state, and local levels of government (see Chapter 6 for more on the structure of the public health system).

National Policy

The federal government oversees national policy and funding, provides expertise, and sets a national agenda (World Health Organization, 2019). Healthy People initiatives identify our nation's health improvement priorities by setting 10-year goals and targets. Since 1990, "Healthy People has established evidence-based national health objectives with clear targets that allow us to monitor progress, motivate action, and guide efforts to improve health across the country" (https://health.gov/our-work/healthy-people/). For example, see Box 28-2 for content areas related to children and adolescents.

State Agencies

The U.S. Constitution bestows states with the responsibility to safeguard the health of their citizens (Turnock, 2016). Much of public health is overseen at the state level. However, the structure of where public health fits into the executive branch of state government varies. The governor appoints a commissioner, or leading health official, to oversee public health and serve as a member of the governor's cabinet.

The purpose of state agencies is to carry forth regulations and policies determined by the federal government (e.g., Medicaid, Medicare, and State Children's Health Insurance Programs). Many of these programs have specific federal requirements but also allow states the ability to personalize the programs to fit each state's individual needs.

BOX **28-2** *HEALTHY PEOPLE 2030*

Content Areas for Children and Adolescents

Healthy People 2030 provides the direction and goals for all community/public health nurses (C/PHNs). *Healthy People 2030* is used to guide prioritizing activities for C/PHNs. Below are the Healthy People 2030 content areas that pertain to the health of children and adolescents.

Access to health
Blood disorders
Cancer
Child and adolescent development
Chronic kidney disease
Chronic pain
Drug and alcohol use
Economic stability
Education access and quality
Emergency preparedness
Environmental health
Family planning
Health care
Heath care access and quality
Health communication
Health insurance
Health IT
Health policy
Hospital and emergency services
Housing and homes
Injury prevention
LGBT
Neighborhood and built environment
Nutrition and healthy eating
Overweight and obesity
Parents or caregivers
People with disabilities
Pregnancy and childbirth
Preventative care
Physical activity
Respiratory disease
Schools
Sensory and communication disorders
Sleep
Sexually transmitted infections
Social and community context
Tobacco use
Transportation
Vaccination
Violence prevention

Reprinted from U.S. Department of Health & Human Services (USDHHS). (2020a). *Healthy People 2030: Browse objectives.* Retrieved from https://health.gov/healthypeople/objectives-and-data/browse-objectives

Local Public Health

Local health departments (LHDs) carry out state laws and policies (Turnock, 2016). They provide the most direct, immediate care to the population while providing the essential public health services at the local level (Moore, Berner, & Wall, 2020) and operate programs with funding from federal and state agencies. LHDs often work with state health departments to ensure that culturally appropriate and population-specific services are delivered to the community.

NURSING ROLES IN LOCAL, STATE, AND FEDERAL PUBLIC HEALTH POSITIONS

Public health nurses are employed at federal, state, and local levels of government. Those working for LHDs are the eyes and ears of their communities (Fig. 28-1).

Assess

An assessment of the situation is the key component to any nursing care. C/PHNs use the nursing process in a variety of ways when they are in the community and when they conduct home visits. Often, the C/PHNs work with other public health personnel when assessing and tracking data. By using data and conducting an assessment, C/PHNs are able to successfully target interventions for populations at risk (Community Tool Box, 2020). See Chapters 12 and 15.

Environmental risks are important to the public's health and are often assessed by C/PHNs. A community positioned next to a factory that emits fumes will have different issues than a rural community 90 miles away from any industry. At the same time, a C/PHN may identify an outbreak of *Escherichia coli* in one town as a risk to a neighboring town. See Chapter 9.

Diagnose

Assessment is key to diagnosing a situation or problem (Box 28-3). For a C/PHN, diagnosis includes identifying priorities for the many concurrent issues which may be present.

As nurses diagnose individual needs, they apply this information and watch for increased or decreased rates (e.g., of disease or injury) among the population. Nurses are in the perfect position to identify issues and trends early (Community Tool Box, 2020).

Constant assessment and diagnosis are tools by which C/PHNs identify critical situations and prioritize issues that must be addressed. Several documents have

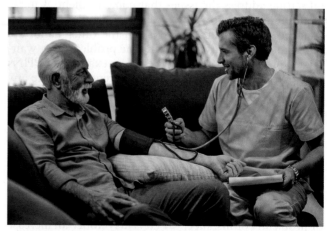

FIGURE 28-1 C/PHNs are the eyes and ears of their community.

BOX 28-3 STORIES FROM THE FIELD

Tuberculosis Exposure (Compare Your Local Response With That Outlined Here)

As a community/public health nurse (C/PHN), you are alerted to a person who has an active TB case. He presents into the health department for a chest x-ray after he failed his tuberculin skin test. The person has recently arrived by plane from another state. He stayed for a few weeks with family members in a small house but now lives with friends in a small apartment. When talking to the patient, you note that he coughs often and does not cover his mouth.

1. *As a C/PHN, what steps would you take to determine exposure? How will you determine who was exposed and will need to be tested? What questions can you ask to help determine when and how the patient was exposed to TB?*
2. *What type of education will you provide to him?*
3. *How can you ensure that the patient is compliant with medication treatment?*
4. *Imagine that you are the school nurse of the patient's 8-year-old daughter, who has also tested positive. What steps would you take?*
5. *What would you do differently if you were a correctional nurse and the patient was an inmate?*
6. *What are the ethical and legal issues related to TB?*

helped C/PHNs prioritize issues, such as *Healthy People* 2030 a guide to identifying many of the nation's top priorities (U.S. Department of Health and Human Services [USDHHS], 2020a). Public health performance standards established by the Centers for Disease Control and Prevention (CDC, 2018a) and the Institute of Medicine (2015) have identified specific leading indicators for improving patient care and health research. See Box 28-4.

Plan and Implement

Once C/PHNs have diagnosed and prioritized the needs of their community, they develop and carry out plans to address those needs. Many interventions require collaborating and working with other agencies and professions. C/PHNs provide preventive health education and serve as advocates to influence those who can make essential policy and funding changes. The interventions are endless, but here are a few examples:

- A nurse conducts home visits to mothers at risk and concurrently conducts family assessments to determine the level of psychological issues and education needed by the family regarding specific needs.
- A community nurse working in risk management develops and teaches an education program about workplace safety and ergonomics and helps to develop policies regarding shift hours and heavy lifting.
- A school nurse serves as an advocate for a program that will help children with special health care needs attend a clinic closer to home.
- A C/PHN develops a campaign for social media sites (e.g., Twitter, Facebook), television, radio, and local newspapers regarding the need to receive a flu shot, including incentives that target older persons in the community, who are at additional risk for developing complications from this illness.
- A C/PHN organizes a health clinic at local shelters that provides foot care and screenings for blood pressure, diabetes, tuberculosis (TB), and cholesterol, as appropriate.
- A school nurse works with schools to educate teens regarding birth control and the impact of teen pregnancy. The nurse includes counseling regarding sexually transmitted diseases (STDs) and works with the community to ensure that a variety of teen-focused activities are available for this population.

BOX 28-4 *HEALTHY PEOPLE 2030*

Public Health Priorities

Leading Health Indicators Framework

The *Healthy People* leading health indicators are selected to communicate high priority health issues and challenges. The focus is on social determinants of health that support quality of life, healthy behaviors, and healthy development across the life stages for all. The leading health indicators are selected and organized using the Health Determinants and Health Outcomes by Life Stages conceptual framework. This approach is intended to draw attention to both individual and societal determinants that affect the public's health and contribute to health disparities from infancy through old age, thereby highlighting strategic opportunities to promote health and improve quality of life for all Americans.

Healthy People 2030

Every decade, the *Healthy People* initiative develops a new set of science-based, 10-year national objectives with the goal of improving the health of all Americans. The development of *Healthy People 2030* includes establishing a framework for the initiative—the vision, mission, foundational principles, plan of action, and overarching goals—and identifying new objectives.

The *Healthy People 2030* framework explains the central ideas and functions of the *Healthy People 2030* initiative. The purpose of the framework is to:

- Provide context and rationale for the initiative's approach
- Communicate the principles that underlie decisions about *Healthy People 2030*
- Situate the initiative in the 5-decade history of *Healthy People*

Leading health indicators will address the lifespan and focus on:

Upstream measures such as risk factors and behaviors
Address issues of national importance
Address high-priority health issues that have an impact on community and public health nursing outcomes
Be modifiable through evidence-based interventions and strategies
Address social determinants of health, health disparities, and health inequity

Source: Office of Disease Prevention and Health Promotion (ODPHP) (2020); U.S. Department of Health & Human Services (USDHHS) (2020b).

- A C/PHN helps identify resources for families without insurance to ensure that well-child and adult screenings are performed regularly to reduce health care costs associated with illness.
- A C/PHN organizes a bicycle fair to educate the community regarding the need for bicycle helmets in hopes of decreasing head injuries, works to develop public policy related to child car seat/booster seat usage, and collaborates with local businesses to provide vouchers for discounts on child restraints for low-income parents.
- A nurse, who is an elected member of the state legislature, sponsors a bill to increase funding for school nurses.

The following interventions are examples of evidence-based practice (see Chapter 4) in public health nursing:

- Media campaigns targeting specific populations to educate and promote healthy lifestyle behavior (Atusingwize, Lewis, & Langley, 2015).
- Improving work-based health literacy through educational programs to improve musculoskeletal pain (Larsen et al., 2015).
- Children with chronic conditions such as asthma are more likely to have anxiety, leading to increased morbidity, including missed days of school and caregiver work time. Asthma education programs along with behavioral building programs may influence mental health, leading to medication compliance and reduced anxiety (McGovern, Arcoleo, & Melnyk, 2020).
- Promoting the use of helmets in an attempt to reduce injuries among motorcyclists in a rural area by adopting a community-based participation approach (Babazadeh, Kouzekanani, Ghasemzadeh, Matlabi, & Allahahverdipour, 2019).

Evaluate

The world in which C/PHNs work is always changing. It is crucial to constantly evaluate programs and interventions to determine whether interventions are effective and desired goals are reached (Box 28-5). The CPHNO supports research studies about the impact that C/PHNs have on improving population health and societal outcomes (Quad Council Coalition, 2018).

BOX 28-5 LEVELS OF PREVENTION PYRAMID

Cervical Cancer in The Community Setting

HEALTH ISSUE: Cervical cancer in the community setting

Tertiary Prevention

Rehabilitation	*Prevention*	
	Health Promotion and Education	*Health Protection*
■ Provide nursing support groups after hysterectomy and other treatment.		

Secondary Prevention

Early Diagnosis	*Prompt Treatment*
■ Promote regular Pap smears ■ Provide Pap smear and high-risk screening counseling at local health fairs	■ Provide resources of medical services available for women diagnosed with cervical cancer

Primary Prevention

Health Promotion and Education	*Health Protection*
■ Promote healthy lifestyle choices that will decrease risk of human papillomavirus (HPV) (use of condoms, decrease tobacco use, food containing vitamin C and beta carotene) ■ Provide HPV vaccine at appropriate age ■ Educate public on risks related to cervical cancer (HPV vaccine, multiple sex partners) ■ Educate women to get regular Pap smears	■ HPV vaccine if eligible ■ Regular screening according to American Cancer Society ■ Use condoms during sex ■ Limit your number of sexual partners ■ Don't smoke

Public Health Nursing Careers

Nurses who work at the state or federal level may:

- Have consultant or oversight-type roles
- Head programs that are specifically funded at the state and/or federal levels (e.g., HIV/AIDS, immunization programs)
- Work in clinics for children with special health care needs
- Provide direct care through ambulatory care clinics
- Be called upon to help during a disaster or communicable disease outbreak (Box 28-6).

BOX **28-6** PERSPECTIVES

A C/PHN Instructor Viewpoint on Community Health Nursing

As an instructor of undergraduate nursing students, I want students to realize that public health nursing is a wonderful and rewarding employment opportunity. Many students often enter the nursing program not knowing much about public health nursing. They may only get minimal exposure to public health and thus do not often understand who or what is involved in public health nursing. In so doing, they miss out on a wonderful opportunity to work with a variety of people. It may be helping new moms, or working with children and adolescents, or the elderly. They may help give vaccinations or prepare for community disasters. They might teach about breast-feeding or conduct cancer-screening clinics. They are out working directly with the people, ensuring the public's health.

Community/public health nurses (C/PHNs) are able to use the science of nursing because they need to understand the pathophysiology, anatomy, human development, and disease transmission. They may not do as many hands-on procedures as hospital nurses, but they still must keep up-to-date in knowledge, as they are often teaching. In addition, they must be quick and receptive thinkers who can work independently and creatively. C/PHNs also are the essence of the "art" of nursing. They must understand and relate to people and grasp social systems and human behavior. They are the voice for the most vulnerable and the champion of all.

Although C/PHNs may not see an immediate reward for their actions, as a nurse who works in the hospital does, C/PHNs make a long and lasting impact not just to an individual but also for an entire society. They have the opportunity to really be a patient advocate. They do this by helping well people stay well and by preventing illness. They also help those who are sick obtain medical access. C/PHNs can also be involved in public policy change that can help an entire community. Public health nursing encompasses the entire art and science of nursing.

Erin M.

Among distinct opportunities at the federal level are those associated with the Department of Veterans Affairs (2020) and the USDHHS (2020c). See Box 28-7.

C/PHNs in these agencies oversee and carry out the initiatives of *Healthy People 2030*, along with other program initiatives. Federally employed C/PHNs at the Health Resources and Services Administration may review state funding proposals for projects and ensure that guidelines are met. They are a resource for state health departments and LHDs and often are called upon as consultants. Nurses working at the National Institutes of Health (NIH) may assist in conducting research or work with legal and bioethics staff in evaluating the impact of research on participants, monitoring patients for adverse reactions, or coordinate care for specific groups of patients (NIH, n.d.).

BOX 28-7 Federal Agencies Employing U.S. Public Health Service Nurses

- Administration for Children and Families (ACF)
- Centers for Disease Control and Prevention (CDC)
- Centers for Medicare and Medicaid Services (CMS)
- Health Resources and Services Administration (HRSA)
- Indian Health Service (IHS)
- National Institutes of Health (NIH)
- Substance Abuse and Mental Health Services Administration (SAMHSA)
- U.S. Department of Agriculture (USDA)
- U.S. Department of Commerce
- U.S. Department of Defense
- U.S. Department of Homeland Security
- U.S. Department of Justice
- U.S. Department of Veterans Affairs (VA)
- U.S. Food and Drug Administration (FDA)
- U.S. Marshals Service

Indian Health Service

C/PHNs working with the **Indian Health Service (IHS)** strive to ensure that comprehensive, culturally acceptable personal and public health services are available and accessible to the 573 federally recognized Tribes that consist of 2.56 million American Indians and Alaska Natives in 170 IHS and tribally managed service units (IHS, 2020). Employment with the IHS allows a C/PHN to live in a variety of rural and urban settings and to work specifically with Native Americans, a vulnerable population. This type of nursing, in remote areas with limited consistent electricity or telephone access, is very challenging but can also be extremely rewarding.

Uniformed Public Health Nursing

Established in 1798, as part of an act to treat sick seamen in Marine hospitals, the **U.S. Public Health Service (USPHS) Commissioned Corps** is a group of more than 6,500 specially trained public health professionals committed to the mission of protecting, promoting, and advancing the health and safety of our nation (Fig. 28-2). As an essential component of the largest public health program in the world, these elite groups of officers are involved in:

- Health care delivery to underserved and vulnerable populations, including immigrants entering the country
- Disease control and prevention, including communicable disease outbreaks
- Biomedical research
- Food and drug regulation
- Mental health and drug abuse services
- Response efforts for natural and man-made disasters, often as first responders, remaining involved until the situation is resolved

The U.S. Surgeon General oversees the Commissioned Corps and supports the officers stationed in more than 20 federal agencies or departments across the nation, filling essential public health leadership and clinical service

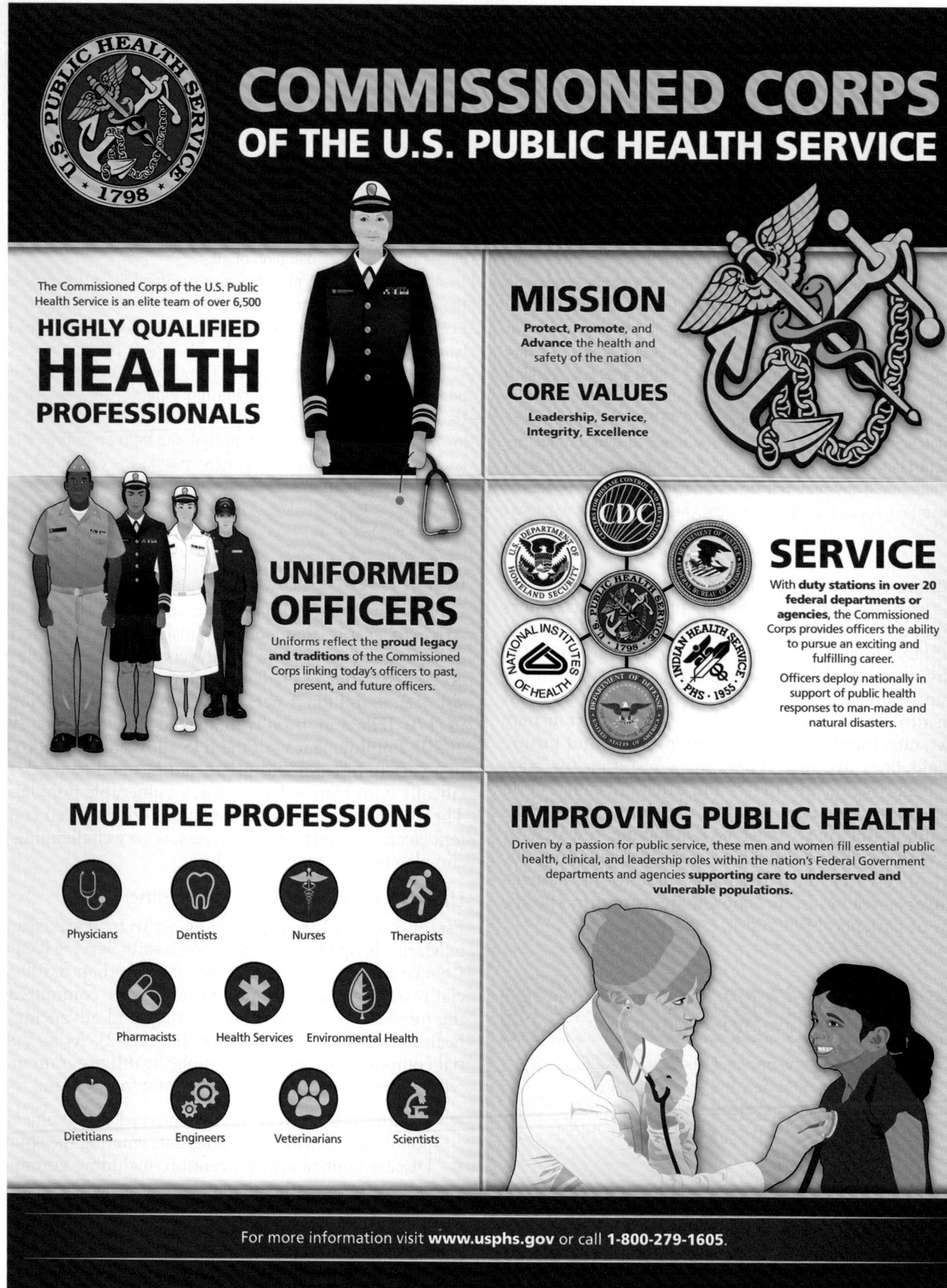

U.S. PUBLIC HEALTH SERVICE 1798
COMMISSIONED CORPS
OF THE U.S. PUBLIC HEALTH SERVICE
The Commissioned Corps of the U.S. Public Health Service is an elite team of over 6,500
HIGHLY QUALIFIED
HEALTH
PROFESSIONALS
MISSION
Protect, Promote, and Advance the health and safety of the nation
CORE VALUES
Leadership, Service, Integrity, Excellence
UNIFORMED
OFFICERS
Uniforms reflect the proud legacy and traditions of the Commissioned Corps linking today's officers to past, present, and future officers.
CDC
SERVICE
With duty stations in over 20 federal departments or agencies, the Commissioned Corps provides officers the ability to pursue an exciting and fulfilling career.
Officers deploy nationally in support of public health responses to man-made and natural disasters.
MULTIPLE PROFESSIONS
Physicians
Dentists
Nurses
Therapists
Pharmacists
Health Services
Environmental Health
Dietitians
Engineers
Veterinarians
Scientists
IMPROVING PUBLIC HEALTH
Driven by a passion for public service, these men and women fill essential public health, clinical, and leadership roles within the nation's Federal Government departments and agencies supporting care to underserved and vulnerable populations.
For more information visit www.usphs.gov or call 1-800-279-1605.
Facebook.com/USPHS
Linked in
Commissioned Corps of the U.S. Public Health Service
CommissionedCorpsUSPHS

FIGURE 28-2 U.S. Public Health Service (USPHS) Commissioned Corps infographic. (From the Commissioned Corps of the USPHS. (2019). *USPHS Commissioned Corps infographic.* Retrieved from https://usphs.gov/aboutus/)

roles within the nation's federal government agencies (USDHHS, n.d.).

The USPHS Chief Nurse Officer is integrally involved with global health care, ensuring that PHS nurses are improving health for the entire community by providing direct care, conducting research, or reviewing new medications. These nurses work in a variety of federal agencies and provide nursing care and health care leadership around the world. Commissioned Corps Officers are on the front line of the COVID-19 response, deploying 400 officers to aid in the response to the coronavirus health emergency (US Food and Drug Administration, n.d.). During the height of the Ebola virus global epidemic, the president of the United States called upon the USPHS Commissioned Corps to deploy to West Africa to provide care to the health care workers who had been exposed to or infected with the Ebola virus (Pierson et al., 2017). Four teams of approximately 70 officers composed of clinicians (physicians, nurses, and behavioral health specialists), pharmacists, infection control and laboratory officers, and administrative management personnel rotated to Liberia for 60 days at a time beginning in October 2014 (Pierson et al., 2017). Upon the departure of these specially trained teams of PHS officers in May 2015, Liberia was declared Ebola-free. Concurrently, smaller teams of PHS officers served to combat the Ebola outbreak in Guinea and Sierra Leone and remained on site educating the community on Ebola treatment and prevention. The president presented the USPHS Commissioned Corps with the Presidential Unit Citation, the highest award for a uniformed service, for their contributions in the fight against Ebola.

More recently Commission Corps officers were sent to Louisiana following catastrophic flooding and heavy rains in 2016 (Iskander et al., 2018). Officers provided round-the-clock medical and behavioral health care for special needs medical shelter residents. In addition, officers coordinated with other shelters and local providers to ensure care for patients with critical health care needs such as dialysis and placement in skilled care facilities (Iskander et al., 2018). For more information on Commissioned Corps deployment: https://www.usphs.gov/

For more information on the USPHS Commissioned Corps in general, visit their Web site at https://dcp.psc.gov/ccmis/

School Nursing

School nursing is a specialized practice of professional nursing that advances the well-being, academic success, and lifelong achievement of students. School nurses are a link between the school, families, community, and health care stakeholders.

History of School Nursing

In 1902, the practice of school nursing began when the New York Board of Education contracted with Lillian Wald's Henry Street Settlement to provide a C/PHN to work with the families and schools to facilitate the return of healthy children to school. The nurse, Lina Rogers, made home visits to follow up on children excluded from school for illness or poor health and was assisted by other Henry Street nurses in providing care, educating families about diseases and the need for hygiene, and working with other organizations to provide needed food, shoes, and clothing (Houlahan, 2018). The board hired 12 more school nurses, and over the next few years, other cities and states began hiring nurses to work in the schools. School nurses have historically advocated for hot lunches, breakfast programs, better social conditions, and the need for increased health education in schools and for families (Houlahan, 2018). See Chapter 3.

School nurses are a professional nursing specialty that serves the school-age population through the age of 21 years, working with students' families and the school community in regular and special education schools, as well as other educational settings (e.g., preschools, court, and other community schools).

- The nationally recommended ratio of one school nurse for every 750 students was adopted to provide accommodations to both disabled and chronically ill students. Increasingly, school nurses are providing care to students with complex social, physical, and emotional needs (Endsley, 2017).
- The National Association of School Nurses (NASN) position statement on safe staffing recommends a 1:225 ratio for populations requiring daily professional nursing services, a 1:125 ratio for populations with complex health care needs, and a 1:1 ratio for students requiring daily professional nursing services (NASN, 2020b).

The role of the **school nurse** has expanded over the years, along with the increase in chronic conditions and challenges in accessing health care (Endsley, 2017). In addition, federal law requires school systems to provide care for children with disabilities. The Individuals with Disabilities Education Act (IDEA, 1975), the Rehabilitation Act (1973), and Title II of the Americans with Disabilities Act (ADA) all mandate equal educational opportunities for all students, including children with complex medical conditions. It is now commonplace for children to attend school accompanied by feeding tubes, catheters, insulin pumps, glucose monitors, and ventilators. There is a growing population of adolescent and preadolescent children who are within 6 months of dying from chronic disease and are routinely attending school (NASN, 2018a). ANA and NASN (2017) defines the role of the school nurse as:

> School nurses, grounded in the ethical and evidence-based practice, are the leaders who bridge health care and education, provide care coordination, advocate for quality student centered care, and collaborate to design systems that allow individuals and communities to develop their full potential (p. 1).

The school nurse role has dramatically changed, as has the student population, in this millennium. Children are affected by poverty, food insecurity, lack of access to medical care, language and cultural barriers, lower socioeconomic status, challenges to basic safety and security, chronic health issues, and discrimination. School nurses play a critical role in promoting the academic success of these and other children in school (Darnell, Hager, &

Loprinzi, 2019). School nurses may be "the only contact a student has with a health care professional"; yet many schools across the United States have one nurse for large populations or no nurse, relying solely on office staff to care for complex medical conditions (Willgerodt, Brock, & Maughan, 2018, p. 232). Today's school nurse performs multiple roles, including care coordination, leadership, quality improvement, and community/public health (NASN, 2018c). See Figure 28-3.

An integrative study looked at the relationship between school nurse interventions and the impact on health and education outcomes of school children. Using the NASN Framework for 21st Century School Nursing Practice, Best, Oppewal, and Travers (2018) categorized school nurse interventions and health outcome measures through a systematic review and meta-analysis of the literature with studies falling under one of the Framework's four areas:

- 54% of the studies were in the area of care coordination, in which nurses provided case management, chronic disease management, collaborative communication with staff and parents, direct patient care, support groups, counseling, and student care plans.
- 18% of school nurse work was in the area of leadership and lifelong learning, in which nurses took classes to support their knowledge and care in areas such as asthma, child protective services, food allergies, and concussions.
- 25% of school nurses provided interventions in the area of health education, screenings, referrals, follow-up on medical issues, and surveillance.
- Less than 3% of the school nurse's time is spent in the area of quality improvement, including documentation and data collection.

School nurses, administrators, teachers, parents, and community stakeholders are all vital in coordinated school health programs and in developing health-promoting schools (Best et al., 2018). The NASN serves as a resource for school nurses across the United States. Their position papers and resources give guidance to nurses in the trenches who typically serve in autonomous positions and may be the only nurse for their district, traveling great distances between schools, especially in rural America. The NASN position papers provide direction for school nurses and include such categories as disaster preparedness, bullying and cyberbullying, chronic absenteeism, individual health care plans, school violence, sexual health education in schools, and telehealth. The full list of position papers can be found at https://www.nasn.org/nasn/advocacy/professional-practice-documents/position-statements (NASN, 2018b).

It is the position of NASN that school nurses play an essential role in keeping children healthy, safe, and ready to learn. The school nurse is a member of a unique discipline of professional nursing and is often the sole health care provider in an academic setting. Twenty-first century school nursing practice is student-centered, occurring within the context of the student's family and school community (NASN, 2016). "It is essential that all students have access to a full-time school nurse all day, every day" (American Academy of Pediatrics [AAP], 2016; NASN, 2018c, p. 3).

Key Roles of the School Nurse

The school nurse's main role is to provide both individual and population health care and coordination for school-age children and adolescents. In providing services, school nurses use their knowledge of:

- Normal growth and development
- Social determinants of health
- Safety and health (including environmental health)
- The educational system
- The connection between health and learning

Other key roles of the school nurse are to (AAP, 2016):

- Promote health among students, families, and staff.
- Provide case management for children with chronic illnesses (e.g., diabetes, asthma, severe allergies).
- Provide immunization monitoring/access.
- Collaborate with parents, teachers, and psychologists in providing appropriate educational plans for students requiring special education services.
- Work with school staff to ensure a healthy and safe environment (e.g., nutrition, physical activity, playground safety).
- Collaborate with community agencies (e.g., public health departments, other health agencies, charitable groups, and service clubs), physicians, dentists, parent groups, and child protective services to meet students' and families' needs.
- Conduct screenings and work with school staff to promote their health and wellness.
- Work with school-based clinics to provide direct health care to children and their families.
- Assist in leading coordinated school health programs.

The NASN (2016) describes the broad role of the school nurse as a "specialized practice of professional nursing that advances the well-being, academic success, and lifelong achievement and health of students" (para. 8). The school nurse (NASN, 2016):

- Facilitates the normal development of students and promotes positive intervention outcomes
- Provides leadership in the areas of health promotion, safety, and a healthy school environment
- Provides high-quality health care and promotes early intervention for actual and potential student health problems
- Uses sound clinical judgment in the provision of case management for students
- Collaborates actively and professionally with others to promote student and family capacity for self-management and adaptation, as well as learning and self-advocacy

The partnership between school nurses and families is important for the child's health outcomes, and the use of problem-based communication strategies helps promote this collaboration (Roberts, Taylor, & Pyle, 2018).

Framework for 21st Century School Nursing Practice™

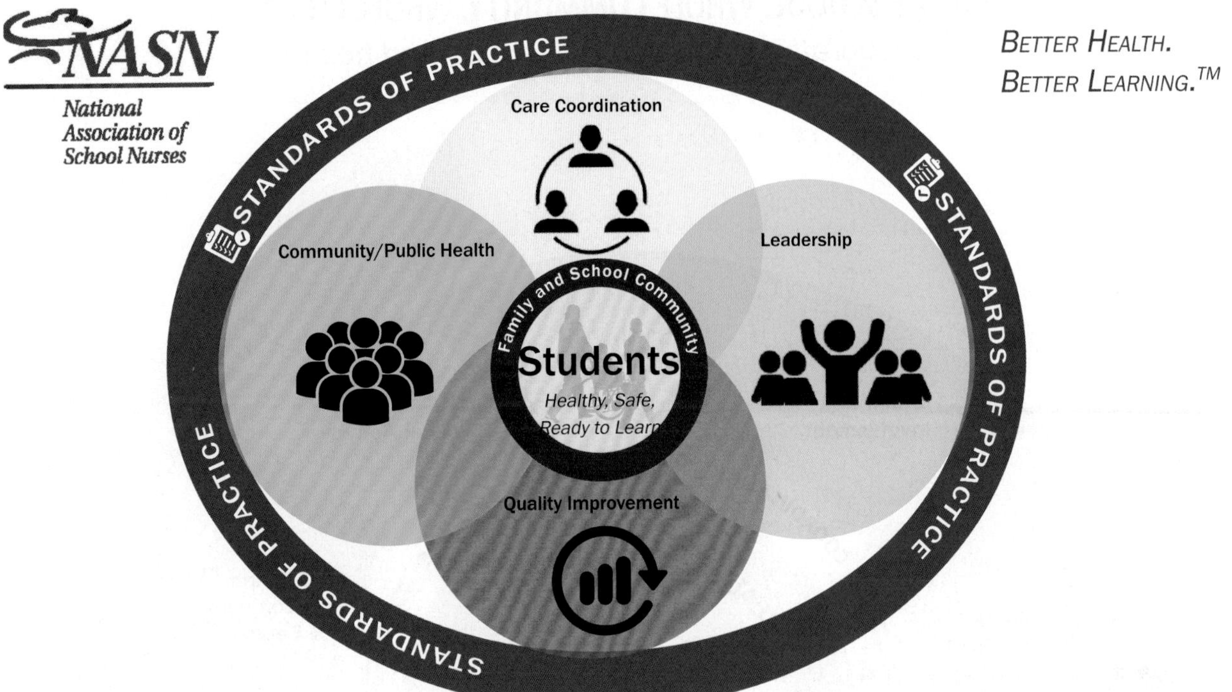

NASN's *Framework for 21st Century School Nursing Practice™* (the *Framework*) provides structure and focus for the key principles and components of current day, evidence-based school nursing practice. It is aligned with the Whole School, Whole community, Whole Child model that calls for a collaborative approach to learning and health (ASCD & CDC, 2014). Central to the *Framework* is student-centered nursing care that occurs within the context of the students' family and school community. Surrounding the students, family, and school community are the non-hierarchical, overlapping key principles of *Care Coordination, Leadership, Quality Improvement,* and *Community/ Public Health.* These principles are surrounded by the fifth principle, *Standards of Practice*, which is foundational for evidence-based, clinically competent, quality care. School nurses daily use the skills outlined in the practice components of each principle to help students be healthy, safe, and ready to learn.

Standards of Practice

- Clinical Competence
- Clinical Guidelines
- Code of Ethics
- Critical Thinking
- Evidence-based Practice
- NASN Position Statements
- Nurse Practice Acts
- Scope and Standards of Practice

Care Coordination

- Case Management
- Chronic Disease Management
- Collaborative Communication
- Direct Care
- Education
- Interdisciplinary Teams
- Motivational Interviewing/ Counseling
- Nursing Delegation
- Student Care Plans
- Student-centered Care
- Student Self-empowerment
- Transition Planning

Leadership

- Advocacy
- Change Agents
- Education Reform
- Funding and Reimbursement
- Healthcare Reform
- Lifelong Learner
- Models of Practice
- Technology
- Policy Development and Implementation
- Professionalism
- Systems-level Leadership

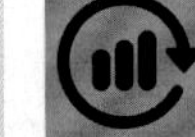

Quality Improvement

- Continuous Quality Improvement
- Documentation/Data Collection
- Evaluation
- Meaningful Health/ Academic Outcomes
- Performance Appraisal
- Research
- Uniform Data Set

Community/ Public Health

- Access to Care
- Cultural Competency
- Disease Prevention
- Environmental Health
- Health Education
- Health Equity
- Healthy People 2020
- Health Promotion
- Outreach
- Population-based Care
- Risk Reduction
- Screenings/Referral/ Follow-up
- Social Determinants of Health
- Surveillance

ASCD & CDC. (2014). *Whole school whole community whole child: A collaborative approach to learning and health.* Retrieved from http://www.ascd.org/ASCD/pdf/siteASCD/publications/wholechild/wscc-a-collaborative-approach.pdf

FIGURE 28-3 Framework for 21st century school nursing practice. (Reprinted with permission from the National Association for School Nurses. (2019). *Framework for 21st century school nursing practice*. Retrieved from https://www.nasn.org/nasn/nasn-resources/professional-topics/framework)

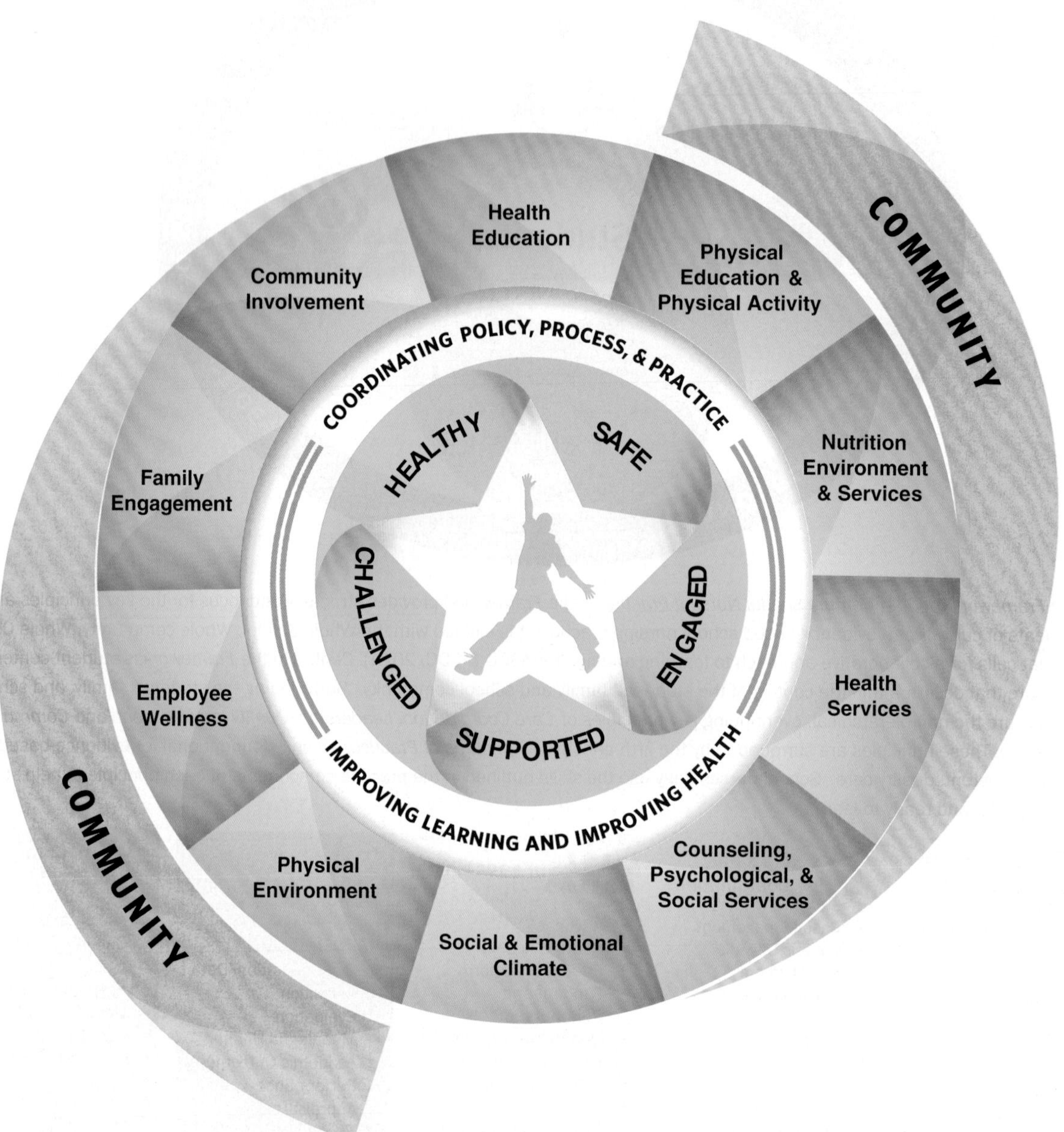

FIGURE 28-4 Whole School, Whole Community, Whole Child model. Reprinted from the Centers for Disease Control and Prevention. (2016). *Whole School, whole community, whole child.* Retrieved from http://www.cdc.gov/healthyyouth/wscc/

Liaison With the Interdisciplinary School Health Team. School nursing services are part of a coordinated school health program that provides school health services, health education, and health promotion programs for faculty and staff (American School Health Association, n.d.). Although the school nurse plays a central role, collaboration with many other individuals is important. School nurses must be familiar with the education setting and work closely with teachers and aides, special education teachers and staff, principals, administrators, school office staff, health aides, psychologists, and speech therapists, as well as parents and families. The Whole School, Whole Community, Whole Child (WSCC) model focuses on the child, emphasizes a school-wide approach, and acknowledges learning, health, and the school as being a part and reflection of the local community (CDC, 2020). The Virtual Healthy School (https://www.cdc.gov/healthyschools/vhs/#!/scene/1) emphasizes the relationship between health and school, highlighting the WSCC model (CDC, 2018b). See Figure 28-4 for the WSCC model.

It includes 10 components:

- Health education
- Physical activity/education

- Nutrition services/environment
- Health services
- Counseling/social/psychological services
- Social/emotional climate
- Physical environment
- Employee wellness
- Family engagement
- Community involvement

Positive Working Relationship With School Team Members. The school principal influences all phases of the school health program by promoting good school health through active support of the school's health services, participation in setting health-related policies, and tapping into community resources. The principal can reinforce positive efforts within the school, ranging from the health teaching in the classroom to the cleaning activities of the custodian. Because of the principal's influential position, it is absolutely essential for the nurse and principal to maintain a positive and cooperative working relationship.

Teachers, whether they are involved in regular instruction, physical education, or special education, play a major role in school health. Because they spend the most time with students, their observations, health teaching, and personal health habits have a profound effect on student health and the quality of school health services.

The school nurse and teachers must collaborate constantly, as the school nurse provides information and guidance to teachers regarding students in their classrooms with specific health conditions and concerns and teachers report on students' health concerns and behaviors. Mink (2019) found that teachers had higher levels of satisfaction when nurses were available on campus full time and appreciated nurses' help with students having chronic conditions, managing medical emergencies, and providing first aid when students were injured. They also found benefits when school nurses followed up on hearing and vision problems, making necessary referrals and getting services for students having problems.

Student study teams (SSTs), where teachers, administrators, psychologists, school nurses (Fig. 28-5), and others meet to discuss students identified as having learning or health problems, were also noted as an important collaborative opportunity (Merced Union High School District, n.d.).

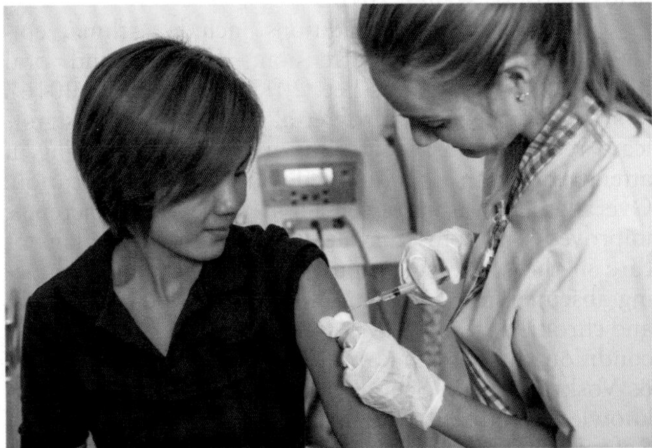

FIGURE 28-5 The school nurse is part of a team providing a coordinated school health program.

Other health team members, such as health educators, health coordinators, psychologists, audiologists, speech therapists, occupational therapists, physical therapists, counselors, health care providers, dentists, dental hygienists, social workers, security and juvenile justice personnel, health aides, and volunteers, may also be involved, depending on size and financial resources of the school. All team members, including students, parents, bus drivers, and custodians, have a specialized role complementary to that of the school nurse.

School-based health centers (SBHCs) provide an access to health care services for youth confronted with barriers to social determinants of health and are often sponsored or funded by public health departments, community health centers, or hospitals. They often provide care for children, and sometimes their families, who otherwise do not have access to health care.

SBHCs provide "significant positive effects on youth health and academic outcomes including high school completion and grade point average, grade promotion, lower rates of hospitalizations, emergency room visits, substance use, and higher rates of contraception use." (Bersamin et al., 2019, p. 11). SBHC are predominantly established in lower socio-economic neighborhood and urban settings. Over the last 3 years, there has been a 20% increase or 2,315 new SBHC across the United States (Bersamin et al., 2019).

Responsibilities of the School Nurse

School nurses address the social determinants of health such as environment, access to health insurance, housing, and income as most health issues are associated with social determinants of health (NASN, 2018c). They bridge health and education preventing illness and promoting and maintaining the health of the school community. The school nurse serves not only individuals, families, and groups within the context of school health but also the school as an organization and its membership (students and staff) as aggregates. The school nurse identifies health-related barriers to learning, serves as a health advocate for children and families, and promotes health while preventing illness and disability (NASN, 2018c).

School nursing activities are varied and is composed of nursing care of children with special health needs, including nasogastric tube feedings, catheterization, insulin pumps, and suctioning; general and emergency first aid; vision, hearing, scoliosis, and TB screenings; height, weight, and blood pressure monitoring; oral health and dental education; immunization assessment and monitoring; medication administration; assessment of acute health problems; health examinations (athletic participation or school entry); and referrals (Best et al., 2018). School nurses also assess and are the frontline providers for identifying communicable diseases, such as outbreaks of influenza or meningitis. Medication administration is another common school nurse duty and includes giving a wide range of medications for acute and chronic issues, as well as delegation of medication tasks:

- 94.3% of school nurses reported giving ADHD medications

- 82.4% gave asthma-related medications
- 64% gave medication for either type 1 or 2 diabetes
- 45.2% gave psychiatric-related medication
- 31.5% of medications were for allergies, 19.6% of medications were for seizures
- 11.2% were for bowel or bladder management (Maughan, McCarthy, Hein, Perkhounkova, & Kelly, 2018).
- Administration of medication can be delegated 77.9% of the time to unlicensed assistive personnel (UAP), such as health aids or school clerks (Maughan et al., 2018).
- Administrators, teachers, and others may also give medications depending upon state laws.

In addition, school nurses perform first aid, help students with inhalers and nebulizer treatments, and some may do gastric tube feedings and ventilator/tracheostomy care. They are responsible for documenting their care, but this can be difficult because of time constraints, educational regulations, and lack of a functional standardized data set or method of collection. Other duties of a school nurse may include training school staff in cardiopulmonary resuscitation (CPR), universal precautions and first aid, as well as overseeing the health and wellness of school staff members. Each school nurse must assess and prioritize how to address the specific needs in each individual school and determine the order. As you can see, there are a wide variety of activities involved in school nursing. This largely autonomous practice requires specific skills and training.

Education: Special Training and Skills of the School Nurse

School nurses operate from one of two administrative bases: the school system or the public health department (NASN, 2016). In most localities, public or private school systems or districts hire school nurses, and they maintain a specialized, school-based practice. Private schools and universities also hire school nurses.

In this specialized role, the nurse can concentrate time and effort solely on the school health program and develop specialized skills in school health assessment and intervention. Today, with the emphasis on delivery of health care at community sites where clients spend most of their time (e.g., schools for children, the workplace for adults), the nurse whose specialty is school health care seems better prepared to meet the complex needs of the school-age population. In contrast, the school nurse who operates under the board of health's jurisdiction provides services to schools as one part of generalized public health nursing services to the community. The community health nurse working through the health department usually devotes only a portion of the workday to the school; she may have additional responsibilities, such as clinic nursing and home visits.

- Depending on the state of residence, a school nurse is usually an RN—frequently with additional education beyond the bachelor's degree in nursing, sometimes including a master's degree—that has primary responsibility for the health care of school-age children and school personnel in an educational setting.
- In some areas of the country, licensed practical nurses (LPNs) or licensed vocational nurses (LVNs) may be hired by school districts, but they must generally work under the supervision of an RN. *School nursing: Scope and standards of practice* (ANA & NASN, 2017) indicates that school nurses should, at minimum, possess a bachelor's degree.

As the needs of school-aged populations become increasingly complex, some states require even more specialized training for school nurses. In California, for instance, school nurses are expected to hold a school health services credential. This credential is obtained through a post-baccalaureate program that includes course work in audiology, guidance and counseling, exceptional children, school health principles and practice, a practicum in school nursing, child psychology, and health curriculum development, in addition to other courses. A national certification is available as well (NASN, 2018d).

Functions of School Nursing Practice

The three main functions of school nursing practice are health services, health education, and promotion of a healthy school environment. Health services include caring for individual students who have chronic conditions, acute situations, and comprehensive care coordination needs while at the same time thinking of the entire population and tracking trends (Willgerodt et al., 2018). For example, the school nurse observes an increase in the number of students diagnosed with asthma and investigates ways to help all students with asthma. One way of doing this may be to organize an *Open Airways* course (American Lung Association, 2018) to assist students in identifying triggers and managing their own care. The goal of this course would be to decrease student asthma attacks.

Health Services for Children With Chronic Conditions. Chronic health conditions are commonly acquired, incurable and conditions lasting longer than 12 months with physical, emotional, functional, developmental, and behavioral conditions (NASN, 2017a). The number of children afflicted with chronic diseases is rising; it is estimated that 25% of children and adolescents in the United States are affected by a chronic condition (Miller, Coffield, Leroy, & Wallin, 2016).

Common chronic conditions include asthma, epilepsy, anaphylaxis, hypertension, diabetes, and oral health (Leroy, Wallin, & Lee, 2017; Miller et al., 2016). A systematic review (Leroy et al., 2017) noted a significant reduction in absenteeism and positive trending in attendance with school-based care and/or education. Overall, there was improvement in medication adherence, improved symptoms, and health care use when plans of care in the school were put in place. Although, reducing absenteeism is a common function for school nurses, and chronic absences have often been linked with chronic conditions like asthma and diabetes (Jacobsen, Meeder, & Voskuil, 2016). School nurses will need to maintain knowledge and training in chronic issues (NASN, 2017a). Refer to content in Chapter 20 and see Box 28-8.

For students in special education programs, school nurses can coordinate **individualized education plans**

BOX 28-8 QSEN: FOCUS ON QUALITY

Patient-Centered Care for Correctional Nurses

Patient-Centered Care: Recognize the patient or designee as the source of control and full partner in providing compassionate and coordinated care based on respect for patient preferences, values, and needs (Cronenwett et al., 2007, p. 123).

(See https://qsen.org/competencies/pre-licensure-ksas/#quality_improvement for the knowledge, skills, and attitudes associated with this QSEN competency.)

Working in a correctional facility is unlike working in any other setting. Prior to being incarcerated, inmates may not have received health care. Custody is always with nurses when providing health care. This may cause problems with patient confidentiality. Nurses must remember not to self-disclose any part of their life outside of work. Instead, develop therapeutic relations by following through with statements made, ask questions, and practice active listening (Nursing @CSU Staff, 2019).

Common health issues with this population are many. Infectious disease includes HIV, STDs, hepatitis B and C, and tuberculosis. Mental illnesses are prevalent. When first arrested, inmates may experience drug or alcohol withdrawal (American Academy of Family Physicians, 2019). Chronic conditions such as hypertension, cancer, diabetes, asthma, and cirrhosis of the liver are seen in the population (USDOJ, 2016). Nurses need to be prepared to care for inmates experiencing a CVA, drug overdoses, or MI. Depression is the most common mental illness seen in this population. Other disorders include bipolar, anxiety, and PTSD (Reingle Gonzalez, & Connell, 2014).

1. *As a new correctional nurse, what concerns/fears might you have when providing patient-centered care to this population?*
2. *Do you think knowing the crime committed would affect the care you provide? Why or why not?*

Source: American Academy of Family Physicians (2019), Cronenwett et al. (2007), Nursing @CSU Staff (2019), Reingle Gonzalez & Connell (2014), U.S. Department of Justice (2016).

(IEPs) with **individualized health plans (IHPs)** to develop health management goals for students. Medically fragile or technology-dependent students, who may require procedures such as suctioning or tube feeding, would have IHPs developed for *specialized physical health care procedures* (Orange County Department of Education, n.d.). Because these students are often hospitalized, interrupting their education, the school nurse needs to assist with transition planning. Collaboration with school psychologists and school and health team members is important to transition planning that is also needed as students move from elementary to middle school, from middle school to high school, and as they move out of public schools and on to other educational or job training settings (NASN, 2018e).

School nurses develop IHPs to ensure that students with special needs (e.g., chronic conditions) have these needs met. If these students attend the regular classroom and do not fall under the IDEA, the plans may be known as **Section 504 plans**, named after the section of the Rehabilitation Act and the accompanying statute, the ADA, that specifically allows for school accommodations with this population. Some examples might include severe peanut allergies that lead to anaphylaxis, serious asthma complications, diabetes, or heart disease.

Students are to be provided with a "free and appropriate public education," and some students may be covered under both IEPs and Section 504 plans (California Code of Regulations 5CCR 3030, n.d.). See Box 28-9 for a list of IEP-eligible disabilities.

Asthma. Asthma is often deemed the most common chronic disease of childhood. Students loose over 13 million missed school days a year from this chronic disease (Everhart, Miller, Leinach, Koinis-Mitchell, 2018). Student symptoms include shortness of breath, tightness of chest, wheezing, and lack of energy (Everhart et al., 2018). School environmental factors (e.g., mold, allergens, indoor air quality) also exacerbate asthma symptoms in children and youth.

Asthma management programs are useful in helping students manage symptoms and reduce asthma triggers. School nurses work with students, their families, and their doctors to develop an *asthma action plan* to control, prevent, or minimize untoward effects of acute asthma episodes. Peak flow meters can be used regularly to determine early signs of asthma problems. Monitoring asthma medications and teaching proper methods of inhaler use are also vital school nursing functions. It often falls to school nurses to ensure that proper protocols and training are in place. It is imperative that school nurses are well versed in the care and treatment of asthma.

In Colorado, a framework for asthma care curriculum was created to guide the continuing education of school nurses and health care team members in their

BOX 28-9 Thirteen Disabilities Eligible for Individualized Education Plans

- Autism
- Deaf-blindness
- Deafness
- Emotional disturbance
- Hearing impairment
- Intellectual disability
- Multiple disabilities
- Orthopedic impairment
- Other health impairment
- Specific learning disability
- Speech or language impairment
- Traumatic brain injury
- Visual impairment, including blindness

Source: Galemore and Sheetz (2015).

state (Cicutto et al., 2017). A Healthy Homes program headed by C/PHNs in Baltimore, Maryland, focused upon home assessments for environmental health risks (lead, asthma triggers, carbon monoxide, pesticide use, environmental tobacco smoke) as well as source of heating in the home. They also included educational sessions to review home environmental health risks and a targeted hazard reduction intervention (U.S. Department of Housing and Urban Development, n.d.). Refer to content in Chapter 20.

Diabetes. Diabetes is another common chronic illness in young people: approximately 208,000 or one in 433 children and adolescents have diabetes (National Diabetes Education Program, 2016). Of these, 87% are diagnosed with type 1 and 11% are diagnosed with type 2 diabetes (NASN, 2017b). It is estimated that there are 18,000 newly found youth under the age of 20 annually diagnosed with type 2 diabetes and over 5,000 newly diagnosed with type 1 diabetes (NASN, 2017b). Both types of diabetes are on the rise in adolescents, leading some scientists to frame it as a major public health crisis caused largely by obesity, sedentary lifestyle, and the predisposition of certain ethnic groups to diabetes (National Institute of Diabetes and Digestive and Kidney Diseases, 2017). Refer to content in Chapter 20.

Working with families and health care providers, school nurses assess and develop a care plan for students with diabetes. School nurses work closely with the family to maintain confidentiality and at the same time ensure that the school is a safe environment for the child:

- A multidisciplinary team approach is needed, with family, school, and physician collaboration.
- Training for teachers and fellow classmates is also important.
- Teachers are often called upon to assist students with their insulin or food management.
- Younger children with type 1 diabetes, especially those who use insulin pumps, may need careful monitoring—something that is not always possible for the school nurse, who may not be present where and when problems arise.
- A student experiencing a hypoglycemic reaction should never be left alone. It is important for school nurses to alert teachers and school personnel to the signs and symptoms (as well as the treatment) of hypoglycemia.
- A current position of NASN, NIH, and CDC is that a *diabetes medical management plan* should be in place to assist in the care of children with diabetes (NASN, 2017b; National Diabetes Education Program, 2016).
- Care coordination, training, and delegation are the roles of the school nurse (NASN, 2017b). However, many school nurses do not feel comfortable delegating tasks such as administration of insulin or glucagon.

Testing blood sugar and taking insulin at school can be frustrating and can cause children to feel different from their peers. Students may be required to administer medication or check blood sugar levels in health offices as well as follow protocol for needle dispensing. Diabetes must be managed 24 hours a day, seven day a week.

Type 2 diabetes cases have been rising, and school nurses can be instrumental in prevention measures and early identification. It is often found more frequently in Native American and Hispanic populations and less frequently among non-Hispanic Whites. Also, obesity is an independent risk factor, with close to a quarter of children and youth being obese. Visceral fat is associated with insulin resistance and impaired glucose tolerance, a pathology linked to type 2 diabetes. Culturally sensitive interventions that include increased physical activity and education on good nutrition, as well as behavior modification and ongoing methods of support (e.g., group meetings, phone/e-mail reminders) were shown to be effective in a systematic review (Brackney & Cutshall, 2015). School nurses should assess their school population and promote interventions that benefit at-risk students, as well as the general school population. Refer to content in Chapter 20.

Seizure Disorders. Seizure disorders are not uncommon in the school-age population. Epilepsy is a disorder of the brain in which neurons sometimes give abnormal signals. For the majority of those diagnosed, seizures can usually be controlled with medication (e.g., antiepileptic drugs specific to the pediatric population), surgical treatment, or a special (e.g., ketogenic) diet (Epilepsy Foundation, 2017; National Institute of Neurological Disorders and Stroke, 2018). It is important for school nurses to develop care plans to address seizure concerns during school hours.

- Care plans include monitoring medication compliance and teaching school staff about first aid measures for seizure victims.
- Children and adolescents with seizure disorders may feel embarrassed or be the victims of teasing or bullying.
- They may exhibit signs of school avoidance. Nurses need to work with these children and to teach all students about the disease process and the need for empathy and understanding.
- Similar to issues related to insulin administration for diabetic students, children with seizure disorders may have an emergency medication ordered by their physician (e.g., Diastat, midazolam, lorazepam, clonazepam). Prescribing providers and school nurses should be aware of the laws regarding the administration of seizure rescue medications, particularly as they pertain to UAP (Hartman, Devore, & Section on Neurology, Council on School Health, 2016).
- The Epilepsy Foundation (n.d.) has advocated for its use in schools, and school nurses are often caught between the rights of students and their parents and their state's nursing practice act. Refer to content in Chapter 20.

Food Allergies and Anaphylaxis. Another leading chronic condition found in school settings is severe food allergies that can lead to anaphylactic shock.

- It is estimated that the 5.9 million school-aged children have food allergies (Food allergy Research and Education [FARE], 2018).

- Such severe allergies result in approximately 200,000 ED visits each year (FARE, 2018).
- Eight common foods account for 90% of severe food allergies. They are fish, shellfish, soy, milk, egg, wheat, peanuts, and tree nuts (e.g., cashews, walnuts).
- Many common foods and school supplies (e.g., play dough) can contain hidden allergens, and care must be taken to prevent exposure.
- School nurses coordinate and work with students and their families, along with school personnel, to raise awareness and enlist caution.
- School nurses also work with families, and health care providers, to ensure that epinephrine via an auto injector (EpiPen) are available for the child in case of emergencies. It is also used for bee sting and other allergies, in addition to food allergies.
- Although many factors are taken into consideration, most pediatric allergists believe students between 12 and 14 years should carry and be able to self-administer their own EpiPen (American Academy of Allergy, Asthma & Immunology, n.d.).
- School nurses should coordinate with teachers and lunchroom personnel to ensure that proper protocol is followed for allergic reactions. School personnel should be made aware of the food allergy, understand an anaphylactic reaction, and be able to verbalize or demonstrate how to use the EpiPen or other needed medication (CDC, 2018c). School nurses need to ensure the Allergy and Anaphylaxis Emergency Plan is completed by the parent and physician to ensure proper treatment for a student with severe allergies while at school (AAP, 2018a). In addition, a 504 or IHP should be completed. Refer to content in Chapter 20.

Behavioral Problems and Learning Disabilities. Other chronic childhood health problems are those of emotional, behavioral, and intellectual development. These are not always easy to detect and measure, and they can be debilitating. Although these problems are not new, awareness and concern have increased as the rates of occurrence for other life-threatening childhood diseases have diminished.

- The National Institute of Mental Health (NIMH) reports that emotional and behavioral disorders affect 10% to 15% of children globally (Kid's Mental Health Portal, 2018).
- Problems such as oppositional defiant disorder, bipolar disorder, and early schizophrenia can affect the school-age population and is a concern to school nurses and staff (Riley, Ahmed, & Locke, 2016).
- The causes of emotional behavioral problems and learning disabilities appear to have genetic, environmental, and cultural influences.
- High-risk children often come from families with a high incidence of child abuse (physical and sexual) and neglect.
- The number of children affected by parental drug use has surpassed that of children with disabilities caused by lead poisoning, another major contributor to developmental problems in children.

Attention-deficit/hyperactivity disorder (ADHD) is a cluster of problems related to hyperactivity, impulsivity, and inattention. Approximately 6.4 million school-age children have been diagnosed with ADHD (National Center for Learning Disabilities, 2017). School nurses must be aware of the signs and symptoms and serve as an advocate for these children and their families. At each stage of development, those with ADHD are presented with distinct challenges. For example, children in elementary school may often have difficulty and conflict with peers, as well as problems organizing tasks. They may be more accident prone and may have more school-related problems, such as grade retention and suspension or expulsion. They often have problems with grooming and with handwriting, and they exhibit difficulty sleeping. ADHD is sometimes found with associated disorders, such as communication or language disorders and learning disabilities. It is estimated that as many as one third of children with learning disabilities also have ADHD (National Center for Learning Disabilities, 2017). Counseling and behavior therapy are often used with these children with a 70% to 80% success rate demonstrated by improved behavior (Substance Abuse Mental Health Services Agency, 2020).

Behavioral and emotional problems of school-age children can stem from many causes. School nurses can be alert to early symptoms and refer families for counseling.

- Collaboration is needed between the child's family, the school, and the child's health care provider to diagnose ADHD and effectively plan appropriate interventions and educational accommodations.
- Numerous checklists and assessment tools are available, and school psychologists typically serve as a source for additional information and resources.
- School nurses can assist parents in recognizing the symptoms of ADHD and obtaining appropriate treatment and follow-up. A multimodal treatment approach may include stimulant medication, usually methylphenidate (Ritalin or Concerta), dextroamphetamine (Dexedrine), and amphetamine (Adderall).
- Family and individual counseling, parent support groups, and training in behavior management techniques, as well as family education about the condition, are also essential features of this method of treatment.
- Not all children and adolescents respond to medication, and medication dosage must be carefully monitored and titrated.
- School nurses and community health nurses can work closely with school staff, parents, and physicians in determining the efficacy of treatment regimens.

The main goal of medication for school-age children is academic improvement. If this does not occur, medication may need to be changed or discontinued. School nurses and community health nurses can work closely with school staff, parents, and physicians in determining the efficacy of treatment regimens (Chan, Fogler, & Hammerness, 2016).

Medication Administration. Medication administration for a variety of conditions has historically been an important responsibility for school nurses (NASN, 2017c). In schools where a nurse is present every day, the nurse can personally oversee medication administration. Unfortunately, many nurses cover more than one school and so other school personnel (e.g., secretaries, health aides) may be tasked with overseeing medication administration. The majority of states have laws allowing teachers or health aides to administer medication. In these situations, school nurses should provide training and audit records to ensure that proper guidelines are followed. In one study, over 800 schools were surveyed and medication administration errors occurred 15% of the time (Maughan et al., 2018):

- 58.4% occurred due to missed dose
- 19% for wrong time
- 18.3% for wrong dose
- 11.2% for wrong medication
- 10.6% for medication not documented
- 9.9% for wrong student
- 8.0% given without authorization

Another issue surrounding medication administration in the school setting is regarding delegation. Each state's individual nurse practice act provides rules on delegation of nursing tasks. School nurses must understand their own state's act and the legal implications regarding their decisions. School districts are responsible for including medication administration guidelines in their policies, and school nurses must comply with established guidelines (NASN, 2017c).

In a landmark case, the ANA filed a lawsuit on behalf of California school nurses to prevent insulin administration by unlicensed personnel. Their argument centered on the state's Nurse Practice Act and the need for licensed nurses to administer this medication (with dosage often checked by two nurses in hospital settings). However, the American Diabetes Association and others argued that not all schools have adequate school nurse coverage, and over one quarter of schools do not employ a licensed nurse. Two courts ruled on the side of the school nurses, but the California Supreme Court ultimately overturned those decisions, making it possible for unlicensed personnel to give medications, including insulin, with parental and medical permission (American Diabetes Association, 2017). The concept of "in loco parentis" instructs school staff to provide care for the student in the parent's place and with their consent (Alliance of Schools for Cooperative Insurance Programs, 2017).

Health Services to Prevent Illness and Injury. School nurses emphasize prevention and focus many of their efforts on prevention of communicable disease (via immunizations) and of injuries.

Immunizations. School immunization rates continue to be high due to vaccine mandates for school entry, yet areas where children remain unvaccinated affect herd immunity rates causing outbreaks of measles and pertussis (NASN, 2020a, 2020b). See Chapter 8 for more on this.

Low immunization levels in many areas, in poor populations, public concern for vaccinations, and increased disease rates signal the need for constant surveillance, outreach programs, and educational efforts. School nurses are deeply involved in each of these preventive activities. Health departments and schools often work collaboratively to provide immunization services. Compulsory immunization laws for school entrance, which vary among states, have enabled public health personnel to carry out these preventive services. All states require children to be vaccinated against certain communicable diseases as a condition for school attendance (CDC, 2018d). Statewide immunization information systems can be beneficial for schools, school nurses, and children and their families. School nurses, like C/PHNs, may have access to not only viewing immunization records but also the ability to update them. This provides ready access for children and parents, as well as school nurses, to check immunization records, track those children whose immunizations are incomplete, and provide critical information during times of disease outbreaks.

School nurses often oversee and ensure that children are in compliance with school entrance laws regarding immunizations. They may call parents directly when they note that the student is out of compliance. They may also arrange to help the student get immunized by facilitating appointments or, in some school districts, by directly providing the immunizations.

The CDC provides information for National Immunization Awareness Month and provides a toolkit for school nurses and others to follow when developing successful immunization outreach programs in schools (CDC, 2018e). School nurses can be effective advocates in helping parents make decisions about vaccines (e.g., HPV for adolescents), especially when they have sufficient knowledge and recognize their role as an opinion leader (Rosen, Ashwood, & Richardson, 2016). See Chapters 8 and 20 for more on parental resistance to vaccines, and current immunization schedules for school-age children and adolescents.

Safety. School nurses are also involved in ensuring that school environments are safe places for students. School safety now incorporates more than just playground equipment. Safety includes the following:

- Safe neighborhood to walk to and from school
- Car safety whether passenger or driver
- Safety from gun violence
- Bullying
- Gangs violence
- Sexual violence
- Firearms, weapons, and mass shootings
- Playground injuries, sport injuries including risk for concussion
- Safety from natural disasters (CDC, 2017a)

Bullying behaviors affect 20% of students in their high school years; bullying includes both in-person and cyberbullying (NASN, 2018f). Cyberbullying occurs on social media sites and can have negative effects on student's health; despite increased attention to this problem students, including, LGBTQ students are at risk for physical, psychological, social, emotional, and academic problems (Byrne, Vessey, & Pfeifer, 2018).

Youth violence is a significant issue and is the third leading cause of death in the United States (CDC, 2016a). The rates and forms of violence vary with gang and violent crimes higher in large cities, LGBTQ and females having a higher prevalence of in-person and cyber bullying, and homicide and physical injuries greatest for racial/ethnic males (CDC, 2016a).

Emergency departments treat more than 800,000 children for concussions yearly; many concussions go undiagnosed (AAP, 2018b). New guidelines have been implemented by the American Pediatric Association using "age appropriate symptom scales to diagnose children and assess their recovery" (AAP, 2018b, para 8). The guidelines were created in response to health care providers asking for more evidence-based guidance, in addition, the guidelines can provide information for families, coaches, and schools (AAP, 2018b).

Another area of growing concern is student safety after natural disasters or emergency situations. Recent earthquakes and potential bioterrorism events may impact schools or not permit children to return home at the end of a school day. School nurses are ideal persons to assist in disaster/emergency relief. Students do spend much of their time in school, and local schools are often designated as shelters in times of disasters (NASN, 2016). School nurses can assist in the development of emergency plans, as well as provide care and comfort to children and their families in times of emergencies.

Health Education and Health Promotion. Another main function of school nursing practice involves education and health promotion. This includes planned and incidental teaching of health concepts and health curriculum development. In some states, school nurses even teach the regular health classes. Education may be one-on-one to help a child obtain better control over asthma or to explain to a newly diagnosed diabetic student what is occurring in his body. As an educator, the school nurse may also teach an entire class regarding a student's severe food allergy or the need for proper hand hygiene. The school nurse explains in simple terms what allergies are and helps students understand that allergies are not contagious, what to do in the case of an allergic reaction, and the importance of not sharing foods that may contain potential allergens (NASN, 2016). The application of research is important in school nursing. See Box 28-10.

Because students trust school nurses, students often listen to them. Educational subjects are limitless but should always apply to the specific needs of the children in the school. The nurse must use creativity and autonomy to identify and prioritize needs. A school nurse may also teach about basic first aid, nutrition, physical exercise, sex education, and seat belt safety, or provide information about careers in the health care professions.

Screenings: Opportunities for Teaching. Most local school districts provide some type of health screening services such as hearing and vision screenings, usually through the school nurse or local health care providers

BOX 28-10 EVIDENCE-BASED PRACTICE

School Nursing

A study by Benjamin-Chung (2018) showed the impact of an elementary school influenza vaccination program to increase vaccination coverage, reduce school absenteeism, and interrupt influenza transmission in an elementary school in California. Outcomes of the study also identified influenza hospitalization numbers were reduced with an indirect effect on elderly hospitalization and nonelementary age groups. An elementary-school influenza program can profoundly impact absentee rates in school-aged children and have an indirect affect in older school-aged children and the community.

Another example of evidence-based practice in school nursing involves testing for high-frequency hearing loss in adolescents (Sekhar et al., 2016). Not all states perform mandated hearing screening, and of those that do, not all test for high frequency hearing loss. This study compared sensitivity of current adolescent hearing screening test results with results from adolescents tested in a sound-treated booth. The researchers felt that if current hearing tests added multiple high frequencies this would improve sensitivity; the inclusion of a two-step screening of initial referrals could then be used to reduce false positives. Results of the study identified that traditional school-based testing methods had poor sensitivity for hearing loss in adolescents. Hearing screenings suggestions from the study include testing at 500, 1,000, 2,000, 4,000, and 6,000 Hz at 20 db HL with adolescents to identify high-frequency hearing loss.

How could you use information from these studies to improve school nursing practice and the health of school-age children?

Source: Benjamin-Chung (2018), Sekhar et al. (2016).

(California School Based Health Alliance, 2020). Although the goal of all screening is to promote early intervention, screening also provides the school nurse many opportunities to teach students and staff. Referral information resulting from screening results is usually given to parents, and school nurses may contact parents to encourage follow-through. Children who are not present for school screenings may not receive the benefits of these screenings (e.g., homeschooled and private school students). School nurses often help to coordinate screening resources and benefits, and they often carry out additional screenings for students who were absent when mass screenings were held.

Vision. School nurses often oversee routine vision screenings at periodic intervals so that vision problems that can interfere with learning may be detected and treated early (e.g., nearsightedness, farsightedness, strabismus, and amblyopia) (NASN, 2017d). School nurses also are involved in follow-up and referral. They often send e-mails or letters to parents, make phone follow-ups, and provide referrals and resources to ensure that corrective eyewear is obtained.

The 2016 School Health Policies and Practices Study (SHPPS) noted that 82.7% of reporting school districts offered vision screening to kindergarten or first-grade students (CDC, 2016b). Local Lions Clubs may be involved in paying for area optometrists to assist with and/or direct screenings, as well as to provide follow-up care (Lions Club, n.d.).

Hearing. Hearing screenings for kindergarten and first-grade students reported 79.5% of districts across the United States offered these services (CDC, 2016b). These mass screenings are done to detect any serious hearing deficits that may be related to recurrent ear infections or noise-induced hearing loss (NIHL), often resulting from loud music, video games, or excessive exposure to noise.

- About 2 to 3 of every 1,000 school-aged children, aged 6 to 19, have some type of detectable hearing loss in one or both ears (National Institute on Deafness and other Communication Disorders, 2016).
- Some have a type of *sensorineural hearing loss*—or one that involves the inner ear or the nerves leading from the inner ear. It is permanent and cannot be surgically or medically corrected (American Speech-Language-Hearing Association, n.d.).
- Similar to vision screening, school nurses screen and refer students with suspected hearing problems to medical specialists (e.g., audiologists, physicians).
- School nurses can use the opportunity afforded by vision and hearing screenings to provide education to students and their parents about preventing problems such as NIHL.

Other Health Screenings. Height, weight, and sometimes blood pressure and cholesterol screenings may be done to monitor normal growth and development and allow for early intervention with populations who are especially susceptible to hypertension and heart disease. In some areas, scoliosis screening is also done, frequently during middle school years, to permit early detection and referral for medical intervention (e.g., bracing, surgery). Scoliosis may be congenital but is often idiopathic, and the efficacy of school screening programs has been questioned. There is much controversy surrounding scoliosis screenings in schools. One study found the lack of referrals, costs, or not having a school nurse to conduct the screenings as concerns. However, the study concluded that school screenings be conducted in the underserved populations that may lack yearly pediatrician visits (Kadhim et al., 2019). A systemic review of school screenings found screenings were successful in detecting problems in the early, treatable stages (Altaf, Drinkwater, Phan, & Cree, 2017).

In Texas, and some other areas of the country, *acanthosis nigricans* (hyperpigmentation from various causes, but sometimes a symptom of diabetes) screenings are being done to look for early markers of type 2 diabetes, especially in high-risk populations (Texas Department of Health Services, 2018).

Pediculosis (or head lice) in school-age children is a continual problem for school nurses. Between 6 and 12 million children aged 3 to 11 each year are estimated to be infected with head lice, and school nurses are often called upon to do "head checks" for pediculosis. Pediculicides (e.g., permethrin, pyrethrins, dimethicone) are helpful in killing lice, and school nurses often provide families with education on prevention and eradication methods (Gunning, Kiraly, & Pippitt, 2019). In addition, a non-chemical based, heat-based treatment has provided families with an alternate option for lice treatment in many communities (Lice Clinics, 2019). See Chapter 20.

Oral and Dental Health: Teaching and Referral. Dental caries affect more than half of school-age children and are the most common chronic disease for that age group. About 20% of 5- to 11-year-olds and 13% of 12- to 19-year-olds have at least one untreated decaying tooth (CDC, 2017b). The percentage of children and adolescents aged 5 to 19 years with untreated tooth decay is twice as high for those from low-income families (25%) compared with children from higher-income households (11%) (CDC, 2017b). School nurses can address dental health issues in a variety of ways.

- At a community level, they can educate the public about the benefits of dental fluoride treatments. They can advocate for fluoridation of drinking water, school-provided fluoride rinses or gels, and dental sealant programs. These are all cost-effective, proven methods of reducing dental caries in school-age children.
- At the classroom level, school nurses can provide dental education and provide toothbrushes, toothpaste, and floss to ensure that students are able to practice good dental hygiene habits.
- Local organizations and businesses often will donate such supplies. Many programs from the American Dental Association, the CDC, and other organizations provide resource materials.
- At an individual level, school nurses can assist in finding resources for those with no dental health insurance.
- Finally, school nurses can successfully educate parents, especially those who are immigrants or have different cultural beliefs, regarding the importance of oral and dental health (Hassmiller, 2016; Reza et al., 2016).

Dental screenings or clinics may be conducted to determine the incidence of dental caries, especially in elementary school children, and to encourage follow-up with local dentists for necessary restorations. At the time of the most recent national survey of schools, only 41.4% of districts reported performing some type of oral health screening (CDC, 2016b). See Chapter 20.

Promotion of a Healthful School Environment. A third function of school nursing practice includes maintaining and promoting a healthful school environment. Promotion of healthful school living emphasizes planning a daily schedule for monitoring healthy classroom experiences, extracurricular activities, school breakfasts and lunches, emotional climate, discipline programs, and teaching methods. It also includes screening, observing, and assessing students to identify needs early and to report illegal drug use, bullying, suspected child abuse, and violations of environmental health standards (NASN, 2017e). Cyberbullying is another area where school nurses can provide education to students, parents, teachers, and school staff, as well as response to warning signs among school-age children and youth (Byrne et al., 2018). Health promotion also involves the nurse in supporting the physical, mental, and emotional health of school personnel by being an accessible resource to teachers and staff regarding their own health and safety.

Proper Nutrition and Exercise. Many factors can affect the school environment—heating, cooling, lighting, safe playgrounds, and policies and practices to limit bullying and social aggression or other forms of school violence. The school cafeteria and physical education activities can promote health or contribute to obesity and sedentary lifestyles.

Obesity. Obesity rates have steadily increased for all children since the 1980s; the rates have doubled for children between ages 2 to 5 and adolescents (ages 12 to 19). Rates have tripled for those between ages 6 and 11 years. Approximately 17% (or 12.7 million) of children and adolescents aged 2 to 19 years are obese (NASN, 2018g).

- American children get less than the recommended 60 minutes daily physical activity and over 90% of children have poor diets (NASN, 2018g).
- Only 58.9% of school districts across the United States assess student achievement of physical education standards (CDC, 2016b).
- Obesity often begins in childhood and becomes a risk factor for cardiovascular disease and diabetes later in life. With the increase in child obesity rates, the number of children diagnosed with type 2 diabetes continues to rise, especially among youth of minority race/ethnicity.
- As children become older, families have less impact on food choices, and peers begin to have more influence.
- Results of the 2017 YRBS indicate that very few high school students eat enough fruits and vegetables—of those surveyed only 13.9% of high school students had consumed more than three servings of vegetables, and only 18% had consumed more than three servings of fruit or 100% fruit juice (CDC, 2018f).

School nurses should play an integral role in the prevention of overweight and obesity, as well as addressing the health needs of overweight and obese students (Box 28-11; NASN, 2018g). Many factors contribute to this health issue: diet, lack of physical activity, genetics, family and social factors, culture, socioeconomic status, and media marketing (NASN, 2018g).

BOX 28-11 LEVELS OF PREVENTION PYRAMID

OBESITY IN A SCHOOL SETTING

HEALTH ISSUE: Obesity in a school setting

Tertiary Prevention

Rehabilitation Move to	Health Promotion and Education	Health Protection
▪ Work closely with the child, family, physician, and teacher to decrease body mass index (BMI)	▪ Continue to promote healthy lifestyle choices and daily physical activity	

Secondary Prevention

Early Diagnosis	Prompt Treatment
▪ Conduct yearly screening of students' heights and weights to calculate BMI ▪ Complete health histories on at-risk children	▪ Initiate referrals for health care provider follow-up in collaboration with parents of students at risk for obesity

Primary Prevention

Health Promotion and Education	Health Protection
▪ Limit passive activities and increase sports and physical activity ▪ Teach children how to make better food choices at fast food restaurants ▪ Educate children and teachers to promote good nutrition and a physically active lifestyle ▪ Promote a change of policy to take junk food out of vending machines	

Homelessness and Hunger. Poor nutrition and obesity are not uncommon among adolescents, whose diets often consist of snacks with limited nutritional value interspersed among unhealthful meals. Homelessness and hunger can also have serious consequences, one being an impact on the academic performance of children.

- Irritability, lack of energy, and difficulty concentrating are only some of the problems that arise from skipped meals or consistently inadequate nutrition.
- Infection and illness (e.g., ear infections, asthma, bronchitis, gastroenteritis) that lead to loss of school days can affect academic progress and interfere with the acquisition of basic skills, such as reading and mathematics.
- Dental caries are frequent.
- Poor nutrition is frequently associated with poverty and hunger, but social pressure to be thin can also spark purposeful malnutrition.
- Homelessness and food insecurity can lead to overreliance on fast food and convenience stores, and lack of stable housing triggers stress and anxiety, which can lead to (Crawford et al., 2015) obesity.

School nurses can help coordinate services for children that are homeless and advocate for better nutritional choices in the lunchroom and vending machines. This may include working for policy changes to limit soft drink sales in public schools. They can also teach all grade levels regarding proper nutrition, and they can educate students and parents alike about nutritious snacks in contrast to snacks with little food value, as well as provide information on community resources (e.g., food banks, health clinics, shelters). School nurses may also work with staff to provide nutrition and exercise programs, support groups, and collaborative efforts to assist families dealing with hunger and homelessness.

Eating Disorders. Eating disorders are another area of concern. Issues with body image and control are at the heart of *anorexia nervosa* and *bulimia nervosa*, common problems for adolescent girls. These diseases have emotional causes that pose complex challenges to treatment. School nurses must be aware of the signs and symptoms of eating disorders and be proactive in identifying students at risk, working collaboratively with other members of the mental health treatment service team to advocate for the child. Scoliosis screenings are an optimal time to also observe for eating disorders, as examination of the spine allows for visualization of the body core. School nurses can work with students to develop a healthier self-concept and identify outside treatment resources (National Eating Disorders Association, 2019).

Adolescent High-Risk Behaviors. Mortality and morbidity rates for adolescents are low overall and demonstrate considerable improvement since the early 1900s. High-risk behaviors that are directly related to morbidity and mortality in youth and young adults: behaviors that lead to unintentional injury and violence, tobacco use, alcohol and drug use, sexual behaviors that leads to pregnancies and sexually transmitted infections, unhealthy dietary behaviors, and lack of physical activity (CDC, 2018g). Many of the health problems faced by adolescents are choices and high-risk activity; for example, sexual activity, substance abuse, injury, and violence are all high-risk behaviors in which adolescents can choose to participate or not. The effects of such choices may not be discovered for many years.

- Suicide is a leading cause of death of adolescents, according to the Youth Risk Behavioral Survey (2007–2017) 17.2% of students had seriously considered attempting suicide.
- Safety while driving or under the influence is other high-risk behaviors. Nationally, 62.8% of student's text while driving, 64.5% of youth drove when they had been using marijuana, 62.6% of students drove while under the influence of alcohol (CDC, 2018f).
- 4,300 youth ages 10 to 24 were victims of homicide, and homicide is the third leading cause of death for this age group (CDC, 2016a). 15.7% of youth carried a weapon (gun, knife, and club) 1 day in the past 30 days, while 3.8% of youth carried a weapon to school (CDC, 2018f). See Chapter 20.

Sexual Activity: Teen Pregnancy and STDs. Sexual activity is a sensitive issue. However, the 2017 YRBSS indicates that 39.5% of students surveyed reported they had had sexual intercourse, and 9.70% had had sexual intercourse with four or more partners in their lifetime (CDC, 2018f).

One in four sexually active adolescent females has an STI (CDC, 2018h). The overall rates of syphilis, gonorrhea, chlamydia, human papillomavirus (HPV), and herpes simplex virus are climbing.

Providing STD services and HIV/AIDS education can be a daunting task. Young people with STDs are often afraid or embarrassed to seek help. Those who have been exposed to the HIV virus may not know that they are infected. Although in some communities, the school-based clinic dispenses condoms, in other areas, school nurses may be restricted in what safer sex products they can provide. However, nurses *can* provide teens with education and with information about resources that are available outside of school property. School nurses can promote, at the local and state level, the HPV vaccine that guards against cervical cancer. They can promote abstinence or delaying sexual initiation, as well as fostering safer sex messages that promote the use of condoms. Sex education is effective at both delaying the onset of sexual activity and decreasing sexual activity in adolescents who are already sexually active. See Chapter 20.

School nurses are sometimes restricted by state and/or district policies from addressing the issues of sex education and STI (including HIV) prevention. However, they can inform students and others in the community about the existence of youth development and family planning programs, which are often stationed strategically in inner cities, near schools, or in school-based clinics. These agencies are empowered to provide birth control information and counseling to young people.

Substance Abuse. Substance abuse among young people was almost unknown before 1950 and rare before 1960. Now, adolescent drug experimentation and use poses serious physical and psychological threats. During the 30 days before being surveyed, adolescent participants in the 2017 Youth Risk Behavior Survey reported that:

- 35.6% tried marijuana.
- 8.8% had smoked tobacco.
- 42.2% had used electronic vapor product. Vaping has increased significantly due to low perceived risk for youth with 12th graders reporting 11% use in 2017 and 21% use in 2018; 10th graders have also showed an increase with 8.2% use in 2017 and 16.1% use in 2018 (National Institute of Drug Abuse, 2018).
- 29.8% of students have had at least one alcoholic drink in the last 30 days (CDC, 2018f).

School nurses can assist in programs targeting all substance abuse. Successful programs focus on protective factors, instead of just high-risk behaviors. The programs focus more on the root causes, or why youth choose high-risk activities. See Chapters 20 and 25.

School nurses can also provide resources for smoking cessation and substance abuse programs. In addition to school-based education, programs of peer leadership and parental education/involvement and community-wide task forces have been developed to lobby for local legislation and strengthen community–school ties. School nurses can be advocates at a community level by lobbying the city council for tougher ordinances controlling advertising content and zoning (especially near schools). School nurses often work in conjunction with law enforcement officials, school district administrators, and other community agencies to ensure compliance with local regulations and prevent or delay tobacco use. Other groups, such as 4-H clubs, religious congregations, the Catholic Youth Organization, and Boy Scouts, use peer counseling to influence young people to assume responsibility for healthy lifestyles, with the goal of developing decision-making skills that lead to healthy lifestyle choices in adolescence and through adulthood. The school nurse participates in and supports existing programs in addition to counseling and referring young people who need help.

Mental Health Issues and Suicide. Depression, schizophrenia, and eating disorders may first appear during adolescence. It is estimated that 13% to 20% of children experience a mental disorder in a given year (NASN, 2018h). Many adolescents are reluctant to seek help for emotional problems or help may not be readily available to them.

- It is estimated that only 10% to 40% of those who need treatment actually receives it (NASN, 2018h).
- Common mental health disorders in adolescence include anxiety, depression, ADHD, eating disorders, bipolar disorder, and schizophrenia (NIMH, n.d.).
- Suicide is the third leading cause of death for young people between ages 15 and 24 years; it is the second leading cause of death in children between ages 5 and 14 years (American Academy of Child & Adolescent Psychiatry, 2017).
- School nurses must be aware of the signs and symptoms of mental illness and suicidal intentions. They can work with school psychologists, social workers, and other mental health workers to address the needs of the students and provide grief counseling to peers after a student commits suicide.
- Recent suicides by youth have been attributed to the students being bullied. School nurses also need to be aware of the increased issues related to bullying in the schools and in cyberspace. The YRBSS states that 19% of children had reported being bullied while at school, and 14.9% had experienced cyberbullying (NASN, 2018f).

Chapters 20 and 25 have more information on adolescent and behavioral health issues.

Abuse and Maltreatment. In 2016, an estimated 676,000 children were victims of abuse and neglect. Of these children, one in four experienced some form of abuse or neglect in their lifetime with one in seven children being abused in the last year; approximately 1,750 children die as a result of child maltreatment (CDC, 2018i).

Child abuse prevention education programs can be found in many school districts as a primary preventive intervention. School nurses are required by law to report suspected or confirmed cases of abuse. In addition, school nurses can educate teachers and other school personnel regarding the signs and symptoms of abuse.

- Early identification of abuse and intervention is critical for the safety of the child. Approximately 18.4% of suspected child abuse reports came from education personnel (NASN, 2018i). It is important to be well versed in subtle signs and symptoms of maltreatment and develop strong collaborative relationships with social service professionals.
- Signs that a child might be maltreated include reports of abuse, a sudden change in behavior, lack of medical treatment follow-through, learning problems of unknown etiology, child responses that are consistently guarded or compliant, and an avoidance of home or certain individuals (NASN, 2018i).

For more information on health problems and issues concerning children and adolescents, see Chapter 20.

School-Based Health Centers

Because of the complex and intertwined emotional, physical, and educational needs of school-age children and adolescents, a more comprehensive interdisciplinary approach to services is needed than the piecemeal approaches attempted previously. School nurses are able to do much to influence school children's health. However, often they need to refer the children to a health care provider. Yet, more parents are working and less available to take care of their children's health care needs during the day. SBHCs provide ready access to health care for large numbers of children and adolescents during school hours, reducing absences from school due to health care appointments. SBHCs provide a variety of services in a user-friendly manner at a convenient location.

- In 2016 to 2017, there were a total of 2,584 SBHCs in the United States, Puerto Rico, and the District of Columbia, providing 6.3 million children with access to school-based health care (School-Based Health Alliance, 2017).
- These clinics are distributed in high schools, middle schools, and elementary schools and are generally established on school grounds. A large majority (81%) of the clinics serve grades 6th through 12th (School-Based Health Alliance, 2017).
- The health care providers consist of nurse practitioners (85%) and physician assistants (20%); 40% of the clinics have physicians (School-Based Health Alliance, 2017).
- Some clinics provide services only to schoolchildren, whereas others extend services to their families and to other neighborhood families with preschool-age children. Most centers are open full-time.
- Many SBHCs in middle schools and high schools offer abstinence counseling, pregnancy testing, sexually transmitted infection diagnosis and testing, and pap tests (School-Based Health Alliance, 2017). SBHCs are staffed by interdisciplinary teams of helping professionals, paraprofessionals, and other staff and can include nurses, nurse practitioners, and social workers. Many hospitals, HMOs, and health departments are sponsors of these school clinics, because it is a cost-effective way to decrease visits to the emergency department and promote health, especially to underserved groups such as adolescents. They help meet the need for patient-centered medical homes, as outlined in the Affordable Care Act. Third-party billing, especially to access Medicaid funding, is increasingly more common among SBHCs, and private foundations have also been instrumental in providing financial and technical support. School nurses support the clinics by referring students who need additional attention. In some areas, school-linked health centers are utilized. These clinics are not on school property but may be nearby or easily accessible through mass transit. Mobile vans also provide access to health services for school-aged children, offering a wide range of services including medical, dental, and behavioral health; in addition, they can assist with health care enrollment (La Clinica, 2019; Metrohealth, 2019).

Evaluation research has demonstrated that SBHCs are effective in increasing student access to health care. This is especially true for adolescents, who often are difficult to reach and do not willingly access health care. Onsite SBHC services are more appealing for adolescents, who have been shown to utilize substance abuse and mental health counseling services, as well as STD and family planning services (School-Based Health Alliance, 2017).

School Nursing Careers

School nurses must be able to work autonomously. They need excellent communication skills and the ability to prioritize and collaborate with many others (professional and nonprofessional). The pay for school nurses depends on location and employer (health department or school district). School nurses save time for teachers and administrators, permitting them to focus on their job of educating students. School nurses positively influence management of student health concerns, student record accuracy, and student immunization rates. Many nursing schools are utilizing schools as clinical sites, with school nurses as preceptors, in an effort to bring more new nurses into this specialty area.

- There are many positive reasons to work as a school nurse: school nurses generally do not work on weekends, many have contracts that give them the summer off, and the daily work schedule and holidays often coincide with those of the nurse's own school-age children, thus allowing a parent to be home with children during off-school hours.
- Finally, for most of those employed as school nurses, it is a wonderful and rewarding experience to work with children whose eagerness and innocence can often refresh the soul. It is an opportunity to protect and heal our future leaders, who may become the ones who will eventually protect and heal the world (Box 28-12).

BOX **28-12** PERSPECTIVES

A School Nurse Viewpoint on Community Health Nursing

A great aspect of being a school nurse is being able to work with many different people. I like being able to work with people who aren't necessarily sick but can benefit from my help. Additionally, school nurses must become familiar with resources and people in the community and surrounding areas. By making friends and connections in facilities, and the community, school nurses can involve local resources and individuals to improve the population. Resources aren't as readily available as they are for other types of nursing. Unlike working in a hospital, where results are apparent in just a few days, school nurses must work tirelessly for long periods of time to see the fruits of their labors.

Being a school nurse requires learning how to get funding for projects. School nurses often don't have a model to work from, because each situation may be unique. They must be innovative, resourceful, and dedicated in order to stick with a project long enough for it to be beneficial to the population.

School nursing is probably the epitome of what nursing was meant to be. It is focused on service and improving the health and well-being of the populace. The focus is on prevention; school nurses seem to get little recognition for their work—because they are saving lives before they are endangered, they are saving teeth before they fall out, and they are saving families before they are lost. I believe their work is pivotal to the improvement of society.

Neil P., school nurse

CORRECTIONAL NURSING

Correctional nurses work within the criminal justice system—in correctional facilities, prisons, jails, detention centers, and substance abuse treatment programs—with clients spanning a range of ages from juvenile to elderly, both male and female (Fig. 28-6; ANA, 2013). Bureau of Justice Statistics dated December 31, 2016, reported an estimated 6,613,500 persons were supervised by U.S. adult correctional systems. The decrease in the incarcerated population was due to a decline in the prison population (down 21,200), while the jail population remained relatively stable (Kaeble & Cowhig, 2018).

About 1 in 38 adults (or 2.6% of persons age 18 or older in the United States) were under some form of correctional supervision at year-end 2016 (Bureau of Justice Statistics, 2018). An estimated 2% to 3% of RNs work in corrections (Correctional Nurse, 2019) as compared to the total national nursing workforce. This appears to be a low number considering there are various career options for working in a correctional setting (e.g., part time, contract service, academic affiliations, etc.) which may impact the total estimations.

History of Nursing in the Correctional Setting

- In the past, the correctional system of prisons and jails has provided minimal, if any, health care to inmates. Historically, nurses involved with prisoner and mentally ill populations included Dorothea Dix, who visited prisons around the country in the 19th century and found prisoners in chains, without proper sanitation, living conditions, nutrition, or clothing (ANA, 2013).
- Prison was viewed as a punishment, and the inmates were seen as not deserving of care that was being paid for through public dollars (Estelle v. Gamble).
- The historic Supreme Court ruling *Estelle v. Gamble* stated that not providing medical services inflicted pain and denied inmates their Eighth Amendment rights (Box 28-13) and led to major reforms in the correctional health system. Medical providers were hired, and inmates' rights were established (Akiyama, Feffer, Von Oehsen, & Litwin, 2018; Dober, 2019).

Although the correctional health system is a relatively new specialty, it is under intense pressure from the courts to ensure that adequate and humane care is provided. Specific issues include the provision of ethically appropriate and timely patient care for inmates, the provision of adequate mental health treatment, prevention of prisoner-on-prisoner violence, maintenance of sanitary and safe conditions, and ending inmate neglect and abuse. Ensuring that inmates' health needs are met amidst the growing number of inmates and their increasing complex health concerns has imposed a huge financial burden on correctional systems.

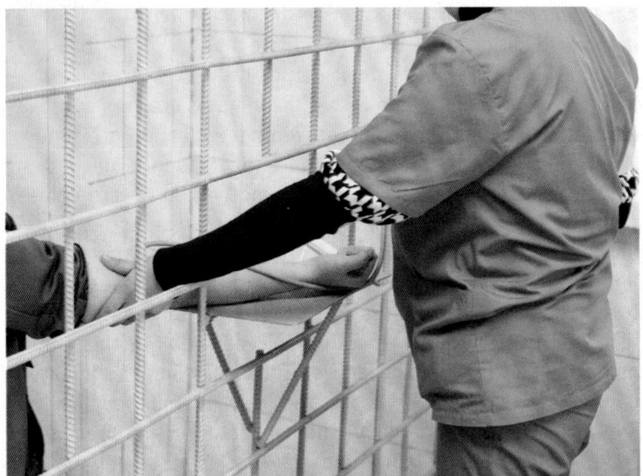

FIGURE 28-6 Correctional nurse taking an inmate's blood pressure.

BOX 28-13 The Rights of Inmates

- Right to humane housing and treatment
- Right to not be a victim of sexual crimes
- Right not to be racially segregated
- Right to complain about conditions
- Rights provided by the American Disabilities Act
- Right to necessary medical care
- Right to necessary mental health care
- Right to a hearing

Source: Findlaw (2020).

Funding for correctional health care derives from public tax dollars and many are contesting that care and expense should be given to incarcerated persons National Commission on Correctional Health Care, 2017). This is an ethical dilemma nurses working in correctional facilities must face every day. In an attempt to decrease costs and save money, several states utilize managed care organizations to provide some services for inmates and are increasingly relying on private prison health care providers and managed care organizations (Pew, 2017).

Correctional nurses must demonstrate nonjudgmental attitudes while at the same time ensuring self-protection from assault. Correctional nurses work in on-site medical units, clinics, or infirmaries housed in criminal justice facilities. These facilities can be local jails or state and federal prison. The care is focused on the individual, immediate, and ambulatory care, emergency needs, and management of chronic conditions, screenings and preventive services. Larger facilities offer ambulatory and inpatient mental health services, and subacute care units for short-term therapies (e.g., IV medications). In addition, the increased female incarceration rates highlight that women's health care concerns must be addressed. As prisoners age, long-term care and end-of-life care must also be provided (Sanders & Stensland, 2018); correctional systems are further challenged with these additional specialty care needs.

Education and Skills Needed

The preferred educational level for correctional nurses is a bachelor's degree. The level of skill, judgment, and autonomy needed by nurses who work in corrections is supported and developed within baccalaureate education. National certification, through the National Commission on Correctional Health Care as a certified correctional health professional-RN (CCHP) (National Commission on Correctional Health Care, 2020) or the American Correctional Association (ACA) as a certified correctional nurse (CCN) (American Correctional Association, n.d.), is available. Some correctional systems employ licensed professional nurses (LPN) and medical assistant technicians (MATs).

Functions of Correctional Nurses

Correctional nurses use public, community, and school health nursing skills, along with skills acquired from the ED, occupational health, mental health, orthopedics, and ambulatory care specialties. In general, primary care interventions are provided for the inmate population with a focus on health promotion and healthful lifestyles during incarceration.

- Nurses assess patients for basic health needs and treat injuries and minor acute medical conditions. As indicated, patients are scheduled for regular appointments to manage chronic conditions of hypertension, diabetes, pulmonary disorders, and mental health.
- The correctional nurses also track and screen for communicable diseases, providing essential related treatment as needed, provide health promotion education, and provide transitional or discharge education and preparation.
- The correctional nurses may encounter a critical medical emergency requiring stabilization before the inmate is transported to an outside treatment facility for complex medical care. Most correctional facilities do not have inpatient acute care medical units, while many have inpatient mental health units for varied behavioral health conditions.

Because correctional facilities operate 24 hours a day, every day of the year, it is vital that correctional nurses have cardiac life support certifications, emergency preparedness, and disaster planning training. To carry out its mission, the Federal Bureau of Prisons follows national preparedness goals; preparedness planning and an emergency operations plan are necessary (Johnson, 2018) (Table 28-1). A seminal study (Taylor & Crianza, 2011) provides vivid examples of natural disasters affecting a large jail system (over 10,000 inmates) and the need to plan for power, water, and telephone outages, as well as housing and moving prisoners under emergency conditions. Many correctional facilities include tabletop exercises in their annual training program, and ensure resources are available to provide adequate supplies to sustain health and wellness for a minimum of 72 hours post the impact of adverse weather. In many situations, nursing and other staff are often asked to remain on-site for extended periods of time and while making arrangements for their own families.

TABLE 28-1 Emergency Preparedness in Correctional Facilities

Prevention	Plan for incidents by assessing threats and processes for response.
Protection	Provide for adequate support and equipment prior to the disaster
Mitigation	Practice and prepare through trainings, drills, and full-scale exercises
Response	Provide necessary response efforts to save lives, and protect property and the community.
Recovery	Assist in the recovery efforts after an incident; learn from the disaster and plan for future crisis.

Source: Johnson (2018).

FEMA Guidelines recommend identifying hazards early and then taking actions to mitigate those hazards before they become major problems (FEMA, 2011). Correctional and medical staff training, and routine facility inspections will enhance correctional disaster management outcomes (Boxes 28-14 to 28-16).

Future Trends

Because of advances in health care, longer prison terms, and more restrictive policies, inmates are older, sicker, and remain in prison longer than they did even 20 years ago. Historically, inmates have not taken good care of them-

BOX 28-14 PERSPECTIVES

A Correctional Nursing Viewpoint on Community Health Nursing

When I completed my graduate nursing program with an MSN and FNP, I planned to work on a mobile clinic/van travelling to several identified underserved communities providing chronic and preventive health care. Instead, I accepted the challenge of a uniformed service enchanted by the mission of providing health care to underserved populations across the nation. Little did I know I would start my NP career working in a federal correctional facility. Honestly, I was a little nervous for the first 3 months as I adjusted to the security restrictions of the setting and the "inmate" population. One day I went to work and told myself "these are individuals coming to the clinic for health care service." They are "patients."

From that time forward, I provided nonjudgmental, holistic nursing care to all the inmates I served for over 10 years. I developed a passion for this special, underserved population and became an advocate for preventive correctional health care and obtained correctional health care certification and a master's degree in criminal justice. What is most surprising about correctional nursing is that the inmates are very appreciative of the health care and preventive education provided. When told they are being empowered to manage their individual medical conditions, there is a motivation toward compliance. When measurable outcomes are presented during chronic care visits or follow-up appointments, the pattern of improvement and compliance is enhanced. It is a great feeling to see the outcomes of one's nursing interventions in this population especially during the chronic care appointments and/or during the release preparation process, when the inmate can explain healthy lifestyle practices learned and they plan to continue. What a validation of the impact of nursing practice!

CAPT Beverly Dandridge, USPHS Commissioned Corps

BOX 28-15 WHAT DO *YOU* THINK?

Potential Botulism Outbreak in Prison Inmates

During sick call today, your correctional nurse colleague notices that four to five inmates from the same housing unit have similar complaints—blurred vision, feeling sick, and some difficulty breathing. It is flu season—could that be the cause?

You know that homemade alcohol is not uncommon in prisons and that it can be easily made from fermented fruit or other food waste. Prisoners call it moonshine, pruno, hooch, brew, raisin jack, and other names. You remember reading about a recent CDC report regarding several outbreaks of botulism in California, Utah, and Arizona prisons. Prisoners there had used potato peels, and the closed containers used to produce alcohol permitted the toxin to grow during fermentation. With no heat used to kill it, the bacteria grew and affected everyone who drank the brew.

With botulism, it is most important to act quickly, as the toxin leads to nerve paralysis, and when it reaches the respiratory muscles, it can cause death. You talk with your colleague and decide to talk with the housing correctional officers and the patients for further information. I think it is better to be safe than sorry! What do you think?

Source: Schoenly (2016a).

BOX 28-16 Correctional System Challenges for Nursing

- Understanding of the population
- Autonomous conditions
- No universal standard for experience/no certifications
- Strict facility protocols for safety and security
- Employee burnout
- Corrections fatigue

Source: Nursing @CSU Staff (2019).

selves, hence, a 50-year-old inmate may have the health of a typical 65 year old in the general public (Schoenly, 2014).

Correctional nurses can increase efforts to improve transitional health care programs, and serve as advocates, and lobby state and federal legislatures to allocate funding for the additional resources needed within the correctional health care systems (Hoke, 2015).

The female inmate population is also increasing. In addition to women's reproductive health issues, females tend to have higher rates of major mental illness, dental problems, insomnia, and chronic medical conditions (Mignon, 2016; Mollard & Hudson, 2016). Previous researcher has found that women in jail have a high risk of cervical cancer and increased rates of abnormal

BOX 28-17 PERSPECTIVES

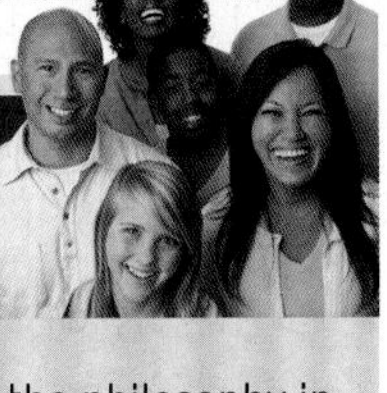

A Supervisor and a Director of Correctional Nursing Viewpoint on Hiring New Nurses

Do you think you might like a job at a prison facility? A Director of Nursing and a Supervisor of Correctional Nursing provide some information on the interview process. Before hiring new correctional nurses, they ask candidates to review the correctionalnurse.net blog and the (Schoenly, 2016b) *Correctional Nurse Manifesto* (Schoenly, 2014). The nurses who are hired receive civilian training and are assigned a preceptor. The process is designed to educate the candidate about the realities and complexities of correctional nursing. As the director notes, "No one dreams of going into correctional nursing, but once you are in, you are hooked because you realize the difference you can make."

The interview process follows the guidelines set forth by the ANA *Correctional Nursing: Scope and Standards of Practice* (2013) and the textbook *Essentials of Correctional Nursing* (Schoenly & Knox, 2013), which provides crucial information such as the ethical, legal, and safety considerations of correctional nursing; common inmate-patient health care concerns and diseases; nursing care processes; and professional role and responsibilities. Also, unlike the nurses hired in the past, newer correctional nurses do provide health care education and health care clinics for chronic diseases on a regular basis. Because of the lack of an inpatient facility, 24-hour nursing care is not provided in some correctional facilities. When 24-hour nursing care is necessary, the inmates are transferred to a correctional facility where such coverage is available or to an acute care facility if more extensive care is required. In addition, the correctional officers are trained to follow procedure and call 911 during an emergency.

Challenges to correctional nursing include the philosophy in the prison setting that "safety comes first," which could result in an inmate missing a sick call. Should this occur, however, their medical needs are taken care of as soon as it is safe and without compromise to their condition, according to both the supervisor and the director of nursing. An emergency that correctional nurses are occasionally faced with is suicide attempts—a situation that is always "scary" even if you have seen it happen before. This situation leads to a lock-down so that all resources can be focused on the suicidal inmate, who sometimes is found hanging and needs to be cut down and resuscitated.

The ability of correctional nurses to deliver medically appropriate care is hindered by the lack of access to preexisting medical records and history. Self-reporting is a far less reliable means for determining an inmate's risk factors and overall wellness. This is one reason that civil litigation by inmates, alleging medical negligence, is a weighty problem for all correctional agencies.

Nurses have an incredible opportunity to improve the health of the inmate population by returning their patients to the community healthier than when they arrived.

Stan, Supervisor of Correctional Nursing
Denise, Director of Correctional Nursing

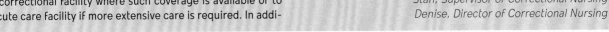

Source: Schoenly (2014, 2016b).

Papanicolaou (Pap) test results (Brousseau, Ahn, & Matteson, 2019).

Researchers have suggested that women in prison need trauma-informed, gender-responsive treatment because of past trauma histories (Mollard & Hudson, 2016). There has been a movement to provide trauma-informed care and gender-responsive programs (GRPs) to women in prison.

One study discovered one third of inmates being released from prison had at least one chronic condition; that number increased to 70% of those 55 years or older (Rosen et al., 2019). Correctional nurses can facilitate chronic disease management by coordinating chronic care education programs and empowering inmates to take better control their chronic conditions. Correctional nurses should also conduct thorough family health histories, as much as possible, as many health conditions tend to have a genetic component and discuss screenings to identify conditions with correctional health care providers to facilitate early intervention and decrease complications and potentially, disease progression.

Ethical and legal issues in correctional nursing often center on the patient (most often someone convicted of a crime, possibly involving violence). Caring for the patient is vital, but custody must also be maintained, and safety is essential. Correctional nurses have an opportunity, to help reduce the burden of disease for communities by providing tri-level preventive health care pre-, intra-, and post incarceration (La Cerra et al., 2017).

CORRECTIONAL NURSING CAREERS

Correctional nurses must have good mental health and assessment skills, strong communication skills, and be strong advocates for nursing and their clients. These nurses work in an intense environment where their safety could be threatened, and they must deal with clients who may be noncompliant, combative, and manipulative. Correctional nurses are also increasingly becoming Certified Correctional Health Care Professionals (Box 28-17; National Commission on Correctional Health Care, 2020).

Correctional nurses usually receive extensive employee benefits and insurance packages as government employees. Correctional nurses have the ability to see recoveries from illnesses and injuries because they work with the same patients for a longer time than hospital-based nurses. Correctional nursing provides an opportunity to work with a vulnerable population and practice the true art and science of nursing. It can be a challenging and rewarding career. See Perspectives about the hiring process for new correctional nurses.

SUMMARY

- ▶ C/PHNs manage a number of issues including communicable diseases, chronic diseases, injuries, maternal child health, immunizations, substance abuse, and disaster response.
- ▶ C/PHNs work with all ages, ethnicities, socioeconomic groups, and populations emphasizing health prevention and promotion.
- ▶ C/PHNs work in several branches of the uniformed services.
- ▶ School nurses work with school populations (elementary, middle, high schools, and college/university levels) including students, their families, and the school staff providing individual care and bridging the gap between medical providers and schools.
- ▶ School nurses provide direct nursing care, first aid, immunizations, environmental assessments, and specialized health care for children with special needs.
- ▶ Correctional nurses work with inmates in federal, state, or local facilities, including drug treatment and juvenile detention centers.
- ▶ Correctional nurses provide individual care in facility clinics and infirmaries while also identifying and developing programs to address major population health concerns of inmates, including mental illness, substance abuse, and communicable diseases.
- ▶ The inmate population is growing older, staying longer, and experiencing more from chronic disease. This, along with an increase in female inmates, brings additional challenges for correctional nurses.
- ▶ All nursing specialty areas provide valuable services which impact the health of our communities. Because of the high level of nursing knowledge, communication skills, autonomy, and leadership needed for professional nursing practice, the educational entry level should be a minimum baccalaureate degree.

thePoint: Everything You Need to Make the Grade!

thePoint® Visit http://thePoint.lww.com/Rector10e for NCLEX-style review questions, journal articles, supplemental materials, study aids for all learning styles, and more!

ACTIVE LEARNING EXERCISES

1. Interview a public health nurse asking the following questions:
   a. Why did you choose public health nursing?
   b. Within what area of public health nursing do you work?
   c. Does an epidemiological background help with your work?
   d. What is the most satisfying part of your job?
2. As a correctional nurse, you will care for people who are accused or sentenced for a variety of crimes. How might a correctional nurse utilize the 10 essential public health services to ensure high standards of health care when working with this vulnerable population?
3. Go to this Web site (https://www.nhlbi.nih.gov/files/docs/public/lung/asthma_actplan.pdf) and print out

a copy of the *Asthma Action Plan*. Discuss this with the parent of a school-age child or adolescent who has asthma. Has a school nurse or public health nurse ever gone over a plan with them? Have they ever been shown how to use a peak flow meter or correctly use an asthma inhaler? What methods have they used to control asthma triggers?

4. Using "Utilize Legal and Regulatory Actions" (1 of the 10 essential public health services; see Box 2-2), consider the following question: Most schools require that children entering school show proof of being fully immunized for a variety of communicable diseases. With a partner, discuss what would happen if schools no longer had this requirement. How would you educate parents who refuse to immunize their child because of the unfounded fear that immunizations cause autism?
5. List five (5) potential areas of employment as a member of the U.S. Public Health Service. What types of services are rendered in each agency? What are benefits of this type of nursing career (uniformed service)?
6. Are prisons and jails appropriate facilities for meeting the needs of individuals with mental health and substance use diseases? Why or why not? If not, what other alternatives may be more effective?

REFERENCES

Akiyama, M., Feffer, R., Von Oehsen, W., & Litwin, A. (2018). Drug purchasing strategies to treat people with hepatitis C in the criminal justice system. *American Journal of Public Health*, *108*(5), 607–608. doi: 10.2105/AJPH.2018.304362.

Alliance of Schools for Cooperative Insurance Programs. (2017). *In loco parentis and district risk*. Retrieved from http://ascip.org/wp-content/uploads/2014/05/Risk-Alert-In-Loco-Parentis-rev-2017.12.20-1A.pdf

Altaf, F., Drinkwater, J., Phan, K., & Cree, A. K. (2017). Systemic review of school scoliosis screening. *Spine Deformity*, *5*(5), 303–309. doi: 10.1016/j.jspd.2017.03.009.

American Academy of Allergy, Asthma & Immunology. (n.d.). *When should children and adolescents assume responsibility for self-treatment of anaphylaxis?* Retrieved from https://www.aaaai.org/conditions-and-treatments/library/allergy-library/children-epinephrine

American Academy of Child & Adolescent Psychiatry. (2017). *Fact sheet: Teen suicide*. Retrieved from https://www.aacap.org/AACAP/Families_and_Youth/Facts_for_Families/FFF-Guide/Teen-Suicide-010.aspx

American Academy of Family Physicians. (2019). *Incarceration and health: A family medicine perspective (Position Paper)*. Retrieved from https://www.aafp.org/about/policies/all/incarcerationandhealth.html

American Academy of Pediatrics. (2018a). *Allergy and anaphylaxis emergency plan*. Retrieved from https://www.foodallergyawareness.org/media/education/AAP_Allergy_and_Anaphylaxis_Emergency_Plan%201.pdf

American Academy of Pediatrics. (2018b). *CDC releases new guidance on diagnosing, managing concussion*. Retrieved from http://www.aappublications.org/news/2018/09/10/concussion091018

American Academy of Pediatrics (AAP). (2016). *Policy statement: Role of the school nurse in providing school health services*. Retrieved from http://pediatrics.aappublications.org/content/pediatrics/early/2016/05/19/peds.2016-0852.full.pdf

American Correctional Association. (n.d.). *What types and levels of certification are available?* Retrieved from http://www.aca.org/ACA_Prod_IMIS/ACA_Member/Professional%20Development/Certification/Certification_Overview/ACA_Member/Certification/Certification_Overview.aspx?hkey=61bb1b2f-6d34-4636-816b-c701570e3b9b

American Diabetes Association. (2017). *California*. Retrieved from https://www.diabetes.org/resources/know-your-rights/safe-at-school-state-laws/CA

American Lung Association. (2018). *Open airways for schools*. Retrieved from https://www.lung.org/lung-health-and-diseases/lung-disease-lookup/asthma/asthma-education-advocacy/open-airways-for-schools/about-open-airways.html

American Nurses Association (ANA). (2013). *Correctional nursing: Scope and standards of practice* (2nd ed.). Silver Spring, MD: Author.

American Nurses Association (ANA). (2015). *Public health nursing: Scope and standards of practice* (3rd ed.) Silver Spring, MD: Author.

American Nurses Association (ANA) and National Association of School Nurses (NASN). (2017). *School nursing: Scope and standards of practice* (3rd ed.). Silver Spring, MD: Author.

American Public health Association. (2013). *The definition and practice of public health nursing*. Retrieved from https://www.apha.org/-/media/files/pdf/membergroups/phn/nursingdefinition.ashx?la=en&hash=331DBEC4B79E0C0B8C644BF2BEA571249F8717A0

American School Health Association. (n.d.). *About the American School Health Association: Core beliefs*. Retrieved from http://www.ashaweb.org/wp-content/uploads/2015/02/ASHA-Core-Beliefs-Combined_2.6.20152.pdf

American Speech-Language-Hearing Association. (n.d.). *Sensorineural hearing loss*. Retrieved from https://www.asha.org/public/hearing/sensorineural-hearing-loss/

Atusingwize, E., Lewis, S., & Langley, T. (2015). Economic evaluations of tobacco control mass media campaigns: A systematic review. *Tobacco Control*, *24*(4), 320–327.

Babazadeh, T. Kouzekanani, K., Ghasemzadeh, S. Matlabi, H., & Allahahverdipour, H. (2019). The role of a community–based intervention in promotion helmet use in a non-probability sample of rural motorcyclists in Iran. *Journal of Community Health*, *44*, 828–835.

Beck, A., & Boulton, M. (2016). The public health nurse workforce in U.S. state and local health departments, 2012. *Public Health Reports*, *131*, 145–152.

Benjamin-Chung, J. (2018). LB20. Impact of school-located influenza vaccination on vaccination coverage, school absenteeism, and influenza hospitalization. *Open Forum Infectious Diseases*, *5*(1), S766. doi: 10.1093/ofid/ofy229.2194.

Bersamin, M., Coulter, R., Gaarde, J., Garbers, S., Mair, C., & Santelli, J. (2019). School-based health centers and school connectedness. *Journal of School Health*, *89*(1), 11–19.

Best, N., Oppewal, S., & Travers, D. (2018). Exploring school nurse interventions and health and education outcomes: An integrative review. *The Journal of School Nursing*, *34*(1), 14–27.

Brackney, D. E., & Cutshall, M. (2015). Prevention of type 2 diabetes among youth: A systematic review, implications for the school nurse. *Journal of School Nursing*, *31*(1), 6–21.

Brousseau, E. C., Ahn, S., & Matteson, K. A. (2019). Cervical cancer screening access, outcomes, and prevalence of dysplasia in correctional facilities: A systematic review. *Journal of Women's Health*, *28*(12). doi: 10.1089/jwh.2018.7440.

Bureau of Justice Statistics. (2018). *U.S. correctional population declined for the ninth consecutive year*. Retrieved from https://www.bjs.gov/content/pub/press/cpus16pr.cfm

Byrne, E., Vessey, J., & Pfeifer, L. (2018). Cyberbullying and social media: Information and interventions for school nurses working with victims, students, and families. *The Journal of School Nursing*, *34*(1), 38–50.

California Code of Regulations 5CCR 3030. (n.d.). *Title 5 education. Division 1 California Department of Education. Chapter 3 individuals with exceptional needs*. Retrieved from http://www.casponline.org/pdfs/pdfs/Title%205%20Regs,%20CCR%20update.pdf

California School Based Health Alliance. (2020). *List of mandated health services*. Retrieved from https://www.schoolhealthcenters.org/start-up-and-operations/school-health-program-models/mandated-health-services/list-of-mandated-health-services/

Center for Disease Control and Prevention (CDC). (2007-2017). *Youth risk behavioral survey*. Retrieved from https://www.cdc.gov/healthyyouth/data/yrbs/pdf/trendsreport.pdf

Center for Disease Control and Prevention (CDC). (2016a). *A comprehensive technical package for the prevention of youth violence and associated risk behaviors*. Retrieved from https://www.cdc.gov/violenceprevention/pdf/yv-technicalpackage.pdf

Center for Disease Control and Prevention (CDC). (2016b). *Results from the school health policies and practices study*. Retrieved from https://www.cdc.gov/healthyyouth/data/shpps/pdf/shpps-results_2016.pdf#page=46

Center for Disease Control and Prevention (CDC). (2017a). *Safe youth, safe schools*. Retrieved from https://www.cdc.gov/features/safeschools/index.html

Center for Disease Control and Prevention (CDC). (2017b). *Oral health in schools*. Retrieved from https://www.cdc.gov/healthyschools/npao/oralhealth.htm

Centers for Disease Control and Prevention (CDC). (2018a). *National public health performance standards*. Retrieved from https://www.cdc.gov/publichealthgateway/nphps/index.html

Centers for Disease Control and Prevention (CDC). (2018b). *The virtual healthy school*. Retrieved from https://www.cdc.gov/healthyschools/vhs/#!/scene/1

Centers for Disease Control and Prevention (CDC). (2018c). *Food allergies in school*. Retrieved from https://www.cdc.gov/healthyschools/foodallergies/index.htm

Centers for Disease Control and Prevention (CDC). (2018d). *Vaccination laws*. Retrieved from https://www.cdc.gov/phlp/publications/topic/vaccinationlaws.html

Centers for Disease Control and Prevention (CDC). (2018e). *Recognizing national immunization awareness month (NIAM)*. Retrieved from http://www.cdc.gov/vaccines/events/niam.html

Centers for Disease Control and Prevention (CDC). (2018f). *Youth risk behavioral survey—2017*. Retrieved from https://www.cdc.gov/healthyyouth/data/yrbs/pdf/2017/ss6708.pdf

Centers for Disease Control and Prevention (CDC). (2018g). *Information on risky behavior for parents with teens (aged 12-19)*. Retrieved from https://www.cdc.gov/parents/teens/risk_behaviors.html

Centers for Disease Control and Prevention (CDC). (2018h). *STDs in adolescents and young adults*. Retrieved from https://www.cdc.gov/std/stats17/adolescents.htm

Centers for Disease Control and Prevention (CDC). (2018i). *Child abuse and neglect prevention*. Retrieved from https://www.cdc.gov/violenceprevention/childabuseandneglect/index.html

Centers for Disease Control and Prevention (CDC). (2020). *CDC healthy schools: Whole school, whole community, whole child*. Retrieved from https://www.cdc.gov/healthyschools/wscc/index.htm

Chan, E., Fogler, J. M., & Hammerness, P. G. (2016). Treatment of attention-deficit/hyperactivity disorder in adolescents: A systematic review. *JAMA, 315*(18), 1997–2008.

Cicutto, L., Gleason, M., Haas-howard, C., Jenkins-Nygren, L., Labonde, S., & Patrick, K. (2017). Competency-based framework and continuing education for preparing a skilled school health workforce for asthma care: The Colorado experience. *The Journal of School Nursing, 33*(4), 277–284.

Community Tool Box. (2020). *Section 7. Ten essential public health services*. Retrieved from https://ctb.ku.edu/en/table-of-contents/overview/models-for-community-health-and-development/ten-essential-public-health-services/main

Correctional Nurse. (2019). *Scope and standards: Prevalence of correctional nurses*. Retrieved from https://correctionalnurse.net/scope-and-standards-prevalence-of-correctional-nurses/

Crawford, B., Yamazaki, R., Franke, E., Amanatidis, S., Ravulo, J., & Torvaldsen, S. (2015). Is something better than nothing? Food insecurity and eating patterns of young people experiencing homelessness. *Australian and New Zealand Journal of Public Health, 39*, 350–354. doi: 10.1111/1753-6405.12371.

Cronenwett, L., Sherwood, G., Barnsteiner, J., Mitchell, P., Sullivan, D., & Warren, J. (2007). Quality and safety education for nurses. *Nursing Outlook, 55*(3), 122–131. doi: 10.1016/j.outlook/2207.02.006.

Darnell, T., Hager, K., & Loprinzi, P. D. (2019). The impact of school nurses in Kentucky Public High Schools. *Journal of School Nursing*, 35(6), 434–441. doi: 10.1177/1059840518785954.

Dober, G. (2019). *Beyond Estelle: Medical rights for incarcerated patients*. Prison Legal News. Retrieved from https://www.prisonlegalnews.org/news/2019/nov/4/beyond-estelle-medical-rights-incarcerated-patients/

Endsley, P. (2017). School nurse workload: A scoping review of acute care, community health, and mental health nursing workload literature. *The Journal of School Nursing, 33*(1), 43–52.

Epilepsy Foundation. (2017). *Ketogenic diet*. Retrieved from https://www.epilepsy.com/learn/treating-seizures-and-epilepsy/dietary-therapies/ketogenic-diet

Epilepsy Foundation. (n.d.). *Diastat 101*. Retrieved from http://www.epilepsy.com/get-help/seizure-first-aid/responding-seizures/diastat-101

Estelle v. Gamble. No. 75-929 (U.S. Supreme Court, 1976).

Everhart, R., Miller, S., Leinach, G., & Koinis-Mitchell, D. (2018). Caregiver asthma in urban families: Implications for school absenteeism. *The Journal of School Nursing, 34*(2), 108–113.

Federal Emergency Management Agency. (2011). *FEMA Funds North Idaho Correctional Facility Retrofit. R10-11-032*. Retrieved from https://www.fema.gov/news-release/2011/09/30/fema-funds-north-idaho-correctional-facility-retrofit

Findlaw. (2020). *Rights of inmates*. Retrieved from https://civilrights.findlaw.com/other-constitutional-rights/rights-of-inmates.html

Food Allergy Research & Education. (2018). *Facts and statistics*. Retrieved from https://www.foodallergy.org/life-with-food-allergies/food-allergy-101/facts-and-statistics

Galemore, C. A., & Sheetz, A. H. (2015). IEP, IHP, and Section 504 primer for new school nurses. *NASN School Nurse, 30*(2), 85–88.

Gunning, K., Kiraly, B., & Pippitt, K. (2019). Lice and scabies: Treatment update. *American Family Physician*, 99(10), 635–642.

Hartman, A. L., Devore, C. D.; & Section on Neurology, Council on School Health. (2016). Rescue medicine for epilepsy in education settings. *American Academy of Pediatrics, 137*(1), e20153876.

Hassmiller, S. (2016). *Why school nurses are the ticket to healthier communities*. Retrieved from http://www.rwjf.org/en/culture-of-health/2016/05/why_school_nursesar.html

Hoke, S. (2015). Mental illness and prisoners: Concerns for communities and healthcare providers. *Online Journal of Issues in Nursing, 20*(1), Manuscript 3.

Houlahan, B. (2018). Origins of school nursing. *The Journal of School Nursing, 34*(3), 203–210. doi: 10.1177/1059840517735874.

Indian Health Service (IHS). (2020). *IHS profile*. Retrieved from https://www.ihs.gov/newsroom/factsheets/ihsprofile/

Individuals with Disabilities Education Act (IDEA). (1975). 20 U.S.C. §§ 1400 et. seq., as amended and incorporating the Education of All Handicapped Children Act (EHA), 1975, P.L. 94-142, and subsequent amendments; Regulations at 34 C.F.R. §§ 300–303 [Special education and related services for students, preschool children, and infants and toddlers].

Institute of Medicine (IOM). (2015). *Genomics-enabled learning health care systems: Gathering and using genomic information to improve patient care and research*. Retrieved from http://www.nap.edu/read/21707/chapter/1

Iskander, J., McLanahan, E., Thomas, J., Henry, B., Byrne, D., & Williams, H. (2018). Public health emergency response lessons learned by rapid deployment force 3, 2006-2016. *American Journal of Public Health*, Online. Retrieved from https://ajph.aphapublications.org/doi/full/10.2105/AJPH.2018.304496

Jacobsen, K., Meeder, L., & Voskuil, V. R. (2016). Chronic student absenteeism: The critical role of school nurses. *NASN School Nurse, 31*(3), 178–185.

Johnson, M. (2018). *How to prepare for emergencies in your correctional facility ahead of time*. Retrieved from https://www.correctionsone.com/products/communications/emergency-response/articles/how-to-prepare-for-emergencies-in-your-correctional-facility-ahead-of-time-xosiXTUrk6gNLwRJ/

Kadhim, M., Lucak, T., Schexnayder, S., King, A., Terhoeve, C., Song, B., & Heffernan, M. J. (2019). Current status of scoliosis school screening: Targeted screening of underserved populations may be the solution. *Public Health, 178*, 72–77. doi: 10.1016/j.puhe.2019.08.020.

Kaeble, D., & Cowhig, M. (2018). *Correctional Populations in the United States, 2016*. U.S. Department of Justice, Office of Justice Programs, Bureau of Justice Statistics. Bulletin NCJ251211. Retrieved from https://www.bjs.gov/content/pub/pdf/cpus16.pdf

Kid's Mental Health Portal. (2018). *Children's behavioral and emotional disorders*. Retrieved from http://www.kidsmentalhealth.org/childrens-behavioral-and-emotional-disorders/#Childrens

La Cerra, C., Sorrentino, M., Franconi, I., Notarnicola, I., Petrucci, C., & Lancia, L. (2017). Primary care program in prison: A review of the literature. *Journal of Correctional Health Care, 23*(2), 147–156. doi: 10.1177/1078345817699801.

La Clinica. (2019). *Mobile health services*. Retrieved from https://laclinicahealth.org/services/mobile-health/

Larsen, A. K., Holtermann, A., Mortensen, O. S., Punnett, L., Rod, M. H., & Jørgensen, M. B. (2015). Organizing workplace health literacy to reduce musculoskeletal plain and consequences. *BMC Nursing, 14*, 46. Retrieved from http://bmcnurs.biomedcentral.com/articles/10.1186/s12912-015-0096-4

Leroy, Z., Wallin, R., & Lee, S. (2017). The role of school health services in addressing the needs of students with chronic health conditions: A systematic review. *The Journal of School Nursing, 33*(1), 64–72. doi: 10.1177/1059840516678909.

Lice Clinics of America. (2019). *Urgent lice treatment for families*. Retrieved from https://www.liceclinicsofamerica.com/how-to-treat-lice/

Lions Club. (n.d.). *Vision screening*. Retrieved from https://lionsclubs.org/en/resources-for-members/resource-center/vision-screening#

Maughan, E., McCarthy, A., Hein, M., Perkhounkova, Y., & Kelly, M. (2018). Medication management in schools: 2015 survey results. *The Journal of School Nursing, 34*(6), 468–479.

McGovern, C., Arcoleo, K., & Melnyk, B. (2020). Sustained effects from a school-based intervention pilot study for children with asthma and anxiety. *Journal of School Nursing*, 1–11. doi: 10.1177/1059840520934178.

Merced Union High School District. (n.d.). *Student study team*. Retrieved from https://www.muhsd.org/business-services/student-support/student-study-team-sst

Metrohealth. (2019). *Enrollment outreach mobile unit*. Retrieved from https://www.metrohealth.org/patients-and-visitors/enrollment-outreach-mobile-unit

Mignon, S. (2016). Health issues of incarcerated women in the United States. *Ciência & Saúde Coletiva, 21*(7), 2051–2060. doi: 10.1590/1413-81232015217.05302016.

Miller, G., Coffield, E., Leroy, Z., & Wallin, R. (2016). Prevalence and costs of five chronic conditions in children. *The Journal of School Nursing, 32*(5), 357 -364. doi: 10.1177/1059840516641190.

Mink, C. A. (2019). *Why the battle to bring back school nurses is such a big deal for health and academics*. Center for Health Journalism. USC Annenberg. Retrieved from https://www.centerforhealthjournalism.org/2019/02/14/why-battle-bring-back-school-nurses-such-big-deal-health-and-academics

Mollard, E., & Hudson, D. B. (2016). Nurse-led trauma-informed correctional care for women. *Perspectives in Psychiatric Care*, *52*(3), 224–230. doi: 10.1111/ppc.12122.

Moore, J. D., Berner, M. M., & Wall, A. N. (2020). *What types of services do local public health agencies provide?* Retrieved from https://www.sog.unc.edu/resources/faqs/what-types-services-do-local-public-health-agencies-provide

National Association of School Nurses (NASN). (2016). *Public health and school nursing: Collaborating to promote health*. Retrieved from: https://higherlogicdownload.s3.amazonaws.com/NASN/3870c72d-fff9-4ed7-833f-215de278d256/UploadedImages/PDFs/Advocacy/2016PHandSN.pdf

National Association of School Nurses (NASN). (2017a). *Chronic health conditions (students with): The role of the school nurse*. Retrieved from https://www.nasn.org/nasn/advocacy/professional-practice-documents/position-statements/ps-chronic-health

National Association of School Nurses (NASN). (2017b). *Diabetes management in the school*. Retrieved from https://www.nasn.org/nasn/advocacy/professional-practice-documents/position-statements/ps-diabetes

National Association of School Nurses (NASN). (2017c). *Medication administration in the school setting*. Retrieved from https://www.nasn.org/nasn/advocacy/professional-practice-documents/position-statements/ps-medication

National Association of School Nurses (NASN). (2017d). *Vision and eye health*. Retrieved from https://www.nasn.org/nasn-resources/practice-topics/vision-health

National Association of School Nurses (NASN). (2017e). *Whole school, whole community, whole child: Implications for 21st century school nurses*. Retrieved from https://www.nasn.org/nasn/advocacy/professional-practice-documents/position-statements/ps-wscc

National Association of School Nurses (NASN). (2018a). *Do not attempt resuscitation (DNAR)—The role of the school nurse*. Retrieved from https://www.nasn.org/advocacy/professional-practice-documents/position-statements/ps-dnar

National Association of School Nurses (NASN). (2018b). *Position statements*. Retrieved from https://www.nasn.org/nasn/advocacy/professional-practice-documents/position-statements

National Association of School Nurses (NASN). (2018c). *Position statement: Role of the 21st century nurse*. Retrieved from https://www.nasn.org/advocacy/professional-practice-documents/position-statements/ps-role

National Association of School Nurses (NASN). (2018d). *National certification*. Retrieved from https://www.nasn.org/nasn-resources/professional-topics/certification

National Association of School Nurses (NASN). (2018e). *IDEA and section 504 teams—the school nurse as an essential team member*. Retrieved from https://www.nasn.org/nasn/advocacy/professional-practice-documents/position-statements/ps-ideia

National Association of School Nurses (NASN). (2018f). *Bullying and cyberbullying—prevention in schools*. Retrieved form https://www.nasn.org/nasn/advocacy/professional-practice-documents/position-statements/ps-bullying

National Association of School Nurses (NASN). (2018g). *Overweight and obesity in children and adolescents in school—the role of the school nurse*. Retrieved from https://www.nasn.org/nasn/advocacy/professional-practice-documents/position-statements/ps-overweight

National Association of School Nurses (NASN). (2018h). *Behavioral/mental health of students—the school nurses role*. Retrieved from https://www.nasn.org/nasn/advocacy/professional-practice-documents/position-statements/ps-behavioral-health

National Association of School Nurses (NASN). (2018i). *Prevention and treatment of child maltreatment—the role of the school nurse*. Retrieved from https://higherlogicdownload.s3.amazonaws.com/NASN/3870c72d-fff9-4ed7-833f-215de278d256/UploadedImages/PDFs/Position%20Statements/2018-ps-child-maltreatment.pdf

National Association of School Nurses (NASN). (2020a). *Position statement: Immunizations*. Retrieved from https://www.nasn.org/advocacy/professional-practice-documents/position-statements/ps-immunizations

National Association of School Nurses (NASN). (2020b). *Position statement: School nurse workload: Staffing for safe care*. Retrieved from https://www.nasn.org/advocacy/professional-practice-documents/position-statements/ps-workload

National Center for Learning Disabilities. (2017). *The state of learning disabilities: Introduction*. Retrieved from https://www.ncld.org/research/state-of-learning-disabilities/

National Commission on Correctional Health Care. (2017). *Position statement: Charging inmates a fee for health care services*. Retrieved from https://www.ncchc.org/charging-inmates-a-fee-for-health-care-services

National Commission on Correctional Health Care. (2020). *Certified correctional health care professional*. Retrieved from https://www.ncchc.org/CCHP-RN

National Diabetes Education Program. (2016). *Helping the student with diabetes succeed: A guide for school personnel*. Retrieved from https://www.diabetes.org/sites/default/files/2020-02/NDEP-School-Guide-Full-508.pdf

National Eating Disorders Association. (2019). *Educator toolkit*. Retrieved from https://www.nceedus.org/wp-content/uploads/2019/01/NEDA-Educator-Toolkit.pdf

National Institute of Diabetes and Digestive and Kidney Diseases. (2017). *Youth with type 2 diabetes develop complications more often than peers with type 1 diabetes*. Retrieved from https://www.niddk.nih.gov/news/archive/2017/youth-type2-diabetes-develop-complications-more-type1-diabetes

National Institute of Drug Abuse. (2018). *Monitoring the future survey results show alarming rise in teen vaping*. Retrieved from https://www.drugabuse.gov/about-nida/noras-blog/2018/12/monitoring-future-survey-results-show-alarming-rise-in-teen-vaping

National Institute of Mental Health (NIMH). (n.d.). *Child and adolescent mental health*. Retrieved from http://www.nimh.nih.gov/health/topics/child-and-adolescent-mental-health/index.shtml

National Institute of Neurological Disorders and Stroke. (2018). *Curing the epilepsies: The promise of research*. Retrieved from https://www.ninds.nih.gov/Current-Research/Focus-Research/Focus-Epilepsy/Curing-Epilepsies-Promise-Research

National Institute on Deafness and other Communication Disorders. (2016). *Quick statistics about hearing*. Retrieved from https://www.nidcd.nih.gov/health/statistics/quick-statistics-hearing

National Institutes of Health (NIH). (n.d.). *National institute of nursing research*. Retrieved from https://www.ninr.nih.gov/

Nursing @CSU Staff. (2019). *What to expect as a correctional care nurse and how to avoid burnout in challenging settings*. Retrieved from https://nursing.usc.edu/blog/correctional-nurse-career/

Office of Disease Prevention and Health Promotion (ODPHP). (2020). *Leading health indicators*. Retrieved from https://health.gov/healthypeople/objectives-and-data/leading-health-indicators

Orange County Department of Education. (n.d.). *Specialized physical health care services*. Retrieved from https://ocde.us/EducationalServices/StudentAchievementAndWellness/Health/Pages/SPHCS.aspx

PewCharitableTrusts.(2017).*Prisonhealthcare:Costsandquality*.Retrievedfrom https://www.pewtrusts.org/~/media/assets/2017/10/sfh_prison_health_care_costs_and_quality_final.pdf

Pierson, J. F., Kirchoff, M. C., Orsega, S. M., Giberson, S. F., Herpin, B. R., Ready, T. W., ... & Kelly, G. G. (2017). Collaboration of the NIH and PHS Commissioned Corps in the International Ebola Clinical Research Response. *Federal Practitioner*, *34*(8), 18–25.

Quad Council Coalition. (2018). *Community/public health nurse competencies*. Retrieved from http://www.quadcouncilphn.org/documents-3/2018-qcc-competencies/

Rehabilitation Act of 1973, Section 504. (1973). *29 U.S.C. §794 et seq., Regulations at 34 C.F.R. §104*. Retrieved from https://www2.ed.gov/policy/rights/reg/ocr/edlite-34cfr104.html

Reingle Gonzalez, J. M., & Connell, N. M. (2014). Mental health of prisoners: Identifying barriers to mental health treatment and medication continuity. *American Journal of Public Health*, *104*(12), 2328–2333. doi: 10.2105/AJPH.2014.302043.

Reza, M., Amin, M. S., Sgro, A., Abdelaziz, A., Ito, D., Main, P., & Azarpazhooh, A. (2016). Oral health status of immigrant and refugee children in North America: A scoping review. *Journal Canadian Dental Association*, *82*, g3.

Riley, M., Ahmed, S., & Locke, A. (2016). Common questions about oppositional defiant disorder. *American Family Physician*, *93*(7), 586–591.

Roberts, D., Taylor, M., & Pyle, A. (2018). Suicide prevention for school communities: An educational initiative for student safety. *NASN School Nurse*, *33*, 169–176. doi: 10.1177/1942602x18766499.

Rosen, B. L., Ashwood, D., & Richardson, G. B. (2016). School nurses' professional practice in the HPV vaccine decision-making process. *Journal of School Nursing*, *32*(2), 138–148.

Rosen, D. L., Thomas, S., Kavee, A., & Ashkin, E. A. (2019). Prevalence of chronic health conditions among adults released from the North Carolina Prison System, 2015-2016. *Noth Carolina Medical Journal*, *80*, 332–337. doi: 10.18043/ncm.80.6.332.

Sanders, S., & Stensland, M. (2018). Preparing to die behind bars: The journey of male inmates with terminal health conditions. *Journal of Correctional Health Care*, *24*(3), 232–242. doi: 10.1177/1078345818780686.

Schoenly, L. (2014). *The correctional nurse manifesto. Professional & Technical Kindle eBooks*.

Schoenly, L. (2016a). *Botulism and prison brew*. Retrieved from http://correctionalnurse.net/?s=botulism

Schoenly, L. (2016b). *Correctional nursing blog*. Retrieved from https://correctionalnurse.net/author/lorryschoenly/

Schoenly, L., & Knox, C. (2013). *Essentials of correctional nursing*. New York, NY: Springer publishing.

School-Based Health Alliance. (2017). *2016-2017 National school-based health care census*. Retrieved from https://www.sbh4all.org/wp-content/uploads/2019/05/2016-17-Census-Report-Final.pdf

Sekhar, D., Zalewski, T., Beiler, J., Czarnecki, B., Barr, A., King, T., & Paul, I. (2016). The sensitivity of adolescent school-based hearing screening is significantly improved by adding high frequencies. *The Journal of School Nursing*, *32*(6), 416–422.

Substance Abuse Mental Health Services Agency. (2020). *Behavioral treatments and services*. Retrieved from http://www.samhsa.gov/treatment/mental-disorders

Taylor, R., & Crianza, S. G. (2011). Lessons learned: How Harris County jail prepares for disasters. *Corrections Today*, *73*(4), 44–46.

Texas Department of Health Services. (2018). *Frequently asked questions: Implementation of laws on screening for type 2 diabetes (acanthosis nigricans screening bill)*. Retrieved from http://www.dshs.texas.gov/schoolhealth/organscreen.shtm?terms=acanthosis%20nigricans%20screening

Turnock, B. J. (2016). *Essentials of public health: What it is and how it works* (6th ed.). Burlington, MA: Jones & Bartlett Learning.

U.S. Department of Health & Human Services (USDHHS). (2020a). *Healthy People 2030: Browse objectives*. Retrieved from https://health.gov/healthypeople/objectives-and-data/browse-objectives

U.S. Department of Health & Human Services (USDHHS). (2020b). *Healthy People 2030 framework*. Retrieved from https://www.healthypeople.gov/2020/About-Healthy-People/Development-Healthy-People-2030/Framework

U.S. Department of Health and Human Services (USDHHS). (2020c). *HHS Careers*. Retrieved from https://www.hhs.gov/careers/job-search

U.S. Department of Health and Human Services (USDHHS). (n.d.). *Why a career at HHS?* Retrieved from http://www.hhs.gov/about/careers/

U.S. Department of Housing and Urban Development. (n.d.). *Healthy homes demonstration grant program*. Retrieved from http://portal.hud.gov/hudportal/HUD?src=/program_offices/healthy_homes/hhi/hhd

U.S. Department of Justice. (2016). *Medical problems of state and federal prisoners and jail inmates, 2011-12*. Retrieved from https://www.bjs.gov/content/pub/pdf/mpsfpji1112.pdf

U.S. Department of Veterans Affairs. (2020). *Office of nursing services*. Retrieved from https://www.va.gov/nursing/

University of Michigan Center of Excellence in Public Health Workforce Studies. (2018). *Public health workforce enumeration, 2014*. Ann Arbor, MI: University of Michigan. Retrieved from https://www.ajpmonline.org/article/S0749-3797(14)00385-7/pdf

US Food and Drug Administration. (n.d.). *FDA commissioned corps officers on the front line of COVID-19 response*. Retrieved from https://www.fda.gov/news-events/fda-voices/fda-commissioned-corps-officers-front-line-covid-19-response

Willgerodt, M., Brock, D., & Maughan, E. (2018). Public school nursing practice in the united states. *The Journal of School Nursing*, *34*(3), 232–244.

World Health Organization. (2019). *National health policies, strategies, plans*. Retrieved from https://www.who.int/nationalpolicies/nationalpolicies/en/

CHAPTER 29

Private Settings

"All Nurses need a plan B. Drastic changes in the health care environment are resulting in a reconfiguration of facilities and threatening job security for many nurses in this country. There is good news[:] there are fantastic opportunities for nurse owned and operated businesses to address these changes and challenges."

—National Nurses in Business Association, n.d., para. 3

KEY TERMS

Case management
Comprehensive primary care center
Entrepreneurial nurse
Faith community nurse (FCN)
Federally qualified health center (FQHC)
Nurse-led health centers/clinics (NLHCs)
Occupational and environmental health nurses
Occupational Safety and Health Administration (OSHA)
Safety-net health care provider
Sustainability
Total Worker Health (TWH)
Transitional care

LEARNING OBJECTIVES

Upon mastery of this chapter, you should be able to:

1. Describe funding sources for nurse-led health centers.
2. Articulate the importance of sustainability for nurse-led health centers.
3. Describe the evolution of faith community nursing.
4. Describe and differentiate among the roles of the faith community nurse.
5. Explain the role of the occupational and environmental health nurse and other members of the occupational health team in protecting and promoting workers' health and safety.
6. Recognize at least three adverse working conditions that impact health status.
7. Discuss the opportunities for nurse entrepreneurship in community/public health practice.

INTRODUCTION

Chapter 28 discussed a wide variety of practice opportunities in the public sector. This chapter examines four unique private sector roles and practice environments available in the United States and in many other countries:

- Nurse-led health centers offer the opportunity for more autonomous practice and present excellent learning venues for nursing students.
- Faith community nursing, begun in the mid-1980s, has gained increasing attention in many religious communities and continues the rich tradition of caring for those in need who may not have access to services.
- Occupational and environmental health is a specialty health practice that focuses on the health and well-being of the working population and therefore covers most of the country's working adults.
- Entrepreneurial roles for nurses offer new venues for meeting the health care needs in communities while providing challenging and autonomous practice.

Each of these areas of practice offers Community/public health nurses an avenue to address health disparities in their communities, increase years of healthy life, and provide holistic, client-centered care to meet the current and emerging health needs in their communities, as indicated in *Healthy People 2030* and Leading Health Indicators (Boxes 29-1 and 29-2).

BOX **29-1** *HEALTHY PEOPLE 2030*

Objectives Related to Private Settings and Occupational Safety and Health

Objectives Relevant to Nurses in Private Settings

AHS-08	Increase the proportion of adults who get recommended evidence-based preventative health care
EH-05	Reduce health and environment risks from hazardous sites
EH-06	Reduce the amount of toxic pollutants released into the environment
AHS-R01	Increase the ability of primary care and behavioral health professionals to provide more high-quality care to patients who need it

Occupational Safety and Health Objectives

OSH-01	Reduce deaths from work-related injuries
OSH-02	Reduce work-related injuries resulting in missed workdays
OSH-03	Reduce work-related skin diseases
OSH-04	Reduce pneumoconiosis deaths
OSH-05	Reduce work-related assaults
OSH-06	Reduce new cases of work-related hearing loss
OSH-D01	Reduce the rate of high blood lead levels in adults exposed at work

Reprinted from U.S. Department of Health & Human Services (USDHHS). (2020). *Healthy People 2030: Browse objectives.* Retrieved from https://health.gov/healthypeople/objectives-and-data/browse-objectives

BOX **29-2** *LEADING HEALTH INDICATORS 2030*

Key Health Indicators Applicable to Nurses Working in Private Settings

Access to Health Services
Medical insurance
Health Care System Quality
Health Care Access
Clinical Preventive Services
Reduce the number of adults with hypertension
Children between the ages of 19 to 35 months receive the recommended doses of DTaP, polio, MMR, Hib, hepatitis B, varicella, and PCV vaccines Determinants of Health Equity

- Environmental Quality
- Environmental health
- General health, health-related quality of life, well-being

Injury
Maternal, infant, and child health
Mental health
Obesity
Oral health
Reproductive and sexual health
Social capital/civic engagement
Serious illness
Social determinants
Substance abuse
Tobacco

Source: The National Academies of Sciences, Engineering, and Medicine (2020).

NURSE-LED HEALTH CENTERS

Nurse-led health centers/clinics (NLHCs), or nursing centers (sometimes referred to as nurse-managed health centers), are organizations that give vulnerable and/or underserved clients access to professional nursing services (Fig. 29-1). NLHCs are found in convenient sites where people live, work, learn, and worship and are overseen by a nurse executive with an advanced degree. Traditionally, targets of service have been those who are least likely to be engaged in ongoing health care services for themselves and their family members. Currently, NLHCs serve population groups of all ages who are uninsured or underinsured.

Historically, the most frequently cited definition of *a nurse-managed health clinic* is the one developed in the mid-1980s by the American Nurses Association (ANA) Nursing Centers Task Force: "a nurse-practice arrangement, managed by advanced practice nurses, that provides primary care or wellness services to underserved or vulnerable populations and that is associated

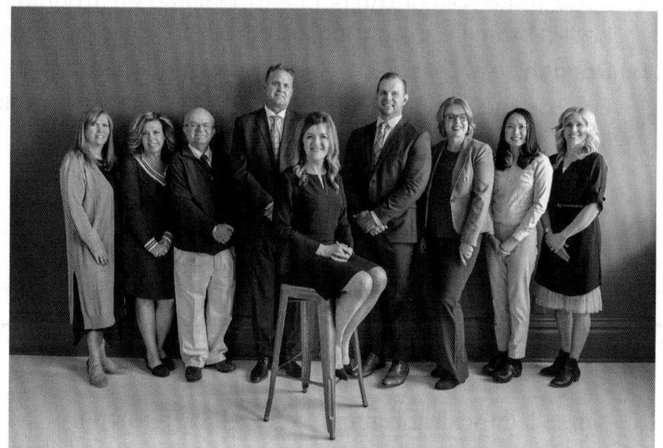

FIGURE 29-1 Bristol Health: an example of a nurse-led health center. Bristol Health has both physicians and nurse practitioners who provide individual, couples, and family counseling and manage medications for mental health conditions. Bristol Health has physicians, nurse Practitioners, counselors, therapists, and psychological testing services. They provide services to children, adolescents, and adults. (Reprinted with permission from Bristol Health. (2019). *Services*. Retrieved from https://bristolhealth.com/)

with a school, college, university or department of nursing, federally qualified health center (FQHC), or independent nonprofit health or social services agency" (Compilation of Patient Protection and Affordability Care, 2010, p. 542). The Compilation of Patient Protection and Affordability Care supports nurse-managed health centers to:

- Improve access to across-the-life span primary health care and wellness services.
- Provide services in medically underserved and vulnerable populations regardless of income or insurance status.
- Serve students as training sites in primary care.
- Establish and enhance electronic methods for effectively collecting patient and workforce data (U.S. Department of Health and Human Services, n.d.).

With an amendment to Title III of the Public Health Service Act (42 U.S.C. 241 et seq.), the Nurse-Managed Health Clinic Investment Act of 2009 of the 111th Congress provides a more present-day definition of an NLHC.

A nurse practice arrangement, managed by advanced practice nurses, that provides primary care or wellness services to an under-served or vulnerable population and is associated with a school, college, university, or department of nursing; FQHC; or an independent nonprofit health or social services agency (Nurse-Managed Health Clinic Investment Act, 2009, p. 2).

NLHCs represent a rising movement of health centers that have emerged as vital safety-net health care providers in America's health care delivery system (Aveling, Martin, Herbert, & Armstrong, 2017; Durovich & Roberts, 2018; Hansen-Turton, Sherman, & King, 2016). Although all NLHCs share the core elements of these definitions, they vary in their practice models. Services offered at NLHCs range from health promotion and wellness to conventional primary care (Aveling et al., 2017; Durovich & Roberts, 2018).

- A **safety-net health care provider** is a provider who, by mandate or mission, organizes and delivers a significant level of health care and other health-related services to the uninsured, Medicaid recipients, and other vulnerable populations (Agency for Healthcare Research and Quality, 2018; Institute of Medicine, 2000; U.S. Centers for Medicare and Medicaid Services [CMS], 2019).
- NLHCs differ from other public health agencies and tertiary medical care facilities. Although some services overlap, the distinctiveness of NLHCs is found in the community orientation of the nurse-managed centers. This model is depicted by Lundeen's comprehensive community-based primary health care model (Hong & Lundeen, 2009; Lundeen, 2005), in which NLHCs are referred to as community nursing centers and are the central figure in this model of health care, which is used at the University of Milwaukee, Wisconsin (Fig. 29-2).

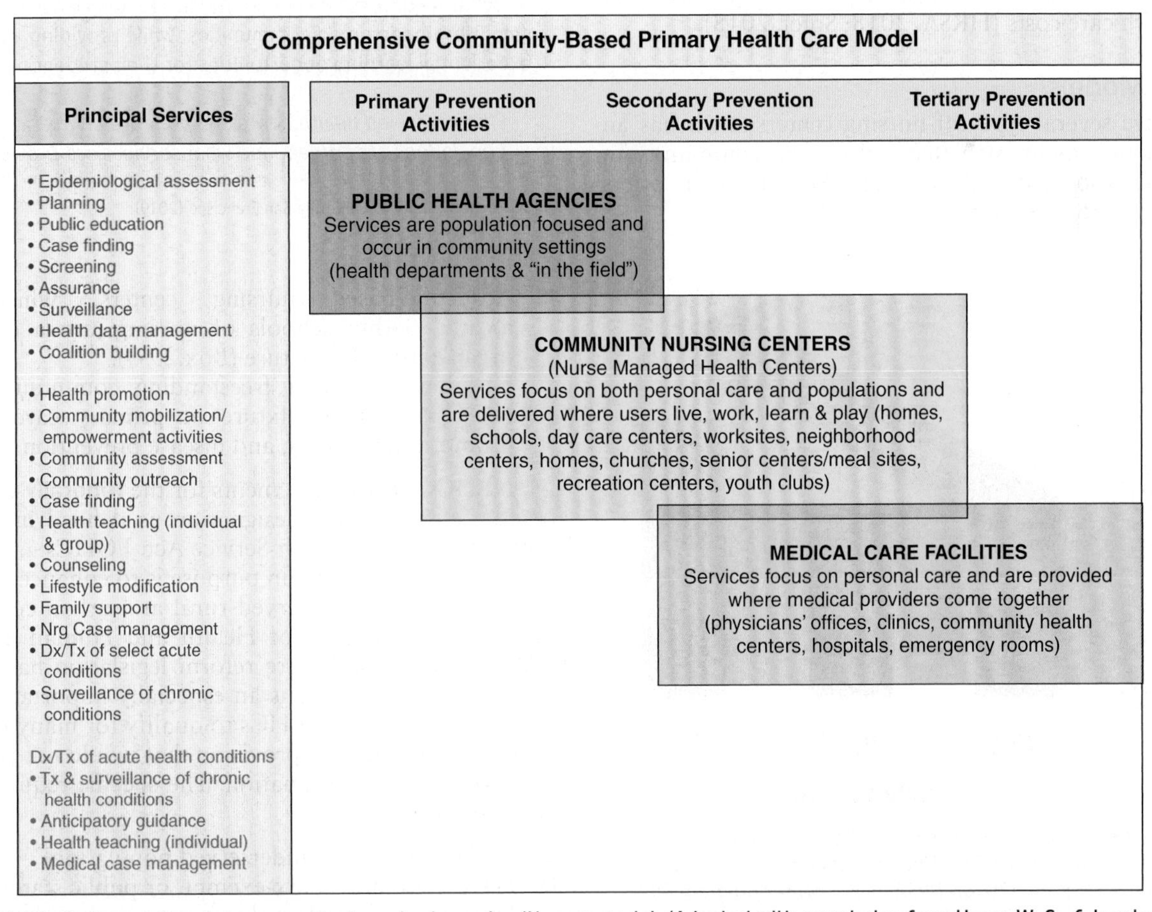

FIGURE 29-2 Comprehensive community-based primary health care model. (Adapted with permission from Hong, W. S., & Lundeen, S. (2009). Using ACHIS to analyze nursing health promotion interventions for vulnerable populations in a community nursing center: A Pilot study. *Asian Nursing Research, 3*(3), 130–138; ©Sally P. Lundeen, RN, PhD, FAAN, UW-Milwaukee College of Nursing, 1993, 2005.)

History of the Nurse-Led Model

Although today's NLHCs trace their roots to changes in national health care laws begun in the mid-1960s, the nursing model of holistic care that focuses on vulnerable populations and integrates primary care and public health dates back to the nineteenth century. Florence Nightingale's passion for at-risk populations, as well as her success related to health reform, provides a model for NLHCs today. Visionaries such as Lillian Wald, who founded the Henry Street Settlement, and Margaret Sanger, who initiated the first family planning clinic, are two examples of nurses providing holistic care to vulnerable populations (see Chapter 3). These nurse activists sought to resolve twentieth century problems caused by immigration, urbanization, and industrialization in the United States (Judd & Sitzman, 2014; Kurtzman et al., 2017).

- Since the late 1970s, in conjunction with the development of educational programs for nurse practitioners, faculties in schools of nursing have established NLHCs. Linkages have provided clinical sites for educating nurses at all levels and settings, as well as for faculty practice opportunities (Resick, Miller, & Leonardo, 2015).
- The Health Resource and Services Administration (HRSA) reports significant increases in the number of patients served in health centers in the past decade (Fig. 29-3). Overall, these health centers have been shown to improve health outcomes while reducing health care costs (HRSA, 2018; Sofer, 2018).

NLHC Models

There are several types of nursing centers; each has an individuality of its own that reflects the community in which it is located and the particular services it offers (Hansen-Turton, Sherman, & King, 2015):

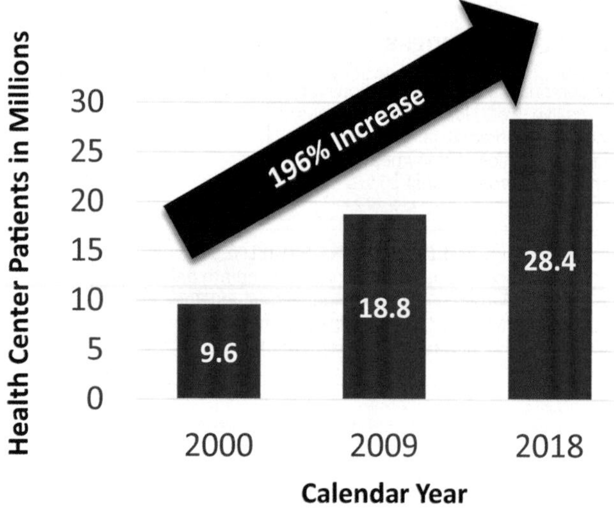

FIGURE 29-3 Increase in numbers of patients served in health centers. (Reprinted from Health Resources and Services Administration (HRSA). (2018). *HRSA health center program fact sheet.* Retrieved from https://bphc.hrsa.gov/sites/default/files/bphc/about/healthcenterfactsheet.pdf)

BOX 29-3 STORIES FROM THE FIELD

Three Nurse-Led Clinics

University of California Los Angeles (UCLA) began providing primary health care services to the homeless and indigent in 1983. It provides access to health care for children and families who have no place else to go—many suffering from the effects of an unstable home life or no home at all. Student nurses participate in the clinic and learn valuable lessons about the challenges of providing care for vulnerable populations. At the same time, the students gain first-hand experience working with resilient individuals who overcome significant hardships. Many students find their experiences in the clinics inspiring. In 2018, UCLA's Health Center at the Union Rescue Mission handled over 8,000 patient visits.

University of California Irvine (UCI) launched the first nurse-managed clinic at El Sol Charter School in Santa Ana. This clinic provides primary care to Orange County's underserved populations, primarily from the Latino community. This clinic is funded by a $1.5 million federal grant and, like the University of California San Francisco (UCSF) clinic, serves the dual purpose of providing care while educating future nurses.

UCSF serves San Francisco's homeless and poor at the Glide Health Services Center in the Tenderloin district. This clinic takes a holistic approach, offering anything from acupuncture to behavioral health, diabetes, and more. The nurse-run clinic accommodates 13,000 visits each year, reaching people who historically felt marginalized by traditional medicine.

All three of these clinics are nurse-led, working in partnership with underserved communities, while providing valuable experiential learning opportunities for their student nurses.

Find nurse-led health centers in your area. What populations are served, and what services are provided?

Source: University of California San Francisco (2019).

- Academic-based nursing centers, which are located within schools of nursing, are a common organizational structure (Box 29-3).
- Hospital-based and freestanding community-based NLHCs offer a mixture of primary care, health promotion, wellness, and disease prevention services.

NLHCs meet requirements for the **federally qualified health center (FQHC)** designation as defined in Section 330 of the Public Health Service Act. FQHCs are safety-net providers whose main purpose is to enhance primary care services in underserved rural and urban communities (U.S. Department of Health and Human Services, CMS, 2018). Health care reform legislation has helped with this funding. This is an especially important designation, as it enables NLHCs to qualify for many funding sources vital to service provision that would not be available without this designation. The specific requirements are that they:

- Serve a medically underserved population.
- Have a nonprofit, tax-exempt, or public status.
- Designate a board of directors, a majority of whom must be consumers of the center's health services.

BOX 29-4 Nurse-Managed Health Center Models

Center Types

- Wellness Center: provides public health as well as health promotion and disease prevention programs and focuses on primary and secondary prevention strategies
- Special Care Centers: provide programs that target specific health conditions such as HIV or diabetes
- Comprehensive primary care center: provides traditional primary care and public health programs

Organizational Structures

- Academic Nursing Center: located within a School of Nursing
- Freestanding Center: independent center with its own governing board
- Subsidiary: part of a larger health care system, such as home health agencies, community centers, schools, and other venues
- Affiliated Center: legal partnership with a health care or human services organization

Adapted from Hansen-Turton et al. (2015); Kinsey and Miller (2016).

- Provide culturally competent, comprehensive primary care services to all age groups.
- Offer a sliding scale fee and provide services regardless of ability to pay.

The variety of nursing center models currently in use and their organizational structures demonstrate the diversity of contemporary NLHCs. Box 29-4 describes the major types of centers, along with the various organizational structures that influence their delivery models.

Role of Students in NLHCs

Undergraduate and graduate students from many disciplines play a vital part in the activities of NLHCs. These disciplines include, but are not limited to, nursing, social work, mental health, dental and oral health, nutrition, speech–language–hearing sciences, and public health. When students engage in NLHC activities for their clinical experience, they become aware of the distinctiveness of nurse-managed centers from other health care delivery systems and the variety of models and organizational structures that exist and are active participants in vital nursing center activities. Most often, students are engaged in primary and secondary prevention strategies via health education, outreach, immunization, and screening programs. Roles that students fulfill are similar to the roles of their staff mentors (Box 29-5):

- Advocate
- Case manager
- Change agent
- Educator
- Referral agent

Faculty roles in NLHC academic models involve clinical supervision and mentorship of undergraduate and graduate students assigned to the nursing center for their clinical experience (American Association of Colleges of Nursing [AACN], 2016).

BOX 29-5 STORIES FROM THE FIELD

Wellness Screening

Public health nurses from an academic wellness NLHC, along with undergraduate student nurses, are conducting blood pressure and glucose screenings at a church-sponsored health fair. This event is conducted on Sundays from 10 AM to 2 PM, before, during, and after church services. Approximately 50% of adults screened have hypertension and/or hyperglycemia. One participant, who was asymptomatic, had severe hypertension (220/154) and was immediately transported to the nearest hospital for evaluation.

1. *What are some feasible referrals that may have been made for those with abnormal screening results?*
2. *What types of primary prevention strategies may benefit those attendees who had normal screening results?*
3. *In what ways do student nurses benefit from participating at a health fair?*

Community Service Learning in NLHCs

Additionally, schools of nursing and NLHCs are an excellent venue to conduct community service learning (CSL) projects with both undergraduate and graduate students. Using a "wall-less" concept of a nursing wellness center, undergraduate and graduate nursing students can participate in CSL activities in a variety of community settings. Outcomes for participating students include (Marquette University, 2019, para. 3):

1. Appreciate people from diverse backgrounds.
2. Exhibit a commitment to social justice.
3. Demonstrate a commitment to be an involved citizen in his or her community.
4. Demonstrate an increased sense of vocation.

One exemplar of a CSL project conducted at urban and rural schools is the "Safety Town" initiative. This CSL project entails educating preschool and early elementary school-age children on indoor and outdoor safety for trauma prevention (Miller & Mest, n.d.). Qualitative feedback from nursing students reveals personal and professional growth regarding primary prevention in pediatric trauma in nontraditional clinical settings within the community.

Funding for NLHCs

As NLHCs vary in their models, so too do they vary in their methods of cost reimbursement, including fee for service, sliding fees, contracts, grant support, third-party payments, and cost-based reimbursement (Hansen-Turton, et al., 2015). Most nursing centers' operational and salary budgets entail a combination of these funding sources.

- In **comprehensive primary care centers**, advanced practice nurses provide primary care services. Such services are usually reimbursable under Medicare, Medicaid, and managed care medical insurance plans (Health Care Provisions in Bipartisan Budget Act of 2018).

- In wellness centers, public health nurses and other interdisciplinary team members provide a range of primary and secondary prevention strategies (Box 29-6). These services are usually not reimbursed by insurance plans but are often covered by grants and contracts (Hansen-Turton, et al., 2015; Resick et al., 2015).

It is important to distinguish between grants and contracts as funding sources for NLHCs. Funding organizations usually release guidelines regarding what initiatives they will fund. Grant guidelines are frequently termed request for proposal (RFP).

- Grants can be a source of initial start-up funding as well as a support for ongoing activities (Torrisi & Hansen-Turton, 2015).
  - A proposal submitted by the NLHC to the funding organization describes how the center would meet the goals and objectives set by the funding organization.
  - Outcomes, or the end results at a specific point in time, are increasingly becoming more important to funders.
  - NLHCs must include measures to collect outcome data and project what outcomes will occur in their submitted proposals.
- Contracts are another source of funding for NLHCs.
  - Contracts are awards for a legal procurement relationship between a funder and a recipient obligating the contractor to furnish a product or service defined in detail by the funder (Find RFP, 2019).
  - A contract has specific goals, objectives, and activities, as well as a time frame during which the activities are to be implemented and evaluated.
  - Contracts are awarded on a noncompetitive basis and often are renewable when goals and objectives are met.

Managing the various funding streams that feed the personnel and operations budgets of an NLHC is an arduous task. To ensure that budgetary dollars are spent in the manner specified by the funding organization, meticulous recordkeeping and itemization of spending is another undertaking that the nurse executive or an operations coordinator of an NLHC must carry out. It is imperative that key personnel from the NLHC maintain precise records and submit accurate quarterly, semiannual, or annual reports as specified in the grant or contract award (Zimmer & Knowlton, 2016).

BOX **29-6** STORIES FROM THE FIELD

Family-Centered Care

Ms. Jones is a 22-year-old mother of three small children who recently moved to an urban area. She brings her oldest child, age 6, to a local comprehensive primary care nurse-managed health clinic for school immunizations. During the course of the history and physical examination, the nurse practitioner becomes aware that this mother also has two younger children, aged 2 and 3, at home. The family rents a small apartment in housing that was built in the mid-1950s. Ms. Jones mentions that her mother (the children's grandmother) also resides with them. The grandmother is the childcare provider, while Ms. Jones works as a local hair salon. The grandmother mother smokes 1.5 to 2 packages of cigarettes daily; Ms. Jones reports that she is a nonsmoker. Upon further questioning, the nurse practitioner learns that the 3-year-old child has a chronic cough and occasional wheezing. Ms. Jones also confides to the nurse practitioner that she recently missed two menstrual periods and is sexually active.

1. *What are some possible health care needs of Ms. Jones? Her mother?*
2. *What screenings should be performed on (a) Ms. Jones, (b) her mother, and (c) her children?*
3. *What other interdisciplinary team members should be involved in this family's health care?*
4. *What are some possible referrals that would benefit this family?*

Sustainability of Nurse-Managed Health Clinics

Sustainability, or the ability to carry on services and health promotion activities, is one of the main challenges of NLHCs. NLHCs have much to offer toward resolving the national health care crisis facing vulnerable populations who are uninsured or underinsured. However, without the ability to maintain fiscal sustainability, NLHCs may fail to reach their full potential for positively influencing the future of health care (Hansen-Turton, et al., 2015). A seminal document by Cutler (2002, p. 23) proposes "critical sustainability questions" that can be used as a preliminary avenue of consideration for organizations such as NLHCs when completing a grant application for funding. The following are some strategies that can be implemented to promote sustainability of NLHCs (Cohn et al., 2017; Sofer, 2018):

- Demonstrate value for money, sometimes measured in terms of cost per client served.
- Track, monitor, and evaluate measurable outcomes that demonstrate the delivery of quality, cost-effective care.
- Hire and develop diverse and effective staff.
- Manage travel costs for serving remote populations through telehealth.
- Utilize technology.
- Develop a sustainability plan.
- Maintain strategic partnerships.

The National Nurse-Led Care Consortium

The National Nurse-Led Care Consortium (NNCC, 2018a) strives to reduce health disparities and meet people's primary care and wellness needs through policy, consultation, programs, and applied research that advance nurse-led health care (Box 29-7). They lead advocacy efforts for nurse-managed health care and support public health initiatives including the Nurse-Family Partnership (NNCC, 2018b). For more information, visit https://www.nurseledcare.org/.

The NNCC conducts a Best Practice Conference, which brings together nurses, staff members, funders, and

BOX 29-7 National Nurse-Led Care Consortium

Mission

To advance nurse-led health care through policy, consultation, and programs to reduce health disparities and meet people's primary care and wellness needs.

Ways NNCC Supports Nurse-Led Care

1. Offering a variety of educational opportunities to build practice, improve quality of care, and promote sustainability.
2. Advocate for policy that supports nurse-led care in Washington, DC, and in state legislature.
3. Provide members with additional resources and discounts on educational opportunities and Annual Conference rates.
4. Build and manage public health programs, providing national models for nursing and public health.

Source: National Nurse-Led Care Consortium (2018a, 2018b).

political leaders to share best practices and participate in networking opportunities. Continuing education credits are available for attendance at scientific sessions.

Nursing Research and NLHCs

NLHCs provide research opportunities for both primary prevention and wellness initiatives (AACN, 2016). Descriptive data have been collected about client demographics, types of service provided, funding methods, and sustainability efforts. The increasing presence of NLHCs had led to an increase in research primarily aimed at determining the quality and cost-effectiveness of care provided (Randall, Crawford, Currie, River, & Betihavas, 2017). NLHCs have been shown to have beneficial effects on patient satisfaction and health outcomes, as well as improved access to care (Sofer, 2018). Other studies include:

- Randall et al. (2017) conducted a systematic review of 15 studies that examined patient satisfaction, patient outcomes, objective clinical measures, access to care, and, to a limited extent, cost-effectiveness. Overall, results were favorable in all areas except for cost-effectiveness (evaluated in only two studies), for which results were mixed.
- Baker and Fatoye (2017) conducted another systematic review of 26 articles that provided data on the clinical and cost-effectiveness of nurse-led care of patients with chronic obstructive pulmonary disease in a primary care setting. Initial results were favorable.

Chan et al. (2018, p. 61) examined outcomes for nurse-led services in an ambulatory community care setting and found some evidence of "better outcomes in terms of health-related quality of life compared to physician-led care." They also noted the lack of cost-effectiveness studies, an area needing further research to help guide future policy.

Future Directions for NLHCs

In 2008, the IOM appointed a committee on the Robert Wood Johnson Foundation Initiative on the Future of Nursing. The purpose of this committee was to produce a report, making recommendations for the future of nursing. This committee developed four key messages regarding the future of nursing (IOM, 2011):

1. Nurses should practice to the full extent of their education and training.
2. Nurses should achieve higher levels of education and training through an improved education system that promotes seamless academic progression.
3. Nurses should be full partners with physicians and other health care professionals in redesigning health care in the United States.
4. Effective workforce planning and policy making require better data collection and information infrastructure.

The main areas of focus for health care reform are prevention and improving the quality of care (Patient Protection and Affordable Care Act [ACA], 2010).

- In NLHCs, advanced practice nurses lead interprofessional teams as critical safety-net providers in America's health care delivery system. Nurses in NLHCs are vital change agents as they partner with the community, interprofessional team members, and students to improve access to care and health outcomes (Randall et al., 2017).
- Community care centers, including NLHCs, have been shown to play a significant role in providing access to care for underserved populations on Medicare (Seo et al., 2019).
- Primary care is being transformed by registered nurses using their skills in coaching, case management, transitional care, chronic disease management, education, and health promotion to help meet the increasing demand for care (Josiah Macy Jr. Foundation, 2016).

Continued expansion of the NLHC model in the next decade and beyond will meet key recommendations from the IOM report on nursing's future and the goals of the ACA (AACN, 2017; Seo et al., 2019). See Box 29-8 for an example of an NLHC that meets the needs of the population served, provides continuity of care, and reduces the use of overcrowded and expensive emergency department services for routine health care.

FAITH COMMUNITY NURSING

A **faith community nurse (FCN)** focuses on the mental, physical, and spiritual health, using a holistic approach to prevention and treatment of illness within the context of a community of faith (Deaconess Nurse Ministry, 2019). Faith community nursing is one of the newest nursing specialties and one of the oldest means of health care delivery.

Historical Background of Faith-Based Nursing

For hundreds of years, deaconesses, sisters, and lay members of religious communities have been involved in ministering to the sick. This tradition was revitalized

BOX 29-8 PERSPECTIVES

Viewpoint of an Executive Director of a Nurse-Led Community Clinic

In fall 2011, in our city of 120,000 in northeast Texas, many health care organizations here held the view that low-income or homeless population were "noncompliant" and did not care about their health. I had learned through volunteering that many barriers to their care existed. These included minimal payment amounts that were too high, service hours that were not convenient to the low-income population, and pre-enrollment criteria that many could not meet. To avoid this, the low-income and/or homeless populations tend to use the hospital EDs for care.

I decided to set up a health clinic that didn't have unrealistic requirements. Individuals needing health services simply have to fill out an income self-declaration. The low-income and homeless populations are very mistrusting of community health and social services. They live day by day. They have to focus on the here and now: Where will my next meal come from? Where will I shower? Where will I launder my clothes? Where will I sleep?

Guided by the understanding that the low-income population has its own culture and very specific needs, the clinic was set up as a caring, compassionate, and supportive environment for this population. Patients of the clinic state that they feel "listened to," even though the length of appointments is still only 20 minutes. Strategies contributing to quality care included:

- Offering clinic hours in the early morning hours, lunch time hours, and evening hours
- Providing behavioral care, counseling, and social services
- Treating patients' anxiety, depression, and other behavioral health conditions
- Building relationships with the patient and family
- Coordinating care and support services to strengthen coping and problem-solving skills

Outcomes of this approach included:

- Ability of patients to manage chronic illnesses
- Increased health-seeking behaviors at the Center rather than the ED
- Positive self-reporting that patients feel "listened to," even though appointments are only 20 minutes long
- Improved ability of patients to seek follow-up care should their situation deteriorate

As a nurse, I find myself constantly advocating for patients and ensuring maximal health for our clients at a lower cost. It is a rewarding experience!

M. Alice Masciarelli, RN, DNP, FACHE, CPHQ
Executive Director, Denton Community Health Clinic, Denton, TX

through the efforts of Reverend Dr. Granger Westberg. As a hospital chaplain and Lutheran minister, Westberg observed a great need for preventive and holistic health services, especially among the underserved, and wrote several books. He launched several church-based holistic health clinics in the 1970s, each staffed by a physician, nurse, and chaplain, that provided health services to the underserved in the community for several years (Westberg Institute for Faith Community Nursing, 2019b). The clinics eventually closed, but the experience led Reverend Westberg to recognize the unique ability of nurses to bridge the disciplines of medicine and religion.

Westberg first coined the term *parish nurse* when he initiated a pilot project in 1984 in which nurses provided holistic, preventive health care for six Christian congregations in the Chicago area. Gradually, more and more churches sought to incorporate a parish nurse into their staff. The term faith community nursing is now commonly used in the United States. The Westberg Institute for Faith Community Nursing (2019b) provides educational programs and resources for nurses who seek to practice as parish nurses and for educators wishing to conduct training programs for parish nursing.

The Health Ministries Association (HMA), along with the ANA, was instrumental in writing the third edition of *Faith Community Nursing: Scope and Standards of Practiced* (ANA & HMA, 2017). The term faith community nursing was defined as "a specialized practice of professional nursing that focuses on the intentional care of the spirit as well as the whole-person health and prevention or minimization of illness" (HMA, n.d., para. 1). Today, nurses who practice in a faith community may be referred to as FCNs, parish nurses, health ministry nurses, congregational nurses, or church nurses depending upon preference and the traditions of the faith community. No matter what title is used, a nurse who practices in a faith community should adhere to the standards of practice, which can be obtained through the ANA at https://www.nursingworld.org/nurses-books/faith-community-nursing-scope-and-standards-of-practice-3rd-edition/.

What Do FCNs Do?

Activities and interventions FCNs implement are as diverse as their faith communities. Some examples include:

- Advocating for the needs of the dying
- Addressing health conditions that are stigmatized, such as HIV
- Supporting patients with mental health issues
- Providing guidance during life transitions such as marriage, divorce, birth, death, illnesses, etc.
- Promoting health education (Faith Community Nursing Health Ministries Northwest, 2019; Nelson, 2018)

FCNs have been instrumental in meeting the educational and health promotion needs of underserved and older adult populations. A few examples of specific programs that have been successful in faith-based settings include:

- University of California, San Diego, offers a comprehensive faith-based wellness program that addresses health disparities in African-American, Latino, and Muslim communities (UC San Diego, 2019).

- The Bronx Health REACH Faith-Based Outreach Initiative provides programs addressing diabetes prevention and management, nutrition, fitness, and health disparities (Institute for Family Health, 2019).
- Abuelas en Acción (Grandmothers in Action) promotes physical activity, nutrition, and stress management in the Latino community (University of Illinois at Urbana Champaign, 2016).
- The "Fit Body and Soul" program strives to prevent diabetes among African American populations (Sattin et al., 2016).

Roles of the FCN

The goal of the FCN is "protection, promotion and optimization of health and abilities; facilitation of healing, alleviation of suffering through the diagnosis and treatment of human responses and advocacy in the context of values, beliefs, and practices of the faith community, such as a church, congregation, parish, synagogue, temple, mosque, or faith-based community agency" (ANA/HMA, 2017, p. 2). Health promotion outcomes may be primary, directed at prevention of disease, illness, or injury; secondary, focused on early detection and appropriate intervention; or tertiary, concerned with promoting a sense of well-being when preventing or curing a condition may not occur. To achieve the goal of faith community nursing, seven diverse nursing roles are central to incorporate into practice (Schroepfer, 2016; Westberg Institute for Faith Community Nursing, 2019c; Zeibarth & Campbell, 2016). The roles of the FCN (Box 29-9) support the development, implementation, and evaluation of faith-based programs.

BOX 29-9 ASSURING CONGREGATIONAL HEALTH AND WHOLENESS

Roles of the Faith Community Nurse

1. Health educator
2. Health counselor
3. Advocate
4. Referral agent
5. Developer of support groups
6. Coordinator of volunteers
7. Integrator of faith and health

Accountability

1. ANA scope and standards of nursing practice
2. ANA scope and standards of faith community nursing
3. Congregational standards
4. Institutional standards
5. ANA social policy statement
6. ANA code of ethics for nurses with interpretive statements
7. State nurse practice act
8. Patients' rights

Source: Dandridge (2014); Schroepfer (2016); Westberg Institute for Faith Community Nursing (2019c).

Health Educator

- A primary role of the FCN is as a health educator. Increasing awareness of health issues through health education is the foundation for health promotion and lifestyle changes. The FCN uses assessment skills to determine the health issues that may be present in the faith community and assesses the educational needs related to these issues.
- The FCN may provide individual and group education strategies such as providing health education materials, leading health education classes, or providing health screenings. The FCN may also develop educational displays or flyers or write educational articles for the faith community newsletter or Web site.

Health Counselor

- In the health counselor role, the nurse seeks to understand the individual's perceptions, fears, and barriers that prevent the person from taking action.
- The FCN may use a five-step health counseling process described as the five A's (Cooper & Zimmerman, 2017; Smoking Cessation Advice, 2018):

1. *Ask* about the person's perceptions related to a specific health concern.
2. *Advise* the person about the health concern and the benefits of taking health-promoting actions.
3. *Assess* the person's readiness to take action.
4. *Assist* in planning ways to address the health concern.
5. *Arrange* follow-up support.

Advocate

- The third role of an FCN is that of an advocate, helping individuals obtain needed services or care whether in the hospital, a long-term care facility, or at home. In the advocate role, the FCN uses knowledge of the health care system and awareness of safe and effective care practices to facilitate appropriate, timely intervention (Mock, 2017).
- Advocacy is indicated when dealing with vulnerable populations, such as older adults, children, or the homeless, who may not have the ability to speak for themselves or may lack the knowledge or awareness of what constitutes safe, effective care. FCNs have actively advocated for those with mental health problems, finding treatment sources and providing referrals and support (Foster, Dawood, Pearson, Manteuffel, & Levy, 2019).

Referral Agent

- The role of referral agent involves several related aspects. First, the nurse needs to develop knowledge of community resources and contacts. Knowledge of what is available, how the service is accessed, eligibility criteria, and limitations of the service is essential.
- Next, the nurse networks with and develops collaborative relationships with community leaders and agencies who provide the services. Through networking with community agencies, the FCN becomes aware of and is able to easily access a variety of community resources to support the client's physical, social, financial, emotional, or spiritual needs (Association of Public Health Nurses, 2016).

Developer of Support Groups

- Receiving emotional support from persons who share similar experiences can provide strength, comfort, knowledge, and a sense of empowerment (Frykedal, Rosander, Berlin, & Barimani, 2016).
- The FCN develops groups tailored to the faith community needs such as coping with loss and grief, cancer, caregiver stress, chronic illness, single parenting, addiction recovery, health promotion, and more (Callaghan, 2016; Grebeldinger & Buckley, 2016).

Coordinator of Volunteers

- The health ministry mission of a faith community typically includes a variety of services and activities to provide holistic support of the physical, social, emotional, mental, and spiritual needs of its members. Such a diverse array of services cannot be provided by the FCN alone.
- In the role of coordinator of volunteers, the FCN recruits, trains, and coordinates other members of the faith community. Volunteers provide or assist with a variety of services such as (Christian Community Health Fellowship, 2019):
  - Home, hospital, or long-term care visitations
  - Respite care
  - Assisting with transportation needs of homebound individuals
  - Calling or sending cards to ill or injured members
  - Assisting with health screenings

Integrator of Faith and Health

- A distinctly unique role of the FCN is as integrator of faith and health (Fig. 29-4). This role emphasizes the holistic relationship between the physical, social, emotional, mental, and spiritual dimensions of the person.
- The FCN helps the person to improve health or enhance wellness by appreciating how the dimensions of the person are interconnected and by helping the person strengthen or support the weaker aspects, as needed.
- The FCN assesses community's strengths and health needs and incorporates an understanding of the connection between faith and health (Brewer et al., 2017; Tettey, Duran, Anderson, & Boutin-Foster, 2017).

Faith Community Nursing Practice

Models of faith community nursing practice are diverse and may be categorized according to volunteer versus salaried positions and institutional versus faith-based sponsorship. The type of practice model adopted depends on variables such as:

- The number of faith community members served
- The existing health ministry services in place
- The faith community's governance structure and financial resources
- Existing health care systems in the community at large

Early in the development of faith community nursing, FCNs were typically part-time volunteers who were members of the faith community they served. This voluntary, part-time status, coupled with the newness of faith community nursing practice, has resulted in limited research on faith community nursing. Nonetheless, studies that have been conducted have validated the effectiveness of FCNs and the programs they have implemented, such as the following:

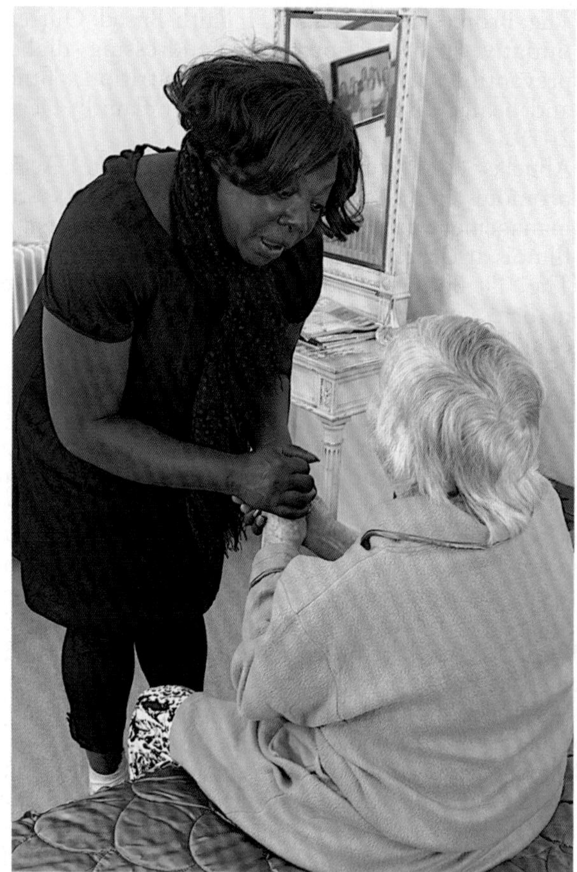

FIGURE 29-4 A faith community nurse provides comfort.

- A faith-based lifestyle intervention was initiated to prevent diabetes among African Americans (Sattin et al., 2016).
- A cardiovascular health education program conducted by trained lay educators in 14 African American congregations found significant reductions in weight and blood pressure (Tettey et al., 2017).
- A 3-month program of coaching and blood pressure self-monitoring, led by 39 FCNs, resulted in decreased blood pressure and improved scores on a lifestyle satisfaction inventory (Cooper & Zimmerman, 2017).
- A gospel rescue mission established a wellness center at a homeless shelter for men and found improved access and treatment adherence (Lashley, 2019).
- A transition of care program led by an FCN reduced 30-day hospital readmission rates by 67% (Strait, Figzgerald, Zurmehly, & Overcash, 2019).
- A breast cancer education program was shown to be effective in improving "general knowledge about breast cancer, higher breast cancer mortality among African American women, warning signs, risks and ways to mitigate risk, and the availability of low-cost or free mammograms" (Brown & Cowart, 2018, para. 4).

There are growing trends in the types of FCN delivery models used today. These include (Sabo et al., 2015):

- Hire salaried full- or part-time staff positions serving one congregation.
- Hire salaried full- or part-time staff positions shared across multiple congregations.
- Maintain a separate health care facility.
- Form partnerships with organizations such as universities or hospitals that agree to provide nursing services to the faith community, possibly involving individual faculty and student groups.
- Invite student nurse participation in service-learning projects that address public health issues in the church setting.

Becoming an FCN

The FCN practices community nursing with a high degree of independence and autonomy. Often, the FCN deals with clients experiencing complex health care situations who may have limited resources and extensive health-related needs. The preferred minimum educational preparation for an FCN includes a bachelor's degree in nursing (ANA/HMA, 2017) and completion of additional education such as the 36-hour Foundations of Faith Community Nursing course offered through the International Parish Nurse Resource Center (The Center for Faith and Community Health Transformation, 2015; Westberg Institute for Faith Community Nursing, 2019a). This course addresses the roles of the FCN and provides information on establishing, promoting, and maintaining an FCN practice. Participants gain experience in resolving complex client situations using scenarios and case studies.

- Several steps are involved in creating an FCN position within a faith community. One of the first things to do is assess the community the nurse plans to serve, identifying the health needs of the faith community and the roles of the FCN that meet those needs through a needs-assessment survey.
- Once the nurse has assessed the needs of the faith community, the next step is to identify how an FCN could help to meet those needs. The FCN uses this information to seek the support of the faith community members and staff.

The Westberg Institute provides information and resources regarding establishing a program, along with the qualifications needed for the nurse. The center also provides an educational program called The Ministry of Church Health to guide the nurse in the many roles that the nurse will have in the community (Westberg Institute for Faith Community Nursing, 2019a).

Web sites for information on Faith Community Nursing include the following:

- International Parish/Faith Community Nursing: https://westberginstitute.org/international-faith-community-nursing/
- HMA: https://hmassoc.org/
- Nurses Christian Fellowship: http://www.ncf-jcn.org/index.php

OCCUPATIONAL AND ENVIRONMENTAL HEALTH NURSING

Business and industry provide another group of settings for community health nursing practice. **Occupational and environmental health nurses** work with employers to cultivate creative and business-appropriate health and safety programs. Program development must consider the business's unique type of work, workforce demographics, and the work/community environments. The practice of occupational health nursing uses an interdisciplinary approach to advocate for the employee's right to have cost-effective, prevention-oriented health and safety programs (Fig. 29-5).

Organizations are expected to provide a safe and healthy work environment in addition to offering insurance for health care. Businesses often choose to hire occupational health nurses (OHNs) because occupational health programs help maximize employee efficiency and decrease costs by effectively reducing work-related injuries, disability claims, and absenteeism and improving employee health and safety.

- Present-day OHNs observe and assess workers' health status, considering the workers' job tasks and hazards. Using their specialized training, education, and experience, they use the nursing process to prevent occupational illness and injury.

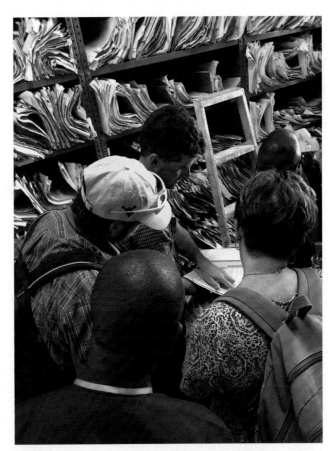

FIGURE 29-5 An environmental health nurse works collaboratively with the community. (Photograph courtesy of the Centers for Disease Control and Prevention. Retrieved from https://phil.cdc.gov/Details.aspx?pid=22796)

- An equally important responsibility is to help organizations maintain compliance with federal, state, and local laws, regulations, and guidelines for workplace health and safety (American Board for Occupational Health Nurses [ABOHN], n.d.).

History of the Occupational and Environmental Health Nurse

Community health nurses have a long history of involvement in occupational health. Early on, the profession primarily focused on providing infant and child health education to the employee families as well as the whole community. World War II showed a marked increase in employment of OHNs. In keeping with the changing times, the OHN's practice broadened to include comprehensive health and safety programs designed to prevent illness and injury for the US workforce. Historic examples include:

- Betty Moulder provided care for coal miners and families in Pennsylvania beginning in 1888 (American Association of Occupational Health Nurses [AAOHN], 2019b).
- In 1895, the Vermont Marble Company hired Ada Mayo Stewart, said to be the first *industrial nurse* in the United States. Stewart provided care for employees and their families, focusing on health promotion and disease prevention (ABOHN, n.d.).

Although occupational and environmental health nursing has been in existence since the late 1800s, the Occupational Safety and Health Act of 1970 led to the proliferation of occupational health nursing employment in the United States. This important legislation established the **Occupational Safety and Health Administration** (**OSHA**, 1970) in the Department of Labor, to ensure a safe working environment for workers in the United States. To ensure that business and industries meet OSHA standards, OHNs monitor the health status of individual workers, workforce populations, and community groups. Other prominent practice guidelines come from:

- US statutes, such as the Genetic Information Nondiscrimination Act
- Family Medical Leave Act
- Americans with Disabilities Act (2000)
- Health Insurance Portability and Accountability Act
- Department of Transportation and U.S. Environmental Protection Agency

OHNs can implement evidence-based interventions to prevent or mitigate negative health effects of the work environment by gathering health and hazard data, evaluating the effects of workplace exposures, and developing workplace prevention programs (ABOHN, n.d.).

Settings for Occupational and Environmental Health Nursing

OHNs work in a variety of settings:

- The manufacturing sector has a strong tradition of employing OHNs, but utility companies, mines, retail store chains (e.g., grocery, department, home improvement), hospitals and medical centers, theme parks, banks, school systems, and government also employ OHNs (ABOHN, n.d.).
- Consulting for companies is a more independent type of employment for about 7% of OHNs, as noted in a seminal study by Harber, Alongi, and Su (2014). Or entrepreneurial nurses may set up an occupational health clinic in areas where many small businesses are located. See Box 29-10 for the perspective of a nurse entrepreneur.

BOX 29-10 PERSPECTIVES

A Nurse Entrepreneur's Viewpoint

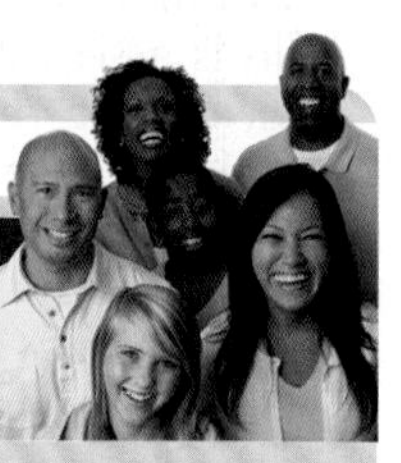

As a newly graduated nurse practitioner, I was excited to step into the role in a small family practice clinic. I worked alongside a family physician who owned the clinic. We took pride in the product we delivered because we made decisions that directly impacted patient care.

A few years later, a corporation bought out that small family practice clinic. Upon the sale of the clinic, the administrative decisions were made by people not only unfamiliar with our patients but unfamiliar with family medicine. Nameless faces on the other end of phone trees addressed my patients' concerns, as the corporation centralized the call centers under the direction of corporate management.

I became frustrated with the dictates of others and the negative impact it had on my patients. This frustration led to my desire to make a change. My first entrepreneurial experience came when an owner of a manufacturing plant approached me about creating and running an on-site clinic for his employees. Together, the company owner and I talked about our vision of the clinic. I created a model where I could run the clinic by myself, with one medical assistant. Care was free to employees, and insurance companies were not involved. The owner of the manufacturing plant paid the overhead. This was a model unlike any other on-site medical clinic in the area.

A few years after starting the on-site clinic, I saw the lack of access my patients had to mental health care in my state. There was a serious shortage of psychiatrists to manage psych meds, so I started a mental health clinic to provide better access to those in my community. I eventually transitioned out of my on-site employee clinic and expanded my mental health clinic to provide a broader array of services. I became a nurse practitioner to help others and make a difference in the world. In order to truly make a difference, I assessed the needs in my community and did what I could to fill the gaps.

—*Kelly Wosnik, DNP, NP-C*

Can you think of something that may frustrate you and see where you might provide a much-needed service, like this nurse entrepreneur?

- Nurse-managed clinics may use OHNs, a nurse practitioner or physician assistant, a physical therapist, a health educator, and a part-time occupational physician.
- A single-nurse unit is a common model of practice in many smaller companies. In a single-nurse unit, OHNs typically build strong networks of colleagues with whom they can discuss professional practice issues.
- Some companies use a medical model of practice, in that a physician determines clinic staffing and the department's approach to clinical practice.

Areas of focus in occupational health nursing could expand to include vulnerable populations, such as immigrant workers, and healthier communities, while continuing to include attending to chronic health conditions and promoting preventive approaches (McCauley & Peterman, 2017).

Roles and Career Opportunities of Occupational and Environmental Health Nurses

There are a wide variety of settings that benefit from OHN programs. In addition to providing first aid for illness and injury that occurs in the workplace, occupational health practices are moving toward a model that provides not only basic occupational health services but also case management, telehealth, care coordination, and primary care (AAOHN, 2019b).

According to the Workforce Management Data Bank, the primary reasons employers establish an on-site clinic are to decrease health care costs, improve workers' quality of life, and improve the company's cost-effectiveness (National Association of Worksite Health Centers, 2019).

Comprehensive occupational worksite programs offer both health protection and health promotion services. After employees are injured or become ill at work, OHNs work to ensure a speedy and functional recovery, frequently helping employees work through the workers' compensation or insurance bureaucracy. Although some companies outsource case management for work-related injuries, many OHNs coordinate and manage cases to ensure the employee's optimum recovery while helping to control costs.

Occupational health nursing practice can be divided into three main categories: compliance, care, and health promotion. There is a wide range of career opportunities for the occupational and environmental health nurse to consider. Examples of the variety of roles and jobs in OHN practice beyond the typical clinical setting include international opportunities, case management, transitional care, and telemedicine.

OHNs practice around the world. There are positions with American companies that have foreign operations as well as with international companies. Depending on the global setting, OHN responsibilities and scope of services may differ from practice in the United States. However, the goals of mitigating factors that may affect a workplace population's health and working to protect and promote safe working conditions are the same. If going abroad sounds appealing, the AAOHN has published an international resource list that outlines the educational and training requirements for countries with an occupational health nursing specialty (Robinson, 2016).

Effective case management is one strategy for employers to not only quantify health care costs but also to demonstrate savings and ensure quality care delivery through coordination of services (Case Management Society of America, 2016; Workplace Health & Safety, 2015).

Case management is the process of assessment, planning, facilitation, care coordination, evaluation, and advocacy for services to meet an individual's and family's comprehensive health needs using resources to promote patient safety, quality of care, and cost-effective outcomes (Case Management Society of America, 2017).

Case management is a care-coordinated strategy that is patient-centered, continuous, and often used in transitional care situations. It is an approach that can be found across many specialties of nursing, from acute care to public health nursing. For example, an employee with asthma may be followed by an OHN for case management, as well as an employee who has been injured on the job. A C/PHN may follow a young mother and her healthy new infant, helping to remind the mother of vaccination clinics and educating on normal child development. If the child develops a chronic condition, such as sickle cell anemia, the C/PHN will help with arrangements for transportation, referrals, and finding resources. A patient may be followed from home to the hospital and back home again, with one nurse as the case manager. This represents the continuum of care. Case management may also be accomplished through a team effort of care collaboration, with physicians, nurses, occupational health specialists, and others involved in coordinating care.

A meta-analysis of studies evaluating the effect of case management on 4,000 patients with type 2 diabetes found statistically significant reductions in hemoglobin A_{1C} and low-density lipoprotein levels, demonstrating the effectiveness of case management over a control group (Zeng, Shuai, Yi, Wang, & Song, 2016). Various methods of case management, from phone consultation to in-person visits, were included in the analysis.

Careful case management can ensure efficient, less fragmented, and more cost-effective use of the health care system, producing better patient outcomes while decreasing costs (Joo & Huber, 2018). It is especially helpful for fragile, vulnerable clients needing an advocate within the health care system.

Transitional care involves managing care from one level to another across the health care spectrum (Naylor et al., 2018). Transitional care strategies have been shown to reduce unnecessary use of health services and improve patient outcomes in chronically ill, injured, and older workers (Social Programs that Work, 2017). There are several models of transitional care (Ortiz, 2019):

- Colman's Care Transitions Intervention Model
- Naylor's Transitional Care Model
- Better Outcomes for Older Adults Through Safe Transitions
- The New York State Department of Health (NYSDH) Transitional Care Model

The NYSDH model is founded on five elements (Ortiz, 2019):

1. Determining the patient's strengths (e.g., emotional/cognitive, physical, medical, economic, abilities, support system)
2. Assessing the patient's functioning before admission to help determine potential resources needed on discharge
3. Informing decision-making through ongoing collaboration among the patient, family, and interdisciplinary transition team
4. Providing both verbal and written information on available options and the range of community services
5. Allowing the patient and family to select preferred providers when possible

One role of the OHN's practice is management of a program to help workers successfully return to work following work-related illness or injury and transition through the often-complex pathway to recovery. Collaboration between all members of the interdisciplinary transitional care team is essential to improve the proportion of employees who successfully return to work (Awang, Shahabudin, & Mansor, 2016).

Transitional care is also found in many nursing specialties and has been especially emphasized since 30-day readmission rates were tied to hospital Medicare payments (see Chapter 6). For example, one large-scale study of over 30,000 patient records found that case management by diabetes educators reduced the 30-day hospital readmission rate from 20.1% to 17.6% over an 18-month period (Drincic, Pfeffer, Luo, & Goldner, 2017).

OHNs can use telemedicine or telehealth (see Chapter 10) to teach, observe processes in distant locations, or provide consultations, to reduce or eliminate OSHA recordable incidents and loss of work time (American Telemedicine Association, 2019). The Chronic Care Act of 2017 expanded the use and reimbursement of telemedicine, addressing complaints by health care providers of their lack (Arndt, 2018).

- In 2018, the U.S. Department of Veteran Affairs (2018) launched an expanded telehealth program that enabled Veterans to access care from their homes, including mental health and suicide prevention programs.
- School nurses have explored the use of telehealth as a means of extending their availability and potential for meeting the health needs of all students, no matter how remote their locations (Reynolds & Maughan, 2015).
- A secondary analysis of a 2017 survey of registered nurses working in Vermont found that almost one fifth of the respondents reported working in telehealth/telephonic nursing. Although there is no real preparation for this skill in nursing school, there are concerns about providing "safe, effective, culturally relevant telehealth, and virtual care" and the need for policy development in this area (Rambur, Palumbo, & Nurkanovic, 2019, p. 64).
- Cost-effectiveness of telemedicine has been demonstrated. Anderson et al. (2018, p. 2031) found that electronic consultations (eConsults) with specialists in dermatology, gastroenterology, endocrinology, and orthopedics at a large, multisite safety-net health center had "average specialty-related episode-of-care costs" that were $82 per month lower than patients having face-to-face appointments.
- Digital health interventions such as short message service, telephone support, mobile applications, video conferencing, telemonitoring with digitally transmitted physiological data, and wearable medical devices were evaluated for cost-effectiveness of cardiovascular disease management interventions in a systematic review of 14 studies published largely between 2015 and 2018 (Jiang, Ming, & You, 2019). Overall, the use of digital health interventions demonstrated higher quality-adjusted years of life (QALYs) while also saving costs in 43% of the studies reviewed. The remainder of the studies had QALY gains but higher costs, making them less cost-effective interventions.

Health Promotion and Wellness

OHNs play a vital role in advocating for health promotion and wellness programs for the workforce they serve. OHNs are in an ideal position to provide guidance, counseling, education, and coaching for employees who want to improve their health. Faced with high health care costs, many employers are turning to worksite health programs to help employees adopt healthier lifestyles and lower their risk of developing costly chronic diseases while improving worker productivity (AAOHN, 2019b).

- The **Total Worker Health (TWH)** initiative is designed to provide holistic approaches to employee wellness. It integrates occupational safety and protection of health along with health promotion to prevent worker injury and illness and improve worker well-being and health (National Institute for Occupational Safety and Health [NIOSH], 2018).
- Because American workers spend a large part of their day at work, the workplace is now considered a social determinant of health; job-related factors include salary, the work environment, time spent at work, physical and psychological stress, employee–employer dynamics, and work–life balance (see Chapters 1 and 11).
- The AAOHN also crafted a position statement that calls for a multifaceted approach to address the rising opioid crisis as it affects the workplace, calling on OHNs to become actively engaged in workplace educational programs and other interventions, such as drug testing policies and procedures (AAOHN, 2018).

The Occupational Health Team

OHNs work in a team environment with a variety of other professionals. Depending on the size of the company, the occupational health team may include the following:

- Safety specialist
- Industrial hygienist
- Ergonomist
- Industrial or organizational psychologist
- Toxicologist
- Physical or occupational therapist
- Physician
- Lawyer
- Employee assistance counselor

Human resources, management, security, and emergency response personnel are also part of the team. The employee is central to the team and is the reason for the team's existence. Team collaboration is essential to the success of the occupational and environmental health program, and the OHN has a key role in ensuring adequate and appropriate communication among the members of the team. Establishing working relationships is paramount to the success of a functional and effective team (OSHA, 2018). Strong interpersonal relationship skills are extremely valuable in a team environment.

Finally, the occupational health team is not complete without the workers themselves. Employees can help identify problems and needs while contributing to decision-making about health programs. Their cooperation in implementing and evaluating programs is essential for an effective health protection and promotion effort.

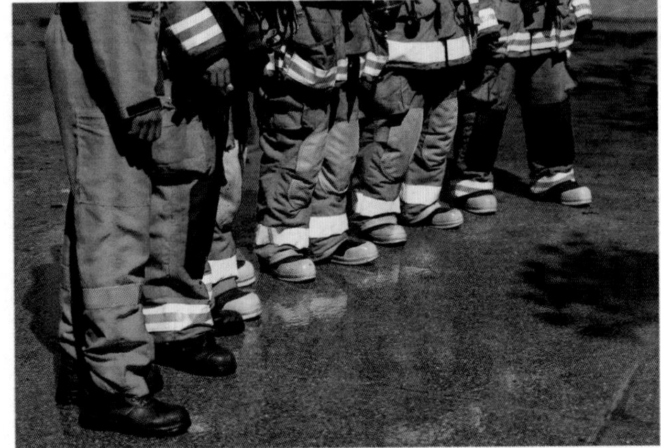

FIGURE 29-6 Example of workplace safety equipment. Firefighters in fireproof uniforms are well prepared to extinguish fires.

Educational Preparation and Evidence-Based Practice

OHNs are the largest group of health professionals working in occupational health (de Castro, Shapleigh, Bruck, & Salazar, 2015). In many work settings, the occupational and environmental health nurse is the only health professional. Independent decision-making is critical. Nurses in occupational settings must also have strong communication skills, including listening, speaking, and writing. The broad knowledge base requirement necessitates a minimum of a bachelor's degree in nursing. During the last two decades, several nursing educational programs (primarily on the graduate level) have developed a specialty focus in occupational and environmental health.

Additionally, OHNs may become certified in this specialty field through ABOHN. Founded in 1972, ABOHN is an independent not-for-profit organization that sets professional standards and conducts occupational health nursing specialty certification. ABOHN is the sole certifying body for OHNs in the United States and has the stated purposes of (ABOHN, 2018):

1. Establishing standards and examinations for professional nurses in occupational health
2. Elevating and maintaining the quality of occupational health nursing service
3. Stimulating the development of improved educational standards and programs in the field of occupational health nursing
4. Encouraging OHNs to continue their professional education

In addition to formal training in occupational health, continuing education plays an important role in keeping abreast with evidence-based practice, as well as maintaining specialty certification. Opportunities range from formal in-person conferences to short, online courses addressing specific topics in occupational health (AAOHN, 2019a).

The Effect of Work on Health

Workers in the United States generally spend more time at work than on any other activity except sleep. Thus, the work environment can have a significant impact on workers' health. A safe and supportive work environment can contribute to the well-being of employees (Fig. 29-6). However, the type of work that people engage in dictates the hazards they encounter. For instance, think about the work of hospital-based nurses. They encounter physical hazards, such as lifting patients in bed without mechanical lifting devices. There are biological hazards associated with blood and body fluids as well as infectious diseases. Some nurses are at risk for chemical exposures, such as those associated with operating room gases or chemotherapy. Radiation hazards may exist when working with patients undergoing radiation therapy.

- Hazardous substances can get into a person's body through inhalation, ingestion, or absorption (percutaneously). Although personal protective equipment (PPE) is available to workers, some may not use PPE consistently, or the equipment may not be entirely effective. Workers exposed to chemicals may not wash their hands sufficiently before eating or smoking, thus providing an opportunity for chemicals to get into their system through ingestion or inhalation. Employers are responsible for training employees (OSHA, n.d.).
- Employees who work in awkward positions or who do repetitive tasks that use the same muscle groups are at risk for musculoskeletal disorders (MSDs). Carpel tunnel syndrome is often associated with repetitive movements, such as typing at a computer keyboard (Hegmann et al. 2016).
    - Workers who compound a workplace exposure with off-work activities that use the same muscle groups in similar actions will accelerate or aggravate a problem. For instance, an office manager may spend hours using electronic devices (cell phone, tablet, computer) in the evenings and on the weekend, so the muscles that are used every day never really get a chance to rest and recover.
    - A research study examining the prevalence of MSDs among office workers found the highest number of MSDs noted in the lower back (almost 50%) and neck (49%) areas (Piranveyseh et al., 2016).

Shift work, particularly rotating shift work, negatively impacts sleep and rest cycles. NIOSH offers a free online course that trains nurses and nurse managers on the risks associated with shift work and long working hours, including training on strategies to reduce such risks (NIOSH, 2018). Insufficient sleep is associated with obesity and diabetes (Gibson-Moore & Chambers, 2019). Low-paying jobs may drive workers to get a second or even a third job to make ends meet. Personal stressors or balancing work and family demands, plus employer expectations at work, can have an adverse effect on worker health (Box 29-11).

- A systematic review of research on workplace mental health interventions found moderate evidence for effectiveness of these programs and their outcomes. Programs that included both physical and mental health interventions and multicomponent interventions had greater evidence of support (Wagner et al., 2016).
- Education to reduce the stigma associated with mental illness has also been shown to be effective in improving worker knowledge and promoting more supportive behavior toward peers with mental health issues (Hanisch et al., 2016).

Future Trends

Future practice considerations for occupational health professionals' center on promoting and maintaining the highest level of physical, social, and emotional health for all workers. Occupational health and environmental nurses play a key role in making positive strides toward this goal by embracing evidence-based research and best practices. Strategic visionaries from the nursing and occupational safety and health (OSH) fields stress the need for working collaboratively (ILO, 2017; 2019a). The Future of Nursing committee of the Institute of Medicine (now named the Health and Medicine Division of the National Academies of Sciences, Engineering, and Medicine) concluded that, "no single profession, working alone, can meet the complex needs of patients and communities" (Lynch, 2015, para. 2). Collaboration with all stakeholders in the health care sector, private industry, government agencies, trade unions, workers, employers, researchers, educators, consultants, administrators, managers, policy makers, technology developers, and human resource professionals is required to advance worker safety and health and create a culture of prevention.

In the progress report, the Future of Nursing committee gave specific recommendations in the areas of removing barriers to practice and care; transforming education; collaborating and leading; promoting diversity; and improving data. The update included progress made to date, remaining challenges, and recommendations towards reaching the goals of The Future of Nursing: Campaign for Action (Campaign for Action, 2019). As nurse specialists, OHNs must keep engaged and abreast of the direction of our nursing profession. The following updates convey highlights of the in-depth work done over the past 5 years. The full report is available for review at https://campaignforaction.org/about/our-story/.

Occupational and environmental health nurse practice will continue to evolve. To respond to these challenges, OHNs need to stay current and connected to the continuously growing body of OSH practices evidence. The International Labour Organization (ILO) is a United Nations agency that is tasked with bringing together "governments, employers and workers representatives of 187-member states, to set labor standards, develop policies and devise programs promoting decent work for all women and men" (ILO, 2019a, para. 1). ILO (2017) outlined five challenges:

1. The need for "OSH data that is reliable and comparable coupled with key indicators that will drive improved performance" (para. 9).
2. Giving priority to "those most vulnerable at work." This requires that "the safety and health of migrant workers must be a global concern" (para. 10).
3. Upgrading OSH within global supply chains. Developing methodologies for "identifying OSH vulnerabilities in the agricultural supply chain and developing targeted interventions" to address them (para. 11).
4. Creating processes for the "global sharing of OSH data, knowledge and expertise and finding the means to sustain such networks" (para. 12).
5. The importance of proactively recognizing the "impact that future jobs and future ways of organizing work will have on the safety and health of workers" (para. 14).

There is still work to be done. The new global estimates on work-related illnesses and injuries represent (ILO, 2019b):

- Costs associated with the illnesses, injuries, and deaths amount to 3.94% of the global gross domestic product per year, or US $2.99 trillion.
- 2.78 million workers continue to die each year from work-related injuries and illnesses.
- 2.4 of the 2.78 million deaths can be attributed to work-related diseases alone.

How the future of nursing is forged will have the greatest impact on this and the next generation of OHNs

BOX 29-11 STORIES FROM THE FIELD

Creating a Safety Culture

A family-owned beverage distributing company with 150 employees is experiencing a higher than average injury rate. This prompted the onsite occupational health team consisting of an occupational health nurse, industrial hygienist, and safety manager to conduct a walkthrough. They identified hazards, such as frayed electrical extension cords, blocked egress (exit) doors, missing machine guarding, and air quality concerns.

1. *What actions should the occupational health nurse take?*
2. *What preventive measures could be put into place to inspire a more proactive safety culture?*
3. *What measures might motivate employees involved to prevent exposure to serious hazards?*

and the populations they serve and protect. It is critical to continue to develop skills and competencies, champion innovation, and collaborate with stakeholders to effect change in an evolving occupational and environmental health landscape. To accomplish this, "the nursing community, must build and strengthen coalitions with stakeholders both within and outside of nursing" (Lynch, 2015, para. 2). The occupational and environmental health nurse will particularly need skills in effective communication, leadership, change management, research, business acumen, and assertiveness. These tools will be crucial for effectively interpreting the OHN's role and promoting future worker population needs.

NURSE ENTREPRENEUR IN COMMUNITY/PUBLIC HEALTH NURSING

C/PHNs often work within an organization to address unmet needs in the community, with the ultimate goal of enhancing service delivery. These positions are often nonexistent until the nurse is able to identify a need and take the necessary steps to start a stand-alone service or to develop a role within an existing agency, often through grant writing. But a growing trend in nursing seeks a more independent practice through entrepreneurship. The National Nurses in Business Association (NNBA, 2018) was first started in 1985 as a grassroots effort for business-minded nurses to connect and share ideas. It has grown into a nursing organization that provides resources for nurses transitioning from traditional nursing positions to self-employment and business ownership. As you think about your own career in nursing, can you envision yourself running a health care business, seeking a small business loan to start a venture, or having the courage to explore other professional options? Independent practice is not for everyone, and nurses are often socialized to view their role as working within a larger organization, such as a health department, a community clinic, or, most often, a hospital. At some point in your career, you may find yourself working with a nurse entrepreneur or becoming one yourself.

- An **entrepreneurial nurse** is one who is willing to take on the risks of starting a new business within a health care or social context. Common examples of nurse entrepreneurs include legal consultants, forensic nurses, home health care agency owners, authors, and nurse consultants in a variety of areas.
- The NNBA (2018) offers membership and resources for those entrepreneurial nurses who are self-employed or small business owners.

For the community/public health nurse, these and many other options offer the independence to provide services in perhaps a new and innovative way. For health care to continue to respond to the changing environment, the innovators are often the ones who have the courage to test those new methods.

Steps to Becoming a Nurse Entrepreneur

One of the first steps to becoming a nurse entrepreneur is to have an idea. It doesn't have to be a new idea or even a "big" idea, but it must address an unmet need within a community. Community/public health nurses are often the first to identify the challenges and needs within a community and to explore solutions. Very often, participation in professional organizations helps to identify health care issues that can be addressed by nurses. The common refrain "why doesn't someone just (invent, build, provide, etc.)?" can often be answered by a nurse. Nurses are problem-solvers, and using the nursing process, they assess the situation, identify the problem, determine a course of action, and evaluate the results. This nursing skill can be leveraged for entrepreneurship (e.g., to start a new business venture, to develop a nonprofit agency, or to create educational tools for use by other health care professionals or the general public).

Entrepreneurial nurses in the community often require skill with grant writing, agency and personnel management, collaboration both inter- and intraprofessionally, fiscal management, and agency promotion. Whatever the health care need, nurses can and do find the solutions. Hahn and Cook (2018) highlight the potential nurse practitioners with full practice authority have as entrepreneurs in their state. These nurse practitioners are finding new ways to practice outside the hospital while addressing gaps in direct patient care systems. They are able to serve vulnerable groups while leveraging reimbursement. Credentialing and payment from private insurance companies can be cumbersome. Legal consultation should be part of every nurse entrepreneur's business plan.

A business plan is essential to starting a business, growing a business, and obtaining financial support. At the very minimum, the business plan should include the description of the business; marketing strategies; competitive analysis, design, and development plan; operations and management plan; and financial factors (Box 29-12).

Opportunities

As the health care needs of the population demand newer, better, and less expensive solutions, nurse entrepreneurs are well positioned to address those needs. Although there are many examples in your own communities of nurse entrepreneurship, the role of the community/public health nurse can serve as a strong base for meeting the health care challenges locally, nationally, and internationally. Some examples of nurse entrepreneurship include (NNBA, 2018):

- Nursing registry and staffing services agency
- Home care agency
- Specialty agencies (vascular, diabetes, dialysis)
- Nurse consultant for local and federal government, and organizations
- Legal, wellness, and coaching consultation
- Elder care managers
- Forensic nursing
- Nurse educators (seminar companies, national speakers, online courses, assisting with accreditation, writing, diabetes educator, podcasts, yoga, wellness, and training programs)
- Retail businesses (patient care products, wellness products, health foods, medical equipment and devices)

BOX 29-12 Small Business Start-Up Information

1. Write a detailed business plans with goals, objectives, and financial costs. Include market research and competitive analysis for your business.
2. Set up the legal business structure. This might require legal consultation.
3. Register your business and obtain a Federal Employee Identification (FEI) number.
4. Obtain start up collateral. Create business or merchant bank account.
5. Determine whether business licensing is required for your business activities. What other government rules and licensing might need to be considered? Be aware of rules in all states you will interact with for business. Will you need business insurance?
6. Establish place of business including all contact and corresponding information.
7. Create a sales and marketing plan. Address marketing for your business including Web site and registered URL, advertising plan, and marketing products. Consider how you will "sell" your product. How will you establish a presence in your community or reach your target audience?
8. Establish accounting and payroll processes.
9. Create internal documents (this can include safety, education, and hiring process within your business).
10. Connect with local small business resources in your community.

Adapted from U.S. Small Business Administration (2018).

- Independent nurse contractor (private care and therapy)
- Nurse practitioner–owned clinic or wellness agency
- Esthetic care
- Adult day care
- Foot care services

One example of a nurse entrepreneur is Barbara Philips, a family nurse practitioner who opened a hypnotherapy practice in Missouri. After years of working in a pain management group in Washington that included use of hypnotherapy, Philips expanded her interest in this area, completing training and certification, and opened her own business in 2016. Her practice assists patients with such health issues as smoking, anxiety, and fibromyalgia. As practice authority can be different in every state, it is prudent to understand the laws affecting your nurse practitioner license and make every effort to practice to your full potential. In addition to Philips's hypnotherapy practice, she also consults on business start-up basics with other nurse entrepreneurs. She says many nurses want to have their own business but don't always consider the whole process. Her suggestions include:

- Know your potential customer.
- Do research and have a business plan.
- Investigate requirements such as regulations and credentialing.
- Have a financial plan.

Philips says that nurses do need to understand the money aspect and that having an expense and income report is a must (personal communication, Barbara Philips, APRN, GNP, FNP-BC, FAANP, NP, business owner).

The opportunities are limitless for nurse entrepreneurship; the only missing piece is the nurse willing to take that leap, come up with an idea, explore the options, create a business plan, garner funding, and make a difference. Community/public health nurses are uniquely qualified to address the ever-growing challenges in our communities. As opportunities in one area of nursing practice recede, other avenues open up. What is needed are nurses who enjoy a challenge and are willing to take risks to provide needed services and improve patient outcomes.

SUMMARY

- Private sector practice opportunities for public health nurses include NLHCs, faith community nursing, occupational and environmental health, and entrepreneurial roles. Each of these areas of practice offers community health nurses an avenue to address health disparities in their communities, increase years of healthy life, and provide holistic, client-centered care.
- NLHCs represent a growing movement of health centers that have emerged as vital safety-net providers in America's contemporary health care delivery system and typically provide care to vulnerable or underserved populations.
- The Health Care Provisions in Bipartisan Budget Act of 2018 and the ACA of 2010 provide funding streams for NLHCs as an avenue to reach vulnerable populations and reduce the burden on traditional health models.
- Faith community nursing is a specialized area of practice that focuses on the care of the spirit as well as the whole-person health.
- The ANA and the HMA have published *Faith Community Nursing: Scope and Standards of Practice*, 3rd edition, which should be used to guide nursing practice in this area.
- FCNs act as health educators, health counselors, advocates, and referral agents. They also establish support groups, coordinate volunteers, and integrate concepts of faith and health.
- The Occupational Safety and Health Act of (1970) led to the proliferation of occupational health nursing employment in the United States and established OSHA, which developed standards for occupational health and monitors the health status of workers and community groups.
- OHNs play a vital role advocating health promotion and wellness programs for the workforce they serve, and OHN duties fall into three categories: compliance, care, and health promotion. OHNs are often involved in case management, transitional care, and telemedicine.

- Occupational and environmental health nurses work with employers to cultivate creative and business-appropriate health and safety programs, using an interdisciplinary approach to advocate for the employee's right to have cost-effective, prevention-oriented health and safety programs. OHNs can become certified in this specialty field through ABOHN.
- The TWH initiative is defined as a strategy that integrates occupational safety and protection of health along with health promotion to prevent worker injury and illness and to improve worker well-being and health through a holistic approach.
- Case management is an approach used in many areas of nursing. It involves assessment, planning, facilitating, care coordination, evaluation, and advocacy for resources to meet client needs. Current research demonstrates cost-effectiveness and better patient outcomes.
- Transitional care is concerned with management of care across the health care system (e.g., hospital to home). Research has shown beneficial effects for patients and cost benefits to hospitals and health care agencies.
- Telemedicine is expanding and being used in a wide variety of settings. It can cut costs and shorten wait time for patients needing to see specialists. Several methods of digital health interventions were discussed (also see Chapter 10).
- There is a growing trend in nursing to seek a more independent practice in health care delivery through entrepreneurship. Common examples of nurse entrepreneurs include legal consultants, forensic nurses, home health care agency owners, authors, and nurse consultants in a variety of areas.
- The NNBA provides valuable resources and guidance on how to establish an independent practice (or health-related business).

ACTIVE LEARNING EXERCISES

1. Using "Enable Equitable Access" (1 of the 10 essential public health services; see Box 2-2) locate a NLHC or a federally qualified health center in your community. Interview a public health nurse or a nurse practitioner employed there. Ask the nurse to describe his or her role and duties. What types of patients are most often seen? What are typical problems or illnesses? If this clinic did not exist, where would those patients get care?
2. Contact a faith community nurse (FCN) in your area and arrange to interview or shadow the nurse. Explore the services offered by FCNs in your area. Identify the knowledge and skills needed to function effectively in the role. Discuss the process the nurse used to establish an FCN practice.
3. Search for current evidence-based practice research articles on case management, transitional care, and telemedicine in nursing practice. Where is most of this research being done (e.g., acute care, public health, ambulatory care, chronic illness care, palliative care)? How can these strategies be effectively employed in public health nursing, faith community nursing, and occupational health nursing and at nurse-led clinics?
4. Research occupational hazards for nurses. You may find that hazards vary depending on specialty areas or geographic locations. Think of the kind of nursing that you see yourself doing after graduation. Identify the occupational risks associated and develop a list of strategies for mitigating those risks. Compare your findings with those of other class members.
5. Think about your clinical experiences in community/public health nursing. Are there unmet needs in the community that could be addressed through a nurse-led business? What elements would you include in a business plan? Locate a nurse entrepreneur and discuss the challenges the nurse met in starting the business; how were those addressed?

REFERENCES

Agency for Healthcare Research and Quality. (2018). *Module 2: Working with safety net practices*. Retrieved from http://www.ahrq.gov/professionals/prevention-chronic-care/improve/system/pfhandbook/mod2.html

American Association of Colleges of Nursing (AACN). (2016). *Advancing healthcare transformation: A new era for academic nursing*. Retrieved from http://www.aacnnursing.org/portals/42/publications/aacn-new-era-report.pdf

American Association of Occupational Health Nurses (AAOHN). (2018). *Position statement: The occupational health nurse's role in addressing the opioid crisis in the workplace*. Retrieved from http://aaohn.org/page/position-statements

American Association of Occupational Health Nurses (AAOHN). (2019a). *Careers: Education*. Retrieved from http://aaohn.org/page/the-occupational-and-environmental-health-nurse-career

American Association of Occupational Health Nurses (AAOHN). (2019b). *What is occupational & environmental health nursing?* Retrieved from http://aaohn.org/page/profession-of-occupational-and-environmental-health-nursing

American Board for Occupational Health Nurses (ABOHN). (2018). *Strategic plan*. Retrieved from https://www.abohn.org/about-abohn/strategic-plan

American Board for Occupational Health Nurses (ABOHN). (n.d.). *Occupational health nursing profession*. Retrieved from https://www.abohn.org/sites/default/files/ABOHNCarGde_032714WEB.pdf

American Nurses Association & Health Ministries Association. (2017). *Faith community nursing: scope and standards of practice* (3rd ed.). Silver Spring, MD: Nursesbooks.org.

American Telemedicine Association. (2019). *Telehealth is access*. Retrieved from https://www.americantelemed.org/policy/

Americans with Disabilities Act (ADA). (2000). *A guide for persons with disabilities seeking employment*. Retrieved from http://www.ada.gov/workta.htm

Anderson, D., Villagra, V., Coman, E., Ahmed, T., Porto, A., Jepeal, N., ... Teevan, B. (2018). Reduced cost of specialty care using electronic consultations for Medicaid patients. *Health Affairs, 37*(12), 2031–2036.

Arndt, R. Z. (February 9, 2018). Chronic Care Act breaks down barriers to telemedicine use. In *Modern healthcare*. Retrieved from https://www.modernhealthcare.com/article/20180209/NEWS/180209899/chronic-care-act-breaks-down-barriers-to-telemedicine-use

Association of Public Health Nurses. (2016). *The public health nurse: Necessary partner for the future of healthy communities. Position Paper*. Retrieved from http://aphn.wildapricot.org/resources/Documents/APHN-PHN%20Value-Position%20P_APPROVED%205.30.2016.pdf

Aveling, E. L., Martin, G., Herbert, G., & Armstrong, G. (2017). Optimizing the community [based approach to healthcare improvement: Comparative case studies of the clinical community model in practice. *Social Science & Medicine*, *173*, 96–103. doi: 10.1016/j.socscimed.2016.11.026.

Awang, H., Shahabudin, M., & Mansor, N. (2016). Return-to-work program for injured workers: Factors of successful return to employment. *Asia Pacific Journal of Public Health*, *28*(8), 694-702. doi: 10.1177/1010539516640354.

Baker, E., & Fatoye, F. (2017). Clinical and cost effectiveness of nurse-led self-management interventions for patients with COPD in primary care: A systematic review. *International Journal of Nursing Studies*, *71*, 125–138.

Brewer, L. C., Balls-Berry, J. E., Dean, P., Lackore, K., Jenkins, S., & Hayes, S. N. (2017). Fostering African-American improvement in total health (FAITH!): An application of the American Heart Association's Life's Simple 7™ among midwestern African-Americans. *Journal of Racial and Ethnic Health Disparities*, *4*(2), 269–281. doi: 10.1007/s40615-016-0226-z.

Brown, M. T., & Cowart, L. W. (2018). Evaluating the effectiveness of faith-based breast health education. *Health Education Journal*, *77*(5), 571–585. doi: 10.1177/0017896918778308.

Callaghan, D. (2016). Implementing faith community nursing interventions to promote healthy behaviors in adults. *International Journal of Faith Community Nursing*, *2*(1), 3.

Campaign for Action. (2019). *The future of nursing 2020–2030*. Retrieved from https://campaignforaction.org/

Case Management Society of America. (2016). *Standards of practice for case management*. Retrieved from http://solutions.cmsa.org/acton/media/10442/standards-of-practice-for-case-management

Case Management Society of America. (2017). *What is a case manager?* Retrieved from http://www.cmsa.org/who-we-are/what-is-a-case-manager/

Chan, R. J., Marx, W., Bradford, N., Gordon, L., Bonner, A., Douglas, C., ... Yates, P. (2018). Clinical and economic outcomes of nurse-led services in the ambulatory care setting: A systematic review. *International Journal of Nursing Studies*, *81*, 61–80.

Christian Community Health Fellowship. (2019). *Introduction to parish nursing*. Retrieved from https://www.cchf.org/resources/h-and-dintroduction-to-parish-nursing/

Cohn, J., Corrigan, J., Lynn, J. Meier, D., Miller, J., Shega, J., et al. (2017). *Community-based models of care delivery for people with serious illness*. [Discussion Paper]. Washington, DC: National Academy of Medicine. Retrieved from https://nam.edu/community-based-models-of-care-delivery-for-people-with-serious-illness/

Compilation of Patient Protection and Affordability Care. [As amended through November 1, 2010] Public Law 111–148; 111th Congress 2nd Session. 2010, 542. Retrieved from https://books.google.com/books?id=6eRqPuV8sBEC&printsec=frontcover&source=gbs_ge_summary_r&cad=0#v=onepage&q&f=false

Cooper, J., & Zimmerman, W. (2017). The effect of a faith community nurse network and public health collaboration on hypertension prevention and control. *Public Health Nursing*, *34*(5), 444–453.

Cutler, I. (2002). *End games: The challenge of sustainability*. Baltimore, MD: Annie E. Casey Foundation.

Dandridge, R. (2014). Faith community/parish nursing literature: Exciting interventions, unclear outcomes. *Journal of Christian Nursing*, *31*(3), 100–106.

de Castro, A. B., Erin Shapleigh, E., Bruck, A., & Salazar, M. (2015). Developing blended online and classroom strategies to deliver an occupational health nursing overview course in a multi-state region in the United States. *Workplace Health & Safety*, *63*(3), 121–126.

Deaconess Nurse Ministry. (2019). *What is faith community nursing?* Retrieved from https://www.faithnurses.org/faith-community-nursing/what-is/

Drincic, A., Pfeffer, E., Luo, J., & Goldner, W. S. (2017). The effect of diabetes case management and Diabetes Resource Nurse program on readmissions of patients with diabetes mellitus. *Journal of Clinical & Translational Endocrinology*, *8*, 29–34.

Durovich, C. J., & Roberts, P. W. (2018). Designing a community-based population health model. *Population Health Management*, *21*(1), 13–19. doi: 10.1089/pop.2017.0015.

Faith Community Nursing Health Ministries Northwest. (2019). *Integrating mind, body, & spirit at all ages*. Retrieved from https://faithcommunitynursingnw.org/

Find RFP. (2019). *Government contracting terminologies*. Retrieved from https://www.findrfp.com/Government-Contracting/Gov-Contract-Term.aspx

Foster, B., Dawood, K., Pearson, C., Manteuffel, J., & Levy, P. (2019). Community health workers in the emergency department—Can they help with chronic hypertension care. *Current Hypertension Reports*, *21*(7), 1–6.

Frykedal, K. F., Rosander, M., Berlin, A., & Barimani, M. (2016). With or without the group: Sweden midwives' and child health care nurses' experiences in leading parent education groups. *Health Promotion International*, *31*, 899–907.

Gibson-Moore, H., & Chambers, L. (2019). Sleep matters: Can a good night's sleep help tackle the obesity crisis? *Nutrition Bulletin*, 44(2), 123–129. doi: 10.1111/nbu.12386.

Grebeldinger, T. A., & Buckley, K. M. (2016). You are not alone: Parish nurses bridge challenges for family caregivers. *Journal of Christian Nursing*, *33*(1), 50–56.

Hahn, J., & Cook, W. (2018). Lessons learned from nurse practitioner independent practice: A conversation with a nurse practitioner entrepreneur. *Nursing Economics*, *36*(1), 18–22.

Hanisch, S. E., Twomey, C. D., Szeto, A. C., Birner, U. W., Nowak, D., & Sabariego, C. (2016). The effectiveness of interventions targeting the stigma of mental illness at the workplace: A systematic review. *BMC Psychiatry*, *16*(1), 1.

Hansen-Turton, T., Sherman, S., & King, E. (Eds.). (2015). *Nurse-led health clinics: Operations, policy, and opportunities*. New York, NY: Springer Publishing.

Harber, P., Alongi, G., & Su, J. (2014). Professional activities of experienced occupational health nurses. *Workplace Health & Safety*, *62*(6), 233–242.

Health Care Provisions in Bipartisan Budget Act of 2018. (February 26, 2018). *Congressional research service*. Retrieved from https://fas.org/sgp/crs/misc/R45126.pdf

Health Ministries Association (HMA). (n.d.). *About us: What we do*. Retrieved from https://hmassoc.org/about-us/what-we-do/

Hegmann, K. T., Thiese, M. S., Kapellusch, J., Merryweather, A. S., Bao, S., Silverstein, B., ... Drury, D. L. (2016). Association between cardiovascular risk factors and carpal tunnel syndrome in pooled occupational cohorts. *Journal of Occupational and Environmental Medicine*, *58*(1), 87–93.

Hong, W. S., & Lundeen, S. (2009). Using ACHIS to analyze nursing health promotion interventions for vulnerable populations in a community nursing center: A Pilot study. *Asian Nursing Research*, *3*(3), 130–138.

Institute for Family Health. (2019). *Bronx health REACH initiative*. Retrieved from https://www.institute.org/bronx-health-reach/our-work/faith-based-outreach-initiative/

Institute of Medicine (IOM). (2000). *America's healthcare safety net: Intact but endangered*. Washington, DC: National Academies Press.

Institute of Medicine (IOM). (2011). *The future of nursing: Leading change, advancing health*. Washington, DC: National Academies Press.

International Labour Organization. (2017). *Director-General Guy Ryder opening address at XXI World Congress on Safety and Health--transcript*. Retrieved from https://www.ilo.org/global/about-the-ilo/how-the-ilo-works/ilo-director-general/statements-and-speeches/WCMS_639102/lang--en/index.htm

International Labour Organization (ILO). (2019a). *About the ILO*. Retrieved from https://www.ilo.org/global/about-the-ilo/lang--en/index.htm

International Labour Organization (ILO). (2019b). *World statistic*. Retrieved from https://www.ilo.org/moscow/areas-of-work/occupational-safety-and-health/WCMS_249278/lang--en/index.htm

Jiang, X., Ming, W. K., & You, J. H. (2019). The cost-effectiveness of digital health interventions on the management of cardiovascular diseases: Systematic review. *Journal of Medical Internet Research*, *21*(6), e13166.

Joo, J. Y., & Huber, D. L. (2018). Scoping review of nursing case management in the United States. *Clinical Nursing Research*, *27*(8), 1002–1016.

Josiah Macy Jr. Foundation. (2016). *Preparing nursing leaders: Annual report*. Retrieved from https://macyfoundation.org/assets/reports/publications/2016_josiah_macy_annual_report_final.pdf

Judd, D., & Sitzman, K. (2014). *A history of American nursing: Trends and eras* (2nd ed.). Burlington, MA: Jones & Bartlett Learning.

Kinsey, K., & Miller, M. E. (2016). The nursing center: A model for nursing practice in the community. In M. Stanhope & J. Lancaster (Eds.), *Public health nursing: Population-centered health care in the community* (9th ed., pp. 455–475). St. Louis, MO: Elsevier.

Kurtzman, E. T., Barnow, B. S., Johnson, J. E., Simmens, S. J., Infeld, D. L., & Mullan, F. (2017). Does the regulatory environment affect nurse practitioners' patterns of practice or quality of care in health centers? *Health Services Research*, *52*, 437–458. doi: 10.1111/1475-6773.12643.

Lashley, M. (2019). An on-site health home for homeless men in addition recovery. *Public Health Nursing*, *36*(2), 184–191.

Lundeen, S. (2005). *Lundeen's comprehensive community-based primary health care model*. Milwaukee, WI: Milwaukee College of Nursing.

Lynch, J., (2015). *IOM releases progress report on Future of Nursing 2020 goals. National nurse leader talks about the campaign's progress, future plans*. Retrieved from https://www.nurse.com/blog/2015/12/10/iom-releases-progress-report-on-future-of-nursing-2020-goals/

Marquette University. (2019). *Service-learning programs*. Retrieved from https://www.marquette.edu/servicelearning/about_mission.shtml

McCauley, L., & Peterman, K. (2017). The future of occupational health nursing in a changing health care system. *Workplace Health & Safety*, *65*(4), 168–173.

Miller, M. E., & Mest, C. (n.d.). My eyes were blind but now I see: Reflections from graduate nursing students about community service and learning and application to graduate nursing education. Unpublished manuscript.

Mock, G. S. (2017). Value and meaning of faith community nursing: Client and nurse perspectives. *Journal of Christian Nursing*, *34*(3), 182–189.

National Association of Worksite Health Centers. (2019). *Benefits of an onsite clinic*. Retrieved from https://www.nawhc.org/What-is-an-Onsite-Clinic

National Institute for Occupational Safety and Health (NIOSH). (2018). *What is total worker health?* Retrieved from http://www.cdc.gov/niosh/twh/totalhealth.html

The National Academies of Sciences, Engineering, and Medicine (2020). Leading Health Indicators 2030: Advancing health, equity and well-being (2020). The National Academies Press. doi: http://nap.edu/25682

National Nurse-Led Care Consortium. (2018a). *About us*. Retrieved from https://www.nurseledcare.org/about/about-us.html

National Nurse-Led Care Consortium. (2018b). *Nurse-led care*. Retrieved from https://www.nurseledcare.org/about/nurse-led-care.html

National Nurses in Business Association. (n.d.). *NNBA*. Retrieved from https://nnbanow.com

Naylor, M. D., Hirschman, K. B., Toles, M. P., Jarrín, O. F., Shaid, E., & Pauly, M. V. (2018). Adaptations of the evidence-based Transitional Care Model in the U.S. *Social Science & Medicine*, *213*, 28–36.

Nelson, L. (2018). *Faith community nurses: Healing across the country*. Retrieved from https://nurse.org/articles/faith-community-nursing/

Nurse-Managed Health Clinic Investment Act of 2009, S.B. 1104/H.R. 2754, 111th Congress. (2009). Retrieved from https://www.congress.gov/bill/111th-congress/house-bill/2754

Occupational Safety and Health Act (OSHA). (1970). *Occupational noise exposure*. Retrieved from http://osha.gov/pls/oshaweb/owasrch.search_form?p_doc_type=STANDARDS&p_toc_level=1&p_keyvalue=1910

Occupational Safety and Health Act (OSHA). (2018). *Occupational health professionals*. Retrieved from https://www.osha.gov/SLTC/healthprofessional/index.html

Occupational Safety and Health Act (OSHA). (n.d.). *Personal protective equipment*. Retrieved from https://www.osha.gov/SLTC/personalprotective-equipment/

Ortiz, M. R. (2019). Transitional care: Nursing knowledge and policy implications. *Nursing Science Quarterly*, *32*(1), 73–77.

Piranveyseh, P., Motamedzade, M., Osatuke, K., Mohammadfam, I., Moghimbeigi, A., Soltanzadeh, A., et al. (2016). Association between psychosocial, organization, and personal factors and prevalence of musculoskeletal disorder in office workers. *International Journal of Occupational Safety and Ergonomics*, *13*, 1–19.

Patient Protection and Affordable Care Act ("PPACA"; Public Law 111–148). (2010). Retrieved from http://housedocs.house.gov/energycommerce/ppacacon.pdf

Rambur, B., Palumbo, M. V., & Nurkanovic, M. (2019). Prevalence of telehealth in nursing: Implications for regulation and education in the era of value-based care. *Policy, Politics, & Nursing Practice*, *20*(2), 64–71.

Randall, S., Crawford, T., Currie, J., River, J., & Betihavas, V. (2017). Impact of community-based nurse-led clinics on patient outcomes, patient satisfaction, patient access and cost effectiveness: A systematic review. *International Journal of Nursing Studies*, *73*, 24–33.

Resick, L., Miller, M. E., & Leonardo, M. E. (2015). Overview of nurse-managed wellness centers and wellness programs integrated into nurse-managed primary care clinics. In T. Hansen-Turton, S. Sherman & E. King (Eds.). *Nurse-led health clinics: Operations, policy and opportunities* (pp. 179–191). New York, NY: Springer.

Reynolds, C. A., & Maughan, E. D. (2015). Telehealth in the school setting: An integrative review. *The Journal of School Nursing*, *31*(1), 44–53.

Robinson, H. (2016). *International resource list*. Retrieved from http://aaohn.org/d/do/130

Sabo, S., de Zapien, J., Teuifel-Shone, N., Rosales, C., Bergsma, L., & Taren, D. (2015). Service learning: A vehicle for building health equity and eliminating health disparities. *American Journal of Public Health*, *105*(S1), S38–S43.

Sattin, R. W., Williams, L. B., Dias, J., Garvin, J. T., Marion, L., Joshua, T. V., … Narayan, K. M. (2016). Community trial of a faith-based lifestyle intervention to prevent diabetes among African-Americans. *Journal of Community Health*, *41*(1), 87–96.

Schroepfer, E. (2016). Professional issues: A renewed look at faith community nursing. *Medsurg Nursing*, *25*(1), 62–66.

Seo, V., Baggett, T. P., Thorndike, A. N., Hull, P., Hsu, J., Newhouse, J. P., et al. (2019). Access to care among Medicaid and uninsured patients in community health centers after the Affordable Care Act. *BMC Health Services Research*, *19*(1), 291. doi: 10.1186/s12913-019-4124-z.

Smoking Cessation Evidence and Resources. Retrieved from https://www.ahrq.gov/evidencenow/heart-health/smoking/index.html

Social Programs that Work. (2017). *Evidence summary for the transitional care model*. Retrieved from https://evidencebasedprograms.org/document/the-transitional-care-model-evidence-summary/

Sofer, D. (2018). Nurse-led health clinics show positive outcomes. *American Journal of Nursing*, *118*(2), 2–12.

Strait, L. A., Fitzgerald, E., Zurmehly, J., & Overcash, J. (2019). A congregation transition of care program using faith community nurses and volunteer faith-based nurses. *Journal of Christian Nursing*, *36*(3), 158–165.

Tettey, N. S., Duran, P. A., Anderson, H. S., & Boutin-Foster, C. (2017). Evaluation of Heart Smarts, a faith-based cardiovascular health education program. *Journal of Religion and Health*, *56*(1), 320–328. doi: 10.1007/s10943-016-0309-5.

The Center for Faith and Community Health Transformation. (2015). *Faith community nursing*. Retrieved from https://www.faithhealthtransformation.org/resources-and-toolkits/faith-community-nursing/

Torrisi, D. L., & Hensen-Turton, T. (2015). Building a nurse-managed clinic. In T. Hansen-Turton, S. Sherman & E. S. King (Eds.). *Nurse-led health clinics: Operations, policy, and opportunities* (pp. 33–66). New York, NY: Springer.

U.S. Centers for Medicare & Medicaid Services. (2019). *What's Medicare?* Retrieved from https://www.medicare.gov/what-medicare-covers/your-medicare-coverage-choices/whats-medicare

U.S. Department of Health and Human Services. (n.d.). *Affordable Care Act Nurse Managed Health Clinics. Frequently asked questions*. Retrieved from https://www.hrsa.gov/sites/default/files/grants/healthprofessions/aca-faq.pdf

U.S. Department of Health and Human Services (USDHHS), Centers for Medicare and Medicaid Services (CMS). (2018). *Federally Qualified Health Center: Rural health fact sheet series*. Retrieved from http://www.cms.gov/MLNProducts/downloads/fqhcfactsheet.pdf

U.S. Department of Veteran Affairs. (2018). *VA expands telehealth by allowing health care providers to treat patients across state lines*. Retrieved from https://www.va.gov/opa/pressrel/pressrelease.cfm?id=4054

U.S. Health Resources & Services Administration (HRSA). (2018). *HRSA health center program fact sheet*. Retrieved from https://bphc.hrsa.gov/sites/default/files/bphc/about/healthcenterfactsheet.pdf

U.S. Small Business Administration. (2018). *Business guide*. Retrieved from https://www.sba.gov/business-guide

University of California San Francisco. (2019). *Community impact: Nurse-run clinics*. Retrieved from https://nursing.ucsf.edu/news/community-impact-nurse-run-clinics

University of California, San Diego. (2019). *Faith-based wellness*. Retrieved from https://ucsdcommunityhealth.org/work/faith-based-wellness/

University of Illinois at Urbana Champaign. (2016). *Faith-based health promotion program successful with older Latinas*. Retrieved from https://www.sciencedaily.com/releases/2016/04/160427165338.htm

Wagner, S. L., Koehn, C., White, M. I., Harder, H. G., Schultz, I. Z., Williams-Whitt, K., … Wright, M. D. (2016). Mental health interventions in the workplace and work outcomes: A best-evidence synthesis of systematic reviews. *International Journal of Occupational and Environmental Medicine*, *7*(1), 1–14.

Westberg Institute for Faith Community Nursing. (2019a). *About faith community nursing*. Retrieved from https://westberginstitute.org/foundations-of-faith-community-nursing/

Westberg Institute for Faith Community Nursing. (2019b). *The mission*. Retrieved from https://westberginstitute.org/history-mission/

Westberg Institute for Faith Community Nursing. (2019c). *Your role as a faith community nurse*. Retrieved from https://westberginstitute.org/faith-community-nursing/your-role/

Zeibarth, D., & Campbell, K. P. (2016). A transitional care model using faith community nurses. *Journal of Christian Nursing*, *33*(2), 112–118.

Zeng, Z., Shuai, T., Yi, L. J., Wang, Y., & Song, G. M. (2016). Effect of case management on patients with type 2 diabetes mellitus: A meta-analysis. *Chinese Nursing Research*, *3*, 71–76.

Zimmer, P. A., & Knowlton, D. L. (April 11, 2016). *Assessing feasibility of nurse practitioner practices: A toolkit for New Jersey communities*. Retrieved from https://thenicholsonfoundation.org/sites/default/files/TOOLKIT_FINAL.pdf

CHAPTER 30

Home Health and Hospice Care

"People from all walks of life agree that someone who is sick deserves, in principle, compassion and care."

—Paul Farmer, American anthropologist and physician

KEY TERMS

Care coordination
Centers for Medicare and Medicaid Services (CMS)
Compassion fatigue
Home health care
Homebound
Hospice
Medicaid
Medicare home health benefit
Medicare hospice benefit
Medicare prospective payment system
Outcome and Assessment Information Set (OASIS)
Palliative interventions
Postacute care
Value-based care
Visiting Nurse Associations

LEARNING OBJECTIVES

Upon mastery of this chapter, you should be able to:

1. Summarize the history and contemporary circumstances of home health and hospice care.
2. Describe reimbursement and payment models for home health care and hospice programs.
3. Explain family caregiver burdens of providing home and hospice care.
4. Describe essential characteristics of home health and hospice nursing practice.
5. Identify unique challenges of home and hospice nurses.
6. Contrast the goals of home health care and hospice.
7. Explain the gaps and future needs of home health care and hospice in the United States.

INTRODUCTION

A home health nurse sits in an upscale condominium with a frail, older man tethered to his home oxygen unit and experiencing air hunger as he struggles to speak of the "good old days" when he was young, full of vigor, and taking on the world. During her next visit to a trailer park, she inspects an infected pressure sore that has become smaller and cleaner with each home visit, as the client's wife carefully follows through with wound care teaching. Next, she monitors the pulmonary and cardiac status of a patient newly discharged to his aging bungalow, detecting early signs of cardiac decompensation and treating him at home in close collaboration with his physician. At that same time, her hospice nurse colleague on arriving at the home of a woman near the end of life finds the patient in pain and vomiting and the family in chaos; by the time this colleague leaves, however, the family is calm and the patient comfortable.

These are the kinds of experiences that make up the daily lives of nurses who work with home care and hospice clients. Indeed, home health and hospice programs allow nurses to practice what some see as the very heart of compassionate and highly skilled nursing care. Home health care and hospice programs are expanding and are the work settings for more and more nurses. Almost 2% of registered nurses work in home health care settings (United States Department of Labor, 2018). This chapter considers the history and current status of home health care and hospice care, how these services are reimbursed, the unique burdens of caregivers in these settings, key aspects of nursing practice in these areas, and expected future trends. (Children and adults with disabilities also receive home health services. Specific care regarding these populations can be found in Chapters 20 and 24, respectively.)

HOME HEALTH CARE

The need for health care at home continues to accelerate as Americans live longer lives. An aging US population means an increasing number of people living with multiple chronic conditions, cognitive impairments such as dementia, and functional limitations that affect daily living. In addition, medical costs continue to escalate despite national insurance programs such as Medicare and Medicaid and expansion of private health insurance options as a result of the Patient Protection and Affordable Care Act (ACA).

- Early hospital discharges resulting from third-party payers' efforts toward cost containment have forced clients to return home quickly to recuperate from surgeries and severe illnesses. Likewise, a growing population survives and yet suffers from complex chronic and life-threatening illness that they struggle to manage at home.
- Advanced technologies such as telehealth monitoring, point-of-care devices, intravenous (IV) antibiotics, chemotherapy, total parenteral nutrition, dialysis, and mechanical ventilation are now routinely provided and maintained in the client's home.

As the population ages, and particularly now that the baby boomers are entering their elder years, home health nursing is challenged to respond. Professional home health care agencies seek to maximize the client's level of independence and to uphold the right to access high-quality health care and supportive services (National Association for Home Care and Hospice [NAHC], 2018). Those most in need of home care services are older adults and those with chronic illnesses. As the number of multiple chronic conditions rises, specifically for older beneficiaries, the need for health care in the home is critical.

Historically, home health care was delivered in the home as a house call (Landers et al., 2016). Today, C/PHNs provide home health care much like their early predecessors, where the focus of care is on maximum independence (Landers et al., 2016). The nurse's role in the home can be extensive. The nurse may be the coordinator of care, managing and providing a plan of care for the patient. The nurse monitors the progress of the patient, makes referrals as necessary, assesses for home safety, provides care such as dressing changes or blood pressure, coordinates communication with the health care team and family members, reviews the medication regime, and educates and advocates for the patient and family. Today's health care system requires nurses to employ a greater understanding of health care cost and reimbursement, a population focus for improving health, and inclusion of quality and satisfaction in the care provided (Landers et al., 2016).

History and Politics of Home Health

As the practice of home health care has evolved, so have the approaches to pay for it and contain its costs.

History of Home Health

Home health, or home-based, care is as old as the nursing profession itself. For centuries, care of the sick and infirm in the home setting was the standard of practice. In the United States, the earliest known organized effort to care for the sick poor at home was made by the Ladies Benevolent Society in Charleston, South Carolina, in 1813 (Fitzgerald, 2016). Later in the 19th century, women were able to receive training to become nurses in the manner of Florence Nightingale, and wealthy women began to hire them as visiting nurses and to sponsor visiting nurse services. **Visiting Nurse Associations** were established in many American cities (Fulmer, 2017). In 1893, Lillian Wald began home visiting in New York City and is famed for professionalizing visiting nursing.

Evolution of the Laws and Models Governing Home Health Coverage

The payment system for **home health care** has changed dramatically over the last 100 years, from the initiation of its coverage by health insurance to today's value-based models of care:

- 20th century insurance companies saw the benefit of home care as a less expensive alternative to hospitals. Private home health agencies evolved as a result of the demand to provide care for chronically ill clients in their homes.
- During the latter half of the 20th century, Medicare and health insurance companies began to cover home health care, allowing patients to rehabilitate in their homes.
- **Medicare home health benefit** was established to provide intermittent home visits in which nurses and therapists would provide services and instruct clients and families in self-care.

Initially, Medicare and other payers required the period of home health care to be brief and the provision of direct skilled care to be temporary. Home health care services were seen as extensions of medical care, with physicians certifying needed services for short-term treatment of sickness.

The number of Medicare-certified home care agencies grew rapidly until enactment of the Balanced Budget Act of 1997 (Public Law 105-33), which explicitly sought to reduce federal payments for home health care. Payment to providers was changed from reimbursement for each visit to the **Medicare prospective payment system**, which determined Medicare payment rates based on patient characteristics and need for services. Most private insurance agencies followed suit and adopted the standards of the Medicare prospective payment system.

- Standardized reimbursement rates forced Medicare-certified home health agency closures. Patients, requiring intensive skilled and personal services, needed to become independent in providing their health care needs at home. The focus of the home health nurse changed from provision of care to education and training, including evaluation of patient progress.
- The enactment of the ACA impacted the provision of home health care through programs and outcome-based quality care:
  - Supplemental payments for rural home care providers were reinstated for 2010–2015 to address the lower ratio of home care professionals in rural areas throughout the United States as compared with more urban areas.
  - The *Community First Choice Option* allowed states to offer home- and community-based services to people with disabilities through Medicaid rather than institutional care in nursing homes.
  - The *Community Care Transitions Program* helped high-risk Medicare beneficiaries who were hospitalized avoid unnecessary readmissions by coordinating care and connecting patients to services in their communities.
- A 2012 ruling by the U.S. Supreme Court (National Federation of Independent Business et al. vs. Sebelius,

Secretary of Health and Human Services, et al., 2012) allowed for states to opt out of the provision in the act to expand Medicaid services. **Medicaid** services are provided primarily to low-income populations. With a growing percentage of payments for home health coming from Medicaid, this is of concern to care providers and consumers of care. Home health care expenditures from Medicaid are expected to exceed Medicare payments in the coming years. The shift in payment source and the limitation that many states may impose on Medicaid coverage is unknown at this time. The **Centers for Medicare and Medicaid Services (CMS)** oversee expenditures and policy implementation.

- The *Improving Medicare Post-Acute Care Transformation Act of 2014* required postacute care facilities to submit standardized data and changed the requirements for home care agency reimbursement. As a result, Medicare-certified agencies must provide outcome-based quality improvement measures for home care services. The Home Health Quality Reporting Program (HH QRP) uses outcome and process measures and considers patient care, avoidable events, utilization, cost, and resources to mitigate costs and improve care (CMS, 2018a).
- It is mandatory for Medicare-certified home health agencies to participate in HH QRP, and their reporting must include data required by both **Outcome and Assessment Information Set (OASIS)** and Home Health Care Consumer Assessment of Healthcare Providers and Systems (CMS, 2018b).
- The Veterans Administration now pays for home- and community-based services for extended care away from nursing homes (Miller et al., 2017).
- The CMS has also implemented the Home Health Value-Based Purchasing Model (Maddox, et al., 2018).

By 2050, the number of people needing home health care services will increase from 15 to 27 million (United States Department of Health and Human Services [USDHHS], 2018). Currently, 40% of Medicare reimbursement dollars are spent on home care services (MedPac, 2017). Today, over 12,000 home care agencies provide skilled, nonskilled, and therapeutic care services; 98% of these agencies are Medicare certified and 78% Medicaid certified. Home health referrals will continue to increase as an alternative to costly hospital stays as cost containment becomes a driving factor for care (Jones et al., 2017).

- Home health care agencies are increasingly relied on to provide postdischarge care as patients prefer to recover in their homes, shortened hospitalization stays become the mainstay, and insurers benefit from cheaper home care costs (David & Kim, 2018).
- Prior to the ACA, home health agencies had little incentive to reduce hospital readmission. With the current focus on cost containment and better patient outcomes, home care agencies are now held accountable for measurement outcomes as they vie for reimbursement dollars.

Value-Based Care and Cost Containment

HH QRP ensures a **value-based care** reimbursement process for home health care, which has the potential to provide better care and improved patient outcomes at a reduced cost. With reduced readmission, a driving force in cost reduction, **postacute care** following hospitalization will need further scrutiny.

A systematic review by Ma, Shang, Miner, Lennox, and Squires (2018) determined that limited research has been done on patients in home health care who are at high risk for hospital readmission. Patients who were readmitted did not always have an identifiable reason documented, although heart failure and respiratory conditions were noted complications. Further studies that identify the reasons for hospital readmission as well as risk factors associated with readmission are needed to mitigate the challenges associated with postacute home care.

Improving patient outcomes through better care transition processes will assist coordination efforts between agencies and providers. In addition, other models associated with cost reduction are being trialed. Home visit program models with practice-extended teams provide care coordination that is organized around patient and consumer engagement. These nurse-led teams show promise in reducing emergency department visits, Medicare expenditures, and hospitalizations through home visits and illness management for older patients and those with stroke, dementia, and late-stage illness (Ruiz et al., 2018).

Care Coordination

The transition from acute care settings to home health requires coordination of services for seamless care. **Care coordination** is defined as "the organization of patient care activities between two or more participants (including the patient) involved in a patient's care to facilitate the appropriate delivery of health care services" (Agency for Healthcare Research and Quality, 2018, para. 1). Care coordination requires effective communication between agencies and health care providers to support the complex needs of patients.

Care coordination is centered on the patient and family, with attention to navigation through the health care system; care is proactive and planned. As health care shifts from acute to population-based care, the focus is not on episodic events but on postacute care, in which a plan of care and quality transition from the hospital to the community is imperative (Allen, Hutchinson, Brown, & Livingston, 2017). Care coordination models that educate and support families and patients, use registry-based information systems, and promote a team-based care delivery system have been shown to have good patient outcomes (Georgiadis & Corrigan, 2017; Noel, Kaluzynski, & Templeton, 2017; Smith & Treschuk, 2018). Currently, home health care is used to provide postacute care and, in many aspects, is considered a continuation of the acute care setting. However, today's community health nurses may find themselves providing increasingly complex care that requires advanced skills in case management, advocacy, and plan of care to support the comprehensive health care needs of patients and their families.

Home Health Agencies

Home health agencies are organizations that provide various home health care services and equipment to patients in their homes, including skilled health care, custodial (unskilled) care, high-technology pharmacy services, and durable medical equipment (DME). These agencies may be nonprofit or for-profit, public or private, community- or hospital-based, and certified or noncertified.

- *Skilled home health care* is care provided by specialists with licenses, certifications, or specific qualifications, such as nurses, social workers, physical therapists, occupational therapists, and home health aides. Home care agencies who offer skilled care typically have internal and external standards that guide the practice of these skilled practitioners. One such external standard is the code of ethics developed by the NAHC (2020), which serves as a guideline for agencies in ensuring that patients and families are treated with a high standard of care and in an ethical manner. Professional home care agencies may receive referrals from hospitals or other facilities for post-acute follow-up. These patients are considered **homebound** and have a plan of care signed by a physician.
- In contrast, *custodial care* involves unskilled or nonprofessional services, such as cleaning and assistance with daily living, and DME includes wheelchairs, commodes, beds, or oxygen. Agencies that provide such services are not held to the same standards as those that offer skilled care.
- *Nonprofit agencies* traditionally have a charitable mission and are exempt from paying taxes. They are financed with nontax funds such as donations, endowments, United Way contributions, and third-party provider payments.
- *For-profit agencies* are expected to turn a profit on the services they provide, either for the individual owners or for their stockholders.
- *Public agencies*, such as city and county agencies, are government agencies created and empowered through statutes enacted by legislation. These agencies include the nursing divisions of state or local health departments, which may or may not combine care of the sick with traditional public health nursing services, including health promotion, illness prevention, communicable disease investigation, environmental health services, and maternal–child care.
- *Private agencies* are those owned and operated not by government but rather by private individuals or large regional or national chains that are administered through corporate headquarters.
- *Community-based agencies* provide services outside of hospitals within a well-defined geographic location.
- *Hospital-based agencies* operate as separate departments within hospitals and may be nonprofit or for-profit. The referrals to such agencies usually come from the hospital staff. Similar agencies may be found as home health departments in rehabilitation and skilled nursing facilities.
- *Certified agencies* are those that have been certified by Medicare and/or Medicaid to provide and be reimbursed for skilled home health care services.
- *Noncertified agencies* remain outside the federal Medicare and/or Medicaid system that reimburses skilled nursing. Such agencies are usually private and derive their funding from direct payment by the client or from private insurers. They may be governed by individual owners or by corporations. For instance, some agencies offer private duty shifts, unskilled assistance in the home with homemaking or housekeeping, and live-in personal care.

Clients and Their Families

The client in home health care is not only the individual patient but also the family and any significant others. The nurse must consider how the environmental, political, emotional, social, economic, cultural, and religious dimensions impact the client's illness and ability to meet the goals outlined in the plan of care. Not all patients in need of home care are able to pay for these services.

Home care recipients are predominantly older patients with acute and chronic health needs. The medical diagnoses coincide with the morbidity rates of the region. Many have chronic conditions that complicate any acute conditions they experience.

- In the United States, home care agencies serve over 5 million patients, with 82% of the patients over the age of 65 years. A majority of patients are women (70%) and non-Hispanic White; half of all clients cared for in home health have a diagnosis of diabetes (USDHHS, 2018).
- Individuals recovering from severe illness or living with debilitating chronic illness rely on family members or other sources of unpaid assistance. Forty-three million people provide informal caregiving for an adult family member or friend (Family Caregiver Alliance, 2018). Seventy percent of all caregivers are women, with an average age of 49.2 years. Family caregiving tasks range from personal care such as bathing and feeding to sophisticated skilled care, including managing tracheostomies or IV lines.

Nurses must assess the home environment and be responsive to family who may exhibit signs of **compassion fatigue**. These informal caregivers assume a considerable physical, psychological, and economic burden in the care of their loved one at home. As a result, caregivers often describe themselves as emotionally and physically drained and may need information about resources to assist them. Frail older caregivers are especially vulnerable to deterioration of their own health because of their caregiving burden. Likewise, the economic cost of providing home care places a significant burden on informal caregivers. Out-of-pocket expenditures include medications, transportation, home medical equipment, supplies, and respite services. These costs may be nonreimbursable and are often invisible, but they are very real to families struggling to provide care on a fixed income. Home health nurses must continually assess the strain on caregivers as they seek to develop a realistic plan of care.

Home Health Care Personnel

Direct care workers (home care aides and personal care attendants) provide a majority of the functional assistance for the home care team and are expected to increase in number by 70% in the next 10 years (Fig. 30-1; Institute of Medicine [IOM], 2015). Wages in this sector of home care are low and have been stagnant for years. Turnover rates are between 60% and 75% and can affect continuity and the quality of care (IOM, 2015).

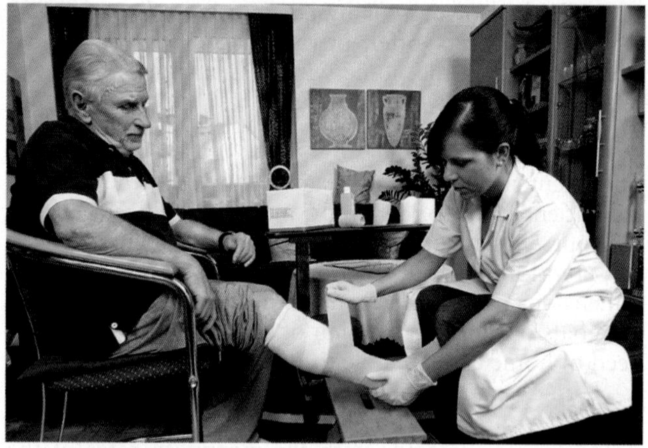

FIGURE 30-1 Skilled care provided in the home setting.

Home care nurses, physical therapy staff, occupational therapists, social workers, and administrative personnel comprise the rest of the home health team. The business and office personnel of a home health agency are critical to the agency's ability to deliver services to clients.

Reimbursement for Home Health Care: Medicare Criteria and Reimbursement

Corporate and governmental third-party payers, as well as individual clients and their families, pay for home health care services. Corporate payers include insurance companies, health maintenance organizations, preferred provider organizations, and case management programs. Government payers include Medicare, Medicaid, the military health system (TRICARE), and the Veterans Administration system. These governmental programs have specific conditions for coverage of services, which are often less flexible than those of corporate payers. For a general description of these reimbursement systems, see Chapter 6. The Medicare policies for home health programs set the precedent for all other reimbursement sources and are discussed below (Fig. 30-2).

Medicare is the largest single payer for home care services in the United States and has set the standard in establishing reimbursement criteria for other payers. Therefore, it is essential that home care nurses seek to understand the complex Medicare home health requirements and rules for determining eligibility for home care

What services are available for America's home health care patients?

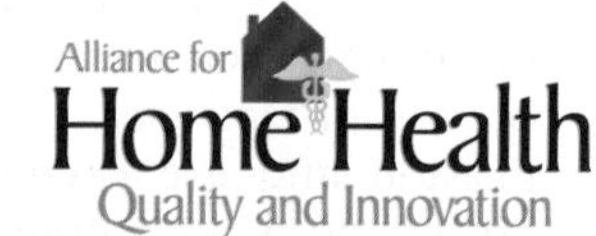

Medicare Home Health Benefit

The **Medicare home health benefit** covers skilled nursing care and therapy services provided to patients in their own residence. The patient must be under the care of a physician, meet the definition of "homebound," and be in need of skilled services on an intermittent basis. Patients receive home health care following an acute care hospital discharge or because they require certain rehabilitation services.

Services include care from highly skilled nurses, physical therapists, occupational therapists, speech-language pathologists, and medical social workers. Home health aides provide personal care services for patients also in need of skilled services.

Medicaid Home Health Benefit

The **Medicaid Home Health benefit** varies by state but is generally broader than the Medicare benefit and commonly provides a combination of highly-skilled medical care and personal care services. States must provide home health services and transportation to care.

Depending on the state in question, states can provide related services, including: pediatric care; physical, occupational and speech therapy; private duty nursing services; personal care; and case management.

Veterans Administration Home Health Care

There are several types of home health services available to Veterans:

Skilled Home Health Care (SHHC) Services, which are short-term services that include nursing care, therapy visits and social work support.

Home Based Primary Care is for Veterans with complex health needs, such as multiple chronic conditions. Care includes primary care visits in the patient's residence, case management services, and mental health services.

Homemaker and Home Health Aide Care is care provided to Veterans to assist them with activities of daily living.

"Home Care" Long-Term Care Provided at Home

"**Home Care**" is a broad term that encompasses all care provided to a person in their residence. Home care reflects Medicare- skilled professionals and their services, skilled or personal care through Medicaid, or care through private pay programs. Home care may also include social services offered through state Area Agencies on Aging, as well as care provided by Private Duty Nurses. In addition to a wide range of services, home care is provided to a diverse group of patients - children, the elderly, the disabled, and U.S. Veterans.

Ultimately, "home care" is an umbrella term used to describe the full spectrum of care, services and equipment provided in a patient's home through various local, state, federal, insurance and private pay options.

Skilled, Clinical Care | Skilled, Clinical Care & Social/Functional Support

Source: Home Health Care Services and Benefits by Payer • Available at www.ahhqi.org WWW.AHHQI.ORG

FIGURE 30-2 Home health care services and benefits by payer. (Reprinted with permission from Alliance for Home Health Quality and Innovation. (2018). *Home health care services and benefits by payer.* Retrieved from http://www.ahhqi.org/images/pdf/what-is-hhc-services-available.pdfFigure)

BOX 30-1 Medicare Home Health Eligibility Criteria

1. The patient must be confined to the home or **homebound**.
2. The patient must need skilled services (from a nurse or therapist).
3. The patient must be under the care of a physician.
4. The patient must receive services under a home health plan of care (POC) that is established and periodically reviewed by a physician.
5. The patient must have had a face-to-face encounter that is related to the primary reason the patient requires home health services with a physician or an allowed NPP (this must be done 90 days prior to the home health start-of-care date or within 30 days of the start of the home health care).

services. It is important to acknowledge that a person may be in dire need of care at home, yet not meet eligibility standards for home health care under Medicare. There are five criteria that must all be met to be eligible for reimbursement by Medicare (CMS, 2019; Boxes 30-1 and 30-2).

The following steps are implemented while the patient is under Medicare-reimbursed home health care:

1. The Medicare prospective payment system pays an agency for a 60-day "episode of care." All services and many medical supplies must be provided under the payment amount adjusted to geographic location and determined by the patient's clinical and functional status at the start of care, as well as the projected need for services over the anticipated 60-day period (CMS, 2018c).
2. When the patient is admitted, the patient is comprehensively assessed using an assessment tool called OASIS. OASIS is used to measure home health quality measures and is the basis for measuring patient outcomes and adherence to best practice for quality improvement.
3. The nurse also completes the Medicare plan of care at admission, and the physician must sign this. It is then used to assess agency compliance with Medicare and state requirements. All follow-up services must match the plan of care.
4. It is a Medicare requirement that patients receiving home health care must be recertified every 60 days. A determination of continued visits is then made based on the objective data obtained (CMS, 2018c). Box 30-3 provides consumer information on quality home care agencies by zip code or city.

BOX 30-3 Compare Home Health Care Providers

The Medicare.gov Web site offers information for consumers about the quality of home health care agencies. It includes data on how frequently best practices are used in patient care and if patients improved in relation to certain aspects of care. It also includes patient feedback about recent home health agency experiences.

You and/or your clients can go to https://www.medicare.gov/homehealthcompare/search.html and enter your zip code (or city, state), and you can see a list of all agencies and the services provided by each (that meet certain criteria). You may select agencies for comparison, and general information is provided, along with the quality patient care information and results of patient surveys. For quality patient care, star ratings are used to denote summaries of 9 out of 29 quality measures, with 4 or 5 stars indicating better performance than other agencies. Star rankings of one or two indicate below-average performance. Most agencies nationwide fall within 3 or 3.5 stars. Survey results include percentages related to how often care was given in a professional manner, how well the team communicated with clients, if they discussed pain, medications, and home safety with clients, how the client rates their overall care from this agency, and would they recommend the agency to family/friends. Overall percentages can be graphed for comparison with state and national averages.

Home Health Nursing Practice

The practice of home health nursing has roots in community/public health nursing (see Chapters 2 and 3). The nurse provides home health nursing care to acute, chronic, and terminally ill clients of all ages in their homes while

BOX 30-2 PERSPECTIVES

A Nursing Instructor's Viewpoint on Medicare Guidelines

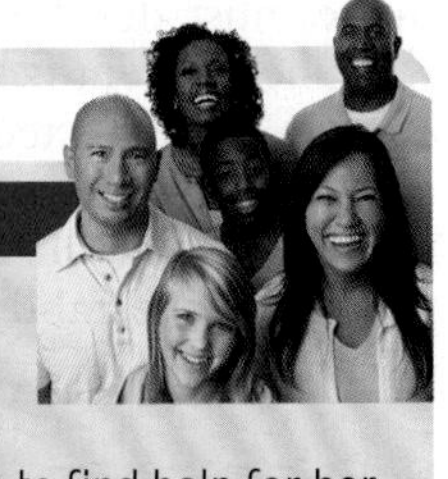

It is vital to develop an expanded vision about the health care needs of frail elders and the kinds of services that are needed in the community. Sometimes, after nurses have been working in Medicare home health for a while, they may begin to identify more with the Medicare guidelines than with their patients. Too often, I have heard experienced home health nurses say about a patient living with severe chronic illness, "She doesn't deserve services. She doesn't have skilled needs."

In contrast, I would hope knowledgeable nurses would say to families and decision makers, "She needs and deserves services, but the Medicare home health benefit will not pay for them. Our agency cannot continue to provide care because of the limits imposed on us. We'll do everything possible to find help for her, but resources are limited." This kind of insight leads to patient advocacy, development of community networks, and becoming outspoken about needed changes in health policy. Visiting nurses witness the struggles of chronically ill people living at home; we must not abandon them.

Beth L., nursing instructor

integrating public health nursing principles that focus on the environmental, psychosocial, economic, cultural, and personal health factors affecting the client's health status and well-being. Home health is a unique field of nursing practice that requires a synthesis of public health nursing principles with the theory and practice of medical/surgical, geriatric, mental health, and other nursing specialties. According to the American Nurses Association (ANA) *Scope and Standards of Practice for Home Health Nursing* (2014), home health nursing goes beyond providing skilled nursing care in the home; it requires the ability of the nurse to coordinate a broad variety of services and professional caregivers to manage patients' complex health problems (the standards of practice are available on thePoint).

Nursing Practice During the Home Visit

A home visit by a home health nurse involves several steps: locating, promoting self-management, detecting, collaborating, mobilizing, strengthening, teaching, and solving problems.

Locating the Client and Getting through the Door. The first step in making a home visit is finding where the person lives. Directions and household identification can be unclear. In rural areas, tracking down clients can involve vague instructions involving barns, bridges, trees, and other colorful local landmarks. When families are unstable, clients may not be staying in households designated on the nurse's paperwork. They may have moved in with relatives or friends or be back home alone despite major care needs (Box 30-4).

Even when the wheels stop at the correct household, there is the challenge of getting through the closed door and making the connection. *Always remember that you are a guest in the home*. Respect and attentive listening are the foundation for establishment of trust between the client and nurse. Agendas must be laid aside initially as the nurse focuses on the concerns and realities of both the client and family. Assumptions and stereotypes are overturned in the process of discovering how clients live, what they believe, and who comprises their family and community. The nurse must take into account the spiritual, cultural, and developmental, as well as environmental, realms of the client in order to be able to develop individualized plans of care to promote health.

The home health nurse is aware that the client is the driver of the plan of care. To have effective outcomes, the nurse must develop a therapeutic relationship in which the client identifies the desired outcomes. Autonomy should be respected, and the family should be empowered by actions recognizing that they are in charge of their lives. The nurse, the patient, and family must work together to establish mutually agreed-upon goals (see Chapter 10).

Hub of the Family Caregiving Wheel: Promoting Self-Management. The practice competencies of home health nurses can be illustrated with the home health nursing caregiving wheel (Fig. 30-3). The hub, or most essential competency, of this wheel is promoting independent self-care and self-management. The challenge to the home health nurse is often assisting the severely chronically ill

BOX 30-4 STORIES FROM THE FIELD

Beyond the Front Door

I received a home visit referral from the VA clinic after the client missed two appointments. The client was a 77-year-old male veteran with a diagnosis of diabetes and right heel ulcer who needed IV antibiotics, and wound care twice a day. I had the address; I circled around the block a couple of times; the house was in a residential neighborhood in the middle of town, a block from an elementary school. The client did not have a phone. I parked close to the address and walked; only then did I see through the 5-foot weeds in front of the house.

I approached the door, knocked, and called for Mr. P a couple of times. He finally answered. An unkempt, unbathed elderly man crawling on his knees (due to his inability to put weight on his right foot), with a toothless smile, let me in and sat in an old chair by the door. Introductions were made.

The home was very dark and dusty; piles of books, magazines, and newspapers were stacked 3 and 4 feet high in between furniture leaving a small maze in which to walk through the house. The VA had sent 2 months of supplies, which were in dozens of boxes by the front door. The house was dark, but the kitchen windows provided some light. I noticed there were no appliances in the kitchen, only piles of books, a Styrofoam ice chest on the floor (inside was warm milk and green lunch meat), and open cans of food in the sink.

Assessment reveals blood glucose of 355, 4-inch diameter stage 3 wound on the right heel, and pain level of 8 out of 10 (had not taken prescribed pain meds). Mr. P is very cooperative and talkative. He has lived alone in the house for over 40 years and never married. Family lives an hour away; he has not seen them in 10 or more years. No friends locally, many have passed on. Mr. P has no car; the closest VA clinic is 90 miles away. He purchases food from the corner grocer but says he has been unable recently to walk to the store.

1. *What are your nursing priorities?*
2. *Reflect on Mr. P's lifestyle. What do you think would have happened to Mr. P. if the nurses did not find him?*
3. *Apply the nursing process to comprehensively identify and prioritize nursing diagnoses and propose interventions. Use Figure 30-3 to guide your care planning.*

Anne Stokman, MSN, RN, CDE

client be able to adapt in the community to be safe and functional. Coordination with other professionals must often be instituted to provide comprehensive quality care. This may include social workers, clergy, physical therapists, occupational therapists, as well as mental health professionals.

Rim of the Home Health Caregiving Wheel: Detecting. Nurses in the home are challenged by an extraordinarily complex environment with much to investigate and continuing assessment process as the nurse seeks to understand the client's health in the context of home. The nurse keeps her ears and eyes "wide open." Who lives in the home? How do they interact? Who are the caregivers,

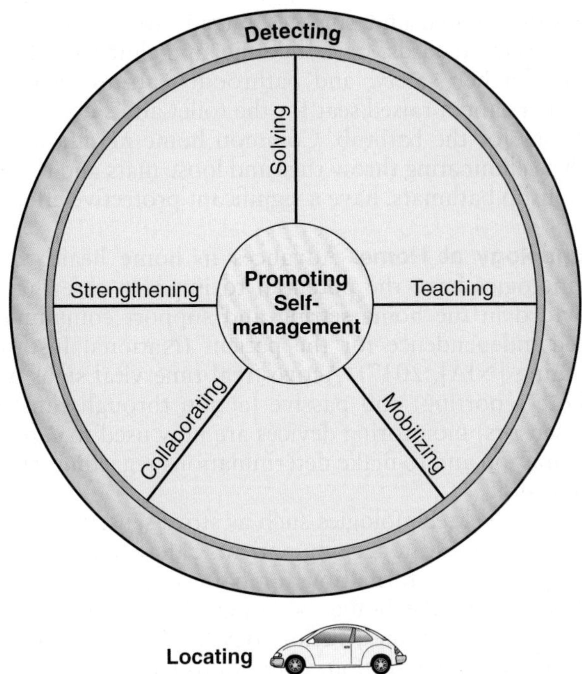

FIGURE 30-3 Home health nursing caregiving wheel.

and how do they care? What is the relevance of culture and religion in the life of the household? How does the physical environment impact patient safety and security? Home visits reveal discoveries that can never be imagined in clinic or hospital settings. Take for example the client whose refrigerator no longer chills and whose impaired vision prevents awareness of the expanding family of roaches in the kitchen.

Spokes of the Home Health Caregiving Wheel: Collaborating, Mobilizing, Strengthening, Teaching, Solving Problems. Home health nursing competencies that radiate from the hub and contribute to promotion of self-care and family care include *collaborating* with multiple team members and *mobilizing resources* in the community that can sustain the client after discharge. The home health care nurse usually is the coordinator of all other home health team members. Working with the social worker, the nurse proposes needed connections with community services. Likewise, *strengthening* involves development of self-management or family caregiving ability. The home health nurse is constantly *teaching* clients and/or family caregivers through concrete explanation, discussion, and modeling behavior. Concerns and relevant feelings must be validated, and the nurse leads the person to consider options for change. The solution develops through a mutual, participatory process. Ultimately, people are responsible for their own health decisions (see Chapter 11).

Finally, home health nursing competency requires flexibility and creativity in *solving* health care problems and the challenges of everyday living. All outcomes of care can be achieved only by adapting to the skills and resources available in the home. Although people of all socioeconomic backgrounds present with severe health problems requiring home health nursing, many families live on the margins. The home health nurse must often be creative in obtaining supplies and adjusting to conditions in the home. For example, how do patients and families with no running water wash their hands before providing care, such as dressing changes? This may lead the home health nurse to contact social agencies in order to provide services or teach the patient and family the use of alcohol-based gels to clean their hands. The home health nurse must be nonjudgmental but work with the patient and family to help them understand the need to keep areas clean.

Home Health Nursing Case Management

The home health nurse is the case manager for each client and responsible for coordination of the other professionals and paraprofessionals involved in the client's care.

The home care nurse is frequently the primary contact with the client's physician, collaborating on the initial plan of care, reporting changes in the client's condition, and securing changes in the plan of care. The nurse may conduct case conferences among team members to share information, discuss problems, and plan actions to affect the best possible outcomes for the client. The nurse case manager also supervises the paraprofessionals, such as home health aides, who also serve the homebound client.

Selected Nursing Challenges in the Home

Working in the home immerses the nurse in challenges unlike anything encountered in controlled institutional environments. Some of these include infection control, medication safety, fall risk, technology at home, and nurse safety (see Chapter 22, Older Adults).

Infection Control. Home health nurses frequently need to work with the family to prevent infection in clients who are debilitated and may be immunocompromised; in addition, many are now dwelling at home with invasive medical devices that make them especially vulnerable to infection. Likewise, nurses are challenged to consider how to protect the home health care team, family, and community from a client with contagious disease. In such cases, all people living in the home will need instruction. Some households have inadequate facilities to control disease transmission. There may be no access to running water, no heating unit to boil equipment, or inadequate facilities to dispose of contaminated equipment. These conditions necessitate the development of creative solutions to control infection.

To guide the nurse, home health agencies have adapted infection control policies and procedures based on the Centers for Disease Control and Prevention's (CDCs) Infection Control Precautions for health care settings with each agency setting up their own specific policy and procedure based upon the standard (CDC, 2018a).

Medication Safety. The home health client taking multiple medications is at particular risk of multiple errors in self-administration, including incorrect medication, dose, time, interval, or route. Often, doses are missed or doubled. Clients may discontinue a drug or not complete the full course. Sometimes, the drug or drugs ordered are inappropriate considering the patient's condition at home.

The home presents risk of medication errors that are different from those found in hospital or nursing home. Every visiting nurse has stories of finding drawers and cupboards filled with multiple prescriptions from various physicians, some current and some outdated for many years. Polypharmacy becomes obvious in the home setting. Clients often have received prescriptions from multiple sources for similar drugs. Also, well-meaning friends often share their prescriptions with the attitude that it "helped them." Even if the client is well organized and taking every drug prescribed, those prescriptions may have originated from several providers over time and may have contradictory side effects. Sometimes, medication errors at home include failure to clearly reconcile hospital or nursing home orders with home discharge orders. Although weekly medication organizers can helpfully put medications in order, they can also confuse new or impaired users. Distraction, visual impairment, forgetfulness, depression, and cognitive impairment are common causes of unintentional medication noncompliance. The home health nurse investigates how the medication is taken by reviewing and reconciling the current list of medications and having the patient explain and demonstrate the process he or she goes through. Intervention requires clear and repeated instruction, updating the medication list, charting or diagramming the schedule for medication taking, and assuring that the client or caregiver knows how to use the medication box.

Risk of Falling. Falls are a serious issue especially for the elderly. Estimates are that one in four adults 65 years and older will fall each year, and falls are the number one cause of injury and death from injuries in the United States (CDC, 2018b). Physiological risk factors include orthostatic hypotension and cardiac dysrhythmias, dizziness, neurologic and musculoskeletal effects on gait and balance, urinary urgency, impaired hearing or vision, alcohol or drug abuse, and medication effects impairing alertness, balance, urinary frequency, and blood pressure. Clients should be observed as they move through their home and carry out activities of daily living (Fig. 30-4). It is important to investigate factors that obstruct movement or threaten balance. The nurse in the home should inspect sidewalks, stairs, and surfaces outside the home; floor, rugs, electrical cords, stairs, lighting, and clutter inside the home; kitchen safety; and bathroom features including grab bars and a raised seat for the toilet and safety modifications for the bathtub. Common home modifications, such as eliminating throw rugs and loose mats and the use of nonslip bathmats, have a significant protective effect.

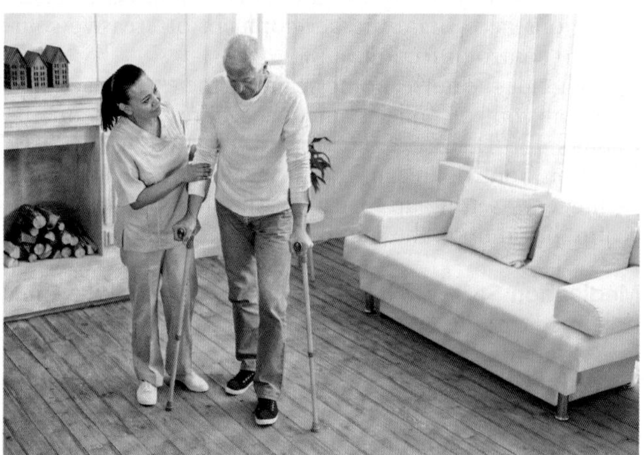

FIGURE 30-4 Fall risk patients need safe home environments.

Technology at Home. Advances in home health care technologies have the potential to improve care that is provided in the home setting and support community-based independence for the patient (National Institute of Aging [NIA], 2017). Active (real-time vital signs and remote reporting) and passive (action through cameras and sensors) monitoring devices are now used to capture information and to make determinations regarding safety and health.

Low-level technologies such as stove sensors or door alarms can assist in keeping patients safe while also providing trended information for patterns and behaviors. Technology in the home can range from using a telephone to smart homes. Technology use has the potential to improve collaboration, care coordination, and communication with providers (NIA, 2017). Data gathered from technology devices can be compiled and used to evaluate patient outcomes and processes for better home care (Box 30-5).

In addition, real-time information is now used in home health to update and change the plan of care. Nurses may use handheld devices to chart. Medical records may be available instantly on the nurse's laptop or tablet, and daily telemedicine monitoring of electrocardiogram, blood pressure, oxygen saturation, and other vital measures can be transmitted electronically to a home health agency or physician office. These assessments can be monitored, and the patient plan of care may be altered based on the analysis. See Chapter 10 for more on technology in the community.

Nurse Safety. Home health nurses face risks not only in driving to their client's homes but also because of environmental hazards: the nurses must be constantly aware of personal safety and surroundings. Client homes are uncontrolled environments, and nurses may face instances of family violence and illegal drug activity, or weapons may be present. The surrounding neighborhood also may pose risks of violence, car theft, vandalism, and robbery. Many home health organizations and their nurses work closely with local law enforcement agencies to identify the wisest process for visiting dangerous neighborhoods and isolated rural areas. Every home health care agency should have a carefully developed program to assure the safety of personnel traveling to homes and training on how to predict aggressive behaviors and diffuse threatening circumstances, along with methods of self-protection if threats escalate (see Chapter 15 for more information on home visits).

The Future of Care in the Home

Home health care has high value as it is patient preferred and low cost and has improved patient outcomes as compared to other postacute care settings (IOM, 2015).

BOX 30-5 PERSPECTIVES

A Home Care Nurse's Viewpoint on Home Care Technology

During my early years in home care, we carried pagers, which resulted in delayed patient care coordination. Today, we have improved patient care transitions and outcomes with advances in home care technology.

I recently visited a 98-year-old man discharged from the hospital with newly diagnosed heart failure. Prior to my visit, a home telehealth device was installed in his home. It was programmed to provide heart failure education daily for 1 year. The patient attaches a blood pressure cuff and O_2 oximeter and steps on a scale, and the device automatically records his blood pressure, pulse, O_2 saturation, and weight. A remote telehealth RN daily reviews his health data. Working from a standard order set, the RN had increased the patient's diuretic dose.

During the visit, the patient provided me health data from his telehealth log, and he had questions about his diuretic therapy. I accessed his clinic and hospital records through my laptop computer using a protected hotspot with my cell phone. I operated a mobile lab device to obtain laboratory results. The patient received immediate information about his diuretic regimen. Technology played an important role in preventing another hospitalization for this high-risk patient.

Janelle Culjis, RN, PhD, ANP

However, the current framework of home health care was not designed to support our aging demographic population.

- Key challenges for home health care include fragmented care coordination, delivery of optimal care with current Medicare restrictions, value over volume, and an infrastructure to support aging in the home (IOM, 2015).
- Rising medical costs support home health care as it is a cost-effective means of delivering care. System reforms that address value-based care, quality of care, cost reduction, and coordination of care are needed. Emerging models for payment and care delivery are starting to address these issues and to realize the full potential of home health for population care.

HOSPICE CARE

Although science and technology have advanced in the world of health care, death is ultimately inevitable for all of us. The contemporary circumstances of death in America are often dehumanizing; most people die in hospitals and long-term care institutions, surrounded by strangers. Uncertainty and denial often prevail during the final stage of life because prognoses are uncertain, and many serious illnesses are now treated aggressively until the last breath. The battle against the "evil" of death seems to be the primary emphasis, with patient, family, and professionals wanting to believe that it is possible to win the final struggle. In the 21st century, fatal conditions have been turned into expensive chronic illnesses. Too often, discomfort is not relieved, and treatment causes further suffering. And as the period of disability extends and the body deteriorates, social isolation develops. In dramatic contrast to the dehumanization of death, the **hospice** movement has developed to humanize the end-of-life experience and provide palliative care. **Palliative interventions** relieve suffering without curing underlying disease. The hospice movement has emphasized four major changes in end-of-life care:

- Care should encompass body, mind, and spirit.
- Death should be discussed and not considered off-limits.
- Medical technology should be used only when absolutely necessary.
- Clients should be actively involved in discussions about treatment decisions.

Table 30-1 contrasts home health with hospice. This section explores the evolution of hospice care in the United States, describes hospice agencies, and examines Medicare criteria for hospice reimbursement. It concludes with an exploration of the unique characteristics of hospice nursing practice.

Evolution of Hospice Care

In medieval Europe, hospices were refuges for the sick and dying. The contemporary hospice movement originated in England, where a physician, Dame Cicely Saunders, founded St. Christopher's Hospice in 1967. Dr. Saunders was credentialed as a nurse, social worker, and physician, and she developed a unique program based both on compassion and skillful relief of physical discomfort through around-the-clock analgesics administered by mouth. It had been previously assumed that only injections, administered sparingly, could be used for terminal pain control. In 1974, the first hospice in the United States was established in Branford, Connecticut. Florence Wald, who was then Dean of the Yale School of Nursing, led this movement. Because even in the 1970s, there was concern about saving money by keeping less critical patients out of the hospital and shortening hospital stays, and hospices in the United States came to focus on providing care in the home. To that end, Congress established the permanent Medicare hospice benefit in 1986, with the intention of keeping people at home, yet receiving comprehensive services that are less expensive than hospitalization (National Hospice and Palliative Care Organization, 2015).

Hospice characteristics have changed over time. Initially, nearly all clients suffered from terminal cancer; presently, people with a variety of end-stage diseases are served. The criteria for being accepted into hospice care are that the patient has been diagnosed with a life-limiting disease and death is likely within 6 months or less. Hospice care is designed not only for the patient but also for support of family members. While cancer remains the top disease qualifying a patient for hospice services, cardiac,

TABLE 30-1 Contrasts Between Home Health and Hospice

Hospice	Home Health
Emphasis is on quality of life and comfort.	Emphasis is on treatment or therapy to restore independence.
Focus is on health of the whole family.	Focus is on health of the client.
Plan of care is guided by client choice.	Plan of care is determined by medical need and client choice.
The nurse is the case manager until death.	The nurse is the case manager until home health discharge.
The client chooses how to live last days.	Priority is given to correcting physiologic imbalances.
Intermittent visits increase in frequency as death becomes imminent.	Intermittent visits decrease in frequency as the client stabilizes.
Nurses are expert in symptom control.	Symptom control is the domain of the physician with some nurses having expertise.
Sedatives and opioids are expertly adjusted to eliminate suffering.	Sedatives and opioids are used hesitantly to reduce suffering.
End-of-life disease course is managed to avoid crises.	End-of-life problems tend to be seen as medical crises.
The goal is for symptoms at end of life to be managed at home if possible. Hospice care is also provided outside of home.	Care provided in client's home. The client must be homebound. The client is brought to a hospital for unmanaged symptoms.
Spiritual care is focus of whole team.	Spiritual needs are met by own clergy.
Survivors have bereavement support.	No bereavement support is provided.

circulatory, and respiratory disorders and dementia are also predominant. Palliative care provided in hospice services is designed to ease pain and suffering and improve quality of life and can be offered in earlier stages of illness, along with continuing medical treatments. With prognoses difficult to predict and denial of death by the patient and family a continuing issue, some hospice referrals are now made very late in the disease process. The National Hospice and Palliative Care Organization (NHPCO) (2020) cites the fact that in 2016, 48% of all Medicare decedents or 1.43 million Medicare beneficiaries had received one or more days of hospice care (p. 3). The NHPCO (2020) also cites the average length of hospice services as 71 days with a median of 24 days of service (p. 4).

Hospice Services and Reimbursement

As in home health care, Medicare has determined the way services are provided. The **Medicare hospice benefit** requires that a client who has a prognosis of 6 months or less must sign up for the comfort-focused hospice benefit and waive regular Medicare health services, except for conditions unrelated to their terminal illness. This mandates that the client acknowledges a terminal prognosis and chooses comfort care instead of life-extending care from a Medicare-approved hospice. When this choice is made, the hospice coordinates care in all settings, functioning both as clinical and financial case manager. The government pays a flat rate to the hospice for each day the patient receives care. There are four payment levels:

- Routine home care with intermittent visits
- Continuous home care when the patient's condition is acute and death is near
- Inpatient hospital care for symptom relief
- Respite care in a nursing home to relieve family members (CMS, 2015)

Hospices coordinate home care and direct inpatient care if needed. The emphasis is on palliative care, with a focus on physical, psychosocial, and spiritual comfort. Palliative care is caring for the patient holistically with an emphasis on improving the quality of life through caring and decreasing the severity of the symptoms of the illness. A strong emphasis is placed on caring for the entire family.

The hospice team includes nurses, physicians, home health aides, physical and occupational therapists, social workers, volunteers, palliative medication and medical equipment specialists, and bereavement counselors. Staff members meet regularly to explore together the challenges of assuring comfort at the end of life. A nurse or physician is available on-call 24 hours a day/7 days a week (CMS, 2015).

Trained volunteers fill an important need in hospice care. They act as companions to the client when the family must be somewhere else or is away for short respite. They run errands for family members, shop, organize hot meals prepared by friends and neighbors, provide childcare, and perform other services as needed.

Hospice and Palliative Care Nursing Practice

The nurse's role is central in the hospice interdisciplinary team. The hospice/palliative care nurse functions as case manager and visits the client more frequently than other members of the team. Nurses work in close collaboration with physicians in the development of a plan of care to assure management of symptoms. This plan of care changes rapidly as the end of life nears. In addition to home visits focusing on palliation and interdisciplinary planning, hospice nurses rotate through 24-hour call 7 days a week to assure continuous availability by telephone and visits for emergent problems reported by the client or family. Hospice nursing competencies and challenges are similar to those described for home health nurses, with the added expertise needed to relieve physical and emotional suffering of terminally ill clients and their families. Hospice and palliative care nurses become expert clinicians in symptom management as they anticipate and treat the physiological and psychological effects of the disease process on the patient. The ANA and the Hospice and Palliative Nurses Association (HPNA) (2014) have established standards of practice for hospice and palliative nursing. Certification of hospice and palliative nursing is available. An overview of palliative care nursing standards encompasses the same general standards as home health nursing standards, with specific competencies delineated (e.g., comfort care, suffering and symptom palliation, support of patient/family throughout illness course, reaffirmation of goals with families during regularly scheduled family meetings, care coordination with interdisciplinary team members).

Nursing practice in hospice settings is a continuation of acute care nursing. The emphasis is on holistic care not curative care. While the nurse has an expert role in pain management, he or she also plans a managerial role in controlling symptoms and adverse effects on the body from the disease process. The ultimate objective is to support the patient while on the journey to a peaceful dignified death (Fig. 30-5). Care is centered on patients and families, generally begins with life-threatening illness, and ends with family bereavement care.

Hospice caregiving can be illustrated as a tree, strongly rooted in the process of nurses deliberately practicing self-care for themselves (Fig. 30-6). This tree has been drawn to explain the expert competencies of hospice nurses who were interviewed to capture the essence of their practice, as described by Zerwekh (1995, 2006).

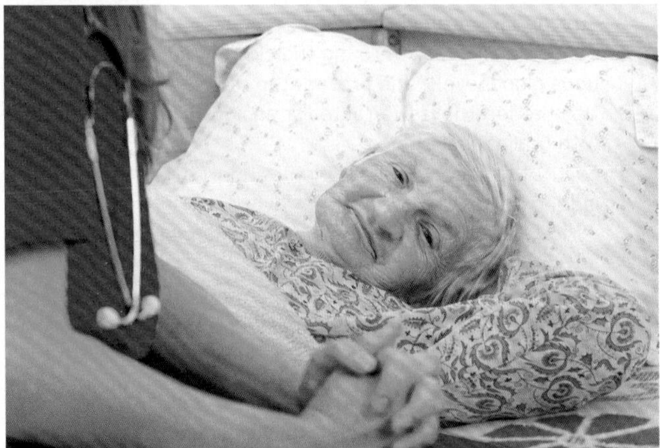

FIGURE 30-5 Providing comfort and emotional support to patients and their families is an essential role of hospice care.

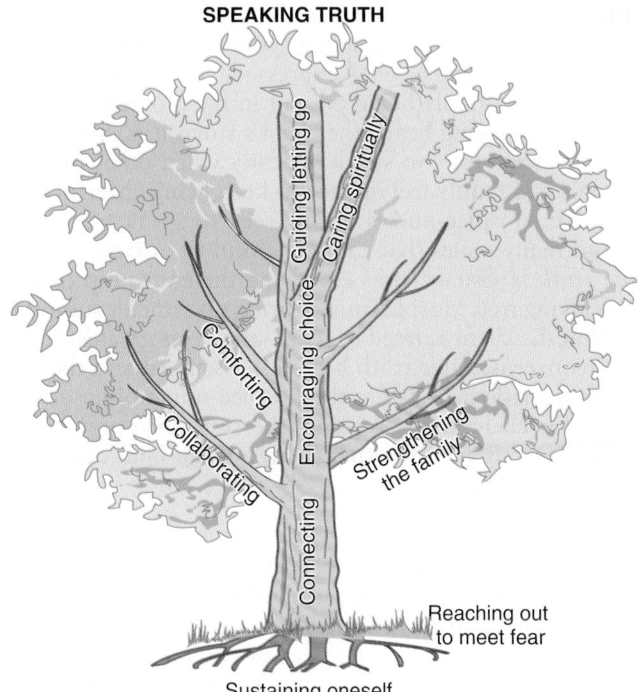

FIGURE 30-6 The hospice caregiving tree.

Each of the hospice nursing practices visualized by the tree diagram is briefly summarized below.

Roots of Hospice Nursing: Sustaining Oneself

Effective hospice nurses understand that to care for others, they must care for themselves. Caring for clients at the end of life can be physically and emotionally draining. The hospice nurse works with clients and families to psychologically prepare for death of a loved one. The nurse often becomes emotionally attached to the dying client and needs to sustain their own emotional well-being to be an effective advocate for the client and family. *Sustaining oneself* requires deliberate effort to maintain one's own physical, emotional, and spiritual well-being. Knowing oneself, identifying sources of stress, and learning how to care for self are important and provide the roots for hospice caring. Expert hospice nurses keep themselves healthy by maintaining a balance between giving and receiving, letting go of predetermined agendas and idealistic hopes to achieve more than is humanly possible, being emotionally open and clear, and deliberately replenishing themselves to restore their energy. Hospice nurses described their emotional challenges as being simultaneously draining and enriching experiences leading to personal and professional growth and development (Ingebretsen & Saghakken, 2016, p. 1).

The Trunk Reaching Upward: Connecting, Speaking Truth, and Encouraging Choice

Rooted in self-care, hospice nurses practice *connecting*, which refers to the centrality of relationships in providing hospice care. The hospice nurse seeks to understand the emotional and spiritual distress common to the end of life, particularly the progressive experience of loss after loss. Guided by that understanding, hospice nurses emphasize attentive listening to understand each individual's unique story. This requires quieting your own thoughts to truly hear what is being expressed. Sometimes, listening involves simply being present in the moment, paying attention. Having heard the client's story, it is important for hospice nurses to speak honestly when other professionals and family feel obliged to keep being cheerful and positive. Hospice nurses openly seek to speak truthfully about many issues that can be painful to discuss. *Speaking truth* is visualized as encircling the entire top of the caregiving tree. Hospice nurses bring up difficult subjects, so that the client is freed to speak about his greatest fears and concerns. After truth has been discussed and the client has made a decision, the hospice nurse often advocates for client wishes against the resistance of various authorities. Remember that these are the final decisions in a dying person's life.

Collaborating

Interdisciplinary teamwork is an essential branch on the tree. The hospice interdisciplinary team members share information and work interdependently. The hospice nurse coordinates the plan of care and day-to-day efforts to provide physical and psychosocial comfort. The hospice nurse supervises licensed and unlicensed personnel in carrying out comfort interventions. The physician is responsible for medical care and serves as liaison with the client's primary care physicians. Social workers, spiritual counselors, physical therapists, pharmacists, and volunteers are integral members of the hospice team as they provide environmental, developmental, and spiritual interventions to aid the patient with psychological peace. The hospice interdisciplinary team is constantly challenged to work creatively together to find solutions for complex end-of-life suffering with emotional, spiritual, and physical components.

Strengthening the Family

The death of a family member causes great disruption for all involved. When family members are in a caregiving role in the home, they experience significant personal suffering. Caregivers are vulnerable to physical and emotional illness themselves. The process of taking care involves managing the illness as well as all practical assistance, seeking information and resources, and preparing for death itself. Family members often are caught up with family issues and struggles with the health care system. An extremely important role in hospice nursing involves supporting family members' abilities as caregivers. Teaching caregiving requires creative teaching methods and flexibility. The hospice nurse often acts as a liaison between the patient and family as well as among family members.

Comforting

Hospice nurses develop extensive expertise in pain and symptom management. The fear of many hospice clients and families is that pain will not be controlled. Most pain can be controlled through careful monitoring and intervention. Box 30-6 lists fundamental palliative principles, and Box 30-7 identifies four important components of pain relief.

BOX 30-6 Fundamentals of Palliative Care

- Make no assumptions about what is wrong.
- Believe the patient's report of symptoms.
- Relieve discomfort to the extent that the patient chooses and finds acceptable.
- Investigate the biologic, psychosocial, and spiritual dimensions of discomfort.
- Anticipate symptoms and relieve them before they occur again.
- Use nursing and complementary (integrative) interventions.
- Become an expert in the use of palliative medication.
- Continually evaluate the effectiveness of interventions.
- Choose the least complex and most manageable interventions that patients and families can manage themselves at home.
- Never give up. Persist in trying different palliative strategies. Remember the patient and caregiver are both involved in treatment.

Spiritual Practice and Letting Go

As death draws near, spiritual needs often intensify as the client searches for meaning and hope. Death is a developmental milestone as well as a spiritual and physical journey. The effect of the journey on the client is impacted by the environmental and cultural habits and customs the client has experienced through the lifetime. Spirituality is a broad concept that the individual client defines as to what has given his or her life meaning and purpose. Religion and spirituality are related in that religion is a system of beliefs and doctrines that aid the client in expressing what gives the client meaning and hope. In a multisite study of quality of life for advanced cancer patients being treated with palliative radiation, researchers found that

BOX 30-7 Essential Components of Pain Relief

1. Continually assess the extent of pain and the relief afforded by interventions.
2. Schedule analgesics around the clock to maintain continuous blood levels, and prevent the return of pain.
3. Use the least invasive route for analgesic administration, with oral as first choice.
4. Follow the World Health Organization (2016) three-step ladder:
   Step 1 for mild pain: Nonopioid (acetaminophen or NSAID) plus adjuvant such as corticosteroid, antidepressant, anxiolytic, or anticonvulsant
   Step 2 for persisting pain: Opioid and nonopioid and/or adjuvant
   Step 3 for moderate to severe pain: Strong opioid and nonopioid and/or adjuvant

Note: The WHO also offers guidelines for persisting pain in children: www.who.int/medicines/areas.quality_safety.guide_perspainchild/en/
Source: World Health Organization (2016).

those who used religious and spiritual coping reported improved quality of life on all outcome measures. Spiritual distress has been long recognized by nurses as a factor that can rob the client of peace. Spiritual peace comes when the client realizes his or her life had meaning, purpose, and hope. Attainment of the spiritual peace calms the patient. Nurses may be called upon to intervene with their patient through prayer and active listening as they help the client to reframe life events and accept love and support from others. *Guiding letting go* is a truly unique nursing practice that involves helping the client to let go of former activities and hopes, including life itself. This involves listening to intense emotions and helping the person and family find resolution (Raingruber & Wolf, 2015). Sometimes, it involves participating in a vigil at the bedside of the dying person and encouraging loved ones to say their final words of farewell. It is this action that often is that one thing that gives the client peace (Box 30-8).

Ethical Challenges in Hospice Nursing

The hospice nurse confronts striking ethical challenges at the end of life. As an advocate for the client, the hospice nurse must integrate his or her own knowledge of the pathophysiology of the disease process with the physiological needs of the dying client while accounting for the psychological and cultural needs of the client and family (Storch, 2015). As client advocates, we, as nurses, must be aware of the ethical challenges surrounding the dying experience. Wide-ranging issues include respect or disregard for client autonomy, relief or disregard for client suffering, and avoidance of killing at the very end of life (Fernandes, 2015). The hospice nurse needs to develop their own knowledge of nursing and medical ethics in order to question the ethical implications of interventions and to advocate for the client and family. An example is patient families will often insist that the patient be fed and given fluids. This may come from the aspect that in our culture food is thought to be comforting. Commonly, a patient close to death will not want to eat or drink; the body no longer needs those nutrients to sustain itself. This refusal on the part of the dying patient stresses the caregivers and the nurse may need to intervene to advocate for the patient's wishes. Ethical unrest in the client, family, as well as the nurse is best addressed through the institutional ethics board. This board consists of various disciplines specializing in health care, ethics, legal, and spiritual care. When the nurse is unsure of the ethical ramifications of decisions by the client or family, it is the nurse's obligation to bring the case before the board following the procedures of the institution. See Chapter 4 for more on ethics. See Box 30-9 for information on how nurses can recognize and manage compassion fatigue.

The Future of Hospice Care

Given a rapidly expanding population of elders living longer with challenging chronic illnesses, home health and hospice care in the home will soon need to transform into a community-based long-term care system that doesn't discharge after an acute episode or admit only at the very end of life. In response to out-of-control medical inflation, federal and state governments have sought to hold down expenses in all areas, including restrictions on home health and hospice care. However, costs keep rising in step with technologic and pharmacologic innovation and marketing. Containing costs will eventually force a shift in services from expensive institutional and high-technology interventions to community-based home services.

The entire model for service provision in the home must change to a health care delivery system that continuously serves those living with disabling and terminal illness to maximize well-being at home, anticipate and prevent crises, and minimize emergent and inpatient interventions. Hospice care is focused on symptom

BOX 30-8 PERSPECTIVES

A Hospice Nurse's Viewpoint on Hospice/Palliative Care Nursing

When I graduated from nursing school, I went directly into the intensive care unit. I loved it! I enjoyed the challenge of working intensely with one or two patients, as well as the supportive work environment with my close-knit group of colleagues.

With marriage and children (my first pregnancy resulted in twins), the 12-hour shifts and full-time schedules were more difficult to balance with family life. At first, I dropped down to working one weekend a month. But, with our growing family, it seemed that I would not be able to remain in the ICU.

I talked to a friend and learned about our hospital's hospice agency; she enjoyed working there, and I thought I would give it a try. It was a perfect fit for me and for our four boys. People always think of hospice/palliative care as depressing, but I find it to be very fulfilling. I think about it as "joining with a family" at their most vulnerable time. The patients let you in, sharing very personal things about their life with you, and they are grateful for your assistance at this time of transition. It can be a very spiritual experience, and I consider it a privilege to be able to share this time with my patients and their families.

The only difficult cases for me are the children; our agency doesn't have a large pediatric hospice, but it is beginning to expand. It is difficult for parents to lose a child, as one would expect. I remember coming home after a long night with a family whose young child lost his long battle with cancer and hosting my 2-year-old's birthday party with family and friends. I couldn't help but think about the contrast—my happy, healthy toddler and the loss of a young boy to cancer. But, I know that I made a difference for that family and child; I am honored to be a hospice/palliative care nurse.

Jessica, hospice RN

BOX **30-9** EVIDENCE-BASED PRACTICE

Nurses and Compassion Fatigue

Do you wonder how hospice nurses sustain compassionate practice as they work every day with suffering patients who always die? Expert hospice nurses embrace the suffering of the client and family and become susceptible to compassion fatigue. Compassion fatigue is often viewed as secondary stress. It is the stress felt by the caregiver from exposure to a traumatization. Nurses often describe this as overload. Although signs of compassion fatigue are individualized, they often include exhaustion and a reduced ability to express empathy for the client. This may result in withdrawal by the nurse emotionally from the client and family, as well as the role of nurse.

Staying psychologically as well as physically healthy as a hospice nurse requires a high level of self-awareness. Nurses must be aware of the signs and symptoms that they may have a tendency to exhibit. Symptoms are individualized based on how a particular nurse adapted to stress in the past and are often subject to developmental, spiritual, cultural, and environmental influences. Recognition of the symptoms allows the hospice nurse to institute stress-relieving activities early in the process. According to the Compassion Fatigue Awareness Project (2017), some symptoms that a nurse may experience include the following:

- Isolating oneself; poor self-care (appearance, hygiene)
- Repressed emotions; apathy; mentally/physically exhausted
- Always finding blame with others; many complaints about job/administration
- Substance abuse; compulsive behaviors (e.g., eating, spending, gambling)
- In debt; legal problems; recurrent flashbacks/nightmares; chronic health problems
- Problems concentrating; feeling preoccupied; denies problems

Compassion fatigue can affect an agency, if enough nurses suffer from the problem and nothing is done to assist them. It can cause problems between nurses and administrators, lead to high turnover and absenteeism, and lead to self-perpetuation. Organizations may exhibit these symptoms:

- Poor teamwork; high absentee rates; continually changing coworker relationships
- Challenging/breaking agency rules; aggression among staff members
- Poor task/assignment completion; unable to meet deadlines; lack of flexibility
- Negative feelings toward management; reluctance toward change
- Poor vision of future; not able to believe that improvements can be made

(Compassion Fatigue Awareness Project, 2017)

Compassion fatigue is not isolated to hospice nurses. All nurses are susceptible to the effects. This may lead to higher rates of turnover and an increase in the nursing shortage as nurses leave the profession.

Often, caregivers experiencing compassion fatigue are unable to identify it in themselves.

1. *What ways can you identify compassion fatigue in others?*
2. *What recommendations can you make to reduce compassion fatigue for yourself?*
3. *How can you transform the organization to reduce compassion fatigue?*

Source: Compassion Fatigue Awareness Project (2017); Upton (2018).

management, not curative interventions. Care revolves around maintenance of quality of life, not necessarily quantity. Clients in hospice care, under Medicare regulations, receive care for symptom management. If care is needed for other health conditions not related to the terminal diagnosis, care is received under their original Medicare benefit. Hospice services should be based on client choice and the reality of a terminal diagnosis. The physician must sign a declaration stating that the terminal diagnosis, if it follows the normal course of the disease process, will cause death in a finite period of time (6 months or less). A sustainable, affordable approach to care in the home requires ongoing case management to coordinate and manage resources with incentives that control cost while assuring quality of life and comfort. The hospice nurse becomes a coordinator of an interprofessional team of health care, spiritual, and community resources. Team members often include volunteers, who, after training, become involved with respite care for the family. Determination of the team members is defined in collaboration with the client and family to allow them independence and minimize the disruption to their individual lifestyle. Although inpatient hospices do exist, the goal of the hospice nurse is to keep the client in their home environment for as long as possible. The purpose of palliative care is symptom control, thereby decreasing stress for the dying client.

Nurses, nurse practitioners, and home visiting physicians will need to have the diagnostic and therapeutic resources to monitor physiologic status and intervene in the home. Telehealth and home monitoring will be essential. The focus must change from doing everything possible to prolong physiologic survival to promoting meaningful and comfortable lives. Nurses will have an active role in this process.

The IOM (2015) report *Dying in America: Improving Quality and Honoring Individual Preferences Near the End of Life* gives direction for needed changes that put the requirements of patients and families first. The report encourages policy changes and serves as a charge for all of us to advocate for improved social, spiritual, and psychological support and care for those of us nearing the end of our lives. As health care providers, we need to strive to provide compassionate, quality-centered, evidence-based care that is consistent with the wishes of our patients and their families (Box 30-10).

BOX **30-10** POPULATION FOCUS

Hospice Care for Children

Although it may be difficult for a family to accept hospice care for their terminally ill child, there is increasing evidence showing that a pediatric palliative care program reduces stress and worry for caregivers. Also, because medical care is received in a stress-free setting, the quality of life as well as length of life may be increased (Gans et al., 2015). Hospice plays an important role in supporting the child and family in the areas of medical, social, spiritual, and psychological support. The value of this service and underutilization justify research in this area. The National Hospice and Palliative Care Organization is committed to care of the child and family who can benefit from hospice care. They provide professional resources and education, as well as patient education information.

Children with life-threatening illnesses are hospitalized more often and spend more days in the hospital than those whose diseases are not life threatening. This causes additional stress on the child as well as the caregivers. Also, the child may be exposed to other diseases, which may affect the quality of their lives. There are many reasons hospice services are underutilized for children. Lack of education on the part of the health care team is a primary cause. Often the health care team is hesitant to recommend hospice until death is imminent on the hope that a curative treatment may be found. Families are often hesitant to commit to hospice as they remain in the denial phase of grieving. Hospice enables care for dying children by a multidisciplinary team supporting the child.

Most important to nursing practice is the limited access to ongoing education and the lack of consistent professional experiences with these children and their families. The National Hospice and Palliative Care Organization (NHPCO) offers palliative care resources for families and professionals at their website. Educating the health care team and family members regarding resources available through hospices services can increase the use, decrease acute care hospitalizations, and increase family satisfaction and coping.

1. *Do you think most nurses working in hospitals are aware of hospice and palliative care services for children?*
2. *What could you do to help communicate the availability and effectiveness of hospice services for children with life-threatening illnesses?*

Source: Gans et al. (2015).

SUMMARY

- Nurses have an important role in working with clients who receive home care or hospice services. As the population continues to age, the need for nurses to work with older adults where they live, as they are discharged from acute care settings earlier and earlier, and, if they are terminally ill, during their final months and days, will only increase. Services are also needed for clients across the lifespan.
- Many types of home care agencies exist: voluntary, proprietary, hospital based, official, homemaker, and hospice. Both formal and informal caregivers provide service. Professional staff members, such as nurses, social workers, therapists, and certified nursing assistants, work in collaboration with family members and, in some situations, with friends and neighbors.
- Medicare covers hospice care without the restrictions experienced by skilled home care clients. Hospice and palliative care programs provide holistic care to clients during the last months of life. Many programs are home based, and they may be offered by a home health agency. In addition to in-home hospices, inpatient hospices exist; these can be located in a freestanding building, in an area of a SNF, or in a section of an acute care facility. The focus of hospice care is not historically aimed at cure, and it employs holistic caregiving practices that involve family members, professionals, and volunteers.
- The nurse provides direct physical nursing care both in home health care and with hospice clients. In addition, the nurse teaches clients, family members, and volunteers; supervises; collaborates with team members; and case manages. Nurse assessment of clients assists in determining plan of care and working toward client management of disease processes in a value-based health model.

ACTIVE LEARNING EXERCISES

1. Search the Internet for home health and hospice agencies in your city or town. Select two agencies and compare services provided and the employment opportunities of each (one nonprofit and one for-profit). How do these job descriptions and the published pay ranges compare to hospitals in your area? What are the benefits of working in home health and hospice? Will the agency hire new graduates, or do they require prior acute care experience? What care is provided by these agencies? Where do you see gaps in services? What type of interventions does the agency utilize to prevent compassion fatigue among its staff?
2. Using "Communicate Effectively to Inform and Educate" (1 of the 10 essential public health services; see Box 2-2), how would you assist the following client? Mr. H is a 72-year-old male who has just been sent home from the hospital following his second stroke and has right-sided weakness. He has a G-tube in place and requires a walker for ambulation. He lives alone but has family in the area. What are your priorities? Using the nursing process, determine a plan of action.

3. Review your personal health insurance policy or that of a family member. What coverage, if any, is provided for home health or hospice care? What restrictions are stated in the coverage—total reimbursement, source of care, or length of service? Do you think this will be adequate to meet your or your family member's needs when these services may be needed? What other options might be available to help defray the cost of this type of care?
4. Interview a home health, hospice, or palliative care nurse to find out the most rewarding part of their job. What things are problematic? Ask about a typical case and home visit. How does this compare to your experiences in your community health nursing clinical course? Do you feel that home health, hospice, or palliative nursing might be something you will consider in the future? What are some safety considerations taken by the home health nurse?
5. Informal caregivers assume additional duties and burdens when caring for a loved one. Find a systematic review or research study on caregiver burden and compare your findings with another classmate's findings. What are the most common issues, and how can the C/PHN address them?

REFERENCES

Agency for Healthcare Research and Quality (AHRQ). (2018). *Care coordination measures atlas update. Chapter 2. What is care coordination?* Retrieved from http://www.ahrq.gov/professionals/prevention-chronic-care/improve/coordination/atlas2014/chapter2.html

Allen, J., Hutchinson, A., Brown, R., & Livingston, P. (2017). User experience and care integration in transitional care for older people from hospital to home: A meta-synthesis. *Quality Health Research, 27(1)*, 24–36.

Alliance for Home Health Quality and Innovation. (2018). *Home health care services and benefits by payer*. Retrieved from https://www.ahhqi.org/images/pdf/what-is-hhc-services-benefits.pdf

American Nurses Association (ANA). (2014). *Scope and standards of practice: Home health nursing* (2nd ed.). Silver Spring, MD: Author.

American Nurses Association (ANA) and Hospice and Palliative Nurses Association (HPNA). (2014). *Scope and standards of practice: Palliative nursing, an essential resource for hospice and palliative nurses*. Silver Spring, MD: Author.

Balanced Budget Act. (1997). *Public Law 105-33*. Retrieved from https://www.gpo.gov/fdsys/pkg/PLAW-105publ33/pdf/PLAW-105publ33.pdf

Buhler-Wilkerson, K. (2016). *Caring for the sick at home*. Retrieved from https://www.ncbi.nlm.nih.gov/pmc/articles/PMC2690354/

Center for Disease Control (CDC). (2018a). *Standard precautions for all patient care*. Retrieved from https://www.cdc.gov/infectioncontrol/basics/standard-precautions.html

Center for Disease Control (CDC). (2018b). *Take a stand on falls*. Retrieved from https://www.cdc.gov/features/older-adult-falls/index.html

Center for Medicare and Medicaid Services (CMS). (2018a). *Impact Act of 2014 Data Standardization & Cross Setting Measures*. Retrieved from https://www.cms.gov/Medicare/Quality-Initiatives-Patient-Assessment-Instruments/Post-Acute-Care-Quality-Initiatives/IMPACT-Act-of-2014/IMPACT-Act-of-2014-Data-Standardization-and-Cross-Setting-Measures.html

Center for Medicare and Medicaid Services (CMS). (2018b). *Home health quality measures*. Retrieved from https://www.cms.gov/Medicare/Quality-Initiatives-Patient-Assessment-Instruments/HomeHealthQualityInits/Home-Health-Quality-Measures.html

Center for Medicare and Medicaid Services (CMS). (2018c). *Home health prospective payment system*. Retrieved from https://www.cms.gov/Outreach-and-Education/Medicare-Learning-Network-MLN/MLNProducts/Downloads/Home-Health-PPS-Fact-Sheet-ICN006816.pdf

Center for Medicare and Medicaid Services (CMS). (2019). *Medicare home health benefit*. Retrieved from https://www.cms.gov/Outreach-and-Education/Medicare-Learning-Network-MLN/MLNProducts/Downloads/Home-Health-Benefit-Fact-Sheet-ICN908143.pdf

Centers for Disease Control and Prevention (CDC). (2015). *Important facts about falls*. Retrieved from http://www.cdc.gov/homeandrecreationalsafety/falls/adultfalls.html

Compassion Fatigue Awareness Project. (2017). *Recognizing compassion fatigue*. Retrieved from https://www.compassionfatigue.org/pages/symptoms.html

David, G., & Kim, K. (2018). The effect of workforce assignment on performance: Evidence from home health care. *Journal of Health Economics, 59*, 26–45.

Family Caregiver Alliance (FCA). (2018). *Caregiver statistics: Demographics*. Retrieved from https://www.caregiver.org/caregiver-statistics-demographics

Fernandes, J. (2015). Assisted dying is a threat to the ethics of palliative nursing. *International Journal of Palliative Nursing, 21*(9), 421–422.

Fitzgerald, C. (2016). *Female benevolent societies*. Retrieved from http://www.scencyclopedia.org/sce/entries/female-benevolent-societies/

Fulmer, H. (2017). History of visiting nurse work in America. *Home Healthcare Now, 35(1)*, 33–42. Reprinted from *The American Journal of Nursing, 2(6)* (1902), 411–425.

Gans, D., Hadler, M., Chen, X., Wu, S., Dimand, R., Abramson, J., ... Kominski, G. (2015). Impact of a pediatric palliative care program on the caregiver experience. *Journal of Hospice & Palliative Nursing, 17*(6), 559–565. doi: 10.1097/NJH.00000000000203.

Georgiadis, A., & Corrigan, O. (2017). The experience of transitional care for non-medically complex older adults and their family caregivers. *Global Qualitative Nursing Research, 4*, 1–9.

Ingebretsen, L., & Saghakken, M. (2016). Hosipce nurses' emtional challenges in their encounters with the dying. *International Journal of Qualitative Studies on Health and Well-being, 1*(11). doi: 10.3402/qhw.v11.31170.

Institute of Medicine. (2015a). *Dying in America: Improving quality and honoring individual preferences near the end of life*. Washington, DC: National Academies Press.

Institute of Medicine (IOM). (2015b). *The future of home health care: Workshop summary*. Washington, DC: Forum on Aging, Disability, and Independence; Board on Health Sciences Policy; Division on Behavioral and Social Sciences and Education; Institute of Medicine; National Research Council. Retrieved from https://www.ncbi.nlm.nih.gov/books/NBK315920/

Jones, C., Wald, H., Boxer, R., Masoudi, F., Burke, R., Capp, R., ... Ginde, A. (2017). Characteristics associated with home health care referrals at hospital discharge: Results from the 2012 national impatient sample. *Health Research and Educational Trust, 52*(2), 879–894.

Landers, S., Madigan, E., Leff, B., Rosati, R., McCann, B., Hornbake, R., ... Breese, E. (2016). The future of home health care: A strategic framework for optimizing value. *Home Health Care Management Practice, 28*(4), 262–278.

Ma, C., Shang, J., Miner, S., Lennox, L., & Squires, A. (2018). The prevalence and risk factors for hospital readmissions among home health care patients: A systematic review. *Home Health Care Management & Practice, 30*(2), 83–92.

Maddox, K., Chen, L., Zuckerman, R., & Epstein, A. (2018). Association between race, neighborhood, and Medicaid enrollment and outcomes in Medicare home health care. *Journal of American Geriatrics Society, 66*(2), 239–246.

MedPac. *Context for Medicare payment policy. Report to the congress: Medicare payment policy.* Retrieved from http://www.medpac.gov/docs/default-source/reports/mar17_medpac_ch1.pdf?sfvrsn=0

Miller, E., Intrator, O., Gadbois, E., Gidmark, S., & Rudolph, J. (2017). VA staff perceptions of the role of the extended care referral process in home and community-based services versus nursing home use posthospital discharge. *Home Health Care Services Quarterly, 36*(2), 63–80.

National Association for Home Care and Hospice (NAHC). (2018). *Mission statement*. Retrieved from https://www.nahc.org/about/mission-statement/

National Association for Home Care and Hospice (NAHC). (2020). Code of ethics. Retrieved from https://www.nahc.org/about/code-of-ethics/

NATIONAL FEDERATION OF INDEPENDENT BUSINESS ET AL. v. SEBELIUS, SECRETARY OF HEALTH AND HUMAN SERVICES, ET AL. (2012). 11-393. 11th Circuit. Retrieved from https://www.supremecourt.gov/opinions/11pdf/11-393c3a2.pdf

National Hospice and Palliative Care Organization (NHPCO). (2020). *History of hospice care*. Retrieved from https://www.nhpco.org/hospice-care-overview/history-of-hospice/

National Institute of Aging (NIA). (2017). *NIH initiative tests in-home technology to help older adults age in place*. Retrieved from https://www.nia.nih.gov/news/nih-initiative-tests-home-technology-help-older-adults-age-place

Noel, M., Kaluzynski, T., & Templeton, V. (2017). Quality dementia care: Integrating caregivers into a chronic disease management model. *Journal of Applied Gerontology, 36*(2), 195–212.

Raingruber, B., & Wolf, T. (2015). Nurse perspectives regarding the meaningfulness of oncology nursing practice. *Clinical Journal of Oncology Nursing, 19*(3), 292–296.

Ruiz, A., Snyder, L., Rotondo, C., Cross-Barnet, C., Colligan, E., & Giuriceo, K. (2018). Innovative home visit models associated with reductions in costs, hospitalizations, and emergency department use. *Health Affairs, 36*(3), 425–432.

Smith, A., & Treschuk, J. (2018). Disconnects and silos in transitional care: Single-case study of model implementation in home health care. *Home Health Care Management & Practice, 30*(3), 1–10.

Storch, J. (2015). Ethics in practice: At end-of-life—Part 1. *Canadian Nurse, 111*(6), 20–21.

United States Department of Health and Human Services (USDHHS). (2018). *Long-term care providers and services users in the United States: Data from the National Study of Long-Term Care Providers, 2013–2014*. Retrieved from https://www.cdc.gov/nchs/data/series/sr_03/sr03_038.pdf

United States Department of Labor. (2018). *National Industry-Specific Occupational Employment and Wage Estimates. NAICS 621600—Home Health Care Services*. Retrieved from https://www.bls.gov/oes/current/naics4_621600.htm

Upton, K. (2018). An investigation into compassion fatigue and self-compassion in acute medical care hospital nurses: A mixed methods study. *Journal of Compassionate Health Care, 5*(7), 1–27. doi: 10.1186/s40639-018-0050-x.

World Health Organization. (2016). *Cancer: WHO's pain ladder for adults*. Retrieved from http://www.who.int/cancer/palliative/painladder/en/

Zerwekh, J. (1995). High-tech home care for nurses. *Home Healthcare Nurse, 13*(1), 9–14.

Zerwekh, J. (2006). *Nursing care at the end of life*. Philadelphia, PA: F.A. Davis.

APPENDIX Quad Council Tier 1 Community/Public Health Nursing Competencies

DOMAIN 1: ASSESSMENT AND ANALYTIC SKILLS

Assessment/Analytic Skills focus on identifying and understanding data, turning data info information for action, assessing needs and assets to address community health needs, developing community health assessments, and using evidence for decision making.

1A1. Assess the health status and health literacy of individuals and families, including determinants of health, using multiple sources of data.

1A2a. Use an ecological perspective and epidemiological data to identify health risks for a population.

1A2b. Identify individual and family assets, needs, values, beliefs, resources, and relevant environmental factors.

1A3. Select variables that measure health and public health conditions.

1A4. Use a data collection plan that incorporates valid and reliable methods and instruments for collection of qualitative and quantitative data to inform the service for individuals, families, and a community.

1A5. Interpret valid and reliable data that impacts the health of individuals, families, and communities to make comparisons that are understandable to all who were involved in the assessment process.

1A6. Compare appropriate data sources in a community.

1A7. Contribute to comprehensive community health assessments through the application of quantitative and qualitative public health nursing data.

1A8. Apply ethical, legal, and policy guidelines and principles in the collection, maintenance, use, and dissemination of data and information.

1A9. Use varied approaches in the identification of community needs (i.e., focus groups, multi-sector collaboration, SWOT analysis).

1A10. Use information technology effectively to collect, analyze, store, and retrieve data related to public health nursing services for individuals, families, and groups.

1A11. Use evidence-based strategies or promising practices from across disciplines to promote health in communities and populations.

1A12. Use available data and resources related to the determinants of health when planning services for individuals, families, and groups.

DOMAIN 2: POLICY DEVELOPMENT/PROGRAM PLANNING SKILLS

Policy Development/Program Planning Skills focus on determining needed policies and programs, advocating for policies and programs; planning, implementing, and evaluating policies and programs, developing and implementing strategies for continuous quality improvement; and developing and implementing community health improvement plans and strategic plans.

2A1. Identify local, state, national, and international policy issues relevant to the health of individuals, families, and groups.

2A2. Describe the implications and potential impacts of public health programs and policies on individuals, families, and groups within a population.

2A3. Identify outcomes of health policy relevant to public health nursing practice for individuals, families, and groups.

2A4a. Provide information that will inform policy decisions.

2A4b. Implement programs and services based on policy decisions.

2A5. Use organizations' strategic plans and decision-making methods in the development of program goals and objectives for individuals, families, and groups.

2A6a. Demonstrate knowledge of laws and regulation relevant to public health nursing services.

2A6b. Plan public health nursing services consistent with laws and regulations.

2A7. Function as a team member in developing organizational plans while assuring compliance with established policies and program implementation guidelines.

2A8. Comply with organizational procedures and policies.

2A9. Use program planning skills and CBPR (i.e., collaboration, reflection, capacity building) to implement strategies to engage marginalized/disadvantaged population groups in making decisions that affect their health and well-being.

2A10. Apply methods and practices to access public health information for individuals, families, and groups.

2A11. Participate in quality improvement teams by using quality indicators and core measures to identify and address opportunities for improvement in services for individuals, families, and groups.

DOMAIN 3: COMMUNICATION SKILLS

Communication Skills focus on assessing and addressing population literacy; soliciting and using community input, communicating data and information; facilitating communications; and communicating the roles of government, health care, and others.

3A1. Determine the health, literacy, and the health literacy of the population served to guide health promotion and disease prevention activities.

3A2. Apply critical thinking and cultural awareness to all communication modes (i.e., verbal, nonverbal, written, and electronic) with individuals, the community, and stakeholders.

3A3. Use input from individuals, families, and groups when planning and delivering health care programs and services.

3A4. Use a variety of methods to disseminate public health information to individuals, families, and groups within a population.

3A5a. Create a presentation of targeted health information.

3A5b. Communicate information to multiple audiences including groups, peer professionals, and agency peers.

3A6. Use communication models to communicate with individuals, families, and groups effectively and as a member of the interprofessional team(s) or interdisciplinary partnerships.

3A7. Describe the role of public health nursing to internal and external audiences.

3A8. Apply communication techniques and models when interacting with peers and other health care team members including conflict management.

DOMAIN 4: CULTURAL COMPETENCY SKILLS

Cultural Competency Skills focus on understanding and responding to diverse needs, assessing organizational cultural diversity and competence, assessing effects of policies and programs on different populations, and taking actions to support a diverse public health workforce.

4A1. Use determinants of health effectively when working with diverse individuals, families, and groups.

4A2. Use data, evidence, and information technology to understand the impact of determinants of health on individuals, families, and groups.

4A3. Deliver culturally responsive public health nursing services for individuals, families, and groups.

4A4. Explain the benefits of a diverse public health workforce that supports a just and civil culture.

4A5. Demonstrate the use of evidence-based cultural models in a work environment when providing services to individuals, families, and groups.

DOMAIN 5: COMMUNITY DIMENSIONS OF PRACTICE SKILLS

Community Dimensions of Practice Skills focus on evaluating and developing linkages and relationships within the community, maintaining and advancing partnerships and community involvement, negotiating for the use of community assets, defending public health policies and programs, and evaluating and improving the effectiveness of community engagement.

5A1a. Use assessments, develops plans, implements, and evaluates interventions for public health services for individuals, families and groups.

5A1b. Assist individuals, families, and groups to identify and access necessary community resources or services through the referral and follow-up process.

5A2. Use formal and informal relational networks among community organizations and systems conducive to improving the health of individuals, families, and groups within communities.

5A3a. Select stakeholders needed to address public health issues impacting the health of individuals, families, and groups within the community.

5A3b. Function effectively with key stakeholders in activities that facilitate community involvement and delivery of services to individuals, families, and groups.

5A4. Build stakeholder capacity to advocate for the health issues of individuals, families, and groups.

5A5. Use community assets and resources, including the government, private, and nonprofit sectors, to promote health and to deliver services to individuals, families, and groups.

5A6. Use input from varied sources to structure public health programs and services for individuals, families, and groups.

5A7a. Interview individuals, families, and groups to identify community resource preferences.

5A7b. Build preferences into public health services.

5A7c. Identify opportunities for individuals, families, and groups to link with advocacy organizations.

5A8. Identify evidence of the effectiveness of community engagement strategies on individuals, families, and groups.

DOMAIN 6: PUBLIC HEALTH SCIENCES SKILLS

Public Health Sciences Skills focus on understanding the foundation and prominent events of public health, applying public sciences to practice, critiquing and developing research, using evidence when developing policies and programs, and establishing academic partnerships.

6A1. Use the determinants of health and evidence-based practices from public health and nursing science, when planning health promotion and disease prevention interventions for individuals, families, and groups.

6A2a. Determine the relationship between access to clean, sustainable water, sanitation, food, air, and energy quality on individual, family, and population health.

6A2b. Assess hazards and threats to individuals, families, and populations and reduce their risk of exposure and injury in natural and built environments (i.e., chemicals and products).

6A3. Use evidence-based practice in population-level programs to contribute to meeting core public health functions and the 10 essential public health services.

6A4. Participate in research activities impacting the health of populations.

6A5. Use a wide variety of sources and methods to access public health information (i.e., GIS mapping, Community Health Assessment, local/state/and national sources).

6A6a. Use research to inform the practice of public health nursing.

6A6b. Identify gaps in research evidence that impact public health nursing practice.

6A7. Demonstrate compliance with the requirements of patient confidentiality and human subject protection.

6A8. Model public health science skills when working with individuals, families, and groups.

DOMAIN 7: FINANCIAL PLANNING, EVALUATION, AND MANAGEMENT SKILLS

Financial Planning and Management Skills focus on engaging other government agencies that can address community health needs, leveraging pubic health and health care funding mechanisms, developing and defending budgets, motivating personnel, evaluating and improvement program and organization performance, and establishing and using performance management systems to improve organization performance.

7A1. Explain the interrelationships among local, state, tribal, and federal public health and health care systems.

7A2. Explain the public health nurse's role in emergency preparedness and disaster response during public health events (i.e., infectious disease outbreak, natural or manmade disasters).

7A3. Implement operational procedures for public health programs and services.

7A4a. Demonstrate knowledge of funding streams to support programs.

7A4b. Select the data for inclusion in a programmatic budget.

7A5. Interpret the impact of budget constraints on the delivery of public health nursing services to individuals, families, and groups.

7A6. Explain implications of organizational budget priorities on individual, groups, and communities.

7A7. Explain public health nursing services and programmatic needs to inform budget priorities.

7A8a. Identify data to evaluate services for individuals, families, and groups.

7A8b. Contribute to the evaluation plan for public health nursing services targeting individuals, families, and groups.

7A9. Deliver public health nursing services to individuals, families, and groups based on reported evaluation results.

7A10. Provide input into the fiscal and narrative components of proposals.

7A11. Use public health informatics skills pertaining to public health nursing services of individuals, families, and groups.

7A12. Provide input for contracts and other agreements for the provision of public health services.

7A13. Organize public health nursing services and programs for individuals, families, and groups within budgetary guidelines.

7A14a. Participate in the implementation of the organization's performance management system.

7A14b. Use self-reflection to identify one's performance in the organization's performance management system.

7A14c. List contributions to the organization's performance management system.

DOMAIN 8: LEADERSHIP AND SYSTEMS THINKING SKILLS

Leadership and Systems Thinking Skills focus on incorporating ethical standards into the organization, creating opportunities for collaboration among public health, healthcare, and other organizations; mentoring personnel; adjusting practice to address changing needs and environment; ensuring continuous quality improvement; managing organizational change; and advocating for the role of governmental public health.

8A1. Demonstrate ethical standards of practice in all aspects of public health and public health nursing as the basis of all interactions with individuals, communities, and organizations.

8A2. Apply systems thinking to public health nursing practice with individuals, families, and groups.

8A3. Participate in stakeholder meetings to identify a shared vision, values, and principles for community action.

8A4a. Identify internal and external factors affecting public health nursing practice and opportunities for interprofessional collaboration.

8A4b. Explain environmental hazards and emergency preparedness to protect individuals, families, and groups.

8A4c. Respond to environmental hazards to protect individuals, families, and groups.

8A5. Use individual, team, and organizational learning opportunities for personal and professional development as a public health nurse.

8A6. Model personal commitment to lifelong learning, professional development, and advocacy.

8A7. Identify organizational quality improvement initiatives that provide opportunities for improvement in public health nursing practice.

8A8. Facilitate the development of interprofessional teams and workgroups.

8A9. Interpret organization dynamics of collaborating agencies.

8A10a. Provide feedback on the organization's mission and vision and the impact on individuals, families, and groups.

8A10b. Influence others to provide feedback on the organization's mission and vision and the impact on individuals, families, and groups.

8A11. Select advocacy strategies to address the needs of diverse and underserved population.

8A12. Identify organizational policies and procedures that meet practice and public health accreditation requirements.

8A13. Influence health as a shared value through community engagement and inclusion of individuals, families, and groups.

INDEX

Note: Page numbers followed by "*f*" indicate figures, "*b*" indicate boxed material, and "*t*" indicate tables.

Y